Alexander's
NURSING
PRACTICE

Commissioning Editor: **Ninette Premdas**

Development Editor: **Sheila Black**

Project Manager: **Frances Affleck**

Designer: **Kirsteen Wright**

Illustration Manager: **Merlyn Harvey**

Alexander's NURSING PRACTICE | 4th EDITION

Edited by

Chris Brooker BSc MSc RGN SCM RNT

Author and Editor, Norfolk, UK

Maggie Nicol BSc(Hons) MSc PGDipEd RGN

Professor of Nursing, CETL Director and FACT Theme Leader, School of Community and Health Sciences, City University, London, UK

Foreword by

Margaret Alexander CBE BSc PhD RN RM RNT FRCN

Emeritus Professor, School of Nursing and Community Health, Glasgow Caledonian University, Glasgow, UK

Illustrations by **Ethan Danielson**

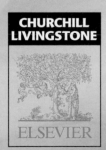

CHURCHILL LIVINGSTONE

ELSEVIER

Edinburgh London New York Oxford Philadelphia St Louis Sydney Toronto 2011

CHURCHILL
LIVINGSTONE
ELSEVIER

CHURCHILL LIVINGSTONE, an imprint of Elsevier Ltd

© Longman Group Limited 1994
© Pearson Professional Limited 1995
© Harcourt Brace and Company Limited 1999
© Harcourt Publishers Limited 2000
© Elsevier Science Limited 2002
© Elsevier Limited 2006
© 2011 Elsevier Limited. All rights reserved.

ISBN 978-0-7020-3152-6

British Library Cataloguing in Publication Data
A catalogue record for this book is available from the British Library

Library of Congress Cataloging in Publication Data
A catalog record for this book is available from the Library of Congress

Notice
Knowledge and best practice in this field are constantly changing. As new research and experience broaden our knowledge, changes in practice, treatment and drug therapy may become necessary or appropriate. Readers are advised to check the most current information provided (i) on procedures featured or (ii) by the manufacturer of each product to be administered, to verify the recommended dose or formula, the method and duration of administration, and contraindications. It is the responsibility of the practitioner, relying on their own experience and knowledge of the patient, to make diagnoses, to determine dosages and the best treatment for each individual patient, and to take all appropriate safety precautions. To the fullest extent of the law, neither the Publisher nor the Editors assumes any liability for any injury and/or damage to persons or property arising out of or related to any use of the material contained in this book.

The Publisher

Printed in China

Contents

SECTION 3   NURSING SPECIFIC PATIENT GROUPS   687

Contributors

Erica S. Alabaster PhD RN MSc DANS RNT DipN WNB Cert FHEA MIFA ILTM
Senior Lecturer and Chair, School of Nursing and Midwifery Studies, University Hospital of Wales, Cardiff and Vale NHS Trust, Cardiff, UK
Chapter 32 Care and rehabilitation of people with long-term conditions

Joan Allwinkle DipDiab RN
Diabetes Specialist Nurse, Department of Diabetes, Royal Infirmary of Edinburgh, University Hospitals Division, NHS Lothian, Edinburgh, UK
Chapter 5 Part 2 Nursing patients with diabetes mellitus

Irene Anderson MSc BSc(Hons) PGCE DPSN RGN LPE FHEA
Principal Lecturer, Tissue Viability; Reader, Learning and Teaching in Healthcare Practice, School of Nursing and Midwifery, University of Hertfordshire, Hatfield, UK
Chapter 23 Tissue viability and managing chronic wounds

Carol Ball PhD MSc RGN
Consultant Nurse Critical Care, Royal Free Hampstead NHS Trust, London, UK
Chapter 18 Recognising and managing shock

Janet Barclay RGN, Independent Prescriber
Diabetes Specialist Nurse, Department of Diabetes, Royal Infirmary of Edinburgh, University Hospitals Division, NHS Lothian, Edinburgh, UK
Chapter 5 Part 2 Nursing patients with diabetes mellitus

Patricia Black MSc(Distinct) PGDip PGCE FHEA RMN RGN
Senior CNS and Lecturer in Palliative Care, School of Nursing, Midwifery and Social Care, Napier University, Edinburgh, UK
Chapter 33 Nursing patients who need palliative care

Jacqueline Bloomfield RN BN MN PGDip PhD
Lecturer, Department of Specialist Care, Florence Nightingale School of Nursing and Midwifery, King's College London, London, UK
Chapter 11 Nursing patients with blood disorders

Chris Brooker BSc MSc RGN SCM RNT
Author and Editor, Norfolk, UK
Chapter 1 Nursing practice – the essence of caring
Chapter 6 Nursing patients with disorders of the immune system

Karen L. Burnet BSc MSc OncCert RGN
CRUK Senior Research Nurse, Cambridge University Hospitals NHS Foundation Trust, Cambridge, UK
Chapter 7 Part 2 Nursing patients with disorders of the breast

Karen Campbell BSc(Hons) RGN PGCE MN
Macmillan Lecturer in Cancer Nursing, Teaching Fellow, School of Nursing, Midwifery and Social Care, Napier University, Edinburgh, UK
Chapter 31 Nursing the patient with cancer

Maggie N. Carson BN(Hons) RGN MSc Cert(Adult End Nurs) PGCE
Lecturer, Nursing Studies, School of Health in Social Science, University of Edinburgh, Edinburgh, UK
Chapter 5 Part 1 Nursing patients with endocrine disorders

Carol Chamley BA MEd CertEd DipN MSSM RSCN ONC RCNT RN(Adult) RNT ENB N51
Senior Lecturer, Faculty of Health and Life Sciences, Coventry University, Coventry, UK
Chapter 19 Pain management

Charmaine Childs PhD MPhil BN RGN HVCert NDNCert
Associate Professor, Alice Lee Centre for Nursing Studies, Yong Loo Lin School of Medicine, National University of Singapore, Singapore
Chapter 22 Maintaining body temperature

Elaine Cole BSc MSc PGDipEd RGN
Senior Lecturer in Emergency and Trauma Care, School of Community and Health Sciences, City University, London, UK
Chapter 27 Nursing the patient who experiences trauma

Jacky Cotton MHS RGN RM
Head of Nursing – Gynaecology, Birmingham Women's
NHS Foundation Trust, Birmingham, UK
*Chapter 7 Part 1 Nursing patients with disorders of the
reproductive systems*

Michelle Cowen BEd(Hons) DipN RN RNT RCNT
Lecturer in Critical Care Nursing, School of Nursing and
Midwifery, University of Southampton, Southampton, UK
*Chapter 20 Maintaining fluid, electrolyte and acid–base
balance*

Patricia Cronin DipN BSc(Hons) MSc PhD RGN RNT
Lecturer, School of Nursing and Midwifery,
Trinity College Dublin, Dublin, Ireland
*Chapter 4 Nursing patients with gastrointestinal, liver and
biliary disorders*

Susanne Cruickshank PGCE MSc BSc ENB A11 ENB
998 RGN
Lecturer in Cancer Nursing, School of Nursing,
Midwifery and Social Care, Napier University,
Edinburgh, UK
Chapter 31 Nursing the patient with cancer

Anita Duffy BSc MSc RNT RGN FFNM RCSI
Lecturer in General Nursing, School of Nursing and
Midwifery, Trinity College, Dublin, Ireland
*Chapter 4 Nursing patients with gastrointestinal, liver
and biliary disorders*

Glenda Esmond BSc(Hons) MSc PGCE RGN
Respiratory Nurse Consultant, Barnet Primary Care
Trust, London, UK
Chapter 3 Nursing patients with respiratory disorders

Josephine (Tonks) N. Fawcett BSc(Hons) MSc RN
RNT ILTM
Senior Lecturer, Nursing Studies, School of Health in
Social Science, University of Edinburgh, Edinburgh, UK
Chapter 17 Stress and anxiety

Jacqui Fletcher BSc(Hons) MSc PGCE RGN
School of Nursing and Midwifery, University of
Hertfordshire, Hatfield, UK
Chapter 23 Tissue viability and managing chronic wounds

Marsh Gelbart BA MA PGCE RN
Lecturer in Adult Nursing, School of Community and
Health Sciences, City University, London, UK
*Chapter 35 Nursing patients with sexually transmitted
infections and HIV/AIDS*

Caroline E. Gibson BSc(Hons) MSc RN
Lecturer in Nursing, Queen Margaret University –
Edinburgh, Musselburgh, UK
Chapter 26 Nursing the patient undergoing surgery

Sue Green BSc MMedSci PhD RN
Senior Lecturer, School of Health Sciences, University of
Southampton, Southampton, UK
Chapter 21 Nutrition and health

Hilary Harkin BSc(Hons) RGN
ENT Nurse Practitioner, Ear, Nose and Throat
Department, St Thomas' Hospital, Guy's and St Thomas'
NHS Foundation Trust, London, UK
*Chapter 14 Nursing patients with disorders of the ear, nose and
throat*

Cheryl Holman RN PhD MSc BEd(Hons) DipN
Adult Nursing Programme Director, School of
Community and Health Sciences, City University,
London, UK
Chapter 34 Nursing older adults

Mark Jones MSc RN BSc(Hons) DipEd DipN
Head of Department, Department of Adult Nursing,
School of Community and Health Sciences,
City University, London, UK
*Chapter 35 Nursing patients with sexually transmitted
infections and HIV/AIDS*

Claire Kilpatrick RN PGDip MSc MFTM RCPS(Glos)
Programme Manager, World Health Organization First
Global Safety Challenge, Geneva, Switzerland
Seconded from Health Protection Scotland, Glasgow, UK
Chapter 16 Infection prevention and control

Andrée le May BSc(Hons) PhD PGCEA RGN
Retired Professor of Nursing and part-time Consultant,
School of Health Sciences, University of Southampton,
Southampton, UK
Chapter 25 Promoting sleep

Brian Lucas RN ENB 219 PhD BA MSc PgDipHe
Lead Nurse – Practice and Innovation, The Queen
Elizabeth Hospital King's Lynn NHS Trust, King's Lynn,
Norfolk, UK
Chapter 10 Nursing patients with musculoskeletal disorders

Ruth E. Magowan BSc(Hons) PGCE RGN RSCN
Lecturer in Nursing, Queen Margaret University –
Edinburgh, Musselburgh, UK
Chapter 26 Nursing the patient undergoing surgery

Breeda McCahill BSc PGDip NBSDip RGN
Nurse Practitioner, Burns Unit, Glasgow Royal Infirmary, NHS Greater Glasgow and Clyde, Glasgow, UK
Chapter 30 Nursing the patient with burn injury

Carol McQuade BSc(Hons) PGDip RGN
Specialist Oncology Breast Nurse Practitioner, Addenbrooke's Hospital, Cambridge University Hospitals NHS Foundation Trust, Cambridge, UK
Chapter 7 Part 2 Nursing patients with disorders of the breast

Maggie Nicol BSc(Hons) MSc PGDipEd RGN
Professor of Nursing, CETL Director and FACT Theme Leader, School of Community and Health Sciences, City University, London, UK
Chapter 1 Nursing practice – the essence of caring

Jill Peters BSc(Hons) MSc DipNP RGN ENB393 A33 NISP
Dermatology Nurse Practitioner, Dermatology Department, NHS Suffolk PCT, Ipswich, Suffolk, UK
Chapter 12 Nursing patients with skin disorders

Jacqui Prieto RN BSc(Hons) BSc PhD PCAP
Senior Clinical Academic Research Fellow, Faculty of Health Sciences, University of Southampton, Southampton, UK
Chapter 16 Infection prevention and control

Allyson Sanderson MA RGN ECP
Senior Lecturer, Teesside University, Middlesbrough, UK
Chapter 13 Nursing patients with disorders of the eye and vision

Helen Singh RGN ENB100 BSc(Hons) MSc
Senior Charge Nurse/Advanced Nurse Practioner Critical Care, Western General Hospital, Edinburgh, UK
Chapter 29 Nursing the critically ill patient

Graeme D. Smith PhD BA RGN
Senior Lecturer, Nursing Studies, School of Health in Social Science, University of Edinburgh, Edinburgh, UK
Chapter 17 Stress and anxiety

Martin Steggall BSc(Hons) MSc PhD RN FHEA
Clinical Nurse Specialist (ED), Barts and The London NHS Trust, Tower Hamlets Primary Care Trust, London; Associate Dean for Pre-registration Undergraduate Nursing and Midwifery, School of Community and Health Sciences, City University, London, UK
Chapter 7 Part 1 Nursing patients with disorders of the reproductive systems
Chapter 8 Nursing patients with urinary disorders

Karen Strickland BSc MSc PGCE RGN
Lecturer in Chronic Illness, Cancer and Palliative Care, School of Nursing, Midwifery and Social Care, Napier University, Edinburgh, UK
Chapter 33 Nursing patients who need palliative care

Sue Stringer BSc(Hons) RGN
Macmillan Head and Neck Nurse Specialist, Sherwood Forest Hospitals NHS Trust (Kings Mill Hospital), Nottinghamshire, UK
Chapter 15 Nursing patients with disorders of the mouth

Christine G. Thom MA MSc OND RGN
Ophthalmic Nurse Practitioner, Ophthalmology Department, St John's Hospital, West Lothian Healthcare NHS Trust, Livingston, UK
Chapter 13 Nursing patients with disorders of the eye and vision

David R. Thompson BSc MA PhD MBA RN FESC FRCN FAAN
Professor of Cardiovascular Nursing, Department of Health Sciences, Department of Cardiovascular Sciences, The University of Leicester, Leicester, UK
Chapter 2 Nursing patients with cardiovascular disorders

Debra Ugboma BN MPhil RN ENB 134
Lecturer in Adult Nursing, Faculty of Health Sciences, University of Southampton, Southampton, UK
Chapter 20 Maintaining fluid, electrolyte and acid–base balance

Susan H. Walker BSc(Hons) MA PGCE RN
Senior Lecturer in Adult Nursing/Clinical Skills, School of Nursing and Midwifery, University of Salford, Manchester, UK
Chapter 24 Maintaining continence

Catheryne Waterhouse BA MSc PGCE
Lecturer/Practitioner, Neuroscience Unit, Royal Hallamshire Hospital, Sheffield Teaching Hospitals NHS Foundation Trust, Sheffield, UK
Chapter 28 Nursing the unconscious patient

Rosemary A. Webster BSc MSc RN
Lead for Education and Practice Development, Glenfield Hospital, University Hospitals of Leicester NHS Trust, Leicester, UK
Chapter 2 Nursing patients with cardiovascular disorders

Sue Woodward MSc PGCEA RGN MAR FIFR
Lecturer, Florence Nightingale School of Nursing and Midwifery, Kings College London, UK
Chapter 9 Nursing patients with disorders of the nervous system

Preface

This extensively updated, full-colour fourth edition will be an invaluable resource, not only for nursing students, but also for nurse educators and qualified nurses, including those returning to practice and those coming to nurse in the UK from other parts of the world. All face the challenge of keeping abreast of new knowledge and technologies, promoting health, providing evidence-based health care in a climate of economic restraint and new roles for registered nurses.

The structure of the book

As in the previous three editions, the book is divided into three sections that are progressive in nature, encouraging the reader to move from the broad approach of Section 1 to a more in-depth appreciation of core nursing issues in Section 2 and the nursing needs of specific patient groups in Section 3. There is extensive cross-referencing between chapters, helping readers to make links and pursue lines of enquiry. This edition benefits from dedicated web-based materials that include:

- additional evidence-based information
- an electronic version of the text that is fully customisable and searchable
- critical thinking questions with outline answers
- over 250 MCQs with answers and feedback
- hot-linked references.

Throughout the text a special icon directs you to the website 🖱 for further information, figures or critical thinking questions.

Section 1 — Care of patients with common disorders

We have decided to continue with the systems approach for this section because of developments in the skills and expertise required by registered nurses. Nurses require a thorough grounding in anatomy, physiology, pathophysiology and medical treatment in order to plan and provide safe and sensitive evidence-based *Nursing management and health promotion*.

It is impossible to include every disease and disorder and so we concentrated on those commonly encountered by nurses in both community settings and hospital. Clearly,

▷ *Nursing management and health promotion* is a crucial part of the chapters of all three sections, reminding readers of the need to make appropriate clinical judgments and decisions in partnership with the individual, having taken account of their unique needs and circumstances.

Section 2 — Core nursing issues

This section builds on the foundations laid in Section 1. The focus is on core nursing issues, which are not merely physiological in origin, but also arise from the subtle, complex interplay of social, psychological and economic factors. Some of these problems have a high profile, such as stress and pain. Others, such as nutrition and sleep, are often relatively neglected, but are very much the concern of nurses. These problems are part of life and may be experienced in many settings and at any time. Throughout the section, both the nurse's and the patient's perspectives have been considered and all interventions are informed by the best available evidence.

Section 3 — Nursing specific patient groups

Some of the most challenging areas of nursing are explored in this section. By addressing these, the broad spectrum and contrasts of adult nursing are revealed. Such challenges, many long-term in nature, often make the greatest demands on the nurse's clinical and interpersonal skills. Section 3 addresses stereotypes and examines values and beliefs, raising awareness of the moral decision-making that underlies so much of day-to-day nursing practice.

Key features

A variety of key features have been used throughout the book and in the electronic ancillaries. These are designed to help you explore the different ways of knowing about nursing and include:

- informative, full-colour illustrations, tables and photographs
- care plans and pathways, which are both educational and useful practice tools
- boxes – many of which are interactive and contain reader activities
  - 《 Reflection – many including accounts of personal 'lived experience'
  - ⓘ Information – providing further information on important topics
  - 🔍 Evidence-based practice – based on research abstracts
- self tests – MCQs with answers and explanations, and critical thinking exercises with outline answers are provided in the electronic ancillaries

- summary of the key nursing issues for each chapter
- ⊖ Reflection and learning – what next? – designed to encourage you to consider how you will use this knowledge in practice and your future learning needs
- references, further reading suggestions and useful websites to enable you to follow up issues raised in each chapter
- appendix of normal biochemical and haematological values that include:
  - arterial blood analysis
  - cerebrospinal fluid
  - reference values in venous serum for the more common analytes
  - reference values for the more common analytes in urine
  - hormones in serum
  - haematological values
- glossary of key words from each chapter.

Norfolk and London, 2011

Chris Brooker
Maggie Nicol

Foreword

It is a joy to welcome the fourth edition of this best-selling nursing textbook, the popularity of which has stood the test of time. Since the initial discussions as to the format, content and ethos of a possible new nursing textbook took place with the publishers, almost 20 years ago now, the book has reflected the essence of nursing, of informed, skilled, compassionate, empathetic caring.

Together with my former co-editors, Josephine (Tonks) Fawcett and Phyllis Runciman, I am delighted to see that, in the hands of the new very competent and experienced editors, Chris Brooker and Maggie Nicol, the recognition of the constantly increasing knowledge and skills for practice is maintained. This fourth edition continues to provide comprehensive up-to-date content and, most importantly, albeit it in a slightly different manner, the inclusion of the lived experience of patients.

The book opens with a summary of the many and significant changes in nurses' roles and the changes in nurse education with the introduction of degree level preparation for all nurses and publication of the new *Standards for pre-registration nurse education* (Nursing and Midwifery Council 2010). Also of importance are the changes in our health care services, not least of which are the impact of the increasing number of older people in our society and the changing expectations of patients. In this edition, the chapters are once again written by currently practising nurses and nurse educators, some of whom are new to the text and others who have continued from previous editions. This book continues to provide a vital resource, not just for student nurses, but also for qualified nurses and nurse educators.

While maintaining the overall structure of three sections established with the previous editions, the editors have introduced a number of innovations, such as dedicated web-based material, and an electronic version of the entire text. There are triggers to encourage the reader to interact with the text, and to reflect on both what a patient feels and how the nurse might respond to a clinical scenario. The Boxes on 'Reflection' provide a stimulus to such thinking. This is complemented by the web-based Critical thinking and Multiple choice questions to which the reader is led by using the 'computer mouse' icon to be found liberally sprinkled throughout the text.

Knowledge for nursing is ever advancing. Where 20 years ago nursing research either did not exist, or was viewed by many with some scepticism, now it is a vital and valued part of nursing. The primacy of evidence-based practice is well illustrated throughout the book. This encourages students and qualified nurses to keep up-to-date with research related to their field of practice, always developing their ability to question practice and to provide the best possible care. The guided access to the web, that is a new feature in this edition, will enable readers to check for advances in research-based knowledge that can be applied in practice.

So yes, knowledge for nursing is growing, in almost every sphere of patient care, and today, for example, patients undergoing major surgery are able to be discharged home much earlier, thus impacting on care in the community. The ways of working with colleagues in health care are changing, and the context for nursing is inevitably influenced by the current times of economic constraint. Nursing cannot take place in isolation from all this, and nurses, whether students or qualified, must keep up-to-date with the developments in technology, treatments and innovations in care, and indeed cope with working in an ever-changing health care system. Many new roles for qualified nurses now exist and the future career pathways for nurses offer many exciting opportunities.

However, amidst all these changes, what must never change is the essence of nursing: the dedication of every nurse to provide compassionate, informed care which is sensitive to the needs of patients, their experiences, their views, their expectations. Nurses' ability to empathise with patients is so important. A measure of success in achieving this can be seen in small examples. When my brother was seriously ill and in hospital, he was moved from the ward with which he was familiar to a single room in another ward. As soon as the porters left him, a student nurse came in, gently took his hand, introduced herself, made sure he had his call bell and knew how to use it, and said that if he felt anxious or wanted anything, he should not hesitate to call them. This was so reassuring for him and for his family members who were there with him. Patients may be anxious or afraid and it is important that, from the first encounter with their nurse, the approach should create a climate of competency and compassion. Every patient is unique, even if the diagnosis may be the same as that of the patient in the next bed. Our approach to each patient must, without fail, be particular to that individual. Nursing is not only about caring *for* our patients, but also caring *with* our patients, and where relevant, their close family or friends. William Blake (1757–1827) wrote that *'art and science cannot exist but in minutely organised particulars'* and it is the demonstration of these minute particulars, examples of which are given above and which are plentiful within the text, that make our patients feel safe, respected and cared for.

As Florence Nightingale said, *'Unless we are making progress in our nursing every year, every month, every week, take my word for it we are going back'* (cited in Skeet 1980: 100). The new editors and all the chapter authors have not only thoroughly updated the content, demonstrating progress in nursing in its many aspects, but also have provided many links to the web, so that regular checks can be made for advances in knowledge and evidence-based practice.

Now it is over to you, to use the knowledge and understandings you have gained from this fourth edition, to ensure that that progress is reflected in practice. As I and my co-editors said in our earlier editions, and as was reiterated by the new editors, knowledge for nursing can never be static. I hope the ways of learning implicit in the approach of this text will encourage you on a journey of life-long learning, of discovery and challenge. Enjoy your journey and never lose the gift of enquiry as you seek to provide the best-quality care for your patients.

Margaret F. Alexander

REFERENCES

Nursing and Midwifery Council: *Standards for pre-registration nurse education*, London, 2010, Nursing and Midwifery Council. Available online http://www.nmc-uk.org.uk.

Skeet M: *Notes on Nursing: the science and the art*, Edinburgh, 1980, Churchill Livingstone.

Acknowledgements

We would like acknowledge the huge contribution made by the editors, Margaret Alexander, Josephine (Tonks) Fawcett and Phyllis Runciman, and the authors and advisers of this highly successful book over the first three editions. We are delighted that Margaret Alexander agreed to write the Foreword for the fourth edition now entitled *Alexander's Nursing Practice*.

The editors would like to thank their families and colleagues for their support and patience throughout the mammoth task and the contributors whose knowledge, skill and hard work made *Alexander's Nursing Practice* possible.

Thanks also to many people at Elsevier who were key to ensuring the book reached publication especially Ninette Premdas, Sheila Black, Frances Affleck, Kirsteen Wright and Merlyn Harvey. Ethan Danielson's clear and attractive full-colour illustrations complement the text.

Nursing practice – the essence of caring

Maggie Nicol, Chris Brooker

Any health system needs nurses who are intellectually able and emotionally aware and who can combine technical clinical skills with a deep understanding and ability to care, as one human to another... As a profession it is our promise to society
  Message from Christine Beasley, Chief Nursing Officer, England (Department of Health 2006)

Introduction

Welcome to the fourth edition of *Alexander's Nursing Practice*, which you will notice has new editors: Chris Brooker and Maggie Nicol. You will also notice the new name: *Alexander's Nursing Practice*. This is to acknowledge the enormous contribution by Margaret Alexander, Josephine Fawcett and Phyllis Runciman in the first three editions. We are honoured to be able to continue their work.

Alexander's Nursing Practice continues to provide evidence-based knowledge and skills to enable students and qualified nurses to deliver competent and holistic care and maintain their professional learning and development against the backdrop of a rapidly changing health care system. The blurring of boundaries between hospital and home has made it essential for nurses to gain and interpret their knowledge and skills in a range of settings. For many patients, a hospital stay may be a very brief life episode; for others, periodic visits to hospital or to and from the primary care team will become a regular, routine part of life. For some, a care home or hospital may replace their own home.

The current challenges for health care

Although the focus of this book is on health care in the UK and the context in which nursing takes place, its content has much wider relevance. As the World Health Organization (WHO 2003) pointed out, health care does not take place in isolation from political, economic and cultural realities within a country. Nurses constitute a major proportion of the health care workforce in many countries, and certainly those of the WHO European Region, of which the UK is a part, and provide nursing care in environments that are touched by these realities. Many of the challenges that face nurses in UK are not dissimilar to those facing nurses in other countries (WHO 2000, 2003).

Health, illness and disease

Health and ill-health are now known to be influenced by a wide range of factors in people's life circumstances – economic, social, cultural, educational, psychological and genetic. Nurses need to be aware of the broader concepts of health currently being debated and at the same time be ready to respond in practical ways to patients' growing desire for more health-related information.

A useful distinction can be drawn between 'illness' and 'disease'. An 'illness' is what the patient experiences; a 'disease' is a description of pathological abnormality, made from the clinician's point of view. As long ago as 1977, Eisenberg drew this distinction between the personal and professional views, stating, 'Illnesses are experiences of changes in one's state of being and social function; diseases are abnormalities in the structure and function of the body organs and systems' (Eisenberg 1977). The concept of 'illness' therefore embraces all the experiential aspects of a disorder: what that patient *lives through*. This book addresses all three concepts: the disease or disorder and its effect on the body; the illness and how this may be manifested; and the nursing care required to restore health. Nursing management and health promotion are inseparable and nurses are in an ideal position to promote health. The aim of health promotion is to provide individuals with knowledge and skills to make healthy choices about their lifestyle and every nursing interaction presents an opportunity for teaching. For example, patients recovering from a heart attack may be interested in reviewing their diet or may wish to stop smoking.

Changing demography

The population of the UK is ageing. In 2008 the percentage of the population aged 65 and over increased to 16% from 15% in 1983, which means an increase of 1.5 million people in this age group. This trend is projected to continue and by 2033 it is predicted that 23% of the population will be aged 65 and over (Office for National Statistics 2009). Nurses will therefore contribute increasingly to health care for older adults and will need a sound understanding of older people's perspectives and of their experiences of illness and disability. Nursing also has a significant role in maintaining health in older age, both for older people who remain fit, and for those who must cope with health-related problems (Audit Commission 2004, WHO 2005).

Although not inevitable, older people are more likely to have long-term illness and because of the ageing population, the number of people in England with a long-term condition is set to rise by 23% over the next 25 years. Whilst just 17% of the under 40s have a long-term condition, 3 out of every 5 people aged over 60 have a long-term condition (Department of Health 2010a). Older adults are also more likely to have a combination of illnesses (e.g. cancer and cardiovascular disease) and are more likely to be admitted to hospital or require long-term care within the community (Scottish Executive 2005). The resurgence of diseases such as tuberculosis the challenge of health care-associated infection and HIV/AIDS affects all age groups.

Changing care provision

There are major technological and medical advances, from which arise both ethical concerns and issues of cost containment. There are challenges associated with the integration of health and social care and with the provision of increasingly complex technical care to support patients who experience early supported discharge schemes and outreach care initiatives. Health care is continually changing in response to new developments in treatments, technologies and research; many treatments, diagnostic processes and even some diseases were unheard of 10 years ago. Technology, for example, has led to significant changes in how people are cared for in their own homes, other community settings and in hospital. Patients are now likely to have more knowledge of their illnesses and treatment options and take more responsibility for their care through self-management.

There are tensions in current approaches to health care delivery, all of which affect nursing practice. For example, there is a mismatch between the need for proactive, integrated and preventive care for people with long-term conditions and a health care system that is perceived as prioritising specialised, episodic care for acute conditions. In the NHS Second Stage Review, Lord Darzi (Department of Health 2008) identified six key goals: tackling obesity, reducing alcohol harm, treating drug addiction, reducing smoking rates, improving sexual health and improving mental health.

In 2010 the new UK Government published its long-term vision for the future of the NHS in England. *Equality and excellence: Liberating the NHS* (Department of Health 2010b) set out the proposed reforms designed to 'put patients at the heart of everything the NHS does'. The focus will be on continuously improving the outcomes of health care and empowering and freeing up clinicians to become more innovative. The importance of shared decision-making is captured in the phrase *no decision about me without me* (Department of Health 2010b, p. 3). As Darzi (Department of Health 2008) pointed out, the public now expects not just services that are there when they need them, and treat them in the way that they want to be treated, but services that they can influence and shape for themselves. Nurses are well placed to respond to these changing demands, with many of the services for long-term conditions now led by nurses.

Changing nursing roles

It is also a time of rapid growth in the range and type of nursing roles and skills and nurse-led initiatives. For example, nurse consultants, nurse endoscopists and advanced nurse practitioners now perform procedures such as angioplasty and minor surgery. A wide range of nurse-led clinics exist for prevention, treatment and rehabilitation in conditions such as coronary heart disease, diabetes mellitus, chronic obstructive airways disease and asthma. Nonmedical prescribing legislation has empowered many nurses to prescribe from the *Nurse Prescribers' Formulary* and some to become independent prescribers, which means they are able to prescribe from the whole *British National Formulary (BNF)*.

Modernising Nursing Careers (Department of Health 2006) recognised that nurses' roles and responsibilities needed to change. In particular it stated that nurses needed to (Department of Health 2006, p. 10):

- organise care around the needs of patients
- ensure patients have a good experience of nursing as patient choice will rest on the reputation of organisations for the quality of the nursing
- work in a range of settings, crossing hospital and community care, and use telemedicine
- develop the skills and competencies to care for older people and people with long-term conditions, who may have both physical and mental health needs
- be able to use preventative and health promotion interventions as well as advanced skills
- work for diverse employers, and take opportunities for self employment where appropriate
- work as leaders and members of multidisciplinary teams inside and outside hospital, and across health and social care teams
- work with new forms of practitioners, for example assistant practitioners and anaesthesia practitioners
- deliver high productivity and best value for money.

Professional accountability

Student nurses are not professionally accountable until they become registered nurses but they are subject to guidance from the Nursing and Midwifery Council (NMC). *Guidance on professional conduct for nursing and midwifery students* (Nursing and Midwifery Council 2010a), which is based on *The Code*, sets out the personal and professional conduct expected of students in order for them to be considered fit to practise. Once registered, *The Code* (Nursing and

Midwifery Council 2008) sets out the standards of conduct, performance and ethics that are expected of nurses and midwives. Professional registered nurses are personally accountable for their actions and omissions in their practice and must always be able to justify their decisions (Nursing and Midwifery Council 2008). Fundamental nursing care is increasingly being delivered by health care assistants and associate practitioners, which means that registered nurses are accountable for care they are not delivering themselves. *The Code* requires that if nurses are delegating care to another professional, health care support staff, carer or relative they must '…delegate effectively and are accountable for the appropriateness of the delegation' (Nursing and Midwifery Council 2008). The NMC (2008, p. 6) states that it is the nurse's responsibility to:

- establish that those to whom they delegate are able to carry out their instructions
- confirm that the outcome of any delegated task meets required standards
- make sure that those for whom they are responsible are supervised and supported.

Thus, as identified in the *Standards for Pre-registration Nursing Education* (Nursing and Midwifery Council 2010b) nurses need to be leaders of nursing as well as care givers. Nurses must be able to justify the decisions they make and therefore require a sound knowledge of the underpinning rationale for their actions. This book is designed to help you. Updated by experts in their field, *Alexander's Nursing Practice* provides a foundation of knowledge on which to build as your career progresses.

Partnerships

Partnership is a key issue in both policy and practice, here in the UK and further afield. Partnership is essential, not only with other health and social care professionals, but also with patients and carers. In the coming decades, the consumer's voice will increasingly be sought and heard in the development and evaluation of health and social care. The emphasis on partnership means that nurses in hospital and in the community must find new ways of working with colleagues in the NHS, social care, public health and in a wider range of service sectors and agencies. Partnership also implies a need for strong clinical leadership. Effective partnerships are fundamental to the aims of clinical governance, with its emphasis on creating an environment in which clinical excellence will flourish. There are references throughout the text which reflect the importance of clinical judgement, decision-making and risk management, all of which require clinical leadership. The NMC recognise the importance of this and identify leadership, management and team working as one of the four domains of competency (Nursing and Midwifery Council 2010b) (Box 1.1).

Reflective practice

Reflective practice is the key to professional development as a nurse. Some of the most sensitive insights of experienced nurses come from their careful, thoughtful analysis of daily work. Much can be learned from patient narratives and the telling of nursing stories, for example 'critical incidents'. Reflection is an important human activity in which people re-capture their experience, mull it over and evaluate it. It

---

Box 1.1 Domains of competency requirements

Professional values

All nurses must act first and foremost to care for and safeguard the public. They must practise autonomously and be responsible and accountable for safe, compassionate, person-centred, evidence-based nursing that respects and maintains dignity and human rights. They must show professionalism and integrity and work within recognised professional, ethical and legal frameworks. They must work in partnership with other health and social care professionals and agencies, service users, their carers and families in all settings, including the community, ensuring that decisions about care are shared.

Communication and interpersonal skills

All nurses must use excellent communication and interpersonal skills. Their communications must always be safe, effective, compassionate and respectful. They must communicate effectively using a wide range of strategies and interventions including the effective use of communication technologies. Where people have a disability, nurses must be able to work with service users and others to obtain the information needed to make reasonable adjustments that promote optimum health and enable equal access to services.

Nursing practice and decision-making

All nurses must practise autonomously, compassionately, skilfully and safely, and must maintain dignity and promote health and wellbeing. They must assess and meet the full range of essential physical and mental health needs of people of all ages who come into their care. Where necessary they must be able to provide safe and effective immediate care to all people prior to accessing or referring to specialist services irrespective of their field of practice. All nurses must also meet more complex and coexisting needs for people in their own nursing field of practice, in any setting including hospital, community and at home. All practice should be informed by the best available evidence and comply with local and national guidelines. Decision-making must be shared with service users, carers and families and informed by critical analysis of a full range of possible interventions, including the use of up-to-date technology. All nurses must also understand how behaviour, culture, socioeconomic and other factors, in the care environment and its location, can affect health, illness, health outcomes and public health priorities and take this into account in planning and delivering care.

Leadership, management and team working

All nurses must be professionally accountable and use clinical governance processes to maintain and improve nursing practice and standards of health care. They must be able to respond autonomously and confidently to planned and uncertain situations, managing themselves and others effectively. They must create and maximise opportunities to improve services. They must also demonstrate the potential to develop further management and leadership skills during their period of preceptorship and beyond.

(Nursing and Midwifery Council 2010a)

needs to take place at a conscious level to allow us to make decisions about our learning (Boud et al 1985).

Nursing students spend half of their pre-registration programme in practice placements. This is where you learn the art and science of nursing by observing expert nurses and, under their supervision, developing your own knowledge and skills. In the *Standards for Pre-registration Nursing Education* (Nursing and Midwifery Council 2010b) the NMC stipulates that nurses must be able to maintain their own personal and professional development and learn from experience, through supervision, feedback, reflection and evaluation. Reflection helps you to look back at your experience and determine what you have learnt, what knowledge and theories you were applying and what you do not yet understand. Thus it is an important skill to develop and throughout this book you are invited to reflect on what you are reading and make links to your clinical experience.

Changes to nursing education

In 2008 a major period of change in nurse education began. In recent years there has been a move towards degree-level nurse education and in 2008 the NMC decided to change the minimum academic level. By 2013 diploma programmes will no longer be offered and all pre-registration nursing programmes will be degree level only.

The NMC (2010c) concluded that degree level nurses would:

- be more independent and innovative and able to use higher levels of professional judgement and decision-making in an increasingly complex care environment
- assess and apply effective, evidence-based care safely and with confidence, managing resources and working across service boundaries
- be members, and often leaders, of multi-disciplinary teams where colleagues are already educated to at least graduate level
- provide leadership in promoting and sustaining change and developing clinical services.

Registered nurses without a degree will retain their registration but will be encouraged to 'top up' their qualifications to degree level.

Standards for pre-registration nursing education

In September 2010, after a period of consultation with higher education institutions, health care providers, individual nurses and patient organisations new standards for pre-registration nursing education were published (Nursing and Midwifery Council 2010b). Currently there are four different programmes leading to qualification as a nurse working with Adults, Children, those with Mental Health problems or those with Learning Disabilities, which are known as 'branches of nursing'. By 2013 this will become one programme with four pathways known as 'fields of practice'. The new standards for pre-registration nursing (Nursing and Midwifery Council 2010b) indicate the knowledge, skills and attitudes that graduate nurses need to demonstrate at the point of registration. There are 34 'generic' competencies, which must be met by all nurses, and a smaller number of 'field specific' competencies that relate to each of the four fields of practice. The competencies are organised into four domains (see Box 1.1).

The new standards (Nursing and Midwifery Council 2010b) have been informed by the Royal College of Nursing definition of nursing as 'the use of clinical judgment in the provision of care to enable people to improve, maintain or recover health, to cope with health problems, and to achieve the best possible quality of life, whatever their disease or disability until death' (Royal College of Nursing 2004).

According to the NMC (2010d), universities will need to work in partnership with health care providers to develop programmes in the context of local health care delivery, addressing national policies across the UK. There may also be local and national strategies to be considered. For example, in England NHS Employers (2010) have produced an implementation guide to prepare employers for the new pre-registration nursing education standards.

Essential skills clusters

The new competencies (Nursing and Midwifery Council 2010b) include revised *Essential Skills Clusters*, which were first introduced by the NMC in 2007. *The Essential Skills Clusters* relate to all nursing fields of practice and identify skills that must be demonstrated at each of three progression points by all students from 2013. There are two progression points during the course of study (end of the first year and end of the second year) and the third is prior to registration. *The Essential Skills Clusters* reflect patient expectations of newly qualified nurses relating to: care and compassion, communication, organisational aspects of care, infection prevention and control, nutrition and fluid maintenance, and medicines management (Nursing and Midwifery Council 2007).

Features of the book

This book seeks to support pre-registration nurses studying for their diploma or degree and those undertaking continuing professional and personal development (CPPD). High quality nursing care will always be fundamental to helping individuals to maintain good health, recover from ill-health, cope with chronic illness and experience dignity and comfort at life's end. High quality nursing care requires high quality nurses and high quality nurses have a good level of evidence-based knowledge to support their actions. This book is designed to help students from all branches/fields of practice to develop and maintain that knowledge.

As editors we hope this book will:

- clearly present the knowledge and skills required to meet the NMC standards for competent, evidence-based practice in the variety of settings in which nurses work
- value the individual 'lived experience' of health and illness, and the importance of listening carefully to the voices of patient and carers
- illustrate the changing context and dynamic nature of health care
- develop ways of thinking, learning and critically discussing the nature of nursing

- encourage reflection and analysis of care
- demonstrate the essential contribution of research in practice.

The book has been completely updated and is now in full colour, which means that the figures and photographs are even better. There is also now a dedicated website, containing supplementary material to support your reading and clinical practice. The website also contains multiple choice quiz questions and critical thinking activities to help you test your knowledge and identify your future learning needs. There are interactive boxes throughout all of the chapters to highlight the latest evidence-based practice and to encourage you to reflect on, and apply new knowledge to, your clinical experience. An icon alerts you to additional materials, such as photographs, charts and tables, on the accompanying website, where you will also find the multiple choice questions and critical thinking exercises for each chapter. The section on normal values in the Appendix provides a handy reference guide; it is crucial that nurses know the normal ranges so that they know when to report abnormal findings. The glossary enables you to check definitions to ensure understanding of the concepts discussed within the chapters.

The book is presented in three sections:

Section 1 – Care of patients with common disorders

This section presents a broad overview of relevant anatomy and physiology and clinical features of disorders of the various body systems. It also includes relevant diagnostic investigations and tests and outlines the principles of medical management. The heart of each chapter is the section entitled *Nursing management and health promotion*. It is here that the unique contribution provided by nurses is discussed with an emphasis on individualised care that is sensitive to patient need. This is important for nurses in all branches or fields of practice.

Section 2 – Core nursing issues

This section focuses on nursing issues that could affect any of our patients, regardless of their illness or condition. The importance of infection prevention and control in health care cannot be over emphasised; we have responded by creating a separate chapter (Ch. 16) for this important topic. Topics such as pain management, shock and wound management are at the heart of every nursing interaction and all nurses need good levels of knowledge to provide effective care.

Section 3 – Nursing specific patient groups

This section addresses the needs of patients with particular care needs such as the critically ill and older adults. All nurses in all specialities are likely to be caring for patients with, for example, long-term conditions or continence problems and it is vital that they are confident and competent to do so. This section will help you to understand the relevant anatomy and physiology, relevant investigations and tests and the specific nursing needs of patient and clients in these groups. The incidence of sexually acquired infections and HIV/AIDS is continuing to rise and we have responded by expanding the chapter on HIV/AIDS (Ch. 35) to include sexually acquired infections.

In conclusion

Practice must never be viewed complacently; the rationale for the care you are giving must always be understood. The knowledge needed for nursing can never be static and those who, as professional nurses, pursue such knowledge will undertake a journey of life-long learning, a journey of discovery and challenge. This is a textbook for enquiring nurses wishing to understand more and improve their practice. Whether you are a student, an experienced nurse or a nurse returning to practice, this book is for you. We hope that you will find it useful, interesting and informative.

REFERENCES

Audit Commission: *Older people – independence and well-being: the challenge for public services*, London, 2004, Audit Commission.

Boud D, Keogh R, Walker D: *Reflection: turning experience into learning*, London, 1985, Kogan Page.

Department of Health: *Modernising nursing careers: setting the direction*, London, 2006, Department of Health.

Department of Health: *High quality care for all: NHS next stage review final report*, London, 2008, Department of Health. Available online http://www.dh.gov.uk/en/Publicationsandstatistics/Publications/PublicationsPolicyAndGuidance/DH_085825.

Department of Health: *Long term conditions*, London, 2010a, Department of Health. Available online http://www.dh.gov.uk/en/Healthcare/Longtermconditions.

Department of Health: *Equity and excellence: Liberating the NHS*, London, 2010b, Department of Health. Available online http://www.dh.gov.uk/en/Publicationsandstatistics/Publications/PublicationsPolicyAndGuidance/DH_117353.

Eisenberg L: Disease and illness: distinction between professional and popular ideas of sickness, *Cult Med Psychiatry* 1(1):9–23, 1977.

NHS Employers: *Preparing for change: implementing the new pre-registration nursing standards*, London, 2010, NHS Employers. Available online http://www.nhsemployers.org/.

Nursing and Midwifery Council: *Circular 07/2002 Introduction of essential skills clusters for pre-registration nursing programmes*, London, 2007, Nursing and Midwifery Council. Available online http://www.nmc-uk.org.uk/.

Nursing and Midwifery Council: *The Code: standards of conduct, performance and ethics for nurses and midwives*, London, 2008, Nursing and Midwifery Council. Available online http://www.nmc-uk.org.uk/.

Nursing and Midwifery Council: *Guidance on professional conduct for nursing and midwifery students*, ed 2, London, 2010a, Nursing and Midwifery Council.

Nursing and Midwifery Council: *Standards for pre-registration nursing education*, London, 2010b, Nursing and Midwifery Council. Available online http://www.nmc-uk.org/.

Nursing and Midwifery Council: *Preparing a future workforce*, London, 2010c, Nursing and Midwifery Council. Available online http://www.nmc-uk.org/.

Nursing and Midwifery Council: *Advice and supporting information for implementing NMC standards for pre-registration nursing education*, London, 2010d, Nursing and Midwifery Council. Available online http://standards.nmc-uk.org/PreRegNursing/non-statutory/Pages/supporting-advice.aspx.

Office for National Statistics: *Latest on ageing*, Newport, 2009, Office for National Statistics. Available online http://www.statistics.gov.uk/cci/nugget.asp?ID=949.

Royal College of Nursing: *The future nurse: the RCN vision*, 2004, Royal College of Nursing. Available online http://www.rcn.org.uk/.

Scottish Executive: *Framework for the future of the NHS*, Edinburgh, 2005, Scottish Executive.

World Health Organization: *Nurses and midwives for health: a WHO European strategy for nursing and midwifery education*, Copenhagen, 2000, WHO Regional Office for Europe.

World Health Organization: *Nurses and midwives: a force for health. WHO European strategy for continuing education for nurses and* *midwives*, Copenhagen, 2003, WHO Regional Office for Europe.

World Health Organization: *Towards age-friendly primary health care*, Geneva, 2005, WHO.

SECTION 1

Care of patients with common disorders

Nursing patients with cardiovascular disorders

Rosemary A. Webster, David R. Thompson

Introduction

The cardiovascular system consists of the heart and blood vessels. It is a closed circuit and is responsible for ensuring that blood flows throughout the body. Heart and circulatory disease, cardiovascular disease (CVD), includes all the diseases of the heart and blood vessels. The two main diseases in this category are coronary heart disease (CHD) and stroke, but CVD also includes congenital heart disease and a range of other diseases of the heart and blood vessels. CVD is the greatest cause of death in the UK, accounting for 34% of the deaths in 2007, a total of over 193 000 people (British Heart Foundation [BHF] 2008). It is the main cause of disability in the UK and as such is likely to be encountered by all nurses, whether hospital- or community-based. CVD also has an immense impact on society in human terms. Bereavement, disability, changing roles within the family and society, and fear are some examples of its consequences. CVD is costly in financial terms, imposing a significant annual burden on the UK economy. CVD cost the health care system in the UK around £3.2 million in 2006 – a cost per capita of just over £50. However, the majority of the costs of CVD fall outside the health care system and are due to illness and death in those of working age and the economic effects on their families and friends who care for them. The overall cost of CVD to the UK economy is estimated to be £30.7 billion per annum (BHF 2008).

Many cardiovascular diseases take the form of progressive debilitating illness, often becoming chronic with intermittent acute episodes. In contrast, a heart attack (myocardial infarction, MI) is often sudden and unexpected, arousing acute distress in the individual and family as they confront a life-threatening crisis. Cardiovascular nursing is evolving as nurses move on from practising the skills of advanced life support, cannulation and phlebotomy, to taking greater responsibility for decisions that influence patient care management. Nursing care has historically ranged from acute care management to long-term support (Ashworth 1992) and includes:

- assessment of symptoms and prioritising acute care management
- providing physical treatment and monitoring for pathophysiological complications
- facilitating lifestyle adjustment and symptom management through developing and evaluating management plans to enable people to attain and maintain a level of health compatible with their personal goals
- assisting people to modify the demands of their activities of living, to balance with their capacity to meet them
- reassuring, supporting and comforting patients and their families.

Government frameworks and standards of care, such as the *National Service Framework for Coronary Heart Disease* (Department of Health [DH] 2000), have resulted in opportunities for nurses to lead and develop CVD services in and between primary, secondary and tertiary care environments. Over the past decade, experienced nurses have increasingly become part of the multidisciplinary team, admitting and discharging patients from specialist units via triage and fast-tracking, prescribing and titrating drug therapies, coordinating specialised clinics and leading rehabilitation and health promotion programmes (Quinn & Morse 2003). For an example of a critical pathway, see website Figure 2.1.

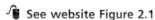 **See website Figure 2.1**

Anatomy and physiology of the heart

The heart is a hollow, four-chambered muscular organ that generates pressure changes resulting in the propulsion of blood around the vascular system. The right side of the heart pumps blood around the pulmonary system where gaseous exchange takes place and then on to the left side of the heart. The left side of the heart operates under much greater pressure to enable it to pump blood around the systemic circulation. The various chambers of the heart are illustrated in Figure 2.1.

The heart is composed of different types of tissue:

- *Pericardium* – a double-layered sac that protects the heart from injury and infection.
- *Epicardium* – the visceral layer of serous pericardium containing elastic fibres, small blood vessels and nerves.
- *Myocardium* – specialised involuntary muscle that forms the main mass of the heart. The atria, which act as filling chambers, have a thin layer of myocardium as they do not, in the fit individual, have to generate high pressures. In the ventricles, the muscular layer is better developed, particularly on the left side, which is larger and thicker than in the right side, as a more forceful contraction is required to pump blood through the systemic circulation.
- *Endocardium* – a thin layer of endothelium and connective tissue that lines the inner chambers of the heart and coats the valves, which open and close to ensure forward blood flow.

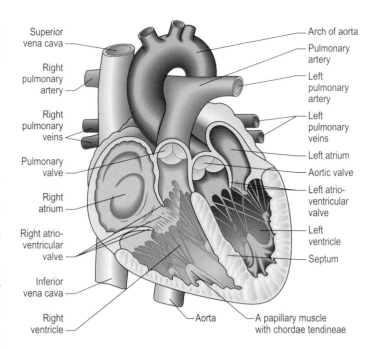

Figure 2.1 The internal anatomy of the heart.

Coronary blood supply

Like all major organs, the heart requires blood flow to maintain cellular activity. It receives its blood supply from the right and left coronary arteries which arise from the aorta just beyond the aortic valve and run over the outer surface of the heart (Figure 2.2).

The left coronary artery runs towards the left side of the heart and divides into two major branches: the left anterior

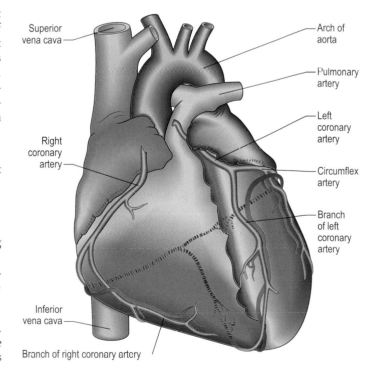

Figure 2.2 The coronary circulation.

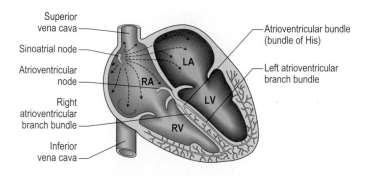

Figure 2.3 The conducting tissues of the heart. LA, left atrium; LV, left ventricle; RA, right atrium; RV, right ventricle.

interventricular branch or left anterior descending artery (LAD) and the circumflex artery (CX). The LAD follows the anterior ventricular sulcus and supplies blood to the interventricular septum and the anterior walls of both ventricles. The CX follows the coronary sulcus and supplies blood to the lateral and posterior regions of the left atrium and left ventricle. The right coronary artery (RCA) runs to the right side of the heart and divides into two branches: the posterior interventricular artery and the marginal artery. The posterior interventricular artery supplies blood to the posterior ventricular walls and the marginal artery supplies the right ventricle. The RCA supplies the sinoatrial (SA) and atrioventricular (AV) nodes in about 60% of cases (Figure 2.3).

After passing through the cardiac capillary bed, the blood drains into the cardiac veins which join to form the coronary sinus on the posterior surface of the heart from where venous blood drains into the right atrium.

Structure and function of cardiac valves

The atrioventricular valves, i.e. the tricuspid and the mitral, function in a similar manner. During ventricular diastole (relaxation), they act as a funnel to promote rapid filling of the ventricles. Most of ventricular filling is passive. During ventricular systole (contraction), intraventricular pressure rises, pushing the cusps, which are restrained by the chordae tendineae, back and up towards the atria, thus preventing backflow of blood during systole.

The semilunar valves, i.e. the pulmonary and the aortic, have three cusps each. These valves are closed during ventricular diastole and intraventricular pressure therefore increases as the ventricles contract. When the pressure in the ventricles becomes greater than that in the aorta and the pulmonary artery the semilunar valves are forced open and blood is ejected. After ventricular systole, the pressure in the aorta and pulmonary artery is greater than that in the left and right ventricles, resulting in retrograde blood flow which fills the valve cusps and snaps them closed. The closure of the valves produces the sounds referred to as heart sounds. Mitral and aortic valve closure produces the first heart sound (S1) which precedes that of the tricuspid and pulmonary valves known as the second heart sound (S2). The second heart sound is normally split because the aortic valve closes before the pulmonary valve, on inspiration, when the right ventricle takes longer to expel the increased venous return.

The conducting system of the heart

The contraction and relaxation of the muscles of the atria and ventricles needs to be coordinated so that filling and emptying of the chambers is controlled and efficient. This occurs as a result of an electrically activated stimulus response system. Specialised automatic cells generate the initial impulse which spreads throughout the myocardium in a coordinated way and triggers a transient release of calcium ions that is responsible for initiating myocardial cell contraction. The automatic cells possess three specific properties:

- automaticity – the ability to generate action potentials, spontaneously and regularly
- excitability – the ability to respond to electrical stimulation by generating an action potential
- conductivity – the ability to propagate action potentials, i.e. spread to other cells.

The main ions (electrically charged particles) involved in the electrical activation of cardiac muscle are sodium (Na^+), potassium (K^+) and calcium (Ca^{2+}). Electrical activity occurs due to the movement of these and other ions in and out of the cells thereby altering the electrical charge of the cell. Cells at rest (known as polarised) are negatively charged on the inside whilst cells that are electrically activated (known as depolarised) are positively charged on the inside. The electrical charge on the surface of an automatic cell leaks away until a certain threshold is reached and spontaneous action potential is generated over the whole cell surface. The automatic cells are found in the cardiac conducting system (see Figure 2.3), which consists of:

- the sinoatrial (SA) or sinus node
- the atrioventricular (AV) junction (the AV node and bundle)
- ventricular conducting tissue (the right and left bundle branches).

The automatic cell with the most rapid leak of charge becomes the principal pacemaking cell and is normally located within the SA node. Both automatic and myocardial cells can transmit impulses, but the specialised cells do so in a more rapid and coordinated way. Electrical activation spreads from the SA node through both atria at a rate of about 1 m/s and reaches the most distant portion of the atria in about 0.08 s. The atria and ventricles are electrically connected via the AV junction, and when the impulse reaches the AV node there is a delay of about 0.04 s to allow blood flow from the atria to the ventricles. From the AV node, the impulse enters the rapidly conducting tissue of the bundle of His and the right and left bundle branches and the entire ventricular mass is depolarised almost simultaneously thereby producing efficient contraction and pumping. Return to the electrical resting state for each cell is called repolarisation and involves active pumping of ions against concentration gradients.

Electrocardiography

Electrocardiography is the graphic recording from the body surface of potential differences resulting from electrical currents generated in the heart (vertical axis) plotted against time (horizontal axis). This recording may be displayed on

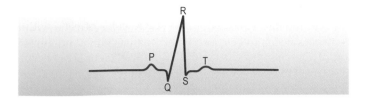

Figure 2.4 ECG of one cardiac cycle.

special graph paper or on an oscilloscope (monitor) and is known as an electrocardiogram (ECG). The main value of the ECG is in the detection and interpretation of cardiac arrhythmias, diagnosis of CHD and assessment of ventricular enlargement (hypertrophy).

The sequence of electrical events produced at each heartbeat has arbitrarily been labelled P, Q, R, S and T (Figure 2.4).

The P wave represents atrial activation and the width of the P wave illustrates the time this takes. The PR interval, measured from the beginning of the P wave to the beginning of the first deflection of the QRS complex, represents the total time taken for atrial activation and AV nodal delay.

The Q, R and S waves are associated with ventricular activation. The first downward deflection after the P wave is always labelled the Q wave and the R wave is the first upward deflection. If a negative deflection follows an R wave, it is labelled an S wave. The width of the QRS complex shows how long the action potential takes to spread through the ventricles.

The ST segment is the line between the S wave and the T wave and represents the early phase of ventricular muscle repolarisation, or recovery.

The T wave represents the electrical recovery or repolarisation of the ventricular muscle. Occasionally, a U wave can be observed following the T wave. The origin of this wave is not well understood, but it is considered significant in a state of hypokalaemia. For more details on the ECG see Riley (2007a) in Further reading.

Cardiac cycle

The cardiac cycle is the cyclical contraction (systole) and relaxation (diastole) of the two atria and the two ventricles. Each cycle is initiated by the spontaneous generation of an action potential in the SA node.

During diastole, which normally lasts about 0.4 s, blood enters the relaxed atria and flows passively into the ventricles. The atria contract fractionally before the ventricles and complete ventricular filling. As the ventricles begin to contract, ventricular pressure increases and for a short time (isometric phase) all four valves are closed and the volume of blood in the ventricles remains constant. Increasing pressure eventually forces the pulmonary and aortic valves to open and blood is ejected into the pulmonary artery and aorta. When the ventricles stop contracting, the pressure within them falls below that in the major blood vessels, the aortic and pulmonary valves close and the cycle begins again with diastole (Figure 2.5).

The normal heart rate is approximately 70 beats/min in the resting adult, with each cardiac cycle lasting approximately

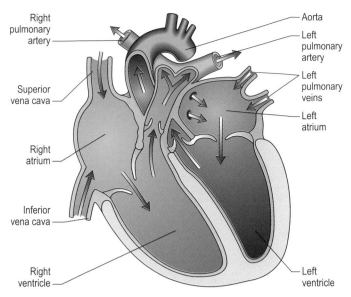

Figure 2.5 Blood flow through the heart.

0.8 s. With each ventricular contraction, 65–75% of the blood in the ventricle at the end of diastole is ejected. This is usually a volume of 70–80 mL of blood and is known as the stroke volume.

Cardiac output is the volume of blood ejected from one ventricle in 1 min. Although cardiac output is a traditional measure of cardiac function, it differs markedly with body size. Thus, a more informative measure is the cardiac index, which is the cardiac output per minute per metre squared of body surface area. Usually it is about $3.2 \, L/m^2$.

The primary factors that determine cardiac output are:

- Preload – the amount of tension on the ventricular muscle fibres before they contract, determined primarily by the end-diastolic volume (EDV).
- Afterload – the resistance against which the heart must pump. It is determined by blood pressure in the aorta, resistance in the peripheral vessels, the size of the aortic valve opening, left ventricular size, contractility of the heart and the heart rate.

Within physiological limits, the volume of blood pumped out by a ventricle is the same as that entering the atrium on the same side of the heart, i.e. cardiac output matches venous return. This principle is often referred to as the Frank–Starling law of the heart. This means that the heart is able to adapt to changing loads of inflowing blood from the systemic and pulmonary circulations. Within certain limits, cardiac muscle fibres contract more forcibly the more they are stretched at the start of contraction. Once the venous return increases beyond a certain limit, the myocardium begins to fail. This regulation of the heart in response to the amount of blood to be pumped is known as intrinsic regulation.

Regulation of cardiac function by the autonomic nervous system

The autonomic nervous system alters the rate of impulse generation by the SA node, the speed of impulse conduction and the strength of cardiac contraction. It regulates the heart through both sympathetic and parasympathetic nerve fibres. The sympathetic fibres supply all areas of the atria and ventricles, and the effects on the heart include increased heart rate, increased conduction speed through the AV node and increased force of contraction. Parasympathetic impulses are conducted to the heart via the vagus nerve and affect primarily the SA node, the AV node and the atrial muscle mass. Parasympathetic stimulation produces decreased heart rate, decreased conduction rate through the AV node and decreased force of atrial contraction.

Sympathetic and parasympathetic control of the heart occurs by reflexes coordinated in the medulla oblongata of the brain. The group of neurones in the brain that affects heart activity and the blood vessels is known as the cardiovascular centre. This centre receives information from various sensory receptors. Baroreceptors, located in the atria, the aortic arch and carotid sinuses, alter their rate of impulse generation in response to changes in blood pressure; chemoreceptors, located for example in the carotid artery, respond to changes in the chemical composition of the blood.

Anatomy and physiology of the blood vessels

Systemic circulation

The systemic circulation is a high-pressure system that supplies all the tissues of the body with blood. It consists of the arteries, arterioles, capillaries, venules and veins. Blood flows through the system because of a downward pressure gradient from the aorta to the superior and inferior venae cavae. Arteries distribute oxygenated blood from the left side of the heart to the tissues, and veins convey deoxygenated blood from the tissues to the right side of the heart. Adequate perfusion resulting in oxygenation and nutrition of body tissues is dependent in part upon patent and responsive blood vessels and adequate blood flow.

Arteries and arterioles

Arteries are thick-walled structures that carry blood from the heart to the tissues. The major arteries leading from the heart branch to form smaller ones, which eventually give rise to arterioles. The walls of the arteries and arterioles are divided into three layers:

- the inner layer provides a smooth surface in contact with the flowing blood
- the middle layer, the thickest, consists of elastic fibres and muscle fibres; the elasticity of the arterial wall enables it to recoil during ventricular relaxation and maintain blood flow
- the outer layer of connective tissue anchors the vessel to its surrounding structures.

Arterioles contain significantly less elastic tissue than the arteries and have a middle layer of predominantly smooth muscle that controls the vessel's diameter. The arterioles are able to respond to local changes in concentrations of oxygen, carbon dioxide and other waste products and changes in blood pressure – a process known as autoregulation which works to maintain adequate blood flow in changing circumstances.

Capillaries

Capillary walls consist of a thin single layer of cells with a large total surface area. The velocity of blood is at its slowest in the capillaries to allow efficient transport of nutrients to the cells and the removal of metabolic wastes.

Veins and venules

Capillaries join together to form larger vessels called venules, which in turn join to form veins. The walls of the veins are thinner and much less muscular than the arteries, allowing them to distend more and permitting storage of large volumes of blood under low pressure. Approximately 75% of total blood volume is contained in the veins. Some veins are equipped with valves to prevent the reflux of blood as it is propelled towards the heart. The sympathetic nervous system can stimulate venoconstriction, thereby reducing venous volume and increasing the general circulating blood volume. This adjustment of the total volume of the circulatory system to the amount of blood available to fill it is part of the process of regulating blood pressure.

Blood pressure

Blood pressure refers to the hydrostatic pressure exerted by the blood on the blood vessel walls and is a consequence of blood flow and vascular resistance. As most of the resistance to blood flow is due to the peripheral vessels, especially the arterioles, it is often described as the total peripheral resistance, as in the equation:

$$\text{mean arterial pressure} = \text{cardiac output} \times \text{total peripheral resistance}$$

Blood pressure varies in different blood vessels. However, clinically the term 'blood pressure' refers to systemic *arterial* blood pressure. It is the pressure of blood that makes the exchange of fluid and nutrients between capillaries and tissues possible.

Arterial blood pressure

Arterial blood pressure fluctuates throughout the cardiac cycle. The maximum pressure occurs after ventricular systole and is known as the *systolic* pressure. Systolic pressure is dependent on the stroke volume, the force of contraction and the stiffness of the arterial walls. Systolic blood pressure normally falls a little on standing and this fall may be particularly marked in those with autonomic failure, taking vasodilator medication or in shock. The level to which arterial pressure falls before the next ventricular contraction is the minimum pressure, known as the *diastolic* pressure. Diastolic pressure varies according to the degree of vasoconstriction and is dependent on the level of the systolic pressure, the elasticity of the arteries and the viscosity of the blood. Normally the diastolic blood pressure rises a little on standing. Alterations in heart rate will also affect diastolic pressure. A slower heart rate produces a lower diastolic pressure as there is more time for the blood to flow out of the arteries. The difference between the systolic and diastolic blood pressures is known as the 'pulse pressure'. The average pressure attempting to push the blood through the circulatory system is known as the 'mean arterial pressure'.

Blood pressure values

There is no such thing as a 'normal' blood pressure, as it varies both from person to person and in individuals from moment to moment, under different circumstances. The optimal blood pressure targets are a systolic blood pressure of less than 120 mmHg and a diastolic blood pressure of less than 80 mmHg (Williams et al 2004). Factors such as age, gender and race influence blood pressure values. Pressure also varies with exercise, emotional reactions, sleep, digestion and time of day.

The predominant mechanisms that control arterial pressure within the 'normal' range are the autonomic nervous system and the renin–angiotensin–aldosterone system. Baroreceptors respond to changes in arterial pressure and relay impulses to the cardiovascular centre in the medulla oblongata. When the arterial pressure is increased, baroreceptor endings are stretched and relay impulses that inhibit the sympathetic outflow. This results in a decreased heart rate and arteriolar dilatation and the arterial pressure returning to its former level. If the blood pressure remains chronically high, the baroreceptors are reset at a higher level and respond as though the new level were normal.

When blood flow to the kidneys decreases, with a fall in blood pressure, renin is released. Renin is an enzyme that acts on the blood protein angiotensinogen, which is converted to angiotensin I in the liver and then, by another enzyme in the kidney, to angiotensin II. Angiotensin II produces an elevation in blood pressure by direct constriction of arterioles. Angiotensin II also directly stimulates the release of the hormone aldosterone from the adrenal cortex which leads to renal retention of sodium and water in the distal convoluted tubules. This increases extracellular volume, which in turn increases the venous return to the heart, thereby raising stroke volume, cardiac output and arterial blood pressure. The kidneys respond to an increase in arterial pressure by excreting a greater volume of fluid. This decreases the extracellular fluid, resulting in a lower venous return and reduced cardiac output until arterial pressure is returned towards normal.

Atherosclerosis

Atherosclerosis is a complex disorder that can affect the muscular arteries throughout the body. It is responsible for most CHD and much peripheral and cerebrovascular disease and is characterised by the progressive accumulation of cholesterol within the arterial intima. It is a disease with phases of stability and instability and is thought to involve endothelial injury, inflammatory processes and the focal distribution of lipids and fibrous tissue in the form of atheromatous plaques, particularly around branching vessels and arterial curvature. These plaques evolve over decades, a mature plaque having a soft, lipid-rich core surrounded by a hard fibrous capsule. There is thickening and hardening of the vessel walls with resultant loss of elasticity (Figures 2.6, 2.7).

With disease progression the lining of the vessel wall may become eroded and, especially if the blood pressure is elevated, the vessel may become permanently dilated and weakened, forming an aneurysm. Vessels may become blocked or stenosed or, as a result of endothelial damage and platelet adhesion, an ulcer-like site can develop, leading to thrombus

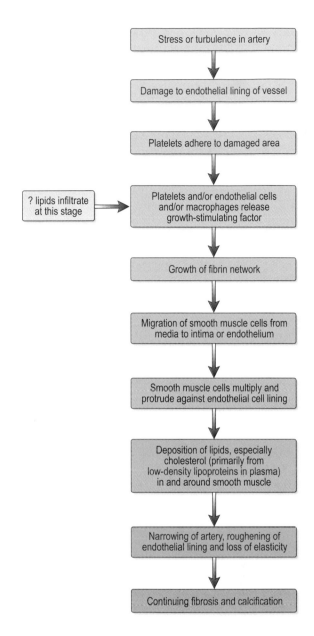

Figure 2.6 Probable course of events in the development of atheroma.

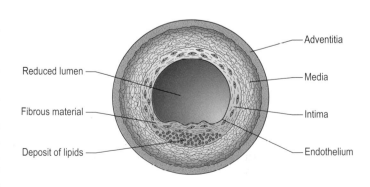

Figure 2.7 Cross-section of an artery.

formation. This thrombus may cause complete obstruction of the artery or may break down spontaneously. This dynamic process occurs over a period of hours to days, preceding an acute coronary event or spontaneous resolution.

For further details of the pathogenesis of atherosclerosis, see Further reading, e.g. Jowett & Thompson (2007).

Ischaemia

Ischaemia is defined as a condition in which there is an imbalance between oxygen supply and demand. Oxygen supply to the tissues of the body varies with blood flow and may be compromised by abnormalities of the vessel wall, the blood flow or the blood itself. Peripheral artery occlusion can occur as a result of an embolus, atherosclerosis, diabetic vascular disease, vasculitis and vasospastic conditions. Myocardial blood supply can be reduced through atherosclerosis, thrombosis and arterial spasm. It is thought that a coronary artery must be narrowed by at least 50% before coronary blood fails to meet the demands of the heart during exertion. Severe anaemia and hypoxia can also result in a decreased oxygen supply. For the myocardium, oxygen demand depends mainly upon heart rate, myocardial contractility and tension in the myocardial wall, with increased oxygen demand occurring in a variety of clinical conditions, including tachycardia, hypertension, valvular stenosis, left ventricular hypertrophy and hyperthyroidism. Localised myocardial ischaemia may be intermittent and have reversible effects, but it inevitably causes decreased myocardial function. Ischaemia results in the build-up of lactic acid, acidosis and the rapid accumulation of potassium in the extracellular space – chemical changes that trigger a pain response. Myocardial ischaemia can produce pain after a minute of ischaemia as the sensory neurones innervating the heart are richly endowed with an ion channel that is opened by the increase in lactic acid concentration.

Risk factors for cardiovascular disease

Epidemiological studies have sought to find associations between CVD and biomedical, behavioural and psychosocial characteristics of a population or individuals. As a result, predictive variables termed 'risk factors' have been defined, which have been shown to be associated with the development of disease. Although, by definition, each risk factor associates positively with increased risk of the disease, it does not follow that risk factors are causal. It is also important to remember that a significant number of patients presenting with CVD do not have identifiable risk factors and that standard risk factors explain less than half the disease.

Non-modifiable risk factors include increasing age, male gender, ethnic origin and a history of premature CVD (Table 2.1). Modifiable biomedical risk factors include: raised serum cholesterol levels/dyslipidaemia (disruption in the amount of lipids in the blood); being overweight/obesity; diabetes/insulin resistance and renal disease. Modifiable behavioural and psychosocial risk factors include tobacco smoking, physical inactivity, poor nutrition, excessive alcohol consumption; anxiety and depression; social isolation and stress.

The known risk factors tend to 'cluster' in individuals with one factor adding to the risk of another, i.e. they are

Table 2.1 Modifiable and non-modifiable risk factors for coronary heart disease

NON-MODIFIABLE RISK FACTORS	MODIFIABLE RISK FACTORS
Age	Blood cholesterol
Gender	Tobacco smoking
Ethnicity	High blood pressure
Genetic predisposition	Overweight and obesity
Low birth weight	Diet
Diabetes mellitus	Alcohol consumption
Hormonal and biochemical factors	Social class Geographical distribution

cumulative, and the impact of any one risk factor needs to be considered in combination with the individual's other risk factors. The risk of a future CVD event can be calculated from a knowledge of an individual's smoking habits and blood pressure and blood cholesterol levels (National Institute for Health and Clinical Excellence [NICE] 2008). These three risk factors are high within the population. It is estimated that approximately 21% of women and 23% of men smoke (BHF 2008). It is estimated that more than a quarter of the world's population have an elevated blood pressure (Kearney et al 2005). The target total cholesterol is less than 4 mmol/L, and it has been estimated that 57% of the population of England have a total cholesterol greater than 5 mmol/L (Joint Health Surveys Unit 2008).

Strategies for managing CVD are linked to the probability or risk of individuals developing the disease over time and many cardiovascular risk assessment tools exist to inform the assessment of overall risk and the most effective and cost effective use of treatment. Cardiovascular risk assessment tools include:

- ASSIGN (Assessing Cardiovascular risk using SIGN) – estimates a 10-year risk percentage of developing CVD in disease-free men aged 30–74. Available at http://assign-score.com
- European Systemic Coronary Risk Estimation (SCORE) – used to estimate fatal cardiovascular events over 10 years in low- and high-risk individuals. Available at http://www.escardio.org/communities/EACPR/toolbox /health-professionals/Pages/SCORE-Risk-Charts.aspx
- Reynolds Risk Score – provides a greater accuracy for assessment of cardiovascular risk in women. Available at http://www.reynoldsriskscore.org/
- UK PDS (Prospective Diabetes Study) – for individuals with type 2 diabetes not known to have CHD. Available at http://www.dtu.ox.ac.uk/.

Coronary heart disease

Coronary heart disease is the most common cause of death in the UK, accounting for 1 in 5 deaths in men and 1 in 7 deaths in women (BHF 2008). There are marked regional variations in death rates. The South of England has the fewest deaths from coronary heart disease, Northern Ireland and Wales are intermediate and the North of England and Scotland have the most (BHF 2008).

There is also a clear difference between socioeconomic groups in the prevalence of CHD, with the lowest incidence among the professional groups and the highest among the unskilled manual group. Ethnic background is also a significant factor. For example, a high mortality from CHD has been found in immigrants from the Indian subcontinent (Khunti & Samani 2004) and a high mortality from hypertension and stroke in immigrants from the Caribbean and Africa (Townsend et al 1992). The annual cost of health service resources for treating CHD in 2006 was around £3.2 billion (BHF Statistics 2008).

Stable angina

Angina is a clinical symptom, rather than a disease, describing discomfort or pain resulting from a transient, reversible episode of inadequate coronary circulation occurring as a result of an imbalance between oxygen supply and demand. It is not associated with myocardial necrosis. Similar symptoms may be caused by disorders of the oesophagus, lungs or chest wall. It is estimated that there are approximately 1.98 million people over 35 years of age living with angina in the UK (BHF 2008). Angina is regarded as stable if it has been recurring over several weeks without major deterioration, although symptoms may be variable depending on environmental temperature and emotion.

PATHOPHYSIOLOGY

Ischaemia usually occurs as the result of reduced coronary artery blood flow following coronary artery obstruction caused by fixed atheromatous deposits in the major epicardial arteries. Spasm or thrombus may also contribute to the obstruction. There is insufficient oxygen delivery for local metabolic demand and this releases lactic acid as cells switch to anaerobic metabolism.

Diagnosis

Angina is diagnosed by the nature of the symptoms, history and examination, the perceived likelihood of coronary artery disease in that individual and the results of various diagnostic tests. Cardiac biomarkers will be negative. Where the diagnosis is in doubt, or where a positive diagnosis of angina would have significant implications, patients should have rapid access to, and be assessed by, a cardiologist within 2 weeks of referral via a rapid access chest pain clinic (DH 2000).

Nature and history of symptoms

The presentation and history may be misleading but is frequently one of discomfort related to specific events. The location, character, duration and any relationship of the symptoms to exertion needs to be determined. Stable angina is typically episodic pain or discomfort occurring centrally in the chest, often described as 'dull', 'aching' or a 'tight band'. It is often confused with indigestion. The discomfort may radiate to the arms, particularly the left arm, jaw or neck. It is often induced by exercise or emotion and relieved by rest and/or glycerine trinitrate (GTN). Typically, the duration of an attack of angina is 2–5 min.

Myocardial ischaemia may also be 'silent', i.e. pain free, due to afferent cardiac nerve damage or nerve impulse inhibition at the spinal or supraspinal level, and the individual may experience breathlessness or palpitations in response to increased oxygen demand. Symptoms may vary from day to day and there is no link between symptom severity and the extent of underlying disease.

History and examination

The history provides subjective information about the presenting symptoms, previous patterns of health and illness, and the activities of living. A family history of coronary heart disease together with risk factor identification and social and psychological background adds to the picture. Physical examination needs to include assessment of body mass index and waist circumference, assessment for vascular disease and other signs of co-morbid conditions. A third or fourth heart sound may be heard during episodes of ischaemia.

Laboratory tests

These should include a fasting lipid profile and a fasting glucose level to give an indication of the risk profile for CHD. These tests should be repeated at least annually.

Non-invasive cardiac investigations

Electrocardiogram (ECG) An abnormal ECG both supports the diagnosis and identifies those with a poor prognosis. The recording is invariably normal between attacks of angina and if possible an ECG should be obtained when there are angina symptoms, when the segment between the end of the QRS complex and the beginning of the T wave may be depressed (ST depression) and the T wave may also be flattened or inverted.

Holter monitoring Continuous monitoring of the ST segments of the ECG can be used to detect transient changes associated with ischaemia.

Exercise tolerance test This is useful for both diagnosis and assessing prognosis. The test is based on the theory that patients with ischaemic heart disease will produce marked ST segment depression on the ECG when exercising. The test is considered negative if there are no significant ECG abnormalities and the patient experiences no significant symptoms. The ECG, heart rate and blood pressure are recorded while the patient engages in some form of physiological stress designed to increase myocardial oxygen demand. Three common methods of exercise testing include climbing stairs, pedalling a stationary bicycle and walking on a treadmill. The patient is monitored for chest pain, fatigue, dyspnoea, excessive heart rate (tachycardia), a fall in blood pressure, ischaemic ECG changes and the development of arrhythmias. The test is stopped if any of these occur, or before, at the patient's request. The patient needs to have the procedure explained in detail before the test and should be advised to avoid a heavy meal prior to the test and to wear loose-fitting clothes. The term 'stress test' is best avoided as it may sound ominous and increase patient anxiety. The procedure takes about 30 min. Using medication rather than exercise (pharmacological stress testing) to induce stress is particularly useful if the patient is unable to exercise. This often involves using intravenous dobutamine, which raises the blood pressure and heart rate and increases myocardial oxygen consumption. Vasodilator agents such as adenosine and dipyridamole are an alternative.

Stress echocardiography involves the imaging of altered myocardial contractility during exercise or pharmacological stress.

Myocardial perfusion scintigraphy is a non-invasive method of obtaining images and assessing myocardial perfusion by intravenous injection of a radioisotope, usually thallium or technetium, which is taken up by the heart and distributed throughout the myocardium in proportion to regional blood flow.

Computed tomography (CT) cardiac imaging is useful for detecting and quantifying coronary calcification.

Invasive techniques to assess cardiac anatomy

Coronary arteriography involves the injection of contrast medium into the heart during cardiac catheterisation. The procedure provides reliable anatomical information to identify the presence of coronary lumen stenosis and inform treatment options. It is justifiable in all cases where the results would alter patient management. It carries a mortality of 0.1–0.2%. Cardiac catheterisation can also be used to determine coronary blood flow, velocity and pressure.

The patient should be fully informed about the procedure (Box 2.1), its findings and their implications. Nurses need to be aware of the possible complications and place particular importance on pain relief. Patients should wait no more than 18 weeks from GP referral to treatment (DH 2005).

Risk stratification

The long-term prognosis of stable angina is variable and estimates for annual mortality range from 0.9 to 1.4% per annum (European Society of Cardiology [ESC] 2006). Risk stratification helps in choosing treatment that reflects the severity of the disease and in informing individuals of their prognosis. Those patients at highest risk are most likely to benefit from more aggressive and early treatment. Risk can be calculated through clinical evaluation, stress testing and assessment of ventricular function and coronary anatomy. The EuroHeart Score is an example of a risk assessment tool for stable angina (Daly et al 2006).

Nursing management and health promotion: stable angina

The major treatment goals are to improve prognosis and to minimise or abolish symptoms. Nursing input into these goals will vary according to the type of contact a person has with health care services. Individuals who develop new symptoms of angina should be assessed by a specialist within 2 weeks of referral and rapid access chest pain clinics, which are frequently nurse led, are examples of how such patients can be seen promptly. Practice nurses and occupational health staff may be the main source of professional information and support for those in the community. Nurses also play a significant role in the care of patients with chronic angina who get limited relief from conventional medical treatment (Stewart 2003). Admission to hospital is

Box 2.1 Information

Cardiac catheterisation

Purpose

Cardiac catheterisation involves the insertion, usually under screening, of a fine, flexible, radio-opaque catheter into one or more of the heart chambers. It is increasingly being performed as a day-case procedure. The catheter is inserted via a peripheral vein or artery under sterile conditions in a cardiac catheterisation laboratory. The femoral artery/vein are the most common entry sites although the radial and brachial are also used. The right and left side of the heart may be investigated separately or together. The procedure is performed to:

- visualise the heart chambers and vessels by means of a radio-opaque substance under X-ray control (angiography), e.g. used in the diagnosis of angina
- measure pressure and record waveforms from the cavity of the heart
- obtain blood samples from the heart
- measure left ventricular function (ejection fraction).

Cardiac catheterisation will always be performed on prospective candidates for coronary artery bypass graft surgery, valve surgery and heart transplantation. It is also used to evaluate the effect of thrombolytic agents and the patency of coronary bypass grafts.

Procedure

The patient must give written informed consent for the procedure. Cardiac catheterisation is usually carried out under local anaesthesia and the patient may be given diazepam as premedication. The patient is usually asked to fast for 4 h to prevent aspiration should cardiac arrest occur. The groin area will be shaved. The procedure is performed by a cardiologist and takes approximately 90 min. The patient will be asked to wear a gown and should be prepared to lie flat on their back on a hard table during the procedure. A needle with a guide wire attached is inserted into the vessel and the needle then removed. A sheath is then threaded over the guide wire, the guide wire removed and the catheter inserted through the sheath. The patient is warned to expect a sudden burning sensation as the dye is injected into the heart. Angina may occur as a result of the catheter blocking the artery and may be treated with sublingual glyceryl trinitrate (GTN) spray, oxygen therapy and intracoronary isosorbide dinitrate.

Following the procedure the patient may require analgesics and should be allowed to rest. Observations are taken and the sheath removed. A pressure dressing will be applied to the wound site, which must be observed for excessive bleeding. The limb should be kept straight for 1–2 h to prevent turbulence of blood flow at the incision site. Patients usually stay in bed for 2 h and most are ready for discharge 2 h later.

Possible complications

Patients may experience transient cardiac arrhythmias and syncope. A reaction to the dye may produce symptoms ranging from a rash to anaphylaxis. There is a 0.5% risk of thrombus formation, leading to a cerebrovascular accident or myocardial infarction, and a 0.1% risk of dying from such a complication. Coronary artery dissection is a rare complication. The patient may experience pulmonary oedema whilst lying flat and this is treated with oxygen, nebuliser therapy and diuretics.

likely to occur only if the angina becomes unstable or further investigation is warranted.

The management of stable angina comprises:

- secondary prevention of cardiac events including risk factor modification
- symptom management
- revascularisation
- rehabilitation and support.

Secondary prevention of cardiac events including risk factor modification

Medication Drug therapy for secondary prevention for those with stable angina includes antiplatelet therapy (aspirin, clopidogrel), lipid-lowering therapy (statin therapy is recommended for all those with clinical symptoms of CHD [NICE 2007]) and the use of angiotensin-converting enzyme (ACE) inhibitors. Blood pressure needs to be controlled, particularly for those with diabetes.

See website for further content

Lifestyle Particular attention should be paid to elements of the patient's lifestyle that could have contributed to the condition and that could affect prognosis. Patients with angina need to have management plans that address modifiable risk factors, in particular smoking, physical activity and dietary habits. Risk factor modification in CHD is discussed in more detail on page 15.

Symptom management

Most patients can reduce their angina symptoms through appropriate management. Patients need to be advised to rest, at least briefly, from the activity that provoked the attack.

Advice in the use of sublingual nitrate for acute relief of symptoms includes:

- sitting down when taking GTN
- awareness of possible side-effects, particularly headache, which may be eased with paracetamol
- knowing to call for help (999) if the symptoms persist after three doses over 15 min
- knowing that GTN is not addictive and will not mask the symptoms of a heart attack
- knowing that GTN can also be taken before doing something known to produce pain.

A range of agents are available for background anti-angina therapy including beta blockers, long-acting nitrates and calcium channel blockers.

See website for further content

Patients need to be advised to continue to take their prescribed medication even if they feel their symptoms have resolved, unless medically advised not to do so.

Patients may be able to reduce the frequency of angina symptoms and improve clinical outcome through regular exercise (Hambrecht et al 2004). They should be advised to avoid situations that trigger the symptoms such as exercising after a heavy meal. The Angina Plan, which encourages a self-management strategy through targeting misconceptions and focusing thoughts and emotions, has been shown to be effective in managing angina (Lewin et al 2002).

Revascularisation

Revascularisation aims to improve survival and/or diminish symptoms; it will not stop the process of atherosclerosis. All procedures can be repeated, but ultimately the blood supply may become insufficient to sustain the ventricle so that cardiac failure ensues. The two well-established approaches to revascularisation for chronic stable angina caused by atherosclerosis are:

- percutaneous coronary intervention (PCI)
- coronary artery bypass grafting (CABG).

Percutaneous coronary intervention (PCI) This treatment is appropriate for patients with limiting angina despite optimal medical treatment and for those with disease (atherosclerosis) of one or two of the coronary arteries. PCI is an umbrella term referring to procedures that involve the introduction of a balloon catheter into the affected coronary artery. Included within this treatment category are:

- *Percutaneous transluminal angioplasty (PTCA)* – involves dilating the narrowed artery with an inflated balloon which is then withdrawn (Box 2.2).
- *Intracoronary stenting* – involves leaving a small cylindrical mesh or coil inside the dilated artery to support the vessel wall. The NICE guidelines (1999) advised routine stenting during PCI for coronary arteries between 2.5 and 3.5 mm, which should make their use appropriate for about 80–90% of procedures.
- *Drug-eluting stenting* – the inserted stent is coated with drugs that are released at the implantation site to have a localised short-term effect on the cell re-growth and vessel narrowing that can occur after stenting. Radiation emitters have also been used to reduce in-stent stenosis, a procedure known as vascular brachytherapy. Laser angioplasty, which uses pulsed ultraviolet light to ablate the plaque, and atherectomy, which involves drilling into the plaque, may also be used.

In Further reading, Levine et al (2003) provide an overview of the management of patients undergoing percutaneous coronary revascularisation.

Coronary artery bypass grafting (CABG) This procedure is appropriate for patients whose angina is severely limiting their lives but whose left ventricle is functioning reasonably. It is particularly appropriate for patients with triple vessel disease. The procedure is described in Box 2.3.

Bypass surgery is a potentially traumatic event, and apprehension about the procedure is common (Lyons et al 2002). Patients awaiting surgery have been found to experience a sense of dependency and impending doom (Lindsey et al 2000). Pre-admission education programmes are now offered at many centres and a visit to the operating theatre and ITU may also help.

After the operation, nursing objectives include:

- pain relief
- fluid management – patients can quickly become dehydrated
- assistance with activities of living
- psychological support – patients may become disorientated and confused and need help coming to terms with the effect of the operation (Laitinen 1996)
- preparation for discharge home.

Box 2.2 Information

Percutaneous transluminal coronary angioplasty (PTCA)

Purpose

PTCA is a technique involving the introduction of a balloon catheter into the coronary artery up to the site of a coronary stenosis, where it is inflated. This process produces compression and redistribution of the lesion and a substantial increase in the size of the lumen. PTCA may be performed to relieve the symptoms of angina if medication is ineffective, or it may be performed soon after successful thrombolysis (see p. 24) to restore perfusion to the ischaemic zone.

Procedure

PTCA is carried out under local anaesthetic in a cardiac catheterisation laboratory. If the procedure is planned, the patient will be admitted to hospital the day before and asked to fast for 4 h prior to the procedure. This is to prevent the risk of complications if bypass surgery is required. The patient will be given 300 mg aspirin prior to the procedure and the preparation is as for cardiac catheterisation.

Usually, two arterial catheters are used: a guiding catheter and a dilating catheter. The guiding catheter is inserted, usually in the leg, and advanced to the coronary artery to be dilated. The dilating catheter is then inserted and manipulated into the stenotic area of the artery. Angiography is performed and heparin administered to avoid clot formation at the catheter site. When the dilatation catheter is placed over the stenosis, it is inflated for 5–6 s and then deflated. Blood flow around the balloon is assessed by angiography. Once it has been decided that maximal dilatation has been obtained, the catheters are removed.

Following this procedure, the patient's cardiac status is usually monitored for 24 h. Peripheral pulses are checked frequently for occlusive thrombus at the insertion site. The patient is advised to rest for 4–6 h, lying as flat as is comfortably possible, to keep the leg used for catheter insertion straight in order to minimise the risk of thrombus formation at the insertion site. The introducer sheath is often left in situ for 2–3 h, until the effects of heparin have been reduced.

The patient should be encouraged to drink extra fluid to help eliminate contrast medium.

Re-stenosis occurs in 15–30% of patients, more frequently within the first few months. Repeat angioplasty may be appropriate for some patients. In an increasing number of patients, a stent is inserted at the time of angioplasty. Drug-eluting stents inhibit smooth muscle migration around the stent and have a low (2–3%) re-stenosis rate. All patients will be commenced on clopidogrel and high-risk patients on glycoprotein IIb/IIIa inhibitors.

Possible complications

Complications tend to be sudden and include:

- myocardial infarction
- chest pain
- vagal reaction
- intimal injury
- bleeding at the puncture site
- occlusive thrombus at the puncture site
- coronary artery spasm
- coronary artery dissection.

 Box 2.3 Information

Coronary artery bypass graft surgery (CABG)

Purpose

Coronary artery bypass graft surgery is a technique in which an occluded or stenosed section of a coronary artery is bypassed using part of a vein or artery from elsewhere in the body. Most commonly the long saphenous vein is used, although increasingly the internal mammary artery is being considered. The objectives of CABG are:

- restoration of perfusion and increased oxygenation to the ischaemic myocardium in the peri-infarction patient
- relief of angina pectoris
- improvement of functional status and quality of life
- prolongation of life.

Surgery is only feasible if the risk of the operation is less than continuing with medical therapy. The procedure tends to be offered to those who have:

- symptoms despite maximal therapy
- triple vessel disease or left main stem coronary artery stenosis
- unstable angina.

Procedure

During surgery, the heart is exposed by median sternotomy, the aorta clamped off and cardiopulmonary bypass maintained via cannulae in the descending aorta. The body temperature may be reduced to 32°C and cardiac arrest induced with a cardioplegic solution.

Revascularisation with arterial grafts is becoming more common, as they last longer (10–15 vs. 5–10 years for veins). The internal mammary artery is biologically superior for grafting compared with the saphenous vein.

The artery or vein to be used is harvested while the chest is being opened. The distal end of the bypass graft is sutured to the required vessels. The aorta is then unclamped, the patient rewarmed if cooling has been used, and normal cardiac rhythm re-established by internal defibrillation. The proximal ends of the grafts are sutured to the ascending aorta and cardiopulmonary bypass is then stopped, the cannulae removed and the chest closed. The whole operation takes up to 4 h.

The patient is normally cared for in an intensive care unit after the procedure and will be ventilated until haemodynamically stable. An arterial line and pulmonary artery flotation catheter will be used to monitor cardiac pressures for 24 h.

The patient will usually be able to eat a normal diet on the first or second day. Activity is increased as tolerated over the first 2 days and early mobilisation is encouraged. Patients are often fit for discharge home after about a week.

Possible complications

Complications include:

- leakage at the incision site, producing discomfort and shock
- hypertension as a result of increased sympathetic activity
- hypotension as a result of reduced cardiac output following hypothermia
- pain at both the graft and incision sites
- post-pump cardiotomy syndrome (up to 3 months)
  - problems with coordination
  - loss of memory
  - loss of sense of taste
  - disturbance of vision
- shortness of breath due to heart failure or chest infection.

Patients will be told to expect some degree of pain from the sternotomy for several weeks, discomfort on coughing or lifting the hands above the head, and leg swelling (Levine et al 2003). Short-term anxiety and depression may occur if patients feel that recovery is slower than anticipated. Partners and other family members will also need ongoing information and support and the patient should be offered cardiac rehabilitation. For further details of nursing management of the cardiac surgical patient see Further reading, e.g. Riley (2007b).

Minimally invasive direct coronary artery bypass surgery (MIDCAP) This is an alternative procedure that does not require cardiopulmonary bypass. It is also termed 'off-pump' or 'beating heart' surgery. It involves revascularisation through a small (10 cm) incision in the anterolateral thoracic wall. For selected patients, this procedure offers a less invasive approach with a faster recovery, less likelihood of infection and an improved cosmetic appearance of the wound. Robotically assisted endoscopic coronary artery surgery is developing with the surgeon performing the operation with videoscopic guidance.

Fast-tracking Patients are increasingly being 'fast-tracked' after cardiac surgery. This focuses on early extubation and a move away from elective overnight ventilation following surgery. The recovery of low-risk patients can therefore be managed without overnight admission to the ITU.

Acute coronary syndrome

The term 'acute coronary syndrome' (ACS) defines a continuum of manifestations of CHD. It includes cases of unstable angina and acute myocardial infarction (NSTEMI and STEMI, see below), which all have a common underlying pathology.

PATHOPHYSIOLOGY

Myocardial cells require a constant supply of oxygen and nutrients in order to generate the high-energy phosphate compounds required for contraction. Generally, myocardial cells are irreversibly injured by 30–40 min of total ischaemia. The pathogenesis of unstable angina and acute myocardial infarction are the same and it is not clear which individuals will develop one or the other.

In *unstable angina,* the coronary artery occlusion tends to be episodic and transient. There is often a fissuring of a plaque with the development of a thrombus, but the thrombus does not completely block the artery and subsequently breaks down with no detectable damage to the myocardium.

In *myocardial infarction* the muscle damage almost always results from total occlusion of a coronary artery by a thrombus, usually at the site of a recently cracked or fissured atheromatous plaque. If the lumen of an artery is blocked for about 20 min, and blood supply by the small vessels of the surrounding collateral circulation is inadequate, infarction may develop. Surrounding the area of necrotic tissue there is usually a zone of injury. This tissue cannot contract but may be salvaged if an adequate blood supply can be quickly established; this is sometimes known as 'hibernating' myocardium. The ischaemic zone separates the zone of injury from undamaged tissue (Figure 2.8). During the first 6 h after the onset of

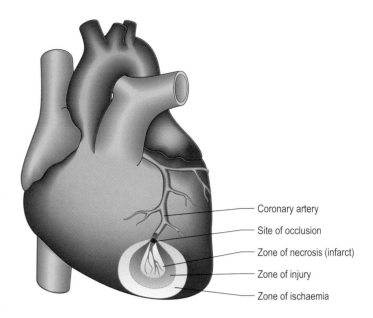

Figure 2.8 Zones of necrosis, injury and ischaemia.

symptoms, the affected myocardium becomes oedematous. There is a shift in the distribution of sodium and potassium ions and an increased risk of arrhythmias. A summary of events following a myocardial infarction is given in Table 2.2. The infarcted area is replaced by fibrous scar tissue over the course of 3–6 weeks. The site of infarction depends on which coronary artery has become occluded. The extent of infarction, and therefore the amount of muscle involved, depends on the artery involved, the previous rate of progression of the disease and the effectiveness of the surrounding collateral circulation. Approximately 50% of MIs are fatal and, in the majority of these cases, death occurs in the first hour after the attack, usually as a result of a cardiac arrhythmia.

Diagnosis

Nature and history of symptoms

Clinical presentation of acute coronary syndrome depends predominantly on whether the obstruction is abrupt or staggered in onset, the site of the occlusion, the resulting loss of

Table 2.2 Events following anterior myocardial infarction (AMI)	
LENGTH OF TIME FOLLOWING AMI	**EVENT**
0–6 h	Cellular breakdown No electrical impulses conducted Necrosis occurs
24 h	Phagocytosis occurs in the infarcted area
5 days	Area infiltrated by fibroblasts, capillaries and collagen tissue Reperfusion of capillaries
2–3 weeks	Fibrosis occurs
2–3 months	Ventricular scarring

Coronary artery
Site of occlusion
Zone of necrosis (infarct)
Zone of injury
Zone of ischaemia

blood flow to the myocardium and whether there is an alternative blood supply to the area in the form of a collateral circulation. Chest pain (angina) is the most common presenting symptom. ACS can occur both in people who are known to have angina and in those who are not. Several clinical presentations have been described (Bassand et al 2007) including:

- prolonged angina at rest lasting for more than 20 min
- new-onset angina that limits ordinary physical activity
- destabilised stable angina with increasing frequency of symptoms and rapidly reduced exercise tolerance
- post-infarction angina occurring in a patient with a recent MI.

The patient should be asked about the location, nature and severity of the pain, any relieving or aggravating factors, and attempted methods of pain relief. As with stable angina, the pain is often described as a tightness, pressure, heaviness or ache and may be mistaken for indigestion. It may occur across the centre of the chest or to one side and can radiate to the arms and/or the throat/jaw, back or shoulder. The pain is not usually affected by movement or breathing in deeply. It may well not be relieved by GTN. Associated symptoms include shortness of breath, nausea, sweating and dizziness. The discomfort and fear around what is causing the symptoms can mean that patients are anxious and distressed. Atypical presentations can make diagnosis unclear; these may include not experiencing any chest pain, sudden loss of consciousness, confusion, profound weakness or arrhythmia.

History and examination

The history provides subjective information about the presenting symptoms, previous patterns of health and illness, and any impact on activities of living. A family history of coronary heart disease together with risk factor identification and social and psychological background adds to the picture. It may be inappropriate to obtain a full history if the patient is in pain, acutely ill, or would benefit from prompt reperfusion therapy. An initial assessment can be enough to set early priorities, without a full physical examination or diagnostic tests.

On examination, patients may appear pale and sweaty and may be clutching their chest. Their blood pressure may be lower than normal with reduced cardiac output or high due to pain and anxiety; slight pyrexia is a common response to muscle damage. Their pulse rate may indicate the presence of an arrhythmia. Changes in respiratory rate can be the first sign of patient deterioration. Dyspnoea may indicate hypoxia or the onset of pulmonary oedema, which is a serious complication. It can also be induced by anxiety. Listening to the chest through a stethoscope (auscultation) may indicate abnormal (turbulent) blood flow which produces an audible murmur. Ventricular septal rupture, mitral regurgitation and aortic stenosis may be picked up in this way. Assessment for the presence of heart failure is also important.

Investigations
Blood tests
- *Serum cardiac markers* (Figure 2.9). The traditional role of biochemical testing has been to provide retrospective confirmation of the presence or absence of myocardial

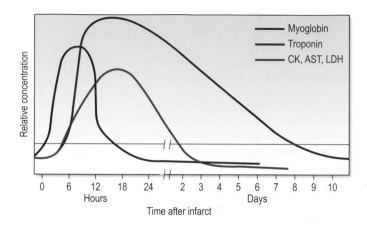

Figure 2.9 Time–activity curves for diagnostic biochemical markers following acute myocardial infarction. CK, creatine kinase; AST, aspartate transaminase; LDH, lactate dehydrogenase.

damage through sequential measurement of serum cardiac markers released into the blood in response to myocardial damage at specific times. Modern analytical equipment now allows for certain markers, in particular the troponins, to be measured in minutes. Bedside analysis is possible, with rapid diagnosis having implications for patient triage and shortening length of hospital stay. Increasingly, measurement of cardiac troponins is allowing cardiac damage to be diagnosed with high sensitivity and specificity. Measurement of cardiac troponin T and cardiac troponin I also allows prognostic risk stratification of patients.
- *White cell count*. This is usually elevated for the first few days following acute myocardial infarction.
- *Erythrocyte sedimentation rate (ESR)*. This usually rises after the first few days and may remain elevated for several weeks.
- *Glucose*. Stress-related hyperglycaemia is common in the acute phase following infarction. Previously undetected diabetes is found in approximately 5% of coronary patients admitted to hospital.
- *Electrolytes*. It is important to know the serum sodium and potassium levels, as these electrolytes can have a major effect on cell excitability.
- *Lipids*. The important lipids in ischaemic heart disease are plasma cholesterol and triglycerides. Total cholesterol should be measured within the first 24 h and a full lipid profile done at 6–8 weeks.
- *Chest X-ray* may show evidence of pulmonary oedema or hypertrophy.
- *ECG*. The standard resting ECG may be normal, at least initially, and repeat ECGs should be performed if the clinical history and presentation suggest that the problem is cardiac. The ECG changes can pinpoint the area of ventricle affected. If there is no myocardial necrosis the ECG may show ischaemic changes (ST depression, T wave inversion) but no ST segment elevation and indicate a possible diagnosis of unstable angina.

There are two categories of ECG findings that indicate myocardial infarction:

1. *Non-ST elevation myocardial infarction (NSTEMI)*. This is when there is some detectable myocardial injury,

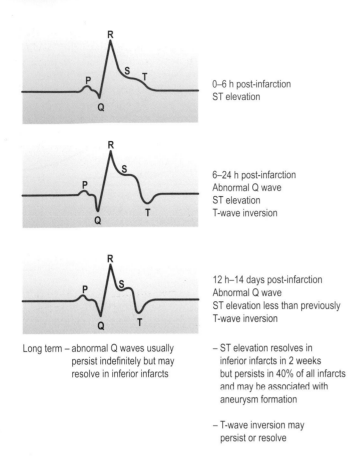

0–6 h post-infarction
ST elevation

6–24 h post-infarction
Abnormal Q wave
ST elevation
T-wave inversion

12 h–14 days post-infarction
Abnormal Q wave
ST elevation less than previously
T-wave inversion

Long term – abnormal Q waves usually
persist indefinitely but may
resolve in inferior infarcts

– ST elevation resolves in
inferior infarcts in 2 weeks
but persists in 40% of all infarcts
and may be associated with
aneurysm formation

– T-wave inversion may
persist or resolve

Figure 2.10 ECG changes in myocardial infarction.

i.e. troponin testing will be positive, but where this damage has not affected the full thickness of the myocardium and hence whilst there may be ischaemic ECG changes there is no ST elevation on the ECG. This condition is potentially unstable and high risk and it may be more appropriate to describe both unstable angina and NSTEMI as 'unstable coronary syndromes'. Both conditions require close observation and admission to coronary care for urgent intervention to prevent progression to transmural (full thickness) myocardial infarction. Without early treatment, around 5–10% of patients will progress to more extensive myocardial damage or death within 30 days (Collinson et al 2000).

2. *ST segment elevation myocardial infarction (STEMI).* This is when there is total occlusion of a coronary artery and transmural (full thickness) muscle damage, i.e. troponin testing will be positive, and there is ST segment elevation on the ECG (Figure 2.10). It is this group of patients who benefit from prompt reperfusion.

Risk stratification

Early risk assessment is required to guide specific treatment to reduce the likelihood of an adverse outcome. The aim is to help identify those patients who need prompt access to specialised care – a challenge for those caring for patients who present with symptoms in the community – and those who are at sufficiently low risk to be discharged or cared for in a low-dependency area. Risk assessment is based on clinical history, observations (heart rate, blood pressure, risk factor profile, ECG changes and biomarkers [troponin levels]). Nurses have a role in identifying patients experiencing an acute cardiac event so that appropriate treatment can be initiated promptly and safely (Kucia et al 2001). Several risk scores for ACS exist, including the TIMI, GRACE and PURSUIT scores, all of which aim to provide guidance for treatment and patient information giving (Yan & Yan 2007).

Nursing management and health promotion: acute coronary syndrome

Nurses caring for ACS patients need to able to support and monitor medical treatments and interventions. They also need to be aware of, and observe for, side-effects and deterioration in a patient's condition alongside providing support, education, comfort and help with activities of daily living as required. Management priorities depend on whether the symptoms are thought to be the result of a thrombus occluding the coronary artery (STEMI) or an unstable coronary syndrome (unstable angina, NSTEMI). Management has historically been divided into three overlapping stages:

*   treatment of the acute attack:
    *   relief of symptoms by analgesics (opiates) plus antiemetic, oxygen and nitrates
    *   monitoring for and treating life-threatening complications
    *   improving blood flow to the myocardium and modification of the affected myocardium
    *   reperfusion with thrombolysis or percutaneous coronary intervention in STEMI
    *   reduction of oxygen demand by rest and beta blockade and alteration of early physiological changes by ACE inhibition
*   risk stratification
*   secondary prevention, including aspirin, and/or clopidogrel, beta blocker, ACE inhibitor and a statin and cardiac rehabilitation.

Patients should ideally be managed in a coronary care unit (CCU) where there can be continuous cardiac monitoring and close observation until the patient is deemed to be stable. These units were first established in the 1960s in order to provide surveillance from skilled personnel with electrocardiographic and resuscitation facilities in a specialised setting.

Possible patient problems include:

*   pain and discomfort
*   fear and anxiety
*   decreased activity levels
*   lack of knowledge and misconceptions
*   altered activities of living
*   loss of control
*   ineffective or inappropriate coping responses e.g. anger, denial.

Immediate priorities

The priorities on admission to hospital include:

*   cardiac monitoring (Table 2.3); ECG
*   establishment of intravenous access
*   relief of pain and associated symptoms

Table 2.3 Observing the cardiac monitor*	
PARAMETER	**ASPECT TO NOTE**
Rate	Is it fast/slow/normal?
Rhythm	Is it irregular/regular?
P waves	Are they present/absent?
QRST complex	Is each complex preceded by a P wave? Is each complex the same?
PR interval	Is it normal/prolonged?
Ectopics (extras)	Are there any extra P waves or extra QRST complexes?

*While observing, note whether the patient is experiencing any symptoms, such as pain, shortness of breath or light-headedness.

- reperfusion therapy where appropriate (see below)
- decrease in the workload of the heart through rest and appropriate medication
- observation for signs of complications/deterioration
- relief of anxiety/information giving and support.
- rehabilitation and recovery.

The patient with an acute coronary syndrome is frequently given oxygen therapy in conjunction with analgesics on admission. However, there is little evidence to support this practice in terms of evidence that oxygen reduces acute myocardial ischaemia (Nicholson 2004).

For a critical care pathway illustrating the management of a patient with a myocardial infarction, see Figure 2.2 on the website.

See website Figure 2.2

Pain control

The patient must be kept free from pain. Pain is a sign of ongoing myocardial ischaemia and should be controlled. Patients should be told of the importance of reporting pain. Accurate pain assessment is essential to ensure that appropriate analgesics are given. Rating scales, where patients rate their pain numerically, can be useful (see Ch. 19). Pain can be difficult to assess and nurses have been shown to be unreliable in assessing cardiac pain (O'Connor 1995), although this can be improved with appropriate education (Thompson et al 1994). Ischaemic pain can easily be confused with pain from other sources, particularly pericarditic or pleuritic pain (Table 2.4). Opiates are the first-line analgesics for ischaemic pain and intravenous diamorphine is the medication of choice. It has immediate effect, reaches its peak effect within 20 min of administration and lasts 3–4 h. Diamorphine produces beneficial effects through:

- decreasing anxiety through action on the central nervous system
- vasodilatation of the peripheral circulation
- central nervous system sedation and primary analgesia through stimulation of opiate receptors.

Guidelines suggest intravenous nitrates for 24–48 h for patients with persistent or recurrent ischaemia or congestive heart failure (ACC/AHA 2006). Patients need to know that they may experience episodes of angina after discharge. They should be aware of the importance of reducing activity if such pain occurs and feel confident to use GTN. Guidance for taking GTN is described in the section on stable angina on page 16.

Reperfusion therapy

Patients with ST elevation myocardial infarction (STEMI) will be potential candidates for reperfusion therapy, i.e. strategies that restore blood flow to the myocardium in order to prevent further myocardial damage and restore myocardial function. The nurse needs to be aware of patient selection criteria and be able to assist in identifying patients who are candidates for therapy (Box 2.4). Awareness of contraindications to therapy and of the importance of initiating therapy as soon as possible after the onset of chest pain are also important, as is monitoring for reperfusion success (a fall in ST segment elevation). The time delay between the onset of symptoms and reperfusion has significant implications for prognosis irrespective of the reperfusion method as

Table 2.4 Characteristics of chest pain*		
DESCRIPTION	**LOCATION**	**MEDICAL DIAGNOSIS**
Tight, like a band around the central chest	Central chest Radiating to jaw, shoulders and arms, usually on left side	Angina pectoris
Precipitated by cold, exercise, large meals, emotion Usually relieved by rest and glyceryl trinitrate (GTN)	May be associated with shortness of breath	
As above, but not relieved by GTN or other measures Lasts longer and is more severe	As above	Myocardial infarction
Stabbing or burning pain Worse on deep inspiration, often relieved by bending forwards	Substernal and often affecting the trapezius muscle and upper abdominal area	Pericarditis
Sudden sharp pain, worsened by inspiration Dyspnoea, cough, cyanosis and possible haemoptysis	Very often lateral	Pulmonary embolus
Excruciating pain 'burning' towards the spine	Intrascapular region	Dissecting aneurysm

*Not all patients present in the manner described above. The description of chest pain is to aid diagnosis and should be used in conjunction with an assessment of the patient's risk of coronary heart disease and a history, physical examination and diagnostic tests.

Box 2.4 Information

Thrombolytic therapy

Purpose

The primary aim in limiting infarct size is the rapid recanalisation of the occluded coronary artery. Occlusion is most often caused by a thrombus at the site of a ruptured atheromatous plaque. The aim of thrombolysis is to induce dissolution of the thrombus through the administration of an intravenous drug in order to establish recanalisation and provide subsequent reperfusion to the ischaemic zone. Thrombolysis is the single most important advance in coronary care since defibrillation, resulting in increased survival and quality of life.

Action

Optimal benefit results when the thrombolytic drug is given promptly after the onset of chest pain, although it is considered worthwhile administering the treatment up to 12 h later. The main thrombolytic drugs currently available are:

- *Streptokinase* – to date, the most widely tested and used, and also the cheapest. It is a bacterial protein whose administration results in a systemic lytic state, with reduced levels of circulating fibrinogen and clotting factors V and VIII. The patient will produce antibodies to streptokinase after its administration and so the medication would be ineffective if given a second time.
- *Recombinant tissue-type plasminogen activator (tPA)* – a naturally occurring human protease that is fibrin-specific and thus works predominantly on the clot, with less risk of systemic bleeding.

- *Reteplase* – a new generation thrombolytic that appears to be as effective as streptokinase. It has the advantage that it can be given as a bolus and is non-antigenic.

Patient selection

Patients considered to be having an acute myocardial infarction, with the onset of symptoms within the previous 12 h.

Contraindications include:

- active or recent bleed
- major surgery or trauma within the previous month
- cerebrovascular accident within the previous 3 months
- severe systemic hypertension.

Reperfusion

Signs and symptoms of reperfusion may include:

- abrupt cessation of chest pain
- reperfusion arrhythmias or conduction disturbances
- rapid return of the ST segment to normal
- improved left ventricular function
- an early peak in cardiac enzymes as a result of enzymes being washed out of the infarct area by the reperfused artery.

Complications

These include:

- bleeding episodes (including rarely cerebral bleeds)
- reperfusion arrhythmias
- allergic reactions
- hypotension.

50% of the myocardium at risk will have died within 3 hours of coronary artery occlusion and 80% within 12 hours (Zeitz & Quinn 2010). Choice of therapy will depend on individual patient characteristics and the availability of facilities.

Thrombolysis

Thrombolytic drugs aim to break down the freshly formed thrombus that is blocking the coronary artery. Mortality in patients given thrombolytic drugs sufficiently early is one third less than in those left untreated and the *National Service Framework for Coronary Heart Disease* (DH 2000) set specific targets for thrombolysis times. The targets are that thrombolysis should be given within 60 min of the call for help and within 30 min of the patient's arrival at hospital. Nurses have successfully taken on the responsibility of initiating and/or prescribing thrombolytic therapy in accordance with agreed protocols (Rhodes 1998, Heath et al 2003). The nurse should explain to the patient the benefits and potential problems of this therapy.

On discharge, people who have received thrombolysis are given a card indicating what medication they received and when. It may be inappropriate for them to have a second treatment with certain thrombolytics. Thrombolysis does not have any effect on the underlying cause of thrombus formation, and reocclusion remains a problem. Heparin, warfarin and aspirin have been used to reduce re-thrombosis. Patients may require subsequent mechanical recanalisation with either rescue angioplasty or surgery.

Primary angioplasty

Angioplasty, which involves inserting a balloon-tipped catheter into the narrowed artery by cardiac catheterisation and then inflating the balloon to open up the artery is an alternative to thrombolytic therapy in acute infarction. It is frequently performed in conjunction with insertion of a metal tube known as a stent at the site of the narrowing to keep the artery opened. Angioplasty results in better patency and causes fewer strokes than thrombolysis and its use as the first-line reperfusion treatment is becoming more established as centres develop the infrastructure and the staff with the skills to undertake the procedure over the 24-h period. The target 'door to balloon' time is 90 min. Patients most likely to gain from this procedure are those with cardiogenic shock or anterior infarcts and older people. It is also an option for patients not eligible for thrombolysis (Kastrati et al 2004). For more on reperfusion therapies see Further reading Zeitz & Quinn (2010).

Complications of acute coronary syndromes

There are a considerable number of complications of acute coronary syndromes which tend to be related to the site and size of damaged myocardium. The most common are listed in Box 2.5. It is not possible to look at each in detail, but the nurse should be able to recognise and report the following major problems and carry out the appropriate nursing intervention.

> ### Box 2.5 Information
>
> #### Complications of acute coronary syndromes
> - Sudden death
> - Arrhythmias
> - Cardiac failure
> - Hypoxia
> - Hypotension
> - Cardiogenic shock
> - Papillary muscle insufficiency
> - Ventricular septal defect
> - Ventricular aneurysm
> - Myocardial rupture
> - Pulmonary embolus
> - Pericarditis
> - Deep vein thrombosis
> - Post-MI syndrome
> - Emotional difficulty

Cardiac arrest

Cardiac arrest may be defined as failure of the heart to pump sufficient blood to maintain cerebral function. It is a term often used synonymously with sudden death, although death is not always the outcome of a cardiac arrest. The three main mechanisms of cardiac arrest are:

- ventricular fibrillation (VF)
- ventricular asystole
- pulseless electrical activity (PEA).

Brain death usually occurs because of the failure of oxygenation of brain cells associated with either failure in ventilation or failure of the heart to pump oxygenated blood to the brain. The brain can tolerate only 4–6 min of anoxia. The signs of cardiac arrest are:

- abrupt loss of consciousness
- absent carotid and femoral pulses
- absent respirations.

A rapidly developing pallor often associated with cyanosis follows. Apnoea, gasping and gagging may occur.

Most in-hospital cardiac arrests are predictable with up to 84% of patients showing signs of deterioration prior to arrest (Kause et al 2004). Monitoring of vital signs and the use of early warning strategies is therefore important (see Ch. 29). The risk of sudden death in myocardial infarction patients is great. In 25% of cases, this occurs within minutes of the onset of pain, before the patient has reached hospital. The nurse must be familiar with resuscitation procedures and equipment within the hospital but should also know how to perform basic cardiopulmonary resuscitation (CPR) without hospital technology. Training programmes in basic CPR for lay people are aimed at reducing this very high early mortality rate, as are the development of trained paramedical staff in ambulances, mobile coronary care units and defibrillators in public places.

To be effective in resuscitation, regular education and training update is necessary, ideally 6-monthly, particularly for those who do not use these skills frequently (Broomfield 1996, Wynne et al 1999).

The risk of sudden death remains high for the first 24 h after infarction, following which it rapidly diminishes. In the CCU, cardiac arrest may be anticipated; in the ward it is often diagnosed by the nurse, who finds the patient unconscious and pulseless. This is an emergency and every nurse is responsible for:

- recognising that cardiac arrest has occurred
- knowing the procedure for summoning help within the hospital
- commencing effective resuscitation.

The priorities of CPR are:

- airway
- breathing
- circulation.

Medical help should be summoned once it has been established that the patient is not breathing. Presence of breathing is assessed by looking for a rise and fall in the chest wall, listening for any breath sounds and feeling for any expelled air. Restoration of an oxygenated blood supply to the brain involves artificial ventilation and external cardiac massage at a ratio of 2:30. At the time of writing the resuscitation guidelines currently recommended by the European Resuscitation Council are being reviewed and new guidelines are expected in October 2010. These guidelines are reviewed on a regular basis and so it is important to visit the website regularly (www.resus.org.uk) to check for new guidance.

Medication

Ideally, all medications used during CPR are best administered through a central line to ensure swift distribution, as circulation time is greatly reduced. CPR should continue for 3 min to allow circulation of the drug. Adrenaline (1 mg i.v.) is given every 3 min during cardiac arrest.

Defibrillation

Defibrillation involves the delivery of a direct current (DC) shock to the heart through the chest wall and is appropriate resuscitation treatment for ventricular tachycardia and fibrillation. Early defibrillation is one of the most important predictors of survival from cardiac arrest (Resuscitation Council 2006) and ideally the first shock should be administered within 90 s of the cardiac arrest. Defibrillation causes depolarisation of all the myocardial cells that are able to respond to a stimulus, thereby terminating the fibrillation and allowing the normal conducting pathways to regain control of the heart. Monophasic defibrillation, with the current going one way through the heart muscle, is increasingly being replaced with equipment that delivers a shock in two directions, biphasic defibrillation. This means that lower energy levels are required and damage to myocardial muscle is reduced. The current can be delivered through hand-held paddles placed over gel pads or via pads stuck to the patient's chest. One pad should be placed below the right clavicle and the other over the apex of the heart in the fifth intercostal space. Precautions should be taken to ensure that floor surfaces are dry and all personnel warned that the shock is about to be delivered. Defibrillators that interpret the patient's heart rhythm and advise about defibrillation are increasingly available in areas where health professionals are less experienced in advanced life support and also in public places such as shopping centres and airports.

After-care

After successful resuscitation, the patient will require skilled nursing care. Full recovery can only be said to have occurred when the patient is fully conscious, with full cardiac, cerebral and renal function. The chances of achieving this are greatly enhanced if the patient is in a CCU where the arrest is witnessed and treatment initiated promptly. Success is less likely in the street where resources are limited.

Several body systems need assessment post arrest, including the cardiovascular, renal, respiratory and central nervous systems. The patient may have been incontinent, have a sore chest and feel exhausted and somewhat embarrassed by their current state. An assessment of their level of orientation, recall, anxiety and general feelings should be made. The psychological support needed will vary. Relatives and witnesses to the arrest and the resuscitation attempt will also need support.

Ethical considerations

Unsuccessful resuscitation attempts do not enhance the dignity that is hoped for when we die. The appropriateness of merely prolonging the process of dying is often the subject of much debate (Cotler 2000). The decision not to attempt resuscitation should involve the patient and the family and be documented to avoid confusion. The decision needs to be reviewed on at least a 24-h basis.

'Do not attempt resuscitation' (DNAR) orders may be a potent source of misunderstanding and dissent amongst doctors, nurses and others involved in the care of patients. Issues surrounding this dilemma include whether resuscitation is appropriate, involvement of the patient and family in the decision-making process and communication difficulties between doctors and nurses once the decision is made (Mason 1996). Increasingly, living wills and advanced directives are being made by patients, and nurses need to be aware of the significance of these when making decisions about resuscitation. It is important that it is understood by all that DNAR orders apply only to the decision whether or not to initiate resuscitation in the event of cardiac or respiratory arrest and should not in any way limit other medical or nursing care (Shepardson et al 1999, Jackson et al 2004).

Cardiogenic shock

Cardiogenic shock is a serious degree of heart failure, precipitated by extensive (>40%) left ventricular damage in which the cardiac output is not sufficient to give an adequate blood pressure to maintain perfusion. The patient develops clinical shock with low urine output, cold clammy skin and hypoxia. Lactic acid is produced in the skeletal muscle beds as the metabolism changes, giving rise to a metabolic acidosis. This process is cyclical, with the heart continually trying to pump harder for an ever falling stroke volume (see Ch. 18).

Clinical features

In the early stages, the patient may be restless and agitated, followed by mental confusion and lethargy as cerebral hypoxia increases. The skin becomes cold and clammy to touch.

Initially, systolic and, later, diastolic pressure will fall. A fall in pulse pressure of more than 30 mmHg may be an indication that shock is developing in the hypertensive patient. The initial response to hypoxia is tachypnoea (rapid respiratory rate), which later becomes shallow and irregular. Most patients benefit from oxygen therapy. Urine output falls as a result of the falling cardiac output, leading to inadequate perfusion of the kidneys. The pulse will initially be rapid and thready as a compensatory response to the falling cardiac output; in the late stages, bradycardia (slow heart rate) develops.

 ## Nursing management and health promotion: cardiogenic shock

The priority when caring for patients with cardiogenic shock is its prevention or early recognition of the signs that shock is developing (O'Neal 1994, De Jong 1999) and subsequently to support the critically ill patient. Nursing management of these patients requires careful observation and recording of response to medication. The treatment priorities are to:

- enhance cardiac output
- restore tissue perfusion
- effect a diuresis through increased renal flow.

Medications commonly used in myocardial infarction such as nitrates, beta blockers, calcium antagonists and opiates may produce hypotension and worsen cardiogenic shock and therefore should be used with caution (Williams et al 2000). The aim is to improve cardiac output using inotropic drugs such as adrenaline, dopamine and dobutamine. These medications, often given via a central line, improve cardiac output by increasing contractility and often heart rate, which increase the demand on the myocardium for oxygen. Cardiac output can also be improved by using vasodilators to reduce afterload. Diuretics are used to induce a diuresis. The patient will require urinary catheterisation to assess hourly urine output and may be haemodynamically monitored using a pulmonary artery flotation (Swan–Ganz) catheter (see Ch. 18). More invasive therapy, such as the intra-aortic balloon pump (IABP) or left ventricular assist device, may be required if pharmacological intervention is ineffective in treating cardiogenic shock. Some patients may be appropriate for PCI (see p. 18).

The outlook for patients developing cardiogenic shock is poor and mortality is high (45–80%), as the process is very difficult to reverse (Goldberg et al 1999). Patients are likely to become increasingly drowsy, confused, immobile and dependent on nursing care for all activities of daily living. They may also be lethargic or semi-conscious. Anxiety and fear need to be recognised and addressed (Williams 1993). Small doses of opiates may promote comfort and rest. The relatives need time spent with them to explain the condition of their loved one and how they can best help. The hospital chaplain or other spiritual advisor may provide comfort for the patient and family at this time.

Myocardial rupture

This very rare complication results in instantaneous death. Necrosis occurs before fibrosis of the myocardium is complete, causing muscle rupture and the pumping of blood into the pericardium. It usually occurs 3–5 days after an extensive infarction in a heart with poor collateral blood flow.

Ventricular septal defect

This occurs more frequently than rupture but in some cases is amenable to treatment. The pathophysiology is the same as that for myocardial rupture, with a hole developing in the septum separating the right and left ventricles. The right ventricle has to cope with increased pressures and blood volumes while the left ventricle suffers a fall in cardiac output. Rapid onset of cardiogenic shock may be the result. Operative repair can be undertaken but the mortality rate is high. If the patient can be supported for 2–4 weeks by aggressive medical management until the septum has become fibrosed, then the surgical results are slightly better.

Papillary muscle rupture

Loss of blood supply to the muscle supporting the mitral valve leads to prolapse and malfunctioning of the valve. If acute rupture occurs, then sudden death may result. Surgical repair can be attempted, but survival rates are low.

Ventricular aneurysm

This occurs when the infarction involves the full thickness of the myocardium. As the necrotic tissue is replaced by fibrous tissue, it is subject to the high pressures in the left ventricle. This fibrous tissue balloons out to form a blood pouch that does not contract. Blood stagnation in this pouch leads to the development of thrombi, and systemic emboli complicate approximately half of cases of left ventricular embolism. If a large area of myocardium is affected it can lead to cardiac failure; if the aneurysm is near the papillary muscle or mitral valve mitral incompetence will result. Surgical resection can be undertaken successfully if the aneurysm is sufficiently small.

Pericarditis

This is thought to be due to an autoimmune reaction in which antigens from the damaged myocardium cause inflammation of the pericardium. The patient presents with pain at any time from 24 h to 1 week after the myocardial infarction. On examination, a 'friction rub' caused by friction between the pericardium and myocardium is often heard, accompanied by an unresolving post-infarction pyrexia. Medical treatment and nursing care involve treating the pain with analgesics and non-steroidal anti-inflammatory agents. Reassurance that the pain is not an extension of the infarction is important.

Emboli

Embolism of a pulmonary or systemic vessel can occur after myocardial infarction. Emboli arise from clots forming in the healing myocardium or from circulatory stasis causing clot formation in the lower limbs. Nursing care involves maintaining passive exercises for the patient, whose mobility is restricted. The use of antiembolism stockings should be considered. All post-myocardial infarction patients and those with known CHD should be given aspirin, which, taken daily, has been shown to be effective in reducing clot formation. In most patients this may be sufficient, but in people with pulmonary emboli or who are known to have mural thrombi, a more aggressive approach to anticoagulation is required.

Secondary prevention and rehabilitation in acute coronary syndrome

The progression of vascular lesions, arterial thrombosis and the occurrence of arrhythmias in those with existing CHD can be influenced by a variety of metabolic and cardiovascular factors. Secondary prevention strategies usually involve specific drug therapies and aim to help people address their risk factors. Secondary prevention needs to be incorporated into cardiac rehabilitation programmes, which should be offered to all patients with ACS. Cardiac rehabilitation should incorporate baseline patient assessment, psychosocial interventions, education and support and exercise training as important components (Balady et al 2007). There is evidence that such strategies can improve survival and quality of life, limit recurrent events and reduce the need for interventional procedures (Jolliffe et al 2005, Smith et al 2006).

Drug therapy

- Blood pressure is treated to a target of under 140/85 mmHg with beta blockers/ACE inhibitors. The target should be <130/80 mmHg in those with diabetes.
- Patients with ACS should be treated immediately with aspirin 300 mg, which is absorbed more quickly if chewed. Aspirin and/or clopidogrel for antiplatelet therapy will continue after discharge. Glycoprotein IIb/IIIa receptor antagonists are likely to be prescribed post PCI.
- Statin therapy should be given to reduce total cholesterol concentrations to <4 mmol/L (LDL-C to below 2 mmol/L) or a 25% reduction in total cholesterol and a 30% reduction in LDL-C, whichever gets the individual to the lowest level (see NICE guidelines 2006b).
- ACE inhibitors reduce afterload and myocardial workload. Benefits are seen in high-risk ACS patients. Post MI, ACE inhibitors reduce mortality and re-infarction but must be avoided in renal impairment.
- Beta blockade reduces contractility, discharge and AV node conduction, which leads to decreased myocardial oxygen demand during sympathetic stimulation. It also increases ejection fraction, improves LV structure and suppresses arrhythmias.
- Nitrates do not reduce mortality but should be used for cardiac pain and heart failure
- Meticulous glycaemic control is required from the time of the acute event for those with diabetes. Blood glucose level in the early stages of ACS is a significant predictor of prognosis with elevated blood sugars being linked with arrhythmias and increased risk of death. A useful indicator of ongoing blood sugar management is the HbA1c blood test, which is a measure of glucose binding with haemoglobin and is an indication of the average blood plasma glucose concentration over several months. The target is an HbA1c of <7%.

Lifestyle targets

- Advice should be given on smoking cessation and the use of nicotine replacement therapy.
- Advice on weight control, diet, alcohol and exercise is necessary.
- The patient should maintain ideal body weight (BMI 20–25 kg/m^2) and avoid excessive weight gain around the abdomen indicative of disproportionate intra-abdominal fat mass – known as central obesity – which is linked to increased risk of CVD (WHO 2008):
  - maintain total intake of fat at <30% of total energy intake; increase intake of monounsaturated fats
  - saturated fats <10% of total fat intake; cholesterol intake <300 mg/day
  - increase intake of fresh fruit and vegetables; regular intake of fish (>2× per week) and other sources of omega-3 fatty acids
  - alcohol intake <21 units/week for men and <14 units/week for women
  - regular aerobic physical activity >30 min/day on most days (see below).

Psychosocial interventions

Individualised educational and behavioural support delivered by cardiac nurses in hospital has been shown to reduce psychological consequences and improve quality of life (Mayou et al 2002). Patients and their families, particularly partners (Moser & Dracup 2004), are likely to be anxious at the time of the acute event, on discharge home from hospital and during recovery. They need individualised and appropriately timed information about what is happening to them and the likely pattern of recovery to enable them to feel more in control and be able to cope. Planned periods of rest and relaxation, graded exercise, instructions on stress management and individual and group support sessions may help.

Physical activity counselling and exercise training

Exercise can be beneficial for recovery and long-term prognosis (Taylor et al 2004) and activity levels need to be built up gradually after the acute event. Activity may be limited initially due to pain, shortness of breath and/or haemodynamic instability and the patient may require assistance with activities of living at this time. Subsequently, a history of the individual's previous physical activity and/or an exercise test should be used to produce a plan for activity levels and an individualised exercise prescription. Exercise should be moderate intensity aerobic activity, such as brisk walking, supplemented by daily lifestyle activities. Discussion about resuming sexual activity needs to be included as appropriate (Jolliffe et al 2005). Attendance at a formal cardiac rehabilitation programme exercise class may help individuals (particularly those at high risk) gain in confidence and stick to their exercise plan.

Service provision varies markedly and many cardiac rehabilitation programmes are focused on select populations resulting in suboptimal referral with issues such as enrolment and completion being poorly addressed. The elderly, women and those from ethnic minorities are underrepresented. The potential for embracing novel methods and the latest technology need to be exploited (Thompson & Clark 2009).

Supervision and follow-up often fail because of a breakdown between primary and secondary services and there is scope for more services with further development of nurse-led risk factor clinics and rehabilitation initiatives.

Arrhythmias

The term 'arrhythmia' is used to imply an abnormality in either electrical impulse formation or electrical impulse conduction within the heart. An arrhythmia may cause an effect by any one of the following changes:

- change in heart rate
- increase in myocardial oxygen requirement
- decrease in myocardial blood flow
- loss of synchronicity of ventricular contraction.

Clinical features

The clinical manifestation of an arrhythmia depends on the ventricular rate, the conduction of the myocardium and the psychological response of the patient. Patient symptoms include:

- palpitations
- dizziness
- faintness
- shortness of breath
- chest pain
- headache
- reduced activity tolerance
- anxiety.

Nursing assessment includes the apparent effect of the arrhythmia on the patient, a history of any past experiences of the problem, knowledge of any relevant medications or other treatments and identification of any possible precipitating factors.

In cardiac disease, the normal sinus mechanism can be altered if the disease affects the heart's specialised conduction tissue. Various conditions result in specific conduction disturbances, and while this chapter cannot deal with them all, it will concentrate on a few of the more common conditions with which the nurse should be familiar. In interpreting heart rhythms, the method used must be systematic and consider all components of the ECG complex.

Normal sinus rhythm should be recognisable to all nurses, as patients requiring cardiac monitors are increasingly nursed on general wards.

Cardiac arrhythmias

The clinical consequences of arrhythmias are extremely variable but are likely to be more pronounced in those with chronic heart disease and be dependent on the ventricular rate, which will determine cardiac output. Treatment usually aims to restore sinus rhythm and prevent recurrence of the arrhythmia. Nursing management involves anticipating and resolving patient problems, monitoring the patient, including their response to treatment, providing information and support and assisting the patient with activities of living that are compromised by the arrhythmias. The nurse's priorities are to:

- recognise and immediately report anything abnormal
- promptly assess the effect of the abnormality on the patient and take the appropriate action.

Sinus arrhythmias

The SA node is under autonomic control, primarily vagal, but is influenced by sympathetic stimulation, temperature, oxygen saturation and other metabolic changes. Sinus arrhythmias are often secondary to these influences.

Sinus arrhythmias are characterised by a constant PR interval but progressive beat-to-beat change in R-R intervals. During expiration, the reflex discharge of the vagal nerve slows the sinus mechanism; during inspiration this influence is diminished, allowing a speeding up of the sinus rhythm. Sinus arrhythmias are not life threatening and resolution of the primary cause resolves the arrhythmia.

Sinus bradycardia

This meets the criteria for sinus rhythm but the rate is less than 60 beats/min. It may result from increased stimulation of the vagus nerve which controls the parasympathetic regulation of the heart, with increased stimulation (often referred to as increased vagal tone) slowing conduction. Sinus bradycardia can also result from hypothermia, certain medications, e.g. beta blockers, raised intracranial pressure and inferior myocardial infarction. Some individuals may experience sinus bradycardia when sleeping. It may be the norm in athletes. Intravenous atropine is given for symptomatic sinus bradycardia.

Sinus tachycardia

This also fits the criteria for sinus rhythm, but the rate is greater than 100 beats/min. It is a direct result of decreased vagal tone and often a response to sympathetic stimulation.

Narrow complex tachycardias

Atrial flutter

This is characterised by rapid and regular atrial excitation at a level above 200 beats/min. The AV node is not capable of conducting atrial rates above this level. The atrial waves form a sawtooth pattern. Ventricular deflections usually occur regularly within the atrial pattern and the block is described as a ratio, e.g. 4:1, which means four P waves per QRS complex. Atrial flutter is not a stable rhythm and often progresses to atrial fibrillation.

Atrial fibrillation

When individual muscle fibres of the atria or ventricles contract independently, they are said to be 'fibrillating'. There is rapid disorganised atrial depolarisation because the atrial tissues have lost synchrony with each other. The atrial waves can occur up to 600 times per minute. Ventricular depolarisation is also irregular as a result of the variable response at the AV node, but the QRS complex is normal. It occurs in congestive cardiac failure and mitral valve disease, and commonly presents with ischaemic changes in old age.

Atrial fibrillation can severely compromise cardiac output, as the loss of the effect of atrial systole can reduce stroke volume by up to 25%. With chronic atrial fibrillation, the danger of thrombi forming in the atria and then embolising is high. Treatment is aimed at reducing the rapid ventricular rate through chemical or DC cardioversion to revert to sinus rhythm. Cardioversion after digoxin therapy may precipitate ventricular fibrillation if large doses of digoxin have been used. Anticoagulation in the form of heparin or warfarin may be prescribed to reduce the risk of thrombi.

Junctional tachycardias

The AV node, unlike the SA node, normally has no pacemaking role but is able to generate impulses. The QRS complex is of normal configuration and duration since the normal conduction pathway is followed below the AV node. Junctional tachycardia is characterised by the sudden onset of tachycardia greater than 150 beats/min. The urgency of treatment depends on symptoms, which tend to be related to the ventricular rate. Carotid sinus massage, which involves gently massaging the carotid artery against the transverse process of the sixth vertebrae for 10–20 seconds by direct pressure, may be performed by appropriately experienced staff. This procedure aims to stimulate the vagus nerve in order to terminate junctional re-entry tachycardias and allows differentiation from atrial flutter.

Supraventricular tachycardia

This term is still often used but is anatomically incorrect because most narrow complex tachycardias incorporate both ventricular and atrial myocardium within the conduction circuit. Medical management of narrow complex tachycardia aims to reduce the rapid ventricular rate using carotid sinus pressure or antiarrhythmic drugs, e.g. amiodarone, adenosine or digoxin. If these measures are unsuccessful then cardioversion may be indicated.

Ventricular arrhythmias

In these rhythms the ectopic focus arises below the AV node.

Ventricular tachycardia

This is a broad complex tachycardia with a QRS complex that looks wide and bizarre. The rate is regular at around 140–200 beats/min. It is generally caused by an irritable or ischaemic myocardium. Treatment, if the patient is symptomatic, is with immediate synchronised cardioversion and/or intravenous lidocaine. Other medication includes amiodarone, flecainide and mexiletine. Persistent episodes of ventricular tachycardia may be treated with override pacing or ablation therapy where the ectopic focus or source of the arrhythmia is identified and removed.

Ventricular fibrillation

In this rhythm, there are no distinguishable complexes on the screen and only an erratic baseline trace is evident. Treatment is by immediate initiation of resuscitation procedures and defibrillation.

▷ Nursing management and health promotion: arrhythmias

Treatment for arrhythmias focuses on treating any underlying cause, controlling the ventricular rate, restoration of normal sinus rhythm (cardioversion) and anticoagulation (to reduce the risk of pooled blood from a less mobile ventricle being ejected into the circulation). It is likely that antiarrhythmic drug therapy will be used as a first-line therapy to attempt to restore sinus rhythm in many patients. This is known as chemical cardioversion.

DC cardioversion (Box 2.6)

The procedure should be fully explained to the patient so that they are aware of what to expect. They will be prepared as for all patients prior to a general anaesthetic. The thought of an anaesthetic and an electric current being put across the heart may be frightening. Care should be taken to ensure that the area is dry and that all personnel are warned that the shock is about to be delivered. The patient is likely to want to know the outcome of the procedure and this should be explained. Topical creams may help to ease any chest soreness caused by the electric shock.

Box 2.6 Information

Cardioversion

Purpose

The term 'cardioversion' is used to mean the delivery of a specific and predetermined amount of energy to the heart, timed (synchronised) in such a way that the shock is delivered well away from the vulnerable period of the T wave on the ECG. It is usually performed electively, with the patient lightly anaesthetised. This differs from defibrillation, which usually involves the delivery of a larger amount of electricity to a patient in ventricular fibrillation without anaesthetic, as the patient is usually unconscious. Elective cardioversion is used to treat supraventricular and ventricular arrhythmias.

Electrical treatment has the advantage that it is free from pharmacological side-effects.

Procedure

Monophasic or biphasic electrical wave forms are used for cardioversion, the latter requiring lower energy settings. Energy levels are titrated upwards if an initial shock is unsuccessful. The patient is asked to remove any dentures or restrictive clothing. An ECG will be performed before and after the procedure, and the patient attached to a cardiac monitor throughout. Oxygen is given both before and after the procedure. A light anaesthetic is usually given and the patient asked to fast for 4–6 h prior to the procedure. Resuscitation equipment needs to be on hand. The defibrillator is set to the required output and the paddles or pads are placed in position, usually with one below the right clavicle and the other over the apex of the heart in order to depolarise an optimal mass of myocardial cells. The patient is usually awake and talking 5–10 min after the procedure; nausea and vomiting are not uncommon, as are a sore throat from the endotracheal tube and chest wall soreness due to the cardioversion. Cardioversion is often performed on a day-case basis and is frequently coordinated and led by nurses (Quinn 1998).

Cardiac electrophysiology studies and ablation processes

Electrophysiology studies involve the introduction of an intravenous or intra-arterial catheter with multiple electrodes positioned at various intracardiac sites for the purpose of recording or initiating electrical activity from specific areas of the atria or ventricles. These studies are performed on patients with arrhythmias that are resistant to medication, in order to identify the nature of the rhythm disturbance – also known as cardiac mapping.

Ablation therapy requires the delivery of a high-energy electric shock through a catheter in order to produce localised tissue damage in the unstable area identified as producing the arrhythmia, e.g. in Wolff–Parkinson–White syndrome. For further information on Wolff–Parkinson–White syndrome and other cardiac arrhythmias see Further reading, e.g. Oldroyd & Kucia (2010).

Implantable cardioverter defibrillators

The implantable cardioverter defibrillator (ICD) is an electronic device used to detect and terminate potentially lethal arrhythmias through the delivery of an electric shock. Current models weigh less than 200 g and are implanted without open chest procedures. They are particularly suitable for patients who have survived one episode of cardiac arrest not thought to be the result of myocardial infarction and for those with recurrent episodes of ventricular tachycardia unresponsive to optimal medication. Appropriate patients are likely to need individualised information and support to enable them to cope with the concept of being dependent on the device (James 2002). For more information on ICDs see Further reading, e.g. James (2007).

Heart block

Heart block occurs when there is a delay or interruption of impulse conduction from the atria to the ventricles at the AV node. Heart block is usually a complication of myocardial infarction. It manifests as:

- first-degree heart block
- second-degree heart block
- third-degree (complete) heart block.

First-degree heart block

This appears as a prolonged PR interval with a mild bradycardia. It is asymptomatic and seldom requires treatment.

Second-degree heart block

This appears as occasional blocking; for example, there may be alternate conducted and non-conducted atrial beats, giving twice as many P waves as QRS complexes. The patient may have no symptoms and require no treatment. If a fall in blood pressure or other signs of reduced cardiac output develop, the heart block is treated by the insertion of a pacemaker (Box 2.7).

Complete heart block

This exists when atrial and ventricular activity are uncoordinated. The atria and ventricles are electrically dissociated and desynchronised, with a subsidiary pacemaker developing in the ventricles. Cardiac output is reduced and the

Box 2.7 Information

Pacemaker insertion

Purpose

Pacemakers are used to gain control over the electrical activity of the heart. They have two basic components:

- a pulse generator containing a power source and electrical circuitry
- one or two pacing leads, each with an electrode on its tip.

Pacemakers may be either temporary or permanent, depending on whether the pulse generator is located externally or implanted. If pacing is planned for a short duration, an external source is used to deliver electricity to the heart via the skin. When long-term control of the heart is required, a permanent pacemaker is implanted. The two most common modes of pacing are:

- demand (ventricular inhibited) – senses intrinsic cardiac rhythm and stimulates myocardial depolarisation and contraction as necessary
- fixed rate – fires at a predetermined rate, irrespective of intrinsic cardiac activity.

Temporary pacing

This is used to maintain cardiac output during episodes of extreme bradycardia, heart block and asystole. It may also be used for the suppression of tachyarrhythmias that are resistant to medication. It is usual for a special room to be set aside for temporary cardiac pacing, with ECG monitoring, fluoroscopy and resuscitation equipment being readily available.

Most commonly, a bipolar catheter is inserted into the subclavian vein, external jugular vein or antecubital fossa under local anaesthesia. The catheter is then passed into the right atrium and thence through the tricuspid valve and into the apex of the right ventricle, where the tip of the catheter is lodged against the ventricular wall. The external end of the catheter is stitched into place at the skin surface. The bipolar catheter is stimulated by the pacemaker's external pulse generator. Verification of pacing is judged from the appearance of a pacing spike preceding the QRS complex of the ECG. Pacing 'threshold' is obtained by determining the lowest voltage needed to elicit a paced beat, ideally less than 0.5 V. The threshold needs to be checked at least every 12 h, as it may increase over time.

Possible complications

These include arrhythmias, failure of the electrode to sense the heart's own electrical activity, failure of the electrode to generate a contraction, abdominal muscle twitching, pneumothorax and infection.

Permanent pacing

The decision to implant a permanent pacemaker is made after careful patient assessment. It is usually offered to patients with symptomatic bradycardias and heart block. The modern pacemaker is a small metal unit weighing between 25 and 30 g. It is powered by a lithium battery with a life of up to 15 years. Two types of pulse generator are currently available:

- single chamber with an electrode placed in either the atrium or the ventricle
- dual chamber with electrodes situated in both chambers.

The pacemaker is usually implanted under local anaesthesia in a cardiac catheterisation laboratory. The pulse generator is implanted in a subcutaneous pocket, usually under the clavicle, axilla or abdominal wall. The procedure is usually performed on a day-case basis.

---

patient is haemodynamically compromised. The ventricles often contract at a rate of less than 40 beats/min and a pacemaker requires to be inserted immediately to restore cardiac output.

 ## Nursing management and health promotion: heart block

The nurse's role is one of observation, reporting and patient support. A pacemaker may be required to gain control over the electrical activity of the heart.

Pacemakers

Indications for pacing vary both nationally and internationally, although the American College of Cardiology, the American Heart Association and the North American Society for Pacing and Electrophysiology (ACC/AHA/NASPE 2002) have produced pacemaker guidelines. Nursing considerations include assessing pacemaker function, ensuring patient comfort and safety, preventing and dealing with complications, and teaching the patient about their condition and its management. The patient needs to be prepared for the procedure, even if it is done as an emergency (see Box 2.7).

Transcutaneous pacing involves stimulating the myocardium through external pads placed on the patient's chest. It has the advantage of being non-invasive, quickly established and initiated by appropriately trained personnel. However, it tends to be used only as a holding measure as it can be uncomfortable and of limited effect.

Transvenous pacing involves inserting a pacing catheter under local anaesthetic into the right ventricle via a large vein. In an acute or emergency situation the pulse generator (pacing box) will remain outside the body and the pacemaker is only in place temporarily. Following pacemaker insertion, the patient should be attached to a cardiac monitor to assess whether the pacemaker is functioning properly. Cardiac output needs to be assessed frequently by recording the patient's blood pressure and asking them to report any symptoms of faintness, dizziness, chest pain or shortness of breath. The ability of the pacing wire to stimulate the myocardium also needs to be checked regularly (threshold check). Limited mobility may make the patient more dependent on nursing care for a while. The patient with a temporary pacemaker should be aware of how long the temporary pacing is likely to continue and appreciate what is likely to happen next. Removal of the temporary pacemaker is performed at the patient's bedside under aseptic conditions.

Permanent pacing involves the pulse generator being placed inside the body cavity. There are pacemaker systems that can stimulate the ventricles, the atria or both (biventricular pacing). Initially, the nursing considerations are similar to those for temporary pacing. Some patients will be helped by a visit from a person who already has a permanent pacemaker, and also by being given an opportunity to handle a pacemaker. The patient needs to be reassured that the pacemaker will not be damaged by day-to-day activities. They should be taught to take their own pulse and be aware of the signs of reduced cardiac output. Signs of infection, such as redness or increased soreness at the implantation site, should also be reported. The importance of follow-up appointments should be explained. It is also useful to warn people that the pacemaker may trigger off alarms at airports. The patient should refrain from driving for 1 month (6 months for LGV and PCV, and re-licensing may be permitted thereafter providing there is no other disqualifying condition).

For further information see Useful websites, e.g. Driver and Vehicle Licensing Agency (DVLA). For further information on the use of pacemakers and implantable internal defibrillators, see Further reading, e.g. ACC/AHA/NASPE (2002) guideline update for implantation of cardiac pacemakers and antiarrhythmia devices.

Heart failure

The term 'heart failure' is used to describe a clinical syndrome that has a characteristic group of signs and symptoms. It results from an inability of the heart to provide an adequate cardiac output for the body's metabolic requirements. It is increasing in prevalence and the prevalence rises steeply with age. Statistical data suggest that after an initial diagnosis of heart failure, 16% of patients die within a year of diagnosis, 40% within the first 2 years and 61% within 5 years (BHF 2008). Patients living with heart failure have been shown to visit their GP on average between 11 and 14 times per year (Gnani & Majeed 2001). Heart failure is often referred to as either acute or chronic. Acute heart failure has been defined as the rapid onset of symptoms secondary to abnormal cardiac function (European Society of Cardiology [ESC] 2005) and it complicates between 25 and 50% of acute coronary syndrome patients.

The clinical condition is often complicated by arrhythmias that reduce the cardiac output further. It may develop suddenly or during the first few hours or days after the infarction. Acute heart failure may resolve with medical therapy as the patient's condition stabilises. However, infarction may result in a long-term reduction of the functional capacity of the myocardium and chronic heart failure. Chronic heart failure can also occur as a result of hypertension, aneurysm, cardiomyopathy, arrhythmias and medication, such as beta blockers and antiarrhythmics, often used in acute cardiac events.

PATHOPHYSIOLOGY

Heart failure can involve either ventricle independently or both together. Pure left or right ventricular failure may not exist for long because of their dependence on each other to maintain adequate blood flow. However, it is useful to look at the heart as two pumps. The left ventricle can cope better with alterations in pressure and the right with alterations in volume. Failure of the left side of the heart causes accumulation of blood in the left ventricle and left atrium with subsequent congestion of the lungs. Right-sided failure, where the right ventricle cannot effectively transfer deoxygenated blood to the pulmonary circulation, subsequently causes congestion of the circulation in the rest of the body (systemic circulation).

Congestive cardiac failure (CCF)

This term describes a state in which there is both right and left ventricular failure with a corresponding combination of systemic and pulmonary symptoms.

Myocardial hypertrophy

In response to the increased workload, the individual myocardial cells enlarge, thus increasing the total amount of contractile tissue. This compensation is usually of a temporary nature, and at this stage the prognosis is poor.

Oedema

Oedema may result when anything increases the movement of fluid from the bloodstream and impairs its return. One of the commonest causes is CCF, where the failure of the pump to move the blood volume forward results in back pressure, which raises the hydrostatic pressure such that it exceeds the colloidal pressure created by plasma proteins. As a result, the excess tissue fluid formed accumulates, exceeding the ability of the lymphatic system to drain the excess away.

In the early stages of heart failure, patients may complain of 'puffy ankles', being unable to fit comfortably into their shoes. There will also be sacral oedema.

Pulmonary oedema As systemic arterial pressure, and therefore afterload, increases, so does pressure in the left heart. Increased left ventricular end-diastolic pressure (LVEDP) results in increased pulmonary pressure and an accumulation of blood in the lungs. If the pulmonary pressure rises above 28 mmHg, there is movement of fluid from the capillaries into the alveoli and interstitial spaces. This causes pulmonary oedema. If this occurs as an acute event, it can lead to death in 30 min. In the congestive failure situation, it is a chronic progressive state where the reduced lung compliance and high pulmonary pressure lead to increased right heart pressures and blood congestion on this side. This further raises pressure in the systemic circulation, making the whole process one of cyclical deterioration. As the systemic pressure rises, there is movement of fluid into the tissues giving rise to peripheral oedema. This is initially gravitational, but as the condition progresses the oedema becomes more widespread (Figure 2.11).

Common presenting symptoms

The presentation and history will depend on which side of the heart is failing. It may present gradually, as occurs in the ageing process, or suddenly, manifesting as acute pulmonary oedema with marked breathlessness, anxiety and tachycardia.

- Fatigue on exertion, dyspnoea (difficulty/laboured breathing) with mild exercise and paroxysmal nocturnal dyspnoea are common early signs of failure of the left ventricle.
- Fatigue, awareness of fullness in the neck and abdomen, and ankle swelling are early signs of failure of the right ventricle.

Features appearing in systemic examination are listed in Table 2.5.

Backward failure
– congestion

Forward failure
– hypotension

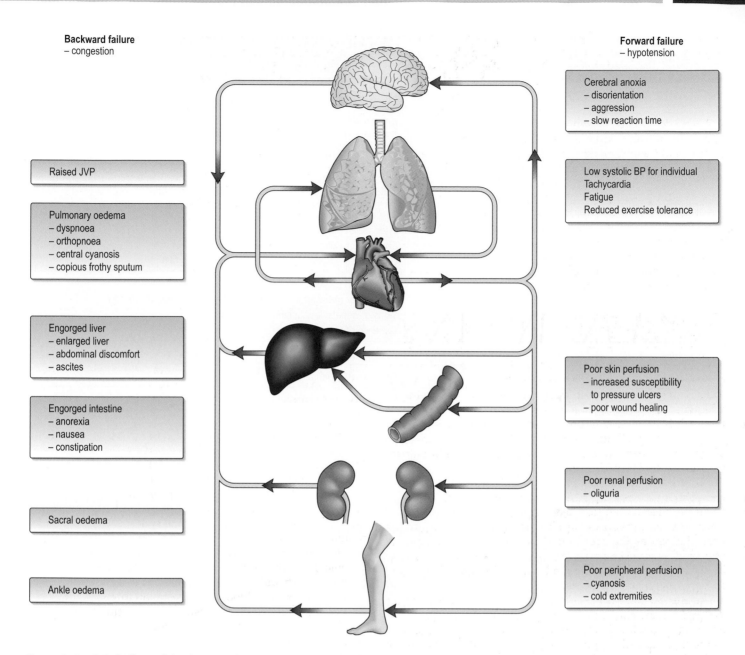

Cerebral anoxia
– disorientation
– aggression
– slow reaction time

Raised JVP

Low systolic BP for individual
Tachycardia
Fatigue
Reduced exercise tolerance

Pulmonary oedema
– dyspnoea
– orthopnoea
– central cyanosis
– copious frothy sputum

Engorged liver
– enlarged liver
– abdominal discomfort
– ascites

Poor skin perfusion
– increased susceptibility
  to pressure ulcers
– poor wound healing

Engorged intestine
– anorexia
– nausea
– constipation

Poor renal perfusion
– oliguria

Sacral oedema

Poor peripheral perfusion
– cyanosis
– cold extremities

Ankle oedema

Figure 2.11 Clinical effects of the decompensatory phase of ventricular failure.

Diagnosis

Heart failure is suspected because of the patient's history, signs and symptoms. This diagnosis is then confirmed or excluded through a 12-lead ECG, which may show left ventricular hypertrophy, ischaemia or infarction; natriuretic peptides – B type natriuretic peptide (BNP) and its end terminal fragment N-BNP where available; a chest X-ray; blood tests, i.e. urea and electrolytes, creatinine, full blood count, thyroid function test, liver function test, glucose and lipids; blood gas analysis, urinalysis and peak flow. Echocardiography is considered essential for the assessment of functional and structural changes of the heart with failure (ESC 2005). Patients with heart failure need a clinical assessment of cardiac output, cardiac rhythm, cognitive function, nutritional status and functional capacity. The patient's fluid balance status should be monitored to assess renal function and the effect of medication.

▷ Nursing management and health promotion: heart failure

The main aims of treatment are:

1. Oxygenation to improve myocardial contractility, maintaining SaO$_2$ within the normal range (95–98%). This may require non-invasive positive pressure ventilation (NIPPV – see Further reading, e.g. Gray et al 2008), continuous positive airways pressure ventilation (CPAP) or bi-level positive airway pressure (BiPAP). See Chapter 3.
2. Rest to reduce cardiac workload – sleeping in a chair, spacing out activities, assistance with activities of daily living.
3. Medication designed to improve cardiac function (see below).

Table 2.5 Systemic examination in heart failure

SYSTEM	POINTS TO NOTE	RATIONALE
Cardiovascular	Chest X-ray	Evaluation of chamber enlargement Indication of primary cardiac abnormality
	Auscultation	Arrhythmia (especially AF) common A prominent third heart sound with a tachycardia (gallop rhythm)
	Vital signs	Venous hypertension common Observe jugular venous pressure
	Presence of oedema	Visible oedema in dependent parts, e.g. ankles, hands and sacrum, in bed-bound patients is a sign of inability to excrete sufficient water
Respiratory	Wheeze, bronchospasm Paroxysmal nocturnal dyspnoea Amount and consistency of sputum Pleural effusion on right side	Possible increased pulmonary fluid Evidence of poor left ventricle compensation Evidence of pulmonary oedema Often found in patients with congestive cardiac failure
Gastrointestinal	Chest X-ray Diet Palpation of abdomen	Recognition of oedema Sodium control is an important part of controlling fluid retention Signs of hepatic and splenic engorgement Presence of ascites
Genitourinary	Micturition	Frequency and amount of urine passed; vital to assess effect of diuretic therapy
Muscular	Physical activity levels	Often severely limited by reduced cardiac reserve
Central nervous	Mental status	Signs of cerebral hypoxia
Skin	Skin integrity	Risk of pressure ulcers and delayed healing

4. Treatment to improve the quality of life – maintaining the 'essence of care' through comfort, nutritional support, personal (including oral) hygiene, appropriate equipment such as commodes and urinals. In addition the patient, who may be seriously unwell, anxious and with limited mobility, will require individualised care that maintains dignity and safety and retains a level of independence and personal choice. It is estimated that the average life expectancy of a patient with chronic heart failure is 4–5 years, and a reduced quality of life and concurrent depression are common. Patients and their families will need information and support to help them retain their independence for as long as possible. There is some evidence that nurse-led care of heart failure patients can increase quality of life for these patients (Mårtensson et al 2005).

5. Minimising complications – venous thromboembolism, respiratory and urinary tract infection, constipation and pressure ulcers.

6. Effective communication, support and information giving to both the patient and family. Effective nurse-led support in the community has been demonstrated to reduce unplanned readmissions (McMurray & Stewart 1998, Yu et al 2006).

Drug therapy

The prime concern for patients with heart failure is to restore haemodynamic stability, using a combination of medications to optimise cardiac function and control fluid loss through the kidneys. The effects of this therapy should be regularly assessed and practice nurses may be involved in monitoring the patient's weight, heart rate and rhythm. Drug therapy includes:

- Diuretics, e.g. furosemide, induce sodium and water excretion, leading to decreased cardiac preload and wall tension, and an effective decrease of symptomatic pulmonary and systemic congestion. However, they have not yet been shown to prolong life in patients with congestive cardiac failure.
- Direct vasodilators, which induce venodilatation, arterial dilatation, or both, i.e. balanced vasodilators, may improve symptoms:
  - venodilators, such as nitrates, exert a venous pooling effect, decreasing cardiac preload and symptoms of congestion
  - arterial dilators, such as diltiazem hydrochloride and hydralazine, decrease afterload and improve cardiac output.
- The ACE inhibitors, e.g. enalapril and captopril, can cause haemodynamic and neurohormonal changes that lead to a reduction of preload and afterload, decreasing symptoms of heart failure. They might also deter the development of overt heart failure in some asymptomatic patients with left ventricular dysfunction.
- Beta blockers are used to reduce the myocardial workload, and myocardial contractility can be enhanced with other drugs such as inotropes. Arrhythmias associated with heart failure need to be treated to maximise cardiac output.

- Opiates are often prescribed for their vasodilator properties and to relieve acute distress.
- Positive inotropic agents including dopamine, dobutamine and the phosphodiesterase inhibitors (e.g. enoximone) are used to improve haemodynamic status.

For further information on the pharmacological management of heart failure, see Further reading, e.g. Gupta (2005).

Other treatment options for heart failure include intra-aortic balloon pump, revascularisation, biventricular pacing/cardiac resynchronisation therapy, valve replacement/repair, ventricular assist devices, cardiomyoplasty, ventricular volume reduction and heart transplant.

The British Heart Foundation, the Department of Health and other national bodies (BHF et al 2003) have set out key aims for the local improvement of heart failure services and provide sources of information and examples of service models designed to help achieve the CHD National Service Framework (NSF) standards (DH 2000), the National Institute for Health and Clinical Excellence (NICE) heart failure guidelines (NICE 2003) and the Scottish Intercollegiate Guidelines Network (SIGN) guidelines (1999). For further information about nurse-led care of the patient with heart failure, see Further reading, e.g. Jaarsma & Stewart (2004), for acute heart failure, e.g. Quinn (2010) and for chronic heart failure, e.g. Oliver et al (2007).

Pericardial disease

PATHOPHYSIOLOGY

Pericardial disease is an umbrella term for clinical conditions affecting the pericardium and pericardial space. It includes:

- *Acute pericarditis* – inflammatory reaction involving the visceral and parietal layers of the pericardium, associated with viral infection, post cardiac surgery and post MI. Produces sudden onset sharp pain that is worse on inspiration, relieved by sitting forward.
- *Constrictive pericarditis* – thickening and fibrosed pericardium impairing ventricular filling and leading to raised elevated coronary heart pressures and reduced cardiac output. Produces symptoms of right and left heart failure, pleuritic chest pain, shortness of breath and fatigue. Temporarily resolved with diuretic therapy, it usually requires surgical pericardiectomy.
- *Pericardial effusion* – accumulation of fluid in the intrapericardial space between the visceral and parietal layers of the pericardium. Fluid accumulation elevates pressure and impairs diastolic relaxation in both ventricles causing cardiac compression and the symptoms of cardiac tamponade – increased restlessness, tachycardia and lowered blood pressure. Treatment requires pericardiocentesis (pericardial tap).

Investigations include 12-lead ECG (concave upwards ST segment elevation in acute pericarditis; AF is common in constrictive pericarditis), echocardiogram and chest X-ray. Left and right heart catheterisation may reveal characteristic features of constriction. Magnetic resonance imaging (MRI) can help to differentiate between constrictive pericarditis and restrictive cardiomyopathy.

 Nursing management and health promotion: pericardial disease

Management involves controlling the symptoms and preventing deterioration. Reducing fever, resolving pain and relieving anxiety are important. Clinical observation needs to include assessing for any deterioration in cardiac function through monitoring blood pressure, and fluid balance is important. Oxygen therapy may be required and positioning of the patient to maximise respiratory function. Close monitoring in response to any heart failure treatment will be important. Patients need to be appropriately prepared for any interventional treatment.

Myocarditis

Myocarditis is an inflammatory process producing a range of symptoms ranging from mild 'flu- like symptoms to heart failure and death. It predominantly affects previously fit young adult males.

PATHOPHYSIOLOGY

Histological changes are non-specific including myocytic necrosis, autonomic nerve injury and dysfunction. The disease process may be localised or widespread across the myocardium. It can produce chronic dilated cardiomyopathy with resulting heart failure and arrhythmias. Patients present with chest pain and shortness of breath. They may develop acute or chronic heart failure, palpitations, fatigue and fever.

Investigations include 12-lead ECG (signs of enlarged heart, ST and T wave changes, AF, bundle branch block), chest X-ray (signs of heart failure, pericardial effusion), echocardiography (dilated ventricles, mitral regurgitation) and MRI scanning to show the extent of inflammation.

 Nursing management and health promotion: myocarditis

The goal is to identify any specific cause and treat, for example with appropriate antibiotic therapy. Symptom management is also important including management of heart failure. Rest and restriction of activity and management of fluid balance play a part. Observation for response to therapy and deterioration (respiration, heart rate, temperature, blood pressure) will be required. The convalescent period is about 6 weeks.

Infective endocarditis

The majority of cases are streptococcal or staphylococcal infections, although an increasing number of infective agents are being isolated due to increasingly invasive medical techniques, such as in dental treatment or urinary investigation. Intravenous drug users also introduce bacteria into their body through use of contaminated needles.

PATHOPHYSIOLOGY

Those who have pre-existing valve disease or congenital lesions are at greater risk of developing bacterial endocarditis, as the underlying structures are already damaged and the blood flow is more turbulent. Certain sites are more favoured than others for bacterial proliferation. When blood flows from a high-pressure to a low-pressure system via a narrow orifice, the organisms tend to gather on the low-pressure side. The vegetations of infective endocarditis are large and can aggregate to form up to 6 cm masses. They have a tendency to embolise and can prolapse into the valve orifice, obstructing flow.

Presentation may be slow and insidious, with general malaise, weight loss, lethargy, intermittent, often low-grade pyrexia, profuse sweating and joint pain. Microembolisation may manifest as splinter haemorrhages of the nail beds. If the infection has eroded tissues within the conduction system there may be evidence of rhythm and conduction disturbances. Evidence of embolisation may be seen in renal, cerebral, pulmonary and gastrointestinal systems. Heart failure secondary to valve failure varies in its severity, depending on the valve affected and the acuteness of onset, and may give rise to shortness of breath and ankle oedema.

Nursing management and health promotion: infective endocarditis

Infective endocarditis should be suspected in ill patients with known cardiac disease or new cardiac murmurs, especially if there is a history of recent dental, invasive diagnostic or surgical treatment and/or signs of embolic or vasculitic complications (Ramsdale & Turner-Stokes 2004). The patient will require intravenous antibiotics and management of symptoms and may need surgery to repair/replace damaged heart valves. Drainage of any abscesses (collections of pus) that may develop in the heart muscle or other parts of the body may be required. The individual should be advised to take prophylactic antibiotics prior to any invasive (e.g. dental) procedure.

Valvular disorders

Adult valvular disease is either congenital or acquired. The effects of congenital problems largely manifest themselves in childhood and so are not discussed here. The major causes of valve pathology are rheumatic heart disease (RHD), infective endocarditis and, to a lesser extent today, syphilis. Disease can cause narrowing (stenosis) of the valve, or regurgitation as a result of failure of the one-way valve, leading to blood backflow through the valve. Major disruption can also result from papillary muscle dysfunction following myocardial infarction or penetrating chest wounds, when onset of symptoms can be sudden and severe.

Valve stenosis and incompetence

Aortic stenosis
PATHOPHYSIOLOGY

The left ventricle becomes progressively hypertrophied, working at a higher pressure to eject blood past the stenosed valve. The chamber size of the ventricle is reduced by the increased muscle mass, which may itself contribute to outflow obstruction. This state is asymptomatic until the orifice is reduced to 0.5–0.7 cm^2 (normal 2.6–3.5 cm^2) when the patient may experience angina, as oxygen supply does not meet demand.

The other major effect is syncope (fainting), as cardiac output fails to rise in response to exercise. Hypertrophy may progress to decompensation and heart failure with rising left ventricular end-diastolic pressure (LVEDP) and pulmonary oedema. There is a link between aortic stenosis and gastrointestinal bleeding, known as Heyde's syndrome. However, the incidence of this is low (Pate & Mulligan 2005) and the problem usually subsides with valve replacement.

Mitral stenosis
PATHOPHYSIOLOGY

In this condition, the left atrium has to eject blood through a resistant valve. Left atrial pressure rises, and the atrium distends and eventually decompensates, with fibrous tissue interspersed between cardiac muscle. Conduction becomes aberrant and atrial fibrillation results, decreasing cardiac output as there is no atrial contribution to ventricular filling. If sinus rhythm persists, evidence of atrial hypertrophy can be seen on ECG. Since conduction takes longer to spread across the enlarged left atrium, the P wave becomes broadened and bifid. Left atrial pressure rises further with the stasis of blood within the chamber. This pressure increase is transmitted to the pulmonary vasculature, where vascular resistance rises with resultant greater right-sided afterload and possible failure. Acute elevations of pressure with exercise, for example, will precipitate pulmonary oedema. Stasis of blood allows the formation of mural thrombus within the atria. The obvious danger is that this may be dislodged and carried forward into the systemic circulation with profound ischaemic consequences for the area supplied by the embolised vessel.

Aortic incompetence
PATHOPHYSIOLOGY

LVEDP is approximately one eighth of the concomitant aortic pressure, and therefore any breach of the valve allows large amounts of blood to flow back into the ventricle. The ventricle dilates to accommodate this volume, LVEDP rises and stroke volume increases, as does systolic pressure. Diastolic pressure within the aorta is low because of regurgitation, and therefore there is a wide pulse pressure, often approximately 140 mmHg (190/50 mmHg). Chronic gradual aortic incompetence (AI) is well tolerated, but if there is an acute onset, left ventricular failure (LVF) quickly develops. AI also occurs when the valve annulus becomes dilated so that the cusps cannot coapt, e.g. in connective tissue disorders, syphilis and aortic dissection.

Mitral incompetence

PATHOPHYSIOLOGY

This allows backflow of blood to the left atrium in systole, where regurgitated blood and the normal atrial volume mix and return to the ventricle during atrial systole. In order to cope with this increased load, the ventricle hypertrophies and then dilates. Forward flow diminishes, with progressive failure of the ventricle and with backflow into the atria at systole. Weight loss and lethargy are marked as the heart can no longer provide the nutrition the blood usually carries. The left atrium dilates, and changes in conduction and rhythm occur.

Tricuspid stenosis and incompetence

PATHOPHYSIOLOGY

These result in increased right-sided pressure, with evidence of stasis and engorgement of the portal and peripheral circulations, e.g. ascites, liver dysfunction and peripheral oedema. If the right atrium becomes hypertrophied due to tricuspid stenosis, the P wave on the ECG will become peaked. The majority of right-sided failure is usually secondary to failure on the left; however, there is an increase in bacterial endocarditis of the right heart, with the increasing use, or abuse, of intravenous medication.

Investigations for valve disorders

These should include ECG, chest X-ray and echocardiography. Cardiac catheterisation is also necessary for those referred for surgery to assess valve function, ventricular function and the patency of coronary arteries.

Valvuloplasty

This involves a catheter being introduced across the stenotic valve. The balloon is then inflated and the calcified stenosis cracked and opened up. It is often carried out prior to surgery. In the mitral position, the approach is across the septum, while with the aortic valve the catheter is introduced retrogradely. Problems include:

- bradycardias
- profound hypotension when the balloon is inflated
- embolisation
- cardiac tamponade (compression of the heart through build-up of blood or fluid in the pericardial space)
- possible myocardial rupture.

The aim of valvuloplasty is to increase the functional area of the valve and therefore cardiac output. It is particularly appropriate for older people with aortic stenosis, for whom a full operation would hold too many risks but whose life expectancy would be short without it. It has the advantage of a short hospital stay and the prompt resumption of normal life.

Valve repair

Preserving the native valve provides improved haemodynamics and reduces the risk of infection, thromboembolic reactions, medical device failure and the need for long-term anticoagulation.

Valve replacement

Valve replacement is required for patients where valvuloplasty is unsuitable or unsuccessful. Valve repair may be considered early on in the disease process before valve replacement is an option. Valve replacement with a mechanical or bioprosthetic valve, made from animal or human tissue, should be performed before the patient is too unwell to tolerate the operation. The choice of valve tends to be determined by the patient's age and the surgeon's preference. The patient undergoes a median sternotomy and valve replacement or repair using cardiopulmonary bypass. Minimally invasive approaches to valve repair are now more frequent with peri- and postoperative care being the same as that for any cardiac surgery patient undergoing such a procedure. The patient who has had a mechanical device fitted needs to become accustomed to hearing it click during each cardiac cycle.

Transcatheter aortic valve implantation (TAVI)

TAVI is a novel therapy that may be used as an alternative to standard surgical aortic valve replacement. The procedure is performed on the beating heart without the need for a sternotomy or cardiopulmonary bypass. It has been used on a select group of patients who are inappropriate for more invasive procedures and is still in the process of being evaluated as a procedure (Thomas 2009).

 Nursing management and health promotion: valvular disease

Treatment centres on managing symptoms and supporting the patient through any invasive procedures to repair or replace the affected valve. Choice of treatment needs to reflect the individual patient's physical condition and circumstances, and guidelines have been produced to facilitate treatment choice (ACC/AHA 2006). Medical treatment should be initiated before symptoms become too severe so that the patient remains well enough for surgery. Patients will need advice about prophylactic antibiotics and the early recognition of symptoms. Heart failure will be controlled with diuretics and vasodilators. Blood pressure will need to be managed to avoid excessive regurgitation through the damaged valve. Anticoagulation will be required if AF is present.

Patients need reassurance about long-term prognosis and encouragement to lead as healthy a lifestyle as possible. Physical activities that produce extreme fatigue will need to be restricted once symptoms appear. After surgery, those with a sternal scar should avoid driving until the wound is healed. For further information on valve disease, see Further reading, e.g. Clare (2007).

Grown-up congenital heart (GUCH) disease

Whilst the demand for health care for children born with congenital heart disease is likely to remain relatively stable, the number of adults with complex congenital heart disease is predicted to increase significantly. The British Cardiac Society (BCS) Working Party on grown-up congenital heart disease estimated that by the year 2010 there would be over 185 000 adults living with congenital heart disease in the UK (BCS 2002) and soon there will be more adults than children living with congenital heart disease. These patients may require admission to hospital for the control of arrhythmias, cardiac catheterisation and the treatment of heart failure. Transition to the adult health care system can be difficult for individuals who have been under the care of one physician for 18 years and should be done gradually and with sensitivity. An accessible and dedicated ward area for these patients is recommended (BCS 2002). Patients in the community may need support and advice on issues such as contraception and pregnancy, the risks of infective endocarditis and general lifestyle advice. It is beyond the scope of this chapter to go into details about specific congenital conditions; however, a comprehensive account is provided in Further reading, e.g. Kennedy (2007).

Hypertension

In adults, hypertension has been defined as persistent raised blood pressure above 140/90 mmHg (NICE 2006a). The optimal blood pressure targets are a systolic blood pressure of less than 120 mmHg and a diastolic blood pressure of less than 80 mmHg (Williams et al 2004). Individuals with blood pressure at the upper limits of the population distribution have an increased incidence of atherosclerotic, thrombotic and haemorrhagic vascular disease and an increased morbidity and mortality due to stroke, myocardial infarction and peripheral vascular disease. The systolic blood pressure is the better predictor of subsequent cardiovascular risk. The World Health Organization (WHO) has estimated that over 50% of CHD in developed countries is due to a systolic blood pressure in excess of the theoretical minimum of 115 mmHg (WHO 2002). In England, 37% of men and 34% of women have hypertension, defined as a systolic blood pressure over 140 mmHg and a diastolic blood pressure over 90 mmHg (BHF 2008).

PATHOPHYSIOLOGY

Although difficult to define in terms of elevated blood pressure, hypertension is commonly classified according to cause:

- Primary or essential hypertension refers to a raised blood pressure where no cause can be found.
- Secondary hypertension is a result of an underlying condition, most commonly:
  - renal disease (see Ch. 8)
  - an adrenaline-secreting tumour, e.g. phaeochromocytoma in the adrenal medulla
  - diseases of the pituitary or adrenal cortex, where there is an elevation of glucocorticoids, e.g. Cushing's disease (see Ch. 5)
  - coarctation (narrowing) of the aorta
  - hyperthyroidism (see Ch. 5).

Hypertension can also be classified according to severity:

- mild – when elevation of blood pressure is only moderate and occurs over a long period of time
- malignant – when there is a sudden and severe blood pressure elevation; the malignancy does not refer to cellular changes but to the fact that this is a life-threatening condition.

Whatever form of hypertension is diagnosed, the concern is always the effect of this high blood pressure on the heart, where the increased demand on its pumping capacity can lead to ventricular hypertrophy, and on the brain, where any elevation of blood pressure could precipitate a cerebral catastrophe (see Ch. 9). Other organs that give rise to concern are the kidneys, where the delicate function of the nephrons can be impaired by constant high pressure, and the eyes, where fine retinal vessels may rupture and significantly impair vision.

Associated factors

Several factors associated with hypertension have been identified:

- obesity – blood pressure has been shown to decrease with weight loss
- sodium intake – results from increased sodium and water retention in the kidneys
- alcohol – blood pressure rises with increased intake
- genetic factors – the kidneys' ability to handle sodium is also thought to be genetically influenced
- smoking – nicotine promotes catecholamine release and so increases heart rate and blood pressure
- stress – this is presumed to relate to increased sympathetic outflow (see Ch. 17).

Common presenting symptoms

People who are aware that they have a condition that predisposes them to hypertension will have been alerted to this potential problem and the symptoms may be more readily appreciated. However, many may be completely unaware of their hypertensive state, either having no symptoms at all or dismissing complaints such as headaches, vertigo, nosebleeds and fatigue.

The elevated blood pressure may only be noticed at a routine examination for another reason, such as insurance cover. A single elevated reading does not justify a diagnosis of hypertension since anxiety about the examination itself may be the temporary cause; however, the person should be reassessed at a later date. Underlying mean blood pressure is traditionally used to diagnose hypertension, although there is emerging evidence that the maximum systolic blood pressure reached and the variability between systolic blood pressure recordings may be significant (Rothwell 2010). Examiners need to be aware of the possible contribution their own technique and instrument calibration may make to errors in estimation, e.g. using inappropriately sized cuffs.

Generally, hypertension is defined by grading, with arbitrary cut-off points according to diastolic pressure.

- Grade 1 hypertension is defined as a systolic blood pressure 140–159 mmHg or diastolic 90–99 mmHg or both.
- Grade 2 hypertension is a blood pressure greater than or equal to 160/100 mmHg (Williams et al 2004). The higher the diastolic pressure, the greater the risk of stroke, renal failure, coronary artery disease and heart failure.

Treatment of hypertension has been shown to reduce the relative risks of cardiovascular mortality and morbidity by 30% (Collins & Peto 1994). The management of the patient with hypertension is generally the responsibility of the primary health care team and hospitalisation is not usually required.

Malignant elevation

At any point in primary hypertension, sudden acute elevation of pressure can occur. This malignant hypertension can rapidly become life threatening. Death can ensue from stroke or from the cerebral oedema of hypertensive encephalopathy. Hypertension generally promotes the progression of atherosclerosis. Sudden increased pressure in vessels already compromised may lead to rupture or embolisation of existing thrombus. The importance of this depends on where the emboli occlude. Further occlusion of the afferent arterioles exacerbates the situation by stimulating increased renin release, which in turn contributes to the hypertensive state. Increased pressure may result in internal haemorrhage or infarction of the kidneys.

The progress of the increasing pressure is mirrored in changes to the vessels of the optic fundus, termed hypertensive retinopathy (see Ch. 13). Once papilloedema (oedema of the optic disc) occurs, intracranial pressure has increased and the individual may complain of blurring of vision.

Investigations

These include:

- blood pressure monitoring – repeat recordings to minimise 'white coat syndrome', correct cuff size, patient sitting down
- chest X-ray and ECG to determine the degree of left ventricular hypertrophy and heart failure
- full blood count, electrolytes, urea or nitrogen and creatinine, to exclude secondary causes and renal effects of the disease process
- urinalysis with microscopy, 24-h collections for creatinine clearance and vanillylmandelic acid (VMA)
- intravenous urogram (IVU) to assess renal perfusion.

Tests for secondary causes of hypertension should include assays for evidence of renal disease, primary aldosteronism, hyperthyroidism and phaeochromocytoma, while urgent assessment and control of blood pressure take place. It may be that the hypertension is a side-effect of other treatment, e.g. oral contraception. Only 4–5% of women taking 'the pill' develop overt hypertension due to oestrogen ingestion, but it may take several months for it to settle. Other forms of contraception should be advised. Hypertension is also one of the signs of pre-eclampsia of pregnancy.

▷ Nursing management and health promotion: hypertension

Management depends largely on how elevated the blood pressure is and the total risk of CVD. All adults should have their blood pressure measured routinely at least every 5 years. Those with 'high normal' systolic blood pressure (130–139 mmHg) or diastolic blood pressure (85–89 mmHg) and those with previously elevated readings should have their blood pressure measured annually (Williams et al 2004). To identify hypertension the patient should be asked to return for at least two subsequent clinics where blood pressure is assessed from two readings under the best conditions available. All hypertensive patients should have a thorough history taken and physical examination.

Drug therapy

Medication is recommended in all patients with a raised cardiovascular risk (10-year risk of CVD of 20% or greater calculated by a recognised cardiovascular risk assessment tool) or existing CVD or target organ damage, diabetes with persistent blood pressure of more than 140/90 mmHg (NICE 2006a). Most people require more than one type of medication to control blood pressure. Care needs to be taken not to lower the blood pressure too far as this may cause feelings of light-headedness and fainting. Beta blockers and ACE inhibitors are the first choice for younger patients. Calcium channel blockers and diuretics are more effective for older patients. The formulation used should ideally be effective for 24 h when taken as a single daily dose and titrated up to the manufacturer's recommendations. Patients should be advised to continue taking their medication even though they feel well or have a 'normal' blood pressure recording.

Lifestyle modification

Certain lifestyle measures can reduce blood pressure (Williams et al 2004), including:

- maintaining a body mass index of 20–25 kg/m^2
- limiting alcohol consumption to three units a day or less for men and two units a day or less for women
- reducing intake of total and saturated fat
- eating at least five portions of fruit and vegetables a day.

Healthy lifestyle advice needs to follow that recommended for CHD secondary prevention (Box 2.8). Dietary changes are aimed at the reduction of obesity, the control of any underlying problem such as diabetes mellitus, and the reduction of the salt content. A diet rich in fruits, vegetables and low-fat dairy food with reduced saturated total fat can substantially lower blood pressure (Cutler et al 1997). It is best to involve the whole family, as it is less socially disruptive if everyone can continue to sit down to the same meals together. Also, the hereditary aspect of hypertension would indicate that it is in the whole family's interest to prevent the problem developing. No salt added at table, or salt substitutes, are advised. The nurse may be able to assist patients in interpreting labels on food products. Moderating alcohol intake is advised. This may be difficult for some, where entertaining forms a great part of their work; however, low-alcohol wines and beers are increasingly available.

 See website Critical thinking question 2.1

Management of malignant hypertension

The aim of medical and nursing management of this life-threatening condition is a controlled reduction in blood pressure, with monitoring of other systems in order to minimise further damage or to prevent it from occurring (Shayne & Pitts 2003). Cerebral function should be assessed continuously. Blood pressure should be monitored, preferably by direct arterial cannulation, at least every 15 min to assess the efficacy of medication. Cardiac demand should be reduced as much as possible by bed rest and sedation. Straining at stool should be avoided. The patient should have urinary catheterisation and frequent observation of urine output. A 24-h urine collection should be commenced for excretory products of catecholamines, such as VMA, levels being twice that of normal in the presence of the

Box 2.8 Evidence-based practice

Secondary prevention for coronary heart disease: How can the service be improved? Do nurses have a significant role?

People with pre-existing coronary heart disease are at particularly high risk of coronary events and death, but effective secondary prevention strategies can reduce admissions to hospital and improve quality of life and the processes of care delivery in the short term. Effective secondary prevention comprises several elements, including pharmaceutical interventions, using antiplatelet agents, statins and beta blockers, and interventions to change behaviour and modify lifestyle, relating to smoking cessation, regular exercise and healthy eating. Most people with coronary heart disease are cared for in the primary care setting and general practitioners have been encouraged to target them for secondary prevention. This has proved difficult and surveys of baseline provision consistently show that secondary prevention is suboptimal.

This research project aimed to evaluate the effects of nurse-led clinics in primary care on secondary prevention, total mortality and coronary event rates after 4 years. It involved 1343 randomly selected patients with a diagnosis of coronary heart disease from 19 general practices in north-east Scotland. Patients in the intervention group were invited to attend nurse-led secondary prevention clinics at their general practice during which their symptoms and treatment were reviewed. The use of aspirin was promoted, lipid management reviewed, lifestyle factors such as exercise assessed and, if appropriate, behavioural changes negotiated. Patients were followed up every 2–6 months. Patients in the control group received the usual care.

Subjects were followed up over a 4-year period by postal questionnaires and review of their case notes. Significant improvements were shown at 1 year in key components of secondary prevention (aspirin, blood pressure management, lipid management, healthy diet), except smoking. These improvements were sustained at 4 years except for exercise. The authors of the report conclude that the improved medical and lifestyle components of secondary prevention produced by nurse-led clinics seem to lead to fewer total deaths and coronary events. They also conclude that nurse-led clinics should be started sooner rather than later.

Murchie P, Campbell NC, Ritchie LD, et al: Secondary prevention clinics for coronary heart disease: four year follow-up of a randomised control trial in primary care, *British Medical Journal* 326:84–87, 2003.

adrenal tumour, phaeochromocytoma. The nurse should also be alert for haematuria or any other sign of blood loss. Complaints of ischaemic chest pain should be investigated and treated as already described. Anxiolytic medication may benefit people whose condition is exacerbated by anxiety.

Aortic aneurysm

An aneurysm is a permanent dilatation of the aorta with a diameter at least 50% greater than would be expected. The aneurysm can be localised or extend along the length of the aorta. The aorta is divided into three segments:

- the ascending aorta
- the arch
- the descending aorta, which consists of abdominal and thoracic portions.

Aneurysms are classified by shape, as being:

- fusiform – involving a complete circumferential section
- saccular – an outpouching from one weakened area.

Saccular aneurysms can be tied off surgically at the neck of the sac, while fusiform types require excision and replacement with a tubular graft. If the graft is required close to the aortic valve, a composite prosthetic valve and tube graft may be employed, with reimplantation of the coronary arteries if necessary.

There are several causes of aneurysm formation:

- *Atherosclerotic disease.* This is the major cause of aneurysms, especially of the descending portion, 75% of the aorta being below the level of the diaphragm. Plaque formation reduces the nutritional supply to the aortic wall by hampering diffusion of nutrients from blood in the lumen.
- *Turbulence around bifurcations.*
- *Hypertension and medial degeneration.* The medial layer of the vessel wall undergoes degenerative changes associated with ageing. Since this is the layer that, due to its elasticity, withstands the most pressure, degeneration allows the wall to dilate. This often occurs without symptoms and may be found on routine examination. The patient is often hypertensive. Increased blood pressure, especially diastolic pressure, reduces the blood flow to the medial layer, which becomes ischaemic and weakened.
- *Cystic medial degeneration* also occurs as a consequence of connective tissue diseases, e.g. Marfan's and Ehlers–Danlos syndromes. These affect the ascending aorta and may cause the annulus of the aortic valve to dilate. This may result in an incompetent valve, as the cusps cannot completely cover the larger area. First presentation may be as a consequence of valvular failure.
- *Infection.* Aneurysms due to syphilis and other infectious causes are less prevalent today; they largely affect the ascending aorta.

Abdominal aortic aneurysm (AAA)

The abdominal aorta is the most frequent site of aneurysm formation, affecting 2–5% of the male population over 60 years with a male to female ratio of 4:1 (Sternbergh et al 1998).

PATHOPHYSIOLOGY

Common presenting symptoms The majority of AAAs are without symptoms, but a pulsating abdominal mass may be felt when lying in bed. Pain relates to compression of neighbouring organs. It is severe, unrelated to movement and radiates through to the low back and possibly down into the thighs and buttocks. Presentation may be due to ischaemia of the end organs whose arterial supply originates within the aneurysmal section. Ischaemia may also be the result of embolisation of thrombus that gathers in the dilated portion due to sluggish blood flow and turbulence around atherosclerotic plaques. Diagnosis is made by ultrasonography, magnetic resonance imaging (MRI) and computed tomography (CT) scanning. Half of the dilatations greater than 6 cm will rupture within a year, so prompt surgical management is called for. Surgical repair involves either a midline incision for a retroperitoneal approach or a transverse approach above the umbilicus if the aneurysm is above the renal arteries and there is renal involvement. The aneurysm is clamped above and below the swelling and the thrombus removed. A synthetic graft is laid within the aneurysmal sac and sutured in place. The sac is trimmed and sewn over the graft. Older or cardiorespiratory-compromised patients may be unsuitable for surgical repair. Endovascular repair involving stent insertion into the affected lumen may be more appropriate for these patients (Ransome 1996). The risk of spontaneous dissection is that severe blood loss, hypotension and death will supervene. Emboli may enter the inferior vena cava and result in pulmonary infarction. Mortality in patients with a ruptured aneurysm is high. Emergency management aims to stabilise blood pressure by large volume infusion of colloid or other volume expanders and by pharmacological support with inotropic medication. Surgical repair should not be delayed. For further information on the care of the patient undergoing surgical repair of an abdominal aortic aneurysm, see Further reading Collins (2003).

Investigations prior to planned surgery include abdominal X-ray, which will highlight any vessel calcification, echocardiography, ultrasound and CT scanning, all of which are non-invasive. Some centres also perform angiography; however, this may precipitate embolisation. Full cardiac investigation is required since atherosclerosis is a diffuse disease. Correction of any coronary insufficiency is recommended prior to surgical non-emergency aneurysm repair, since postoperative mortality is largely due to myocardial infarction.

Thoracic aneurysms

The aetiology is similar to aneurysms in the abdomen. False thoracic aneurysms can be secondary to blunt or penetrating injury to the chest in road traffic accidents, although they are more often associated with true rupture of the aorta, from which mortality is high. Some thoracic aneurysms are stabilised by surrounding tissue which can allow time for the patient to present at cardiothoracic services.

PATHOPHYSIOLOGY

Atherosclerosis affects the arch and descending thoracic aorta, while cystic medial degeneration and infections are found as causative agents in the ascending portion.

Common presenting symptoms depend on the site of occurrence. Chest X-ray shows a widened mediastinum. Dilatation causes pressure on other structures: bronchospasm may result from deviation of the trachea, secretion retention and alveolar collapse from obstruction, shortness of breath and haemoptysis if erosion occurs into the left main bronchus. Obstruction of the oesophagus may present as dysphagia, while fainting may be the result of reduced cardiac output due to obstruction of the superior vena cava.

Dissecting aortic aneurysms
PATHOPHYSIOLOGY

Tears in the intima due to the forces of hypertension, and the degenerative changes already discussed, allow a column of blood to enter and disrupt the media, creating a false lumen.

Classification is by site of the tear. In addition to previously discussed predisposing diseases, there is a higher, but as yet unexplained, incidence of dissection among pregnant women.

Common presenting symptoms depend upon the site and severity of the rupture. Severe anterior chest pain can be mistaken for acute myocardial infarction, but it is often described as tearing in nature. Pain may migrate as the dissection progresses. Alterations of neurological function may reflect involvement of the vessels originating from the arch of the aorta. As the dissection progresses, loss of peripheral pulses and palpable blood pressure will track its course. Renal artery dissection or occlusion will result in acute renal failure, exacerbated by the effects of profound hypotension. Alterations in rhythm or degrees of heart block may result from septal disruption as a consequence of aortic valve regurgitation. Leakage into the pericardium manifests as compression known as tamponade. The signs of cardiac tamponade are:

- hypotension
- tachycardia
- raised central venous pressure/jugular venous pressure
- oliguria
- peripheral vascular constriction
- fall in peripheral temperature.

If uncorrected, i.e. by pericardial aspiration of blood, this will lead to the state of pulseless electrical activity (PEA), cardiac arrest and death.

Investigations are identical to those used to detect AAAs.

 ## Nursing management and health promotion: dissecting aortic aneurysm

Pain control is an important aim of nursing care for these patients. The pain is often described as ripping or tearing in nature. Its location varies according to the section of artery affected and may progress as the dissection progresses. Intravenous opioids are the analgesia of choice because of their associated sedative effect and the slight vasodilatation achieved, both of which encourage a reduction in blood pressure. Operative correction is urgently required. If hypertension persists, this should be controlled by the use of arterial vasodilators, intensively and invasively monitored. If hypotension and collapse have supervened, then intervention is as for AAAs. The prospect of surgery is extremely frightening, whether emergency or elective, and this should be acknowledged by nurses. Operations carry high risks, but there is often no alternative intervention. Surgery is likely to require invasive monitoring and the specialist nursing skills of the intensive care unit, and the patient should be moved to such a unit as soon as is feasible. This may mean a journey of several hours by road or air, a daunting prospect for patient and escorting staff alike. It often necessitates the separation of the patient from their family at a time of great stress, so every effort should be made to ensure effective communication. The management of cardiogenic shock is described in Chapter 18. Postoperative care is similar to that following cardiac surgery.

The need for spiritual care must be recognised. There may be times when a dignified, peaceful death is more appropriate than surgery. For further information on the care of the patient with an abdominal aortic aneurysm see Further reading, e.g. Young & Daniels (2007).

Peripheral vascular disease

Peripheral vascular disease includes pathological processes affecting both the arterial and venous circulations. Arterial and venous peripheral disease can occur alone or together and it is important to be able to differentiate between the two.

Arterial disease

Arterial occlusions

Atherosclerosis is the commonest cause of arterial disease. It is characterised by the development of atherosclerotic plaques within the intima of the artery wall which inhibit arterial blood flow (see p. 14). Symptoms of impaired blood supply may be slow to appear if collateral circulation has had time to develop.

Arteriosclerosis obliterans

PATHOPHYSIOLOGY

This is the state of chronic occlusive atheroma of the arteries supplying the extremities. Turbulence at bifurcations, as occurs in larger vessels, predisposes to intimal changes. There is also a degenerative element in its development. The same process is found in the cerebral and visceral arteries. The factors influencing its development have been discussed in the section on CHD. It is typically a disease of middle-aged to older men, who may be hypertensive, diabetic, have a diet high in lipids, and smoke, resulting in greater risk of atherosclerosis.

The result of increasing occlusion of the vessels, with medial calcification and loss of elastic fibres, is the slowing of blood flow. The blood becomes hypercoagulable. Thrombosis of the deep veins may occur, secondary to sudden arterial thrombosis. The ischaemia of surrounding tissue is evidenced by skin and muscle atrophy, loss of subcutaneous fat deposits and ischaemic neuropathy.

Severe occlusion can result in gangrene, usually first seen at the toes, then extending into the foot and leg. At the boundary between viable and necrotic tissue, an area of inflammation is often seen. The extent of the ischaemia will depend on how quickly occlusion developed and how extensive collateral circulation has become. Gangrene occurs when insufficient oxygen is conveyed to the tissue to sustain its life. This can be exacerbated by any other superimposed demand, e.g. infection, when oxygen demand rises but cannot be sustained by an impaired blood flow. Diabetic patients are more prone to infected ulceration in association with gangrene (see Ch. 5). Vasoconstriction should be avoided if at all possible.

Common presenting symptoms

These may occur gradually or with sudden acute thrombosis, which may be the first indication of a process that has been silently progressing for some time (Table 2.6).

Table 2.6 Presenting features of arterial and venous peripheral vascular disease		
ASSESS	**ARTERIAL DISEASE**	**VENOUS DISEASE**
Pain	Acute: sudden, severe pain, peaks rapidly Chronic: intermittent claudication, rest pain	Acute: little or no pain; tenderness along course of inflamed vein Chronic: heaviness, fullness
Impotence	May be present with aortoiliac femoral disease	Not associated
Hair	Hair loss distal to occlusion	No hair loss
Nails	Thick, brittle	Normal
Skeletal muscle	Atrophy may be present; may have restricted limb movement	Normal
Sensation	Possible paraesthesia	Normal
Skin colour	Pallor or reactive hyperaemia (pallor when limb elevated; rubor [red] when limb dependent)	Brawny (reddish-brown); cyanotic if dependent
Skin texture	Thin, shiny, dry	Stasis dermatitis; veins may be visible; skin mottling
Skin temperature	Cool	Warm
Skin breakdown (ulcers)	Severely painful; usually on or between toes or on upper surface of foot over metatarsal heads or other bony prominences	Mildly painful, with pain relieved by leg elevation; usually in ankle area
Oedema	None or mild; usually unilateral	Typically present, usually foot to calf; may be unilateral or bilateral
Pulses	Diminished, weak, absent	Normal
Blood flow	Bruit may be present; pressure readings lower below stenosis	Normal

Adapted from Bright & Georgi (1992).

Pain: intermittent claudication The term 'claudication' comes from the Latin 'claudicare' meaning to limp. Intermittent claudication is the commonest symptom of vascular disease and describes exercise-induced pain in muscle groups distal to the occluded vessel. Its nature varies from a numb cramp to severe pain. It is a manifestation of increased oxygen demand with exercise and the subsequent accumulation of metabolic wastes. It is relieved by rest. The calf muscles are the most commonly affected, but thigh and buttock muscles can also be involved, depending on the site of occlusion. The distance the individual can walk on the flat before onset of symptoms, the claudication distance, is an indication of the progress of the disease. Pain may eventually occur at rest, most often in the toes and foot and particularly at night, when limbs become warm and oxygen demand increases, thus interfering with sleep. Pain may become severe and difficult to contain if the patient develops gangrene. Neuropathy reduces sensation and may make the person unaware of the progressive gangrenous changes. Any exercise that can be tolerated should be encouraged.

Investigations

Pulses should be assessed at rest in a warm room. They will remain intact until two thirds of the lumen is occluded. Posterior tibial, popliteal and femoral pulses should be included in the examination; dorsalis pedis pulses are not consistently present in all people. The volume of the pulses should be compared, as well as simple presence or absence. Many people find it difficult to differentiate between their own pulse and the patient's; increasing the examiner's heart rate by exercising immediately before the examination can make it easier to distinguish their own pulse. The noise of turbulent blood flow (bruit) may also be heard as a murmur or abnormal sound when a stethoscope is placed over areas of turbulence in arteries that are still pulsating.

Colour and temperature As occlusion develops, the feet, and especially the toes, may be red in colour. This can later develop into bluish mottled areas or areas of pallor. With sudden occlusion, pallor may be marked. Elevation of legs with severe occlusion results in deathly pallor. Once legs return to the dependent position, colour normally returns. Superficial veins normally refill within 15 s, but in these cases it may take a minute or more. In severe cases, the limbs may become a cyanotic red colour (rubor). Temperature changes accompany reduced blood flow with cool pale extremities.

X-rays will show calcification of the vessel wall.

Doppler ultrasound When low-intensity sound is directed through the tissue towards a blood vessel, sound waves strike moving blood cells and are transmitted back. The frequency of these sound waves reflects changes in proportion to the velocity of the blood. Sound waves diminish in arterial occlusion and stenosis. Doppler ultrasound is used to assess the ankle brachial pressure index (ABPI) which decreases with arterial occlusion. Duplex scanners offer a sensitivity of 80% and are more reliable than angiography for detecting femoral and popliteal disease (Figure 2.12).

Helical or spiral computed tomography is a minimally invasive technique for vascular imaging which scans large areas in a short period of time, thereby reducing motion artefact.

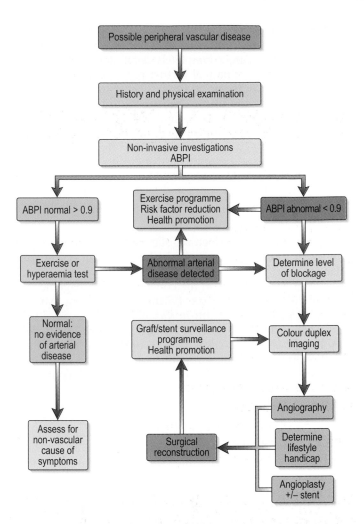

Figure 2.12 The management of peripheral vascular disease. (Adapted from Murray 2003.)

Exercise testing will assess the functional limitations of arterial stenosis and differentiate occlusive arterial disease from other causes of exercise-induced lower limb symptoms.

Arteriograms are usually performed in order to assess occlusion prior to surgery.

Other examinations include ECG, a full blood count, urea, electrolytes and blood sugar estimation.

Treatment

Underlying disease states such as diabetes mellitus and infection should be as well controlled as possible. Advice aimed at minimising symptoms and the risk of extending atherosclerosis should be given, as follows:

- Modify the diet to reduce lipid intake and reduce weight.
- Avoid the following which lead to vasoconstriction:
  - cigarette smoking
  - tight clothing
  - cold temperature.
- Avoid direct use of heat because of the risk of burns in a limb with decreased sensation.
- Avoid using hot water bottles, sitting too close to fires or radiators, taking hot baths and soaking the feet in hot water.

- Promote increased blood supply by a generally warm environment and elevation of the head of the bed.
- Avoid maintaining a completely dependent position since the resultant oedema will further reduce circulation.
- Encourage exercise up to the limit of pain. This is to maintain joint and muscle function and to promote collateral circulation (Leng et al 2005). Walking 3–4 times a day will decrease ischaemic time, and pain control can also be improved by increasing blood flow; however, ischaemic pain is notoriously difficult to manage and may require opiate analgesics and night sedation.
- Avoid trauma to the impaired limb.
- Avoid wearing ill-fitting shoes; referral to a chiropodist may be required.

Patients will be prescribed regular aspirin or other antiplatelet medication to reduce the risk of coronary or cerebrovascular events.

For more information on the conservative management of intermittent claudication see Further reading, e.g. Murray (2003); on promoting health in vascular nursing, e.g. Litchfield (2003); and on patients' experiences on living with peripheral vascular disease, e.g. Gibson & Kenrick (1998).

Following assessment, sympathectomy may be considered to increase blood flow by obliterating neural control of vasoconstriction.

Percutaneous transluminal balloon angioplasty (PTBA) is a minimally invasive treatment for patients with atherosclerotic peripheral vascular disease. This surgical technique involves placing an intra-arterial balloon within an obstructing arterial lesion and forcibly dilating the balloon under fluoroscopy. In selected patients, the use of an intravascular stent may be an alternative to traditional bypass. Intravascular brachytherapy, whereby radiation is applied directly to the lesion, can inhibit re-stenosis (narrowing) of the vessels (Hansrani et al 2005).

If the occlusion is sudden and acute and the viability of the limb is in question, then surgical intervention, using either saphenous vein or prosthetic material, e.g. a femoropopliteal bypass, will be required to bypass the occlusion. Endarterectomy of the vessel may be performed first to core out the atheroma of the vessel.

Prior to surgery, the patient may undergo arteriography and should be rehydrated and have blood coagulation status assessed. There is a strong association with CHD, so full cardiac assessment is required prior to operation.

If the lesion is localised and accessible, embolectomy under local anaesthesia may be sufficient to reperfuse the limb. In this procedure, a catheter is inserted into the artery up to the level of the occlusion when the balloon at the end is inflated, aiming to fracture the plaque. Inflammation and re-endothelialisation occur secondary to this. Fibrinolytic drugs can be infused at the site of the occlusion. The advantage of embolectomy is that general anaesthesia can be avoided; however, reocclusion occurs more frequently than with bypass grafting. For further information on peripheral artery bypass see Further reading, e.g. Galloway et al (2005).

Pain may become so severe and gangrene so advanced that the limb is no longer viable and amputation may become unavoidable. Bypass grafting may minimise the extent of amputation by restoring circulation, e.g. to a foot, but losing some of the toes. Amputation of a limb is traumatic for anyone but may be accepted as a means of relief from intolerable pain. It may, however, require skilled counselling before this fact can be faced by the patient and the full support of rehabilitation and limb-fitting services postoperatively is accepted (see Ch. 10). For further information on the care of a patient faced with the prospect of an amputation see Further reading, e.g. Donohue (1997a–d).

Thromboangiitis obliterans or Buerger's disease

This chronic occlusive inflammatory disease has no known cause. It manifests in a younger population than atherosclerosis, is predominant in men and is strongly associated with smoking. It is postulated that carbon monoxide has a toxic effect on the arterial wall and nicotine has vasoconstrictive effects. In contrast to atherosclerosis, it affects small and medium vessels of the extremities. It is not a diffuse disease since only segments of arteries develop lesions. Thrombosis is a secondary feature. The lumen may become occluded and the intima thickened but the medial wall structure remains intact, in contrast to atherosclerotic disease. The diagnosis can often be made on the basis of a careful history and physical examination. A patient may present with cold hypersensitive fingers and toes on two or more limbs. Investigations aim to exclude other causes of ischaemia. Occasionally, arteriography is warranted to confirm the diagnosis. The patient is strongly advised to stop smoking. Besides the general treatment approaches used in ischaemic diseases of the limbs, including antibiotics, antirheumatics and corticosteroids, some specific surgical procedures may be considered.

Raynaud's disease

This is episodic vasospastic ischaemia of the small arteries and arterioles in the most distal part of the extremities in response to cold or, less commonly, emotional stress. It usually occurs in young women and is more prevalent in cool, damp climates. A distinction should be made between Raynaud's phenomenon, which results in no permanent damage, and Raynaud's disease, the more advanced condition associated with permanent damage. The fingers become pale and cold, but pulses are intact. Cyanosis may also be a feature. Pain is not always present, but function may be lost. Similar episodes of vasospasm can be found secondary to scleroderma, some neurological conditions and in some occupational groups, e.g. those that use pneumatic vibrating tools. Treatment includes avoiding situations that trigger the problem. This may mean a change in occupation, giving up smoking and keeping warm. Vasodilating medication, including calcium channel blockers (e.g. nifedipine), prostaglandin therapy and sympathectomy have been tried as means of improving the circulation. The nurse's primary role is patient education so that the onset of symptoms associated with this disease can be identified and minimised.

▷ Nursing management and health promotion: arterial disease

Almost all the activities of life are affected by the distress of arterial disease. A healthy lifestyle should be encouraged as discussed in the section on secondary prevention of CHD.

The person's home and work circumstances can be considered, and hazards minimised. Useful advice includes the following points:

- Toenails may be best cut by the chiropodist in case soft tissue injury is inflicted, especially as some people with atherosclerotic disease, with or without diabetes, may also have poor sight.
- Caution should be exercised with electric blankets, hot water bottles, open fires and hot baths, as burns may not be felt.
- Cold can also be damaging.
- Constrictive clothing, e.g. tight underwear, is best avoided.
- Sitting cross-legged causes constriction of lower limb circulation.
- Remaining in one position for any length of time puts pressure on one area of tissue, allowing ischaemic changes to occur.

Pain management

The pain of claudication is relieved by rest; however, exercise to the limit of pain is to be encouraged in the hope of developing increased perfusion and collateral circulation. Controlling ischaemic pain is essential and will often require the use of opiate analgesics, which may cause drowsiness as a side-effect. Keeping warm, especially for people affected by vessel spasm, and positioning the affected limb in a dependent position from time to time are also advised. Anti-inflammatory medications are used in diseases with an inflammatory response. Distraction techniques can also be helpful (see Ch. 19).

Discharge planning

After successful surgery, it is important to consider how vascular improvement can be maintained to ensure a reasonable quality of life and prevent further hospital admissions.

Venous disease

Venous insufficiency

Venous disease results from:

- obstruction, by thrombus or thrombophlebitis
- incompetence of valves in the veins.

Some diseases, such as varicose veins, may seem trivial but can contribute to day-to-day discomfort and absence from work. Other venous diseases are associated with chronic health problems, such as venous ulcers, or a sudden medical emergency, such as pulmonary embolus following venous thromboembolism.

Venous thromboembolism

Venous thromboembolism (VTE) is a condition in which a blood clot (thrombus) forms in a vein. It occurs most commonly in the deep veins of the legs, known as deep vein thrombosis (DVT) (NICE 2010). The thrombus may dislodge and travel around the body in the blood as an embolism with the risk that it may travel to the lung as a potentially fatal pulmonary embolism. Thrombus formation is more likely to occur when flow is reduced within the veins. This can occur due to obstruction and stasis but is also associated with increased blood viscosity, slower flow and damage to the endothelial wall of the vessel. Hypercoagulability may be a feature of dehydration or malignant disease. It seems that there is also an imbalance between fibrinolysis and coagulation in postoperative patients, which predisposes them to DVT. Trauma may be mechanical or chemical. The increasing use of vascular cannulae predisposes the patient in hospital to the irritant effects of pharmacological preparations, the plastic of the cannula itself and the possibility of intimal trauma at insertion.

Any reduction in blood flow allows clotting factors that normally would be cleared from the circulation on movement to remain active for longer. The effects of the muscle pumps of the leg and negative intrathoracic pressure during inspiration normally promote venous return. Any situation that reduces their action predisposes to stasis of the venous circulation. Immobility and the recumbent position are frequently features of the postoperative patient and the older person. There has also been much debate about the risks arising from sitting still for long periods during long-haul flights and passengers are now encouraged to wear antiembolus socks and exercise their limbs regularly.

Muscle relaxant medications used during surgery abolish the muscle pump, and breathing is under positive pressure when ventilated mechanically. Stasis is more common in the dilated portions of varicosities. Mechanical obstruction to flow can be seen in pregnancy and abdominal tumours. Women taking oral contraception run a slightly increased risk of DVT, especially if there is a family history of thrombosis. If a DVT was to develop, then oral contraception would be discontinued and another form adopted. For further information on assessing patients at risk of DVT see Further reading, e.g. Autar (1998).

Assessment

Clinical assessment includes the use of Homan's sign, which involves sharply dorsiflexing the foot when the patient is lying flat with their legs straight. The test is positive if pain is felt in the calf. Alternatively, the knee can be slightly flexed and the gastrocnemius muscle compressed against the tibia. Again if pain is felt, the test is positive. More than 25% of DVTs produce no symptoms and are only detected on screening. In other cases, the affected area will be tender, swollen and hot. Compression ultrasonography has become a first-line investigation with the measurement of circulating D-dimer concentrations. D-dimer, a by-product of fibrin production, is a useful adjunct to ultrasonography, with a 98% sensitivity for DVT and a high negative predictive value (Gorman et al 2000). Venography, plethysmography (use of infrared light to assess relative changes in blood volume) and isotope scanning may also be used (Figure 2.13).

Once diagnosed, treatment includes pain relief and anticoagulation, first with heparin and later with warfarin. Prophylactic subcutaneous heparin is almost a routine postoperative prescription. Leg elevation, with some flexion at the knee, will be necessary until swelling and pain subside. Avoidance of dehydration, external pressure, immobility in those at risk and careful observation are all part of the preventive management. Home management is cost effective and likely to be preferred by patients (Schraibman et al 2001).

See website Critical thinking question 2.2

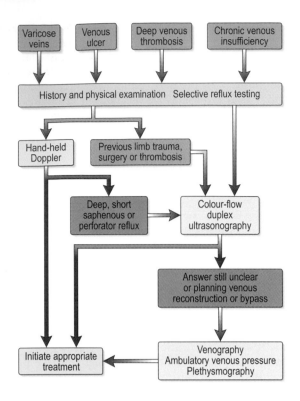

Figure 2.13 Investigation pathway for patients presenting with venous disease. (Adapted from Murray 2003.)

Chronic venous insufficiency

Of those suffering from chronic venous insufficiency, most will have had episodes of DVT previously. Pressure within the venous system remains high, resulting in increased capillary pressure and allowing chronic oedema to develop. The valves and elastic fibres of the vein wall are also destroyed by thrombophlebitis, aggravating the situation. Accumulation of interstitial fluid increases pressure locally. Eczema may occur secondary to this, possibly with pruritus. Owing to stasis, red blood cells may be trapped and haemolysed. This manifests as areas of brown pigmentation (haemosiderin). Melanin may also be deposited. Prolonged oedema reduces the nutrition available to subcutaneous tissue, which then fibroses. This induration further prevents drainage of any oedema.

Venous ulcers

Ulceration may follow trauma or dermatitis of such an area. Ulcers are commonly seen around the internal malleolus and tend to recur in the same place, as the scar tissue is atrophic.

Infection of ulcers is common. Venous ulceration is a major problem, particularly in older people, with district nurses spending a significant amount of time treating them. Compression therapy is considered to be the most appropriate non-invasive treatment of leg ulcers, although appropriate patients may benefit from surgery. Prompt and correct treatment of thrombophlebitis helps to prevent chronic venous insufficiency. Pain is worse in the dependent position, so elevation of the limb when seated and regular walking should be advised. Prolonged standing should be avoided.

Oedema is treated by elevation during bed rest. Once it is reduced, support stockings should be fitted. Any infection should be isolated and treated with appropriate medication. If varicose veins contribute to ulceration, they may be dealt with surgically. Chronic ulcers may have to be skin-grafted. For information on the care and management of leg ulcers, see Chapter 23.

Varicose veins

Varicosities are tortuous, dilated and incompetent veins, partly due to the effects of gravity. Dilatation causes the valves to become incompetent and retrograde flow is no longer prevented. It has a genetic component: about half the sufferers will have a family history of varicosities. The hormonal changes in pregnancy also reduce venous tone, while the obstruction to venous return by the gravid uterus combines to increase pregnant women's susceptibility. Obesity has a similar obstructive effect. Standing for prolonged periods maximises the force of gravity. Thrombophlebitis of the deep veins increases venous pressure, while inflammation destroys valve tissue. This increase in pressure is transmitted to the superficial veins which, being relatively less supported by surrounding structures, dilate. Most people complain of dull aching in their legs. Trauma may result in significant blood loss and should be guarded against. Ulcers are rare. Some individuals are concerned by appearance. Elevation and use of support stockings may reduce the aching and oedema.

Assessment involves history taking, examination and investigation for reflux, including the Brodie–Trendelenburg test, which means selective clinical testing for reflux, which can identify sites of perforation or junctional incompetence in either the long or short saphenous system. Continuous wave Doppler or colour flow duplex ultrasonography is also used (see Figure 2.13). Conservative treatment involves patient education, control of risk factors, advice on camouflage techniques and cosmetic treatments, e.g. laser therapy, microsclerotherapy. Support hosiery should be worn as routine.

If symptoms persist, the most common management is the surgical stripping and ligation of the varicosed vein. For some, the injection of a sclerosing agent would be considered. Treatment is increasingly being carried out on a day surgery basis and this has an impact on nursing care priorities both in hospital and at home. There is potentially less time for providing accurate information to patients about the disease process, treatment options and interventions for its prevention. For further information on surgical intervention, see Chapter 26. Patients can usually return to driving in a week and to work between 1 and 3 weeks after the procedure. Some 20–30% of patients will develop recurrent varicose veins within 10 years (London & Nash 2000). For a review of the treatment and prevention of varicose veins see Further reading, e.g. Vowden & Vowden (2003).

▷ Nursing management and health promotion: venous insufficiency

Nursing care focuses on pain management, encouraging activities that minimise disease progression and promoting health and independence. Bed rest or limb elevation reduces the throbbing pain of venous insufficiency. Mobility should be maintained as much as possible. Walking rather than standing is advisable. Supportive antiembolism stockings, by aiding venous return, reduce the feeling of pressure in the legs. However, they can be hot and uncomfortable. Once any oedema has reduced, the patient should be measured again, to ensure that the stockings fit properly and are still therapeutic. Similarly, swollen legs should not be squeezed into elastic stockings that have become too small. Anti-inflammatory medication may be prescribed to settle the inflammatory process of thromboembolism.

Patients should be advised to elevate the legs when sitting, in order to increase venous return and reduce oedema, and to avoid standing for long periods. Occupations that involve standing for long periods, e.g. shop assistants, may present a problem. After an operation for ligation of varicosities, measures to prevent DVT should be considered. The patient will be advised to:

- walk a prescribed distance of perhaps 2 miles daily
- avoid standing for long periods
- always elevate the feet when sitting.

Adequate hydration and balanced nutrition assist flow and maintain vessel integrity. A diet deficient in fibre has been thought to predispose to varicose veins. Constipation and straining at stool can cause compression and dilatation of both the superficial and deep veins in the leg. Some supplementation of vitamins, trace elements and iron may have to be considered in the older person. Avoidance of trauma and infection is important, as in arterial disease. Blood loss can be severe, even from venous circulation. Prophylactic use of support hose by at-risk groups may be advised by the occupational health nurse.

The cosmetic effect of these problems can prove very upsetting, as wearing thick white stockings is far from attractive. Trousers and opaque-coloured tights may make them more acceptable. The perfect compression stocking, which would be easy to put on, comfortable to wear, give adequate graduated compression and look fashionably sheer, has not yet been invented!

SUMMARY: KEY NURSING ISSUES

- Cardiovascular disease (CVD) is the greatest cause of death in the UK. It is the main cause of disability in the UK and as such likely to encountered by all nurses, whether hospital- or community-based.
- Cardiovascular nursing is evolving as nurses move on from practising the skills of advanced life support, cannulation and phlebotomy, to taking greater responsibility for decisions that influence patient care management.
- Government frameworks and standards of care, such as the *National Service Framework for Coronary Heart Disease* (DH 2000) have resulted in opportunities for nurses to lead and develop CVD services in and between primary, secondary and tertiary care environments.
- The main value of the ECG is in the detection and interpretation of cardiac arrhythmias, diagnosis of CHD and assessment of ventricular enlargement (hypertrophy).
- There is no such thing as a 'normal' blood pressure, as it varies both from person to person and in individuals from moment to moment, under different circumstances. The optimal blood pressure targets are a systolic pressure of less than 120 mmHg and a diastolic pressure of less than 80 mmHg (Williams et al 2004).

Factors such as age, gender and race, exercise, emotional reactions, sleep, digestion and time of day influence blood pressure values.

- Coronary heart disease is the most common cause of death in the UK, accounting for 1 in 5 deaths in men and 1 in 6 deaths in women (BHF 2008).
- The term 'acute coronary syndrome' defines a continuum of manifestations of CHD. It includes cases of unstable angina and acute myocardial infarction which all have a common underlying pathology.
- In unstable angina, the coronary artery occlusion tends to be episodic and transient. In myocardial infarction (MI) the muscle damage almost always results from total occlusion of a coronary artery by a thrombus.
- Approximately 50% of MIs are fatal and in the majority of these cases death occurs in the first hour after the attack, usually as a result of a cardiac arrhythmia.
- Cardiac arrest may be defined as failure of the heart to pump sufficient blood to maintain cerebral function. It is a term often used synonymously with sudden death, although death is not always the outcome of a cardiac arrest.
- Most in-hospital cardiac arrests are predictable with up to 84% of patients showing signs of deterioration prior to arrest (Kause et al 2004). Monitoring of vital signs and the use of early warning strategies is therefore important.
- To be effective in resuscitation, regular education and training update is necessary, ideally 6-monthly, particularly for those who do not use these skills frequently.
- Cardiogenic shock is a serious degree of heart failure, precipitated by extensive (>40%) left ventricular damage in which the cardiac output is not sufficient to give an adequate blood pressure to maintain perfusion.
- Cardiac rehabilitation should incorporate baseline patient assessment, psychosocial interventions, education and support and exercise training as important components (Balady et al 2007). There is evidence that such strategies can improve survival, quality of life, limit recurrent events and reduce the need for interventional procedures (Jolliffe et al 2005, Smith et al 2006).

➲ REFLECTION AND LEARNING – WHAT NEXT?

- **Test** your knowledge by visiting the website 🖱 and answering the multiple choice questions and critical thinking questions.
- **Consolidate** your learning by looking at some of the further reading suggestions, references and specialist websites.
- **Revisit** some of the additional material on the website.
- **Consider** what you have learnt and how this will help your professional development.
- **Reflect** on how you can apply this knowledge to the care of your patients.
- **Discuss** your learning with your mentor/supervisor, lecturer and colleagues.

REFERENCES

ACC/AHA: Guidelines for the management of patients with valvular heart disease, *Circulation* 114:84–231, 2006.

ACC/AHA/NASPE: Guideline update for implantation of cardiac pacemakers and antiarrhythmia devices, *J Cardiovasc Electrophysiol* 13:1183–1199, 2002.

Ashworth P: Cardiovascular problems and nursing. In Ashworth PM, Clarke C, editors: *Cardiovascular intensive care nursing*, Edinburgh, 1992, Churchill Livingstone.

Balady GJ, Williams MA, Ades PA: Core components of cardiac rehabilitation/secondary prevention programmes: 2007 update: a scientific statement from the American Heart Association Exercise, Cardiac Rehabilitation and Prevention Committee, the Council on Clinical Cardiology; the Council on Cardiovascular Nursing, Epidemiology and Association of Cardiovascular and Pulmonary Rehabilitation, *Circulation* 115:2675–2682, 2007.

Bassand JP, Hamm CW, Ardissino D, et al: Guidelines for the diagnosis and treatment of non-ST elevation acute coronary syndromes: the task force for the diagnosis and treatment of non-ST-segment elevation acute coronary syndromes of the European Society of Cardiology, *Eur Heart J* 28:1598–1660, 2007.

Bright LD, Georgi S: Peripheral vascular disease: is it arterial or venous? *Am J Nurs* 92(9):34–47, 1992.

British Cardiac Society: Grown up congenital heart (GUCH) disease: current needs and provision of service for adolescents and adults with congenital heart disease in the UK, *Heart* 88:I1–I14, 2002.

British Heart Foundation (BHF): *Coronary heart disease statistics*, London, 2008, British Heart Foundation. Available online http://www.heartstats.org/homepage.asp.

British Heart Foundation (BHF), National Institute for Health and Clinical Excellence, Department of Health, NHS Modernisation Agency, Coronary Heart Disease Collaborative: *Developing services for heart failure*, London, 2003, DH.

Broomfield R: A quasi-experimental research to investigate the retention of basic cardiopulmonary resuscitation skills and knowledge by qualified nurses following a course in professional development, *J Adv Nurs* 23:1016–1023, 1996.

Collins R, Peto R: Antihypertensive drug therapy: effects on stroke and coronary heart disease. In Swales JD, editor: *Textbook of hypertension*, Oxford, 1994, Blackwell Scientific.

Collinson J, Flather M, Fox KA, et al: Clinical outcomes, risk stratification and practice patterns of unstable angina and myocardial infarction without ST elevation, *Eur Heart J* 21:1450–1457, 2000.

Cotler M: The 'do not resuscitate' order: clinical and ethical rationale and implications, *Med Law* 19:623–633, 2000.

Cutler TM, Windhausser MM, Lin PH, Jaranja N: A clinical trial of the effects of dietary patterns on blood pressure. DASH Collaborative Research Group, *N Engl J Med* 336:1117–1124, 1997.

Daly C, Clemens F, Lopez Sendon JL, et al: Predicting prognosis in stable angina – results from the EuroHeart survey of stable angina: prospective observational study, *Br Med J* 332:262–267, 2006.

De Jong: Cardiogenic shock: changes in vital signs may signal impending circulatory collapse, *Am J Nurs* 97:40–41, 1999.

Department of Health (DH): *National Service Framework for coronary heart disease*, London, 2000, DH.

Department of Health (DH): *The coronary heart disease national service framework. Leading the way. Progress report 2005*, London, 2005, HMSO.

European Society of Cardiology (ESC): Executive summary of the guidelines on the diagnosis and treatment of acute heart failure. Task Force on acute heart failure, *Eur Heart J* 26:384–416, 2005.

European Society of Cardiology (ESC): Task Force on the Management of Stable Angina Pectoris of the European Society of Cardiology. Guidelines on the management of stable angina pectoris: full text, *Eur Heart J* 2006.

Gnani S, Majeed A: Co-existing conditions of health services associated with heart failure: a general practice based study, *Health Stat Q* 12:27–33, 2001.

Goldberg RJ, Samad NA, Yarzebski J, et al: Temporal trends in cardiogenic shock complicating myocardial infarction, *N Engl J Med* 340:1162–1168, 1999.

Gorman WP, Davis K, Donnelly R: Swollen lower limb – 1: general assessment and deep vein thrombosis. In Donnelly R, London N, editors: *ABC of arterial and venous disease*, London, 2000, BMJ Books.

Hambrecht R, Walther C, Morbius-Wiunkler S, et al: Percutaneous coronary angioplasty compared with exercise training in patients with stable coronary artery disease: a randomised trial, *Circulation* 109:1371–1378, 2004.

Hansrani M, Overbeck K, Smout J, et al: Intravascular brachytherapy for peripheral vascular disease (Cochrane Review). In *The Cochrane Library*, Issue 2, Chichester, 2005, Wiley.

Heath SM, Baine RJ, Andrews A: Nurse initiated thrombolysis in the accident and emergency department: safe, accurate and faster than fast track, *Emerg Med J* 20:418–420, 2003.

Jackson EA, Yarzebski JL, Goldberg RJ, et al: Do not resuscitate orders in patients hospitalized with acute myocardial infarction: the Worcester heart attack study, *Arch Intern Med* 164:776–783, 2004.

James J: Management and support of patients with internal cardioverter defibrillators. In Hatchett R, Thompson D, editors: *Cardiac nursing: a comprehensive guide*. Edinburgh, 2002, Churchill Livingstone.

Joint Health Surveys Unit: *Health Survey for England 2006. Cardiovascular disease and risk factors*, Leeds, 2008, The Information Centre.

Jolliffe JA, Rees K, Taylor RS, Oldridge N, Ebrahim S: Exercise-based rehabilitation for coronary heart disease. In *Cochrane Heart Group (Cochrane Review). Cochrane Library. Issue 3*, Oxford, 2005, Update Software, 2001.

Kastrati A, Mehilli J, Nekolla S, et al: A randomized trial comparing myocardial salvage achieved by coronary stenting versus balloon angioplasty on patients with acute myocardial infarction considered ineligible for reperfusion, *J Am Coll Cardiol* 43:734–741, 2004.

Kause J, Smith G, Prytherch D, et al: A comparison of antecedents to cardiac arrest, deaths and emergency care admissions in Australia and New Zealand and the United Kingdom – the ACADEMIA study, *Resuscitation* 62:275–282, 2004.

Kearney PM, Whelton M, Reynolds K, et al: Global burden of hypertension: analysis of worldwide data, *Lancet* 365:217–223, 2005.

Khunti K, Samani N: Coronary heart disease in people of south-Asian origin, *Lancet* 364:2077–2078, 2004.

Kucia A, Taylor KTN, Horowitz JD: Can a nurse trained in coronary care expedite the emergency department management of patients with acute coronary syndromes? *Heart Lung* 30:186–190, 2001.

Laitinen H: Patients' experience of confusion in the intensive care unit following cardiac surgery, *Intensive Crit Care Nurs* 12:79–83, 1996.

Leng GC, Fowler B, Ernst E: Exercise for intermittent claudication (Cochrane Review). In: *The Cochrane Library, Issue 1*, Chichester, 2005, Wiley.

Levine GN, Kern MJ, Berger PB, et al: Management of patients undergoing percutaneous coronary revascularisation, *Ann Intern Med* 139:123–136, 2003.

Lewin RJP, Furze G, Robinson J, et al: A randomised controlled trial of a self-management plan for patients with newly diagnosed angina, *Br J Gen Pract* 52:194–196, 2002.

Lindsey GM, Smith LN, Hanlon P, Wheatley DJ: Coronary artery disease patients' perceptions of their health and expectations of benefit following coronary artery bypass grafting, *J Adv Nurs* 36:1412–1421, 2000.

London NJM, Nash R: Varicose veins. In Donnelly R, London N, editors: *ABC of arterial and venous disease*, London, 2000, BMJ Books, pp 42–45.

Lyons A, Fanshaw C, Lip GYH: Knowledge, communication and experiences of cardiac catheterization: the patient's perspective. Psychology, *Health Med* 7:461–467, 2002.

Mårtensson J, Strömberg A, Dahlström U, et al: Patients with heart failure in primary health care: effects of a nurse-led intervention on health-related quality of life and depression, *Eur J Heart Fail* 7:393–403, 2005.

Mason S: The ethical dilemma of the do not resuscitate order, *Br J Nurs* 6:646–649, 1996.

Mayou RA, Thompson DR, Clemens A, et al: Guideline-based early rehabilitation after myocardial infarction. A pragmatic randomised controlled trial, *J Psychosom Res* 52:89–95, 2002.

McMurray JJV, Stewart S: Nurse-led multidisciplinary intervention in chronic heart failure [editorial], *Heart* 80:430–431, 1998.

Moser D, Dracup K: Role of spousal anxiety and depression in patients' psychosocial recovery after a cardiac event, *Psychosom Med* 66:527–532, 2004.

Murchie P, Campbell NC, Ritchie LD, et al: Secondary prevention clinics for coronary heart disease: four year follow-up of a randomised control trial in primary care, *Br Med J* 326:84–87, 2003.

Murray S: Chronic ischaemia. In Murray S, editor: *Vascular disease: nursing and management*, London, 2003, Whurr, pp 238–269.

National Institute for Health and Clinical Excellence (NICE): *Coronary artery stents in the treatment of ischaemic heart disease*, 1999, NHS HTA Programme, West Midlands Development and Evaluation Service, University of Birmingham.

National Institute for Health and Clinical Excellence (NICE): *Chronic heart failure. National clinical guideline for diagnosis and management in primary and secondary care*, Guideline No 5. London, 2003, Royal College of Physicians of London.

National Institute for Health and Clinical Excellence (NICE): *Hypertension: Management in Adults in Primary Care*, NICE Clinical Guideline 34, London, 2006a, NICE.

National Institute for Health and Clinical Excellence (NICE): *Statins for the prevention of cardiovascular events*, London, 2006b, NICE.

National Institute for Health and Clinical Excellence (NICE): *Clopidogrel in the treatment of non-ST-segment-elevation acute coronary syndrome*, Technology appraisal 80, London, 2007, NICE.

National Institute for Health and Clinical Excellence (NICE): *Lipid Modification*, NICE Clinical Guideline 67. London, 2008, NICE.

National Institute for Health and Clinical Excellence (NICE): *Venous Thromboembolism: reducing the risk of venous thromboembolism (deep vein thrombosis and pulmonary embolism) in patients admitted to hospital*, NICE Clinical Guideline 92, London, 2010, NICE.

Nicholson C: A systematic review of the effectiveness of oxygen in reducing acute myocardial ischaemia, *J Clin Nurs* 13:996–1007, 2004.

O'Connor L: Pain assessment by patients and nurses, and nurses' notes on it, in early acute myocardial infarction, *Intensive Crit Care Nurs* 11:183–191, 1995.

O'Neal PV: How to spot early signs of cardiogenic shock, *Am J Nurs* 94 (5):36–41, 1994.

Pate GE, Mulligan A: An epidemiological study of Heyde's syndrome: an association between aortic stenosis and gastrointestinal bleeding, *J Heart Valve Dis* 13:713–716, 2005.

Quinn T: Early experience with nurse led elective cardioversion, *Nurs Crit Care* 3:59–62, 1998.

Quinn T, Morse T: The interdisciplinary interface in managing patients with suspected cardiac pain, *Emerg Nurse* 11:22–24, 2003.

Ramsdale DR, Turner-Stokes L: On behalf of the Advisory Group of the British Cardiac Society Clinical Practice Committee and the RCP Clinical Effectiveness and evaluation unit. Prophylaxis and treatment of infective endocarditis in adults: concise guidelines, *Clin Med* 4:545–550, 2004.

Ransome P: Transluminal aortic stenting, *Nurs Stand* 23(11):52–53, 1996.

Resuscitation Council: *Advanced Life Support*, ed 5, London, 2006, Resuscitation Council (UK).

Rhodes MA: What is the evidence to support nurse-led thrombolysis? *Clinical Effectiveness in Nursing* 2(2):29–77, 1998.

Rothwell P: Limitations of the usual blood-pressure hypothesis and importance of variability, instability, and episodic hypertension, *Lancet* 375:938–948, 2010.

Schraibman IG, Milne AA, Royle EM: Home versus in-patient treatment for deep vein thrombosis (Cochrane Review). In *The Cochrane Library*, Issue 2, Chichester, 2001, Wiley.

Scottish Intercollegiate Guidelines Network (SIGN): *Diagnosis and treatment of heart failure due to left ventricular systolic dysfunction*, Edinburgh, 1999, SIGN.

Shayne PH, Pitts SR: Severely increased blood pressure in the emergency department, *Ann Emerg Med* 41:513–529, 2003.

Shepardson LB, Younger SJ, Speroff T, et al: Increased risk of death in patients with do not resuscitate orders, *Med Care* 37:722–726, 1999.

Smith SC, Allen J, Blair SN, et al: AHA/ACC guidelines for secondary prevention for patients with coronary and other atherosclerotic vascular disease: 2006 update: endorsed by the National Heart, Lung and Blood Institute, *Am J Cardiol* 47:2130–2139, 2006.

Sternbergh WC, Gonze MD, Garrad CL, et al: Abdominal and thoracoabdominal aortic aneurysm, *Surg Clin North Am* 78:827–834, 1998.

Stewart S: Refractory to medical treatment but not to nursing care: can we do more for patients with chronic angina pectoris? *Eur J Cardiovasc Nurs* 2:169–170, 2003.

Taylor RS, Brown A, Ebrahim DM, et al: Exercise-based rehabilitation for patients with coronary heart disease: systematic review and meta-analysis of randomized controlled trials, *Am Heart J* 116:682–692, 2004.

Thomas M: Transcatheter aortic valve implantation (TAVI). How to interpret data and what data is required, *EuroIntervention* 5:25–27, 2009.

Thompson DR, Clark AM: Cardiac rehabilitation: into the future, *Heart* 95:1897–1900, 2009.

Thompson DR, Webster RA, Sutton TW: Coronary care unit patients' and nurses' ratings of intensity of ischaemic chest pain, *Intensive Crit Care Nurs* 10:81–88, 1994.

Townsend P, Davidson N, Whitehead M: *Inequalities in health: the Black Report and the health divide*, Harmondsworth, 1992, Penguin.

Williams A: A case for emotional support and human contact. Management of cardiogenic shock, *Prof Nurse* 8:520–523, 1993.

Williams B, Poulter NR, Brown MJ, et al: British Hypertension Society guidelines for hypertension management 2004: (BHS-IV) summary, *Br Med J* 328:634–640, 2004.

Williams G, Wright DJ, Tan LB: Management of cardiogenic shock complicating acute myocardial infarction: towards evidence-based medical practice, *Heart* 83:621–626, 2000.

World Health Organization (WHO): *The World Health Report 2002. Reducing risks – promoting healthy life*, Geneva, 2002, WHO.

World Health Organization (WHO): *Cardiovascular Disease Risk Factors*, World Heart Federation, 2008. Available online http://www.world-heart-federation.org/cardiovascular-health/cardiovascular-disease-risk-factors/.

Wynne GA, Gwinnutt C, Bingham B, et al: Teaching resuscitation. In Colquhoun MC, Handley AJ, Evans TR, editors: *ABC of resuscitation*, London, 1999, BMJ Books.

Yan AT, Yan RT: Risk scores for risk stratification in acute coronary syndromes: useful but simpler is not necessarily better, *Eur Heart J* 28:1072–1078, 2007.

Yu DS, Thompson DR, Lee DT: Disease management programmes for older people with heart failure: crucial characteristics which improve discharge outcomes, *Eur Heart J* 27:596–612, 2006.

Zeitz CJ, Quinn T: Reperfusion strategies. In Kucia AM, Quinn T, editors: *Acute cardiac care: a practical guide for nurses*, Oxford, 2010, Wiley-Blackwell.

FURTHER READING

ACC/AHA/NASPE: Guideline update for implantation of cardiac pacemakers and antiarrhythmia devices, *J Cardiovasc Electrophysiol* 13:1183–1199, 2002.

Autar R: Calculating patients' risk of deep vein thrombosis, *Br J Nurs* 7:7–12, 1998.

Clare C: Valve disorders. In Thompson D, Hatchett R, editors: *Cardiac Nursing. A Comprehensive Guide*, Edinburgh, 2007, Churchill Livingstone.

Collins F: Abdominal aortic aneurysm repair. In Murray S, editor: *Vascular disease: nursing and management*, London, 2003, Whurr.

Donohue SJ: Lower limb amputation 1. Indications and treatment, *Br J Nurs* 6:970–972, 974–977, 1997a.

Donohue SJ: Lower limb amputation 2. Once the decision to amputate has been made, *Br J Nurs* 6:1048–1052, 1997b.

Donohue SJ: Lower limb amputation 3. The role of the nurse, *Br J Nurs* 6:1171–1174, 1187–1191, 1997c.

Donohue SJ: Lower limb amputation 4. Some ethical considerations, *Br J Nurs* 6:1311–1314, 1997d.

Galloway S, Bubela N, McKibbon A, et al: Symptom distress, anxiety, depression and discharge information needs after peripheral artery bypass, *J Vasc Nurs* 13(2):35–40, 2005.

Gibson JME, Kenrick M: Pain and powerlessness: the experience of living with peripheral vascular disease, *J Adv Nurs* 27(4):737–745, 1998.

Gray A, Goodacre S, Newby DE: Non-invasive ventilation in acute cardiogenic pulmonary oedema, *N Engl J Med* 359:142–151, 2008.

Gupta SK: *The pharmacotherapy of heart failure*, Tunbridge Wells, 2005, Anshan.

Jaarsma T, Stewart S: Nurse-led management programmes in heart failure. In Stewart D, Moser DK, Thompson DR, editors: *Caring for the heart failure patient*, London, 2004, Martin Dunitz, pp 161–180.

James J: Management and support of patients with implantable cardioverter defibrillators. In Thompson D, Hatchett R, editors: *Cardiac Nursing. A Comprehensive Guide*, Edinburgh, 2007, Churchill Livingstone.

Jowett NI, Thompson DR: *Comprehensive coronary care*, ed 4, London, 2007, Baillière Tindall.

Kennedy F: Congenital heart disease in adults. In Thompson D, Hatchett R, editors: *Cardiac Nursing. A Comprehensive Guide*, Edinburgh, 2007, Churchill Livingstone.

Levine GN, Kern MJ, Berger PB, et al: Management of patients undergoing percutaneous coronary revascularisation, *Ann Intern Med* 139:123–136, 2003.

Litchfield B: Promoting health in vascular nursing. In Murray S, editor: *Vascular disease: nursing and management*, London, 2003, Whurr.

Murray S: Chronic ischaemia. In Murray S, editor: *Vascular disease: nursing and management*, London, 2003, Whurr.

Oliver J, Rogers A, Addington J: Chronic heart failure. In Thompson D, Hatchett R, editors: *Cardiac Nursing. A Comprehensive Guide*, Edinburgh, 2007, Churchill Livingstone.

Olroyd C, Kucia AM: Arrhythmias. In Kucia A, Quinn T, editors: *Acute Cardiac Care. A practical guide for nurses*, Edinburgh, 2010, Wiley-Blackwell.

Quinn T: Acute heart failure. In Kucia A, Quinn T, editors: *Acute Cardiac Care. A practical guide for nurses*, Edinburgh, 2010, Wiley-Blackwell.

Riley J: The ECG: Its role and practical application. In Thompson D, Hatchett R, editors: *Cardiac Nursing. A Comprehensive Guide*, Edinburgh, 2007a, Churchill Livingstone.

Riley J: Nursing management of the cardiac surgical patient. In Thompson D, Hatchett R, editors: *Cardiac Nursing. A Comprehensive Guide*, Edinburgh, 2007b, Churchill Livingstone.

Vowden K, Vowden P: Venous disorders. In Murray S, editor: *Vascular disease: nursing and management*, London, 2003, Whurr.

Wilkinson IB, Cockcroft J, Waring S: *Hypertension: Your Questions Answered*, Edinburgh. 2002, Churchill Livingstone.

Young J, Daniels L: Aortic aneurysm. In Thompson D, Hatchett R, editors: *Cardiac Nursing: A Comprehensive Guide*, Edinburgh, 2007, Churchill Livingstone.

Zeitz CJ, Quinn T: Reperfusion strategies. In *Acute Cardiac Care. A practical guide for nurses*, Edinburgh, 2010, Wiley-Blackwell.

USEFUL WEBSITES

British Heart Foundation: www.bhf.org.uk

British Heart Foundation statistics: www.heartstats.org/homepage.asp

Driver and Vehicle Licensing Agency (DVLA): www.dvla.gov.uk

Peripheral Vascular Diseases Group (useful pictures and animated clips): www.link.med.ed.ac.uk/pvd

www.heartcentreonline.com

Society of Heart Valve Disease: www.shvd.org

YourHeart (information for cardiac patients and their families): www.yourheart.org.uk

Nursing patients with respiratory disorders

Glenda Esmond

Introduction

The respiratory system is one of the most vital systems in the human body. In health, it functions automatically and usually without our awareness. However, there are several diseases, both acute and chronic, which have a disruptive effect on the respiratory system. The most common causes of respiratory disease are related to smoking, infection, allergens, genetics and poverty. Respiratory disease affects approximately 8 million people in the UK, resulting in one in five people dying of respiratory disease. The burden of respiratory disease on the National Health Service (NHS) is steadily increasing. It is the single most common reason why people consult their general practitioner (GP) and accounts for over a million bed days a year in England (British Thoracic Society 2006a). The impact on the individual is more difficult to measure, although it has been recognised that disability is a frequent consequence of respiratory impairment.

Respiratory nursing encompasses roles within primary, community and acute care. Nurses are developing new independent and interdependent roles to meet the demands of new approaches to health care delivery. Increasingly, they are being employed in community and specialist clinics to screen, advise, immunise and treat patients and to promote disease prevention and health education. At the same time, technological and medical advances are demanding a higher level of clinical nursing skills.

This chapter will review the anatomy and physiology of the respiratory system and address two of the major principles of nursing management of respiratory disorders: disease prevention and health promotion. It will explore the nursing care and assessment skills required when caring for patients with respiratory disorders and the psychological and social impact of chronic respiratory illness upon the individual, their family and friends. It will also identify and evaluate strategies to promote respiratory treatment concordance and explore the function of specialist nurses and the interprofessional team in providing holistic respiratory care. Although the emphasis is on nursing management, the implicit assumption is always that nurses work in close collaboration with other health care professionals and, in many instances, will be responsible for coordinating the work of the whole team.

Anatomy and physiology – overview

This section is intended as an overview of the most relevant points relating to normal respiratory function. For a more detailed discussion please consult a biology text book such as Ross and Wilson (Waugh & Grant 2006).

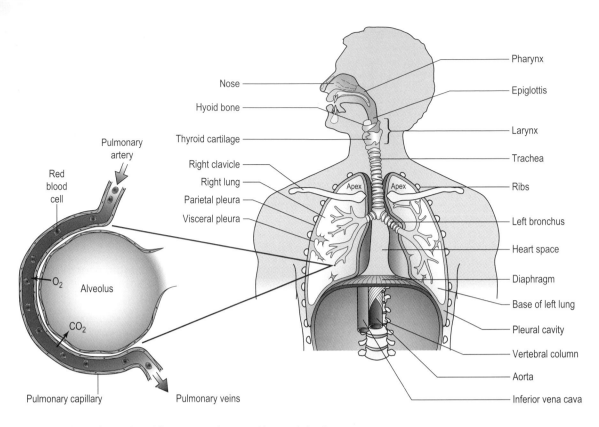

Figure 3.1 Respiratory system. (Reproduced from Esmond 2001 with permission.)

The respiratory system comprises the upper and lower airways and the thoracic cage (Figure 3.1).

The upper airway includes the nose, mouth, nasopharynx, oropharynx, laryngopharynx and larynx and has a protective role. The nasopharynx filters, warms and moistens the air before it enters the lungs, protecting the lung from exposure to microorganisms, toxic gases and particulates larger than 10 µm (microns) in diameter. Any particles that are deposited in the airways are propelled upwards towards the oropharynx by the mucociliary system. The mucus traps the particles and the cilia (microscopic hair-like projections) sweep the mucus upwards so that it can be expectorated. Ciliary movement can be impaired by tobacco smoke, pollution and excessive mucus production. The larynx protects the lower airways by closing during swallowing to prevent food entering the lower airways. It is also responsible for initiating the cough reflex, as it is sensitive to particles that cause irritation.

The lower airways include the trachea, bronchi, lungs, bronchioles, which are conducting air passages, and the alveoli, which are small grape-like sacs that extend from alveolar ducts, responsible for the passage of gases between the lungs and bloodstream. These structures work in combination with the thoracic cage, which includes the ribs, sternum and vertebrae, in affecting the exchange of oxygen and carbon dioxide in the lungs.

Control of breathing

The rate and depth of breathing, which is mostly involuntary, is controlled by complex interactions between many physiological processes to allow an adequate exchange of oxygen and carbon dioxide.

Respiratory centre

The medullary respiratory centre, situated in the medulla oblongata in the brain stem, primarily controls breathing through stimulating the contraction of the diaphragm and the external intercostal muscles, which expand and contract the thoracic cavity. During inspiration the diaphragm contracts and flattens causing the thoracic cavity to lengthen, whilst the external intercostal muscles contract to expand the chest. This creates a negative intrapulmonary pressure. During expiration the diaphragm rises and the intercostal muscles relax, resulting in a positive intrapulmonary pressure. Air pressure differences allow the movement of air in and out of the lungs. All gases move from an area of greater pressure to one of lesser pressure. During inspiration, air is drawn into the lungs. It flows through the bronchi and then into the bronchioles, alveolar ducts and alveolar sacs until it reaches the alveolar capillary membrane. The lungs are able to expand and move easily because the visceral pleura that lines the lungs and the parietal pleura that lines the mediastinum and chest wall creates a potential space, known as the pleural cavity. It contains a small amount of lubricating fluid that allows easy movement between the pleura when the lungs expand.

Pulmonary stretch receptors

Pulmonary stretch receptors are located in the smooth muscle of the bronchi and bronchioles and respond to inspiration by sending impulses through the vagus nerve to the medullary respiratory centre when the lungs are filled with air, inhibiting further inflation of the lungs. This is known as the Hering–Breuer reflex and prevents over-inflation of the lungs.

Chemoreceptors

Peripheral chemoreceptors located in the aorta at the aortic arch (aortic body) and at the carotid bifurcation (carotid body) send impulses by sensory nerves to the medullary respiratory centre in response to a decrease in oxygen and pH, and an increase in carbon dioxide in the blood. The chemoreceptors in the carotid bodies are the main oxygen sensors and are stimulated to increase the breathing rate when there is a significant decrease in oxygen levels, i.e. below 90% or 8 kPa.

The normal stimulus to breathe is the rising level of carbon dioxide that easily crosses the blood–brain barrier into cerebrospinal fluid where it hydrates to form carbonic acid and then dissociates into bicarbonate and hydrogen ions. The hydrogen ions stimulate the central chemoreceptors in the medulla oblongata to send impulses to the medullary respiratory centre to increase the respiratory rate, thereby eliminating excess carbon dioxide.

Gas transport

The main function of the respiratory system is the transfer of gases, principally oxygen and carbon dioxide. Gas transfer occurs by diffusion and includes the movement of oxygen from the alveolar capillary membrane to the mitochondria within the cells, and the movement of carbon dioxide from tissue capillaries to the alveolar capillary membrane. There are millions of alveoli, each surrounded by pulmonary capillaries and lined by a single layer of epithelium. This allows maximal gas exchange because the barrier between the gas in the alveoli and the blood in the capillaries is very thin (0.5 µm thick).

Oxygen transport

During inspiration, air containing 21% oxygen is taken into the lungs and passes down the trachea and bronchi and into the alveoli, where it comes into contact with the pulmonary circulation. Once the oxygen diffuses across the alveolar capillary membrane it is carried in arterial blood to the heart and pumped around the body in two ways. Approximately 3% dissolves in the plasma, with the remaining 97% being carried in the red cells, bound to haemoglobin. Each haemoglobin molecule can reversibly bind (i.e. can give up again) four molecules of oxygen to form oxyhaemoglobin. The maximum amount of oxygen that can chemically combine with haemoglobin is called the oxygen capacity. The oxygen capacity, plus the oxygen carried as dissolved oxygen, is termed the oxygen content.

Carbon dioxide transport

Carbon dioxide, the waste product of metabolism, is transported in the blood in three forms: dissolved carbon dioxide, bicarbonate ions and carbamino compounds (carbaminohaemoglobin). The carbon dioxide diffuses from the blood capillaries across the alveolar capillary membrane to the alveoli to be exhaled. Because of the properties of haemoglobin,

the unloading of oxygen and the loading of carbon dioxide are reciprocal events. When the carbon dioxide levels rise the affinity of haemoglobin for oxygen decreases.

Ventilation and perfusion

Adequate alveolar ventilation and perfusion are required for normal gas exchange. Alveolar ventilation ($\dot{V}$) is the volume of gas that reaches the alveoli per minute and is approximately 4 L/min. The perfusion ($\dot{Q}$) is the amount of blood that flows through the pulmonary capillaries per minute and is approximately 5 L/min. The normal $\dot{V}/\dot{Q}$ ratio is $\dot{V}$ minus $\dot{Q}$ which is 0.8, although this will change in various parts of the lung due to gravitational forces. In healthy individuals these gravitational differences do not affect adequate gaseous exchange; however, in lung disease the mismatch is wider and is the most common cause of low oxygen levels in arterial blood (hypoxaemia). With effective ventilation and perfusion, oxygen is able to diffuse from the alveoli into the blood to achieve a partial pressure (PaO_2) of between 10 and 13 kPa.

Acid–base balance

The respiratory system also has an important role in maintaining acid–base balance. The regulation of acid–base balance is expressed as pH, which measures acidity and alkalinity, or hydrogen ion ($H+$) concentration in the body. The normal pH of arterial blood is 7.35–7.45. A fall in pH (<7.35) indicates an increase in hydrogen ions causing an acidosis. In respiratory disease this is due to raised carbon dioxide levels, caused by alveolar hypoventilation. This situation can be corrected through increasing ventilation, but if the respiratory acidosis continues, the action of buffers and the renal system will be activated to maintain homeostasis. Buffers (bicarbonate, proteins and phosphate) combine with the acid to prevent excessive changes in hydrogen ion concentration. The kidneys contribute to the regulation of acid–base balance by increasing or decreasing the bicarbonate concentration. This is the most efficient mechanism; however, it takes several hours or even days for the renal system to change the plasma bicarbonate level.

Pulmonary function

Lung volume capacity and compliance

The volume of air breathed in and out and the number of breaths per minute vary from one individual to another according to age, size and activity. Normal, quiet breathing gives about 15 complete cycles per minute in the adult. Lung volume can be assessed in the following terms (Figure 3.2):

- Tidal volume (TV) – this is the amount of air that passes in and out of the lungs during each cycle of quiet breathing (approximately 500 mL in the adult). Exchange of gases takes place only in the alveolar ducts and sacs. The rest of the air passages are known as 'dead space' and contain about 150 mL of air.
- Inspiratory capacity – this is the amount of air that can be inspired with maximum effort. This consists of tidal volume plus the inspiratory reserve volume (IRV).
- Functional residual capacity (FRC) – this is the amount of air remaining in the air passages and alveoli at the end of quiet respiration; it is composed of expiratory reserve

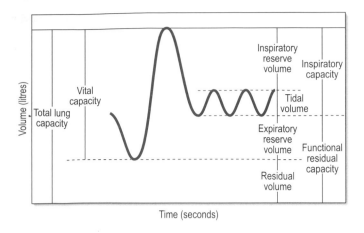

Figure 3.2 Lung volumes and capacity. (Reproduced from Esmond 2001 with permission.)

volume (ERV) and residual volume (RV). The RV prevents collapse of the alveoli and makes continuous gaseous exchange possible as the alveolar gas mix remains constant.

- Vital capacity (VC) – this is the TV plus the IRV and ERV.
- Total lung capacity (TLC) – with maximum effort the adult lungs can hold 4–6 L of air. Most of this can be forcibly expelled, leaving an RV of about 1 L.

Lung expansion and recoil

Elastic fibres in lung tissue and the surface tension of the fluid lining the alveoli give the lungs their natural recoil tendency. Ease of expansion and recoil depends on normal compliance and elasticity and on the presence of surfactant in the fluid lining the alveoli. Compliance can be reduced by the stiffening of normally soft alveolar tissue due to pulmonary oedema or to the ageing process. Conversely, compliance can be increased by extreme softening due to loss of lung tissue, as in emphysema.

Principles of nursing management in the prevention and treatment of respiratory disorders

There are two main nursing priorities:

- health promotion and disease prevention
- developing clinical skills in order to ensure competent care.

Health promotion and disease prevention

Promoting health and preventing disease are vital to the social and economic well-being of our society and their importance is reflected in government legislation and the development of large-scale screening and health education programmes (Donaldson et al 2005). With the cost of health care soaring, it makes good sense to prevent disease where possible rather than just treating the consequences.

Tobacco smoke, which contains nicotine, tar, carbon monoxide and 4000 chemicals, is currently the leading cause of respiratory ill health and premature death. In susceptible

individuals smoking may affect the respiratory system and cause:

- recurrent infections in the airways
- damage and loss of efficiency in the lungs
- lung cancer
- chronic bronchitis and emphysema.

Fletcher & Peto (1977) demonstrated that smoking accelerates the normal decline in lung function due to the ageing process from about 30 mL per year to 45 mL per year (Figure 3.3). The consequence of this increased loss of lung function is that functional impairment occurs leading to fatigue and breathlessness which impacts on the individual's ability to perform normal activities of daily living (ADL). Furthermore, smoking in pregnancy leads to an increased risk of spontaneous abortion, premature birth, smaller babies and sudden infant death syndrome. Children who are subject to passive smoking from parental smoking are more likely to experience acute respiratory illness, chronic middle ear infection, asthma, chronic cough and wheezy chest.

Nurses are well placed in their many roles in the hospital and community to have an active and expanding role in the area of primary health prevention through health promotion activities in relation to tobacco control (Buck 1997).

Smoking cessation

Of the 13 million smokers in the UK, over 68% (General Household Survey – Office for National Statistics 2005) say they want to stop and this has often been directly related to specific reasons, for example a life event, health reasons, social pressure or financial reasons. Of this 60%, only half intend to stop in the next year, only a third of these make an attempt and only 2% succeed on their own. Stopping smoking requires motivation, effort, commitment and stamina to be successful, therefore it has to be the right time for the smoker to make an attempt. Helping people to stop smoking is a challenge faced by many nurses as it requires facilitating change and supporting patients through the process rather than actively providing care. Behaviour change required for smoking cessation is complex, with nicotine

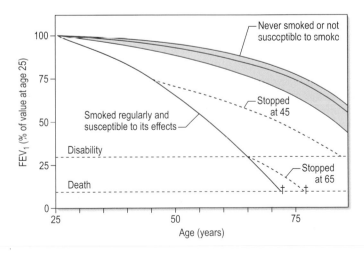

Figure 3.3 The effects of smoking on the decline in lung function. (Reproduced from Fletcher and Peto 1977 with permission.)

addiction as well as many other factors including social and psychological influences playing their part. Evidence-based smoking cessation guidelines have been developed to assist health care professionals to develop smoking cessation strategies that fit in with the overall tobacco control (National Institute for Health and Clinical Excellence [NICE] 2006a, 2008a, West et al 2000).

Nurses are in an ideal position to encourage and enable smokers to quit the habit through applying the five As for anybody who smokes:

- Ask about smoking.
- Assess the smoker's motivation to stop smoking.
- Advise all smokers to stop smoking.
- Assist motivated smokers in stopping smoking.
- Arrange follow-up.

This approach is supported by NICE (2002, 2008b) and it will ensure that patients are referred to smoking cessation services, often run by practice nurses or specially trained smoking cessation advisors. There are two main strategies used in smoking cessation: pharmacological interventions and lifestyle behavioural change.

Pharmacological interventions The use of pharmacological agents has been shown to double the chances of success of smokers wishing to quit (West et al 2000) and, provided they are used in sufficient quantity and for a long enough period of time, to reduce the withdrawal symptoms as outlined in Table 3.1.

Currently there are three pharmacological preparations that can be used for smokers who have been assessed as being ready to quit:

- nicotine replacement therapy
- varenicline (Champix®)
- bupropion (Zyban®).

Pharmacological interventions should be used as part of a programme that includes advice and support from a health care professional which will assist with lifestyle behavioural changes.

Further reading (British National Formulary, NICE smoking cessation guidance) is recommended for familiarisation with medication doses, side-effects and the advantages and disadvantages of each of the products.

Lifestyle behavioural change Smoking is a complex habit and dealing with the nicotine withdrawal alone may not be sufficient to quit smoking. Emphasis needs to be placed on the psychological and social aspects of the habit as well as the management of the nicotine withdrawal symptoms if smoking cessation is to be achieved. The most commonly used approach to behavioural change for smoking cessation is based on the Prochaska & DiClemente (1984) model of change, which assumes that the individual attempting to change behaviour will follow a series of five stages:

1. pre contemplation – not interested in considering a change in behaviour
2. contemplation – considering a change in behaviour but not yet made the decision
3. preparation – made a commitment to change behaviour but not planned to do so
4. making a change – implementation of plan that will change behaviour
5. maintenance – continuing to make changes to behaviour and maintaining the healthier lifestyle.

Being able to assess a person's stage of change will allow the nurse to use appropriate strategies to help the individual to quit the habit of smoking. Furthermore, helping smokers to understand the effects of smoking on the body and how stopping smoking can improve health can motivate the smoker to quit. Table 3.2 demonstrates the withdrawal effects which Hatsukami et al (1984) showed were of rapid onset following stopping smoking.

Respiratory assessment and investigations

While causative factors, organisms and irritants differ, the clinical manifestations can appear similar. Therefore an important aspect to respiratory care is assessment and specialised investigations to enable a differential diagnosis to be made and the severity of symptoms identified.

Nursing assessment of respiratory status

The assessment of respiratory status is important in determining the severity of the respiratory problem in order to prioritise care. During the acute phase of respiratory illness (i.e. acute asthma 'attack' or acute infective exacerbation of chronic obstructive pulmonary disease [COPD]) the emphasis is placed on physiological assessment in order to detect life-threatening situations that require immediate treatment. However, the impact of the respiratory problem on ADLs, as a consequence of breathlessness, and the psychosocial aspects are equally important if the patient and family are to cope with the consequences of chronic respiratory illness. Respiratory assessment requires observation, communication and clinical skills and should include assessment of

Table 3.1 Withdrawal symptoms		
SYMPTOMS	**DURATION**	**PREVALENCE**
Irritability/aggression (nicotine withdrawal)	– 4 wks	50%
Depression	– 4 wks	60%
Restlessness	– 4 wks	60%
Poor concentration	– 2 wks	60%
Cough (clearing lungs out)	– 2 wks	60%
Increased appetite (food tastes better)	+ 10 wks	70%
Light headedness (more oxygen to brain)	– 48 h	10%
Night-time awakenings	– 1 wk	25%
Urges to smoke	+ 2 wks	70%
Anxiety	– 1 wk	50%

– 4 wks, in the first 4 weeks; + 10 wks, after 10 weeks.

Table 3.2 The effects once you give up smoking begin as soon as the cigarette is stubbed out

Short term (7–14 days)

Nicotine levels in the blood begin to fall
20 minutes
Stimulation of adrenaline and noradrenaline ceases and blood pressure and heart rate return to normal
2 hours
Nicotine levels continue to fall in the blood
8 hours
Carbon monoxide and nicotine levels in the blood are reduced by half
Oxygen levels return to normal
24 hours
Carbon monoxide will be eliminated from the body
A CO reading will be at normal levels
3–4 days
Smooth muscle in the bronchioles begins to relax
Breathing improves
Energy levels increase
5–14 days
Mucus glands no longer being over-stimulated
Mucus clearance begins

Medium term (2–12 weeks)

Circulation, sense of smell and taste improve
3–9 months
Respiratory symptoms improve
Nasal congestion, cough and sputum production reduce
12 months
Risk of small cell lung cancer halved
Lung function cannot be reversed after years of damage; however, stopping smoking means that the rate of decline reverts to the age decline of a non-smoker (30 mL per year) and prevents further damage. The reduction in mucus production helps to reduce exacerbations

---

physiological factors, mental state, causative factors, symptoms, impact on ADLs and psychosocial factors.

Respiratory rate, rhythm and depth

Normal breathing should be regular and appear effortless with a respiratory rate in adults between 12 and 20 breaths per minute. The majority of patients with underlying respiratory disease will have an elevated respiratory rate (>20 breaths per minute) to facilitate adequate oxygenation and ventilation. Respiratory depression (<12 breaths per minute) may occur due to exhaustion and fatigued respiratory muscles caused by the work of breathing. The use of sedatives and opioid analgesics may also cause respiratory depression. Observation of the rhythm and depth of breathing should be assessed, as this will indicate the quality of each breath. Slow, shallow breathing is a sign of respiratory depression and indicates that there is an insufficient number and quality of breaths to sustain adequate ventilation. Equally, a rapid, irregular breathing pattern which does not allow expansion of the lower lobes of the lungs will also result in ventilatory failure.

Chest movement

The chest movements should be symmetrical and are best observed by standing in front of the patient rather than to one side. If one side of the chest is not expanding as well

as the other this may indicate a collapsed lung due to pnuemothorax (air in the pleural space) or the presence of bronchial obstruction. The patient's use of accessory muscles in the neck and shoulders (the sternocleidomastoid and trapezius muscles) should also be noted as this indicates that the patient is unable to use the diaphragm and external intercostal muscles sufficiently to maintain ventilation.

Oxygen levels

Observation of skin colour and pulse oximetry (oxygen saturation) will indicate whether the patient is receiving adequate oxygenation. The patient's skin should be observed for blueness of the lips, tongue and oral mucosa, as this indicates the presence of central cyanosis caused by hypoxaemia (low oxygen levels in arterial blood). In patients with dark skin it may not be possible to see changes in lip colour and therefore the oral mucosa and tongue should always be examined. Hypoxaemia will also be detected through performing pulse oximetry as this will measure oxygen saturation levels. According to the British Thoracic Society (2008) the normal ranges are:

- 94–98% for adults <70 years of age
- 92–98% for adults >70 years of age.

When examining the skin, the presence of peripheral oedema should be noted as this may indicate the presence of cor pulmonale (right ventricular hypertrophy and failure) due to vasoconstriction of the pulmonary circulation as a result of local hypoxia in the lungs. Another sign of chronic tissue hypoxia is finger clubbing, which is where the terminal phalanges of the fingers become enlarged and the base of the nail feels spongy.

Mental state

Respiratory assessment should include assessment of mental state because confusion and disorientation may be a sign of severe hypoxia resulting in a reduced supply of oxygen to the brain. Asking relatives and friends if they have noticed a change in mental state may be helpful when the nurse has not previously known the patient. The patient's level of alertness also needs to be assessed as drowsiness may indicate hypercapnia (raised levels of carbon dioxide in arterial blood).

Causative factors

Factors that influence the patient's respiratory health status, such as allergens, the environment and smoking, should be identified so that potential health education strategies can be implemented. As smoking is a major cause of respiratory illness a thorough smoking history should include current and past smoking habits, with the total pack years of smoking being estimated. The number of pack years can be calculated as follows:

Pack years = (number of cigarettes smoked per day
× number of years smoked) divided by 20

The patient's present and past occupation may indicate exposure to toxic substances, such as asbestos and industrial chemicals. Through identifying exposure as the causative factor of respiratory disease the patient and their family may be eligible for compensation.

Symptoms

The most common symptom associated with respiratory disease is breathlessness, although wheeze – often described by patients as chest tightness, cough and muscular chest pain – can be equally troublesome. Through assessing symptoms at regular intervals it is possible to monitor treatment effectiveness. Assessment for the presence of infection is important as it causes much respiratory disease, such as pneumonia and tuberculosis. A raised temperature and pulse rate, a raised white blood cell count, positive blood cultures and a productive cough with yellow or green sputum indicate the presence of infection.

Impact on activities of daily living

Assessing the impact of breathlessness on all the activities of daily living will allow the nurse to plan care effectively, identifying the need for referral to occupational therapy, physiotherapy, dietetics and social services as appropriate. Particular attention to mobility and nutritional status is essential, as breathlessness has been shown to cause immobility, and malnutrition due to increased energy requirements and poor appetite (Margereson & Esmond 1997). Patients with underlying respiratory disease should be observed for increasing breathlessness and oxygen desaturation (lowering of oxygen levels) on exertion, as this may indicate the need for supplementary oxygen to prevent complications of immobility. Assessment of the patient's nutritional status should include body mass index (BMI, see Ch. 21), identification of recent significant weight loss, eating habits and changes in appetite. Patients found to have a BMI less than 20 or those with a recent weight loss greater than 10% should be referred to a dietitian.

Psychosocial factors

The chronic nature of much respiratory disease can affect the patient's psychological state and relationships with family and friends. Through assessing the patient's perceptions and concerns, coping strategies, such as relaxation techniques to alleviate fear and anxiety or activity pacing to allow greater mobility, can be identified to assist with adaptation to chronic respiratory illness. The introduction of nurse-led clinics, usually run by practice nurses or respiratory nurse specialists, has assisted those suffering from chronic respiratory illness to feel at ease to discuss psychosocial issues. This is usually achieved through the nurse building a therapeutic trusting relationship with the patient over a period of time so that a profile of perceptions and concerns can be developed. Consideration of current social issues and need for referral to social services or community nursing should be continually assessed so that interventions can be identified at the earliest opportunity.

Respiratory investigations

The symptoms of breathlessness, wheeze, chest tightness and cough can be associated with many different respiratory conditions. Respiratory investigations are used to determine the cause of respiratory symptoms, allowing appropriate treatment to be commenced, to monitor disease progression, and to assess treatment effectiveness. The most commonly used respiratory investigations are:

- lung function tests
- pulse oximetry

- chest X-ray
- sputum microscopy, culture and sensitivity
- bronchoscopy.

Lung function tests

Lung function tests assess the functioning of the lungs and can be used to confirm a diagnosis through measuring flow rates and lung volumes. They include the following, which are collectively called spirometry:

- *Peak expiratory flow (PEF)*, commonly referred to as 'peak flow', is measured in litres per minute and is an objective measure that detects airflow obstruction in the larger airways. If the airways are narrowed then the rate of expiration is limited and the PEF will be lower than the predicted normal value for the person's age, height and sex. To ensure the measurement is accurate, the patient must be taught how to perform the test (Figure 3.4). The patient must be standing or sitting in an upright position and is required to make a seal with his/her lips around the mouthpiece before exhaling forcibly. The test is repeated three times and the highest result recorded.
- *Forced expiratory volume in 1 second and forced vital capacity.* Forced expiratory volume in one second (FEV_1) determines the amount of air that is exhaled in the first second of a forced expiration. Forced vital capacity (FVC) is the total amount of air exhaled from maximal inspiration to maximal expiration. A spirometer is the instrument used to measure FEV_1 and FVC and can detect obstructive patterns of breathing which occur in asthma, COPD, cystic fibrosis and bronchiectasis, and restrictive patterns of breathing due to fibrosing alveolitis, sarcoid, asbestosis, kyphoscoliosis and muscular dystrophies.
- *Reversibility testing.* Respiratory function tests can also be used to determine the extent to which airflow obstruction can be reversed with bronchodilators. The respiratory function test is performed before and 15 minutes after administration of a bronchodilator, and the two results compared. An increase in FEV_1 or PEF of greater than 15% is representative of a positive response and indicates the presence of asthma. This is not the case in COPD where the airflow is fixed and the respiratory function test will either show limited (<15%) or no reversibility following bronchodilators.

Pulse oximetry

Pulse oximetry is a simple, non-invasive way of measuring peripheral oxygen saturation of arterial blood (SpO_2) to determine whether the values are within the normal range (see p. 56). A probe consisting of a small light-emitting diode on one side and a light detector on the other is placed on the patient's finger. The technique works because of the light-absorbing characteristics of haemoglobin. In hypoxaemia the 'blueness' of the blood will be measured by the pulse oximeter. Although clearly useful, pulse oximetry has its limitations. It is unable to detect changes in carbon dioxide levels (Esmond & Mikelsons 2009) and produces inaccurate readings at saturation levels below 82% (Carter 1998), and so may not be reliable in severe respiratory disease. Inaccurate readings may also be due to a number of other factors including:

1. Fit disposable mouthpiece to peak flow meter

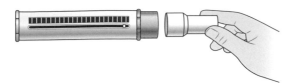

2. Ensure patient stands up or sits upright and holds peak flow meter horizontally without restricting movement of the marker. Ensure the marker is at the bottom of the scale

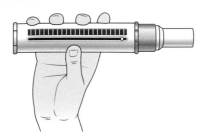

3. Ask patient to breathe in deeply, seal lips around mouthpiece and breathe out as quickly as possible

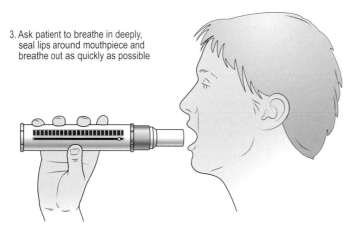

4. Repeat steps 2 and 3 twice more. Choose and record the highest of the three readings

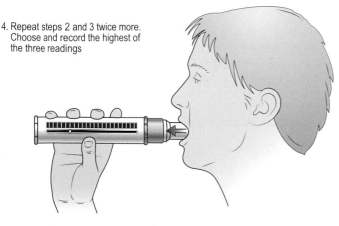

Figure 3.4 Measuring PEFR using a peak flow meter. (Reproduced from Brooker & Nicol 2003 with permission.)

- peripheral vasoconstriction (insufficient perfusion to detect pulse)
- anaemia (if vasoconstriction occurs)
- movement, i.e. shivering or fitting (affects the ability of the light to travel from the light-emitting diode (LED) to the photodetector)
- nail varnish/false nails (blockage of the light detector)

- dark skin pigment (blockage of the light detector)
- intravenous dyes (reduce readings by absorbing light)
- severe hypoxaemia (not accurate below 82%)
- high levels of carboxyhaemoglobin due to smoking (due to vasoconstriction)
- exposure to carbon monoxide.

Chest X-ray

Chest X-ray is a valuable aid to diagnosis of respiratory disease and will show the lung fields, pleura, rib cage, diaphragm shape and size of the heart. Chest X-ray is usually performed when patients present with persistent cough, chest pain, unexplained breathlessness, haemoptysis (coughing up blood), weight loss and pyrexia.

Sputum

The observation of sputum colour, viscosity, odour and amount is vital in order to monitor the effectiveness of antibiotic treatment. Patients who are producing sputum require:

- a sputum pot with a lid, as swallowing the sputum may cause nausea
- tissues to wipe excess secretions from the mouth and nose
- mouthwash/regular mouth care as sputum is often foul tasting
- encouragement with fluid intake as dehydration will increase the viscosity of the sputum.

The diagnosis of respiratory infections can be achieved through microbiological analysis of sputum. A specimen of mucopurulent or purulent sputum, not saliva, should be collected in a sterile container, to prevent contamination, prior to the commencement of antibiotic therapy. Sputum should never be left for long periods before being transferred to a laboratory otherwise an overgrowth with Gram-negative organisms may occur. The patient should be asked to rinse their mouth before the specimen is obtained to prevent contamination of the sputum with food, which renders it unusable by the laboratory. The laboratory will perform microscopy, culture and sensitivity to antibiotics.

Bronchoscopy

Flexible fibreoptic bronchoscopy is an invasive procedure that is commonly used to diagnose:

- lung cancer
- tuberculosis
- pneumonia and other respiratory infections.

Bronchoscopy and related procedures (lung biopsy, brushing and lavage) are usually performed under sedation and local anaesthetic to the throat. Sedatives, such as midazolam, may cause respiratory depression, hypoventilation and hypotension, and local anaesthetics applied to the throat may lead to laryngospasm and bronchospasm. The patient therefore needs careful monitoring during the procedure and for 6–8 hours afterwards as bronchoscopy can cause bronchospasm, hypoxaemia, fever, pneumonia, pneumothorax and haemorrhage. On discharge, the patient should be given information (usually a post-bronchoscopy leaflet) explaining how they should feel during the first 12 hours and detailing what to do if prevailing symptoms worsen or new symptoms develop. It is not usually necessary to admit patients to hospital following bronchoscopy unless significant post-bronchoscopic bleeding, pneumothorax and/or respiratory distress occur.

Common respiratory disorders

Asthma

Asthma is a common chronic inflammatory condition of the airways, characterised by bronchospasm, severe dyspnoea, wheezing, chest tightness and expiratory exertion. As a result of inflammation, the airways are hyper-responsive and narrow easily in response to a wide range of provoking stimuli.

PATHOPHYSIOLOGY

Immunoglobulin E (IgE) is present in small amounts in normal blood but in increased amounts in asthma sufferers. In allergic extrinsic asthma, the disease process involves inhalation of antigens (allergens) which are absorbed by the bronchial mucosa and trigger production of IgE antibodies. These antibodies bind to mast cells and basophils around the bronchial blood vessels. When the allergen is encountered again, the antigen–antibody reaction releases histamines and bradykinin, resulting in bronchial muscle spasm, oedema and excessive secretion of thick mucus. In many cases, the severity of attacks lessens with age and good treatment, unless other factors are involved. There are various theories of the pathogenesis of intrinsic asthma. Allergens may be implicated (http://www.allergyuk.org). Whatever the cause, the bronchi and bronchioles are chronically inflamed, oedematous, full of mucus and subject to bronchospasm.

Clinical features are produced in response to the narrowing of the airways and include wheeze, chest tightness, dry, non-productive cough and breathlessness. Symptoms of uncontrolled asthma are often worse at night and early morning.

Investigations are used to confirm the diagnosis based on clinical presentation and past history and will include spirometry (FEV_1, FVC, PEF). Furthermore, once a diagnosis has been established, PEF using a peak flow meter will be used to monitor asthma. Skin sensitivity tests and a history of exposure to specific allergens may help in isolating and avoiding triggering factors.

Treatment

The aim of treatment is to control symptoms and prevent asthma 'attacks', thus treatment needs to be targeted at prevention and control of inflammation and bronchoconstriction. The British Guidelines on Asthma Management (British Thoracic Society and Scottish Intercollegiate Guidelines Network [SIGN] 2008) recommend a stepwise approach that corresponds to the severity of asthma based on symptoms and peak flow measurements (Figure 3.5). The main treatments used to control asthma are bronchodilators and corticosteroids. For further information on asthma medication see http://www.brit-thoracic.org.uk/ClinicalInformation/Asthma/.

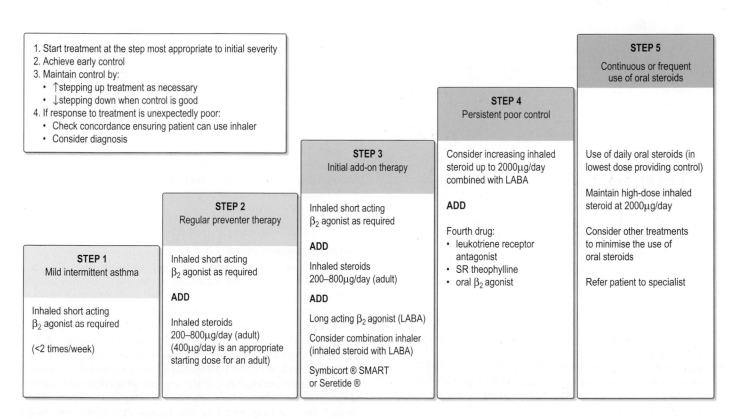

Figure 3.5 Stepwise asthma management.

Acute severe asthma

It is important that both patient and nurse are able to detect acute severe asthma as delay in recognising deterioration may be fatal. Table 3.3 outlines the symptoms of acute asthma and classifies them into acute severe asthma, life-threatening asthma and near fatal asthma.

The aim of treatment is to prevent hypoxia and to reduce bronchoconstriction and inflammation of the airway, and therefore the patient will immediately require:

- high-flow oxygen (40–60%)
- nebulised bronchodilators delivered via an oxygen supply (6–8 L/min) (see below)
- oral prednisolone (40–60 mg) or intravenous hydrocortisone (100 mg) (British Thoracic Society/SIGN 2008).

Patients with an acute exacerbation of their asthma *must* be given high concentrations of oxygen (40–60%) using a high-flow mask, such as the Hudson or non-rebreathing mask. Unlike patients with COPD there is little risk of precipitating hypercapnia (PCO_2 >6.0 kPa) with high-flow oxygen. Hypercapnia may occur due to exhaustion and fatigue of respiratory

muscles, and may lead to respiratory arrest if not reversed. Nebulised β_2 agonists (e.g. salbutamol) and anticholinergics (ipratropium bromide) in high doses will be administered to ensure bronchoconstriction is alleviated as quickly as possible. The decision to use oral or intravenous corticosteroids will depend on the patient's clinical state.

Asthma mortality

There are several factors that have been identified as increasing the risk of premature death from asthma (British Thoracic Society/SIGN 2008). They are:

- inadequate treatment with inhaled or oral steroids – as asthma control will be poor
- non-compliance with treatment and monitoring – as signs of deterioration may be ignored
- failure to attend appointments and self-discharge – this may indicate denial about the life-threatening consequences of uncontrolled asthma
- mental health problems, which include psychiatric illness, current or recent tranquilliser use, deliberate self-harm and alcohol or drug abuse
- learning disabilities – because symptoms are often under reported.

When assessing a patient it is important to consider whether the patient with acute asthma has any additional risk factors so that discharge planning can be as effective as possible. For example, early discharge would not be appropriate for the high-risk patient as they are unlikely to complete the course of treatment.

 ## Nursing management and health promotion: asthma

The role of the nurse in asthma care will depend on the severity of the patient's symptoms. The majority of people with asthma are cared for by practice nurses in the community who provide preventative asthma care. This is achieved by:

- monitoring symptoms
- peak flow monitoring (Figure 3.4)
- checking inhaler technique (Figure 3.6)
- providing allergy avoidance advice
- identification of acute severe asthma requiring emergency treatment
- developing a self-management plan.

Self-management plans

Patients with acute severe asthma will require hospital admission as this is life threatening. Respiratory nurse specialists should be involved with discharge planning as they provide liaison between primary and secondary care to ensure that continuity of care is achieved. They will also continue to monitor severely asthmatic patients in nurse-led asthma clinics where they provide education and support in developing individualised self-management plans. Self-management has become an integral part of asthma management (British Thoracic Society/SIGN 2008) and empowers the patient to make changes to their own treatment without consulting a health care professional. The

Table 3.3 Levels of severity of acute asthma	
Near fatal asthma	Raised $PaCO_2$ and/or requiring mechanical ventilation with raised inflation pressures
Life-threatening asthma	Any one of the following in a patient with severe asthma: • PEF <33% best or predicted • SpO_2 <92% • PaO_2 <8 kPa • Normal $PaCO_2$ (4.6–6.0 kPa) • Silent chest • Cyanosis • Feeble respiratory effort • Bradycardia • Dysrhythmia • Hypotension • Exhaustion • Confusion • Coma
Acute severe asthma	Any one of: • PEF 33–50% best or predicted • Respiratory rate ≥25/min • Heart rate ≥110/min • Inability to complete sentences in one breath
Moderate asthma exacerbation	• Increasing symptoms • PEF >50–75% best or predicted • No features of acute severe asthma
Brittle asthma	• Type 1: wide PEF variability (>40% diurnal variation for >50% of the time over a period >150 days) despite intense therapy • Type 2: sudden severe attacks on a background of apparently well-controlled asthma

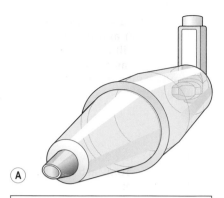

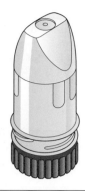

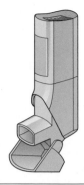

Ⓐ

How to use:
- Remove cap and shake inhaler and place into spacer
- Gently breathe out
- Make seal with lips around mouthpiece
- Press the canister once to release dose of drug
- Breathe in and out slowly and gently (tidal breathing) five times. This will make a clicking sound as the valve opens and closes

Ⓑ

How to use:
- Unscrew and remove cap
- Hold the device upright
- Twist the grip forwards and backwards. A click should be heard
- Gently breathe out
- Make seal with lips around mouthpiece
- Breathe in steadily and deeply through the mouthpiece
- Remove inhaler from mouth and hold breath for at least 10 seconds

Ⓒ

How to use:
- Shake the inhaler and remove cap
- Gently breathe out
- Hold the inhaler upright and do not occlude air holes
- Make seal with lips around the mouthpiece
- Once inhaler is activated take a deep breath
- Hold breath for at least 10 seconds
- Close the cap

Figure 3.6 Inhaler delivery devices. (Reproduced from Brooker & Nicol 2003 with permission.)

nurse has an important patient education role, as acquisition of knowledge and skills is necessary for the patient to have the confidence and ability to take control of their asthma care. For a self-management plan to be developed it is necessary that the patient:

- has knowledge of the disease process
- is able to perform and interpret peak flow measurements
- is able to recognise symptoms
- has the confidence to adjust medication
- has sufficient insight to know when professional advice is required.

Asthma UK produces pre-printed self-management plans that can be individualised for the patient but this will only be successful when combined with education, support and agreement between the health care professional and patient.

 See website Critical thinking question 3.1

Chronic obstructive pulmonary disease

Chronic obstructive pulmonary disease (COPD) is defined by the World Health Organization (WHO) as: 'a disease state characterized by airflow limitation that is not fully reversible. The airflow limitation is usually both progressive and associated with an abnormal inflammatory response of the lungs to noxious particles or gases' (Global Initiative for Chronic Obstructive Lung Disease [WHO GOLD] 2007). Tobacco smoke is the most important risk factor for the development of COPD, although occupational exposure (e.g. coal mining and welding) and α_1-antitrypsin deficiency can also cause COPD.

PATHOPHYSIOLOGY

COPD is a term used to describe a number of overlapping conditions:

- chronic bronchitis – chronic inflammation of the membranes of the trachea and bronchi resulting in a productive cough on most days for at least three months in at least two consecutive years
- emphysema – abnormal, permanent enlargement of the terminal airspaces due to destruction of the alveolar wall
- chronic asthma that has become unresponsive to treatment.

Clinical features

The clinical features will depend upon disease severity but usually include chronic cough, wheeze and breathlessness. In advanced cases the slightest physical activity can cause severe respiratory distress and cyanosis. Abnormal ventilation results in chronic hypoxaemia (low oxygen), hypercapnia (high CO_2) and polycythaemia (raised red blood cell count), which cause cyanosis and facial flushing, because CO_2 is a vasodilator. The patient is weakened by constant respiratory effort and becomes unable to tolerate normal basic activities of living.

Investigations

Lung function tests (spirometry, see p. 57) are used to confirm the diagnosis based on history, symptoms and clinical examination. Spirometry (FEV_1, FVC, FEV_1/FVC), blood gas analysis and chest X-ray will confirm the stage and effects of the disease and influence treatment.

▷ **Nursing management and health promotion: COPD**

The aim of treatment is to prevent further deterioration in lung function, control unpleasant symptoms, increase physical activity and improve the individual's quality of life.

The majority of treatment will take place in the community or outpatient setting. It is during acute exacerbations, usually as a consequence of respiratory infection, that patients may require hospital intervention or admission, although some acute exacerbations can be managed through 'hospital at home' schemes.

The management of COPD is dependent on the severity of the disease process and the associated symptoms. Figure 3.7 outlines the treatments used to manage each stage of COPD, based on the National Institute for Health and Clinical Excellence (NICE) COPD guidelines (NICE 2010) and GOLD guidelines (WHO 2007).

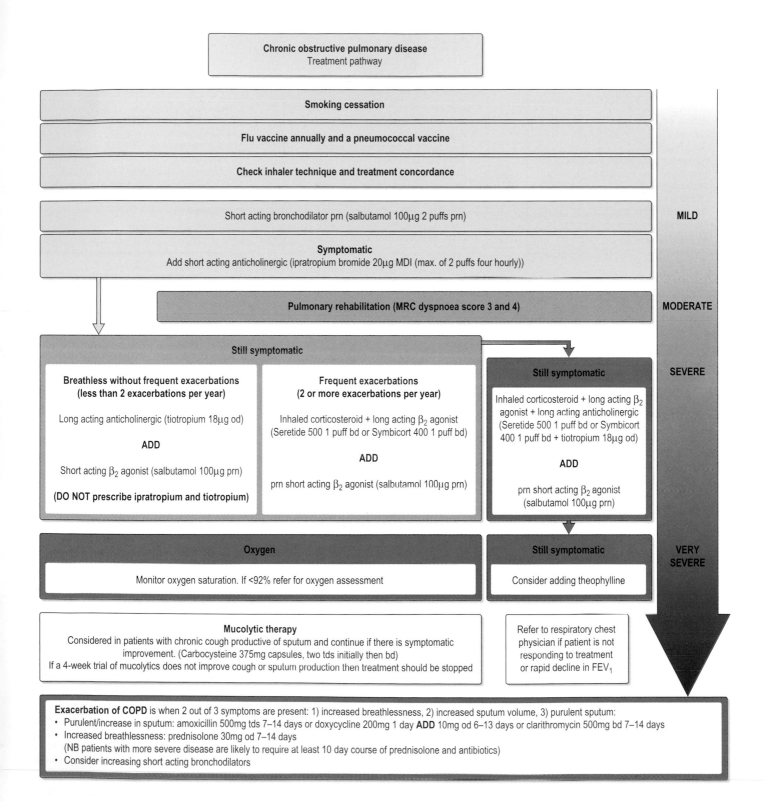

Figure 3.7 COPD treatment guidance.

As well as medication the other mainstay treatments for severe COPD are:

- smoking cessation (see p. 54)
- long-term oxygen therapy
- pulmonary rehabilitation (see p. 63).

Long-term oxygen therapy

The use of long-term oxygen therapy in patients with chronic hypoxaemia (PaO_2 <7.3 kPa) due to COPD has shown an increase in survival of approximately 5 years when 28% oxygen was administered for 15–16 hours per day (Nocturnal Oxygen Therapy Trial Group 1980, Medical Research Council Working Party 1981). The reason for low concentrations of oxygen being administered to COPD patients is that they develop sensitivity to falling oxygen levels in the blood rather than raised levels of carbon dioxide. If a higher percentage of oxygen is administered this may reduce the stimulus to breathe and lead to carbon dioxide retention.

Long-term oxygen therapy is delivered by an oxygen concentrator rather than oxygen cylinders. This frees the patient from relying on the delivery of the cylinders, allows the patient to be more mobile around the home and eliminates the need for storage of numerous cylinders. Patients who need to use oxygen outside the home can be provided with portable oxygen cylinders, although not all patients are willing to wear nasal cannulae in public. According to the British Thoracic Society's Home Oxygen Guidance (British Thoracic Society 2006b) the patient newly started on long-term oxygen therapy should have written instructions and outpatient or community follow-up so that the following aspects of care can be addressed:

- safe use of oxygen (e.g. fire risk and smoking, falls due to tubing)
- oxygen saturation (SaO_2) monitored to ensure that oxygen therapy is correcting hypoxaemia (SaO_2 >92%)
- psychological and social concerns and issues that may prevent the patient complying with the oxygen therapy
- monitoring of patient's condition and observation for signs of deterioration (e.g. peripheral oedema).

Respiratory nurse specialist

The respiratory nurse specialist is often the most appropriate person to provide the education, support and follow-up required for patients recently commenced on long-term oxygen therapy as they have clinical expertise and a liaison role.

Pulmonary rehabilitation

Pulmonary rehabilitation is different from rehabilitation offered to patients with other conditions (e.g. cardiac or musculoskeletal rehabilitation); there is no cure and the patient does not have the potential to return to a pre-disease state because the lung damage is not reversible. It is all about the patient achieving their own maximum potential within the limits of their disease and being able to live with and cope with a respiratory disability.

The aim of pulmonary rehabilitation is to reduce respiratory symptoms, increase exercise tolerance, improve psychological coping and improve overall quality of life (Garrod 2004). The common components of pulmonary rehabilitation programmes include:

- *Education* – increasing the patient's knowledge so that they are empowered to make decisions about their health needs, including modification of high-risk behaviours such as smoking.
- *Exercise* – the majority of rehabilitation programmes use interval training which consists of 2–3 minutes of high-intensity training (e.g. bicycle or step-ups) alternating with equal periods of rest. This allows the patient to exercise safely and learn how to control their dyspnoea whilst exercising.
- *Breathing control* – patients are taught breathing techniques using their diaphragm, designed to slow respiratory rate while increasing their tidal volume.
- *Psychosocial interventions* – patients with COPD have a high incidence of depression and anxiety and therefore need to develop coping strategies to deal with the impact of respiratory disability on their lives.
- *Nutritional intervention* – patients with COPD require nutritional advice and support as they are at high risk of malnutrition. Both the practical aspects of preparing meals as well as the physiological barriers, such as breathlessness and reduced appetite due to infection, need to be addressed. Usually, small regular high-calorie meals or snacks are better tolerated than two large main meals per day (see Ch. 21).

For pulmonary rehabilitation to be successful a multi-professional approach is essential (Garrod 2004). The team should include a respiratory nurse specialist, physiotherapist, dietitian, psychologist, occupational therapist and respiratory doctor. Organisation of the programme is usually undertaken by the respiratory nurse and/or the respiratory physiotherapist, with input from the other disciplines as appropriate.

Management of acute respiratory exacerbation of COPD

A patient with an acute exacerbation of COPD presents with worsening symptoms of a previously stable condition and two of the following three symptoms:

1. increased breathlessness
2. increased sputum volume
3. purulent sputum.

As the underlying cause of the acute exacerbation is usually infection, the patient is usually commenced on antibiotic therapy. If breathless, patients will also start oral corticosteroids and be given increased doses of bronchodilators, often nebulised (see Box 3.1).

During acute exacerbations COPD patients are at risk of either type I respiratory failure (low oxygen levels in arterial blood) or type II respiratory failure (low oxygen and high carbon dioxide levels in arterial blood). It is therefore necessary to monitor arterial blood gases and treat with oxygen therapy and, if necessary, non-invasive ventilation (see Ch. 32).

Patients may require admission to hospital during an acute exacerbation; however, increasing numbers of patients are being cared for at home by respiratory nurses providing 'hospital at home' or early supported discharge (British Thoracic Society 2007). Patients assessed as suitable for home treatment will be provided with an oxygen concentrator, nebuliser and home visits from the respiratory nurses who will monitor progress and provide advice and support. Once

Box 3.1 Information

Nebulisers

A nebuliser is a device that administers medication (i.e. bronchodilators, antibiotics) by converting a liquid into a mist that can be inhaled into the lungs. It is commonly used in treating patients with cystic fibrosis or acute asthma and during exacerbations of COPD. The jet nebuliser is the most widely used device. Compressed gas (oxygen or air) is forced through a narrow opening in the base of the nebuliser unit creating the negative pressure required to draw up the drug solution from its reservoir. When the liquid collides with the jet of gas, it fragments into droplets that then impact on a baffle. The smallest particles form a therapeutic mist for the patient to inhale, while larger particles return to the reservoir and are recycled until the prescribed dose has been given, usually about 10 minutes. A flow rate of 6–8 L/min produces 50% of the particles at a diameter of less than 5 μm which allows deposition of the drug in the lungs.

Compressed air is the most common source for driving a nebuliser unless a high rate of inspired oxygen (i.e. asthmatic patients) is indicated and prescribed. To prevent worsening of carbon dioxide retention, patients at risk of carbon dioxide retention (i.e. COPD patients) should use compressed air to drive the nebuliser. The use of nasal cannulae to deliver the prescribed flow rate of oxygen during nebulisation will prevent hypoxaemia (Esmond 1998).

recovered from their acute exacerbation the patient will be discharged back into the care of the GP and community nurses (i.e. community matron).

 See website Critical thinking question 3.2

Respiratory failure

If impending respiratory failure is recognised early, the actual state can be avoided; nurses should be alert for the following clinical signs:

- restlessness and confusion
- increase in respiratory rate with laboured ventilatory effort and use of ancillary respiratory muscles (sternocleidomastoid and abdominal muscles)
- forced and abnormal movement of the diaphragm
- pronounced flaring of the nostrils with each breath
- pale or deeply cyanosed and clammy skin.

Where impending respiratory failure is suspected arterial blood gases (ABGs) will be taken to confirm if the patient has respiratory failure and whether it is:

- type I respiratory failure – PaO_2 <8 kPa
- type II respiratory failure – PaO_2 <8 kPa, $PaCO_2$ >6 kPa
- respiratory acidosis – PaO_2 <8 kPa, $PaCO_2$ >6 kPa, pH <7.35.

Untreated, the condition will worsen steadily, and increasingly difficult ventilatory effort will leave the patient exhausted and hypoxic, which will eventually lead to the patient becoming comatose and to death. However, respiratory support techniques can be used for patients with impending respiratory failure. The treatment options are:

Type I respiratory failure:
- oxygen therapy (high flow 40–100%)
- continuous positive airway pressure (CPAP) (see Ch. 29).

Type II respiratory failure:
- oxygen therapy (low flow 24–28%)
- non-invasive ventilation (NIV)
- endotracheal intermittent positive pressure ventilation (IPPV) (see Ch. 29).

Oxygen therapy

The aim of oxygen therapy is to increase the fractional inspired oxygen (FiO_2) above 21% (air) to ensure adequate saturation of haemoglobin.

In the presence of type I respiratory failure oxygen therapy must be prescribed at a level which will correct hypoxaemia, and a patient with severe asthma or pulmonary embolism may require 60–100% oxygen initially to prevent hypoxia, until specific disease management is initiated.

In the presence of type II respiratory failure, the low levels of oxygen are providing the respiratory drive, i.e. the stimulus to the respiratory centre in the medulla. High percentages of oxygen can reduce the hypoxic respiratory drive causing carbon dioxide retention and a respiratory acidosis. This is because patients with underlying respiratory disease such as COPD develop sensitivity to falling oxygen levels in the blood rather than raised levels of carbon dioxide. If a higher percentage of oxygen is administered, this may reduce their stimulus to breathe and lead to carbon dioxide retention. If the rising levels of carbon dioxide remain untreated, narcosis, disorientation and ultimately death due to respiratory acidosis will occur. These patients require low percentage oxygen (24–28%) initially. The oxygen can be gradually increased on the basis of repeated arterial blood gases whereby carbon dioxide levels can be monitored. Patients with COPD can receive more than 28% oxygen, provided arterial blood gases indicate that there is no evidence of carbon dioxide retention (hypercapnia). Bateman & Leech (1998) found that only 10–15% of COPD patients are at risk of hypercapnia but it is unusual to administer more than 35% oxygen to patients with type II respiratory failure.

Oxygen delivery devices

A variety of oxygen devices are available. They can be categorised into two types:

- *Variable performance devices* (nasal cannula, Hudson mask and any system that does not incorporate a 'Venturi' mechanism) deliver a percentage of oxygen that varies according to the rate and depth of the patient's respirations.
- *Fixed performance devices* include in the delivery circuit a 'Venturi' coloured adaptor or the use of the Venturi principle incorporated in the humidification delivery device (e.g. Respiflow humidification system). The 'Venturi' supplies oxygen to the patient at a precise flow rate that causes mixing of the oxygen with air drawn into the system through holes in the adaptor. This system is more accurate and is not dependent on the patient's rate and depth of respirations. During acute respiratory episodes these are the masks of choice as they provide accurate concentrations of oxygen and prevent patients re-breathing their own carbon dioxide.

Humidification of oxygen

When oxygen is delivered at low flow rates of <4 L/min and in the absence of respiratory tract infections, the oropharynx or nasopharynx may be able to provide adequate humidification. However, oxygen is very drying and therefore humidification should be considered for patients with:

- flow rates above 4 L/min
- respiratory infections
- tracheostomy (see Ch. 14)
- nasal discomfort/dryness.

Nursing management and health promotion: oxygen therapy

As well as ensuring the patient is receiving the prescribed percentage of oxygen using an appropriate oxygen device, the nurse needs to consider the comfort of the patient. As oxygen can cause mucosal drying, the development of mouth ulcers is not uncommon in patients receiving continuous oxygen therapy. The nurse needs to offer/perform regular mouth care to prevent the development of mouth ulcers as the resulting pain and difficulty with eating and drinking can have a significantly adverse effect on the patient's recovery. The use of humidification helps to counteract the drying effect, and is indicated if the patient complains of discomfort or there are signs of mouth ulceration. An oxygen mask creates a barrier when speaking and the noise of the oxygen may interfere with the patient's ability to hear, which means that some patients may have difficulty with communication. Facing the patient, taking time and speaking clearly can improve communication, prevent isolation and facilitate the patient to express concerns and care needs. The nurse also needs to be aware that pressure ulcers can occur under the straps of the oxygen mask and therefore regular inspection behind the ears for redness and ulceration is necessary. If the straps are causing pressure and/or discomfort, padding behind the ears may help.

Continuous positive airway pressure (CPAP)

Oxygenation can be enhanced by using continuous positive airway pressure (CPAP) which increases lung volume and keeps the alveoli open at the end of each breath to allow more time for gaseous exchange. A full-face mask is strapped in position and needs to be tight fitting, as any leaks will reduce the effectiveness of the positive pressure. The aim of treatment is to increase functional lung capacity and compliance, decrease the work of breathing, improve ventilation and perfusion, increase oxygen saturations, mobilise secretions, and re-expand collapsed alveoli. CPAP relies on the patient's own respiratory effort and therefore is indicated for treatment of type I respiratory failure when there is:

- a restrictive pattern of breathing (e.g. fractured ribs, pain)
- atelectasis (collapse of lung tissue affecting part or all of one lung) often secondary to pneumonia
- increased work of breathing due to the respiratory effort required to maintain adequate oxygen levels
- difficulty with clearing secretions, particularly when the cough reflex is reduced due to fatigue.

CPAP needs to be used with caution and by experienced practitioners as it is contraindicated in patients with pneumothorax, bullae (air cysts inside the lung), lung abscess, haemoptysis and hypotension. The majority of patients receiving CPAP will be cared for in a critical care environment, such as the high-dependency unit (HDU) or intensive care unit (ICU) (see Ch. 29).

Non-invasive ventilation (NIV)

Non-invasive ventilation (NIV) is a form of ventilation using a well-fitting nasal or full-face mask, and unlike CPAP does not rely on the ability of the patient to breathe spontaneously as the machine has an inspiratory and expiratory phase. It is used to treat patients in type II respiratory failure and has the advantages of being non-invasive, able to provide adequate oxygen levels with carbon dioxide clearance, and able to decrease work of breathing and improve quality of sleep. For it to be successful the patient must be able to cooperate with treatment, have normal swallowing reflexes and haemodynamic stability and the ability to clear bronchial secretions. Nurses caring for patients receiving NIV need to be skilled so that they are able to troubleshoot problems such as mask problems, dry nose, air leaks, eye irritation and gastric distension. Patients will require psychological support to deal with the effects of altered body image due to needing to wear a facial mask. For further information about respiratory support techniques see Esmond & Mikelsons (2009).

Infections of the respiratory system

Infections of the upper respiratory tract are addressed in Chapter 14. This chapter will focus on pneumonia and tuberculosis.

Pneumonia

Pneumonia is an infection of the lung caused by bacteria, viruses or fungi. There is parenchymal/alveolar inflammation and the alveoli fill with fluid which leads to consolidation and exudation.

PATHOPHYSIOLOGY

Pneumonia may be acquired in the community or in hospital, when it is known as a nosocomial infection (hospital acquired) as it has been acquired from other patients, the environment or health care workers. The type of pneumonia is determined by the causative organism, e.g. pneumococcal pneumonia, *Streptococcus pneumoniae* and *Pneumocystis* pneumonia (PCP).

Pneumonia can occur in previously healthy people although there is a higher incidence amongst the elderly and those with co-morbidities. Complications of pneumonia include meningitis, empyema (pus in the pleural space), lung abscess and septicaemia. Death occurs most often in the elderly and those with debilitating chronic conditions, especially when pneumonia is secondary to recent influenza.

Clinical features

Clinical presentation will vary in severity depending on the overall condition of the patient but includes varying degrees of pyrexia, cough with copious purulent sputum, breathlessness and tachypnoea (rapid respiratory rate).

Investigations

Investigations will include chest X-ray, sputum microscopy, culture and sensitivity, blood cultures, white cell count (WBC), pleural fluid microscopy, culture and sensitivity, pneumococcal antigen tests and serological tests.

Treatment

The aim of treatment is to identify the cause of the pneumonia, deliver appropriate treatment and rule out other causes of disease. Pneumonia will require treatment with antibiotics that are effective against the causative organism. In accordance with the British Thoracic Guidelines on management of pneumonia (British Thoracic Society 2009), a broad spectrum antibiotic will be prescribed initially, until sputum microbiological results are available. The choice of the oral or intravenous route will depend on the severity of presenting features.

 Nursing management and health promotion: pneumonia

The needs of the patient with pneumonia will be determined by the causative factors and symptoms experienced by the patient but most patients will require the following care:

- Monitoring temperature, pulse, respirations, BP, peak flow rate and oxygen saturation and reporting changes.
- Positioning the patient in an upright position supported by pillows or leaning against a bed table will help to alleviate dyspnoea by allowing effective lung expansion.
- Administration of oxygen to manage hypoxaemia (low oxygen levels). The dryness of oxygen will restrict the expectoration of sputum so it is advisable to use humidified oxygen therapy and offer frequent drinks or mouth washes.
- Assistance with sputum clearance and encouraging the patient to expectorate the sputum. Chest physiotherapy will also be initiated to assist with airway clearance and usually consists of postural drainage, percussion and breathing control.
- The patient with pyrexia requires sufficient fluid intake to replace fluid lost in sweat; this will assist with excretion of toxins from the body. An antipyretic, such as paracetamol, may be used to control body temperature and make the patient more comfortable (see Ch. 22).
- Additional analgesia may be required, as paracetamol alone may be insufficient to manage pleuritic chest pain, which is caused by inflammation of the pleura.
- Nutritional support, as pyrexia and pain may have an adverse effect on nutrition.
- Psychological support, as having pneumonia can be a very frightening experience. Listening to fears and anxieties can be very supportive. During severe breathless episodes, the patient may be reassured by the presence of the nurse or family member.

Prevention of pneumonia

A pneumococcal vaccine is available and is recommended for high-risk groups such as the elderly and those with underlying respiratory disease (Department of Health 2006).

Box 3.2 Reflection

Identify a patient you have cared for with an underlying respiratory condition and reflect on the care provided considering the following aspects:

- What are the key physiological changes that have occurred?
- What evidence-based clinical guidelines are available to guide practice?
- What health promotion activities need to be included in the care plan and how would you action these?
- What medication is used in the management of the patient and what are the dose, route and side-effects?
- What is the role of the nurse in caring for the patient?
- Who are the other members of the multidisciplinary team and what are their roles?
- Consider what you have learnt and what your future learning needs are.

The polyvalent vaccine is usually a single 'one-off' injection. Vaccination against influenza ('flu' vaccine) is also recommended and needs to be administered annually. In addition, causative risk factors such as poverty, poor housing, malnutrition, environment exposure to pollutants, smoking (both active and passive) and excessive alcohol consumption need to be addressed if mortality rates are to be reduced (Box 3.2).

Tuberculosis

Tuberculosis (TB) is a notifiable disease, which in accordance with the Public Health Act (Department of Health 1984) requires individuals diagnosed with TB to be notified to the Consultant in Community Diseases Control (CCDC) or Director of Public Health who is responsible for TB surveillance and control of spread of TB within the local community.

PATHOPHYSIOLOGY

Tuberculosis is a chronic infectious disease caused by the tubercle bacillus, *Mycobacterium tuberculosis*. It mainly affects the lungs as it is transmitted by inhalation of infected droplets of sputum coughed up by someone with active TB. However, other parts of the body (extrapulmonary) can be affected, through the bacterium entering the bloodstream through the lymphatic system. The most common forms of extrapulmonary disease are lymphadenopathy, pleural effusion, pericardial TB, miliary TB and TB meningitis.

Most people infected with *Mycobacterium tuberculosis* never develop active disease as the body's immune system makes the bacterium dormant. Soon after the primary infection enters the lung, the inflammatory response occurs and a calcified lesion is left. The primary infection remains dormant but may be reactivated (post-primary infection) to become active TB if the immune system is weakened.

The risk factors for developing active TB are associated with exposure to infectious TB and immune system weakening; this includes immunodeficiency (i.e. HIV), close contact with someone newly diagnosed with infectious TB, homelessness, particularly with a history of alcohol misuse and malnutrition, the elderly and those with chronic respiratory disease.

Clinical features of TB are those associated with infection: chronic cough, pyrexia, weight loss, night sweats, general malaise and haemoptysis (blood in the sputum).

Investigations will include a chest X-ray, a tuberculin skin test to detect past or present tuberculosis infection and sputum microbiological analysis; acid-fast bacillus (AFB) in sputum indicates that the patient has active (smear positive) TB. A smear negative result cannot exclude the presence of TB until the sputum culture, which takes approximately 8 weeks, also proves negative.

Treatment

The National Institute for Health and Clinical Excellence (2006b) produced guidelines on the treatment and management of TB in the UK. Currently, first-line treatment for tuberculosis consists of a 6-month treatment regimen of rifampicin, isoniazid, pyrazinamide and ethambutol or streptomycin for 2 months and then rifampicin and isoniazid for a further 4 months. The fourth drug, ethambutol or streptomycin, can be omitted when patients have a low risk of developing resistance to isoniazid.

Multi-drug resistant TB

Pulmonary tuberculosis is a treatable condition but multi-drug resistant tuberculosis (MDR-TB) can develop for the following reasons:

- inadequate initial therapy (single drug therapy or low dose)
- failure to complete the course of antibiotics because of poor adherence to treatment
- patients become asymptomatic after 2–4 weeks of treatment and so believe they no longer need the medication
- lack of knowledge and understanding of TB and its treatment
- inability to access health care, which is prevalent amongst the homeless and minority ethnic groups if there are language problems.

▷ Nursing management and health promotion: tuberculosis

Treatment of TB usually takes place at home; only those with severe illness, secondary complications (e.g. pleural effusion or adverse drug reactions) or social problems are admitted to hospital. The nursing priorities are:

- *Prevention* – based upon public health education and on screening and vaccination to protect those at risk. Specialist TB nurses, working closely with health visitors, public health nurses, school nurses, GPs, microbiologists and CCDCs are key in the prevention and control of TB.
- *Infection control* – when a patient with suspected TB is admitted to hospital they should be nursed in a single room so that isolation precautions for airborne infections can be implemented. If the patient needs to leave their room they should wear a face mask. Once the patient has commenced TB treatment and has three consecutive smear negative sputum results, they can be nursed in an open ward. Patients with, or suspected to have, MDR-TB should be cared for in a negative pressure room and, because of the serious consequences of contracting MDR-TB, staff caring for the patient should wear dust mist-fume masks as these provide greater protection (see Ch. 16).

- *Contact tracing* – people who have been in close contact with the person diagnosed with TB (index or source case) will be contacted and screened for TB. Contact screening is usually done by the TB nurse specialist who will screen close contacts (people living in same house and very close associates such as boyfriend/girlfriend) of the index or source case.
- *Treatment supervision* – adherence to therapy is essential if TB is to be controlled and MDR-TB is to be prevented. Baker (2001) suggests that placing the emphasis on supporting rather than monitoring patients is likely to improve treatment completion rates, as it allows exploration of factors that may lead to patients not adhering to treatment. These may include lack of knowledge, social problems, health beliefs, cultural beliefs and chaotic lifestyle. By working in partnership with the patient, strategies to improve adherence can be individualised.
- Directly observed therapy (DOT) is where the patient is observed taking their therapy by a health care professional (World Health Organization 2003). This strategy is labour intensive and often difficult to achieve; in the UK it is only implemented if the patient is assessed to be at high risk of non-adherence. Homeless people are a group at high risk of non-adherence as they have difficulty accessing health care and obtaining medication. Incentives such as provision of meals and taxis have been used in association with DOT to encourage homeless people to attend appointments.

Cystic fibrosis

Cystic fibrosis (CF) is the most common life-threatening genetic disorder in the UK. It affects approximately 1 in 2500 live births because 1 in 25 Caucasians in the UK are carriers of the CF gene. As it is a recessive genetic disorder, when both parents are carriers of the abnormal gene there is a 1 in 4 chance of each pregnancy producing a child with CF.

PATHOPHYSIOLOGY

CF involves a basic dysfunction of the exocrine glands ducts due to altered sodium and chloride channel function at the epithelial cell surface. This results in the production of abnormally concentrated secretions that tend to block exocrine ducts. CF is a multi-system disorder that primarily affects the respiratory and digestive system, although there are often associated problems of liver disease, cystic fibrosis related diabetes (CFRD), arthropathy and male infertility. The main cause of morbidity and mortality in CF is bacterial lung infections (Döring et al 2004). A background of chronic lung sepsis, usually due to *Staphylococcus aureus*, *Haemophilus influenzae* or *Pseudomonas aeruginosa*, is punctuated at increasingly frequent intervals by acute infective exacerbations. In response to persistent inflammation, pulmonary fibrosis and bronchiectasis (collection of necrotic material and bronchial secretions in dilated bronchi) progress, culminating in respiratory failure and death.

Investigations

The diagnosis of CF is based on history and clinical examination and will be confirmed by a sweat test and genotyping. Once the diagnosis is made, the severity will be determined by performing spirometry, chest X-ray, sputum cultures and pancreatic function tests.

Treatment

Treatment is aimed at delaying progression of the disease by maintaining lung function through preventing and controlling lung infections (Kerem et al 2005). This involves:

- physiotherapy to assist mucus clearance from the lungs
- administration of a combination of oral, nebulised and intravenous antibiotics to control infection
- nebulised bronchodilators (e.g. salbutamol)
- anti-inflammatory medication (i.e. oral or inhaled steroids)
- nutritional support consisting of pancreatic enzyme supplementation, fat-soluble vitamin supplementation and 20–50% increased calorie intake
- monitoring disease progression (FEV_1, FVC, SpO_2 and weight)
- aggressive treatment of acute exacerbation to prevent loss of lung function.

▷ Nursing management and health promotion: cystic fibrosis

CF puts many demands on the individual and their family. The treatment regimen can be demanding, symptoms unpleasant, and coping with emotions associated with a life-threatening chronic illness often stressful. The cystic fibrosis nurse has an important role in supporting the patient and family and is often the person they contact for support. The CF nurse also has a coordinating role within the multidisciplinary team and often acts as the patient's advocate.

Bronchiectasis

Bronchiectasis is a chronic dilation of the bronchi caused by inflammation. Collections of necrotic material and bronchial secretions in the dilated bronchi result in inflammation that causes secondary bacterial infection and fibrosis in the lung. This will result in recurrent and persistent lower respiratory tract infections causing production of large amounts of purulent sputum, bronchoconstriction, cough and haemoptysis. The main causes of bronchiectasis are:

- childhood infections (i.e. bronchiolitis)
- immunodeficiency syndromes (i.e. hypogammaglobulinaemia)
- allergic bronchopulmonary aspergillosis (ABPA)
- pneumonia
- cystic fibrosis

- tuberculosis
- α_1-antitrypsin deficiency.

Treatment

The principles of treatment are the same as cystic fibrosis.

Lung cancer

Lung cancer can be of primary origin or can occur as secondary metastatic spread from other primary sources.

PATHOPHYSIOLOGY

Lung cancer is classified according to basic cell type, i.e. squamous cell adenocarcinoma (the most common), undifferentiated carcinoma and large and small cell carcinoma. The tumour may present as a cauliflower-shaped mass which slowly infiltrates the lung parenchyma. Because this form of cancer is difficult to detect in the early stages, it has a high potential for metastatic spread before being discovered.

Clinical features include a persistent cough of several months' duration which may be accompanied by haemoptysis (bloodstained sputum), chest pain, hoarseness and breathlessness. There may also be weight loss, anaemia, pleural effusion and bone pain. The patient will look generally unwell.

Investigations

Diagnosis is confirmed by clinical examination, chest X-ray or CT scan and sputum cytology. A bronchoscopy may be performed to enable a small piece of lung tissue (biopsy) to be taken via the bronchoscope and sent for pathology.

Treatment

A full explanation of the diagnosis and prognosis will be given to the patient and family so that an informed decision can be made regarding treatment. Approximately 15% of primary lung tumours can be treated successfully by surgical removal. This will involve either lobectomy (removal of the affected lobe) or pneumonectomy (removal of the whole lung) followed by cytotoxic chemotherapy. Where there is invasive and metastatic spread, the treatment is usually conservative, involving chemotherapy, radiotherapy, intervention to alleviate symptoms and pain control (see Ch. 31).

Pneumothorax

A pneumothorax occurs when the integrity of either layer of the pleura is breached, allowing air to enter the pleural cavity leading to lung collapse. There are two types of pneumothorax (Gallon 1998):

- Spontaneous pneumothorax – occurs as a result of the rupture of small blebs, cysts or bullae (air cysts inside the lung).
- Traumatic pneumothorax – caused by blunt chest trauma or a penetrating injury (e.g. stab wound or fractured rib, central line insertion). Trauma, particularly with

penetrating injuries, can also cause blood to enter the pleural cavity and this is known as a haemothorax.

Tension pneumothorax

Both spontaneous and traumatic pneumothorax can develop into a tension pneumothorax. This is a life-threatening event because air enters the pleural space on inspiration but cannot leave on expiration. The increased pressure causes the mediastinum to shift, moving the heart towards the opposite side.

Signs and symptoms

The first sign of pneumothorax is the sudden onset of dyspnoea with unilateral chest pain that may radiate to the shoulder or arm and becomes worse on inspiration. On physical examination there is hyper-resonance and decreased breath sounds on the affected side and chest movement is asymmetrical. Severe dyspnoea, cyanosis, hypotension and tachycardia signify a tension pneumothorax, requiring immediate treatment.

A chest X-ray will confirm the presence and the amount of air in the pleural cavity and will be performed before initiation of treatment unless there is a tension pneumothorax, in which case the treatment is required immediately. The chest X-ray along with the signs and symptoms will determine the management of the pneumothorax.

Treatment

The size of a pneumothorax along with the symptoms will guide treatment. According to the British Thoracic Society guidelines (Henry et al 2003) a pneumothorax is described as small (<2 cm) or large (>2 cm). Treatment options for pneumothorax include:

- observation for a small closed pneumothorax without significant breathlessness
- simple needle aspiration for a small (<2 cm) pneumothorax not associated with breathlessness
- intercostal chest drain for a large (>2 cm) pneumothorax, or small (<2 cm) when associated with breathlessness (Box 3.3)
- pleurodesis or pleurectomy when the lung has failed to re-expand after insertion of intercostal chest drainage or after two or more recurrences.

SUMMARY: KEY NURSING ISSUES

- Lung disease affects around 8 million people in the UK and results in tens of thousands of deaths annually with a higher incidence of respiratory disease in the lower socio-economic groups.
- The overwhelming cause of respiratory disease is tobacco smoking.
- Breathlessness is the main cause of disability associated with respiratory disease and impacts on the individual's ability to perform activities of daily living.
- Due to the chronic nature of much respiratory disease, self-management skills need to be taught so that individuals are empowered to manage their condition and make decisions about their health.
- Nurses have an important role in improving the quality of life of people with respiratory disease through holistic care.
- Respiratory nurse specialist roles provide continuity of care and a focal point for patients to seek advice and support.

REFLECTION AND LEARNING – WHAT NEXT?

- **Test** your knowledge by visiting the website 🖰 and answering the multiple choice questions and critical thinking questions.
- **Consolidate** your learning by looking at some of the further reading suggestions, references and specialist websites.
- **Revisit** some of the additional material on the website.
- **Consider** what you have learnt and how this will help your professional development.
- **Reflect** on how you can apply this knowledge to the care of your patients.
- **Discuss** your learning with your mentor/supervisor, lecturer and colleagues.

Box 3.3 Information

Nursing management of an underwater-sealed chest drain

The underwater-sealed drainage system acts as a one-way valve, allowing air to bubble out through the water during expiration, but because the end of the tube is under water, air is prevented from being drawn back into the pleural cavity during inspiration (Avery 2000). If at any point the seal is broken, air can enter the pleural cavity causing the lung to collapse again. The nurse has an important role in caring for patients with a chest drain as many of the potential complications can be prevented if principles of chest drain management are understood and implemented. The nurse needs to ensure that:

- the water level in the chest drain bottle covers the end of the tube
- connections are secure and not leaking
- the chest drain bottle is kept below the chest level to prevent fluid entering the pleural cavity
- the chest drain remains patent by checking that the water in the tube is 'swinging' and 'bubbling' as the patient breathes
- tubing is not routinely clamped (unless the connection becomes disconnected) because this prevents air escaping and may lead to lung collapse
- infection is prevented by adhering to asepsis and checking that the drain site dressing is kept clean and dry
- when removing the chest drain, air is prevented from re-entering the pleural cavity by getting the patient to take a deep breath and hold it while the drain is pulled out and the 'purse-string' suture tied to seal the wound.

REFERENCES

Avery S: Insertion and management of chest drains, *Nurs Times* 96:3–6, 2000.

Baker T: Tuberculosis returns, *Nurs Times* 97:56–57, 2001.

Bateman NT, Leech RM: ABC of oxygen: acute oxygen therapy, *Br Med J* 317:798–801, 1998.

British Thoracic Society: *The Burden of Lung Disease*, 2006a. Available online http://www.brit-thoracic.org.uk.

British Thoracic Society: *Clinical Component for the Home Oxygen Service in England and Wales*, 2006b. Available online http://www.brit-thoracic.org.uk/Portals/0/Clinical%20Information/Home%20Oxygen%20Service/clinical%20adultoxygenjan06.pdf.

British Thoracic Society: *Intermediate Care – Hospital-at-Home in Chronic Obstructive Pulmonary Disease Guideline*, 2007. Available online http://www.brit-thoracic.org.uk/ClinicalInformation/IntermediateCareHospitalatHomeforCOPD/IntermCareHospitalatHomeforCOPDGuideline/tabid/261/Default.aspx.

British Thoracic Society: *Emergency Oxygen Use in Adult Patients*, 2008. Available online http://www.brit-thoracic.org.uk/ClinicalInformation/EmergencyOxygen/tabid/219/Default.aspx.

British Thoracic Society: Guidelines for the management of community acquired pneumonia in adults, *Thorax* 64(Suppl III):iii1–iii55, 2009.

British Thoracic Society and Scottish Intercollegiate Guidelines Network: *The British Guidelines on Asthma Management*, 2008. Available online http://www.brit-thoracic.org.uk/ClinicalInformation/Asthma/AsthmaGuidelines/tabid/83/Default.aspx.

Brooker C, Nicol M: *Nursing adults: The practice of caring*, Edinburgh, 2003, Mosby.

Buck D: The cost-effectiveness of smoking cessation interventions: what do we know? *Int J Health Educ* 35(2):44–51, 1997.

Carter BG: Accuracy of two pulse oximeters at low arterial hemoglobin oxygen saturation, *Crit Care Med* 26:1128–1133, 1998.

Department of Health: *Public Health (Control of Disease) Act*, London, 1984, The Stationery Office.

Department of Health: *Immunisation against infectious disease, 'The Green Book'*, 2006. Available online http://www.dh.gov.uk/en/Publicationsandstatistics/Publications/PublicationsPolicyAndGuidance/DH_079917.

Donaldson GC, Wilkinson TM, Hurst JR, Perera WR, Wedzicha JA: Exacerbations and time spent outdoors in chronic obstructive pulmonary disease, *Am J Respir Crit Care Med* 171(5):446–452, 2005.

Döring G, Høiby N, for the Consensus Study Group: Early intervention and prevention of lung disease in cystic fibrosis: a European consensus, *J Cyst Fibros* 3:67–91, 2004. Available online http://www.elsevier.com/framework_products/promis_misc/2004.pdf.

Esmond G: Nebuliser therapy update, *Prof Nurse* 14(1):39–43, 1998.

Esmond G: *Respiratory Nursing*, Edinburgh, 2001, Baillière Tindall.

Esmond G, Mikelsons C: *Respiratory Support Techniques: Oxygen, Non Invasive Ventilation, CPAP*, Oxford, 2009, Wiley.

Fletcher CM, Peto R: The natural history of chronic airflow obstruction, *Br Med J* 1:1645–1648, 1977.

Gallon A: Pneumothorax, *Nurs Stand* 13:35–39, 1998.

Garrod R: *Pulmonary Rehabilitation: a multidisciplinary approach*, Oxford, 2004, Wiley-Blackwell.

Hatsukami DK, Hughes JR, Pickens RW, Svikis D: Tobacco withdrawal symptoms: An experimental analysis, *Psychopharmacology* 84:231–236, 1984.

Henry M, Arnold T, Harvey J, on behalf of the BTS Pleural Disease Group: British Thoracic Society guidelines for the management of spontaneous pneumothorax, *Thorax* 58(Suppl 2):ii39–ii52, 2003. Available online http://www.brit-thoracic.org.uk/ClinicalInformation/Pneumothorax/tabid/114/Default.aspx.

Kerem E, Conway S, Elborn S, Heijerman H: for the Consensus Committee: Standards of care for patients with cystic fibrosis: A European consensus, *J Cyst Fibros* 4:7–26, 2005. Available online http://www.elsevier.com/framework_products/promis_misc/2005.pdf.

Margereson C, Esmond G: Chronic obstructive pulmonary disease. The role of the nurse, *Nurs Times* 93(20):5–8, 1997.

Medical Research Council: Long term domiciliary oxygen therapy in hypoxemic cor pulmonale complicating chronic bronchitis and emphysema: Report of the Medical Research Council working party, *Lancet* 1:681–686, 1981.

National Institute for Health and Clinical Excellence: *Smoking cessation – bupropion and nicotine replacement therapy*, 2002. Available online http://www.nice.org.uk/TA039/guidance.pdf.

National Institute for Health and Clinical Excellence: Chronic Obstructive Pulmonary Disease. National clinical guideline on management of chronic pulmonary disease in adults in primary and secondary care, *Thorax* 59(Supp 1):1–232, 2004.

National Institute for Health and Clinical Excellence: *Brief interventions and referral for smoking cessation in primary care and other settings*, 2006a. Available online http://www.nice.org.uk/guidance/index.jsp?action=byID&r=true&o=11375#documents.

National Institute for Health and Clinical Excellence: *Clinical diagnosis and management of tuberculosis, and measures for its prevention and control*, 2006b. Available online http://www.nice.org.uk/guidance/index.jsp?action=byID&r=true&o=10980.

National Institute for Health and Clinical Excellence: *Smoking cessation services in primary care, pharmacies, local authorities and workplaces, particularly for manual working groups, pregnant women and hard to reach communities*, 2008a. Available online http://www.nice.org.uk/nicemedia/pdf/PH010guidance.pdf.

National Institute for Health and Clinical Excellence: *Varenicline for smoking cessation*, 2008b. Available online http://www.nice.org.uk/Guidance/TA123/Guidance/pdf/English.

Nocturnal Oxygen Therapy Trial Group: Continuous or nocturnal oxygen therapy in hypoxaemic chronic obstructive pulmonary disease: a clinical trial, *Ann Intern Med* 93:391–398, 1980.

Office for National Statistics (ONS): *Social and Vital Statistics Division (2005) General Household Survey*, London, 2005, The Stationery Office.

Prochaska JO, DiClemente C: *The transtheoretical approach: Crossing traditional foundations of change*, Homewood, IL, 1984, Don Jones/Irwin.

Waugh A, Grant A: *Ross and Wilson Anatomy and Physiology in Health and Illness*, ed 10, Edinburgh, 2006, Churchill Livingstone.

West R, McNeill A, Raw M: Smoking cessation guidelines for health professionals: an update, *Thorax* 55:987–999, 2000.

World Health Organization: *Treatment of tuberculosis: Guidelines for national programmes*, Geneva, 2003, WHO.

World Health Organization: *Global initiative for chronic obstructive lung disease guidelines*, 2007. Available online http://www.goldcopd.com/.

USEFUL WEBSITES

Asthma UK: www.asthma.org.uk

British Lung Foundation: www.lunguk.org

British National Formulary: www.bnf.org

British Thoracic Society: www.brit-thoracic.org.uk

Department of Health: www.dh.gov.uk

Global Initiative for Chronic Obstructive Lung Disease: www.goldcopd.com

National Institute for Health and Clinical Excellence: www.nice.org.uk

Thorax (the journal of the British Thoracic Society): www.thorajnl.com

World Health Organization: www.who.int/health

Nursing patients with gastrointestinal, liver and biliary disorders

Patricia Cronin, Anita Duffy

Introduction

As gastrointestinal disorders continue to be the number one complaint requiring medical attention in a variety of settings, anatomical and physiological knowledge of the gastrointestinal (GI) system is essential for nursing practice. In 2007 Dinsdale reported that deaths from diseases of the GI system had increased by 25% over the previous ten years (Dinsdale 2007). Therefore, as the demand for medical care rises there is an increased need for knowledgeable and competent nurses to assess, plan, implement and evaluate the sometimes complex and challenging nursing care patients require.

Because the GI system comprises a large number of organs with a range of interrelated functions, disorders can produce diverse and often distressing symptoms such as pain, dysphagia, anorexia, weight loss, dyspepsia, nausea and vomiting, constipation and diarrhoea causing considerable embarrassment and activity restrictions in patients' lives.

Disorders of the GI system may present as acute, life-threatening emergencies or chronic illnesses, requiring long-term management and sometimes admission to hospital for more intensive treatment and/or surgical intervention. Although the specific needs of patients vary, there are general principles of pre-operative and postoperative care that are standard and require skilled nursing care. Nurses are in an ideal position to provide explanations of investigations, treatments, diagnosis and prognosis, and to follow up any information given by medical colleagues. When providing nursing care to patients with GI disorders a process of continuous assessment, planning, intervention and evaluation should be undertaken. This process should be flexible, allowing priorities to be changed as the patient's condition and circumstances evolve.

This chapter begins with an overview of the basic anatomy and physiology of the GI tract and related structures, describing the basic functions of the system and how the specialised organs and tissues contribute to effective functioning. Readers are encouraged to read Waugh & Grant (2006) Chapter 12 for a more in-depth discussion of the anatomy and physiology of the GI system. The disorders of the GI system, liver and biliary tract most commonly encountered by nurses in hospital or community settings are described and the essential nursing care these patients require is detailed. Nursing patients with disorders of the mouth and its related structures is addressed in a separate chapter (Ch. 15).

ANATOMY AND PHYSIOLOGY OF THE GASTROINTESTINAL TRACT

The gastrointestinal tract begins at the mouth and ends at the anal canal and includes the oesophagus, stomach, duodenum and small and large intestines. The ancillary organs of digestion – the liver, pancreas and gall bladder – are connected to, but not part of the digestive tract. The digestive tract is responsible for the ingestion of food and fluids at the mouth, breaking the food into pieces of a manageable size, moving the food along the canal before digestion and absorption of the nutritional content of the food occurs, and finally expelling residues and waste products by defaecation. This section will briefly describe the structure and function of the different components of the digestive tract.

The mouth

The mouth has three functions in the process of digestion: mastication (the mechanical chewing of food), salivation (moistening of the food) and deglutition (swallowing of the food) (see Ch. 15 and Figure 15.1).

The tongue, composed mainly of skeletal muscle covered with mucous membrane, manoeuvres and shapes food within the mouth for swallowing. The tongue is also a sensory organ, allowing the taste, texture and temperature of food and fluids to be perceived. The upper surface of the tongue is covered with filiform papillae or taste buds, housing the relevant sensory nerve endings (Drake et al 2005).

Saliva, composed of 99.5% water and 0.5% solutes, is released from three pairs of glands: the parotid, the submandibular and the sublingual glands located outside the mouth around the lower jaw. The submandibular glands secrete about 70% of saliva in the absence of a food stimulus to keep the mucous membranes moist and lubricate the tongue and lips during speech. However, the sight, smell or presence of food in the mouth will stimulate the parotid glands also to secrete saliva. In digestion, saliva helps to lubricate food prior to swallowing and also initiates the digestion of starch (Waugh & Grant 2006).

Swallowing

There are three stages of swallowing or deglutition. After food has been sufficiently chewed, it is formed into a bolus between the palate and the tongue. The tongue rolls the bolus and pushes it into the pharynx. This is a voluntary reaction and known as the buccal stage of swallowing. The bolus then passes over the glottis at the entrance of the larynx and trachea. When swallowing occurs a small flap of cartilage, the epiglottis, covers the glottis. This stage of swallowing is referred to as the pharyngeal stage and is involuntary. Once the bolus has passed safely over the epiglottis and involuntarily entered the oesophagus, this stage of swallowing is known as the oesophageal stage of swallowing (Waugh & Grant 2006). For more information see Chapter 15.

The oesophagus

The oesophagus is a muscular tube connecting the pharynx to the stomach. It is composed of three layers of tissue: an inner mucosal layer with an underlying submucosal layer, a middle muscular layer and an outer connective tissue layer. The mucosal layer contains glands that secrete mucus for the lubrication of food as it passes down the oesophagus. The submucosal layer provides a nerve and blood supply. The muscles of the middle layer are arranged both circularly and longitudinally. The composition of this layer changes throughout the length of the oesophagus in such a way that there is more striated, or voluntary, muscle at the pharyngeal end. Towards the stomach end, the muscle becomes predominantly and then entirely smooth, or involuntary.

The propulsion of food towards the stomach is achieved by peristalsis, a series of relaxations and contractions of the muscles that force the bolus along the oesophagus. Peristalsis is brought about by waves of contraction of the circular muscle, narrowing the lumen and thereby compressing the bolus of food. This action is preceded by a contraction of the longitudinal muscles to widen the lumen in order to receive the bolus of food. Peristalsis is entirely under involuntary control. Relaxation of the lower oesophageal sphincter allows food to enter the stomach (Drake et al 2005).

The stomach

The stomach is a J-shaped enlargement of the GI tract connecting the oesophagus to the duodenum (Norton et al 2008). It is made up of four parts: cardia, fundus, body and pylorus (including the pyloric antrum and pyloric canal). Between the pyloris and the duodenum is the pyloric sphincter. The stomach wall is composed of four layers, similar to the remainder of the GI tract: mucosa, submucosa, muscularis and serosa. The basic structure of the stomach is illustrated in Figure 4.1.

Digestion continues in the stomach when the bolus of food enters through the lower oesophageal sphincter. On the inner surface of the stomach, the mucosal layer of tissue is supplied with blood vessels and lymph glands by the underlying submucosal layer. Between the mucosal layer and the outermost peritoneal layer lies a muscular layer that is composed of three layers: an inner layer of oblique fibres, a middle layer of circular fibres and an outer layer of longitudinal fibres. These layers of muscle allow increasingly stronger waves of contraction in three directions to mix the food in the stomach and allow maximal contact with gastric juice. Innervation of the stomach is from a branch of cranial nerve X (vagus) providing parasympathetic nerve endings that stimulate the secretory cells of the stomach. The internal surface area of the stomach is increased by the arrangement of rugae in the lining (Waugh & Grant 2006).

Gastric juice

Cells in the mucosa of the stomach produce mucus, hydrochloric acid and pepsinogen. This mixture is referred to as 'gastric juice' and, when combined with food in the stomach,

is known as 'chyme'. Hydrochloric acid helps to maintain the acidity of the stomach at a pH of about 2. At this level of acidity, pepsinogen, an inactive precursor, is converted to pepsin, a protein-digesting enzyme that works optimally at this pH level. The stomach is mainly responsible for initiating protein digestion, although some carbohydrate digestion can continue by the action of any salivary amylase that has not yet become inactivated by the acidity of the stomach.

Release of gastric juice by the stomach mucosa is stimulated by the sight, smell and thought of food, referred to as the cephalic phase of digestion. The gastric phase of digestion begins when food reaches the stomach and continues until chyme enters the duodenum where the intestinal phase of gastric digestion begins. The length of time taken to empty the stomach is variable and depends on the composition of the meal eaten. The average time for emptying of the stomach after a meal is about 4 h. Emptying takes place through the pylorus. The pyloric region holds about 30 mL of chyme; with each wave of contraction in the stomach about 3 mL of chyme is released into the duodenum. This process is regulated by the pyloric sphincter (Waugh & Grant 2006).

Digestion

Digestion in the stomach is controlled by several factors. The presence of food in the stomach stretches the stomach wall, activating stretch receptors and stimulating the release of gastric juice. The hormone gastrin is released by the stomach walls, also stimulating the release of gastric juice. The presence of food substances such as protein and caffeine further stimulates gastrin release. Waves of contraction in the stomach are increased by stretching of the stomach wall and by the presence of protein. However, low pH inhibits gastrin release. Both the cephalic and gastric phases of digestion can also be inhibited by emotional factors. The stomach is not involved in the main process of absorption, although some water, alcohol and certain medications such as aspirin are absorbed in the gastric phase.

The intestinal phase of digestion begins when chyme enters the duodenum. The main effect on gastric digestion of the entry of food into the duodenum is inhibitory. The enterogastric reflex, mediated via the medulla, leads to the inhibition of gastric secretion. Enterogastrone relates to any hormone secreted by the mucosa of the duodenum that inhibits the forward movement of the contents of chyme. The enterogastric reflex is one of the three extrinsic reflexes of the gastrointestinal tract. When it is stimulated the release of the hormone 'gastrin' from the G-cells in the antrum of the stomach is inhibited, thereby further inhibiting gastric motility and secretion of gastric acid. In addition, the presence of food in the duodenum stimulates the release of three hormones, namely secretin, cholecystokinin and gastric inhibitory peptide, all of which inhibit gastric juice secretion and reduce gastric motility (Figure 4.2).

The small intestine

Extending from the pyloric sphincter to the ileocaecal valve, the small intestine is responsible for the completion of digestion, the absorption of nutrients and the reabsorption of most of the water that enters the digestive tract. The duodenum is the first section of the small intestine and is approximately 25 cm in length. Secretions from the gall bladder and

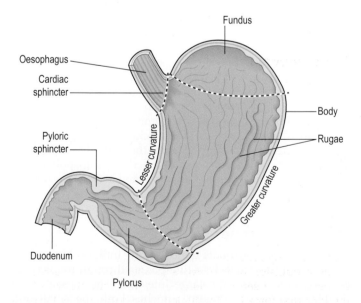

Figure 4.1 Longitudinal section of the stomach. (Reproduced with permission from Waugh & Grant 2006.)

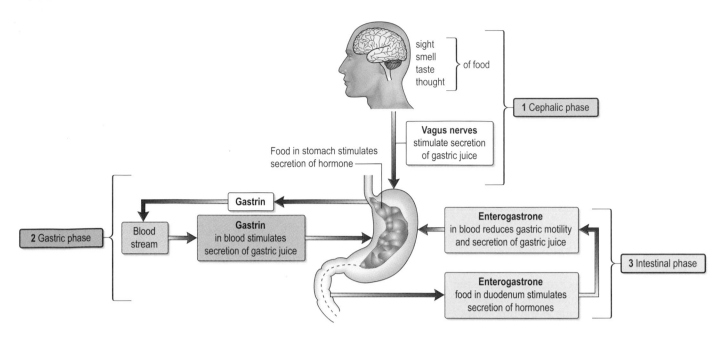

Figure 4.2 The phases of secretion of gastric juices.

the pancreas are mixed with chyme and enter the duodenum through the ampulla of Vater, the joining of the common bile duct and the pancreatic duct. The emptying of the gall bladder is regulated by the sphincter of Oddi (Waugh & Grant 2006).

The duodenum

In common with the remainder of the small intestine, the duodenum has a mucosal layer, a submucosal layer, a muscular layer and a peritoneal layer (Drake et al 2005). However, unlike the remainder of the small intestine, the duodenum is relatively immobile. Its regulatory role is fulfilled when the stimulus of chyme entering the duodenum triggers the enterogastric reflex as well as stimulating the release of gastrin, secretin, cholecystokinin and gastric inhibitory peptide. Secretin also stimulates the cells of the liver to secrete bile, and cholecystokinin stimulates the release of digestive enzymes by the small intestine.

Chyme is very acidic (with a pH of about 2) because of its high concentration of hydrochloric acid. When chyme enters the duodenum it becomes neutralised by the effect of alkaline bicarbonate released by the pancreas. The bile emulsifies fats in the chyme, breaking up fat globules into smaller particles. The enzymes of pancreatic juice can then begin to digest respective food substances in the duodenum. This action is continued as the chyme is passed down the small intestine (Waugh & Grant 2006).

The jejunum and ileum

The first two fifths of the small intestine after the duodenum is the jejunum, and the remaining three fifths, the ileum. Two types of movement, known as segmentation and peristalsis, mix and move food along the small intestine. Secretory cells of the mucosa of the small intestine release a slightly alkaline juice containing mainly water and mucus. The remaining enzymes of digestion in the GI tract are located on the microvilli, microscopic finger-like projections of the cell membrane.

The enzymes of the small intestine complete the digestion of all components of the diet, including protein, fat, carbohydrate and nucleic acids (Norton et al 2008).

Absorption of nutrients

Absorption takes place along the full length of the small intestine and 90% of all the products of digestion are absorbed here. The products of digestion are amino acids and peptides from protein, fatty acids and monoglycerides from fats, hexose sugars from carbohydrates, and pentose sugars and nitrogen-containing bases from nucleic acids. About 7.5 litres of water are secreted into the small intestine daily and 1.5 litres ingested. As only about 1 litre enters the large intestine, the major portion of the water is reabsorbed in the small intestine. Absorption occurs by two main processes: diffusion and active transport. Absorption takes place at the villi. Each villus contains an arteriole and a venule connected by a capillary network, and a central lacteal, a projection of the lymphatic system (Figure 4.3). Short-chain fatty acids, amino acids and carbohydrates are absorbed directly into the bloodstream. Triglycerides form structures called chylomicrons, which are also absorbed into the lacteals and then enter the bloodstream where the thoracic lymphatic duct empties into the left subclavian vein. Monosaccharides, amino acids, fatty acids and glycerol are actively transported into the villi. Disaccharides, dipeptides and tripeptides are also actively transported into the enterocytes and digestion is completed before transfer into the capillaries of the villi (Waugh & Grant 2006).

The large intestine

With most of the nutrients removed, the indigestible residue of food from the small intestine passes through the ileocaecal valve and enters the large intestine. The mesentery, a double layer of peritoneum, attaches both the small and large intestines to the rear wall of the abdomen and provides both with their blood supply.

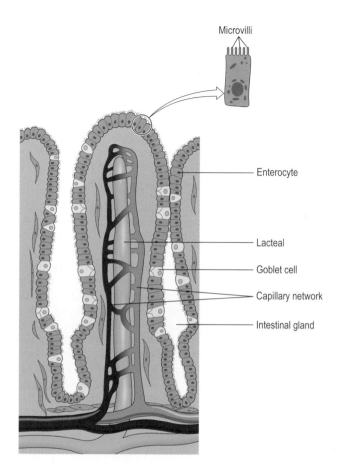

Figure 4.3 A highly magnified view of one complete villus in the intestine. (Reproduced with permission from Waugh & Grant 2006.)

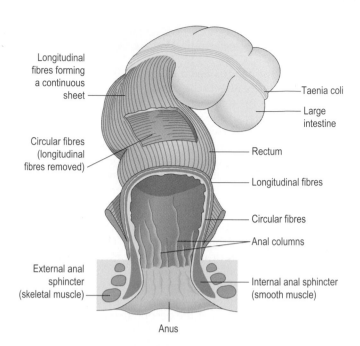

Figure 4.4 The arrangement of muscle fibres in the colon, rectum and anus (sections have been removed to show layers). (Reproduced with permission from Waugh & Grant 2006.)

The large intestine is divided into four portions: the ascending, transverse, descending and sigmoid colon. The curves joining the ascending with the transverse colon and the transverse with the descending colon are referred to as the hepatic and splenic flexures respectively. Two features can be identified near the ileocaecal valve: the caecum, a pouch below the ileocaecal valve, and the appendix, a finger-like projection of the caecum. The descending colon leads to the sigmoid colon, terminating in the rectum. Three muscular bands called the taeniae coli run the length of the large intestine. These maintain a slight longitudinal tension in the large intestine and give the colon its characteristic segmented appearance. The rectum stores food residue as faeces before expulsion via the anus. The anal canal opens externally at the anus, controls evacuation and has an internal anal sphincter of smooth muscle and an external anal sphincter of skeletal muscle (Drake et al 2005).

In common with the small intestine, the large intestine has mucosal, submucosal, muscular and peritoneal layers, but differs in appearance from the small intestine in that there are no villi. The large intestine is designed mainly for the absorption of water and the lubrication of food residue as it is passed by the mass action of food entering at the ileocaecal valve to the rectum. Any nutrients that enter the large intestine are broken down by commensal bacteria, causing the gases methane, hydrogen, carbon dioxide and sulphur dioxide to be produced. Food can sometimes take up to 24 h to pass through the large intestine.

Defaecation

When faeces reach the rectum, a reflex is initiated whereby stretch receptors in the wall of the rectum send signals to the brain informing it of the presence of faeces. However, defaecation can be suppressed until the time and place are appropriate. When it is appropriate to defaecate, the internal anal sphincter automatically relaxes and the external anal sphincter, under voluntary control, is relaxed. Intra-abdominal pressure is increased as the individual breathes in and holds the breath against a closed glottis (Valsalva's manoeuvre), and faeces are expelled from the rectum via the anal canal (Waugh & Grant 2006) (Figure 4.4).

DISORDERS OF THE GASTROINTESTINAL TRACT

Disorders of the mouth

The mouth and tongue are often examined during clinical examination, as local abnormalities or indications of disease elsewhere can often be detected in this manner. For example, a dry, furred tongue can indicate the presence of a digestive problem or dehydration.

Patients with gastrointestinal and liver disease require meticulous attention to oral hygiene as the mouth can be affected directly, as in Crohn's disease, and indirectly, as in vitamin and iron deficiency in malabsorption and GI haemorrhage. Patients on steroid and immunosuppressive therapy are also prone to infections of the mouth and oesophagus.

The principles of mouth care and the treatment of a range of disorders affecting the mouth and related structures are described in detail in Chapter 15. For further reading on oral care, see Nicol et al (2008).

Disorders of the oesophagus

Because the oesophagus has a relatively narrow lumen, any obstruction rapidly affects the passage of food. The two most common symptoms experienced by patients with disease of the oesophagus are dysphagia and pain. The term dysphagia refers to difficulty in swallowing. This can present in varying degrees, ranging from slight and intermittent difficulty in swallowing solid food to total occlusion of the oesophagus, preventing the patient even from swallowing saliva. Oesophageal pain can be extremely severe and should not be underestimated. There are three main presentations:

- A burning pain (known as 'heartburn') felt high in the epigastrium and behind the sternum. This is usually due to the reflux of gastric contents and sometimes radiates to the neck and to one or both arms.
- A deep, boring, gripping pain across the front of the chest which may radiate to the back, neck or arms. This is usually due to spasm of the oesophageal muscle and is similar in nature to the pain of angina pectoris (see Ch. 2).
- Pain behind the sternum on swallowing, especially hot liquids. This is usually due to oesophagitis.

Gastro-oesophageal reflux disease

Gastro-oesophageal reflux disease (GORD) is an increasingly prevalent condition where the reflux of the contents of stomach causes troublesome symptoms that can have a significant impact on the physical, social and emotional life quality of those living with it (Box 4.1). The prevalence of GORD worldwide is estimated to be between 5 and 20% with the highest incidence being found in Europe and the USA (van Baalen 2008).

Although there is considerable variation in the severity and frequency of symptoms, and less than half of those who have endoscopy show evidence of oesophageal injury, prolonged and severe reflux can lead to erosive oesophagitis, oesophageal ulcer, peptic stricture, haemorrhage, Barrett's columnar-lined oesophagus (CLO) (Box 4.2) and a predisposition to malignant changes and the development of oesophageal cancer (Morcom 2008).

Box 4.1 Information

Clinical features of GORD (Morcom 2008, Norton et al 2008)

- Heartburn
- Belching
- Regurgitation of food, acid or bile
- Asthma – commonly nocturnal, where the reflux can lead to a minimal inhalation of stomach contents
- Water brash (excessive production of saliva)
- Painful swallowing (odynophagia)
- Food sticking (dysphagia – difficulty in swallowing), resulting from oesophagitis or stricture
- Chest pain, which can be difficult to distinguish from angina

Box 4.2 Information

Barrett's columnar-lined oesophagus (CLO)

Barrett's columnar-lined oesophagus (CLO) is generally accepted to be a pre-malignant condition for oesophageal adenocarcinoma and has been defined as 'an oesophagus in which any portion of the normal squamous lining has been replaced by metaplastic columnar epithelium which is visible macroscopically' (British Society of Gastroenterology 2005.

PATHOPHYSIOLOGY AND RISK FACTORS

Normally, the action of swallowing stimulates the relaxation of the lower oesophageal sphincter (LOS), which permits the passage of food into the stomach. In GORD, however, there is prolonged or inappropriate relaxation of the LOS, which results in reflux of gastric contents into the oesophagus. Fox & Forgacs (2006) suggest that those with mild to moderate GORD do not necessarily have more transient LOS relaxations but structural changes at the gastro-oesophageal junction reduce the resistance to reflux during these events. Therefore, as structural changes become more marked the risk of reflux rises and the reflux volume increases, extending further up the oesophagus. As the stomach is highly acidic with a pH of 1–4, regurgitation of contents is abrasive to the oesophageal lining resulting in the characteristic symptoms of GORD.

Hiatus hernia

In those with severe GORD symptoms, a hiatus hernia, which is a condition whereby a portion of the stomach protrudes upwards into the chest through an opening in the diaphragm, is often present (Fox & Forgacs 2006). In this condition, a large amount of gastric contents pass unhindered into the hiatal sac with ensuing severe symptoms. Hiatus hernias occur most frequently from middle age onwards. They are four times more common in women than in men and are often found in association with obesity. However, they can also result from a congenital abnormality presenting in early infancy. Hiatus hernias are described as 'sliding' or 'rolling' (para-oesophageal), the former being the more common. In sliding hernias, the oesophageal sphincter mechanism is defective, causing reflux of acid-peptic stomach contents and, as their name suggests, the herniated stomach tends to slide back and forth into and out of the chest. In the less common 'rolling' or para-oesophageal hernia, the gastro-oesophageal junction remains where it belongs but part of the stomach is squeezed up beside the oesophagus. These hernias remain in the chest at all times.

Although the primary cause of GORD is the compromised functioning of the LOS, genetic, environmental, behavioural and co-morbid risk factors are thought to be associated with the development of the condition (Dent et al 2005). Whilst lifestyle factors such as smoking, alcohol consumption and drugs that impair sphincter pressure (anticholinergics, theophylline, nitrates, calcium channel blockers, progestogens, nicotine replacement therapy) do not cause GORD, they can worsen the symptoms. Obesity has also been associated with GORD, particularly where there is a tendency to consume larger meals and rich, energy-dense foods, which increase the risk of reflux. Although Dent et al (2005) found no clear association between certain foods and GORD, some patients report that fatty foods, citrus fruits, coffee, chocolate, etc. may trigger an episode and therefore they avoid them (Fox & Forgacs 2006). Reflux is also very common in pregnancy due to the effect of progesterone in relaxing the gastro-oesophageal sphincter smooth muscle and also the increased pressure on the stomach as the fetus grows.

Diagnosis

Traditionally, diagnosis of GORD focused on the notion of a continuous spectrum of disease and the presence of objective evidence of reflux and injury to the oesophagus (Fox & Forgacs 2006, Morcom 2008). For example, absence of oesophageal injury was associated with mild disease whilst Barrett's CLO was classified as a severe form of GORD. However, recent evidence suggests that this idea of progression from mild to severe disease is rarely seen and the new conception of GORD has its basis in a global definition that focuses on symptoms rather than injury. What this means is that while heartburn and regurgitation constitute the cardinal symptoms of GORD, evidence of oesophageal injury is not necessary to confirm a diagnosis. What is considered important is that treatment and management options are based on patients' reports of symptoms and the impact on their lives.

A significant outcome of this change is that pharmacological and lifestyle management are the first line of treatment and routine endoscopic investigation is not considered necessary for those who do not present with 'alarm' symptoms. However, urgent referral for endoscopic investigation is recommended (Box 4.3) in cases where alarm features are present. These include gastrointestinal bleeding, iron deficiency anaemia, unexplained and unintentional weight loss, progressive dysphagia, persistent vomiting, palpable epigastric mass, a family history of gastrointestinal cancer, previous documented peptic ulcer or suspicious imaging results (National Institute for Health and Clinical Excellence [NICE] 2005a).

Treatment options

Lifestyle modifications alone are not considered effective for the relief of GORD symptoms and are generally recommended as an adjunct to pharmacological therapy, which is the mainstay of non-surgical intervention. Nonetheless, based on the assumption that certain factors such as smoking, alcohol

> **Box 4.3 Information**
>
> ### Endoscopy in GI medicine
>
> Endoscopy refers to the visualisation of the interior of the body cavities and hollow organs by means of a flexible fibreoptic instrument (endoscope). The use of this technique has contributed greatly to diagnosis and therapy in many areas of medical practice. For use in the gastrointestinal tract, the endoscope is variously designed to view the oesophagus, the stomach, the duodenum, the colon and the rectum. It is also possible, by a modification of the gastroduodenoscope, to visualise the pancreatic and common bile duct; this is called endoscopic retrograde cholangiopancreatography (ERCP). Although most endoscopes are flexible, a rigid instrument may be used for a sigmoidoscopy. For further information see Cotton & Ackerman (2003).

> **Box 4.4 Reflection**
>
> ### Lifestyle choices and GORD
>
> Mrs Mary Smith, a 56-year-old, obese woman with a BMI of 35, is admitted to the endoscopy unit. She has been treated with PPIs for the last three months but her GORD symptoms recurred when her medication was stopped. She has been booked for an oesophagogastroduodenoscopy (OGD). On arrival to the unit Mrs Smith states she is very anxious about having this test.
>
> **Activity**
>
> - Reflect on what lifestyle choices may have impacted on Mrs Smith's symptoms.
> - See the website for Critical thinking question 4.1 in relation to this case.
>
> 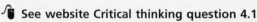 **See website Critical thinking question 4.1**

consumption and obesity can contribute to frequency and severity of symptoms, modifications are often recommended. Dietary adjustments such as avoiding alcohol and foods that appear to trigger symptoms are strategies adopted by patients. Avoiding large meals and eating several hours before going to bed is suggested. For those who are overweight or obese, weight loss can be effective in ameliorating symptoms, and elevating the head of the bed is also helpful for some (Morcom 2008). Smoking cessation is advised (Box 4.4).

In those with a hiatus hernia and whose symptoms are considered mild, additional advice and education include taking small meals more frequently, wearing loose clothing and avoiding bending over from the waist. Sleeping well supported by pillows is also helpful.

Pharmacological interventions

Pharmacological intervention forms the mainstay of treatment.

Proton pump inhibitors (PPIs) Those with reflux symptoms are given initial treatment with proton pump inhibitors (PPIs) for one month. PPIs (e.g. omeprazole, lansoprazole) are effective acid suppressants and heal reflux oesophagitis in many patients. There is a high rate of symptom recurrence in GORD when PPIs are discontinued, and when this happens long-term and maintenance therapy is required (van Baalen 2008). PPIs are considered to be safe and effective and are not associated with the development of abnormal cells or neoplasms (Fox & Forgacs 2006). In a minority of patients where PPI therapy is ineffective, altering the medication and dosage must be undertaken in order to achieve a level of symptom control.

Histamine H_2-receptor antagonists (H_2RAs) Although histamine H_2-receptor antagonists (H_2RAs) such as cimetidine and ranitidine also suppress acid, they are seen as less effective than PPIs in healing oesophagitis and maintaining remission from mucosal symptoms and injury (Fox & Forgacs 2006). However, they are sometimes used before bed if GORD symptoms are prominent at night.

Prokinetics such as metoclopramide and domperidone offer some symptom relief and healing of oesophagitis. They stimulate gastrointestinal motility, thus increasing gastric emptying, and so reduce the exposure to acid reflux. However, their impact is modest and their usefulness is limited by some unpleasant side-effects such as fatigue, headache, insomnia, confusion and vision changes. They also have the potential for interaction with other drugs such as narcotic analgesics, sedatives, hypnotics and tranquillisers and have been known to affect the absorption of digoxin and the rate of absorption of insulin.

Gastroprotective agents such as alginates and antacids (e.g. Gaviscon, Maalox Plus) are widely used because of their over the counter availability and they provide instant and temporary relief from symptoms. However, their value in symptom relief is extremely limited and they have no effect on the healing of oesophagitis (Morcom 2008).

Surgical interventions

The vast majority of patients with GORD respond to pharmacological therapy and lifestyle adjustments or modifications. However, for a minority they are ineffective and surgery is an option that offers a permanent resolution for symptoms. Surgery is also recommended for those who have volume reflux, respiratory symptoms (e.g. cough/asthma) and Barrett's CLO. Before surgery is considered, however, diagnostic investigations include visual assessment of the oesophagus (gastroscopy) in order to determine whether there is evidence of physical damage (oesophagitis, hiatus hernia, Barrett's CLO). In addition, 24-h oesophageal manometry and motility studies may be performed to establish the extent of the acid reflux and the severity of the disease and to identify those best suited to surgery (van Baalen 2008).

The purpose of anti-reflux surgery is to recreate the LOS and surgery is commonly performed laparoscopically as this enables a more rapid recovery and reduced hospital stay. It is also associated with reduced pain as there is no abdominal or chest incision and improved respiratory function postoperatively (van Baalen 2008). Essentially, laparoscopic anti-reflux surgery (LARS) mobilises the lower end of the oesophagus, reduces the oesophageal hiatus using sutures, and wraps the fundus of the stomach partially or completely around it (fundoplication).

Nursing management and health promotion: GORD

Most patients who present with GORD are managed in primary and secondary care settings. In many instances the patient may be managed solely by their GP. However, community or practice nurses may have the opportunity to provide information and education in order to ensure the patient understands the role of medication management. Taking time to assess the patient's understanding will not only ensure medication is taken appropriately but is also likely to enhance patient adherence to any regimen. Health promotion may involve educating the patient about lifestyle modifications such as dietary choices and management and smoking cessation.

PRE-OPERATIVE MANAGEMENT

Preparation for LARS surgery will be as for elective abdominal surgery on the GI tract as described in Chapter 26 (see p. 695). In addition, the patient must be given information about the surgery and the risks associated with it. The short- and long-term effects of the surgery and the changes in diet that are required should be explained in sufficient detail so that the patient has a clear understanding of the implications and is making an informed choice to undergo the procedure.

POSTOPERATIVE MANAGEMENT

Those who have LARS surgery normally remain in hospital for approximately 48 h post surgery. Nursing management in the postoperative period centres on early detection of and minimising the risk of complications (Box 4.5).

Monitoring of vital signs (temperature, pulse, respirations, blood pressure, oxygen saturation), assessment and management of postoperative pain and nausea and vomiting are central in reducing the potential for complications. Vital sign monitoring should be undertaken half-hourly in the immediate postoperative period, gradually reducing the frequency to 4-hourly if the patient's vital signs remain within normal parameters.

Pain assessment and documentation should be undertaken using a pain assessment tool such as the visual analogue scale (see Ch. 19). Opiates are commonly used to control pain and are usually administered intravenously. Should the patient have patient controlled analgesia (PCA), it does not remove the need for evaluation of the effectiveness of pain relief. This should be undertaken at the same time as vital sign monitoring. Sedation level must also be monitored. The patient should also be given antiemetics intravenously as it is important to minimise the risk of nausea and vomiting. The patient remains nil by mouth on the day of surgery, and monitoring for signs of dysphagia is undertaken. To maintain hydration, intravenous fluids are administered. Oral fluids and a liquid diet are normally introduced the day after surgery.

Dietary advice

If the patient's vital signs are within normal limits, signs of dysphagia are absent and postoperative pain is well controlled, the patient is discharged with written information about lifestyle and dietary modifications. Early dysphagia is common following LARS and patients are advised to adhere to a liquid diet initially. As symptoms resolve and patients no longer experience food sticking they can progress towards a normal diet. In a small number of cases, symptoms persist and may require oesophageal dilatation or surgical revision of the fundoplication.

Box 4.5 Information

Complications and side-effects of LARS (van Baalen 2008)

Complications of LARS	Side-effects of LARS
Dysphagia (early and late)	Inability to belch
Para-oesophageal hernia	Early feeling of fullness
Gastrointestinal perforation	Bloating
Pneumothorax	Increased flatulence
Pulmonary embolism	
Injury to major vessels	

Patients are advised to eat small, frequent meals in the first few weeks following surgery to counter early feelings of fullness. This feeling usually lessens over time. Patients who have this type of surgery also lose the ability to belch and therefore have a tendency to increased bloating and flatulence. They should be advised to chew their food thoroughly and avoid excessive swallowing while chewing. Eating large meals should be discouraged and 'fizzy' drinks are not recommended. Nausea, vomiting and coughing should be prevented where possible as this increases abdominal pressure and may result in herniation of the stomach into the chest. Antiemetics are used to reduce this risk. Additionally, patients should avoid heavy lifting, straining and excessive exercise in the early postoperative period.

Carcinoma of the oesophagus

The majority of carcinomas of the oesophagus occur in older people with a male to female ratio of 2:1 (Cancer Research UK 2009a). The incidence of oesophageal cancer has increased and according to Cancer Research UK (2009a) it is the ninth most common cancer in the UK. This form of cancer is extremely unpleasant and distressing, with surgery on its own or in conjunction with chemotherapy offering the only possibility of cure. However, the prognosis remains poor and the 5-year survival rate is less than 30%. This has been associated with the late presentation of symptoms in this condition (Cancer Research UK 2009a).

PATHOPHYSIOLOGY AND RISK FACTORS

Squamous cell carcinoma and adenocarcinoma make up the majority of malignant oesophageal tumours. Globally, squamous cell carcinoma remains the most common, although the incidence of adenocarcinoma has been rising in recent years (Griffin & Dunn 2008). This is thought to be associated with the increase in chronic acid and bile reflux arising from lifestyle factors such as those cited below, which causes dysplasia (abnormal maturation/development of cells) of the epithelium of the oesophagus. Squamous cell carcinoma generally occurs in the middle and upper part of the oesophagus, whilst adenocarcinoma tends to arise in the lower third. The primary tumour can spread locally, up or down the oesophagus, and through its wall to the trachea, bronchi, pleura, aorta and lymph vessels. Distant metastases may occur in the liver and lungs.

Several predisposing factors for oesophageal cancer have been identified:

- Lifestyle factors such as smoking, alcohol consumption and a diet high in fat (van Baalen 2009).
- Barrett's CLO is associated with a 40-fold increased risk of developing adenocarcinoma of the oesophagus.
- Achalasia of the cardia (an obstruction that develops in the terminal oesophagus just proximal to the cardio-oesophageal junction and the upper oesophagus becomes dilated and filled with retained food), gastro-oesophageal reflux, Paterson–Kelly (Plummer–Vinson) syndrome and previous trauma are all associated with an increased risk of oesophageal cancer.
- A high incidence of squamous cell carcinoma of the oesophagus in developing countries has been linked to poverty and malnutrition (van Baalen 2009).

Clinical features of oesophageal cancer

The most prominent presenting feature is dysphagia. In the initial stages, this symptom will occur only occasionally and the individual will probably not seek medical help. However, as the tumour increases in size it occludes the lumen of the oesophagus. Dyspepsia after eating can also occur. Although pain on swallowing or reflux is less common, their occurrence tends to indicate a spread of the cancer. Poor oral intake due to dysphagia and cancer cachexia causes weight loss. Many patients develop a cough due to pressure on the bronchus, and a chest infection due to aspiration of oesophageal contents. Haematemesis (vomiting of blood which may appear bright red or dark and blackish) and melaena (abnormally dark tarry faeces containing blood) occasionally occur as a result of bleeding from an ulcerated tumour. The patient will rapidly become emaciated due to difficulty in eating and drinking, and skilled nursing care is essential to comfort and support the patient in coping with these and other effects of the illness.

Diagnosis

Where oesophageal carcinoma is suspected an urgent referral for gastrointestinal endoscopy is recommended (NICE 2005b) Disease staging is undertaken using computed tomography (CT) and endoscopic ultrasound (EUS). According to van Baalen (2009), contrast-enhanced spiral CT scanning of the chest and abdomen provides information regarding the location and size of the primary tumour, whether or not it is operable and whether or not metastatic disease exists. If the tumour is deemed to be operable EUS is used to assess and stage the tumour. Bronchoscopy may be performed if the tumour is in the upper zone. This will identify whether the bronchus has been invaded and will have a bearing on treatment and care.

Treatment options

Despite the generally poor prognosis, there are a number of treatment options for those with oesophageal cancer. These include: surgery and chemotherapy; surgery alone; endoscopic resection; chemotherapy; chemoradiotherapy and palliative care. These options depend primarily on the location, histology and spread of the tumour as well as patient characteristics and the existence of co-morbidities. Each patient is carefully assessed as to the extent of the disease before a treatment plan is chosen and commenced. Surgery remains the standard treatment where the tumour is localised or operable. However, chemotherapy is now commonly administered pre-operatively as it has been demonstrated not only to improve outcome in respect of survival but also helps in reducing the tumour size, improving tumour-related symptoms, and improving nutritional status and weight gain (van Baalen 2009). Chemoradiotherapy is administered if the tumour is radiosensitive, i.e. a squamous cell carcinoma. This treatment is usually used for tumours of the upper third of the oesophagus, but is also sometimes used for the relief of pain. For those with inoperable carcinoma of the oesophagus, the focus of palliative treatment is on symptom relief. Malignant dysphagia may be relieved by oesophageal dilatation, endoscopic or open insertion of a stent, or tumour ablation with laser, heat, diathermy or injection of cytotoxic substances (Griffin & Dunn 2008).

Nursing management and health promotion: oesophageal carcinoma

Nursing management will depend on whether treatment is surgical or non-surgical.

SURGICAL: PRE-OPERATIVE MANAGEMENT

In addition to the standard pre-operative preparation for all patients who are undergoing gastrointestinal surgery (see Ch. 26) there are particular considerations that must be attended to in the patient who is to have an oesophagectomy. There are several types of oesophagectomy (Box 4.6), the choice of which is determined by the location and size of the tumour as well as the patient's age, build and level of fitness to tolerate what is physically demanding surgery. Oesophagectomy is not only procedurally difficult but, as it involves the cardiovascular system, carries with it a significant morbidity (van Baalen 2009). Therefore, thorough physiological assessment and preparation must be undertaken in order to minimise the impact for the patient.

In patients who are experiencing nutritional deficits due to dysphagia, nutritional assessment using a tool such as the Malnutrition Universal Screening Tool (MUST) (Elia 2003) is fundamental and it is essential that any deficiencies are addressed pre-operatively. This can be undertaken by encouraging the patient to sip nutritional supplements or, where deemed necessary, through the use of fine-bore nasogastric tube feeding.

Psychological and emotional preparation is extremely important for these patients and their families. Patients should be educated as to what to expect in the immediate postoperative period but should also be counselled as to the impact on lifestyle and quality of life in the medium and long term.

POSTOPERATIVE MANAGEMENT

In addition to standard postoperative care (see Ch. 26) there are specific management considerations for patients following oesophagectomy. Given the significant risk of a number of complications, patients are nursed in intensive care for approximately 2 days after surgery. Intensive cardiopulmonary monitoring is undertaken as the risk of respiratory complications is high. Physiotherapy, humidified oxygen for several days and nursing the patient in a semi-upright position are some additional strategies that are used to reduce the incidence of respiratory complications. Given the nature and complexity of the surgery, pain intensity is high following oesophagectomy.

Box 4.6 Information

Types of oesophagectomy (for further information see van Baalen 2009)

- Two-phase subtotal oesophagectomy via a right thoracotomy (Ivor-Lewis)
- Three-phase subtotal oesophagectomy (McKeown)
- Left-sided subtotal oesophagectomy
- Transhiatal oesophagectomy

Failure to adequately control pain can contribute to poor inspiration and ventilation, which increases the likelihood of respiratory problems. Thus, epidural analgesia (see Ch. 19) is the most favoured method of pain control (van Baalen 2009). Careful assessment and monitoring of the patient's wound(s) and wound drains must also be undertaken.

Nutrition

Oral fluids and diet are withheld for the first 7 days following surgery. The patient will have a nasogastric tube on free drainage to ensure the stomach remains decompressed in order to facilitate healing. In order to combat further nutritional depletion, enteral feeding is commenced using a feeding tube such as a jejunostomy that can be inserted at the time of surgery. Feeding continues until the patient is able to take sufficient oral intake. Fluids are given intravenously whilst the patient is nil by mouth. Careful monitoring and accurate recording of fluids and enteral feeding are required throughout. Van Baalen (2009) outlines the need for a water-soluble barium swallow prior to recommencing oral intake, to ensure there is no leak from the anastomosis. Once a leak has been discounted the patient will commence on fluids only and gradually progress to a soft and finally a normal diet.

Psychological support

In addition, in the initial postoperative period the nurse will be required to provide considerable assistance to the patient with meeting their activities of living. The patient can expect to remain in hospital for up to 2 weeks. However, convalescence and recovery are slow and it can take the patient several months to adjust to the negative physical, psychological and social effects of the surgery. Verschuur et al (2006) found that physical issues were perceived by patients as most problematic and were cited as early satiety (fullness), eating problems, fatigue, constipation/diarrhoea, pain and weight loss. Because of physical problems, patients can find it difficult to return to normal social activity. Fear of a return of the cancer or the development of metastases tends to cause patients to have low moods associated with an unpredictable future. Patients can also feel frustrated at being dependent on others or being unable to resume normal activities.

It is essential therefore that continued support either through specialist nurse follow-up and/or community nurse should form part of the overall care of patients following oesophagectomy. Education and advice regarding strategies for management of physical problems should continue in the follow-up period. Moreover, patients should be given the opportunity to discuss the psychological and social implications of the surgery. Given the ultimately poor prognosis, it is important that patients and their families feel supported throughout.

NON-SURGICAL MANAGEMENT

Many patients with this form of cancer will be very distressed and emaciated, their life dominated by the symptoms of the disease and by the thought that there is no cure. However, by adopting a caring and sensitive approach, the nurse can do much to alleviate the patient's physical and emotional suffering (Hodgson 2006).

Nutrition and weight loss

Some patients experience significant weight loss, for example several kilograms over a period of months (Nicklin & Blazeby 2003). Weight should be recorded weekly and noted in relation to pre-illness weight. An accurate account of daily dietary intake should be recorded with the dietitian's help. Consistency of food is important and the patient should avoid large pieces of meat, 'stringy' foods such as oranges, and 'stodgy' foods such as scones and pastries, as these food choices may lead to blocking of the oesophageal lumen. The patient should be encouraged to take fluids with meals and to chew foods thoroughly, for example, twice as long as normal. In order to ensure adequate nutrition it may be necessary to provide a liquidised diet.

As the disease advances, the patient will be able to swallow liquids only and should be supplied with a variety of nutritionally supplemented liquids. Supplementary drinks are now available in a variety of sweet and savoury flavours. Eventually, total dysphagia will occur. It cannot be overemphasised how distressing this is for the patient and family. See Chapter 21 for more information on nutritional care.

Oesophageal stent

In the case of a bolus obstruction, it may be necessary to perform an endoscopy to relieve the obstruction. The insertion of a stent is often used to relieve dysphagic symptoms. The oesophagus is dilated at endoscopy and the tube inserted. Following this procedure, the patient will lose the action of the gastro-oesophageal sphincter and will therefore suffer from reflux. The head of the bed should be elevated at all times. The patient will be prescribed an H_2 blocking agent, e.g. cimetidine, to help prevent reflux oesophagitis. This should be given in syrup form. Encouragement should be given to eat a semi-solid diet and to chew food well. The patient should take carbonated drinks, e.g. soda or tonic water, with every meal as this helps keep the stent clear.

Immediately after the insertion of a stent, the patient may suffer quite severe discomfort and analgesics may be necessary. A chest X-ray will be performed and the patient should not be allowed any food or fluid until this has been done in case perforation of the oesophagus has occurred.

Pain

In the earlier stages of oesophageal cancer, if pain is present, mild analgesics such as paracetamol given in dispersible form may be all that is necessary. As the disease advances, opiates may be required. Initially, the patient may be able to swallow a morphine suspension, but if total occlusion of the oesophagus occurs, it may be necessary to give the morphine by injection. The most effective and convenient way of administering this is by the subcutaneous route via using a syringe driver. This delivers a constant level of opioid and allows for a 'booster' dose to be given as necessary, to avoid the distress of breakthrough pain. If circumstances allow, the patient will be able to be at home with a community nurse visiting daily to change the syringe. If necessary, an antiemetic can also be added to the syringe driver.

Time must be set aside to allow these patients to express their thoughts, fears and anger, which may be directed towards either the distressing nature of their symptoms or the poor prognosis of the disease, or perhaps both. In the final stages of the disease, every effort should be made to allow the patient to die in the environment of their own choosing. If the patient's choice is to remain at home, a Macmillan or Marie Curie nurse can provide the support and care required.

Disorders of the stomach and duodenum

Disorders of the stomach and duodenum are the most common organic disorders of the GI tract. They are considered together here because disorders of one organ commonly affect the other.

Gastritis

Gastritis is an inflammatory condition of the stomach that may be acute, a sudden inflammation of the lining of the stomach, or chronic, inflammation of the lining of the stomach that occurs gradually and persists for a long time.

PATHOPHYSIOLOGY AND RISK FACTORS

Acute gastritis is commonly caused by injury to the protective mucosal barrier by ingestion of an irritant such as drugs (aspirin, ibuprofen, indomethacin), chemicals (alcohol), or *Helicobacter pylori*, which is an infection that can cause pain, nausea, vomiting and inflammation. Chronic gastritis can be found in patients with pernicious anaemia, autoimmune disorders, chronic alcohol abuse, peptic ulceration and gastric cancer, and following gastric surgery. Chronic gastritis is usually classified as Types A–C. Type A (fundal) is rare and is associated with hypersensitivity or autoimmune responses, while *Helicobacter pylori* is a major causative factor in Type B (chronic antral gastritis). Type C is drug related and usually caused by non-steroidal inflammatory medication (NSAIDs).

Clinical features

The outstanding presenting symptom in gastritis is abdominal pain, either before or after the consumption of food. Other common symptoms include epigastric tenderness, indigestion, flatulence, nausea and vomiting. Less common features include malaena, haemetemesis, weight loss and iron-deficiency anaemia (Banning 2006). However, in chronic gastritis, the patient is often asymptomatic. Where symptoms are present, these are the same as those found with acute gastritis, pain being associated with eating and often being described as 'indigestion'.

Diagnosis

Diagnosis is made endoscopically by gastric biopsy. *Helicobacter pylori* is found in the biopsy of many patients with chronic gastritis.

Treatment options

An antacid may be prescribed to relieve discomfort and an H_2 blocker such as cimetidine prescribed to prevent histamine from stimulating the gastric parietal cells to secrete hydrochloric acid. Most important is dietary advice, as the patient should avoid causative agents such as alcohol and highly spiced foods. If the patient is found to have *Helicobacter pylori*, combined/triple therapy of antibiotics and proton pump inhibitors (PPIs) will be commenced (see below).

▷ Nursing management and health promotion: gastritis

In the very acute stage, if vomiting is present, an antiemetic will be prescribed and intravenous fluid replacement therapy may be necessary for a short time. Frequent mouthwashes will promote patient comfort and an appropriate diet should be gradually reintroduced. The opportunity should be taken to explore the patient's dietary habits and to promote a healthy eating pattern. This is particularly important where the problem of alcohol abuse has been identified.

Peptic ulcer

Peptic ulceration is a common gastrointestinal disorder that can affect up to 15% of the population at any one time. A peptic ulcer occurs in those parts of the digestive tract that are exposed to gastric secretions, namely the stomach and duodenum. In the past, peptic ulcer disease was thought to be a chronic relapsing condition that required long-term acid suppression therapy and often major surgical intervention. There was also an associated mortality due to major gastro-intestinal haemorrhage and development of gastric cancer. The identification of the *Helicobacter pylori* bacterium by Marshall and Warren in 1984, and its association with peptic ulcer disease, radically altered the management of this condition from the 1990s, especially with the shift in focus in the NHS from secondary to primary care.

PATHOPHYSIOLOGY AND RISK FACTORS

Peptic ulcer formation requires both the presence of gastric acid and damage to the mucosal defence barrier. *H. pylori* is known to be a major factor in causing this damage and is present in over 95% of all patients with duodenal ulcers and 80–90% of those with gastric ulcers (Banning 2006). Gastric irritant medications such as aspirin and non-steroidal anti-inflammatories (NSAIDs) are also known to cause mucosal damage. Cigarette smoking is considered to be a causative influence in the development of peptic ulcers and there is growing evidence that smoking prevents the healing of gastric and duodenal ulcers (Haslett et al 2002). The exact mechanisms by which this occurs are not clear, but it is known that long-term smoking increases gastric secretion and interferes with the actions of H_2-receptor antagonists.

The gastric mucosa is protected, in part, by being buffered by food but erratic dietary habits may contribute to ulcer formation. There is conflicting evidence as to whether emotional factors such as stress and anxiety are also causative factors.

In *H. pylori* infection, the bacteria burrow beneath the mucosal layer and release a toxin that results in a local inflammatory and systemic immune response. Consequently there is inhibition of the release of somatostatin, a gastric hormone that inhibits gastric acid formation, and oversecretion results. *H. pylori* survives in this acid climate by enzymatically creating an alkaline microenvironment.

Chronic peptic ulcers penetrate through the mucosa to the muscle layers and may damage blood vessels, causing bleeding. In the duodenum, they are found immediately beyond the pylorus and in 10–15% of cases are multiple. The resulting fibrosis can lead to pyloric stenosis, which in turn can lead to gastric outlet obstruction. Gastric ulcers are found on the lesser curvature of the stomach in 90% of cases.

Clinical features

The person with a chronic peptic ulcer will describe a pattern of episodic pain and dyspepsia. Pain is a classic symptom and is described as a burning or boring pain in the epigastrium; often patients point directly to where the pain is felt. The pain is sometimes more diffuse or radiates through to the back. Patients sometimes experience 'water brash', which is saliva filling the mouth.

While studies show the relationship to food and mealtimes is variable, the person with a duodenal ulcer is more likely to feel pain and 'hunger feelings' about 2–3 h after a meal, whereas with a gastric ulcer pain is felt about 30–60 min after a meal and is not relieved by more food. Sometimes patients admit to inducing vomiting in an attempt to relieve the pain. Persistent non-induced vomiting of large amounts indicates an obstruction to the pylorus: pyloric stenosis. Other common features are belching and regurgitation which causes heartburn.

Diagnosis

An accurate diagnosis of peptic ulceration is made by endoscopy and/or barium meal. A full blood count is taken for haemoglobin estimation. Diagnosis of *H. pylori* infection is commonly made using the non-invasive ^{13}C-urea breath test. *H. pylori* produces urease as a source of protection from the harmful effects of gastric hydrochloric acid. The breath test detects isotopic carbon dioxide after ingestion of radiocarbon-labelled urea. The *H. pylori* enzyme splits the carbon from the urea. It is then carried as carbon dioxide via the blood to the lungs, where it can be detected in exhaled breath. This test is specific and has 80–90% sensitivity as no other bacterium is known to produce the urease enzyme. Moreover, the test can be undertaken in a GP's surgery and reduces patient discomfort and distress associated with an endoscopy.

Alternatively, diagnosis of *H. pylori* infection can be made by blood or serum tests for antibodies, and at endoscopy by taking a biopsy from the stomach lining and subjecting it to the rapid urease test, which detects the enzyme that *H. pylori* produces.

Treatment options

Treatment is dependent on the cause and severity of the ulcer. Removal of the causative factor followed by healing of the ulcer is the main aim of treatment, e.g. eradication therapy in *H. pylori* or discontinuation of NSAIDs or aspirin, followed by acid-suppressing medication.

Advice should be given about avoiding known aggravating factors such as smoking and erratic dietary patterns. Patient adherence to medication regimens is crucial to the success of *H. pylori* eradication and ulcer healing. Therefore, patient education is essential (Box 4.7).

Box 4.7 Reflection

Identifying priorities of care for the patient with a duodenal ulcer

Mr R, who lives alone, has been diagnosed as having a duodenal ulcer. He is 54 years old. He has lost a lot of weight over the last few months as a result of vomiting and does not eat much now. He is very thin and is also very anxious. He admits that he smokes 30–40 cigarettes a day and has difficulty sleeping.

Activity

- Reflect on what the priorities of care may be for Mr R.

Pharmacological therapy may include:

- A proton pump inhibitor (PPI), e.g. omeprazole, to inhibit the release of hydrochloric acid from the parietal cells.
- H2-receptor antagonists, e.g. cimetidine and ranitidine. These assist in ulcer healing by preventing histamine from stimulating the gastric parietal cells to secrete hydrochloric acid.
- Antacids for the relief of dyspepsia. Many preparations are based on magnesium and may result in a degree of diarrhoea.
- Misoprostol 2–4 times a day. Misoprostol inhibits gastric acid secretion by acting directly on the parietal cells. It is also used to prevent the gastric damage that can occur from long-term use of NSAIDs.
- Where the existence of *H. pylori* is confirmed, eradication therapy (combined/triple therapy) is the first-line treatment. It is given for a period of 7 days and consists of:
  - a proton pump inhibitor (e.g. lansoprazole/ omeprazole) twice daily in conjunction with two antibiotics, commonly:
  - clarithromycin three times a day and/or
  - amoxicillin three times daily and/or
  - metronidazole three times daily.

In patients with penicillin allergy, it is common practice to use clarithromycin instead of amoxicillin. Substitution is also necessary where bacterial resistance is suspected, particularly to metronidazole (>25%). This regimen is effective in eradicating *H. pylori* in 75–90% of cases and can be assessed by a resolution of the symptoms and confirmed with a repeat ^{13}C-urea breath test. If the test is still positive a further course of eradication therapy should be given but with different antibiotics.

In some cases of *H. pylori* antisecretory treatment (proton pump inhibitors or H_2-receptor antagonists) is continued for 4–8 weeks to ensure ulcer healing. Long-term acid-lowering therapy may be required if there are complicating factors such as NSAID therapy. Confirmation of ulcer healing should be undertaken by a repeat endoscopy. For further information, see the European Helicobacter Study Group (2000) and Banning (2006).

Surgical intervention may be necessary for patients with peptic ulcer and the indications are as follows:

- failure to respond to medical therapy
- recurrence
- development of complications such as perforation, haemorrhage and pyloric stenosis.

The aim of surgical intervention is to reduce acid and pepsin secretion. This is achieved by interrupting the vagus nerve or by resection of the gastric acid-producing section of the stomach.

Nursing management and health promotion: peptic ulcer

Since the introduction of H_2-receptor antagonists in the 1970s and with the identification of *H. pylori*, surgery for peptic ulceration is rarely necessary and is used only for complications. Although the incidence of perforation is decreasing, duodenal ulcers perforate more often than gastric ulcers and usually into the peritoneal sac causing peritonitis. Surgery is performed to close the perforation and drain the abdomen. In recurrent uncontrolled haemorrhage the bleeding vessel is ligated. Conservative management using nasogastric suction, intravenous fluids and antibiotics is occasionally used in the elderly and very sick patients.

PRE-OPERATIVE MANAGEMENT

The patient who is to undergo an elective procedure may be admitted 1 day prior to surgery or, if otherwise healthy, may be requested to attend a pre-admission clinic. This allows time for medical examination to be made regarding the individual's fitness for the operation and a general anaesthetic. A blood sample is required for grouping and cross-matching in case blood transfusion is required.

A full nursing assessment is made and a care plan formulated to meet the specific needs identified and to fulfil standard pre-operative nursing requirements (see Ch. 26). Explanations are given of the timescale for the preparation that will take place. If the patient is a smoker, the importance of smoking cessation is emphasised and support to do so is offered.

Preparation of the GI tract will include nil orally for 4–6 h pre-operatively. On the morning of the operation, the patient is prepared for theatre. A nasogastric tube is passed perioperatively. Prior to emergency surgery, regular vital signs recordings are made in order to detect any deterioration in the patient's condition. Analgesics are given for pain relief, and clear, concise explanations are given to the patient and the relatives regarding treatment.

POSTOPERATIVE MANAGEMENT

On the patient's return to the ward, the nurse will monitor and/or observe the following:

- Airway, respiratory rate, skin colour, blood pressure, pulse, temperature, oxygen saturation level and bleeding/drainage from the wound and the wound drain if present. Careful monitoring of these is important during the first 24–48 h, decreasing in frequency as haemodynamic stability is regained.
- Nasogastric aspirate. The nasogastric tube is usually left on free drainage between aspirations to allow air to escape. The aspirate should be observed for colour and amount. Normally the volume of aspirate reduces and bowel sounds are heard within 24–48 h. Should large amounts of

aspirate continue, this would indicate that absorption from the stomach is not occurring; it may also indicate the onset of paralytic ileus (see Ch. 26). Care should be taken that the nasogastric tube is positioned comfortably and well supported. Nasal care is given as required.

- Intravenous infusion and cannula site. The intravenous infusion must be maintained as prescribed, to preserve fluid and electrolyte balance and to prevent dehydration while oral fluids are not being taken.
- Urinary output. Renal function is a good indicator of tissue perfusion (see Ch. 18).

Nutrition and hydration

Fluids are withheld for at least 24 h, after which period, if bowel sounds have returned, sips of water or ice chips may be given. Fluids may then be given at hourly intervals, beginning with 30 mL and gradually increasing until free amounts of fluid are well tolerated. Light, easily digested food is gradually introduced and the patient is encouraged to eat, but is asked to avoid drinking fluids for at least 30 min after meals (see 'dumping syndrome' below). Oral hygiene is also important and the patient's mouth should be kept clean and moist using mouthwashes or by brushing the teeth if the patient can tolerate this.

Mobilisation

Following surgery, patients should be encouraged to sit up, get out of bed and take a few steps as soon as possible. They should also be encouraged to breathe deeply and cough regularly to clear the lungs of anaesthetic gases and excess mucus. These measures will help to prevent chest infection. Regular gentle leg activity, even when in bed, can also help to prevent the development of deep vein thrombosis. Adequate analgesia and holding the wound firmly when moving or coughing will encourage the patient to cooperate actively with postoperative therapy.

Dumping syndrome (rapid gastric emptying)

Dumping syndrome is a postoperative complication of gastric surgery that may occur following eating. It can be separated into early and late forms according to how soon it occurs after eating a meal. Dumping syndrome occurs when the undigested contents of the stomach are transported or 'dumped' too quickly into the small intestine. The sudden emptying of hyperosmolar solutions into the small bowel results in rapid distension of the jejunal loop anastomosed to the stomach and a withdrawal of water from the circulating blood volume into the jejunum to dilute the high concentration of electrolytes and sugars. Symptoms of early dumping include nausea, vomiting, bloating, cramping, diarrhoea, dizziness and fatigue. They tend to occur within 10–15 min of eating and usually settle within 30–60 min. Symptoms of late dumping include weakness, sweating and dizziness. Many people have both types (Norton et al 2008).

In order to delay stomach emptying and minimise the occurrence of dumping symptoms, patients should be educated to eat with their head at a 15–45 degree elevation. They should eat small meals more frequently and where possible these should be of a dry consistency. Fluids should be consumed up to 1 h before or after eating but should not be taken with meals. Concentrated sources of carbohydrate such as high-energy snacks and drinks should be avoided but fat can be consumed as tolerated. After meals patients should lie down for 20–30 min or until symptoms subside. If symptoms persist, changes in dietary intake and further surgery may eventually be indicated.

Discharge planning

Patients who have undergone surgery for peptic ulceration are generally fit to be discharged within a week of the operation. However, older patients and those with concurrent disease may need a longer period in hospital. Therefore, it is important for the nurse to be fully aware of the patient's social circumstances so that from the time of admission adequate preparation for discharge can be made and potential problems anticipated. Early communication with the patient's family or friends is essential in planning for discharge.

An outpatient follow-up appointment may be arranged to ensure that a satisfactory recovery has been achieved, to discuss any ongoing management and to monitor the patient's rehabilitation. The GP is always given details of the patient's surgery and discharge and of any special aftercare that may be required. If continuing care of the wound is required, this should be arranged with the community nursing team or practice nurse prior to discharge.

Complications of peptic ulceration

The three major complications of peptic ulcer are:

- haemorrhage
- perforation
- pyloric stenosis.

See the website for the management of the complications of peptic ulceration.

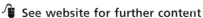 **See website for further content**

Carcinoma of the stomach

Gastric carcinomas are the seventh most common cancer in men in the UK and the 14th most common in women (Cancer Research UK 2009b) although the incidence has more than halved since the 1970s. The highest incidence is in eastern Asia and the lowest in western and northern Africa. Ninety-five per cent of gastric cancers are in those over the age of 50. Although the incidence of H. pylori is declining, it remains a major cause of gastric cancer. Smoking is also associated with the condition in approximately 1 in 5 people in Europe (Cancer Research UK 2009b). Consuming a diet high in salt and carbohydrates and low in fat, fresh fruit and vegetables is thought to predispose to gastric cancer; fruit and vegetables and high dietary vitamin C seem to have a protective effect (Hicks 2001). Having a parent or sibling with gastric cancer also increases the risk as does pernicious anaemia, chronic gastritis and gastric surgery.

PATHOPHYSIOLOGY AND RISK FACTORS

Gastric carcinomas are almost always adenocarcinomas derived from the mucus-secreting cells of the gastric glands; 60% occur at the pylorus or in the antrum, 20–30% in the body of the stomach and 5–20% in the cardia. The tumour spreads along the gastric wall to the duodenum and oesophagus and through the wall to the peritoneum. Adjacent organs become infiltrated. Metastatic spread may occur locally to neighbouring organs within the peritoneal cavity, or via the lymphatic or blood vessels to the liver, lungs and bones. The 5-year survival rate varies noticeably according to the stage of the cancer with advanced disease having a rate as low as 10% in Western countries (Wan & Allum 2008).

Clinical features

In the initial stages, symptoms do not differ significantly from indigestion or a feeling of having an 'upset stomach'. Individuals report feeling full or distended after eating. Common symptoms include anorexia, loss of weight and epigastric pain. These are often tolerated despite the distress they cause, with the result that there may be considerable delay before the patient seeks medical help. Nausea and vomiting may also occur whilst weakness, anaemia, retrosternal back pain, darkened stool or melaena have also been reported. By the time the person seeks medical help the disease may be well advanced and may have spread to adjacent organs. Tumours that are located in the cardia or fundus of the stomach can cause dysphagia among other symptoms (Hicks 2001). If a tumour obstructs the pylorus the individual will experience dramatic weight loss and dehydration and is likely to vomit small amounts of undigested food on a regular basis.

Diagnosis

Diagnosis can be made by medical history, clinical examination and a barium meal, usually confirmed by CT scanning. Fibreoptic gastroscopy allows direct inspection and a biopsy to be taken.

Treatment options

The prognosis for those with gastric cancer is poor. Surgery still offers the best hope of a cure and even in more advanced stages is undertaken to relieve symptoms. A partial or total gastrectomy, which is either palliative or so-called 'curative', depending on the extent of the tumour, may be undertaken. The results of a large clinical trial on operable tumours (the MAGIC trial) examined the benefits of chemotherapy before and after surgery. It was found that chemotherapy before surgery reduced the size of the tumour making it easier to resect. Similarly, in patients with what are initially considered to be inoperable tumours, resection can be made possible with chemotherapy (Cancer Research UK 2009b). In patients with advanced disease, palliative chemotherapy may be used to shrink or slow down progression of the tumour or relieve symptoms. Radiotherapy may also shrink a tumour and is used to relieve pain or stop bleeding (Cancer Research UK 2009b).

 ## Nursing management and health promotion: carcinoma of the stomach

PRE-OPERATIVE MANAGEMENT

For details of peri-operative nursing priorities in abdominal surgery see Chapter 26.

Similar to those undergoing surgery for oesophageal cancer, there are particular considerations that must be attended to in the patient who is to have a partial or complete gastrectomy. In addition to the thorough physiological assessment needed prior to surgery, these patients may require nutritional support pre-operatively. Nutritional assessment using a tool such as MUST (Elia 2003) is essential in order to identify actual and potential deficiencies such as weight loss, nausea and vomiting, dietary changes or impediments to sufficient calorific intake. Changes to elimination pattern should also be assessed. Where the patient is found to be debilitated or undernourished, parenteral nutrition should be considered.

Psychological and emotional preparation is a fundamental aspect of care as these patients are undergoing major surgery whilst already living with a traumatising diagnosis. Primarily, some effort should be directed at allaying the patient's fears and anxieties about the impending surgery. Time should be taken to answer questions and the patient and their family should be encouraged to verbalise their fears and concerns. Patients and their families will require explanations and discussion of what to expect in the immediate postoperative period.

POSTOPERATIVE MANAGEMENT

Partial or total gastrectomy is major surgery and intensive monitoring of vital signs is required in the immediate postoperative period. Pain management and evaluation of the effectiveness of analgesia is fundamental. Where the patient has a PCA pump it should not be assumed that it is effective. Pain relief should be sufficient to enable the patient to mobilise, perform deep breathing and coughing and undertake leg exercises (see Ch.19).

The patient will have a nasogastric tube and strict monitoring of the type and amount of drainage is required. Some bloody drainage for the first 12 h is expected, but excessive bleeding should be reported. Drainage is less following a total gastrectomy as there is no longer a reservoir. Ensure the tube is secured to prevent dislocation as this would result in increased pain and distension.

Parenteral nutrition may already be in place or commenced following surgery to meet the patient's calorific needs, to replace fluids lost through drainage and vomiting, and to support the patient metabolically until oral intake is adequate. Patients who have had abdominal surgery will experience paralytic ileus following handling of the bowel (see Ch. 26). Therefore, oral intake will not be resumed until bowel sounds return and the patient will require supplementary intravenous fluids. After the return of bowel sounds and removal of the nasogastric tube, fluids may be commenced. Food in small portions should be gradually introduced and added until the patient is able to eat six small meals a day and drink 120 mL of fluid between meals.

Following gastrectomy, patients may have a urinary catheter in situ in order to accurately measure kidney function and output. Depending on the type of gastrectomy performed, patients may have a thoracic and/or abdominal incision. The dressing should be observed for signs of bleeding and output from wound drains strictly monitored and recorded.

Patients should be assisted with mobilising as soon as possible postoperatively. Whilst in bed, the patient should be positioned in a low Fowler's position (head elevation 15–45 degrees) to promote comfort and aid gastric emptying.

Complications of gastric surgery include dysphagia, gastric retention, bile reflux, dumping syndrome (see above) and vitamin and mineral deficiencies. Gastric retention causes abdominal distension, nausea and vomiting and it may be necessary to reinstate nil by mouth status and nasogastric drainage. Regurgitation may occur if the patient eats too much or too quickly. At times, oedema along the suture line may prevent fluids and food from moving into the intestinal tract. It is important that pressure remains low in the remaining portion of the stomach or the pouch to avoid disrupting the sutures.

Discharge planning

Detailed information about diet, pain management and monitoring for the onset of complications should be given in verbal and written form when preparing the patient and their family for discharge. Teaching the patient about dietary self-management is essential. The nurse should ensure that the patient understands the strategies for prevention and management of dumping syndrome (see above). In addition, patients should be encouraged to eat a diet that is high in protein with reduced sugar and salt. They should also be encouraged to monitor their weight. Anaemia is common in those who have had a total gastrectomy as there is a reduction in gastric acid production and a deficiency of intrinsic factor. These patients will require vitamin B_{12} injections at 3-monthly intervals.

Patients and their families should be informed of the signs and symptoms of complications such as bleeding, obstruction and perforation and should have impressed upon them the importance of seeking medical help where symptoms worsen or do not resolve.

Long-term care after palliative surgery

After the patient has been discharged home, it is very likely that the symptoms of the cancer will gradually increase. Skilful and sensitive nursing care will be required to help the patient to remain as comfortable and as free from anxiety as possible.

Pain from the tumour, metastases and ascites can be relieved initially by oral morphine sulphate (MST), progressing, as the need arises, to the judicious use of opioid analgesics, usually diamorphine, given subcutaneously via a syringe driver. Such delivery gives a consistent level of analgesia and is often the key factor in enabling the patient to be pain-free and to remain at home.

Dietary intake may prove a problem. Persistent nausea and vomiting may develop and be difficult to control. Regular and pre-emptive antiemetic medication can be most beneficial. Meals should be small and attractively served at times when the effect of antiemetics is at its optimal level. Nutritious drinks such as Ensure® and Enlive® can help to supplement nutrition without extra effort on the part of the patient.

Diarrhoea and constipation can both occur. A common side-effect of opiate analgesics is constipation, for which an oral laxative should be prescribed. Orally or rectally administered medications can help to control these symptoms, as can dietary advice.

Mouth infections such as candidiasis are very common and occur in all malignant disease. Nystatin lozenges or suspensions may be given after meals and oral hygiene and dental/denture care must be meticulously maintained.

For some patients there may be the added distress of ascites, which is an accumulation of serous fluid within the peritoneal cavity that can cause pressure on other abdominal organs and the respiratory system. Abdominal paracentesis (see Box 4.19), whereby the ascitic fluid can be drained off, may be preferred to relieve the symptoms. Diuretics may also be used.

Patients with incurable gastric cancer are likely to experience psychological distress. The support of the community nursing team and where possible the Macmillan or Marie Curie nursing services can prove indispensable in giving the patient the confidence to remain at home rather than in hospital. The daily visits of such a nurse, as well as ensuring that the practical aspects of care are achieved, give the patient and the family the opportunity to talk about fears and worries. The visiting nurse is in an ideal position to monitor the well-being of both parties and to recognise when plans of care should be reviewed. Chapters 31 and 33 explore many ways in which a sensitive continuity of care can be achieved, whether in hospital, at home or in a hospice.

Disorders of the small and large intestines

Unlike disorders of the upper GI tract, in which the major problem is that of ingestion of nutrients, disorders of the small and large intestines result in problems of absorption of nutrients or the transit and elimination of bowel contents. People suffering from such problems complain of varying degrees of abdominal pain and discomfort, diarrhoea and/or constipation. Often the symptoms are insidious and/or embarrassing, such that they are ignored or tolerated and not mentioned even to close relatives.

Malabsorption syndromes

Malabsorption is a consequence of impaired digestion or absorption of nutrients from the intestinal lumen.

PATHOPHYSIOLOGY AND RISK FACTORS

Malabsorption is caused by a number of conditions. These include:

- lack of digestive enzyme activity, as in chronic pancreatitis and hypolactasia
- lack of bile salts, as in common bile duct obstruction and liver disease
- loss or damage to the absorptive area, as in coeliac disease, extensive bowel resection or Crohn's disease
- failure of adequate removal from the interstitial fluid of absorbed nutrients, as in obstruction of lymphatic drainage.

Clinical features

Whatever the cause, the presenting signs and symptoms of malabsorption are essentially the same. Patients may complain of frothy, greasy and bulky stools that are difficult to flush away (steatorrhoea), diarrhoea, weight loss and abdominal distension.

Vitamin and mineral deficiencies due to malabsorption may result in anaemia, lack of iron, folate and vitamin B_{12}, bleeding disorders and purpura due to lack of vitamin K, and peripheral neuropathy due to lack of vitamins A and B. Protein deficiency can result in oedema and the musculoskeletal system may also be affected by osteopenia due to lack of calcium, vitamin D and phosphate, and tetany due to lack of calcium.

Diagnosis

When a careful history and clinical examination suggest malabsorption, the following diagnostic tests will be carried out to determine the cause:

- faecal fat estimation
- glucose and lactose tolerance tests
- haematological studies
- radiological and barium studies
- endoscopic examination and biopsy.

Treatment options

The form of treatment offered will clearly depend upon the cause of the malabsorption. In coeliac disease, where there is sensitivity to gluten, or in lactose intolerance, the advice seems simple: avoid foods containing the offending element. However, for the individual, such advice is not always easy to follow and the condition can potentially cause disruption and stress in everyday life, undermining the sense of well-being. Where malabsorption is part of, or has resulted from, some other disorder, nutritional supplementation may be required on a temporary or permanent basis.

 Nursing management and health promotion: malabsorption syndromes

The assessment and planning of care will necessarily focus on the problems of nutritional impairment, diarrhoea and any associated feeling of embarrassment, anger or despair. For some, pain will be a distinctive feature, in which case providing analgesics must be a priority.

A full nutritional assessment should be made with the assistance of the dietitian. While assessing elimination function, efforts should be made to minimise the physical misery and embarrassment caused by diarrhoea. Attention to hygiene and the provision of soothing creams for any excoriation can make all the difference. Ensuring rest and relaxation can help general malaise. This is not always easy, as the investigations may be many and frequent. Supporting the patient through such tests and ensuring full understanding will help in maintaining a positive attitude.

Counselling and teaching will be a priority once the diagnosis and management have been determined. This is especially important as discharge approaches and the patient

begins to take responsibility for dietary modification. The community nurse, GP and self-help groups can give support in the community, but probably the best support can be gained from those closest to the patient. The involvement of family and significant friends in any teaching and health promotion programme should be encouraged.

Irritable bowel syndrome

Irritable bowel syndrome (IBS) is the name for a group of unexplained symptoms related to disturbance of the large bowel. IBS is a chronic, relapsing and often lifelong condition (NICE 2008) and at any one time between 10 and 20% of people living in Western countries meet the diagnostic criteria (Gut Trust 2010). The condition commonly affects those in the 20–30 age group with twice as many women being affected than men. Recent trends also suggest there is a notable prevalence among older adults (NICE 2008).

Clinical features

Individuals with IBS characteristically complain of abdominal pain or distension (bloating), which can be linked to or relieved by defaecation, and/or an alteration in bowel habit. People with IBS present with a wide range of symptoms but there is a tendency to be either 'diarrhoea dominant' or 'constipation dominant' or altering (NICE 2008). Some people also experience nausea, backache and lethargy. Many find the symptoms distressing and/or embarrassing and are often reluctant to discuss them with others.

Diagnosis

According to the NICE guidelines for irritable bowel syndrome (NICE 2008), any person presenting with abdominal pain or bloating or a change in bowel habit for a period of longer than 6 months should be assessed for IBS. However, organic bowel disease must be excluded when making the diagnosis. Unintentional or unexplained weight loss, rectal bleeding, a family history of bowel or ovarian cancer, anaemia, abdominal or rectal masses, markers for inflammatory bowel disease and an altered bowel habit that includes more frequent and/or looser stools in a person over the age of 60 years require referral for further investigation (NICE 2008).

In making the diagnosis, it is important that the level of distress and frequency of symptoms are assessed, particularly in relation to altered bowel habit or stool passage. NICE (2008) recommends the use of the Bristol Stool Form Scale (Box 4.8) to assist the individual with stool descriptors. Diagnosis of IBS is made on the basis of the clinical features presented above. Investigations in those who meet the criteria for IBS include a full blood count, erythrocyte sedimentation rate (ESR), C-reactive protein and antibody testing for coeliac disease.

Treatment options

Once the diagnosis of IBS is confirmed, time is spent discussing the symptoms and findings and reassuring the patient that there is no underlying pathology. The focus of treatment for IBS is aimed at control of the predominant symptoms. This is primarily directed towards dietary and

Box 4.8 Information

Bristol stool form chart (Lewis & Heaton 1997)

Type 1   Separate hard lumps, like nuts (hard to pass).

Type 2   Sausage-shaped, but lumpy.

Type 3   Like a sausage but with cracks on its surface.

Type 4   Like a sausage or snake, smooth and soft.

Type 5   Soft blobs with clear cut edges (passed easily).

Type 6   Fluffy pieces with ragged edges, a mushy stool.

Type 7   Watery, no solid pieces. Entirely liquid.

lifestyle changes but at times supplemented by pharmacological therapy and psychological interventions.

Pharmacological therapy is based on the nature and severity of the symptoms being experienced. Antispasmodics are used sometimes in conjunction with dietary and lifestyle management. For those with constipation, laxatives should be considered but lactulose is contraindicated in IBS because of the increased risk of abdominal symptoms (e.g. abdominal cramping and diarrhoea) (NICE 2008). Loperamide is the drug of choice for those with diarrhoea. Where pain management is unsuccessful with antispasmodics, laxatives and loperamide, tricyclic antidepressants may be considered.

Psychological interventions such as cognitive behavioural therapy (CBT), hypnotherapy and/or psychological therapy should be considered if the person does not respond to pharmacological treatments after 12 months.

Nursing management and health promotion: irritable bowel syndrome

Once a diagnosis of IBS has been made, the majority of those with the condition are managed within the community setting. For the most part, the focus of care should be on education to promote and enhance self-management. The focus of education is related to diet, lifestyle, physical activity and medication to manage their symptoms.

Nutritional assessment should be undertaken and the person should be advised to eat regularly and avoid long gaps between meals. At least eight cups of water and non-caffeinated drinks should be consumed daily, and coffee, tea, alcohol and carbonated drinks should be reduced. Avoiding processed foods, limiting high-fibre foods and confining fruit to three portions a day may also help. The use of oral aloe vera should also be avoided by those who have IBS because of its laxative effects and the potential for abdominal cramps and diarrhoea (NICE 2008). Where necessary, the person should be referred to a dietitian.

The person's level of physical activity should also be assessed and advice given where there is an identified need to increase activity levels. In addition, the person should be encouraged to identify leisure time and take time to relax.

Patients who are receiving pharmacological therapy require education to develop an understanding that medication doses should be adjusted in order to achieve a soft well-formed stool.

The nurse should discuss a range of coping strategies with the person but should be realistic as alternative therapies are

not readily available on the NHS and can be very expensive. However, alternative therapies such as hypnotherapy have been shown to have significant and long-term value in symptom control in IBS (Gonsalkorale et al 2003). Acupuncture and reflexology are not recommended due to a lack of evidence to support their efficacy (NICE 2008). For further information on the management of IBS refer to the NICE guideline http://www.nice.org.uk/nicemedia/pdf/IBSFull Guideline.pdf

Inflammatory bowel disease: Crohn's disease and ulcerative colitis

Inflammatory bowel disease is the term used to describe two chronic and debilitating conditions: Crohn's disease (CD) and ulcerative colitis (UC). Although they are often described together, each has its own unique pathology, characteristics and treatments (Box 4.9). Both disorders are relatively common in developed countries and usually affect people in young adulthood. The incidence of both conditions has risen in Western populations over the last century. As yet no definitive cause has been found but it is currently believed that a combination of genetic susceptibility and environmental factors such as bacteria, drugs, smoking and perhaps diet is implicated (Carter et al 2004).

PATHOPHYSIOLOGY AND RISK FACTORS

In UC, inflammatory changes occur in the mucosa and submucosa. These changes are diffuse, with widespread superficial ulceration. The rectum is almost always involved (proctitis) and a variable amount of the rest of the colon, although the entire colon can be affected. The extent of the disease is generally divided into four categories (Box 4.10). The inflammatory process primarily affects the mucosa and is continuous. Initially, there is reddening and oedema of the mucosa with bleeding points. This is followed by ulceration. In acute disease, especially of the transverse colon, there may be gross dilatation (toxic dilatation) causing the bowel wall to become thin and rupture. In chronic disease, the colon becomes shortened and narrowed.

Box 4.9 Information

Distinguishing features of inflammatory bowel disease

Ulcerative colitis	Crohn's disease
Colon only	Any part of the gut (from the mouth to the anus)
Rectum is involved	Rectum is usually spared
Usually starts in the rectum	Not continuous with alternating normal areas in between diseased areas
Deep layers of the gut not involved – mucosa and submucosa only	Full thickness – affects all layers
Bleeding is evident	Up to 1/3 have no bleeding
No perianal disease	Perianal disease
No granuloma	Granuloma

Box 4.10 Information

Ulcerative colitis – extent of the disease (Norton et al 2008)

- Distal disease – affecting the rectum (proctitis) or the rectum and sigmoid colon (proctosigmoiditis).
- Left-sided disease – affecting up to the splenic flexure (left-sided colitis and distal colitis (affects 33% of patients in the UK).
- Pancolitis – affecting the whole colon (19% of patients in the UK).
- Proctitis – affects the rectum only (48% of patients in UK).

In CD, the inflammatory changes affect isolated segments of all layers of the intestinal tract. The damaged mucosa develops granulomas, which give the bowel a cobblestoned appearance. Fibrosis and narrowing of the tract can occur and the transmural damage can lead to fistula formation whereby abnormal passageways develop between loops of the bowel.

Clinical features

Bloody diarrhoea with frequency, urgency and abdominal cramping is characteristic of UC. Pain may be relieved by defaecation. Pus and mucus may be present in the stool. Attacks vary in severity from being troublesome to life threatening (Box 4.11).

The symptoms of CD depend on the site of inflammation and as with UC, the severity of the attacks varies. In small

Box 4.11 Information

Clinical features of ulcerative colitis and Crohn's disease

Ulcerative colitis	Crohn's disease
Characterised by relapses and remissions	Characterised by episodes of remission and relapse, which are unpredictable
Lifelong condition that is treatable	Symptoms are dependent on the site, severity and pathological process of the disease
Bloody diarrhoea	Diarrhoea and/or bleeding (altered bowel habits)
Frequency, urgency, abdominal cramps (usually pre-defaecation)	Cramping abdominal pain
Passing mucus rectally	Anorexia and weight loss
May be pus in the stools	Pyrexia (fever)
Loss of appetite (anorexia)	Anal and perianal lesions
Blood loss can vary from mild to causing shock	Slowed growth in children
Malaise (lethargy)	Malaise (lethargy), anorexia
Tenesmus	Subacute GI obstruction
Malodorous flatus	Susceptible to extra-intestinal manifestations

bowel disease the patient may present with nausea and vomiting, bloating/abdominal distension, canker sores (a type of oral ulcer that presents inside the mouth or upper throat and is caused by a break in the mucous membrane) and duodenal ulcers. Patients may also experience abdominal pain and an abdominal mass is sometimes palpable, particularly in the right iliac fossa. In large bowel disease patients can experience severe diarrhoea, rectal bleeding or passing mucus rectally. In perianal Crohn's disease patients can experience varying bowel habits from diarrhoea to constipation and severe rectal pain. They may also develop recurrent fistulae, abscesses and skin tags (Norton et al 2008) (see Box 4.11).

Both conditions may be associated with extra-intestinal symptoms that include arthritis, skin lesions and eye inflammation. Whilst both conditions have minimal mortality rates they can have a substantial negative impact on quality of life (Rowlinson 1999).

Sometimes the disease is in quite an advanced state before help is sought. In such situations, the symptoms may reflect the more serious complications of rectal abscesses, fissures, fistulae or even obstruction and perforation, which will constitute an abdominal emergency.

Diagnosis

History and examination suggesting inflammatory bowel disease prompt hospital admission for diagnostic tests. There are no specific blood tests for IBD but haematological studies may support a diagnosis. These can reveal a raised white cell count (WBC), a raised erythrocyte sedimentation rate (ESR) and C-reactive protein, a raised platelet count and lowered haemoglobin (Hb), B_{12} and zinc. There is often hypoproteinaemia.

Other investigations will include:

- examination of the diarrhoea for blood, fat and infective agents
- radiological and barium examination to reveal characteristic features of inflammatory bowel disease
- endoscopic examination – proctoscopy, sigmoidoscopy and colonoscopy; great care must be taken with such examinations, which are in fact contraindicated in fulminating disease due to the risk of perforation of the bowel
- ultrasound and CT scanning to determine the presence of abscess formation.

Treatment options

As there is no real cure for inflammatory bowel disease, with the exception of total colectomy in UC, the aim of treatment is to bring about remission of active disease and maintain this for as long as possible. This may involve the initial correction of fluid and electrolyte imbalance (see Ch. 20), malnutrition and anaemia, and relief of abdominal pain as well as pharmacological interventions (Box 4.12). Please refer to the website and http://www.bsg.org.uk for additional information on pharmacological management in UC and CD.

See website for further content

Close observation will be required for signs of obstruction or perforation.

Box 4.12 Information

Non-surgical treatment in inflammatory bowel disease

Ulcerative colitis	Crohn's disease
Pharmacological treatments (corticosteroids, aminosalicylates, thiopurines, infliximab)	Pharmacological treatments (corticosteroids, aminosalicylates, thiopurines, methotrexate, infliximab) Antibiotics e.g. metronidazole
Fluid replacement/blood transfusion	Nutritional assessment and nutritional replacements/supplements
Local disease – topical therapy of salicylates and steroid enemas	Elemental diet
20–30% of patients require surgery	50% of patients will require surgery in the first 10 years

In fulminating disease, enteral nutrition may not be possible and parenteral nutrition will be required (see Ch. 21). If enteral nutrition is possible, an elemental diet free of residue may be necessary for a short while before a low-residue diet can be reintroduced. As the inflammation settles, dietary restrictions can be reduced. During any quiescent phase, a 'normal' healthy diet is recommended. Such a diet should have sufficient kilocalories to restore and maintain weight, as well as being high in protein and carbohydrate and low in fat. Supplements of vitamins, iron, folic acid, zinc and potassium may be required.

SURGICAL MANAGEMENT

Surgery is required in 20–30% of patients with ulcerative colitis and up to 50% with Crohn's disease, but it is always preferred that any surgery be postponed for as long as possible. As a result, living with this condition can mean living with the constant anxiety that symptoms will become severe and complications arise. Surgery becomes unavoidable when:

- acute episodes become more frequent or fail to respond to medical treatment and there is a deterioration, leading to generalised debility, malnutrition, fluid and electrolyte disturbance and anaemia
- obstruction is acute and/or fails to resolve by conservative means
- perforation occurs
- toxic megacolon occurs – the colon hypertrophies, dilates and could rupture
- fistulae develop – these may be internal or enterocutaneous
- abscesses fail to respond to intensive treatment
- malignant changes are considered to be a risk.

The choice of operation will depend on the extent and severity of the disease. It is generally accepted that the emergency operation of choice is colectomy (removal of the colon) with terminal ileostomy (opening into the ileum) and preservation of the rectum. Preserving the rectum means that it may be possible to have the ileostomy reversed in the future.

In recent years, ileal-anal pouch surgery (formation of a pouch/reservoir from the ileum that is joined to the anus) (Williams 2008) has changed greatly the treatment of ulcerative colitis and it has become standard care for those with the condition. Patients are advocates of this type of surgery as it removes the necessity of having a stoma. Further information on ileal-anal pouch surgery can be found on the website.

 See website for further content

In CD, the patient may undergo more than one operation over many years, as surgery may initially be limited to resection of the affected segments of the bowel. However, because the disease affects the total GI tract, alternatives to stoma formation are less easily achieved.

▷ Nursing management and health promotion: inflammatory bowel disease

The nursing care of patients with inflammatory bowel disease is essentially symptomatic and must be individualised. Assessment and nursing management will focus on nutritional status, pain and discomfort, bowel function, patient knowledge and ability to cope with the condition, body image and self-esteem, and work and social implications. Education and inclusion of the patient in their care is essential throughout their hospitalisation both in terms of enabling them to cope with the stress of undergoing a range of often exhausting investigations for which fasting and bowel preparation is required and in preparing them to live with the condition (Box 4.13).

Box 4.13 Reflection

The person living with Crohn's disease

Margaret is a 23-year-old hotel receptionist who was diagnosed with Crohn's disease when she was 17 years old. Margaret has been in and out of hospital regularly due to her condition. Margaret attended an outpatient appointment and was admitted to the GI ward after her appointment. When Margaret met her admitting nurse she burst into tears, explaining how she had developed an embarrassing and 'horrible' faecal discharge from her vagina and uncontrollable diarrhoea. On admission, Margaret was pyrexial with a temperature of 38.4°C, pale, clammy and very distressed. The nurse offered her a single room as she was obviously distressed by her diarrhoea.

Her consultant suggested a fistula was the cause of Margaret's problem and advised that the best plan of action would be to surgically repair it. Margaret was also informed that there was a possibility she would require a defunctioning stoma or proctectomy. Margaret was unable to sleep and spent most of the night talking to the night nurses about her condition and her options. She also told the nursing staff that she had ended her relationship with her boyfriend of two years because of her present condition.

Refer to website Critical thinking question 4.2 in relation to this case.

 See website for further information on faecal incontinence and Critical thinking question 4.2

Nursing monitoring should focus on early detection of deterioration in the patient's condition, particularly any elevation in temperature or pulse rate or signs of impending shock. During fulminating episodes, the patient may be acutely ill. Abdominal pain can be severe and diarrhoea unremitting and the presence of fissures, fistulae and rectal abscesses may make the symptoms worse. The patient will be prone to infection, and the nurse should be alert for signs of pyrexia and tachycardia that may indicate the presence of infection. Alteration in vital signs in conjunction with increasing abdominal tenderness could also indicate the advent of colonic dilatation, toxic megacolon or perforation.

Accurate intake and output recording is essential as these patients are prone to dehydration from fluid and electrolytes lost through diarrhoea. Muscle weakness, cramps, tachycardia and pyrexia can indicate electrolyte imbalance. Dehydration and electrolyte imbalance must be corrected, usually through the intravenous route. Patients should also be observed for signs of prolonged bleeding such as lethargy, tiredness, breathlessness and pale mucosa.

Patients with IBD experience loose frequent stools, sometimes with the presence of blood and mucus, up to 20 times per day. These episodes are often accompanied by abdominal pain and cramps that are made worse by food and fluids. These patients are not only incapacitated by these episodes, they are often embarrassed and self-conscious about odours. Ideally they should have easy access to a toilet or commode, and privacy should be ensured. Advice on good perianal care is essential as the area is prone to excoriation and patients should be encouraged to maintain a high standard of personal hygiene. A barrier cream may be helpful. Patients may request a continence pad as a precautionary measure. A stool chart should be maintained to record number and character of bowel movements (Box 4.8), including the presence or absence of blood/mucus. Although antidiarrhoeal medication should not be given in the acute phase, antispasmodics are sometimes helpful.

Nutritional assessment and management is fundamental for patients with IBD. They are often malnourished or afraid to eat for fear of exacerbating already debilitating symptoms. A nutritional assessment tool such as MUST (Elia 2003) should be maintained. There is no definitive advice regarding what foods to eat but patients should be encouraged to eat small, regular meals and supplements may be beneficial. Small snacks between meals will help to increase calorie intake. The provision of regular oral hygiene and antiseptic mouthwashes is essential to prevent candidiasis. For some, particularly those with Crohn's disease, supportive therapy in the form of nasogastric, enteral or parenteral feeding may be required to correct malnutrition (Carter et al 2004).

In order to offer education and support that is individualised it is important that the nurse gets to know the patient's lifestyle, likes and dislikes, and to identify any sources of stress in their daily life. Fatigue will be a constant feature and the patient should be encouraged and facilitated to rest. A tactful approach when disturbing an exhausted patient in order to carry out essential care is helpful in gaining cooperation, despite the patient appearing unappreciative of the nursing care being carried out.

The patient will have to accept the reality of a condition that is with them for life. Time must be spent on a regular basis helping them to adjust and to plan positively for the future. The National Association for Colitis and Crohn's Disease (NACC) can offer a great deal of support to both patients and their families (see Useful websites, p. 124). Psychological and social adjustment is central to successful self-management in the person with IBD. The impact on self-esteem and body image of the condition can be devastating. Not only does the patient have to cope with the indignity of having faecal urgency and the risk of soiling themselves, they can also experience negative changes in their physical experience as a result of malnutrition, prolonged steroid use or surgery (e.g. formation of a stoma). There are also actual and potential work and social implications. People may refuse certain employment or their ability to sustain their job might be affected by the cyclical nature of remissions and acute phases of the condition. Social implications include the potential for isolation due to a lack of willingness to engage in social activities or intimate relationships.

PERI-OPERATIVE MANAGEMENT

The principles of peri-operative care are discussed in Chapter 26. In inflammatory bowel disease there are additional concerns of which the nurse must be aware. Many patients are physically debilitated and, should they present as an abdominal emergency, it may not be possible to improve this state prior to surgery. The psychological preparation for surgery that may involve stoma formation is essential, even if time is limited. Patients and their families are likely to already have conceptions or misconceptions about life with a stoma and may be distressed. If optimal time is available, preparation, in which the stoma nurse specialist plays a key role, centres on assessment of the person's ability to live with the stoma postoperatively. This preparation encompasses both physiological and psychological factors that include assessment of the person's emotional well-being, their knowledge levels regarding surgery, the impact of the surgery on sexual functioning and activity, their physical abilities (e.g. existence of co-morbidities, eyesight, and manual dexterity), cultural considerations and the positioning of the stoma. Further information on the role of the stoma nurse specialist can be found on the website.

See website for further content

For more information about pre- and postoperative care of a patient with a stoma, see Burch (2005), and for the psychological, sexual and cultural issues that must be considered when caring for such a patient, see Black (2004).

Stoma care

Postoperatively, the nurse must maintain close observation of the stoma to ensure that it is viable and has a good blood supply. The stoma should be pink; if it darkens in colour this indicates that the blood supply is threatened. Initially the stoma will be oedematous, but this should reduce over a few days. A clear drainage stoma bag should be used to allow good observation of the stoma. Daily assessment should include:

- observation of the mucocutaneous junction (where the mucosa of the bowel joins the skin) for signs of separation

- assessment of the condition of the peristomal skin for redness, inflammation and broken areas
- monitoring the surrounding area for any indication that the stoma is receding into an indentation or crease on the abdomen (Porrett 2005, Vujnovich 2008).

If an ileostomy has been formed, digestive enzymes will be present and fluid faeces will become copious; care must be taken that the skin is protected by the correct application of the stoma bags. The stoma is formed so that it is approximately 3.5 cm long, thus protecting the surrounding skin. However, care is still necessary to protect the skin and position the appliance. No pressure should be put on the stoma during care.

The patient should be reassured that the output from the stoma will reduce and become more 'paste-like' in consistency as the small intestine recovers and adjusts. The stoma nurse specialist can demonstrate the various appliances available so that the patient has a supply of those most suitable prior to discharge. Initial care of the stoma is given by the nursing staff, with the patient gradually taking over under supervision and then performing care independently before going home.

It is fundamental that the patient has knowledge and understanding of the potential adjustments to lifestyle that may need to be made in respect of food, medications, maintenance of general health, work life and hobbies. Moreover, there may be implications for sexual functioning depending on the type of surgery that has been undertaken as well as the parallel issues of the impact on body image and self-esteem (Black 2004).

Dietary advice should be given by the dietitian and the stoma nurse specialist before discharge, and the patient and family should be advised of the likely protracted recovery and adjustment time that will be required before a return to good health and a full lifestyle can be achieved. Continuity of care is key to supporting and enabling the patient and their family and is provided in the community by the primary health care team and the stoma nurse specialist. For further reading see Williams (2006a,b), Fulham (2008), Vujnovich (2008) and Borwell (2009). For reading on the numerous implications and complications of stoma formation see Black (2004, 2009).

Diverticular disease

Diverticular disease presents as small hernias or outpouchings of the mucosa through the muscular wall of the bowel. These occur predominantly in the sigmoid and descending colon. The presence of uncomplicated diverticula with minimal or no symptoms is known as diverticulosis and is present in at least 50% of people in their 50s, rising to 67% of those in their 80s, with an equal prevalence between men and women (Janes et al 2006). However, three quarters of these people remain asymptomatic throughout their lives. In the presence of symptoms the condition is referred to as diverticular disease. When inflammation occurs, it is known as diverticulitis and, if persistent, is considered a chronic inflammatory disease.

PATHOPHYSIOLOGY AND RISK FACTORS

Although the pathogenesis of diverticular disease is not fully understood, studies have shown that there is an inverse relationship between its incidence and fibre content in the diet (Janes et al 2006). Research has indicated that people with diverticular disease have diets low in fresh fruit and vegetables, brown bread and potatoes, and high in meat and milk products. Chronic constipation and the excessive use of purgatives may also cause diverticular disease by raising intraluminal pressure.

It is thought that a low volume of colonic content leads to a reduction in the diameter of the colon. Increased luminal pressure during segmentation causes herniation of the mucosa through the muscle wall. Faeces may collect in the hernia(e), causing inflammation, perforation and abscess formation, the formation of fistulae into the small intestine, bladder or vagina, and peritonitis. Repeated attacks can eventually lead to obstruction.

Clinical features

Clinical features include the presence of intermittent grumbling, spasmodic pain in the left iliac fossa or suprapubic region, and a mass that is palpable on abdominal or rectal examination. Constipation, intermittent constipation or intermittent diarrhoea is common. The majority of patients with diverticular disease are asymptomatic.

Diagnosis

Diagnosis is made by barium enema. Flexible sigmoidoscopy (visualisation of the rectum and sigmoid colon) is undertaken to exclude cancer. Colonoscopy (visualisation of the colonic mucosa) is indicated when there is rectal bleeding or where a carcinoma is suspected. Most individuals are treated in the community by their GP.

Treatment options

The main treatment is dietary. The individual should be encouraged to increase fibre intake, including unprocessed bran, wholemeal bread, fruit and vegetables, and should drink plenty of water. Antispasmodics such as propantheline bromide can be used. It must be emphasised that stimulant laxatives should not be used, as they increase the pressure in the muscular wall of the colon and can cause more herniation of the mucosa.

In severe exacerbations, admission to hospital may be necessary if there is marked abdominal pain and pyrexia. Treatment will include broad-spectrum antibiotics, intravenous infusion and nasogastric aspiration until the inflammation subsides. Although many people who live with diverticular disease feel able to cope and have no difficulty adhering to dietary advice, complications do occur in about 25% of sufferers and surgical intervention will be required. Depending on the nature and severity of the problem, resection and temporary or permanent stoma formation may be necessary.

Surgical procedures for diverticular disease might include:

- colectomy (removal of the entire colon)
- Hartmann's procedure (formation of an end colostomy through surgical resection of the descending or sigmoid colon with closure of the rectal stump and formation of a colostomy)
- transverse loop colostomy (formation of a colostomy in the right upper quadrant – may be a temporary measure).

Appendicitis

The vermiform appendix is a blind-ended, worm-like tube that projects into the caecum in the right iliac fossa. It has a large amount of lymphoid tissue in its walls and is covered by the peritoneum. The appendix is described as vestigial in that it constitutes the remnant of a structure whose function is no longer required. In adulthood it is about the size of an adult little finger (5–6 cm) (Figure 4.5).

Inflammation of the appendix is the most common cause of abdominal sepsis in developed countries. The concern is always that the inflamed appendix might rupture, causing peritonitis. Appendicitis is a life-threatening condition and constitutes a surgical emergency.

PATHOPHYSIOLOGY AND RISK FACTORS

Although in many people the appendix has virtually disappeared by their middle years, appendicitis can occur at any age. It is rare in infancy and less common in later life, but in the UK can affect 12–15% of those aged 8–15 years. Its prevalence is thought to be closely related to refined Western diets where faecolith (hard faecal matter) residues may be retained in and obstruct the lumen of the blind-ended appendix. The incidence of appendicitis does appear to have fallen significantly over the past 10 years, perhaps reflecting the promotion of a healthier diet that is high in fibre. Less commonly, viral infections, contaminated food and intestinal (tape) worms can precipitate appendicitis.

When the lumen of the appendix becomes obstructed, bacteria proliferate and cause an acute inflammatory response. The local end-arteries become thrombosed and gangrene sets in. This in turn leads to perforation and localised

peritonitis. If left untreated, this becomes generalised peritonitis (Box 4.14).

Clinical features

For many, appendicitis occurs suddenly, but for others symptoms of colic and fever may 'grumble' on for some time before an acute episode occurs. In such cases, the obstruction has perhaps been partial and the inflammation transitory. These recurrent episodes can result in adhesions forming which can cause further problems (for detail on adhesions see the website).

🖱 **See website for further content**

Because of the mobile position of the appendix (see Figure 4.5), clinical presentation can vary. Typically, however, the patient experiences central abdominal pain localising to

 Box 4.14 Information

Peritonitis (inflammation of the peritoneum)
Acute peritonitis

Acute peritonitis is commonly caused by irritating substances, often bacterial in nature, entering the abdominal cavity due to:

- perforation of an organ by either trauma or disease, e.g. a penetrating injury, a perforated appendix, duodenal ulcer, or ruptured fallopian tube as a result of an ectopic pregnancy
- gangrene of an organ such as might occur in a strangulated hernia
- septicaemia, which may have originated in another part of the body.

The peritoneum becomes inflamed, inciting a dramatic increase in the production of serous fluid. This rapidly becomes infected and purulent in the presence of bacteria (typically *Escherichia coli* and *Bacteroides*). Toxins are absorbed from the inflamed and oedematous peritoneum and large amounts of fluid are lost into the peritoneal cavity, leading to paralytic ileus, abdominal distension, hypovolaemia, fluid and electrolyte imbalance and loss of protein.

Immediate and intense pain is felt at the site, followed by vomiting, pyrexia, extreme weakness and shock. Diagnosis is essentially clinical, supported by X-ray examination to detect the presence of free air, fluid levels, abdominal masses and perforations.

Treatment is by a combination of surgery, intravenous antibiotic therapy and specific intervention for the underlying cause. The peritoneal cavity may need to be opened to remove the toxic material and allow drainage of the peritoneal cavity. Supportive therapy includes intravenous fluids to maintain fluid and electrolyte balance, nasogastric aspiration to relieve distension, oxygen therapy and analgesics. If the patient continues to remain pyrexial, tachycardic and in pain, an abdominal abscess should be suspected as a complication.

Chronic peritonitis

This is far less common than acute peritonitis but may occur in association with tuberculosis or as a complication of some long-standing irritant such as peritoneal dialysis or a foreign body. Symptoms are less severe and include low-grade fever, vague pain and malaise. Treatment will depend on the cause.

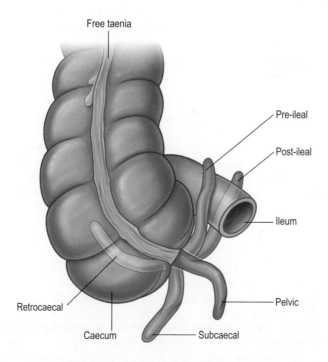

Figure 4.5 Position of the appendix. (Reproduced with permission from Drake et al 2005.)

Free taenia

Pre-ileal

Post-ileal

Ileum

Retrocaecal

Pelvic

Caecum

Subcaecal

the right iliac fossa in the first few hours. There may be rebound tenderness and guarding of the abdomen. The patient may experience nausea and vomiting, have a mild pyrexia, furred tongue and/or unpleasant smelling breath.

Diagnosis

Following a careful history and examination, only essential investigations will be carried out to confirm diagnosis. If this is in doubt, an ultrasound scan may be undertaken.

Treatment options

Surgical appendicectomy, either through an open incision or laparoscopically, is the treatment of choice. The appendix is removed and the remaining stump is sutured. The cavity will be irrigated and a drainage tube inserted if any infected material is evident.

 ## Nursing management and health promotion: appendicitis

PRE-OPERATIVE MANAGEMENT

As appendicitis so often presents as an emergency, the patient may have to be prepared quickly for surgery. Nonetheless, safe physical preparation must be attended to with appropriate psychological and emotional support being offered. The pre-operative nursing assessment should focus on establishing baseline data and identifying factors that may increase the potential for postoperative complications. Vital signs should be monitored to assess if there is infection (peritonitis) or signs of septic shock. Pain assessment is important in determining whether the patient's condition is deteriorating and should be undertaken using a pain assessment tool. Enemas or aperients must not be given as induced peristalsis can cause a perforation of the bowel. Heat should not be applied directly over the area of the pain as it may cause the appendix to rupture and peritonitis to develop. In the past, withholding analgesia has been standard practice in those suspected of having appendicitis. However, Zimmerman (2008) reports on findings from American studies that demonstrate that diagnostic accuracy and physical findings did not differ in adults who were prescribed morphine pre-operatively.

POSTOPERATIVE MANAGEMENT

In the majority of cases, postoperative recovery will be uneventful and rapid. In addition to the standard postoperative care of all patients following surgery (see Ch. 26), patients who have had an appendicectomy should be placed in a semi-sitting position to reduce tension on the incision thus helping to reduce pain. Pain assessment and management should be undertaken and opiates such as morphine administered if the patient does not have PCA. Vital signs should be monitored for signs of complications. Diet and fluids can be commenced when bowel sounds are present.

Discharge is usually early if the surgery was uncomplicated. The patient should be advised on meeting their hygiene needs and caring for the wound and/or

laparoscopic puncture sites. Where necessary, arrangements should be made for sutures to be removed. The nurse should ensure the patient understands the need for a gradual return to normal activity within 2–4 weeks but that heavy lifting must be avoided in that period.

Complications

Should perforation and peritonitis occur (see Box 4.14), the patient may become seriously ill. Intestinal peristalsis will be halted and the risks of dehydration, electrolyte imbalance and septic shock are very real. Treatment will involve the removal of the appendix and toxic material, drainage of any abscess and the administration of systemic antibiotics. Oxygen therapy may be necessary and vascular volume will be restored and maintained intravenously. Opiate analgesics will be given to ensure that pain is not allowed to exacerbate an already serious situation. With effective and prompt intervention, the mortality rate of such complications is low (Box 4.15).

Abdominal hernias

A hernia is the protrusion of an organ through the structures that normally contain it. Abdominal hernias occur where there is an acquired or congenital weakness in the muscle wall of the abdomen, allowing an outpouching of peritoneum to form a sac. Acquired weakness can occur in any condition that may result in chronically raised intra-abdominal pressure, e.g. chronic cough, constipation or heavy lifting, or where abdominal muscle weakness has developed, e.g. obesity, old age, illness or pregnancy.

An untreated hernia may progress to contain peritoneal contents, typically the small or large bowel. The major concern is that, due to twisting and/or constriction at the neck of the sac, the blood supply may become impaired at that site. Unless this is immediately resolved, all of the symptoms of intestinal obstruction will occur (Box 4.16).

PATHOPHYSIOLOGY AND RISK FACTORS

The most commonly occurring types of abdominal hernia may be described as follows:

Inguinal hernia may be indirect or direct, the former being the more common. In indirect inguinal hernia, congenital abdominal weakness causes the hernial sac to protrude through the inguinal ring and follow the round ligament or spermatic cord. A direct inguinal hernia protrudes directly through the posterior ring. Inguinal hernias are far more common in men than in women.

 Box 4.15 Reflection

Identifying the nursing care of a patient with appendicitis

Read the case history of an adolescent with appendicitis on the website and answer the Critical thinking question.

 See website Critical thinking question 4.3

Box 4.16 Information

Intestinal obstruction

Intestinal obstruction occurs when the normal transit of intestinal contents is impeded due to mechanical obstruction, vascular occlusion or impaired innervation. Obstruction may be partial or complete.

Mechanical obstruction

- Intraluminal causes
- Neoplasms
- Strictures
- Foreign bodies
- Faeces
- Intussusception: a telescoping of one part of the bowel into another part

Extramural causes

- Adhesions
- Strangulated hernia
- Volvulus: twisting of the bowel
- Neoplasms outwith the intestinal tract

When the obstruction occurs, the affected intestine becomes distended with GI secretions (as much as 8 litres is formed each day). As the fluid accumulates, the pressure rises and the bowel responds by attempting to propel the contents forward. This serves only to increase secretions; eventually, the increase in pressure increases capillary permeability and fluid is forced out into the peritoneal cavity. The distension may cause respiratory embarrassment. Severe abdominal colic is experienced. If the obstruction is in the small bowel, vomiting occurs. Obstruction in the large bowel results in distension with air and faeces, and the eventual increase in pressure results in necrosis and the threat of perforation. The outcome of unresolved obstruction will be electrolyte imbalance, hypovolaemia and possibly peritonitis.

Vascular occlusion

Obstruction may occur if there is vascular occlusion of the major mesenteric blood supply by a thrombus or embolus. It is the resulting ischaemia that leads to obstruction. Although there is pain, there is no distension. As the condition deteriorates, the pain may actually decrease. If undiagnosed, gangrene and bacteraemia develop as toxins from the lumen invade the peritoneum and are absorbed into the bloodstream. If surgical intervention is not prompt, death may result. It should also be noted that any mechanical obstruction (e.g. strangulation) that impairs blood supply carries with it a significant mortality risk.

Impaired innervation: paralytic ileus

Paralytic ileus will occur when trauma, inflammation or pain in the thoracolumbar region interferes with the normal innervation of the bowel. It can therefore be a complication of such conditions as back and chest injury, renal pathology and peritonitis. Temporary (paralytic) ileus that follows the necessary handling of the bowel in certain abdominal surgical procedures usually resolves in 12–48 hours (see Ch. 26). Paralytic ileus will result in marked distension, causing discomfort and respiratory embarrassment.

Treatment

Treatment will involve the correction of fluid and electrolyte imbalance, the relief of the distension and pain, and surgical intervention to address the cause.

Femoral hernia is considered to be acquired, resulting from herniation through the femoral canal. This canal is wider in women, making such herniation more commonly a female complaint. Femoral hernias also have a greater risk of complications.

Umbilical hernia Many infants are born with an umbilical hernia. This normally disappears in the first year of life without surgical repair. Acquired umbilical hernias can develop in overweight individuals or in those with abdominal ascites.

Incisional hernia Following abdominal surgery, the incision site is a point of potential weakness. This becomes a problem if the patient experiences postoperative problems such as impaired healing, especially if drainage of the wound has been required, abdominal distension or generalised debility.

Reducible and irreducible hernias

In the early stages a hernia may often be reducible, i.e. with manual palpation or a change to standing posture the sac will return to the abdominal cavity. However, as the hernia becomes larger and adhesions form, reduction becomes impossible and the hernia is described as irreducible or incarcerated. If the blood flow is then impaired and obstruction occurs, the hernia is described as strangulated.

See the website for the clinical features, treatment options and nursing management and health promotion of patients with abdominal hernias.

 See website for further content

Colorectal cancer

Cancers that occur in the large bowel, rectum and anus are collectively referred to as colorectal cancers. Colorectal cancer is the third most common cancer after breast and lung (Cancer Research UK 2009a). Although it can affect all age groups, it is uncommon in those under 50 years but thereafter risk increases with age. It can affect any part of the large bowel but is most common in the sigmoid colon and rectum (NICE 2004).

PATHOPHYSIOLOGY AND RISK FACTORS

Colorectal cancer is more common in relatives of those who have the disease than those who do not. Genetic syndromes such as familial adenomatous polyposis (FAP) and hereditary non-polyposis colorectal cancer (HNPCC) cause colorectal cancer. People who have FAP tend to develop hundreds of polyps and by the age of 40 years most will have cancer unless the colon is surgically removed (NICE 2004). Inflammatory bowel disease is also associated with an increased risk, particularly where the condition has been present for more than 10 years. Colorectal cancer is increasingly associated with lifestyle and environmental factors, particularly in developed countries. Those that have been identified include a high consumption of processed meat, low consumption of vegetables, very low intake of fibre, alcohol consumption, obesity and smoking (Norton et al 2008).

More than 90% of cases of colorectal cancer are adenocarcinomas, where the tumours arise from the epithelial cells of glandular tissue. As they grow, they progressively obstruct the bowel by extending into the lumen or spreading circumferentially to form a ring-like stricture. Metastatic spread is by direct infiltration of local tissues and organs via the lymphatic and portal circulation, or by implantation during surgery.

Clinical features

The symptoms are subtle, gradual and easily ignored or explained away and unfortunately, patients tend not to present until the disease is at an advanced stage. Symptoms will vary somewhat according to the site of the tumour. Those with right-sided tumours may experience anaemia, weight loss, ill-defined abdominal pain, alteration in bowel habit and perhaps a felt abdominal mass. Those who have left-sided tumours can have abdominal cramping and an alternating bowel habit, i.e. constipation alternating with diarrhoea with or without the presence of mucus or blood. In people with rectal tumours, bright red blood in the stool, tenesmus (feeling of the need to evacuate) and a change in bowel habit may occur. Pain is not a common feature in the early stages and, perhaps due to this, medical advice is often not sought until either the patient is anaemic and debilitated or the symptoms associated with obstruction are marked. More rarely, patients may present with a fistula, bowel obstruction, haemorrhage or even perforation of the bowel.

Diagnosis

Many patients will present with a palpable mass that can be detected on abdominal or rectal examination. Specific investigations to confirm diagnosis will include barium studies, sigmoidoscopy, colonoscopy and biopsies. CT scan, chest X-ray and ultrasound scan will be necessary to seek out metastases, particularly in the lung and liver. For the latter, liver function tests will also be carried out.

Staging

The staging of the carcinoma is based on histological examination of a resected specimen. For colorectal cancer, Dukes' staging is the most widely used and, at its simplest, it describes four stages (Box 4.17).

Treatment

Surgical removal of the tumour is the only effective management and is curative in 50% of patients diagnosed with colon cancer (Norton et al 2008). The type and extent of surgery will depend on the site of the tumour (Box 4.18) but during

Box 4.17 Information

Dukes' classification of bowel cancer

Stage A	The cancer is only affecting the innermost lining of the colon or rectum or slightly growing into the muscle layer.
Stage B	The cancer has grown through the muscle layer of the colon or rectum.
Stage C	The cancer has spread to at least one lymph node in the area.
Stage D	The cancer has spread to somewhere else in the body, like the liver or lung. Some doctors prefer to call this cancer Stage 4, or advanced bowel cancer.

Box 4.18 Information

Surgery for colorectal cancer

TYPE/LOCATION OF COLORECTAL CANCER/TUMOURS	TYPE OF SURGERY
Right colon (caecum, ascending, proximal transverse colon)	Right hemicolectomy
Transverse colon	Transverse hemicolectomy
Left colon	Left hemicolectomy
Sigmoid colon	Sigmoid hemicolectomy
High rectum or low sigmoid colon	Anterior resection – a colonic pouch is created to enable the patient to have a normal bowel function or a temporary colostomy or ileostomy to allow the anastomosis to heal and to prevent complications
Lower rectum	Abdominoperineal resection – results in the formation of a permanent colostomy. In some cases it is possible to preserve the sphincter muscles and reconstruct the rectum in tumours situated above 5 cm from the anal verge

resection a segment of the bowel is removed and includes margins above and below the location of the tumour, the vascular supply to the area and the part of the mesentery including lymphatics and lymph nodes. It may be possible for resection and end-to-end anastomosis to be performed, but often stoma formation is necessary on a temporary or permanent basis.

Radiotherapy and chemotherapy are also used either alone or in conjunction with surgery (either before or after) to control recurrence or reduce the size of the tumour before/after surgery, as a means of controlling symptoms and improving quality of life in patients whose condition is advanced.

Nursing management and health promotion: colorectal cancer

Psychological support

The realisation that seemingly minor ailments are actually symptoms of cancer is most stressful for any individual. The patient is usually shocked, bewildered and frightened and will rely on family members or carers for emotional support. From the moment a patient is referred, as an outpatient or inpatient, a sensitive and tactful approach is of paramount importance. Psychological care needs to include the family and significant others in order to develop a trusting relationship. The beneficial effect of spending time to allow fears to be expressed and explanations and support to be given cannot be overstated.

PERI-OPERATIVE MANAGEMENT

The principles of peri-operative nursing care are discussed in Chapter 26. If surgery is to include stoma formation this will present a further source of stress. A cooperative team approach by the various health care professionals involved will greatly assist the patient's physical and psychological recovery and adjustment to what may prove to be major and perhaps only palliative surgery. See the website for the specific input of the stoma nurse specialist.

🖱 **See website for further content**

Discharge planning

For those patients for whom cure is not a possibility, planning for discharge and home care should aim to maximise their independence and quality of life for as long as possible. This requires the coordination and integration of hospital and community services, and a respect for the wishes of both the patient and the family. See Chapter 31 for a detailed discussion of the care of the patient with cancer.

Health promotion

Great efforts are being made to detect colorectal cancer early, when its prognosis is so much more favourable. The 5-year survival rate for localised lesions is 80–90%. This rate drops to 35–65% once the disease has spread to adjacent structures and lymph nodes. Factors being addressed include fostering awareness of early warning signs and information for those especially at risk. Preventive measures also include providing advice concerning diet and health screening. In the UK, the NHS Bowel Cancer Screening Programme has been rolled out, with men and women between the ages of 60 and 69 being invited for screening every 2 years.

Anorectal disorders

Anorectal conditions such as haemorrhoids, abscesses, fissures, fistulae and sinuses are relatively common and always distressing, but are often tolerated for many months or even years before professional help and advice are sought.

Haemorrhoids

Haemorrhoids, commonly called 'piles', are generally considered to be varices of the superior haemorrhoidal veins occurring as a result of congestion of the venous plexus.

PATHOPHYSIOLOGY AND RISK FACTORS

It would seem that a lack of dietary fibre is the most important predisposing factor. The resulting chronic constipation and straining during bowel movements raises intra-abdominal pressure, leading to venous plexus engorgement (Box 4.19). The bulging mucosa is dragged down and, as the condition worsens, the haemorrhoids prolapse into the anal canal. Other conditions that can lead to or aggravate the congestion are pregnancy, where the development of haemorrhoids is often neglected, tumours and cardiac failure.

Haemorrhoids may be internal or external. Internal haemorrhoids are classified according to the degree to which they prolapse into the anal canal. External haemorrhoids occur outside the anal canal and are less common.

Clinical features

Commonly the patient complains of 'fresh' blood in bowel movements, which at first may be thought to be due simply to the passing of constipated motions. The experience of prolapse, at first transient, becomes increasingly frequent and is associated with pain, the discharge of mucus and pruritus (intense itching). Often such symptoms have been managed by over-the-counter remedies such as creams to reduce the itching and pain. Education of the patient in order to achieve the passing of soft bulky stools with minimal effort often yields more relief in the long term than conventional treatments. The addition of supplementary dietary fibre and ensuring an adequate fluid intake are often seen as more acceptable (Norton et al 2008). However, many people find the adjustment of diet too much of a change in lifestyle. Should the haemorrhoidal vessels thrombose, pain is always severe and it may only be at this stage that the patient seeks help.

Diagnosis

Diagnosis is confirmed by:

- history and examination to exclude other pathologies, particularly a carcinoma
- rectal examination, proctoscopy and/or sigmoidoscopy.

Treatment options

If the haemorrhoids are identified in their early stages, management requires no more than attention to the patient's diet and perhaps a bulk laxative. If the constipation is corrected, the problem will usually resolve but the patient must understand this and feel confident in diet alteration. The practice nurse can play an important part in patient education and in arranging a follow-up appointment to monitor the patient's well-being.

SURGICAL MANAGEMENT

The following surgical treatments may be used to resolve haemorrhoids that do not respond to conservative management:

- *Injection* – for haemorrhoids in the early stages, injection of the haemorrhoidal veins with an irritant solution provokes fibrosis and atrophy with minimal discomfort.
- *Band ligation* – bands are applied to the mucosa-covered haemorrhoidal pedicle, constricting the vessels, which eventually shrink.
- *Infrared coagulation* – infrared radiation is applied in pulses to the haemorrhoid by means of a fibreoptic probe, causing coagulation and shrinkage.
- *Haemorrhoidectomy*. The above interventions are the most commonly used and can be carried out on an outpatient basis. If, however, the haemorrhoids are not amenable to such therapies, haemorrhoidectomy to ligate and excise the haemorrhoids may be required. If thrombosis has occurred, this procedure will be required immediately.

Box 4.19 Information

Constipation

Constipation may be defined as difficult and infrequent defaecation. The following factors can contribute to its development.

Diet

A diet that is low in fibre and bulk predisposes to small faecal bulk. A low fluid intake also contributes to small bulk. Small bulk predisposes the GI tract to reduced peristaltic action and slow passage of contents along the colon. Epidemiological studies indicate that low-fibre diets contribute to many of the GI diseases found in the Western world, such as diverticulosis, appendicitis and haemorrhoids.

Exercise

Lack of exercise contributes to reduced peristalsis, due to reduced muscle tone of the bowel and abdominal muscles. Individuals who take less exercise include the older person and those who are ill or have a physical disability. Hospital patients are, in general, restricted in their mobility, given their environment and their medical condition, and investigations and treatment often predispose patients to constipation.

Elimination habits

Neglecting to empty the rectum when the stimulation caused by faeces therein (the 'call to stool') is ignored results in constipation. If this occurs repeatedly, faecal impaction can result. Watery diarrhoea, caused by the breakdown of faecal material proximal to the hard impacted mass, can bypass the mass. Impacted faeces can press on the urethra and cause retention of urine.

Socioeconomic factors

Nutritional and dietary intake is determined by eating patterns formed in childhood and influenced by familial and social norms and income levels. A low income can result in the exclusion from the diet of fresh fruit and vegetables, which can be relatively expensive. Low-income families and older people living alone may have to make difficult choices in spending their limited resources on food, heating and clothing. Lack of transport or reduced mobility can also limit shopping expeditions and therefore the choice of foods. The older person living alone may be less likely to cook nutritious meals for a number of reasons, e.g. lack of motivation, poor appetite and limited mobility.

Medication

Many medications have side-effects that cause constipation; these include ganglion-blocking drugs, psychotropic drugs, muscle relaxants, and morphine and its derivatives.

Dentition

Poor dentition makes chewing difficult, especially where there has been dental clearance and dentures do not fit well or comfortably. This can result in the avoidance of fresh fruit and vegetables, and an emphasis on soft, easily chewed foods that do not add fibre to the diet.

Motility of colon

Eating results in increased colonic motor activity that may be perceived by the individual as an urge to defaecate, but lack of mobility or regular exercise decreases gut motility and may contribute to constipation.

The bowel may become obstructed by a growth, a hernia or by adhesions following surgery. In addition, spasticity can occur in inflammatory conditions such as appendicitis or diverticulitis.

Rectal conditions

Local conditions such as haemorrhoids or anal fissure, which cause pain on defaecation, can result in avoidance of defaecation with eventual constipation.

Prevention and treatment

Dietary advice is important in the prevention of constipation. Wholemeal bread, fresh fruit and vegetables, and cereals such as porridge oats and All Bran are important. Unprocessed bran can also be added to soups or stews. The individual should be advised to drink plenty of fluid throughout the day. Older people who have urinary incontinence tend to take inadequate fluid in an attempt to avoid being incontinent of urine.

The importance of emptying the bowel regularly and of not ignoring the call to stool should be emphasised. The individual should be encouraged to take as much physical exercise as possible.

The initial treatment of constipation can include the use of laxatives. Bulk-forming preparations such as Fybogel and stimulant laxatives such as bisacodyl by mouth or by rectum may be used initially. Where there is a faecal mass, rectally administered faecal softeners such as arachis oil may be necessary.

Any condition, such as haemorrhoids, anal fissure or diverticulosis, which is predisposing the individual to constipation, should be treated.

 ## Nursing management and health promotion: haemorrhoids

Whether it is the cause or the effect, it is most important that difficulty with defaecation is effectively corrected. Measures to achieve this include:

- increasing dietary fibre
- maintaining a high fluid intake (2–3 L/day)
- prescribing a stool softener to facilitate water and fat absorption into the faeces
- ensuring sufficient exercise and activity.

In addition, nursing priorities must include measures to alleviate pain and itching, to ensure good personal hygiene, to provide appropriate privacy in a hospital setting and to prevent infection.

PRE-OPERATIVE MANAGEMENT

If surgery is required, the aim of nursing care in the pre-operative period is to control the acute symptoms and to ensure that the patient feels comfortable and free from any distress when defaecating. One of the major postoperative fears in any form of anorectal surgery is the pain that might be experienced upon the first bowel movement. Time is well spent explaining postoperative care and how any pain and discomfort will be relieved or minimised. Patients are very often comforted merely by the fact that the nurse understands their fears and has the knowledge and skill to help them to manage the problem.

POSTOPERATIVE MANAGEMENT

Care priorities in the postoperative period include:

- relief of pain and promotion of comfort
- prevention of postoperative haemorrhage

- prevention of postoperative urinary retention
- prevention of infection
- promotion of optimal faecal elimination
- patient education prior to discharge regarding lifestyle and diet.

For other common anorectal disorders and principles of nursing care for patients undergoing perianal surgery, refer to the website.

🖱 **See website for further content**

THE HEPATOBILIARY SYSTEM

Anatomy and physiology of the liver

The liver, weighing approximately 1.5 kg, is the largest single gland in the body and is located mainly in the upper right quadrant of the abdomen just below the diaphragm. The liver is a compact lobular organ with large right and left lobes and two smaller caudate and quadrate lobes (Figure 4.6). Blood is supplied to the liver by the hepatic artery and the hepatic portal vein which carry blood containing the products of digestion from the small intestine directly to the liver. The hepatic portal system also collects blood from the lower oesophagus, the stomach, the spleen and the large intestine.

Each lobe of the liver is subdivided into functional units called lobules. In these lobules, branches of the hepatic artery, the hepatic portal vein and a bile duct run concurrently in a structure known as the portal triad. All of the blood entering the liver mixes in spaces called sinusoids and then drains into a central vein. The multiple functions of the liver are carried out mainly by two types of cells: the parenchymal cells or hepatocytes, which release substances into bile canaliculi, into blood and lymph channels, and the

Kupffer cells which form a part of the lining of blood sinusoids and are phagocytic.

Functions of the liver

Due to its size and unique structure the liver has both endocrine and exocrine functions. The exocrine functions include the production of bile consisting of water, inorganic electrolytes and bile salts. Bile assists in the neutralisation of acid chyme in the duodenum. The endocrine functions of the liver include the detoxification of drugs and other noxious substances, carbohydrate metabolism, protein and fat metabolism, synthesis of plasma proteins and most blood clotting factors from amino acids, the breakdown of erythrocytes and defence against microbes, the inactivation of hormones including insulin, glucagons, cortisol, aldosterone, the thyroid and sex hormones (Waugh & Grant 2006), production of heat and the storage of glycogen, fat-soluble vitamins (A, D, E and K), iron, copper and vitamin B_{12}.

Anatomy and physiology of the gall bladder

Lying beneath the liver, the gall bladder is a pear-shaped sac approximately 10 cm long attached to the posterior surface of the liver. It has a middle muscular layer comprising of smooth muscle under vagal and hormonal control. Vagal stimulation causes the gall bladder to contract. The mucosal surface area of the gall bladder is increased by the presence of rugae, promoting the reabsorption of water and a 10-fold concentration of the bile that enters from the cystic duct. As the muscular walls of the gall bladder contract, bile is expelled, the sphincter of Oddi (also known as the hepatopancreatic sphincter) relaxes and bile is ejected via the bile duct into the duodenum (Figure 4.7). The functions of the gall bladder include storing bile and

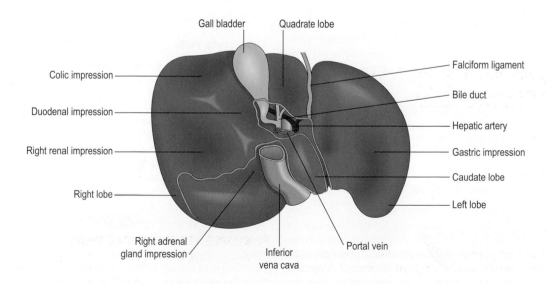

Figure 4.6 The liver. (Reproduced with permission from Waugh & Grant 2006.)

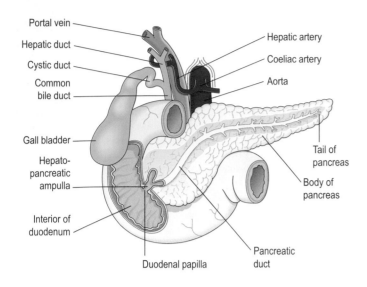

Figure 4.7 The gall bladder and related structures. (Reproduced with permission from Waugh & Grant 2006.)

releasing the stored bile. Bile is composed principally of bilirubin, derived from the breakdown of haemoglobin from erythrocytes, and bile salts, formed from excess steroid hormones. The release of bile is stimulated by cholecystokinin and secretin.

DISORDERS OF THE HEPATOBILIARY SYSTEM

Disorders of the liver

Liver disease is the fifth biggest killer in the UK after cardiac disease, cancer, stroke and respiratory disease (Office for National Statistics 2008). The liver, because of the large number of functions it performs, is essential to life and can be affected by a number of diseases. Consequently, the nursing care of a patient with liver disease is complex. The onset of illness can be acute, as in an acute attack of viral hepatitis, or chronic, where the disease processes have been progressing for many years before symptoms become evident, i.e. liver cirrhosis. As a result of the liver's large blood supply, it has notable regenerative properties. The liver can compensate for a significant amount of damage, but eventually a threshold is reached and liver functions decline, resulting in liver decompensation. For clinical features associated with the development of liver decompensation see Box 4.20.

Manifestations of liver disease

Liver disease can manifest in many ways. In the early stages patients can be asymptomatic or symptoms can be vague and may be disregarded. Non-specific indications such as flu-like symptoms, anorexia, nausea, lethargy, malaise and vomiting are common. Weight loss also occurs in chronic liver disease, most notably in malignant disease. More specific features include enlargement of the liver

Box 4.20 Information

Clinical features of liver decompensation

- Abnormal excretion of bile, leading to an accumulation of bilirubin in the blood, producing jaundice.
- Abnormal clearance of proteins absorbed through the intestinal tract, leading to ammonia retention and hepatic encephalopathy.
- Ascites, leading to fluid accumulation in the abdomen that becomes more difficult to manage.
- Portal hypertension, where scarred liver tissue acts as a barrier to blood flow and causes increased portal blood pressure. A major consequence is the rupture of oesophageal varices, causing massive and potentially fatal haemorrhage.

(hepatomegaly), portal hypertension with associated ascites and splenomegaly, jaundice, pruritus, right upper quadrant pain, fever, dark urine, pale stools, oesophageal varices and hepatic encephalopathy or coma.

Assessment of liver disease

Patient history

A comprehensive history from the patient and sometimes a family member is required, especially due to the stigma often associated with liver disease such as chronic alcohol consumption in relation to cirrhosis, and sexual behaviour or intravenous drug use with hepatitis. Hence, the patient may not give an accurate history (Sargent 2005). The nurse should ask direct questions to identify any risk factors in a sensitive manner. It is important to ascertain information regarding any history of intravenous drug use, sexual history and orientation, alcohol consumption, medication history including herbal remedies and/or recreational drug use. Past medical and surgical history and previous blood or blood product transfusion are important and a family history can indicate possible hereditary liver disease. The patient's recent travel history should be established, as should their occupational history to exclude causes from occupational hazards. A general physical examination of the patient may reveal signs of liver disease (Figure 4.8).

Laboratory tests

Laboratory tests can detect liver disease and estimate the severity of the disease, as elevated liver enzymes are usually the first sign of liver damage. Liver function tests are primarily carried out to estimate hepatic injury. The enzyme tests aminotransferases, alanine aminotransferase (ALT) and aspartate aminotransferase (AST) are the most common liver function tests carried out. A full blood count, virology screen and urinalysis is also useful. For further reading on liver function tests see Sargent (2005).

Liver biopsy

A liver biopsy may also be ordered by the physician as liver biopsy is a key tool in diagnosing and evaluating liver disease. A small piece of tissue is removed from the liver for histology, cytology or microbiological examination. A biopsy may be percutaneous, guided by ultrasound, CT or MRI, or alternatively transjugular. The percutaneous route is the

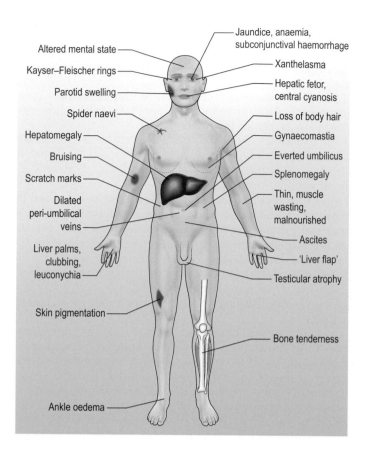

Altered mental state

Kayser–Fleischer rings

Parotid swelling

Spider naevi

Hepatomegaly

Bruising

Scratch marks

Dilated peri-umbilical veins

Liver palms, clubbing, leuconychia

Skin pigmentation

Ankle oedema

Jaundice, anaemia, subconjunctival haemorrhage

Xanthelasma

Hepatic fetor, central cyanosis

Loss of body hair

Gynaecomastia

Everted umbilicus

Splenomegaly

Thin, muscle wasting, malnourished

Ascites

'Liver flap'

Testicular atrophy

Bone tenderness

Figure 4.8 Signs of liver disease. (Reproduced with permission from Bacon et al 2006.)

most widely used procedure. Three types of needles can be used to obtain the biopsy tissue under local anaesthetic: suction needles, cutting needles or the automated spring-loaded biopsy gun. According to Karamshi (2008), studies identified the cutting needle to be the most popular choice, mainly due to ease of use and ability to cut through liver tissue resulting in better preservation of tissue.

Prior to the procedure informed consent is obtained from the patient. If the patient is taking prescribed drugs such as aspirin or non-steroidal anti-inflammatory drugs these need to be discontinued at least 2 days before the biopsy. Warfarin should be discontinued 5 days prior to the procedure. The patient's prothrombin time and platelet count are measured and the patient's blood group is determined. If the patient has a clotting disorder, vitamin K is given parenterally. Prophylactic antibiotics are administered to patients at risk of bacteraemia. In some cases a premedication of midazolam and fentanyl may be given if the patient is extremely anxious. Fasting is not required.

A baseline of the patient's vital signs is recorded. The patient lies in the supine position and is asked to raise their right hand and rest it on their head. The physician prepares the biopsy site with an antiseptic solution and administers a local anaesthetic. The patient is then requested to exhale and hold their breath while the physician inserts the biopsy needle. Immediately following the procedure a dry dressing is placed on the puncture site. The specimen is placed in 4% formaldehyde in a specimen jar. The jar is then correctly labelled and sent to the laboratory.

Approximately 10–20% of patients experience discomfort in the upper right quadrant region or shoulder during the procedure, with post procedure pain occurring up to 3 h following the biopsy. Analgesia should be used with caution with liver disease because NSAIDs can cause gastric mucosal and haemodynamic complications. In addition, the side-effects of narcotic analgesia, such as mental status changes, constipation and hypotension mimic the symptoms of hepatic encephalitis. Severe pain occurring in the right hypochondrium is likely to indicate a subcapsular accumulation of blood or bile, and the sudden occurrence of very severe pain is a sign of biliary peritonitis. Intramuscular opioid/narcotic analgesia may be prescribed and administered to manage severe pain.

Bed rest is required for 6–8 h after the procedure and the patient's vital signs must be recorded at intervals of 15 min for 2 h, 30 min for 2 h, and hourly for the next 2 h to observe for signs of haemorrhage. The biopsy site should also be checked for signs of haemorrhage or bile leakage. The mortality risk following a liver biopsy is 0.01% due to complications such as haemorrhage, bacteraemia, bile peritonitis, haemothorax and subcutaneous emphysema. After 8 h of monitoring the patient may be discharged home if their vital signs are stable and they have someone to care for them. For further information see Karamshi (2008).

Hepatitis

Hepatitis denotes inflammation of the liver that may be acute or chronic. Globally, viruses are the most common cause of acute hepatitis, but the disease may also be a response to certain medications (Box 4.21) and alcohol.

PATHOPHYSIOLOGY AND RISK FACTORS

All types of hepatitis will cause similar symptoms, ranging from slight to severe and possibly life threatening, as in fulminant hepatic failure, which is very rare. Many patients with acute hepatitis will not require hospitalisation and some will not even contact a doctor. The clinical features are described in three phases (Box 4.22).

All the hepatitis viruses can cause a similar initial illness. The differences between them would appear to be their modes of transmission and progression of disease. The most common viruses in acute viral hepatitis are A, B and C.

Box 4.21 Information

Medication-induced hepatitis

Hepatitis may be caused by any drug, but the more common culprits include analgesics such as paracetamol taken in excess, psychotropic drugs such as the phenothiazines, antibiotics such as erythromycin, and anaesthetics such as halothane. Any patient with hepatitis should be questioned regarding medication taken recently, including those taken without medical advice, and including herbal remedies.

In most incidences of medication-induced hepatitis, the biopsy shows changes as for viral hepatitis. However, some medications will also cause fatty changes in the liver cells.

Box 4.22 Information

Clinical features of acute hepatitis

Pre-icteric phase

Flu-like symptoms last from 2 to 7 days in hepatitis A virus (HAV) and slightly longer in hepatitis B virus (HBV). Symptoms include headache, low-grade fever (37.5–38.5°C), nasal congestion, sore throat, anorexia, lethargy, mild upper abdominal pain or discomfort in the right hypochondrium, arthralgia and arthritis. As the liver has no sensory innervation, pain is caused by stretching of the liver capsule. In inflammatory conditions such as hepatitis, pain is usually perceived as a dull ache in the right upper quadrant.

Icteric phase

Prodromal or early symptoms usually disappear. Jaundice of varying intensity occurs but rarely causes plasma bilirubin to rise above 200 mmol/L. Jaundice is a yellowing of the sclera, skin and mucous membranes caused by the deposition of bile pigments. Jaundice occurs when the bilirubin level in the blood exceeds 50 mmol/L. There are three distinct types:

- *Hepatocellular jaundice* – hepatocyte destruction renders the liver unable to transport bilirubin; this is the type of jaundice seen in viral hepatitis.
- *Haemolytic jaundice* – caused by excessive red cell destruction (see Ch. 11).
- *Cholestatic jaundice* – caused by obstruction to the flow of bile through the liver ducts due to cirrhosis or malignancy. Obstruction of the larger extrahepatic ducts may be caused by gall stones or cancer of the head of pancreas (Fawcett & Smith 2004).

The convalescent phase

This occurs approximately 2 weeks after the onset of jaundice. Jaundice lessens and eventually disappears. Other symptoms resolve.

Hepatitis is referred to as chronic when the patient continues to have clinical symptoms or abnormal liver function tests 6 months after the onset of the illness. The main causes of chronic hepatitis are hepatitis B, C and D viruses, autoimmune hepatitis and alcohol and drug-related liver disease.

Viral hepatitis

Further information about each of the viruses that cause hepatitis is provided on the website.

 See website for further content

 ## Nursing management and health promotion: hepatitis

There is no specific treatment for acute hepatitis although advice can be given to help the patient cope with the illness. Management focuses on the relief of symptoms and supportive therapy. Should the patient require nursing support, a nursing care plan should be devised to include education and information on coping with the physical side-effects of the condition. Because the patient may be asymptomatic on admission it is important to obtain baseline measurements of the vital signs in case the patient's condition deteriorates during hospitalisation or following treatment. The patient's vital signs should be recorded and the colour of the skin, mucous membrane and sclera should be observed for signs of jaundice. If the patient has jaundice, antihistamines, warm emollient baths and calamine lotion may help relieve the symptoms of itch or pruritus.

The patient should also be monitored for signs of anaemia. Urine, faeces and gums should be observed for signs of bleeding and the patient's full blood count should be monitored.

Flu-like symptoms such as acute fever can be managed by regular paracetamol, i.e. 1 g four times a day. Infection control universal precautions must be maintained with all patients, not only those diagnosed with hepatitis. Nonetheless, if the patient has diarrhoea and requires nursing assistance, plastic gloves and aprons must be used for all procedures. Linen and disposable wipes must be disposed of as per local policy and thorough handwashing must be carried out after patient contact.

It is important to maintain adequate fluid and nutritional intake. An intravenous line may be inserted on admission. Intravenous fluids may be necessary if the patient is dehydrated or unable to tolerate oral fluids. The patient's intake and output must be monitored as renal complications or hepatorenal syndrome are common with patients with disorders of the liver (Whitman & McCormick 2005). Antiemetic drugs such as metoclopramide may be prescribed to manage nausea or vomiting.

A high-calorie, high-protein diet is recommended in the form of small regular meals. Fatty foods should be avoided and the patient should be advised to refrain from consuming alcohol. Daily weights should be recorded and if necessary a referral to a dietitian may be made. Vitamin K may be required parenterally.

It is advisable for the patient to rest as much as possible and to avoid strenuous exercise. Fatigue should be managed by promoting bed rest and limiting the number of visitors the patient has whilst in hospital. A referral to a medical social worker may be required if the patient is unable to work.

The patient's blood analysis should be monitored for signs of liver dysfunction. LFTs, platelet count, prothrombin time and international normalised ratio (INR) all increase with impaired liver function, while albumin decreases.

Observe for signs of anxiety or depression and allow the patient to discuss their concerns in an open manner. The patient may request a referral to a counsellor. If the patient has an alcohol dependency, referral can also be made to an alcohol counsellor for appropriate support.

Education and advice for the patient and their family regarding the spread of infection is essential. Lifestyle choices and changes that can prevent further complications should be discussed. Where appropriate, patients should be advised to avoid sexual practices that may result in damage to the skin and mucous membranes. Alcohol, drug use and herbal supplements should also be discouraged. Any identified cause should be stopped, and no medication should be taken without medical advice. It is important the patient knows to notify their GP and other health care workers, i.e. dentists, of their hepatitis status (Box 4.23).

Box 4.23 Reflection

Care of an individual following a needlestick injury

A colleague sustains an accidental needlestick injury following the administration of an intramuscular injection.

Activities

- Identify possible risks to the nurse following a needlestick injury.
- What is the correct procedure following this event? (See website for further information.)

 See website for further content

Non-viral hepatitis

Autoimmune hepatitis

Autoimmune hepatitis is rare and its cause is unknown but it is thought to be immune mediated whereby the body's immune system attacks liver cells. Prognosis is dependent on the severity of the inflammatory activity. Patients with severe multilobular necrosis on biopsy generally develop cirrhosis within 5 years. For further information on clinical features, diagnosis and treatment options see the website.

 See website for further content

Alcohol-induced hepatitis

Alcoholic hepatitis is an acute inflammatory liver disorder generally caused by heavy alcohol consumption (Sargent 2005). Alcoholic hepatitis usually occurs after years of alcohol abuse and often following a recent prolonged bout of heavy drinking.

Clinical features

Alcoholic hepatitis is characterised by an enlarged liver, jaundice, fever and lethargy. Elevated liver enzymes are often the first sign of liver disease. The patient usually presents with anorexia, vomiting, lethargy, diarrhoea and upper abdominal pain. A fever may be present and the patient will appear generally unwell and malnourished. There may be signs of chronic liver disease, i.e. ascites and oedema, encephalopathy, jaundice and the dilated capillaries of spider telangiectases. Gastrointestinal bleeding may occur from erosions or peptic ulceration or as a result of bleeding tendencies due to the liver's inability to synthesise adequate clotting factors.

Diagnosis

The diagnosis is made from an accurate picture of the patient's alcohol intake, liver function tests and liver biopsy, provided the patient's clotting time and platelet count are satisfactory.

Treatment options

Patients presenting with alcoholic hepatitis may have mild or severe liver damage. They may present with severe complications associated with portal hypertension such as ascites, oesophageal varices and hepatic encephalopathy, all of which will be discussed further in this chapter. Patients must be advised to refrain from consuming alcohol, and chlordiazepoxide (Librium) orally may be prescribed in anticipation of alcohol withdrawal symptoms. The patient will require a high-protein, high-carbohydrate diet, and in some cases enteral nutritional support may be prescribed. Alcoholic hepatitis usually improves over time if the patient abstains from alcohol. For patients who develop liver cirrhosis controversy exists regarding liver transplantation and patients must have abstained from alcohol for at least 6 months prior to receiving a liver transplant.

Medication-induced hepatitis

Paracetamol or acetaminophen is the most common cause of drug-induced hepatitis representing one third of self-poisoning either deliberately or accidently. Paracetamol is found in over-the-counter preparations with a variety of other medications such as decongestants, caffeine and codeine. While paracetamol is safe when used in therapeutic doses it can be fatal following an overdose. Hepatotoxity and liver failure have been well linked to paracetamol poisoning with Wallace et al (2002) reporting between 100 and 200 deaths per year as a consequence.

Diagnosis

Hepatitis usually begins within 24–48 hours following a paracetamol overdose and liver enzymes dramatically rise. Prothrombin time and INR become raised. For further information see Hartley (2002).

Treatment options

Intravenous *N*-acetylcysteine (Parvolex) is the antidote of choice and is very effective when given within 8 h of ingestion. Hepatic and renal function needs to be closely monitored. Early contact with a liver unit is advisable and if there is no improvement in the patient's condition within 3–5 days liver failure and/or death may occur. In patients who do survive, the liver regenerates quickly with liver function tests returning to normal within 3 weeks. Refer to Sargent (2009) for further information.

Cirrhosis of the liver

Cirrhosis or scarring of the liver is an irreversible progressive condition and an escalating health problem. There are many clinical manifestations, varying with the severity and duration of the disease.

PATHOPHYSIOLOGY AND RISK FACTORS

Alcohol- and drug-induced hepatitis are the commonest causes of cirrhosis, with others being viral hepatitis, primary biliary cirrhosis, autoimmune hepatitis, haemochromatosis and Wilson's disease. Biliary disorders such as biliary stones (see p. 110), malignancy, primary biliary cirrhosis or sclerosing cholangitis can also lead to the development of cirrhosis by obstructing the biliary tree and causing elevation of the liver enzymes (Sargent & Fullwood 2008). Prolonged low-grade inflammation causes progressive scarring and destruction of the liver cells. In an attempt to repair the damaged cells the remaining liver cells proliferate to form nodules and fibrous tissue with the result that the liver becomes irregular and distorted in shape. The blood vessels are also destroyed, thus resistance to the flow of blood increases, which in turn leads to portal hypertension (Kelso 2008).

Clinical features

As the disease progresses, the patient feels increasingly fatigued and lethargic. Anorexia, nausea and weight loss are common. Jaundice, bruising, spider telangiectases and finger clubbing are also evident. Pruritus is common and is probably caused by bile salt deposition in the skin. Endocrine abnormalities such as gynaecomastia (enlargement of male breasts), impotence in males and amenorrhoea and infertility in females can also develop. The major complications of cirrhosis, resulting from hepatocellular failure, portal hypertension and portal systemic shunting, are ascites, gastrointestinal bleeding, hepatic encephalopathy, renal dysfunction and hepatocellular carcinoma. Thus, the medical and nursing management of patients diagnosed with liver cirrhosis is complicated and challenging.

Treatment options

The aim of treatment is the removal of any identifiable cause such as alcohol abuse and the management of the major symptoms and complications. Liver transplantation may be considered when earlier treatment fails. Considerable counselling and support may also be required to eliminate an alcohol problem and improve nutrition.

 Nursing management and health promotion: cirrhosis of the liver

Nursing Care Plan 4.1 summarises the care required for a man with liver failure due to alcoholic cirrhosis.

Complications of liver cirrhosis

Ascites

The term 'ascites' refers to a marked increase in the volume of fluid in the peritoneal cavity. This is usually due to an underlying disease in which the total body fluid is increased. Ascites is the abnormal accumulation of extracellular fluid within the peritoneal cavity (Sargent 2006a) and results from a combination of the following factors:

- raised portal pressure
- increased lymphatic pressure in the liver

Nursing Care Plan 4.1 Care plan for a man with liver failure due to alcoholic cirrhosis		
PROBLEM (ACTUAL/POTENTIAL)	**REASON**	**NURSING ACTION**
1. Anxiety, anger and fear	Due to: lack of knowledge, fear of the unknown and perhaps denial of the reality of his condition	Encourage fears to be expressed and questions to be asked. Explain all procedures and maintain a non-judgemental approach. Confidence will be restored and he will feel better able to cope
2. Loss of self-concept: • body image • role performance • self-identity • self-esteem	Due to: • physical alteration resulting from jaundice, ascites and weight loss • loss of libido, impotence and gynaecomastia due to retention of oestrogens normally broken down in the liver	• Restore optimal liver function • Provide a trusting relationship • Refer to a specialist counsellor as appropriate
3. Pain and discomfort	Due to: • the enlarged liver that stretches the liver capsule (the liver itself has no sensory nerve innervation) • biliary obstruction secondary to the cirrhosis • gastritis due to alcohol abuse • oedema, ascites, bowel disturbance, dyspepsia and itching	Relieve pain and discomfort via: • comfort measures such as positioning, gentle movement and distraction techniques • medication for pruritus: – sodium bicarbonate baths – calamine lotion – colestyramine which binds the bile salts in the intestines – antihistamine • analgesics, used with caution to avoid hepatotoxic effects
4. Insomnia	Due to: pain, anxiety, dyspnoea induced by ascites, itching and the strange environment	• Relieve pain, anxiety, dyspnoea and itching (see above) • Provide optimal peace and quiet when appropriate
5. Nutritional impairment: anorexia, anaemia and weight loss	Due to: • the inability of the liver to perform its metabolic functions and the reduction in production of bile • reduction in iron, vitamin B_{12} and red blood cells • fetor hepaticus (a bad taste in the mouth and bad breath) • previous dietary neglect due to alcohol excess	• A diet high in calories: – protein to restore plasma proteins – glucose, thought to aid liver cell recovery • Supplements, e.g. vitamins and iron • Low salt to reduce oedema • Controlled fat intake according to degree of jaundice

Nursing Care Plan 4.1 Care plan for a man with liver failure due to alcoholic cirrhosis – cont'd

PROBLEM (ACTUAL/POTENTIAL)	REASON	NURSING ACTION
		• Small tempting meals • Oral hygiene • Monitoring of weight • If anaemia becomes severe, blood transfusion and oxygen therapy may be required
6. Fluid and electrolyte imbalance and impaired tissue perfusion	Due to: • reduced arterial flow, portal hypertension, ascites • salt retention due to loss of detoxification of aldosterone and the triggering of the renin–angiotensin mechanism	• Reduce salt intake to no added salt (NAS) or less as necessary • Fluid restriction (1–1.5 L/day) if hyponatraemia develops • Gentle use of diuretics • Manage the care of the patient requiring paracentesis (Box 4.24)
7. Infection	Due to: loss of Kupffer cell function and lymphocyte production and exacerbated by nutritional, circulatory and respiratory impairment	• Hygiene maintained at a high standard. Strict asepsis with any invasive techniques. Regular monitoring of vital signs • Chest physiotherapy as appropriate • Infection screening as appropriate • Antibiotics if necessary but used with caution
8. Impaired skin integrity	Due to: oedema, loss of protein, jaundice, weight loss and bleeding tendency (see problem 11)	• Regular relief of pressure • Sensitive care of the skin, nails and when shaving • Use of emollients • Optimal positioning and repositioning
9. Immobility	Due to: malaise, weakness, ascites, dyspnoea and perhaps confusion	• Ensure optimal activity and rest. Provide companionship • Relieve symptoms as described
10. Impaired detoxification of natural and medicinal substances	Due to: liver cell damage	• Careful and tactful enforcement of abstinence from alcohol • Vigilance with all medications
11. Tendency to bleed that might be insidious or dramatic leading to hypovolaemic shock	Due to: • portal hypertension and development of oesophageal varices • gastritis • loss of clotting factors • inadequate absorption of vitamin K • reduced reserves of blood in the liver	• Regular monitoring of vital signs • Monitoring of any vomit for blood, fresh or digested • Skin and mucous membranes observed for bruises or bleeding • Give vitamin K as necessary • Manage hypovolaemic shock should severe bleeding occur (see gastrointestinal bleeding)
12. Encephalopathy • lethargy • flapping tremor (asterixis) • irrational behaviour • aggression • loss of ability to perform daily duties	Due to: inability of the liver to convert ammonia to urea. Ammonia levels rise to such a level that cerebral cell damage occurs due to nitrogenous neurotoxins Note: **1.** A GI bleed constitutes a 'high-protein meal' and will exacerbate encephalopathy **2.** Infection will exacerbate encephalopathy by inducing a catabolic state **3.** Hypoxia will exacerbate encephalopathy	• Careful monitoring of behaviour and ability to communicate effectively • Observe for precipitating factors, e.g. 1, 2 or 3 • Manage encephalopathy: – reduce protein intake – give rectal and colonic washouts, if necessary, to remove blood from bowel – give oral lactulose, an osmotic laxative, to reduce ammonia by acidification of bowel environment and to help evacuate bowel contents, *and/or* – give oral neomycin (poorly absorbed from the gut) to reduce intestinal flora – monitor level of consciousness (LOC) – ensure safety and comfort

- low plasma protein – albumin
- sodium retention.

PATHOPHYSIOLOGY AND RISK FACTORS

Hepatic cirrhosis accounts for over 80% of cases but ascites can also be caused by cardiac failure, nephrotic syndrome, malignancy in the peritoneum or infection such as tuberculosis. In health, serous fluid is continually produced in the peritoneal cavity and is sufficient to provide lubrication only. Ascites occurs when fluid enters the peritoneal cavity more quickly than it can be returned to the circulation by the capillaries and lymphatics. Fluid normally leaves a capillary at its arteriolar end and returns at its venous end but, in cirrhosis, portal hypertension causes more fluid to be produced in the hepatic sinusoids which are unable to drain via impaired hepatic lymphatics. The failing liver cannot synthesise enough of the plasma protein, albumin, and the resulting hypoalbuminaemia lowers the osmotic pressure of the blood, reducing the amount of peritoneal fluid reabsorbed at the venous end.

This picture is further complicated by sodium and hence water retention. The presence of ascites in liver disease is a poor prognostic sign as it implies poor liver function. Severe ascites can cause great discomfort: dyspnoea, anorexia and the ability to eat only small meals; inhibited mobility and discomfort when lying in bed or sitting upright in a chair. If pain occurs, it is often felt in the back. Many of the symptoms correspond to the discomfort of full-term pregnancy. Increased intra-abdominal pressure also leads to hernias, especially at the umbilicus.

Ascitic fluid in cirrhosis is usually straw-coloured; blood-stained ascites indicates malignant disease; bile staining indicates a communication with the biliary system; and cloudy fluid denotes infection. Chylous ascites, which has a milky appearance, is caused by lymphatic obstruction.

Clinical features

Abdominal swelling can occur over a number of weeks or rapidly over a few hours. In order to detect ascites there must be at least 1.5 L of fluid in the peritoneal cavity, confirmed by abdominal percussion. Other clinical features include abdominal pain, anorexia, nausea and sometimes difficulty in breathing. The patient often presents with other features of portal hypertension and cirrhosis as mentioned above.

Treatment options

The main elements of treatment include restriction of sodium and fluid intake, administration of diuretics and abdominal paracentesis (Box 4.24) in refractory ascites. Pleural effusions are also common with ascites, especially right-sided effusions. Draining fluid from the pleural space or peritoneal cavity by paracentesis can improve respiratory function and patient comfort. Dietary sodium restriction is essential. The patient should be recommended the liver disease diet (Palmer 2004), which includes the following:

- daily weights and abdominal girth measurements
- high-carbohydrate diet: the major source of calories in this diet
- moderate fat intake: the increased carbohydrate and fat help in preserving the protein in the body and prevent muscle wasting

Box 4.24 Information

Abdominal paracentesis

In intractable ascites, i.e. when sodium restrictions and diuretic therapy have little effect, it is possible to drain the fluid from the peritoneal cavity by means of a catheter inserted through the abdominal wall. This procedure is known as abdominal paracentesis. Such patients are already hypoproteinaemic and the sudden loss of fluid and protein by paracentesis is likely to lead to a shift of both from the rest of the body into the abdominal cavity, sometimes with consequent hypovolaemia, shock and even death. The protein is therefore replaced at the time of paracentesis by an infusion of salt-poor albumin.

The patient's blood pressure should be monitored closely and the fluid drained no more quickly than at a rate of approximately 2 L/h. Strict aseptic technique should be used when inserting the catheter to avoid introducing infection that can lead to bacterial peritonitis. This procedure requires cooperation from the patient to lie relatively still in bed while the catheter is in situ over several hours. Help will be required from the nursing staff to maintain comfort over this period. Any leakage on removal of the catheter can be collected in a drainable bag until the puncture site heals (usually within 48 h).

Nursing management of a patient during paracentesis

Monitor and record vital signs for baseline data prior to the procedure. Vital signs should be recorded every 15 min during the procedure, thereafter 15–30 min for the first hour, and hourly for the following 2 h until the patient is cardiovascularly stable. The paracentesis catheter may be in place for 4–6 h. Monitor neurological signs for signs of increased confusion, i.e. hepatic encephalopathy. Monitor for signs of infection. Record intake and output including ascitic drainage, replacement albumin if required and urine output. Notify the physician/medical team if any signs of deterioration occur. The INR, prothrombin time and platelet counts should be checked and corrected prior to large-volume paracentesis (LVP) (Yeung & Wong 2002). Patients may require LVP every 2–4 weeks, and the procedure can be performed in the outpatient setting (Ginès et al 2004).

- high-protein diet
- vitamin B supplements
- low-salt diet
- abstain from alcohol
- small frequent meals as tolerated
- referral to a dietitian.

If the patient is unable to tolerate oral diet then enteral or parenteral feeding may be commenced (see Ch. 21). Patients requiring rehydration are commenced on an intravenous infusion of colloids rather than sodium chloride due to the patient's inability to cope with excess sodium. Generally patients with compromised liver function have a central line inserted and aseptic techniques must be maintained in such circumstances (Sargent 2005).

 ## Nursing management and health promotion: ascites

For these patients, pain may be mild and responsive to non-opioid analgesics. However, in malignant disease it can be severe and difficult to control. Strong analgesics and small doses of prednisolone are used to control severe pain.

Bed rest should be promoted and the patient should be assisted into a comfortable position. Where possible the patient should maintain a semi-prone position to improve kidney perfusion and venous return to the heart, which in turn promotes diuresis. The patient's legs should be elevated to help reduce peripheral oedema. Pressure ulcer risk assessment should be undertaken and vigilant pressure area care provided. This assessment is vital because oedema may compromise skin quality and the patient may be reluctant to move and is likely to experience difficulty in moving.

Vital sign monitoring should be undertaken as a baseline before commencing treatment, i.e. paracentesis (see Box 4.24). Recording daily weight and abdominal girth is also important to monitor the extent of ascites and oedema. Fluid loss is measured by weighing the patient at the same time each day in similar clothes, with an empty bladder.

The patient should be encouraged to eat a diet very low in salt. Daily sodium intake must be restricted to 60 mmol, and to 40 mmol in severe ascites. It is important to ensure that the patient manages the restriction in fluid intake and understands why the restriction is necessary. The nurse should help the patient to 'pace' the fluid intake throughout the day. It is also important that the patient's family and friends are made aware of diet and fluid restrictions. Diuretics should be administered as prescribed. Spironolactone is the medication of choice because of its potassium-sparing properties.

Gastrointestinal bleeding

Gastrointestinal bleeding is the direct result of portal hypertension and may be slow and insidious, as in portal hypertensive gastropathy, or sudden and catastrophic, as in major oesophageal or gastric variceal rupture.

PATHOPHYSIOLOGY AND RISK FACTORS

Portal hypertension is defined as portal venous pressure exceeding 10 mmHg (Koti & Davidson 2003). Portal hypertension occurs when there is an obstruction in the intra- or extrahepatic circulation. Cirrhosis is the commonest cause of portal hypertension.

Varices are caused by the dilatation of the collateral veins and the formation of new veins in the upper stomach and the oesophagus. Thirty to fifty per cent of patients with portal hypertension will develop varices (Norton et al 2008). However, only one third of these patients will bleed from the varices. The risk of bleeding from oesophageal varices is about 25% within 2 years of diagnosis and between 3 and 30% from gastric varices (Koti & Davidson 2003). The collateral vessels are most problematic at the gastro-oesophageal junction where they can rupture and cause massive haemorrhage.

Clinical features

The cardinal signs of portal hypertension (increased pressure in the venous system) include:

- caput medusae – dilated veins in the anterior abdominal wall with blood flow away from the umbilicus
- ascites – fluid retention in the abdominal cavity

- splenomegaly – an enlarged spleen
- jaundice – yellow discolouration of the skin
- spider naevi or angiomas – a red central spot, with small veins extending outwards similar to spider legs, often found on the face, neck and upper part of the body
- palmar erythema – reddening of the palms of the hands
- asterixis or tremor
- gynaecomastia – male breasts
- testicular atrophy – reduction in the size of the testicles
- impotence and loss of libido in men and amenorrhoea in women.

Diagnosis

Portal hypertension is diagnosed by medical history, palpation of the abdomen, and ultrasound when splenomegaly is demonstrated. Angiography of the portal venous system will determine the cause and site of the obstruction. Endoscopy will demonstrate gastro-oesophageal varices.

Treatment options

Presenting symptoms are treated. Non-selective beta blockers, i.e. propranolol, reduce portal flow by reducing cardiac output and splanchnic arterial flow, thereby halving the risk of a first bleed. Sclerotherapy is a treatment for oesophageal varices that involves the injection of an irritant solution causing thrombosis and obliteration of the varicosed veins. Endoscopic band ligation should also be considered in the early stages, particularly if beta blockers are contraindicated (Mirza & Aithal 2006). Banding is an alternative for the long-term treatment of varices as it has fewer complications than sclerotherapy. Bleeding from oesophageal varices is treated by blood transfusion and by variceal eradication. This can be done endoscopically either by injection sclerotherapy or band ligation.

Balloon tamponade (compression of the varices using inflated balloons) and medication such as vasopressin are used only to stop active bleeding until variceal eradication treatment is commenced. Patients who do not respond to endoscopic management of their varices will be treated with a transjugular intrahepatic portosystemic stent (TIPSS). TIPSS is a radiological intervention whereby a metal stent is inserted in the liver to connect the portal and systemic veins. It is effective in lowering the portal pressure and thus controlling variceal bleeding and re-bleeding. It is associated with a low complication and mortality rate. For further information see Christensen (2004).

▷ Nursing management and health promotion: gastrointestinal bleeding

It is important to note that there is a 50% mortality rate from the first major bleed in high-risk patients. The patient will present with hypovolaemic shock, hence blood pressure, pulse and oxygen saturations should be monitored every 15 min. The patient's level of consciousness should be carefully observed and recorded.

Treatment is with intravenous fluids and blood transfusions and an accurate record of all fluid intake and output is kept. In addition, any clotting disorders should be corrected prior to endoscopic therapy (Norton et al 2008). If the patient is vomiting profusely from bleeding oesophageal varices, a high-flow suction catheter is required for intermittent suction and maintenance of a clear airway.

Intravenous infusion of a vasoconstricting agent such as vasopressin may be used to constrict the splanchnic arterioles supplying the viscera and so reduce the blood loss at source. Intravenous vitamin K may also be administered. A urinary catheter is passed and urine output measured hourly during the acute phase, as underperfusion of the kidneys due to shock can result in renal impairment (see Ch. 18).

A balloon tamponade tube may be passed nasogastrically to control haemorrhage and save the patient's life. A Sengstaken or Minnesota tube is passed into the stomach and the gastric balloon inflated to approximately 300 mL of air. Gentle but firm traction is applied to maintain the balloon at the oesophago-gastric junction. The oesophageal balloon is inflated only if bleeding persists, as it carries a risk of oesophageal perforation. Great care is required when inflating the oesophageal balloon (no more than 30 mL of air) and it must be deflated for 30 min every 4 h. The nurse will monitor the inflation pressures and times and move the tube from side to side in the mouth every hour to prevent pressure ulcers from forming there. The tube should be in position for no more than 48 h, and immediate treatment such as endoscopic eradication or transjugular intrahepatic portosystemic shunting (TIPSS) is required on removal because of the risk of re-bleeding.

The patient is nil by mouth prior to transfer to theatre for endoscopic eradication of varices. Standard pre-operative preparation is followed (see Ch. 26) and on return to the ward a clear airway and no oral fluids must be maintained until sensation and the ability to swallow have returned. The nurse will observe closely for recurrence of bleeding.

Because of the experience of either vomiting blood or passing melaena the patient may be extremely anxious. A calm approach and clear explanations of treatment and care are essential in order to help relieve the natural fears that extensive bleeding causes. Anxiety and agitation can be relieved by small intravenous doses of a benzodiazepine sedative such as midazolam. As patients with liver disease are very sensitive to sedatives, the benzodiazepine antagonist flumazenil should be immediately available. Antiemetics such as metoclopramide can be given if the patient is nauseated and retching, as vomiting could cause further haemorrhage.

Hepatic encephalopathy

Hepatic encephalopathy (HE) is a neuropsychiatric syndrome that occurs only in the presence of significant liver disease. It may be overt or subclinical and is potentially fully reversible (Sargent 2007).

PATHOPHYSIOLOGY AND RISK FACTORS

The subclinical form can be difficult to diagnose but the overt form can lead to bizarre and even violent behaviour. The exact cause is unclear, but one popular theory is that ammonia generated from the muscles, kidneys and small and large bowel, which the failing liver has been unable to neutralise, crosses the blood–brain barrier and causes changes in cerebral neurotransmission (Sargent 2007). Because nitrogen products can mimic neurotransmitters,

Box 4.25 Information

Hepatic encephalopathy

Grade I	Lack of awareness, euphoria, short attention span and impaired ability for simple arithmetical calculations.
Grade II	Increased drowsiness, lethargy, apathy, disorientation in time and place, personality change and inappropriate behaviour.
Grade III	Very drowsy, semi-stupor, somnolence, confusion and gross disorientation.
Grade IV	Coma: (a) arousal to painful stimuli; (b) unresponsive to painful stimuli.

neurological symptoms often result (Norton et al 2008). HE is classified into four grades (Box 4.25).

Clinical features

Some patients experience fetor hepaticus – a sour, faecal smell in the breath – and often there is a 'flapping' tremor or asterixis that can be seen by asking the patient to hold their arms outstretched with their fingers separated. Other physical manifestations seen in HE are exaggerated deep tendon reflexes, a positive Babinski's sign (neurological reflex where, when the sole of the foot is firmly stroked, the big toe extends and flexes towards the top of the foot while the other toes fan out) and ankle clonus (involuntary extension and flexion of the foot) (Sargent 2007).

Treatment options

Medical treatment is generally aimed at limiting the production of ammonia by colonic bacteria. Laxatives such as lactulose are prescribed, which is especially beneficial following GI bleeding, as it alters bowel pH, which then modifies colonic bacterial metabolism so that less ammonia is produced. Good nutrition is required and for patients with severely compromised liver function the gastroenterologist may suggest limiting the intake of protein. However, protein restriction is rarely recommended these days as most patients with liver failure are malnourished due to ill health or alcohol abuse.

▷ Nursing management and health promotion: hepatic encephalopathy

Early detection and management of HE can be largely nurse-led. The better the nurse–patient relationship the easier it will be to detect subtle changes in the patient's condition and reverse the encephalopathy before coma develops.

Bed rest should be promoted and the patient should be assisted into a comfortable position. Vigilant pressure area care should be undertaken. The nurse must observe for further complications of prolonged bed rest such as the development of deep venous thrombosis, pulmonary embolism and chest infection, loss of muscle strength and contractures, and depression. A safe environment must be maintained at all times as the patient is at risk of becoming confused and unsteady. A call bell should be placed within easy reach of the patient. The patient should be nursed in a room close to the nurses' station as the patient's condition may deteriorate rapidly with few warning signs.

The patient's neurological status and vital signs (temperature, pulse, respirations, blood pressure and oxygen saturation) must be recorded at least four times daily. If the patient's condition changes, the nurse will need to monitor neurological and vital signs closely, sometimes as frequently as every 15 min.

Good dietary advice is essential, not only to avoid protein excess but also to maintain a high calorie intake to avoid tissue catabolism. If the patient is unable to tolerate oral diet then enteral or parenteral feeding may be commenced. Intravenous colloids may be prescribed for patients who are dehydrated. It is very important that a bowel chart is maintained, and constipation should be avoided. Lactulose can be used to promote one to two bowel movements per day.

Close monitoring of fluid balance and daily weight is also important to avoid dehydration, especially in patients on diuretic therapy or undergoing abdominal paracentesis (see Box 4.24). A urinary catheter is inserted and output measured hourly as patients with hepatic disorders may develop renal failure or hepatorenal syndrome. Strict aseptic technique should be used for all invasive procedures and any indications of infection must be reported and treated promptly.

Psychological care is also a nursing priority. Body image issues should be discussed with the patient and fears and anxieties considered in an open, uncritical, empathetic manner. The patient may be offered counselling to assist with sexuality issues that occur following liver disease.

Patients with a severely compromised liver should be nursed in an intensive care unit or a liver unit with specialist nurses experienced in caring for the complex complications related to liver disease. For further information see Sargent (2007).

End-stage liver disease is irreversible without a liver transplant. If a patient is not a candidate for transplantation, end-of-life issues should be addressed with the patient and family, especially if a life-threatening complication or a sudden deterioration of liver function develops.

Cancer of the liver

Tumours of the liver can be either primary or secondary growths. The liver is the most common site for metastatic spread and patients often present with symptoms from the secondary rather than the primary lesion.

Primary tumours

Hepatocellular carcinoma is the principal primary tumour found in the liver. It is one of the major cancers of the world but the incidence varies greatly between countries. The highest-risk populations are in sub-Saharan Africa and eastern Asia, and males are more commonly affected than females (Chen et al 1997).

PATHOPHYSIOLOGY AND RISK FACTORS

Chronic hepatitis B and C virus infections are the main causes of the cancers in high-incidence areas. Hepatocellular carcinomas also occur in haemochromatosis (a condition caused by excess iron in the body) and alcoholic cirrhosis of the liver.

Clinical features

Often, early symptoms are vague, but in the later stages the patient presents with weight loss, loss of appetite, nausea, lethargy, abdominal pain, jaundice and ascites. Typically, the liver is enlarged and hard. The tumour is highly vascular and occurs most frequently in the right lobe. It may invade the hepatic and portal veins with the obstruction to these vessels resulting in portal hypertension. The cardinal signs of portal hypertension may also occur. There may be local spread to the peritoneum or metastatic spread to the lungs or lymphatic system. In the early stages, unless the cancer is blocking the bile ducts, the person has mild or no jaundice. In the late stages of the disease patients may develop HE.

Diagnosis

A very high serum alpha-fetoprotein (AFP >500 ng/mL; normal: <10 ng/mL) is diagnostic. Ultrasound-guided fine-needle aspiration or biopsy at laparoscopy is performed to obtain cells for histological examination. Ultrasound, CT scan and angiography are needed to define the extent of liver involvement and venous invasion prior to a decision being taken on treatment.

Treatment options

The first objective is to establish whether the tumour in the liver is sufficiently localised to be resected surgically. Treatment depends on the size and stage of the tumour: small tumours up to the size of 5 cm or up to three small tumours less than 3 cm can be resected surgically or removed by a lobectomy. Resection of liver tumours constitutes major surgery. Complete removal of the tumour may be possible, depending on the site and size of the tumour and on liver function. Resection is contraindicated in patients with extensive liver cirrhosis. Because the liver has a good capacity to regenerate, the prognosis is relatively good following small hepatic lobectomy if the entire tumour has been resected. More extensive resections carry a higher mortality rate. The nursing management of a patient following major liver surgery is intensive and should be carried out in a specialist unit. Unfortunately, surgery is usually impossible, either because liver involvement is too extensive or because metastasis to other organs has occurred. Some patients may benefit from chemotherapy or radiotherapy or chemoembolisation (the injection of anticancer drugs directly into blood vessels feeding the tumour). Medical therapy also aims for palliative relief of symptoms such as pain or ascites.

Secondary tumours

These are the most common malignant liver tumours and can originate from a primary cancer growth in any part of the body.

PATHOPHYSIOLOGY AND RISK FACTORS

The histology of the liver cells may indicate the primary site. However, the cancer cells may be anaplastic, giving no indication of their origin.

Clinical features

Clinical features are as for primary malignant tumours, with signs of associated cirrhosis. Pain is often the most common symptom for which the patient seeks medical help. The abdomen will become distended due to the enlarged liver, peritoneal invasion and ascites. The patient will have difficulty in bending over and is usually anorexic.

Diagnosis

Diagnosis is by fine-needle aspiration under ultrasound imaging to obtain cells for histology. If the primary site is unknown and causing no symptoms but there are metastatic deposits in the liver, the patient is not subjected to investigations to locate the primary tumour, as outcome is determined by the spread to the liver.

Treatment options

Treatment is generally restricted to symptom control, although occasionally a localised metastasis from the colon can be resected.

Nursing management and health promotion: cancer of the liver

Nursing management of the patient with either primary or secondary liver cancer is generally aimed at symptom control as well as providing the emotional support patients require when facing a terminal illness (see Chs 31, 33).

The World Health Organization (2002) defines palliative care as the active total care of patients whose disease is not responsive to curative treatment. Hence the aim of palliative care is to relieve the symptoms and promote patient comfort throughout the disease trajectory. Palliative care requires the nurse to attend to the physiological, psychological, spiritual and social aspects of the patient's well-being.

Time should be spent with the patient, allowing an opportunity to express thoughts, fears and anger. As the prognosis for liver cancer is so poor, patients may be left with a very short time to put their affairs in order and to prepare for impending death. Family and friends will also need support from nursing medical staff and palliative care team.

Initially, the patient may be able to attend personal needs, and may also be able to return home. However, repeated admission may be necessary for abdominal paracentesis (see Box 4.24). As the disease advances, there may be progressive dependence on nurses and/or relatives for care.

Due to extreme weight loss, much attention is required in maintaining intact pressure areas. Oral hygiene is important in the hope of preventing candida or oral thrush infection. Small sips of fluids may be given and small chips of ice or frozen juice may be refreshing in the mouth. A cool, moist washcloth on the forehead may also increase physical comfort.

If the patient develops signs of hepatic encephalopathy (HE) (see p. 108), safety is an issue and the patient should be nursed in a room close to the nurses' station. At this point, the patient and family may appreciate the privacy of a single room. Keep the patient comfortable and pain free. A subcutaneous infusion of morphine via a syringe pump may be commenced. Maintain the patient's dignity and comfort in the palliative stage of the disease. For further reading refer to Ahmed & Lobo (2007).

Disorders of the biliary system

Cholelithiasis

Cholelithiasis or the presence of gallstones is very common. It is estimated that approximately 5.5 million people in the UK have gallstones (Peate 2009).

PATHOPHYSIOLOGY AND RISK FACTORS

Gallstones are formed from the constituents of bile salts. Stones vary in size and shape, and may be solitary or multiple. Their colour can vary from yellow to dark brown. There are three main types:

- pure cholesterol stones (a 'solitaire' that fills the gall bladder): 10%
- pigmented stones ('jack stones', black and shiny): 2–3%
- mixed stones (mainly cholesterol, often with some calcium): 80%.

Gallstones are more prevalent among women than men and their incidence appears to be increasing. It is estimated that 1.5% of men and 6.1% of women will have gallstones by the age of 40 (Karanjia & Ali 2007). Until about 20 years ago, the most likely person to develop gallstones was said to be an obese woman in her 40s with fair skin ('fair, fat, fertile, female and 40'). This categorisation is now considered outdated as, for unknown reasons, gallstones are affecting people at a much younger age. Other factors related to the development of gallstones include the use of oral contraceptives, diabetes mellitus and genetic history. Of patients found to have gallstones during screening there is a 2% chance per year of these patients developing symptoms. It is believed that only 10–30% of gallstones become symptomatic. More often they cause biliary colic or an acute or chronic cholecystitis.

Biliary colic is caused by a transient obstruction of the gall bladder from an impacted stone or stones leading to severe spasms of the gall bladder and/or biliary ducts. Cholecystitis can less commonly be caused by trauma and, even more rarely, by tumours.

Clinical features

The patient complains of a sudden onset of severe gripping pain in the right hypochondrium that often radiates to the back. The pain, referred to as 'biliary colic', may vary in intensity and can last for several hours. The pain will ease when the stone either passes into the common bile duct or falls back into the gall bladder. Nausea and vomiting is also common.

Diagnosis

Tests that may be used to establish a diagnosis include:

- blood tests – liver function tests, serum amylase and white blood count
- ultrasound
- CT scanning
- endoscopic retrograde cholangiopancreatography (ERCP)
- intravenous cholangiogram (used occasionally)
- oral cholecystogram (less common).

Ultrasound is now the main investigative procedure for patients with suspected gallstones. It is non-invasive and causes minimal discomfort to the patient. Ultrasound can identify stones in the gall bladder, thickening of the gall bladder wall and both intra- and extrahepatic duct dilatation.

Nursing management and health promotion: cholelithiasis

Pain management is the main nursing priority. Using a pain scale, assess the patient's pain score and administer a prescribed intramuscular opioid/narcotic analgesia and an antiemetic. The effect of the analgesia should be evaluated. Following investigations the patient may require a cholecystectomy (see below).

If the patient refuses surgery or if it is contraindicated (e.g. first trimester of pregnancy), lifestyle changes and dietary modifications are advised. Small meals that are low in fat are advised in order to allow the gall bladder to rest and prevent painful spasms. Red meats should be avoided and high-starch foods such as potatoes, bread and rice are recommended. Fibre intake should be increased by eating fruit and vegetables and an increased intake of vitamin C should be encouraged as it converts cholesterol to bile acid. Refined sugar intake should be reduced and convenience foods that may contain hidden fats should be avoided. In patients who are overweight, rapid weight loss is not recommended as it can increase the risk of stone formation. Patients should be advised to lose weight slowly by increasing physical activity and monitoring calorie consumption.

Acute cholecystitis

Cholecystitis is inflammation of the gall bladder.

PATHOPHYSIOLOGY AND RISK FACTORS

The usual cause of acute cholecystitis is impacted gallstones in the cystic duct or Hartmann's pouch causing severe biliary colic.

Clinical features

The patient presents with an acute illness that is severe in nature and may be in hypovolaemic shock due to vomiting and pain. The pain is typically described as severe, in the right hypochondrium and frequently radiating to the right scapula. On examination, an abdominal mass may be felt and Murphy's sign, a catching of the breath at the height of inspiration when the gall bladder is palpated, is usually positive. There may also be tenderness and guarding of the whole abdomen and sometimes the patient may not be able to tolerate a physical examination. Sweating and pallor may also be present. Patients often present with a pyrexia and tachycardia due to infection. Jaundice can occur, especially if there is an obstruction of the common bile duct. Frequently, patients describe a history of pale stools and dark urine. Also, they may complain of fatty intolerance and describe pain after eating a fatty meal.

Treatment options

Cholecystectomy is indicated in patients with biliary colic or acute cholecystitis and may be carried out as an urgent case. In the past, surgeons preferred to treat patients with cholelithiasis with intravenous fluids and analgesia and perform an elective procedure approximately 6 weeks after an acute episode. Nowadays, surgeons are more likely to operate on patients sooner as an 'early' cholecystectomy means the patient is not at risk of further attacks of acute cholecystitis while awaiting elective surgery.

Open cholecystectomy was performed commonly in the past but since the introduction of laparoscopic cholecystectomy in 1978, the use of open cholecystectomy has fallen sharply. However, it is extremely important that the patient also understands and gives consent for an open laparotomy procedure as laparoscopic removal may not be possible. Operating on an acutely inflamed gall bladder carries a risk of conversion to open surgery due to challenges identifying the biliary tree, common bile duct, cystic duct and cystic artery (Graham 2008). Furthermore, patients who have pre-existing medical conditions may not be suitable for laparoscopic surgery.

Removal of gallstones can also be performed by endoscopic retrograde cholangiopancreatography (ERCP) and sphincterotomy and less commonly by extracorporeal shock wave lithotripsy (ESWL) to break up the stones. Occasionally, bile acid therapy is offered to patients who are unsuitable for surgery. Nonetheless, most patients nowadays will be prepared for laparoscopic surgery as gallstones almost never spontaneously disappear, except when they are formed under special circumstances, such as pregnancy or sudden weight loss.

The advantages of laparoscopic cholecystectomy include:

- reduced stay in hospital
- early mobilisation with lower risk of complications
- minor nature of surgical wounds
- reduced need for opioid analgesics
- quick return to normal life.

Nursing management and health promotion: acute cholecystitis

PRE-OPERATIVE MANAGEMENT

If the patient requires surgery, pre-operative preparation must be undertaken (see Ch. 26). Pre-operatively, pain must be assessed and managed as a priority. Opioid/narcotics such as pethidine and NSAID medications such as diclofenac have been found to be effective for pain management. An antiemetic also should be prescribed and administered. Vomiting can be severe and distressing, hence a nasogastric tube may be passed and aspirated hourly to promote patient comfort.

Hourly monitoring and recording of the patient's vital signs should be undertaken. The patient should be nil orally and intravenous fluids should be commenced to maintain hydration. Fluid and electrolyte balance should be monitored carefully. The patient should also be prescribed and administered an intravenous broad-spectrum antibiotic prior to surgery.

Nurses should provide assistance with personal hygiene to keep the patient comfortable, particularly as excessive perspiration commonly occurs with acute cholecystitis. Oral hygiene is also a nursing priority as the patient is nil per mouth, may be vomiting and may have a nasogastric tube in situ.

The patient may be restless and uncomfortable due to the severity of the pain and possibly due to fear. It is important to reassure the patient and relieve anxiety by explaining that the condition can be treated and the pain relieved. If the patient is expected to have a laparoscopic cholecystectomy the nurse should explain that the patient may experience shoulder and neck pain for 2–3 days postoperatively. This is due to phrenic nerve irritation from the carbon dioxide gas used to inflate the peritoneum in laparoscopic surgery. This pain can be eased by moving position, physiotherapy and applying hot packs. Some patients find the symptoms improve by taking peppermint water.

If the patient is due to have an open cholecystectomy, the nurse should explain the importance of deep breathing exercises postoperatively. Preparation of the patient for the immediate postoperative period also includes explanations regarding intravenous fluids, management of the nasogastric tube, the T-tube and the possibility of having an indwelling urinary catheter. The patient should be informed and educated about the postoperative pain management plan and the use of patient controlled analgesia (PCA) (see Ch. 19).

POSTOPERATIVE MANAGEMENT

Immediate postoperative nursing care for patients following a laparoscopic cholecystectomy is similar to the initial care provided for all other patients following other abdominal surgery requiring general anaesthesia (see Ch. 26). Typically, patients are discharged 8 hours postoperatively and most can resume normal activities, such as returning to work, after 2 weeks.

Following open laparotomy surgery analgesia is vital so that the patient can perform deep breathing and coughing exercises in order to prevent atelectasis and pneumonia. Opioid patient controlled analgesia (PCA) is regularly used to manage postoperative pain. The patient should also be assisted to an upright sitting position and encouraged to perform deep breathing exercises to prevent pulmonary complications.

Intravenous fluids are prescribed and administered until the patient is able to tolerate oral fluids (30–60 mL/h). When bowel sounds return, usually after 24 h, and if tolerated, free fluids may be given. Diet can then be introduced gradually and increased to normal over the next 3 days.

Early removal of the indwelling catheter, usually the morning following the surgery, is recommended to reduce the likelihood of the patient developing a urinary tract infection.

Sometimes, the patient returns to the ward with a T-tube inserted to maintain patency and prevent stricture of the biliary duct. The 'T' part of the T-tube is in the common bile duct and the long leg of the tube is brought out through a stab wound in the abdominal wall and connected to a drainage bag. In the first 24 h the T-tube usually drains approximately 300–500 mL of bile. The drainage will reduce over the consecutive days, to approximately less than 200 mL. The nurse should check for bile leakage from around the tube and wound site. Furthermore, it is vital that the T-tube is not removed accidentally. A T-tube cholangiogram is carried out 8–10 days postoperatively to check the patency of

the bile duct and the flow of bile into the duodenum prior to the removal of the T-tube. If the ducts are stone free, the tube will be removed.

Following removal of the tube, the nurse should observe the amount of bile leakage and apply a sterile dressing to the wound. Observation of the patient for any signs of biliary peritonitis should be made for 24 h. Wound sutures, if present, are removed when the wound is healed, generally 5–7 days postoperatively, unless an absorbable subcutaneous suture is used. If wound sites are dry the wound can be left exposed.

Postoperative complications

Occasionally postoperative complications can occur and it is very important that nurses are aware of the symptoms that indicate their onset. Bile duct injury is one such complication that is more common after laparoscopic surgery. Symptoms include persistent pain accompanied by pyrexia of 38°C or above, abdominal distension and jaundice. The patient may need ERCP to locate the injury and may need to return to theatre for surgical repair. Paralytic ileus can also occur postoperatively (see Ch. 26). If paralytic ileus does occur, the patient should be kept fasting, a nasogastric tube passed and the stomach kept empty. Intravenous antibiotics are usually given for 5 days and then discontinued. The nurse must inform the surgical team if any of the above symptoms occur.

Depending on the patient's fitness and age, discharge home normally occurs within 6–10 days. Discharge plans will need to be discussed with relatives or carers. The patient must be instructed to avoid lifting heavy objects and to avoid driving for 4–6 weeks to prevent wound herniation. Explain to the patient that faeces pass quicker through the bowel following a cholecystectomy and bile binders such as colestyramine may be required for chronic diarrhoea. Normal diet is encouraged. In an uncomplicated recovery, the patient should be fit to return to work in 4–6 weeks. A detailed discharge summary will be sent to the GP. A follow-up appointment will be given for 4 weeks after discharge. See Box 4.26 to reflect on the nursing care of a patient following a laparoscopic laparoscopic cholecystectomy. For further information in relation to the nursing care of patient undergoing cholecystectomy surgery see Thomas (2009) and Graham (2008).

Chronic cholecystitis/choledocholithiasis

See the website for information relating to the pathophysiology and risk factors, clinical features and nursing management and health promotion of patients with chronic cholecystitis and choledocholithiasis.

See website for further content

Tumours of the biliary tract

Tumours may present in the gall bladder or bile duct (cholangiocarcinoma).

Cancer of the gall bladder

PATHOPHYSIOLOGY AND RISK FACTORS

This is a rare cancer and is nearly always related to gallstones. It is more common in females than in males.

Box 4.26 Reflection

Care of a patient following a laparoscopic cholecystectomy

Anne Black is a 52-year-old woman admitted to the GI ward complaining of severe gripping pain radiating to her right shoulder. She is very nauseated and was vomiting on admission. However, the vomiting has subsided following an intramuscular injection of prochlorperazine 12.5 mg. She was also given 75 mg of pethidine intramuscularly for pain relief 30 min before her arrival to the ward. She informs the nursing staff that the pain is slightly improved but still distressing. Her vital signs are recorded on arrival (BP 140/80, pulse rate 86 beats per minute, respiration rate 24 breaths per minute, oxygen saturations 98% on air, temperature 37.6°C). On examination, her sclera are slightly jaundiced, she is guarding her abdomen and has a positive Murphy's sign. The nursing staff prepare the patient for a laparoscopic cholecystectomy.

Activities

- Describe the potential advantages and disadvantages of laparoscopic surgery over an open laparotomy.
- Describe the postoperative nursing care Mrs Black should receive following laparoscopic surgery.
- What discharge advice should the nursing staff give to Mrs Black?

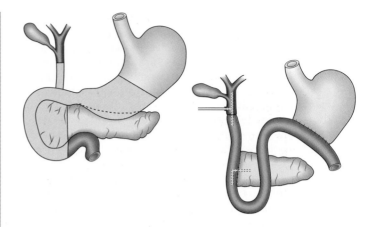

Figure 4.9 Whipple's procedure.

Clinical features

Signs and symptoms are consistent with those for gallstones, and a history of persistent obstructive jaundice may be present. A mass may be palpable.

Treatment options

In most cases, surgery is not a chosen treatment and survival rates are poor. Eighty per cent of gall bladder tumours are adenocarcinomas. As with other tumours, the involvement of lymph nodes and the presence of metastases will determine the patient's prognosis.

Cancer of the bile duct (cholangiocarcinoma)

PATHOPHYSIOLOGY AND RISK FACTORS

The cause of bile duct cancer is unknown although there are strong associations with inflammatory bowel disease and primary sclerosing cholangitis. It is more common in older people, and men are affected more than women. It is a rare cancer but its incidence appears to be increasing. Tumours can arise from the intra- or extrahepatic biliary tree. Direct spread and metastases are present in at least 50% of the patients who go for surgery.

Treatment options

As cancer of the bile ducts carries a very poor prognosis, treatment is usually in the form of palliative therapy. For some patients, palliation can be achieved by the insertion of a stent, either by ERCP or by percutaneous transhepatic techniques, e.g. percutaneous transhepatic cholangiography (PTC). In a few cases, where the tumour is at the lower end of the common bile duct, a radical resection in the form of a Whipple's procedure may be possible (Figure 4.9). This is major surgery and should be considered only if the tumour is localised and the patient is fit for surgery.

Tumours of the upper biliary tract are resectable in only 10% of cases. Following resection of the tumour, a Roux loop of jejunum is anastomosed to the biliary tract or, in some cases, the left hepatic duct. A hepaticojejunostomy then restores the continuity of the small intestine. It can also be performed to bypass the tumour and achieve palliation. Radiotherapy and chemotherapy have not been shown to improve survival.

Nursing management and health promotion: cholangiocarcinoma

The patient with a diagnosis of cholangiocarcinoma will require specialised nursing care. Only a few of these patients will be considered for major resection, following which they are cared for in a high-dependency ward for approximately 48 h. In some cases, the patient is prepared for major resection but at the time of surgery it is discovered that only a bypass of the tumour may be carried out safely. These patients are usually devastated by this turn of events and require a great deal of support. Following palliation, jaundice will subside and the patient's appetite will improve. For a few months patients may feel so well that they become unrealistic about the prognosis. Few patients survive more than a year following palliation. Following resection, the outlook is better. Good family support is necessary. It is important to take an honest approach and to give explanations to the patient and family as they request them. It will be necessary to spend time with the patient and the relatives to answer their questions and offer support. Close communication with the GP is also important so that community care can be provided when necessary.

THE PANCREAS

The pancreas has both exocrine and endocrine functions and lies below and behind the stomach, in the epigastric and left hypochondriac region of the abdominal cavity (see Figure 4.7). The function of the exocrine gland is to produce and release pancreatic juice containing enzymes that digest protein, carbohydrate, fat and nucleic acids, and bicarbonate. The exocrine secretory functions of the pancreas are under vagal and hormonal control. The initial stimulus for the release of pancreatic juice is food entering the duodenum and stimulating the release of cholecystokinin and secretin. Cholecystokinin is responsible for stimulating the release of the pancreatic enzyme portion of pancreatic juice and secretin is responsible for the release of bicarbonate. The pancreatic duct, which delivers pancreatic juice to the duodenum, and the common bile duct join at the ampulla of Vater. Release of bile and pancreatic juice into the duodenum is controlled by the sphincter of Oddi. This sphincter, a ring of smooth muscle, is relaxed by cholecystokinin.

The endocrine function of the pancreas is concerned with the secretion of the hormones insulin and glucagon directly into the bloodstream in response to fluctuating blood glucose levels. The islets of Langerhans contain the endocrine hormone producing cells. Insulin and glucagon are synthesised and secreted by the beta cells and alpha cells, respectively. For further information on the endocrine role of the pancreas see Chapter 5.

DISORDERS OF THE PANCREAS

Pancreatitis

Broadly speaking, inflammation of the pancreas is classified as either acute or chronic with the essential difference being that the gland returns to normal after an acute attack. In chronic pancreatitis, the inflammatory process is continuous leading to irreversible damage to the gland and impairment of function. Both types appear to be increasing due to a rise in alcohol consumption and a higher incidence of gallstones (Sargent 2006b).

Acute pancreatitis

Acute pancreatitis can be life threatening and in its most severe form has a mortality rate of 25% (Sargent 2006b). In the UK, gallstones account for approximately 50% of cases whilst excessive alcohol consumption is said to be a factor in 20–25% of occurrences (UK Working Party on Acute Pancreatitis 2005). Other identified causes include infection, e.g. mumps, abdominal trauma, medication, e.g. corticosteroids, hypercalcaemia, hyperlipidaemia, pancreatic cancer, endoscopic retrograde cholangiopancreatography (ERCP) and hereditary factors. In approximately 10% of cases there is no known cause (idiopathic).

PATHOPHYSIOLOGY AND RISK FACTORS

The exact process by which pancreatic necrosis occurs is unclear. However, it is thought that premature activation of the enzyme trypsin is the initial step in the process. It is normally activated in the small intestine and causes early activation of other enzymes in the pancreas resulting in autodigestion of pancreatic tissue. This autodigestion leads to varying degrees of oedema, haemorrhage and necrosis, and abscess and cyst formation in and around the pancreas. Spasm of the sphincter of Oddi with reflux of duodenal contents into the pancreatic duct is thought to be an important factor in this enzyme activation. Gallstones block the papilla of Vater, which in turn blocks the main secretory duct from the pancreas and the common bile duct. The pancreatic enzymes are then backed up. Passage of stones down the common bile duct may also promote reflux of infected bile along the pancreatic duct when these ducts form a common channel to the papilla of Vater. Although not clear, it is thought that ethanol (alcohol) either has a generalised impact on cell physiology or a specific effect on pancreatic enzymes.

Activated enzymes such as trypsinogen and chymotrypsinogen, phospholipase, elastase and catalase are responsible for increased capillary permeability. This permits large volumes of fluid to escape into the peritoneal and retroperitoneal cavity, causing damage to the surrounding tissue. This severe loss of circulating fluid leads to hypovolaemic shock and predisposes the individual to acute renal failure, which may result from local intravascular coagulation in the renal vascular bed. Development of pulmonary oedema with left-sided pleural effusion may result from release of toxins. The release of lipase causes fat necrosis in the omentum and areas adjacent to the pancreas. Calcium soaps become sequestered in areas of fatty necrosis, which may result in the development of hypocalcaemia. In 10–20% of cases systemic inflammatory response syndrome (SIRS) occurs, which predisposes to multi-organ failure and/or pancreatic necrosis.

Clinical features

The clinical presentation of acute pancreatitis varies and may be influenced by factors such as age, the presence of co-morbidities and the severity of the attack. However, abdominal pain located in the epigastrium and often radiating to the back is the most common clinical feature, occurring in over 95% of patients (Sargent 2006b). The pain can be unbearably severe, reaching maximal intensity in approximately 30 min, and is resistant to attempts at relieving it. The pain is often accompanied by nausea and vomiting and eating fatty foods or consuming alcohol can exacerbate it. The patient may be very distressed and anxious due to the pain and may be sweating visibly.

Acute pancreatitis is often associated with severe shock. There may be signs of dehydration with rapid pulse and respiration rates, hypotension and pyrexia. Marked abdominal tenderness is usually present in the upper abdomen, which may appear distended. Bruising around the umbilicus (Cullen's sign) and in the loin region (Grey Turner's sign) are rare late manifestations of acute pancreatitis due to petechial bleeding into the retroperitoneal space.

Diagnosis

Investigations will include blood analysis, urinalysis, X-ray, ultrasound and, in cases where diagnosis is inconclusive, a CT scan. In acute pancreatitis, there is an elevated plasma concentration of pancreatic enzymes. Serum amylase and/or serum lipase should be more than or equal to three times the upper limit of normal. Although both are used, serum lipase is one of the most reliable markers of acute pancreatitis as its half-life is longer than amylase and the pancreas is the only source of lipase. It rises within 4–8 h of onset, peaks within 24 h and returns to normal within 8–14 days.

Plain X-ray films of the abdomen can reveal distended loops of small bowel with paralytic ileus but can be a poor prognostic tool given the difficulty with visualising the pancreas. Ultrasound can reveal dilated pancreatic ducts, ascites and gallstones in patients with biliary-induced disease (Fawcett & Smith 2005). Chest X-ray may indicate the presence of a left-sided pleural effusion. Urea and electrolyte levels are important indicators of the state of hydration and are necessary for the correct management of the patient. A raised white blood cell count ($9–20 \times 10^9$) reveals an active inflammatory process. Hyperglycaemia and glycosuria are often present but are transient. Arterial blood gases may reveal severe hypoxia. CT scanning, although not used routinely, is indicated where a deterioration in clinical status, signs of sepsis or persistent organ failure are evident (Sargent 2006b).

It is important that patients with a severe attack are identified early as they need admission to a high-dependency or intensive care unit. For this reason, a number of scoring systems have been developed to predict the severity of attack, e.g. Modified Glasgow Scoring System, Ranson's criteria, APACHE II, Atlanta Classification. See Hughes (2004) and Sargent (2006b) for a more detailed discussion of the systems most commonly in use.

Treatment options

The overall goal in the management of acute pancreatitis is to provide supportive therapy, treat complications (Box 4.27) as they occur and limit the severity of the inflammatory response (Sargent 2006b). Acute pancreatitis is usually managed conservatively, and in mild attacks treatment is generally symptomatic. The principles of management are as follows:

Pain relief This is usually provided in the form of opiates/narcotics. Intravenous administration using PCA is the preferred option. Although epidural analgesia has been effective in some patients it should be used with caution, particularly in patients with altered coagulation (see Ch. 19).

Correction of shock If haemorrhagic pancreatitis is diagnosed, shock is treated by intravenous administration of large volumes of crystalloids, plasma, dextran or blood in order to maintain circulatory blood volume and adequate urine output. Oxygen therapy is essential to correct the associated hypoxia. PO_2 saturation levels should be monitored. Hypoxaemia may develop insidiously such that respiratory failure (ARDS) can develop. Arterial blood gases are closely monitored in case ventilatory support is required (see Chs 3, 29).

Box 4.27 Information

Major complications of acute pancreatitis

Pancreatic pseudocyst

Pancreatic pseudocysts may develop following acute and chronic pancreatitis and are described as such because they are lined with granulation tissue whilst true cysts are lined with epithelium. A pseudocyst is a sac containing pancreatic juice, debris and blood that may be confined initially to the pancreatic parenchyma. They may regress spontaneously, persist with or without symptoms or result in complications. They can rupture with the result that liquefied necrotic tissue becomes evident and can involve adjacent structures where they can cause pain, nausea, vomiting, haemorrhage following erosion of blood vessels, infection and biliary obstruction (Smith & Fawcett 2006). Further complications include pancreatic fistulae or pancreatic ascites. Ultrasound scan can be used in diagnosis and monitoring. Surgery may be necessary if the cyst is symptomatic, since there is a danger that it may rupture or precipitate haemorrhage. Large cysts can resolve with percutaneous aspiration or drainage but those that communicate with the main pancreatic duct require surgical intervention (Smith & Fawcett 2006).

Pancreatic abscess

A pancreatic abscess is an intra-abdominal collection of pus, usually near or around the pancreas. They arise as a consequence of acute pancreatitis, usually a few weeks after the attack has started. This is a serious complication of acute pancreatitis. The patient is usually very ill, with pyrexia, a raised white blood cell count and tachycardia. Early diagnosis by CT scanning and the use of aggressive surgical intervention have improved mortality rates. Surgery consists of extensive drainage and debridement of infected tissues. Multiple large drains are used to drain the abscess cavity. Peritoneal lavage with normal saline 0.9% warmed to body temperature can be used to irrigate the cavity. Adequate nutrition following surgery is vital. Most surgeons establish a feeding jejunostomy and gastrostomy tube during surgery.

Pancreatic necrosis

This complication is a major cause of death in acute pancreatitis with a mortality rate of between 15 and 50% depending on the severity and course of the disease (Sargent 2006b). Early differentiation between non-infected (sterile) or infected pancreatic necrosis is essential in order to determine the most appropriate treatment (Sargent 2006b). This can be done using CT or fine-needle aspiration (Werner et al 2005). The mortality associated with non-infected necrosis is low and it can be treated conservatively. In infected necrosis, the patient often fails to improve with conservative management. A persistent pyrexia, raised white blood cell count, tachycardia, hypotension and poor respiratory function are ominous signs. There is some controversy over the use of radiological drainage or surgical debridement for pancreatic necrosis. However, at laparotomy, necrotic tissue is removed, peritoneal lavage is carried out and the pancreatic bed adequately drained. A feeding jejunostomy and gastrostomy tube may be inserted.

In some cases, the surgeon may opt to leave the wound open to allow for packing of the wound and to minimise the need for repeated laparotomies to deal with recurrent intra-abdominal sepsis.

Duodenal ileus

Due to persistent pancreatic inflammation, duodenal ileus may persist. Nutritional status will need to be maintained either by parenteral means or by jejunostomy feeding. A gastroenterostomy may need to be performed.

Haemorrhage

Severe bleeding may occur from gastric or duodenal ulceration. Prophylactic intravenous cimetidine is given to patients with acute pancreatitis. On rare occasions, haemorrhage may occur into a pseudocyst or by erosion of a blood vessel by the inflammatory process.

Suppression of pancreatic function The patient is kept nil by mouth to decrease stimulation of pancreatic enzymes and a nasogastric tube is passed to drain gastric secretions and prevent them from entering the duodenum, thus reducing stimulation. The role of nutrition has been contentious but recent guidelines suggest that where nutritional support is required enteral feeding may be given via a nasogastric tube if tolerated (UK Working Party on Acute Pancreatitis 2005).

Controlling infection Bacterial infection of necrotic pancreatic tissue is a major cause of morbidity and mortality. However, the use of antibiotics as prophylaxis is controversial and the guidelines indicate that they should not be used beyond 7–14 days without evidence of bacterial growth on culture (UK Working Party on Acute Pancreatitis 2005). When there is evidence of infection, a broad-spectrum antibiotic is prescribed.

Monitoring blood glucose levels This is required because secondary diabetes mellitus can sometimes develop, requiring insulin therapy.

Monitoring cardiac status This will be required if electrolyte derangement is such as to cause potentially lethal dysrhythmias.

For the majority of patients this supportive treatment will settle the acute attack and surgical treatment will not be necessary. If there is any doubt about the diagnosis, a laparotomy will exclude other causes of peritonitis such as perforated peptic ulcer and mesenteric ischaemia.

Surgical intervention

At an early stage in management, gallstones as a cause of the acute attack are excluded by ultrasound scanning. Cholecystectomy during the course of the patient's admission is now advocated to avoid recurrent problems following discharge. Patients with gallstone pancreatitis can usually be identified by their slow clinical progress and by the use of various clinical and biochemical prognosis factors.

Early ERCP may demonstrate the presence of stones in the common bile duct, which can be extracted by a small balloon catheter or basket following sphincterotomy. The complication of peripancreatic necrosis or abscess can be detected by radiological imaging. Most patients will require necrosectomy, i.e. the removal of necrotic tissues, and drainage at laparotomy. It may be wise to put in place a gastrostomy and jejunostomy tube at this time, as recovery is slow and the patient may require prolonged nutritional support (see Ch. 21).

 Nursing management and health promotion: acute pancreatitis

Care of patients with acute pancreatitis will vary according to the severity of the attack. Whilst those with a severe attack of acute pancreatitis will be nursed in a high-dependency unit or intensive care, most will be nursed on the ward. It should be borne in mind that the severity of the attack is not always easily judged by an initial assessment. Therefore, it is imperative that nurses caring for these patients are vigilant in their monitoring in order to detect any deterioration in the patient's condition. The priorities of nursing care include:

Management of fear and anxiety The sudden onset of pain and the sheer severity of the pain are very frightening for these patients. Added to this, few people will have heard of pancreatitis and the patient is likely to have no knowledge of the condition. Attempts to reduce anxiety and fear through continuity of care, information giving and good pain management are important. It is important to explain the rationale of all procedures and investigations in order to alleviate anxiety. Showing the patient diagrams can be very helpful. Communication with the family is vital and nurses and medical staff should give a full explanation of what has occurred to the patient and relatives where applicable.

Respiratory monitoring Patients who are in pain are more likely to have reduced respiratory depth evidenced by shallow breathing. In addition, patients with acute pancreatitis may suffer respiratory distress due to inadequate gaseous exchange and shock. Strict respiratory monitoring should be undertaken including rate and depth of breathing, oxygen saturation, and colour of skin, nail bed and peripheries. If tolerated, the patient should be positioned in bed so as to promote ventilation. Chest physiotherapy should be undertaken and deep breathing and coughing of secretions encouraged although this may be very difficult for the patient if the pain is intense. Humidified oxygen therapy may be administered. Good oral hygiene should be maintained and mouth care given where necessary.

Cardiovascular monitoring Cardiovascular monitoring should include blood pressure, pulse, temperature, skin temperature and colour recording as well as central venous pressure (CVP) monitoring where a central line has been inserted. Patients with acute pancreatitis are also at risk of developing thrombi and for this reason antiembolism stockings should be worn and/or low molecular weight heparin administered.

Pain management The pain from acute pancreatitis increases metabolic activity, which in turn increases the release of pancreatic enzymes. Therefore, good pain management and the promotion of patient comfort are essential. Pain should be assessed and evaluated using a recognised pain assessment tool such as a visual analogue scale (VAS). Intravenous administration of opiates/narcotics such as morphine or fentanyl using a PCA system is the preferred option. As respiratory depression is the main side-effect of opiate analgesia, respiratory, cardiovascular and sedation level monitoring are important. Some protocols dictate that oxygen is administered while the PCA is in progress. Regardless of whether or not the patient is being administered oxygen, oxygen saturation rates must be recorded.

Monitoring fluid status and elimination Intravenous access is established early in those with acute pancreatitis, and in severe cases a central line is inserted. The choice of intravenous fluids will depend on the patient's haemodynamic status. The nurse must ensure that strict monitoring of fluid input and output is undertaken. A urinary catheter may be inserted to assist with accurate output measurement. Urinalysis should be performed daily. Patency of the intravenous infusion is essential and monitoring for redness, inflammation and signs of extravasation must be undertaken. Bowel movements and the presence of flatus should be observed.

Blood sugar monitoring In acute pancreatitis, persistent hyperglycaemia can be an indication of a poor prognosis (Sargent 2006b). Therefore, close monitoring of blood glucose is necessary. Capillary testing should be undertaken making sure that testing sites are rotated to prevent fingers becoming sore. If blood glucose levels become unstable then insulin therapy using a sliding scale (variable regimen) may be required.

Maintaining nutrition Traditionally, patients with acute pancreatitis are nil by mouth in order to 'rest' the pancreas. A nasogastric tube is normally inserted to drain gastric secretions and prevent them from entering the duodenum, thus reducing stimulation. Drainage must be recorded accurately and frequent oral care must be undertaken to promote patient comfort. In addition, it is important that the nasogastric tube is properly secured to reduce 'drag' and nasal care should be undertaken. In the presence of nausea and vomiting, antiemetics should be administered. Where nutritional support is required enteral feeding may be given via a nasogastric tube if tolerated (UK Working Party on Acute Pancreatitis 2005). Where there is evidence of gastric ileus, jejunal feeding may be the route of choice. Care and observation of the insertion site is important and includes observation for signs of inflammation, excoriation and leakage. Parenteral nutrition should only be commenced when attempts at enteral feeding have failed (Sargent 2006b). As the patient's general condition improves, clear oral fluids can be introduced, gradually progressing to a light diet.

Maintaining skin integrity and hygiene needs As many of these patients are acutely ill, they will require assistance and support in maintaining personal hygiene. Skin should be kept clean and dry, especially if the patient is pyrexial or sweating excessively. Particular attention should be paid to the skin and hygiene needs of those who may develop jaundice due to obstruction of the common bile duct. This can be accompanied by discomfort and itching of the skin. Cool sponging and the application of calamine lotion may help. In addition, during the acute phase when the patient is most incapacitated, it is important that assessment of susceptibility to pressure ulcer development is undertaken. During periods of intense pain, patients may be reluctant to move and the nurse should ensure that continuous assessment of the skin and regular repositioning are undertaken. Early mobilisation should be encouraged.

Discharge planning following acute pancreatitis will be determined by the patient's individual situation and the perceived cause of the attack. For patients who have gallstones, treatment must be planned to prevent recurrence. This may involve an open or laparoscopic cholecystectomy with an operative cholangiogram or, for patients who are not fit for surgery, an ERCP and sphincterotomy. The timing of this treatment will depend on the severity of the attack of acute pancreatitis. In the interim, these patients should be referred to a dietitian for advice on a low-fat diet.

Where alcohol is implicated in the onset of acute pancreatitis, the advice is that the person should abstain permanently or risk a life-threatening recurrence. In a person with alcohol dependency this can be extremely challenging and without appropriate support and counselling they are likely not to succeed. Therefore it is imperative that nurses broach the subject in a non-judgemental manner ensuring that the patient has sufficient information and time to consider referral for counselling. Many hospitals now employ alcohol nurse specialists to provide support and advice on abstinence. Continued supports in the community should also be explored.

Advice regarding return to work is important. The patient often feels tired and in many cases it is advisable not to return to work for perhaps 4–6 weeks. The patient may be very worried about work, family and financial situation, and a visit from the social worker may be of value. The patient will be reviewed in the outpatient clinic initially at 3–4 weeks. For further information see Fawcett & Smith (2005) and Sargent (2006b).

Chronic pancreatitis

Although chronic pancreatitis remains a relatively rare condition in the UK its incidence is rising, which it has been suggested is due in part to increased alcohol consumption worldwide. Nonetheless, the actual mechanism by which alcohol damages the pancreas is poorly understood. It has been proposed that genetic predisposition is an important factor in the development of chronic pancreatitis in light of the fact that only a minority of people with alcohol dependence (approximately 10%) develop the condition. Therefore, alcohol could be described as a co-factor in susceptible human beings (Etemad & Whitcomb 2001). Other risk factors include: metabolic (hypercalcaemia, hyperlipidaemia, chronic renal failure, cystic fibrosis and hyperparathyroidism); genetic and hereditary predisposition; idiopathic (no known cause); nutritional or tropical pancreatitis; and obstructive (post-traumatic ductal strictures, pseudocysts, tumours, pancreatic divisum).

PATHOPHYSIOLOGY AND RISK FACTORS

Chronic pancreatitis leads to permanent damage of the gland, with replacement of the cells by fibrotic tissue and calcification. The ducts become narrowed and the flow of pancreatic juice is obstructed. The cells slowly stop secreting pancreatic juice. The obstructed ducts can give rise to recurrent attacks of pancreatitis. Irreversible structural damage may have taken place long before the person with chronic pancreatitis develops clinical signs and symptoms of exocrine and endocrine dysfunction. In advanced disease peripancreatic fibrosis can occur that involves the portal and splenic veins. As a result portal hypertension and occlusion of the lymph nodes develops (Smith & Fawcett 2006). Endocrine dysfunction and the development of diabetes mellitus occur later in the process of pancreatic cell destruction. Furthermore, those who are diagnosed with chronic pancreatitis can develop pancreatic pseudocysts (see Box 4.27) and are at increased risk of developing pancreatic cancer (Cavestro et al 2003).

Clinical features

Although its presentation varies from person to person, pain, either persistent or episodic, is the symptom with which the patient usually presents and has been described as the most distressing. It is classically located in the epigastrium, radiates to the back and can be relieved by sitting forward. The pain is associated with oral intake, and nausea and vomiting may also be present. A history of recent alcohol abuse may be given.

The gradual destruction of the pancreas leads to impairment of endocrine and exocrine function although clinical signs such as malabsorption and steatorrhoea may only appear after significant destruction has taken place. In steatorrhoea, the stool is pale, offensive and difficult to flush away and is due to a high undigested fat content. Steatorrhoea accompanied by weight loss provides evidence of advanced structural damage of the pancreas. It is often a distressing feature for the patient.

Endocrine insufficiency manifests itself by the development of diabetes mellitus. In those who develop diabetes (up to 30%), severe hypoglycaemia is a particular risk. Its management in chronic pancreatitis is similar to that of other diabetic patients except that it usually requires treatment with insulin. Transient jaundice may be present due to inflammation of the head of the pancreas, which obstructs the common bile duct.

Diagnosis

Due to the complexity of the disease diagnosing chronic pancreatitis in the early stages is difficult, particularly when trying to differentiate between acute relapsing and chronic pancreatitis. Moreover, in the early stages of the illness there may not be any clinical signs of pancreatic destruction. As a result investigations may not detect chronic pancreatitis unless the condition is at an advanced stage. If the attack that prompts the patient to seek medical help is severe then blood analysis for serum amylase and lipase may show elevations seen in acute pancreatitis. However, they are not reliable markers for the presence of chronic pancreatitis. A plain abdominal X-ray may show speckled calcification of the pancreas whilst ultrasound scan may show an enlarged, swollen gland. CT gives good detail but only in the advanced stages of the disease. Direct tests of pancreatic and duodenal juice via ERCP are more definitive but these are considered invasive and expensive (Smith & Fawcett 2006). ERCP is also performed to outline the pancreatic duct if surgery is contemplated. Faecal fat estimation, although used less often now, may reveal malabsorption. Fasting blood sugars are assessed and a glucose tolerance test may be necessary.

Treatment options

Management of chronic pancreatitis is mainly symptomatic. The patient should be advised to stop drinking alcohol and may need professional counselling to this end. Replacement of pancreatic enzymes with a commercial preparation may help to alleviate the steatorrhoea and reduce pain. Good control of diabetes will be necessary.

Pain control can be difficult, since some of these patients may become addicted to opiates (Haslett et al 2002). Management advice from a pain control specialist is invaluable. In a small number of patients in whom severe pain persists, surgery will be indicated. It may be necessary to resect the head of the gland (Whipple's procedure; see Figure 4.9) or the body and tail (distal pancreatectomy). Adequate drainage of the duct (pancreatojejunostomy) may be undertaken

where ERCP shows the pancreatic duct to be dilated. A total pancreatectomy is rarely undertaken due to the resulting permanent diabetes mellitus and exocrine insufficiency.

 ## Nursing management and health promotion: chronic pancreatitis

Nursing management of an acute attack in chronic pancreatitis is similar to that for acute pancreatitis.

Pain Pain is often constant in nature, radiating through to the back. It is often described as being like a sharp knife twisting in the gut and presents a major challenge to pain control. Pain assessment, using a recognised pain assessment tool, should be undertaken. The analgesic ladder is also an effective tool for determining the level at which the pain is controlled. NSAIDs such as diclofenac sodium (Voltarol) in suppository form can be of value. It is often necessary to use opioid analgesics to alleviate pain and a pain specialist or pain management team can be invaluable in advising about management of what is often intractable pain (see Ch. 19). Assisting the patient into a comfortable position may help. The patient may find that bending forward while leaning on a bed table helps. The use of a heat pad to the back may give some relief.

Alcohol dependency Alcohol dependence is commonly implicated in the onset of chronic pancreatitis. Total abstinence may help reduce the severity of the pain but it does not always resolve it. If the patient has a known dependency sudden withdrawal may precipitate delirium tremens. Mild sedation is frequently used to prevent this. Expert help and continued support may assist the patient to overcome an alcohol problem.

Nutrition The patient diagnosed with chronic pancreatitis is at risk of being nutritionally compromised and many experience significant weight loss as, at times, they are reluctant to eat for fear of exacerbating the pain. In addition, as the function of the pancreas deteriorates, they can experience dyspepsia, malabsorption and steatorrhoea. Therefore, nutritional assessment must be undertaken. Once the acute attack is resolved a dietitian consultation will provide the appropriate information and education about pancreatic enzyme replacement therapy and maintaining a well-balanced diet low in fat and high in carbohydrates. Pancreatic enzyme supplements can be prescribed and taken prior to meals to aid absorption of nutrients. This should also help alleviate the steatorrhoea. Concurrent administration of H_2-receptor antagonist or protein pump inhibitors (PPIs) may improve the efficacy of these supplements. Close monitoring of blood glucose should be undertaken and in the event of the development of diabetes mellitus, the input of a diabetic nurse specialist will provide invaluable assistance.

Health promotion Information and education about the implications of living with chronic pancreatitis are fundamental in order to facilitate lifestyle adjustments, particularly in respect of maintaining nutritional status and abstaining from alcohol. Smoking cessation is also advocated since smoking is thought to be implicated in increasing the risk of developing pancreatic cancer. For those who do not have an alcohol dependency or where the cause is not known there is a sense of helplessness associated with not knowing why they have developed this condition. Depending on the severity of the symptoms chronic pancreatitis can have a significant impact on the quality of life of those living with it. Symptoms can be debilitating leading to attendant psychosocial problems, loss of work, reliance on narcotics to manage the pain and significant periods of time spent in hospital. Integrated support across acute and community based services is essential in enabling these patients to maximise self-management of this lifelong condition. Caring for these patients can present a professional and personal challenge to members of the multidisciplinary team, who may feel inclined to blame the patient for the illness.

Cancer of the pancreas

The cause of pancreatic cancer is unknown, but cigarette smoking, pre-existence of diabetes mellitus, chronic or hereditary pancreatitis, stomach ulcer, IBD, previous cancers, family history, diet, being overweight and physically inactive have all demonstrated an increased risk (Cancer Research UK 2010). It is relatively rare in those under the age of 50 years but increases dramatically with age (Hayes 2006). It is the fifth most common cause of death from cancer in the UK with 7781 deaths in 2008 and a lifetime risk of 1:86 for both men and women (Cancer Research UK 2010).

PATHOPHYSIOLOGY AND RISK FACTORS

Tumours of the pancreas can arise from exocrine or endocrine tissue and can be malignant or benign although the latter are very rare; adenocarcinomas of the exocrine pancreas account for approximately 95% of malignant tumours and nearly all arise from the ductal tissue (Cancer Research UK 2010). Endocrine tumours also exist and arise from the islets of Langerhans. Tumours of the head of the pancreas account for more than two thirds of pancreatic cancers. Lesions frequently obstruct the pancreatic duct, causing chronic pancreatitis. The carcinoma can also obstruct the bile duct, giving rise to obstructive jaundice. Cancer of the pancreas carries a very poor prognosis because the disease has often spread to nearby organs by the time a diagnosis is made. Surgical resection has not been shown to improve the rate of survival. However, cancer of the duodenum, lower bile duct and peri-ampullary regions often presents earlier with obstructive jaundice, and surgical resection offers a much better prognosis.

Clinical features

Clinical features will vary according to the location, size in relation to nearby structures, and the specific anatomical location of the tumour (Hayes 2006). Many of the early symptoms are non-specific and tend to go unrecognised with the result that diagnosis occurs at an advanced stage. However, obstructive jaundice is often the symptom with which the patient first presents to the GP. The urine is dark in colour, the stool pale and fatty, and the skin and sclera have a yellowish tinge. Severe itch can be a very distressing symptom. Severe weight loss (approximately 2–3 kg per month) and anorexia are associated with vague epigastric

pain, often radiating to the back. Initially pain is intermittent, but gradually it becomes constant and severe.

Diagnosis

Blood is taken for liver function tests and to check for the presence of a coagulation defect. The most frequently used biomarker for pancreatic cancer is carbohydrate antigen 19-9 (CA 19-9). In addition, it can help with predicting prognosis, assessing treatment response in advanced disease or determining the risk of recurrence following surgery (Hayes 2006). Dual-phase CT scanning is a sensitive and non-invasive diagnostic tool that has a degree of specificity in detecting a pancreatic mass, local invasion by tumour, or metastases. An ultrasound scan will detect a dilated biliary tree and exclude the presence of gallstones. Pancreatic tissue may be obtained for cytology by using CT scan or ultrasound-guided fine-needle aspiration. ERCP can be used to define the site of obstruction and obtain biopsies.

Treatment options

Relief of obstructive jaundice and pain control are all that can be offered to the majority of patients with pancreatic cancer. ERCP with stenting of the biliary tree can relieve obstructive jaundice and may reduce the necessity for surgical intervention. Chemotherapy is used but appears to have little long-term clinical benefit or effect on survival. Where the tumour is not resectable radiotherapy has been shown to reduce local progression and has an effect on survival time and metastatic spread (Hayes 2006). Surgery is usually palliative but jaundice may be relieved by cholecystojejunostomy or choledochojejunostomy.

In a minority of cases (15–20%) where the tumour is deemed to be resectable, a Whipple's procedure (pancreatoduodenectomy) (see Figure 4.9) may be considered if the tumour is less than 2 cm in diameter and confined to the head of the pancreas. However, this surgery is highly complex with variable results and a high rate of peri-operative mortality, although this is improving particularly in hepatobiliary specialist centres. However, the 5-year survival rate remains less than 10%. For further detail on Whipple's procedure and the pre- and postoperative nursing care for these patients see Hayes (2006).

▷ Nursing management and health promotion: cancer of the pancreas

Investigative procedures are extensive, and surgery in the majority of cases offers palliation only. The nurse has a very important role in helping both the patient and the family to cope as the prognosis is one of the worst and the condition dramatically affects the patient's quality of life (Hayes 2006).

Anxiety Patients with pancreatic cancer are usually very anxious. They may have no previous history of illness and often deny the diagnosis. They may have difficulty coming to terms with the diagnosis and are often angry and withdrawn, especially with close family members. Relatives often feel shut out and helpless. The nurse can help by offering support and advice to the patient and family members, who should be given opportunities to discuss the illness and its implications.

If surgery is to be undertaken extensive discussion with the patient and relatives is necessary. Some patients are prepared for a Whipple's procedure but then at surgery it is found that the disease is more extensive than expected and a bypass is all that can be safely attempted. This is devastating for the patient and family, who will have built up hopes for recovery.

Pain Pain is often persistent, particularly when the disease is at an advanced stage. Oral opioids may be given and titrated to the patient's specific needs. Progression to subcutaneous diamorphine may be necessary as the disease advances and an oral laxative will also be given to prevent the side-effect of constipation. As the disease advances, pain may become more difficult to control. A coeliac plexus nerve block may also be of benefit.

Close monitoring of the effectiveness of pain control is essential to ensure that the best possible quality of life can be maintained for the patient (see Ch. 19). If the patient is discharged home, liaison with the primary health care team is essential to ensure that full continuity of care is achieved. Referral to a hospice should be made to ensure that the patient and their family receive the best possible care as the condition deteriorates (see Ch. 33).

Jaundice Jaundice is usually persistent and accompanied by severe itching (pruritus). The itching is usually all over the body and the patient may scratch until the skin bleeds. Patients may be so distressed by itch that they feel they are being driven mad. Every effort should be made to relieve itching that is believed to be caused by a deposition of bile salts in the skin. Antihistamines are used but they can cause sedation. A twice-daily bath with added sodium bicarbonate is very effective. Calamine lotion or Eurax cream applied locally may help. Night sedation is important, as itching is often worse at night. For further reading on pruritus see Bosonnet (2003).

Following ERCP and stenting, the jaundice and itch will subside over 7–10 days. The patient will feel much better as soon as the itch disappears and as the jaundice fades. Patients should be actively encouraged to drink extra fluids. This helps the jaundice to abate by flushing bilirubin and bile salts out of the blood and tissues.

Anorexia and weight loss Poor appetite and subsequent weight loss are further distressing aspects of the disease. Meals should be small and attractively presented. Liaison with the dietitian is necessary. High-protein drinks between meals may be tolerated well. If weight loss is severe, special care should be taken to prevent the development of pressure ulcers. Malaise associated with anorexia and weight loss will increase the patient's dependency and nurses and other carers will need to offer more and more assistance with many aspects of daily life (see Ch. 31).

THE SPLEEN

The spleen (Figure 4.10) is the largest lymph organ in the body and lies in the upper left quadrant of the abdomen, between the fundus of the stomach and the diaphragm. It is richly supplied with blood via the splenic artery. Blood flow through the spleen is slowed down by the fact that blood

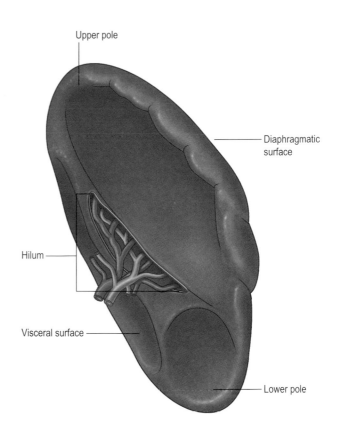

Figure 4.10 Surface and hilum of the spleen. (Reproduced with permission from Drake et al 2005.)

must pass through sinuses in which the monophage/macrophage system scavenges old erythrocytes and pathogenic particles and passes the breakdown products on to the liver via the hepatic portal system. The main functions of the spleen include phagocytosis, storage of blood, immune activation in the presence of antigens and erythropoiesis.

DISORDERS OF THE SPLEEN

Splenic trauma

The spleen is highly vascular and is one of the organs most frequently damaged by abdominal trauma. Fractures of the lower ribs following trauma are often implicated in splenic injury, with an estimate of up to 20% (Herbert & Sartorelli 2006). These are not always identifiable from an abdominal ultrasound. Furthermore, the spleen is particularly susceptible to injury when it is pathologically enlarged.

PATHOPHYSIOLOGY AND RISK FACTORS

Injury to the spleen can result in rupture, evulsion from its pedicle or tearing beneath the capsule, with possible formation of a subcapsular haematoma. Delayed rupture of the spleen occurs in about 5% of patients and is thought to be caused by haematoma bursting through the capsule wall. This usually occurs within 2 weeks of injury, but in a few cases can be delayed for months or even years.

Clinical features

Rupture and evulsion of the spleen causes immediate intraperitoneal bleeding. As blood spreads throughout the peritoneal cavity, signs of haemorrhage and hypovolaemic shock (see Ch. 18) may develop. Patients generally present as an acute abdominal emergency. The patient experiences abdominal pain with particular tenderness in the left upper quadrant and percussion dullness of the left flank (Ballance's sign). Referred pain is often felt in the left shoulder tip (Kerh's sign). Bruising to the abdomen is not always evident.

Not all patients with splenic injury present in such a dramatic way. Sometimes, patients may require a splenectomy following lymphatic malignancy, sickle cell disease or malignancy causing infarction of the spleen or due to splenic injury during or as a consequence of surgery.

Treatment options

If a diagnosis is difficult to establish and splenic injury is suspected, vigilant and careful observation of the patient is vital. Injury to the spleen is an indication for splenectomy, provided the organ cannot be conserved. Preference is given to conserving splenic tissue if at all possible by suturing capsular tears or by performing a partial splenectomy as there is a risk of systemic infection following splenectomy (Forrest et al 1995).

Nursing management and health promotion: splenic trauma

Following splenic injury, the patient's pain should be monitored, noting the site, type and duration. Whether the pain is increasing or decreasing may be relevant. There is no evidence to support withholding pain relief until a diagnosis is confirmed, hence opioid analgesia should be prescribed and administered. The patient will be nil per mouth during this acute period and so oral hygiene needs will be a nursing priority.

The patient's vital signs should be monitored. Any changes in the patient's condition should be reported immediately as, following rupture, temporary improvement in the patient's condition may precede sudden deterioration.

Intravenous access should be established and intravenous fluids, blood and blood products should be administered as required. Oxygen therapy may be commenced to raise the circulating levels and a urinary catheter is inserted to assess renal function. Blood pressure, pulse, respirations and PO_2 saturations should be closely monitored and any changes reported immediately. A nasogastric tube may be passed to empty the stomach contents and prevent aspiration.

The nurse should provide reassurance as the patient may be distressed and anxious pre-operatively. Relatives should be kept informed and comfort and support should be given during this stressful and worrying time.

PRE-OPERATIVE MANAGEMENT

In preparation for splenectomy, a full assessment of the patient's blood count and coagulation status must be made. In the presence of any bleeding tendency, a transfusion of blood or platelets may be administered. In patients with thrombocytopenia, platelets should be made available for use to cover the intra- and postoperative phase. *Haemophilus influenzae* type B vaccine is also given prophylactically. Preparation for surgery is as for abdominal surgery requiring general anaesthesia (see Ch. 26).

POSTOPERATIVE MANAGEMENT

Postoperative care is as described for abdominal surgery requiring general anaesthesia (see Ch. 26). The patient will usually be nursed in a high-dependency area until stable enough to return to a general ward.

Nursing observations include monitoring the patient's vital signs and pain levels. The use and effectiveness of the PCA and prescribed antiemetics should be monitored. Ensure the patient's comfort throughout.

The wound should be monitored for signs of inflammation. If wound drains are present output should be monitored and they should be removed when drainage is minimal. Fluid intake and output should be carefully recorded and oral fluids should be encouraged when the patient is able to tolerate them.

In the postoperative period, an anti-pneumococcal vaccine is given to prevent or minimise the risk of developing a chest infection. These patients are more susceptible to chest infection because of the role of the spleen in immune activation. Furthermore, because the spleen is located close to the left lung there is an increased risk of collapse of the left lower lobe following splenectomy. Therefore, chest physiotherapy is essential. The nurse must also encourage the patient to perform deep breathing exercises and aid expectoration between physiotherapy sessions. Low-dose heparin should be prescribed due to a transient increase in platelet and leucocyte levels. The nurse should perform passive leg exercises whilst the patient is on bed rest and encourage movement and early ambulation. Antiembolism stockings should be worn to prevent the development of postoperative deep venous thrombosis.

Pancreatitis caused by the handling and bruising of the tail of the pancreas during surgery is a complication of splenic surgery. Injury to the pancreas occurs in 1–3% of patients who undergo a splenectomy (Herbert & Sartorelli 2006). The serum amylase and lipase should be monitored for 2–4 days postoperatively. Nurses should observe for the signs and symptoms of the development of pancreatitis, i.e. nausea and vomiting, severe abdominal pain and abdominal distension. The nurse must be alert to any increase or change in the nature of the patient's pain.

Due to the loss of lymphoid tissue, there is an increased risk of infection following splenectomy. As most infections occur within 3 years of surgery, prophylactic penicillin for this period or even longer may be prescribed. Antibiotic cover is mandatory when the patient is a child (Garden et al 2002).

Persistent haemorrhage occurs in less than 1% of patients following a splenectomy and usually occurs in those who have had surgery for the treatment of thrombocytopenia. It is important that the patient is educated about the complications that can occur following a splenectomy and any lifestyle changes that they may need to consider.

Hypersplenism

Hypersplenism is a syndrome consisting of splenomegaly (enlargement of the spleen) and pancytopenia (reduced red cells, granular white cells and platelets in the blood) and is common in patients with cirrhosis and associated portal hypertension. The bone marrow is normal and no autoimmune disease is present. In the context of gastrointestinal nursing, the nursing care of the patient with hypersplenism will be as for a patient with cirrhosis (see p. 103). Further information on the pathophysiology and clinical features can be found on the website.

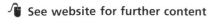 **See website for further content**

SUMMARY: KEY NURSING ISSUES

- The predominant function of the GI and hepatobiliary system is to digest food in order to generate energy for the body.
- Because the GI and hepatobiliary system comprises a large number of organs with a range of interrelated functions, disorders can produce diverse and often distressing symptoms, such as pain, dysphagia, anorexia, weight loss, dyspepsia, nausea and vomiting, constipation and diarrhoea, causing considerable embarrassment and activity restrictions in patients' lives.
- Both surgical and conservative management of patients with GI and hepatobiliary conditions constitute interventions that can result in decrement in the patient's life quality.
- Deaths from diseases of the GI system have increased by 25% over the last 10 years. Malignancies of the GI and hepatobiliary system are among the most common and, given their relationship with nutrition, digestion and excretion, can cause significant suffering for patients and their families.
- In order to provide effective care, nurses must have a good knowledge and understanding of the anatomy and physiology of the gastrointestinal and hepatobiliary system.
- Nurses have a key role in health promotion such as screening, advising about lifestyle changes, providing educational support, promoting and enabling self-care and monitoring the patient's physical, psychological and social functioning.
- Pain assessment and management are essential nursing skills as pain is severe for many patients presenting with disorders of the GI and hepatobiliary systems.
- A non-judgemental approach is vital when supporting patients suffering from disorders that are linked to obesity, alcohol and drug abuse and cigarette smoking.
- Nurses specialising in gastrointestinal nursing need a wide variety of skills and knowledge in order to assess, plan, implement and evaluate the sometimes complex and challenging nursing care required by patients with gastrointestinal, hepatobiliary, pancreatic and splenic disorders.
- Nurses specialising in gastrointestinal nursing are now performing diagnostic and therapeutic endoscopy, GI tract manometry and siting gastrostomy tubes. These advances are in line with evolving technology and the increased demand for rapid access to health care services and it is likely that the role will continue to evolve and grow to meet the needs of a modern health service.

REFERENCES

Ahmed I, Lobo D: Malignant tumours of the liver, *Surgery (Oxford)* 25 (1):34–41, 2007.

Bacon BR, O'Grady JG, Di Bisceglie AM, Lake JR: *Comprehensive Clinical Hepatology*, ed 2, St Louis, 2006, Mosby.

Banning M: *Helicobacter pylori*: pathophysiology, assessment and treatment, *Gastrointestinal Nursing* 4(8):28–33, 2006.

Black PK: Psychological, sexual and cultural issues for patients with a stoma, *Br J Nurs* 13(12):692–697, 2004.

Black P: Managing physical postoperative stoma complications, *Br J Nurs (Stoma Care Supplement)* 18(17):S4–S10, 2009.

Borwell B: Rehabilitation and stoma care: addressing the psychological needs, *Br J Nurs (Stoma Care Supplement)* 18(4):S20–S25, 2009.

Bosonnet L: Pruritus: scratching the surface, *Eur J Cancer Care (Engl)* 12 (2):162–166, 2003.

British Society of Gastroenterology: *Guidelines for the diagnosis and management of Barrett's columnar-lined oesophagus*, 2005. Available online http://www.bsg.org.uk/images/stories/docs/clinical/guidelines/oesophageal/Barretts_Oes.pdf.

Burch J: The pre- and postoperative nursing care for patients with a stoma, *Br J Nurs* 14(6):310–318, 2005.

Cancer Research UK: *CancerStats*, 2009a. Available online http://publications.cancerresearchuk.org/WebRoot/crukstoredb/CRUK_PDFs/CSOESOPHKEYFACT09.pdf.

Cancer Research UK: *Stomach Cancer*, 2009b. Available online http://www.cancerhelp.org.uk/type/stomach-cancer/index.htm.

Cancer Research UK: *Pancreatic Cancer*, 2010. Available online http://www.cancerresearchuk.org/cancerstats/types/pancreas/riskfactors/index.htm.

Carter MJ, Lobo AJ, Travis SPL (on behalf of the IBD section of the British Society of Gastroenterology): Guidelines for the management of inflammatory bowel disease in adults, *Gut* 53(Suppl V):v1–v16, 2004.

Cavestro G, Comparato G, Nouvenne A, Sianesi M, Di Mario F: The race from chronic pancreatitis to pancreatic cancer, *Journal of Pancreas (online)* 4(5):165–168, 2003.

Chen C, Yu M, Liaw Y: Epidemiological characteristics and risk factors of hepatocellular carcinoma, *J Gastroenterol Hepatol* 12(9–10):294–308, 1997.

Christensen T: The treatment of oesophageal varices using a Sengstaken-Blakemore tube: considerations for nursing practice, *Nurs Crit Care* 9(2):58–63, 2004.

Cotton P, Ackerman U: *Practical gastrointestinal endoscopy: the fundamentals*, ed 5, Oxford, 2003, Blackwell Science.

Dent J, El-Serag HB, Wallander MA, Johansson S: Epidemiology of gastro-oesophageal reflux disease: a systematic review, *Gut* 54:710–717, 2005.

Dinsdale P: Indispensable skills, *Nurs Stand* 21(17):24–25, 2007.

Drake RL, Vogl W, Mitchell AWM: *Gray's Anatomy for students*, Philadelphia, 2005, Elsevier.

Elia M: *Screening for Malnutrition: A Multidisciplinary Responsibility: Report by Malnutrition Advisory Group*, Maidenhead, 2003, BAPEN. Available online http://www.bapen.org.uk/the-must.htm.

Etemad B, Whitcomb D: Chronic pancreatitis: diagnosis, classification and new genetic developments, *Gastroenterology* 120(3):682–707, 2001.

European Helicobacter Study Group: *Current concepts in the management of Helicobacter pylori infection*, 2000. The Maastricht 2–2000 consensus report. Available online http://www.helicobacter.org.

Fawcett TM, Smith GD: Jaundice: its causes and care, *Gastrointestinal Nursing* (1):23–27, 2004.

Fawcett TM, Smith GD: Acute pancreatitis: pathophysiology and patient care, *Gastrointestinal Nursing* 3(8):31–39, 2005.

Forrest APM, Carter DC, McLeod IB: *Principles and practice of surgery*, ed 3, Edinburgh, 1995, Churchill Livingstone.

Fox M, Forgacs I: Gastro-oesophageal reflux disease, *Br Med J* 332 (7533):88–93, 2006.

Fulham J: A guide to caring for patients with a newly formed stoma in the acute hospital setting, *Gastrointestinal Nursing* 6(8):14–23, 2008.

Garden OJ, Bradbury AW, Forsyth J: *Principles and practice of surgery*, ed 4, Edinburgh, 2002, Churchill Livingstone.

Ginès P, Cárdenas A, Arroyo V, Rodés: Management of cirrhosis and ascites, *N Engl J Med* 350(16):1646–1654, 2004.

Gonsalkorale W, Miller V, Afzal A, Whorwell P: Long term benefits of hypnotherapy for irritable bowel syndrome, *Gut* 52(11):1623–1629, 2003.

Graham L: Care of patients undergoing laparoscopic cholecystectomy, *Nurs Stand* 23(7):41–48, 2008.

Griffin MS, Dunn L: Oesophageal cancer, *Surgery (Oxford)* 26 (11):458–462, 2008.

Gut Trust: *Irritable bowel syndrome*, 2010. Available online http://www.theguttrust.org.

Hartley V: Paracetamol overdose, *Emerg Nurse* 5(2):17–24, 2002.

Haslett C, Chilvers ER, Boon NA, College NA: *Davidson's Principles and practice of medicine*, ed 19, Edinburgh, 2002, Churchill Livingstone.

Hayes C: Pancreatic cancer: an overview for allied healthcare practitioners, *Gastrointestinal Nursing* 4(8):12–21, 2006.

Herbert JC, Sartorelli KH: Spleen. In Lawrence PF, Bell RM, Dayton MT, editors: *Essentials of general surgery*, ed 4, Baltimore, 2006, Lippincott Williams and Wilkins, pp 427–439.

Hicks SJ: Gastric cancer: diagnosis, risk factors, treatment and life issues, *Br J Nurs* 10(8):529–536, 2001.

Hodgson T: Oesophageal cancer: experiences of patients and their partners, *Br J Nurs* 15(21):1157–1160, 2006.

Hughes E: Understanding the care of patients with acute pancreatitis, *Nurs Stand* 18(18):45–52, 2004.

Janes SEJ, Meagher A, Frizelle A: Management of diverticulitis, *Br Med J* 332(7536):271–275, 2006.

Karamshi M: Performing a percutaneous liver biopsy in parenchymal liver disease, *Br J Nurs* 17(12):746–752, 2008.

Karanjia N, Ali T: Gallstones, *Surgery (Oxford)* 25(1):16–21, 2007.

Kelso LA: Cirrhosis: caring for patients with end-stage liver failure, *Nurse Pract* 33(7):24–31, 2008.

Koti RS, Davidson BR: Portal hypertension, *Surgery (Oxford)* 1(5):113–117, 2003.

Lewis SJ, Heaton KW: Stool form scale as a useful guide to intestinal transit time, *Scand J Gastroenterol* 32(9):920–924, 1997.

Mirza M, Aithal G: Portal hypertension and ascites, *Surgery (Oxford)* 25(1):28–33, 2006.

Morcom J: Understanding GORD from a primary care nurse perspective, *Gastrointestinal Nursing* 6(1):12–20, 2008.

National Institute for Health and Clinical Excellence (NICE): *Improving outcomes in colorectal cancers – manual update*, 2004. Available online http://www.nice.org.uk.

National Institute for Health and Clinical Excellence (NICE): *Management of Dyspepsia in Adults in Primary Care (Amended from 2004)*, Clinical Guideline 17, 2005a. Available online http://www.nice.org.uk.

National Institute for Health and Clinical Excellence (NICE): *Referral Guidelines for Suspected Cancer*, Clinical Guideline 27, 2005b. Available online http://www.nice.org.uk/CG027.

National Institute for Health and Clinical Excellence (NICE): *Irritable Bowel Syndrome in Adults*, Clinical Guideline 61, 2008. Available online http://www.nice.org.uk.

Nicklin J, Blazeby J: Anorexia in patients dying from oesophageal and gastric cancers, *Gastrointestinal Nursing* 1(7):35–39, 2003.

Nicol M, Bavin C, Cronin P, Rawlings-Anderson K: *Essential Nursing Skills*, ed 3, Edinburgh, 2008, Mosby.

Norton C, Williams J, Taylor C, Nunwa A, Whayman K, editors: *Oxford Handbook of Gastrointestinal Nursing*, Oxford, 2008, Oxford University Press.

Office for National Statistics: *Health Service Quarterly* 40(Winter):59–60, 2008.

Palmer M: *Hepatitis and liver disease, what you need to know*, New York, 2004, Avery Publishers.

Peate I: Caring for the person with biliary disorders: gallstones, *British Journal of Healthcare Assistants* 3(2):61–65, 2009.

Porrett T: The immediate postoperative period. In Porrett T, McGrath A, editors: *Stoma Care*, Oxford, 2005, Blackwell Publishing, pp 65–76.

Rowlinson A: Inflammatory bowel disease 3: importance of partnership in care, *Br J Nurs* 8(15):1013–1018, 1999.

Sargent S: The aetiology, management and complications of alcoholic hepatitis, *Br J Nurs* 14(10):556–562, 2005.

Sargent S: Management of patients with advanced liver cirrhosis, *Nurs Stand* 21(11):48–56, 2006a.

Sargent S: Pathophysiology, diagnosis and management of acute pancreatitis, *Br J Nurs* 15(18):999–1005, 2006b.

Sargent S: Hepatic nursing. Pathophysiology and management of hepatic encephalopathy, *Br J Nurs* 16(6):335–339, 2007.

Sargent S: Drug-induced liver injury. In Sargent S, editor: *Liver Diseases: An essential Guide for Nurses and Health Care Professionals*, Oxford, 2009, Wiley-Blackwell, pp 256–270.

Sargent S, Fullwood D: Diagnosing and treating a patient with primary biliary cirrhosis, *Br J Nurs* 17(9):566–570, 2008.

Smith G, Fawcett T: Chronic pancreatitis: pathophysiology and patient care, *Gastrointestinal Nursing* 4(7):20–26, 2006.

Thomas BR: Cholecystectomy: take a look at two options, *Nursing* 39 (2):36–39, 2009.

UK Working Party on Acute Pancreatitis: UK guidelines for the management of acute pancreatitis, *Gut* 54:1–9, 2005.

van Baalen C: Managing gastro-oesophageal reflux the surgical way, *Gastrointestinal Nursing* 6(2):24–29, 2008.

van Baalen C: Pre- and postoperative management of patients with oesophageal cancer, *Gastrointestinal Nursing* 7(7):26–32, 2009.

Verschuur EML, Steyerberg WE, Kuipers EJ: Experiences and expectations of patients after oesophageal cancer surgery: an explorative study, *Eur J Cancer Care (Engl)* 15(4):324–332, 2006.

Vujnovich A: Pre and post operative assessment of patients with a stoma, *Nurs Stand* 22(19):50–56, 2008.

Wallace CI, Dargan PI, Jones AL: Paracetamol overdose: an evidence based flowchart to guide management, *Emergency Medical Journal* 19:202–205, 2002.

Wan A, Allum WH: Gastric cancer, *Surgery* 26(11):439–443, 2008.

Waugh A, Grant A: *Ross and Wilson: Anatomy and Physiology in Health and Illness*, ed 10, Edinburgh, 2006, Elsevier.

Werner J, Feuerbach S, Uhl W, Buchler M: Management of acute pancreatitis: from surgery to interventional intensive care, *Gut* 54(3):426–436, 2005.

Whitman K, McCormick C: When your patient is in liver failure, *Nursing* 34(4):58–63, 2005.

Williams J: Stoma care part 1: choosing the right appliance, *Gastrointestinal Nursing* 4(6):16–19, 2006a.

Williams J: Stoma care part 2: choosing appliance accessories, *Gastrointestinal Nursing* 4(7):16–19, 2006b.

Williams J: Thirty years of ileal-anal pouch and beyond, *British Journal of Nursing (Stoma Care Supplement)* 17(17):S20–S23, 2008.

World Health Organization: *National cancer control programmes: policies and managerial guidelines*, ed 2, Geneva, 2002, World Health Organization. Available online http://www.who.int/cancer/media/en/408.pdf.

Yeung E, Wong F: The management of cirrhotic ascites, *Medscape Gastroenterology eJournal* 4(4): 2002. Available online http://www.medscape.com/viewarticle /442364_1.

Zimmermann P: Is it appendicitis? *Am J Nurs* 108(9):27–31, 2008.

USEFUL WEBSITES

British Liver Trust: www.britishlivertrust.org.uk

Coeliac UK: www.coeliac.co.uk

Colostomy Association: www.colostomyassociation.org.uk

Ileostomy and Internal Pouch Support Group: www.the-ia.org.uk

National Association for Colitis and Crohn's Disease (NACC): www.nacc.org.uk

National Institute for Health and Clinical Excellence (NICE): www.nice.org.uk

Patients on Intravenous and Naso-gastric Nutrition Therapy (PINNT): www.pinnt.com

Scottish Intercollegiate Guidelines Network: www.sign.ac.uk

UK Transplant: www.uktransplant.org.uk

Nursing patients with endocrine and metabolic disorders

Maggie N. Carson
Part 1   Nursing patients with endocrine disorders

Joan Allwinkle, Janet Barclay
Part 2   Nursing patients with diabetes mellitus

PART 1 NURSING PATIENTS WITH ENDOCRINE DISORDERS

Introduction

Endocrinology is the study of hormones – chemical messengers secreted by endocrine glands and neurones. Hormones, usually travelling in the bloodstream, maintain homeostasis by acting on and coordinating activity within target organs or tissues.

Endocrinology is a rapidly growing field (Wilson 2005). Considerable progress is being made, with important implications for other areas of medicine, e.g. neuroendocrinology, which in turn has important applications within psychiatry. Advances are constantly being made and current research is adding to knowledge of genetic causes of many endocrine conditions. Genetic research is an area from which future treatments of endocrine disease will come.

Another area of considerable interest within endocrinology is the effects of cancer therapies on pituitary and thyroid function. One third of the UK population develops cancer, which is increasingly becoming a curable chronic disease; at the end of 2008 there were 2 million cancer survivors in the UK (3.3% of the total population and 10% of those over the age of 65). The overall survival following childhood cancer is 70–90% but 60–70% of these individuals have one or more ongoing medical problems and the most frequent conditions encountered are endocrine in nature.

Apart from diabetes mellitus (see pp. 149–175) and thyroid disorders, endocrine problems are not common. Many endocrine disorders are rarely seen and may be difficult to diagnose without complicated and exhaustive testing. As a result, patients may be referred by their general practitioner or local hospital to specialist centres for diagnosis. For the patient, this has the advantage of offering highly specialised care. It also means that relatively few nurses have the opportunity to care for people with these disorders. However, given the wide-ranging effects of endocrine dysfunction, it is important that all nurses have a general understanding of endocrinology. Endocrine diseases can affect every system of the body, sometimes causing disfigurement and a change in body image and quality of life (QoL) and even occasionally posing a threat to life. These disorders can seriously affect the patient's psychological outlook, either as a direct result of the illness or by virtue of the individual's reaction to it.

It is well documented that individuals react differently to being ill. Anger may be directed at family members or at nursing and medical staff. This situation may be exacerbated by an unstable mental state, mood swings, depression or frank psychosis, which may, in fact, be sequelae of the disorder, e.g. Cushing's syndrome. The nurse must be aware of this possibility and react accordingly, offering support and understanding to the patient and their relatives. Identifying the patient's worries and concerns, providing factual information and educating the patient about their condition and its management will all help to minimise psychological distress. Explanations that the underlying illness may be influencing the patient's mood may help them and their relatives to cope.

As the tests and investigations required to diagnose some of the rarer endocrine conditions are often long and exhausting, clear explanations are essential so that the patient understands the need for them and the procedures that will be followed. This will help to reduce anxiety and increase the patient's confidence in the health care team. The psychological support that the nurse can offer this group of patients is vitally important. Many benefit from referral to a support group (see Useful websites) and the contact this brings with other patients who have the same condition. Often these patients are young and probably otherwise in good health, and therefore the impact of endocrine disease on their body image and/or self-esteem should not be underestimated. For example, patients experiencing sexual dysfunction may feel embarrassed to talk to and seek support from family members and friends –in such cases, support from the health care professional is crucial.

Anatomy and physiology

The nature of the endocrine system, being one of control, means that it has far-reaching effects throughout the body on various target organs. This section provides a brief outline of hormonal action and outlines the anatomy and physiology of individual endocrine glands and structures (see Further reading, e.g. Montague et al 2005). The gonads, ovaries and testes are described in Chapters 7 and 8.

Hormones

The endocrine system is one of the two major control systems of the body, the other being the nervous system. The nervous system mediates endocrine activity. The endocrine glands/structures produce hormones, which are secreted into the bloodstream for transport to their respective target organs (Figure 5.1). Hormones are either lipid-based (e.g. glucocorticoids) or peptides (e.g. adrenaline [epinephrine], insulin).

Action

Hormones affect only those cells or organs upon which they have an excitatory or inhibitory action. This system allows individuals to respond to changes in their environment and is important in controlling growth and development, sexual maturation and homeostasis.

Many hormones are bound to proteins within the circulation. Only unbound or free hormones are biologically active, and that binding serves as a buffer against very rapid changes in plasma levels of a hormone. This principle is important in the interpretation of many tests of endocrine function.

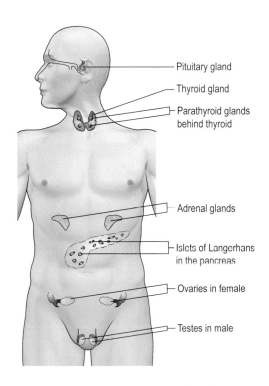

Figure 5.1 The endocrine glands/structures and their location in the body.

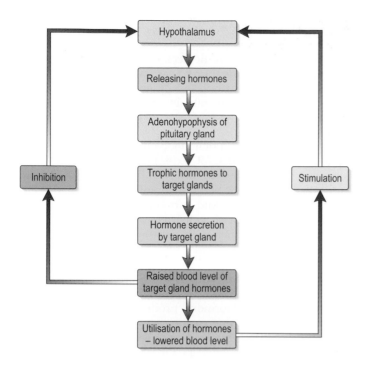

Figure 5.2 Negative feedback regulation of the secretion of anterior pituitary hormones.

Control

Most hormone systems are controlled by a negative feedback system which ensures that hormone levels, whilst fluctuating, remain within a preset range (see Appendix – normal values). Figure 5.2 illustrates how negative feedback operates in the hypothalamic–pituitary–thyroid axis.

Pattern of secretion

Hormone secretion is either continuous or intermittent. An example of continuous secretion is thyroxine by the thyroid gland, in which hormone levels over a day, month or year show very little variation. Intermittent secretion is seen in three forms: circadian, menstrual and pulsatile.

Other factors which affect hormone secretion include stress, disease, trauma, surgery or emotional upset. As in any complex regulatory system, it is likely that disequilibrium in endocrine function will have important consequences. Disorders of the endocrine system may be categorised most simply as those involving overproduction (hypersecretion) and those involving underproduction (hyposecretion).

Pituitary

The pituitary gland lies immediately below the hypothalamus (part of the floor of the third ventricle of the brain) in the pituitary fossa. It is connected to the hypothalamus by the pituitary stalk and comprises two lobes which function independently of each other (Figure 5.3). During fetal life the glandular anterior lobe develops from the oropharynx to become the adenohypophysis. The neural posterior lobe is a down-growth from the forebrain, which becomes the

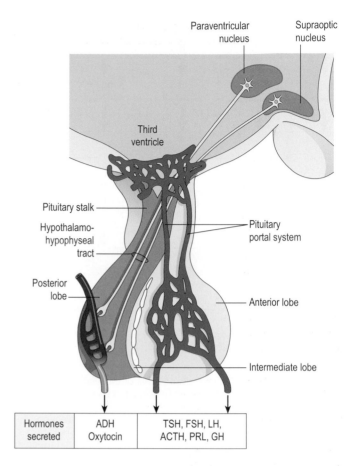

Figure 5.3 The pituitary gland and its relationship with the hypothalamus. ACTH, adrenocorticotrophic hormone; ADH, antidiuretic hormone; FSH, follicle-stimulating hormone; GH, growth hormone; LH, luteinising hormone; PRL, prolactin; TSH, thyroid-stimulating hormone. (Reproduced from Waugh & Grant 2006 with permission.)

neurohypophysis. The posterior pituitary receives nerve fibres from hypothalamic nuclei via the hypothalamohypophyseal tract in the pituitary stalk.

The hypothalamus contains specialised cells or nuclei (paraventricular and supraoptic) which synthesise the hormones antidiuretic hormone (ADH) (also known as arginine vasopressin [AVP] or vasopressin) and oxytocin. The hypothalamus also produces releasing/inhibiting hormones that regulate the secretion of anterior pituitary hormones (Figure 5.4). The hypothalamus also controls many centres for functions such as appetite, thirst, temperature regulation, sexual activity and sleep/wake cycles.

The pituitary stalk carries blood to both lobes of the pituitary in a portal system by which the hypothalamic releasing/inhibitory hormones are carried to the anterior pituitary. The trophic hormones produced in the anterior pituitary stimulate the other endocrine glands. ADH and oxytocin are stored in the posterior pituitary until released. Table 5.1 outlines the hormones secreted by the pituitary gland.

The optic chiasm sits just above the pituitary fossa. Therefore, an expanding lesion from the pituitary or the hypothalamus may result in a defect in the visual fields because of pressure on the optic nerve or optic chiasm.

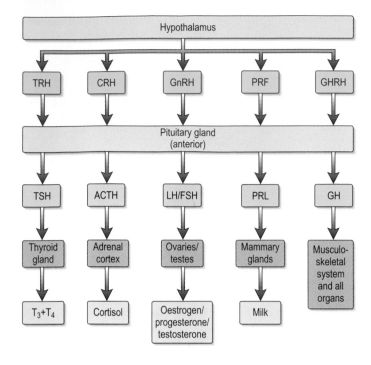

Figure 5.4 Schematic diagram showing some of the relationships between the hypothalamus, the anterior pituitary gland and their target organs. ACTH, adrenocorticotrophic hormone; CRH, corticotrophin-releasing hormone; GH, growth hormone; GHRH, growth hormone releasing hormone; GnRH, gonadotrophin-releasing hormone; LH (ICSH)/FSH, luteinising hormone/follicle-stimulating hormone; PRF, prolactin-releasing factor; PRL, prolactin; TRH, thyrotrophin-releasing hormone; TSH, thyroid-stimulating hormone.

Thyroid

The thyroid is a gland in the neck sited anteriorly to the larynx and attached to the thyroid cartilages and the trachea. It comprises two lobes connected by an isthmus (Figure 5.5). Structures in close proximity include the oesophagus, the parathyroid glands, the recurrent laryngeal nerves and the carotid arteries.

The thyroid receives a rich blood supply from the superior thyroid arteries (branch of external carotid arteries) and from the inferior thyroid arteries (branch of subclavian arteries). Each lobe is filled with follicles, which produce and store two of the thyroid hormones. Between the follicles are parafollicular cells (C cells) which secrete the hormone calcitonin; this, together with parathyroid hormone (PTH) from the parathyroid glands, regulates calcium and phosphate homeostasis.

The hormones, thyroxine (T_4) and some circulating tri-iodothyronine (T_3), are synthesised and secreted by the thyroid gland. Thyroid hormone production is dependent on the availability of iodine in the diet (see Ch. 21). More T_4 than T_3 is produced, but T_4 is converted in some tissues to the more biologically active T_3. Over 99% of all thyroid hormone is bound to plasma thyroid-binding proteins. Only the free hormone is available for use by the tissues. If the levels of T_4 and T_3 in the blood fall, the hypothalamus releases thyrotrophin-releasing hormone (TRH). As the levels of TRH rise, the pituitary gland secretes thyroid-stimulating hormone (TSH) which stimulates the thyroid gland to produce more T_4 and T_3. The principal effect of thyroid hormones is to influence the metabolism of cells and, therefore,

Table 5.1 Hormones of the pituitary gland and their action	
HORMONE	**ACTION**
Anterior lobe	
Growth hormone (GH) (*syn.* somatotrophin)	Pulsatile release. Does not have a single target gland but acts on a variety of tissues, e.g. bone, viscera and soft tissues. It is particularly important in children to stimulate growth. Action in adults recently thought to involve maintenance of cardiovascular activity, fat deposition and muscle development
Prolactin (PRL)	Main action is to stimulate lactation in females; also stimulates the corpus luteum of the ovary to secrete progesterone
Adrenocorticotrophic hormone (ACTH)	Secreted under circadian rhythm. Stimulates the adrenal cortex to secrete corticosteroids
Luteinising hormone (LH) known as interstitial cell-stimulating hormone (ICSH) in men (gonadotrophins)	In women LH promotes ovulation; stimulates formation of the corpus luteum. In men ICSH stimulates the production of the androgen hormone testosterone
Follicle-stimulating hormone (FSH) (a gonadotrophin)	FSH stimulates the production of sex hormones and contributes to regulation of the menstrual cycle in women. In women, stimulates the production of ovarian follicles and secretion of oestrogen; in men, stimulates spermatogenesis
Thyroid-stimulating hormone (TSH)	Stimulates the thyroid to release the hormone thyroxine
Posterior lobe	
Antidiuretic hormone (ADH) (also known as arginine vasopressin [AVP] or vasopressin)	Controls water homeostasis in the body by regulating water reabsorption from the distal convoluted tubules of the kidney
Oxytocin	Induces uterine contraction during labour (unusually controlled by a positive feedback mechanism) and ejection of milk from breasts postpartum

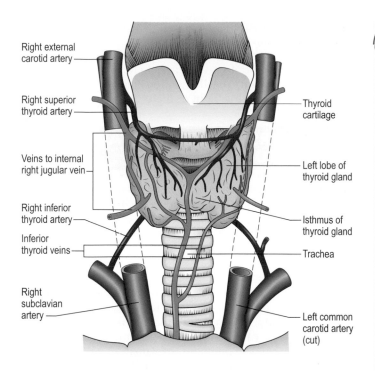

Right external carotid artery

Right superior thyroid artery

Veins to internal right jugular vein

Right inferior thyroid artery

Inferior thyroid veins

Right subclavian artery

Thyroid cartilage

Left lobe of thyroid gland

Isthmus of thyroid gland

Trachea

Left common carotid artery (cut)

Figure 5.5 The thyroid gland and associated structures.

the metabolic rate. Low levels of hormone are associated with a low temperature, i.e. patients will complain of feeling cold, slow heart rate, weight gain, poor concentration and low mood whereas patients with high concentrations of thyroid hormones experience a rapid heart rate, heat intolerance, anxiety and weight loss despite increased appetite.

Parathyroids

The parathyroid glands are usually situated on the posterior lobes of the thyroid gland. They are usually four in number; however, 6% of people have more than four glands. The blood supply is from the inferior and superior thyroid arteries.

The glands secrete parathyroid hormone (PTH), which is the most important hormone involved in calcium and phosphate homeostasis. PTH maintains plasma calcium levels within normal limits (2.12–2.62 mmol/L). It acts predominantly on

the renal tubules to increase reabsorption of calcium but also increases gut absorption of calcium and mobilises it from bone. Plasma calcium will therefore rise, and in turn suppress PTH secretion; conversely, a fall in plasma calcium will stimulate the secretion of PTH.

Vitamin D and calcitonin are also involved in calcium metabolism (Box 5.1).

Adrenals

The adrenal glands are situated one on the upper part of each kidney (Figure 5.6A). They are highly vascular and derive their blood supply from the renal arteries, the inferior phrenic arteries and directly from the aorta; they are drained by the suprarenal veins.

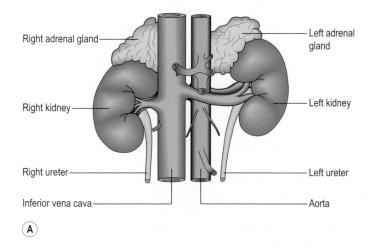

Right adrenal gland

Right kidney

Right ureter

Inferior vena cava

Left adrenal gland

Left kidney

Left ureter

Aorta

Ⓐ

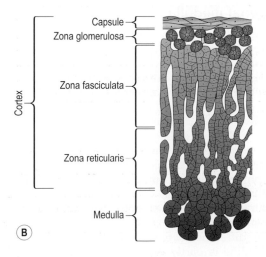

Capsule

Zona glomerulosa

Zona fasciculata

Cortex

Zona reticularis

Medulla

Ⓑ

Figure 5.6 A. The adrenal glands and associated structures. B. Layers through the adrenal gland.

The adrenal glands have a composite origin. The cortex, the outer part, has the same embryonic site of origin as the gonads. The medulla, the inner part, is derived from neural crest cells which have migrated from the developing neural tube and have become enclosed within the cortex. The latter can arguably be considered part of the nervous system. The secretions, and therefore the actions, of the two separate parts of the glands are quite different and will be discussed separately.

Adrenal cortex

The adrenal cortex has three layers (Figure 5.6B) that produce different hormones, collectively termed corticosteroids:

- mineralocorticoids (in the zona glomerulosa, the outer layer)
- glucocorticoids (in the zona fasciculata, the middle layer)
- adrenal sex hormones (androgens) and some glucocorticoids (in the zona reticularis, the inner layer).

Glucocorticoids such as cortisol, the principal glucocorticoid, have varied and wide-ranging actions, many of which are not fully understood. They are essential to life and, in their absence, blood sugar, blood pressure and blood volume fall, sodium excretion increases and muscle contractility decreases. If present in excessive amounts, an opposite set of changes occurs: blood volume expands, blood pressure rises, potassium falls, glycogen storage is increased, blood sugar levels rise, connective tissue is reduced in quality and strength, and immunity is impaired. Wound healing and the inflammatory process are also inhibited.

Mineralocorticoids The most important of the mineralocorticoids is aldosterone, which is the most potent regulator of sodium and potassium and is important in maintaining acid–base balance. Aldosterone acts on the distal convoluted tubules of the kidney and stimulates the cells to reabsorb and thus conserve sodium (see Chs 8, 20).

Adrenal androgens The adrenal cortex, in addition to the gonads, produces male sex hormones. The effects are appropriate in the male, but in the female excessive production may have a virilising effect.

Adrenal medulla

The catecholamines adrenaline (epinephrine), noradrenaline (norepinephrine) and dopamine are secreted by the adrenal medulla. Eighty per cent of adrenomedullary secretion is adrenaline, most noradrenaline and dopamine being secreted by neurones and functioning as neurotransmitters.

In normal secretion, adrenaline probably has some effect on mean blood pressure; although it increases systolic pressure, it decreases diastolic pressure. When secreted under the control of the sympathetic nervous system (Ch. 9) it causes tachycardia, decreased gut motility and the closure of sphincters in the gut, pupil dilatation, bronchodilatation and piloerection.

Noradrenaline raises both systolic and diastolic blood pressure.

The difference between the effects of adrenaline and noradrenaline is partly explained by the presence of different receptors (α- and β-adrenoreceptors) on the surface of effector cells. Noradrenaline is most active at α-adrenoreceptors and adrenaline at β-adrenoreceptors.

The main effect of the catecholamines is on the cardiovascular system and the central nervous system, and on carbohydrate and lipid metabolism. Together, adrenaline and noradrenaline prepare the body for the 'fight or flight' response.

DISORDERS OF THE PITUITARY AND HYPOTHALAMUS

Disorders of the endocrine system result in either oversecretion or undersecretion of a hormone. Therefore, in principle, treatment should be straightforward, either replacing the missing hormone or removing, or suppressing the source of, the oversecretion, though in reality this is sadly not always the case. Advances have made the treatment of the wide range of endocrine disorders more successful, and the outlook for those affected is becoming ever more hopeful. However, patients with pituitary disease still have a greater mortality due to cardiovascular, cerebrovascular and respiratory causes than the general population and women have a worse outcome than men.

Hypersecretion of a hormone usually arises from a so-called 'functioning' pituitary adenoma. As this adenoma grows, it is likely to disrupt the normal function of other areas of the pituitary, and as a result progressive hypopituitarism occurs. This failure of the pituitary hormones occurs in a characteristic sequence (Boon et al 2006) – first GH is lost, followed by the gonadotrophins LH/ICSH and FSH, ACTH and then TSH. PRL deficiency is rare except as seen postpartum in Sheehan's syndrome.

Hypersecretion of anterior pituitary hormones

Cushing's disease caused by an excess of glucocorticoid hormones stimulated by an ACTH-producing adenoma of the pituitary is discussed in a later section (see p. 142).

Hypersecretion of growth hormone: acromegaly

Acromegaly is a rare condition caused by prolonged, excessive secretion of GH from a benign tumour of the pituitary gland occurring after fusion of the epiphyses of the long bones. It affects both sexes equally. The mean age at diagnosis is between 40 and 50 years, although excessive secretion of GH can occur at any age. In children where epiphyseal fusion has not yet occurred, it leads to gigantism. Acromegaly leads to a reduction in life expectancy with a two- to four-fold increase in mortality rate (Colao et al 2004).

PATHOPHYSIOLOGY

Clinical features The onset of acromegaly is insidious, leading on average to a delay in diagnosis of around 8 years from the onset of signs and symptoms, which include:

- excessive sweating, seen in >80% of patients
- headaches

- enlargement of the hands and feet
- tiredness and lethargy
- joint pain and osteoarthritis
- coarse facial features, frontal bossing, enlarged nose, protruding jaw and increased interdental separation
- oily skin
- deep voice
- tongue enlargement
- soft tissue swelling
- goitre and other organ enlargement
- features of hyperprolactinaemia (increased prolactin in the blood)
- visual field defects.

Complications include:

- hypertension
- insulin resistance, impaired glucose tolerance and diabetes mellitus
- obstructive sleep apnoea
- increased risk of colonic polyps and colorectal cancer
- ischaemic heart disease
- congestive cardiac failure
- cerebrovascular disease.

Common presenting signs/symptoms The patient may notice an increase in shoe size or that they have had to have a ring enlarged. Along with their family and friends they may notice a change in their facial appearance. Women often feel very self-conscious about this, and also about their deepening voice, as they may be mistaken for men on the telephone. The major events that prompt a consultation with their GP are usually headache and sweating. Visual symptoms may be identified by their optometrist (ophthalmic optician), or their dentist may notice changes to dentition. Therefore patients may be referred to an endocrinologist by a number of routes.

MEDICAL MANAGEMENT

Investigations

Diagnosis can be confirmed following clinical examination and pituitary function testing. On clinical examination, some or all of the symptoms listed above may be present. Magnetic resonance imaging (MRI) usually shows the pituitary tumour and whether there is enlargement of the pituitary fossa. If acromegaly is suspected, a blood sample should be obtained and an insulin-like growth factor 1 (IGF-1) and random GH level measured. If the IGF-1 level is 'normal', when compared to the age-adjusted range, and GH <0.5 mU/L, the diagnosis of acromegaly can be excluded (Trainer 2002). Otherwise, the patient should proceed to have an oral glucose tolerance test (OGTT). The OGTT has been the gold standard for the diagnosis of acromegaly for many years. False positives may occur if the patient has diabetes mellitus, renal or liver disease, or anorexia nervosa. In acromegaly, measurement of GH levels during the OGTT are consistently elevated and fail to suppress to <2 mU/L in response to a 75 g oral glucose load. Normally, the level of GH would be undetectable. Acromegaly is therefore diagnosed on the basis of an elevated IGF-1 and failure to suppress GH during the OGTT. Further pituitary function tests may be performed to assess whether the remainder of the pituitary gland has been compromised. Prolactin is co-secreted in 30% of tumours.

Treatment

In untreated acromegaly, the mortality is nearly twice that of the normal population; early treatment is therefore essential. The aim is to relieve and, if possible, resolve symptoms associated with elevated GH and IGF-1 levels and the local effects caused by the tumour mass itself, and to prevent co-morbidity by lowering mean GH and IGF-1 levels to accepted 'safe' levels with minimal disruption to the patient's lifestyle. Treatment may take the form of surgery, radiotherapy or medication. Until recently, surgery and radiotherapy were used in conjunction, with medical therapy then used to control residual excess GH secretion, as radiotherapy only lowers GH levels gradually. Today, medical therapy may also be used pre-operatively to control symptoms or to attempt to shrink a large tumour prior to surgery (Ben-Shlomo & Melmed, 2008). In patients unfit for surgery, medical therapy alone may be used.

Surgery is currently regarded as the first-line therapy for acromegaly and, when performed by a pituitary surgeon, remains the treatment of choice. Hypophysectomy via the trans-sphenoidal route, which has a low morbidity and mortality, is the surgical procedure most commonly used. It results in a rapid fall in GH levels, often with no loss of any other pituitary hormones. Surgery is both rapid and inexpensive when compared to medical therapies. In patients with microadenomas <1 cm diameter it is curative in ~80% of cases. With macroadenomas >1 cm diameter it is nearer 40% (Kaltsas et al 2001).

Radiotherapy Conventional external beam radiotherapy (25 fractions over 5 weeks delivered daily Monday–Friday) results in a delayed fall in GH and IGF-1 levels over the following decade which is paralleled by the development of hypopituitarism. After 5 years, 63% of patients have a normal IGF-1 (Jenkins et al 2006). Although used less often nowadays, it is safe, and radiation-induced visual damage is extremely rare. Patients may feel tired during the period of treatment and may experience some temporary hair loss at the site of entry of the beams. It is a useful treatment for patients in whom surgery is contraindicated or if GH/IGF-1 levels are not too high and/or there is a large tumour or residual tumour postoperatively, or where medical therapy fails to control GH/IGF-1 levels. Another form of radiotherapy is stereotactic radiotherapy, which may be single fraction radiosurgery or linear accelerator based stereotactic radiotherapy (multiple fraction). The expense is greater than conventional radiotherapy but is a 'one-off' cost. Long-term data are required, but early results suggest that GH and IGF-1 levels fall more rapidly after radiosurgery than with conventional radiotherapy and there is less damage to surrounding tissues, which may reduce the incidence of radiotherapy-induced hypopituitarism (Swords et al 2003). These two forms of radiotherapy can be given following conventional radiotherapy but cannot be used if the tumour is close to the optic chiasm.

Medication has changed radically in recent years. It is now possible to control GH and IGF-1 levels in more than half of patients with a somatostatin analogue, a synthetic compound which acts on the somatostatin (syn. growth hormone-release inhibiting hormone) receptors of the tumour and suppresses the secretion of GH, e.g. lanreotide or octreotide. These analogues are given by deep intramuscular or subcutaneous (s.c.) injection by a nurse every 7–14 or 28 days and are the most widely used form of medical therapy. If the patient is resistant to this class of medication, pegvisomant, a GH receptor antagonist, i.e. it binds to GH receptors, blocking the impact of excessive circulating GH which in turn causes IGF-1 levels to fall, can be used. It is given by a once daily s.c. injection. However, it is very expensive and is currently used only for patients with active disease who have failed to respond to other medical therapies.

 ## Nursing management and health promotion: acromegaly

Change in body image is an important feature of this disorder. The patient may have considerable difficulty in coming to terms with their changed appearance and may be anxious about the investigations they must undergo and the treatment that may be required. Their QoL may be affected.

It is important to create as relaxed an environment as possible and to reduce anxiety by spending time with the patient and their family, explaining the reasons for their changed appearance, the effect of therapy and the expected treatment outcome. They will be reassured to hear that biochemical cure may result in a return to a more normal appearance, although the degree will depend on the stage of the disease at the beginning of treatment. Some symptoms, such as sweating, may be cured almost immediately, while others, e.g. soft tissue swelling, may take longer to resolve. Bony changes are usually not reversible.

There are now specific validated QoL assessment tools for acromegaly. The ACROQoL is useful in assessing the impact of the disease on a patient's QoL (Badia et al 2004).

Some patients benefit from meeting other patients who have been treated successfully and, if the patient wishes, nursing staff should try to arrange this either directly or through a local patient support group (see Useful websites, e.g. The Pituitary Foundation).

Prolactin hypersecretion

Hyperprolactinaemia is a common abnormality (Boon et al 2006). However, a wide variety of medications and diseases can cause high prolactin levels. Before carrying out extensive investigations for pituitary disease, it is important to exclude causes such as hypothyroidism and to take a detailed medication history. Medications that block the dopamine receptor and so elevate prolactin levels include tranquillisers, e.g. chlorpromazine; antiemetics, e.g. metoclopramide; and some antidepressants, e.g. amitriptyline and fluoxetine. The other key differential diagnosis is a hypothalamic or suprasellar space-occupying lesion which interferes with dopamine production. Dopamine is the natural prolactin inhibitory factor and therefore, in its absence, hyperprolactinaemia ensues; due to the mechanism this is known as disconnection hyperprolactinaemia.

PATHOPHYSIOLOGY

Hyperprolactinaemia causes galactorrhoea (abnormal/inappropriate flow of milk) and amenorrhoea in women; raised prolactin level suppresses gonadotrophin-releasing hormone (GnRH) secretion within the hypothalamus, leading to gonadotrophin deficiency (LH and FSH) and then oestrogen deficiency, resulting in infertility. In men, galactorrhoea is much less frequent, but elevated prolactin lowers ICSH and FSH levels which in turn lowers testosterone levels, resulting in a reduced libido, erectile dysfunction and infertility. Prolactinomas are almost always benign.

Common presenting signs/symptoms in premenopausal women include menstrual disturbances, e.g. amenorrhoea, oligomenorrhoea (infrequent menstruation) and infertility. Galactorrhoea occurs in about 80% of these women (Schlechte 2003). The majority of prolactinomas in women are small (referred to as microprolactinomas) at the time of diagnosis, so headaches and neurological deficits are rare. Men, on the other hand, may present with headache, visual loss, cranial nerve defects and/or hypopituitarism due to the mass effect of the tumour which tends to be larger at the time of diagnosis (referred to as a macroprolactinoma). In both men and women elevated levels of prolactin over a long period can lead to low bone density which increases when prolactin levels are normalised but does not return to normal.

MEDICAL MANAGEMENT

Investigations

When other causes have been excluded, prolactin levels should be measured in the unstressed patient. Because venepuncture is stressful, an intravenous cannula is sited in the patient's arm and the patient allowed to rest for 30 min prior to the blood sample being taken. The patient should not smoke or drink tea or coffee in this period. If the prolactin levels are raised, an MRI scan is performed. If this shows a large pituitary tumour, tests of other pituitary functions should be done to detect any other pituitary hormone deficits. Visual field tests may also be needed to assess if the tumour mass is causing pressure on the optic chiasm. Pituitary MRI will usually show even a small tumour of only a few millimetres in size.

Treatment

The aim for microprolactinomas is to lower the excessive prolactin levels, thereby restoring gonadal function. In macroprolactinomas, the aim is tumour reduction, preventing tumour expansion and restoring gonadal function. Reduction of tumour size and lowering of hormone levels may be achieved by medication alone. Consequently, this is the treatment of choice and trans-sphenoidal surgery is usually performed only in patients who are resistant to or cannot tolerate dopamine agonists.

Prolactinomas respond well to dopamine agonists, e.g. bromocriptine, cabergoline or quinagolide, resulting in reduced prolactin levels (which return to normal in over 90% of cases) and significant reduction in tumour size (in over 75% of cases). This in turn results in the restoration of gonadal function and cessation of galactorrhoea, usually within a few weeks of starting treatment. In most women menstrual cycles resume and fertility is restored. Patients must therefore be given appropriate contraceptive advice. Dopamine agonists are usually stopped once a woman has become pregnant but this can result in tumour regrowth in some patients who may require surgical debulking of the tumour, restarting the dopamine agonist or delivery if the pregnancy is far enough advanced.

Irradiation of the pituitary gland results in a reduction in prolactin secretion, but this takes many years to achieve. Dopamine agonists are therefore continued while waiting for the effects of radiotherapy to occur, but the need for this treatment should be reassessed regularly.

Nursing management and health promotion: prolactin hypersecretion

Specific nursing care is aimed at ensuring that the medication regimen is followed correctly in order to avoid side-effects. Dopamine agonists, especially bromocriptine, often cause nausea, vomiting, constipation and postural hypotension mediated by dopamine release. Consequently, there should be a slow increase in dosage, the first doses being given whilst eating and on retiring to prevent the common symptoms of postural hypotension and gastric irritation. The dosage can then be gradually increased. Cabergoline, a longer acting dopamine agonist, need only be taken once or twice a week. It is more potent than bromocriptine and has a lower profile of side-effects (Webster 2000). (See Further reading, e.g. Besser & Thorner 2002, Liu & Couldwell 2004.)

Hyposecretion of anterior pituitary hormones

Hypopituitarism

Hypopituitarism is a partial or total deficiency of anterior pituitary hormone secretion. It may be associated with pathology that destroys the pituitary itself or with disturbance of hypothalamic control of the pituitary. Total failure of all hormone production is termed panhypopituitarism.

Hypopituitarism is most commonly caused by a pituitary tumour. These are frequently benign. Pituitary cancer is very rare. Benign microadenomas having no clinical effects are surprisingly common and are found in up to 23% of people at postmortem. Other common causes include head injury and (para-)sellar radiotherapy or surgery.

PATHOPHYSIOLOGY

Tumours can vary greatly in size and may extend outside the pituitary fossa to compress surrounding structures. They are generally classified as functioning or non-functioning, depending on whether they produce a hormone, e.g. GH.

Common presenting signs/symptoms Effects caused by local compression may arise (see Ch. 9), but people usually present with signs of pituitary hormone deficiency. Presentation may vary and depends on which hormones are deficient (Table 5.2).

Table 5.2 Signs and symptoms of anterior pituitary hormone hyposecretion

HORMONE DEFICIENCY	SIGNS AND SYMPTOMS
GH	*Children* Growth retardation, short stature *Adults* Lethargy Muscle weakness Increased fat mass
Gonadotrophins (LH/ICSH, FSH)	*Men* Reduced libido, erectile dysfunction Reduced need to shave Loss of axillary/pubic hair Later gynaecomastia (breast development) Infertility *Women* Oligomenorrhoea, amenorrhoea Infertility 'Hot flushes' Dyspareunia Breast atrophy Loss of axillary/pubic hair
ACTH	Weakness, tiredness Hypotension Dizziness on standing Hyponatraemia Pallor Hypoglycaemia
TSH	*Children* Growth retardation *Adults* Apathy Constipation Intolerance to cold Dry skin Weight gain

(Adapted from Boon et al 2006.)

MEDICAL MANAGEMENT

Investigations

Diagnostic investigations include visual field testing and biochemical investigation to determine the severity and degree of pituitary failure and to distinguish between isolated hormone failure and complete anterior pituitary failure. MRI is also performed.

Treatment

The choice of treatment will depend on the diagnosis of the cause of the pituitary failure and will aim to relieve the clinical effects and symptoms experienced by the patient. Treatment may involve surgery, radiotherapy to reduce the tumour and medication to replace the deficient hormones (see below).

Nursing management and health promotion: hypopituitarism

Effective nursing intervention depends upon the establishment of an effective therapeutic relationship in a friendly environment. As the effects of hypopituitarism can be widespread, causing diverse physical and psychological changes which can be difficult to comprehend, it is important to ensure that all of the patient's questions are answered in a way that is understood. Open and frank discussion about changes in body image and sexuality is essential to the individual concerned. Clear, ongoing explanations of the extensive and possibly uncomfortable investigations will help to relieve the patient's anxiety. The presence of a nurse known to the patient during these investigations can be reassuring.

Neurosurgery or radiotherapy is a frightening prospect for most people. Pre-operative preparation must include an explanation of procedures, the nature of immediate postoperative care and the expected long-term outcome. Reminding the patient that many of their symptoms will be relieved by surgery, radiotherapy and/or hormone replacement therapy will be of considerable psychological benefit.

Supporting the patient taking ongoing replacement therapy

Replacement of deficient hormones should alleviate many symptoms, allowing the patient to lead a near normal life. It is essential that the individual feels free to contact the appropriate doctor or specialist nurse at any time to discuss their condition or any related anxieties. As pituitary disease is a lifelong condition that will require ongoing monitoring, hospital attendance will continue on at least an annual basis for many years, giving the doctor or nurse the opportunity to build therapeutic relationships with their patients. Encouraging concordance by educating the patient as to the importance of correctly taking their replacement medication is vital (Box 5.2).

Box 5.2 Reflection

Hormone replacement therapy for hypopituitarism

Clare has hypopituitarism caused by a benign tumour. You and your mentor are admitting Clare when she asks about hypopituitarism and the different drugs used to replace the deficient hormones.

Activities

- Access the resources below and find out:
  - about the medications used to replace the anterior pituitary hormones
  - information about the pituitary gland/disorders written for patients.
- Discuss with your mentor how you might use the website material to help Clare understand her condition and its management.
- Reflect on how the need to take medication to replace several hormones may affect Clare's quality of life.

Resources

The Pituitary Foundation – Hormone Replacement Therapy (Updated 2006) http://www.pituitary.org.uk/content/view/61/72

(*Medical information*)

The Pituitary Foundation – The Pituitary Gland Its Disorders & Hormones Explained (Updated 2009) http://www.pituitary.org.uk/content/view/74/

(*Patient information*)

Anterior pituitary hormone replacement

Cortisol Hydrocortisone in tablet form is given for ACTH deficiency. It directly replaces the missing hormone and is rapidly absorbed with a short half-life (<2 hours). It is usually taken on waking, at midday and in the early evening. Alternative preparations include cortisone acetate, which is metabolised to cortisol, and synthetic preparations, e.g. prednisolone and dexamethasone. It is important to monitor cortisol levels regularly, as over-replacement can be associated with hypertension, hyperglycaemia and hyperinsulinaemia, as well as reduced bone mineral density (BMD). The omission of even one dose may have serious consequences. Patients should be advised to carry a blue 'steroid' card and to wear a MedicAlert® bracelet at all times, indicating they are cortisol deficient. Patients should also be given an emergency hydrocortisone pack to keep at home containing a vial of hydrocortisone for i.m. injection which they have been shown how to use. The nurse should demonstrate how to use this and ensure that the patient has practised and is competent.

See website Critical thinking question 5.1

Thyroxine Levothyroxine (thyroxine sodium) is given in tablet form, usually one dose in the morning. In the older people or in patients with known heart disease doses should be reduced. Levothyroxine replacement should not be started until ACTH deficiency has been excluded or treated as otherwise there is a risk of worsening the cortisol deficiency. As levothyroxine has a very long half-life, the occasional missed dose is not critical. Thyroxine levels can be monitored by the patient's GP who should perform thyroid function tests regularly. Excessive doses of levothyroxine over a long period should be avoided as there is an increased risk of osteoporotic fractures and atrial fibrillation.

Growth hormone Until 1989 the sole indication for GH therapy was in children with GH deficiency and it was claimed that low levels of GH had little or no effect in adults. Studies have shown that replacement GH therapy in patients with adult onset GH deficiency has profound effects on patients' QoL, vascular morbidity and cardiovascular mortality (Brooke & Monson 2003). It is now apparent that GH replacement is associated with favourable changes in body composition, bone density, lipid metabolism, physical performance and cardiovascular function (Mukherjee & Shalet 2004). The National Institute for Health and Clinical Excellence (NICE) (2003) produced guidance for the prescription of GH in England and Wales which was subsequently ratified for use in Scotland. Eligibility for GH replacement is dependent on patients fulfilling several criteria, which include biochemical evidence of GH deficiency, and demonstrating a reduced QoL, judged by their responses to a disease-specific questionnaire, the Adult Growth Hormone Deficiency Assessment – Quality of Life (AGHDA–QoL). Continuation of therapy is dependent on demonstrating that symptomatic benefit, based on improvement in questionnaire score, has been achieved (NICE 2003). GH is replaced by a daily s.c. injection which patients are taught to self-administer using a special pen device. Needle-free delivery devices are available. The normal starting dose is 0.3–0.5 mg daily titrated over a 3-month period. During this time IGF-1 levels are checked every 6 weeks with the aim of keeping the levels within the age-matched reference range. The dosing schedule is adjusted to maximise benefits and minimise side-effects, which can include transient oedema, arthralgia and headaches. Older patients, women and those with a higher body mass index (BMI) can be more prone to side-effects. Patients on GH replacement should be reassessed annually for blood lipids and glucose, body composition (waist circumference, lean body mass and BMD), exercise endurance and well-being using the AGHDA–QoL questionnaire. (See Further reading, e.g. Piersanti 2004.)

Gonadotrophins Testosterone replacement therapy has been available for many years – various forms developing from s.c. implants in the 1940s, i.m. injections, oral tablets to transdermal patches and gels in the 1990s (Schubert et al 2004). Replacement can result in an improvement in sexual function, an increase in BMD and improvements in body composition, e.g. increased lean body mass/decreased fat mass in hypogonadal men. In addition, positive changes are seen in erythropoiesis, prostate size and lipid profiles. Testosterone replacement is usually commenced when the diagnosis of hypogonadism is established and serum testosterone levels fall below a normal age-matched reference range.

Many testosterone preparations with differing routes of administration are available. Replacement depends on the formulation and there are advantages and disadvantages to each. Most preparations have unfavourable pharmacokinetics which result either in sub- or supra-physiological and/ or fluctuating levels of testosterone. Testosterone replacement can be by i.m. injection, implants every 3–6 months, transdermal patches including scrotal patches, transdermal gel, oral tablets or buccal tablets. Testosterone levels are monitored either immediately prior to an injection/implant or 8 h after the application of a patch.

Intramuscular injections have, for many years, been the most widely used and accepted form of testosterone replacement in the UK but these can be uncomfortable, are disruptive as the patient must make an appointment to see their GP or practice nurse every 3–4 weeks and can cause fluctuations in mood, energy levels and sexual function due to the changing levels of testosterone, which are high immediately post-injection but then fall off over the next 2–3 weeks. Transdermal patches (scrotal or non-scrotal) and transdermal gels mimic the normal physiological and diurnal variations of testosterone resulting in more stable levels of testosterone (Swerdloff et al 2000). Both the patch and the gel are self-applied, making them a popular choice, but both frequently cause skin irritation often causing discontinuation. Other options include testosterone implants. Pellet insertion requires minor surgery every 3–6 months and may be complicated by local infection, extrusion and scarring. Oral replacement requires frequent dosing (2–4 times/day) and often does not achieve normal levels of testosterone due to variable absorption.

Ultimately, the choice of testosterone replacement therapy should be made by the patient once they have the information required to make an informed decision. Younger patients are more likely to choose a long-acting preparation whereas men over the age of 50 should be advised to opt for a short-acting one. This is to ensure that if the preparation has to be stopped due to a contraindication to testosterone replacement therapy, e.g. prostate cancer, levels of serum testosterone will immediately fall.

Whatever the replacement therapy chosen, testosterone levels should always be closely monitored to ensure they remain within physiological parameters.While suboptimal dosing can negatively affect a patient's QoL and sexual function, supra-physiological dosing can promote secondary polycythaemia and progression of prostate cancer (see Chs 8, 11). Patients on testosterone replacement should therefore always have their haemoglobin and prostate specific antigen (PSA) levels monitored regularly as well as an annual rectal examination of their prostate gland.

Disorder of posterior pituitary/ hypothalamus: abnormal antidiuretic hormone (ADH) secretion

Diabetes insipidus

Diabetes insipidus (DI) is defined as the passing of large amounts (>3 L/24 h) of dilute urine (osmolality <300 mOsmol/kg) and exists in two main forms:

- cranial DI – reduced hypothalamic secretion of ADH
- nephrogenic DI – resistance of the renal tubules to ADH.

Causes of both types may be familial or acquired and include pituitary tumours, meningitis, encephalitis, tuberculosis, sarcoidosis, head injury, neurosurgery, Sheehan's syndrome, sickle cell disease, chronic renal disease, hyper/ hypocalcaemia, hyperglycaemia and some medications (lithium). Primary polydipsia may be psychological.

PATHOPHYSIOLOGY

Clinical features Deficiency of ADH leads to polyuria, nocturia and a compensatory polydipsia. Urine output may reach 10–15 L or more per day, leading to severe dehydration if the individual's fluid intake is restricted in any way.

MEDICAL MANAGEMENT

Investigations

Diagnosis is often made by single paired urine and plasma osmolality, obviating the need for the more stressful and prolonged water deprivation test. Plasma osmolality will show high concentration and urine will be dilute. However, sometimes the results are equivocal and a water deprivation test is required to make the diagnosis.

Treatment

Administration of desmopressin (DDAVP), a synthetic vasopressin (see below).

 Nursing management and health promotion: diabetes insipidus

During diagnosis and any further investigations, the nurse's interventions will include accurate recording of fluid balance with the full cooperation and participation of the patient. It is essential for the patient to have easy access to toilet facilities. Samples of urine will be required for osmolality assessment.

The nurse will also be involved in medication administration and education of the patient with regard to self-administration of their DDAVP, continued measurement of fluid balance and regular weight recording. Most patients rapidly become aware if their DDAVP is no longer effective and will contact their GP or the doctor or specialist nurse.

Posterior pituitary hormone replacement desmopressin (DDAVP) is available orally, sublingually, intranasally and parenterally and should be started as a low dose and gradually increased until urine output is controlled. Doses can vary enormously between individual patients. Blood sodium levels should be checked after starting or altering treatment to detect hyponatraemia.

DISORDERS OF THE THYROID

Simple goitre

A goitre is an enlargement of the thyroid gland. It can occur without over- or underactivity of the gland. The term 'simple goitre' is a paradox as its cause is poorly understood. In young adults the gland is soft and diffuse, enlarged two to three times its normal size. Thyroid hormones and TSH levels are normal and there is no evidence of autoimmunity. If the stimulus to goitre formation remains, whatever it is, the gland becomes further enlarged and nodular over the ensuing 20 years or so (euthyroid [normal thyroid function] multinodular goitre) and people 60 years of age or beyond may develop hyperthyroidism (toxic multinodular goitre).

Hypersecretion of thyroid hormones

Hyperthyroidism or overactive thyroid (previously known as thyrotoxicosis), is characterised by high levels of circulating thyroid hormones. The most common cause of hyperthyroidism is intrinsic thyroid disease; pituitary-driven hyperthyroidism is extremely rare. Hyperthyroidism mainly affects women aged between 30 and 50 years, but can occur at any age in either gender.

Graves' disease

Graves' disease is the most common form of hyperthyroidism. It is an autoimmune disorder in which anti-TSH receptor autoantibodies behave like TSH, stimulating thyroid hormone production and in some cases thyroid enlargement or goitre. Graves' disease tends to run in families and may be associated with eye features (Box 5.3). The ophthalmopathy of Graves' disease, which affects the majority of patients to some extent, is also autoimmune in aetiology. There are changes in the retro-orbital space, with water accumulation and enlargement of the extraocular muscles and increased fat. The increased pressure behind the eye pushes the eye forward (exophthalmos) and the swollen muscles work inefficiently, causing double vision (diplopia). Vision may be threatened. Swelling of the eyelids is due to prolapse of retrobulbar fat and poor lymphatic and venous drainage. Lid

> **Box 5.3 Reflection**
>
> ### Thyroid eye disease (TED)
>
> Thyroid eye disease can impact significantly on a patient's quality of life.
>
> #### Activities
>
> - Access the resources below and find out about the effects of TED.
> - Reflect on how it might feel to have TED.
> - What support would you want to offer a patient with TED?
>
> #### Resources
>
> Beigi B, Greenwood R 2003 The management of Thyroid Eye Disease. Focus Occasional Update from The Royal College of Ophthalmologists, Issue 26 Summer 2003. Available online http://www.rcophth.ac.uk/docs/members/focus-collegenews/FocusSummer03.pdf
>
> British Thyroid Association – Thyroid Eye Disease Patient Information http://www.british-thyroid-association.org/info-for-patients/Docs/ptinfo-TED.pdf
>
> Patient UK Thyroid eye disease http://www.patient.co.uk/doctor/Thyroid-Eye-Disease.htm
>
> Thyroid Eye Disease Charitable Trust (TEDct) http://www.tedct.co.uk/

retraction and lid lag is a feature. In mild cases artificial tear drops can help combat the symptoms of dry and gritty eyes. Attaching prisms to glasses can help with double vision. In more severe cases, corticosteroids or radiotherapy are used to reduce swelling. Patients may also undergo surgery to reduce the pressure behind the eyes, or to remove excess tissue.

Toxic multinodular goitre

As mentioned above, this is often the outcome of the simple diffuse goitre in the young adult. It is the second most common cause of hyperthyroidism after Graves' disease. Older people with hyperthyroidism may present with cardiovascular effects, e.g. atrial fibrillation, predominating.

Toxic adenoma (solitary nodule)

Toxic adenoma causes about 5% of hyperthyroidism. In these patients, the thyroid nodule acts autonomously and produces excess levels of thyroid hormone, leading to suppression of the normal thyroid gland.

Other causes of hyperthyroidism

These include:

- Thyroiditis (infection or inflammation of the thyroid gland). Occurring after a viral infection, postpartum (usually in the first 6 months after childbirth) or may be autoimmune.
- Overtreatment of hypothyroidism with levothyroxine.

PATHOPHYSIOLOGY

In hyperthyroidism, high levels of circulating thyroid hormones stimulate cell metabolism, resulting in a high metabolic rate. TSH secretion is suppressed. There is tachycardia and, in older patients, atrial fibrillation and cardiac failure. Patients complain of general fatigue, although for short spells they may become more active, and find that they are restless.

Common presenting symptoms There is increased irritability, with mood swings or aggressive behaviour and inability to relax and sleep, heat intolerance with hot moist skin and excessive sweating, palpitations and tachycardia, and sometimes a feeling of shakiness and a fine tremor of the hands. By far the most common symptom, however, is weight loss, despite an increased appetite. Patients often complain of excessive watering and grittiness of the eyes. There may also be diarrhoea, thirst, oligomenorrhoea/amenorrhoea and pruritus. Enlargement of the gland may have been noticed.

MEDICAL AND NURSING MANAGEMENT

Investigations

Clinical examination will confirm tachycardia and atrial fibrillation, goitre and eye signs. Diagnosis is usually confirmed by elevated serum T_4 and suppressed TSH.

Treatment

Treatment approaches for hyperthyroidism are:

- antithyroid drugs (ATDs)
- surgery
- radioactive iodine therapy.

Medication is usually the first line of treatment. Carbimazole or propylthiouracil is used in one of two ways. The first, known as 'block and replace', occurs when drugs are used to completely inhibit the synthesis of thyroid hormones. Levothyroxine is then added to this regimen as a 'replacement' dose to achieve a euthyroid state. Treatment usually continues for 6 months. Fewer blood tests are required, thyroid function tests are more stable and there is less likelihood of the thyroid gland becoming overactive again once the drugs are stopped or reduced.

The second regimen, known as 'dose titration', occurs when the patient is commenced on drugs until a euthyroid state is achieved. The dose is titrated so that the amount of hormone being produced by the overactive thyroid gland is reduced to normal. Thyroid function tests (serum T_4 and TSH) are performed every 4–8 weeks and the drug dose is adjusted to ensure that the patient remains euthyroid and to avoid over- or under-medication. Treatment usually continues for some 18 months, with regular outpatient visits. Side-effects (see below) are less common because of the lower drug doses and concordance increased as patients only have to remember to take one drug.

ATDs are usually well tolerated. Occasionally patients may complain of gastrointestinal symptoms or an altered sense of taste or smell. The most common adverse reaction is an urticarial rash which occurs in about 2% of patients. Other side-effects include fever and arthralgias, usually within the first few months of starting therapy, and are more common in patients treated with higher doses. Patients are asked to report unexplained fever or sore throat as the major side-effect of ATDs, which is rare, is agranulocytosis, which

occurs in approximately 1 in 300–500 patients (see Ch. 11). Should fever or sore throat occur, they are forewarned to stop taking their medication immediately and to seek medical advice.

Symptomatic control of tachycardia is obtained by administration of beta-blockers, such as propranolol, given until thyroid hormone levels are normal.

Surgical intervention Indications for surgery include:

- suspicious or malignant thyroid nodule
- pregnant women not adequately controlled on drugs or who develop serious allergic reactions
- patients who refuse radio-iodine
- poor patient concordance
- patients who are not well controlled by antithyroid drugs
- patients with severe Graves' ophthalmopathy or relapsed Graves' disease.

Partial thyroidectomy is performed only after ATDs have produced a euthyroid state. In some centres, the patient is given potassium iodide for 1–2 weeks before surgery, which will inhibit thyroid hormone release, reduce the size and vascularity of the gland and reduce the risk of peri- and postoperative haemorrhage. Approximately 80% of patients are cured by surgery, with the best surgical centres achieving <4% recurrence. Partial thyroidectomy is also a useful treatment for patients with large/unsightly goitres.

Specific complications of surgery include:

- compromise of airway
- postoperative haemorrhage
- recurrent laryngeal nerve palsy
- thyroid crisis
- tetany due to damage/removal of parathyroid glands
- hypothyroidism (affecting 10–20% of patients within 10 years).

A Critical thinking question on the website provides an opportunity for you to consider the early postoperative complications following partial thyroidectomy.

See website Critial thinking question 5.2

Radioactive iodine therapy Iodine-131 (^{131}I) destroys functioning cells or inhibits cell replication. It is usually administered orally as a single capsule taken with water or as a drink on an outpatient basis. Patients are advised to avoid eating for 3–4 h after administration to allow adequate absorption of the iodine; they are also advised to drink at least 2 L of fluid over the next 24 h and to pass urine frequently in order to excrete free circulating radioactive iodine as rapidly as possible. Transient side-effects include nausea, anterior neck pain and increased thyroid hormone levels which can exacerbate heart failure.

Patients present a radiation hazard for approximately 1 week following this treatment and should have no close contact (<1 metre) with children under the age of 11 during this time (see p. 138). This type of therapy is used to treat multinodular goitres and relapsed Graves' disease or when surgery is not appropriate, but is not usually offered to women of child-bearing age or patients with Graves' ophthalmopathy as it can exacerbate symptoms, especially in patients who smoke.

Cancer of the thyroid gland

Thyroid cancer is rare in the UK, comprising less than 1% of all cancers (Cancer Research UK 2009). It is three times more common in women than men; of the 1933 cases diagnosed in 2006, 1421 were women (Cancer Research UK 2009).

The five main types of thyroid cancer are:

- papillary (most common type, accounts for ~80% of all thyroid cancers)
- follicular (less common, usually found in older people)
- anaplastic (rare, more common in older people)
- lymphoma (usually non-Hodgkin lymphoma)
- medullary cell (rare, may run in families).

Papillary and follicular thyroid cancers are differentiated cancers (i.e. the cancer cells retain histological features typical of normal thyroid cells).

PATHOPHYSIOLOGY

Papillary or follicular cancers usually present with a lump which can cause hoarseness or difficulty in swallowing. At night, patients can notice difficulty breathing. Metastatic spread from follicular cancer commonly involves the brain, liver, lungs and bones.

Common presenting symptoms Often the patient will have noticed a painless small nodule or swelling in the neck. Patients may be euthyroid or may have symptoms of either hyper- or hypothyroidism.

MEDICAL MANAGEMENT

Investigations

T_3, T_4 and TSH levels are measured and an ultrasound scan of the neck is undertaken. Fine-needle biopsy or aspiration is necessary to distinguish cancer from benign pathologies, to give a firm diagnosis and to differentiate between the types of thyroid cancer. Radioactive isotope scanning, using technetium or iodine, is a painless procedure which involves injecting the radioactive isotopes intravenously and then, after 20 min rest, scanning the thyroid gland with a gamma camera. As cancer cells do not absorb the radioactive liquid as well as normal thyroid cells, any cancer cells will generally appear as 'cold areas' or 'cold nodules' on scanning. However, only 10% of such cold nodules are malignant. Many turn out to be cysts, and surgery may be avoided if aspiration cytology is normal.

Patients with papillary and follicular cancers will be commenced on levothyroxine which decreases the rate of growth of the cancer.

Staging (see Ch. 31)

Staging is the process by which a cancer is described in terms of tumour size (T), spread to lymph nodes (N) and metastatic spread (M).

The basic TNM stages for thyroid cancer are:

- tumour size – T1, T2, T3, T4a and T4b
- nodal spread – either N0 (no spread), or nodal spread N1a, N1b
- metastatic spread – either M0 (no spread), or metastatic spread M1.

Some types of thyroid cancer are staged using number stages. The number of stages used, 2 or 4, depends upon the cancer type and whether the patient is under or over 45 years of age.

Staging information is required by the clinician in order to select the most appropriate treatment. (See Cancer Research UK 2009 Macmillan Cancer Support 2009.)

Treatment

Surgery, radioactive iodine (^{131}I) or radiotherapy may be given alone or in combination. The treatment chosen will depend on several factors including the patient's age, general health, and the type and stage of the tumour. The treatment of choice is near-total thyroidectomy. This is usually followed by a large dose of ^{131}I to ablate any thyroid remnant. Any tissue showing radio-iodine uptake subsequently must be assumed to be recurrent disease, and further ^{131}I may be taken up therapeutically by the tumour tissue. Follow-up is important and will usually be carried out at 6-monthly intervals initially. At follow-up the tumour marker, serum thyroglobulin (Tg), is measured. It should not be detectable in a patient who has had a total thyroidectomy, ^{131}I ablation of remnant and is taking levothyroxine in a dose sufficient to suppress serum TSH. If detectable, further surgery or ^{131}I therapy may be required.

 # Nursing management and health promotion: the patient receiving ^{131}I therapy

Before ^{131}I ablative therapy the patient will have discontinued thyroid hormones for 4–6 weeks to allow TSH to rise, which ensures better uptake of ^{131}I. In those in whom a period of hypothyroidism is best avoided, e.g. an older patient with coronary heart disease, high TSH levels in the blood can be achieved by giving thyrotropin alfa (recombinant human rhTSH). Thyrotropin alfa is given as two i.m. injections 24 h apart, prior to commencement of ^{131}I, and negates the need to discontinue thyroid hormone replacement.

The patient and family should be given clear explanations regarding the effect of ^{131}I, the reasons for the patient being nursed alone with restricted access for staff and visitors, and procedures to be followed in the handling of body fluids. It should be explained to the patient that they cannot be discharged until their radiation level is safe.

Measures should be taken to prevent constipation, as this inhibits the subsequent excretion of radioactive material. A high fluid intake should be encouraged to promote a good urinary output. Commodes and bedpans should be designated for the patient's exclusive use. All body fluids will be highly radioactive following ^{131}I administration and the patient should be encouraged to bathe or shower regularly to remove contaminated perspiration.

The patient should be nursed in a single room containing a minimum of equipment. Dosimeters should be worn at all times by staff members to indicate radiation exposure. Duties should be coordinated so that each staff member spends a minimum amount of time with the patient.

As with all endocrine disease, prompt treatment should result in complete alleviation of all signs and symptoms; the patient should be reassured of this whilst undergoing treatment. Follow-up after treatment is essential. Nursing staff should encourage the patient to attend outpatient or GP clinics as advised. The patient should be reassured that, particularly with localised disease from a papillary cancer, the probability of 'cure' is extremely high. (See Further reading, e.g. Schafer 2005.)

Hyposecretion of thyroid hormones

Underactivity of the thyroid gland may be primary (70%), resulting from disease of the thyroid, or secondary, due to pituitary failure.

Aetiology and epidemiology

Primary hypothyroidism resulting from autoimmune disease is the commonest cause of thyroid underactivity. It may be associated with other autoimmune disease. It is six times more common in women than in men and the mean age of diagnosis for women is 57.

Hypothyroidism (also known as myxoedema) may also be iatrogenic, i.e. caused by previous treatment for hyperthyroidism by surgery or radioactive iodine.

Iodine deficiency, a major public health issue across the world, is another cause of hypothyroidism and is due to insufficient dietary iodine (see Further reading, e.g. de Benoist et al 2004). This leads to reduced thyroid hormone production. Goitre is a common feature of this condition. The most devastating effects of iodine deficiency are increased perinatal mortality and impaired mental development. Iodine deficiency is the biggest cause of preventable brain damage in childhood. Endemic hypothyroidism is occasionally seen in areas where iodine levels in the water supply are low, usually inland areas far from the sea or in mountainous regions. It is still seen in some areas of the world, such as parts of central Africa, central Asia and central and eastern Europe as well as in the Andes and the Himalayas (Delange & Dunn 2005). It has also reappeared in developed countries like New Zealand where the population has heeded public health advice about the dangers of too much salt in the diet and reduced their intake (Mann & Aitken 2003).

Some medications may also induce hypothyroidism, for example lithium carbonate (used in bipolar disorders) and amiodarone (an anti-arrhythmic agent) (Boon et al 2006).

Congenital hypothyroidism occurs in approximately 1 in 2500–3000 live births, resulting in approximately 200 new cases per year, and usually results from congenital absence of the thyroid gland; it can also be caused by certain enzyme defects. If congenital hypothyroidism is not detected and treated early the infant/child will not develop fully either mentally or physically and this can lead to reduced intellectual ability and impaired work capacity. Routine neonatal screening is performed in most developed countries at 5–7 days and is a good example of how endocrinology has significantly contributed to improving the public health of the nation.

PATHOPHYSIOLOGY

In primary hypothyroidism, insufficient T_4 is produced by the thyroid gland. Serum T_4 is low and levels of TSH are high. The onset is slow and insidious. Because the affected individual is often an older person, it may be accepted as a normal part of ageing and it may be some time before a medical opinion is sought. The patient may report sensitivity to cold, weight gain, a general slowing down of body functions, lethargy, depression and an inability to 'think quickly'. The face will be puffy in appearance and hair sparse, coarse and brittle. In severe hypothyroidism, the patient may be admitted in a coma and perhaps be thought to be suffering from hypothermia. This represents a medical emergency in which intensive treatment and care are essential. Diagnosis of hypothyroidism is confirmed by low plasma levels of T_4 and raised TSH levels.

MEDICAL MANAGEMENT

Treatment

Hypothyroidism is treated with replacement doses of levothyroxine commencing with a low dose of 50 µg (25 µg if there is a history of heart disease/angina) and increasing by increments every 3–4 weeks until serum TSH is normal. There are currently 1 800 000 adults taking thyroxine replacement in the UK (Leese et al 2008). Levothyroxine has a stable 24-hour profile and is easy to monitor. A typical adult dose would be 100–200 µg daily. There is an increased requirement during pregnancy. Care should be taken not to over-replace thyroxine as this can result in an increased risk of osteoporosis and/or atrial fibrillation.

Levothyroxine is only partly absorbed after ingestion and foodstuffs (especially those rich in calcium or iron), other minerals, other drugs and tablet composition can all influence its absorption. Conditions such as coeliac disease and nephrotic syndrome will also affect the dose required. Tablets should be taken in the morning on an empty stomach and as a single daily dose. Symptomatic relief should become apparent 2–4 weeks after starting replacement therapy with improvements to puffy eyes and a reduction in weight often noticed in this time. However, it will take some 6–8 weeks for a steady state of thyroid hormones to be achieved.

▷ **Nursing management and health promotion: hypothyroidism**

The nurse should advise the patient and their family that there will only be a gradual improvement in symptoms until the steady state is reached. Until then, it is important to remind the patient and their family that symptoms of lethargy and mental slowness are part of the disease process. Improvement to hair and skin texture can take 3–6 months. In an attempt to reduce constipation patients should be advised to eat a high-fibre diet. It is usual to treat patients in the community with a 6-monthly or annual hospital review, often at a specific nurse-led thyroid clinic. Community nursing teams should follow up medical treatment and explanations and ensure that patients understand the reasons for T_4 replacement therapy and the importance of attending for regular check-ups and blood tests to ensure that a euthyroid state is achieved and maintained. The patient should be advised that they will need to take T_4 replacement therapy for life.

Patients requiring lifelong replacement therapy are entitled to free prescriptions, including all other prescribed medication as well as T_4. At the time of writing all prescriptions are free in Wales, and both Northern Ireland and Scotland are reducing prescription charges ready to abolish them in 2010 and 2011 respectively. Exemption certificates are obtained in England by completing form FP92A (currently ES92A in Scotland,) obtained from GPs or pharmacists.

Patients often forget to take long-term medications routinely and poor concordance with thyroid replacement is not uncommon. Patients can feel despondent if the T_4 does not make them feel as they did before the onset of their disease and consequently not adhere to their treatment. As the half-life of T_4 is 6–7 days patients may not notice any changes if they miss the odd tablet and consequently bad habits can develop.

Condition-specific questionnaires have been designed and validated for use with patients with hypothyroidism: the Underactive Thyroid-Dependent Quality of Life Questionnaire (ThyDQoL) and the Underactive Thyroid Treatment Satisfaction Questionnaire (ThyTSQ) (McMillan et al 2006). The ThyDQoL has 18 domains covering QoL measures such as energy levels, physical capabilities, motivation, physical appearance and weight together with other aspects of life affected by hypothyroidism (McMillan et al 2004). It is an individualised measure of the perceived impact of hypothyroidism on the patient's QoL and is a useful tool to use when assessing a new patient or evaluating the benefits of treatment.

DISORDERS OF THE PARATHYROIDS

This section outlines hypersecretion and hyposecretion of parathyroid hormone.

Hypersecretion of the parathyroids

Hypercalcaemia

In most instances, raised plasma calcium levels are caused by primary hyperparathyroidism or are secondary to malignancy. Other causes include myeloma, vitamin D poisoning, tuberculosis and thiazide diuretics. Mild hypercalcaemia, which is often asymptomatic, occurs in about 1 in 1000 of the population (Kumar & Clark 2009).

PATHOPHYSIOLOGY

Hypercalcaemia impairs renal function by reducing the glomerular filtration rate and by causing nephrogenic diabetes insipidus leading to an inability to conserve water. The resulting dehydration augments sodium reabsorption, leading to enhanced calcium reabsorption and impairing the kidney's ability to excrete the unwanted calcium.

Even mild symptoms can lead to an early diagnosis, due to advanced chemical analysis techniques; this means that it is now extremely rare to see the severe renal and skeletal problems associated with hypercalcaemia that occurred in the past.

Common presenting symptoms Patients may present with symptoms of malignancy or of hypercalcaemia including:

- vague malaise (very easily missed)
- weakness
- depression
- drowsiness, coma
- nausea, vomiting
- anorexia
- constipation
- nocturia
- polydipsia, polyuria
- psychosis.

MEDICAL MANAGEMENT

Investigations

Diagnosis is based on medical history, clinical examination and tests to ascertain the cause though initial treatment is often started before all tests are completed.

Treatment

Hypercalcaemia caused by malignancy is usually seen only in patients with advanced cancer when bony metastases have occurred and signifies a poor prognosis. If possible, it should be treated, as this may improve the patient's QoL. Adequate hydration is of great importance and, in itself, is often enough to relieve the symptoms of the hypercalcaemia. Patients should be rehydrated with up to 3 litres of 0.9% sodium chloride/day. However, it is now established that bisphosphonates, e.g. disodium pamidronate, are highly effective in lowering malignant hypercalcaemia. These are administered by an intravenous infusion, but oral preparations, e.g. sodium clodronate or ibandronic acid, can be used in the long term to prevent a recurrence of hypercalcaemia. Other treatments include oral phosphate and corticosteroid therapy.

Primary hyperparathyroidism

This condition is caused by the overproduction of PTH, such as by a parathyroid adenoma. It affects more women than men and its incidence increases with age.

MEDICAL MANAGEMENT

Treatment

Surgery is indicated for the management of hypercalcaemia due to excessive PTH secretion, as no long-term medication is available. However, asymptomatic hypercalcaemia requires no surgical intervention and can be treated conservatively with simple monitoring of calcium levels on an intermittent basis by the patient's GP or the hospital outpatient department.

Following parathyroidectomy, hypocalcaemia of either a transient or permanent nature may ensue. This should be treated promptly to prevent tetany. If severe hypocalcaemia occurs, i.v. calcium gluconate (10 mL of 10%) should be given immediately. Vitamin D and oral calcium supplements will be required. Calcium levels should be monitored closely until they have stabilised.

▷ Nursing management and health promotion: primary hyperparathyroidism

The investigations for diagnosis of hypercalcaemia may require hospital admission, particularly if the hypercalcaemia is severe and/or is thought to be secondary to malignancy. The patient will probably have been unwell for some time and will be feeling very tired and weak on admission.

Careful explanations of the investigations and treatment are required. These will include a 24-h urine collection for calcium. As it is particularly important for the accuracy of this test that the urine collection is completed properly, it is essential that this is explained clearly and is fully understood by the patient. If surgery is undertaken, the perioperative care is the same as for thyroidectomy (see p. 137). In addition, regular assessment for latent tetany due to hypocalcaemia is undertaken – Chvostek's and Trousseau's signs (Box 5.4).

Secondary and tertiary hyperparathyroidism

Secondary hyperparathyroidism occurs due to disease processes that cause hypocalcaemia, e.g. in vitamin D deficiency or in renal disease. The parathyroid glands strive to keep the calcium levels up, while calcium remains normal or is low. Rarely, this can lead to autonomous secretion of parathyroid hormone, leading to permanent hypercalcaemia, termed tertiary hyperparathyroidism. This is often seen in patients with renal failure.

Hyposecretion of the parathyroids

Hypocalcaemia

The most common cause of hypocalcaemia is artefactual due to low albumin levels, i.e. the calcium is normal when the low albumin is corrected for by the laboratory. Other relatively common causes include hypomagnesaemia, renal failure and vitamin D deficiency (Box 5.1, p. 129). Autoimmune hypoparathyroidism is rare, but iatrogenic hypoparathyroidism following neck surgery is more common, usually presenting within 24–48 hours of surgery.

Treatment

If hypocalcaemia is mild and the patient asymptomatic, oral calcium replacement should be given. Severe or symptomatic hypocalcaemia should be treated with i.v. calcium gluconate and vitamin D added if the patient requires i.v. calcium for more than two days.

Rickets and osteomalacia

These are diseases of calcium and phosphorus metabolism resulting from a deficiency in vitamin D intake and synthesis. As these conditions are usually seen and treated by endocrinologists, as opposed to other physicians, they are considered here.

Vitamin D deficiency during growth produces abnormalities in the growing skeleton known as rickets. In childhood, rickets produces soft, painful bones. The weight-bearing bones bend and may give rise to gross deformities. In the adult, where bone growth is completed, osteomalacia is the result; symptoms are generally diffuse bone pain and myopathy.

Rickets is not now commonly seen in the UK, due to better nutrition and, possibly, to a reduction in industrial pollution which allows more sunlight through. It is, however, sometimes seen in the communities who tend to cover up and avoid exposing themselves to sunlight, particularly those individuals with an increased vitamin D requirement, e.g. babies, children and pregnant women.

Treatment is by vitamin D replacement, and prevention is the aim, particularly targeted to known vulnerable groups.

DISORDERS OF THE ADRENALS

This section outlines hypersecretion of the adrenal medulla and cortex, cortical hyposecretion and congenital adrenal hyperplasia.

Hypersecretion of the adrenals

Adrenal medulla – phaeochromocytoma

Phaeochromocytoma is a very rare condition which causes about 1 in 1000 cases of secondary hypertension (Kumar & Clark 2009). A tumour of the adrenal medulla produces excessive adrenaline and noradrenaline. The tumour is small, with about 10% being multiple tumours and 10% being malignant.

PATHOPHYSIOLOGY

Clinical features The tumour produces the clinical effects of excessive catecholamine secretion which include hypertension and palpitations.

Box 5.4 Information

Chvostek's and Trousseau's sign: tests for latent tetany due to hypocalcaemia

Chvostek's sign

The nurse can test for this sign by tapping the person's facial nerve about 2 cm anterior to the ear lobe. If hypocalcaemia (or hypomagnesaemia) is present, unilateral twitching of facial muscles, especially around the mouth, may be observed.

Trousseau's sign

This is tested by inflating a sphygmomanometer cuff on the upper arm to a pressure above systolic pressure for 2–3 min. The constrictive effect of the inflated blood pressure cuff exacerbates the hypocalcaemia in the limb distal to the cuff. Spasm of the forearm muscles (contraction or twitching) will be observed in the limb concerned.

Common presenting symptoms Patients may present with anxiety, tachycardia, palpitations and panic attacks. Headaches, sweating and pallor may also occur. There may be a history of high blood pressure, which may be labile. Patients may present as an emergency with a hypertensive crisis or may be asymptomatic.

MEDICAL MANAGEMENT

Investigations

A careful history and clinical examination may lead the physician to suspect a phaeochromocytoma. Investigations include 24-h urine collections for urinary free noradrenaline (norepinephrine NE) and adrenaline (epinephrine E) and dopamine or their two major metabolites, metanephrine and vanillyl-mandelic acid (VMA). Normal levels of NE/E and catecholamine secretion usually exclude a diagnosis of phaeochromocytoma. Abdominal X-rays and a computed tomography (CT) scan may show a tumour of the medulla.

Treatment

This includes surgical removal of the tumour and administration of α- and β-adrenoreceptor blocking medications, e.g. phenoxybenzamine and propranolol.

Nursing management and health promotion: phaeochromocytoma

The first priority of care is to limit anxiety as much as possible and to nurse the patient in a quiet, non-stressful environment. Clear, concise explanations of the reasons for the symptoms will help to relieve the anxiety.

Blood pressure and pulse should be recorded 4-hourly and any sweating or flushing noted. Antihypertensive medication must be maintained as the risk of postoperative hypotensive collapse is reduced by adequate preparation with adrenoreceptor blocking medication.

A care plan should be devised such that the patient can be as independent as possible in self-care tasks. Pre-operative preparation is as for general abdominal surgery (see Ch. 26). Specific postoperative care includes ½-hourly recording of blood pressure to observe for immediate postoperative hypotensive collapse brought on by the reduced blood volume characteristic of chronic vasoconstriction. Specialist medication such as sodium nitroprusside, a potent vasoconstrictor, should be available to control blood pressure in a hypotensive crisis.

Adrenal cortex – Cushing's syndrome/disease

Cushing's syndrome/disease is caused by the excessive and inappropriate circulation of glucocorticoids. It most commonly occurs when synthetic corticosteroids are prescribed.

See website for further content

Spontaneous causes of Cushing's syndrome are extremely rare. The major causes, excluding iatrogenic causes, are (Kumar & Clark 2009):

- pituitary-dependent disease (Cushing's disease)
- ectopic ACTH production
- adrenal adenoma or cancer
- alcohol-induced.

PATHOPHYSIOLOGY

Clinical features Increased plasma cortisol levels have wide-ranging clinical effects on most systems of the body, i.e. altered fat and carbohydrate metabolism, diabetes mellitus, central obesity, muscle wasting, sodium retention leading to hypertension, oedema, immunosuppression and osteoporosis. Comprehensive coverage of the signs and symptoms is provided in Table 5.3.

Common presenting symptoms Because of the wide-ranging clinical effects of Cushing's syndrome/disease, the patient can present with varying symptoms. Frequently, the patient will complain of infections which will not resolve, weight gain, bruising and discoloration of the skin.

Table 5.3 Signs and symptoms of Cushing's syndrome/disease	
SYMPTOMS OR SIGN	**AETIOLOGY**
Muscle wasting which can be demonstrated by the patient being unable to stand from a squatting position	Catabolic effect of the corticosteroids
Osteoporosis which can be so severe as to result in spontaneous fracture of vertebrae or ribs	Protein loss from the skeletal matrix
Skin thinning and purple striae, plethora, easy bruising and purpura	Atrophy of the elastic lamina allows disruption of the dermis so capillaries can be seen below the surface. Weakening of the capillaries leads to easy bruising (often without trauma)
Oedema	Weakening of the capillaries
Poor wound healing, immunosuppression	The lymphocytes are destroyed, lowering the ability to fight infection. Signs of infection, e.g. swelling and redness, are masked
Obesity and 'buffalo hump' (pad of fat across shoulders)	Altered metabolism of fat. Fat is laid down over the trunk. Lipid levels may be raised
Hypertension	Sodium-retaining properties of glucocorticoids
Diabetes mellitus	Alteration in the normal metabolism of carbohydrate and the increased conversion of protein to carbohydrate
Depression, euphoria and frank psychosis	Unknown
Change in libido, erectile dysfunction, oligomenorrhoea and infertility	Due to the general hormone imbalance that is occurring
Excess hair growth, hair loss (particularly of the male pattern type in women)	This is seen in Cushing's disease/ syndrome but is not solely due to cortisol overproduction

MEDICAL AND SURGICAL MANAGEMENT

Investigations

Diagnosis is confirmed by radiological (e.g. CT or MRI scan of head and pituitary fossa) and biochemical (e.g. dexamethasone suppression test) investigations.

🖱 **See website for further content**

The differential diagnosis between pituitary disease, ectopic ACTH production and primary adrenal hypersecretion is important as the treatment and management will vary considerably.

Treatment

Metyrapone is commonly used to lower cortisol levels. An alternative approach is to remove completely endogenous cortisol by adrenalectomy and to supplement levels with an oral corticosteroid.

Trans-sphenoidal surgery is used to remove an ACTH-producing pituitary tumour. Ketoconazole (antifungal medication) may be used, as it inhibits the cortisol synthesis pathway. Surgical removal of a benign adrenal adenoma offers a good chance of cure, but adrenal cancer carries a poor prognosis. The medication mitotane is licensed for the symptomatic treatment of adrenal cortical cancer.

Following adrenalectomy patients will require lifelong hydrocortisone and mineralocorticoid replacement therapy. They must always wear a MedicAlert® bracelet and carry a 'steroid' card, and be informed of the dangers of hypocortisolaemia, a life-threatening condition.

Ectopic ACTH syndrome

This condition most often occurs in patients with an oat cell cancer of the lung. The cancer cells themselves produce ACTH and give rise to Cushing's syndrome. Care is as for cancer, taking into account the additional complications of Cushing's syndrome. A subgroup of patients with ectopic ACTH production from less malignant carcinoid tumours present with more classical Cushing's syndrome and may survive for many years with appropriate treatment.

 ▷ **Nursing management and health promotion: Cushing's syndrome**

The main aim of nursing care is to relieve the symptoms of the disease. On admission, a full nursing history is taken and the patient's needs thoroughly assessed to provide a basis for a care plan (Nursing Care Plan 5.1). The story of Jenny who has Cushing's syndrome is available on the companion website, which you might want to use for discussion with your mentor.

🖱 **See website for further content**

A major consideration will be the psychological impact of the illness, e.g. related to a change in body image. Providing clear ongoing explanations of the hormonal changes that the patient is experiencing, the investigations and the subsequent treatment that they will undergo helps provide optimal psychological support.

Ongoing follow-up after discharge from hospital is essential. Initially, 3-monthly tests will be carried out, gradually reducing to an annual check. If adrenalectomy or pituitary surgery has been performed, precautions will need to be taken regarding hydrocortisone replacement; this must be explained in detail. An information leaflet can be useful as a reference for the patient when at home. This should tell the patient when to increase the therapy, e.g. during illness, and when to seek medical advice.

Hyposecretion of the adrenals

Addison's disease

Addison's disease is a rare condition in which there is total destruction of the adrenal cortex and failure of cortisol secretion. It may occur at any age, though the most common age of onset is between 40 and 60 years and it is more common in females. Autoimmune adrenalitis is the most common cause in the developed world and is responsible for 80–90% of cases. Adrenal destruction by medication (e.g. mitotane), TB, HIV or cancer is a rare cause.

PATHOPHYSIOLOGY

Clinical features High levels of ACTH result in pigmentation of the skin and mucosae. The production of all three types of cortical hormones is reduced. Plasma levels of proteins and sodium are low and that of potassium is high, with serum urea being elevated due to volume depletion.

Common presenting symptoms The onset of the disease is usually insidious, often starting with a feeling of general malaise and weakness. Non-specific symptoms can make it difficult to distinguish from depression. Skin discoloration may have been noticed, especially in the palmar creases and on the inside of the lips and cheeks. Postural hypotension, salt cravings, hyperpigmentation, unexplained weight loss, nausea/abdominal pain and persistent fatigue are all grounds for suspicion, and the primary care team are vital in the prompt detection of Addison's and subsequent treatment of emergencies. Approximately 6% of patients every year will require hospital treatment, usually because of a severe episode of vomiting and diarrhoea. Some patients will first present as medical emergencies with an addisonian crisis (see below). Untreated, this can be fatal.

MEDICAL MANAGEMENT

Investigations

Diagnosis is by clinical examination and blood tests to confirm high levels of ACTH and low levels of cortisol. In the short Synacthen® test (SST), tetracosactide (synthetic ACTH) is given i.v. or i.m., and blood samples for plasma cortisol taken at 0, 30 and 60 min after its administration will show a failure of the adrenal glands to respond to the stimulus of the parenteral ACTH. Once this has been demonstrated, the cause of the adrenal failure needs to be identified. The most common cause, i.e. autoimmune, can be diagnosed from an assay to detect the presence of 21-hydroxylase antibodies. If there are no antibodies present, other causes are investigated. Tests will include an MRI of the adrenal glands and screening for TB, HIV and cancer.

Nursing Care Plan 5.1 Care of a patient with Cushing's syndrome

NURSING CONSIDERATIONS	ACTION	RATIONALE	EXPECTED OUTCOME
1. Pain from fractured vertebrae or ribs as a result of osteoporosis	• Provide immediate pain relief. Administer as prescribed, noting the efficacy • Handle and position the patient carefully	Pain and discomfort will increase anxiety. Pain relief will reduce this. Fractured ribs will cause shallow breathing which increases the risk of chest infection. Gentle handling will reduce distress and prevent further fractures	The patient should be pain-free and comfortable and anxiety reduced
2. Infection as a result of immunosuppression	• Make 4-hourly recordings of temperature, pulse, respiration and blood pressure. Report any variation from the normal range immediately	Death from overwhelming infection can occur. Signs of infection will be masked, so infection may be advanced before signs are seen	Any infection will be identified early and correct treatment commenced
3. Damage to skin as a result of skin thinning and oedema or poor wound healing	• If the patient is immobile, care of pressure areas will be required to prevent tissue damage. Legs will need to be elevated to relieve the oedema and any wounds will require aseptic technique when dressed	Tissue will be rapidly broken down and slow to heal, so preventive measures are essential. Susceptibility to infection requires precautions to prevent introduction of infection	Further tissue damage will be prevented and any present source of infection removed as rapidly as possible
4. Hypertension	• Record blood pressure 4-hourly after 10 min lying flat and 1 min standing. Report levels beyond the normal range or postural deficit	Increasing blood pressure may lead to stroke or heart failure and if persistently high will need to be treated with drugs. Postural deficit will indicate a problem with sodium excretion or retention	Blood pressure levels will remain within acceptable limits
5. Diabetes mellitus as a result of abnormal carbohydrate metabolism	• Record pre- and postprandial blood sugar levels and possibly perform daily urinalysis	Persistently high blood sugars will lead to the complications of diabetes mellitus and may need to be treated with insulin	Blood sugar levels will remain within the normal range
6. Psychosis and mental health problems	• Ascertain the patient's mental status early on. A psychiatric opinion should be obtained. Mood swings and bizarre behaviour should be reported. The patient may be so disturbed as to require 24-h mental health nurse observation	The patient's psychological state may change rapidly and close observation for this is necessary. Some patients can express suicidal ideation	The patient will not be a danger to themselves or others and patient safety is maintained at all times

Treatment

Treatment is by long-term replacement doses of glucocorticoid and mineralocorticoid. This should lead to an improvement in the patient's well-being. Glucocorticoid replacement is with hydrocortisone (in two or three divided doses throughout the day; on waking, at lunchtime and before 6pm) and levels of hydrocortisone should be checked regularly to ensure the dose is correct by performing a hydrocortisone day curve. Mineralocorticoid replacement with fludrocortisone (taken as a single morning dose) should be checked by regular blood pressure readings, which should show no postural hypotension, and by measurement of plasma renin.

Early administration by the patient or a family member of i.m. hydrocortisone will often stabilise an acute episode of vomiting and diarrhoea. Patients should be provided with emergency hydrocortisone packs and educated in their use (see below).

Addisonian crisis

This is a life-threatening event. It occurs in such situations as injury, infections, anaesthesia and surgical procedures where, unlike in the healthy individual, the stress response does not occur. The absence of the cortisol surge to a major stressor results in severe shock. Addisonian crisis requires immediate intervention. Symptoms may include:

- sudden penetrating pain in the abdomen, legs or lower back
- fever
- severe vomiting and diarrhoea leading to dehydration
- hypotension
- hypoglycaemia
- altered consciousness.

Treatment aims to restore steroid, sodium and glucose levels to within normal range by i.v. administration of 100 mg hydrocortisone, and i.v. infusion of 0.9% sodium chloride given quickly with dextrose if glucose levels are low. Hydrocortisone is then given i.v. or i.m. 6-hourly until the patient is stable, following which steroid replacement can be given orally and mineralocorticoids introduced.

 Nursing management and health promotion: Addison's disease

Careful observation of temperature, pulse, and standing and lying blood pressure should be made. A raised temperature will indicate signs of infection which the patient may not be

Box 5.5 Reflection

MedicAlert®: increasing patient safety

The use of MedicAlert® bracelets is a vital part of increasing the safety of patients with a variety of disorders.

Activities

- Find out what advice about MedicAlert® is available for patients with Addison's disease in your area.
- How do patients obtain a MedicAlert® bracelet?
- Which other groups of patients should be encouraged to become MedicAlert® members?
- Reflect on the need to wear a bracelet and carry a steroid card – how would you feel?

Resource

MedicAlert® Foundation www.medicalert.org.uk

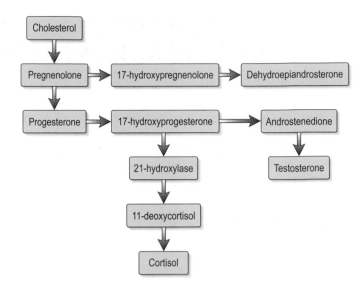

Figure 5.7 Simplified schematisation of cortisol synthesis.

able to fight effectively. Any postural drop in blood pressure should be reported immediately.

The corticosteroid replacement therapy should be administered with the patient's full involvement so that they have a full knowledge of dosage and timing and techniques for self-administration before discharge. The patient should be given a 'steroid' card and advised to carry this and to wear a MedicAlert® bracelet on their wrist or ankle at all times (Box 5.5). They should be provided with a thorough education of the 'sick day rules' that they must follow in case of an intercurrent illness or other stressful life events.

An emergency hydrocortisone pack should be kept at home in case of serious illness or trauma. Ideally it should be self-administered by the patient, or the GP or community nurse called to administer it. It may be sensible also to teach a member of the family how to do this.

See website Critical thinking question 5.1

It is vital that the patient and family have a thorough understanding of their condition and the symptoms associated with complications. This will help to restore confidence and enable the patient to return to a full and active life.

Congenital adrenal hyperplasia (CAH)

This is a group of inherited disorders caused by a deficiency of one of the five enzymes involved in cortisol synthesis. It is one of the most common autosomal recessive disorders with a prevalence in the USA and Europe of approximately 1:15 000–16 000 (van der Kamp & Wit 2004).

PATHOPHYSIOLOGY

To understand CAH it is necessary to understand the biosynthesis of steroids (Figure 5.7). The most common deficiency (accounting for 95% of cases; Labarata et al 2004) occurs if the enzyme 21-hydroxylase (CYP21) is absent because of a gene defect; cortisol will not be produced in sufficient quantity. By means of the negative feedback system, ACTH production will be increased to stimulate cortisol production. This in turn leads to hypertrophy of the adrenal cortex and elevated levels of 17-hydroxyprogesterone, androstenedione and testosterone – the hormones occurring before the enzyme block. This will result ultimately in virilisation.

CAH disorders can be divided into three main groups:

- severe or classic – with or without salt wasting (SW)
- moderate/less severe – simple virilising (SV)
- mild – non-classic (NC).

Common presenting signs and symptoms

Classical CAH presents at birth or in early infancy with sexual ambiguity and salt-wasting due to mineralocorticoid deficiency. Life-threatening vomiting and dehydration, resulting in hyponatraemia and hyperkalaemia, and collapse can occur in the neonatal period. In the female infant, the high level of androgens present cause clitoral hypertrophy and fusion of the labial folds resulting in ambiguous genitalia. Internal genitalia may develop normally. The syndrome may not be recognised in the male infant, who will have normal genitalia. If a diagnosis is not made at birth, a genotypical female (XX) may be labelled male. Gender assignment should therefore wait until adequate anatomical and biochemical information is available.

Moderate or simple virilising CAH is typically recognised by signs of virilisation in prepubertal children. Effects can include premature development of pubic hair (precocious puberty), advanced bone age, accelerated growth velocity and diminished final height in both sexes as a result of premature fusion of the bony epiphyses.

Mild or non-classic CAH, because prenatal virilisation does not occur, presents in late childhood or early adulthood (Labarata et al 2004). Symptoms of androgen excess include hirsutism, severe acne, temporal baldness and infertility in adolescents and adult women. Menarche may be normal or delayed and secondary amenorrhoea is common. Polycystic ovarian syndrome (PCOS) may also be present. In young men, early beard growth, acne and a growth spurt may prompt the diagnosis. Men may also present with oligozoospermia or diminished fertility despite appearing asymptomatic and are only diagnosed when efforts to conceive fail.

MEDICAL MANAGEMENT

Investigations

These include blood tests to confirm high levels of ACTH and 17-hydroxyprogesterone. In the infant a thorough physical examination together with an abdominal ultrasound should be performed to ascertain the presence of internal female reproductive organs.

Treatment

Replacement of the glucocorticoid is usually given in the form of prednisolone to suppress the ACTH production and thereby reduce the overstimulation of the adrenals. Other requirements frequently include mineralocorticoids, e.g. fludrocortisone. Reconstructive surgery for females is usually initiated between the ages of 3–6 months and, while specific to each child's individual anatomy, may involve clitoroplasty, labioscrotal reduction and vaginal exteriorisation.

 Nursing management and health promotion: congenital adrenal hyperplasia

Information should be given regarding corticosteroid replacement therapy (see p. 145). Nursing care should concentrate on the psychological support which will be required by both the parents and the child, and for individuals diagnosed during adulthood.

The psychosocial and psychosexual implications of CAH are considerable and formal counselling and psychotherapy should be made available. In female patients, hirsutism and acne can be especially distressing. Antiandrogens, e.g. cyproterone acetate, are now the treatment of choice. Other important issues for women which need discussion include menstruation, sexuality, fertility and the possible need for plastic surgery, as some effects of virilisation are not reversible by medication (Hagenfeldt 2004). This is particularly important as the patient approaches adulthood, as sexual intercourse may be rendered difficult, painful or impossible. Prevention of subfertility should be implemented as a treatment goal from the start of puberty. Effective transition of care for the patient from the paediatric to adult endocrinologist is of utmost importance.

THE GONADS – DISORDERS OF SEXUAL DIFFERENTIATION

In normal development, gonadal and phenotypic sex follow an orderly process of development determined by chromosomal sex at the moment of conception.

During the early stages of fetal life the gonad has the potential to develop female or male characteristics. In the presence of another X chromosome (i.e. 46, XX) or the absence of another chromosome (i.e. 45, XO), development will follow the female pattern. The presence of two X chromosomes is, however, necessary for normal ovarian function.

By the second month of fetal development the genital organs are undifferentiated duct systems, termed the müllerian (paramesonephric) and wolffian (mesonephric) ducts. In the normal female, as development progresses, the wolffian system regresses and the müllerian system develops to form the uterine tubes, the uterus and the upper vagina. The external genitalia undergo little change.

In the male, the müllerian system regresses and the wolffian system develops to form the testes, vas deferens, prostate and seminiferous tubules. The genital tubercle present in both systems forms the clitoris in the female and the penis in the male.

There is evidence to suggest that the normal development of a male fetus is hormone-dependent. It appears that testosterone inhibits the regression of the wolffian duct and stimulates its development into the male sexual structures. In contrast to this, the ovary is unaffected by hormones in utero.

Abnormalities of sexual differentiation may present with abnormal genitalia at birth, growth disturbance in childhood or abnormal secondary sexual development.

Abnormalities of gonadal development

True hermaphroditism, i.e. the presence of both male and female sexual characteristics in the same individual, is extremely rare. It occurs when both the müllerian and wolffian systems continue to develop. Diagnosis requires a high index of suspicion for subtle abnormalities of the genitalia. Ovotestes may exist or an ovary on one side and a testis on the other.

Chromosomal abnormalities

There are several chromosomal abnormalities that affect sexual differentiation. This section outlines four such disorders.

Klinefelter's syndrome is a condition in which phenotypical males have one or more extra X chromosomes and one Y chromosome. Eighty per cent of patients display the classic karyotype (47, XXY) but additional X or Y chromosomes may be present. The greater the number of additional chromosomes present, the greater the severity of the condition. It is the most prevalent sex chromosome disorder in men with an incidence of 1 in 600 male newborns (Kamischke et al 2003). Symptoms and presentation depend on when the diagnosis is made as this can be antenatal, during childhood or adolescence, or late into adulthood.

See website for further content

Adult patients present with low testosterone and elevated LH and FSH, often during investigations for infertility or following an unexpected fracture. Men with Klinefelter's syndrome are typically tall with long legs compared to upper body length, due to delayed epiphyseal closure of their long bones, exhibit excessive fat, especially around the trunk, and are infertile. They may exhibit a varying degree of interstitial (Leydig) cell failure resulting in testosterone deficiency (Bojesen et al 2004). Almost 40% of patients show some degree of intellectual dysfunction. Adolescence can be a particularly stressful time as boys have to come to terms with hormone replacement therapy, possible breast development and infertility. Counselling should be offered and information provided about support groups.

Turner's syndrome is a condition in which the individual is phenotypically female but has the genotype XO, i.e. complete or partial absence of one X chromosome. It is the most commonly occurring chromosomal abnormality in females, with an incidence of approximately 50 in 100 000 (Gravholt 2004). Affected individuals have short stature with a 'web neck' and low-set ears and may have widely spaced nipples and peripheral oedema. The ovaries are atrophic and serum LH and FSH levels are elevated. These individuals are prone to a variety of serious cardiac problems including coarctation of the aorta and aortic dissection. Women with Turner's syndrome are thought to have a reduced life expectancy, mainly due to these serious cardiac problems, but they may also have multiple co-morbidities, which can include hypothyroidism, deafness, osteoporosis, oestrogen deficiency and infertility (Ostberg & Conway 2003).

Kallman's syndrome In this condition there is a normal karyotype but a genetic defect in the pathway leading to gonadotrophin secretion; thus there is a deficiency of gonadotrophins and therefore sex steroid secretion is reduced. This condition is sometimes termed congenital hypogonadotrophic hypogonadism. Typically, the individual has anosmia (absence of the sense of smell). Normal gonadal function can be restored with replacement of LH and FSH, meaning that fertility is possible. Otherwise, treatment is either oestrogen or testosterone replacement (The Pituitary Foundation 2006).

Testicular feminisation This is a syndrome of androgen resistance or complete androgen insensitivity (CAI syndrome) caused by mutations in the androgen receptor gene. While the karyotype is male (46, XY), the phenotype is female. Testes are present, but because of tissue resistance to circulating androgens but not oestrogen at puberty, breast tissue develops although pubic hair does not (Skordis et al 2005). Regression of the müllerian system occurs due to tissue insensitivity but the wolffian system does not develop and a blind-ended vagina results. The gonads may become malignant and are usually removed at the onset of adult life.

Nursing management and health promotion: disorders of sexual differentiation

Whilst disorders of the gonads are rarely life threatening or require admission to hospital, the psychological and social implications for the individual and their family cannot be overemphasised.

The role of the nurse in the investigation and treatment of these conditions is to offer psychological support to the individual, and, if they agree, their family, in an environment which is both relaxed and supportive.

Counselling on an informal and formal basis is essential during investigations, when complete privacy must be ensured. Feelings of inadequacy regarding sexuality and low self-esteem are common. An approach which demonstrates empathy with the individual helps to create a positive image during the initial examinations and investigations and during subsequent treatment.

SUMMARY: KEY NURSING ISSUES

- The endocrine system is one of the major control systems of the body, the other being the nervous system.
- As endocrine diseases are not common, patients may have had a long 'journey' before receiving a diagnosis and may have seen many different health professionals before they come to you.
- Altered body image is an important feature of endocrine disease and some patients may have considerable difficulty in coming to terms with their changed appearance. Providing opportunities to talk about such matters is an important part of the nurse's role.
- A patient's QoL can be severely affected by endocrine disease. Many disease-specific questionnaires are available to assess the impact of disease on patients and to monitor response to treatment. Together with a careful assessment of patients these can provide valuable information for the nurse when planning care.
- Many patients benefit from joining a local support group specific to their condition and the contact with others with similar histories.
- The majority of patients, once diagnosed, will require long-term follow-up. Establishing an ongoing nurse–patient relationship built on trust is therefore crucial.
- Nurses have an important role in ensuring that patients are aware of the importance of correctly taking their hormone replacement therapy and other prescribed medications. Ensuring patient concordance with treatment is a key nursing role to ensure optimal benefit to the patient and reduce the possibility of side-effects or emergencies. This is especially true for patients on hydrocortisone replacement who must be made aware of the 'sick day' rules and be trained in the emergency self-administration of i.m. hydrocortisone. All patients should also be encouraged to become members of MedicAlert®.
- Nursing initiatives within endocrinology include nurse-led clinics, telephone help-lines and the auditing of services to ensure best practice.
- All nurses working in endocrinology should ensure they keep up-to-date with advances in their field by regularly attending local, national or international conferences. They should strive to disseminate their local knowledge and expertise by presenting at these meetings and by publishing their research, audit or patient cases.
- Good links and effective communication between primary and secondary care teams are important to ensure that patients feel well supported by both their GP/Practice Nurse and their specialist endocrine team, thus ensuring that care is streamlined.

REFLECTION AND LEARNING – WHAT NEXT?

- **Test** your knowledge by visiting the website and answering the multiple choice questions and critical thinking questions.
- **Consolidate** your learning by looking at some of the further reading suggestions, references and specialist websites.
- **Revisit** some of the additional material on the website.
- **Consider** what you have learnt and how this will help your professional development.
- **Reflect** on how you can apply this knowledge to the care of your patients.
- **Discuss** your learning with your mentor/supervisor, lecturer and colleagues.

REFERENCES

Badia X, Webb SM, Prieto L, Lara N: Acromegaly Quality of Life Questionnaire (AcroQoL), *Health Qual Life Outcomes* 2(13), 2004. Available online http://www.pubmedcentral.nih.gov/picrender.fcgi?artid=404471&blobtype=pdf.

Ben-Shlomo A, Melmed S: Somatostatin agonists for treatment of acromegaly, *Mol Cell Endocrinol* 286:192–198, 2008.

Bojesen A, Jun S, Birkbaek N, Gravholt CH: Increased mortality in Klinefelter's syndrome, *J Clin Endocrinol Metab* 89(8):3830–3834, 2004.

Boon NA, Colledge NR, Walker BR: *Davidson's Principles and Practice of Medicine*, ed 20, Edinburgh, 2006, Churchill Livingstone.

Brooke AM, Monson JP: Adult growth hormone deficiency, *Clin Med* 3:15–19, 2003.

Cancer Research UK: *UK Thyroid Cancer incidence statistics*, 2009. Available online http://info.cancerresearchuk.org/cancerstats/types/thyroid/incidence/.

Colao A, Ferone D, Marzullo P, Lombardini G: Systemic complications of acromegaly: epidemiology, pathogenesis and management, *Endocr Rev* 25(1):102–152, 2004.

Delange FM, Dunn JT: Iodine deficiency. In Braverman LE, Utiger RD, editors: *Werner and Ingbar's the thyroid: a fundamental and clinical text*, ed 9, Baltimore, 2005, Lippincott, Williams and Wilkins, pp 264–288.

Gravholt CH: Long-term follow-up of Turner's syndrome, *International Growth Monitor* 14(4):2–6, 2004.

Hagenfeldt KB: Congenital adrenal hyperplasia due to 21-hydroxylase deficiency – the adult woman, *Growth Horm IGF Res* (Suppl A):S67–S71, 2004.

Jenkins PJ, Bates PR, Carson MN, et al: Conventional pituitary irradiation is effective in lowering serum growth hormone and insulin-like growth factor-1 in patients with acromegaly, *J Clin Endocrinol Metab* 91(4):1239–1245, 2006.

Kaltsas GA, Isidoi AM, Florakis D, et al: Predictors of the outcome of surgical treatment in acromegaly and the value of the mean growth hormone day curve in assessing post-operative disease activity, *J Clin Endocrinol Metab* 86:1645–1652, 2001.

Kamischke A, Baumgardt A, Horst J, Nieschlag E: Clinical and diagnostic features of patients with suspected Klinefelter's syndrome, *J Androl* 24(1):41–48, 2003.

Kumar P, Clark M: *Clinical medicine*, ed 7, Edinburgh, 2009, Saunders.

Labarata JI, Bello E, Ruiz-Echarri M, et al: Childhood onset of congenital adrenal hyperplasia: long-term outcome and optimization of therapy, *J Pediatr Endocrinol Metab* 17(Suppl 3):411–422, 2004.

Leese GP, Flynn RV, Jung RT, et al: Increasing prevalence and incidence of thyroid disease in Tayside, Scotland: the Thyroid Epidemiology Audit and Research Study (TEARS), *Clin Endocrinol (Oxf)* 68(2):311–316, 2008.

Macmillan Cancer Support: *Staging of thyroid cancer*, 2009. Available online http://www.cancerbackup.org.uk/Cancertype/Thyroid/Causesdiagnosis/Staging.

Mann J, Aitken E: The re-emergence of iodine deficiency in New Zealand? *N Z Med J* 116(1170):351–355, 2003.

McMillan C, Bradley C, Woodcock A, et al: Design of new questionnaires to measure quality of life and treatment satisfaction in hypothyroidism, *Thyroid* 14(11):916–925, 2004.

McMillan C, Bradley C, Razvi S, Weaver J: Psychometric evaluation of a new questionnaire measuring treatment satisfaction in hypothyroidism: the ThyTSQ, *Value Health* 9(2):132–139, 2006.

Mukherjee A, Shalet SM: Overview of growth hormone deficiency in adults. In Abs R, Feldt-Rasmussen U, editors: *Growth hormone deficiency in adults; 10 years of KIMS*, Oxford, 2004, Oxford Pharmagenesis, pp 51–61.

National Institute for Health and Clinical Excellence (NICE): *Growth hormone deficiency (adults) – human growth hormone Technology appraisal TA64*, 2003. Available online http://guidance.nice.org.uk/TA64.

Ostberg JE, Conway GS: Adulthood in women with Turner's syndrome, *Horm Res* 59(5):211–221, 2003.

Schlechte JA: Prolactinoma, *N Engl J Med* 349:2035–2041, 2003.

Schubert M, Minnemann D, Hubler D, et al: Intramuscular testosterone undecanoate: pharmacokinetic aspects of a novel testosterone formulation during long-term treatment of men with hypogonadism, *J Clin Endocrinol Metab* 89:5429–5434, 2004.

Skordis N, Lumbroso S, Penkleous M, et al: Complete androgen insensitivity syndrome caused by the R855H mutation in the androgen receptor gene, *J Pediatr Endocrinol Metab* 18(3):309–313, 2005.

Swerdloff RS, Wang C, Cunningham G, et al: Long-term pharmacokinetics of transdermal testosterone gel in hypogonadal men, *J Clin Endocrinol Metab* 85:4500–4510, 2000.

Swords FM, Allan CA, Sibtain A, et al: Stereotactic radiosurgery XVI: a treatment for previously irradiated pituitary adenomas, *J Clin Endocrinol Metab* 88:5334–5340, 2003.

The Pituitary Foundation: *Kallman's syndrome*, 2006. Available online http://www.pituitary.org.uk/content/view/176/123/.

Trainer PJ: Acromegaly – consensus. What consensus, *J Clin Endocrinol Metab* 87:3534–3536, 2002.

Van der Kamp HJ, Wit JM: Neonatal screening for congenital adrenal hyperplasia, *Eur J Endocrinol* 151(Suppl 3):U71–U75, 2004.

Waugh A, Grant A, editors: *Ross and Wilson Anatomy and physiology in health and illness*, ed 10, Edinburgh, 2006, Churchill Livingstone.

Webster J: Cabergoline and quinagolide therapy for prolactinomas, *Clin Endocrinol (Oxf)* 53:549–550, 2000.

Wilson JD: The evolution of endocrinology, *Clin Endocrinol (Oxf)* 62(4):389–396, 2005.

FURTHER READING

Azziz R: Diagnostic criteria for polycystic ovary syndrome: a reappraisal, *Fertil Steril* 83(5):1343–1346, 2005.

Besser GM, Thorner MO: *Comprehensive clinical endocrinology*, Edinburgh, 2002, Mosby.

Braverman LE, Utiger RD, editors: *Werner and Ingbar's the thyroid: a fundamental and clinical text*, ed 9, Philadelphia, 2004, Lippincott Williams and Wilkins.

Carson MN: Assessment and management of patients with hypothyroidism, *Nurs Stand* 23(18):48–56, 2009.

de Benoist B, Andersson M, Egli I, et al, editors: *Iodine status worldwide. WHO Global Database on Iodine Deficiency*, 2004. Available online http://www.ceecis.org/iodine/01_global/01_pl/01_01_who_%20status_worldwide_04.pdfhttp://www.who.int/vmnis/iodine/status/summary/severity_color.pdf.

Liu JK, Couldwell WT: Contemporary management of prolactinomas, *Neurosurg Focus* 16(4):E2, 2004.

Montague SE, Watson R, Herbert R: *Physiology for nursing practice*, ed 3, Edinburgh, 2005, Baillière Tindall.

Perros P, Kendall-Taylor P: Medical treatment for thyroid-associated ophthalmopathy, *Thyroid* 12:241–244, 2002.

Piersanti M: Growth hormone replacement for patients with adult onset growth hormone deficiency – what have we learned? *Neurosurg Focus* 16(4):E12, 2004.

Schafer J: *My story, thyroid papillary carcinoma*, 2005. Available online http://oncolink.upenn.edu/types/article.cfm.

USEFUL WEBSITES

ACTH: www.cushingsacth.co.uk

Addison's Disease Self Help Group (ADSHG): www.addisons.org.uk

AMEND (Association for Multiple Endocrine Neoplasia Disorders): www.amend.org.uk/

British Thyroid Foundation: www.btf-thyroid.org/

Climb: Congenital Adrenal Hyperplasia UK Support Group: www.livingwithcah.com/

eXtra (Klinefelter's Syndrome Association) UK: www.ksa-uk.co.uk/

The Pituitary Foundation: www.pituitary.org.uk/

Thyroid Eye Disease Charitable Trust (TEDct): www.tedct.co.uk/

PART 2 NURSING PATIENTS WITH DIABETES MELLITUS

Introduction

Diabetes mellitus is defined as a metabolic disorder of multiple aetiology. It is characterised by chronic hyperglycaemia (increased blood glucose) with disturbances of carbohydrate (CHO), protein and fat metabolism which results from defects in insulin secretion, insulin action or both (World Health Organization [WHO] 1999). Diabetes UK (2008) estimates that there are around 2.3 million people diagnosed with the condition in the UK and there are more than half a million individuals who are unaware that they have diabetes. Diabetes is associated with several long-term complications that include sight impairment, renal failure, neuropathy and cardiovascular diseases. The care of people with diabetes represents a large proportion of health resources (Box 5.6)

The terms insulin-dependent and non-insulin-dependent diabetes have been replaced by the WHO classification (WHO 1999) which recognises the main types of diabetes as follows:

- type 1 diabetes (formerly insulin-dependent diabetes)
- type 2 diabetes (formerly non-insulin-dependent diabetes)
- gestational diabetes
- impaired glucose regulation
- other specific types.

The chapter briefly outlines the anatomy and physiology of the pancreas and the hormonal regulation of blood

Box 5.6 Reflection

Numbers of people with diabetes worldwide set to increase

The International Diabetes Federation (IDF) (2008) estimates there are 246 million people affected by diabetes worldwide with the highest prevalence in developed countries, and that the figure will reach 380 million by 2025.

Activity

- Reflect on why diabetes has a high prevalence in developed countries and discuss your reasons with your mentor.

Diabetes UK (2008) considers diabetes to be 'one of the biggest health challenges facing the UK today'.

Activity

- Consider the statement from Diabetes UK. Discuss with colleagues the implications for health care systems if diabetes, especially type 2, continues to increase.

glucose levels (see Further reading, e.g. Tortora & Derrickson 2009). The types, pathophysiology, clinical presentation, medical management and the acute metabolic and chronic complications of diabetes are covered. Key issues of nursing management and health promotion of diabetes and its complications are discussed in some depth.

Anatomy and physiology

The pancreas

The pancreas has both endocrine and exocrine function. The endocrine function of the pancreas is concerned with the secretion of several hormones. The hormone-secreting islets of Langerhans are found scattered throughout the pancreas. There are four types of cell contained within the islets. Alpha (α) cells secrete glucagon and beta (β) cells secrete insulin; each has a key role in regulating blood glucose. Other islet cells include those that secrete pancreatic polypeptides and delta (δ) cells that secrete somatostatin (also known as growth hormone release-inhibiting hormone [GHRIH]) which contributes to the regulation of a variety of hormones throughout the body, including insulin and glucagon.

Exocrine tissue is responsible for the secretion of digestive enzymes that leave the pancreas in ducts to enter the duodenum (see Ch. 4).

Blood glucose regulation

Within a 24-hour period, the healthy human will alternate between the fed state and the fasting state several times. Two hours following a meal, blood glucose will tend to rise as absorption of nutrients takes place. This is the postprandial or fed state. Once glucose has been taken up into the cells, blood glucose levels will tend to fall and will not rise again until the next meal is taken. This is the preprandial or fasting state. In health these fluctuations are slight, as insulin is secreted at a low (basal) level throughout the whole day, only rising to an increased stimulated level at mealtimes. Insulin and glucagon are principally (but not exclusively) responsible for blood glucose regulation.

Insulin

Insulin, an anabolic hormone, is secreted in response to a rising blood glucose level. Insulin has effects on the metabolism of carbohydrate, fat and protein. Its physiological effects in different tissues include:

Carbohydrate
- Increased glucose uptake by the cells
- Increased glycolysis (breakdown of glucose)
- Increased glycogenesis (conversion of glucose to glycogen for storage in the liver and skeletal muscle)
- Decreased glycogenolysis (breakdown of glycogen back into glucose)
- Decreased gluconeogenesis (formation of glucose from non-CHO sources, e.g. amino acids, lactate, glycerol).

Fat
- Increased lipogenesis (formation of triglycerides from glucose and amino acids before storage in adipose tissue)
- Decreased lipolysis (breakdown of stored fat for energy)
- Increased synthesis of low density lipoproteins and cholesterol.

Protein
- Increased protein synthesis
- Decreased protein breakdown.

All of these effects have the effect of preventing an abnormal rise in blood glucose during the postprandial period.

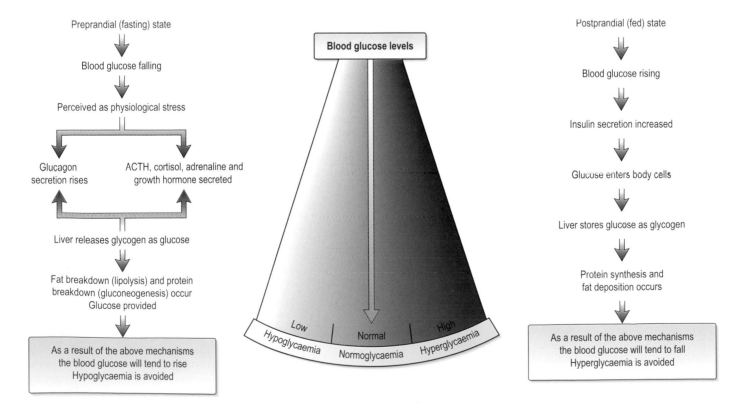

Figure 5.8 The regulation of blood glucose in health.

Insulin secretion is highest in the fed state and lowest in the fasting state (Figure 5.8).

Glucagon

Glucagon, a catabolic hormone, is secreted in response to a falling blood glucose level and its physiological effects include:

- increased glycogenolysis and the release of glucose from the liver
- increased fat and protein breakdown in order to provide an alternative source of glucose via lipolysis and gluconeogenesis
- influence on the production of ketone bodies (ketogenesis); in total or near-total insulin lack, these weak acids are produced as a result of the chemical processes involved in fat breakdown.

The actions of glucagon and the other counter-regulatory hormones are all geared towards preventing an abnormal fall in blood glucose (hypoglycaemia). Glucagon secretion is highest in the fasting state and lowest in the fed state (Figure 5.8).

Other influences on blood glucose regulation

Anterior pituitary gland The pituitary hormones influencing glucose regulation include:

- Growth hormone (somatotrophin) – this hormone tends to raise blood glucose. It is diabetogenic in action and anti-insulin in effect. It influences blood glucose in two main ways – by increasing glycogenolysis and by inhibiting muscle glycogen storage.
- Adrenocorticotrophic hormone (ACTH) – this hormone stimulates the adrenal cortex to release the glucocorticoid hormone cortisol (see below). A negative feedback mechanism operates in response to the circulating levels of cortisol in the blood.

Adrenal cortex secretes a group of glucocorticoid hormones, the most significant of which is cortisol. Cortisol is a catabolic hormone. Secretion is increased during prolonged periods of physical or psychological stress (see Ch. 17), when its effect is to raise the blood glucose level in order to meet the additional metabolic demands of the stressed state. Cortisol increases glycogenolysis, lipolysis and the breakdown of protein to provide amino acids for gluconeogenesis, providing an alternative source of glucose to meet cell energy needs.

Adrenal medulla secretes the catecholamines adrenaline (epinephrine) and noradrenaline (norepinephrine). These 'fight or flight' hormones are catabolic in their action. In response to stress, they place the body and brain in a state of high alert, causing blood glucose to rise as glycogen stores are released and fat/protein breakdown occurs. This increases the amount of available glucose and helps to prepare the body to meet increased energy demands.

Liver and skeletal muscle About 60% of absorbed nutrients are stored as reserves in order to meet energy demands during fasting. Under the influence of insulin, the liver and, to a lesser extent, skeletal muscle can store glucose in the form of glycogen. The liver is also involved in protein and fat synthesis for subsequent storage.

During fasting or in response to stress, glucagon (and other stress hormones) will increase glycogenolysis in the liver and skeletal muscle to release glucose (Figure 5.8).

Type 1 diabetes

The pathogenesis of type 1 diabetes is complex and has been the subject of extensive research. It is currently thought that a genetic predisposition to the disease, possibly combined with environmental triggers, activates an autoimmune attack on the pancreatic islet β cells. Insulin secretion is virtually absent.

PATHOPHYSIOLOGY

Islet cell destruction probably begins very early in life and is known to start several years before onset of diabetes (Holt & Kumar 2010). Individuals may present with initial symptoms when the demand for insulin has been increased, e.g. in response to a physical or psychological stress such as illness, trauma, surgery or pregnancy. Additional metabolic demands posed by the stressed state can no longer be met by the failing pancreas and symptoms of diabetes become evident for the first time.

Once insulin therapy is commenced, the remaining β cell mass can temporarily provide sufficient insulin to meet the body's demands. In this case the exogenous insulin can be reduced, and, on occasion, stopped. This remission or 'honeymoon period' is short lived. As the β cell mass reduces further, symptoms of hyperglycaemia will reappear, necessitating lifelong treatment with insulin.

Clinical presentation In general terms, the lack of insulin means that body cells are unable to use glucose for metabolism. The signs, symptoms and clinical features of type 1 diabetes can best be explained in terms of the specific effects of insulin lack, as follows:

- Hyperglycaemia – glucose is unable to enter cells and accumulates in the blood, causing an abnormally high blood glucose level.
- Glycosuria (glucose in the urine) – increased amounts of glucose are filtered in the glomeruli. The capacity of the kidneys to reabsorb glucose is exceeded and glucose appears in the urine.
- Polyuria (excretion of excessive volumes of urine) – this occurs because glucose is highly osmotic and as glucose is lost in the urine, large volumes of water are lost with it.
- Polydipsia (excessive thirst) – as fluid loss continues, signs and symptoms of fluid imbalance occur (see Ch. 20) and copious drinking is noted in response to severe thirst.
- Cell glucose requirements are unmet. The counter-regulatory response is increased secretion of glucagon and other stress hormones in an attempt to increase glucose availability. Under the influence of these hormones there is:
  - glycogenolysis
  - gluconeogenesis.
- Increasing blood glucose – the efforts to meet the cellular demands for glucose have the combined effect of raising the blood glucose even higher.
- Polyphagia (increased appetite) – caused by cell requirements for glucose being unmet (see above).

- Weight loss – occurs due to the depletion of body fat and protein stores. This, along with cell deprivation of glucose and fluid and electrolyte imbalance, causes muscle weakness and exhaustion.
- Ketonaemia (ketone bodies in the blood) and ketonuria (ketone bodies in the urine) – without insulin, there is fat breakdown which results in the formation of ketone bodies – β-hydroxybutyric acid, acetoacetic acid and acetone (a process known as ketogenesis). The ketone bodies accumulate in the blood and are excreted in the urine.
- Characteristic sweet 'pear drop' odour on the breath – caused by the excretion of acetone by the lungs.
- Metabolic acidosis (see Ch. 20) – ketone bodies are weak acids and release hydrogen ions [H⁺] causing disruption to blood pH (normally maintained within a narrow range). The processes leading to acidosis cause the accumulation of excess acid in the blood (acidaemia) resulting in an abnormally low blood pH.
- Kussmaul's respiration (hyperventilation: rapid deep respiration) – acidaemia leads to increased respiratory buffering in an attempt to correct acidaemia by removing more acidic carbon dioxide through increased rate and depth of respiration.
- Diabetic ketoacidosis (DKA) – a life-threatening situation, which without urgent treatment will progress to coma and ultimately to death (see p. 160). Uncontrolled lipolysis in the absence of insulin, gluconeogenesis, ketogenesis and glycogenolysis combine to raise the blood glucose level still further, increase osmotic diuresis, and exacerbate fluid imbalance and metabolic acidosis. As a result of these profound biochemical disturbances, the patient may experience nausea and vomiting and unexplained colicky abdominal pain.

Onset and progress of type 1 diabetes

Although the onset of type 1 diabetes may appear abrupt, the patient may have had signs, such as glycosuria, in the absence of overt symptoms over many months. Once symptoms appear, the condition will usually have a rapid progression. However, there will be variations in severity, some patients being much more acutely ill than others at the time of diagnosis.

Although most patients are referred to hospital, admission is not automatic. The majority of newly diagnosed patients with type 1 diabetes will be managed as outpatients. All adults with diabetes will receive high quality care and support throughout their lifetime, to optimise the control of their blood glucose, blood pressure and other risk factors for developing complications of diabetes (Department of Health [DH] 2001, 2008).

More recently, care of people with type 1 diabetes has focused on diabetes centres and patients require admission to hospital less often, unless particularly unwell. The central objective of care is to help the patient acquire the knowledge and skills needed to resume an independent lifestyle. The patient will usually be asked to attend the diabetes outpatient clinic at specified intervals or, if unable to do so, may be visited at home by the diabetes specialist nurse. This is essential for the ongoing care, treatment supervision and evaluation of progress of these patients.

Type 2 diabetes

Type 2 diabetes seems likely to have a multifactorial aetiology. Although these factors are not fully understood, they differ from those thought to cause type 1 diabetes.

Type 2 diabetes has a strong genetic component, in families and between racial groups. Glucose metabolism becomes less efficient from the third or fourth decade of life onwards and this deterioration accelerates in people over 60 years of age. Whilst this alteration in glucose tolerance may not in itself be pathological, when compounded by other factors it can contribute to the onset of symptoms of diabetes.

Tissue sensitivity to insulin may decline in type 2 diabetes. The result is that hyperglycaemia can occur even when the circulating levels of insulin are normal or raised. Several reasons have been suggested for the development of insulin resistance: these include resistance in peripheral tissues in obesity, the effects of ageing and the presence of anti-insulin antibodies in the blood.

Whatever the cause, the result is inefficient use of available insulin.

Specific factors in the development of type 2 diabetes

β cell deficiency There is a markedly reduced first phase insulin secretion in response to glucose and, in established diabetes, an attenuated second phase. Insulin pulsatility is also abnormal, thereby reducing tissue insulin sensitivity (Williams & Pickup 2004).

Obesity Obesity is known to induce insulin resistance in body cells. However, only a minority of obese people develop type 2 diabetes and only around 60% of people with the disorder are obese. Glucose tolerance decreases as weight increases and can be reversed as weight loss occurs. Fat distribution appears to be significant in that there is a relationship between central obesity and diabetes. Research by Wei et al (1997) indicates that waist circumference is the best central obesity-related predictor of type 2 diabetes, suggesting that distribution of body fat, especially abdominal localisation, is a more important determinant than total body fat (see Further reading, e.g. Ashwell 2009, Hadaegh et al 2006). Up to 80% of type 2 diabetes is preventable by adopting a healthy diet and increasing physical activity (International Diabetes Federation [IDF] 2008).

Racial and environmental factors There are wide geographical variations in the incidence of type 2 diabetes. The IDF estimates that in Europe in 2007, 8.4% of adults aged 20–79 had diabetes (IDF 2008). A study by Massó-González et al (2009) found that in the UK the incidence of type 2 diabetes increased during the period 1996 to 2005, while the incidence of type 1 diabetes remained comparatively steady during the same period. They also reported that more patients diagnosed with type 2 diabetes between 1996 and 2005 were obese (an increase from 46% to 56%). In certain societies, incidences of up to 40% have been reported, e.g. among the Pima Indians of North America and the Nauru Islanders of the Pacific, where obesity is also very common. These remarkably high prevalences are probably due to the exposure of genetically isolated, diabetes-predisposed populations to influences such as a 'Western' diet and reduced physical activity. The prevalence for diabetes for all age groups worldwide is predicted to be 4.4% in 2030 (Wild et al 2004).

PATHOPHYSIOLOGY

Type 2 diabetes usually presents in those over the age of 40 and most commonly in people over 60. The signs, symptoms and clinical features of type 2 diabetes, although still marked, are less severe than those of type 1 diabetes and are due to the more gradual onset and the effects of hyperglycaemia arising from a relative deficiency of insulin. There is still some insulin being secreted; as a result, ketogenesis is inhibited and, as the hyperglycaemia is less severe, dehydration is also much less common.

Clinical presentation The effects of a relative lack of insulin include:

- Hyperglycaemia-related symptoms – nocturia, polyuria and polydipsia may develop gradually. The patient, who is often obese, may initially be gratified to note that weight loss is occurring.
- Genital or oral fungal infections – candidal infections are common and result in the distressing symptoms of pruritus vulvae in the female and balanitis in the male. The sugar-rich urine around the genitalia appears to provide the microorganism with favourable conditions in which to multiply.
- Staphylococcal skin infections – these commonly result in boils and abscesses, and may provide the initial stimulus for the patient to visit their GP.
- Non-specific symptoms – such as tiredness and lethargy – are also frequently reported. The cause is uncertain, but altered fluid and electrolyte balance may be responsible. Visual disturbance may occasionally be reported, as hyperglycaemia may cause lens opacity and accommodation may be affected by alterations of the lens fluid.

Onset and progress of the disease At the time the patient first seeks medical attention, evidence of vascular and neurological complications such as proteinuria, sexual dysfunction, retinopathy and peripheral neuropathy may already have developed. Such patients have probably had asymptomatic diabetes with persistent hyperglycaemia for several years prior to diagnosis. A diagnosis will usually be made on the evidence of glycosuria and a fasting or random venous plasma blood glucose concentration of ≥ 7.0 mmol/L and ≥ 11.1 mmol/L, respectively.

Ketonuria is not a feature of type 2 diabetes, as ketogenesis is inhibited by the presence of even small amounts of insulin.

Asymptomatic glycosuria may be discovered as an incidental finding, e.g. during a routine medical examination. Such a finding would normally prompt capillary and then venous blood glucose analysis. In the absence of symptoms, these results should be confirmed by repeat testing on a different day.

The WHO (1999) has set glucose values for diagnosing diabetes (Table 5.4).

Table 5.4 Diagnostic glucose concentrations

DIAGNOSIS	VENOUS WHOLE BLOOD (MMOL/L)	CAPILLARY WHOLE BLOOD (MMOL/L)	VENOUS PLASMA BLOOD (MMOL/L)
Diabetes mellitus			
Fasting	≥ 6.1	≥ 6.1	≥ 7.0
2 h postprandial	≥ 10.0	≥ 11.1	≥ 11.1
Impaired glucose tolerance (IGT)			
Fasting and	<6.1 and	<6.1 and	<7.0 and
2 h postprandial	≥ 6.7	≥ 7.8	<11.1
Impaired fasting glycaemia (IFG)			
Fasting and	≥ 5.6 and <6.1	≥ 5.6 and <6.1	≥ 6.1 and <7.0
2 h postprandial	<6.7	<7.8	<7.8

In the absence of symptoms, abnormality in both 2 h postprandial and fasting blood sugar is required to establish the diagnosis of diabetes mellitus. The 2 h postprandial test should be performed following the oral glucose tolerance test using 75 g glucose load (WHO 1999).

Impaired glucose tolerance and impaired fasting glycaemia

Impaired glucose tolerance (IGT) and impaired fasting (hyper) glycaemia (IFG) are recognised as stages in the natural history of diabetes rather than as a class of diabetes (WHO 1999). It is not clear why some people may have blood glucose results at or just above the upper limit of normal. Inconclusive results in the absence of symptoms may not necessarily be judged abnormal. It is known that some people with IGT or IFG will go on to develop diabetes mellitus and that they may have a greater risk of developing atherosclerosis.

Onset and progress of the disease Although it is clearly desirable that people should be spared the negative consequences of being inappropriately labelled as 'having diabetes', they should nonetheless have access to regular medical screening. Health promotion should be carried out, usually by the practice nurse or the GP, or the patient may also be asked to attend a diabetes clinic for an annual review.

IGT has implications for women who are planning to conceive. Current evidence suggests that it is important to correct hyperglycaemia and ensure tight control of blood glucose prior to conception to reduce the risk of fetal abnormality (Williams, 2003). Pre-conception advice should be made available and the woman's blood glucose brought within normal limits before conception and closely monitored throughout pregnancy. This care may be provided at a combined diabetes obstetric clinic.

Diabetes mellitus secondary to other conditions

Pancreatitis and cancer of the pancreas (see Ch.4) may greatly reduce the number of functioning β cells and result in impaired insulin secretion. Chronic liver disease will have considerable consequences for the metabolism of nutrients. Glycogenesis and glycogenolysis may both be impaired and consequently hyper- and hypoglycaemia frequently feature in chronic disorders of the liver. Chronic renal failure can cause impaired glucose tolerance and insulin resistance, although the underlying mechanism by which this occurs remains unclear.

Some drugs, notably corticosteroids, have a diabetogenic effect. The thiazide group of diuretics have been known to worsen established diabetes and in some older patients may actually hasten the onset of the disease. Excess secretion or administration of glucocorticoids, aldosterone, catecholamines or growth hormone will have a diabetogenic effect and can result in hyperglycaemia. Diabetes may therefore be a feature of Cushing's syndrome/disease, phaeochromocytoma, primary aldosteronism and acromegaly (see Ch. 5, Part 1).

There are other rare genetic disorders which give rise to secondary diabetes (Williams & Pickup 2004). Friedreich's ataxia, an inherited disorder of balance and movement, is one example. Another is Wolfram syndrome with autosomal recessive inheritance. This disease is generally referred to as DIDMOAD (diabetes insipidus, diabetes mellitus, optic atrophy and deafness).

MANAGEMENT STRATEGIES IN DIABETES MELLITUS

Diabetes care in the UK and Europe has been strongly influenced by the St Vincent declaration (Krans et al 1992). Countries concerned pledged to deploy resources for its resolution and to intensify research into prevention and cure of diabetes and its complications.

Diabetes management requires a multidisciplinary approach. For patients who are not acutely ill at the time of diagnosis, management may be provided entirely within the community or outpatient setting. However, many patients are more acutely ill at the time of onset and require hospital care to allow close monitoring of the effects of early treatment.

The diabetes care team share common goals, each contributing expertise in accordance with the patient's individual needs. The patient is the most important member of the diabetes care team, and full participation by the patient is necessary to achieve the following aims:

- attaining and maintaining normoglycaemia (blood glucose within the normal range)
- monitoring response to therapy
- preventing and detecting the acute metabolic complications of diabetes
- preventing and detecting the chronic complications of diabetes
- facilitating self-care through education
- promoting social and psychological adjustment.

Attaining and maintaining normoglycaemia

There are three main therapeutic approaches:

- dietary therapy – nutritional advice
- non-insulin therapy
- insulin therapy.

Nutritional advice for people with diabetes

Appropriate dietary advice is essential in the effective management of diabetes. The aim is to give people with diabetes information to enable them to make informed choices about the type and quantity of food they eat. It is important that all newly diagnosed patients should be offered a consultation with a registered dietitian at the time of diagnosis. Dietitians are skilled in translating nutritional guidelines into practice. Dietary recommendations are the same as those given to the general population (see Ch. 21) (Box 5.7).

Carbohydrate

All food that contains carbohydrate (CHO) will cause blood glucose levels to rise. The extent of the glycaemic response (the rise in blood glucose after eating) caused by food varies. This is affected by the amount of food consumed, the source of the CHO such as glucose or starch, the cooking method and other components of the meal.

The glycaemic index (GI) explains some of the differences caused by different CHOs on blood glucose levels. It allows the glycaemic effect of foods to be ranked against a standard such as glucose (Box 5.8). Foods with a high GI cause a rapid rise in blood glucose levels. Lower GI foods cause a more gradual glycaemic response and if taken as part of a meal can lower the glycaemic effect of the whole meal (Dyson 2004).

Box 5.7 Reflection

Eating well

Eating a healthy balanced diet as recommended for the general population is also important in the management of both type 1 and type 2 diabetes and the prevention of complications.

Activities

- Access the resources below and consider the nutritional advice offered to people with type 1 and type 2 diabetes.
- Reflect on the benefits of such a diet, for example better blood glucose control, and discuss with your mentor how you might use the resources when educating people newly diagnosed with diabetes.

Resources

Diabetes UK 2009 Ten steps to eating well. For people with Type 1 diabetes. Available online http://www.diabetes.org.uk/Guide-to-diabetes/Food_and_recipes/Eating-well-with-Type-1-diabetes/Ten-steps-to-eating-well/

Diabetes UK 2009 Ten steps to eating well. For people with Type 2 diabetes. Available online http://www.diabetes.org.uk/Guide-to-diabetes/Food_and_recipes/Eating-well-with-Type-2-diabetes/Ten-steps-to-eating-well/

Box 5.8 Information

Glycaemic index (GI) examples

Low GI	
Porridge	Couscous
Most fruit	Sucrose
Granary bread	Full fat ice cream
Pasta	**High GI**
Beans	Cornflakes
Pulses	White/wholemeal bread
Yoghurt	Chips
Intermediate GI	Jelly babies
Croissants	Cornchips
Potatoes	Honey
Pineapple	Glucose

Table 5.5 Sources of fat

TYPE OF FAT	FOOD SOURCE
Saturated fat	Fatty meat, meat pies, sausages Butter, lard, suet, ghee, coconut oil, palm oil Cocoa butter – chocolate Cheese Cream Pastries, cakes, biscuits made with saturated fats Savoury snack foods
Monounsaturated fat	Olive oil Rapeseed oil Peanut oil (groundnut oil) Some soft margarines
Polyunsaturated fat	Sunflower oil and seeds Flaxseed oil and seeds Corn oil Soybean oil Some soft margarines Oily fish Poultry Eggs from hens fed a special diet

Sucrose (a disaccharide – ordinary table sugar) is no longer considered to be any more harmful to blood glucose levels than other CHOs. However, it is an empty calorie source, harmful for teeth and should be taken sparingly as part of a meal.

Fructose (a monosaccharide present in some fruit and vegetables and in honey). Fruit consumption should be encouraged as fructose has a low glycaemic effect. People with diabetes should be encouraged to eat five servings of fruit and vegetables per day. However, excessive fruit intake can significantly increase blood glucose levels and therefore a sensible intake level should be encouraged. These foods are a good source of soluble fibre, which is also found in oats, pulses, nuts and grains.

Carbohydrate restriction is not recommended but some measure of control may be discussed, particularly in those with type 1 diabetes. Historically, dietitians advised people to measure their intake in 10 g exchanges to rigidly control their intake. This became less common in the 1980s when advice focused more on healthy eating guidelines. Quantifying CHO is now being used more frequently in view of the Dose Adjustment for Normal Eating (DAFNE) project findings (DAFNE Study Group 2002). The DAFNE education programme teaches people to adjust their insulin injections to fit their lifestyle, instead of adjusting their lifestyle to a particular insulin regimen, thus improving glycaemic control and quality of life in people with type 1 diabetes. However, the emphasis is markedly different, with the educated patient adjusting the amount of insulin given for the amount of CHO consumed, irrespective of the source of CHO.

Fat

Fat intake should not be overlooked when providing dietary advice to people with diabetes. A reduction in intake is generally necessary for weight control. People with diabetes should generally be encouraged to eat less fat and, where possible, to choose fats from monounsaturated sources, e.g. olive oil (Table 5.5).

Weight management

Obesity increases insulin resistance and therefore correction of obesity can increase the sensitivity of cells to insulin. Weight reduction alone may bring the blood glucose down within normal limits. Weight management is particularly important in people with type 2 diabetes, where obesity is a well-recognised problem. Losing weight is notoriously difficult. Social attitudes can lead to overweight people feeling stigmatised. As a result, guilt or low self-esteem may affect the patient's response to dietary advice. Drugs for the treatment for obesity have been developed (orlistat, sibutramine) and must be used according to national guidelines (see Useful websites, e.g. British National Formulary, NICE, SMC).

Weight is not a sensitive indicator of glycaemic control. However, the negative significance of rapid weight loss accompanied by thirst, glycosuria and ketonuria should be recognised. Similarly, it can be a positive sign if the patient's weight is stable and within an acceptable range. Body mass index (BMI) calculation can provide a picture of the patient's weight in relation to their height and thereby an indication of whether they are overweight or obese (see Ch. 21). A patient is considered to be overweight if their BMI is $>25 \, \text{kg/m}^2$ and obese if it is $>30 \, \text{kg/m}^2$ (see p. 152 for information about monitoring central obesity). It is important that nurses involved in monitoring the patient's weight in the home, clinic or hospital adopt a sensitive approach. For hospital inpatients, weekly weighing should be adequate. Routine weighing at each outpatient clinic appointment is advisable. Frequency of self-weighing by a patient at home will be at the patient's discretion and in relation to the advice offered and the goals which have been set. On the whole, weighing more frequently than once a week is neither psychologically desirable nor valuable as a monitoring tool.

Advice on increasing physical activity should also be included.

Alcohol

It is not necessary to avoid alcohol completely with diabetes. As with the adult population in general, a maximum of 14 units of alcohol per week for women and 21 units for men should not be exceeded. Those treated with insulin should avoid hypoglycaemia when consuming alcohol by ensuring adequate CHO intake.

Non-insulin therapies

Non-insulin therapies are only effective if cells are capable of secreting some insulin. These forms of therapies are used exclusively for patients with type 2 diabetes.

In the absence of persistent symptoms, dietary treatment should continue for at least 3 months before drug therapy is commenced. Oral hypoglycaemic therapy would then be reserved for those with type 2 diabetes who have persistent hyperglycaemia despite a period of dietary adjustment (United Kingdom Prospective Diabetes Study Group (UKPDS) 1998a, Department of Health 2001, National Institute for Health and Clinical Excellence [NICE] 2009, SIGN 2010) (Table 5.6).

Sulphonylureas

Drugs such as gliclazide stimulate β cells of the pancreas to secrete more insulin in response to blood glucose levels, increase insulin sensitivity and reduce liver metabolism of insulin.

Side-effects The most common side-effect is hypoglycaemia. This can be minimised by starting on the lowest dose possible and gradually increasing the amount over a period of weeks. It is essential that both the patient and carers are aware of the risks of hypoglycaemia. Sulphonylureas should be taken 20–30 min before food. The relationship between exercise, medication and diet will form an important part of the patient education programme.

Weight gain, gastrointestinal disturbance and skin rash can occur. Facial flushing following alcohol ingestion can occur with chlorpropamide. The effect of sulphonylureas is potentiated by other protein-bound medication, e.g. warfarin. This interaction increases the amount of available sulphonylurea and may therefore cause hypoglycaemia.

Biguanides

The drug metformin reduces glucose absorption in the gut, reduces peripheral insulin resistance and inhibits liver gluconeogenesis. Guidelines recommend first-line use of metformin following UKPDS findings of a survival benefit in this group (UKPDS 1998a, SIGN 2010).

Side-effects Gastrointestinal upset is the most common. Medication-induced hypoglycaemia is very uncommon with biguanide therapy, as is vitamin B_{12} malabsorption. Lactic acidosis is a rare occurrence but should be noted and metformin is contraindicated in patients with renal, liver and severe cardiovascular disease or serious systemic illness.

Table 5.6 Non-insulin agents	
DRUG GROUPS AND EXAMPLES	**POINTS TO NOTE**
Sulphonylureas	
Gliclazide Glipizide Glimepiride Gliquidone Tolbutamide	Stimulation of β cells to produce insulin and increase insulin sensitivity
Chlorpropamide Glibenclamide	Avoid use in older people – risk of hypoglycaemia
Biguanides	
Metformin	Inhibition of liver gluconeogenesis. Increases peripheral uptake of insulin Treatment of choice for overweight patients with type 2 diabetes. Contraindicated in renal, liver and cardiac disease
Dipeptidyl peptidase 4 inhibitors (DPP-4 inhibitors)	
Sitagliptin Vildagliptin Vildagliptin/metformin	Do not need to be taken with food. Given twice daily
Glucagon-like peptide-1 (GLP-1) mimetics (similar glucoregulatory actions to those of the incretin GLP-1)	
Exenatide	Must be injected subcutaneously twice daily up to 1 hour before 2 meals in the day, at least 8 hours apart, i.e. breakfast and evening meal. Can cause hypoglycaemia when used with sulphonylureas. Contraindicated in severe gastrointestinal disease
Prandial glucose regulators	
Nateglinide Repaglinide	β cell stimulation. Shorter acting than sulphonylureas – fewer 'hypos'. Take only at meals
Thiazolidinediones	
Pioglitazone	Combats insulin resistance. Increases insulin sensitivity. Increases peripheral uptake of glucose. Reduces liver production. Contraindicated in heart failure and poor liver function. Used in conjunction with other agents
Alpha-glucosidase inhibitor	
Acarbose	Delays carbohydrate absorption. Poorly tolerated due to gastrointestinal side-effects

Dipeptidyl peptidase 4 inhibitors (DPP-4 inhibitors)

These are a relatively new form of oral agents, e.g. sitagliptin. They improve glycaemic control by increasing the levels of active incretin peptide hormones, e.g. glucagon-like peptide 1 (GLP-1), in the intestine. They can be used in combination with other oral hypoglycaemic agents.

Side-effects These include gastrointestinal disturbances, peripheral oedema and upper respiratory tract infection. They may cause hypoglycaemia if used with a sulphonylurea.

Glucagon-like peptide-1 (GLP-1) mimetics

GLP-1 mimetics, e.g. exenatide, increase the secretion of insulin from the pancreas on a glucose-dependent basis. Exenatide has similar glucoregulatory properties to the incretin hormone GLP-1 (Drucker et al 2008). These drugs are injected subcutaneously.

Side-effects Gastrointestinal disturbances are most common in the first few days of starting treatment and usually subside. If used with sulphonylureas, there may be a risk of hypoglycaemia. Other side-effects include decreased appetite, headache and increased sweating. Observe injection sites for any local reaction.

Prandial glucose regulators

These drugs, e.g. repaglinide, are designed to stimulate extra insulin release to coincide with meal digestion. They should be taken up to 15 min before each meal and are rapidly absorbed. As they are also quickly eliminated from the body the insulin effect is short lived, thus reducing the risk of hypoglycaemia.

Side-effects Side-effects are uncommon but can include gastrointestinal upset, nausea and skin rash.

Thiazolidinediones

The thiazolidinediones (glitazones), e.g. pioglitazone, tackle insulin resistance and act by increasing insulin sensitivity within the peripheral tissue, increasing peripheral glucose uptake and reducing liver glucose production. They are used in conjunction with other oral agents.

Side-effects can include weight gain, headache and fluid retention. Use of thiazolidinediones is therefore not advised in patients with cardiac failure or poor liver function.

Alpha-glucosidase inhibitor

The drug acarbose can be used alone or in combination with other oral agents. Acarbose acts by delaying the breakdown of starch and sucrose into monosaccharides which can be absorbed in the small intestine. The effect is to reduce the postprandial peak in blood glucose. Acarbose is poorly tolerated due to prominent side-effects and is now less commonly used.

Side-effects The most common side-effects are flatulence and diarrhoea.

Insulin therapy

In type 1 diabetes, insulin therapy is essential to maintain life, and will be required throughout life. Insulin cannot be given orally as its amino acid structure would be inactivated by digestive enzymes. Parenteral administration is absolutely necessary and usually takes the form of subcutaneous (s.c.) injection.

In type 2 diabetes, glycaemic control deteriorates as the condition progresses and 30% of patients will eventually require insulin therapy (UKPDS 1998a). Others may require insulin therapy during periods of stress or illness but this does not change the classification of diabetes.

The objectives of insulin therapy are to:

- maintain blood glucose within normal limits
- relieve hyperglycaemia-associated symptoms
- correct metabolic/biochemical disturbances
- prevent diabetes-associated complications.

In the past, all insulin preparations were derived from beef (bovine) and pork (porcine) sources. Recombinant DNA technology and other advanced techniques have resulted in the production of biosynthetic human insulin and purified or highly purified porcine and bovine insulin.

Types and duration of action

There are many insulin preparations on the market. These may be categorised as rapid-acting analogue, short-acting, intermediate-acting, long-acting (including long-acting analogue) and biphasic (Figure 5.9).

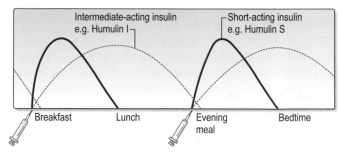

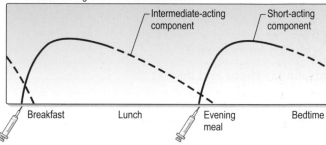

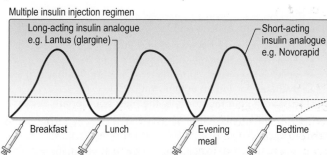

Figure 5.9 Duration of action for short-, intermediate- and long-acting insulins and rapid- and long-acting analogue insulins.

Rapid-acting analogue insulin (insulin lispro, insulin aspart, insulin glulisine) These are clear, colourless solutions. They have a rapid onset of action and therefore should be injected 0–15 min before meals. They are also licensed to be given up to 15 min after a meal.

Short-acting insulin (soluble insulin) These are clear solutions. The onset of action is delayed for 30 min when injected s.c.; their maximal effect occurs in 3–4 h but can last up to 8–10 h.

Intermediate-acting insulin (isophane insulin) These are cloudy in appearance. Their onset of effect is delayed for 1–2 h. The intermediate-acting insulins achieve maximum effect in 4–6 h and have a duration of action of 12–20 h.

Long-acting analogue insulin (insulin glargine, insulin detemir) This is slowly absorbed, providing a continuous level of insulin over a 24-h period. It is a true basal insulin with a peakless action profile, which therefore reduces the risk of hypoglycaemia. It may also be used in conjunction with oral hypoglycaemic agents in the treatment of people with type 2 diabetes.

Biphasic insulin These ready-mixed insulins include a combination of short-acting, or rapid-acting analogue and intermediate-acting insulin in set ratios. Examples include Humulin M3® and NovoMix 30® (insulin aspart and insulin aspart protamine).

Administering insulin

The overall aim in administering insulin therapy is to achieve the best possible control of blood glucose throughout the 24-h period. The treatment should mimic the physiological response to normal variations in blood glucose. Patients can self-administer insulin using an insulin injecting device in the form of a syringe or pen device with a pen needle attached (Box 5.9). There are also insulin pumps available to those who meet NICE guidance criteria for pump therapy. Self-administration of insulin can be quick and

discreet, enabling adaptability for the day-to-day changes in the patient's activity levels, eating pattern and lifestyle.

Timing and frequency of injections

Long-acting analogues must be administered once daily, every 24 hours. This can be at any time of the day to fit in with the patient's life. For many patients, twice-daily injections remain the preferred regimen. These are administered with breakfast and with evening meal. Older patients, who have perhaps been required to progress to insulin from diet and/or oral therapy, may be more willing to accept once-daily injections.

To mimic normal blood glucose fluctuations, a single injection of insulin with a 24-h period of action could be given once daily in combination with rapid-acting insulin with a short (4–5 h) duration of action, with each meal. This multiple injection system has considerable advantages, giving flexibility of mealtimes and meal size. This system is most effective if blood glucose levels are regularly monitored and patients are taught to adjust diet, exercise and insulin accordingly. It does, however, not suit everyone.

Injection sites

Insulin is given by s.c. injection. Common sites for injection are the upper thighs and the abdominal wall. The outer aspect of the upper arms and buttocks can also be used, but this may prove difficult when attempting to pinch up the skin. Overuse of one site can lead to lipohypertrophy, loss of sensitivity and impaired or erratic absorption of insulin. For this reason injection site rotation is advised (Figure 5.10).

Injection technique

Cleansing the skin with alcohol prior to injection is unnecessary. The site must be visibly clean. Insulin syringes and pen needles currently in use in the UK have a variety of needle lengths and gauges, and it is important to select the appropriate needle for the body weight of the patient to ensure a s.c. injection. A mound of skin should be gently pinched up to avoid intramuscular injection. The skin should not be pinched if a 4 mm, 5 mm or 6 mm needle is used. The syringe or pen device should be held as illustrated in the appropriate device leaflets and the needle inserted straight into the subcutaneous tissue at a 90° angle. The insulin should be injected steadily and the needle held in position for a further count of at least 6 s before withdrawing smoothly. (See Useful websites, e.g. BD Medical – Diabetes Care for information on injection technique and pen use.)

Box 5.9 Reflection

Insulin injections and devices

Some people newly diagnosed with type 1 diabetes, or people with type 2 diabetes who need to transfer to insulin therapy will be apprehensive about injecting insulin.

Activities

- Reflect on the aspects of injecting insulin that might cause people anxiety.
- Access the resource below and find out:
  - how 'needle phobia' is addressed
  - what devices (pens, auto-injectors, needle-free devices) are available for insulin administration.
- Discuss with your mentor how the most appropriate device can be selected for a person's circumstances.

Resource

Diabetes UK http://www.diabetes.org.uk/Guide-to-diabetes/Treatment__your_health/Treatments/Insulin/Worried_about_injecting/

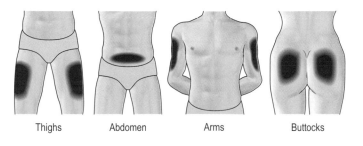

| Thighs | Abdomen | Arms | Buttocks |

Figure 5.10 Suitable injection sites for insulin.

Monitoring response to therapy

The methods used for monitoring glycaemic control include:

- glycated (glycosylated) haemoglobin (HbA_{1c})
- self blood glucose monitoring (SBGM)
- continuous glucose monitoring system (CGMS)
- blood ketone monitoring
- urinalysis
- body weight monitoring.

Glycated (glycosylated) haemoglobin estimation (HbA_{1c})

Glucose in solution is bound to the proteins of haemoglobin. The rate at which proteins bind to glucose is directly related to the current glucose concentration in the blood. It gives an indication of control over a period of time, normally 2–3 months, and not merely a one-off recording as in plasma glucose estimation. Anything which interferes with normal haemoglobin levels, such as haemorrhage or anaemia, could potentially distort glycated haemoglobin results. Similarly, conditions which influence serum albumin levels, such as renal or hepatic disease, may result in problems in interpreting glycated albumin results.

HbA_{1c} should be below 7.5% in patients with type 1 diabetes. In type 2 diabetes, individual targets should be set between 6.5% and 7.5%. Other risk factors such as vascular complications and hypoglycaemia risk should be taken into consideration. This result should be discussed with the patient, to be actively encouraged to manage their diabetes effectively (NICE 2009).

Changes to HbA_{1c} measurements

HbA_{1c} testing will be standardised and reported in mmol/mol (correct scientific value) in line with the International Federation of Clinical Chemists (IFCC) reference method. This change will occur worldwide. For example, an HbA_{1c} of 7% will now be reported as 53 mmol/mol. Most laboratories will give results in both mmol/mol and percentages from April 2011. (See Useful websites, e.g. International Diabetes Federation.)

Self blood glucose monitoring (SBGM)

SBGM is the most widely used method of testing glucose levels. It provides a simple and, if performed correctly, reliable method of monitoring glycaemic control. Results may be downloaded from a blood glucose meter or written into the patient's monitoring diary. Training by the diabetes specialist nurse or other trained health care professional must be given to the patient. Importantly patients should agree their individual target levels with the diabetes team; Diabetes UK (2009) offers some targets as a guide. Diabetes UK (2009) currently recommends that people with diabetes should keep blood glucose levels as near normal as possible (in the range of a person without diabetes, i.e. 3.5–5.5 mmol/L before meals [preprandial] and less than 8 mmol/L two hours after meals [postprandial]). (See Useful websites, e.g. Diabetes UK.)

Near-patient blood glucose testing in hospital requires a standardised system throughout, with a quality assurance programme in place involving internal and external quality control. Results are recorded on a chart and should be regularly monitored.

(See Useful websites for information on blood glucose meter systems.)

Advantages

Blood glucose monitoring offers increased patient involvement in diabetes management and helps to improve day-to-day glycaemic control. It is used by patients to adjust their insulin levels, assess if blood glucose level is acceptable for driving or exercise, and monitor the effect of certain amounts and types of food eaten (DAFNE 2002). It can also give warning of impending metabolic crisis and guide subsequent intervention.

Blood glucose meters are inexpensive and often provided by NHS diabetes clinics. Each model has different functions to suit the individual patient's capabilities. Some have integrated test strips with capillary-fill dosing, most have a large memory store for downloading results. Quality control solution is supplied with some meters to check the accuracy of the meter. For visually impaired individuals, there are talking meters. Intensive training is required from a diabetes specialist nurse in the use of these devices.

Disadvantages

Blood glucose monitoring requires a fair degree of manual dexterity, visual acuity, cognitive ability and motivation (Box 5.10). There may be cost implications for test strip prescriptions in some countries. However, a consensus statement (Owens et al 2005), offering guidelines as to the appropriateness of SBGM, has been published.

Frequency

For patients with type 1 diabetes, preprandial and pre-bedtime tests, with the occasional postprandial test, can provide important feedback and aid learning for all seriously motivated people with diabetes and can be an essential tool in achieving tight diabetic control (Holt & Kumar 2010).

Continuous glucose monitoring system (CGMS)

Some patients with excessively fluctuating blood glucose levels may require continuous glucose monitoring. This uses a sensor inserted under the skin in the abdomen, measuring

Box 5.10 Reflection

Monitoring blood glucose: physical problems

Think about some physical problems (such as arthritis affecting the hands, a tremor caused by Parkinson's disease or a stroke affecting the dominant hand) leading to poor manual dexterity that make it difficult for a patient who needs/wants to monitor blood glucose as part of managing their diabetes.

Activities

- Use the Useful websites to investigate whether there are blood glucose meters that meet the needs of people with poor manual dexterity. Discuss your findings with a Specialist Nurse or another member of the diabetes care team.

interstitial glucose every 10 seconds. This gives a 6-day profile of blood glucose. Results can be interpreted by the diabetes team and discussed with the patient, suggesting ways to improve glucose levels.

Blood ketone monitoring

The ketone body β-hydroxybutyrate can be measured with a blood ketone meter. It can be detected quickly and simply by using a blood ketone meter and test strips (the same principles as the blood glucose meter). Patients with newly diagnosed or established type 1 diabetes can be taught to test for blood ketones at home, in times of stress and illness in particular, along with 'sick day rules'. This is useful as insulin treatment can be altered to eliminate ketones with the assistance of the diabetes team. If ketone levels are too high, this can lead to DKA, requiring hospital admission. There is one meter available in the UK that measures both blood glucose and blood ketones (Optium Xceed™, Abbott Laboratories).

Urinalysis

Urine can be tested to detect the presence of glucose and ketones. However, with the increasing use of blood glucose meters for glycaemic control, the use of urine testing is declining. Testing the urine for glucose is not completely accurate as it does not reflect the current blood glucose level. If there is any reason to suspect that the patient is suffering from, or is at risk of, episodes of hypoglycaemia, then instruction in blood glucose monitoring should be considered. Urine ketone testing can aid in initial diagnosis of type 1 diabetes, or to monitor ketone production in illness or stress.

A potential renal complication (diabetic nephropathy) associated with diabetes can be detected by the presence of very small amounts of albumin in the urine (microalbuminuria). Commercial dipstick strips are available that detect the low level of albumin that would not be revealed by a standard dipstick.

Chemically impregnated dipsticks are the usual means of screening for various conditions on admission to hospital. The manufacturer's instructions for use and storage of urine testing materials must be followed precisely. Results of urinalysis should be accurately recorded in the appropriate chart.

Body weight monitoring

See nutritional advice for people with diabetes.

Preventing and detecting acute metabolic complications of diabetes

The acute metabolic complications arising from diabetes are:

- diabetic ketoacidosis (DKA)
- hyperosmolar hyperglycaemic state (HHS)
- hypoglycaemia.

Diabetic ketoacidosis

DKA is characterised by uncontrolled hyperglycaemia and uncontrolled lipolysis caused by an insulin deficiency, accompanied by dehydration and acidosis. Individuals with longstanding diabetes can usually recognise the signs and symptoms of impending ketoacidosis and will seek medical help at a much earlier stage in its development. Those newly diagnosed with type 1 diabetes are taught how to recognise and respond to indications of hyperglycaemia and ketoacidosis.

Epidemiology

In the UK, DKA is the most common cause of death for people with diabetes below the age of 20 years. There is very little recent research showing the incidence of DKA, although it is thought that this has not declined significantly through the decades despite increasing knowledge and more sophisticated management in specialist units (Dave et al 2004). These patients will be at risk of cerebral oedema, and must be managed in a high dependency environment.

Aetiology

Newly presenting diabetes may lead to DKA where there may have been a delay in diagnosis. In patients with established diabetes, DKA can be precipitated by infection, myocardial infarction, stroke or physical or emotional trauma, as these increase stress hormone secretion. Stress hormones raise the blood glucose and increase insulin requirements. DKA is caused by an inadequate dosage of insulin being taken during intercurrent illness or other major stress, or by insulin being omitted altogether. Inadequate concordance with treatment regimens can be a particular contributing factor, often associated with repeated hospital admissions.

PATHOPHYSIOLOGY AND PRESENTATION

Symptoms of DKA are a consequence of the combined effect of insulin lack and increased secretion of catabolic, counter-regulatory stress hormones. As a result, two major biochemical disturbances occur simultaneously:

- Increased lipolysis results in the formation of ketone bodies which are weak acids and cause metabolic acidosis
- Accelerated gluconeogenesis and glycogenolysis cause hyperglycaemia, which in turn results in osmotic diuresis, dehydration and electrolyte imbalance with a loss of sodium (hyponatraemia) and potassium (hypokalaemia).

Note that hyperkalaemia may be evident in the very early stages due to severe metabolic acidosis, but once rehydration is underway, hypokalaemia is usual and may be severe.

Box 5.11 provides further information about the development, presentation and effects of DKA.

MEDICAL MANAGEMENT

Reversing hyperglycaemia Short-acting, soluble insulin is administered to lower blood glucose. Initially, 50 units of short acting insulin in 50 mL of sodium chloride 0.9% (1 unit/mL) are administered intravenously via syringe driver infusion at 6 units/h. The insulin dose will later be varied in accordance with the blood glucose level; the aim should be a gradual reduction in blood glucose over a period of 12 hours.

Capillary blood glucose should be checked hourly and venous blood glucose and plasma potassium are measured at appropriate intervals by the laboratory.

Box 5.11 Information

The development of diabetic ketoacidosis

The key precipitating factors for DKA are inadequate supply of insulin and increased demand for insulin, often in combination. These are often triggered by:

- newly presenting type 1 diabetes
- infection, especially respiratory, urinary or abscesses
- trauma or surgery
- severe illness, e.g. myocardial infarction or stroke
- failure to take sufficient insulin – this may be accidental or deliberate. Patients can discover that ketosis will cause rapid weight loss.

As a result of reduced insulin and increased stress hormone levels, cells will be unable to utilise glucose, glycogen will be converted to glucose, gluconeogenesis provides glucose from non-CHO sources (such as protein) and lipolysis occurs, releasing ketone bodies. The combined effects of these events are:

- hyperglycaemia and hyperketonaemia
- osmotic diuresis
- fluid and electrolyte imbalance (see Ch. 20)
- catabolism/wasting
- acid–base imbalance – acidaemia caused by the process of metabolic acidosis (see Ch. 20).

As a result the patient will present with the following signs and symptoms:

Presentation – signs and symptoms

- Polyuria progressing to oliguria
- Polydipsia
- Lethargy/weakness
- Nausea/vomiting
- Abdominal colic
- Muscle cramps
- Blurred vision
- Hyperglycaemia
- Glycosuria
- Ketonuria
- Ketone breath (sweet 'pear drop' fruity odour)
- Weight loss
- Electrolyte imbalance – hypokalaemia, hyponatraemia
- Hypotension and tachycardia
- Acidaemia (a high level of acid (hydrogen ions) in the blood
- Rapid, deep (Kussmaul's) respirations
- Evidence of intercurrent infection/illness
- Skin flushed and warm
- Hypothermia may develop
- Confusion and drowsiness progressing to coma.

Complications

- Cerebral oedema
- Adult/acute respiratory distress syndrome (ARDS)
- Thromboembolism.

Rehydration Rapid restoration of circulating fluid volume is necessary, followed by gradual correction of the interstitial and intracellular deficit. Sodium chloride (NaCl) 0.9% is given by i.v. infusion with potassium chloride (KCl) included if hypokalaemia is present or anticipated (see below). When blood glucose falls to approximately 10 mmol/L, the sodium chloride is replaced by i.v. glucose 5%, but the insulin infusion continues (British National Formulary 2009).

Replacing potassium Derangements in plasma potassium can vary. Hyperkalaemia may be evident in the very early stages due to severe metabolic acidosis, but once rehydration is underway, hypokalaemia is usual and may be severe. Intravenous potassium chloride is prescribed in accordance with the blood biochemistry. This must be administered by a regulated infusion delivery system.

Monitoring The patient will be closely monitored for the following:

Cardiac monitoring should be commenced and a 12-lead ECG is performed to detect cardiac arrhythmias associated with an imbalance of serum potassium.
Monitoring acidaemia (caused by metabolic acidosis) Arterial blood gases (ABGs) are checked initially, but venous bicarbonate levels are adequate for monitoring 1- to 2-hourly thereafter.
Monitoring fluid and electrolyte imbalance Blood urea, electrolytes and osmolality.

Response to fluid and potassium replacement Blood pressure and pulse are measured hourly as a guide to blood volume. Central venous pressure (CVP) or pulmonary artery occlusion pressure (PAOP) (also known as pulmonary capillary wedge pressure [PCWP]) may be initiated and measured in the older patient or those with renal or heart failure.
Monitoring ketosis and renal function Urine is tested for glucose, ketones and protein.
Oxygen therapy Oxygen will be prescribed and administered in accordance with blood gas results.
Nasogastric aspiration may be necessary to protect the airway if the patient is vomiting, drowsy or unconscious.
Investigating underlying infection A chest X-ray is performed. Blood cultures, full blood count, urine and sputum specimens are sent to microbiology.
Observation of vital signs Temperature, pulse, blood pressure, pulse oximetry, colour and respiration are recorded hourly. Fluid intake and output is measured and recorded.

Additional therapy which may be required in the management of DKA includes:

Alkaline – sodium bicarbonate This is not routinely used as it may exacerbate tissue hypoxia and hypokalaemia. As overcorrection may result in alkalosis, sodium bicarbonate is usually reserved for the treatment of very severe acidosis, and then only if the patient does not respond to adequate treatment with fluids and insulin.

Broad-spectrum antibiotics These may be given only if infection is suspected.

Anticoagulants Low-dose heparin 5000 IU s.c. twice daily may be given as standard venous thromboembolism prophylaxis.

Urinary catheterisation It may be necessary to facilitate the hourly measurement of urinary output as severe dehydration carries a risk of acute renal failure. However, catheterisation should be avoided if possible because of the risk of urinary tract infection (see p. 168).

▷ Nursing management and health promotion: diabetic ketoacidosis

The biochemical disruption of DKA is profound and life threatening. Each patient admitted with DKA will have unique problems and needs. The newly admitted patient with DKA is vulnerable in a variety of ways. Once the patient's condition is stable, every effort should be made to establish the cause of DKA and, where appropriate, the patient should be referred to the diabetes specialist nurse to discuss any changes to medication and issues of self-management in an effort to prevent recurrence. For many patients, however, the experience of DKA is what first makes them aware that they have diabetes.

Priorities for nursing care will be strongly influenced by the prescribed medical therapy and the need for complex monitoring (see above) and many hospitals have adopted DKA protocols to ensure fluids and insulin are initiated for these patients within a certain timeframe, and ongoing management is monitored.

Whilst the nurse must draw upon technical skills in such a situation, it is vitally important to maintain a holistic approach to care. The nurse should be sensitive to the vulnerability of the patient and try to accommodate individual needs when planning and implementing care.

Katie's story and Part 1 of her Nursing Care Plan for the first 24 h after admission is provided as an example of how a patient may present with severe DKA and how nursing priorities may be met following admission and until consciousness is regained (Box 5.12). Although Katie was unconscious on admission, the vast majority of patients presenting with DKA will not be unconscious.

Part 2 of Katie's Nursing Care Plan is presented as a Critical thinking question on the companion website and provides an opportunity for you to complete the remaining nursing considerations and related care.

 See website Critical thinking question 5.3

Further information relevant to the subsequent care of a patient with DKA is provided with that required by a patient with HHS (see pp. 164–165).

Hyperosmolar hyperglycaemic state (HHS)

HHS refers to the serious metabolic disruption characterised by marked hyperglycaemia (>33 mmol/L) in the absence of diabetic ketoacidosis (DKA) in addition to high serum osmolarity. It was previously known as hyperosmolar non-ketotic coma (HONK). However, it is recognised that a minor degree of ketosis and acidosis could also occur, hence the revision of the term hyperglycaemic hyperosmolar non-ketotic state or coma.

PATHOPHYSIOLOGY

HHS is a consequence of relative deficiency of insulin in conjunction with the rise in counter-regulatory stress hormones (cortisol, adrenaline, glucagon and growth hormone) with the resultant increase in liver glucose output and decreased peripheral glucose uptake. Rise in blood glucose levels leads to glycosuria, osmotic diuresis and dehydration with ensuing hyperosmolarity and hypernatraemia. The underlying reason for the lack of ketosis in HHS remains unclear. HHS typically presents in individuals with type 2 diabetes and therefore patients tend to be older than those with DKA. Unlike DKA, osmotic symptoms could have evolved over several days or weeks. Mental obtundation (blunting, reduced alertness and pain sensation) or altered consciousness is more frequent due to hyperosmolarity. Focal neurological signs or seizures may be a clinical feature in some patients. Physical examination reveals signs of dehydration, tachycardia and hypotension.

ℹ️ Box 5.12 Information

Katie's story and part 1 of her nursing care plan

Katie is a lively 18-year-old and the eldest of three children. She lives with her family but is soon to leave home to start university some 30 miles away.

Katie and her two brothers have recently had gastroenteritis. The boys are now fully fit but Katie is far from well. She has been passing an excessive amount of urine and is constantly thirsty. She has lost weight and has recently been complaining of feeling tired all the time.

This morning she is very drowsy. Her skin feels hot and dry and she looks flushed. She has vomited several times and has complained of abdominal pain and cramps in her limbs. Her breath has a peculiar sweet smell and her mouth is very dry. She has also been complaining of blurred vision.

Her parents are alarmed and have called the GP to request an urgent visit. Alerted by the 'acetone breath', her symptoms and the history of recent illness, the GP checks Katie's capillary blood glucose and finds it to be greater than the upper limit on his blood glucose meter (33.3 mmol/L). She is too drowsy to produce a urine specimen to check for ketones but the GP is in little doubt about the diagnosis. An ambulance is summoned and Katie and her parents are taken to hospital. The ward is alerted to expect an unconscious patient with DKA.

On admission, Katie is acutely ill and has complex care requirements. A nurse who has the appropriate levels of knowledge and skill is assigned to care for her. She has prepared for Katie's admission and will subsequently assess her nursing needs and plan and evaluate her care.

Part 1 of Nursing Care Plan for Katie during the first 24 h after admission

NURSING CONSIDERATIONS	ACTION	RATIONALE	EVALUATION
Impaired consciousness	• Position and support Katie in semi-prone or lateral position • Keep artificial airway in position until voluntarily expelled • Perform oropharyngeal suction if secretions are audible • Provide nasogastric (NG) aspiration • Continuously monitor colour, pulse oximetry and respiration • Administer oxygen as prescribed, ensuring that fire safety rules are observed • Monitor neurological status hourly. Record/report findings	To prevent asphyxia and prevent aspiration of secretion/vomitus Due to unconscious state and recent vomiting To correct hypoxia and prevent oxygen combustion To detect change in conscious level	Skin colour and respirations are normal Risk factors eliminated Blood gases improving Katie is progressively more responsive
Hyperglycaemia and ketonaemia	• Administer prescribed short-acting insulin i.v. by infusion pump • Monitor capillary blood glucose hourly: record/report findings	To correct hyperglycaemia and ketonaemia To evaluate response to insulin therapy and prevent hypoglycaemia	Trends indicate blood glucose returning towards the normal range
Fluid deficit/replacement	• Administer i.v. fluids as prescribed. Observe venepuncture site for redness, swelling or extravasation. Record all fluids in fluid balance chart • Monitor CVP, BP, breathing, temperature: observe neck veins, skin colour and urine volume • Catheterisation usually prescribed if unconsciousness persists and if patient is oliguric • Test urine hourly for ketones: record results	To correct hypovolaemia To monitor effects of fluid replacement To monitor renal function and detect renal insufficiency (urine <30 mL/h)	No discomfort or swelling of venepuncture site Vital signs are returning to normal ranges Urine volume >30 mL/h Ketonuria diminishing
Electrolyte imbalance/replacement	• Observe effects of potassium replacement; provide continuous cardiac monitoring • Report tall peaked T wave on ECG (indicates hyperkalaemia) • Report flattened or inverted T wave (indicates hypokalaemia) • REPORT ECG CHANGES PROMPTLY	Overzealous potassium replacement can cause ventricular fibrillation, and cardiac arrest Persistent hypokalaemia due to inadequate potassium replacement can result in heart block, which may lead to cardiac arrest	Potassium should be 3.3–4.7 mmol/L Cardiac monitor should display normal tracing
Probable current infection/potential risk of infection	• Collect throat swab, catheter specimen of urine and, when consciousness returns, a specimen of sputum. Monitor TPR. Take venous blood specimen for culture and full blood count • Administer prescribed antibiotics and note/report side-effects • Reduce risks of infection by high standards of nursing care (e.g. personal, hand and catheter hygiene)	To detect/monitor current infection To safely administer therapy To prevent healthcare-associated infection	Specimen analysis. Blood culture results and TPR normal Patient infection-free

The commonest precipitating factor of HHS is infection. Other precipitating factors include myocardial infarction, stroke, and non-concordance with treatment, pancreatitis or medications particularly corticosteroid therapy. Mortality rate remains high (15%), reflecting in many cases the underlying causes and the advanced age at presentation.

MEDICAL MANAGEMENT

Insulin therapy and blood glucose monitoring Insulin infusion of 50 units of soluble insulin in 50 mL of sodium chloride 0.9% should be commenced. High doses of insulin are rarely needed. An insulin rate of 0.3 U/h is reasonable although the rate may have to be reduced further if the fall of blood glucose is too rapid. Capillary blood glucose monitoring should be performed hourly to monitor response to insulin and also to avoid hypoglycaemia. However, capillary blood glucose measurement may not be accurate in severe hyperglycaemia and dehydration. Therefore, venous samples should be sent to the laboratory during the initial phase of treatment.

Rehydration The fluid deficit is considerable with estimated fluid deficit of 8–12 L. Fluid replacement in HHS should be slower and must be approached with a degree of caution taking into consideration coexisting conditions and the age of the patient.

0.9% sodium chloride is the most appropriate initial fluid. Colloid should be considered in hypotensive patients with systolic blood pressure <100 mmHg. If plasma sodium is higher than 155 mmol/L after initial fluid replacement, 0.45% sodium chloride should be considered. 5% dextrose should be initiated once blood glucose is less than <15 mmol/L. 0.9% saline should be continued at a slower rate to complete rehydration.

Replacing potassium Potassium replacement should commence once hyperkalaemia is excluded or reversed with rehydration and insulin therapy. Hyperosmolarity causes a shift of potassium from within the cells to the extracellular space.

Cardiac monitoring should be commenced and a 12-lead ECG is performed to detect cardiac arrhythmias associated with serum potassium lack or excess.

Oxygen therapy This will be administered in accordance with blood gas results.

Monitoring level of consciousness This is vitally important as there is a risk of a stroke (cerebral thrombosis) and cerebral oedema. Cerebral oedema can develop with rapid fall in osmolality, particularly with the use of 0.45% sodium chloride.

Additional therapy which may be required in the management of HHS includes:

Anticoagulants Low-dose heparin 5000 IU s.c. twice daily may be given as standard venous thromboembolism prophylaxis.

Urinary catheterisation It may be necessary to facilitate the hourly measurement of urinary output as severe dehydration carries a risk of acute renal failure. However, catheterisation should be avoided if possible because of the risk of urinary tract infection (see p. 168).

Nasogastric tube to protect the airway if the patient is unconscious or drowsy and vomiting.

Treatment of the coexisting morbidity or the underlying precipitating factors

Nursing management and health promotion: subsequent care in DKA and HHS

When the patient is alert and able to respond, the focus of care will change. The nurse will work with the patient, the dietitian and the medical staff to stabilise blood glucose and to monitor the effects of therapy. The subsequent care of the patient with a hyperglycaemic crisis, whether due to DKA or HHS, will be similar in many respects. Appropriate nursing interventions will be required to ensure the patient's safety and comfort, such as meeting hygiene needs. The patient is likely to be vulnerable due to an impaired level of consciousness, dehydration, electrolyte imbalance, the hazards of immobility and diabetes-associated risk factors. The level of consciousness in HHS is important as there is a risk of cerebral thrombosis due to combined effects of immobility, dehydration and diabetes-associated atherosclerosis. A patient with DKA may not necessarily be unconscious. The nurse should promptly report any evidence of deterioration in the patient's level of consciousness or any neurological function (see Ch. 9).

Restoration of self-care The diabetes specialist nurse, ward nurses, dietitian and medical staff will initiate the process of preparing the patient to assume responsibility for self-care, along with the contribution made by the community nurses and GP once the patient returns home.

Patient education The newly diagnosed patient will require information about how a balance between activity, food and medication can be achieved with the help of frequent blood glucose monitoring. This is especially important for patients with type 1 diabetes.

Once the crisis has passed, perhaps the most important aspect of care is to prevent further episodes of DKA or HHS. This involves identifying the events which led up to the crisis and discussing with the patient where action might have been taken to avert the crisis or obtain help at an earlier stage. Glycated haemoglobin estimation can provide useful information about glycaemic control over the preceding weeks, as can the patient's record of blood glucose or urinalysis results.

Providing psychological support The experience of a hyperglycaemic crisis can cause great distress, not only to the patient but also to family and friends. Adopting a warm empathic approach and accepting the fears of the patient is important if trust and rapport are to be established. The nurse should first ascertain the level of the person's existing knowledge and provide essential information using brief, clear explanations, checking that these are understood. Access to medical staff and information about the ward should be provided.

It is all too easy to be wise after the event and it is unhelpful for the patient to feel that they were to blame for any episode of DKA or HHS. The main aims should be to help the patient understand their diabetes and have confidence in its management; therefore time should be spent re-assessing their knowledge and addressing any issues which may help to prevent further episodes of illness. If severe underlying emotional distress or disturbance has precipitated the metabolic crisis, then the patient's difficulties may need to be sensitively explored. In accordance with the patient's wishes, appropriate counselling facilities may be provided. The newly diagnosed patient will require emotional support in meeting the immediate practical demands imposed by the condition. Information about the services and publications provided by Diabetes UK can be very useful.

Hypoglycaemia

Hypoglycaemia is a common complication of insulin treatment and occurs when blood glucose falls below 4 mmol/L. Of people with insulin-treated diabetes, 25–30% suffer one or more severe hypoglycaemic episodes every year (Williams & Pickup 2004).

There are several causes of hypoglycaemia. The three main causes are:

- excess insulin
- insufficient food
- increased exercise/activity.

Box 5.13 outlines the classification, causes and risk factors for hypoglycaemia.

Box 5.13 Information

Hypoglycaemia: classification, causes and risk factors

Classification

- *Asymptomatic* – biochemical hypoglycaemia without symptoms
- *Mild* – easily recognised and corrected by the patient
- *Moderate* – patient conscious but requiring help from others
- *Severe (leading to loss of consciousness)* – cerebral function severely affected by glucose lack

Causes

- Excess insulin
- Wrong type of insulin
- Inappropriate combination of insulin
- Excess dosage of oral sulphonylureas
- Delayed or missed meal
- More than usual amount of exercise
- Alcohol ingestion, especially when hungry
- Stress, such as hypothermia

Risk factors

- Impaired awareness of hypoglycaemia
- Strict glycaemic control
- Excess alcohol consumption
- Drug misuse

PATHOPHYSIOLOGY AND PRESENTATION

Symptoms are idiosyncratic, developing over a very short period of time (5–15 min).

Endocrine/autonomic response Glucagon and counter-regulatory hormones are secreted in response to falling blood glucose and act to restore blood glucose to normal. Activation of the autonomic nervous system in response to the stress of hypoglycaemia provokes autonomic symptoms of hypoglycaemia (MacAuley et al 2001). These hormones potentiate the effects of the sympathetic nervous system to cause the following symptoms:

- pounding heart and palpitations
- sweating
- trembling
- sensation of hunger
- sensation of anxiety.

Central nervous system response As brain cells are unable to metabolise alternatives to glucose for energy, a fall below the normal blood glucose will cause neuroglycopenic symptoms, including:

- lack of concentration
- dizziness
- unsteady gait
- slurred speech
- tingling around the lips.

Other non-specific symptoms, including headache and nausea, can occur. In addition, observers may notice abnormalities such as:

- pallor
- irrational behaviour
- muscle twitching/seizures
- extreme drowsiness or coma.

Some of these symptoms and signs could, with disastrous consequences, be mistakenly attributed to excess intake of alcohol.

Loss of sensitivity to symptoms Recently diagnosed patients may rely on autonomic symptoms such as sweating, tremor and pounding heart to alert them to a fall in blood glucose. However, after some years, patients may become less sensitive to these symptoms and come to rely on neuroglycopenic features to alert them to impending hypoglycaemia.

In longstanding insulin-treated diabetes, perception of the onset of symptoms of hypoglycaemia may become blunted, due to autonomic neuropathy or the effect of intensified insulin treatment (Williams & Pickup 2004). The patient may remain asymptomatic even when the blood glucose falls below 2 mmol/L, although at this level some signs may be obvious to others. This is known as impaired awareness of hypoglycaemia. Symptoms can also be masked by the following:

- Alcohol – if the patient is known to have consumed alcohol or smells of alcohol, this can lead to mistaking hypoglycaemia for intoxication, particularly as many symptoms and clinical features are similar.
- Ageing – in older people hypoglycaemia may cause neurological disturbances and the presenting symptoms

can be mistaken for failing mental function or transient ischaemic attacks (cerebrovascular disease).

- Time of day – hypoglycaemia during sleep can be asymptomatic. It is often not detected although features such as night sweats, restlessness, nightmares, snoring and headaches on waking may give the patient an indication of its occurrence. Rebound hyperglycaemia can occur and is attributed to an increase in the release of counter-regulatory hormones during the night to correct the hypoglycaemia. This is known as the Somogyi phenomenon.

- Sulphonylurea-induced hypoglycaemia – chlorpropamide and glibenclamide, even at normal therapeutic doses, have been implicated in severe, prolonged hypoglycaemic coma. This risk is increased in older people, particularly when they may be unwell and not eating, and in those with poor renal function. Subsequent prolonged hypoglycaemia may be fatal.

MEDICAL MANAGEMENT

Treatment of hypoglycaemia is simple and the effects are usually dramatic and gratifying. Nevertheless, the risks posed by hypoglycaemia and the importance of early detection and intervention must be stressed.

Hypoglycaemia can be treated with oral carbohydrate, s.c. or i.m. glucagon, or i.v. glucose depending on the stage and severity.

The conscious patient should be given rapidly absorbed glucose as a glucose drink or as sweets, followed by a more gradually absorbed form of carbohydrate, e.g. glucose tablets or a glass of fruit juice, followed by biscuits or a sandwich. Hypoglycaemia can recur if food is not consumed after initial treatment with glucose.

The confused or drowsy patient If the patient cannot eat or drink safely, glucagon by i.m. injection can be given. This will have the effect of raising the blood glucose. Where possible, relatives should be taught how to administer glucagon.

The unconscious patient Medical help should always be sought for the unconscious patient, although if hypoglycaemia is known to be the problem, glucagon i.m. should be given while the paramedic or doctor is awaited and the patient should be placed in the recovery position until consciousness returns. Nothing should be given orally whilst the patient is unconscious (MacKinnon 2002).

If glucagon is unavailable, or fails to bring a response within 10–15 min, i.v. dextrose in a dose of 30–50 mL of glucose 50% is required, which will usually raise the blood glucose sufficiently for consciousness to be regained. When coma persists, hospital admission will be necessary.

The hospitalised patient with hypoglycaemia Unconscious hypoglycaemia in the hospitalised patient may be treated by i.v. dextrose as first-line treatment. Venous blood must be taken for laboratory estimation of blood glucose. Continuous i.v. infusion of dextrose 10–20% will be commenced and the patient's response monitored by regular measurement of blood glucose. Approximately 1–2% of patients with hypoglycaemic coma fail to respond promptly to parenteral therapy. For these patients, other causes of coma such as

alcohol or drug overdose, hypothermia or cerebral haemorrhage should be excluded. Cerebral oedema can accompany prolonged hypoglycaemia; an i.v. infusion of mannitol (a hyperosmotic fluid that acts as an osmotic diuretic) may be required and oxygen therapy administered.

▷ Nursing management and health promotion: hypoglycaemia

In hypoglycaemic coma the period of unconsciousness and extreme vulnerability tends to be short. The nurse must:

- ensure the airway is clear
- monitor conscious level
- administer prescribed therapy
- monitor capillary blood glucose
- explore the possible cause of the hypoglycaemic coma
- provide information and encouragement for the patient to help improve diabetes management.

The acute metabolic complications of diabetes vary in cause, severity and outcome. All indicate a lack of stability of diabetes management requiring further assessment and investigation. Modification of treatment or lifestyle with the assistance of the diabetes team should be offered.

Preventing and detecting the chronic complications of diabetes

The Diabetes Control and Complications Trial (DCCT) conducted in the early 1990s (Diabetes Control and Complications Research Group 1993) is considered to be one of the most important pieces of diabetes research in recent years. It demonstrated that tight control of blood glucose prevented or delayed the onset of complications in type 1 diabetes, particularly retinopathy, neuropathy and nephropathy. However, the risk of severe hypoglycaemic attacks increased three-fold.

In 1998, the United Kingdom Prospective Diabetes Study Group (UKPDS) reported their findings in relation to the reduction of long-term complications in patients with type 2 diabetes. It was found that, through tight control of blood glucose and maintenance of blood pressure within normal limits, the risk of deaths related to diabetes could be reduced. Long-term complications of diabetes such as heart disease and stroke and the loss of sight and kidney damage could also be reduced (UKPDS 1998a,b).

Chronic complications of diabetes mellitus have important implications for the planning of nursing care. Whatever the setting, the nurse should carefully assess the individual's nursing needs, giving special consideration to risks associated with impaired circulation and sensation, increased risk of infection and delayed healing. Recognition of these risk factors will enable care to accommodate the patient's particular vulnerabilities and will help to ensure that suitable educational support is provided.

This section outlines the following chronic complications associated with diabetes:

- atherosclerosis (see Ch. 2)
- cardiovascular disease (see Ch. 2)

- cerebrovascular disease (see Ch. 9)
- diabetic retinopathy (see Ch. 13)
- diabetic nephropathy (see Ch. 8)
- diabetic neuropathy.

Atherosclerosis

Although atherosclerosis is not peculiar to diabetes, it is known that myocardial infarction, stroke and peripheral vascular disease leading to gangrene are relatively frequent complications and are major causes of death in people with diabetes. Atherosclerosis develops at a much younger age in people with diabetes. This is most noticeable in females.

Both types of diabetes carry increased risk, but those with type 2 diabetes show the strongest tendency to develop atherosclerosis. This is potentially due to age-related factors and the effects of longstanding asymptomatic hyperglycaemia prior to diagnosis. In type 1 diabetes, microvascular disease such as retinopathy usually precedes evidence of atherosclerosis.

Aetiology

Up to 70% of adults with type 2 diabetes have raised blood pressure and more than 70% have abnormal cholesterol levels (Department of Health 2001). Risk factors for coronary artery disease are (Kirby 2003):

- increased concentrations of low density lipoprotein (LDL) cholesterol
- decreased concentrations of high density lipoprotein (HDL) cholesterol
- hypertension
- hyperglycaemia
- smoking.

People with diabetes should focus on managing these risk factors.

Onset and progress of the disease

The development and vascular distribution of atherosclerosis in diabetes are similar to that found in the non-diabetic population, except the more severe peripheral arterial involvement which may affect the lower limbs of some people with diabetes.

Cardiovascular disease

Compared with the general population, diabetes in men is associated with a two- to three-fold risk of developing coronary heart disease. In premenopausal women this is increased to four to five times the risk if the woman has diabetes.

Myocardial infarction

Atherosclerosis of the coronary arteries causes narrowing which can impair oxygen delivery to the myocardium, resulting in angina pectoris or myocardial infarction (MI). Due to the effects of autonomic neuropathy the patient with diabetes may develop a cardiac arrhythmia and may have a 'silent' (painless) MI. Indeed, MI is more often fatal in people with diabetes compared with MI in those without diabetes (Stevens et al 2004).

Cerebrovascular disease

The incidence of stroke in patients with diabetes is also high, and mortality following stroke is increased compared to the non-diabetic population. Hypertension is probably the most important of those factors which contribute to the development of atherosclerosis.

Retinopathy

Diabetic retinopathy is one of the leading causes of blindness in people aged between 30 and 65 years in industrialised countries (Frier & Fisher 2006). By 20 years after the onset of diabetes, almost all patients with type 1 diabetes and over 60% of patients with type 2 diabetes will have some degree of retinopathy.

Retinopathy results from changes in the basement membrane of small blood vessels of the retina (retinal microangiopathy) and can take two forms:

- background (non-proliferative) retinopathy including maculopathy
- proliferative retinopathy.

Background retinopathy and maculopathy

Background retinopathy rarely causes a major threat to vision unless the macula is affected. In the early stages of retinopathy, the capillaries of the retina become more permeable. This can cause fluid exudation (hard exudates) into the retina.

See website Figure 5.1

Retinal veins swell at localised spots, giving the appearance of 'beading'. Microaneurysms can develop; these can rupture, causing small bleeds. Arteriolar occlusions cause retinal infarcts or 'cotton wool spots' on the retina. More spots occur in rapidly developing retinopathy or where there is coexisting hypertension. Evidence of venous bleeding and 'cotton wool' spots suggests progression to pre-proliferative retinopathy. Maculopathy can cause severe loss of central vision and is most common in type 2 diabetes. In this condition, oedema, haemorrhages and exudates are concentrated on the macular area of the retina.

Proliferative retinopathy

Microvascular disease of the retina can result in areas of hypoxia. As a compensatory development, new, abnormal blood vessels (neovascularisation) grow forward from the retina to invade the vitreous body.

See website Figure 5.2

These new vessels are fragile and poorly supported; consequently, haemorrhages into the vitreous body are common. Progressive traction on the retina can result in retinal detachment. Proliferative retinopathy and retinal detachment will seriously threaten vision.

MEDICAL MANAGEMENT

The main priorities in the treatment of diabetic retinopathy are to reduce the risk of haemorrhage and to limit new vessel growth into the vitreous body. Photocoagulation by means of laser technology can be used to treat proliferative and pre-proliferative retinopathy.

Screening Retinal photography should be carried out annually. Many health authorities are using mobile units to carry out retinal screening in the community. Annual ophthalmoscopic examination for those with no identified retinopathy and 6-monthly for those with background retinopathy is strongly advised. This will enable swift and appropriate treatment to help prevent blindness. Where glycaemic control is poor, or where hypertension or renal involvement is more frequent, eye examinations may be recommended. Referral to an ophthalmologist should be made for maculopathy, proliferative and pre-proliferative retinopathy, a reduction in visual acuity, retinal detachment or rubeosis iridis (development of new, abnormal blood vessels on the front of the iris).

🖱 **See website Figure 5.3**

Prevention The patient should be aware of the established link between poor blood glucose control and retinopathy and of the importance of promptly reporting changes in vision. The risks of retinopathy increase if the patient is hypertensive.

Other eye disorders

Although retinopathy poses an important threat to vision in diabetes, approximately 50% of visual loss in people affected by type 2 diabetes will be due to other causes that include cataract, age-related macular degeneration, glaucoma, optic neuropathy and occlusion of retinal blood vessels (Frier & Fisher 2006) (see Ch. 13).

Sadly, many patients with diabetes do ultimately suffer partial or total blindness. Maintaining independence in relation to diabetes management and general self-care will present quite a challenge but patients may be referred to local visual impairment services and the Royal National Institute of Blind People (RNIB). Allwinkle (2002) describes various devices which can enable the blind or partially sighted patient to administer insulin and monitor blood glucose. The nurse and the visually impaired patient with diabetes should work together to seek out ways of reducing the patient's dependence on others.

Diabetic nephropathy

Approximately 30% of patients with type 1 diabetes develop diabetic nephropathy after a disease duration of 20 years (Frier & Fisher 2006) and up to 40% of patients with type 2 diabetes will eventually develop diabetic nephropathy, the incidence of which is related to the duration of their diabetes (Molitch 1997). Between 10% and 20% of patients with type 2 diabetes who have diabetic nephropathy will eventually progress to end-stage renal failure (Cooper 1998).

AETIOLOGY AND PATHOPHYSIOLOGY

The kidneys of people with diabetes are vulnerable with respect to the following:

- Microvascular changes – damage to the capillaries in the glomeruli can occur. The basement membrane initially thickens and, in the later stages, nodules of glycoprotein are deposited in the glomerular capsule. As a result, the filtering capacity of the glomeruli is reduced.
- Macrovascular changes – atheromatous changes in renal vessels can lead to poor renal perfusion which will ultimately impair renal function.
- Hypertension – a common feature in diabetes, hypertension can contribute to kidney damage and, conversely, can also result from kidney damage.
- Urinary tract infection (UTI) can occur for several reasons that include:
  - diabetes-associated predisposition to infection
  - damaged renal tissue vulnerable to infection
  - the need for catheterisation during metabolic crisis
  - atonic bladder associated with autonomic neuropathy, causing urinary stasis and ascending UTI.

MEDICAL MANAGEMENT

All patients with diabetes should be screened for early renal damage.

Screening involves the measurement of urinary albumin concentration and serum creatinine at regular intervals, usually annually, and this should be measured using an early morning urine sample. Urinary albumin:creatinine ratio should be measured by a laboratory method or a 'near-patient' test specific for albumin at low concentration. Any abnormal result should be confirmed by a further sample (SIGN 2010).

Microalbuminuria is defined as a rise in urinary albumin loss of between 30 and 300 mg/day. This is the earliest sign of diabetic nephropathy and predicts increased total mortality, cardiovascular mortality and morbidity and end-stage renal failure (SIGN 2010).

All patients with proteinuria should have their blood pressure measured at every clinic or surgery visit. The UKPDS demonstrated that reducing blood pressure from 154/87 mmHg to 144/82 mmHg in type 2 diabetes led to a risk reduction of 8% in developing microalbuminuria over 6 years (UKPDS 1998b). In the Heart Outcomes Prevention Study (HOPE) study (2000) angiotensin-converting enzyme (ACE) inhibitor therapy for 4.5 years in type 2 diabetes was associated with an absolute risk reduction of developing proteinuria of 2%. Therefore, tight blood pressure control (<140/80 mmHg) in patients with type 2 diabetes should be maintained (SIGN 2010). Both the Diabetes Control and Complications Trial (DCCT) (Diabetes Control and Complications Research Group 1993) and UKPDS (1998b) have shown that a reduction in mean HbA_{1c} (glycated haemoglobin) was associated with a reduction in the occurrence of microalbuminuria and proteinuria.

Established diabetic renal disease is treated in the same way as renal disease in the non-diabetic population (see Ch. 8).

Treatment choices for the patient in end-stage renal failure include haemodialysis, continuous ambulatory peritoneal dialysis (CAPD) or renal transplant using live or cadaver donors.

Renal transplantation using a live donor offers the best treatment for suitable patients. Careful selection of patients is important, given that other major diabetes-related complications usually coexist with the renal disease. Virtually all patients with end-stage renal failure have retinopathy, and 20–30% are blind. Retinopathy alone would not militate against active treatment by dialysis or renal transplantation but the presence of widespread cancer, advanced dementia or severe cerebrovascular disease may do so.

Due to the danger of lactic acidosis, the oral hypoglycaemic drug metformin (a biguanide) should not be used for patients with renal impairment. Chlorpropamide (a sulphonylurea) should also be avoided as it is mainly excreted by the kidneys and in renal failure can accumulate in the blood, causing serious hypoglycaemia. For some patients in renal failure, whose diabetes was previously controlled by oral medication, insulin therapy may be indicated.

 ## Nursing management and health promotion: diabetic nephropathy

Diabetes control should be closely monitored by regular blood glucose measurement. Measurement and recording of fluid intake and output and body weight may be required to monitor renal function. Dietary and fluid restrictions may be necessary. Patients and their families should be made aware of the vital importance of these measures.

Prevention of renal failure

By identifying early renal impairment by screening for microalbuminuria, making efforts to improve diabetes control and detecting and treating hypertension, it is possible to prevent or delay the progression of renal disease (Diabetes Control and Complications Research Group 1993).

Nursing and medical staff should exercise extreme caution in the introduction and subsequent care of urinary catheters in order to prevent infection. Prompt treatment of any established UTI will normally be required to minimise damage. (See Further reading, e.g. see Hasslacher 2001.)

Diabetic neuropathy

Although the cause of diabetic neuropathy is uncertain, it is known that neural function in the diabetic patient deteriorates in response to pressure, metabolic changes and ischaemia (Watkins et al 2003). Incidence of diabetic neuropathy is known to rise in line with duration of diabetes and increasing age. A popular theory is that nerve damage occurs as a result of the accumulation of metabolites of glucose, causing osmotic swelling and subsequent damage to the nerve cell. Ischaemia as a cause of diabetic neuropathy, however, remains controversial but must be considered a contributory factor (Watkins et al 2003).

PATHOPHYSIOLOGY

Structural damage to the neurones affecting the Schwann cells causes segmental areas of demyelination to appear, thus impairing conduction of the nerve impulses. There is no widely accepted classification of diabetic neuropathy, but a number of clinical syndromes are recognisable.

🖱 **See further content on the website**

Peripheral neuropathy This is a distal symmetrical neuropathy, principally affecting the lower extremities and playing a major part in the aetiology of diabetic foot problems. It affects either sensory or motor nerves and the patient's symptoms will reflect this.

Polyneuropathy This is widespread neuropathic changes affecting many nerves. Again, the lower extremities are often affected (peripheral polyneuropathy).

Mononeuropathies Single nerves or their roots are affected. The condition is often of rapid onset and reversible, suggesting an acute vascular origin rather than chronic metabolic disturbance (Williams & Pickup 2004). Examples of mononeuropathy include ptosis (drooping eyelid) and diplopia (double vision) which can occur as a result of damage to the oculomotor nerves (cranial nerve III).

Autonomic neuropathies Damage to autonomic nerves causes numerous abnormalities in many areas of the body. Common manifestations are abnormal sweating, postural hypotension, diarrhoea and erectile dysfunction. Less common are gastroparesis (delayed gastric emptying due to poor motility) and bladder dysfunction (Williams & Pickup 2004).

MEDICAL MANAGEMENT

Prevention of diabetic neuropathy is important and major benchmark studies such as the DCCT and UKPDS have shown that strict glycaemic control can decrease the risk of complications, including neuropathy. Other sensible measures such as avoiding smoking and tight control of blood pressure, blood cholesterol and triglycerides are advised (see Ch. 2).

Diabetic neuropathy affects many systems of the body. Management, which is essentially symptomatic, may involve the multidisciplinary efforts of the diabetes care team. A variety of treatment approaches may be adopted, including medication, surgery and physiotherapy.

 ## Nursing management and health promotion: diabetic neuropathy

Meeting the particular comfort needs of the patient will be a central focus for nursing care. Reducing the risk of accidental tissue damage arising from severe sensory impairment will also be a priority.

Neuropathies can seriously interfere with lifestyle and emotional well-being. An example of this is erectile dysfunction which affects up to 35% of all men with diabetes. Erectile dysfunction can be devastating for both the patient and his partner. Many men with diabetes and erectile dysfunction would like help for this problem but are reluctant to seek advice. Once the diagnosis has been made, there are several treatment options available, including professional sexual counselling, vacuum devices, penile injections and oral agents such as sildenafil (see Ch. 7). The choice of treatment will depend on local circumstances, personal experience and, most importantly, the patient's own preference (Mills 2003).

The diabetic foot

People with diabetes are at particular risk of foot problems, either neuropathic or caused by ischaemia. People with diabetes must be screened, at least annually, for foot disease. Based on UK population surveys, diabetic foot problems are a

Table 5.7 Clinical signs of the diabetic foot

SIGN	NEUROPATHIC FOOT	ISCHAEMIC FOOT
Temperature	Warm	Cool
Peripheral pulses	Present	Absent
Pain	Loss of sensation	Intermittent claudication and rest pain
Skin	Dry cracking skin	Blanches on elevation
Deformity	Present	Absent
Position of ulcer	Plantar surface, toes or high pressure areas	Margins of foot and toes

common complication of diabetes, with prevalences of 23–42% for neuropathy, 9–23% for vascular disease (ischaemic foot) and 5–7% for foot ulceration (SIGN 2010) (Table 5.7). Education of the patient is vital to prevent problems (Box 5.14).

Screening Foot examination by trained professionals should consist of foot inspection for appearance and footwear, and assessment of sensation using a 10 g monofilament. Palpation of foot pulses and use of Doppler ultrasound should be undertaken if possible.

Painful peripheral neuropathy can be a major problem for many people, particularly at night. It can be treated with some success by tricyclic antidepressants such as amitriptyline. Gabapentin has also been shown to be effective, with fewer side-effects. Topical capsaicin should also be considered for localised neuropathic pain.

Deformity of the foot can lead to ulceration, particularly in the absence of protective pain sensation and with the contribution of unsuitable footwear. Early detection can initiate properly fitting shoes before ulceration occurs.

Charcot foot/Charcot joint is a neuroarthropathic syndrome with osteoporosis, fracture, acute inflammation and disorganisation of foot architecture (SIGN 2010). Signs and symptoms include a hot, red and swollen foot with, or often without, pain. Immobilisation of the limb, usually by casting of the foot, and reduction of stress by decreasing the amount of weight-bearing on the affected limb through use of crutches are the current mainstays of treatment. However, other treatment options are being considered, including drug intervention.

Management of ulcers

Neuropathic ulcers are most frequently caused from callus build-up and potentially thermal injury, e.g. stepping into hot water, and chemical injury, such as from use of corn plasters. The injury is usually not perceived by the patient, due to loss of pain sensation. The treatment aim is to redistribute plantar pressures by some form of cast or cradled insole. However, in the neuroischaemic foot, the aim is to protect the vulnerable margins of the foot such as by the use of a wide-fitting shoe.

The ulcer will require initial debridement and management of exudate with an appropriate wound dressing product (see Ch. 23). Biological debridement using larval therapy can be very effective. The larvae (maggots) of the sterile blowfly (*Lucilia serricata*) are applied to the wound where the enzymes they produce remove slough and necrotic tissue thereby providing more favourable conditions for healing (see Ch. 23).

Box 5.14 Information

Measures to protect the feet in diabetes

General measures

- Do not smoke.
- Eat a healthy balanced diet.
- Try to maintain body weight within normal limits.
- Try to keep active; this will help improve the circulation.
- Have blood pressure and blood lipids checked regularly.

Footwear

- Ensure correctly fitting shoes – ask for feet to be measured when buying shoes. Break in new shoes very gradually. Don't buy shoes that cause pain/discomfort in the shop.
- Ensure that socks or tights/stockings fit comfortably – avoid constrictions around ankles and avoid socks with thick seams.
- Change footwear as soon as possible if wet.
- Avoid walking barefoot – wear slippers and beach shoes to prevent injury.
- Do not wear sandals if there is any loss of sensation in the feet.

Foot care

- Bathe feet daily using lukewarm (not hot) water and soap/soap substitute.
- Pat feet dry gently; pay special attention to the area between the toes.

- Apply a moisturising cream daily to avoid dryness and keep the skin supple.
- Avoid exposing feet to excess heat or cold.
- Avoid sunburn to the feet and legs.
- Cut nails according to the shape of the toes while they are still soft from bathing but do not dig down the side of the toenails.
- Inspect feet daily for blisters, corns, calluses, cracks or redness (using a mirror to view the underside of the foot).
- Do not burst blisters.
- If a minor cut or abrasion does occur, wash thoroughly and cover with a clean dressing. See your doctor if the cut has not healed in 48 h.
- Your podiatrist should be consulted for treatment of ingrown toenails, corns or calluses. Do not attempt the physical removal of corns or other abnormalities, or use home remedies or over-the-counter (OTC) products such as corn plasters.
- Your general practitioner should be consulted for the treatment of verrucas.
- A doctor or nurse should be consulted if foot problems such as tingling, numbness, swelling, pain or loss of feeling develop.
- Ensure you have your feet inspected annually by a trained health professional.

Stimulation of wound healing can be improved by topical preparations such as becaplermin (a recombinant human platelet-derived growth factor) which may be used for neuropathic, diabetic ulcers. Living human tissue replacement therapy can also be used for persistent wounds (SIGN 2010).

Infection The use of broad-spectrum antibiotics is vital to help improve healing. A wound swab for culture should be taken before antibiotics are commenced. Progression to cellulitis and osteomyelitis will require hospital admission for administration of i.v. antibiotics, immobilisation and appropriate wound management. Stress hormones are released in response to severe infection, causing hyperglycaemia. The resulting increase in insulin demand will present an increased challenge to the pancreas, increasing the risk of metabolic crisis. Intravenous fluids and insulin may be required.

Necrosis The ischaemic foot results from atherosclerotic changes in the distal arteries of the legs. Revascularisation of the infected neuroischaemic foot should be explored. Angioplasty is indicated in the treatment of single or multiple stenosis or short segment occlusions of blood vessels. If angioplasty is not possible because of long arterial occlusions, bypass should be considered. Patients with a neuropathic foot in which there is necrosis will probably require surgical debridement. However, severely affected patients may eventually require digital amputation or, in even more serious cases, a below knee amputation (see Ch. 10).

Nurses involved in the care of people with diabetes should undertake regular monitoring of the patient's feet and commence appropriate and timely treatment whenever necessary (Edmonds et al 2008).

Facilitating self-care through education

In both hospital and community settings, overall coordination of patient learning is undertaken by the diabetes specialist nurse working closely with the specialist dietitian and the patient's physician. Care of patients, with type 2 diabetes in particular, will be undertaken by community and hospital nurses who are not specialists in diabetes care. All such nurses may be required to undertake a teaching role and must therefore ensure that their own knowledge base is adequate.

Assessment

By establishing a rapport with the patient and family, the nurse will be equipped to assess the patient's needs in relation to:

- current level of knowledge about diabetes
- understanding of the reasons for prescribed treatment
- knowledge and skills required for self-care
- emotional response to the diagnosis
- social support from family and friends
- barriers to learning, e.g. sensory loss, mobility and manipulation problems, language difficulties, reading and writing difficulties and intellectual impairment.

See website Critical thinking question 5.4

Planning a teaching programme

Staff members must show consistency in the information they provide. Any member of the diabetes care team may be involved in coaching the patient and family in diabetes management. It is likely that the majority of this will rest with the nursing staff, including the diabetes specialist nurse who will work in partnership with the patient and family. The most important team member is of course the patient. Guidance published by NICE in 2003 suggests principles of good practice rather than recommendations on the type, setting and frequency of education (Avery 2003).

Sessions should be short and information presented in small, easily assimilated and integrated sections with teaching points categorised into lists. Ordering presentation so that the most important point is always raised first can help the patient to prioritise information. Being direct and specific will aid retention, as will using simple words and brief sentences. Clarifying points and ensuring comprehension before moving to a new topic is very important. Interactive participation is encouraged, although not everyone will feel comfortable with this approach.

Adopting a friendly manner and taking time to talk about non-medical matters can relax the patient and set the scene for a more productive session. It is important to consider the age group for which teaching materials have been designed in order to avoid giving inappropriate information.

An impressive array of informative and attractive booklets is available, many of which are sponsored by manufacturers and written by diabetes health care professionals. These provide back-up for teaching and discussion and aide memoires for patients. Conversation maps, patient orientated websites and DVDs can be sourced for patients to view individually or in groups. Dose Adjustment For Normal Eating (DAFNE) in type 1 diabetes and Diabetes Education and Self Management for Ongoing and Newly Diagnosed (DESMOND) in type 2 diabetes are structured education packages used throughout the UK (Box 5.15).

Box 5.15 Reflection

DAFNE and DESMOND

Both DAFNE and DESMOND are incorporated into the multidisciplinary approach to management of diabetes.

Activities

- Access the websites below and find out what publications, structured education packages, courses and programmes are available.
- Discuss with a diabetes specialist nurse or your mentor how the structured education packages are used locally in patient education.

Resources

Diabetes Education and Self Management for Ongoing and Newly Diagnosed (DESMOND) http://www.desmond-project.org.uk/

Dose Adjustment For Normal Eating (DAFNE) http://www.dafne.uk.com/

The programme

The teaching programme should be tailored to suit the patient's individual needs but is likely to include some of the following topics:

- what is diabetes? – type 1 and type 2
- treatment of diabetes
    - oral hypoglycaemics
    - insulin therapy
- why insulin and how does it work?
- types of insulin
- storage and administration of insulin
- diet–insulin–exercise balance – insulin dose adjustment (Box 5.16)
- monitoring blood glucose
- recognising and treating hypo- and hyperglycaemia
- what to do during illness
- testing for ketones
- avoiding complications
- health screening
- lifestyle factors – sport, alcohol, smoking, illicit drugs, driving, travel, pregnancy and sexual health.

Promoting psychological and social adjustment

A diagnosis of diabetes has an emotional impact on those affected. The shock of a diagnosis of diabetes has been likened to the experience of bereavement (Everett & Kerr 1998). People newly diagnosed with diabetes may experience the following responses:

- shock and disbelief of diagnosis
- anxiety about different aspects of managing the condition
- confusion about all the information given at diagnosis

- fear about the future and possible development of complications
- anger that it has happened and a feeling of 'why me?'
- sadness at the loss of the person before diagnosis
- stress at not being able to cope.

Psychosocial factors influencing self-management of diabetes

Diabetes self-management has been estimated to be seen as over 98% the patient's responsibility (Anderson & Funnell 2002). This is an enormous demand on the person with diabetes and their family. One of the purposes of diabetes education is to impart knowledge and skills that enable the person with diabetes to make informed decisions about how they are going to lead their life with diabetes. However, there are other determinants of behaviour which can influence behavioural choices. These include health beliefs, the person's locus of control (Peyrot & Rubin 1994), self-efficacy, behavioural intentions, quality of life (Everett & Kerr 2001) and emotional well-being and depression (SIGN 2010). (See Further reading, e.g. Naidoo & Wills 2009.)

Behaviour changes

The empowerment model (Funnell et al 1991) is the model of choice which acknowledges the patient's expertise, their personal responsibilities in self-management and their right to informed choice (see Further reading, e.g. Naidoo & Wills 2009).

Lifestyle implications

The charity Diabetes UK works to raise funds for diabetes research and to increase the awareness of diabetes and its implications. Vitally it also provides information and advice for people with diabetes and professionals involved in their

---

Box 5.16 Information

Exercise and people with diabetes

Exercise and increasing activity can provide many health benefits for the person with diabetes, such as improving insulin sensitivity, weight management and reduction, heart and circulatory protection, strengthening of joints and bones and many other benefits. Exercise will reduce blood glucose levels, and a clear understanding of the role of exercise in blood glucose control is essential for every patient with diabetes. The nurse must find a way of explaining this role that is appropriate to the learning needs of individual patients. The analogy of 'fuel intake' (food) and 'energy output' (activity/exercise) is often useful for the purposes of illustration.

What happens during exercise?

When energy output is low, the demand for fuel in the form of glucose is also low. However, during bursts of physical activity the demand for glucose will rise and it is then drawn from the glycogen reserves in the liver and muscles. The rate at which glucose is taken up by the cells is influenced by medication (insulin or tablets). If available supplies of glucose are depleted and are not replaced, the patient's blood glucose will fall and may continue to fall for several hours after prolonged or intense exercise, thus increasing the risk of hypoglycaemia.

Avoiding exercise-induced hypoglycaemia

Insulin-treated patients should be advised to monitor blood glucose before and after exercise and when to take extra carbohydrate to avoid hypoglycaemia. A quickly absorbable form of glucose such as glucose tablets or a glucose drink may be used to augment diet and help prevent an abrupt fall in blood glucose. Another strategy to avoid exercise-induced hypoglycaemia is for the insulin dose to be reduced prior to planned and prolonged strenuous activity. Insulin dose adjustment in relation to exercise is an important aspect of the patient's education programme when commencing insulin therapy. Blood glucose should then be monitored to gauge the effects of any reduction. Patients controlled with oral hypoglycaemic therapy may, less frequently, also experience exercise-induced hypoglycaemia and consequently may need to adjust their carbohydrate intake to meet the additional energy demands imposed by the exercise.

Patients with type 1 diabetes should also be made aware that hyperglycaemia (blood glucose >14.0 mmol/L) with ketonuria is an absolute contraindication to exercise as this can indicate that there is a lack of circulating insulin and that the patient is metabolically unstable. Exercise in this situation could cause higher blood glucose levels and a risk of DKA (Burr & Dinesh 1999).

care. It is a national organisation with local branches throughout the UK. Different sections cater for particular groups, e.g. teenagers and those with visual impairment. Diabetes UK offers help and advice on a wide variety of topics such as monitoring and treatment approaches, insurance, holidays and travelling abroad.

Employment

In view of the risk of hypoglycaemia, people with diabetes who are treated with insulin are excluded from some areas of employment, e.g. those which involve certain categories of vocational driving (see below), airline piloting and air traffic control, deep sea diving, working on offshore oil rigs, working down coal mines, at heights or near dangerous moving machinery. Diabetes would also exclude an applicant from joining the UK armed forces or the police. However, in many cases, if diabetes develops while in the job, it is sometimes possible to continue employment. (See Useful websites, e.g. Diabetes UK.)

Driving and motor vehicle insurance

The UK Driver Vehicle Licensing Authority (DVLA) must, by law, be informed when a driver is diagnosed as having diabetes and is receiving treatment with insulin or oral or injected non-insulin therapies. When a licence is issued it will be for a period of 1–3 years to allow periodic review by the DVLA. A medical practitioner may be required to advise on the stability of the driver's diabetes control prior to re-licensing. The DVLA must be informed if any problems or diabetic complications develop which may affect safety.

Different regulations apply to different groups of vehicles, for example the medical standard is more stringent for a group 2 licence covering Large Goods Vehicle (LGV) and/ or a Passenger Carrying Vehicle (PCV). People will have their group 2 licence removed when they commence insulin therapy. There are also restrictions on lighter goods and smaller passenger vehicle licences. Hypoglycaemia is the main danger when driving. People with diabetes should receive education about how to avoid and effectively manage hypoglycaemia when driving.

Patients whose diabetes is treated with medication must inform their insurer. Failure to notify the insurer can result in withdrawal of insurance cover, invalidate any claim and lead to the offence of driving without third party insurance.

The regulations concerning driving and mandatory third party insurance for people with diabetes are complex and readers are directed to the helpful information produced by Diabetes UK (see Useful websites, e.g. Diabetes UK Diabetes Information Driving and Diabetes [reviewed 2009], UK Driver Vehicle Licensing Authority).

Travel

Altered mealtimes, travelling across different time zones, and dietary and climatic changes may all have an effect on diabetes management. It is essential for the person with diabetes to monitor their diabetes closely whilst travelling. They must seek specific advice from their GP or the diabetes team regarding insulin adjustment. All medication and monitoring equipment should be carried in hand luggage to allow for ready access and to reduce risk of loss. Also, the extremely low temperature of the cargo hold can adversely affect the action of insulin. A doctor's letter detailing the need to carry injecting equipment and blood glucose monitoring equipment in their hand luggage is required for air travel. (See Useful websites, e.g. Fit for Travel.)

Eating out

Flexible insulin regimens, insulin pen devices and SBGM have simplified eating out for people with diabetes. People having insulin therapy are advised as to appropriate insulin adjustment to allow more freedom of choice when eating out.

Smoking

Having diabetes increases the risk of developing vascular and neuropathic disorders. Smoking compounds these risks. The diabetes team should encourage smoking cessation and should discuss the availability of resources to provide support whilst the patient is trying to stop smoking (Haire-Joshu et al 2003). However, it must be accepted that the patient may decide to continue to smoke against advice.

Identification

Patients should be strongly advised to carry a card or wear a MedicAlert® pendant or bracelet to identify themselves and give details of the type of diabetes they have and its management.

Future developments

Research in diabetes care is at an exciting stage. Combined kidney and pancreas transplants are now undertaken in a number of centres in the UK for those with renal failure as a complication of type 1 diabetes. Successful transplantation allows the patient to be free of the restrictions of renal dialysis as well as daily injections of insulin.

Pancreatic islet cell transplantation offers people with type 1 diabetes hope for a cure. This is the subject of intensive research trials. Islet cells are isolated from the donor pancreas and injected into the liver of the recipient. The cells develop a blood supply and begin to produce insulin, a process called the Edmonton protocol. New combinations of immunosuppressive agents prevent the body rejecting the transplanted islet cells, eliminating the need for corticosteroid therapy which could damage the newly transplanted cells. A major drawback to the increasing availability of this advance is that the equivalent of two donated pancreases is required to provide sufficient islet cells for transplantation.

Over the years, feasibility studies into the effectiveness of non-enteral routes of delivering insulin have been attempted. These have included ocular, buccal, rectal, vaginal, oral, nasal and uterine delivery systems. A body of evidence suggested that inhaled insulin was an effective, well-tolerated, non-invasive alternative to s.c. soluble insulin for patients with type 2 diabetes (Cefalu 2003). Inhaled insulin became available on prescription to patients in the UK in 2006, but was discontinued in 2007 due to economic reasons.

Research is ongoing into the closed loop system or 'artificial pancreas'. It consists of a continuous glucose meter and an insulin pump, allowing communication between the devices. It is hoped to develop a system that will automatically check blood glucose and administer an appropriate dose of insulin thus allowing more freedom and greater diabetes control for the user.

The ultimate hope is that diabetes will at some future date be preventable. Researchers continue to seek definitive answers to the questions surrounding aetiological factors, with a view to finding ways of manipulating these factors to prevent the disease developing.

Trends in diabetes care provision

Over recent years there have been significant changes in the structure and function of the primary care team and a shift of focus with more health care provided in community settings. Emphasis has been on developing further the role of the diabetes specialist nurse who 'can transform the standard of diabetic care, achieving liaison between hospital, general practitioner and patients at home and offering a wide range of clinical and educational expertise' (Watkins et al 2003).

The growth in the number of practice nurses has made it possible for many GP practices to run their own clinics for people with diabetes. In some areas, dietitians and podiatrists are available in the health centres where clinics are run.

Community nurses and health visitors may find themselves taking high-quality diabetes care directly into the patient's home. Effective hospital–community liaison will become especially important to ensure continuity for the patient in 'shared care'.

Whatever the care setting, it is important that the patient has access to facilities for estimation of glycated haemoglobin and microalbuminuria and for screening for retinopathy and foot-threatening neuropathic or vascular disease. It appears likely that integrated hospital and community care will offer the best use of resources for diabetes screening. However, dealing with a severe metabolic crisis such as DKA will remain the province of the hospital.

Continuing education for all members of the diabetes care team must be a priority. National standards and guidelines and frameworks are necessary to create best practice through a firm research base and to support provision of the highest possible quality of care for people with diabetes. Diabetes specialist nurses and community diabetes facilitators make a significant contribution in the education of their colleagues. Providing education and support which will enable the patient to move away from the despondency and fear which frequently accompany diagnosis, towards independence and autonomy, is surely both the science and the art of nursing care in diabetes.

SUMMARY: KEY NURSING ISSUES

- Diabetes is often referred to as an 'epidemic'. Diabetes UK (2008) considers diabetes to be 'one of the biggest health challenges facing the UK today'. The International Diabetes Federation (IDF) (2008) estimates there are 246 million people affected by diabetes worldwide with the highest prevalence in developed countries.

- Diabetes is a metabolic disease which results from defects in insulin secretion, insulin action or both (WHO 1999). The two main types are type 1 and type 2.

- All nurses, wherever they practise, will encounter people with diabetes.

- Nurses have a vital health promotion role in the prevention and early detection of type 2 diabetes.

- Diabetes specialist nurses are key in the education of people diagnosed with diabetes so they can understand and manage their condition.

- Lifestyle and healthy eating are the cornerstones of effective glycaemic control. Patient-centred care is paramount.

- Acute life-threatening complications, e.g. hyperglycaemia leading to diabetic ketoacidosis, can occur.

- Diabetes is associated with several long-term complications that include sight impairment, renal failure, neuropathy and cardiovascular diseases.

- People with diabetes require tailored care to reduce complications.

- Diabetes management is constantly evolving, as new evidence emerges. Research continues into the possibility of manipulating aetiological factors to prevent diabetes developing.

⊖ REFLECTION AND LEARNING – WHAT NEXT?

- **Test** your knowledge by visiting the website 🖱 and answering the multiple choice questions and critical thinking questions.

- **Consolidate** your learning by looking at some of the further reading suggestions, references and specialist websites.

- **Revisit** some of the additional material on the website.

- **Consider** what you have learnt and how this will help your professional development.

- **Reflect** on how you can apply this knowledge to the care of your patients.

- **Discuss** your learning with your mentor/supervisor, lecturer and colleagues.

REFERENCES

Allwinkle J: Blood glucose monitoring for visually impaired people with diabetes, *The Journal of Diabetes Nursing* 6(5):157–159, 2002.

Anderson RM, Funnell MM: Using the empowerment approach to help patients change behaviour. In Anderson BJ, Rubin RR, editors: *Practical psychology for diabetes clinicians*, Alexandria, VA, 2002, American Diabetes Association.

Avery J: NICE guidelines on the use of patient education models [editorial], *Journal of Diabetes Nursing* 7(7):258, 2003.

British National Formulary (BNF): 2009. Available online http://www.bnf.org/bnf/.

Burr B, Dinesh N: *Exercise and sport in diabetes*, Chichester, 1999, Wiley.

Cefalu WT: Novel routes of delivery for patients with Type 1 or Type 2 diabetes, *Ann Med* 33(9):579–586, 2003.

Cooper ME: Pathogenesis, prevention and treatment of diabetic nephropathy, *Lancet* 352:213–219, 1998.

DAFNE Study Group: Training in flexible, intensive insulin management to enable dietary freedom in people with Type 1 diabetes: dose adjustment for normal eating (DAFNE) randomised controlled trial, *Br Med J* 325:746–749, 2002.

Dave J, Chatterjee S, Davies M, et al: Evaluation of admissions and management of diabetic ketoacidosis in a large teaching hospital, *Practical Diabetes International* 21(4):149–153, 2004.

Department of Health: *National Service Framework for diabetes: standards*, 2001. Available online http://www.dh.gov.uk/en/Publicationsandstatistics/Publications/PublicationsPolicyAndGuidance/DH_4002951.

Department of Health: *Five years on: delivering the diabetes national service framework*, 2008. Available online http://www.dh.gov.uk/en/

Publicationsandstatistics/Publications/PublicationsPolicyAndGuidance/ DH_087123.

Diabetes Control and Complications Research Group: The effect of diabetes on the development and progression of long term complications in insulin dependent diabetes, *N Engl J Med* 329:977–986, 1993.

Diabetes UK: *Shocking new statistics*, 2008. Available online http://www. diabetes.org.uk/en/About_us/News_Landing_Page/Shocking-new-statistics/.

Diabetes UK: *Blood glucose. Blood glucose targets*, 2009. Available online http://diabetes.org.uk/Guide-to-diabetes/Monitoring/Blood_glucose/ Blood_glucose_targets/.

Drucker DJ, Buse JB, Taylor K, et al: DURATION-1 Study Group 2008 Exenatide once weekly versus twice daily for the treatment of type 2 diabetes: a randomised, open-label, non-inferiority study, *Lancet* 372 (9645): 1240–1250.

Dyson P: Diet and diabetes – the new recommendations, *Journal of Diabetes Nursing* 8(4):127–131, 2004.

Edmonds ME, Foster AVM, Sanders L: *A Practical Manual of Diabetic Foot Care*, ed 2, Oxford, 2008, Wiley-Blackwell.

Everett J, Kerr D: A picture of the impact of newly diagnosed Type 2 diabetes, *Journal of Diabetes Nursing* 2(6):170–175, 1998.

Everett J, Kerr D: Measuring quality of life in diabetes, *Journal of Diabetes Nursing* 5(2):53–55, 2001.

Frier BM, Fisher M: Diabetes mellitus. In Boon NA, et al, editor: *Davidson's principles and practice of medicine*, ed 20, Edinburgh, 2006, Churchill Livingstone, pp 805–847.

Funnell MM, Anderson RM, Arnold MS, et al: Empowerment: an idea whose time has come to diabetes education, *Diabetes Educ* 17:37–41, 1991.

Haire-Joshu D, Glasgow RE, Tubbs TL: Smoking and diabetes, *Diabetes Care* 26:s89–s90, 2003.

Holt T, Kumar S: *ABC of diabetes*, ed 6, Oxford, 2010, BMJ Books Wiley-Blackwell.

HOPE (Heart Outcomes Prevention study): Effects of ramipril on cardiovascular and microvascular outcomes in people with diabetes mellitus. Results of the HOPE study and MICRO-HOPE sub-study, *Lancet* 355:253–259, 2000.

International Diabetes Federation (IDF): *Diabetes prevalence*, 2008. Available online http://www.idf.org/diabetes-prevalence.

Kirby M: Lipid management in people with diabetes, *Diabetes and Primary Care* 5(4):152–157, 2003.

Krans HMJ, Porta N, Keen H, editors: *Diabetes care and research in Europe. The St Vincent Declaration action programme*, Copenhagen, 1992, World Health Organization Regional Office for Europe.

MacAuley V, Deary IJ, Frier BM: Symptoms of hypoglycaemia in people with diabetes, *Diabet Med* 18(9):690–705, 2001.

MacKinnon M: *Providing diabetes care in general practice*, ed 4, London, 2002, Class Publishing.

Massó-González EL, Johansson S, Wallander M, García-Rodríguez LA: Trends in the Prevalence and Incidence of Diabetes in the UK – 1996 to 2005, *Epidemiol Community Health*. Published online first: 24 February 2009, doi:10.1136/jech.2008.080382.

Mills LS: Erectile dysfunction: assessment and treatment in diabetes, *Journal of Diabetes Nursing* 7(4):146–149, 2003.

Molitch ME: Management of early diabetic nephropathy, *Am J Med* 102:392–398, 1997.

National Institute for Health and Clinical Excellence (NICE): *Guidance on the use of patient education models for diabetes. Technology appraisal TA60*, London, 2003, NICE.

National Institute for Health and Clinical Excellence (NICE): *Type 2 Diabetes – newer agents (partial update of CG66) Clinical guidelines CG87*, 2009. Available online http://www.nice.org.uk/guidance/index. jsp?action=byID&o=12165.

Owens D, Pickup J, Barnett A, Frier B, et al: The continuing debate on self-monitoring of blood glucose in diabetes, *Diabetes and Primary Care* 7(1):9–21, 2005.

Peyrot M, Rubin RR: Structure and correlates of diabetes-specific locus of control, *Diabetes Care* 17(9):994–1001, 1994.

Scottish Intercollegiate Guidelines Network (SIGN): *Management of diabetes*, 2010, No. 116. Available online http://www.sign.ac.uk/ guidelines/fulltext/116/index.html.

Stevens RJ, Coleman RL, Adler AI, et al: Risk factors for myocardial infarction: case fatality and stroke case fatality in Type 2 diabetes, *Diabetes Care* 27(1):210–1206, 2004.

United Kingdom Prospective Diabetes Study Group: Intensive blood glucose control with sulphonylureas or insulin compared with conventional treatment and risk of complications in patients with Type 2 diabetes (UKPDS 33), *Lancet* 352(9131):837–853, 1998a.

United Kingdom Prospective Diabetes Study Group: Tight blood pressure control and risk of macrovascular and microvascular complications in Type 2 diabetes (UKPDS 38), *Br Med J* 317:703–713, 1998b.

Watkins PJ, Amiel SA, Howell SL: *Diabetes and its management*, ed 6, Oxford, 2003, Blackwell Publishing.

Wei M, Gaskill SP, Haffner SM, Stern MP: Waist circumference as the best predictor of non-insulin dependent diabetes mellitus (NIDDM) compared to body mass index, waist/hip ratio and other anthropometric measurements in Mexican Americans: a 7 year prospective study, *Obes Res* 5(1):16–23, 1997.

Wild S, Roglic G, Green A, et al: Global Prevalence of Diabetes, *Diabetes Care* 27(5):1047, 2004.

Williams G, Pickup JC: *Handbook of diabetes*, ed 3, Oxford, 2004, Wiley-Blackwell.

Williams J: Overview of the care of pregnant women with pre-existing diabetes, *Journal of Diabetes Nursing* 7(1):12–15, 2003.

World Health Organization (WHO): *Values for diagnosis of diabetes mellitus and other categories of hyperglycaemia*, 1999. Available online http:// www.who.int/diabetesactiononline/diabetes/basics/en/index4.html.

FURTHER READING

Alexander WD: Treatment of erectile dysfunction in men with diabetes, *Diabetes and Primary Care* 5(2):64–69, 2003.

Ashwell M: Obesity risk: importance of the waist-to-hip ratio, *Nurs Stand* 23(41):49–54, 2009.

British National Formulary: Available online http://www.bnf.org.

Department of Health (DH): *Five Years on Delivering the Diabetes National Framework*, 2008. Available online http://www.dh.gov.uk/en/ Publicationsandstatistics/Publications/ PublicationsPolicyAndGuidance/DH_087123.

Diabetes UK: *Recommendations for the management of pregnant women including gestational diabetes*, London, 2004, Diabetes UK.

Dunning T: *Care of People with Diabetes: A Manual of Nursing Practice*, ed 3, Oxford, 2009, Wiley-Blackwell.

Edmonds ME, Foster AVM, Sanders L: *A Practical Manual of Diabetic Foot Care*, ed 2, Oxford, 2008, Wiley-Blackwell.

Fisher M: *Heart disease and diabetes*, London, 2003, Martin Dunitz.

Frier BM, Fisher M: *Hypoglycaemia in clinical diabetes*, ed 2, Oxford, 2007, Wiley-Blackwell.

Hadaegh F, Zabetian A, Harati H, Azizi F: Waist/height ratio as a better predictor of type 2 diabetes compared to body mass index in Tehranian adult men – a 3.6-year prospective study, *Exp Clin Endocrinol Diabetes* 114(6):310–315, 2006.

Hasslacher C: *Diabetic nephropathy*, Oxford, 2001, Wiley-Blackwell.

Moshe H: *Textbook of diabetes and pregnancy*, London, 2003, Taylor and Francis.

Naidoo J, Wills J: *Foundations for Health Promotion*, ed 3, Edinburgh, 2009, Baillière Tindall.

Nathan DM, Zinman B, Cleary PA, et al: Modern-Day Clinical Course of Type 1 Diabetes Mellitus After 30 Years' Duration. The Diabetes Control and Complications Trial/Epidemiology of Diabetes Interventions and Complications and Pittsburgh Epidemiology of Diabetes Complications Experience (1983–2005). Diabetes Control and Complications Trial/Epidemiology of Diabetes Interventions and Complications (DCCT/EDIC) Research Group, *Arch Intern Med* 169(14):1307–1316, 2009.

Royal College of General Practitioners (RCGP): *Clinical guidelines for Type 2 diabetes. Prevention and management of foot problems*, London, 2000, RCGP.

Scanlon P, Aldington S, Wilkinson C, Matthews D: *A Practical Manual of Diabetic Retinopathy Management*, Oxford, 2009, Wiley-Blackwell.

Snoek FJ, Skinner TC: *Psychology in diabetes care*, ed 2, Oxford, 2005, Wiley-Blackwell.

Tortora GJ, Derrickson B: *Principles of anatomy and physiology*, ed 12, New York, 2009, John Wiley & Sons Inc.

USEFUL WEBSITES

Abbott Diabetes Care (Abbott Laboratories): www.diabetesnow.co.uk

Aventis Pharma UK: www.aventis.co.uk

Insulin and mode of action

Bayer plc: www.bayerdiag.com

Urine glucose monitoring

Becton Dickinson (UK) Ltd BD Medical – Diabetes Care: www.bddiabetes.co.uk

Measurement of insulin and injection technique

British National Formulary: www.bnf.org

Diabetes Education and Self Management for Ongoing and Newly Diagnosed (DESMOND): www.desmond-project.org.uk

Diabetes in Scotland: www.crag.scot.nhs.uk/topics/diabetes/main.htm

Diabetes UK: www.diabetes.org.uk

Diabetes and the body 2009: www.diabetes.org.uk/Guide-to-diabetes/Introduction-to-diabetes/What_is_diabetes/Diabetes-and-the-body/

Diabetes Information Driving and diabetes (reviewed 2009): www.diabetes.org.uk/upload/How%20we%20help/catalogue/DrivingandDiabetes_Final_ToUpload.pdf

Dose Adjustment For Normal Eating (DAFNE): www.dafne.uk.com

Eli Lilly & Co Ltd: www.lilly.co.uk

Fit for Travel: www.fitfortravel.nhs.uk/advice/advice-for-travellers/diabetes.aspx

International Diabetes Federation: www.idf.org

Lifescan UK: www.lifescan.co.uk

Blood glucose monitoring

National Institute for Health and Clinical Excellence (NICE): www.nice.org.uk

NHS Diabetes: www.diabetes.nhs.uk

Novo Nordisk Pharmaceuticals Ltd: www.novonordisk.co.uk

Roche Diagnostics Ltd: www.roche.com

Royal National Institute of the Blind (RNIB): www.rnib.org.uk

Scottish Intercollegiate Guidelines Network (SIGN): www.sign.ac.uk

Scottish Medicines Consortium (SMC): www.scottishmedicines.org.uk/smc/CCC_FirstPage.jsp

UK Driver Vehicle Licensing Authority (DVLA): www.dvla.gov.uk

World Health Organization (WHO) About Diabetes: www.who.int/diabetesactiononline/diabetes/basics/en/index4.html

The status of all drugs, including those used for type 2 diabetes, are subject to change. For example, the marketing authorisation for rosiglitazone-containing anti-diabetes drugs was suspended by the European Medicines Agency in September 2010. Readers are advised to check such status, availability and current safety issues by accessing the Medicines and Healthcare products Regulatory Agency (MHRA) website (www.mhra.gov.uk).

Nursing patients with disorders of the immune system

Chris Brooker

Introduction

The immune system is a complex, diverse and diffuse collection of cells, tissues, organs and molecules (e.g. interferons [IFNs]). It is programmed to respond to the many challenges presented to it by foreign particles and cells, microorganisms such as bacteria, viruses, fungi and protozoa, and cancer cells. Various defence mechanisms function to protect the body from harm, and in order to carry out this function it must be able to recognise 'self' from 'non-self'.

The defence mechanisms providing immunity include: physical, chemical and microbiological barriers, second-line non-specific defences and specific immune responses (Storey & Jordan 2008). These can be categorised as first-, second- and third-line defences (Figure 6.1):

- *first-line* – natural (innate), non-specific barriers to invasion by foreign substance, for example, the intact skin and mucosae, antimicrobial substances in body fluids and the microorganisms forming the normal flora (see Ch. 16)
- *second-line* – natural (innate), non-specific defences which limit microbial spread; the inflammatory response, phagocytosis and immunological surveillance
- *third-line* defences – when first- and second-line barriers are breached or compromised the adaptive (acquired), specific immune responses come into play; humoral immunity (B lymphocytes/B cells and antibodies [immunoglobulins]) and cell-mediated immunity (T lymphocytes/T cells).

Although immunity is generally described as being either natural non-specific immunity or adaptive specific immunity, the functions are inextricably linked. Moreover, the interdependence and interactions between humoral and cell-mediated immunity are increasingly recognised.

For the most part the immune system functions to protect individuals from microbes and infection (see Ch. 16), and natural killer (NK) cells (a type of lymphocyte) undertake immunological surveillance in order to detect and destroy foreign, infected, damaged or cancerous cells. However, abnormalities may occur and immune responses may be excessive (hypersensitivity), may fail to function properly (immunodeficiency) or may fail to recognise 'self' leading to an immune attack on body cells (autoimmune disorders).

This chapter outlines immune responses, concentrating on adaptive immunity, and describes the nursing management of some immune response disorders: hypersensitivity, immunodeficiency and autoimmune conditions. It will come as no surprise that problems of the immune system impact on all body systems. Nurses working in all areas of practice may encounter people with immune disorders. Readers are provided with cross references to relevant chapters (e.g. Chs 5, 11, 16, 31), and suggestions for further reading.

Currently, there are many developments in the management of immunological disorders, transplantation and the use of targeted immunological-based treatments for conditions such as cancer. The use of monoclonal antibodies, cytokines and cancer vaccines, for example, is of increasing importance and will impact on nursing practice.

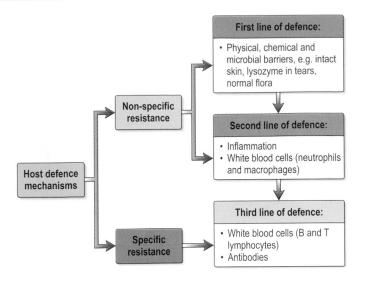

Figure 6.1 Overview – first-, second- and third-line defence mechanisms. (Reproduced from Rennie-Meyer 2007.)

reaches maximum size at puberty, thereafter becoming smaller as lymphoid tissue is replaced by fat.

B lymphocytes undergo processing in the bone marrow. During maturation, T and B lymphocytes acquire the surface receptors that enable them to recognise antigens (foreign cells/substances that stimulate a specific immune response in the host, including the production of antibodies).

Spleen, lymph nodes and MALT

The spleen is the largest lymphoid organ and is situated in the left upper abdomen (left hypochondriac region). It has a capsule, is vascular and contains both lymphatic and reticular tissue. Immune functions include the 'filtering' of blood and removal of worn-out blood cells and microbes by phagocytosis and providing a site for lymphocyte proliferation and antibody production.

The lymph nodes are small accumulations of lymphoid tissue found at strategic locations throughout the body (e.g. in the axillae and the cervical nodes in the neck). Lymph nodes filter the lymph, trapping extraneous particles such as microbes, cancer cells and damaged or worn-out cells. The trapped material is phagocytosed by macrophages (derived from monocytes) and the action of antibodies. In addition the lymph nodes provide a site for B and T lymphocyte proliferation and antibody production.

MALT containing both B and T lymphocytes is present in the respiratory, gastrointestinal and genitourinary tracts, all of which are exposed to the external environment. MALT, such as the tonsils and Peyer's patches in the ileum (small intestine), assists to detect pathogenic microorganisms entering the body.

See Further reading (e.g. Montague et al 2005, Waugh & Grant 2010) or consult your own anatomy and physiology textbook for more information.

Components and features of the immune system – an overview

The diverse and widespread cells, tissues, organs and molecules that form the immune system include the lymphatic system – lymph capillaries and vessels that convey lymph, lymph nodes, the spleen, the thymus gland, the mucosa-associated lymphoid tissue (MALT) such as the tonsils and that found in the gastrointestinal tract, the bone marrow and B and T lymphocytes.

Bone marrow and thymus

Lymphocytes develop in the bone marrow (see Ch. 11) but require further processing to form the two functionally different groups, B and T lymphocytes. The T lymphocytes are so called because they are processed in the thymus gland, which lies behind the sternum in the mediastinum and extends into the neck. Well developed in infants, it

Types of immunity

This part of the chapter outlines natural non-specific immunity and considers both types of adaptive specific immunity. Table 6.1 contrasts the features of natural and adaptive immunity. As mentioned earlier there is considerable

Table 6.1 Contrasting the features of adaptive and natural immunity (adapted from Staines et al 1993)

FEATURE	NATURAL NON-SPECIFIC IMMUNITY	ADAPTIVE SPECIFIC IMMUNITY
Resistance	Unaltered response on further exposure to the antigen. No 'memory'	Improved by repeated infection, i.e. has 'memory'
Sensitivity	Generally effective against all organisms. Cannot recognise specific antigens	Specific for the stimulating antigen
Major cell types	Phagocytes – neutrophils, monocytes, macrophages Natural killer (NK) cells	B and T lymphocytes (macrophages act as APCs in cell-mediated immunity)
Important chemicals	Complement proteins Lysozyme (antibacterial enzyme) Cytokines, e.g. interferons (IFNs) Acute phase proteins Inflammatory mediators, e.g. histamine, bradykinin	Antibodies (immunoglobulins) Other cytokines produced by lymphocytes (sometimes called lymphokines)

Note. Natural non-specific immunity is more primitive in evolutionary terms, and the mechanisms of adaptive specific immunity are directed to amplifying and increasing the efficiency of the mechanisms of natural immunity.

Box 6.1 Information

Cellular and chemical components of the immune responses

Cells – white blood cells (leucocytes) (see Ch.11 for further information)

Leucocytes are classified as:

- granular polymorphonuclear leucocytes – neutrophils, eosinophils and basophils
- non-granular (agranulocytes) – monocytes, macrophages (derived from monocytes), and lymphocytes.

The major phagocytic leucocytes (neutrophils, monocytes and macrophages) are able to recognise foreign material and to engulf and digest microorganisms by a process called phagocytosis.

- *Neutrophils* – the major phagocytes against bacteria and fungi.
- *Eosinophils* are capable of phagocytosis, but their main functions include defence against infestation by parasites and participation in allergic reactions.
- *Basophils and tissue-based mast cells* contain histamine (an inflammatory mediator), heparin and other chemicals. Released when basophils degranulate, the chemicals have a role in the inflammatory response, hypersensitivity and, in extreme situations, anaphylaxis (p. 185).
- *Monocytes and macrophages* – phagocytes present in the blood before they move into tissue sites where they develop into macrophages. Apart from being powerful phagocytes, tissue macrophages act as APCs for T lymphocytes in adaptive cell-mediated immunity.
- *Lymphocytes* include B lymphocytes (humoral immunity) which produce antibodies, T lymphocytes (cell-mediated immunity) and natural killer (NK) cells (immunological surveillance). B- and T-lymphocyte function is discussed in the section about adaptive specific immunity (see pp. 179–182).

Chemicals

- *Acute phase proteins* – serum proteins produced by the liver, e.g. C-reactive protein (CRP) and lactoferrin. Produced early in the inflammatory response, they may act to promote phagocytosis.
- *Antibodies (immunoglobulins)* – proteins known collectively as immunoglobulins (Igs) with specific antigen-binding properties. Five classes of antibody – immunoglobulin G (IgG), IgA, IgM, IgD and IgE – are produced by plasma cells (derived from B lymphocytes).
- *Complement* – a group of over 20 serum proteins. Cascading systems (where one component activates the next and so on), for example the antibody-mediated classical pathway and the alternate pathway, converge to form a multi-part membrane attack complex capable of cytolysis. Complement is involved in:
  - inflammation by causing vasodilatation and increasing the permeability of the capillary endothelium
  - preparation of antigens by opsonisation; 'tagging' antigens for phagocytic cells to recognise and ensuring that the antigen adheres to the surface of the phagocytic cell, thereby promoting phagocytosis
  - cytolysis (cell breakdown) and anaphylaxis.
- *Cytokines* – a large group of protein intercellular signalling molecules. Examples include the interferons (IFNs), interleukins (ILs), tumour necrosis factors (TNFs) and colony stimulating factors (CSFs). They act on several cells of the immune system including monocytes, B and T lymphocytes.
- *Histamine* – an inflammatory mediator released by mast cells when they degranulate after adhering to a microorganism. This gives rise to increased vascular permeability, arteriolar dilatation, smooth muscle contraction in the respiratory and alimentary tracts, and increased secretion of respiratory mucus. Other inflammatory mediators such as prostaglandins (from platelets) and bradykinin (released by neutrophils) are also released during the inflammatory response.

interaction between natural and adaptive immunity, and between both parts of adaptive immune responses. For example, tissue macrophages engulf antigens and act as antigen-presenting cells (APCs), which stimulate T-lymphocyte responses.

Information about the numerous cells and chemicals involved in immune responses is provided in Box 6.1.

Natural non-specific immunity

Natural non-specific immunity represents first- and second-line body defences (see Figure 6.1) and includes: intact skin/mucosae, specialised epithelial surfaces, body secretions containing antibacterial substances such as lysozyme and immunoglobulins (Storey & Jordan 2008) (Box 6.2) and the microorganisms that comprise the normal flora. The processes of inflammation (see Ch. 23) and phagocytosis (engulfing and destroying foreign particles by white blood cells) are also included (see Further reading, e.g. Waugh & Grant 2010). These defences can be breached in a number of situations, for example when skin is inflamed or damaged (see Ch. 12).

Additionally, natural killer (NK) cells, a type of large granular lymphocyte (LGL) that detects and destroys damaged or malignant cells and virus-infected cells, undertake non-specific immunosurveillance. NK cells are activated by various chemicals including interferons (IFNs), which have a role in increasing cell resistance to viral infection.

Adaptive specific immunity

Adaptive immune responses involve specially programmed cells (B and T lymphocytes, also called B and T cells) that respond to recognised antigens. There is specificity of response as each lymphocyte is equipped to recognise only one antigen. Once contact has been made with that antigen and it has been destroyed, some '*memory*' cells remain in the body. If the same antigen is encountered again (perhaps many years later), the remaining progeny of that memory cell are stimulated to replicate (clonal expansion), and this second response is both faster and more intense.

The adaptive specific immune response comprises the humoral (antibody-mediated) immune response, initiated by B lymphocytes, and the cell-mediated response, initiated by T lymphocytes. The humoral (antibody-mediated) response

Box 6.2 Information

Host defences: first-line mechanisms

Skin and mucosae

- Intact skin/mucosae
- Sloughing and constant renewal of skin and other epithelial surfaces
- Low pH of the skin – the 'acid mantle'
- Low water content
- Antibacterial lysozyme and immunoglobulin A (IgA) in sweat
- Normal flora.

Eyes and ears

- Eye lashes and blink reflex
- Blinking moving tears across the eyeball
- Antibacterial lysozyme and IgA in tears
- Ear secretions trapping foreign particles and containing IgA.

Gastrointestinal tract

- Saliva containing antibacterial lysozyme
- Hydrochloric acid in gastric juice
- Gastric mucus protecting the gastric lining from acid damage
- Mucosa-associated lymphoid tissue (MALT)
- Peristalsis
- Vomiting reflex when 'bad' food is ingested
- Normal flora.

Female genital tract

- Normal flora of the vagina producing an acid environment (pH 4.5) during the reproductive years

- Stratified squamous epithelial lining protecting the vagina from trauma
- Regular shedding of the outer layer of the endometrium (stratum functionalis) during menstruation.

Urinary tract

- Regular and complete voiding of urine
- Position of the kidneys and length of ureters
- Length of the male urethra
- pH of urine
- Mucosa-associated lymphoid tissue (MALT).

Respiratory tract

- Nasal secretions containing antibacterial lysozyme
- Nasal hairs
- Shape of the upper respiratory tract
- Normal flora of nasopharynx
- Sneeze and cough reflexes
- Mucosa-associated lymphoid tissue (MALT)
- Mechanisms that protect the larynx during swallowing
- Mucus production and ciliated epithelium – microbes and other foreign particles are trapped in mucus. The mucociliary escalator/transport moves the mucus upwards and out of the lungs.

Body secretions

- Secretions such as breast milk, tears and those produced by the ear, urinary, genital, respiratory and gastrointestinal tracts contain immunoglobulins (Storey & Jordan 2008).

deals mainly with extracellular organisms through the production of antibodies (immunoglobulins), whereas cell-mediated responses are important for dealing with intracellular organisms such as viruses.

Humoral (antibody-mediated) immune response

B lymphocytes produce antibodies (immunoglobulins). The antigen receptor on their surface is specific for one antigen only. B lymphocytes are capable of memory and are specialised to deal with microorganisms which do not, of their own accord, enter host cells, e.g. circulating bacteria. Following contact with an antigen the B cell either differentiates into a plasma cell which produces an antibody, or becomes a memory cell.

Antibodies (immunoglobulins)

Antibodies are globular proteins with the ability to recognise and bind to a specific antigen, usually a microorganism. They are produced by plasma cells and, once formed, circulate in the blood and other body fluids. Antibodies are characteristically Y-shaped, with two identical heavy chains, each connected to two identical light chains (Figure 6.2).

They have many roles that include:

- binding to a specific antigen, which causes antigen agglutination (clumping together), thus improving conditions for subsequent phagocytosis

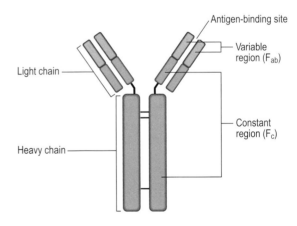

Figure 6.2 Antibody (immunoglobulin) structure – the heavy chain determines the class of antibody, e.g. IgG, IgA, etc. (Reproduced from Boon et al 2006 with permission.)

- acting as an opsonin to tag the antigen for destruction by phagocytes
- activating the complement pathway (interaction between natural and adaptive immunity)
- enhancing the ability of other cells, e.g. eosinophils and NK cells, to destroy foreign or abnormal cells (interaction between natural and adaptive immunity).

Although antibodies function in many different ways, all involve joining with the antigen to produce an immune complex.

Box 6.3 Information

Classes of antibodies (immunoglobulins)

- *IgM* – only found in blood. The first immunoglobulin to appear in the bloodstream in the primary immune response to infection. It functions in complement activation and agglutination of antigens. Since it disappears quickly after the antigen disappears, it is an indicator of current or very recent infection.
- *IgG* – the most plentiful immunoglobulin. Produced in large quantities in both the primary and secondary immune responses, particularly important in the secondary response. Levels in the blood give an indication of recent infection. Functions to neutralise toxins. It is also important as a defence against infection in the first few weeks of life, being the only immunoglobulin that crosses the placenta to the fetus.
- *IgA* – secreted onto the mucosal surfaces of the respiratory, gastrointestinal and genitourinary tracts and present in body secretions.
- *IgE* – normally found on the surface membrane of basophils (in the skin, mucosae and the lungs) and mast cells. It is associated with hypersensitivity (allergic) reactions and is active in parasite infestations.
- *IgD* – present in small quantities bound to B lymphocytes where it aids in the immunological 'memory' function.

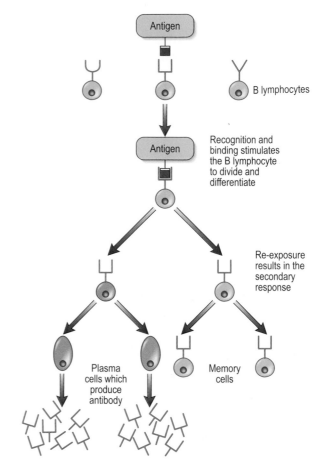

Figure 6.3 The primary immune response.

Each of the five classes may be produced with specificity for a single antigen. Their structure varies according to function and they are present in different amounts in the blood and other body fluids (Box 6.3).

Primary and secondary antibody-mediated immune response

When a specific antigen is encountered for the first time it takes approximately 2 weeks for a corresponding antibody to be detected in the blood. The production of this antibody is called the primary response. Although the immune system reacts immediately to antigens, the synthesis of antibody takes some time. However, on subsequent exposures to the specific antigen the matching specific antibody is produced much faster.

Primary response During this process the antigen binds to its specific receptor on the surface of the B lymphocyte, triggering the following sequence of events:

- The B lymphocyte is stimulated to differentiate into a plasma cell and to undergo multiple divisions so that identical plasma cells are formed.
- Plasma cells synthesise the specific antibody.
- Meanwhile, some B lymphocytes differentiate to become memory cells, which persist and replicate in the body long after the invading antigen has been destroyed (Figure 6.3).
- Once sufficient quantities of specific antibody have been produced to destroy the antigen, the plasma cells die, leaving memory cells ready to respond to any future encounter with that antigen.
- Antibodies bind to the antigen activating the events outlined above to produce an immune complex.

The time interval occurring between contact with the antigen and the production of IgM may allow disease to develop in the individual due to the effects of the antigen, e.g. microbial infection.

Secondary response occurs when a person encounters an antigen for the second time. The memory cells respond rapidly by producing plasma cells, which then secrete the specific antibody. This response occurs within a few days and, together with any residual antibody from the primary response, usually prevents disease from developing. In other words, the person has developed immunity.

Cell-mediated immune response

Cell-mediated immunity comprises T-lymphocyte-dependent responses directed against foreign cells/tissue (such as in transplant rejection), microorganisms that invade the host cells (viruses, fungi, parasites), phagocytosis-resistant bacteria and cancer cells. T lymphocytes are described as being thymus dependent (see p. 178). They are also antigen specific, have an antigen receptor and are capable of 'memory'.

There are several subsets of T lymphocytes (cells):

- T-helper cells (helper T cells)
- T-cytotoxic cells (cytotoxic T cells)
- T-suppressor cells
- delayed hypersensitivity T cells.

Box 6.4 Information

T-cell subsets (adapted from Brooker 2010 with permission)

- *T-helper cells (helper T cells) CD4+* – have a key role in the immune response, both cell mediated and antibody mediated. Their role includes the production of cytokines and the activation of B cells.
- *T-cytotoxic cells (cytotoxic T cells) CD8+* – destroy certain cells, such as malignant cells and virus-infected cells.
- *T-suppressor cells CD8+* – slow or stop the activity of other T cells and B cells once the antigen is dealt with.
- *Delayed hypersensitivity T cells* – T cells involved with macrophages and other T cells in cell-mediated delayed hypersensitivity and chronic inflammation.

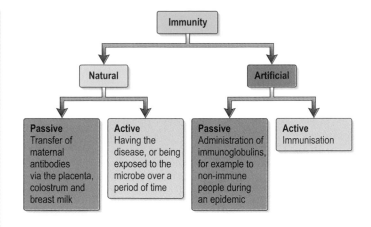

Note:

1. *Passive immunity* tends to be short-lived because the recipient's immune system is not stimulated.
2. *Active immunity* is usually of longer duration because it involves stimulation of the immune system to produce a specific antibody or T lymphocyte.

Figure 6.4 Natural and artificial immunity.

Box 6.4 provides further information on the T-cell subsets.

T-cell subsets are also classified according to their surface molecules, i.e. the glycoproteins CD4 or CD8. T-helper cells are designated CD4+; T-cytotoxic cells and T-suppressor cells are CD8+. The level of CD4+ cells and the ratio of CD4+ to CD8+cells are used when assessing the immune system in people with HIV disease (see Ch. 35) or other viral infections and following organ transplant.

T cells function in a variety of ways:

- Some produce cytokines to stimulate other immune responses, such as adaptive immune activity.
- Some collaborate with B cells to enhance antibody production.
- Others kill foreign cells directly.

Once all the antigen has been destroyed, the immune response is 'switched off' by the T-suppressor cells until the next time the antigen is encountered.

Immunity against infectious disease

Immunity to a specific infectious disease may be due to inherited qualities. Otherwise immunity develops by natural processes or is achieved by artificial means, i.e. vaccines. Both natural and artificial immunity may be passive or active (Figure 6.4).

Natural immunity may be passive where maternal IgG crosses the placenta to the fetus and following birth is transferred in colostrum and breast milk. This type of passive immunity is short-lived but helps to protect the infant until their own immune responses are sufficiently developed.

Active natural immunity is acquired if the person has the specific infection. Because this involves the production of a specific antibody or T lymphocyte, active immunity tends to be of longer duration (see primary and secondary response, p. 181).

Artificial immunity involves processes whereby immunity is initiated or augmented. Passive artificial immunity is achieved by the administration of immunoglobulins (usually obtained from the plasma of immune individuals). There are normal immunoglobulins produced from pooled plasma and disease-specific immunoglobulins including those for rabies, tetanus, hepatitis B and varicella-zoster. Immunoglobulins are used in disease outbreaks, e.g. measles, to protect non-immune individuals, or in the prophylaxis and/or management of specific diseases such as for people with tetanus-prone wounds. Passive immunity is short-lived because the person's immune system is not stimulated to produce specific antibodies (see Further reading, e.g. Health Protection Agency 2008, Provan et al 2008). *Note.* Immunoglobulins obtained from animals (antisera) can result in serious allergic reactions, including serum sickness, and have largely been replaced by human immunoglobulins.

Active artificial immunity is achieved by immunisation and, because this involves the production of a specific antibody or T lymphocyte, tends to be of longer duration (see primary and secondary response, p. 181).

Immunisation

Many countries offer some type of routine immunisation programme to infants, children and young people. Across the UK there is considerable variation in the uptake of immunisation between areas and specific groups. Recent guidance from the National Institute for Health and Clinical Excellence (NICE) (2009) aims to increase immunisation uptake.

Additionally, special groups including health and social care workers, unpaid carers and people travelling to certain countries are offered relevant immunisation. Some vaccines, such as the annual influenza and pneumococcal vaccines, are provided to people at increased risk of infection, e.g. those aged 65 years or over and people with chronic heart, respiratory and kidney disease, diabetes and following splenectomy.

Immunisation invokes a primary immune response to a particular antigen so that when the antigen is subsequently encountered, the individual will be immune to it. The principle of immunisation is to introduce attenuated (weakened) microorganisms or inactive products into the body so that the person mounts an immune response without developing the disease. Depending on the type of vaccine, an initial dose may be followed by a course of doses. Booster doses may be required months or years after the first dose to maintain an adequate level of memory cells. The types of vaccines used include:

- *Live vaccines.* Strains of microorganisms that have been attenuated. They retain their antigenicity but not their pathogenicity so are capable of stimulating an immune response without causing the disease. Examples include bacille Calmette–Guérin (BCG), used to prevent tuberculosis, and the measles, mumps and rubella (MMR) vaccine.
- *Inactivated (killed) vaccines.* These are preparations in which the organisms have been inactivated; the seasonal influenza vaccine is one example.
- *Detoxified or extracts of bacterial exotoxins.* An example is tetanus toxoid.

Box 6.5 provides an opportunity for you to explore issues around immunisation.

Box 6.5 Reflection

Immunisation

During a public health placement you are invited to accompany your mentor (a health visitor) to an 'immunisation question and answer' session at the local health centre.

Activities

- Think about the questions that might be asked by: people expecting their first baby, those with older children and teenagers, people aged 65 years or over and people caring for relatives with chronic diseases. What type of fears might be expressed?
- Use the resources provided to find answers to the following:
  - What vaccines are given and when does the immunisation schedule start?
  - Why are some vaccines given as a course over several weeks?
  - Why are booster doses needed?
  - What minor and major side-effects can occur?
  - When is vaccination contraindicated?
  - Which vaccines are offered to healthy people aged 65 years or over?
- Find out which vaccines are under consideration for addition to the list of those routinely offered.

Resources

British National Formulary (BNF) 2010 – http://www.bnf.org (section 14.1, Active immunity, is particularly informative)

Department of Health 2006 (updated 2008) A quick guide to childhood immunisation. Available online http://www.dh.gov.uk/en/Publicationsandstatistics/

Department of Health 2006 (modified Dec 2009) Immunisation against infectious disease – 'The Green Book'. Available online http://www.dh.gov.uk/en/Publichealth/Healthprotection/Immunisation/Greenbook/DH_4097254

Department of Health 2010 Immunisation. Available online http://www.dh.gov.uk/en/Publichealth/Immunisation/index.htm

Disorders of immunity

Disorders of immunity can be classified as:

- hypersensitivity and allergic reactions
- immunodeficiency
- autoimmune disease
- transplantation and graft rejection.

This chapter will concentrate on the first three disorders. Transplantation and graft rejection is beyond the scope of this chapter and readers are directed to Further reading, (e.g. Colledge et al 2010, Ch. 4 and Rich et al 2008, Ch. 80 – an advanced text).

Hypersensitivity and allergic reactions

Hypersensitivity is an abnormal and excessive immune response following contact with an antigen (also known as an allergen). Its effects range from local tissue damage to life-threatening anaphylaxis. Hypersensitivity reactions are classified as: immediate – types I, II and III which are antibody mediated; and delayed – type IV which is cell-mediated by antigen-specific T cells and macrophages.

Type I antibody-mediated (anaphylactic) hypersensitivity

In this type of immune response, excessive IgE production results in IgE binding to mast cells which, when the antigen is encountered, degranulate to release histamine and other inflammatory mediators, giving rise to an acute inflammatory reaction. The response usually develops within minutes of exposure to the antigen and will recur on subsequent encounters.

The reaction can be local, as in asthma (see Ch. 3), bronchospasm, rhinitis, conjunctivitis, hay fever and skin conditions such as urticaria and eczema (see Ch. 12 for allergy testing), or it can be systemic, as in anaphylaxis (see below). Typical antigens include:

House dust mite and pollen associated with asthma and hay fever (see Chs 3, 14).

Insect venom Stings by wasps and bees.

Foodstuffs such as fish and shellfish, eggs, milk, soy products, peanuts (a legume vegetable) and tree nuts such as almonds and walnuts. Note that peanut oil may be called arachis or groundnut oil.

Many people describe themselves as having a food allergy when they actually have a non-immune food intolerance. Notably, a true food allergy has an immunological basis – either IgE-mediated or cell-mediated. The majority of allergic responses to food are immediate IgE-mediated reactions, whereas cell-mediated responses, such as occur in coeliac disease, may take hours or days to develop (McKevith & Theobald 2005). According to Sicherer & Sampson (2010), around 5% of young children and 3–4% of adults in westernised countries experience abnormal immune responses to foods and the prevalence appears to have increased. Fox et al (2009) suggest that sensitisation to peanuts in infants is linked to the level of exposure to peanuts in the home, with high levels of exposure appearing to promote sensitisation.

Drugs such as antibiotics (e.g. penicillin), some anaesthetic agents, angiotensin converting enzyme (ACE) inhibitors. *Note.* Other substances, including aspirin, opiates and iodine-based radiographic contrast media, can cause mast cell degranulation without IgE binding. Iodine-based contrast media may cause both immediate and non-immediate hypersensitivity reactions (Brockow et al 2009).

Latex Latex rubber is present in a multitude of household items and medical devices (Box 6.6). Although latex allergy is uncommon in the general population, the risk of allergy is higher in patients who undergo repeated invasive procedures using latex-containing devices and for health care staff (Pollart et al 2009) (Box 6.7).

The nature of the symptoms will depend on whether the antigen is encountered locally or systemically, or absorbed via the intestine.

The term 'atopy' describes the tendency of 10–15% of the population to suffer from allergic conditions such as asthma, eczema, hay fever, urticaria and food allergy. There is often a familial (genetic) disposition to this condition.

Box 6.6 Information

Examples of products containing latex (reproduced from Rennie-Meyer 2007 with permission)

Household objects	Medical devices
• Adhesive tape and bandages	• Ambu bags
• Balloons	• Blood pressure cuffs (bladder and tubing)
• Camera eyepieces	• Condom urinary collection devices
• Carpet backing	
• Computer mouse pads	• Elastic bandages
• Condoms and diaphragms	• Electrode pads
• Dummies and baby bottle teats	• Enema tubing
• Elastic	• Gloves
• Erasers	• Goggles
• Handgrips, e.g. kitchen utensils, bicycles	• Haemodialysis equipment
• Hot-water bottles	• Injection ports on intravenous infusion tubing and fluid bags
• Household rubber gloves	
• Paint	• Stretcher canvasses
• Racquet handles	• Protective sheets and pillow covers
• Raincoats	
• Rubber bands	• Stethoscope tubing
• Rubber toys	• Sticking plasters
• Shoe soles and waterproof footwear	• Tourniquets
• Shower curtains and bathmats	• Trolley wheels
	• Urinary catheters
• Swimming fins and goggles	• Vial stoppers
• Tyres	• Wound drains and tubes

Box 6.7 Reflection

Latex allergy: staff and patients

Both health care staff and patients are at risk of developing an allergy to latex. Latex allergy can cause an urticarial skin rash, asthma (bronchospasm), rhinitis, conjunctivitis and rarely life-threatening anaphylaxis.

Activities

• Access the resource and consider the measures recommended to protect people with latex allergies.
• Reflect on polices/procedures in your placement regarding:
  – the use of latex products
  – the availability of substitute products
  – the identification of people with latex sensitivity
  – ways of ensuring that all staff know which patients are latex sensitive.

Resource

NHS National Patient Safety Agency 2005 (last modified 2009) Protecting people with allergy associated with latex. Available online http://www.npsa.nhs.uk/

Type II antibody-mediated (cytotoxic) hypersensitivity

This occurs when antibodies (IgM or IgG) bind to antigens on the surface of body cells. As a result the cell can be damaged or destroyed by several mechanisms involving phagocytosis, activation of the complement proteins, direct cell lysis and a process of extracellular killing by enzymes, free radicals and other molecules that results in lysis. Examples of cytotoxic hypersensitivity include a mismatched (ABO) blood transfusion (see Ch. 11) or a transplant.

Type III antibody-mediated (immune-complex) hypersensitivity

This is an exaggerated form of the natural immune mechanism caused by the deposition of many large immune complexes (products of antigen–antibody reaction) within the tissues or in the capillary endothelium of the kidney, joints, skin and other sites. The excess immune complexes may activate complement and attract phagocytes, resulting in mast cell degranulation and a pathological inflammatory response. This may be local (Arthus reaction), such as occurred with non-human insulin before the recombinant human insulin analogues were introduced (see Ch. 5), or cause widespread inflammation (known as serum sickness, previously common when horse antisera were in use, see p. 182). The damaging inflammation may cause conditions that include glomerulonephritis, extrinsic allergic alveolitis, arthritis, skin rashes and lymphadenopathy. This type of hypersensitivity occurs when the person has contact with an antigen, such as foreign antigens including microorganisms, over a long time span. It may also be associated with some autoimmune disorders.

Type IV cell-mediated or delayed (24–72 hours) hypersensitivity

Type IV hypersensitivity involves antigen-specific T cells and macrophages. The sensitised T cells, on repeat contact with an antigen, release cytokines that attract the phagocytic macrophages. These reactions cause chronic and sometimes extensive inflammation and are apparent a few hours after exposure to the antigen. Examples of type IV hypersensitivity include the Mantoux skin test, which is used to ascertain whether a person has tuberculosis or has immunity to tuberculosis, and contact dermatitis (see Ch. 12). It also contributes to graft rejection.

Anaphylaxis (anaphylactic shock)

Anaphylaxis is a sudden severe allergic reaction that is potentially life threatening (Finney & Rushton 2007). It is a form of type I hypersensitivity but involves an exaggerated response to an antigen such as a foodstuff (e.g. peanuts), an antibiotic or other medication, a vaccine or a bee sting (Ferns & Chojnacka 2003, Reading 2004). The incidence of anaphylaxis is increasing (Simons 2009). A pilot study by Clark et al (2009) reported a therapeutic intervention used for a small number of subjects with severe peanut allergy, whereby tolerance to peanut protein was increased using peanut oral immunotherapy (OIT). A larger 3-year trial is planned.

PATHOPHYSIOLOGY

Anaphylaxis occurs due to an IgE-mediated release of inflammatory mediators, such as histamine, from mast cells causing a massive inflammatory response.

Common presenting signs and symptoms Anaphylaxis can present in a variety of ways and health professionals must always be alert to the possibility of it occurring. People with anaphylaxis may present with some or all of the following:

- urticaria
- pruritus
- angioedema
- airway obstruction and stridor
- difficulty swallowing and/or speaking
- bronchospasm and wheeze
- chest tightness
- pulmonary oedema
- respiratory distress
- abdominal pain, diarrhoea and vomiting
- vascular collapse
- tachycardia
- hypotension and shock
- altered consciousness
- anxiety and fear
- pallor.

MEDICAL MANAGEMENT

Anaphylaxis is a medical emergency and an accurate diagnosis must be made rapidly in order to preserve life. Treatment is based on the administration of adrenaline (epinephrine) to support cardiovascular and respiratory function, chlorphenamine (an antihistamine) to counter the harmful effects of the histamine, hydrocortisone, oxygen and intravenous (i.v.) fluids. The Resuscitation Council UK (2005a) publishes guidelines in the form of an anaphylaxis algorithm.

 See website Figure 6.1

Cardiopulmonary resuscitation (CPR) may also be required (see Ch. 2).

Details of the drugs regimen (adrenaline, chlorphenamine and hydrocortisone), including age-related doses and frequency of administration to be used for anaphylaxis in community settings, are provided in the *British National Formulary* (2010).

 ## Nursing management and health promotion: anaphylaxis (anaphylactic shock)

It is vital that nurses are able to recognise anaphylaxis and take urgent action to safeguard the person's life (Finney & Rushton 2007). Initiating the appropriate management in a timely manner increases the chance of a swift recovery. Without effective management at the onset there is a very real risk of death.

Nurses may be faced with a person with anaphylaxis in a variety of situations – on duty in the community, clinic, ward/unit, in a meeting or moving between departments, or off duty out shopping or jogging in the park. It is possible that the nurse will be required to provide initial care, especially in circumstances where emergency facilities are not available. Nurses have a professional duty, both on and off duty, to provide assistance in an emergency situation (Nursing and Midwifery Council [NMC] 2008). However, if the nurse chooses to offer assistance when off duty she/he also accepts a legal duty of care (NMC 2008).

Maintenance of the airway, breathing and circulation is paramount and the nurse should be prepared to commence CPR (see Ch. 2). The Resuscitation Council UK (2005b) publishes guidelines entitled *Anaphylactic reactions – Initial treatment* (Figure 6.5); the advanced *Anaphylaxis algorithm* is available on the companion website.

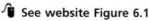 **See website Figure 6.1**

During initial treatment the nurse must be calm and endeavour to reduce the person's anxiety (Box 6.8). Once the person is stabilised the nurse will need to provide a fuller explanation and continue to reduce anxiety. The question of how to prevent a similar occurrence will need to be explored, the cause of the reaction investigated and the necessity of future antigen (allergen) avoidance dicussed. People with frequent, unpreventable attacks should have a MedicAlert® card or bracelet, and the person and relatives should be supplied with adrenaline, and taught how to manage and administer it, using, for example, the autoinjector pre-filled adrenaline (epinephrine) pens – Anapen®, Epipen® (Box 6.9). It is important for the person and their family to have an individual emergency plan to deal with any recurrence of anaphylaxis (Simons 2009).

See website Critical thinking question 6.1

Immunodeficiency

Immunodeficiency is a state of defective immune responses, leading to increased susceptibility to infection, autoimmune diseases and cancer. Recurrent infections are an indication of an immunodeficiency.

See website Table 6.1

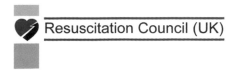

Resuscitation Council (UK)

Anaphylactic reactions – Initial treatment

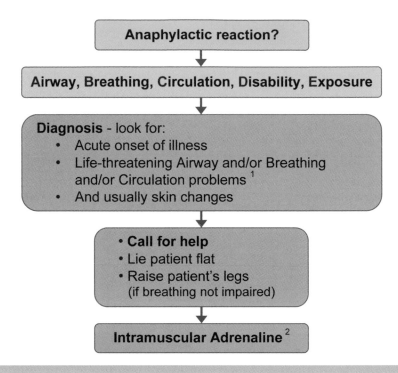

| Anaphylactic reaction? |

| Airway, Breathing, Circulation, Disability, Exposure |

Diagnosis - look for:
- Acute onset of illness
- Life-threatening Airway and/or Breathing and/or Circulation problems [1]
- And usually skin changes

- **Call for help**
- Lie patient flat
- Raise patient's legs (if breathing not impaired)

Intramuscular Adrenaline [2]

---

[1] Life-threatening problems:

Airway:	swelling, hoarseness, stridor
Breathing:	rapid breathing, wheeze, fatigue, cyanosis, SpO_2 < 92%, confusion
Circulation:	pale, clammy, low blood pressure, faintness, drowsy/coma

[2] Intramuscular Adrenaline

IM doses of 1:1000 adrenaline (repeat after 5 min if no better)

• Adult	500 micrograms IM (0.5 mL)
• Child more than 12 years:	500 micrograms IM (0.5 mL)
• Child 6 -12 years:	300 micrograms IM (0.3 mL)
• Child less than 6 years:	150 micrograms IM (0.15 mL)

Figure 6.5 Anaphylactic reactions – Initial treatment. (Reproduced from the Resuscitation Council UK 2005b with permission.)

Immunodeficiency may be a primary disorder or much more commonly secondary to other conditions or treatments, such as chemotherapy. Immunodeficiency may result from impaired humoral and/or cell-mediated immune responses.

Primary immunodeficiency

The many primary immunodeficiencies are rare and complex conditions and can be difficult to classify, thereby requiring specialist diagnosis, management and care. An overview of some disorders is provided here and readers requiring more

Box 6.8 Reflection

'A wasp sting might have killed me'

'I was out for a run and something flew into my mouth. I spat it out and then realised that it was a wasp as it had stung me on the tongue. The pain was really bad and my tongue was swelling. No mobile phone and miles from anywhere – I was alone on the fen and there was no-one in sight. How did I feel? Panicky and terrified – what should I do, how could this happen, was I going to die? The pain was increasing and spreading to my throat and teeth. I tried to remain calm and quickly ran back home with a mounting sense of panic.'

Activity

- Reflect on the person's feelings of fear and panic and consider how you might feel in similar circumstances
- Discuss with your mentor or colleagues how the nurse can help to reduce fear and anxiety in such a situation

Box 6.9 Reflection

Self-administration of adrenaline

People at risk of anaphylaxis must always have access to their adrenaline (epinephrine) autoinjectors. This means carrying one in a bag or pocket, or having a well-labelled pack available in a specific place at home, work or college/school.

Activities

- Reflect on how having to always have an adrenaline autoinjector available may impact on normal life:
  - thinking about the need to check that packs are in date and arranging replacements
  - feeling confident about using the autoinjector
  - ensuring that family, friends, work colleagues or lecturers/teachers know where the packs are located and, if necessary, can administer the adrenaline
  - requirement to have a letter from your GP before you can travel by air with the autoinjector in hand baggage.

Resources

Allergy UK (previously known as British Allergy Foundation) – http://www.allergyuk.org

British National Formulary 2010 – http://www.bnf.org

detailed information are directed to Further reading (e.g. Nairn & Helbert 2007, Rich et al 2008, Colledge et al 2010).

Primary phagocyte problems

These include:

- problems with phagocyte migration to areas of inflammation; a deficiency in cell adhesion molecules (CAM) prevents the phagocytes from moving out of the blood vessels
- defects affecting cytokines or their receptors
- chronic granulomatous disease.

The presentation is with recurrent bacterial and fungal infections. Treatment includes appropriate antibiotics,

prophylactic antibiotics and antifungal drugs and in some cases haematopoietic stem cell transplantation (HSCT) (see Ch. 11).

Complement deficiencies

Genetically determined deficiencies can affect many of the complement proteins. Depending on which complement protein and which pathway is involved there may be infection with encapsulated bacteria if the complement membrane attack complex (see p. 179) is impaired, or autoimmune conditions such as systemic lupus erythematosus (SLE, see pp. 190–191). A lack of the regulatory C1 inhibitor is associated with angio-edema (hereditary angioedema [HAE] and acquired).

See website Figure 6.2

For further information see Useful websites (e.g. Primary Immunodeficiency Association).

No specific treatment exists but those affected should be offered prophylactic penicillin and immunisations against *Haemophilus influenzae* B, pneumococcus and meningococcus.

Combined B- and T-lymphocyte deficiencies

Severe combined immune deficiency (SCID) comprises a group of genetic immunodeficiency disorders caused by an inability to produce normal mature B and T lymphocytes. Both parts of the adaptive immune response are affected, thereby leaving the infant without humoral and cell-mediated responses. Affected infants have recurrent infections (bacterial, viral and fungal) and diseases such as measles and chicken pox can become life-threatening. SCID is generally fatal unless a haemopoietic stem cell transplantation (HSCT) is undertaken. Developments in gene therapy may provide an effective treatment in the future.

T-lymphocyte deficiencies

These present as recurrent infections caused by fungi, protozoa and viruses. There are several types of T-lymphocyte problems (Figure 6.6), including:

- autoimmune lymphoproliferative syndrome in which lymphocytes are not destroyed naturally by apoptosis (cell death), leading to autoimmune disorders
- bare lymphocyte syndromes in which certain HLA (human leucocyte antigen) molecules are not expressed in the thymus gland and particular lymphocytes do not develop/mature; this defect is also associated with other problems such as vasculitis
- DiGeorge's syndrome (thymic–parathyroid aplasia) which is caused by a failure of the thymus to develop and may be associated with other congenital defects.

There may also be problems with antibody function because some T cells collaborate with B cells to enhance antibody production.

The management of T-cell deficiencies will depend on the specific deficiency but may include:

- prophylactic antimicrobial agents
- treatment of specific infections
- depending on the deficiency – HSCT or bone marrow transplant (BMT), thymic tissue transplant, replacement immunoglobulins.

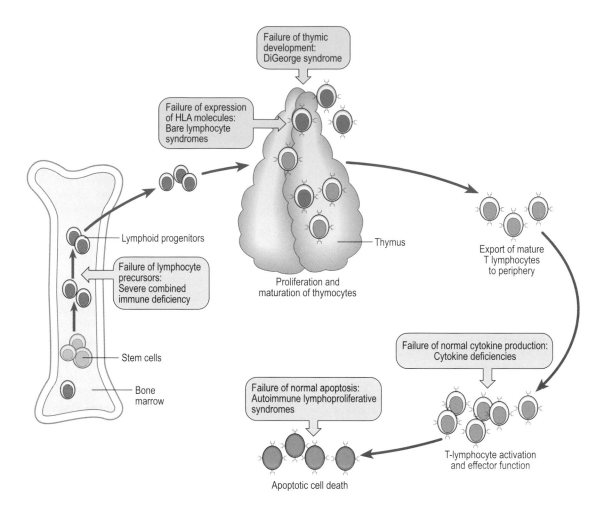

Figure 6.6 T-lymphocyte function and dysfunction. (Reproduced from Boon et al 2006 with permission.)

Antibody deficiencies (primary)

These are associated with bacterial infections, particularly those caused by *Streptococcus pneumoniae* and *Haemophilus influenzae*. There are several genetically determined defects of antibody production, some of which present during infancy once the passive immunity from maternal IgG diminishes. They include:

- Combined variable immunodeficiency (CVID). Presenting in adulthood, there is a failure to produce IgG, leading to recurrent infections such as chronic sinusitis. There is also an increased risk of autoimmune conditions such as autoimmune haemolytic anaemia (see Ch. 11) and some cancers.
- Selective IgA deficiency. Common in Northern Europe (Marshall 2006). Those affected may have recurrent but mild infections, or the deficiency may be detected incidentally during a routine blood test.
- Specific IgG deficiency.

Management includes intravenous immunoglobulin (IVIG) replacement therapy (Deane et al 2009) which is often self-administered at home. Antibiotics are used to treat infection and as prophylaxis.

Secondary immunodeficiency

This occurs as a result of some altered state, condition or its treatment. Common causes include:

- extremes of age
- malnutrition
- stress
- chronic conditions such as diabetes mellitus, cancer
- chemotherapy
- radiotherapy
- long-term high-dose corticosteroid therapy
- drugs that suppress gastric acid production
- immunosuppression following transplants
- HIV/AIDS.

See Chapters 5, 17, 21, 31, 34, 35.

Autoimmune disorders

Normally the body is able to differentiate between self and non-self, an ability known as tolerance, which develops during fetal life (Farley & Hendry 2002). Autoimmune disorders occur when this normal tolerance to 'self' breaks down and autoantibodies against 'self antigens' develop so that the immune system fails to recognise self. The inheritance of particular HLA genes is associated with autoimmune disorders, such as DR3/DR4 with type 1 diabetes. Change in normal immune tolerance may be spontaneous or caused by external factors such as drugs and microorganisms. Autoimmune conditions, of which there are many, range from

Box 6.10 Information

Examples of autoimmune disorders

- Addison's disease – Ch. 5
- Anti-GBM disease (Goodpasture's syndrome, a type of glomerulonephritis) – Ch. 8
- Autoimmune haemolytic anaemia – Ch. 11
- Autoimmune hepatitis – Ch. 4
- Bullous skin disorders (e.g. pemphigus, pemphigoid) – Ch. 12
- Graves' disease hyperthyroidism – Ch. 5
- Hypoparathyroidism – Ch. 5
- Hypothyroidism – Ch. 5
- Idiopathic thrombocytopenic purpura (ITP) – Ch. 11
- Multiple sclerosis – Ch. 9
- Myasthenia gravis (see below)
- Pernicious anaemia – Ch. 11
- Rheumatoid arthritis – Ch. 10
- Some types of male infertility
- Sympathetic ophthalmitis/ophthalmia – Ch. 13
- Systemic lupus erythematosus (SLE) (see pp. 190–191)
- Thyroiditis hyperthyroidism – Ch. 5
- Type 1 diabetes mellitus – Ch. 5

organ-specific disorders such as myasthenia gravis (below) to generalised manifestations such as systemic lupus erythematosus (SLE) (pp. 190–191) (Box 6.10). They are characterised by periods of remission and 'flares' (relapse) and are more common in women (Colledge et al 2010). They may also involve a hypersensitivity reaction, whether immediate or delayed.

There are several mechanisms whereby autoantibodies are formed including:

- exposure of body proteins previously 'hidden' from the immune system; for example spermatozoa which are only formed long after immunocompetence is achieved (may occur following inflammation of the testes) or the lens proteins of the eye which are 'shown' to the immune system following eye injury
- an extrinsic agent, such as a microorganism (e.g. certain streptococcal infections), drug (e.g. halothane) or other chemical, can change the 'self' antigens so that the immune system recognises them as foreign
- genetic mutations which alter immune cells.

This chapter outlines two autoimmune disorders, myasthenia gravis and SLE.

Myasthenia gravis

Myasthenia gravis is a rare autoimmune disease affecting the neuromuscular junction. It is associated with a disorder of the thymus gland; some patients (approximately 15%) have a thymoma while most of the others have thymic hyperplasia (Allen et al 2006). It usually occurs in individuals aged between 15 and 50 years.

PATHOPHYSIOLOGY

Acetylcholine (a neurotransmitter) normally facilitates transmission of impulses from the motor nerves to voluntary muscle (see Chs 9, 10). In myasthenia gravis there are autoantibodies to the acetylcholine receptors in the neuro-muscular junction. These block neuromuscular transmission and instigate complement activation (see p. 179), leading to inflammation with loss of acetylcholine receptors and further damage.

Common presenting signs and symptoms There is progressive fatigable weakness in which some muscle groups tire more quickly (Kittiwatanapaisan et al 2003). Movement may be powerful at first but quickly weakens. Localised symptoms include diplopia (double vision) or ptosis (lid droop) (see Ch. 13) due to weakness of the extraocular muscles. There are particular problems in chewing, swallowing (dysphagia), talking and moving the limbs. The muscles around the shoulder girdle are those most commonly affected.

Symptoms are often worse at the end of the day or after exercise. Diplopia or progressively quieter speech may be early symptoms. Respiratory muscles may be affected, resulting in a weakened cough, aspiration and the distinct possibility of respiratory failure. Relapses sometimes occur after infections or following emotional upsets and stressful events.

MEDICAL MANAGEMENT

History, investigations and diagnosis The person presents with a history of muscle weakness and inability to sustain muscle power. There are difficulties with activities above shoulder level, e.g. pulling on a jumper or brushing hair. Anti-acetylcholine receptor antibodies (AchRA) can be detected in the serum. A computed tomography (CT) scan of the chest is performed to rule out thymoma. Investigations for other autoimmune disorders, e.g. autoimmune thyroid disease, are undertaken.

Diagnosis is assisted by an intravenous injection of the short-acting anticholinesterase, edrophonium. This allows acetylcholine to accumulate. Muscle power usually improves within 30 seconds of the injection and often persists for 2–3 minutes as a result of the temporary increase in acetylcholine at the damaged neuromuscular junction.

Treatment The aims of therapy are to increase acetylcholine activity at the neuromuscular junction and to decrease the immune responses responsible for damage to the motor end plates.

Acetylcholine activity is increased with anticholinesterase inhibitors (acetylcholinesterase is an enzyme that breaks down acetylcholine), e.g. pyridostigmine. These drugs can cause muscarinic side-effects such as diarrhoea.

Immunological treatments include:

- thoracoscopic thymectomy
- corticosteroids
- plasma exchange (plasmapheresis) to remove autoantibodies
- intravenous immunoglobulin
- immunosuppressant medication such as azathioprine.

Plasmapheresis or immunoglobulin may be effective in the early stages of treatment or later during an exacerbation (Richman & Agius 2003). Some drugs, including aminoglycoside antibiotics, can cause deterioration.

Nursing management and health promotion: myasthenia gravis

Nurses need to work with the person and their family to identify actual and potential problems and their need for information and teaching. The person and their family are informed about sources of help and information, for example the Myasthenia Gravis Association (see Useful websites).

Conditions such as myasthenia gravis are best managed by a multidisciplinary team (MDT) including nurses (community and hospital based), medical staff, speech and language therapists (SLT), occupational therapists (OT), physiotherapists and pharmacists.

Emergency situations associated with myasthenia gravis

There are two potential life-threatening situations: myasthenic and cholinergic crises.

- A myasthenic crisis reflects a sudden exacerbation of the condition with respiratory muscle weakness. It is distinguished from cholinergic crisis by improvement following a small dose of intravenous edrophonium.
- A cholinergic crisis may occur as a consequence of overdosage of an anticholinesterase drug. Muscle weakness and fasciculation, paralysis, excess salivation, pallor and sweating, constricted pupils and possibly respiratory failure may occur. This is a result of excessive acetylcholine, which causes hyperstimulation of the acetylcholine receptors.

Both conditions are life-threatening and require urgent medical intervention. The consequences of myasthenic or cholinergic crisis are life threatening. Paralysis of the respiratory muscles can rapidly lead to severe hypoxia; consequently, the patient may require resuscitation and ventilation (see Ch. 29).

Ongoing care and support

Most people with myasthenia gravis live independently at home for as long as possible. Nursing care, when required, will depend on the severity of their symptoms. The person will experience varying degrees of fatigue and muscle weakness and the OT can teach them how to conserve energy in order to make best use of limited energy. Lack of energy may mean that help is needed with activities of living: eating, drinking, mobility, washing and dressing. If blinking is impaired the person may need eye care including eye drops to prevent corneal drying (see Ch. 13).

Dysphagia can lead to choking and the person must be referred to the SLT for assessment and advice regarding oral intake including food texture and thickened fluids. Advice on a balanced nutritious diet is particularly important where chewing and swallowing are impaired. Family and nurses can encourage the person to take small mouthfuls of food and concentrate on chewing slowly and then swallowing. If oral intake is insufficient the dietitian is consulted as enteral feeding may be required (see Ch. 21).

If respiratory muscle fatigue makes breathing difficult, the person is helped to maintain a position that aids breathing, such as sitting up in a chair, or propped up in bed. The nurse will observe for signs of deterioration (e.g. increasing distress, cyanosis) and monitor oxygen saturation and measure peak expiratory flow rate as appropriate. The physiotherapist will be able to advise the person about how to breathe more effectively and also to maximise coughing to expectorate bronchial secretions.

Reduced mobility may increase the risk of pressure ulcers and the nurse should assess the level of risk (see Ch. 23). Again, the physiotherapist can advise regarding mobility and supply mobility aids.

Systemic lupus erythematosus

Systemic lupus erythematosus (SLE) is a multisystem disorder affecting connective tissue. Presentation is characterised by a wide variety of signs and symptoms which depend upon the system attacked by the autoantibodies. Most of those affected are women (Doherty et al 2006) and onset usually occurs in young adulthood.

PATHOPHYSIOLOGY

The cause of SLE is not yet fully understood. Box 6.11 provides an explanation by Doherty et al 2006.

Common presenting signs and symptoms The presentation is often vague and non-specific. There may be:

- joint symptoms – arthralgia, arthritis
- mouth ulcers
- pleurisy, pericarditis, myocarditis, alveolitis
- skin rashes – usually on areas exposed to sunlight; characteristically, a 'butterfly rash' across the nose and cheeks

See website Figure 6.3

- Raynaud's phenomenon

See website Figure 6.4

- kidney involvement with proteinuria due to glomerulonephritis, which may progress to renal failure
- fatigue, confusion, seizures or mental health problems
- haematological problems – reduction in circulating blood cell numbers, e.g. neutropenia, or haemolytic anaemia
- lymphadenopathy, weight loss and fever.

See website Critical thinking question 6.2

 Box 6.11 Information

Aetiology and pathogenesis of SLE

'At least 50 antigen targets for autoantibody production are described in SLE. However, none of the diverse manifestations of SLE can be attributed to a single antigenic stimulus, and it is likely that this wide spectrum of autoantibody production results from polyclonal B- and T-cell activation. Many autoantigens in SLE are components of the intracellular and intranuclear machinery. In normal health these antigens are "hidden" from the immune system and do not provoke an immune response. Although the triggers that lead to autoantibody production in SLE are unknown, one mechanism may be exposure of intracellular antigens on the cell surface during apoptosis. This hypothesis is supported by the fact that environmental factors that associate with flares of lupus – such as sunlight and artificial ultraviolet (UV) light, pregnancy and infection – increase oxidative stress and subsequent apoptosis.' (Doherty et al 2006, p. 1132)

Note: People with the specific antiphospholipid antibody have an increased risk of venous thromboembolism (VTE) and may require anticoagulants such as warfarin.

MEDICAL MANAGEMENT

History, examination and investigations As the symptoms of SLE are both diverse and variable, a thorough history is essential. There may be external signs of tissue damage such as skin rash, which may assist diagnosis. Antinuclear antibodies (ANA) will be found in the serum of most people with SLE. Some will also have detectable anti-DNA antibodies. A full blood count (FBC) may identify anaemia, leucopenia and thrombocytopenia (see Ch. 11).

Treatment This aims to relieve symptoms and prevent organ damage. Analgesics and non-steroidal anti-inflammatory drugs (NSAIDs) may help to alleviate joint pain and other symptoms. Hydroxychloroquine, an antimalarial drug, is sometimes used to reduce the frequency of exacerbations of skin and joint lesions. A short course of corticosteroids, e.g. prednisolone, is used for rashes, joint and other problems. In acute life-threatening situations, such as brain or kidney involvement, high-dose corticosteroids are given intravenously or orally with cyclophosphamide. Other immunosuppressants, e.g. ciclosporin, azathioprine, tacrolimus, may also be used in the management of SLE.

 ## Nursing management and health promotion: SLE

The specific care of people with SLE depends very much on the stage of the disease and on the systems involved. In any event, the aim is to alleviate symptoms as they present (Sohng 2003). As with people with other autoimmune conditions the nurse works with the person and their family to identify actual and potential problems and their need for information and teaching. Other members of the MDT are involved as appropriate, such as the physiotherapist and OT for joint involvement, and specialist nurses will provide support, advice and monitoring. For example specialist renal nurses will monitor renal function – urinalysis for microalbuminuria, blood tests and blood pressure; anticoagulant specialist nurses will monitor those people who are prescribed warfarin to reduce the risk of VTE. The person and their family should be informed about sources of help and information, for example the Arthritis Research UK (see Further reading).

Ongoing care and support

As fatigue is common, the person with SLE should be encouraged to have adequate rest. SLE is a multisystem condition and those affected may need help from the nurse for a range of issues, such as seizures, confusion, low mood or fears about prognosis. The person and their family should be offered opportunities to discuss their fears and feelings about the condition. Emotional support will be needed as this is a chronic disease of uncertain progression.

Poor peripheral circulation leading to cold hands and feet may occur and people should be advised to avoid the cold and trauma to the fingers and be encouraged to wear appropriate clothing. There is also an increased susceptibility to infection due to the debilitating effects of the disease process and treatment with immunosuppressant drugs (see Chs 11, 31).

People should be given advice about photosensitivity in order to reduce rashes and skin damage which will include:

* avoiding sunlight and other forms of UV light
* use of high-SPF creams or lotions
* covering the skin and wearing wide-brimmed sun hats.

Some may be self-conscious about facial rashes and benefit from a chance to discuss their anxieties and ways of minimising the appearance of the rash.

Pregnancy and the oral contraceptive are associated with 'flares' of SLE. During pregnancy the woman should be cared for by an MDT that includes a specialist in the care of SLE.

SUMMARY: KEY NURSING ISSUES

* The three lines of body defence are: *first line* natural, non-specific barriers such as intact skin; *second line* natural, non-specific defences, such as inflammation and phagocytosis; and *third line* adaptive, specific immune responses – humoral (antibody) and cell-mediated immunity.
* Although immunity is divided into natural and adaptive responses, numerous interactions and collaboration occur between different components of the immune system.
* Nurses in all areas of practice will care for people with disorders affecting the immune system – ranging from life-threatening allergies through to varying degrees of immunodeficiency and autoimmunity.
* Knowledge and understanding of the complexity of immunological processes and disorders is still incomplete and many exciting developments can be anticipated in the future. The use of immunological treatments for diseases such as cancer will expand over the next decade.

REFLECTION AND LEARNING – WHAT NEXT?

* **Test** your knowledge by visiting the website 🖱 and answering the multiple choice questions and critical thinking questions.
* **Consolidate** your learning by looking at some of the further reading suggestions, references and specialist websites.
* **Revisit** some of the additional material on the website.
* **Consider** what you have learnt and how this will help your professional development.
* **Reflect** on how you can apply this knowledge to the care of your patients.
* **Discuss** your learning with your mentor/supervisor, lecturer and colleagues.

REFERENCES

Allen CM, Lueck CJ, Dennis M: Neurological disease. In Boon NA, Colledge NR, Walker BR, editors: *Davidson's Principles and Practice of Medicine*, ed 20, Churchill Livingstone, 2006, Edinburgh, p 1252.

Boon NA, Colledge NR, Walker BR, editors: *Davidson's Principles and Practice of Medicine*, ed 20, Edinburgh, 2006, Churchill Livingstone.

British National Formulary (BNF): *Medical emergencies in community – Anaphylaxis*, 2010. Available online http://bnf.org/bnf/bnf/current/200070.htm?q=%22anaphylaxis%22#_hit.

Brockow K, Romano A, Aberer W, et al: Skin testing in patients with hypersensitivity reactions to iodinated contrast media – a European multicenter study, *Allergy* 64(2):234–241, 2009.

Brooker C, editor: *Mosby's Dictionary of Medicine, Nursing and Health Professions*, Edinburgh, 2010, Mosby.

Clark AT, Islam S, King Y, et al: Successful oral tolerance induction in severe peanut allergy, *Allergy* 64(8):1218–1220, 2009.

Colledge NR, Walker BR, Ralston SH: *Davidson's Principles and Practice of Medicine*, ed 21, Edinburgh, 2010, Churchill Livingstone.

Deane S, Selmi C, Naguwa SM: Common variable immunodeficiency: Etiological and treatment issues, *Int Arch Allergy Immunol* 150(4):311–324, 2009.

Doherty M, Lanyon P, Ralston SH: Musculoskeletal disorders. In Boon NA, Colledge NR, Walker BR, editors: *Davidson's Principles and Practice of Medicine*, ed 20, Edinburgh, 2006, Churchill Livingstone, p 1132.

Farley A, Hendry C: Autoimmune disorders, *Nurs Stand* 16(41):38–40, 2002.

Ferns T, Chojnacka I: The causes of anaphylaxis, *Br J Nurs* 12(17):1006–1012, 2003.

Finney A, Rushton C: Recognition and management of patients with anaphylaxis, *Nurs Stand* 21(37):50–57, 2007.

Fox AT, Sasieni P, du Toit G, et al: Household peanut consumption as a risk factor for the development of peanut allergy, *J Allergy Clin Immunol* 123(2):417–423, 2009.

Kittiwatanapaisan W, Gauthier DK, Williams AM, et al: Fatigue in myasthenia gravis patients, *J Neurosci Nurs* 35(2):87–93, 2003.

Marshall SE: Immunological factors in disease. In Boon NA, Colledge NR, Walker BR, editors: *Davidson's Principles and Practice of Medicine*, ed 20, Edinburgh, 2006, Churchill Livingstone, p 74.

McKevith B, Theobald H: Common food allergies, *Nurs Stand* 19(29):39–42, 2005.

National Institute for Health and Clinical Excellence (NICE): *Reducing differences in the uptake of immunisations (including targeted vaccines) among children and young people under 19 years*, 2009. Public health guidance 21. Available online http://guidance.nice.org.uk/PH21.

Nursing and Midwifery Council: *Duty of Care*, 2008, (June). Available online http://www.nmc-uk.org/

Pollart SM, Warniment C, Mori T: Latex allergy, *Am Fam Physician* 80(12):1413–1418, 2009.

Reading D: Managing anaphylaxis, *Practice Nurse* 28(3):28–31, 2004.

Rennie-Meyer J: Preventing the spread of infection. In Brooker C, Waugh A, editors: *Foundations of Nursing Practice: Fundamentals of holistic care*, Edinburgh, 2007, Mosby, pp 398, 406.

Resuscitation Council UK: *Anaphylaxis algorithm*, 2005a. Available online http://www.resus.org.uk/.

Resuscitation Council UK: *Anaphylactic reactions – Initial treatment*, 2005b. Available online http://www.resus.org.uk/.

Richman DP, Agius MA: Treatment of autoimmune myasthenia gravis, *Neurology* 61(12):1652–1661, 2003.

Sicherer SH, Sampson HA: Food allergy, *J Allergy Clin Immunol* 125:S116–S125, 2010.

Simons FE: Anaphylaxis: Recent advances in assessment and treatment, *J Allergy Clin Immunol* 124(4):625–636, 2009.

Sohng KY: Effects of a self-management course for patients with systemic lupus erythematosus, *J Adv Nurs* 42(5):479–486, 2003.

Staines N, Brostoff J, James K: *Introducing immunology*, ed 2, London, 1993, Mosby.

Storey M, Jordan S: An overview of the immune system, *Nurs Stand* 23(15–17):47–56, 2008.

FURTHER READING

Arthritis Research UK: *Lupus (SLE) Information Booklet*, 2009. Available online http://www.arc.org.uk/arthinfo/patpubs/6023/6023.asp.

Colledge NR, Walker BR, Ralston SH: *Davidson's Principles and Practice of Medicine*, ed 21, Edinburgh, 2010, Churchill Livingstone.

Department of Health: *Immunisation against infectious disease – 'The Green Book'*, 2006 (modified December 2009). Available online http://www.dh.gov.uk/en/Publichealth/Healthprotection/Immunisation/Greenbook/DH_4097254.

Health Protection Agency: *Immunoglobulin Handbook*, 2008. Available online http://www.hpa.org.uk.

Male D, Brostoff J, Roth DB, et al: *Immunology*, ed 7, Edinburgh, 2006, Mosby.

Montague SE, Watson R, Herbert R: *Physiology for Nursing Practice*, ed 3, Edinburgh, 2005, Baillière Tindall.

Nairn R, Helbert M: *Immunology for Medical Students*, ed 2, Edinburgh, 2007, Mosby.

Provan D, Chapel HM, Sewell WA, et al: UK Immunoglobulin Expert Working Group. Prescribing intravenous immunoglobulins: summary of Department of Health guidelines, *BMJ* 337:a1831, 2008.

Rich R, Fleisher T, Shearer W: *Clinical Immunology: Principles and Practice*, ed 3, Edinburgh, 2008, Mosby.

Waugh A, Grant A: *Ross and Wilson Anatomy and Physiology in Health and Illness*, ed 11, Edinburgh, 2010, Churchill Livingstone.

USEFUL WEBSITES

Allergy UK (previously known as British Allergy Foundation): www.allergyuk.org

Arthritis Research UK: www.arthritisresearchuk.org/

British National Formulary (BNF): www.bnf.org/

Myasthenia Gravis Association: www.mga-charity.org/

NHS National Patient Safety Agency: www.npsa.nhs.uk/

Primary Immunodeficiency Association: www.pia.org.uk/

Resuscitation Council (UK): www.resus.org.uk/

Severe Combined Immunodeficiency (SCID): www.ich.ucl.ac.uk/gosh_families/information_sheets/immunodeficiency_scid/immunodeficiency_scid_families.html

World Health Organization: www.who.int/immunization/en/

Nursing patients with disorders of the breast and reproductive systems

Jacky Cotton, Martin Steggall
Part 1 Nursing patients with disorders of the reproductive systems

Karen Burnet, Carol McQuade
Part 2 Nursing patients with disorders of the breast

Introduction

Any threat to an individual's reproductive capacity affects that person's body image, self-esteem and gender identity. Since these are influenced by personal attitudes, social customs and cultural background, people respond differently to such a threat. Attitudes towards sexual reproduction, underlying beliefs held and feelings experienced are influenced by cultural, social and religious values, background, lifestyle and parental and peer pressure.

Reproduction and the ability to procreate are important issues, evidenced by the incidence of subfertility in the UK and the growing development of reproductive technologies. While the physiological aspects of reproduction are concerned with continuance of the species, the psychosocial aspects of reproduction are of significance to the feelings of health and well-being for both men and women. For some people, having their own children and raising a family are vital parts of their role in life. For others, these are inconsequential and for some this may be desirable but if not possible may cause sadness and regret.

Disease prevention rather than disease control/treatment is a fundamental philosophy of health care. Health care professionals, in particular practice nurses, have an important role in advising and encouraging good health awareness and in facilitating and conducting screening and health monitoring. However, screening is not always possible and some diseases can be far advanced before diagnosis.

When a person's quality of life is affected by the disease, intervention is required and developments in techniques and technology now mean that recovery is often much quicker. Minimally invasive techniques have the advantage of a shorter general anaesthetic, or the use of conscious sedation or local anaesthetic, thus allowing some treatments to be performed in the community, in outpatients, as a day case or a shorter inpatient stay in hospital. This has implications for nursing and patient care following treatment to adapt to the dynamic nature of nursing in a changing society.

This part of the chapter explores areas of women's health, men's health and infertility.

Anatomy and physiology of the female reproductive system

The primary function of the reproductive system is the propagation of the human species. Sexual drive and anticipated pleasure help to meet the reproductive need. The female reproductive system produces gametes (secondary oocytes; strictly speaking these are not known as ova until penetration by a spermatozoon), receives the male penis during sexual intercourse and facilitates the passage of male gametes (spermatozoa). It supports the growth and development of the embryo/fetus during pregnancy and expels the fetus during labour (Figures 7.1, 7.2). See pages 248–249 for anatomy and physiology of the breast. The events occurring at the start of and the end of a female's reproductive life, the menarche (the first menstruation) and the climacteric and menopause, are outlined.

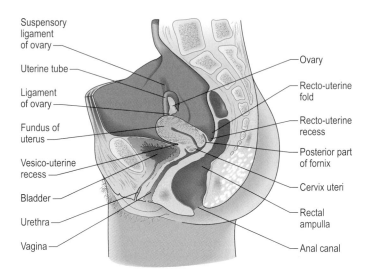

Figure 7.1 The relationship of the female reproductive organs: sagittal section.

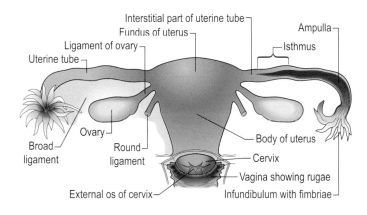

Figure 7.2 The organs of the female reproductive system and attachments.

The female reproductive system consists of:

- internal genitalia
  - ovaries (2)
  - uterus
  - uterine (fallopian) tubes (2)
  - vagina
- external genitalia
  - vulva.

Ovaries

There are two ovaries, the size and shape of large almonds, one on either side of the uterus. The surface of the ovary consists of a single layer of germinal epithelium surrounding connective tissue that forms the stroma of the ovarian cortex and medulla. The ovarian follicles develop in the cortex. Female infants are born with approximately 100 000 primordial follicles, which may fall to approximately 30 000 by adolescence. Each follicle contains a secondary oocyte. The medulla consists of connective tissue, blood vessels and nerves.

The ovary has two functions:

- secondary oocyte production
- hormone secretion.

Oocyte (ovum) production

Ovarian cycles begin at puberty; a cycle lasts around 28 days (range 21–35 days) and has two phases follicular (days 1–14) and luteal (days 14–28). Follicles begin to mature under the influence of the follicle-stimulating hormone (FSH) and luteinising hormone (LH), released by the anterior pituitary gland (see Ch. 5). During the cycle, follicles can pass through five stages (Figure 7.3):

- primary follicle – each oocyte is surrounded by a thin layer of epithelial cells
- developing follicle – the follicular epithelium proliferates, the oocyte moves to a side position, and a fluid-filled cavity develops within the epithelium
- mature (Graafian) follicle – the follicle reaches its maximum size
- corpus luteum – a yellow body forms in the ovarian follicle after ovulation
- corpus albicans – scar tissue on the surface of the ovary when the degenerated corpus luteum atrophies.

The maturing follicle is surrounded by a layer of ovarian tissue, known as the theca. Several follicles may develop together but usually only one will become the dominant follicle and mature fully. The mature (Graafian) follicle ruptures at the surface of the ovary and discharges the oocyte and fluid into the peritoneal cavity – a process called ovulation. Wafting movements of the fimbriated (finger-like) ends of the uterine tubes assist the transfer of the oocyte into the uterine tube. It is thought that fertilisation of the oocyte usually occurs in the ampulla of the uterine tube.

The ruptured follicle contracts around leaked blood after ovulation. The epithelial cells (granulosa) multiply and the corpus luteum is formed under the influence of LH. The corpus luteum synthesises sex hormones for at least 8–10 days. If the oocyte is not fertilised, the corpus luteum degenerates,

hormone production ceases and a scar forms near the surface of the ovary. If the ovum is fertilised, the corpus luteum continues to develop, increasing its size and hormone production for about 2 months.

Hormone secretion

Ovarian sex hormone secretion is influenced by hypothalamic gonadotrophin-releasing hormone, which stimulates the pituitary gland to release FSH and LH (see Ch. 5). FSH stimulates the initial development of ovarian follicles and their secretion of oestrogen; LH stimulates further follicular development, initiates ovulation and stimulates ovarian hormone production. FSH and LH control the secretion of two ovarian steroid hormones – oestrogens and progestogens.

Oestrogens The effects of oestrogens include:

- development of female secondary sexual characteristics
- pubertal growth spurt
- development and functioning of female reproductive structures – oogenesis and maturation of follicles
- metabolic effects including protein anabolism, calcium homeostasis, lipid metabolism and fluid and electrolyte balance.

The oestrogen secreted by the theca interna cells of the developing follicle is oestradiol, and its metabolite (waste product) is oestriol. Many other oestrogens may be identified in the urine. Oestradiol is also produced by theca interna cells that invade the corpus luteum.

Progestogens The main progestogen is progesterone (the 'gestation' hormone); it is produced by the luteinised cells of the corpus luteum. The metabolite of progesterone is pregnanediol, which is also excreted in the urine.

Uterus

The uterus is a hollow, muscular pear-shaped organ approximately 7.5 cm long. It has three main parts:

- fundus (top)
- body
- cervix (cervix uteri or uterine cervix).

See Figures 7.1, 7.2.

The uterine tubes enter the uterus at its upper outer angles or cornua. The body of the uterus narrows towards the cervix, an area known as the isthmus. The cavity of the uterus connects with the cervical canal at the internal os. The cervical canal opens into the vagina via the external os. The cervix occupies the lower third of the uterus and half of the cervix projects into the vagina. The uterus normally lies in an anteverted position, almost at right angles to the vagina (see Figure 7.1).

Structure

The uterus has three coats:

- endometrium – specialised mucous lining
- myometrium – smooth muscle
- perimetrium – outer serous coat (parietal peritoneum).

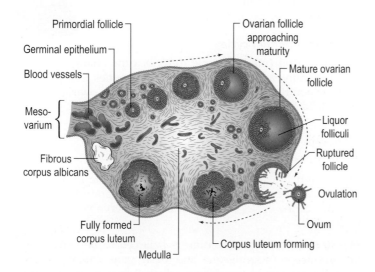

Figure 7.3 Sequence of development of the ovarian cycle.

Primordial follicle
Germinal epithelium
Blood vessels
Meso-varium
Fibrous corpus albicans
Fully formed corpus luteum
Medulla
Ovarian follicle approaching maturity
Mature ovarian follicle
Liquor folliculi
Ruptured follicle
Ovulation
Ovum
Corpus luteum forming

Endometrium The lining mucosa of the uterus is highly vascular and contains many tubular glands. The layers of the endometrium are:

- outer layer – which is shed during menstruation (stratum functionalis)
- inner layer – permanent layer responsible for the regeneration of the endometrium after menstruation (stratum basale).

The thickness of the endometrium varies from 0.5 mm just after menstrual flow to about 5 mm near the end of the menstrual (uterine) cycle (see below and p. 197).

Myometrium The myometrium comprises three interlocking layers of smooth muscle fibres:

- an outer layer of longitudinal fibres
- an intermediate layer, in which fibres run irregularly, transversely and obliquely
- an inner layer of circular fibres.

Perimetrium Parietal peritoneum forms the external coat of the uterus but does not cover the lower anterior quarter of the uterus and the cervix.

The cervix consists mainly of fibrous tissue. The endocervical canal is lined with columnar epithelium but this changes to stratified squamous epithelium in the ectocervix (the part that protrudes into the vagina) (see pre-invasive cervical cancer, p. 211).

Blood supply

The blood supply to the uterus is from the uterine artery, a branch of the internal iliac artery. Veins accompany the arteries and drain into the internal iliac veins. Tortuous arterial vessels enter the layers of the uterine wall and divide into capillaries between endometrial glands.

Nerve supply

Innervation of the uterus and the uterine tubes comprises parasympathetic fibres from the sacral outflow and sympathetic fibres from the lumbar outflow.

Supporting structures

The uterus is maintained in an anteverted and anteflexed position in the pelvis by fascia and muscle structures (Figure 7.4). The uterine ligaments are the:

- broad ligament – a fold of peritoneum and fibromuscular tissue extending from the uterus to the pelvic side wall
- cardinal ligaments (transverse cervical or Mackenrodt's ligaments) – formed by dense fascia at the base of the broad ligaments, from the cervix to lateral walls of the pelvis
- round ligaments – extend from the anterior cornua of the uterus forwards and down through the inguinal canal to the subcutaneous fat of the labia majora
- uterosacral ligament – passes from the cervix and cardinal ligaments backwards to the sacrum, dividing to pass around the rectum
- pubocervical ligament – passes from the anterior cervix forwards to the pubic bone, dividing to pass around the urethra.

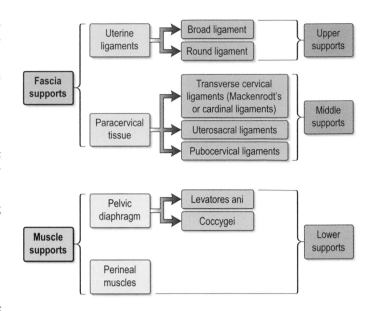

Figure 7.4 The supports of the uterus.

These ligaments support the position of the uterus within the pelvis. Paracervical tissue, fatty and connective tissue form a supportive sling, allowing the uterus to pivot either backwards or forwards. This gives the uterus mobility anteriorly and posteriorly. Lateral and downward movements are limited by the muscles of the pelvic floor.

Functions

The functions of the uterus are:

- menstruation – sloughing off of the stratum functionalis layer of endometrium with loss of blood from torn vessels; an outline of the menstrual (uterine) cycle is provided below
- maintenance of pregnancy – implantation of the ovum in the uterine lining and retention of the embryo/fetus during growth and development
- initiation of labour – the uterine muscle develops powerful, rhythmic contractions which shorten and dilate the cervix and expel the infant.

Menstrual (uterine) cycle

The menstrual (uterine) cycle describes the changes in the endometrium caused by the ovarian hormones (see p. 195). It corresponds to the hormonal events of the ovarian cycle and can be divided into three phases:

- proliferative phase (follicular or pre-ovulatory)
- secretory phase (luteal or post-ovulatory)
- menstrual phase.

Although the menstrual phase occurs at the end of the cycle, by convention the first day of menstruation is counted as day 1 of the cycle, as it provides an observable landmark (Figure 7.5).

Menstrual phase Menstruation is believed to be caused by low levels of progesterone and oestrogens causing vasospasm of arteries to the endometrium. The menstrual phase usually lasts for 3–6 days and is characterised by bleeding

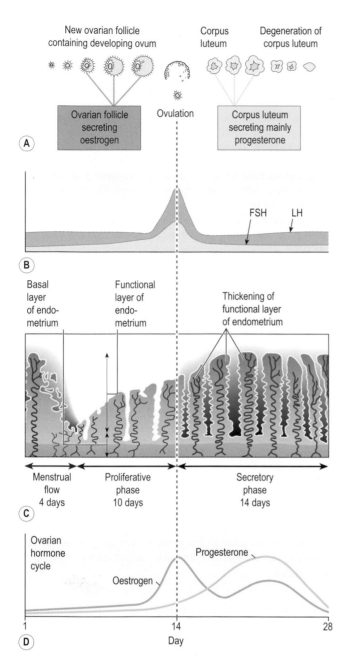

New ovarian follicle
containing developing ovum

Corpus
luteum

Degeneration of
corpus luteum

Ovarian follicle
secreting
oestrogen

Ovulation

Corpus luteum
secreting mainly
progesterone

(A)

FSH   LH

(B)

Basal
layer
of endo-
metrium

Functional
layer of
endo-
metrium

Thickening of
functional layer
of endometrium

Menstrual
flow
4 days

Proliferative
phase
10 days

Secretory
phase
14 days

(C)

Ovarian
hormone
cycle

Progesterone

Oestrogen

1   14   28

(D)   Day

Figure 7.5 Summary of one menstrual cycle. A. Ovarian cycle; maturation of follicle and development of corpus luteum. B. Anterior pituitary; LH and FSH levels. C. Menstrual cycle; menstrual, proliferative and secretory. D. Ovarian cycle hormones: oestrogen and progesterone levels. (Reproduced from Waugh & Grant 2006 with permission.)

vessels and connective tissue produces thickening of the endometrium. This phase extends to the 14th or 15th day of the cycle, when ovulation occurs.

Secretory phase This commences after ovulation. Progesterone produced by the corpus luteum promotes the secretory phase. The endometrial glands become enlarged, the arteries coil, connective tissue hypertrophies and tissues rich in glycogen become oedematous. At 7–8 days following ovulation, the endometrium is 5–6 mm in depth and is in a state of readiness to implant a fertilised ovum.

If implantation occurs, the corpus luteum continues to produce progesterone and maintains the pregnancy until the placenta is sufficiently developed (fully functioning by 10 weeks). In the absence of implantation, the corpus luteum degenerates and production of oestrogen and progesterone declines. The endometrial stroma starts to disintegrate, oedema disappears and the endometrium shrinks. Vasoconstriction occurs. The endometrium begins to slough and menstruation begins again 14 (±1) days after ovulation. This time relationship is constant.

Fluctuations in the length of the cycle occur in the preovulatory phase, as follicles may not mature at the same rate each month. Although this may result in variation in the time of onset of menstruation, most women establish a regular pattern.

Uterine tubes

The uterine tubes (10–14 cm long) turn posteriorly as they extend laterally from the cornua (or horns) of the uterus towards the lateral pelvic wall. The ends open as funnel-shaped structures with fimbriae (finger-like projections) (Figure 7.2). The broad ligament of peritoneum forms the outer serous layer of the tubes. The middle coat, of muscular tissue, is arranged in two layers: an outer longitudinal layer and an inner circular layer. The lining mucosa, comprised mainly of ciliated columnar epithelium and secretory cells, lies in folds. The lumen of the tube is narrow. The ends of the tubes are mobile and at ovulation the fimbriae enfold the adjacent ovary to take up the released oocyte.

Functions

The uterine tubes convey oocytes from the ovary to the uterus. They are the site of fertilisation of the oocyte by a spermatozoon. Passage of the oocytes or ova along the tube is facilitated by the action of cilia and peristalsis.

Vagina

The vagina is a fibromuscular channel extending downwards and forwards from the cervix to the labia. The endocervix protrudes into the upper end of the vagina, known as the vault. This creates anterior, posterior and lateral fornices (Figure 7.1). The anterior wall of the vagina is approximately 7.5 cm and the posterior wall about 9 cm in length. The vagina is composed mainly of smooth muscle with a lining mucosa arranged in folds or rugae. Until first sexual intercourse, a fold of mucous membrane, the hymen, forms a border around the external opening of the vagina, partially closing the outlet. Normally the anterior and posterior walls

from the uterus, with 50–60 mL of blood being lost at each menstrual period when necrotic parts of the stratum functionalis slough away, leaving a thin, bleeding area of tissue. By the third day of menstruation new epithelial cell growth has begun to cover the disorganised stratum basale of the endometrium; by the fifth day, epithelium covers the whole surface.

Proliferative phase During this phase the stratum functionalis regrows, under the control of oestradiol from the maturing follicle. The growth of epithelium, glands, blood lie in apposition but the vagina is capable of considerable distension during intercourse and childbirth.

The vagina is kept moist during the reproductive years by mucus from the cervix and transudation of fluid through the vaginal wall. Glycogen produced in the vagina is fermented by the bacterium *Lactobacillus* (Döderlein's bacillus) (part of the normal flora of the vagina) to produce lactic acid. This maintains a slightly acid environment in the vagina, inhibiting the growth of some other microorganisms.

Functions

The vagina:

- receives semen, deposited in the posterior fornix during sexual intercourse
- provides an outlet for menstrual flow, the fetus and other products of conception (POC)
- has an acid environment as part of the non-specific (innate) defences against infection.

Vulva

The vulva comprises the external genitalia, consisting of:

- mons pubis
- labia majora
- labia minora
- clitoris
- fourchette
- urinary orifice
- vaginal orifice
- greater vestibular glands (Bartholin's glands)
- vestibule (Figure 7.6).

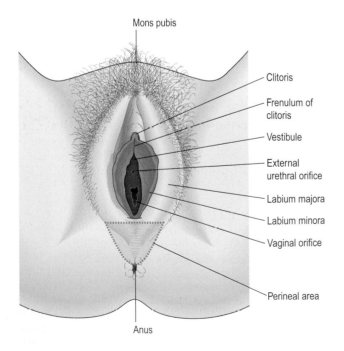

Mons pubis
Clitoris
Frenulum of clitoris
Vestibule
External urethral orifice
Labium majora
Labium minora
Vaginal orifice
Perineal area
Anus

Figure 7.6 Female external genitalia. (Reproduced from Waugh & Grant 2006 with permission.)

Pelvic floor

The pelvic floor is formed by tissues that fill the pelvic outlet and support the pelvic organs.

- The *levator ani muscles* form a broad muscular sheet extending from the pubic bone to the sacrum and coccyx and laterally to the pelvic walls. The urethra, vagina and rectum perforate this muscular sheet.
- The *superficial perineal muscles* lie under the levator ani muscles. They pass from the pelvic side walls, the pubis and the sacrum to unite centrally between the vagina and the rectum, where they form the superficial part of the perineal body.
- The *perineal body* consists of wedge-shaped muscle and fibrous tissue lying between the lower vagina and lower rectum.

The menarche

The menarche describes the first menstruation. In Western countries, this usually occurs between 9 and 16 years of age. Nutrition and body weight and composition influence menstruation and sexual development. The onset of menstruation may be delayed by excessive physical activity.

Some oestrogen synthesis stimulates early secondary sexual characteristics to occur some time before the menarche. There may be follicular growth and some oestrogen withdrawal bleeding to give the early periods of the first few months. These cycles are anovular (without ovulation) and such periods are painless. More discomfort may be experienced with menstruation that follows ovulation. A rise in basal temperature may be a guide to whether ovulation has occurred.

Variation in menstrual cycle length occurs in response to significant life events. Excitement, stress, anxiety or change of environment can delay the maturing of a follicle, ovulation and menstruation. Excessive exercise, as in athletes, can result in irregular periods, anovulatory cycles and amenorrhoea.

The climacteric and menopause

The climacteric describes the normal changes that occur leading up to the menopause (cessation of menstruation). The process of the climacteric is usually gradual and may extend over several years. Most women experience the climacteric or perimenopause over a period of 2–3 years, but it may extend longer. During this time the body adjusts to less oestrogen.

The ovaries 'age', resulting in ripening of fewer follicles and decreased stimulation by the pituitary hormones. The ovaries atrophy and less oestrogen is released into the circulation. Initially this reduced oestrogen level in the blood results in excessive production of FSH from the anterior pituitary gland, and this feedback mechanism can continue for several years. The withdrawal of oestrogen and the increase in pituitary hormone contribute to the changes associated with the climacteric.

The menopause is marked specifically by the date of the last menstrual period so can only be identified in retrospect some months after the event. The menopause is only one effect of the climacteric. Events occurring after menstruation has stopped for at least a year are termed postmenopausal.

The menopause signifies the end of a woman's reproductive capacity. This normally occurs between 45 and 58 years of age and in the UK the average age when periods stop is 51 years.

A premature menopause is one which occurs before the age of 40 years. This can occur naturally or may be induced iatrogenically. The age of menarche, socioeconomic factors, race, use of oral contraceptives and number of pregnancies appear to have no effect on whether a woman has an early or a late menopause (Abernethy 2005).

The fluctuations in oestrogen production, while following a gradual decline, alter the menstrual pattern in many women, showing considerable variation amongst women until the menopause.

After the menopause there is continued secretion of oestradiol and oestrone, although in varying and declining amounts. Oestrone becomes the predominant oestrogen. Small amounts of oestrogen can be found in the blood and urine of postmenopausal women.

Information about the disorders associated with oestrogen withdrawal and hormone replacement is outlined in a later section (see pp. 206–208).

Uterine bleeding patterns

The climacteric is characterised by irregular menstruation. Periods may become scanty, or bleeding may be heavy. The menstrual cycle shortens, associated with a decrease in oestradiol secretion. As this continues, LH levels rise and then menstrual cycles lengthen. Anovulatory cycles result in oestrogen-withdrawal bleeding patterns, irregular cycles with intermittent and prolonged spotting (low oestrogen profile) or prolonged amenorrhoea followed by sudden, profuse bleeding (high oestrogen profile).

Somatic changes

Somatic changes are caused by a decrease in oestrogen and an increase in gonadotrophins. Since the diurnal secretion of oestrogen varies from woman to woman, the changes experienced vary in severity but are progressive.

The ovaries atrophy and follicles disappear or fail to respond to gonadotrophins. Other internal reproductive organs become thinner and atrophy. Vaginal mucosa atrophies with a loss of rugae, elasticity and lubrication, and an increase in pH. Vaginal dryness can result in pruritus and dyspareunia. Loss of the acidic environment allows microorganisms to multiply more easily. There is an increase in connective tissue, causing narrowing and shortening of the vagina. The vagina is more prone to ulceration and bleeds easily to touch. Vaginitis may occur in older women. The labia thin and lose their sexual responsiveness. Pubic hair growth decreases with advancing years. The pelvic floor loses tone and elasticity, and become less effective in supporting the pelvic contents. The urethral mucosa may also show atrophic changes, resulting in symptoms of urethritis and cystitis, in the absence of bacteriuria.

Physiological changes, resulting in lack of lubrication, loss of libido and dyspareunia, can contribute to sexual problems for the woman. Hormone replacement therapy (HRT) may be a possible treatment option or psychosexual counselling may be of benefit. Many factors contribute to a satisfying sex life – satisfaction in a relationship, psychological well-being and emotional security can all make a significant contribution, illustrating the need for a holistic approach.

Vasomotor disturbances

Vasomotor disturbances commonly accompany the climacteric. The frequency and intensity of these vary between individuals. Hot flushes/flashes are the most common but perspiration, headache, fainting and palpitations may also be experienced. Hot flushes can start with a sensation of extreme warmth in the chest, quickly followed by flushing of the face and neck. The flush may be accompanied by sweating and palpitations. Dizziness and nausea may also be experienced. Shivering is often reported after the flush, probably due to compensatory constriction of the blood vessels. While vasomotor symptoms will eventually subside with no long-term effects, hot flushes and sweats are embarrassing, uncontrollable and can be distressing for many women. Porter et al (1996) report on a survey of 6096 women aged 45–54 years and note that 84% experienced at least one of the classic symptoms associated with the menopause and 45% of the women reported one or more symptoms as a problem. Randomised controlled trials (RCTs) have indicated the value of oestrogen in reducing the severity of vasomotor symptoms when compared with placebo.

In addition to oestrogen therapy, other treatments, such as vitamin E and/or B_6, clonidine, phytoestrogens, propranolol and oil of evening primrose (contains gamma linoleic acid), have been used. Progestogens have been shown to alleviate hot flushes. Phytoestrogens, found in soya products, have been suggested as a remedy for menopausal symptoms. While some women do find them valuable, there is controversy about advocating them as a therapy for menopausal symptoms (Naftolin & Stanbury 2002).

Emotional changes

These can include anxiety, poor concentration, dizziness, a bloated feeling and depressive feelings after the menopause. In addition to hormonal changes occurring at the perimenopause, women may also be facing other psychosocial changes such as children leaving home which can affect their emotional state.

Menstrual disorders

Amenorrhoea

Amenorrhoea (absence of menstruation) is either primary or secondary. Primary amenorrhoea is the non-appearance of menstruation in a female by the age of 16 years. There may be an anatomical fault or some disturbance in hormonal secretions. Delayed puberty may be familial or constitutional. Secondary amenorrhoea is the absence of menstruation for a period of time which is twice the length of the normal menstrual cycle for a woman who has previously menstruated, i.e. missing two or more menstrual periods. This may result in the woman waiting some time before seeking investigation.

Amenorrhoea is physiological before puberty, during pregnancy and lactation, and after the menopause. Inheritance, race, climate and general nutrition influence the menarche (see above).

Before puberty

A teenage girl may be seen by her GP because of delay in the onset of menstruation. The doctor may undertake a general physical examination to determine if other secondary sex characteristics are present; if so, menstruation will follow in due course. If secondary sex characteristics or menstruation fail to develop, the doctor will refer the patient to a consultant gynaecologist and endocrinologist for investigation.

During pregnancy

Following ovulation, cells of the ovarian follicle are stimulated by LH to develop the corpus luteum which produces progesterone. This hormone stimulates the endometrium and its secretory glands in readiness to receive the fertilised ovum from the uterine tube. When the fertilised ovum embeds in the lining of the uterus (now known as the decidua), it produces the hormone human chorionic gonadotrophin (hCG). This hormone supports the corpus luteum to continue producing progesterone until the placenta is established and producing hormones. The presence of the growing fetus and the continued production of progesterone prevent the loss of endometrium and the menstrual flow.

Amenorrhoea is frequently one of the first symptoms that lead a woman to suspect that she is pregnant. Levels of hCG in the urine provide a positive diagnosis when undertaking a urinary pregnancy test. This can be confirmed by the presence of fetal heart pulsation seen on ultrasound scan (USS) from 5 to 6 weeks' gestation onwards.

During lactation

Women who totally breast feed their baby may not ovulate or menstruate during the first 6 months after childbirth or until weaning commences. Breast feeding therefore exerts a measure of birth control, but must not be recommended as an effective contraceptive.

Total nipple stimulation is important for suppression of ovarian function. The suckling stimulus to the nipple leads to a neurohormonal reflex production of prolactin by the anterior pituitary gland which inhibits gonadotrophin hormone release, preventing ovulation and menstruation.

Suppression of the ovaries declines where supplements comprise more than 50% of the diet of the baby who is breast feeding. The incidence of ovulation and the risk of pregnancy then rise rapidly.

A poor state of nutrition in the woman can inhibit ovulation, particularly in developing countries. To ensure contraception during the period of lactation, the woman may be advised to use a barrier method. The progestogen-only pill is considered safe during lactation since it does not affect the milk supply and only insignificant quantities enter the milk. However, the combined oral contraceptive pill inhibits lactation.

After the menopause

The menopause, the date of the final menstrual period, may not be fully acknowledged until a year without periods has passed.

Pathological amenorrhoea

There are a number of pathological causes of amenorrhoea.

Uterine lesions, congenital abnormalities

PATHOPHYSIOLOGY

Examples include:

- congenital absence of uterus and vagina
- primary deficiency of endometrium – the endometrium may be absent, deficient or fail to be stimulated by oestrogen.

Ovarian lesions

Failure of normal ovarian development is rare. Chromosomal abnormalities such as Turner's syndrome may occur (see Ch. 5).

PATHOPHYSIOLOGY

Turner's syndrome is a condition that results from the absence of one female sex chromosome. It is characterised by infantile development of the genitalia, absence of breasts, short stature and a webbed neck. There may be associated congenital cardiac lesions.

MEDICAL MANAGEMENT

Chromosomal studies confirm the diagnosis. Early diagnosis is important and investigations can usually be initiated before puberty, suspicion being aroused by the short stature of the child. Treatment, such as ethinyl oestradiol 0.01 mg twice daily, in 3-week cycles, given for several months, then norethisterone added for the last 10 days of each cycle, can be used to stimulate development of the breasts and uterus. Menstruation may occur with this treatment.

Pituitary disorders

Disorders of the pituitary gland may result in the secretion of abnormal levels of hormones which affect the sensitive feedback mechanism ultimately affecting hormones of the menstrual cycle (see Ch. 5).

Other endocrine disorders

These include:

- congenital adrenal hyperplasia (also known as adrenogenital syndrome)
- Cushing's syndrome/disease
- Addison's disease
- hypothyroidism
- hyperthyroidism
- diabetes mellitus.

See Chapter 5 for further information.

Emotional stress

Emotional disturbance is likely to affect menstrual function through the hypothalamic–pituitary axis. Emotional distress caused by some traumatic event may contribute to amenorrhoea.

MEDICAL MANAGEMENT

Discussion with a health professional will help the patient understand and be reassured about the effects of stress on menstruation. Physical and mental relaxation will help her deal with the stress and will promote a spontaneous return of menstruation.

Eating disorders

Eating disorders such as anorexia nervosa can affect the menstrual cycle.

PATHOPHYSIOLOGY

Anorexia nervosa is associated with distortion of body image which results in disordered eating behaviour that includes dieting and extreme exercise routines and misuse of laxatives. There is extreme weight loss and dislike for foods, particularly carbohydrates. There is failure in hypothalamic stimulation of LH release and amenorrhoea occurs.

MEDICAL MANAGEMENT

Girls and women with anorexia nervosa are usually reluctant to accept they have a problem or to seek help. Their weight loss may be being investigated or they may present to their GP with another problem but when a diagnosis is made, care is usually maintained by mental health services. Positive physical and psychological changes can promote a return to menstruation.

Serious mental health illness

Psychotic illness may be a cause of amenorrhoea and the woman may not menstruate for many months or years.

PATHOPHYSIOLOGY

A life crisis can contribute to disturbances in the activity of neurotransmitter catecholamines in the brain or the chemistry of the hypothalamic–pituitary axis may be disrupted.

MEDICAL MANAGEMENT

It is essential to ascertain that the patient is not pregnant. A reliable source of information will be needed, whether the patient herself or her partner. Once the acute symptoms of the patient's illness have been treated and the body chemistry becomes more stable, a return to normal menstruation would be expected

Severe systemic illness

PATHOPHYSIOLOGY

The stress of severe illness may induce ineffective functioning in multiple body organs and may temporarily suppress menstrual function. Stress, as experienced by prisoners of war or refugees, associated with malnutrition, minimal protein and vitamin intake, leads to amenorrhoea.

MEDICAL MANAGEMENT

When amenorrhoea is secondary to general illness, the medical condition must be treated before the amenorrhoea can be relieved. The influences of emotional and physical stress are complex, and sometimes assisting the patient to relax and lower anxiety levels may promote menstruation before the general illness is fully relieved.

 Nursing management and health promotion: amenorrhoea

The nursing care for a patient with amenorrhoea is commonly undertaken in the community.

Assessment As part of the routine assessment, the nurse should take a detailed history including:

- the date of the last menstrual period
- any problems with menstruation
- knowledge from the woman about the reason for amenorrhoea
- does the woman perceive amenorrhoea as a problem?

Assessment should take account of her lifestyle, including nutrition, eating pattern, body weight, level of exercise and any stressful life events.

Planning care The nurse should discuss with the patient reasons for amenorrhoea and how these relate to the patient. The patient's level of anxiety should be noted and the nurse may recommend simple relaxation techniques or suggest relaxation audiotapes.

If, following a medical assessment, puberty is deemed to be delayed, reassurance and counselling are part of nursing care. Nurses can encourage optimism, provide general information about diet, exercise and lifestyle, and offer support, but in some cases skilled counselling may also be of value.

Evaluating care The patient's long-term goal of 'return of menstruation' may not be achievable within the early weeks of care and expectations should be realistic. This may include an evaluation of the level of the patient's anxiety. The patient should be asked to report menstruation. Achievement of such a long-term goal may occur as a result of medical treatment, particularly if hormonal or anxiolytic drugs have been prescribed.

Dysmenorrhoea

Dysmenorrhoea is pain associated with menstruation. Many women experience minor discomfort, but dysmenorrhoea is more disabling. Before the start of bleeding, the breasts may feel larger and ache; women may also experience abdominal distension and bloating, constipation and feeling generally unwell. The symptoms may persist for 1–2 days and be relieved or replaced by backache, urinary frequency and loose stools once menstruation occurs.

For some women, the first hours or the first day are the most painful. Dragging sensations from the umbilical area down to the groins and thighs may be experienced, or the pain may be severe, colicky or spasmodic in nature across the abdomen and back. The pain may be so distracting as to interfere with the woman's usual daily activities: 45–95% of menstruating women can be affected (Proctor & Farquhar 2006). Absenteeism from work and school is common due to symptoms of dysmenorrhea.

Two types of dysmenorrhoea are described:

- primary dysmenorrhoea (spasmodic) is due to physiological processes of menstruation, with muscle contraction
- secondary dysmenorrhoea (congestive) is associated with organic pelvic disease.

Primary dysmenorrhoea

Primary dysmenorrhoea is seen in young women in their late teens and early 20s. At first they may have anovulatory pain-free menstruation. Later, when ovulation becomes established, they experience pain 24 h before the flow begins. The pain is severe and colicky over the lower abdomen, often radiating to the thighs and back, and lasts for at least 12 h. Nausea, fainting and diarrhoea may accompany the acute phase and the girl looks tense, pale and drawn.

PATHOPHYSIOLOGY

Dysmenorrhoea is associated with an increased production of endometrial prostaglandins, resulting in intense uterine

Box 7.1 Reflection

Dysmenorrhoea

You are on a community placement and currently working with the school nurse. She asks you to prepare some information about primary dysmenorrhoea and self-help measures for girls in the early years at high school.

Activities

- Reflect on how dysmenorrhoea can affect the quality of life in girls aged 12–14 years.
- Access the resources below and use them to prepare a short talk that includes information about primary dysmenorrhoea and self-help measures.

Resources

NHS Choices Your health, your choices: www.nhs.uk/conditions/periods-painful/Pages/Introduction.aspx.

Women's Health Concern Period pain (review): 2007. www.womens-health-concern.org/help/factsheets/fs_periodpain.html.

contractions. Uterine arterioles can go into spasm and the resulting muscle ischaemia produces uterine pain.

Misunderstandings about the physical changes of menstruation and the nature of dysmenorrhoea may underlie ineffective management. Education about the nature of dysmenorrhoea and its effective management should therefore be addressed with young girls and their parents as appropriate (Box 7.1).

Rarely, dysmenorrhoea may be due to an obstruction to the flow of blood as a result of a clot being lodged in the cervix. Other possible causes include pelvic inflammatory disease (PID), endometriosis (ectopic endometrium present in the muscle wall, ovaries or elsewhere in the pelvic cavity) and congenital abnormalities.

MEDICAL MANAGEMENT

Detailed interviews may be carried out with the girl and her mother. In this way, shared and differing attitudes to the subject can be identified and problems defined. Vaginal examination may be carried out.

Efforts are made to educate the girl and her mother, as necessary, about normal menstrual function. A period of rest and the application of warmth to the abdomen or back may be helpful. Dysmenorrhoea should not be used as an excuse for avoiding school or work. Regular exercise, the avoidance of constipation and the prevention of anxiety are emphasised. Exercise encourages the release of endogenous endorphins which have natural analgesic properties. A series of exercises to stretch the ligaments that support the uterus in the pelvis may relieve menstrual pain. Attention should be paid to maintaining good posture.

Treatment Treatment for dysmenorrhoea aims to relieve pain or symptoms either by affecting the physiological mechanisms behind menstrual pain (such as prostaglandin production) or by relieving symptoms. Treatments using simple analgesics such as paracetamol, aspirin, and non-steroidal anti-inflammatory drugs (NSAIDs) work by inhibiting prostaglandin production. An oral contraceptive may be indicated as these inhibit ovulation. A levonorgestrel releasing intrauterine system may also be of use. Slow release of levonorgestrel into the uterine cavity prevents thickening of the endometrium. Women may experience amenorrhoea with resultant reduction in dysmenorrhoea. The levonorgestrel releasing intrauterine system has also been shown to be effective in reducing dysmenorrhoea in women with endometriosis after one year (Vercellini et al 2003).

In severe cases, hysteroscopy (endoscopic examination of the uterine cavity) may be necessary to exclude uterine pathology. A laparoscopy may be required to exclude endometriosis. A pregnancy and vaginal delivery may improve or cure primary dysmenorrhoea.

Nursing management and health promotion: primary dysmenorrhoea

Assessment An assessment should be made of the patient's general health. The patient's description of the nature of her painful periods should be recorded along with any observations about her physical and emotional symptoms on particular days of the cycle. Any medication used for pain relief or contraception, and its effectiveness, should be noted. Dietary habits and exercise activities are also relevant. Sensitive questioning of the patient will reveal any anxieties or stressors which may be contributing to symptoms.

Planning care Care should be developed with the patient. Helping the girl/woman recognise signs of impending menstruation will allow her to take analgesics in time to prevent pain. A holistic approach to strategies to relieve pain should be discussed. Useful information includes:

- a simple explanation of how hormones function in the menstrual cycle and the effects of excessive prostaglandins
- discussion of the beneficial effects of a diet adequate in fibre, vitamins and polyunsaturated fats, and low in salt
- discussion of the patient's present level of physical exercise and the benefits of exercise and good posture in stimulating organs and the release of pain-relieving endorphins (see Ch. 19)
- teaching simple relaxation exercises with referral to massage and local heat application
- discussion about drugs that inhibit prostaglandin secretion.

Evaluating care A pain verbal rating scale could be used by the patient (see Ch. 19). If optimal pain relief is not achieved it may be necessary to amend analgesic regimens. Relaxation exercises should be used while the effects of analgesics are awaited. The achievement of the patient's goals will be her first step in a change of lifestyle. Further support and encouragement may be given by her mother, friend, partner, a school or practice nurse or the GP.

Secondary dysmenorrhoea

Secondary dysmenorrhoea is experienced in later menstrual life by women in their mid-20s after years of painless menstruation.

PATHOPHYSIOLOGY

Women usually complain of a dragging pain in the lower abdomen, pelvic area and breasts, accompanied by headache. The pain occurs some days before the menstrual flow and may continue throughout bleeding.

The condition is usually associated with pelvic pathology, although anxiety or depression can be an aggravating factor:

- Adenomyosis (infiltration of the myometrium by endometrial cells) – increased tension in the uterine muscle, as blood accumulates in the cystic spaces.
- Fixed retroversion of the uterus can cause severe pain, especially if associated with a low-grade pelvic infection.
- Partial stenosis of the cervix, following cautery or surgery.
- Endometriosis interferes with normal rhythmic uterine contractions.
- Pelvic congestion, due to increased blood supply to the uterus, and menorrhagia (see below).
- Pelvic inflammation, particularly salpingitis, might contribute to pain.
- Fibromyomata ('fibroids') and polyps interfere with normal rhythmic uterine contractions and cause muscular spasms as the uterus attempts to empty itself of the abnormal tissue.

MEDICAL MANAGEMENT

History and examination A detailed history of the problem is recorded and a full physical examination including vaginal examination is undertaken to assess underlying causes. An accurate history of the pain is important, noting the age of onset, and the site, radiation, duration, character and time of onset in the menstrual cycle. The doctor seeks information about any related symptoms, possible abnormal uterine bleeding, pain on sexual intercourse (dyspareunia), pruritus and premenstrual tension.

Treatment Investigations may involve hysteroscopy and endometrial biopsy. A laparoscopy may be performed if endometriosis is suspected. The presence of fibroids or polyps will be treated appropriately (see pp. 208–210). Pelvic inflammation can be treated by antibiotics. An analgesic drug can be prescribed that is suitable for inhibiting prostaglandin synthesis, e.g. mefenamic acid.

 Nursing management and health promotion: secondary dysmenorrhoea

On assessment, pain will be identified as a problem. Goals and interventions will be similar to those described for primary dysmenorrhoea, particularly encouraging personal health messages. Additional problems will be identified and appropriate nursing interventions planned depending on the specific underlying pathology and the treatment interventions recommended.

Pre- and postoperative care planning will be needed if surgical procedures are planned (see Ch. 26). At the time of discharge the patient's future prospects for an improved pattern of menstrual cycles should be better.

Abnormal uterine bleeding

Abnormal uterine bleeding is described according to the rhythm or pattern of blood loss:

- menorrhagia – heavy or profuse menstrual bleeding; bleeding occurs at normal intervals but is increased in amount or duration
- polymenorrhea – menstruation occurring with a frequency of less than 21 days
- polymenorrhagia – periods that are both heavy and frequent
- metrorrhagia – irregular or unusual uterine bleeding between periods
- dysfunctional uterine bleeding – abnormal uterine bleeding for which no organic cause is identified.

Abnormal uterine bleeding with the passing of blood clots is significant. The bleeding is greater than normal if the usual anti-clotting agents released by the endometrium are unable to control the volume or rate of blood loss.

Menorrhagia

Menorrhagia may be ovarian or uterine in origin.

PATHOPHYSIOLOGY

Ovarian There is hormonal imbalance (of oestrogen and progesterone secretion) usually due to the oversecretion of gonadotrophins. Emotional stress may contribute to this oversecretion.

Ovarian lesions are of two types:

- Polycystic growths – may disturb the normal production of ovarian hormones and excessive endometrial growth occurs.
- Immature follicles – may fail to result in ovulation. The corpus luteum fails to form, so progesterone cannot be produced. Oestrogen levels continue to rise and there is a proliferation of the endometrium.

Uterine Lesions include:

- Fibroids – increase the endometrial surface area, thereby increasing bleeding. Fibroids may prolong the flow by restricting or disturbing contractions.
- Polyps – increase endometrial surface area.
- Adenomyosis – interferes with muscle contractions.
- Multiparity – reduced tone in the uterine muscle fibres caused by replacement by fibrous tissue will interfere with normal contractions.
- Developmental anomalies, e.g. a bicornuate, septate or duplicated uterus – may impede contractions.
- Endometriosis – is accompanied by increased blood supply to the uterus.
- Tumour formation – increases blood supply and bleeding.
- Intrauterine contraceptive devices – cause endometrial irritation. Excessive bleeding may be problematic during the first 3 months after insertion.
- Tubal ligation – involves some alteration in the course of blood vessels that increases uterine blood supply.

MEDICAL MANAGEMENT

Medical examination will try to establish whether bleeding is a problem of quantity or rhythm, or both. Pelvic examination may reveal tenderness, masses or irregularities. If no pelvic abnormality is found, then a provisional diagnosis of dysfunctional uterine bleeding is made.

Investigations A full blood count will identify anaemia. Other endocrine imbalances may be important so thyroid function tests may also be done. An USS will help identify the presence of fibroids or masses. Hysteroscopy and endometrial biopsy may also be undertaken based on results of examination and USS.

Treatment will depend on the amount of blood lost. Any anaemia identified should be corrected as appropriate. Mefenamic acid 500 mg or tranexamic acid 1 g, three times daily on the first day of the period and on other days with a heavy flow is often helpful, for a period of 3 months, followed by review.

Hormone therapy may be given. Progesterone may be prescribed to balance oestrogen secretion and reduce excessive endometrial growth. This may be in the form of the levonorgestrel releasing intrauterine system described under treatment of dysmenorrhoea. One of the combined contraceptive pills may be given to suppress hormone production. Progestogen administration will modify flow for patients with heavy but regular cycles.

Endometrial ablation is another treatment option for menorrhagia and is one of several minimally invasive procedures developed over recent years. It is undertaken as a day case procedure and is increasingly done as an outpatient procedure (Clark & Gupta 2005). This involves destroying the endometrium, preventing its cyclical regeneration. For many women the associated physical, social and psychological implications make it preferable to more extensive surgery such as hysterectomy. Different techniques have developed but they are based on the same principle which involves the introduction of instruments to destroy the endometrium using heat via a hysteroscope. These include:

- Balloon endometrial ablation – a special catheter is introduced via the cervix into the endometrial cavity. Water distends the catheter balloon so that it comes into direct contact with the endometrial lining. The water is then superheated to 87°C and left in situ for 8 minutes. The heat produced effectively destroys the endometrium.
- Electrical energy – a newer technique involves a similar procedure but uses a triangular mesh device which is introduced to the uterine cavity and expands to conform to the endometrial lining. Electrical energy is then delivered to destroy the endometrium as above, but only takes 90 seconds instead of 8 minutes.
- Freezing.
- Laser.

Following the procedure slight vaginal bleeding can be expected for a few days. Menstruation will become lighter or may cease, but dysmenorrhoea and premenstrual symptoms may continue. This procedure may require to be repeated at a later stage or a hysterectomy may eventually be necessary.

When a hysterectomy is deemed necessary it may be possible to undertake this without major surgery by means of laparoscopic surgery. This requires insertion of a number of small trocars through the abdominal wall, providing entry sites for instruments. The viewing laparoscope is inserted below the umbilicus, two other insertion sites will be positioned just above the pubic hair line and accessory insertion sites will be used for electrosurgical techniques, a stapling device or to insert sutures via the abdominal cavity. The woman can be discharged from hospital within 2 days.

If large fibroids or endometriosis exist, an abdominal hysterectomy is required. Alternatively, in the case of fibroids, a myomectomy may be appropriate, particularly if the woman wants to retain her uterus. Here the fibroids are shelled out of the myometrium.

Metrorrhagia

PATHOPHYSIOLOGY

- Lowered oestrogen level may occur just prior to the formation of the corpus luteum, resulting in vaginal blood spotting at the time of ovulation.
- Cervical pathology, e.g. inflammation, erosion, polyps or cancer, may cause slight bleeding, especially after intercourse or vaginal examination.
- Vaginal pathology, e.g. inflammation, infection, ulceration and atrophy, may cause bleeding.
- Endometrial cancer is a major cause of irregular bleeding.
- Complications of an early pregnancy – as a fertilised ovum embeds into the endometrium, slight bleeding may occur. This loss may be repeated during several months of the pregnancy. Haemorrhage might also occur in a pregnant woman due to placenta praevia (placenta implanted abnormally low in the uterus).

MEDICAL MANAGEMENT

Investigations The vulva, vagina and cervix should be inspected closely. Colposcopy examination, whereby the cervix is examined under magnification, will identify any abnormalities including pre-cancer or cancer. If abnormal cells are identified, biopsies of the cervix may be taken for histological examination.

Liquid-based cytology smear tests have replaced Papanicolaou (Pap) smears as the routine investigation to evaluate changes in cells obtained from the cervix (see p. 212). A high vaginal swab (HVS) will allow the identification of infection (bacterial or fungal) or parasitic infestations. Where endometrial bleeding is suspected it is important to perform a hysteroscopy and endometrial biopsy to rule out cancer.

Treatment depends on the cause. Bacterial infections of the reproductive tract will be treated with the appropriate antibiotic, e.g. metronidazole or clindamycin for bacterial vaginosis. Vaginal candidiasis is treated with an antifungal, e.g. clotrimazole or nystatin pessaries. Trichomonal infections are treated with metronidazole or tinidazole.

In ovulation spotting, small quantities of oestrogen may be given for 6–7 days, 3 days before ovulation.

Any malignant changes identified will be treated appropriately by surgical excision, radiotherapy or cytotoxic medication.

Premenstrual syndrome

Premenstrual syndrome (PMS) refers to physical and psychological symptoms occurring in the latter half of the cycle, 2–12 days prior to menstruation, subsiding once menstruation commences. There is a symptom-free week following menstruation. The symptoms vary between women but can also vary from cycle to cycle in individuals.

Most women will experience some symptoms during their reproductive life but 40% of women are thought to suffer from true PMS, with about 5–10% experiencing symptoms that are severe enough to disrupt their lives (Andrews 2005).

Symptoms of PMS frequently start after discontinuing the oral contraceptive pill or after a pregnancy, and become progressively worse with age.

Signs and symptoms are varied but include:

- mood swings, feeling upset, irritability and anxiety
- fluid retention, weight gain, swollen extremities, breast tenderness, abdominal bloating and pelvic pain
- headache, food craving, increased appetite, palpitations, fatigue and dizziness or fainting
- depression, forgetfulness, confusion, crying and insomnia.

PATHOPHYSIOLOGY

Numerous theories have been suggested to explain PMS, but the precise cause remains unknown.

Prostaglandins exert sedative effects on the central nervous system and affect both aldosterone and antidiuretic hormone (ADH) activity.

Fluid retention or redistribution Redistribution of body fluids in intracellular and extracellular compartments.

Hypoglycaemia Abnormalities of glucose metabolism in the luteal phase of the menstrual cycle that exaggerate blood glucose swings might account for premenstrual hypoglycaemic symptoms.

Vitamin B_6 (pyridoxine) deficiency Vitamin B_6 increases inhibitory amines such as dopamine and 5-hydroxytryptamine (serotonin), and also acts as a coenzyme in converting excitatory amino acids to corresponding inhibitory amino acids, with sedative effects. Vitamin B_6 can reduce the excitatory amines.

Progesterone withdrawal PMS may be due to deficiency of progesterone production. Many PMS patients have been shown to have adequate corpus luteum functioning, suggesting that it may be the rate of fall of progesterone level during the late luteal phase causing PMS rather than a deficiency.

Endorphin withdrawal Endorphins appear to be important in the physiology of pain and mood change. It has been suggested that endorphin levels decrease in the week preceding menstruation which may affect ovarian function.

Serotonin (5-hydroxytryptamine) Serotonin acts as a neurotransmitter that influences mood, appetite and behaviour. In women with PMS it can be significantly lower in the luteal phase of the menstrual cycle than in control subjects.

While researchers have been keen to find one reason for PMS, it is more likely that it is a combination of physical, psychological and social factors.

MEDICAL MANAGEMENT

Recommended treatment focuses on identifying and controlling individual symptom clusters. Drug treatments are used cautiously. The patient–doctor relationship is thought to be an important influence on some women, relieved that their condition is being taken seriously.

Investigations A thorough examination is required to diagnose PMS accurately and identify any underlying pathology. Other medical, mental health and gynaecological conditions must be excluded or be identified as coexisting with PMS.

Estimations of oestrogen, progesterone, prolactin, gonadotrophin or electrolytes are not usually helpful in making a diagnosis of PMS.

Treatment A complete cure does not yet exist but an integrated treatment programme can be adopted whereby women are asked to record, on a daily basis, personal experiences in mood, behaviour and physical discomforts for at least 3 months. This will identify symptom clusters and appropriate strategies to improve the severity of symptoms.

Women should be advised to:

- exercise regularly
- avoid coffee, tea and chocolate
- eat a diet low in sugar, fat and salt, and high in protein
- take supplements of vitamins B_6 and E_1, and magnesium
- limit fluid intake
- chart their weight daily
- avoid alcohol and smoking
- avoid stress.

It is important the woman understands that no single treatment will work for everyone and they may need to try a combination of treatments before they find one that suits them. Choice of treatment will depend on types and severity of symptoms and possible side-effects. All treatment options should be discussed fully with the GP.

General relaxation techniques may be helpful for some symptoms such as headache or fluid retention.

Drug treatments used in PMS will depend on the particular cluster of symptoms experienced.

Hormonal treatment Women may already have tried over-the-counter (OTC) remedies.

Hormonal treatment of PMS aims to interrupt the 'normal' menstrual cycle and associated hormone production by the body. Oral contraceptives will stop ovulation and help stabilise hormone levels but can cause side-effects. Progesterone or progestogen may also be used. In severe cases analogues of gonadotrophin-releasing hormone (GnRH), such as buserelin, will inhibit the release of gonadotrophins and so suppress follicular development, ovulation and the endocrine changes of the cycle. This creates a 'medical oophorectomy' but the woman may suffer unpleasant menopausal symptoms and this treatment should not be used on a long-term basis.

Diuretics Women can now obtain these as OTC preparations at pharmacies. By reducing the excess fluid in the body, these can relieve feelings of bloatedness and sore breasts.

Analgesics Abdominal cramps, sore breasts, headaches, muscular and joint pain can be relieved by NSAIDs but they can make fluid retention worse.

Selective serotonin reuptake inhibitors (SSRIs) may be the most effective treatment for severe PMS. SSRIs such as fluoxetine and sertraline are antidepressants and can help relieve tiredness, sleep problems, food cravings and low mood. However, they may have negative side-effects which may outweigh their benefits.

Psychological support Having their symptoms taken seriously by a health professional can provide great support. Techniques to improve coping skills and stress management may also be helpful. Vitamin B_6 up to a dose of 100 mg/day can be helpful for premenstrual depression and other symptoms.

Surgery In cases of severe PMS or those compounded by other gynaecological problems, hysterectomy with bilateral salpingo-oophorectomy (BSO) followed by HRT may be considered. Oophorectomy must be included to prevent the ovarian cycle, otherwise the cyclical problems will persist.

 Nursing management and health promotion: PMS

Assessment Nurses may encounter women who experience PMS symptoms not discussed with their doctors. Nurses have opportunities to provide such women with information suggesting daily recording of physical changes, discomforts, emotional feelings and behaviour.

Planning care A supportive–educative approach combines the giving of information and advice, also allowing the woman to look at achieving the aims for her particular circumstances. Advice should be based on the areas previously outlined in treatment.

A counselling approach by the nurse can encourage the woman to verbalise her preferred choices. Information should be given to the patient about the nature of any drugs prescribed. The possible value of self-help groups can also be discussed with the woman, but the value of family support, emphasised in some cultures, should not be undermined.

Evaluating care It is important that the woman records the effect of treatment. Some symptoms may have greatly improved, whilst others have shown no improvement. The woman must appreciate that not all treatments suit everyone. Each planned action should be reviewed and alternative therapies tried. Evidence of a sustained low mood or other severe symptoms should be referred to the GP or PMS specialist.

Disorders of the climacteric/menopause

Physiological, psychological and social changes associated with the climacteric/menopause have been described earlier. This section outlines the long-term effects of oestrogen withdrawal on women's health.

Decreased oestrogen is associated with the development of osteoporosis and cardiovascular disease, resulting in an increased risk of fragility fractures, coronary heart disease and stroke (Chs 2, 9, 10). Factors contributing to an increased risk of osteoporosis and cardiovascular disease include:

- inherited factors
- sedentary lifestyle
- low calcium intake/absorption
- low body mass index (BMI) – less than 22 kg/m^2 (National Institute for Health and Clinical Excellence [NICE] 2008)
- early menopause
- cigarette smoking
- excessive stress
- excessive salt intake
- high protein intake
- moderate to excessive alcohol intake
- caffeine intake
- pre-existing disorders of the kidney or thyroid, Crohn's disease, rheumatoid arthritis and diabetes.

Osteoporosis

Osteoporosis is a disease characterised by a decrease in bone density, predisposing to bone fragility and fractures. It is estimated that annually there are 180 000 osteoporosis-related symptomatic fractures in England and Wales. These include:

- 70 000 hip fractures
- 25 000 clinical vertebral fractures
- 41 000 wrist fractures (NICE 2008).

The disease is age related but more common in women due to the effects of reduced oestrogen levels. The World Health Organization (WHO) defines osteoporosis as bone mineral density (BMD) T-score of more than −2.5 standard deviations below the mean value for young adults (WHO 1994). This definition has been used to diagnose osteoporosis based on BMD assessed at the hip and spine using dual energy X-ray absorptiometry (DEXA).

Oestrogens play an important part in achieving maximum BMD. In early adult life, the rate of bone formation exceeds that of resorption, thus increasing BMD. When oestrogen levels decline, bone resorption increases and bone loss accelerates after the menopause.

Cardiovascular disease

Coronary heart disease (CHD) is a leading cause of death in women. In the UK it accounts for 1 in 7 deaths in women (British Heart Foundation 2008). Conflicting study results have caused confusion over whether oestrogen helps prevent CHD. The British Menopause Society (Rees & Stevenson 2007) has produced a consensus statement on up-to-date evidence relating to HRT. The Women's Health Initiative (WHI) trial (Rossouw et al 2002) has shown that the timing of starting HRT is important and that oestrogen may have a protective role in preventing CHD in women aged 50–59 years.

MEDICAL MANAGEMENT: MENOPAUSE
Hormone replacement therapy (HRT)

This is an area that has been extensively researched but the results of two major studies have provided additional information. The WHI randomised controlled trial examined various strategies for primary prevention and control of some of the commonest causes of morbidity and mortality amongst healthy postmenopausal women aged 50–79 (Rossouw et al 2002). The Million Women Study (MWS) was an observational study that studied a range of HRT regimens for women (aged between 50 and 64 years) who attended the UK breast screening programme. In response to the findings of the two studies, the British Menopause Society (2008) produced a consensus statement on managing the menopause.

Clinicians should discuss the risks and benefits with every woman on an individual basis before prescribing HRT. It effectively relieves vasomotor symptoms and can be effective in preventing osteoporosis (Medicines and Healthcare products Regulatory Agency [MHRA] 2007). However, because of risks associated with long-term use, it is only recommended for prevention of osteoporosis for women unable to use other treatments such as bisphosphonates.

Unopposed oestrogen therapy for women with an intact uterus increases the risk of endometrial hyperplasia and cancer (Beral et al 2005) so progestogens are given for 12–14 days per month on a cyclical basis, resulting in a withdrawal bleed. Tibolone is a synthetic steroid with properties of oestrogens, progestogens and androgens; if taken continuously it should not cause a withdrawal bleed (Box 7.2).

Box 7.2 Evidence-based practice

Providing information about HRT

Postmenopausal women with an intact uterus who use oestrogen-only HRT are at increased risk of endometrial cancer. Many women taking HRT who have an intact uterus use combined oestrogen–progestogen preparations or tibolone to reduce this risk. Limited information is available on the incidence of endometrial cancer in users of these therapies.

The Million Women Study recruited from 1996 to 2001 over 700 000 postmenopausal women in the UK who had no previous history of cancer or hysterectomy. During the study, 1320 cases of endometrial cancer were diagnosed in this group.

The findings showed that oestrogens and tibolone increase the risk of endometrial cancer. Progestogens counteract the adverse effect of oestrogens on the endometrium and this effect is greater the more days each month that they are added to oestrogen and the more obese the woman is. However, combined oestrogen–progestogen HRT causes a greater increase in breast cancer than the other therapies do. Thus, when endometrial and breast cancers are added together, there is a greater increase in total cancer incidence with use of combined HRT, both continuous and cyclic, than with use of the other therapies. A woman's BMI significantly affected these associations, such that the adverse effects of tibolone and oestrogen-only HRT were greatest in non-obese women, and the beneficial effects of combined HRT were greatest in obese women.

Activities

- Access the study by Beral et al (2005) and the Million Women Study Collaborators and consider the results in full.
- Consider how you would convey the information in this study to a postmenopausal woman asking advice about starting HRT.

Short-term HRT may be prescribed for specific menopausal symptoms such as hot flushes and atrophic vaginitis, for as long as treatment is required. Long-term HRT may be prescribed for women under 40 years who have had a premature menopause occurring naturally, as a result of surgery or iatrogenically.

While HRT can provide benefits in easing the adverse effects of the menopause, it can also have side-effects, and there are risks particularly with long-term use. Treatment may be abandoned by women because of either the side-effects or the fear of the risks. Possible side-effects include:

- breast pain/tenderness
- leg cramps
- vaginal discharge/bleeding
- fluid retention/bloating
- mood changes
- increased appetite.

Such side-effects might be reduced or eliminated by changing to a different preparation. However, women are encouraged to persist with one form of therapy for at least 3 months as some of the early side-effects can be temporary.

The link between HRT and breast cancer has been the subject of research for some time. Beral (2003) confirmed earlier findings that the present use of HRT is associated with an increase in breast cancer. However, the Women's Health Initiative Steering Committee (2004) describe results indicating that the risk of breast cancer in women taking only oestrogen was lower than in its placebo group. It is generally agreed that further research is required on this issue. Contraindications to HRT are usually described as absolute or relative. Absolute contraindications generally include:

- pregnancy
- undiagnosed endometrial bleeding
- endometrial or breast cancer
- severe active liver disease
- porphyria.

If individual women wish to take HRT for severe acute symptoms, they should be referred to a specialist centre for advice and monitoring.

Possible contraindications are identified to highlight potential complications, to ensure that underlying disorders are treated or monitored, and to monitor the appropriate therapy, which may differ from uncomplicated cases. Caution is therefore required in prescribing HRT for women with:

- endometrial hyperplasia, endometriosis or fibroids
- hypertension – treat prior to HRT
- coagulation problems – refer to a haematologist
- diabetes – liaise with diabetes team in case insulin requirements change
- gallstones – may increase the risk of disease (Cirillo et al 2005)
- otosclerosis – referral to an ENT specialist may be indicated.

Menopause clinics Some GPs prescribe HRT directly, whereas others refer women to hospital menopause clinics staffed by nursing and medical staff.

Nursing management and health promotion: postmenopausal women

Women should be encouraged to make an informed choice about HRT. However the media present reports on a regular basis with contradictory information on risks and benefits. The nurse is instrumental in providing up-to-date information enabling women to come to an informed decision on whether it is appropriate for them and reassuring them about risks.

It is important to warn about the early side-effects of the sudden rise in oestrogen levels when starting HRT. Women should understand that there are a range of medications, doses and types of HRT, so if one type is unacceptable, another regimen may be tried.

The following is a guide for nurses interviewing women facing the menopause:

- Provide information and advice according to individual needs/concerns and any ongoing postmenopausal symptoms.
- Encourage healthy lifestyles and health awareness.
- Encourage the selection of low-fat, calcium-rich foods; explain links to cardiovascular conditions and the maintenance of BMD.
- Ask women about their usual physical exercise pattern; reinforce the need for regular weight-bearing exercise.
- Discuss the benefits and possible side-effects of HRT.
- Explain about breast awareness/self-examination and attending for routine screening.
- Check the woman's understanding of the information given by encouraging feedback.
- Provide information from unbiased organisations (see Useful websites, e.g. The British Menopause Society) or booklets provided by health organisations.
- Provide contact details in the event of any problem occurring.

DISORDERS OF THE FEMALE REPRODUCTIVE SYSTEM

This section outlines some benign and malignant tumours, displacements of the reproductive organs, salpingitis, problems of early pregnancy (ectopic and miscarriage), family planning services, termination of pregnancy and infertility.

Benign ovarian tumours

Ninety per cent of all ovarian tumours are benign and many will resolve spontaneously (Campbell & Monga 2006). Management focuses on excluding malignancy or treating symptoms that may develop.

Dermoid cyst (benign cystic teratoma)

Dermoid cysts arise from embryonic tissue. They may develop at any age but are more common in young women.

PATHOPHYSIOLOGY

Dermoid cysts are usually unilocular cysts containing ectodermic structures. The cyst is thick-walled, whitish-yellow in colour and lined with skin, hair follicles, hair and sweat glands. Teeth may be found emerging from primitive sockets, and bone, cartilage, lung and intestinal epithelium can be identified within the cyst.

MEDICAL MANAGEMENT

The majority are asymptomatic but sometimes the cyst may undergo torsion and the patient may present with abdominal pain. Patients are referred to a gynaecologist for further investigations and treatment.

Malignant change may occur in any of the primitive tissues of the cyst.

Investigations A vaginal and abdominal examination will be undertaken. USS can identify the ovarian cyst and cervical cytology may also be checked. Any malignant cells present might be associated with an ovarian cancer.

Treatment Surgery is by laparoscopy or laparotomy. The extent of surgery will vary according to the age of the woman. In women of reproductive age, the benign cyst alone may be shelled out, leaving the normal functioning ovarian tissue. Both ovaries will be assessed, as the cysts are often bilateral.

Women who have completed their family or are over 50 years of age would be advised to have the ovary removed (oophorectomy). In the event of malignancy of the dermoid cyst, both ovaries and the uterus would be removed. Metastatic spread to the peritoneum requires further management by an oncologist.

 ## Nursing management and health promotion: dermoid cyst

General pre- and postoperative care is required (see Ch. 26). Specific nursing care will depend upon the extent of the surgery undertaken; for example patients may have day-case laparoscopic surgery, and those having an oophorectomy will usually have a very short hospital stay. Nurses must provide information and advice before discharge and support this with written material (Box 7.3 outlines discharge advice for day-case gynaecological surgery).

Benign uterine tumours

Endometrial polyps

Polyps are benign growths of the endometrium. They may develop from an overgrowth of endometrial glands and stroma. The polyp may produce a stalk and may descend towards the vulva. Single or multiple polyps may occur commonly in women of any age group. Slight vaginal bleeding (metrorrhagia) occurs between menstrual periods or following coitus. Polypectomy will be undertaken by twisting it off at its stalk either in an outpatient clinic or under anaesthetic depending on site and size. Any tissue removed must undergo histological examination to exclude malignant change.

Box 7.3 Information

Discharge advice following day-case gynaecological surgery (adapted from Cotton 2003 with permission)

- The woman should have tolerated fluids and light diet before discharge.
- She must have passed urine prior to leaving the unit/ward.
- An explanation is given that the anaesthetic may take 24–48 hours to be cleared from the body.
- A responsible adult must accompany the woman home.
- A responsible adult must be present in the woman's home during the night after surgery in case she is taken ill during the night. She should not be alone with young children for this reason.
- The woman must have ready access to a phone overnight and contact numbers, should help or advice be needed, such as for increasing pain or heavy vaginal loss.
- She must be told that extra care should be taken for 24–48 hours after the operation, as the anaesthetic can affect coordination and reflexes and that she should not drive, drink alcohol or operate machinery.
- The woman should arrange to have some pain-killers in the house such as paracetamol or ibuprofen.

- Women who have undergone laparoscopy must be warned of potential referred shoulder pain as well as abdominal pain. This is due to carbon dioxide used during the operation collecting under and irritating the diaphragm.
- Advice should be given about wound care, what type of skin closures have been used and, if they need removing, when she should visit her practice nurse for this.
- There is likely to be some vaginal loss and women should be advised not to use tampons initially because of the risk of infection. Increasing vaginal loss or discharge with an offensive odour should be reported to her GP. This is particularly relevant if she has had any surgery to the cervix. In this instance, she should be advised to refrain from sexual intercourse and using tampons for 6 weeks.
- She may be able to return to work after 2–3 days depending on the type of surgery carried out. Often women who have undergone laparoscopy require up to a week to recuperate fully and she should be warned that she might feel tired for a few days due to the anaesthetic.
- Women should be given information about when test results will be available and the date of any follow-up appointments.

Fibromyomata

Fibromyomata or fibroids are benign uterine tumours comprising fibrous and muscle tissue. They can occur in women between 35 years of age and the onset of the climacteric. The growth of fibroids is stimulated by ovarian hormones, particularly oestrogens. Childless women are more liable to develop fibroids.

PATHOPHYSIOLOGY

Fibroids are spherical in shape and firm in consistency. Some fibroids are small, while others may grow large enough to fill the abdominal cavity. They have a capsule which contains the blood vessels supplying the fibroid. As it grows, the centre of the fibroid becomes less vascular and liable to degenerative change.

Multiple fibroids may be present, giving the uterus an irregular shape (Figure 7.7) or causing displacement of the uterus and uterine vessels.

Common presenting symptoms Menorrhagia often occurs when there are fibroids in the uterus. If the fibroids are submucous then menstruation may become irregular and there may be metrorrhagia, but this is not common. Pain may result as the uterus strongly contracts to attempt expulsion of the fibroid. Pressure upon pelvic nerves may cause back or leg pain; pressure on pelvic organs may lead to:

- frequency of micturition
- retention of urine
- intestinal obstruction
- oedema of a leg.

A fibroid may become infected and necrotic, causing a purulent vaginal discharge.

The most noticeable change is that of increasing abdominal girth; rapid increase may indicate that malignant change has taken place in the fibroid. Fibroids can be a cause of

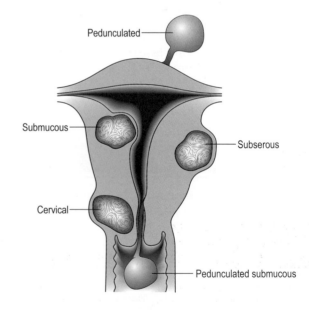

Figure 7.7 Common sites of fibromyomata in the uterus.

infertility by interfering with spermatozoa transit or ova implantation.

MEDICAL MANAGEMENT

On pelvic examination, the uterus is usually found to be symmetrically enlarged. It feels harder than it does in pregnancy. The uterus may feel nodular due to the presence of multiple fibroids. The lower part of a fibroid may be felt through the cervix and the difference between fibroid and cervical cancer may be difficult to ascertain.

Investigations Pelvic USS may assist with diagnosis of fibroids. Endometrial biopsy may be performed to exclude endometrial cancer.

Treatment Small fibroids may not need treatment and any symptoms should disappear with the menopause. Medical treatment may be prescribed in the interim to relieve symptoms. A gonadotrophin-releasing hormone analogue may be prescribed which affects oestrogen secretion. In a woman whose family is not complete it may be appropriate to shell out the fibroids from the myometrium (myomectomy); an older woman may be treated by hysterectomy. If the fibroids are small, a vaginal hysterectomy may be possible. Submucous fibroids can be removed hysteroscopically.

Embolisation of uterine arteries is a relatively new alternative treatment to hysterectomy (NICE 2004). This involves cannulating the right femoral artery under local anaesthetic. Under screening control, a catheter is passed through the arterial system to the right and then left uterine arteries which are individually embolised with polyvinyl alcohol solution. Contrast medium is injected to ensure effective arterial occlusion. Women require effective opiate pain control following this procedure, but once pain is controlled they can be discharged.

Nursing management and health promotion: fibromyomata

Nursing care will be prioritised depending upon the type of surgery completed. Observations of pulse, blood pressure and vaginal blood loss are recorded to monitor bleeding from the operation site. Pain assessment and administration of effective analgesia are required.

Care following hysterectomy will be similar to that described for invasive cervical cancer (see pp. 214–217), but without the anxieties linked to cancer.

Trophoblastic tumours

Trophoblastic tumours arise from the primitive tissues destined to develop into the placenta. They may be benign or malignant.

Hydatidiform mole (vesicular mole)

A hydatidiform mole results in swelling of chorionic villous tissue, destined to become the placenta when the fertilised ovum implants. The uterus fills with grapelike vesicles which produce large quantities of human chorionic gonadotrophin (hCG). No fetus develops.

PATHOPHYSIOLOGY

A benign tumour mass of chorionic cells forms in the uterus and exists as though it were a developing pregnancy. Ovarian follicles are enlarged and there is an increase in blood and urine levels of hCG. The uterus increases in size, sometimes faster than in a pregnancy.

Common presenting symptoms A woman may complain of loss of fresh or altered blood vaginally which does not seem like normal menstruation. She may be feeling unwell with some nausea and vomiting that resembles early pregnancy. It may be diagnosed if a woman suffers problems associated with early pregnancy.

MEDICAL MANAGEMENT

A general physical and vaginal examination will be performed. The uterus may be increased in size. A 'blighted ovum' might be suspected but the watery vesicles of the mole, if identified or reported, will alert the doctor to the condition.

Investigations Urinary pregnancy tests are positive, although there is no embryo/fetus present. The diagnosis is confirmed by USS and by the finding of high levels of hCG in urine or serum.

Treatment Molar tissue must be removed either by surgical evacuation or medically by administering oxytocin. Thorough follow-up of the woman is necessary. In the UK, women are registered in a national follow-up programme. Blood and urine levels of hCG are monitored on a 2-weekly basis. The duration and type of follow-up depend on how quickly hCG levels fall.

Complications A rising level of hCG with negative curettings of the uterine cavity suggests that the mole has invaded the myometrium and may even erode through the uterine wall. Deposits of molar tissue may be found in other parts of the body, in the peritoneum or in the lungs, and may cause death. Progression to malignant choriocarcinoma can occur following hydatidiform mole.

Choriocarcinoma

Choriocarcinoma is a malignant tumour of chorionic cells and occurs following a normal pregnancy, miscarriage or evacuation of a hydatidiform mole. Choriocarcinoma occurs in 3–10% of hydatidiform moles (Campbell & Monga 2006).

PATHOPHYSIOLOGY

The uterus becomes ulcerated, with invasion of the myometrium which can result in perforation. Metastatic spread of the cancer is speedy and extensive; the brain, lung, liver and other organs may be involved. Early deterioration is expected if the condition is not treated early.

Diagnosis is difficult but confirmed by hCG estimations in urine and plasma.

MEDICAL MANAGEMENT

Follow-up arrangements after mole removal are usually stringent and take place in a specialist centre. There are greater risks of disease progression if a woman delays consultation.

Investigations A choriocarcinoma produces large amounts of hCG, which is used as a tumour marker and also used to monitor the response to therapy.

Treatment Choriocarcinoma is highly chemosensitive to single-agent chemotherapy although women at high risk may require multi-agent chemotherapy. Methotrexate is given intramuscularly, with oral folinic acid to protect the bone marrow, with almost 100% success.

If there is metastatic disease, methotrexate may be combined with other cytotoxic agents. Four per cent of patients may have cerebral metastases at the time of diagnosis (Hydatidiform Mole and Choriocarcinoma UK Information and Support Service. Charing Cross Hospital Trophoblast Disease Service 2009). For most women an appropriate regimen of intrathecal chemotherapy will be effective in treating cerebral metastases.

Women are advised not to become pregnant within 2 years of treatment. However, depending on the stage of disease, some women will require a hysterectomy.

 ### Nursing management and health promotion: hydatidiform mole/ choriocarcinoma

Hydatidiform mole

Nursing care following evacuation of hydatidiform mole will be similar to that following evacuation of the uterus. Patients should recover quickly from anaesthetic and the patient will become self-caring soon after returning to the ward. Postoperatively, the nurse should check the level of vaginal blood loss, which should be minimal within 24 h.

Minimal abdominal discomfort should be experienced by the patient. A mild analgesic will be prescribed, if necessary. If a patient experiences more severe pain, she should be closely observed in case of uterine perforation. A series of postoperative urine and blood specimens will be required to estimate hCG levels. The patient must be registered with one of the specialised centres in the UK for appropriate follow-up.

Choriocarcinoma

In the event of persistently high levels of hCG, a diagnosis of choriocarcinoma would require the woman's transfer to a specialist centre for chemotherapy. The woman may be very anxious, having to face up to the seriousness of her illness and the urgency of treatment. The nurse should reassure and support her with information about future treatment.

The partner should be fully involved and can accompany the woman to the treatment centre.

Special facilities are available to protect her from infection as chemotherapy progresses and her immune system is compromised (see Ch. 16). Physical, psychological and social aspects of nursing care will be of primary concern. Many weeks of treatment may be involved before recovery is achieved and the patient returned to normal life. Follow-up and further hCG monitoring are essential.

Gynaecological cancer

The organs of the female reproductive system are susceptible to malignant tumours. Information about the characteristics and effects of benign and malignant tumours is provided in Chapter 31. The cervix, endometrium, ovary and vulva are potential sites for primary cancers (see Further reading, e.g. RCN 2005). A rapid referral system whereby women suspected of having cancer are seen by specialists within 14 days of referral has been introduced through the NHS Cancer Plan (Department of Health [DH] 2000).Women suffering with rarer cancers such as those of ovary or vulva must be treated in a cancer centre where specialist medical and nursing skills are available.

Cervical cancer

In the UK 2873 new cases of cervical cancer were diagnosed in 2006, accounting for 2% of female cancers (Cancer Research UK 2009a). There were 949 deaths from cervical cancer during 2006 in the UK (Cancer Research UK 2009a). Women aged between 30 and 50 years of age are most at risk of cancer of the cervix, which is preceded by a pre-invasive condition that can be simply and effectively treated if identified by cervical cytological screening.

Studies have shown that 99.7% of cervical cancers are caused by the human papilloma virus (HPV) (Walboomers et al 1999), particularly subtypes 16, 18, 31, 33 and 45. This infection is acquired through sexual activity. Other risk factors include:

- age of first sexual intercourse
- number of sexual partners
- smoking
- less affluent lifestyle.

A vaccination programme against HPV was introduced across the UK for girls aged 12–13 years in 2008. Girls aged 17–18 years were also offered the vaccine in 2008. A catch-up programme for girls aged 13–18 years old was put in place. A further development was a catch-up programme whereby all girls born on or after 1 September 1990 could have the vaccine by the end of the academic year 2009/10 (NHS Cervical Screening Programme 2008). It is anticipated that this will further reduce cervical cytology abnormalities in this generation.

Pre-invasive cervical cancer

PATHOPHYSIOLOGY

The area where the columnar epithelium of the endocervix joins with the stratified squamous epithelium of the ectocervix is called the squamocolumnar junction (SCJ). Columnar cells migrate down to the ectocervix, moving the SCJ to a new position and causing a red area of columnar epithelium around the cervical os. The area where columnar cells are replaced with squamous cells is called the transformation zone and is most commonly where precancerous changes occur. Cells are removed from this area when a cervical smear is taken. Pre-invasive changes identified early are curable.

In England, all women during their reproductive years should have a regular smear test from age 25 until 65 (NHS Cervical Screening Programme 2008) (Box 7.4). If a

---

 Box 7.4 Information

NHS Cervical Screening Programme

- Approximately four million women invited for screening annually in UK.
- Failsafe recall system in place to encourage women to attend for screening and subsequent treatment if required.
- In England the current programme is:
  - age 25 years receive first invitation for screening
  - age 25–49 years smears repeated 3 yearly
  - age 50–64 years smears repeated 5 yearly
  - age 65 years or over – only women who have not been screened since 50 years of age or who have recent abnormal cytology.

woman has an abnormal result, the frequency is increased. At the time of writing the Independent Advisory Committee on Cervical Screening (ACCS) is reviewing the evidence to ascertain whether women aged 20–24 years should be offered routine screening for cervical cancer in England.

All women registered with a GP are included in the screening programme. However, there are women from some hard-to-reach communities such as travellers or some immigrants who do not participate in the programme. These women must be encouraged to enter the screening programme and given appropriate information so they can appreciate the benefits of this.

Common presenting symptoms The earliest knowledge of cervical changes may be from a report on a cervical smear test. In some cases irregular vaginal bleeding may be associated with prolonged menstruation, occur between periods, follow sexual intercourse, or be postmenopausal.

MEDICAL MANAGEMENT

Investigations These will include:

- cervical smear
- colposcopy and biopsy of cervical tissue.

Papanicolaou (Pap) smear test Papanicolaou and Traut showed the value of smears in detecting cervical cancer as early as 1941, but it was not until 1964 that cervical screening was introduced in the UK. Pap smears involved scraping a layer of cells from the SCJ using a wooden spatula which were then spread and fixed on a microscope slide before being examined microscopically. This procedure has now been replaced across the UK by liquid-based cytology (LBC) which provides more accurate results and has reduced the number of smears showing borderline nuclear abnormality.

Liquid-based cytology LBC is a newer method of preparing the sample. Samples are collected from the woman as for a Pap test but a brushlike device is used instead of a spatula. The head of the collecting device is rinsed or broken off into a small container of preservative fluid. In the laboratory the sample is prepared and a thin layer of cervical cells is placed on a microscope slide and stained for examination by a cytologist (NICE 2003). Advantages of LBC over the Pap smear are:

- improved slide preparation, allowing a more homogeneous sample for examination
- increased sensitivity and specificity
- improved handling procedures for laboratory samples.

Abnormalities in cervical cytology indicating pre-invasive disease are described as cervical intraepithelial neoplasia (CIN) – CIN1, CIN2 or CIN3 (Box 7.5).

A woman who has had a total hysterectomy performed for pre-cancer or cancer will require subsequent vault smears. Routine cervical smears are required following a subtotal hysterectomy. Women may be asked to have a smear test repeated where there is an inconclusive diagnosis or if minor cytological abnormalities are detected.

Colposcopy and biopsy Colposcopy involves examining the cervix and surrounding tissue under binocular magnification. Women with abnormal cytology are referred either by GPs or by direct referral from cytology laboratories.

Box 7.5 Information

Histology of cervical intraepithelial neoplasia (CIN)

Current terminology for CIN describes three grades of change as part of a continuum of pre-invasive disease:

- CIN1 corresponds to mild dysplasia – affects one third thickness of cervical epithelium.
- CIN2 corresponds to moderate dysplasia – affects two thirds thickness of cervical epithelium.
- CIN3 corresponds to severe dysplasia and carcinoma in situ (CIS) – affects two thirds to full thickness of cervical epithelium.

Increasingly nurses are trained to perform colposcopy to diagnose and treat abnormalities.

Saline may be applied to the cervix to identify blood vessel patterns. Acetic acid is applied to the transformation zone, mucus is removed with a cotton wool ball or a swab and the area is carefully examined for abnormal epithelium. Iodine can be used to outline abnormalities. A diagnostic biopsy may be taken for histological examination to confirm pre-invasive disease. More commonly an excision biopsy is taken which also treats the abnormality.

Treatment options

Conservative treatment In the early days of screening all instances of abnormal cervical cytology were treated. However, the majority of borderline abnormalities will revert to normal and so initially repeat smears will be used to monitor the woman.

Destructive treatment Several treatments have been developed that work on the same principle of destroying tissue either by heat or cold. However, the commonest treatment undertaken now is excision of the transformation zone. This procedure can be performed using laser or a diathermy loop. The latter method is easier to perform and more economical in terms of time. Large loop excision of the transformation zone (LLETZ) may be performed under colposcopic guidance by low-voltage diathermy. This is performed under local anaesthetic in the colposcopy department. A bloodstained vaginal discharge usually follows for 1–2 weeks. Secondary haemorrhage may occasionally occur.

 ## Nursing management and health promotion: pre-invasive cervical cancer

Treatment is provided as an outpatient or as a day patient under general anaesthetic if the patient is particularly anxious or the abnormal cells extend up the cervical canal and a large loop excision is required.

This is a particularly anxious time for women and the nurse will need to ensure the patient understands the procedures planned and the expected outcome. Sensitive approaches are required to help the woman to express her feelings. Following the procedure, the woman must be given the following information:

- A bloodstained vaginal discharge should be expected for 1–2 weeks post procedure.
- The woman should refrain from sexual intercourse or using tampons for 4–6 weeks to allow the cervix to heal.

- She should contact her GP or the colposcopy department if bleeding becomes heavy, bright red or offensive which may indicate an infection.
- Details of when and how she will receive results of her tests.
- Future follow-up arrangements.

Information should also be given about the effects of lifestyle, and the woman should be encouraged to refrain from smoking and limit sexual partners.

 See website Critical thinking question 7.1

Invasive cervical cancer

PATHOPHYSIOLOGY

Squamous cell cancers account for 80–85% of cervical cancer (Jefferies 2008). Adenocarcinomas account for 15% of cancers. Squamous cancers develop from the outer layer; adenocarcinomas develop from glandular cells, often in the cervical canal, and so can be more difficult to detect by screening. An ulcer may develop on the cervix with tissues becoming eroded and infected producing an unpleasant vaginal discharge.

The cancer spreads by direct infiltration of surrounding tissues and via lymphatic vessels. The prognosis for cervical cancer relates to the extent of the growth at the time of diagnosis rather than to the histological type of the cancer. Box 7.6 outlines the International Federation of Gynecology and Obstetrics (FIGO) (2006) classification of cervical cancer.

Common presenting symptoms A woman may have no particular symptoms but a cervical smear result may confirm the presence of cervical cancer. However, she may have experienced postcoital bleeding. On vaginal examination, there may be an abnormal appearance to the cervix such as an ulcerated area or overgrowth of tissue.

As the disease progresses, vaginal discharge becomes more continuous; a thin bloodstained loss may change to a thicker, brown, offensive discharge or heavier bleeding episodes. Lower abdominal pain develops as the growth increases in size and exerts pressure on surrounding structures. Very severe lower back and sciatic pain may occur

and lymphatic nodes adhere to the sacral plexus. Pressure on the pudendal nerve and blood vessels causes obstruction to the venous return and oedema of the legs.

Incontinence of urine and faeces may occur if there is spread of tumour to the bladder and rectum or as a later reaction to radiation side-effects. Ureters may become blocked and renal failure may ensue.

MEDICAL MANAGEMENT

Investigations Treatment depends on the stage of the disease so a number of investigations are required for staging of the disease. Radiological investigations will include a chest X-ray or computed tomography (CT) of the chest and magnetic resonance imaging (MRI) scan of the abdomen to determine the presence of any metastases.

A general physical and pelvic examination is undertaken. An examination under anaesthetic (EUA) is undertaken to assess the vagina, rectum and bladder to identify extent of spread and lymph node involvement.

Tumour-derived/associated markers in the plasma of patients with cervical cancer may be useful to support other clinical findings. Marker measurement values tend to increase with the stage of disease and decrease with effective treatment. However, histological examination provides a more definitive diagnosis on which to plan treatment.

Treatment

This depends on the extent of the disease and age of the woman. The woman will be cared for by a multidisciplinary team including gynaecological and medical oncologist, radiologists, clinical nurse specialists and pathologists in a gynaecology cancer centre.

Surgery The extent of surgical excision will depend on the progression of the disease. When the cancer is confined to the cervix, cone biopsy of the endocervical tissue is appropriate, although if the woman has completed her family, a total abdominal hysterectomy (TAH) is preformed. Where there is extension of the growth into the vagina a trachelectomy (removal of the cervix and upper 2–3 cm of the vagina) or radical hysterectomy may be performed. Pelvic lymph nodes may be removed laparoscopically. A radical (Wertheim's) hysterectomy involves removal of cervix, uterus, upper third of vagina, parametrial tissue and bilateral pelvic lymph nodes. Concurrent radiotherapy and chemotherapy is indicated if lymph node involvement is confirmed.

Pelvic exenteration This is only undertaken where there is extensive recurrent disease. It involves removal of all the reproductive organs and the urinary bladder. If the rectum is also removed, a terminal colostomy is formed. This extremely radical surgery may be combined with cytotoxic drug therapy using cisplatin and other chemotherapeutic agents.

Radiotherapy Radiotherapy is indicated in cases where lymph nodes removed surgically show involvement of disease or if the patient is unfit for surgery. It may also be used to reduce tumour size, inhibit its growth and reduce its blood supply before surgical removal by hysterectomy. Stages III and IV of cervical cancer are usually inoperable. Palliative irradiation therapy is then indicated. Radiotherapy will also affect healthy cells (see Ch. 31). The bladder and

---

 Box 7.6 Information

International Federation of Gynecology and Obstetrics (FIGO) (2006)

Classification of cancer of the cervix

Stage 0	Pre-invasive cancer, also known as carcinoma in situ (CIN3)
Stage I	Cancer confined to cervix
Stage II	Involvement of vagina except the lower third or infiltration of parametrium. No involvement of side wall
Stage III	Lower third of the vagina is involved or the parametrium with extension to pelvic side wall
Stage IV	Spread of growth to organs beyond the reproductive tract

rectal tissue may become friable or fibrosed and a fistula may develop. The woman may become distressed by urinary problems or diarrhoea. Vaginal stricture may occur which creates sexual dysfunction. Symptoms are relieved as they occur. The patient's general comfort is of prime importance.

Nursing management and health promotion: hysterectomy for cervical cancer

Pre-operatively the assessment process will identify the patient's gynaecological details and her previous medical history will be documented to ensure she is fit for surgery and anaesthetic (general, epidural or spinal).

The woman's individual problems (actual or potential) and need for nursing assistance and support are identified. These include:

Anxiety The woman may experience considerable anxiety related to the anaesthetic, surgery and her condition. She may be anxious about a change in body image and sexuality and its effect on her relationship with her partner. Anxiety may focus on family members at home as the woman is often the caring head of the family. She may be worried that her illness will affect her ability to work and support the family in future. The nurse should be supportive and encourage her to express these concerns.

Information needs In preparation for surgery, the patient will need information about what to expect in both the lead-up to the operation and the recovery period. The benefits of planned information giving pre-operatively are accepted (see Ch. 26). An information booklet explaining

the operation and its resultant internal changes should be provided to support verbal advice given. This provides a record of discussions and reinforces her understanding.

It is usually recommended that sexual intercourse should not be resumed for about 6 weeks postoperatively to allow internal healing and reduce the incidence of infection. If appropriate the patient will benefit from knowing that sexual pleasure is achievable even though the uterus has been removed. Appropriate information at this stage will help recovery (Box 7.7).

Immobility

Patients will have limited mobility in the first 24 h after a hysterectomy. There is a risk of venous thromboembolism (VTE) and possibly pressure ulcer development. They will be taught leg exercises pre-operatively and encouraged to practise leg exercises pre- and postoperatively. Women will be fitted with antiembolic hosiery/stockings and subcutaneous heparin is prescribed prophylactically unless contraindicated. Patients will also benefit from being given information about deep-breathing and coughing exercises and how to move effectively with minimal assistance postoperatively.

Protection from hazards

The doctor is responsible for obtaining written informed consent from the patient. The nurse checks that the woman has consented and confirms her identity before she leaves the ward for surgery. The perioperative team will transfer the patient safely to the operating theatre where the checks on identity and consent are repeated.

Postoperative care

The patient's individual needs and actual problems will be identified in her postoperative care plan. This focuses on monitoring the patient's condition to identify complications at an

---

Box 7.7 Evidence-based practice

A study of self-concept and social support after hysterectomy

Although a woman may be happy to have a hysterectomy to alleviate symptoms affecting her quality of life, it can affect her feelings of self-worth and sexuality. Webb & Wilson-Barnett (1983) studied depression, self-concept and sexual life in 128 women during recovery from hysterectomy as part of a nursing study. The women were interviewed 1 week and 4 months after the hysterectomy. The results showed that women felt physically and emotionally much better, were less tired and irritable, had gone back to work and had resumed leisure and social activities. Responses showed that:

- 94% were happy to have no more periods.
- 84% were glad they could no longer become pregnant.
- 90% of those who were sexually active said their sex life was now as good as, or even better than, previously.
- 92% were glad they had the operation.

The small numbers who gave 'negative' replies to these questions were still not completely recovered and gave this as the reason for their answers. They referred to physical complications of wound, urinary or vaginal infections which delayed recuperation rather than the psychological problems suggested in medical studies.

The greatest area of dissatisfaction was in the lack of information from medical and nursing staff. Women would have liked guidance on what they could do, how they might feel as they progressed and what symptoms or complications could occur.

Webb C, Wilson-Barnett J: Self concept, social support and hysterectomy, *Int J Nurs Stud* 20(2):97–107, 1983.

Activities

- Access the research by Webb & Wilson-Barnett and think about how their findings have influenced the nature of information provided to women having a hysterectomy.
- Consider information that a woman having a hysterectomy will require under the following headings:
  - procedure/consent
  - preparation for admission
  - nursing procedures pre-operatively
  - nursing procedures postoperatively
  - information on recovery period to return to normal lifestyle.
- Reflect on the most appropriate timing of the information, e.g. in outpatient clinic before being booked for hysterectomy, at pre-admission assessment, pre-operatively on the ward or prior to discharge, and the format, e.g. verbal, written, telephone help line, web-based.

early stage (see Ch. 26 for general care of a patient following major abdominal surgery). These could include haemorrhage, urinary retention and fluid imbalance (Nursing Care Plan 7.1).

The nurse has a vital role in providing the woman with advice prior to discharge 3–4 days following surgery (Box 7.8).

Endometrial cancer

Endometrial cancer is more common with advancing age, the median age being just over 60 years (Campbell & Monga

2006). Risk factors for developing the disease include obesity, nulliparity, late menopause and unopposed oestrogen therapy. An excess of oestrogen is common to all the risk factors. As women are living longer, the present rate is expected to increase.

PATHOPHYSIOLOGY

The cancer arises in the columnar epithelium lining the endometrial glands; the growth is usually an adenocarcinoma. The cancer penetrates the endometrium, spreads laterally and

Nursing Care Plan 7.1 Care of a patient following a hysterectomy

POTENTIAL PROBLEMS	EXPECTED PATIENT OUTCOMES	NURSING CARE	RATIONALE
1. Irregularity in vital signs	• Pulse and BP measurements are within acceptable limits for the patient • Blood loss through wound, vagina or drainage tubes is minimal in any 24 h	Record BP and pulse Inspect wound/drains for excessive bleeding Observe for any vaginal loss. Record temperature	Haemorrhage caused by loss of haemostasis at operation site would result in hypovolaemia, requiring blood transfusion Appropriate drainage tube is in position in wound Pyrexia may occur due to infection, e.g. chest, urinary tract, wound or veins
2. Fluid imbalance	• No signs of dehydration or fluid overload • Patient is adequately hydrated • Signs of fluid overload are detected from fluid balance record	Maintain intravenous therapy as prescribed Observe i.v. cannula site for signs of inflammation or fluid extravasation Record fluid intake and output	Major surgery depletes body potassium, sodium and water levels Fluid and electrolyte replacement is needed by the intravenous route until patient can tolerate sufficient volumes orally
3. Patient to have restricted oral intake	• Intestinal peristalsis returns within 48 h	Patient to be given oral fluids when able to tolerate, starting with water. Light diet to be given on the 1st postoperative day. IVI can be discontinued once oral fluids tolerated Record any bowel activity	Intestinal peristalsis decreases or stops when the abdomen is opened and the gut is handled. Food and fluid, if taken, could not pass through the GI tract. Peristalsis returns after surgery and an early return to normal eating habits will ensure patient's GI tract returns to normal pattern quickly
4. Urinary bladder may be drained by a self-retaining catheter **Risk of bladder dysfunction after catheter removal** **Risk of urinary tract infection**	• Urine drains freely to minimise pressure on operation sites • Urine is clear and has low bacterial count	Observe and record urinary output Obtain catheter specimen of urine for microscopy, culture and sensitivity Meatal hygiene requires daily washing with soap and water Remove catheter when advised – usually 24–48 h postoperatively Ensure patient self voids urine after catheter removed. Perform bladder scan after self voiding to check for residual urine left in bladder	During hysterectomy, the ureter may be partially dissected to allow resection of the medial portion of the cardinal ligament, or more extensively dissected to sever the cardinal ligament at the pelvic side wall. There may be oedema and bruising of posterior urethral wall. Diminished bladder sensation, reduced bladder compliance and stress incontinence may occur. Urinary tract infection is a risk with a catheter in the urinary bladder
5. Possibility of patient becoming distressed or uncomfortable due to postoperative pain	• Patient expresses verbally or by body language that pain has decreased to an acceptable level on a pain scale of 1 = 'low' to 5 = 'high'	Remind the patient of the availability of analgesia Supervise the patient-controlled analgesia system (PCA) Reposition the patient as necessary for comfort Assess effectiveness of analgesia with patient using pain scale 1 = 'low' to 5 = 'high' Amend prescription if required	Patients have different pain tolerance levels. It may not be possible to keep the patient pain-free at all times A degree of pain control that is acceptable to the patient should be planned

Continued

Nursing Care Plan 7.1 Care of a patient following a hysterectomy – cont'd

POTENTIAL PROBLEMS	EXPECTED PATIENT OUTCOMES	NURSING CARE	RATIONALE

6. Limited mobility with risk of:
  • **venous stasis leading to VTE**
  • **pressure ulcers**
	• No limb tenderness, pain, swelling or redness during hospital stay
	
	• Moves safely within limits allowed
	
	• Pressure areas remain intact
		Supervise limb exercises whilst patient in bed, Patient encouraged to move position in bed to relieve pressure over bony prominences: 2-hourly
		Antiembolism hosiery/stockings to be worn until discharge
		Assist with mobilisation – mobilise on 1st postoperative day: get out of bed and mobilise around bed area. Assist with shower by day 2
		Administer heparin as required
			The patient who is immobilised by major surgery and in bed may lack the lower limb muscular contraction required to aid venous return to the heart. Venous blood flow in the limbs is slowed down, increasing the potential for blood clot formation, inflammation of the vein and surrounding tissues (phlebitis and cellulitis) with accompanying swelling and pain and possible thromboembolism. Body pressure exerted over pressure areas for more than 2 h will result in compromise of the blood supply to the tissues and increase the risk of the development of pressure ulcers
			Exercising of limb muscles, early mobilisation and the use of antiembolism hoisery/stockings are preventive measures that reduce risk
			Measures to relieve pressure over pressure areas are effective in preserving skin and other tissue integrity

7. Information needs in readiness for discharge (see Box 7.8)	• With information patient will continue recovery once discharged from hospital, usually on 3rd–4th day post op	Ensure patient is given appropriate advice to prepare for discharge to include: • Exercise/activity/lifting levels over next few weeks • When to resume sexual activity (when vaginal vault healed, usually 6 weeks post op) • When to return to work – after 6 weeks • When to commence driving (once able to do an emergency stop)	Depending upon progress during the hospital stay, the patient will need advice and counselling in areas of the activities of living Personal care, including wound management, the importance of exercise and restricting of lifting activity, should be related to the surgical removal of ligaments and supporting structures in the pelvis and the slow healing of abdominal muscle and other tissues The patient will need to know what to do if problems occur, and who to contact: GP or hospital. The patient should be encouraged to ask questions and talk about any concerns Information about local support groups should be provided if the patient feels in need of support and social contact Advice to be given about when sexual intercourse may be resumed

grows slowly. With time it penetrates the myometrium, reaching the perimetrium, and the lymph nodes become involved. Secondary deposits may affect pelvic and aortic lymph nodes and the ovary. Blood-borne metastatic spread to the lung, bone, liver or brain may occur. The International Federation of Gynecology and Obstetrics (FIGO) (2006) has developed a classification of the different stages (Box 7.9).

Common presenting symptoms From the age of 45 years, women expect changes in the menstrual cycle. The early signs of endometrial cancer may be difficult to distinguish from the changes of the climacteric. Post-menopausal bleeding (PMB), any unexpected or irregular vaginal bleeding, is a significant sign. The majority of women presenting with PMB will have benign endometrial pathology (Clark & Gupta 2005). However, as 75–80% of women with endometrial cancer present with PMB (Campbell & Monga 2006) investigations must be undertaken urgently to obtain a differential diagnosis.

MEDICAL MANAGEMENT

Investigations Sometimes a routine cervical smear test may yield the first evidence of malignant endometrial cells. Initial investigations include a transvaginal scan (TVS) and endometrial biopsy. If the endometrial biopsy is insufficient for histological identification of malignancy or if there is thickening of

Box 7.8 Information

Discharge advice following major gynaecological surgery (adapted from Cotton 2003 with permission)

The advice and information given to women being discharged after major surgery such as hysterectomy or vaginal repairs will depend on the type and extent of surgery, but will include:

- That she will be reviewed either in the outpatient clinic or, increasingly, at her own GP's surgery 6 weeks after her operation to ensure healing is complete. This appointment should be arranged before she leaves.
- Any drugs she needs to continue at home, such as a course of antibiotics, should be prescribed and given to the woman with a full explanation about how she should take them. Any of her own drugs she has brought in with her should be returned to her.
- Advice about the care of her wound is important, and in clean, healing wounds there is usually no need to wear a dressing. However, the area should be carefully dried after bathing. She should be warned that the wound may itch for several months and if she is worried to contact the practice nurse. Arrangements should be made for removing sutures if there are any still in situ.
- Alteration to diet, reduction in normal pattern of exercise and analgesia containing codeine increase the risks of the woman becoming constipated. It may be painful if she has to strain at stool and can cause damage to surgery such as posterior vaginal repairs. Advice should be given about drinking sufficient water, taking a high-fibre diet and being alert for the development of constipation.
- It is important that the woman does not return home and become an invalid. She should continue abdominal/pelvic floor exercises

as advised by the physiotherapist. Exercise should be encouraged in small amounts, increasing on a regular basis, as she feels stronger. Walking is an excellent mode of exercise but the woman should be advised not to walk too far at first, as she will have to walk back home when she may feel extremely tired. If she participates in regular exercise such as aerobics or tennis, she will be able to return to these by 6 weeks. Swimming should be avoided until the wound has healed completely because of the risk of infection.

- Driving a motor vehicle should not be attempted until the woman is able to sit comfortably in the driver's seat and undertake an emergency stop, at least 2–3 weeks after she has gone home. However, her gynaecologist may give her a specific time period before she should drive. The woman should check with her insurance company whether there are any restrictions on her policy whilst she is convalescing.
- After 6 weeks, most major surgical sites have healed completely. However, after a hysterectomy some women will still feel tired and, if they have a physically demanding job, may require up to 10–12 weeks away from work to convalesce fully.
- Sexual intercourse should be avoided for 6 weeks if there has been vaginal surgery, particularly to the vaginal vault as in TAH. When the woman does resume sexual relations, she should be encouraged to take the lead and feel in control, as she may be apprehensive about discomfort.
- It is important that she returns to normal life as soon as possible. However, she should be advised against any heavy lifting or vacuuming for at least a month, but can then start to increase the activities as she is able.

Box 7.9 Information

International Federation of Gynecology and Obstetrics (FIGO) (2006)

Classification of cancer of the corpus uteri (endometrial)

Stage I	Tumour confined to the corpus (body)
Stage II	Tumour invades the cervix but does not extend beyond the uterus
Stage III	Local and/or regional spread: tumour has extended outside the uterus but not outside true pelvis
Stage IV	Tumour extends outside true pelvis and has involved the mucosa of bladder and/or bowel

the endometrium shown on the TVS (indicative of pathology), the diagnosis can be confirmed by a hysteroscopy with endometrial biopsy.

Treatment

Total abdominal hysterectomy and bilateral salpingo-oophorectomy (TAH and BSO) Endometrial cancer usually requires the removal of the uterus, cervix, uterine tubes and ovaries. Radiotherapy may be necessary if there has been invasion through the myometrium.

Radical hysterectomy A radical hysterectomy also includes removal of pelvic lymph nodes. Surgical treatment may be combined with radiotherapy to the pelvic wall. Alternatively, the

uterine tumour may be irradiated to shrink it and deplete its blood supply before surgery or if the patient is unfit for surgery.

Hormonal treatments Although there is a lack of randomised studies, it is felt by some that progestogens may prevent recurrence of early stage disease.

The 5-year survival rate in women with stage I endometrial cancer is around 85% whereas it is only 25% in women diagnosed with stage IV (Cancer Research UK 2009b).

Nursing management and health promotion: endometrial cancer

The nursing care of the patient with endometrial cancer involves general pre- and postoperative care and specific care for hysterectomy. Care will be individualised but will be similar to that outlined for a woman with cervical cancer (see pp. 214–216 and above).

Following TAH and BSO most women will have normal bladder function postoperatively. Sometimes, however, a self-retaining urethral catheter may be used initially, to avoid distending the urinary bladder and exerting pressure on the posterior urethral wall, which may be swollen and bruised.

The woman will need information about her progress at regular intervals in the postoperative period. Of particular concern may be the need to have radiotherapy at an early, vulnerable stage after major surgery (see Ch. 31). Psychological support from the nurse should help the patient to view the radiotherapy as the final safety net in the treatment process.

Positive improvements should be seen within 3 months of treatment being completed. Medical follow-up is essential to monitor progress and identify early signs of recurrent disease.

Ovarian cancer

In the UK, ovarian cancer is the fourth most common cancer in women. In 2006, 6596 women were diagnosed with ovarian cancer in the UK, and in 2007 the disease caused the deaths of 4317 women (Cancer Research UK 2009c).

Ovarian cancer is more common in developed countries (Campbell & Monga 2006). A relationship is said to exist between multiple ovulation in women in well-nourished communities and the incidence of ovarian cancer. Pregnancy and the oral contraceptive pill have a protective effect. The condition is more common in infertile and nulliparous women and in women who are celibate. There is also a 3–5% genetic risk whereby women with the BRCA1 and 2 genes are at risk (Easton et al 1995). The peak incidence is between 50 and 70 years of age (Blake et al 2008).

At the time of writing, there is no UK screening programme, but research is ongoing (see Ch. 31). The tumour is often widespread before symptoms appear. As a result, late detection of the condition prohibits effective treatment and the mortality rate is higher than for other genital malignancies.

PATHOPHYSIOLOGY

Ovarian tumours may occur unilaterally or bilaterally. Occasionally they arise from metastatic spread from a cancer in adjacent organs. However, more commonly they develop as a primary tumour and are divided into epithelial, sex chord stromal tumour or germ cell tumours. Ovarian cancer spreads via lymph and blood vessels. Box 7.10 outlines the International Federation of Gynecology and Obstetrics (FIGO) (2006) staging classification of ovarian cancer.

Ovarian cancer is histologically classified according to the type of cell from which it originates, the most common source being surface epithelium (formed from embryonic mesothelium). The three commonest types of tumour are:

- serous (tubal)
- endometrioid (endometrial)
- mucinous (endocervical).

Serous papilliferous cancer The malignant serous tumour is the commonest type of primary ovarian cancer and often affects both ovaries. Tumour cells are disseminated into the peritoneal cavity to form multiple seedling metastases. In most cases there is rapid spread in the peritoneal cavity with ascites (fluid in the peritoneal cavity).

Mucinous cancer Approximately 10% of ovarian cancer is classified as mucinous (Campbell & Monga 2006). Many of these tumours are identified at an early stage of growth, which gives a better prognosis for the patient. These are amongst the largest of ovarian tumours, often reaching up to 25 cm in diameter.

Endometrioid cancer This type of ovarian cancer resembles an endometrial adenocarcinoma. The tumour consists of endometrial tubular gland cells. It may be secondary to uterine disease or a primary ovarian growth that coexists with endometrial cancer.

Germ cell tumours Similar tumours may arise in the germ cells of either gender and may be benign or malignant. Benign conditions are very common; malignancy is rare. The commonest type of germ cell tumour is the dermoid cyst (see p. 208) or cystic teratoma. Dermoid cysts usually occur in the ovary but are very rare in the testes; malignant teratoma is more common in the testes.

Malignant germ cell tumours include dysgerminoma and choriocarcinoma (see pp. 210–211). The former is highly malignant and metastasises via the blood and lymphatics.

MEDICAL MANAGEMENT

Ovarian cancer is insidious in its growth and the woman may have no discomfort or suspicion of disease until an advanced stage. Approximately 70% of women have the disease diagnosed when it has spread beyond the ovaries (Blake et al 2008). Late symptoms are related to increased pressure in the abdominal venous channels, causing oedema in the legs and pain from pressure on nerves to the legs. Metastatic growth in the peritoneum will contribute to extensive ascites, abdominal pain, urinary frequency, nausea, vomiting, emaciation and breathlessness. A thrombosis may form in an iliac vein or in the inferior vena cava. If growth has spread to other organs there may be symptoms, such as intestinal obstruction (see Ch. 4).

Investigations A full pelvic examination is necessary, with palpation of the ovaries. Ultrasound and CT scanning of the abdomen and pelvis is indicated. Further CT or MRI scans are performed to assess the extent of lymph node involvement and other metastatic spread. A chest X-ray may identify metastatic spread to the lungs, or pleural effusion.

An intravenous urogram (IVU) may be performed if obstruction of a ureter is suspected.

A full blood count, serum biochemistry and serum Ca-125 tumour markers are required. Ovarian tumours are always surgically removed and the final diagnosis is confirmed histologically. It is important that the ovary and peritoneal cavity should be fully assessed to define the spread of the disease.

Treatment This will depend on the extent of the disease. When ovarian cancer is diagnosed, laparotomy is undertaken with a TAH, BSO, pelvic lymph node removal and omentectomy (removal of the omentum, part of the peritoneum) as it is important to achieve macroscopic clearance. As much malignant tissue as possible will be removed. Adjuvant chemotherapy is normally given except in early

Box 7.10 Information

International Federation of Gynecology and Obstetrics (FIGO) (2006)
Classification of ovarian cancer

Stage I	Tumour limited to ovaries
Stage II	Tumour involves one or both ovaries and extends beyond the ovaries but is confined within the pelvis
Stage III	Tumour involves one or both ovaries with intraperitoneal metastases and/or regional lymph node involvement.
Stage IV	Other distant metastases beyond the peritoneal cavity

stages of the disease. Radiation is generally confined to palliation. In advanced stages, palliative treatment only may be possible (see Chs 31, 33), for example, abdominal paracentesis to drain ascites to relieve the pain and breathlessness.

At the time of writing, there are trials of poly(ADP-ribose) polymerase (PARP) inhibitors involving women with advanced ovarian or breast cancer linked to BRCA1 and 2 genes (Cancer Research UK 2009d).

 ## Nursing management and health promotion: ovarian cancer

In addition to physical care (see pp. 214–217), the patient with ovarian cancer and her family will need much psychological support from the nurse. Anxieties associated with investigations, diagnosis and the effects of hysterectomy and chemotherapy will need to be anticipated and managed in all aspects (see Ch. 31). The patient may make a full recovery quite quickly or, if metastatic disease remains, may be debilitated for longer. Oncology nurse specialists perform a pivotal role in supporting patients at this time.

The nurse will work towards helping the patient make physical and emotional adjustments. Attention will be given to the relief of pain, nausea and vomiting after surgery and chemotherapy. As physical problems are relieved, the patient may cope better emotionally, but when the prognosis is poor, time is needed to adjust to the sad news. Jefferies (2002) demonstrated the positive impact nurses can have both at the time of diagnosis and throughout the course of the disease. Chapter 33 provides detailed information about palliative care, symptom relief, end-of-life care and bereavement care.

Uterine displacement and prolapse

Cervicovaginal prolapse

The cervix can become prolapsed and elongated by the opposing forces of pull of the transverse cervical and uterosacral ligaments against prolapsed vaginal walls. Importantly, in this situation the cervix prolapses but the uterus stays in the pelvis.

Types of prolapse

Anterior vaginal wall prolapse

- *Cystocele* – a prolapse of the bladder and upper anterior vaginal wall (Figure 7.8A).
- *Urethrocele* – a lower vaginal wall prolapse with urethral descent.

Posterior vaginal wall prolapse

- *Rectocele* – a prolapse of the rectum and the middle third of the posterior vaginal wall. If the lowest part of the vaginal wall prolapses, the perineal body is involved rather than the rectum (Figure 7.8B).
- *Enterocele* – if the upper part of the posterior vaginal wall prolapses, the rectouterine recess/pouch is elongated and a loop of small bowel or omentum may descend.

Both anterior and posterior vaginal walls may be involved in the prolapse. When a large cystocele is present, bladder

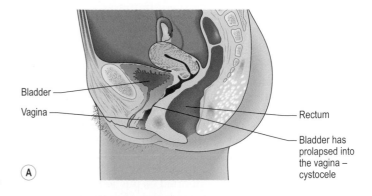

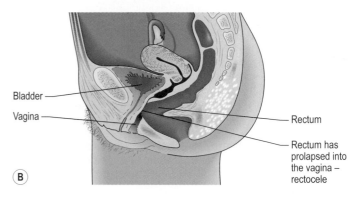

Figure 7.8 Uterovaginal prolapse. A. Cystocele; B. rectocele. (Reproduced from Cotton 2003 with permission.)

emptying tends to be incomplete, causing bladder hypertrophy. There is a lump, urinary frequency, dysuria and stress incontinence (see Ch. 24). The uterus may become distorted, leading to reflux of urine and, ultimately, renal damage. Urinary tract infection is common.

A woman with a rectocele may notice a lump and experience difficulty during defecation.

Uterovaginal prolapse

When the structures supporting the uterus and vagina become ineffective, the genital tract descends, prolapses or herniates through the gap between the muscles of the pelvic floor.

The uterus descends in the axis of the vagina taking the vaginal wall with it. This prolapse is essentially but not exclusively a postmenopausal condition.

Three degrees of uterine prolapse are described:

- *first degree* – the cervix is still within the vagina
- *second degree* – the cervix appears at the introitus
- *third degree* – the uterus and vagina are completely prolapsed and lie outside the vulva.

Rectal prolapse may also occur. This is sometimes called complete procidentia.

Contributing factors are:

- stretching of tissues from repeated child-bearing
- injury to the pelvic floor during childbirth
- the long-term maintenance of an upright, erect body position that strains the transverse ligaments (the chief support of the uterus)

- increased intra-abdominal pressure associated with obesity, chronic cough or heavy lifting work.

MEDICAL MANAGEMENT

History The woman may be overweight, complains of backache and describes a feeling of 'something coming down' when she is in an upright position. There is urinary frequency, incomplete bladder emptying and the residual urine is a focus for infection. Stress incontinence may be a major problem for some women (see Ch. 24). There may be difficulty in voiding urine and in defecation. The cystocele or rectocele may have to be supported or pushed upwards vaginally before urine can be passed or the bowel evacuated.

Examination Severe prolapse may be diagnosed by inspecting the vulva with the patient lying on her back and straining downwards. A vaginal speculum is used to allow direct vision of a prolapsed anterior vaginal wall and any rectocele or enterocele formed by a prolapsed posterior vaginal wall. A rectal examination is needed to confirm the latter type of displacement. The degree of uterine prolapse is usually assessed before surgery when the patient is anaesthetised.

Investigations A diagnosis of uterine displacement can be made on examination. Pre-operative assessment will involve investigations to assess the woman's general health prior to general anaesthetic.

Treatment Surgical treatment is curative for prolapse but is not suitable for all women. Some may be unfit for surgery due to poor physical condition or may not have completed their family. The uterus may be supported by the use of a polyethylene or flexible vinyl ring pessary. Such pessaries can cause local inflammation and are changed every 4–6 months when the vaginal walls can be examined for inflammation or ulceration. A course of vaginal oestrogen may be prescribed to diminish atrophic changes, inflammation, infection and discharge.

Surgical repair of uterine displacement and prolapse This may involve removal of the uterus vaginally and reconstruction of the supporting pelvic floor muscles between the anus, vagina and bladder, and approximating the medial borders of the pubococcygeus muscles. Childbirth can result in supporting structures being torn, separated and overstretched. Repair of cystocele is known as anterior colporrhaphy supporting the urethra and urethrovesical junction. A rectocele is repaired by a posterior colpoperineorrhaphy, the repair of the perineal body. Bladder, perineum and vulva have an excellent capacity for repair, related to a rich blood supply and good venous drainage. Surgery is usually very successful.

 ## Nursing management and health promotion: uterine displacement

Pre-operative care

Pre-operative assessment and care of women for major gynaecological operations has been discussed earlier in the chapter. Care is always individualised according to needs, but some problems and interventions are similar.

Information Information about procedures before and after surgery will increase patient understanding and cooperation and reduce anxiety.

Potential embarrassment A woman admitted for repair of prolapse may experience embarrassment due to stress incontinence and the need for some type of protection. The nurse will ensure that her special requirements are met discreetly.

Evacuating the lower bowel before surgery The woman's lower bowel may be emptied before surgery and an oral laxative, or suppositories or evacuant microenema may be prescribed.

Identification of sexual activity Whilst embarrassing for some women, it is important to identify if the woman is still sexually active. This will influence the amount of vaginal tissue removed during surgery.

Postoperative care

Risk of strain on internal suture lines from a full bladder An indwelling catheter on continuous drainage is required. Precautions are taken to prevent the introduction of infection when the closed urinary drainage system is breached when collecting specimens or changing drainage bags.

Loss of bladder tone This is possible after catheter removal. Residual amounts of urine retained in the bladder after voiding should be assessed. This can be done by a non-invasive bladder scan or by catheterisation. A residual urine of less than 60 mL is satisfactory.

Risk of wound infection Regular perineal cleansing can minimise the risk of infection.

Constipation This will potentially strain the repaired posterior vaginal wall. A stool-softener laxative can be prescribed to promote easy defecation.

Pre-discharge counselling An opportunity is created for the patient to discuss her feelings and worries about the level of recovery from surgery, bladder functioning, future return to sexual activity and work. In particular the woman is advised to avoid jarring or lifting activities for 2 months to prevent straining the healing tissues. Contact numbers should be given if problems arise once home (Box 7.8, p. 217).

Infections of the female reproductive tract

Infections of the female reproductive tract include vaginitis, cervicitis, endometritis, salpingitis and pelvic inflammatory disease (PID), oophoritis and toxic shock syndrome (TSS), some of which are sexually transmitted (see Ch. 35). This chapter concentrates on salpingitis and PID and readers are directed to Further reading, e.g. Collins et al 2008, Gupta et al 2009.

Salpingitis and pelvic inflammatory disease

Inflammation/infection of the uterine tubes, salpingitis, usually affects both tubes simultaneously. It may result from ascending infection from the vagina, cervix or uterus or it can occur directly from appendicitis, a pelvic abscess or other site of inflammation such as diverticulitis. The ovaries may also be involved in the inflammatory process. Salpingitis may therefore be part of generalised PID.

Acute salpingitis may follow childbirth, miscarriage or termination, diagnostic or operative procedures involving the uterus, or the insertion of intrauterine devices.

PATHOPHYSIOLOGY

Ascending salpingitis is most commonly caused by the organism *Chlamydia trachomatis*. Gonococcal infection, which is sexually transmitted, may also be the cause. Streptococcal and staphylococcal salpingitis may follow miscarriage or termination, childbirth or the insertion of an intrauterine device. These causes may reflect reactivation of pre-existing disease. Intestinal tract commensals, *Escherichia coli* or *Streptococcus faecalis*, may be involved if the infection is linked to appendicitis or bowel infection. The blood-borne *Mycobacterium tuberculosis* may unobtrusively inflame the reproductive organs.

The uterine tubes become engorged and swollen, possibly filled with pus (pyosalpinx). The ciliated epithelial lining is damaged, thus reducing the ability to move oocytes/ova and spermatozoa within the tubes.

Common presenting symptoms The patient feels generally unwell, with:

- pyrexia, sweating
- nausea, vomiting
- aching joints
- severe pelvic and abdominal pain.

MEDICAL MANAGEMENT

Women usually present with symptoms of generalised PID, or salpingitis may be identified for the first time during laparoscopy where the tubes are inflamed, distended and blocked. Adhesions may form between the tubes and other pelvic structures and peritonitis may be evident.

Tenderness will be felt over the uterine cornua on pelvic examination. There may not be obvious vaginal discharge so this cannot be relied upon for diagnosis. Infection spread via the genital tract will affect the lumen of the uterine tube, creating a purulent, foul discharge that is drained through the vagina. Scar tissue may form, causing narrowing or closure of the tube which will affect fertility. Adhesions may form between the inflamed tubes and the peritoneum. Peritonitis may occur if pus leaks out of the tubes into the peritoneal cavity. Rarely, an abscess may form in the pelvis or on the ovaries.

Investigations High vaginal or cervical swabs are taken and sent for microbiological culture and sensitivity to antibiotics. During surgery, samples for microbiological samples may be obtained.

Laparoscopy is not indicated in the acute phase as this may cause further spread of infection unless an abscess requires drainage or ectopic pregnancy is suspected.

Treatment Antibiotic therapy is prescribed along with analgesia.

 Nursing management and health promotion: salpingitis/PID

Nursing care will be planned to relieve symptoms, particularly pain, nausea, vomiting and potential fluid and electrolyte imbalance (see Chs 19, 20). Analgesics and antibiotic drugs are administered often intravenously for 24 hours. Information will need to be shared with the woman about the prevention of infection, the risk of infertility and the possibility of an ectopic pregnancy following salpingitis/PID.

Disorders of early pregnancy

Ectopic pregnancy

An ectopic pregnancy occurs when the fertilised ovum implants and develops outside the uterus. In the UK several studies indicate that the incidence is rising. Lewis (2007) reported 11.1 ectopic pregnancies per 1000 pregnancies. The Royal College of Obstetricians and Gynaecologists (RCOG) (2006) recommends using the term 'pregnancy of unknown location' where no identifiable pregnancy is seen on scan but there is a positive β-hCG.

PATHOPHYSIOLOGY

A delay occurs in the passage of the fertilised ovum through the uterine tube. This may be due to ciliary damage, obstruction in the tube or adhesions from an earlier infection. The pregnancy implants in the muscle wall of the tube and erodes into blood vessels. Increased tension in the tube will cause pelvic pain and may lead to rupture which can result in massive intraperitoneal haemorrhage.

Common presenting symptoms The woman experiences the early signs of pregnancy.

The trophoblast slowly erodes the tubal wall, which results in gradual or sudden rupture of the tube. The woman experiences abdominal pain. Urgent attention should be paid if the woman complains of shoulder pain due to referred pain from the diaphragm, which is irritated by blood in the abdomen.

Tubal rupture causes severe localised pain, which is followed by intense, more generalised abdominal pain. The POC are expelled into the peritoneal cavity and there is haemorrhage from the tubal placental site. This leads to hypovolaemic shock (Ch. 18), with rapid, feeble pulse rate, hypotension and pallor – an acute abdominal emergency exists and the woman must be treated as a gynaecological emergency. Despite medical advances in the past decade, there has been no decrease in the number of women dying from an ectopic pregnancy. There were 10 reported pregnancy deaths due to ectopic pregnancy from 2003 to 2005 (Lewis 2007).

MEDICAL MANAGEMENT

Investigations

Pregnancy tests Standard immunological pregnancy tests are unhelpful as a tubal pregnancy may not produce enough hCG to give a positive result. Estimation of the β subunit of hCG (β-hCG) is undertaken which is accurate 2 weeks after conception. Absence of β-hCG excludes pregnancy. In ectopic pregnancy the levels are lower than those at a comparable gestation in a normal intrauterine pregnancy. At a titre of 1000–1500 iu/L, it should be able to detect an intrauterine sac on a transvaginal scan, but levels above 1500 iu/L in the presence of an empty uterus may indicate an ectopic pregnancy.

Repeat blood tests may be required after 48 hours to assess both the amount and rate of increase of β-hCG levels.

USS By the sixth or seventh week of pregnancy, a gestational sac can be identified within the uterus on ultrasound scanning. A pregnancy outside the uterus often cannot be identified on scan. Consequently the presence of a raised β-hCG level combined with the lack of an identifiable intrauterine pregnancy indicates an ectopic pregnancy.

Treatment

Surgical An ectopic pregnancy always requires urgent surgery by laparoscopy or laparotomy. During laparoscopy under general anaesthetic, an incision is made into the tube and the pregnancy removed – the tube then heals spontaneously or the damaged tube is removed (salpingectomy). A laparotomy may be required if the tube has ruptured. Recovery after salpingectomy is usually rapid and uncomplicated.

Medical Non-surgical techniques have been developed. These include the puncture and aspiration of the ectopic sac or the local injection of embryotoxic drugs, such as methotrexate or potassium chloride (Campbell & Monga 2006). The need for a general anaesthetic with its associated risks is removed but careful follow-up is required to monitor the effects on the woman and the pregnancy.

A ruptured ectopic pregnancy quickly results in hypovolaemia and intravenous fluids are essential. The patient may need resuscitation but immediate surgery and treatment of the cause of bleeding is essential.

Women who are rhesus negative and are not sensitised should be given anti-D immunoglobulin following an ectopic pregnancy (RCOG 2002).

A woman who has suffered one ectopic pregnancy is at risk of developing a similar pregnancy in the second tube. However, the woman should be reassured she may be able to have a normal pregnancy via the remaining tube.

Nursing management and health promotion: ectopic pregnancy

Pre-operative care

Risk of hypovolaemia The nurse assesses and monitors the patient's physical state intensively from the time of admission to the ward. If the tubal pregnancy ruptures, the patient may suffer hypovolaemic shock and cardiac arrest. Vital signs are recorded every 15 min. Tachycardia, hypotension and increasing pain are indications that urgent medical intervention is required.

Pain The patient will experience pain which may be moderate, but may become intense and intolerable if the pregnancy ruptures. Analgesia is given as prescribed.

Preparation for general anaesthesia Emergency surgery will be required and fasting for an appropriate time may not be possible (see Ch. 26). Therefore, it is important for the anaesthetist to know when the patient last ate or drank and of any vomiting. It may be necessary to introduce a nasogastric tube prior to surgery to reduce the risk of regurgitation and inhalation of gastric contents when the patient is anaesthetised.

Anxiety and the need for information The patient may be anxious about the operation and distressed about losing a pregnancy. She will need information about the surgery and postoperative care, and needs to be encouraged to talk about any worries she may have. The nurse must show empathy and understanding of the patient's feelings and concerns.

Postoperative care

Postoperative care will be individualised according to patient need (see Ch. 26). Her condition will begin to stabilise as soon as the ectopic pregnancy is removed, bleeding is controlled and blood volume restored. Her main problems will be similar to those of other patients who have had open abdominal surgery, plus those associated with pregnancy loss as follows:

- *Change in vital signs.* The nurse monitors pulse rate, blood pressure, respiration rate and body temperature. Wound site and vaginal blood loss are observed for more than minimal drainage. Primary and secondary haemorrhages are risks.
- *Postoperative pain.* The level of pain can be assessed using a verbal rating scale (see Ch. 19). Analgesics are prescribed and administered to control pain.
- *Post-anaesthetic nausea.* This problem may be prevented or treated by giving an antiemetic medication with analgesics as prescribed.
- *Fluid and electrolyte imbalance.* Intravenous fluid and electrolyte replacement therapy is administered as prescribed, until oral intake is resumed. Fluid intake and output are recorded.
- *Risk of venous thromboembolism.* The patient is actively encouraged to exercise her legs hourly whilst confined to bed. Antiembolism hosiery/stockings will be fitted preoperatively and worn until discharge. Early mobilisation is usual and encouraged.
- *Personal care.* Whilst intravenous therapy is in situ, assistance will be given to maintain the patient's preferred standard of personal care until fully mobile.
- *Loss and grieving.* It must be acknowledged that the woman has lost a pregnancy and she must be given opportunities to talk about her feelings and emotions freely. Information should be shared about the possibility of future pregnancies. Details of local support groups for those who suffer loss should be given. The effect on future fertility should be acknowledged and the nurse should give the woman and her partner appropriate support and information about assisted conception services as required.

Miscarriage and termination of pregnancy

The legal definition of the term 'abortion' refers to the premature delivery of a non-viable fetus, spontaneously or by induction. The term 'miscarriage' is recommended when the pregnancy loss is spontaneous and is generally more acceptable to women who lose a wanted pregnancy (RCOG 2006). Currently, in the UK, a fetus is considered viable from the 24th week of pregnancy. This viability is recognised and safeguarded in the Infant Life (Preservation) Act 1929 and its amendment under the Human Fertilisation and Embryology Act 1990. However, debate continues around reducing the gestational age of viable pregnancies due to the technological developments increasingly available to support very premature infants. Spontaneous miscarriage refers to all types of naturally occurring miscarriages. Induced 'abortion' refers to interventional termination of pregnancy (TOP).

A spontaneous miscarriage is a response to a naturally occurring phenomenon such as hormonal problems, uterine abnormality, cervical problems, a genetic malformation in the embryo/fetus or psychological factors. Miscarriage occurs in 10–20% of clinical pregnancies (RCOG 2006). Miscarriages in the early weeks of the second trimester of pregnancy may be due to a cervix that dilates in response to the increasing weight of the fetus. The cervical os dilates, the membranes rupture and the pregnancy is lost. The woman will be distressed by the loss of the pregnancy and will need psychological support from the nurse, encouraging her and her partner to express their feelings.

To counteract recurrence of miscarriage, it is necessary to identify the pregnancy and any incompetence of the cervix at an early stage. In the case of cervical incompetence, a purse-string (Shirodkar's) suture can be inserted surgically, closing the internal os. The suture is removed at 38 weeks' gestation or when labour commences, to enable delivery to occur.

Miscarriage may be categorised by the:

- level of certainty of the miscarriage occurring
  - threatened
  - inevitable
  - missed
  - induced
- degree of expulsion of the POC
  - incomplete
  - complete.

See Figure 7.9.

The care of women having a miscarriage is increasingly undertaken in outpatient settings or in the community.

Threatened miscarriage

PATHOPHYSIOLOGY

A threatened miscarriage is when a woman known to be pregnant develops vaginal bleeding during the first 24 weeks of gestation. Some lower abdominal pain related to uterine muscle contractions may be experienced at the time of bleeding, but there may be no uterine contractions and no pain. The blood loss may be brown or red.

It is not unusual for a show of blood to coincide with the woman's regular date of menstruation. This type of bleeding is due to the fertilised ovum becoming more deeply implanted in the uterine wall. There is little risk of loss of the pregnancy if the bleeding settles quickly (Figure 7.9A).

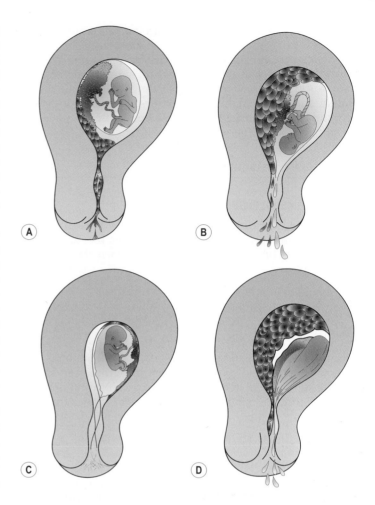

Figure 7.9 The types of miscarriage. A. Threatened miscarriage. B. Inevitable miscarriage. C. Missed miscarriage. D. Incomplete miscarriage.

MEDICAL MANAGEMENT

The presence of bleeding, slight uterine contractions and a closed cervical os established by examination assist in identifying threatened miscarriage; 70–80% of women can be expected to continue to full-term pregnancies.

Treatment While the woman is continuing to lose blood vaginally, it is recommended that she does not undertake strenuous activities. Bed rest is unlikely to influence the outcome but the woman may blame herself if she goes on to miscarry following strenuous activity.

Women who are rhesus negative and are not sensitised should be given anti-D immunoglobulin if they have a threatened miscarriage:

- over 12 weeks' gestation or
- with heavy vaginal bleeding or associated with pain before 12 weeks' gestation (RCOG 2002).

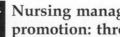 **Nursing management and health promotion: threatened miscarriage**

The woman and her partner will be very concerned about the possible loss of the pregnancy. This may result in tearfulness, anxiety, irritability and feelings of frustration. The woman may be apprehensive of pain and uncertain of what to expect.

Nursing care aims to reduce anxiety by providing accurate information about likely outcomes and support and reassurance for the couple. Vaginal bleeding will be monitored closely and abdominal discomfort or pain will be assessed. The supportive, counselling contact time with the nurse will be appreciated by the woman and her partner.

Inevitable miscarriage

PATHOPHYSIOLOGY

A threatened miscarriage can become inevitable if vaginal bleeding continues. A miscarriage becomes inevitable, with no possibility of saving the pregnancy, when the following are present:

- heavy vaginal blood loss often with clots
- strong uterine contractions
- pain
- dilatation of the cervix.

Contractions will increase, the fetal sac membranes rupture and the uterine contents move through the cervical os. Part or all of the POC will be voided from the uterus (Figure 7.9B). An inevitable miscarriage may be complete if all POC are voided, or incomplete if some products are retained.

MEDICAL MANAGEMENT

Estimation of blood loss and assessment of pulse, blood pressure, respiration and appearance of the patient will indicate whether hypovolaemic shock is developing. Intravenous fluids may be required and analgesics are administered as necessary.

Fetal tissue that has been expelled is retained and examined to assess whether the fetal sac and contents are intact or whether remnants have been retained. USS can be useful to determine the type of miscarriage (complete, incomplete, missed, etc.) and, based on this, appropriate information can be given to the woman about the likely outcome and therapeutic options. Following a complete miscarriage, the uterus will contract and the complex interlocking layers of smooth muscle fibres of the myometrium will exert pressure on blood vessels to restrict blood loss. If any of the POC are thought to have been retained, the uterus cannot contract fully and bleeding will continue. Retained POC may also provide a locus for infection. Several treatment options are available and the woman must be involved in the choice of approach. They are:

- evacuation of the retained products of conception (ERPC) from the uterus, an invasive procedure; in the UK a general anaesthetic is usual, but in many countries local anaesthetic or sedation is used (RCOG 2006)
- medical management with the use of a prostaglandin analogue such as misoprostol
- expectant management ('wait and see'), but women must be aware that it may take several weeks for complete resolution.

Women who are rhesus negative and are not sensitised should be given anti-D immunoglobulin if they have a miscarriage over 12 weeks' gestation, or have an ERPC or medical management (RCOG 2002).

Nursing management and health promotion: inevitable miscarriage

The nurse must monitor vaginal blood loss extremely closely whichever form of management is undertaken. The patient may be distressed by the blood loss, pain, and the anguish of losing a pregnancy particularly if planned. The nurse has an important role to provide support for both the woman and her partner at this time, encouraging them to talk through their feelings of loss. In this respect, time and empathy from the nurse will be appreciated. If a fetus has been passed, the woman should be supported in viewing the fetus if she wishes and photographs should be taken to provide a record which the woman may want either at the time or later. Information about support groups, such as the Miscarriage Association, can be helpful.

Missed miscarriage

PATHOPHYSIOLOGY

A missed miscarriage is one in which the embryo/fetus dies, but is not expelled. The size of the uterus fails to increase during the first trimester, the fetus does not develop and the expected signs of a normally developing pregnancy will be missing. In some cases a fertilised ovum fails to develop further than embryonic stages. The death of the embryo/fetus may occur at any week of gestation. Some placental tissue survives to produce progesterone and prevent expulsion (Figure 7.9C).

MEDICAL MANAGEMENT

Following a positive pregnancy test, the woman may have stopped feeling pregnant. She may experience a brown vaginal discharge. Some hCG may still be present but levels fall.

Investigations An USS of the uterus will indicate a gestational sac smaller than that expected for the gestational age and the absence of a fetal heart.

Treatment Once a missed miscarriage has been diagnosed, treatment options should be discussed with the woman. These include:

- ERPC (see above).
- Medical management with the administration of mifepristone (an antiprogesterone) orally then misoprostol vaginally 24–48 hours later. This induces the uterine muscles to contract and the woman experiences labour.
- Expectant/conservative management where nature is allowed to take its course; however, this can take several weeks and some women cannot cope with the thought of carrying their dead baby in utero during this time. The woman must also be provided with 24-hour contact details in case of haemorrhage following expulsion of the POC.

As discussed earlier, the administration of anti-D immunoglobulin may be needed for unsensitised women who are rhesus negative.

Nursing management and health promotion: missed miscarriage

If ERPC is planned, the woman will need the usual preparation to undergo anaesthesia safely (see Ch. 26). Following treatment, observations of vital signs and vaginal blood loss will be required to assess recovery.

If medical management is planned the nurse must be available to observe the patient's vital signs and need for pain relief and provide support during the 'labour' phase. The patient should be nursed in a single room but must not feel isolated during this time. Patients and their partners cope emotionally in different ways but the nurse can anticipate that couples may feel sad and angry about the lost pregnancy. They must be given opportunities to express their needs and feelings freely.

Incomplete miscarriage

An incomplete miscarriage is one in which only part of the POC are expelled from the uterus (Figure 7.9D).

PATHOPHYSIOLOGY

Portions of placenta and membranes are retained, some bleeding continues and could possibly be heavy. Retained products can become infected so the aim should be to remove them.

MEDICAL MANAGEMENT

The residual products may be voided spontaneously by the woman but otherwise they will need to be removed either by surgical evacuation using vacuum aspiration or by the administration of misoprostol, previously described for inevitable miscarriage.

Women who are rhesus negative and are not sensitised should be given anti-D immunoglobulin if they have a miscarriage over 12 weeks' gestation, or have an ERPC or medical management (RCOG 2002).

Nursing management and health promotion: incomplete miscarriage

The patient's symptoms will depend on the amount of tissue retained. She may experience moderate to severe abdominal pain while the uterus contracts trying to expel the retained POC. Nursing care involves administering analgesics and monitoring their effect. Vaginal blood loss must be monitored, as heavy, continuous blood loss may reduce circulating blood volume, resulting in hypovolaemic shock. Observations of vital signs will facilitate early recognition of shock and prompt correction of the condition by intravenous fluid replacement. A supportive approach must be used as for other forms of miscarriage (Box 7.11).

Recurrent miscarriage

Recurrent miscarriage refers to spontaneous miscarriage that occurs in three or more successive pregnancies at a similar gestational age. Many factors may contribute to recurrent miscarriage.

Box 7.11 Reflection

Pregnancy loss

Failure of a fertilised embryo to develop into a successful pregnancy resulting in a live baby can occur at many different stages of the pregnancy.

Activity

- Think about the different types of pregnancy loss that can happen.
- Reflect on how the woman and her partner may be feeling after the loss of a pregnancy and what you might say to the couple to support them.

PATHOPHYSIOLOGY

Genetic, hormonal, anatomical, infectious and immunological factors have been implicated in the causation of recurrent miscarriage. However, the underlying mechanisms are poorly explained, largely speculative and require further investigation.

MEDICAL MANAGEMENT

This depends on the reason for recurrent miscarriage. There is insufficient evidence for many treatments previously thought to have been useful, e.g. leucocyte transfusions (RCOG 2003). Surgery to correct uterine abnormalities should be considered carefully as postoperative scarring may affect future fertility.

Nursing management and health promotion: recurrent miscarriage

Physical and psychological care are paramount at the time that the miscarriage occurs. Referral to a specialist unit where further chromosomal testing can be undertaken should be offered to the couple.

Termination of pregnancy

An unwanted pregnancy creates emotional anguish for a woman. She may experience feelings of conflict about both wanting and rejecting the pregnancy. She may fear having to explain it to others. Family standards of behaviour, cultural norms and religious beliefs may appear to be violated both by the pregnancy and by the possibility of termination. The woman may feel very alone, indecisive and under pressure from a partner who may reject the pregnancy. The conditions of the Abortion Act require decision making to be completed early in the pregnancy.

The Abortion Act 1967 and 1990 amendments

In the UK, the Abortion Act 1967 became law in 1968 and applies to England, Wales and Scotland but not Northern Ireland. The Act states that the termination of pregnancy by a registered practitioner is not illegal under certain conditions. Notification of a termination must be given on a prescribed form to the Chief Medical Officer of the Department of Health within 7 days of the termination. The

Abortion Act 1967 was amended by the Human Fertilisation and Embryology Act 1990, recognising viability of the fetus at 24 weeks' gestation.

Conditions of the Act and statutory grounds

A legally induced termination must be:

- performed by a registered medical practitioner
- performed, except in an emergency, in a National Health Service hospital or in a place for the time being approved for the purpose of the Act
- certified by two registered medical practitioners as necessary on any of the following grounds:
  - the continuance of the pregnancy would involve risk to the life of the pregnant woman greater than if the pregnancy were terminated
  - the continuance of the pregnancy would involve risk of injury to the physical or mental health of the pregnant woman greater than if the pregnancy were terminated
  - the continuance of the pregnancy would involve risk of injury to the physical or mental health of any existing child(ren) in the family of the pregnant woman greater than if the pregnancy were terminated
  - there is a substantial risk that if the child were born it would suffer from such physical or mental abnormalities as to be seriously handicapped
- in emergency, certified by the operating practitioner as immediately necessary:
  - to save the life of the pregnant woman
  - to prevent grave permanent injury to the physical or mental health of the pregnant woman.

Conscientious objection and the Abortion Act 1967

The Act states that no-one shall be under any legal obligation to participate in any treatment authorised by the Act to which he or she has a conscientious objection unless the treatment is necessary to save the life or prevent grave permanent injury to the physical or mental health of a pregnant woman. The conscience clause does not only apply to members of a particular religion or faith and the objector must participate in emergency care of the patient should it be necessary. This is affirmed in The Code: Standards of conduct, performance and ethics for nurses and midwives (Nursing and Midwifery Council [NMC] 2008 modified 2009).

Counselling of the pregnant woman requesting termination

A woman who requests a termination of pregnancy will be referred for counselling to discuss any contraindications to termination and provide evidence for the final decision making. If possible she should be seen with her partner although they may not want to be involved. All women/girls, even those under the age of 16 years, are entitled to complete confidentiality when requesting termination and partners or parents are not informed without the woman's consent. However, those under 16 years of age are encouraged to speak to their parents. Adolescent girls may be accompanied by parents who may be angry and there is a risk the girl passively acts in accordance with her parents' wishes.

The counselling service ensures that adequate assessment and advice are provided for the woman who seeks a termination. It is suggested that in this way she will experience less regret, guilt or long-term psychological problems.

MEDICAL MANAGEMENT

All non-sensitised rhesus negative women having a termination of pregnancy should have anti-D immunoglobin (RCOG 2002).

Methods used for termination

Suction termination This is the most commonly used method for early termination of pregnancy. It may be performed with a local or general anaesthetic, or conscious sedation. Pre-operatively the patient may have vaginal misoprostol to soften the cervix. The cervix is dilated, a flexible cannula is inserted and the contents of the uterus are aspirated by suction. The uterus is then curetted to ensure total removal of the POC.

Surgical dilatation and evacuation This can be used in the second trimester of pregnancy. The cervix is dilated and the POC are removed using forceps and suction, usually under general anaesthetic. Pre-operatively the patient may have vaginal misoprostol to soften the cervix and facilitate easier dilatation.

Medical termination (unlicensed regimens). The specific regimen depends on the period of gestation, but is based for example on oral mifepristone 200 mg followed by vaginal misoprostol 800 µg after a period of time (1–3 days up to 9 weeks' gestation; 36–48 h for pregnancies 9–24 weeks' gestation).

Following administration of misoprostol the patient remains under observation for a further 6 h. Before discharge, arrangements are made for the patient to return in 5–9 days to assess the outcome.

If the POC have not been expelled 4 h following the misoprostol in pregnancies over 7 weeks' gestation up to 9 weeks, a second dose of misoprostol 400 µg (oral or vaginal) may be administered.

For pregnancies of 9–13 weeks' gestation, a further four doses of misoprostol 400 µg (oral or vaginal) can be given at intervals 3 h apart if needed. In later terminations of 13–24 weeks' gestation, should further doses of misoprostol 400 µg be needed it is administered orally.

While this method of terminating a pregnancy has its advantages – not least that there is no anaesthetic or surgical intervention – there are also potential problems of which the woman should be made aware. These include:

- a chance that the termination will be unsuccessful/incomplete, resulting in the need for surgical intervention; excessive vaginal bleeding may occur
- the possibility of pain, necessitating powerful analgesics
- possible psychological distress for the woman seeing the expelled fetus.

Other methods involving the administration of prostaglandins, for example intravenously, extra-amniotically or intra-amniotically, are now rarely performed.

Complications of pregnancy termination

- Pelvic infection – inflammation of the endometrium (endometritis) and salpingitis.

- Perforation of the uterus – caused accidentally during cannula insertion or use of the curette.
- Haemorrhage – bleeding should not be more than a normal menstruation.
- Laceration of cervix, cervical incompetence and recurrent miscarriage.
- Ectopic pregnancy – related to previous salpingitis.
- Incomplete removal of uterine contents.
- Hydatidiform mole.
- Delayed menstruation.
- A live fetus at the time of delivery.
- Possible susceptibility to subsequent pregnancy loss and premature births.
- Infertility.

With improved services, the numbers of complications associated with termination of pregnancy can be greatly reduced.

▷ Nursing management and health promotion: termination of pregnancy

Care before the procedure

The procedure is generally completed on an outpatient basis or as a day patient in hospital. The nurse must demonstrate a non-judgemental attitude and provide support and information for the woman. Blood tests such as ABO grouping and the rhesus factor are necessary precautions prior to the procedure.

Care following the procedure

Vital signs related to bleeding, i.e. pulse and blood pressure, and abdominal cramping pain must be observed by the nurse. Vaginal loss must be monitored closely. Pyrexia may indicate the onset of infection. Mild analgesics may be ordered to relieve cramping pain and also for their antipyretic properties. Nurses should be aware of those women who require anti-D immunoglobulin.

Women are advised to avoid the use of tampons, strenuous activities or sexual intercourse for 2 weeks to reduce the risk of infection and aid healing. Appropriate contraception must be discussed to prevent a further unwanted pregnancy. However, the nurse must be sensitive to the fact that some couples decide to terminate a wanted pregnancy due to serious fetal abnormalities.

Family planning services

Free contraceptive services are now available from general practitioners, family planning clinics in hospitals and the community, and voluntary organisations such as the FPA and Brook Advisory Centres who receive grants from central government or from purchasing commissioners. Male and female sterilisations are available in NHS facilities but must be considered permanent. Vasectomies may be performed in some large family planning clinics and by some GPs in the surgery.

Postnatally, community midwives, health visitors and GPs routinely discuss birth control methods with the new mother. This is invaluable in reminding women of their fertility and the possibility of another early pregnancy if precautions are not taken when resuming sexual activities.

The contraceptive needs of young people

Provision of extra contraceptive services for young people after puberty, under 16 years and up to 20 years of age, is controversial and, in the past, was given a low priority. With more recent concern about sexually transmitted infections (see Ch. 35) and unacceptably high teenage pregnancy rates, young people have been specially targeted for health education and advice about their sexual behaviour. Specialist services are now delivered through many health and voluntary services such as Brook which specifically aim at reaching and meeting the needs of teenagers.

Infertility

While some couples living together choose not to have children, the majority clearly do raise a family. For many people this is an important role, and when childlessness is a reality it brings disappointment. In addition, many other feelings, associated with social and cultural expectations and religious beliefs, may be experienced.

Some couples choose to delay having children but later may experience difficulty in conceiving. One in six couples will seek specialist help for a fertility problem. In one third of couples experiencing subfertility the problem lies with the woman, in one third with the man, and in the remaining third both the man and the woman contribute some causative factor.

 See website for further content

A couple is said to be subfertile if they have been having unprotected sexual intercourse for 12 months without conception occurring. Primary subfertility describes cases where a pregnancy has never occurred, and secondary subfertility those cases where there has been a previous pregnancy, irrespective of the outcome.

In 5–10% of cases no obvious cause for the infertility is found (Adamson & Baker 2003).

MEDICAL MANAGEMENT

The diagnosis and management of subfertility is complex. The couple may require to undergo a variety of tests and investigations which can cause embarrassment and stress.

See website for further content

Female subfertility

Female subfertility may be due to failure to produce oocytes or a patent system for a fertilised ovum to travel to and implant in the endometrium. This may be due to failure to ovulate, irregular ovulation, tubal obstruction, hostile cervical mucus, endometriosis or uterine conditions which inhibit implantation. Fertility declines with the age of the female and sharply so after 37 years. This is becoming more important as many couples are deferring starting families until later in life due to careers and personal choice. They may then encounter difficulties which need investigating and treating, providing extra pressure due to time constraints.

Ovulation disorders

These are among the commonest causes of subfertility. Failure to ovulate is linked with the functioning of hormones from the hypothalamus, pituitary and ovary (HPO axis).

- Hypothalamic disorders – abnormal levels of GnRH. There may be over- or underproduction resulting in anovulation.
- Pituitary disorders – abnormal secretion of prolactin resulting in anovulation and amenorrhoea.
- Ovarian causes – in polycystic ovary syndrome (PCOS), multiple small follicles partly develop but none reaches maturity, resulting in small cysts on the ovary. Often associated with obesity and hirsutism (see Ch. 5, Part 1).

Treatment seeks to remedy problems from imbalances in the HPO axis. Ovulation induction is aimed at encouraging development of more than one follicle. Clomiphene citrate stimulates gonadotrophin release. It can be prescribed for up to six cycles. This is also often effective for women with PCOS.

For women who do not respond to clomiphene therapy, human menopausal gonadotrophin (hMG) may be used for direct ovarian stimulation. Careful monitoring of the dose is required to reduce the risk of multiple pregnancy and ovarian hyperstimulation syndrome.

If a woman has hyperprolactinaemia, bromocriptine, a powerful dopamine agonist, inhibits prolactin release and may be an appropriate therapy.

Tubal disorders

A tubal disorder may prevent spermatozoa reaching the oocyte or, if fertilisation does occur, the ovum may not reach the uterine cavity for implantation. Tubal surgery may be advised to attempt to restore normal anatomy and function. However, the risks of further adhesions developing must be balanced against proposed benefits. Diagnostic procedures will include laparoscopy and hysterosalpingography for full assessment of the condition.

Treatment Surgical procedures used to treat tubal infertility include fimbrioplasty, salpingostomy and tubal cannulation. However, a successful outcome of such surgery depends on the degree of tubal damage and the adequacy of the surgery performed. Many patients will decide to opt for assisted conception techniques such as in vitro fertilisation (IVF), embryo transfer (ET) and gamete intrafallopian transfer (GIFT) rather than undergo further surgery.

Endometriosis

The association between endometriosis and infertility is complex (Mahutte & Arici 2002). Many women with the condition conceive successfully without intervention.

Treatment There is controversy over the treatment of infertile women with endometriosis without distortion of the pelvic viscera. Treatment using minimal access surgical techniques is usually only indicated for women suffering with other symptoms such as pelvic pain.

Male subfertility

Iammarrone et al (2003) suggest an increasing incidence of male reproductive problems. Impaired semen quality and spermatozoa dysfunction can occur as a result of many factors. The cause may be unknown, but it may be associated with a previous infection or factors such as stress, excessive smoking or alcohol intake or rise in scrotal temperature. Obstruction of the deferent duct (vas deferens) will result in ejaculate without spermatozoa. Anti-spermatozoa antibodies which attack spermatozoa or inhibit their motility may be present in semen.

Common presentations are:

- oligozoospermia – reduced number of spermatozoa
- asthenozoospermia – reduced motility
- tetratozoospermia – reduced normal morphology
- oligoasthenotetratozoospermia – a combination of the above three
- azoospermia – absence of spermatozoa.

Semen analysis includes an assessment of volume; sperm concentration, motility and morphology; and the number of white cells present. Spermatozoa and cervical mucus interaction can be examined in a postcoital test.

Men presenting with subfertility should be fully investigated to ascertain the type and identify any related health issues requiring independent treatment.

Treatment should be aimed at achieving natural conception. When natural conception is not possible, assisted conception techniques are offered. IVF involves fertilisation using male and female gametes under laboratory conditions. The fertilised embryo is then transferred into the uterus – a procedure known as embryo transfer (ET). This procedure is carried out in cycles of ovarian stimulations to produce several mature follicles at the same time. This principle has now been developed for other assisted conception techniques. These include:

- gamete intrafallopian transfer (GIFT) – gametes are introduced into the uterine tube for fertilisation in vivo
- donor insemination (DI) – donor spermatozoa used in cases of azoospermia
- subzonal insemination (SUZI) – used in cases of oligozoospermia or tetratozoospermia
- intracytoplasmic sperm injection (ICSI) – small amounts of viable sperm required
- testicular sperm aspiration (TESA)
  - percutaneous sperm aspiration (PESA) – used in cases where an obstruction prevents spermatozoa travelling along the deferent duct; spermatozoa are aspirated from the testes through the scrotum
  - microsurgical epididymal sperm aspiration (MESA) – as for PESA.

Chromosomal screening is required to exclude conditions such as cystic fibrosis and check karyotyping.

Provision of information and counselling

Investigations and treatments for subfertility can be intrusive and stressful for couples already anxious about not being able to conceive. It is essential that couples are given appropriate information about risks, benefits and alternatives of investigations and proposed treatments. Emotional support and counselling must be available to support the couple through the roller coaster of emotions they will experience. The importance of this is recognised by most assisted conception units, who employ specialist counsellors to provide this service.

In vitro fertilisation and embryo transfer

The pioneering work of Edwards and Steptoe in 1978 led to the first human birth after conception in vitro. In the intervening decades the success rate of IVF has improved as a result of advances in ovulation induction regimens, oocyte retrieval, embryo culture, embryo transfer and improved facilities of cryopreservation. IVF is now widely accepted as a form of treatment for unexplained subfertility. However, certain inclusion factors must be considered (Box 7.12).

The estimated live birth rates per cycle are reported to be between 13 and 28% but effectiveness of IVF has not been properly evaluated against other treatments (Pandian et al 2005).

In the UK the Human Fertilisation and Embryology Authority (HFEA) licenses and regulates assisted conception centres. The HFEA was established by the Human Fertilisation and Embryology Act 1990 (Department of Health [DH] 1990). A further Human Fertilisation and Embryology Act 2008 was introduced to amend the earlier Act because of 'technological developments, such as new ways of creating embryos that have arisen since 1990, and changes in society' (DH 2008). For example, one of the key provisions of the 2008 Act is to 'ensure that all human embryos outside the body – whatever the process used in their creation – are subject to regulation' (DH 2008).

The Human Fertilisation and Embryology Act has a conscientious objection clause. Consequently anyone who can show a conscientious objection to any of the activities governed by the Act is not obliged to participate in them. Nurses must make known any conscientious objection to the appropriate person as soon as possible (Nursing and Midwifery Council [NMC] 2008 modified 2009).

Box 7.12 Information

Indications for selection into IVF programmes
- Both partners are generally healthy.
- Ovaries are accessible.
- The uterus is functioning normally.
- Menstrual function is normal or correctable.
- Age below 40 years – units are able to set their own age limits so may be lower.
- The couple have an uncorrected problem, e.g.:
  - tubal blockage
  - inadequate spermatozoa for normal reproduction
  - endometriosis
  - cervical hostility
  - immunological
  - anovulation
  - undiagnosed by available methods.

Ovarian stimulation Various protocols are in use to achieve controlled hyperstimulation of the ovaries. Agents used include clomiphene citrate, purified FSH, exogenous gonadotrophin and gonadotrophin-releasing hormone agonists (GnRHAs). Modifications to protocols depend on the patient's response.

Commonly daily injections of FSH or hMG are used until dominant follicles have reached 18–20 mm in diameter. The ovaries are scanned regularly to monitor the size of follicles. A condition known as ovarian hyperstimulation syndrome can develop whereby the ovaries are overstimulated and additional symptoms develop. In severe cases, fluid passes out of the circulatory system resulting in ascites and haemoconcentration. It can be life threatening and if signs are detected during treatment cycle, that cycle should be abandoned.

Once follicles have developed to an appropriate size, hCG is administered and oocyte collection is undertaken 24–36 h later. The timing is important; if left too long the woman may ovulate spontaneously but if undertaken too soon it may be difficult to harvest follicles that are mature enough.

Oocyte harvesting Oocytes for fertilisation can be recovered from mature ovarian follicles by:

- ultrasound-guided follicle needle puncture and aspiration; can be performed under light general anaesthetic or sedation
- laparoscopy and needle aspiration; requires a general anaesthetic.

Each mature follicle is carefully aspirated and the oocytes are collected in the culture tube.

Laboratory procedures The aspirate is immediately passed to the embryologist for examination and identification of oocytes. Once sufficient suitable oocytes have been identified, they are placed in an incubator.

Close coordination between the embryology and surgical services is essential for treatments to be effective.

Fertilisation A fresh specimen of semen is required and this is often produced in the department, which can be embarrassing and stressful for the man. The sample is centrifuged to separate spermatozoa from seminal fluid. In IVF, the spermatozoa and oocytes are mixed together. Between 16 and 20 h later the oocytes are examined for fertilisation and once fertilisation has been established the embryos are returned to culture in fresh medium for another 24 h. In GIFT the oocytes and prepared spermatozoa are placed into a catheter to be inserted into the fimbrial end of the uterine tube, where the gametes are deposited for fertilisation. In ICSI, a spermatozoon is injected into the oocyte.

Embryo transfer This occurs 2–3 days after oocyte retrieval when the embryos are at the two- or four-cell stage. Embryo transfer into the uterus is a delicate procedure that does not necessarily result in successful implantation and pregnancy. The incidence of pregnancy increases with the number of embryos replaced; the HFEA *Code of Practice* 2009 provides guidance on reducing the risk of multiple pregnancy.

If menstruation does not occur the woman will undergo a urinary pregnancy test to confirm if a pregnancy has been achieved.

Pre-implantation diagnosis of genetic disease (PGD)

This technique has been developed for embryos produced through IVF. A single cell is removed for genetic testing. This is particularly useful for couples who carry genetic defects that can affect the well-being of the child. However, the benefits must be weighed against the potential damage removal of the cell may cause to the developing embryo.

Gamete intrafallopian transfer

GIFT offers an alternative treatment to IVF when women have at least one patent tube. It is primarily used in patients who have unexplained subfertility and cervical hostility. It is contraindicated in women with severe endometriosis, active infection and intrauterine abnormalities.

The technique involves ovarian stimulation and harvesting of oocytes as in IVF. The oocytes are then mixed with the freshly donated spermatozoa and transferred into the fimbriated ends of the tube(s) (Figure 7.10). GIFT is normally performed laparoscopically.

Zygote intrafallopian transfer (ZIFT)

The oocytes are fertilised in vitro before transfer to the uterine tube. In this treatment, therefore, fertilisation is known to have occurred and embryos have the opportunity to benefit from the tubal environment and to enter the uterine cavity naturally.

Nursing management and health promotion: IVF

The couple may have experienced many investigations and surgical interventions before being offered the opportunity to seek pregnancy by IVF, and, though always hopeful for success, must recognise that this is not guaranteed.

Pre-laparoscopy care

Reducing anxiety

Pre-treatment counselling provides a realistic picture of the chances of cumulative success rather than encouraging the couple to focus on success of the first cycle (Anderson & Alesi 1997).

The nurse must ensure that couples have appropriate information about the various stages of treatment and procedures to provide reassurance during a highly stressful time.

Self-care in the follicular stage

The woman's role in maintaining self-care can be explained – collecting her urine for laboratory testing, and administering injections at specified times crucial to her ovarian stimulation. The woman should understand that there are

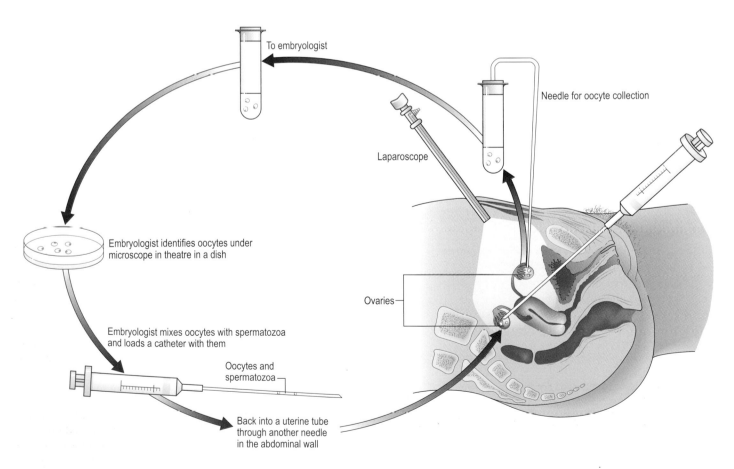

To embryologist

Needle for oocyte collection

Laparoscope

Embryologist identifies oocytes under microscope in theatre in a dish

Ovaries

Embryologist mixes oocytes with spermatozoa and loads a catheter with them

Oocytes and spermatozoa

Back into a uterine tube through another needle in the abdominal wall

Figure 7.10 The GIFT treatment.

differences in need between individual women and the nurse's explanations can alleviate concerns.

Preparation for oocyte recovery

Explanation should be given about USS monitoring of follicular development. Once proposed ovulation has been estimated, preparation should be made for harvesting of oocytes. If this is to be done laparoscopically, the woman will be starved for a minimum of 6 h before general anaesthetic and will be prepared as for any other surgery. However, it can also be done under sedation vaginally with ultrasound guidance.

Post-laparoscopy care

Recovery from the laparoscopy is rapid and the woman will be ready for discharge a few hours after the procedure. Mild analgesics such as paracetamol may be prescribed for relief of pain. The couple will be keen to know whether the laparoscopy was successful and how many oocytes were recovered.

Sometimes the time of ovulation has been misjudged and the follicles have already ruptured prior to laparoscopy or the recovered oocytes are too immature to be viable. Adhesions may obscure the ovarian tissue, thus negating the procedure.

The nurse should adopt a sensitive approach when informing the couple of the outcome of the procedure, particularly if suitable oocytes have not been successfully collected. In this case details of possible re-entry to another treatment cycle may be required by the couple.

Preparation for embryo transfer

As described above, the oocytes are matured in the laboratory for up to 2–3 days. The embryos are observed in the laboratory as they develop to a two- or four-cell stage prior to transfer. Failures may also occur at this delicate laboratory stage and this is a further worrying time for the couple.

Once it is confirmed there are suitable embryos for transfer, the woman attends the unit. In theatre, the woman is positioned in a modified lithotomy (Trendelenburg) position for the procedure of embryo transfer. Following embryo transfer the woman can resume her normal activities.

Continuing need for support and counselling

Nurses working in all settings will be required to utilise their counselling skills with couples who are involved in subfertility treatment. Treatment may not be successful or the resulting pregnancy may result in a miscarriage. Couples may continue to need to talk about their feelings of inadequacy or failure and to be allowed to grieve for their losses.

Some couples may have to accept that they will not have children of their own. Other possibilities such as adoption should be sensitively discussed.

DISORDERS OF THE MALE REPRODUCTIVE ORGANS

This section outlines some common conditions affecting the testes and penis, and sexual dysfunction. The anatomy and physiology of the male reproductive system and disorders affecting the prostate, urethra and urinary function are described in Chapter 8.

Testicular disorders

Undescended testes (cryptorchidism)

PATHOPHYSIOLOGY

This is a condition in which one or both testes have not descended into the scrotum within 12 months of birth. It is a common condition, seen in approximately 1% of boys after their first year, and may be self-correcting or require surgery in the form of orchidopexy. Normal descent keeps the testes cooler in the scrotum and avoids germ cell degeneration caused by the higher temperature in the abdomen, which carries a risk of malignancy. Types of undescended testis are:

- a mobile testis that is normally in the scrotum but can move up and down
- an ectopic testis which does not descend from the inguinal canal into the scrotum
- an undescended testis (possibly abnormal): remains in the abdomen and fails to enter the inguinal canal and pass into the scrotum.

MEDICAL MANAGEMENT

Treatment aims to promote normal testicular function. Treatment should be completed by the boy's second year, before the testis starts functioning. Untreated cryptorchidism results in sterility, since the cells involved in the initial development of sperm cells are destroyed by the higher temperature within the body. The testis may migrate spontaneously, or require an orchidopexy to bring the testis into the scrotum. During orchidopexy the testis is fixed in the scrotum with non-absorbable sutures.

More extensive surgery may be needed with removal of the abnormal testis (orchidectomy) and repair of an inguinal hernia if present. In addition to the risk of infertility, there is also a high risk of malignancy if the testes are left in the abdomen.

Testicular torsion

This is an acutely painful condition caused by the twisting of the testis on its spermatic cord resulting in obstruction to the blood supply. It may occur spontaneously or as the result of strenuous exertion. It commonly occurs in adolescents aged 10–16 years and is uncommon in men over 30 years. This condition is a surgical emergency requiring immediate treatment.

PATHOPHYSIOLOGY

Testicular torsion results when an abnormality of the tunica vaginalis (outer, double membrane around a testis) allows increased mobility of the testis and axial rotation of the spermatic cord above. The resulting ischaemia can lead to cell damage and infection within approximately 6 h.

Common signs and symptoms There will be sudden onset of acute pain in the groin, often radiating to the scrotum and abdomen. The scrotum is swollen and red. Exercise may be the precipitating factor, but the onset of pain can also occur at rest. Nausea and vomiting are common.

MEDICAL MANAGEMENT

The patient may give a history of previous, less severe episodes which resolved spontaneously. Testicular examination may be hampered by the severity of the pain. The affected testis will be elevated, but abnormal mobility may be present in the other testis.

Treatment is by immediate surgery to relieve the torsion and secure testicular fixation. However, if the torsion is detected at an earlier stage, it may be possible by gentle external manipulation to rotate the twisted testis in the appropriate direction. This may immediately resolve the emergency, but the testis should later be surgically secured to prevent recurrence.

 ## Nursing management and health promotion: testicular torsion

The patient will normally be young and fit and his stay in hospital brief. Although the surgery is not considered major, the acute onset of pain and the nature of the problem may cause considerable anxiety and embarrassment. Giving the patient adequate information will help to relieve anxiety and promote recovery. He should be informed that analgesics can be given immediately and that the acute pain will cease once the operation has been performed.

Postoperatively, the patient will have a small inguinal wound and perhaps some scrotal swelling. He will normally be able to return to school or to work in about 2 weeks, at which point he should feel comfortable walking and sitting. Lifting, heavy work and sports involving running, jumping or stretching should be avoided for about 6 weeks. An athletic support should always be worn when sports activities are resumed.

The patient who has received treatment in good time should also be reassured that no impairment to sexual function or fertility will result.

Hydrocele

PATHOPHYSIOLOGY

A hydrocele is a collection of serous fluid in the tunica vaginalis surrounding the testes. It may occur spontaneously or it may be secondary to an inflammatory condition of the testis or epididymis. The hydrocele usually occurs on one side only (although it can be bilateral), is painless, and can swell to a considerable size. It may accompany a condition that causes oedema, such as congestive heart failure or nephrotic syndrome.

Common signs and symptoms Hydrocele is usually asymptomatic, but an increase in scrotal size and associated discomfort will often prompt the man to seek advice. The embarrassment caused by the swelling may be such that the individual curtails social activities, swimming, sunshine holidays and sexual relations.

MEDICAL MANAGEMENT

The presence of fluid within the scrotal sac makes it dull to percussion and provides a red glow on transillumination. As a hydrocele can form around a testicular cancer, the possibility of cancer should be excluded.

Treatment The condition may be reducible by the wearing of a scrotal support, but may require aspiration under local anaesthetic, although patients need to be aware that fluid can reaccumulate. Bleeding and infection are common complications, and recurrence at 6–15 weeks is common.

Varicocele

A varicocele occurs when the veins draining the testes become distended and tortuous. This may cause enlargement of the spermatic cord. Palpation of the scrotum reveals a mass of enlarged varicose veins. Varicoceles are classified as:

- grade 1 – subclinical and detectable only using Doppler ultrasound
- grade 2 – palpable when the patient is standing
- grade 3 – visible scrotal swelling and palpable when lying down.

A persistent varicocele may raise the temperature within the scrotum due to the increased blood supply and contribute to a subfertile state (see p. 228).

MEDICAL MANAGEMENT

The dragging discomfort felt in the scrotum may be relieved by the wearing of a scrotal support. If the condition is more severe, ligation of the veins may be needed. A small length of vein may be removed.

Epididymitis (inflammation of epididymis)

PATHOPHYSIOLOGY

A bacterial infection causes acute inflammation of the epididymis. The microorganisms responsible include *Chlamydia trachomatis* and *Neisseria gonorrhoeae* which are sexually transmitted (see Ch. 35) and *Escherichia coli*; rarely it may be caused by *Mycobacterium tuberculosis*.

Common signs and symptoms The testes are swollen, tender and painful. The man is pyrexial and may complain of general aches and pains. He may experience nausea and vomiting.

MEDICAL MANAGEMENT

It is vital to rule out testicular cancer or torsion of the testes as this requires urgent surgery. Doppler ultrasound can be used to differentiate between epididymitis and testicular torsion.

Treatment This includes:

- bed rest
- extra oral fluids
- analgesia
- antibiotics
- scrotal support or elevation and possibly cold packs applied locally.

Possible complications of epididymitis include:

- abscess development
- chronic epididymitis
- infarction of the testis
- reduced fertility.

Orchitis (inflammation of the testes)

PATHOPHYSIOLOGY

Orchitis is usually caused by a viral infection, especially mumps occurring after puberty.

The complications include atrophy of the testes, and if both testes are affected it can cause reduced fertility.

MEDICAL MANAGEMENT

Orchitis is usually unilateral and the testis is painful and swollen. The inflammation usually resolves without treatment in about 10 days, but men will need the same supportive measures outlined for epididymitis.

Testicular cancer

Testicular cancer is relatively rare (less than 1% of all cancers in the UK), but is the most common cancer in males aged 15–44 years (Cancer Research UK 2009e). It is unusual in prepubertal boys and commonly occurs in the mid-20s. However, testicular cancer should not be thought of only as a 'young-man's' disease; men in their 50s can also develop testicular cancer due to an increased incidence of lymphoma (O'Flynn & Pearce 2005). There were 2065 cases of testicular cancer diagnosed in the UK during 2006, and 58 deaths in 2007 (Cancer Research UK 2009e). However, the mortality from testicular cancer has steadily declined (McCullagh & Lewis 2005).

Testicular cancer is one of the most curable solid tumours. Improvements in survival for men with testicular cancer have been ascribed to effective diagnosis, use of improved tumour markers, changes in surgical procedures and highly effective chemotherapy.

There is a worldwide increase in testicular cancer. This increase is particularly seen in white males in the industrialised countries of Western and Northern Europe (Cancer Research UK 2009e).

PATHOPHYSIOLOGY

The risk factors implicated in the development of testicular cancer include:

- undescended testes
- orchidopexy
- inguinal hernia
- carcinoma in situ (CIS)
- testicular torsion, although trauma has not been proven to cause testicular cancer
- mumps associated orchitis (inflammation of a testis) after puberty
- genetics – Rapley et al (2000) noted that the presence of a newly discovered gene (TGCT1) increases susceptibility to development of certain testicular tumours.

These risk factors are themselves influenced by:

- Age (see above) – different types of tumours occur in different age groups. For example, germ cell tumours are common in the 20–45-year age group and seminomas occur in men aged 35–45 years. Yolk sac tumours have been diagnosed in boys under the age of 10 years, and lymphomas are diagnosed in older men.

- Racial group – white men are more likely to develop testicular cancer than black men. For example, in the USA during the period 2002–2006 the incidence for white men was 6.3 per 100 000, whereas for black men it was 1.3 per 100 000 (National Cancer Institute 2009).
- Genetics – Nicholson & Harland (1995) reported that one third of all testicular cancer patients are genetically predisposed to the disease, possibly related to a homozygous (recessive) inheritance of a single predisposing gene. Around 2–3% of testicular cancers are bilateral, developing either simultaneously or successively.
- Suboptimal androgen – a low level of androgen hormones may be related to the development of testicular cancer (James 2000).

There are several cell types in the testes, any of which may develop one or more tumour types. It is vital to differentiate between these tumour types as their prognosis and treatment differs. Testicular cancers are grouped as:

Germ cell tumours The majority of testicular cancers (95%) develop in the germ cells (McCullagh & Lewis 2005). There are two main types of germ cell tumours (GCTs) in men – seminomas and non-seminomas – but many testicular tumours contain features of both types. The growth, spread and response to treatment of these 'mixed tumours' is such that they are regarded as being non-seminomas.

Invasive testicular germ cell cancers generally start as non-invasive CIS or intratubular germ cell neoplasia.

- **Seminoma** Some 50% germ cell cancers of the testis are seminomas, which develop from the spermatozoa-producing germ cells of the testis. These tumours are classified as either typical (or classic) seminomas or spermatocytic seminomas. The majority of seminomas are typical. Most spermatocytic tumours grow very slowly and usually do not spread (see Ch. 31).
- **Non-seminoma germ cell cancer** These tumours generally occur at an earlier age than seminomas, usually affecting young men in their 20s. Non-seminoma germ cell cancers include embryonal carcinoma, yolk sac carcinoma, choriocarcinoma and teratoma. These tumours may be mixed and involve various cell types, but all non-seminomatous germ cell cancers are treated the same way, i.e. orchidectomy followed by chemotherapy, which means that the exact histological type of this form of testicular cancer is not always important.
  - **Embryonal carcinoma** About 20% of testicular tumours are embryonal tumours. Microscopically these tumours can resemble tissues of very early embryos. This type of non-seminoma tends to be aggressive, increasing the likelihood of metastatic spread.
  - **Yolk sac carcinomas** (also known as endodermal sinus tumours, infantile embryonal carcinoma, or orchidoblastoma). Yolk sac carcinoma is the most common form of testicular cancer in infants and young boys. When these tumours occur in young children, they are often successfully treated, but in adults they are more dangerous, especially if they are 'pure', i.e. they do not contain other types of non-seminoma cells.

– **Choriocarcinoma** This is a very rare and aggressive type of adult testicular cancer. Such cancers are likely to spread rapidly to distant organs of the body.
– **Teratomas** There are three main types: mature teratoma, immature teratoma, and teratoma with malignant transformation. Mature teratomas are benign tumours formed by cells similar to cells of adult tissues. Immature teratomas are cancers that may spread to other organs.

Stromal tumours Cancers occurring in the stroma of the testes (supportive and hormone-producing tissues) are described as gonadal stromal tumours. The cancer can affect the Sertoli cells or the Leydig (interstitial) cells. They are uncommon cancers accounting for 4% of adult testicular cancer and 20% of childhood testicular tumours.

- **Sertoli cell tumours** Sertoli cells support and nourish the spermatozoa-producing germ cells. These tumours are usually benign but once spread occurs they are likely to be resistant to radiotherapy and chemotherapy.
- **Leydig cell tumours** These tumours develop from the normal Leydig cells of the testis. These are the cells that normally produce androgen hormones (such as testosterone). Leydig cell tumours may develop in adults (75% of cases) or children (25% of cases). They frequently produce androgen hormones and sometimes the cancers produce oestrogens (female sex hormones). Most Leydig cell cancers do not metastasise and are cured by orchidectomy, but a small proportion do spread from the testis. Metastatic cancers have a poor prognosis, as they are not very responsive to chemotherapy or radiotherapy.

Secondary testicular cancer can result from, for example, lymphoma, colon and prostate cancers which can metastasise to the testis (Han et al 2000). Among men over 50 years of age, testicular lymphoma is more common than primary testicular tumours, and prognosis depends on the type and stage of lymphoma (see Ch. 11). Treatment, like other forms of testicular cancer, is orchidectomy, supported by radiotherapy and/or chemotherapy.

Other cancers, for example melanoma and those of the lung and kidney, can metastasise to the testes. Prognosis is usually poor because these cancers can metastasise widely to other organs.

Disease progression A summary of disease progression is as follows:

- Rarely there is spontaneous regression.
- GCTs should be considered malignant.
- Lymphatic spread can occur in all types of testicular cancer.
- Local spread from the testis to the epididymis or spermatic cord can occur. This increases the chances of metastasis via the lymph or blood.
- Distant metastasis occurs from either direct blood vessel invasion or cancer cell emboli from lymphatic metastasis.

With the exception of seminoma, the growth rate among germ cell tumours tends to be high.

Staging

The staging of a cancer is needed to determine the extent of spread and inform treatment choices. There are different ways of staging testicular cancer – the number system and the tumour, nodes, metastasis (TNM) classification (see Further reading, e.g. International Union Against Cancer).

Number staging uses four basic stages, but some stages have further classification criteria. The basic stages are:

- Stage 1 – the cancer is confined to the testis.
- Stage 2 – there is spread to pelvic or abdominal lymph nodes. This is subdivided into 2A, 2B or 2C depending on the size of the lymph nodes involved.
- Stage 3 – there is spread to the lymph nodes above the diaphragm or supraclavicular nodes.
- Stage 4 – there is metastatic spread to other organs.

Tumour, nodes, metastasis (TNM) staging This is based on the three criteria: tumour size (T), lymph node involvement (N) and metastasis to distant sites (M). In common with the number system, each of the three TNM criteria has several stages.

- T stage – has five incremental stages ranging from CIS up to spread of the cancer to the scrotum. The T stage is determined after histological examination of the entire testis following orchidectomy.
- N stage – has four stages ranging from no lymph node involvement to the presence of a lymph node >5 cm in diameter. Lymphatic spread occurs via the testicular vessels that drain to the para-aortic (close to the aorta) lymph nodes; computed tomography (CT) scanning can be used to assess lymph node involvement.
- M stage – has three stages ranging from no metastasis up to spread to organs such as the liver. Early venous spread occurs, for example to the liver, lungs and bone, if early embryonic cells (trophoblasts) are present.

In addition, the levels of various tumour markers in the blood are used as a further refinement in staging (see below).

Common signs and symptoms

There is usually a lump or painless swelling in a testis, which is discovered incidentally or during testicular self-examination (TSE) (Box 7.13). Presentation may include:

- a lump, swelling or area of hardness in the testis
- a heavy dragging sensation or dull ache felt in the lower abdomen, anal or scrotal area
- in some men, gynaecomastia (male breast development), inflammation of the testis or back ache/pain (Blandy & Kaisary 2009)
- for around 10% of men pain is the main symptom
- rarely, men present with infertility (Ritchie 1998).

MEDICAL MANAGEMENT

General physical examination is undertaken along with a thorough examination of the testes.

During palpation a 'normal' testis has a smooth consistency, is mobile and is separate from the epididymis. A hard, firm or fixed area within the testis should raise suspicions and should be removed as a matter of urgency.

Investigations include blood assay, ultrasound scan (USS), CT scan and surgical exploration. USS can exclude other testicular problems, e.g. hydrocele or epididymitis (inflammation of the epididymis) and should be used in all men with suspect

Box 7.13 Reflection

Testicular self-examination (TSE) (adapted from Steggall 2003)

Nurses have an important role in providing information about TSE and encouraging men to examine their testes regularly to find abnormalities that could be potential cancers, thereby ensuring diagnosis at an early stage of the cancer and prompt treatment.

Advice for men

It is easiest to examine your testes after a warm bath or shower has relaxed the scrotal tissues.

- Support your scrotum in the palm of one hand. Note the size and weight of your testes. This will help you to detect any changes in the future. It is normal for one testis to hang slightly lower than the other.
- Examine each testis in more detail by rolling it between your fingers and thumb. Press firmly but gently to feel for any lumps, swellings or changes in firmness.
- Do not worry if you find the epididymis, a tube that carries sperm to the penis. This can be felt at the top and back of each testis.

It is a good idea to do TSE about once every month or two. It is also important not to become obsessed with TSE – remember testicular cancer is uncommon. But if you do find anything unusual, don't wait for it to disappear or start throbbing – see your doctor as soon as possible.

Activities

- Locate some resources that promote TSE: leaflets, posters or web-based information.
- Reflect on the resources you located – was the information easily accessible? Were there resources for non-English speakers, or that met the needs of marginalised groups such as men with learning difficulties, homeless men or serving prisoners?

signs/symptoms. A CT scan may be used to identify metastatic spread to lymph nodes and lung, although many patients will undergo chest X-ray to identify metastases.

The tumour markers routinely used are:

- alpha fetoprotein (AFP) – produced by yolk sac cells
- lactate dehydrogenase (LDH) – a marker of tissue destruction
- β human chorionic gonadotrophin (β-hCG) – secreted by yolk-sac cells and trophoblastic cells.

Of patients with non-seminomatous testis tumour, approximately 50–60% will have increased AFP and approximately 30–35% increased β-hCG (Dearnaley et al 2001).

The overall sensitivity of any test or marker will vary with the degree of tumour burden. Determinations of AFP and β-hCG, along with other staging modalities, help to achieve accurate staging of the tumour.

Treatment Treatment modalities are:

- surgery – partial or total orchidectomy
- chemotherapy
- radiotherapy.

The cryopreservation (using extreme cold) of spermatozoa should be discussed as it must be undertaken before surgery, even if the man is expected to have unilateral

orchidectomy, because subsequent chemotherapy or radiotherapy can affect his fertility. The availability of testicular prostheses must also be discussed pre-operatively.

 See website Critical thinking question 7.2

Orchidectomy may be curative in early-stage testicular cancer, but the addition of chemotherapy or radiotherapy is curative in over 95% of men (Cancerbackup 2009).

Further treatment choices will depend on specific tumour histology. Chemotherapy and radiotherapy can be used alone or in combination. Tumours discovered to be benign tumours need no further treatment following orchidectomy.

Usually, the survival of men with GCTs depends on the stage at presentation and therefore the quantity of tumour burden and the efficacy of later treatment choices.

A characteristic of testicular cancers that influences the usefulness of treatment is that they originate from germ cells, which are generally sensitive to radiotherapy and a variety of chemotherapeutic agents.

Despite the speed of disease progress, usually there is a predictable spread pattern that assists in diagnosis, but of significance is that testicular cancer mainly affects young men who are otherwise healthy and can tolerate multimodal treatment (Ritchie 1998).

Decisions about treatment options will be informed by the relative advantages and disadvantages of different regimens. Successful outcomes have been ascribed to combination therapy, but accurate cancer staging and the ability to know that treatment is ineffective by using 'simple' investigations such as USS and AFP/β-hCG, mean that the man's progress can be monitored and new therapy commenced quickly if necessary.

Since more than half the men with testicular tumours already have metastatic disease on presentation, it is usual for other treatment modalities to be used after orchidectomy. Where para-aortic node enlargement remains following chemotherapy, dissection of retroperitoneal lymph nodes may be curative (Brewster 2001). However, this form of treatment may leave the man with erectile dysfunction and ejaculatory disorders.

Post orchidectomy, treatment is determined by tumour histology, risk factors associated with the cancer stage and the prognosis for advanced disease.

Cure rates are exceptionally good for stage 1 and 2 cancer, whatever treatment is used. However, for metastatic disease, survival is dependent on individual clinical factors and treatment choices (Laguna et al 2001).

Chemotherapeutic regimens frequently used in testicular cancer include a combination of bleomycin, etoposide and the platinum-based cisplatin (PEP). The use of these drugs is associated with risks, for example dose-related side-effects with bleomycin, which must be considered against the high cure rate (see Ch. 31). The durations of chemotherapeutic regimens depend on the class of drug prescribed.

Radiotherapy to para-aortic lymph nodes can be used in metastatic seminoma.

▷ Nursing management and health promotion: testicular cancer

All men will have a unilateral orchidectomy, but some will need chemotherapy or radiotherapy depending on the stage of the cancer.

Nurses have an important role in the early diagnostic stages because staging of this cancer can only be made once the testis has been removed. Nurses should anticipate that men will experience major anxieties about their prognosis and recovery that will not be answered until the histology is known. Many men will experience disbelief and find it difficult to absorb and retain information given during consultation. Consequently, nurses should plan time with these men after they have had their histology report explained to them. This allows for clarification and reiteration of points explained by their consultant/doctor. This contact can be within a clinic or by telephone. Nurse/patient conversations are best supported with literature (pamphlets).

Moynihan (1996) suggests that at diagnosis, fear of dying was the most frequently expressed anxiety by men. A nursing care priority is the support of men and their families by providing information and allowing time for them to discuss their uncertainties, anxieties and fears.

Many men now access web-based information on a variety of health problems. This can be overwhelming and confusing, as there is a mix of semi-professional and research literature. The nurse can recommend appropriate and reputable websites that provide more detailed information than pamphlets. The nurse should also explain that whilst statistics summarise populations of men, every case is unique and their treatment and care will also be unique to them. Examples of men's experiences of testicular cancer diagnosis and treatment are available at http://www.checkemlads.com/.

Nursing care comprises several phases which include preoperative preparation, managing pain, prevention of postoperative complications such as wound infection (see Ch. 26), and longer-term aspects including the cancer diagnosis, changes to sexual function and fertility, altered body image and health promotion (by encouraging regular TSE of the unaffected testis, see Box 7.13, p. 235).

Postoperatively, men will need the opportunity to express feelings about having cancer and the treatment, particularly their perception of body image changes. The word cancer still 'strikes fear' so any cancer diagnosis will provoke fears of death, disfigurement and ability. Therefore the man experiences loss attached to the psychological self. Testicular cancer is also coupled to fear of embarrassment because the cancer involves the genitalia and sexual function.

In all definitions of altered body image there is a central/core theme – the impact of change on the body taken in context within the society in which the person lives. Watson (1980) describes elements of the 'self' that may change as the loss of physical self, psychological self and sociocultural self. Blackmore (1989) suggests that testicular cancer and its treatment involve all three 'losses'.

Fear of infertility/change in sexuality may have profound effects on men who have not yet fathered a child or would like more children. Clark et al (2000) contend that men have concerns regarding future health, employment, relationships, sexual activity and fertility. Sexual function can therefore be impaired after treatment; although recovery can occur, it can take time (Van Basten et al 1999).

Surgery will not inevitably lead to reduced sexual function or fertility but there is evidence that points to changes in fertility. Fosså & Kravdal (2000) reported that men with testicular cancer had reduced fertility before and after diagnosis.

Men should understand the importance of attending follow-up appointments aimed at early diagnosis of recurrence or spread of the cancer and prompt reporting if they have signs or symptoms. If further treatment, such as chemo/radiotherapy, is required, the man and his family should be informed of the risks and side-effects. Many men will benefit from the long-term support provided by patient support groups, and information should be provided; some men may need referral to a professional counsellor.

Vasectomy

Couples who have used a range of birth control methods over the years may decide that permanent surgical sterilisation would now be preferable. Vasectomy is one of the most reliable and cost-effective permanent methods of contraception.

Pre-operative counselling

Before such a decision is taken the couple should meet with their GP or family planning counsellor to discuss their needs and circumstances and their reasons for considering permanent sterilisation. The counsellor should provide information about both female and male sterilisation and the risks, side-effects and failure rates of the procedures available. The long-term effects and prospects for reversal of the sterilisation should be explained. The couple should also be encouraged to consider the implications of a breakdown of their marriage or partnership, or the loss by death of one of the couple or of any existing children.

A man contemplating vasectomy may have particular anxieties about the effect of the procedure on his masculinity and sex drive. He must be assured that, as the testes will not be removed, his hormone production, virility and sex drive will be unaffected. The nature of the operation should be described with the aid of a simple diagram. He can be reassured that vasectomy is usually performed under local anaesthetic as a day case and there should be little disruption to his usual routine. Men are advised to avoid strenuous exercise for 48 h. Initially there may be swelling and bruising but this should soon subside. Simple analgesics such as paracetamol are usually sufficient for any mild pain/discomfort experienced. If scrotal swelling increases, pain becomes prolonged or severe, or there is discharge from the site the man should contact his GP or out of hours service.

It should be explained that eventually the ejaculate will contain no spermatozoa and that spermatozoa are still produced but are broken down and reabsorbed. However, it is essential that the man must be aware that:

- Vasectomy may be irreversible.
- There is a small risk of spontaneous late recanalisation of the deferent duct, potentially resulting in unexpected conception.
- Spermatozoa may appear in ejaculate up to 3 months after vasectomy, so alternative barrier contraception must be considered until two semen analyses have shown no spermatozoa.

- If spermatozoa persist in ejaculate, the procedure may need to be redone.
- There is a chance of wound infection and a 1% risk of scrotal pain (Brewster 2001).

Disorders of the penis

Phimosis and paraphimosis

PATHOPHYSIOLOGY

Phimosis refers to a condition where tightness of the prepuce (foreskin) of the penis prevents it being retracted over the glans penis. There may be problems in passing urine. Phimosis may be present at birth, but much more commonly it is associated with repeated balanitis (see below) which leads to scarring.

Paraphimosis occurs when the prepuce can be retracted behind the glans penis but cannot be easily returned. In this situation the circulation to the glans penis is compromised, and there is pain and swelling. This requires urgent treatment as it could lead to gangrene.

Importantly, paraphimosis can occur if the prepuce is not returned after patient/client hygiene or urinary catheterisation (Box 7.14).

MEDICAL MANAGEMENT

It may be possible to reduce a paraphimosis manually under local anaesthetic or light general anaesthesia. However, if this is not successful the man will need an emergency circumcision. An elective circumcision may be necessary for men with phimosis, paraphimosis or recurrent episodes of balanitis. The complications associated with circumcision include bleeding, pain and oedema (Box 7.15). Further information about phimosis, paraphimosis and circumcision is provided in Chapter 8.

Balanitis

The term balanitis refers to inflammation of the glans penis; if the prepuce is also involved it is known as balanoposthitis.

PATHOPHYSIOLOGY

The causes/contributing factors of balanitis include:

- inadequate hygiene
- bacterial infection – including some sexually transmitted infections (STIs), e.g. chlamydia, gonorrhoea

Box 7.14 Information

Preventing paraphimosis (adapted from Steggall 2003)

The prepuce is routinely retracted to allow cleansing of the glans penis, limiting the chance of irritation and infection, but if it is not returned to its normal position during bed bathing or following catheterisation, paraphimosis easily occurs. Nurses must ensure that self-caring patients, health care assistants and other carers are aware of the importance of repositioning the prepuce after retracting it to facilitate washing and drying of the glans penis.

Nurses need to observe for signs of inflammation such as redness or swelling and report any difficulty in repositioning the prepuce.

Box 7.15 Information

Complications of circumcision (adapted from Steggall 2003)

- Pain – requires a local anaesthetic, such as lidocaine-based gel, or systemic analgesia.
- Erection – may require a benzodiazepine to limit the likelihood of erection, e.g. diazepam.
- Oedema – the penis should remain upright; the man should wear close-fitting underwear with a non-absorbent dressing.
- Bleeding – frequent wound checks for blood loss; excessive blood loss may require a return to theatre.
- Wound infection – observation of wound site; nature and colour of any discharge and raised temperature should be considered suspicious and reported immediately.

- fungal infection – candidiasis, which can be associated with diabetes (see Ch. 5)
- allergy
- skin conditions
- phimosis.

Common signs and symptoms There is inflammation with redness, soreness, irritation and sometimes a discharge. Balanitis associated with a STI may be accompanied by dysuria.

MEDICAL MANAGEMENT

It is important to differentiate between balanitis and penile cancer (see below).

Treatment includes advice about hygiene – retracting the foreskin and washing the glans penis at least daily. A swab of any discharge is sent for microscopy, culture and sensitivity and the appropriate antibacterial or antifungal drug is prescribed. If phimosis is a problem it may be that circumcision will be needed. Further investigations should be considered if diabetes, allergy or other skin condition is suspected.

Penile cancer

Penile cancer is an uncommon but devastating tumour for the individual (Rippentrop et al 2004). It is a relatively rare tumour, especially in North America and Europe, but has a higher incidence in African, Asian and South American countries (Mobilio & Ficarra 2001). The increase in incidence in these latter countries is thought to be related to ambient temperature.

In the UK around 400 men are diagnosed with penile cancer each year (Cancer Research UK 2009f).

Prevention of penile cancer

Prevention of penile cancer is achieved through neonatal circumcision or good personal hygiene. Circumcision needs to be performed in early childhood for the benefits of avoiding penile cancer in later life. However, the procedure is not without risks (and costs). Rickwood et al (2000) estimate that £5 million would be released for other purposes if neonatal circumcision was reserved for those who clinically needed the procedure.

Although circumcision is a relatively common operation, there are very few medical indications. The surgery is often performed for cultural/religious reasons or because parents believe that it is more hygienic, will reduce the (already very low) risk of cancer, or avoid the prospect of having to perform the surgery later.

At birth the foreskin normally adheres to the surface of the glans penis. The adhesion spontaneously separates over time, allowing mobility and retraction of the foreskin, therefore circumcision is rarely required unless a phimosis is present. Phimosis is entirely normal in very young boys and is not an indication for circumcision in boys less than 10 years old (Rickwood et al 2000). At 6 years of age approximately 8% of boys have a non-retractile foreskin, whereas at 16 years only 1% have a non-retractile foreskin (Lissauer & Clayden 1997).

The foreskin should never be forcibly retracted; once the foreskin is mobile and retractile, boys should be taught how to clean the foreskin. This will further reduce the chances of developing penile cancer.

PATHOPHYSIOLOGY

Cancer of the penis has been attributed to chronic irritation of the glans penis caused by smegma and to phimosis (see above), which makes washing difficult if the prepuce is not easy to retract.

The incidence of the disease is also thought to be related to cultural/religious practices; circumcision at birth is thought to confer complete immunity from this malignancy (Schoen et al 2000), whereas adult circumcision is thought not to confer any protection.

The incidence of penile cancer is higher where neonatal circumcision is not routinely performed. However, this is not a recommendation that all male babies be circumcised to prevent penile cancer. On the contrary, there are several medical groups in the UK, USA and Australia that offer substantial support for guidelines that recommend that circumcision is *not* performed.

Men who present with penile growths may have high anxiety about the prospect of having a potentially lethal cancer; however, not all growths will be cancerous. Some penile tumours (usually squamous cell carcinoma) are strictly benign, whereas others have the potential to become malignant. Penile cancer is more common in men over 60 years of age, but it can affect younger men.

Most cancers develop on the glans penis or the prepuce. Palpable lymph nodes are found at diagnosis in 58% of men (Ornellas et al 1994).

Risk factors for penile cancer include:

- **Age** – penile cancer is rare below the age of 40 (Brewster 2001).
- **Premalignant lesions** – lesions appearing on the glans penis as chronic painless red or pale patches are premalignant.
- **Prepuce present** – penile cancer is rare in men circumcised at a young age. Chronic irritation with smegma and balanitis in men with inadequate hygiene are contributory.
- **Human papilloma virus (HPV)** – HPV wart infection, especially with types 16, 18 and 21, has been implicated (Brewster 2001). Those men with HPV are more likely to develop cancer of the penis (Cancer Research UK 2009f). Using a sheath contraceptive or limiting sexual partners can reduce the risk of contracting penile cancer.
- **Tobacco use** – Harish & Ravi (1995) found that all forms of tobacco products significantly and independently increased the incidence of penile cancer (as well as lung cancer).

There are several types of penile lesions. However, a key element in determining whether penile cancer is present or not is to determine the normal colours/features of the penis and what are benign lesions. This is usually achieved by referring the man to his GP, urologist or uro-oncology nurse specialist.

Types of lesions include:

- **Benign lesions** – benign tumours include linear, curved or irregular rows of conical or globular excrescences, varying from white to yellow to red, arranged along the coronal sulcus
- **Premalignant skin lesions** – various types, including balanitis xerotica obliterans (BXO), have potential to become malignant lesions (Lynch & Pettaway 2002) (Table 7.1). Premalignant lesions of the glans penis or prepuce spread locally before attacking the corpus cavernosum of the penis and the urethra. There will eventually be spread into the perineum and pelvic cavity. Spread to the inguinal lymph nodes is slow, and distant spread to the liver or lungs via the blood is uncommon.
- **Viral-related lesions** – some penile lesions have been related to the HPV. Other viral-related lesions include classic Kaposi's sarcoma.
- **Squamous cell carcinoma** – squamous cell carcinoma is the most common tumour of the penis (Kroon et al 2004). CIS is called erythroplasia of Queyrat if it involves the glans penis, prepuce or penile shaft, or Bowen's disease if it involves the remainder of the genitalia or perineal region (Lynch & Pettaway 2002). Erythroplasia of Queyrat is identified by a red or velvety lesion on the glans penis, or on the prepuce of the uncircumcised male. The lesion can ulcerate, which causes urethral discharge and pain (Lynch & Pettaway 2002).

Table 7.1 Premalignant lesions of the penis (adapted from Lynch & Pettaway 2002)

TYPE	INCIDENCE	FEATURES
Cutaneous horn	Rare	Usually develops over an existing skin lesion, e.g. wart, naevus, traumatic abrasion or malignancy
Keratotic balanitis	Rare	Hyperkeratotic growths on the glans, with similar features to verrucous carcinoma
Balanitis xerotica obliterans (BXO)	Relatively common	A white patch on the prepuce or glans, involving the urethral meatus
Leukoplakia	Rare	Solitary or white plaques involving the urethral meatus

MEDICAL MANAGEMENT

Investigations and diagnosis Penile cancers often present as a hard painless lump on the glans penis. The lump can be large because it may have been ignored or gone unnoticed, particularly if it is underneath the prepuce. Some lesions bleed, giving rise to potential confusion with haematuria (Brewster 2001). A chronic red or pale patch on the glans warrants further investigation by a urologist.

Usually there is little doubt of the diagnosis of penile lesions, since individuals often delay seeking treatment and the lesions are clearly visible (Blandy & Kaisary 2009). Phimosis, or a tight prepuce, can mask colour changes in the glans penis, although other signs, such as odour, discharge and bleeding may be present and therefore provide an indicator that a lesion exists. Delaying diagnosis allows the tumour to spread into the local lymph nodes, worsening the clinical picture due to metastasis of the tumour.

A biopsy of the affected area will confirm diagnosis and indicate the degree of invasion and spread. Most penile tumours are squamous cell carcinomas and imaging of the inguinal lymph nodes is required to establish the degree of any metastasis, particularly if inguinal lymph nodes are palpable. The man may have a chest X-ray, CT scan and bone scan to detect metastatic spread.

Staging It is important to assess tumour grade, depth of invasion and tumour configuration since these relate to prognosis and subsequent treatment. There is no universally accepted staging of penile cancer, therefore the tumour, nodes, metastasis (TNM) system is most commonly used.

Tumours of the penis are given a grade based on histopathological features:

- GX – grade of differentiation cannot be assessed
- G1 – well differentiated
- G2 – moderately differentiated
- G3–4 – poorly differentiated/undifferentiated.

The grade is used when determining the extent of additional treatment required; growth patterns are particularly useful in determining the 'aggressiveness' of a tumour (Blandy & Kaisary 2009).

Treatment The traditional options for treatment are radiotherapy (which includes external beam radiation, brachytherapy and iridium), chemotherapy (with 5-fluorouracil, cisplatin, etc.) or surgery (Pow-Sang et al 2002). However, therapies such as laser, cryotherapy (intense cold), photodynamic, neoadjuvant and sentinel node mapping are also used in some centres (Singh & Khaitan 2003). Combination therapies are frequently used with some good results, but data required to evaluate treatment regimens are sparse owing to the low incidence of penile cancer (Singh & Khaitan 2003).

Chemotherapeutic agents, e.g. topical 5-fluorouracil, have been used although individuals often also need radiotherapy. Data for chemotherapy are limited, often due to the fact that the tumours are rare.

Radiotherapy may be considered in individuals who are young, with small (2–4 cm), superficial tumours or in patients who refuse surgery, or those men with metastasis who do not wish to undergo a disfiguring penectomy (amputation of the penis).

Normally the man will have a circumcision to reduce further irritation and to quantify the degree of the premalignant or malignant lesions. In some cases, where the cancer is confined to the prepuce, circumcision may be the only treatment needed.

Where tumours are too extensive for radiotherapy alone, a penectomy (partial or total) will be needed. A partial penectomy preserves part of the penis. A total penectomy, however, is radical surgery in which the entire penis is excised along with the scrotum and the creation of a urostomy. Lymph node dissection is required where nodes are involved followed by radio- or chemotherapy, and penile reconstruction.

Reconstructive surgery of the penis, using tissue from the forearm and an implant, is possible once there is confirmation that there is no residual cancer. The forearm site is used because it is comparatively sensitive, has little hair and is well vascularised.

If the tumour has not invaded the lymph nodes, 5-year survival rates are between 65 and 90%; however, if there is metastatic squamous cell carcinoma, 5-year survival rates fall to less than 10% (Ritchie et al 2004).

 ## Nursing management and health promotion: penile cancer

Changes to the colouration of the glans penis may be an incidental finding on urethral catheterisation or during routine teaching of catheter care. Discolouration should be noted and the relevant medical team informed for further advice. As the commonest presentation of penile cancer is as a painless lump, nurses should be aware that even an interview question about men's genitalia and urinary symptoms could lead to an early detection of penile cancer.

Partial or total penectomy will result in a profound change in the man's body image. The man will need time to accept the diagnosis of cancer, its implications in terms of treatment and the long-term changes that will occur in his relationship. The nurse should ensure that the man is in contact with a psychosexual counsellor and the erectile dysfunction team who will help him to cope with issues surrounding body image and sexual function that accompany penectomy. It is vital that this referral occurs as soon as possible in order to reduce the level of anxiety he and his partner will experience.

After a penectomy, men will require time to express feelings and thoughts regarding their diagnosis and treatment, especially their change in body image and sexual function.

Nurses need to be aware of the specific postoperative complications of partial/total penectomy and the nursing actions required. The complications include (Donat et al 2002):

- Haemorrhage – check the wound dressing and bedding for blood loss; regular vital signs observations and colour until stable.
- Infection – assess the wound for signs of infection (e.g. redness, discharge, pain) and record regular temperature measurement; ensure that urinary meatus and catheter are cleaned daily during usual hygiene.
- Oedema – a supportive dressing is used for at least 24 hours; the wound is checked daily for swelling.

Box 7.15, page 237, outlines the complications following circumcision.

Sexual dysfunction

Erectile dysfunction

Erectile dysfunction (ED) is a common male sexual dysfunction with an estimated incidence of 5.8% of men (Mercer et al 2003). ED is the inability to achieve and maintain an erection sufficient for sexual intercourse. ED commonly has profound negative impact on quality of life in the patient (and his partner), resulting in poor self-image and self-confidence, and depression (Fugl-Meyer et al 1997).

PATHOPHYSIOLOGY

The common causes of ED have traditionally been classified as either 'organic' or 'psychogenic'. Organic causes include some antihypertensive drugs, diabetes mellitus with associated acceleration of atherosclerosis, postsurgical intervention (Hendry 1995) or radiotherapy, etc. Psychological or 'psychogenic' causes include change in body image following illness/surgery, relationship difficulty or breakdown, etc. There is growing evidence linking ED and cardiovascular disease (Thompson et al 2005). Risk factors for both diseases include obesity, diabetes mellitus, physical inactivity, hypertension, dyslipidaemia and tobacco use (Ponholzer et al 2005) and ED is now thought to be a harbinger of cardiovascular disease in younger men (<60 years) (Speel et al 2003). The mean time between onset of ED and a cardiac event is approximately 3 years (Montorsi et al 2003) although this becomes longer if risk factors are modified by changing diet and increasing physical activity (Hatzichristou et al 2002). An additional risk factor for development of ED is low or low-normal testosterone, which is also associated with diabetes mellitus and the metabolic syndrome (Maggio & Basaria 2009).

The introduction of phosphodiesterase type-5 inhibitors, particularly sildenafil, encouraged some men to raise their concerns of their sexual function. Recent evidence from Wagner et al (2002) suggests that the majority of men with ED still do not seek advice from their GP. Evidence from Steggall & Gann (2002) indicated the average length of time that men had ED before seeking treatment was 5 years (range 3 months to 28 years), indicating that even those with organic causes to their ED undergo a lengthy period of anxiety and fear of embarrassment. This exacerbates their ED. Most ED is multifactorial with organic and psychological elements often affecting the quality of the man's erection (Ralph & McNicholas 2000). Psychogenic ED is the commonest type in younger men; unfortunately every time the man fails to achieve an erection there is increased anxiety which perpetuates the cycle of failure. ED in middle age and in older men is usually secondary to an organic pathology.

Epidemiology and aetiology Current epidemiological evidence indicates that 8% of men in their 40s report moderate or complete ED and this increases to 40% in men aged 60–69 years (McKinlay 2000). As stated above, the causes of ED had been classified as either organic (i.e. drugs/conditions that influence blood supply and innervation) or psychogenic where 'stress' plays a part. As recently as the 1980s it was thought that psychogenic causes were responsible in as many as 90% of cases of ED. The current view is that blood flow changes are the key factor in ED, particularly changes to penile blood flow.

The exact effects of lifestyle and medical factors on ED still need further clarification. Potential risk factors such as smoking, hypertension, abnormal blood lipids, vascular disease and diabetes mellitus have been proposed given their effects on the cardiovascular system (Table 7.2).

A number of common medical conditions, for example diabetes mellitus and treatment for hypertension, are known to cause ED. Treatment for hypertension lowers blood pressure, therefore making it more difficult to gain an erection. Diabetes mellitus accelerates atherosclerosis, thereby narrowing arteries. Since the corpus cavernosum of the penis is made up of small arteries, these are more likely to become blocked due to atheroma, resulting in ED.

The precise relationship between blood supply and nerve supply is unknown, but an additional key element is that of desire.

MEDICAL MANAGEMENT

Currently, opinion and treatment options focus on improving penile blood flow. Clearly, any medication or medical conditions that affect arterial tone or diameter can affect the strength of the erection. Drugs implicated in the development of ED (Jackson et al 1999) include:

- cardiovascular
  - angiotensin converting enzyme (ACE) inhibitors
  - β-blockers
  - calcium antagonists
  - centrally acting agents, e.g. methyldopa
  - digoxin
  - lipid-lowering drugs
  - thiazide diuretics

Table 7.2 Organic and psychogenic risk factors for erectile dysfunction (adapted from Steggall 2003)

EXAMPLES OF ORGANIC FACTORS	EXAMPLES OF PSYCHOGENIC FACTORS
• Diabetes mellitus	• Stress
• Smoking	• Low mood
• Excessive alcohol consumption	• Anxiety
• Hypertension	• Bereavement
• Antihypertensive and other drugs	• Relationship difficulties
• Post myocardial infarction	• Pressure to perform
• Following urological treatment, e.g. radical prostate surgery	• Fear of failure
• Chronic renal failure	• Iatrogenic
• Renal dialysis and following renal transplant	• Personality
• Neurogenic causes/diseases (e.g. multiple sclerosis, Parkinson's disease)	
• Hypogonadism (with reduced libido)	
• Spinal injury	
• Pelvic injury	

- endocrine
  - antiandrogens
  - luteinising hormone-releasing hormone (LHRH)
  - oestrogens
  - testosterone
- psychoactive
  - anxiolytics, hypnotics
  - selective serotonin reuptake inhibitors (SSRIs)
  - tricyclic antidepressants (TCAs)
- miscellaneous
  - carbamazepine
  - H_2-receptor antagonists
  - metoclopramide
  - all recreational drugs.

Investigations and diagnosis Diagnosis of ED is often determined by the patient himself. The inability to penetrate is frequently the main precipitating factor. However, individuals may also complete one of the erectile function assessment scores (see International Index of Erectile Function (IIEF) – Rosen et al 2002). A thorough organic and psychogenic

assessment is required to determine the type of ED and inform subsequent treatment choices (Table 7.3).

Specific investigations include:

- Blood pressure.
- Hormone profile, e.g. testosterone, luteinising hormone (LH), follicle stimulating hormone (FSH), sex hormone binding globulin (SHBG) and prolactin. If testosterone is 12 nmol/L or less, repeat between 9.00 and 11.00 h; if testosterone remains low, consider referral to an endocrinologist or testosterone supplementation.
- Fasting blood lipids and fasting glucose.
- Prostate specific antigen (PSA) in older men.

Treatment The common treatment options are summarised in Table 7.4. The efficacy can be variable and dependent on frequency of dosing and the strength of the medication.

Successful treatments can be dependent on patient motivation, patient training, the frequency of administration (Heaton et al 2002) and the quality of information giving. However, the estimated efficacy is approximately:

Table 7.3 Assessment for erectile dysfunction (adapted from Steggall 2007)

ASSESSMENT	RATIONALE	IMPLICATION FOR TREATMENT
Surgical history	Clues to organic causes of ED, i.e. damage to nerves or blood supply, or altered body image	Assess blood supply or nerve damage
Medical history	Clues to organic causes of ED, i.e. specifically assessing whether there is known physiological dysfunction	Assess blood or nerve damage
Current medication	Clues to organic causes of ED, i.e. antihypertensives nearly always cause ED	Check for contraindications
Allergies	Interaction with treatment	Interaction with treatment
Tobacco	Assess vascular damage	Give lifestyle advice
Alcohol (or illicit drugs)	Desensitises the individual to stimulation	Potential to effect success of treatment
Specific history		
Description of the problem	Erection failure, loss of desire, or rapid ejaculation, duration of problem	Guides management and treatment
Gradual or sudden onset?	Organic or psychogenic causes?	Gradual suggests an organic causes whereas sudden onset suggests a psychogenic cause
Early morning tumescence	Is the blood supply intact?	May need locally acting medication if blood flow is poor
Libido	Assess desire	Often absent in long-term ED; possible compensatory mechanism
Is penetration possible?	Assess strength of erection	Assesses blood flow; may indicate 'strength' of medication required
Current sexual relationship	Need to know if there is some sexual activity	Absence of intimacy is important – for the medication to work some type of sexual stimulation is required
Psychological factors		
Social problems (particularly prior to onset of problem)	Anxieties inhibit function	Feelings of 'impotence' in other areas will be reflected in sexuality – need to resolve underlying problem
Performance anxiety	Maintains problem	Break cycle of failure/restore confidence
Does the partner know of their visit?	Status of relationship	Address unresolved issues with both partners

Table 7.4 Summary of treatments available for erectile dysfunction (adapted from Steggall 2007)

TREATMENT	DOSAGE GUIDE	CONTRAINDICATIONS	MODE OF ACTION
Sildenafil citrate (Viagra®)	25–100 mg, need 6–10 doses before benefits seen; regular dosing helps to reduce performance anxiety	Concurrent use of nitrates; recent myocardial infarction, unstable angina or stroke; ischaemic optic neuropathy, hypotension; do not use with nicorandil (lowers BP), some antibiotics, and grapefruit juice	Phosphodiesterase type-5 inhibitor, increases blood flow to penis
Tadalafil (Cialis®)	10–20 mg, need 6–10 doses before benefits seen; regular dosing helps to reduce performance anxiety	As above	As above
Vardenafil (Levitra®)	5–20 mg, need 6–10 doses before benefits seen; regular dosing helps to reduce performance anxiety	As above	As above
Medicated Urethral System for Erections (MUSE®): intraurethral alprostadil (prostaglandin E_1)	250–1000 µg Essential to massage the intra-urethral medication for up to 10 minutes	Sickle cell disease, or bleeding disorders	Increases blood flow to penis
Intracavernosal injection of alprostadil (prostaglandin E_1) – Caverject®, Caverject® dual chamber or Viridal Duo®	2.5–60 µg Essential to provide full teaching of injection technique and support/discuss patient anxieties	Warfarin, bleeding disorders	Increases blood flow to penis
Vacuum devices	Important to teach correct technique and reinforce that the vacuum needs to be inflated slowly	None, but must be competent to remember to remove the constriction ring within 30 minutes	Non-pharmacological, drawing blood into the corpus cavernosum under pressure. Blood held in place by constriction band
Surgery (prostheses)	Various prostheses available	Depends on fitness for surgery	Prosthesis – artificial implants replace the corpus cavernosum. Erection then possible 'on demand'
Psychosexual therapy (behavioural programme with counselling of underlying issues)	Weekly or regular attendance with 'homework'	Lack of acceptance, culturally unacceptable	Breaks pattern of failure, removes anxiety and restores confidence

- 70% for phosphodiesterase type-5 inhibitors (there is some variation in efficacy between the phosphodiesterase type-5 inhibitors)
- up to 50% for MUSE®
- 90% for intracavernosal injections
- 90% for vacuum devices.

Nursing management and health promotion: erectile dysfunction

Erectile dysfunction is a common problem for men. There is a strong association between vascular disease and erection failure, and therefore all men with cardiovascular risk factors are at risk of ED. The key to treatment is that of communication; men do not know which words to use to broach the subject, and are therefore hopeful that it will be discussed at some point during their care. An excellent opportunity for raising the profile of ED is simply to have a poster in the waiting/clinical area, with advice to talk to a GP or clinical nurse specialist about the problems. To facilitate conversation, perhaps during a medication review or when giving patients tablets to take away (TTAs), it is useful to make a comment such as 'Some men who are taking blood pressure/diabetic medication, or who have had a recent stay in hospital, can have trouble with their sex lives. If you find that you experience problems, talk to your GP or ask to be referred to a clinical nurse specialist who deals with this problem'.

Priapism

Priapism is a prolonged painful erection, not associated with sexual desire. After 2–3 h, the erection becomes increasingly painful as a result of ischaemia. It is a urological emergency because of irreversible ischaemic damage and corporal fibrosis if left for more than 6 h (Reynard 2001). Detumescence is achieved by aspirating one of the corpora with a butterfly cannula. For further information refer to Reynard (2001).

Ejaculation dysfunction

This section outlines premature ejaculation and retrograde, delayed or absent ejaculation.

Premature ejaculation

Premature ejaculation (PE) is defined as persistent or recurrent ejaculation with minimal stimulation that causes marked interpersonal distress; the estimated prevalence is 22.7% (Porst et al 2007). Premature ejaculation is often attributed to anxiety; ejaculation and orgasm take place too quickly due to poor control during sexual activity although there is a growing consensus that there may be a neurobiological cause to PE (Waldinger 2007). Some studies indicate that the skin of the penis is hypersensitive in men who experience premature ejaculation.

MEDICAL MANAGEMENT

The most widely used definition of rapid ejaculation is that of the *Diagnostic and Statistical Manual – IV* (DSM-IV) criteria for premature ejaculation (American Psychiatric Association 1994):

- **Criterion A** – persistent or recurrent ejaculation with minimal sexual stimulation before, on or shortly after penetration and before the person wishes it. Factors such as age, novelty of the sexual partner or situation and recent frequency of sexual activity must be taken into account.
- **Criterion B** – the disturbance causes a marked distress or interpersonal difficulty.
- **Criterion C** – premature ejaculation is not exclusively the result of the direct effects of a substance (e.g. withdrawal of opiates).

However, contemporary understanding of PE is moving towards a biomedical rather than a psychological causation, which is dependent on ejaculatory latency time (ELT). Based on ELT measures, Waldinger (2007) has proposed a new classification of a PE syndrome rather than a pathology or disease, incorporating the four types of the complaint. These are summarised with suggested interventions below:

- Lifelong PE – neurobiological or genetic cause. Medication is suggested.
- Acquired PE – medical or somatic cause. Psychotherapy is suggested.
- Natural-variable PE – caused by normal variation. Reassurance and psycho-education is suggested.
- Premature-like ejaculatory dysfunction – psychological cause. Psychotherapy.

Recently, the definition of lifelong PE has been the subject of a consensus committee of the International Society for Sexual Medicine (McMahon et al 2008). The consensus agreement is that lifelong PE is characterised by:

- ejaculation which always or nearly always occurs before or within about one minute of vaginal penetration, and
- the inability to delay ejaculation on all or nearly all vaginal penetrations, and
- negative personal consequences, such as distress, bother, frustration and/or the avoidance of sexual intimacy.

The 1 minute intravaginal ELT (IELT) threshold is not in itself an absolute criteria for diagnosis, as approximately 10% of lifelong premature ejaculators have ELTs between 1 and 2 minutes (McMahon et al 2008).

Diagnosis The features considered in a diagnosis of PE are:

- When premature ejaculation started (onset) or how long it has been happening (duration) – has the man always had premature ejaculation (lifelong) or did it start sometime after he became sexually active (acquired)?
- When does it happen – is it a generalised occurrence (in every situation) or situational (occurs in some situations but not in all)?

The normal estimated ELT range is from 6.9 minutes to 13.6 minutes after vaginal penetration.

Treatment The treatment options for PE are behavioural therapies (from Masters & Johnson 1970), which include sensate focus, stop-start and squeeze techniques (Lipsith et al 2003), lidocaine or lidocaine-based creams or sprays, constriction devices that compress the urethra, desensitising bands (Jan Wise & Watson 2000), selective serotonin reuptake inhibitors (SSRIs) (Waldinger et al 2001), atypical antidepressants or tricyclic antidepressants (TCAs). Only behavioural therapy and lidocaine-based sprays are currently approved or licensed for treatment of premature ejaculation.

Behavioural therapies involve solitary and/or mutual masturbation, which can present the participant with particular religious/cultural problems; therefore the behavioural therapy programmes can be unsuccessful. De Amicus et al (1985) reported that 3 months after cessation of treatment only a few of the patients maintained their immediate post-treatment progress. Hawton (1988) reported that 75% of patients with premature ejaculation rated their problem as unresolved at an average of 3 years after treatment.

The use of SSRIs has been extensively reported (Waldinger 2004) to markedly delay ejaculation from baseline levels. However, they do not produce long-term benefit in all men: often the individual returns to pre-treatment ELT levels on cessation of medication. Paroxetine 20 mg daily has been found to be superior in delaying ejaculation compared to other SSRIs (Waldinger 2004).

Gupta (1999) describes a combined model, offering sensate focus assignments and couple work (especially communication), with a medication prescription of SSRIs early in the treatment programme. Currently, the use of SSRIs has been found to delay ejaculation without affecting mood, although with variable efficacy (Waldinger et al 1998).

Delayed, retrograde or absent ejaculation

Delayed ejaculation can be divided into congenital anorgasmia (without orgasm), which may be related to negative behavioural messages about sexual activity (Hendry 1995) and delayed or absent ejaculation due to medication (Wang et al 1996). For example, excess alcohol consumption, some antidepressants (e.g. SSRIs) and recreational drugs can delay ejaculation.

Retrograde ejaculation, where semen is discharged into the bladder, can occur following prostate, bladder or testicular surgery, and is associated with diabetic neuropathy (see Ch. 5).

Treatment for delayed ejaculation includes behavioural therapy and psychotherapy. Alternative strategies include the use of vibro-tactile stimuli to bombard the pudendal nerve increasing the amount of stimulation, which may also allow ejaculation. Irrespective of cause, however, treatment is difficult. If fertility becomes the main issue, alternative methods of semen harvest are possible (see Infertility). Individuals are not always necessarily infertile.

CULTURAL AWARENESS IN REPRODUCTIVE HEALTH

Socioeconomic factors and liberal attitudes to expression of beliefs and values have encouraged people from all over the world to settle in the UK. Whilst this has resulted in vibrant multicultural societies, people moving between cultures will inevitably bring aspects of their own culture with them, including practices and beliefs that shape their approach to their way of life. It is important that nurses are aware of how the attitudes of people from different cultural backgrounds influence their approach to sexuality and reproductive health.

Communication can be a problem if English is not the patient's first language. Although family members may be able to speak English and their mother tongue, it is not appropriate to use them as interpreters. In the past children have often been used when discussing reproductive health issues or intimate problems and it can be intensely embarrassing for the patient to reveal these details to their offspring. In addition, if there are any tensions between a couple, the nurse cannot be sure that all appropriate information is communicated. Consequently accredited interpreters should be used who have an understanding of health and treatments.

Many examinations of a patient's reproductive system involve intimate procedures such as vaginal or testicular examination which can be intensely embarrassing. Often a same-gender health professional will be requested and clinicians should respect these wishes and do their utmost to support these requests. Often, due to pressures on available medical staff, this may not be possible and this should be explained sympathetically to the patient. Staff should also be aware of the effect investigations for subfertility can have on men from different cultures.

Although illegal in the UK, female circumcision and female genital mutilation is widely practised in some groups in Africa and Egypt, in parts of the Middle East and in South East Asia. Health professionals who encounter women who have undergone this must be able to provide appropriate support or refer to other agencies. Often the first time the woman may present is in pregnancy and a care plan must be developed with a consultant obstetrician to ensure safe delivery for both mother and child.

Nurses and other health care professionals must ensure that they adopt an open and non-judgemental attitude towards all patients/clients. They need to make a rapport quickly during relatively brief interactions in order to provide reassurance and support. Whilst this is important for all patients, it is particularly relevant for men and women from different cultural backgrounds. The nurse should have a good awareness of cultural aspects and, whilst they may not have an in-depth knowledge of particular cultural beliefs, they should know what resources they can access when required.

Educating, advising and counselling people who have quite different beliefs, values and attitudes concerning health issues from those of the health professionals providing help and support requires tact and sensitivity. Understanding and empathy can help nurses to appreciate what others consider to be important. A balance is required between giving sound advice and respecting the social, cultural and religious views of others.

SUMMARY: KEY NURSING ISSUES

- Reproductive structures and function are very closely linked to an individual's feelings of self-worth, attractiveness and sexuality.
- Reproductive tract conditions and subsequent examination and investigation can be acutely embarrassing. Embarrassment may cause the individual to delay seeking help.
- People may present in a very emotional state. The nurse must adopt a sensitive and non judgemental attitude at all times. Often the nurse will have to discuss intimate details with the person at the first meeting and so must be able to establish a rapport and trust quickly, thereby ensuring that patients feel comfortable and able to discuss their issues and anxieties.
- The nurse must have a good level of knowledge underpinning their practice so that they are able to give explanations in a way the patient understands but also to provide answers to any queries the patient has. It is unrealistic to expect the nurse to be able to deal fully with all queries but they must know how to access further information and be able to direct the patient to recognised websites providing accurate up-to-date information.
- Privacy and dignity of the patient is particularly key whilst carrying out nursing procedures. Procedures should be conducted in a private area where there will be no interruptions as this will help the patient to relax, reducing the discomfort of any procedures.
- Nursing patients with reproductive system disorders can be challenging but is extremely rewarding, particularly when the nurse has contributed to improving the patient's quality of life.

➡ REFLECTION AND LEARNING – WHAT NEXT?

- **Test** your knowledge by visiting the website 🖱 and answering the multiple choice questions and critical thinking questions.
- **Consolidate** your learning by looking at some of the further reading suggestions, references and specialist websites.
- **Revisit** some of the additional material on the website.
- **Consider** what you have learnt and how this will help your professional development.
- **Reflect** on how you can apply this knowledge to the care of your patients.
- **Discuss** your learning with your mentor/supervisor, lecturer and colleagues.

REFERENCES

Abernethy K: The menopause. In Andrews G, editor: *Women's sexual health*, ed 3, Edinburgh, 2005, Elsevier, pp 451–484.

Adamson GD, Baker VL: Subfertility: causes, treatment and outcome, *Best Pract Res Clin Obstet Gynaecol* 17(2):169–185, 2003.

American Psychiatric Association: *Diagnostic Criteria from DSM-IV*, Washington, DC, 1994, American Psychiatric Association.

Anderson J, Alesi R: Infertility counselling. In Kovacs G, editor: *The Subfertility Handbook*, Cambridge, 1997, Cambridge University Press, pp 90–106.

Andrews G: Premenstrual Syndrome. In Andrews G, editor: *Women's sexual health*, ed 3, Edinburgh, 2005, Elsevier, pp 425–450.

Beral V: Breast cancer and hormone-replacement therapy in the Million Women Study, *Lancet* 362(9382):419–427, 2003.

Beral V, Bull D, Reeves G: Million Women Study Collaborators: Endometrial cancer and hormone-replacement therapy in the Million Women Study, *Lancet* 365:1543–1551, 2005.

Blackmore C: Altered images, *Nurs Times* 85(2):36–39, 1989.

Blake P, Lambert H, Crawford R, editors: *Gynaecological oncology: a guide to clinical management*, ed 2, Oxford, 2008, Oxford University Press.

Blandy J, Kaisary A: *Lecture notes on Urology*, ed 6, Oxford, 2009, Wiley-Blackwell.

Brewster S: Urological oncology. In Brewster S, Cranston D, Noble J, Reynard J, editors: *Urology: a handbook for medical students*, Oxford, 2001, Bios Scientific Publishers Ltd, pp 128–164.

British Heart Foundation: *Coronary Heart Disease Statistics 2008*, 2008. Available online http://www.heartstats.org/temp/2008.Chaptersp1.pdf.

British Menopause Society (BMS): *Managing the Menopause. Hormone replacement therapy*, 2008, BMS Council Consensus Statement. Available online http://www.thebms.org.uk/statementpreview.php?id=1.

Campbell S, Monga A, editors: *Gynaecology by Ten Teachers*, ed 18, London, 2006, Edward Arnold.

Cancer Research UK: *UK Cervical Cancer Statistics*, 2009a. Available online http://info.cancerresearchuk.org/cancerstats/types/cervix/incidence/

Cancer Research UK: *Uterus Cancer survival statistics (updated 2006)*, 2009b. Available online http://info.cancerresearchuk.org/cancerstats/types/uterus/survival/

Cancer Research UK: *UK Ovarian Cancer incidence statistics*, 2009c. Available online http://info.cancerresearchuk.org/cancerstats/types/ovary/incidence/

Cancer Research UK: *Experimental drug may work in many cancers*, 2009d, National Cancer Research Institute Press Release (6th Oct 2009) Available online http://info.cancerresearchuk.org/news/archive/pressreleases/2009/october/parp-inhibitor-drug?utm_campaign=6331596&utm_content=30070606591&utm_medium=email&utm_source=Emailvision_PG#.

Cancer Research UK: *UK Testicular Cancer Statistics*, 2009e. Available online http://info.cancerresearchuk.org/cancerstats/types/testis/

Cancer Research UK: *Penis Cancer*, 2009f. Available online http://info.cancerresearchuk.org/cancerandresearch/cancers/penile/

Cancerbackup: *Treatment for testicular cancer*, 2009. Available online http://www.macmillan.org.uk/Cancerinformation/Cancertypes/Testes/Treatingtesticularcancer/treatingtesticularcancer.aspx.

Cirillo DJ, Wallace RB, Rodabough RJ, et al: Effect of estrogen therapy on gallbladder disease, *J Am Med Assoc* 293(3):330–339, 2005.

Clark A, Jones P, Newbold S, et al: Practice development in cancer care: self-help for men with testicular cancer, *Nurs Stand* 14(5):41–46, 2000.

Clark TJ, Gupta JK: *Handbook of Outpatient Hysteroscopy*, London, 2005, Hodder.

Cotton J: Nursing patients with sexual health and reproductive problems. In Brooker C, Nicol M, editors: *Nursing Adults: The practice of caring*, Edinburgh, 2003, Mosby, pp 738–739.

De Amicus LA, Goldberg DC, LoPiccolo J, et al: Clinical follow-up of couples treated for sexual dysfunction, *Arch Sex Behav* 14:467–490, 1985.

Dearnaley DP, Huddart RA, Horwich A: Managing testicular cancer, *Br Med J* 332(7302):1583–1588, 2001.

Department of Health (DH): *Human Fertilisation and Embryology Act 1990*, 1990. Available online http://www.opsi.gov.uk/acts/acts1990/Ukpga_19900037_en_1.

Department of Health (DH): *The NHS Cancer Plan: a plan for investment a plan for reform*, 2000. Available online http://www.dh.gov.uk/en/Publicationsandstatistics/Publications/PublicationsPolicyAndGuidance/Browsable/DH_4098139.

Department of Health (DH): *Human Fertilisation and Embryology Act 2008*, 2008. Available online http://www.dh.gov.uk/en/Publicationsandstatistics/Legislation/Actsandbills/DH_080211.

Donat SM, Cozzi PJ, Herr HW: Surgery of penile and urethral carcinoma. In Walsh PC, Reyik AB, Vaughan ED, Wein AJ, editors: *Campbell's Urology*, ed 8, Philadelphia, 2002, W B Saunders, pp 2983–2999.

Easton DF, Ford D, Bishop DT: Breast and ovarian cancer incidence in BRCA1-mutation carriers, *Am J Hum Genet* 56(1):265–271, 1995.

Fosså SD, Kravdal Ø: Fertility in Norwegian testicular cancer patients, *Br J Cancer* 82:737–741, 2000.

Fugl-Meyer AR, Lodnert G, Branholm IB, et al: On life satisfaction in male erectile dysfunction, *Int J Impot Res* 9:141–148, 1997.

Gupta M: An alternative combined approach to the treatment of premature ejaculation in Asian men, *Sexual and Marital Therapy* 14(1):71–76, 1999.

Han M, Kronz JD, Schoenberg MP: Testicular metastasis of transitional cell carcinoma of the prostate, *J Urol* 164(6):2026, 2000.

Harish K, Ravi R: The role of tobacco in penile carcinoma, *Br J Urol* 75:375–377, 1995.

Hatzichristou D, Hatzimouratidis K, Bekas M, et al: Diagnostic steps in the evaluation of patients with erectile dysfunction, *J Urol* 168:615–620, 2002.

Hawton K: Erectile dysfunction and premature ejaculation, *Br J Hosp Med* 40:428–436, 1988.

Heaton JP, Dean J, Sleep DJ: Rapid communication: Sequential administration enhances the effect of apomorphine SL in men with erectile dysfunction, *Int J Impot Res* 14(1):61–64, 2002.

Hendry WF: Iatrogenic damage to male reproductive function, *J R Soc Med* 88(10):579–584, 1995.

Human Fertilisation and Embryology Authority (HFEA): *Code of practice*, ed 8. Available online http://www.hfea.gov.uk/

Hydatidiform Mole and Choriocarcinoma UK Information and Support Service. Charing Cross Hospital Trophoblast Disease Service: 2009. Available online http://www.hmole-chorio.org.uk/index.html.

Iammarrone E, Balet R, Lower AM, et al: Male infertility, *Best Pract Res Clin Obstet Gynaecol* 17(2):211–229, 2003.

International Federation of Gynecology and Obstetrics (FIGO): Benedet JL, editor: *Staging Classifications and Clinical Practice Guidelines for Gynaecological Cancers*, 2006. Available online http://www.figo.org/

Jackson G, Betteridge J, Dean J, et al: A systemic approach to erectile dysfunction in the cardiovascular patient: a consensus statement, *Int J Clin Pract* 53(6):445–451, 1999.

James WH: A possible cause of testicular cancer, *Br J Cancer* 82(12):2022–2023, 2000.

Jan Wise ME, Watson JP: A new treatment for premature ejaculation: case series for a desensitising band, *Sexual and Relationship Therapy* 15(4):345–350, 2000.

Jefferies H: Ovarian cancer patients: are their informational and emotional needs being met? *J Clin Nurs* 11(1):41–47, 2002.

Jefferies H: Cervical Cancer Part 1: An overview of screening and diagnosis, *Nurs Times* 104(44):26–27, 2008.

Kroon BK, Horenblas S, Nieweg OE: Contemporary management of penile squamous cell carcinoma, *J Surg Oncol* 89(1):43–50, 2004.

Laguna MP, Pizzocaro G, Klepp O, et al: EAU Guidelines of Testicular Cancer, *Eur Urol* 40(2):102–110, 2001.

Lewis G, editor: *The Confidential Enquiry into Maternal and Child Health. Saving Mothers' Lives: Reviewing maternal deaths to make motherhood safer – 2003–05*, Seventh Report of the Confidential Enquiries into Maternal Deaths in the United Kingdom, 2007. Available online http://www.cmace.org.uk/

Lipsith J, McCann D, Goldmeier D: Male psychogenic sexual dysfunction: the role of masturbation, *Sexual and Relationship Therapy* 18(4):447–471, 2003.

Lissauer T, Clayden G: Abnormalities of the penis. In *Illustrated Textbook of Paediatrics*, London, 1997, Mosby, p 211.

Lynch DF, Pettaway CA: Tumours of the Penis. In Walsh PC, Reyik AB, Vaughan ED, Wein AJ, editors: *Campbell's Urology*, ed 8, Philadephia, 2002, W B Saunders, pp 2945–2981.

Maggio M, Basaria S: Welcoming low testosterone as a cardiovascular risk factor, *Int J Impot Res* 21:216–224, 2009.

Mahutte NG, Arici A: New advances in the understanding of endometriosis related infertility, *J Reprod Immunol* 55(1–2):73–83, 2002.

Masters WH, Johnson VE: *Human Sexual Inadequacy*, Boston, MA, 1970, Little Brown.

McCullagh J, Lewis G: Testicular cancer: epidemiology, assessment and management, *Nurs Stand* 19(25):45–53, 2005.

McKinlay JB: The worldwide prevalence and epidemiology of erectile dysfunction, *Int J Impot Res* 12(Suppl 4):S6–S11, 2000.

McMahon CG, Althof S, Waldinger MD, et al: An evidence-based definition of lifelong premature ejaculation: report of the International Society for Sexual Medicine Ad Hoc Committee for the Definition of Premature Ejaculation, *British Journal of Urology International* 102:338–350, 2008.

Medicines and Healthcare products Regulatory Agency (MHRA): *Drug Safety Update* 1(2):2–4, 2007.

Mercer CH, Fenton KA, Johnson AM, et al: Sexual functioning problems and help seeking behaviour in Britain: National probability sample survey, *Br Med J* 327:426–427, 2003.

Mobilio G, Ficarra V: Genital treatment of penile carcinoma, *Current Opinions in Urology* 11:299–304, 2001.

Montorsi F, Briganti A, Salonia A, et al: Erectile dysfunction prevalence, time of onset and association with risk factors in 300 consecutive patients with acute chest pain and angiography documented coronary artery disease, *Eur Urol* 44:360–365, 2003.

Moynihan C: Psychosocial assessments and counseling of the patient with testicular cancer. In Horwich A, editor: *Testicular cancer*, ed 2, London, 1996, Chapman and Hall Medical.

Naftolin F, Stanbury MG: Phytoestrogens: are they really oestrogen mimics? *Fertil Steril* 77(1):15–17, 2002.

National Cancer Institute: *Surveillance Epidemiology and End Results (SEER) Stat Fact Sheet – Testis*, 2009. Available online http://seer.cancer.gov/statfacts/html/testis.html.

National Institute for Health and Clinical Excellence (NICE): *Guidance on the use of liquid-based cytology for cervical screening*, Technology Appraisal TA 69, 2003. Available online www.nice.org.uk/nicemedia/pdf/TA69_LBC_review_FullGuidance.pdf.

National Institute for Health and Clinical Excellence (NICE): *Uterine artery embolisation for the treatment of fibroids*, Interventional Procedure Guidance 94, 2004. Available online www.nice.org.uk/nicemedia/pdf/ip/IPG094guidance.pdf.

National Institute for Health and Clinical Excellence (NICE): *Alendronate, etidronate, risedronate, raloxifene and strontium ranelate for the primary prevention of osteoporotic fragility fractures in postmenopausal women*, Technology Appraisal TA 160, 2008. Available online www.nice.org.uk/nicemedia/pdf/TA160.

NHS Cervical Screening Programme: *Cancer screening programmes*, 2008. Available online http://www.cancerscreening.nhs.uk/cervical/index.html.

Nicholson PW, Harland SJ: Inheritance and testicular cancer, *Br J Cancer* 71(2):421–426, 1995.

Nursing and Midwifery Council (NMC): *The Code: Standards of conduct, performance and ethics for nurses and midwives*, 2008 (Modified 2009). Available online http://www.nmc-uk.org/.

O'Flynn KJ, Pearce I: Testicular tumours, *Trends in Urology Gynaecology and Sexual Health* 10:20–23, 2005.

Ornellas AA, Seixas AL, Marota A, et al: Surgical treatment of invasive squamous cell carcinoma of the penis: retrospective analysis of 350 cases, *J Urol* 149:492–497, 1994.

Pandian Z, Bhattacharya S, Vale L, Templeton A: In vitro fertilisation for unexplained subfertility, *Cochrane Database Syst Rev* (2):CD003357, 2005.

Ponholzer A, Temmi C, Mock K, et al: Prevalence and risk factors for erectile dysfunction in 2869 men using a validated questionnaire, *Eur Urol* 47:80–86, 2005.

Porst H, Montorsi F, Rosen R, et al: The Premature Ejaculation Prevalence and Attitudes (PEPA) survey: prevalence, co-morbidities, and professional help-seeking, *Eur Urol* 51(3):816–824, 2007.

Porter M, Penney G, Russell D, et al: A population based survey of women's experience of menopause, *Br J Obstet Gynaecol* 103:1025–1028, 1996.

Pow-Sang MR, Benavente V, Pow-Sang JE, et al: Cancer of the penis, *Cancer Control* 9(4):305–314, 2002.

Proctor M, Farquhar C: Diagnosis and management of dysmenorrhoea, *Br Med J* 332(7550):1134–1138, 2006.

Ralph D, McNicholas T: UK Management guidelines for erectile dysfunction, *Br Med J* 321:499–503, 2000.

Rapley EA, Crockford GP, Teare D, et al: Localisation to Xq27 of a susceptibility gene for testicular germ-cell tumours, *Nat Genet* 24:197–200, 2000.

Rees M, Stevenson J: *Primary prevention of coronary heart disease in women*, 2007, British Menopause Society Council Consensus Statement. Available online http://www.thebms.org.uk/.

Reynard J: Urological emergencies and trauma. In Brewster S, Cranston D, Noble J, Reynard J, *Urology: a handbook for medical students*, Oxford, 2001, Bios Scientific Publishers Ltd, pp 15–34.

Rickwood AM, Kenny SE, Donnell SC. Towards evidence based circumcision of English boys: survey of trends in practice, *Br Med J* 321:792–793, 2000.

Rippentrop JM, Joslyn SA, Konety BR: Squamous cell carcinoma of the penis, *Cancer* 101(6):1357–1363, 2004.

Ritchie AW, Foster PW, Fowler S: Penile cancer in the UK: clinical presentation and outcome in 1998/99, *British Journal of Urology International* 94(9):1248, 2004.

Ritchie JP: Neoplasms of the Testis. In Walsh PC, Retik AB, Darracott Vaughan E, Wein AJ, editors: *Campbell's Urology*, ed 7, Philadelphia, 1998, W B Saunders, pp 2411–2452.

Rosen RC, Cappelleri JC, Gendrano N: The International Index of Erectile Function (IIEF): a state of the science review, *Int J Impot Res* 14(4):226–244, 2002.

Rossouw JE, Anderson GL, Prentice RL, et al: Risks and benefits of estrogen plus progestin in healthy post-menopausal women; principal results from the Women's Health Initiative randomised controlled trial, *J Am Med Assoc* 288(3):321–333, 2002.

Royal College of Obstetricians and Gynaecologists (RCOG): *Green-top Guideline 22 Anti-D Immunoglobulin Rh Prophylaxis*, 2002. Available online http://www.rcog.org.uk/womens-health/clinical-guidance/use-anti-d-immunoglobulin-rh-prophylaxis-green-top-22.

Royal College of Obstetricians and Gynaecologists (RCOG): *Green-top Guideline No 17 The Investigation and Treatment of Couples with Recurrent Miscarriage*, 2003. Available online http://www.rcog.org.uk/files/rcog-corp/uploaded-files/GT17RecurrentMiscarriage2003.pdf.

Royal College of Obstetricians and Gynaecologists (RCOG): *Green-top Guideline No 25 The Management of Early Pregnancy Loss*, 2006. Available online http://www.rcog.org.uk/files/rcog-corp/uploaded-files/GT25ManagementofEarlyPregnancyLoss2006.pdf.

Schoen EJ, Oehrli M, Colby CJ, Machin G: The highly protective effect of newborn circumcision against invasive penile cancer, *Pediatrics* 105(3):36–40, 2000.

Singh I, Khaitan A: Current trends in the management of carcinoma of the penis – a review, *Int Urol Nephrol* 35(2):215–225, 2003.

Speel TG, van Langen H, Meuleman EJ: The risk of coronary heart disease in men with erectile dysfunction, *Eur Urol* 44:366–370, 2003.

Steggall MJ: Nursing patients with sexual health and reproductive problems. In Brooker C, Nicol M, editors: *Nursing Adults The practice of caring*, Edinburgh, 2003, Mosby, pp 749, 752–753.

Steggall MJ: Erectile dysfunction: physiology, causes and patient management, *Nurs Stand* 21(43):49–56, 2007.

Steggall MJ, Gann SY: Assessing patients with actual or potential erectile dysfunction, *Prof Nurse* 18(3):155–159, 2002.

Thompson IM, Tangen CM, Goodman PJ, et al: Erectile Dysfunction and Subsequent Cardiovascular Disease, *JAMA* 294(23):2996–3002, 2005.

Van Basten JP, Ven Driel MF, Hoekstra HJ, et al: Objective and subjective effects of treatment for testicular cancer on sexual function, *British Journal of Urology International* 84(6):671–678, 1999.

Vercellini P, Frontino G, De Giorgi O, et al: Comparison of a levonorgestrel-releasing intrauterine device versus expectant management after conservative surgery for symptomatic endometriosis: a pilot study, *Fertil Steril* 80(2):305–309, 2003.

Wagner G, Claes H, Costa P, et al: The Lyon Arms Group: A shared care approach to the management of erectile dysfunction in the community, *Int J Impot Res* 14:189–194, 2002.

Walboomers JM, Jacobs MV, Manos MM, et al: Human papillomavirus is a necessary cause of invasive cervical cancer worldwide, *J Pathol* 189(1):12–19, 1999.

Waldinger MD: Lifelong premature ejaculation: from authority-based to evidence-based medicine, *British Journal of Urology International* 93:201–207, 2004.

Waldinger MD: Evolution of the understanding of premature ejaculation: historical perspectives, *Eur Urol* (Suppl 6):762–767, 2007.

Waldinger MD, Hengeveld MW, Zwinderman AH, Olivier B: Effect of SSRI antidepressants on ejaculation: a double-blind, randomised, placebo-controlled study with fluoxetine, fluvoxamine, paroxetine, and sertraline, *J Clin Psychopharmacol* 18(4):274–281, 1998.

Waldinger MD, Zwinderman AH, Aeilko H, Olivier B: Antidepressants and ejaculation: a double-blind, randomized, placebo-controlled, fixed-dose study with paroxetine, sertraline, and nefazodone, *J Clin Psychopharmacol* 21(3):293–297, 2001.

Wang R, Monga M, Hellstrom WJ: Ejaculatory dysfunction. In Comhaire FH, editor: *Male Infertility: Clinical Investigation, Cause Evaluation and Treatment*, London, 1996, Chapman Hall, pp 205–221.

Watson J: In Brown MS, editor: *Nursing and the concept of Loss*, New York, 1980, John Wiley and Sons.

Waugh A, Grant A: *Ross and Wilson Anatomy and Physiology*, ed 10, Edinburgh, 2006, Churchill Livingstone.

Women's Health Initiative Steering Committee: Effects of conjugated equine estrogen in postmenopausal women with hysterectomy: the Women's Health Initiative randomised controlled trial, *J Am Med Assoc* 291(14):1701–1712, 2004.

World Health Organization: *Assessment of fracture risk and its application to screening for postmenopausal osteoporosis*, 1994. Available online http://whqlibdoc.who.int/trs/WHO_TRS_843.pdf.

FURTHER READING

Andrews G, editor: *Women's sexual health*, ed 3, Edinburgh, 2005, Elsevier.

Collins S, Arulkumaran S, Hayes K, et al, editors: *Oxford Handbook of Obstetrics and Gynaecology*, ed 2, Oxford, 2008, Oxford University Press.

Dunleavey R: *Cervical Cancer: A Guide for Nurses*, Oxford, 2008, Wiley-Blackwell.

Gupta S, Holloway D, Kubba A: *Oxford Handbook of Women's Health Nursing*, Oxford, 2009, Oxford University Press.

Hughes C: Cervical cancer: prevention, diagnosis, treatment and nursing care, *Nurs Stand* 23(27):48–56, 2009.

International Union Against Cancer (UICC): *TNM Classification of Malignant Tumours*, ed 7, 2009. Available online http://www.uicc.org/

Royal College of Nursing (RCN): *Gynaecological cancer. Guidance for nursing staff*, 2005. Available online http://www.rcn.org.uk/__data/assets/pdf_file/0007/78649/002518.pdf.

Royal College of Nursing (RCN): *Competences: an integrated career and competence framework for nurses and health care support workers working in the field of menopause*, London, 2009, RCN.

Royal College of Obstetricians and Gynaecologists (RCOG): *Patient information. About abortion care: what you need to know*, 2004. Available online http://www.rcog.org.uk/womens-health/clinical-guidance/about-abortion-care-what-you-need-know.

Wein A, Kavoussi L, Norvick A, et al, editors: *Campbell-Walsh Urology*, ed 9, Philadelphia, 2007, Saunders.

USEFUL WEBSITES

British Menopause Society: www.thebms.org.uk/index.php

Brook Advisory Services: www.brook.org.uk

Cancer Counselling Trust: www.cancercounselling.org.uk

Cancer Research UK: http://info.cancerresearchuk.org

Cancerbackup/Macmillan: www.cancerbackup.org.uk

FPA (putting sexual health on the agenda): www.fpa.org.uk/Homepage

Human Fertilisation and Embryology Authority (HFEA): www.hfea.gov.uk

Miscarriage Association: www.miscarriageassociation.org.uk

NHS choices Your health, your choices: www.nhs.uk

Orchid (Fighting male cancer): www.orchid-cancer.org.uk

Royal College of Obstetricians and Gynaecologists: www.rcog.org.uk

Sexual Dysfunction Association: www.sda.uk.net

Women's Health Concern: www.womens-health-concern.org

Introduction

Breasts (mammary glands) fulfil different functions and mean different things to a woman throughout her lifetime. Physiologically they are organs of lactation, developing in puberty to enable a mother to feed her offspring, but in psychological and social terms they symbolise femininity and sexuality. Images of females with perfectly formed breasts are often used in the media as symbols of sexual desirability, promoting an idealistic beauty which few women can attain. It is not surprising therefore that breast disease often has profound implications, not only for a woman's physical health but also for her social and familial roles, body image and self-confidence. Women who suffer any alteration or disfigurement to their breasts often experience anxiety, depression and loss of sexual satisfaction.

This chapter outlines the anatomy and physiology of the breast before considering benign disorders of the breast, such as mammary dysplasia, fibroadenomas, mastalgia, breast infections and the rare condition of gynaecomastia that affects men.

Breast cancer and its detection and treatment are covered in detail as breast cancer is the most common cancer in the UK (Cancer Research UK 2009a) (see Figure 31.2, p. 794). Related issues including breast reconstruction and the presence of cancer genes in some families who are at high risk for breast cancer are discussed in the chapter, with further information provided on the companion website.

The chapter discusses the vital role of the nurse in promoting breast health and the early detection of disease. The importance of involving the woman and her family in making informed treatment choices and in carrying out subsequent self-care is stressed. The significance of breast disease for a woman's psychological well-being is discussed.

Anatomy and physiology

Structure of the breast

The breast comprises glandular, fatty and fibrous tissue which is covered by skin. Men and women both have breast tissue, but normally in the male it remains rudimentary and, unlike the female breast, does not develop in puberty.

Medially, the breasts reach the sternal edge and laterally the mid-axillary line and extend up into the axilla forming the triangular shaped axillary tail. The breast lies on a thick layer of fascia, underneath which are the pectoralis major and the serratus anterior muscles. Behind the pectoralis major is the pectoralis minor muscle. Its function is to stabilise the shoulder girdle, serratus anterior and the latissimus dorsi muscles from the base and back of the axilla respectively. These structures and their nerve supply are important considerations when axillary lymph node surgery is required for the treatment of breast cancer (Figure 7.11).

The nipple and areolar complex are situated centrally but actual positioning varies with the size of the breast. The nipple can project above the areolar skin and is constructed of smooth muscle. This becomes erect when stimulated, allowing the baby to suckle more easily during breast feeding. The pigmented skin of the areola has a number of small protuberances (Montgomery's tubercles), which lubricate the areolar skin during breast feeding.

The glandular tissue of the breast is divided into 12–20 lobes or segments (Figure 7.12). Each segment is made up of hundreds of lobules or alveoli which are activated during pregnancy to produce milk. They are connected by terminal ducts which join to form lactiferous ducts before ending in approximately 10 openings in the nipple. These tree-like structures are lined with ductal and alveolar (lobular) epithelium and are surrounded by contractile myoepithelial

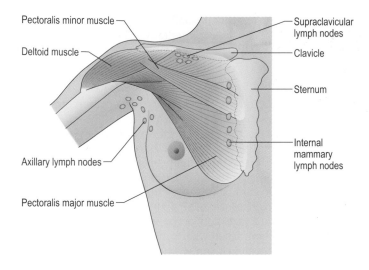

Figure 7.11 The breast and associated structures.

cells. These cells contract in response to the hormone oxytocin to facilitate the ejection of milk during breast feeding.

Breast tissue is supported by Cooper's ligaments, fibrous bands which connect the skin of the breast to the underlying fascia. These ligaments may contract when affected by cancer, causing dimpling of the skin (peau d'orange). With increasing age and weight, these ligaments stretch, causing the breasts to droop.

Blood and lymph vessels

The breast is highly vascularised. It receives arterial blood from the thoracic branches of the axillary artery, branches of the internal mammary artery (from the subclavian artery) and branches from the internal thoracic artery.

Venous drainage is from the subareolar complex draining to the intercostal, axillary and internal thoracic veins.

The lymphatic drainage is of great significance in the potential spread of breast cancer. Most lymph drainage of the breast comes from the breast parenchyma and the subareolar region which then drains to the axillary lymph nodes. Further drainage occurs in the subcapsular and interpectoral node groups. Drainage from the medial part of the breast is via the internal mammary nodes which lie beneath the ribs and lateral to the sternum.

Nerve supply

Most of the breast innervation is via the sensory and autonomic nerves accompanying the blood vessels. Branches of three thoracic nerves containing sympathetic fibres innervate the breast parenchyma. The area around the nipple has many sensory nerve endings. When touched, these cause reflex erection and, during breast feeding, milk release.

Normal breast changes

Natural changes occur at puberty, during the menstrual cycle, pregnancy and lactation and with normal ageing and the climacteric.

Puberty

Breast development begins at puberty. Under the control of the hypothalamus the pituitary gland produces the gonadotrophins, FSH and LH. These hormones stimulate ovarian follicles and the release of oestrogens, which in turn cause the increase in the breast connective tissue, a lengthening of the ducts in the breast and the formation of the breast lobules. Complete development of the lobules is achieved only with adult levels of progesterone.

Menstrual cycle

At the start of each menstrual cycle, rising oestrogen levels cause breast ducts and lobules to enlarge. After ovulation,

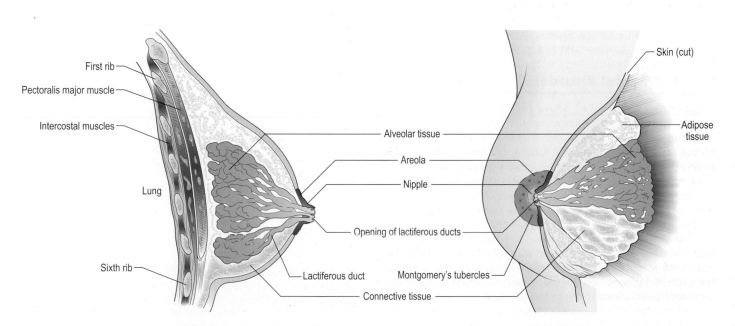

Figure 7.12 Lateral cross-section of the breast.

the corpus luteum produces progesterone which causes further breast changes. At this time, some women experience breast tenderness and heaviness. If pregnancy does not occur, hormone levels fall, ducts and lobules regress, and the breasts lose their tenderness and swollen feeling. This usually precedes the onset of menstruation.

Pregnancy

If pregnancy does occur, the levels of oestrogen and progesterone continue to rise, causing the ducts and lobules to increase in size and number in preparation for lactation. The enzymes necessary for milk production are stimulated by prolactin (see Ch. 5) and by placental lactogen, but milk production is suppressed during pregnancy by high progesterone levels. Further information about lactation is provided on the companion website.

 See website for further content

Climacteric

As a woman approaches the menopause (last menstruation), changes in ovarian function and a subsequent drop in hormone levels cause breast glandular epithelium and adjacent connective tissue to regress and be replaced by fat. This process of involution causes the breasts to become softer and less lumpy. Consequently, the breasts are easier to examine and assess by mammography (X-ray of the breast).

Benign breast disorders

Benign breast disorders account for approximately 90% of all breast problems. The most prominent group of benign disorders results from 'anomalies of normal development and involution' (ANDI). The largest group of ANDI disorders is developmental and can occur before birth, and during pre-pubertal and pubertal breast development. Aberrations of involution or changes in the structure of breast tissue can occur during the perimenopause and menopausally. Other ANDI disorders include benign mammary dysplasia and papillomas. Other benign breast disorders covered in this section include breast pain and breast infection.

Developmental disorders

It is estimated that about 1% of men and 5% of women are born with one or more extra nipples (polythelia). The most common site for the location of extra nipples is along the milk line or the ectodermal ridge. Extra breasts can also develop and mostly occur in the lower axilla.

Abnormalities of breast development include the absence (amastia) or underdevelopment (hypoplasia) of one breast.

There is usually some difference in breast size for a woman, the left breast being larger than the right, but the difference should not be extreme. If it is, then surgical intervention involving augmentation of one breast and reduction of the other breast can be offered by many plastic surgeons.

Pre-pubertal breast enlargement is quite common and only requires investigation if it is associated with other signs of premature sexual development. Otherwise known as juvenile hypertrophy, the overgrowth of breast tissue can occur in adolescent girls whose breasts develop normally during puberty

but then continue to grow. Usually, no hormone abnormality can be detected. Treatment is usually a reduction mammoplasty (removal of tissue from each breast).

Fibroadenomas

A fibroadenoma can be considered as an aberration of normal breast tissue growth. It usually presents as a dense mass comprising both fibrous and glandular breast tissue. It grows as a centrifugal nodule that is usually well circumscribed and freely movable within the surrounding breast tissue. Fibroadenomas are very common (13% of all palpable breast lesions), and in women aged 20 years or less, they account for 60% of breast masses (Dixon & Thomas 2006) (Box 7.16). Juvenile or giant fibroadenomas are rare and occur in adolescence. They are often a fast-growing lesion that can grow up to 5 cm in size and will distort the breast. For women who present with a presumed fibroadenoma a biopsy will be performed to confirm the diagnosis and to discount breast cancer.

 See website Figure 7.1

Aberrations of involution

A variety of benign breast disorders occur during normal involution.

Sclerosis

Aberrations of stromal involution include the development of localised areas of excessive fibrosis or sclerosis of the breast tissue.

Cysts and nodularity

Diffuse lumpiness or thickening of breast tissue occurs, which may contain single or multiple cysts. Commonly, it is bilateral, although it may affect a single breast. Premenstrual tenderness is often experienced coinciding with an increase in nodularity. Cysts are distended, fluid-filled lobules and usually develop around the perimenopause. They present as tender, fluctuant entities which, when examined under ultrasound, are shown to be fluid-filled. They may increase in size, stay the same or disperse.

> **Box 7.16 Reflection**
>
> **Finding a breast lump**
>
> Aasiya is 18 and has found a palpable, smooth breast lump in her right breast. Although very worried that it is breast cancer, it was 6 weeks before she plucked up courage to see her GP. She is given an appointment to be seen at her local breast unit for a definitive diagnosis.
>
> **Activities**
>
> - Reflect on the feelings that may have influenced her delay in seeking help.
> - Which tests and investigations will Aasiya undergo?
> - The results confirm the lump to be a fibroadenoma. How can this be explained to Aasiya to give her reassurance?
> - Discuss with your mentor how you would introduce the topic of breast awareness with Aasiya.

Duct ectasia

Duct ectasia occurs during breast involution when the major subareolar ducts dilate and shorten. By the age of 70 years it is estimated that 40% of women have duct dilatation or duct ectasia. Normal breast secretions can be retained behind these blocked ducts. Presentation of duct ectasia includes nipple discharge, nipple retraction, inflammation or a palpable mass. Indications for surgery are problems with discharge, or if the woman wants reversal of nipple retraction.

Epithelial hyperplasia

This is a common condition amongst women of all ages but particularly in the age group 30–55 years. It is often called 'fibrocystic disease' but this term is misleading as is not a disease but a natural occurrence in women as they approach the climacteric/menopause. It is thought to be caused by the incomplete involution of breast tissue during each menstrual cycle, causing an increase in numbers of cells lining the terminal duct lobular unit. This, in turn, leads to cystic changes, fibrosis and nodularity. Histologically, the cells show hyperplasia, but with unaltered individual cellular appearance. However, where atypical hyperplasia is present, the risk of cancer developing in the breast is raised and regular screening may be advised.

Other disorders of breast structure

Some other disorders of breast structure are outlined in Box 7.17.

 Box 7.17 Information

Other disorders of breast structure

Duct papillomas

These are benign wart-like lesions in the lactiferous duct wall. Most occur beneath the areola. Papillomas present with pain or bloody discharge and are usually soft and difficult to locate. They are usually surgically resected.

Lipomas

When examined, these fatty lumps can be mistaken for cysts within the breast tissue. They do not cause major problems and diagnosis by ultrasound and cytology should be all that is needed.

Mondor's disease

This is caused by a superficial thrombosis of a breast vein. It is usually very painful, requiring analgesics. Malignancy should always be excluded, but no other treatment should be necessary and the condition usually resolves in 6 months.

Galactocele

This cystic breast lesion occurs during pregnancy or lactation. Once diagnosed, treatment is by aspiration. This may have to be performed on several occasions to allow the walls of the cyst to adhere.

Fat necrosis

Presenting as a painful mass, fat necrosis can imitate breast cancer and should be diagnosed with care. About half of the cases of fat necrosis are caused by breast trauma, although the other cases have no history of trauma. The mass is usually excised to ensure that it is not cancerous.

MEDICAL MANAGEMENT OF BREAST LUMPS/LUMPINESS

Investigations Assessment of a woman who complains of a lump or lumpiness within her breasts might involve clinical examination, mammography, ultrasound scan (USS) and sometimes fine-needle aspiration (FNA) cytology, core biopsy or a newly developed therapeutic vacuum-assisted biopsy, depending on her age and the clinical findings. Cystic fluid is usually sent for examination if the fluid is blood-stained, as this may indicate cancer.

Follow-up examinations are not usually required unless histology reveals atypical hyperplasia in a younger woman or if there is a family history of breast cancer.

Nodularity is sometimes aggravated by oral contraceptives or the intrauterine contraceptive device. If this appears to be the case, a change in method of contraception may be recommended.

 Nursing management and health promotion: excision biopsy of breast lesions and fibroadenomas

Assessment

Surgery is not usually undertaken for benign lesions unless a diagnosis is not possible. Fibroadenomas are not usually removed unless they are large, increasing in size or of particular concern to the woman. Nursing assessment should include the presenting symptoms and, in particular, discomfort and any aggravating or alleviating factors. The nurse should determine the woman's knowledge about her condition, her fears and concerns, and whether the condition is affecting her life.

Perioperative care

For general pre- and postoperative care see Chapter 26. Reassurance that this is not cancer may be needed but the nurse should not give false reassurance where doubt exists as to the nature of the lump. As postoperative recovery is usually rapid, surgery is frequently performed on a day case basis or may require an overnight stay in hospital. Postoperatively, the nursing priorities are wound management and pain control. Because the breast is very vascular, there may be bruising even though the surgery is minor. A wound drain is rarely needed, but, if used, is usually removed the following morning.

The breast is likely to be very painful for several days. Paracetamol or a non-steroidal anti-inflammatory drug (NSAID) is usually sufficient for pain relief, but if bruising and oedema are very extensive, a stronger opiate-based analgesic may be required. Wearing a supportive bra is usually advised for at several weeks postoperatively to improve comfort and avoid strain being placed on the wound. The woman should be encouraged to bring a well-fitted bra into hospital with her so that she may wear it very shortly after the surgery.

Patient education

The nurse should take the opportunity to promote breast health by discussing breast screening and breast awareness. It may be appropriate to discuss how breast comfort can be enhanced by a correctly fitted bra of the right size. Women who have premenstrual breast discomfort may find reducing salt or omitting caffeine from their diet helpful. Others find that a course of evening primrose oil brings relief.

Breast pain

Breast pain (mastalgia) has been reported in over 50% of women who attend benign breast disease clinics (Iddon 2006). For most women, some breast discomfort is accepted as a part of the normal breast changes of the menstrual cycle. However, some women suffer more intense pain affecting quality of life, usually from mid-cycle onwards and often relieved by menstruation. The pain can differ from cycle to cycle and can continue for many years. Gamma linolenic acid (GLA), found in evening primrose oil, taken daily for 3 months and reducing caffeine and fat intake have been found to benefit some patients. Hormone manipulation using the oral contraceptive can also help. If, despite using GLA, the breast pain continues, danazol, bromocriptine or tamoxifen may be considered. Such drug interventions should be medically supervised at a specialist benign breast disease clinic (Purushotham et al 2000).

Non-cyclical breast pain, usually experienced by women over 40, is the most common mastalgia. Often localised within the breast, non-cyclical mastalgia can be relieved by infiltrating the area with local anaesthetic and a corticosteroid. For both cyclical and non-cyclical mastalgia, wearing a firm, well-fitted bra can help.

Breast infections

PATHOPHYSIOLOGY

Breast infections, such as mastitis, are relatively common, and present with swelling, redness, tenderness and pain, which may be associated with a breast abscess or nipple discharge. Breast abscesses are commonly seen during or following lactation. Infection may arise from a cracked nipple, but often there is no apparent cause. Staphylococcal infections are common.

MEDICAL MANAGEMENT

Pus is aspirated from a palpable breast abscess with a wide-gauge needle following local anaesthesia. The pus is sent for microscopy, culture and sensitivity. Flucloxacillin is usually prescribed until the culture and sensitivity result is available. A persistent abscess may require surgical drainage and excision of the surrounding capsule. A persistent nipple discharge may be treated by a microdochectomy (removal of a major duct behind the nipple), or a duct clearance (removal of the major duct system behind the nipple). The surgery can usually be performed on a day case basis.

 Nursing management and health promotion: breast abscess

Until the presence of infection has been established, fear of a more serious problem, particularly cancer, may remain. An explanation of the nature and possible cause of infection will help to reassure the woman, particularly as recurrent infections are quite common and may cause distress.

The discomfort and pain accompanying a breast infection are usually the most distressing features of the condition. A supportive bra, applications of heat or cold 'packs' and padding to protect a sore nipple may all reduce discomfort, but mild to moderate analgesia is usually necessary to control pain.

Where surgical excision of the abscess is required, nursing management will be similar to that for a woman undergoing an excision biopsy (see above). The nurse must be particularly vigilant in observing for signs of wound infection.

Gynaecomastia (overdevelopment of male breast tissue)

PATHOPHYSIOLOGY

Gynaecomastia is a rare benign disorder resulting from oestrogen production either in puberty (30–60% of boys aged 10–16 years) or at a later age. This may be due to excess oestrogen, e.g. some testicular cancers, liver disease, to decreased testosterone, e.g. in Klinefelter's syndrome (see Ch. 5), or to drugs, including risperidone, methyldopa, diltiazem, spironolactone, atazanavir or oestrogen.

MEDICAL MANAGEMENT

Surgery is not usually recommended, as 80% of cases resolve within 2 years. If the condition has arisen as a side-effect of drug administration, medication review can be considered. Hormonal manipulation may be needed where gynaecomastia is due to the oversecretion of oestrogen.

 Nursing management and health promotion: gynaecomastia

Overdevelopment of breast tissue in a boy or man will cause an altered body image and emotional distress. Some men with gynaecomastia believe they have lost their masculinity and experience anxiety and depression as a result. When gynaecomastia occurs in adolescence, such feelings may be particularly acute.

The nurse must be sensitive to such feelings and show understanding. It may be difficult for a boy or man to express these feelings to a female nurse, but he is more likely to do so within a trusting professional relationship. A clear explanation of why the breast tissue has developed and of any treatment that may be given is essential (see Further reading, e.g. Dixon 2006, Burnet 2001).

Breast cancer and potential sequelae

Incidence and mortality

During 2006 breast cancer was diagnosed in 45 500 women and 300 men (Cancer Research UK 2009a). Breast cancer is the second most common cause of cancer death in women after lung cancer (Cancer Research UK 2009b). In 2007 there were 11 990 deaths from breast cancer in women and 90 in men (Cancer Research UK 2009b). In the UK approximately one in nine women will develop breast cancer at some time in their lives. Figure 7.13 shows the incidence and mortality in England 1971–2007. Survival from breast cancer is

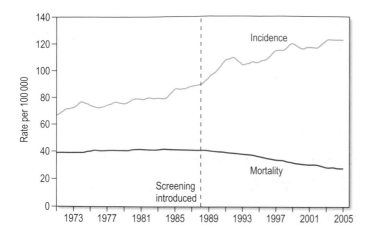

Figure 7.13 Female breast cancer incidence and mortality, England, 1971–2007 (from UK National Statistics).

improving and the estimated 5-year survival rate is approximately 80%.

Risk factors (Box 7.18)

Increasing age Breast cancer in women is very rare below the age of 35 years; 80% of cases occur in women aged 50 years or over. Age is the most significant risk factor for breast cancer.

Previous breast cancer Those already diagnosed with breast cancer are at an increased risk of developing another one. However, treatments given for the first breast cancer, such as tamoxifen, can reduce this risk by up to 40%.

Family history If several female members of a woman's family have breast cancer the chances are increased for other females in that family. The National Institute for Health and Clinical Excellence (NICE) (2006a) has categorised the specific risk of familial breast cancer.

When compared to the general population a woman may have an increased risk of breast cancer if she has one of the following:

- a mother or sister diagnosed with breast cancer before the age of 40
- two close relatives from the same side of the family diagnosed with breast cancer, one being a mother, sister or daughter

 Box 7.18 Information

Factors increasing the risk of early breast cancer

- Increasing age
- Previous breast cancer
- Family history
- Benign breast disease
- Hormone-related factors and hormone replacement therapy (HRT) use (particularly oestrogen combined with a progestogen)
- Weight
- Alcohol intake
- Radiation exposure

- three close relatives with breast cancer at any age
- a mother or sister with breast cancer diagnosed at any age
- a mother or sister with breast cancer in both breasts, diagnosed before the age of 50
- one close relative with ovarian cancer and one with breast cancer diagnosed at any age and at least one to be a mother, sister or daughter.

See website for further content

These criteria should be enough to prompt the woman to see her GP for a discussion about her risk category and referral to a dedicated breast unit.

Benign breast disease Much benign breast disease does not predispose to breast cancer unless the problematic area contains atypical cells which are not cancer but are abnormal in appearance. However, an overproliferation of normal cells can increase the risk of breast cancer by 1.5–2 times.

Lobular carcinoma in situ (LCIS) describes some changes to the breast cells which have not yet demonstrated malignant tendencies. Whilst LCIS is not a cancer it does increase the risk of breast cancer.

Hormone-related factors Women who have their first child after the age of 35, those who experience early menarche and those who have a late menopause have a slightly increased rate of breast cancer.

Hormone replacement therapy It has been shown that HRT increases the risk of breast cancer. Combined HRT (oestrogen and progestogen) used over 10 years leads to 5 extra breast cancers for every 1000 women (Million Women Study Collaborators 2003). The decision to take HRT is a personal one and one that needs to be discussed in detail with the woman's GP, considering the risks and benefits to that individual.

Weight Overweight, postmenopausal women have increased risk of breast cancer.

Alcohol intake An increased risk of breast cancer correlates with the amount of alcohol that women drink. It is estimated that there could be three extra cases of breast cancer for every 200 women who drink alcohol compared to those who do not.

Exposure to radiation Being exposed to large amounts of radiation such as a radiation accident can cause breast cancer. Traditionally, treatment for Hodgkin's lymphoma (see Ch. 11) included radiation to the chest and this has increased the risk of breast cancer for those young women who were treated in puberty or their early 20s.

Prevention and early detection

The focus of primary prevention is on the identification of risk factors and at-risk individuals (see Ch. 31). Survival rates for breast cancer have improved since the 1970s, when the 5-year survival was only 50%, compared to the current overall 5-year survival rate of 80%. However, this survival rate varies according to the stage of the cancer at diagnosis: 90% for stage I down to 10% for stage IV cancers (Cancer Research UK 2009a). Therefore, taking measures to detect breast cancer earlier is important in reducing breast cancer mortality.

Breast awareness

For many years there has been debate as to the value of monthly breast self-examination (BSE) in the detection of early breast cancer. Research has been unable to demonstrate that it alters survival from the disease. However, a woman who is aware of any changes that occur in her breast and, if she wishes, practises self-examination, is more likely to notice any changes. This may aid diagnosis when a cancer is small, so enabling a wider choice of surgical treatment options to be offered. It also encourages an individual to participate in their own health care.

Breast awareness is about the woman knowing what is normal for her and detecting the following changes:

- change in breast size, noticeably smaller or larger
- newly inverted nipple or a nipple that has changed its shape
- discharge from one or both nipples
- change in colour of the breast skin
- a new lump or thickening in the breast or axilla that feels different from the rest of the breast tissue
- a rash or eczema-like changes around the nipple
- pain in one part of the breast or in the axilla
- puckering or dimpling of the skin of the breast (peau d'orange).

If any lumps, thickening or other changes are noticed, the woman should contact her GP immediately for an examination and advice.

Breast cancer screening

In 1986, the Forrest Report (Department of Health and Social Security [DHSS] 1986) recommended the introduction of a national breast screening programme and this was implemented in 1988. The UK programme invites women aged between 50 and 70 years to attend for free screening using mammography (X-ray of the breast). Research is ongoing to assess full field digital mammography as an alternative for an X-ray mammogram.

The aim of screening using mammography is to detect breast cancer at an earlier stage than is possible by clinical examination or BSE, i.e. before a lump is palpable in the breast. In addition, it is hoped that pre-invasive disease (in situ) cancer will be detected before the cancer cells have shown any evidence of spread. Because of the huge costs involved with a national screening programme, constant review of the service continues. A research study was developed by Tabar et al (2003) questioning the effectiveness of the mammography and screening programme in Sweden. In their 20-year review of the service before and after its introduction they found that screening contributed to substantial reductions in breast cancer mortality. The NHS-funded service continues and the programme is being extended to include women aged 47–73 years by 2012 (NHS Breast Screening programme [NHSBSP] 2009), with the provision for older women to be screened on request.

Mammography will detect 85–90% of all breast cancers in the women examined. It is most effective in postmenopausal women in whom breast tissue has been largely replaced by fat. For young women, in whom breast tissue is dense, and detection of abnormalities therefore more difficult, mammography is usually used in conjunction with breast ultrasound.

The success of the national screening programme depends on a high uptake of the service. If fewer women attend, the cost per life saved increases and, although some women will clearly benefit, the cost-effectiveness of the programme will be called into question (Box 7.19). Duffy et al (2005) make the point that breast cancer should be detected and treated in the preclinical phase in order to save lives, and with 'broader adherence to the screening programme' even greater reductions in breast cancer mortality would be achieved.

Procedures Screening may take place in static or mobile units. Screening involves taking two X-ray views of each compressed breast. Mammograms are repeated every 3 years and, although the screening starts from age 50, a woman may not be called until she is 53. The woman is notified of her result by letter. If an abnormality is detected, the letter will ask her to attend for re-screening at an assessment centre (Figure 7.14). Here, a fresh two-view diagnostic mammogram may show the detected lesion to be merely an overlapping of normal structures or a benign lesion requiring no intervention. In some instances, further assessment of the suspicious area using an USS and FNA cytology or a core biopsy may be required.

Psychological considerations Most women who present for breast screening are asymptomatic: apparently healthy people who, on the whole, come to be reassured that all is well. Inevitably, screening reminds the individual that breast

---

Box 7.19 Reflection

Breast screening uptake

Poor attendance for breast screening may result from various factors, such as GP registers not being up to date, fear of cancer, fears of discomfort or radiation exposure, lack of awareness of screening (perhaps because the publicity is not provided in the woman's language or poor literacy skills), or a lack of understanding of the value of mammography, so it is essential that women fully understand what breast screening is about.

To further explain breast screening, all women invited into the programme are sent a leaflet entitled *Breast Screening – The Facts* (NHSBSP revised 2009).

However, 3 in 10 women do not take up the invitation for breast screening; in 2008, of the 2.2 million invitations sent out, around 73% of women attended (Cancer Research UK 2009c).

Activities

- Access the leaflet *Breast Screening – The Facts* (NHS Breast Screening Programme revised 2009) and reflect on why 3 in 10 women choose to ignore the invitation for screening.
- Find out if leaflets are available in a variety of languages.
- Discuss with your mentor how well known it is that women older than the screening age range can request screening and consider how awareness could be increased.

References

Cancer Research UK: *Charity concerned that one third of women ignore breast screening invite*. September 2009c: Press release. Available online http://info.cancerresearchuk.org/news/archive/pressrelease/2009-09-30-breast-screening-uptake.

NHS Breast Screening Programme Breast Screening – The Facts (NHSBSP revised): 2009. Available online http://www.cancerscreening.nhs.uk/breastscreen/publications/ia-02.html.

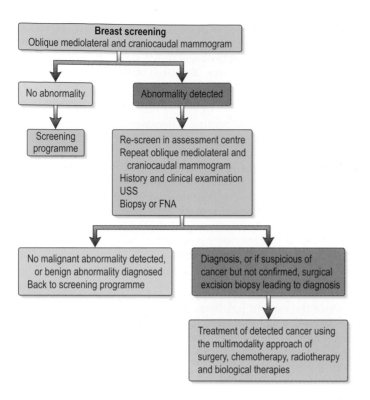

Figure 7.14 Flow diagram of breast cancer screening procedure.

cancer is a potential threat. It is therefore important that efforts are made to reduce women's anxiety where possible. It is particularly important that results are sent quickly. If the first screening is a positive experience, the woman will be more likely to attend 3 years later and may urge her friends to do likewise.

The nurse's role At the inception of the breast screening programme, the Forrest Report (DHSS 1986) recommended that qualified nurses should be available to support women undergoing screening. The report stressed the importance of having specialist nurses with an in-depth knowledge of breast disease and its treatment and good communication skills to give support to women recalled to assessment centres following the detection of an apparent abnormality. However, all nurses have a role in promoting health and should take every appropriate opportunity to raise women's awareness of the availability and benefits of screening programmes. Community nurses in particular can encourage women to attend for screening and can answer queries or discuss worries as part of their general health promotion on an individual basis or through group discussion, e.g. in well women clinics.

PATHOPHYSIOLOGY

Breast cancers may be classified according to the type of tissue from which they arise and their appearance under the microscope. The histological type of a cancer is often relevant to the choice of treatment. Ductal carcinomas arise from the epithelial cells of the ducts and account for the majority of all breast cancers (Sainsbury et al 2006). Medullary, colloidal and tubular carcinomas are all types of breast cancer arising from ductal tissue. They are usually localised, but can be multifocal. They are rarely bilateral. Cancers arising from cells of the breast lobules are known as lobular carcinomas. These account for approximately 15% of breast cancers and are more commonly multifocal and bilateral compared to ductal carcinomas (Crowe & Lampejo 1996).

In Paget's disease of the nipple, malignant cells are found in the epidermis of the nipple and are usually associated with small multifocal areas of ductal carcinoma behind the nipple and deep in the breast. Other breast cancer types, such as squamous cell or inflammatory carcinomas, are less common. Sarcomas and lymphomas may also arise in the breast, as may metastatic cancer tumours, although these are rare.

Breast cancers are classified as non-invasive or in situ (confined to the ducts or lobules) or invasive (able to invade the basement membrane of the duct or lobule). This distinction has a bearing on prognosis and treatment. Ductal carcinoma in situ (DCIS) represents a very early stage of breast cancer which is often seen as microcalcifications on a mammogram. It cannot be predicted when, or if, a non-invasive breast cancer will become invasive.

Cellular differentiation, i.e. the degree to which cancer cells resemble their tissue of origin, is another important prognostic factor: cells are described as well differentiated, moderately differentiated or poorly differentiated, or grades I, II or III. Poorly differentiated cancers tend to be more aggressive, with the ability to metastasise at an earlier stage, and hence carry a poorer prognosis.

Common presenting signs and symptoms The discovery of a non-tender, hard, usually irregular lump or thickening in the breast is the most common presentation of breast cancer. Increasingly, it is also diagnosed after a solid mass or microcalcifications are seen on a mammogram during routine screening.

Pain is not usually a presenting feature, but sometimes a sharp, pricking pain may be the first symptom experienced. A change in breast size or shape may be noticed. Signs of inflammation and tissue oedema may also be present, and superficial veins can dilate and become more visible if partially obstructed by tumour. If the tumour is advanced at the time of presentation, it may be fixed to the muscles beneath the breast. There may also be large palpable axillary lymph nodes or ulceration of the tumour through the skin, causing an infected, weeping, malodorous wound, although most women are sufficiently well informed to present to their GP before this advanced stage. Oedema of the arm may result if the cancer in the axilla is blocking the drainage of blood and lymph from the arm.

MEDICAL MANAGEMENT

Investigations

Once a breast abnormality has been detected, further diagnostic investigation will be carried out following referral to a specialist. This may involve:

- breast examination
- mammography

🖥 **See website Figure 7.2**

- USS to distinguish solid from cystic lesions
- FNA to drain cysts and obtain samples for cytology
- biopsy of the suspicious area for cytology.

FNA cytology A syringe with a small-bore needle is inserted into the breast mass and the contents withdrawn, placed on a slide and sent to the laboratory for cytological studies. Where a mass is found to be a cyst and a large amount of fluid is aspirated, it is usually discarded, unless it is found to be bloodstained, in which case a sample will be sent for examination. Cytological results are graded C0–C5:

- C0 – insufficient specimen
- C1 and C2 – benign cells
- C3 and C4 – cells suspicious of carcinoma
- C5 – carcinoma.

FNA cytology is a useful diagnostic tool but is not conclusive alone. A benign result may simply indicate that the needle missed the target; where other signs are suspicious, a biopsy will still be recommended. This method of gaining a provisional diagnosis can be very fast and is often used in clinics where the woman (or man) is given a diagnosis by the end of the clinic visit.

Biopsy Biopsy of the suspicious area is a widely used method to achieve a diagnosis. The types include:

- Core biopsy – removal of a core of tissue using a special large bore needle. When guided by ultrasound, it can accurately obtain good specimens of the suspicious lesion. It can be undertaken in the outpatient department using a local anaesthetic and the patient returns for the result several days later. The information obtained from a biopsy, including the type of cancer, is very important when planning treatment.
- Vacuum-assisted biopsy – an X-ray-guided outpatient biopsy, useful for the investigation of breast calcifications. Many tissue samples can be taken from a defined area.
- Excision biopsy – excision of the lump in its entirety, usually under general anaesthesia, as a day case.
- Localisation biopsy – where a mammographic abnormality has been detected but there is no associated palpable mass. A wire may be inserted into the abnormal area under X-ray or ultrasound control. This tissue, once surgically excised from the breast, will be X-rayed to ensure that the surgeon has removed the area of abnormality.

The tissue obtained is sent for a histological diagnosis.

Overview of treatment

Once a histological diagnosis has been confirmed then treatment is decided at a multidisciplinary meeting (MDM). The MDM provides a broad base of expert knowledge to manage the patient with breast cancer, and should comprise core personnel who meet weekly. The core members should include consultant radiologist, surgeon, pathologist, clinical oncologist, medical oncologist and breast care nurse. Other professionals may also join the MDM, including a reconstructive/plastic surgeon, physiotherapist, therapy radiographer, geneticist/genetics counsellor, psychologist and social worker. The MDM reviews the pathology and formulates a treatment plan for the individual patient. Decisions are based on several factors, including the:

- size, position and tumour type
- spread of the disease
- woman's general health
- woman's priorities and wishes.

Staging of the cancer is determined (see Ch. 31). There are two ways of staging breast cancer: the number system and the tumour, nodes, metastasis (TNM) classification (see Useful websites, e.g. Cancer Research UK). The purpose of staging breast cancer is to:

- Plan treatment.
- Act as a prognostic index. There are various indexes available but the two mainly used in the UK are the Nottingham Prognostic Index (NPI) and Adjuvant online (see Useful websites). The NPI is the most widely used index and incorporates three prognostic factors: tumour size, node status and histological grade. Adjuvant online is a computer-based tool used to determine baseline prognosis and the efficacy of chemotherapy and hormone therapy after surgery.
- Evaluate results of treatment.
- Facilitate the exchange of information between oncology centres.

Once the patient has been assigned an index and her case has been discussed at the MDM, a treatment package will be developed to treat her optimally and to meet her individual needs. This process would also apply to men diagnosed with breast cancer.

In order to standardise the care for breast cancer, treatment usually follows a set of protocols devised by the treating breast unit. In England these guidelines are informed by documents that include Department of Health (DH) *The NHS Cancer Plan* (2000), Department of Health (DH) *NHS Cancer Reform Strategy* (2007) and guidelines from the National Institute for Health and Clinical Excellence (2009a,b).

A woman diagnosed with breast cancer has the right to be told of all the possible treatment options and to decide which, if any, of these options she will take. She may wish to seek a second opinion from another specialist and to gather information to help her make a decision as to which is the best treatment for her. Research about particular aspects of treatment including drug trials is becoming the norm in breast cancer care and most women being treated for cancer will be approached about entering one or more studies. In this event the study should be clearly explained and written information given as back-up. The woman must be assured that she has the absolute right to refuse entry or to leave the study without incurring any detrimental effect to her future care.

Treatments for breast cancer can be divided into two categories – *local* and *systemic*.

Local treatments are surgery and radiotherapy, and systemic treatments include chemotherapy, hormonal (endocrine) therapy and targeted therapies. All of these treatments can be given before surgery (neoadjuvant) or after surgery (adjuvant). Surgery is the usual first line treatment for breast cancer and will be considered in most cases.

Surgical interventions

The extent and nature of the surgery is dependent on the type of cancer and an accurate pathological diagnosis is obtained before the definitive surgical technique is decided.

Surgical procedures are as follows:

- **Vacuum-assisted biopsy or surgical biopsy** – used to remove small lesions within the breast such as atypical ductal hyperplasia or lobular carcinoma in situ. They are mostly performed as an outpatient procedure, usually in a dedicated breast unit. The area of suspect tissue is removed, examined by the pathologist and, if there is no evidence of disease, regular outpatient follow-up will be organised, perhaps including mammography to monitor the breast.

- **Lumpectomy** – removal of the breast lump but with very little surrounding normal tissue. This can be the equivalent to an excision biopsy and is used for the treatment of smaller areas of DCIS as long as a margin of at least 5 mm of normal breast tissue is around the lesion.
- **Wide local excision** – usually used for an invasive breast cancer. This involves the removal of the abnormal areas together with a 1–2 cm margin of normal tissue around the lesion to reduce the possibility of leaving microscopic cancer cells behind.
- **Re-excision** – may be recommended if, after pathological examination, the margins around the cancer are not clear. The amount of tissue removed in this operation can be considerable, depending on the size and location of the tumour in relation to the breast, and may leave the breast smaller and altered in contour.
- **Partial mastectomy** – surgical technique often used for Paget's disease which involves removal of a portion of the breast, usually the nipple and areolar complex. Inevitably, the breast is left smaller and its contour is changed.
- **Mastectomy** – complete removal of all the breast tissue, overlying skin and the nipple. The pectoralis major and minor muscles remain and the axillary skin fold remains intact. The scar is oblique but less extensive than with a radical mastectomy.
- **Radical or Halsted's mastectomy** – rarely used nowadays unless there is extensive local spread of the breast cancer. This operation involves the removal of the pectoralis major and minor muscles, as well as the breast tissue and overlying skin, the nipple and the axillary lymph nodes. A long, oblique scar remains. The axillary skin fold is usually removed and, as a result, the chest wall may appear concave and the ribs more prominent.
- **Axillary dissection** – usually performed if the patient has a confirmed *invasive* breast cancer or, in cases of extensive DCIS in the breast, to determine whether the cancer has spread to the lymph nodes. The presence of cancer cells in the lymph nodes indicates that micrometastatic spread is likely and that additional adjuvant drug therapy is indicated. Where possible, axillary dissection (removal of some or all of the axillary lymph nodes) may be undertaken through the same incision as that made for the breast surgery. This would include some mastectomy and wide local excision procedures. Axillary dissection can lead to chronic swelling, or lymphoedema (see pp. 259, 266–268), of the affected arm.
- **Sentinel lymph node biopsy (SLNB)** – developed to avoid compromising the lymphatic system, SLNB is becoming an accepted, standard procedure used to determine whether there is spread of cancer cells to the axillary lymph nodes. SLNB requires the removal of only 1–3 sentinel lymph nodes (those draining closest to the breast) for close review by the pathologist. If the sentinel nodes do not demonstrate cancer cells, this eliminates the need to dissect additional axillary lymph nodes. However, if cancer cells are present in the sentinel nodes the patient will undergo a formal axillary dissection.

Breast reconstruction procedures are discussed on page 266.

Nursing management and health promotion: breast cancer surgery

Pre-treatment

For the patient, the period prior to admission to hospital is usually characterised by anxiety and uncertainty. Diagnosis has often been confirmed by biopsy so the patient's concerns are focused on her cancer, how far it has spread and the physical effects on her body of the impending surgery and any follow-up treatment. A breast care nurse specialist will usually be involved with her care and should have been present when the patient received her malignant diagnosis. Nursing intervention at this time will include assessing the patient's personal situation, helping her to cope with anxiety, providing psychological support and information and assisting her in making informed choices with regard to treatment options.

Assessment

There may be limited time available for assessment at this stage, but where possible the nurse should try to identify the following:

- the woman's reaction, and that of her family, to the diagnosis or potential diagnosis of breast cancer
- any major fears and concerns of the woman and her family
- the woman's feelings about body image changes, and her views about reconstructive surgery
- the woman's knowledge of breast cancer and cancer generally, the information she has been given by medical staff, how much she has understood and how much she wants to know
- whether the woman has previous experience of family or friends having breast cancer or any other kind of cancer
- the support available to the woman through family and friends (Box 7.20)
- any concurrent stressors, e.g. bereavement
- previous anxiety/depression; Watson (1991) found that women who had experienced previous anxiety/depression were more likely to re-experience this following diagnosis and treatment.

The psychological impact of breast disease

Nurses have a particularly important role in supporting patients through the traumatic experience of breast cancer. Although many women with breast cancer will face similar problems, no two individuals will respond to their diagnosis and treatment in the same way. Ongoing assessment is key to providing psychological and emotional support that is genuinely responsive to each woman's needs and priorities.

For most women, a diagnosis of breast cancer is devastating. They may have to face the prospect of mutilating surgery to a body part associated with sexuality and motherhood, the prospect of months of intensive treatment and the possibility

Box 7.20 Evidence-based practice

Early psychological adjustment in breast cancer patients: a prospective study

In a study by Nosartis et al (2002), the presence of social support was cited as a predictor for a more successful adjustment to a diagnosis of breast cancer.

Many patients will suffer significant psychological morbidity in the first year after their diagnosis of breast cancer. This study aimed to identify and understand the risk factors for developing this morbidity. Eighty-seven patients aged 40–75 years were assessed psychologically prior to their diagnosis of breast cancer, 8 weeks after the beginning of their breast cancer treatment and again 9 months after their first follow-up. Assessments included standard psychological instruments for measuring morbidity and coping, symptom attribution, beliefs about breast cancer, social support, sociodemographic and clinical variables and the General Health Questionnaire (GHQ-12) and Mental Adjustment to Cancer (MAC) questionnaire.

A total of 85.1% of patients completed both follow-ups. Results showed that a significant proportion of patients had considerable psychological morbidity before they received their definitive diagnosis of breast cancer, especially those who thought they had breast cancer. At first follow-up those who had significant psychological morbidity included those with pre-diagnostic morbidity as well as a lack of social support and feelings of 'personal responsibility/avoidance'. Those at second follow-up with considerable psychological morbidity could be predicted by their lack of social support alone.

Conclusions were that psychological morbidity is higher before, rather than following, a definitive diagnosis of breast cancer. Early reactions of this kind are predictive of post-treatment adjustment. Only the presence of social support in this study seems to be associated with successful adjustment in the first year after a breast cancer diagnosis. Women who have poor social support can thus be identified and cared for with this in mind.

Activities

- Access the study by Nosartis et al (2002) and think about how you could use their findings in the assessment of women undergoing surgery for breast cancer.
- Discuss with your mentor how a lack of social support might be strengthened for women, for example a lone mother with two primary school-aged children newly moved to an area away from family, or a single woman in her late 70s with no family.

Reference

Nosartis C, Roberts JV, Crayford T, et al: Early psychological adjustment in breast cancer patients: a prospective study. *J Psychosom Res* 53(6):1123–1130, 2002.

The fear may be based on misconceptions about cancer treatments. Nurses, especially those in community practice, should dispel myths about cancer therapy, raise awareness of the success rate of breast cancer treatment and emphasise the importance of early detection.

Some women who undergo surgery for breast cancer initially experience euphoria that the cancer has 'gone'. Others deny the removal of their breast or are unable to discuss it or to look at the scar. Much research has been carried out into the psychosocial sequelae of breast surgery. It has been reported that one third of women develop severe anxiety or depression within a year of their diagnosis (Maguire & Hopwood 2006). It was thought that this was related mainly to the altered body image of mastectomy, but Fallowfield et al (2000) found that women who had a wide local excision had levels of anxiety and depression similar to those experienced by women who had chosen mastectomy. Dorval et al (1998) found that having a partial or total mastectomy did not significantly affect quality of life but that the individual's response to the surgery was affected by her age. They suggested that having a partial mastectomy may have lessened the negative effect of breast cancer for younger women.

Following diagnosis and surgery, a period of adjustment occurs with fluctuating emotions. Northouse (1989) found that post mastectomy the major concern for most women and their partners were about survival, extent of the cancer and the possibility of recurrence. Other worries may include lifestyle changes, treatment regimens and side-effects as well as altered appearance. For the majority of women who have undergone breast surgery, anxiety begins to reduce after several months and normal life will be resumed. Some women, however, will continue to experience great anxiety, show signs of depression, withdraw from social contact or have sexual problems. These women are likely to benefit from more in-depth counselling and psychological support. Nurses, particularly those in the community and in outpatient departments, should recognise emotional problems and, where necessary, suggest referral to a counsellor, psychiatrist or psychologist via the GP or hospital medical staff.

Survivorship, or living with the diagnosis of breast cancer, can be problematic for the patient and her family. Concurrent stressors including effects of long-term hormone therapy or chemotherapy, resources of the patient and her family and the meaning of illness to the family were all found to have an effect on the experience of living with the diagnosis of breast cancer (Mellon et al 2006). Being diagnosed with breast cancer is a life-changing event, and the changed future this represents for the individual must be taken into account when caring for them.

Supporting information needs

Being a recipient of the bewildering treatments for breast cancer can decrease the woman's self-determination and this can lead to psychological morbidity. Research has shown that many patients find that information helps them to make sense of their situation, and hence to feel more in control, less vulnerable and less anxious (Fallowfield et al 2000). Most women have some knowledge of breast cancer, but may not be familiar with the details of the tests or treatments being discussed. Many will, in fact, have misconceptions about breast cancer and its prognosis. Research by Macleod et al (2004) demonstrated that different groups of women

---

that they may eventually die of the disease. Some women will discover a lump when washing or during BSE whilst others are unaware that anything is wrong but find out following routine breast screening. Acute anxiety and panic with palpitations, loss of concentration and insomnia may be experienced in the period when a medical opinion is sought and a diagnosis awaited. Some women describe this time of flux as the most agonising period of their illness. For some women, the fear of cancer or its treatment is so great that they deny the presence of a lump or delay seeking medical help.

receive differing amounts of information from the available sources, the affluent group accessing more information than the deprived group. They state that health care professionals need to be aware that there may be greater psychological distress in the deprived group of women, perhaps exacerbated by the lack of informational support.

Nurses must be sensitive to the specific information needs of each woman. Women and their families will vary in the amount of detailed information they want about their disease or treatment. As too much information can increase confusion and anxiety, it is important for nurses to ascertain what each individual wants to know, and to clarify what has been understood. It is also important to remember that, in times of stress, information is more difficult to assimilate and remember. It is often necessary for the nurse to provide information in stages and to repeat information.

Where nurses are unable to answer questions, they should arrange for a specialist breast care nurse or a member of the medical staff to see the woman as soon as possible.

Treatment phase

Assessment

On the patient's admission to hospital, the nurse should undertake a more comprehensive assessment, including medical history, family history and a full physical and psychological assessment. In particular, the factors relevant in the pre-treatment phase should be reassessed to determine if the woman's needs and concerns have changed. It is important to assess pre-operative shoulder function if axillary surgery is planned; early involvement of the physiotherapist will improve postoperative function. Good communication between the patient, ward nurses and the specialist breast care nurse will help to identify any particular issues important to the patient that may affect her coping abilities and recovery from the surgery. See Chapter 26 for a detailed discussion of general pre-operative care.

Giving psychological support

The nurse should give each patient the opportunity to discuss her fears but must respect her wishes if she prefers not to disclose her feelings.

See website Critical thinking question 7.3

Where possible, a private room should be available for patients to spend some time in solitude or to talk privately with staff or family members.

A relaxed but professional atmosphere on the ward will assist, as will encouraging women to remain in their day clothes, open visiting if practical, and the opportunity to go out, e.g. for meals.

Patient education

The pre-operative routine should be explained, including the approximate time of surgery and the timing of any medication to be administered.

The woman is told that she may have drainage tubes in situ on return from theatre, sometimes in the breast wound and usually in the axilla to prevent the collection of blood and serous fluid beneath the suture line. She should be advised that the drains will not affect mobility

and reassured that it is difficult to dislodge the tubing as it is sutured in place. Sutures to the breast and axillary wound are usually subcutaneous and dissolvable, with 'paper stitches' such as 3M™ Steri-strips™ holding the wound edges together. A light dressing is all that is needed to cover the breast scar, although surgeons may have dressing preferences. It is worth telling the woman what sort of dressing to expect as she may think that the breast wound will be exposed on her return from theatre, which might be distressing.

A patient undergoing axillary dissection is warned that she may experience discomfort on moving her arm for a few weeks postoperatively. The nurse should stress the importance of postoperative exercises and work with the physiotherapist who can assess shoulder function preoperatively and teach exercises that can be used postoperatively. Written information about arm exercises is provided so that the woman can continue them following discharge. Because surgery may compromise the axillary lymphatics, nurses should provide information about the risk of lymphoedema and preventative measures (Box 7.21).

The possibility of an intravenous infusion, or more rarely, a blood transfusion postoperatively should also be explained so that the patient is not alarmed at finding one in place.

Patients often find it helpful to be told of the expected appearance of the wound and scar. Wound size and position, and wound closure to be used can be mentioned. Drawings, photographs and DVDs/videos may be helpful aids. It is important to warn the patient that, because the breast is so vascular, bruising and swelling are expected postoperatively. She should be reminded of this when she

Box 7.21 Information

Practical advice on avoiding the complications of lymphoedema

The British Lymphology Society recommends the following advice:

- Take care not to develop infection in the affected arm by avoiding injections and vein puncture in that arm. An infection in the arm could further compromise the lymphatic system by causing localised swelling and inflammation.
- Avoid using the affected arm when blood pressure is manually recorded.
- Try to avoid cuts and scratches in the arm. If damage to the arm does occur, wash the area carefully with soap and apply an antiseptic cream to the wound.
- Report any signs of infection to the GP or the hospital.
- Wear protective gloves when gardening.
- Avoid insect bites by using insect repellent.
- Use a thimble for sewing.
- Avoid the use of a wet-shave razor for removal of underarm hair by using depilatory cream or an electric razor instead.
- Take care not to burn in the sun and use protective sun cream.
- Use the arm as normally as possible as regular movement will help lymph drainage.

Resources

The British Lymphoedema Society (BLS) and The Lymphoedema Support Network http://www.lymphoedema.org.

first looks at the scar. Women who are not having immediate reconstruction should be informed about the availability of prostheses.

Information given verbally may be reinforced with printed material or various web-based sources of reliable information, such as Cancer Research UK and Macmillan Cancer Support (see Useful websites).

Postoperative care

For general postoperative nursing care see Chapter 26. The following discussion focuses on considerations that are particularly relevant to breast surgery.

Wound management (see Ch. 23)

The size and position of the wound will depend on the operation performed. Generally, a low-suction drain is placed beneath the breast wound and in some cases another in the axillary region to reduce the likelihood of a collection of serous fluid (seroma) forming. Initially, the drains and the wound dressing should be observed frequently for signs of excessive blood loss. Undue blood loss should be reported to medical staff immediately.

The wound drains will remain in situ for 2–5 days until the wound drainage is minimal, usually less than 50 mL/day. The nurse should ensure that the drains are patent and that, unless informed otherwise, suction is maintained; drainage volume should be recorded. Removal of the drains can be painful; this should be explained to the patient and removal should be preceded by the administration of oral analgesics or inhalation of Entonox®.

Some units permit patients to go home with the axillary drain still in situ. The woman, and a member of her family, are given instructions about managing the wound and drain. Community nurses should be involved in the patient's early discharge, and will empty and finally remove the drains at home. Close contact is usually maintained with the hospital and patients are asked to notify the hospital should the drain become loose or blocked or cause pain. Research shows that, with good support, early discharge with axillary drains in situ is safe and does not cause any greater psychological distress for patients (Chapman 2001).

The wound should also be observed for signs of infection, i.e. redness, swelling, pain and discharge. Temperature, pulse and respiration should be monitored 4–6-hourly and a raised temperature brought to the attention of the medical staff.

Wound dressings should be changed only if they are saturated by wound exudate. Unnecessary dressing changes slow wound healing and increase the risk of infection. The wound dressing can be removed 48 h postoperatively if the wound is clean and dry. The patient can have a shower or bath at this point, providing that the wound is not soaked and the patient carefully pats the area dry with a clean towel.

The nurse must also consider other factors, such as nutritional intake, medication, stress and concurrent illness (e.g. diabetes mellitus), which may affect wound healing and resistance to infection (see Ch. 23).

Managing pain

Pain from the wound will always be experienced to some degree, but pain on shoulder movement is often more of a problem. Pain is sometimes more intense a day or so after the operation when the initial numbness has faded. Patients should be encouraged to take analgesics regularly for the first 48 h, but many women find that the wound is less painful than they had expected and require oral analgesics infrequently beyond this period. It should be stressed, in any event, that it is preferable to take analgesics and continue arm exercises than to take no analgesics and avoid the exercises.

The experience of pain is influenced by many factors, such as anxiety and emotional distress (see Ch. 19), and must be considered by the nurse when promoting comfort postoperatively.

Women who have had a mastectomy may experience phantom breast and nipple sensations at some point. This may be very distressing and requires the nurse to reassure that these sensations will not continue for long. In rare cases nerve damage may occur during surgery. If the nerve has only been bruised, patients may complain of an uncomfortable tenderness (neuropraxia) but this sensation should fade over a period of weeks to months. Referral to a physiotherapist and a review of the patient's oral analgesics may help. As the bruising subsides, so will the symptoms of pain and altered sensation.

Promoting shoulder movement

Patients whose surgery involved dissection of the axillary lymph nodes are at risk of developing problems with shoulder movement. Postoperative exercises will help to ensure that a full range of shoulder movement is attained following surgery. Ideally, exercises should be taught by a physiotherapist. The nurse must know what they involve, however, so that she can encourage the patient to practise them. Generally, gentle exercises are begun on the first or second postoperative day and gradually increased in extent and frequency as drainage from the wound diminishes and the axillary drain is removed.

Preparing the patient for discharge

Looking at a breast scar for the first time is often very difficult and may confirm a woman's fears about breast loss and intensify her grief. However, others find the scar neater and less distressing than they had imagined. Women who have wide local excisions may have a similar range of reactions.

The nurse should encourage a woman to look at her scar sooner rather than later, as this represents a significant step in rehabilitation. The woman may wish to be accompanied by her partner or a nurse when first seeing her scar and this may also be the first time she talks about the loss/alteration of her breast. The woman must never be forced to look at her wound and it may not be until the first outpatient visit that she is able to take this step.

Rehabilitation proceeds at different rates, but the nurse should explain to each woman that it may take several months before she feels that her energy has returned to normal. Persistent fatigue may cause frustration and may give rise to anxiety that the cancer has returned. Fatigue is more likely if chemotherapy or radiotherapy is given postoperatively, but where it is profound, depression should also be considered as a possible contributing factor.

Most women can begin driving again in 2–3 weeks, providing they feel confident, their arm movement is not too uncomfortable and the seat belt is not pressing on the scar line. They must be confident enough to perform an emergency stop if necessary. Light household duties can be undertaken when the woman feels well enough, usually 2–3 weeks postoperatively, and she may return to work at around 6 weeks. This will, of course, depend on the extent of the surgery, the particular individual and the type of work she does.

Pain and discomfort from the wound will steadily reduce, but some discomfort often remains for 2–3 months. Paraesthesia around the scar and axilla may fade over several months, but some may always remain and can be made a little worse by local radiotherapy.

A collection of serous fluid (seroma) in the breast wound or the axilla may occur postoperatively. Some women believe that the large lump they can feel is cancer that has suddenly grown after surgery. Prior explanation of this and the possibility of seroma formation is likely to reduce any anxiety. The problem can be resolved by the aspiration of the fluid and may be performed in outpatients. Many specialist breast care nurses and nurse practitioners have been trained to carry out aspiration and patients should be informed who to contact should this problem arise.

Lymphoedema is a possible long-term complication that can occur in anyone who has axillary surgery or radiotherapy. Women should have access to a breast care nurse to provide information (verbal and written) before or at the time of cancer treatment. This includes advice regarding care of a potentially swollen limb or other area and to contact the breast care nurse if swelling occurs, so that they can then refer to the appropriate service. Some units in the UK require patients to attend their GP for a referral to the local lymphoedema service. Lymphoedema following breast surgery is discussed on pages 259, 266–268.

Prior to discharge, any woman who has had a mastectomy or a significantly wide local excision without immediate breast reconstruction should be given a temporary prosthesis, shown how to position it in her bra and alter its shape, and advised how to wash it (Box 7.22).

Adjuvant local treatments

Radiotherapy (see Ch. 31) Following surgery for early breast cancer, radiotherapy reduces the risk of local relapse by 70% and of breast cancer mortality by 17% (START Trialists Group 2008). Radiotherapy is offered to all patients following breast conserving surgery and to selected patients after mastectomy, depending on grade, size and nodal involvement.

In the UK most radiotherapy is administered by linear accelerator machines. A course of radiotherapy is given in daily doses, known as fractions; a course is given in either 15 or 25 fractions. Radiotherapy is usually given to the breast/chest wall over a period of 3–6 weeks, three to five times a week. In most units radiotherapy is planned using a non-diagnostic computed tomography (CT) scan to enable more accurate delivery of radiation and avoidance of the underlying organs such as lung and heart (for left-sided tumours).

There have been several technological advances in the delivery of radiotherapy over the last decade. These aim to increase accuracy and reduce the side-effects from radiation and include:

- **Intensity modulated radiotherapy (IMRT)** – a multileaf collimator (tube of overlapping metal leaves) which

Box 7.22 Information

Breast prostheses

The fitting of a breast prosthesis is an integral part of the rehabilitation following mastectomy or partial mastectomy without immediate breast reconstruction. The aim of the prosthesis is to match as closely as possible the woman's other breast in terms of size, shape, weight and feel, so that she may look normal and feel confident in clothing. This is important in helping her to resume her normal social activities and regain a healthy body image.

Temporary prostheses

A temporary prosthesis (sometimes known as a 'cumfie') is fitted as soon as the wound drains from the mastectomy scar have been removed and is worn until a permanent prosthesis can be fitted. It is soft, light and washable, and can be pinned securely into the cup of a bra. If a bra cannot be worn because of discomfort, the prosthesis can be pinned into a camisole or slip. The woman may find that wearing loose clothing helps to achieve an even appearance. However, it is important that the nurse spends time fitting this prosthesis well, as it is with this that the woman will first face the outside world again.

Permanent prostheses

A permanent prosthesis is usually fitted 5–6 weeks after surgery or 2 weeks after the completion of radiotherapy, when the wound is well healed. Every woman should be given a fitting appointment prior to leaving hospital. The fitting may be undertaken by a specialist nurse, surgical appliance officer or visiting prosthesis company fitter. A private room with a full-length mirror is necessary and it is essential that each woman is treated with respect and sensitivity.

Today most permanent prostheses are made of silicone gel which feels soft and comfortable next to the skin and takes on the body's temperature. Many shapes and sizes are available; it should be possible for all women to be fitted with a prosthesis that gives a balanced appearance in a bra. Partial prostheses are available for women who have breast conservation. Silicone prostheses generally last for 2–3 years, but a woman is entitled to a replacement whenever it begins to show signs of wear and tear or if she loses or gains weight or changes shape.

Special 'mastectomy bras' are not necessary, but the bra does need to be supportive and of the correct cup size, covering all of the tissue of the remaining breast. It is helpful if the nurse can give basic advice about bras and instruct a woman where she may be fitted for a bra locally, if her previous bras are now inappropriate. Volunteer organisations give helpful advice about bras, swimwear and other clothing (see Useful websites, e.g. Breast Cancer Care).

focuses the radiation beam is part of newer linear accelerators. This allows the shape of the beam to be adjusted, thus reducing the exposure of healthy tissue to radiation. In addition the dose intensity can be modulated across the beam in such a way as to remove localised overdosage (hot spots) that was common in traditional techniques.

- **Intra-operative radiotherapy (IORT)** – uses a portable electron beam driven device which has the advantage of delivering partial breast irradiation during surgery. This avoids outpatient visits for external beam irradiation and spares adjacent normal tissue, thus minimising local skin reactions. However, it is not widely used within the UK as further investigation and evaluation are necessary to determine the optimum role and indications for its use (Orecchia et al 2005).

- **Brachytherapy** – typically involves the insertion of radioactive implants, usually iridium wires, into the space within the breast where the cancer has been removed. The implants are usually remotely afterloaded by the radiotherapist or physicist so reducing the risk of radiation exposure to staff and visitors to the ward. The iridium implants are withdrawn from the patient after the daily dose of radiation has been given.
- **MammoSite® Radiation Therapy System (RTS)** – brachytherapy in which a single catheter is inserted into the cavity from where the breast cancer was removed. A balloon at the end of the catheter is inflated. The high dose rate brachytherapy pellet is placed in the centre of the balloon, and the surrounding tissue is irradiated. This treatment also takes 5 days, has the same benefits as regular breast brachytherapy and is currently under trial in some centres.

Side-effects of radiotherapy Side-effects are classified as early and late onset (see Ch. 31 for a detailed account). Early effects of radiotherapy can include erythema and soreness of the skin over the treated area and tiredness towards the end of the treatment period.

Photosensitivity of the skin can occur and the skin should be protected, such as with products with high sun protection factor (SPF). Rarely, moist desquamation of the skin may occur.

Late onset effects of radiotherapy include radiation pneumonitis, which presents with a cough, fever and dyspnoea; however, this is quite rare and affects approximately 1% of irradiated breast cancer patients. Other late effects can include damage to the myocardium and the coronary arteries which has long been recognised as a side-effect of radiotherapy to the left side of the chest. Every effort is made to individualise treatment plans to reduce the amount of cardiac tissue subjected to radiation to minimise this toxicity.

Late skin effects can include the development of telangiectasia (dilatation of small blood vessels), which has no physical effects but the permanent mark on the skin is an enduring reminder of the radiotherapy that the woman has been given.

Systemic treatments

Systemic therapy has become increasingly important in the management of breast cancer as women with breast cancer often develop disseminated disease from undetectable micrometastases present at diagnosis. The aim is to destroy micrometastases before they become clinically apparent and this is achieved by using treatments that treat the whole body and not just the primary cancer. Treatments include chemotherapy (using cytotoxic drugs), hormone manipulation therapy and therapies that target cancer cells.

Neoadjuvant (primary) chemotherapy For women presenting with a tumour greater than 3 cm in size, many UK breast units will offer neoadjuvant chemotherapy in order to shrink the tumour prior to surgery (Abraham et al 2005). In some circumstances, often for older women, hormone therapy is used to achieve the same result. Any micrometastases that may have spread from the original tumour are also systemically treated by the chemotherapy or hormone therapy.

Throughout the chemotherapy (up to eight courses), the tumour size will be assessed clinically. However, this can be very subjective so a more accurate assessment can be undertaken using ultrasound or magnetic resonance imaging (MRI). When the optimum response to the medication has been achieved, surgery is performed and in some cases breast conservation can be achieved. Sometimes, at the end of the chemotherapy, the tumour is no longer detectable radiologically, but surgery in the previous location of the tumour is always recommended as small lesions are not always seen radiologically. Radiotherapy is then given to the breast or the chest wall to complete the local treatment.

Adjuvant chemotherapy (in addition to surgery) has now become the standard treatment in early breast cancer and has resulted in significant survival benefit. The Early Breast Cancer Trialists' Collaborative Group (EBCTCG 1998) has re-confirmed this survival benefit with the addition of anthracycline-containing regimens over the gold standard cyclophosphamide, methotrexate and 5-fluorouracil (CMF) regimen. These studies have resulted in anthracycline-based chemotherapy being adopted as the standard adjuvant chemotherapy for breast cancer in the UK, which continues to show a modest 4% improvement in absolute 10-year survival compared with non-anthracycline containing regimens (EBCTCG 2005). Indications are that taxane chemotherapy drugs may have an additional survival advantage in adjuvant treatment for moderate and high risk younger patients. Research continues in this area.

The woman can usually have adjuvant chemotherapy administered intravenously over a 4–12-month period as an outpatient. In addition, some 20% of women having chemotherapy will also require treatment with the targeted monoclonal antibody trastuzumab; this is also administered intravenously.

Hormonal therapies Adjuvant hormonal therapies are used to prevent breast cancer cells from receiving stimulation from endogenous oestrogen. Many breast cancers are thought to be stimulated by female sex hormones, particularly oestrogen, and are known as oestrogen receptor positive, or ER positive. Hormonal therapies act by inhibiting oestrogen synthesis, or blocking its effect on cells. They include:

- **Ovarian suppression** – is particularly relevant for premenopausal women who have an oestrogen-positive tumour. Suppression may be achieved by bilateral oophorectomy or radiation ablation of the ovaries. For younger women who have not had a child, luteinising hormone releasing hormone (LHRH) agonists such as goserelin can be used. Goserelin given as a subcutaneous (s.c.) bolus injection every 28 days prevents ovarian oestrogen production. Once goserelin is discontinued, the effect is usually reversed. However, the optimum duration of LHRH agonists is not yet known, and the current recommendation is for 2 years of goserelin (Abraham et al 2005).
- **Tamoxifen** – a selective oestrogen receptor modulator (SERM) that inhibits the growth of breast cancer cells by competitive antagonism of oestrogen at the ER receptor site. Tamoxifen also exhibits partial oestrogen agonist

activity which can be both beneficial and detrimental. Tamoxifen prevents bone demineralisation but does increase the risk of endometrial cancer and venous thromboembolism (VTE). In addition to reducing rates of disease relapse and death, tamoxifen also reduces the risk of developing a contralateral breast cancer. Treatment should continue for 5 years as this has been shown to be more beneficial than 2 years (Belfiglio et al 2005). Tamoxifen is given orally and can be used for both pre- and postmenopausal women. Women should be informed about the side-effects that include menopausal signs and symptoms with hot flushes, night sweats, vaginal dryness/discharge and increased risk of VTE. However, these effects are outweighed by the benefits of treatment.

- **Aromatase inhibitors (AIs)** – drugs that markedly reduce the concentration of circulating oestrogen levels in postmenopausal women. They work by inhibiting or inactivating aromatase, the enzyme required to synthesise oestrogens from androgenic substrates. In contrast to tamoxifen, these drugs lack agonist activity (Smith & Dowsett 2003). They are ineffective in premenopausal women and should only be given to women who are postmenopausal. AIs may be non-steroidal or steroidal. Anastrozole and letrozole are in the non-steroidal group and both agents have been evaluated extensively in women with metastatic breast cancer and approved in Europe for the first line treatment of ER-positive metastatic breast cancer (see p. 262). The steroidal AI exemestane is approved for hormonal therapy in women with metastatic breast cancer after disease progression. Preclinical studies have suggested that it may have a different toxicity profile to the non-steroidal agents; however, these findings have yet to be confirmed in definitive clinical studies.

Targeted therapies These are treatments directed against specific molecular targets considered to be involved in the development of cancer cells (Giaccone & Soria 2007), that is, therapies that target specific characteristics of cancer cells that allow them to grow in a rapid or abnormal way. The main targets are the human epidermal growth factor receptor-2 (HER2), tyrosine kinases and angiogenesis (formation of new blood vessels). Targeted therapies aim to limit toxicities whilst selectively acting against cancer cells. Cancers which are HER2 positive have been found to be more aggressive which leads to a poor prognosis. Overexpression of HER2 can result in inappropriate cellular responses such as deactivation of normal apoptosis (cell death) involved in cellular migration, which can lead to distant metastases. Two methods for evaluating the level of HER2 have evolved to discover whether cancer cells overexpress these receptors: immunohistochemistry which is used to determine HER2 overexpression, and fluorescence in situ hybridisation (FISH) which is used to determine the HER2 copy number.

One of the most successful targeted therapies for breast cancer has been trastuzumab, a humanised monoclonal antibody specifically able to block the function of HER2. Trastuzumab has been shown in several large randomised controlled trials to be highly effective in reducing the risk of relapse.

The Herceptin® Adjuvant (HERA) trial study was designed to assess the efficacy of trastuzumab compared with observation alone in women with node-positive (regardless of tumour size) or node-negative HER2-positive breast cancer (Piccart-Gebhart et al 2005). A meta-analysis by NICE (2006b) showed that the addition of trastuzumab led to a 33% relative improvement in overall survival and a 50% relative improvement in disease-free survival. Unfortunately, studies also showed a relative increase in cardiac toxicity, therefore careful monitoring of the patient's cardiac function should be observed. At present, most oncology units are following the HERA study protocol, i.e. cardiac monitoring every 12 weeks.

▷ Nursing management and health promotion: adjuvant therapy

Postoperatively, the woman will probably attend a surgical outpatient clinic where she will hear the results of her surgery, i.e. number of lymph nodes involved with cancer, the size and grade of the tumour and its oestrogen status, all factors that will determine the need for adjuvant treatment. These results are discussed at an MDM where decisions will be made about an appropriate treatment plan.

Breast cancer mortality has declined since 1995, attributable in part to changes in treatments available and the delivery of these treatments (Abraham et al 2005).

Information about radiotherapy and drug therapies should be given, as relevant, both verbally and in writing. The woman should understand why adjuvant treatment has been advised, for what period and at what intervals it will be administered, and what the side-effects may be. At this point the woman may be invited to join a research study, as several current national trials looking into effectiveness of different types of chemotherapy and hormone therapy are ongoing. The timing of this decision may put yet another strain on a woman who is already coping with having cancer, so the support and information she receives from her oncologist, ward nurse and breast care nurse will be crucial at this time.

Radiotherapy

All patients should be given clear advice about skin care during their radiotherapy treatment. They should be encouraged to use aqueous cream or E45® to moisturise the area that is receiving the radiotherapy and should wash or shower the area during the treatment period using tepid water and a very mild soap. Patients should wear loose-fitting, cotton clothing next to their skin and avoid wearing underwired bras. Towards the end of treatment some women may need to wear a loose T-shirt or an unstructured bra support. The College of Radiographers (2001) has produced guidelines for minimising, assessing and care of skin reactions.

🔖 **See website Critical thinking question 7.4**

Psychologically it may be quite distressing for the woman to attend a radiotherapy department several times a week, as this is a continual reminder that she has had breast cancer.

Chemotherapy

Several different chemotherapy regimens are used and the woman may have already received chemotherapy preoperatively. Chemotherapy may be administered through a temporary venous cannula or a central venous access device (CVAD) of some type (see Ch. 31 and Further reading, e.g. Dougherty 2006).

Vascular access in patients receiving chemotherapy can be difficult due to the multiple cannulations required to administer a course of adjuvant chemotherapy. Regular venepuncture and cannulation can lead to thrombophlebitis, particularly as the chemotherapy practitioner will be advised to use only one arm to avoid compromising the skin and lymphatics of the arm affected by the breast surgery. Infusion thrombophlebitis can occur at any stage during the lifetime of a short peripheral cannula (Jackson 2003). It is essential therefore that nurses are aware of the importance of assessing the vein and adhering to local policies on venous assessment.

The alternative to temporary venous cannulation is to use a semi-permanent venous access device. CVADs are used mainly to overcome poor peripheral venous access, or for prolonged courses of intravenous chemotherapy.

Outline of side-effects (see Chs 11, 31)

The woman should be reassured that adjuvant chemotherapy regimens used in breast cancer tend to have milder side-effects than those used for other cancers and can usually be managed by the outpatient department.

Nausea is commonly experienced but is normally mild and can be controlled by antiemetics, including 5-HT_3 antagonists such as ondansetron or granisetron. Vomiting should be rare.

Breast cancer chemotherapy regimens containing an anthracycline such as adriamycin or epirubicin will cause total alopecia which can be very stressful for women. Scalp cooling using ice caps can restrict the amount of chemotherapy reaching the hair follicles and so may prevent complete hair loss, although the hair may thin and become drier and of poorer quality. Gentle shampoos should be used, and perms, colourants and the use of heated tongs should be avoided.

Myelosuppression (bone marrow suppression) occurs with all cytotoxic drugs, but it is rare for neutropenia to be severe or for septic shock to result. Nevertheless, every patient should be advised about good oral hygiene and the avoidance of obvious sources of infection. If the woman's temperature rises above normal she is usually advised to contact the hospital (see Chs 11, 31).

Fatigue is the most common problem and can be quite debilitating for the woman. Generally it is worst in the middle of a month's treatment cycle, when blood counts are at their lowest level.

Stomatitis/mucositis and a susceptibility to mouth ulcers can be helped by pain relief, using a soft toothbrush, bactericidal mouthwashes and antifungal drugs.

Menstrual cycle disruption is usual, with menstruation becoming irregular or stopping, and this is yet another assault on the woman's body. Menopausal symptoms, e.g. hot flushes, may be experienced, but if the woman is in her early 30s there is a 90% chance of menstrual cycles returning after chemotherapy finishes. Women in their early 40s are much more likely to have an early climacteric/menopause (see pp. 206–208).

Endocrine therapy

For most of the endocrine therapies pre- and postmenopausal women will usually experience menopausal symptoms, which can be very distressing. These may include fatigue, hot flushes, night sweats, joint pain, headaches and insomnia. Preparations containing gamma linolenic acid can help with such symptoms; otherwise the woman's consultant or GP can prescribe medication to reduce the hot flushes. Unfortunately these remedies are not without side-effects and many women prefer to manage without such intervention.

Gastric upsets are uncommon but may occur, particularly if the tamoxifen tablets are not taken with food. Very occasionally, thrombocytopenia occurs and women should be advised to report increased bruising or bleeding from the gums. A small increase in VTE is associated with tamoxifen use and women must inform their clinician of any new pain and swelling in their calves or sudden and unusual shortness of breath. Many women complain about an increase in weight, particularly around the abdomen, soon after starting the tablets. This may be due in part to fluid retention and in part to a reduction in physical activity following surgery. Other rare and more serious side-effects include endometrial cancer and cataract formation. Any abnormal vaginal bleeding should be investigated as well as any rapid deterioration in eyesight.

As AIs lower endogenous circulating oestrogen levels a consequence for some women is osteoporosis. Women receiving an AI should be assessed for risk factors for osteoporosis, including a family history, fragility fractures, calcium intake, smoking and alcohol use, body mass index and exercise. Bone density should be measured at baseline and women with T-scores greater than −2.5SD (osteoporosis) should receive calcium/vitamin D, and a bisphosphonate (see Ch. 10). They should also be advised on weight bearing exercise. Women with bone densities between −1.5 and −2.5SD (osteopenia) should have an adequate intake of calcium and vitamin D with regular bone density measurements as an essential, ongoing assessment.

Targeted therapies

The biological therapy trastuzumab can cause several side-effects for some, but not all, patients. These include fatigue, which certainly occurs during the treatment but can continue for up to a year, a flu-like reaction of fever, chills, rash and nausea, headache, breathlessness, wheezing, diarrhoea and myalgia. Side-effects occur in 50% of women after the first treatment but usually decrease after the first few treatments. Diarrhoea can affect about a third of the people who receive this treatment but is usually mild and can be helped with anti-diarrhoeal tablets. Congestive cardiac failure is a rare side-effect but the drug should not be given to a patient with congestive cardiac failure or angina that requires treatment.

Follow-up for asymptomatic women

The aims of follow-up should be to detect and treat local recurrence and adverse effects of therapy (NICE 2002). Intensive follow-up, designed to detect metastatic disease before symptoms develop, is not beneficial and routine tests to detect metastatic cancer are not necessary because they do not improve quality of life or survival.

Many breast units within the UK now adhere to this and have developed systems for patient-led follow-up where women no longer attend an outpatient breast clinic but have access to breast care nurses who will arrange an appointment if there is any cause for concern. The NICE (2002) document also suggests that routine follow-up should not continue for more than 3 years unless women are involved in trials where the protocol requires long-term follow-up.

Special populations and breast cancer

Breast cancer can affect both sexes and all ages, although it is predominantly a disease of women over 50 years of age. This section outlines the needs of special populations including men, older women, young women, and women from black and ethnic minority groups.

Male breast cancer

Male breast cancer (MBC) is rare and accounts for less than 1% of all breast cancers (Cancer Research UK 2009c). Male breast anatomy is the same as that of the female breast; it is the absence of hormonal stimulation which accounts for the developmental and physiological differences. However, the disease is similar in both male and female. It is generally accepted that male and female breast cancers are the same disease. All histological types reported among women also occur among men, and BRCA2 gene mutations have been reported with the same frequency in the tumour tissue of both men and women. However, the aetiology of male breast cancer is still obscure. Klinefelter's syndrome (see Ch. 5) has been reported to increase the risk of MBC, but this rare syndrome accounts for only a small proportion of all MBCs. Previous breast or testicular disease and gynaecomastia have also been reported. Other studies suggested an increased risk in occupational exposure to high temperature and electromagnetic fields (Johnson et al 2002). Although several risk factors for MBC have been identified, increasing age remains relevant as MBC is usually diagnosed in men aged between 60 and 70 years (National Cancer Institute 2008).

Diagnosis of MBC is made by triple assessment as in symptomatic women. The majority of MBCs are invasive ductal carcinomas which are ER positive, and treatment for male breast cancer is similar to that of females. Surgery is the mainstay of treatment and mastectomy the treatment of choice due to the paucity of breast tissue in males. Diagnosis is often at a later stage where the skin and underlying fascia is involved (Souhami & Tobias 2005). Adjuvant radiotherapy, chemotherapy, endocrine therapy and targeted therapies are also used.

It is important that nurses recognise the particular problems that men may experience when they are diagnosed and treated for breast cancer. Information about breast cancer is aimed at women which can make it difficult or embarrassing for men to talk about what is primarily a female condition. Hormone therapy causes similar side-effects such as hot flushes or reduced libido. This can threaten a man's sexuality and will require particular support from the nurses who care for him (Burnet 2001).

Breast cancer in older women

Older women account for more than half of new cases of breast cancer. Breast cancer is a major health problem in older women. Around 30% of all breast cancers occur in patients aged more than 70 years, and 48% in those aged over 65 years. These percentages are likely to increase in line with the ageing population (Wyld & Reed 2003). The biology of breast cancers in women aged 70 years or over differs from other age groups: oestrogen receptor positivity increases with age, HER2 expression reduces and tumours tend to be of a lower grade (Wyld 2007). This indicates that breast cancer survival in the older woman is similar to survival rates for the general population. However, chronic co-morbidities increase with age and breast cancer is not always the most significant threat to life in this age group (Aapro 2002). It is therefore necessary to evaluate co-morbidities and tumour biology prior to making treatment decisions. As a result, breast cancer treatments in older women show reduced rates in surgery, radiotherapy and chemotherapy as well as targeted therapies. Surgery is the mainstay of treatment, but for older women with co-morbidities and ER-positive tumours it may provide little benefit for those who have had a good response to endocrine therapy alone. However, women who are fit and healthy should be offered standard surgical therapies.

Most chemotherapy trials exclude women aged 70 years or over, therefore it is difficult to evaluate the effectiveness of chemotherapy in this age group. However, the ACTION trial in the UK aims to establish whether chemotherapy is of benefit in older women (Wyld 2007).

Caring for older women with breast cancer can pose a challenge which emphasises the importance of designing a care plan that takes into account the individual's health status, wishes, desires and needs for quantity plus quality of life.

Breast cancer in young women

Approximately 20% of breast cancer cases occur in women under 50 years of age. It is the commonest cancer diagnosed in women under 35 years of age; however, there are very few women diagnosed in their teens or early 20s (Cancer Research UK 2009c). Young women tend to have larger tumours at diagnosis than older women. This is in part because they have denser breast tissue, which makes it difficult to detect a lump, and also because breast tissue is influenced by cyclical hormonal changes making diagnosis more difficult. Compared to older women, breast cancer in young women is usually more aggressive, often of a higher grade and tending to be ER negative. Their HER2 status is similar or slightly increased compared to older women (Wyld 2007). Treatment for breast cancer in younger women includes the multimodality treatments of surgery, chemotherapy, radiotherapy, endocrine and targeted therapies. Due to the adverse prognostic features displayed by these tumours, young women are much more likely to be treated with chemotherapy, which has significantly contributed to improved survival in younger women but is also associated with acute and long-term side-effects such as a chemically induced menopause and infertility (Knobf 2006). These issues raise questions about reduced bone density caused by loss of circulating oestrogen and whether the young woman wants to become pregnant or not after treatment. Young women can have a significantly poor prognosis, in part due to the more aggressive tumour. Premature menopause,

Box 7.23 Reflection

A young woman with breast cancer

Lucy is a 33-year-old single woman in a long-term relationship. She has just been diagnosed with breast cancer and will require adjuvant chemotherapy after her surgery. Adjuvant chemotherapy has contributed to the overall survival in women with early breast cancer, but it is also associated with long-term side-effects, often causing temporary (and for some, permanent) menopause.

Activities

- Think about the symptoms of a temporary menopause and how you could explain them to Lucy.
- Reflect on how nurses might help Lucy and her partner to deal with a breast cancer diagnosis and treatment and its effects as well as her recovery.

sexual dysfunction, infertility and adverse body image are well-documented effects of systemic cancer therapy. Therefore, good information, communication, counselling and support are essential interventions for young women treated for breast cancer (Box 7.23).

Breast cancer in black and ethnic minority women

A study by Jack et al (2009) involving 35 000 women identified some significant differences in breast cancer incidence, stage at diagnosis, treatment and survival in women belonging to different racial/ethnic groups. Box 7.24 provides readers with an opportunity to consider these differences and reflect on how the care of black and ethnic minority women can be improved.

Breast reconstruction

There are several surgical procedures but these usually involve silicone breast implants or the transfer of a skin and tissue flap from another part of the woman's body (autologous).

Box 7.24 Evidence-based practice

Breast cancer in black and ethnic minority women

Jack et al (2009) report that black and Asian women are significantly more likely than white women to be diagnosed with breast cancer at a stage where cancer cells have spread to other areas of the body. Evidence of cancer spread at diagnosis was found in 17% of Pakistani women and in 15% of black African women, whereas spread had occurred in 7% of white women.

Activities

- Access the study by Jack et al (2009) and consider the reasons why black and Asian women are more likely to present with more advanced breast cancer.
- What differences in the type of breast cancer and age at presentation between groups are identified in the study?
- Consider with your mentor how you would raise awareness of breast cancer symptoms in black and Asian women and increase the uptake of screening.

See website for further content

Reconstruction is undertaken for several reasons: cosmetic, when the woman feels her breasts are too small; where one breast has failed to develop at puberty; when the woman has a bilateral prophylactic mastectomy due to genetic predisposition to breast cancer; or following breast cancer surgery in which a significant part, or all, of a breast was removed.

Immediate reconstruction can be undertaken with the mastectomy, or as a delayed reconstructive procedure. Reconstruction following breast cancer surgery aims to create a breast form which resembles the woman's other breast as closely as possible in size, shape and consistency. Complete symmetry when the woman is naked is not possible to achieve but the aim of the surgery should be that any differences are slight when she is wearing a bra.

Every woman should be offered the opportunity of breast reconstruction, immediate or delayed, if she needs a mastectomy as part of her breast cancer treatment (NICE 2002). Breast reconstruction may help to reduce the psychological or emotional problems experienced by women after surgery or it may enable a woman to undergo a mastectomy which she would have otherwise found intolerable (Hart 1996).

The presence of bone metastases should not prohibit a woman from having reconstructive surgery if she perceives that this will improve her quality of life and she is generally well enough to undergo surgery. Only uncontrolled metastatic breast cancer should be considered an absolute contraindication to breast reconstruction (see Further reading, e.g. Harmer 2003).

Fungating breast tumours

Rarely, a breast tumour recurs at the original site, or the woman presents with a cancer that has invaded the skin surface to cause ulceration. The resulting wound may be deep or superficial but will be unsightly and distressing for the patient. As the cancer outgrows its blood supply there is central tissue necrosis and possible infection with excessive wound exudate, bleeding and unpleasant odour. Nerve involvement can cause pain and itching, again very distressing for the patient and presenting a care challenge.

Because of better treatments and public understanding of breast cancer the associated signs and symptoms of a fungating tumour are an unusual occurrence, but it is something that nurses should be aware of as much can be done to alleviate the suffering and to manage these rare but unpleasant open wounds (see Ch. 23).

Medical management would consider any previous surgery and radiotherapy but both can be used again with great success to control the disease locally. Also, hormone treatment and chemotherapy can be used for systemic disease control and to control the active tumour (see Useful websites, e.g. Macmillan Cancer Support).

Breast cancer related lymphoedema

Lymphoedema can occur at any time after the diagnosis and treatment of breast cancer. It may be related to the presence of tumour or subsequent surgery and radiotherapy. Lymphoedema is the accumulation of protein-rich fluid in the interstitial spaces in the tissue of a limb or other body area.

It is worth considering it in some depth as it is a condition that has been greatly improved by better understanding and nursing intervention.

PATHOPHYSIOLOGY

Lymphoedema results from defective lymph drainage due to tissue fibrosis, disease or a congenital disorder. Those affected may have an uncomfortable, unsightly and functionally impaired arm, often with some swelling of the adjacent chest and back (Pain et al 2005). Understandably, this condition can cause considerable physical and psychological distress (Woods 2003).

The aetiology of breast cancer related lymphoedema (BCRL) is poorly understood and multifactorial although it is thought that BCRL is caused by surgical damage to the axilla that leads to interruption of lymph vessels draining the arm.

Axillary surgery to remove some or all of the axillary lymph nodes, or axillary radiotherapy, increases the risk of lymphoedema of the limb on the affected side. Scarring from these treatments will occlude or narrow many lymph vessels thereby reducing lymph drainage from the arm. For most women, the drainage remains adequate and collateral vessels may develop to increase drainage. However, lymphoedema may develop weeks, months or years after surgery or radiotherapy, sometimes following a wound complication, cording, infection or injury, but often without an obvious reason. It may remain mild or gradually progress until the arm is so heavy that it is difficult to lift and to use. Over time, fibrosis within the tissue of the arm may occur, causing hardness. There is also a higher risk of infection and cellulitis, as the protein-rich fluid is an ideal culture for bacteria.

Disease within the axillary region which obstructs lymph flow will also cause lymphoedema, such as recurrent cancer or late presentation with advanced cancer of the breast. Signs of venous obstruction are sometimes seen, commonly as colour changes of the arm and distended veins visible on the upper arm and chest wall.

Brachial plexus nerve damage is rarely seen but may also result from radiation fibrosis or cancer infiltration of the nerve plexus, causing weakness, paraesthesia or nerve pain.

MEDICAL MANAGEMENT

Treatment options are limited and depend on whether the lymphoedema has been caused by fibrosis or by axillary disease. Assessment may include CT scanning and colour Doppler ultrasound to determine the amount of scarring, venous obstruction or disease.

Where venous obstruction is due to a thrombosis, anticoagulation therapy should be initiated. In the case of axillary disease, surgery to remove as much of the cancer as possible may be of use by reducing the obstruction of lymph and venous flow. However, chemotherapy or endocrine therapies, which cause less disruption to normal structures than surgery, are more likely to be used. Analgesics ranging from paracetamol to opiates will be used as required. If, however, the pain is due to brachial plexus damage, it is unlikely to respond adequately to opiates since nerve pain is only partly opiate responsive. Other drug groups may be required (e.g. anticonvulsants, antidepressants, corticosteroids and NSAIDs) for nerve pain (see Ch. 19).

The risk of infection in a swollen limb is high and can result in cellulitis. A small cut or insect bite may provide an entry point for infection and potentially severe cellulitis requiring intravenous antibiotics (Box 7.21, p. 259). If cellulitis is recurrent, patients are often given a prescription or a supply of antibiotics to ensure treatment as soon as infection occurs.

 ## Nursing management and health promotion: lymphoedema

Treatment effectiveness is measured in terms of the reduction in size and weight of the arm, and for most women this is possible. However, sometimes all that can be done is to increase the softness and movement of the arm and to reduce the discomfort, but these improvements can represent a substantial increase in the quality of life for the patient.

Nursing interventions must be preceded by an assessment to identify the physical and psychosocial needs of the individual patient.

Nursing interventions

Nursing interventions aim to:

- reduce arm size
- improve the use of the arm
- improve the comfort of the arm
- improve the shape of the arm.

There are now four recognised elements to the management of lymphoedema:

- skin care
- exercise and movement
- lymph drainage
- external containment.

It is very important to explain clearly the aim of treatment and to promote a realistic expectation of outcome. Although therapy is aimed at control rather than cure, the patient who is given sufficient information and is encouraged to participate in treatment is likely to adopt a more positive attitude towards her situation and compliance can therefore be maintained.

Skin care The emphasis is on the importance of skin hygiene and care. Advice given at the time of the axillary surgery should be re-emphasised. The skin of the arm should be moisturised as dry skin is less supple and tiny breaks in the skin occur through which bacteria can enter, increasing the risk of infection.

Exercise and movement Lymph drainage can be promoted through movement and appropriate exercise of the arm as muscle contraction enhances lymph drainage (Woods 2003).

Lymph drainage Manual lymph drainage (MLD) is a specialised massage technique carried out by trained MLD therapists. Simple lymphatic drainage (SLD) has been developed from MLD for use by women and their relatives. The aims of SLD as with MLD are to:

- stimulate normal lymph drainage
- 'milk' fluid away from the congested areas
- improve superficial lymph drainage (Woods 2003).

SLD massage is light, aiming to stimulate the lymphatic vessels in the skin. Deeper massage increases blood flow to the muscles, causing more fluid to accumulate in the tissues, and would thus be counterproductive.

Lymph tape is another form of lymph drainage whereby a special tape is applied to the affected area. A thin, porous cotton fabric tape applied correctly will lift the skin to increase the space between the skin and muscle. Muscle contraction and relaxation promotes lymph flow and decreases pain. The tape is left on for 3–5 days and is helpful in decreasing swelling of difficult and stubborn areas, especially the breast following radiotherapy. The therapist initially applies the tape and then teaches the woman to do this independently.

External containment (compression sleeves or bandages)
External containment restricts lymph build-up and promotes absorption of fluid. It supports muscles to maximise the pump action and thereby increases lymphatic drainage.

For women with severe lymphoedema, lymphorrhoea (leakage of lymph), skin problems or difficulty using a sleeve, compression bandaging is the treatment of choice.

Low-stretch bandages are used to bandage the fingers and hand before the arm is encased. The pressure applied should be graduated, greater pressure being applied at the lower end of the limb. The bandages should be reapplied daily. Due to the size of the arm and of the bandages required, the woman may need to be admitted to hospital which also affords an opportunity for physiotherapy, occupational therapy and psychological support. However, community nurses experienced in this technique can undertake compression bandaging in the patient's home. This is particularly helpful for women with advanced disease and those who feel unwell. Bandaging of a large arm may provide great comfort and relief from pain even if it is unlikely to reduce arm size.

Several ready-made compression sleeves are available for lymphoedema management. Compression must be fairly strong (around 40 mmHg) if it is to be effective. Supports such as Tubigrip® are not adequate. Sleeves may be difficult to put on but once fitted are supportive and comfortable. They should be worn during the day when the patient is most active. The sleeves should not be allowed to form creases, as this will cause ridging in the swollen tissue. The sleeve, easily laundered, may need to be worn for several weeks, during which time the patient must be monitored regularly to assess progress. If the oedema is modest, it may be possible for the arm to return to its normal size.

Previously, attempts to reduce the size and weight of the arm by surgical removal of tissue have had very little success and have frequently caused further problems with infection, swelling and pain as well as extensive scarring. Liposuction has been used for limb lymphoedema; however, it is important to note that liposuction does not correct the lymphatic failure and patients will still require compression hosiery.

Metastatic breast cancer

Approximately 10% of women diagnosed with breast cancer have metastatic disease at clinical presentation, but metastasis can also occur months or years after presentation.

The majority of patients who relapse do so within the first two years of diagnosis. In the UK we have chosen not to screen for metastatic disease at the time of diagnosis or at subsequent follow-up visits unless there are clinical indications.

If there is suspicion of metastatic disease, positron emission tomography (PET) and CT scanning are recommended if plain X-rays and ultrasound are not diagnostic (NICE 2009b).

Once breast cancer has metastasised systemically the disease is no longer considered curable and the aim of treatment is to increase the woman's survival whilst providing the best quality of life possible.

PATHOPHYSIOLOGY

Breast cancer appears to spread by direct invasion into the surrounding tissue and via the lymphatic and arteriovenous systems to distant areas. If untreated, local invasion of the breast cancer will cause ulceration, fixation to the chest wall and oedema of the arm. It may also, in extreme circumstances, erode blood vessels, causing haemorrhage, and invade the ribs or lungs and pleura, causing pleural effusion. Invasion of the brachial plexus can cause severe pain with functional and sensory loss in the arm. Invasion of the cutaneous nerves causes irritation and burning pain in the affected area. Because such aggressive local disease is not necessarily accompanied by metastatic spread, a woman may survive for many years with these problems.

Spread to distant sites is common but may not become apparent for months or many years after the initial diagnosis and treatment. Metastases can occur anywhere and do not follow a systematic course. However, metastatic spread may be first discernible in the axillary, and then supraclavicular lymph nodes, following the pattern of lymphatic drainage from the breast. The most common sites of distant metastases are bone, lungs, liver and brain. Less frequently, metastases occur in the ovaries and mediastinum and, rarely, in the oesophagus, stomach, intestine and pericardium. Breast cancer has a predilection for spreading to bone, and bone metastasis is one of the major causes of increased morbidity and eventual mortality in breast cancer patients. Table 7.5 outlines some common problems associated with metastatic breast cancer (see Ch. 33).

MEDICAL MANAGEMENT

Management involves the use of both local and systemic measures that control and/or palliate symptoms and improve quality of life (see Ch. 33). The first choice of treatment is one that is the least toxic but has the highest response rate. This strategy aims to achieve optimal disease control and maintain remission for as long as possible.

Local treatments include surgery and radiotherapy, and systemic treatments include endocrine therapy, chemotherapy, targeted therapies and the use of bisphosphonates.

Local treatments

Surgery Surgery is rarely used in the management of metastatic breast cancer but can help with locally recurrent disease. If the disease occurs locally following breast conserving surgery and radiotherapy then mastectomy may be indicated provided that the cancer is limited to breast tissue and has not invaded the skin.

Table 7.5 Common problems associated with metastatic breast cancer

SITE OF DISTANT SPREAD	PROBLEMS
Bone	Bone pain Pathological fractures *Hypercalcaemia *Spinal cord compression (SCC)
Bone marrow	Pancytopenia – neutropenia (infection), anaemia and thrombocytopenia (bleeding, bruising)
Lung/pleura	Pleural effusion Reduced lung expansion/dyspnoea with persistent cough
Liver	Right upper quadrant abdominal pain 'Squashed stomach' syndrome Nausea and vomiting Ascites
Skin	Ulceration/fungation Pain/irritation
Central nervous system – cerebral metastases	Confusion, headaches, nausea, vomiting, altered behaviour, seizures, altered consciousness *Cerebral oedema, raised intracranial pressure
Mediastinum	*Superior vena cava (SVC) obstruction
Axilla/supraclavicular fossa	Lymphoedema Brachial plexus pain and paraesthesia/paralysis of arm

*Oncological emergencies

Radiotherapy Radiotherapy is sometimes used to relieve bone pain and in the oncological emergencies such as spinal cord compression (SCC), cerebral oedema and superior vena cava obstruction, where tumour pressure must be reduced quickly. Corticosteroids, usually dexamethasone, are used with radiotherapy to reduce the oedema in tissues surrounding the tumour and hence relieve pressure further.

Systemic treatments

Hormonal therapies Women who have ER-positive breast cancer survive longer after recurrence than women with ER-negative breast cancer. Tissue from the recurrent tumour should be tested for ER status where possible. Hormonal therapies that may be used include those also used as adjuvant treatment for early stage breast cancer (see pp. 262–263).

Tamoxifen may be indicated, but there is evidence that anastrozole (an AI) may have superior efficacy and tolerability in the first line treatment for postmenopausal women with advanced breast cancer (Nabholtz et al 2003). Although AIs are not to be used for premenopausal women, tamoxifen can be used in both pre- and postmenopausal women.

Goserelin, a luteinising hormone releasing hormone (LHRH) agonist, may be used to suppress oestrogen production in premenopausal women. Side-effects are the symptoms of the climacteric/menopause, e.g. amenorrhoea and hot flushes.

Aromatase inhibitors are used to prevent the conversion of adrenal androgens to oestrogens. This occurs in several tissues and organs and is the main source of oestrogen in postmenopausal women. The side-effects most commonly reported with the use of AIs include menopausal symptoms and bone loss. Bone loss appears to increase during the first two years of therapy with declining loss thereafter. It is therefore essential that careful monitoring of bone density is undertaken for the early recognition and treatment of osteoporosis.

Chemotherapy (see pp. 262, 264) Chemotherapy is used for women who have had a relapse within two years of diagnosis and are ER negative, or have aggressive disease in the liver or lungs. There are many different chemotherapy drugs used to treat metastatic breast cancer, which can either be used as single therapy or as combination therapy.

Treatment is given as outpatient infusions in a series of treatments known as cycles. The frequency of administration varies. Treatment response is measured, for example, by CT scan, bone scan or X-ray. The decision to continue, change or stop treatment is based on response and the woman's tolerance to treatment.

Chemotherapy can cause unpleasant side-effects (see Ch. 31), but for women with metastatic breast cancer it can also relieve the cancer symptoms thereby improving quality of life.

Targeted therapies (see pp. 263–264) There are currently two different types of targeted therapies used for HER2-positive metastatic breast cancers: trastuzumab (a monoclonal antibody) and the newer lapatinib (a tyrosine kinase inhibitor).

The current recommendations from NICE (2009b) are for women with HER2-positive metastatic breast cancer to have trastuzumab in combination with taxanes (e.g. docetaxel), or monotherapy. Trastuzumab can be given weekly or every 3 weeks and is given as an infusion.

Lapatinib interferes with communication between cancer cells thereby affecting the cancer's ability to develop. Lapatinib is licensed for use in combination with capecitabine in the treatment of advanced or metastatic HER2-positive breast cancer in patients who have previously had therapy with anthracyclines, taxanes and with trastuzumab (British National Formulary [BNF] 2009).

Bisphosphonates Bone is commonly the site for metastatic breast cancer. Once metastatic spread to bone occurs the disease is no longer curable. It can cause weakening of bone structure, pain and pathological fractures with potential disability.

Bisphosphonates are a group of synthetic analogues of pyrophosphate which bind to calcium. Bisphosphonates help to strengthen bone and reduce the risk of fractures. They can also help to relieve bone pain and have reduced the need for radiotherapy in managing bone pain. Often such pain is poorly localised and is described as a burning, aching, gnawing or stabbing which is unrelieved by rest. Other sequelae of metastatic bone disease (MBD) are SCC caused by pathological fractures of the vertebrae and hypercalcaemia, both of which are oncological emergencies.

The bisphosphonates usually prescribed for MBD in breast cancer are zoledronic acid and ibandronic acid.

Zoledronic acid is given by intravenous infusion, once a month or so. However, this is given on an outpatient basis and careful monitoring of renal function is required prior to administration.

Ibandronic acid can be given orally, or by intravenous infusion. Patients are advised that they should sit or stand upright to take the tablet, which should be swallowed whole with ample water. The tablet is taken on an empty stomach before breakfast. The patient needs to be in an upright position (standing or sitting) and fast for at least 30 min or 60 min depending on the dose (BNF 2009).

Patients need to be advised that there might be a temporary increase in bone pain, known as tumour flare, following intravenous administration and they may require analgesics until this subsides. Very rarely, bisphosphonates can cause jaw necrosis and patients are advised to inform their dentist that they are being treated with bisphosphonates. There are several other side-effects associated with bisphosphonates and readers are directed to the BNF or their own national formulary.

Bisphosphonates are usually given for as long as they are working. If the bisphosphonate is given to reduce high levels of calcium in hypercalcaemia it may only be given when required.

 ## Nursing management and health promotion: metastatic breast cancer

Nurses are paramount to the care of patients with metastatic breast cancer and should be involved in a holistic assessment which should address the physical, psychological and social impact of the disease, with particular consideration of the patient's own perception of these problems. The difficulties faced by the patient are likely to be determined in part by the site(s) of cancer spread. It should be remembered that medical priorities will not necessarily match the personal priorities of the patient, and the decision to treat should be discussed carefully.

The reaction of the patient and her family to the news of progressive disease should be sensitively explored, and the nurse should assess how well they are coping. For many, the discovery of metastatic disease is more devastating than the original diagnosis of breast cancer, as the realisation dawns that treatment is now aimed at controlling rather than curing the illness. The patient and her family may once again experience shock, anger, denial, depression and despair as they try to come to terms with the implications of the diagnosis. They may feel that they had 'paid the price' at the time of the original diagnosis and that disease recurrence is very unfair. Even where cure is no longer possible, the philosophy of rehabilitation and health promotion will remain at the centre of care, so that the highest quality of life can be maintained for as long as possible.

Palliative care

Despite remarkable advances in screening, early detection, diagnosis and treatment of breast cancer it remains a disease with significant mortality. Nursing and medical staff have a responsibility for the provision of individual care for patients approaching the end of life and their families (see Ch. 33).

The role of the clinical nurse specialist in breast care

The role of the clinical nurse specialist (CNS) in breast care has developed largely in response to the recognition that women with breast cancer benefit from the support and expertise of nurses specialising in this area (NICE 2002). It must be stressed that the CNS provides an additional service to that provided by hospital and community nursing staff, and not an alternative to that service. The CNS functions as a resource for patients, their families and other nurses.

Ideally, the clinical involvement of the CNS with the patient will begin at the time of diagnosis and prior to hospital admission. This may involve meeting patients in screening assessment units, and requires the cooperation of outpatient nurses and doctors in informing the nurse specialist of new patients. Many CNS follow a limited intervention strategy of seeing patients in hospital before and after their surgery and then visiting them at home or making contact by telephone postoperatively to assess how they are coping. Where problems arise, referral for more in-depth psychological support can be made, but the nurse is likely to continue her involvement with the patient and her family. Because of the increasing complexity of the treatments available, the larger centres may employ more than one nurse specialist, and each is then able to focus her expertise on different aspects of the woman's care.

The CNS also provides a contact point for patients and their family should they require advice or support at any time. She should facilitate communication between the community care team and the hospital but should also be able to use discretion on the patient's behalf if a large number of carers become involved. She will resume contact with patients should metastatic breast cancer develop. Many breast care nurse specialists also provide breast prosthetic and lymphoedema services.

In some breast units across the UK the traditional role of the breast care nurse, which was firmly based in the psychological care of patient with breast cancer, has developed into the nurse practitioner. This newer role incorporates the psychological care of the patient with some physical care of the patient, including the physical assessment and examination of new patients and the follow-up assessment of patients who have finished their initial treatment for breast cancer. The role of the CNS in breast care will continue to develop and respond to the changes in the care and treatment of patients diagnosed and treated for breast cancer.

SUMMARY: KEY NURSING ISSUES

- Nurses need to be aware that breasts have physical, social and emotional aspects and these need to be recognised when caring for a woman with breast disease.
- Breasts are organs of lactation that develop in puberty under the influence of hormones. They can be subject to benign and malignant disease.
- The gold standard treatment for breast cancer incorporates a multidisciplinary approach involving surgery, radiotherapy, chemotherapy, hormonal and targeted biological therapies.
- Breast surgery and specifically breast reconstruction are developing areas of breast cancer treatment.

- The medical treatments for breast cancer aim to treat the local disease and act systemically for any cancer cells that have spread. These treatments are constantly under review, being researched and developed to improve their efficacy and to reduce their side-effects.

- Being diagnosed with breast cancer is a profound experience that affects individuals in different ways, taking into account that individual's context. It is a complex disease and a condition that the individual should, with good nursing care, learn to manage.

⊙ REFLECTION AND LEARNING – WHAT NEXT?

- **Test** your knowledge by visiting the website 🖱 and answering the multiple choice questions and critical thinking questions.

- **Consolidate** your learning by looking at some of the further reading suggestions, references and specialist websites.

- **Revisit** some of the additional material on the website.

- **Consider** what you have learnt and how this will help your professional development.

- **Reflect** on how you can apply this knowledge to the care of your patients.

- **Discuss** your learning with your mentor/supervisor, lecturer and colleagues.

REFERENCES

Aapro M: Progress in the treatment of breast cancer in the elderly, *Ann Oncol* 13:207–210, 2002.

Abraham J, Palmer C, Basu B, et al: Systemic adjuvant therapies for breast cancer. In Querci Della Rovere G, Warren R, Benson JR, editors: *Early Breast Cancer Care. From Screening to Multidisciplinary Management*, ed 2, London, 2005, Taylor & Francis, pp 440–455.

Belfiglio M, Valentini M, Pellegrini F, et al: Twelve year mortality results of a randomized trial of 2 versus 5 years of adjuvant tamoxifen for post menopausal, early stage breast carcinoma patients (SITAM -01), *Cancer* 104(11):2334–2339, 2005.

British National Formulary: 2009. Available online http://bnf.org/bnf/.

Burnet K: *Holistic Breast Care*, London, 2001, Baillière Tindall.

Cancer Research UK: *UK CancerStats Key Facts on Breast Cancer*, 2009a. Available online http://info.cancerresearchuk.org/cancerstats/types/breast/?a=5441.

Cancer Research UK: *UK Cancer Mortality Statistics for Females*, 2009b. Available online http://info.cancerresearchuk.org/cancerstats/mortality/females/.

Cancer Research UK: *UK Breast cancer incidence statistics*, 2009c. Available online http://info.cancerresearchuk.org/cancerstats/types/breast/incidence/.

Chapman D: There's no place like home, *Nurs Stand* 16(11):18–19, 2001.

College of Radiographers: *Summary of intervention for acute radiotherapy induced skin reactions in cancer patients*, 2001. Available online http://www.sor.org/public/document-library/sor_summary_intervention_acute_radiotherapy.pdf.

Crowe DR, Lampejo OT: Malignant tumours of the breast. In Blackwell RE, Grotting JC, editors: *Diagnosis and management of breast disease*, Oxford, 1996, Blackwell Science, pp 200–300.

Department of Health (DH): *The NHS Cancer Plan: a plan for investment, a plan for reform*, 2000. Available online http://www.dh.gov.uk/en/Publicationsandstatistics/Publications/PublicationsPolicyAndGuidance/DH_4009609.

Department of Health (DH): *NHS Cancer Reform Strategy*, 2007. Available online http://www.dh.gov.uk/en/Publicationsandstatistics/Publications/PublicationsPolicyAndGuidance/DH_081006.

Department of Health and Social Security: *Breast cancer screening: the Forrest report*, London, 1986, HMSO.

Dixon JM, Thomas J: Congenital problems and aberrations of normal breast development and involution. In Dixon JM, editor: *The ABC of breast diseases*, ed 3, Oxford, 2006, Wiley-Blackwell/BMJ Publishers, pp 8–14.

Dorval M, Maunsell E, Deschenes L, Brisson J: Type of mastectomy and quality of life for long term survivors, *Cancer* 15(10):2130–2138, 1998.

Duffy SW, Smith RA, Gabe R, et al: Screening for breast cancer, *Surg Oncol Clin N Am* 14(4):671–697, 2005.

Early Breast Cancer Trialists' Collaborative Group (EBCTCG): Polychemotherapy for early breast cancer: an overview of the randomised trials, *Lancet* 352:930–942, 1998.

Early Breast Cancer Trialists' Collaborative Group (EBCTCG): Effects of chemotherapy and hormonal therapy for early breast cancer on recurrence and 15-year survival: and overview of the randomised trials, *Lancet* 365(9472):1687–1717, 2005.

Fallowfield LJ, Hall A, Maguire GP, Baum M: Psychological outcomes of different treatment policies in women with early breast cancer outside a clinical trial, *Br Med J* 301:575–580, 2000.

Giaccone G, Soria J-C: *Targeted Therapies in Oncology*, London, 2007, Informa Healthcare.

Hart D: The psychological outcome of breast reconstruction, *Plast Surg Nurs* 16(3):167–171, 1996.

Iddon J: Breast pain. In Dixon J, editor: *The ABC of breast diseases*, ed 3, Oxford, 2006, Wiley-Blackwell/BMJ Publishers, pp 15–19.

Jack RH, Davies EA, Møller H: Breast cancer incidence, stage, treatment and survival in ethnic groups in South East England, *Br J Cancer* 100:545–550, 2009.

Jackson A: Reflecting on the nursing contribution to vascular access, *Br J Nurs* 12(11):657–665, 2003.

Johnson K, Pan S, Mao Y: The Canadian Cancer Registries Epidemiology Research Group: Risk factors for male breast cancer in Canada, 1994–1998, *Eur J Cancer Prev* 11(3):253–263, 2002.

Knobf M: Reproductive and hormonal sequelae of chemotherapy in women: Premature menopause and impaired fertility can result, effects that are especially disturbing to young women, *Am J Nurs* 103(3):60–65, 2006.

Macleod U, Ross S, Fallowfield L, et al: Anxiety and support in breast cancer: is this different for affluent and deprived women? A questionnaire study, *Br J Cancer* 91:879–883, 2004.

Maguire P, Hopwood P: Psychological aspects. In Dixon J, editor: *The ABC of breast diseases*, ed 3, Oxford, 2006, Wiley-Blackwell/BMJ Publishers, pp 87–92.

Mellon S, Northouse LL, Weiss LK: A population-based study of the quality of life of cancer survivors and their family caregivers, *Cancer Nurse* 29(2):120–131, 2006.

Million Women Study Collaborators: Breast cancer and hormone replacement therapy in the Million Women Study, *Lancet* 362(9382):419–427, 2003.

Nabholtz JM, Bonneterre J, Buzdar A, et al: Anastrozole (Arimidex) versus tamoxifen as first-line therapy for advanced breast cancer in postmenopausal women: survival analysis and updated safety results, *Eur J Cancer* 39(12):1684–1689, 2003.

National Cancer Institute: *Male Breast Cancer Treatment (PDQ®)*, 2008. Available online http://www.cancer.gov/cancertopics/pdq/treatment/malebreast/Patient.

National Institute for Health and Clinical Excellence (NICE): *Guidance on Cancer Services. Improving Outcomes in Breast Cancer (Manual update)*, 2002. Available online http://www.nice.org.uk.

National Institute for Health and Clinical Excellence (NICE): *Familial Breast Cancer. Clinical Guideline CG41*, 2006a. Available online http://www.nice.org.uk/nicemedia/pdf/CG41fullguidance.pdf.

National Institute for Health and Clinical Excellence (NICE): *Trastuzumab for the adjuvant treatment of early-stage HER2-positive breast cancer*, Technology Appraisal Guidance, 2006b. Available online http://www.nice.org.uk/nicemedia/pdf/TA107guidance.pdf.

National Institute for Health and Clinical Excellence (NICE): *Early and locally advanced breast cancer: diagnosis and treatment.* Clinical guidelines CG80, 2009a. Available online http://www.nice.org.uk/nicemedia/pdf/CG80FullGuideline.pdf.

National Institute for Health and Clinical Excellence (NICE): *Advanced breast cancer: diagnosis and treatment.* Clinical guidelines CG81, 2009b. Available online http://www.nice.org.uk/nicemedia/pdf/CG81FullGuideline.pdf.

NHS Breast Screening Programme (NHSBSP): *What does the NHS Breast Screening Programme do?*, 2009. Available online http://www.cancerscreening.nhs.uk/breastscreen/index.html.

Northouse L: The impact of breast cancer on patients and husbands, *Cancer Nurs* 12(5):276–284, 1989.

Orecchia R, Luini A, Gatti G: The role of intraoperative radiotherapy in the conservative management of early stage breast cancer. In Querci Della Rovere G, Warren R, Benson JR, editors: *Early Breast Cancer Care. From Screening to Multidisciplinary Management*, ed 2, London, 2005, Taylor & Francis, pp 422–432.

Pain S, Vowler S, Purushotham A: Axillary vein abnormalities contribute to development of lymphoedema after surgery for breast cancer, *Br J Surg* 92(3):311–315, 2005.

Piccart-Gebhart MJ, Procter M, Leyland-Jones B: Trastuzumab after adjuvant chemotherapy in HER2-positive breast cancer, *N Engl J Med* 353(16):1659–1672, 2005.

Purushotham AD, Britton P, Bobrow L: Benign breast disease. In Borgen PI, Hill A, editors: *Breast diseases*, Georgetown, TX, 2000, Landes Bioscience, pp 192–200.

Sainsbury JRC, Ross GM, Thomas J: Breast cancer. In Dixon J, editor. *The ABC of breast diseases*, ed 3, Oxford, 2006, Wiley-Blackwell/BMJ Publishers, pp 36–42.

Smith I, Dowsett M: Aromatase inhibitors in breast cancer, *N Engl J Med* 348(24):2431–2442, 2003.

Souhami R, Tobias J: *Cancer and its management*, ed 5, Oxford, 2005, Wiley-Blackwell.

START Trialists Group: The UK Standardisation of Breast RT (START) Trial B of RT. Hypofractionation for the treatment of early breast cancer: a randomised trial, *Lancet* 371:1098–1107, 2008.

Tabar L, Yen MF, Vitak B, et al: Mammography service screening and mortality in breast cancer patients: 20 year follow-up before and after introduction of screening, *Lancet* 26:1405–1410, 2003.

Watson M: Breast cancer. Ch 10. In Watson M, editor: *Cancer patient care: psychosocial treatment methods*, Cambridge, 1991, Cambridge University Press.

Woods M: Lymphoedema and breast cancer. In Harmer V, editor: *Breast cancer, nursing care and management*, London, 2003, Whurr, pp 214–232.

Wyld L: Management of breast cancer at the extremes of age, *Breast Cancer Forum* (14), 2007.

Wyld L, Reed M: The need for targeted research into breast cancer in the elderly, *Br J Surg* 90(4):388–399, 2003.

FURTHER READING

Autier P, Boniol M, La Vecchia C, et al: Disparities in breast cancer mortality trends between 30 European countries: retrospective trend analysis of WHO mortality database, *BMJ* 341:c3620, 2010.

Beral V, Peto R: Editorial. UK cancer survival statistics, *BMJ* 341:c4112, 2010.

Borgen PI, Hill A, editors: *Breast diseases*, Georgetown, TX, 2000, Landes Bioscience.

Burnet KL: *Holistic Breast Care*, London, 2001, Baillière Tindall.

Dixon J, editor: *ABC of Breast Diseases*, ed 3, Oxford, 2006, Wiley-Blackwell/BMJ Publishers.

Dougherty L: *Central venous access devices: Care and Management*, Oxford, 2006, Wiley-Blackwell.

Harmer V: *Breast Cancer. Nursing Care and Management*, London, 2003, Whurr Publishers.

Sampson V, Fenlon D: *The Breast Cancer Book. A Personal Guide to Help You Through it and Beyond*, London, 2002, Vermillion.

USEFUL WEBSITES

Adjuvant online – www.adjuvantonline.com

Breast Cancer Care – www.breastcancercare.org.uk

Cancer Research UK – www.cancerresearchuk.org.uk

    (a) TNM breast cancer staging – www.cancerhelp.org.uk/type/breast-cancer/treatment/tnm-breast-cancer-staging

    (b) Number stages of breast cancer – www.cancerhelp.org.uk/type/breast-cancer/treatment/number-stages-of-breast-cancer

Macmillan Cancer Support – www.macmillan.org.uk

NHS Breast Screening Programme – www.cancerscreening.nhs.uk/breastscreen/

Nursing patients with urinary disorders

Martin Steggall

Introduction

This chapter begins with a brief overview of the anatomy and physiology of the urinary system and of the male reproductive organs. With respect to the latter, this chapter complements the anatomy and physiology described in Chapter 7. Common disorders of the kidneys and the rest of the urinary tract and their treatment and nursing care are then described, including infections, significant renal disorders, obstructive disorders and disorders of the bladder. With regard to the male urinary system and reproductive organs, only prostatic disorders and conditions primarily affecting the urethra are considered here. Conditions more directly affecting reproductive and sexual function, such as erectile dysfunction (ED) and testicular cancer, are discussed in Chapter 7.

ANATOMY AND PHYSIOLOGY

The urinary system comprises the kidneys, the ureters, the urinary bladder and the urethra. Its function is to excrete the waste products of metabolism in the form of urine.

The urinary tract

The kidneys – structure

The kidneys are paired organs which lie on the posterior abdominal wall, extending from the twelfth thoracic vertebra to the third lumbar vertebra. Because of the position of the liver, the right kidney is normally slightly lower than the left. Three layers of supportive tissue surround each kidney: an inner fibrous capsule, a middle fatty layer and an outer fascia. This fatty encasement is necessary for maintaining the kidneys in their normal position. Beneath this, a dark outer cortex surrounds a paler medulla, which consists of pale conical striations called the renal pyramids (Figure 8.1).

At the hilus, i.e. the concave medial border of the kidney, blood vessels, lymph vessels and nerves enter and leave the organ. Medial to the hilus is the flat, funnel-shaped renal pelvis, which is continuous with the ureter leaving the hilus. Extending from the pelvis into the medulla are the cup-shaped calyces; these receive from the renal papillae the urine that has been formed in the nephrons and has passed through the collecting tubules. From the calyces

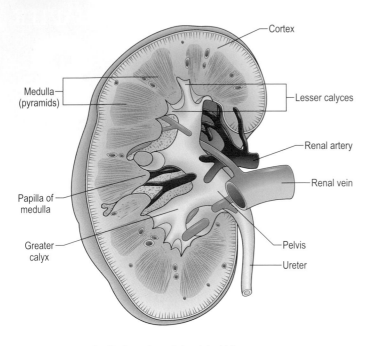

Figure 8.1 Longitudinal section of the right kidney.

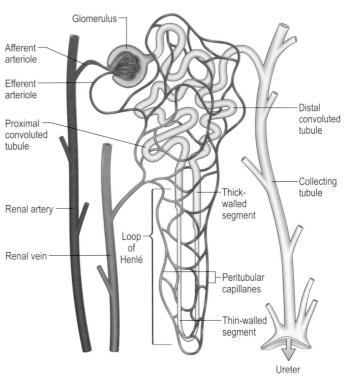

Figure 8.2 Nephron with long loop of Henlé (deep nephron).

the urine passes into the renal pelvis, which acts as a reservoir.

Each kidney receives approximately 625 mL of blood per minute from branches of the renal artery (the two kidneys receive around 25% of cardiac output) and are a key organ in maintaining homeostasis with the functions of:

- production of urine by glomerular filtration, reabsorption (selective) of substances needed by the body such as glucose, and tubular secretion of waste products and other substances in order to maintain fluid, electrolyte and acid–base balance
- control and maintenance of fluid balance (see Ch. 20)
- maintenance of acid–base balance (see Ch. 20)
- control and maintenance of electrolyte balance (see Ch. 20)
- renin production – initiates the renin–angiotensin–aldosterone system concerned in the control of blood pressure (see Ch. 20)
- erythropoietin production, a hormone that stimulates red blood cell production in the bone marrow (erythropoiesis)
- control of calcium reabsorption and vitamin D hydroxylation.

The nephron The functioning units of the kidneys are the nephrons, of which there are two types: cortical and juxtamedullary. The cortical nephrons have their glomeruli in the cortex and have short loops of Henlé, and the juxtamedullary nephrons, with long loops of Henlé, are located in the medulla. Eighty-five per cent of the nephrons are cortical.

A nephron comprises a convoluted tubular system and a tuft of capillaries known as the glomerulus (Figure 8.2). The glomerulus is enclosed in the cup-shaped upper end of the tubule (glomerular or Bowman's capsule). The tubule has three sections: the proximal convoluted tubule (PCT), the loop of Henlé, and the distal convoluted

tubule (DCT). The DCTs merge to form straight collecting tubules; these ultimately terminate at the renal papillae.

Blood supply The renal arteries (see above) branch into smaller and smaller vessels, ultimately becoming wide-bore afferent arterioles which lead into the glomeruli. These capillaries then merge again to form a narrower-bore efferent arteriole which leaves the capsule and subdivides into a second network of peritubular capillaries which supply the renal tubule, and a specialised capillary network (the vasa recta) associated with the loop of Henlé. The capillaries merge into venules and then veins, eventually joining the renal vein, which in turn flows into the vena cava.

Formation of urine

The first process in the production of urine is *filtration*. Arterial blood arriving in the wide-bore afferent arteriole enters the glomerulus within the Bowman's capsule, where substances that are between 3 and 7 nanometres can pass through holes in the capsule endothelium called fenestrations. Note that in health, blood cells and large molecules such as proteins with a molecular weight of 69 000 or above do not pass through the glomerular filtration barrier into the tubule. Once inside the body of Bowman's capsule, the material that has been filtered, which is called filtrate, enters the first section of the PCT, which is the main site of *reabsorption* in the nephron. To maintain a flow of blood into the glomerulus, and therefore to maintain filtration, blood must enter at a constant pressure and constant volume. This is achieved by two structures that line the afferent arteriole, the macula densa and the juxtaglomerular apparatus (JGA). When the blood volume and pressure falls, perhaps as a result of blood loss during surgery, the diameter of the arteriole is reduced, thereby maintaining perfusion pressure. This situation cannot last, i.e. the arteriole cannot continue to get smaller because this would limit the kidney's ability to remove waste products and maintain fluid balance. The constriction of the arteriole is achieved by release of renin. Renin combines with angiotensinogen to form angiotensin I, which is converted by angiotensin-converting enzyme (ACE) into angiotensin II, which is a strong vasoconstrictor. In addition, it stimulates the release of aldosterone (a hormone from the adrenal cortex), which promotes sodium reabsorption, which therefore enhances water reabsorption (see Ch. 20). This, in conjunction with antidiuretic hormone (ADH; also known as arginine vasopressin [AVP] or vasopressin), helps to increase water reabsorption and water intake, and accounts for the fact that urine would normally be expected to be concentrated, i.e. have a specific gravity towards 1.035, in states where fluid loss and dehydration had occurred (see Ch. 20).

Further material covering kidney function – glomerular filtration, selective reabsorption and tubular secretion – is available on the companion website.

See website for further content

See also Thibodeau and Patton (2007) in Further reading.

The functions occurring in the nephron have been summarised in Table 8.1.

The ureters

Urine is conveyed from the pelvis of each kidney to the bladder via the ureters (Figure 8.3). The ureters are tubular structures approximately 25–30 cm long, ranging in diameter from 2 to 8 mm at various points along their length.

Each ureter descends behind the peritoneum from the kidney to the bladder and comes obliquely through the bladder wall before opening into the bladder cavity on its posterior inner surface. This arrangement is such that, when the bladder fills or empties, it is compressed, closing the distal ends of the ureters; in this way, there is no back-flow into the ureters.

Each ureter is composed of three layers of tissue:

- an outer fibrous layer
- a middle layer of smooth muscle; contraction of the muscle layer produces peristaltic movement of urine along the ureter into the bladder
- an inner mucosa of transitional epithelium (urothelium).

The bladder

The bladder is a muscular sac which acts as a reservoir for urine before it is expelled from the body. It lies behind the peritoneum in the pelvic cavity, with its anterior surface located just behind the symphysis pubis. In males, the bladder lies in front of the rectum and is superior to the prostate gland and the urethra. In females, it lies just anterior to the ureters and the superior section of the vagina.

Table 8.1 Summary of processes occurring in the nephron	
LOCATION IN THE NEPHRON	**PROCESSES**
Proximal convoluted tubule (PCT)	The PCT is the site of most *selective reabsorption* – the vast majority of filtrate is reabsorbed in the PCT. Specifically specialised cells that line the PCT reabsorb water (H_2O), electrolytes including bicarbonate (HCO_3^-), glucose and other substances, returning them to the circulation via the vasa recta. Substances such as the waste products urea and creatinine are not reabsorbed as they need to be excreted. At the end of the PCT the filtrate contains water, waste and some electrolytes
Loop of Henlé	The cells change their structure in the loop of Henlé, allowing selective reabsorption of water and sodium (Na^+)
Distal tubule (DCT)	Sodium and chloride (Cl^-) can be reabsorbed here. The hormone aldosterone facilitates the reabsorption of sodium (and with it water) and chloride, but the hormone ADH is required for any reabsorption of water. The cells of the DCT are also concerned with the reabsorption and/or secretion of hydrogen (H^+) and potassium (K^+) ions into the filtrate. This last process, known as *tubular secretion*, is vital in the maintenance of acid–base balance
Collecting duct	Once the filtered fluid gets to the collecting ducts only in exceptional circumstances can water and sodium chloride (NaCl) be reabsorbed. ADH is required to make the collecting ducts more permeable to water in order to produce concentrated urine

The bladder is composed of four layers:

- an outer fibrous adventitia (except where the peritoneum covers the superior surface)
- a muscular layer consisting of smooth muscle arranged in inner and outer longitudinal layers and a middle circular layer
- a submucosal layer of connective tissue
- a mucosal layer of specialised transitional epithelium.

The muscle layer is called the *detrusor* and is an exceptionally strong muscle that contracts during micturition (passing urine). The interior of the bladder has three orifices, two for the ureters and one for the opening of the urethra. This forms a triangle called the trigone (Figure 8.4).

The nerve supply to the bladder is both sensory and motor. Sympathetic nerves arise from T9 to L2 and parasympathetic and somatic nerves from S2 to S4. The motor innervation involves the parasympathetic supply to the detrusor muscle and the sympathetic supply to the trigone. Pudendal nerves under voluntary control supply the external sphincter and muscles of the perineum.

In adults the normal bladder holds around 200–400 mL of urine before the urge to pass urine becomes too great. However, in some patients this volume can be more than 1 L.

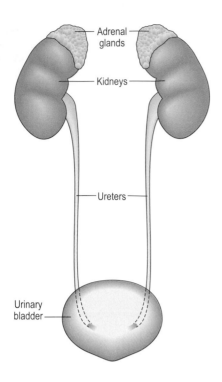

Figure 8.3 The ureters and their relationship to the kidneys and the bladder.

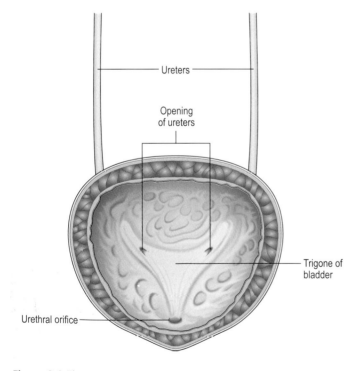

Figure 8.4 The trigone of the bladder.

This is often caused by a blockage in the urinary system or some nerve damage to the spinal cord that controls the bladder. If patients are unable to control the bladder, renal failure can ensue if pressure (i.e. volume) is allowed to build in the bladder.

Micturition is a complex process that involves exchange of nerve information from the brain to the detrusor, coordinating

muscle contraction and opening of the internal and external urinary sphincters, so that urine can flow down the urethra.

Babies are incontinent because the nerve supply from the bladder to the spinal cord is incomplete until the age of around 2 years. This is referred to as the spinal reflex arch.

The urethra

The urethra is the tube that carries the urine from the bladder to the outside world. It has an outer layer of smooth muscle continuous with that of the bladder. Beneath this lies a thin, spongy layer supplied with blood vessels, lymph vessels and nerves. The innermost layer is a lining of mucous membrane continuous with that of the bladder.

In males, the urethra is around 20–25 cm long, has several curves and must pass through the prostate gland. In addition to carrying urine the male urethra also carries semen. It has an internal sphincter composed of smooth muscle which responds to parasympathetic and sympathetic stimulation. The external urethral sphincter lies at the point where the urethra leaves the prostate; this sphincter is composed of skeletal muscle and is hence under voluntary control.

The female urethra is approximately 3–5 cm in length, is straight and is not involved in reproduction. It runs behind the symphysis pubis, opening at the external urethral orifice (the meatus) located between the clitoris and vagina. The passage of urine from the bladder through the urethra is governed by two sphincter muscles. At the opening from the bladder is an internal sphincter composed mainly of elastic tissue and smooth muscle and controlled by autonomic nerves. Near the external urethral orifice the smooth muscle is replaced by striated muscle to form an external sphincter under voluntary control.

The male reproductive organs

The male reproductive organs are those structures responsible for the production, maturation and delivery into the female reproductive tract of spermatozoa necessary for the fertilisation of secondary oocytes (immature ova). The essential organs of this system are the two testes, in which spermatogenesis (spermatozoa production and maturation) occurs (Figure 8.5). The accessory organs which support the reproductive process include:

- ducts – the epididymis, deferent ducts (vas deferens), ejaculatory ducts and urethra, which convey spermatozoa to the exterior
- glands – the seminal vesicles, the prostate gland and the bulbourethral (Cowper's) glands, which produce fluid as a vehicle for sperm
- supporting structures – the scrotum, penis and spermatic cords (Figure 8.5).

The testes

The testes are paired oval organs suspended in the scrotum by the spermatic cords and are encased in three layers of tissue. The complex two-stage process of spermatogenesis (*spermatocytogenesis* – production of haploid spermatids, and *spermiogenesis* – a maturation stage) required to produce mature viable spermatozoa takes place in the testes. The testes also produce androgens (masculinising hormones), the

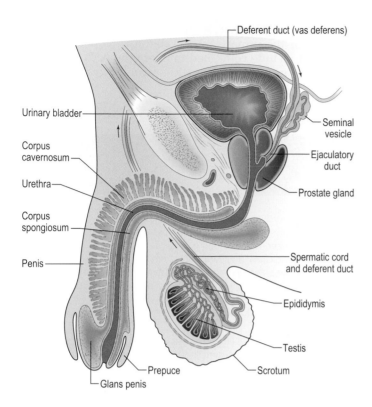

Deferent duct (vas deferens)

Urinary bladder

Corpus cavernosum

Urethra

Corpus spongiosum

Penis

Seminal vesicle

Ejaculatory duct

Prostate gland

Spermatic cord and deferent duct

Epididymis

Testis

Prepuce

Glans penis

Scrotum

Figure 8.5 Section of male reproductive structures. Arrows show the structures through which the spermatozoa pass.

most important of which is testosterone, which is produced by interstitial cells (Leydig's cells). Testosterone promotes:

- maleness and male sexual behaviour
- the development and maintenance of male secondary sex characteristics and the functions of the accessory structures
- protein anabolism
- growth of bone and skeletal muscle and closure of the bony epiphyses
- a mild stimulant effect on the kidney tubule, with reabsorption of sodium and water and excretion of potassium
- inhibition of anterior pituitary secretion of the gonadotrophins follicle-stimulating hormone (FSH) and interstitial cell-stimulating hormone (ICSH). FSH stimulates the seminiferous tubules of the testes to produce spermatozoa. A negative feedback mechanism operates whereby when testosterone levels are high, FSH and ICSH production is inhibited.

The ductal system

The epididymis is the first part of the ductal system and forms a collection of tubules arising from the testis. The deferent duct (vas deferens), which is continuous with the epididymis, loops through the inguinal canal and joins the ejaculatory ducts, which pass through the prostate gland and lead into the urethra. Spermatozoa undergo further maturation as they pass through the ductal system before ejaculation. They remain in the deferent duct (vas deferens) for varying periods of time, depending upon the frequency of ejaculation.

The accessory glands

The seminal vesicles secrete a thick, nutritive alkaline fluid that mixes with sperm on ejaculation. This fluid accounts for 30% of the volume of the seminal fluid and contains fructose and protein, which are essential to sperm motility and metabolism.

The prostate gland is a lobulated structure which lies in the pelvic cavity in front of the rectum and behind the symphysis pubis, surrounding the uppermost part of the urethra. It is palpable on rectal examination. The prostate gland secretes a thin, milky, alkaline fluid that makes up 60% of the seminal fluid; this fluid creates an environment more hospitable to sperm by giving protection from the normally acidic environment of the male urethra and female vagina. A neutral or slightly alkaline medium also increases sperm motility.

The prostate begins to enlarge after the age of 40 years, which, because the urethra passes through it, can lead to urinary symptoms, such as difficulty emptying the bladder (see p. 292).

The bulbourethral glands are two pea-sized glands opening onto either side of the urethra. They produce a lubricating alkaline mucus that is expressed into the urethra during ejaculation, further reducing its typically acidic state, and contribute less than 5% to the volume of seminal fluid.

The supporting structures

The penis is a pendulous, soft tissue structure with a root and a body. There is erectile tissue supported by fibrous tissue and covered with skin. The three elongated masses include the corpus spongiosum containing the urethra, and two parallel columns, the corpora cavernosa, which provide the organ's main structural support.

The expanded distal end of the penis, the glans penis, surrounds the urethral meatus. The covering of skin folds upon itself at the glans penis to form a movable double layer called the prepuce.

The scrotum is divided into two compartments and each contains one testis, one epididymis and the testicular end of the spermatic cord. The temperature of the testes is 2–3°C below body temperature, which helps to preserve sperm viability.

Spermatic cords Leading from each testis is a spermatic cord consisting of a testicular artery, a testicular venous plexus, lymph vessels, a deferent duct (vas deferens) and nerves.

DISORDERS OF THE URINARY SYSTEM

This section covers a range of investigations and disorders of the kidney and other parts of the urinary system. The nursing management is discussed along with an outline of the medical and surgical treatment. Readers who require more detail about treatment are directed to Further reading suggestions, e.g. Colledge et al 2010, Garden et al 2007, Levy et al 2009, and Reynard et al 2008, 2009.

General investigations of the renal and urinary tract

Disorders of the renal and urinary system can be detected using various tests and investigations. Some pathologies, for example, prostate enlargement and prostate cancer, have similar signs and symptoms, and therefore in practice, multiple tests and investigations can be used to aid diagnosis. The common tests and investigations have been divided into those testing urine (Table 8.2), those testing blood (Table 8.3) and those that examine the structure of the urinary tract (Table 8.4). Other investigations used include computed tomography (CT) scan, magnetic resonance imaging (MRI) scan and radionuclide studies.

Table 8.2 Urine tests

TYPE OF TEST/ INVESTIGATION	INDICATION/ASSOCIATED PATHOLOGY	SIGNIFICANCE OF FINDINGS
Urinalysis a. Specific gravity (SG) b. Glucose c. Blood d. Protein e. Nitrites and/or leucocytes f. Ketones	All	a. Range 1.001–1.035 indicates degree of hydration b. Glycosuria may indicate diabetes mellitus, use of corticosteroids. If positive result, need fasting blood glucose c. Haematuria indicates infection, calculi, renal damage, tumour. A positive result for blood warrants further (specific) investigation d. Proteinuria or albuminuria indicates infection or renal damage; further investigation, e.g. MSU, needed e. Indicates urinary tract infection (UTI) f. Ketonuria indicates breakdown of fats and suggests starvation or possibly uncontrolled diabetes mellitus; further (specific) investigations needed (Steggall 2007)
Midstream urine (MSU) or catheter specimen of urine (CSU)	UTI – cystitis, acute pyelonephritis and chronic pyelonephritis (reflux nephropathy) Prostatic enlargement Renal failure	Detects presence of infection; ensure aseptic technique to avoid contaminants and false-positive results. Microbiological examination of the specimen will indicate the presence of and the types of infective organism
24-hour urine analysis e.g. calcium, phosphate, oxalate	Urinary calculi	Measures the substances excreted in the urine in different types of urinary calculi
Urine cytology	Bladder cancer	Detects presence of tumour cells. Not diagnostic but used in combination with other tests
Urinary flow rate	Prostatic enlargement/cancer	Determines the speed of bladder emptying, volume voided and time taken to empty the bladder. Used to determine the extent of prostate/urethral compression
Post-void residual volume	Urinary retention/prostatic enlargement	Determines the volume of urine in the bladder

Table 8.3 Blood tests

TYPE OF TEST/INVESTIGATION	INDICATION/ASSOCIATED PATHOLOGY	SIGNIFICANCE OF FINDINGS
Urea and electrolytes (U/Es)	All	Elevations in urea and creatinine indicate decreased renal function
Full blood count (FBC)	All	Low haemoglobin may indicate blood loss; anaemia. Increase in white cell count may indicate infection
Serum creatinine clearance (used to estimate GFR) 🖰 See website Figure 8.1	Renal failure and conditions affecting renal function, e.g. diabetic nephropathy	Estimate of renal function. Monitoring patients with reduced renal function
Erythrocyte sedimentation rate (ESR)	Nephritis	Non-specific test that detects inflammation/infection Erythrocytes sediment more quickly in individuals in whom disease is present
Prostate specific antigen (PSA) (a screening test, also used to monitor response to treatment of prostatic cancer)	Prostatic cancer	PSA result <4 ng/mL is within normal range; PSA result 4–10 ng/mL indicates an intermediate risk of prostate cancer; PSA >10 ng/mL indicates a high risk of prostate cancer

Table 8.4 Tests of urinary tract structure/function

TYPE OF TEST/ INVESTIGATION	INDICATION/ ASSOCIATED PATHOLOGY	SIGNIFICANCE OF FINDINGS
Intravenous urogram/ pyelogram (IVU/IVP)	Renal failure, calculi, recurrent UTI, trauma	Indication of structural abnormality or obstruction
Urethrogram; endoscopy: urethroscopy, cystoscopy, nephroscopy	Calculi, obstruction	Indication of presence of calculi or mass
X-ray or ultrasound (U/S, USS) of kidneys, ureter and bladder (KUB)	Prostate, calculi, UTI	Imaging of renal tract may indicate presence of calculi
Biopsy	Kidney, prostate, bladder	Diagnostic for pathology, e.g. cancers, causes of renal failure, types of glomerular disease, etc. Determines the stage of the disease

Table 8.5 Classification of common urinary tract infections by site

SITE	TYPE OF INFECTION	CAUSES/SIGNS
Kidney	a. Acute pyelonephritis	a. Chills, fever, flank pain; accompanied by bacteriuria and pyuria
	b. Chronic pyelonephritis (reflux nephropathy)	b. Chronic bacterial infection of the kidney associated with vesicoureteric reflux (VUR) (reflux of infected urine from the bladder into the ureters); causes scarring on the kidney
Bladder	Cystitis	Dysuria (pain on passing urine), frequency, urgency, cloudy urine that may have a strong odour and sometimes haematuria, suprapubic or back pain. There is inflammation of the bladder which can be bacterial or non-bacterial
Urethra	Urethritis	As cystitis but it is inflammation of the urethra

Urinary tract infections (UTIs)

Urinary tract infections are a common problem across the lifespan; they are more common in females than males, except in the neonatal period. For most patients with a normal urinary tract, UTIs are easily treated by antibiotic therapy, although early identification and treatment of patients with complicated infections are essential.

Urinary tract infections are defined as an inflammatory response of the urothelium (cells lining the urinary tract) to bacterial invasion that is usually associated with bacteriuria and pyuria (Steggall 2007).

Normally the urine does not contain bacteria; the presence of bacteria in the urine is termed bacteriuria. Bacteriuria can be symptomatic or asymptomatic. Pyuria is the presence of pus (white blood cells [WBCs]) in the urine, indicating an inflammatory response of the urothelium to bacterial invasion. Bacteriuria without pyuria suggests bacterial colonisation not infection. Pyuria without bacteriuria warrants evaluation for renal tuberculosis, stones or cancer. Infections are generally defined clinically by their presumed site of origin.

Most bacteria enter the urinary tract through the urethra into the bladder. This is enhanced in individuals with significant soilage of the perineum with faeces and patients with intermittent or indwelling catheters. Depending on the location of the infection, there are further classifications of UTI (Table 8.5).

Recurrent urinary tract infections are commonly due to reinfection or bacterial persistence; reinfection is especially common in women.

Pathogens

Most UTIs are caused by facultative anaerobes (bacteria that can grow in the presence or absence of oxygen) that generally come from bowel flora.

The most common cause of UTI is the bacterium *Escherichia coli* (*E. coli*), accounting for 85% of community-acquired and 50% of hospital-acquired infections. Other Gram-negative Enterobacteriaceae include *Proteus mirabilis* and *Klebsiella*, and Gram-positive *Enterococcus faecalis* and *Staphylococcus epidermidis*.

Hospital-acquired infections are frequently caused by *E. coli* and *Enterococcus faecalis* as well as by *Enterobacter, Klebsiella* and *Pseudomonas aeruginosa*.

In patients with diabetes mellitus, the most common infection is by *Klebsiella* spp; less common organisms such as *Gardnerella vaginalis, Mycoplasma* spp and *Ureaplasma urealyticum* may infect patients with intermittent or indwelling catheters.

Defences against UTI

The main defences against infection are the flow of urine and the acidity of urine. Normally urine is acidic, which inhibits bacterial growth. In addition, the urine contains urea and organic acids that make the conditions less favourable for bacterial survival. Other factors that protect against UTI include the antibacterial effects of bladder mucosa, as well as neutrophils and the cytokines interleukin IL-6 and IL-8.

For women, the vaginal flora is an important host defence against UTI since it is an acidic environment. Lactobacilli make up the majority of the vaginal flora in healthy, premenopausal women; sexual intercourse, use of antibiotics and intravaginal antimicrobials can reduce the normal *Lactobacillus*-dominant vaginal flora, increasing susceptibility to UTI. One way in which to reduce the likelihood of getting a UTI after sexual activity is to pass urine after intercourse.

Pyelonephritis

Pyelonephritis, or inflammation of the renal pelvis and renal tissue, may occur in one or both kidneys. Bacteria may enter the urinary tract, especially the kidneys, via the bloodstream or, more commonly, the bladder. Most organisms causing urinary tract infection – *E. coli, Klebsiella* spp, *Proteus, Pseudomonas, E. faecalis* and *S. epidermidis (S. albus)* – are found in the bowel and the perineum. There are two types of pyelonephritis, acute and chronic (often called reflux nephropathy as it can result from vesicoureteric reflux [VUR]), but the presenting features are different (Table 8.5).

Investigations for acute and chronic pyelonephritis (reflux nephropathy)

- Collection of a midstream specimen of urine (MSU) for microscopy examination, culture for evidence of a causative organism and antibiotic sensitivity.
- A full blood count and urea and electrolyte estimation. A raised white blood cell count and erythrocyte sedimentation rate (ESR) may be revealed in response to *E. faecalis* and *S. epidermidis* infection.
- An ultrasound scan (U/S, USS) or sometimes an intravenous urogram (IVU) is performed to locate any obstruction in the urinary tract (Box 8.1).
- Specific investigations to demonstrate the presence of VUR, for example a micturating cystogram.

Treatment of acute pyelonephritis

The main aim of treatment is to eradicate the infection by means of antibiotic therapy (often i.v.). This may be commenced even before organism sensitivities are known. A more specific antibiotic can then be used following urine culture results. Analgesics, antiemetics and antipyretics may be prescribed. Oral fluids are recommended, up to 3 L/24 h.

Further investigations may be needed to identify the underlying cause of the condition. Where inflammation persists, renal impairment may progress to end-stage renal failure requiring treatment by dialysis (pp. 286–289).

Cystitis

Cystitis may be chronic or acute and is characterised by severe inflammation of the bladder walls. More commonly affecting women, cystitis may also result from predisposing factors such as the presence of foreign bodies or stones, obstruction, tuberculosis, carcinoma in situ, chronic urinary infection and schistosomiasis (disease caused by flukes). Features of cystitis include burning on micturition, urinary frequency and urgency, and possibly incontinence. The results of MSU may be needed to treat any infection, although there is no need to wait for the results before commencing antibiotic therapy. Persistent infections warrant further investigations, for example IVU, and may be treated with long-term antibiotic therapy. A key feature in treatment should be increased fluid intake to help flush the urinary system. In addition to increasing fluid intake there is a range of self-help

Box 8.1 Information

Intravenous urogram or pyelogram (IVU/IVP)

This investigation, which involves the intravenous injection of an iodine-based contrast agent which is then excreted by the kidneys, allows a series of X-ray images of the kidneys, ureters and bladder to be taken.

The IVU radiograph may demonstrate a variety of pathologies:

- absence of kidney
- congenital abnormalities affecting the urinary tract, e.g. duplex ureter, horseshoe kidney
- renal trauma
- obstruction of the kidney, e.g. a large calculus in the renal pelvis, or scarring from repeated UTIs caused by VUR
- obstruction of the ureter – within the lumen, in the wall or arising from outside the ureter, such as late stage cervical cancer
- irregularities of the bladder wall – causes include bladder cancer, calculi, diverticulum (an abnormal pouch in the wall) or a foreign body.

Before, during and following an IVU

Where there are no contraindications the patient is given a laxative to clear the bowel and thus ensure a clear image of the contrast agent on the X-ray. The patient may be requested to abstain from food and fluids for a period of time before the start of the X-ray examination. The patient should void beforehand to make sure that the contrast agent remains concentrated as it is excreted into ureter and bladder, thus providing high quality images. Voiding just beforehand is also important for patient comfort as the examination can take 40–60 min. Prior to the intravenous injection of the contrast agent, a control X-ray of the kidneys, ureters and bladder (KUB) is taken. Patients should be informed that some people experience a warm feeling and some may be aware of a metallic taste in their mouth following the administration of contrast agent; they can be reassured that it is short-lived. Rarely patients have an allergic reaction to the iodine-based contrast agents; they should tell the radiographer at once if they have difficulty breathing or their skin feels itchy. Following the investigation, the patient is allowed to eat and drink again. The contrast medium will be passed when the patient voids urine, with no after-effects or change in the colour of the urine.

Note: in some situations such as an emergency (e.g. suspected kidney trauma), the examination can be undertaken without withholding fluid.

measures available to women who suffer from recurrent cystitis, for example attention to personal hygiene, passing urine frequently during the day and not 'holding on', emptying their bladder just before going to bed, cranberry juice, etc. (Boxes 8.2, 8.3). Nurses providing information to patients should be aware that cranberry juice may possibly increase the action of coumarin anticoagulants, e.g. warfarin.

Obstructive disorders of the urinary tract

There are many disorders that cause obstruction to the flow of urine, for example prostate enlargement, calculi or tumours (Figure 8.6). Although the early stages may cause only mild

Box 8.2 Reflection

Self-help measures to prevent cystitis

Rosa has had several bouts of cystitis requiring a course of antibiotics. You meet her when you are on a placement with the practice nurse in the health centre. Rosa tells you that she is really fed up with the discomfort and having to pass urine every few minutes; it is very inconvenient to take time off work to attend the health centre and she loses a day's pay.

Activities

- Reflect on the physical problems experienced by Rosa and the disruption to her life.
- Using the resources below, investigate the advice on self-help measures and discuss their suitability with your mentor or lecturer.

Resources

Bupa factsheet Cystitis: prevention of cystitis, http://hcd2.bupa.co.uk/fact_sheets/html/cystitis.html.

The Cystitis and Overactive Bladder Foundation: www.cobfoundation.org.

Box 8.3 Evidence-based practice

Effectiveness of cranberry juice in preventing UTI

Following articles and news items in the general media, the view that cranberry juice prevents UTI is widely held by members of the public.

Activities

Access the Cochrane Review 'Cranberries for preventing urinary tract infections' by Jepson & Craig and consider their findings.

- In which group of people may cranberries prevent UTIs?
- Is it effective in people with a urinary catheter?
- Consider the authors' conclusions.
- Assess the strength of evidence for recommending cranberries to patients; discuss this with your mentor.
- Search the literature for other studies on the efficacy of cranberries in preventing UTIs.

(From Jepson & Craig 2008.)

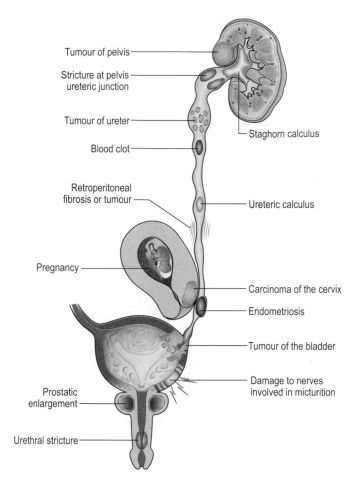

Figure 8.6 Conditions causing obstruction to the urinary tract.

symptoms which are easily ignored, the progressive damage caused by abnormal pressure, infection and stone formation can lead to renal failure. The importance of early detection and intervention cannot be overemphasised.

Urinary stones (renal calculi)

The formation of stones or calculi in the urinary tract is common in Europe, North America and Japan; there are many aetiological factors involved in their formation. Renal stones are more common in men than in women (M:F = 3:1).

PATHOPHYSIOLOGY

Urinary calculi are formed by the aggregation of mineral crystal deposits in the urine (Steggall & O'Mara 2008). The main types of stone are calcium oxalate, although other compositions of stone occur (Steggall & O'Mara 2008). The frequency of different types of stone varies between countries and is probably related to diet, environmental factors and possibly genetic factors (Goddard et al 2006). The risk factors for developing calculi are stasis of urine, chronic urinary infection and excess excretion of stone-forming substances. The most common presenting feature is pain and haematuria, caused by movement of the calculi, although this is not a universal symptom. Stones lodged in the renal pelvis (e.g. 'staghorn' calculus) tend to be immobile and so the presenting features are urinary tract infection and pyrexia.

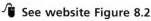 See website Figure 8.2

MEDICAL MANAGEMENT AND TREATMENT

Stones less than 5 mm in diameter may pass unobstructed through the urinary tract and be excreted in the urine. In some cases an alpha-blocker (e.g. tamsulosin) can be used to aid the passing of a stone. Increasing fluid intake to increase fluid output is not recommended in the acute phase of management because it will result in further distension of the urinary system; a normal fluid intake should be encouraged. For further information see Further reading, e.g. Reynard et al 2008, 2009.

Management of acute renal colic

Information about investigations is provided in Tables 8.2, 8.3 and 8.4.

The patient with renal stones may be acutely ill, suffering from excruciating pain arising in the loin and radiating to the groin (and the testis or labium), which can last 5–6 h. Pain is caused by small calculi being moved along the ureter by peristaltic movements, by impaction and by obstruction of urine. Bed rest, warmth to the site of pain (Boon et al 2006) and analgesics are the first line of treatment.

Medications include the opioid morphine intramuscularly. Pethidine should be avoided as it is associated with a higher incidence of vomiting (Holdgate & Pollock 2004). Diclofenac sodium (per rectum, usually at night) is a prostaglandin synthetase inhibitor which reduces renal blood flow and urination. It has an antispasmodic and anti-inflammatory effect and is long acting. Nausea may be relieved by an antiemetic such as i.m. prochlorperazine.

Flush-back of calculi and stenting (Box 8.4) This procedure affords temporary relief when a calculus causes obstruction and pain in the ureter. The stone is flushed back to the pelvis of the kidney. A small silicone tube called a stent is positioned in the ureter from the pelviureteric junction (PUJ) to the bladder. This stent is left in position to hold the stone in place. Further treatment to remove the stone can now be planned. The stent should not be left for more than 6 weeks. If the planned treatment cannot be carried out by the end of this period, the stent should be changed.

Insertion of a nephrostomy tube is indicated when obstruction in the kidney or the ureter cannot be relieved by flush-back and stenting (Figure 8.7).This is carried out under X-ray control, usually with a local anaesthetic. A small silicone tube is placed percutaneously into the collecting system of the kidney. The tube is held in place by a suture and connected to a closed-system drainage bag.

Ureteroscopic removal of calculi This procedure is suitable in the treatment of small calculi in the ureter. The ureteric orifice is dilated cystoscopically and a ureteroscope, to which a 'stone basket' is attached, is introduced into the ureter. The basket is opened out to ensnare the stone. The basket and stone are then withdrawn.

Box 8.4 Information

Stenting

The stents used by most surgeons are called 'double-J' or 'pigtail' stents and have small holes down most of the length of their tubing. These stents are self-retaining and must be removed endoscopically.

Some surgeons use an infant feeding tube as a stent following pyeloplasty (reconstructive surgery on the renal pelvis), pyelolithotomy or ureterolithotomy (removal of a stone from the renal pelvis and ureter respectively). Infant feeding tubes are self-retaining to a degree, but the patient will need a urethral catheter in situ to keep the tube in place.

When the catheter is removed the patient may pass the feeding tube without intervention. If this does not happen within 24 h, endoscopic removal will be required.

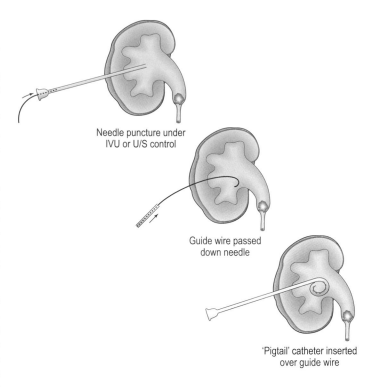

Needle puncture under IVU or U/S control

Guide wire passed down needle

'Pigtail' catheter inserted over guide wire

Figure 8.7 Percutaneous nephrostomy.

Rigid ureteroscopes are now available which can be inserted under direct vision. The surgeon is able to see the stone and can disintegrate it in situ (using mechanical means or laser) before removing the smaller fragments in a 'basket' (Underwood et al 2003).

Extracorporeal shock wave lithotripsy (ESWL) This procedure is the treatment of choice for the majority of patients with calculi, both renal and ureteric (Downey 2000). It effectively treats 70–80% of cases. Large calculi are broken up by means of this technique before percutaneous removal.

There are several lithotripsy centres in the UK, but some patients have to travel some distance for this treatment. Second-generation lithotripsy machines allow most patients to be treated without anaesthetic. Depending on the density of the stone more than one treatment may be required. The patient lies on a special table which allows shock waves produced by the lithotriptor machine to pass through it.

See website Figure 8.3

The force of the shock waves causes the stone to disintegrate and fragment. The position of the patient on the table is dependent on the location of the stone. The whole procedure is performed under specialised X-ray and ultrasonic control. The disintegrated or powdered calculus is then allowed to pass down the ureter over the next few days.

Percutaneous nephrolithotomy (PCNL) This procedure is used to remove calculi lying within the kidney. Large staghorn calculi may need to be broken up first, using ESWL. PCNL is performed under X-ray and ultrasound control. The patient will normally have a general anaesthetic. The kidney is punctured and the tract into the kidney is dilated to allow the nephroscope and a variety of grasping instruments to be inserted (Figure 8.8). The stone can then be

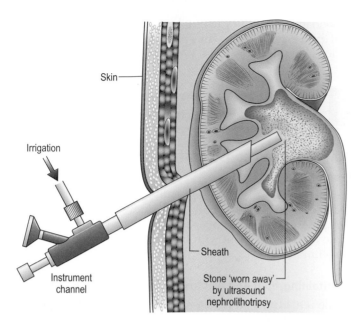

Skin

Irrigation

Instrument channel

Sheath

Stone 'worn away' by ultrasound nephrolithotripsy

Figure 8.8 Percutaneous stone removal.

removed or broken down into fine powder by ultrasonic probes. This powder can be aspirated through the centre of the probe.

Sometimes an electrohydraulic probe is used. This produces shock waves in the irrigating fluid to the kidney and results in the stone splitting into several fragments.

At the end of the procedure, a large nephrostomy tube with a smaller tube running down its centre is left in position to allow drainage and to prevent haematoma formation. This also allows access for a nephrogram 24–48 h postoperatively to assess the effectiveness of treatment.

No anaesthetic is required for a nephrogram X-ray. A contrast agent is injected down the smaller inner tube of a nephrostomy tube into the kidney. X-rays can then be taken and any fragments of calculi identified. Provided that there are no fragments left, the tubes can be removed.

Ureterolithotomy This open surgery (rarely used) is appropriate in the treatment of calculi occurring mid-ureter and causing obstruction that cannot be dealt with in any other way. An X-ray to identify the position of the stone will determine the incision to be made. The ureter is exposed and opened and the stone removed. The ureter is repaired either by removing a small section or by suturing the opening. A stent is usually left in place, positioned along the length of the ureter. This allows the ureter to heal and prevents leakage. A wound drain will be left in position to prevent haematoma formation. The stent will normally be removed after 7 days.

Pyelolithotomy This open surgery (rarely used) can be used for the removal of calculi in the renal pelvis or kidney which are causing an obstruction that cannot be removed by ESWL or PCNL. The procedure involves first exposing the affected kidney and then opening the renal pelvis to remove the stone. Sometimes it is not possible to remove all of a staghorn calculus in this way, in which case further incisions into the surrounding renal tissue (nephrolithotomy) are necessary. A stent will be left in place for 7 days.

▷ Nursing management and health promotion: acute renal colic

Major nursing considerations

A patient admitted with renal colic can often do little more than cope with the excruciating pain, and is often unable to answer questions or to follow advice and instructions until the pain is relieved.

🖱 **See website Critical thinking question 8.1**

Once the acute attack has subsided, the patient should be allowed to rest since only then will it be possible to absorb all the necessary explanations relating to investigations and treatment.

Priorities in postoperative nursing care depend on the procedure undertaken, but care following interventions to remove renal or ureteric calculi includes (see Ch. 26 for general perioperative care):

- Record observations, temperature, pulse, respirations and blood pressure and observe for signs/symptoms of infection, such as dark coloured, cloudy urine with an abnormal odour.
- Monitor fluid intake and urine output and record volume and colour of urine on the fluid chart. A decrease in volume may indicate obstruction. Haematuria may indicate trauma, but some haematuria is to be expected (but it should reduce, becoming less red).
- Encourage a fluid intake of 3 L daily to prevent infection.
- Administer analgesics if the patient is in pain. Severe pain must be reported to medical staff as this may indicate trauma, a misplaced stent or return of obstruction.

Discharge advice The patient should be advised:

- to continue to drink 3 L daily
- to take mild analgesics such as paracetamol or co-proxamol if in pain
- to seek help from the GP if urine output is bloodstained or they experience discomfort or a burning sensation on voiding urine.

The patient should also be advised when follow-up treatment will take place and what this will entail. If treatment is not within 6 weeks, it must be impressed upon the patient that it is very important to have the stent changed. If it is not changed, sediment and crystals will build up around it and form more calculi.

Renal disorders

This section of the chapter outlines a range of conditions that affect the kidney including glomerulonephritis, nephrotic syndrome, acute renal failure (ARF) and chronic renal failure (CRF).

Glomerulonephritis

Glomerulonephritis is a group of disorders usually characterised by inflammation of the glomeruli of the kidney, but some are not associated with inflammation. The disorder may be primary to the glomeruli (e.g. minimal change nephropathy, IgA nephropathy), post infection (an immune response to streptococcal infection), autoimmune (e.g. anti-GBM disease or Goodpasture's syndrome), or secondary to a systemic disorder (e.g. systemic lupus erythematosus, amyloidosis). There are acute and chronic types with varying prognosis.

Proteinuria, haematuria, hypertension, nephrotic syndrome (see below) and renal impairment characterise this disorder but the severity of these effects will vary between individuals. Presentation is usually described in terms of a range of clinical syndromes, but accurate diagnosis requires histological investigation. (For further information see Further reading, e.g. Feehally et al 2007.)

PATHOPHYSIOLOGY

Histological examination of renal tissue will demonstrate inflammation in the majority of cases, but it is also possible to find minimal change and no evidence of an inflammatory process. The disease process results from a defect in the immune response, such as a hypersensitivity to an exogenous antigen. The antigen–antibody reaction results in the formation of insoluble immune complexes that circulate in the blood and, instead of being ingested by macrophages, reach the kidney, where they become 'trapped' and set up a damaging inflammatory reaction in the delicate filtration structure. As a result of this:

- large molecules such as proteins and red blood cells are able to pass through the filtration fenestrations into the PCT
- the osmotic pressure of the blood plasma falls, leading to oedema
- sodium and water are retained, as are waste products and potentially toxic substances.

Many cases of acute glomerulonephritis occur 1–3 weeks after a streptococcal infection such as tonsillitis or otitis media, most commonly in children or adolescents; however, only 5% of these infections lead to glomerulonephritis. It is rare in developed countries as a result of better hygiene and the appropriate use of antibiotics. The disease can range from a mild, transitory, asymptomatic condition to a very severe form that precipitates acute renal failure (ARF), cardiac failure and seizures.

MEDICAL MANAGEMENT

Tests and investigations

Investigations include:

- urinalysis
- MSU
- full blood count and urea and electrolyte estimation
- antistreptolysin O (ASO) titre
- throat swab
- chest X-ray
- ECG
- ultrasound scan
- renal biopsy.

Treatment

Treatment will vary according the type of glomerulonephritis, but broadly the aim of treatment is to reduce renal

workload, restore and maintain fluid and electrolyte status and prevent uraemia. Thus management aims to prevent serious complications from occurring.

 Nursing management and health promotion: glomerulonephritis

Major nursing considerations

Promoting rest

Bed rest is a necessity, especially in the early period, to reduce the workload of both the kidneys and the heart. This can pose quite a challenge in the care of younger patients. Time needs to be spent with the patient, explaining why rest is so important.

Maintaining fluid and electrolyte balance (see Ch. 20)

While renal function is impaired and fluid overload poses a very real problem, fluid and sodium intake must be restricted. Potassium levels in the blood must be closely monitored and, if necessary, dietary modification made or ion exchange resins given. If hypertension is marked, antihypertensive medication may be required.

Preventing uraemia

While renal function is impaired, the waste products of metabolism will build up in the blood. To prevent this, a protein-restricted diet will be necessary. Calorie intake can be maintained with carbohydrates, and vitamin supplements can be given. This diet must also be low in salt and many patients find meals unpalatable. The dietitian can contribute greatly to the patient's well-being by ensuring that the restricted diet includes at least some of the patient's favourite foods.

Preventing infection

If a link to a recent streptococcal infection is confirmed, penicillin may be prescribed. All patients with renal impairment are prone to infection. All infection prevention and control measures must be adhered to.

Promoting convalescence and the maintenance of health

Most patients make a full recovery, but convalescence may take as long as 2 years. The acute condition can resolve fairly rapidly, and the majority of people recover normal renal function within a couple of months. Such patients often feel better quite quickly and it can be hard to persuade them that restrictions are still needed. Proteinuria can persist and regular monitoring will be necessary. After discharge, support for the patient and family will ensure that necessary lifestyle adjustments are made for the initial months. Exercise should be gentle and energetic sports activities avoided. Any infection should be treated seriously and medical advice sought.

Incomplete resolution and permanent glomerular damage can result in chronic glomerulonephritis and all the associated symptoms of renal impairment. Decreasing renal function may require renal replacement therapy such as dialysis (pp. 287–289).

Nephrotic syndrome

The nephrotic syndrome encompasses a group of signs and symptoms including proteinuria, hypoalbuminaemia (low serum albumin), oedema and lipidaemia. It can be a manifestation of certain forms of glomerulonephritis but may also occur as a complication of diabetes mellitus or amyloidosis, whereby insoluble starch-like deposits occur in kidney tissue. Often no cause can be found.

PATHOPHYSIOLOGY AND CLINICAL FEATURES

The glomerular filtration membrane is normally impermeable to blood cells and macromolecules such as proteins with a molecular weight of 70 000 or above. In the nephrotic syndrome increased glomerular permeability occurs, and protein molecules such as albumin enter the filtrate within the tubules. When the capacity of the tubule to reabsorb protein is exceeded, protein is lost in the urine. A low plasma albumin reduces plasma osmotic pressure and fluid leaks into the extracellular compartment. The resultant oedema occurs in dependent areas and may give rise to ascites (free fluid in the peritoneal cavity) in severe cases. Intravascular volume is maintained in many cases. How this occurs is not fully understood, but activation of the renin–angiotensin–aldosterone mechanism is thought likely.

This syndrome is characterised by heavy proteinuria (especially albumin) and hypoalbuminaemia leading to oedema. These patients generally have a low urine output and low urine sodium. Derangement of lipoproteins is evident and loss of fibrinogen in the urine can occur. Infection and thrombosis are common complications.

MEDICAL MANAGEMENT

Treatment

The main aim of treatment is to reduce oedema. Diuretic therapy can be adjusted according to the severity of the oedema and small maintenance doses can be administered when the oedema is under control. Severe oedema may also be treated by the administration of salt-poor albumin to temporarily increase plasma osmotic pressure. Patients are advised to adhere to a diet free from added salt.

Identification of the underlying disease process, possibly by renal biopsy and histological examination, will dictate the nature of ongoing treatment. In many patients, chronic renal failure will eventually develop.

Acute renal failure

Acute renal failure (ARF), sudden and severe reduction in normal renal function, may result from primary renal disease but is more frequently associated with other organ failure. Failure is often reversible, but should the kidneys fail to recover, permanent replacement treatment will be required.

A mortality rate of up to 50% is associated with ARF, the actual risk depending on patient factors, the cause of failure and other organ involvement (Thomas 2008). Where death occurs, renal failure is often not the primary cause.

PATHOPHYSIOLOGY

Causes

The causes of acute renal failure may be classified into three categories – prerenal, renal and post-renal – each having a different physiological location.

Prerenal causes are those in which a loss or decrease in renal perfusion results in renal ischaemia. They include:

- extracellular depletion, resulting from large gastrointestinal tract loss such as vomiting, diarrhoea, drainage or nasogastric aspiration; urinary loss due to polyuria or diuresis; loss from the skin, e.g. sweating or burn injury (see Chs 20, 30)
- circulating volume loss, as in haemorrhage or hypoalbuminaemia
- reduced cardiac output, as in cardiac arrest, valvular disease, cardiac tamponade
- vascular disease, e.g. renal artery thrombosis or embolism.

Renal causes include conditions that impair renal function by damaging the structure of the kidney (tubules, interstitium, glomeruli or capillaries). If tubular damage occurs, this is termed acute tubular necrosis (ATN). ATN is often caused by prolonged pre- and post-renal events.

Nephrotoxic substances can also result in acute failure. These include:

- medications – aminoglycoside antibacterial drugs (e.g. gentamicin) and non-steroidal anti-inflammatory drugs (NSAIDs)
- exogenous chemicals, e.g. heavy metals, phenols, carbon tetrachloride, chlorates, ethyl glycol
- bacterial toxins, particularly those released by Gram-negative microorganisms responsible for septicaemia (see Ch. 18).

Post-renal causes are mainly attributed to obstruction. The most common of these is bladder output obstruction which may be due to prostatic hypertrophy, tumours or calculi.

Clinical features

ARF proceeds through four phases: onset, oliguric, diuretic and recovery. The onset phase is the time from the initial renal insult to the onset of oliguria. The oliguric phase is characterised by a urine output of less than 400 mL/24 h; however, some patients may be anuric. The oliguria is accompanied by abnormal plasma levels of creatinine, urea and electrolytes. The effects of acute fluid overload and hyperkalaemia ($K^+ > 6$ mmol/L) can result in sudden death.

The patient may complain of anorexia, nausea and vomiting. Increased respiration due to pulmonary oedema and acidosis can occur. Drowsiness, confusion and coma may follow.

MEDICAL MANAGEMENT

Tests and investigations

These will depend on the suspected cause and on the immediacy of the presentation but may include:

- full blood count, urea and electrolyte estimation, serum creatinine clearance (used to estimate GFR)

- urinalysis, MSU, 24-h collections of urine for creatinine clearance
- X-ray of kidneys, ureters and bladder
- ultrasound
- renal biopsy.

Treatment

The goal is to restore biochemical balance and prevent ARF progressing. The onset of renal failure must be identified early to minimise damage and, if possible, prevent the necessity for dialysis. The priorities of treatment are as follows.

Treating the cause, e.g. correcting hypovolaemia and increasing renal perfusion, managing sepsis and relieving any urinary obstruction.

Reversing, restoring and maintaining fluid and electrolyte status (see Ch. 20)

- *Hyperkalaemia.* Immediate measures may be required to correct hyperkalaemia, which could cause fatal dysrhythmias. Cardiac monitoring is essential, in particular observing for any changes in cardiac rhythm. Hyperkalaemia can be corrected in the short term by i.v. insulin-glucose infusion or sodium bicarbonate, either of which will shift potassium into the cells. Other measures include the administration of ion exchange resins, which when administered orally or rectally remove potassium ions.
- *Hyponatraemia and hypernatraemia.* In the oliguric state there is a danger of hyponatraemia, due to the risk of fluid overload and to the failure of the damaged tubules to reabsorb sodium. However, hypernatraemia can also be a problem in prerenal ARF, as mechanisms instituted retain sodium in order to restore blood volume. Fluid intake must be restricted to the equivalent of insensible loss plus the previous day's urinary output. Sodium intake must be monitored closely.
- *Uraemia.* The inability to excrete the nitrogenous waste products of metabolism is managed by dietary restrictions, but ensuring adequate calorie intake to prevent the patient becoming catabolic (see Ch. 21). Parenteral nutrition may be necessary and potassium intake will be restricted.
- *Metabolic acidosis.* The loss of the kidneys' buffering function, the electrolyte imbalance and the increased anaerobic respiration by damaged renal cells all result in acidosis. In the short term, this is managed by i.v. sodium bicarbonate.

If acute renal failure is very severe, persists or worsens, dialysis will be necessary.

 Nursing management and health promotion: acute renal failure

Major nursing considerations

The care of patients with ARF will involve a large multidisciplinary team and may be carried out either in an intensive care setting or on a ward, depending on the condition of the patient. Priorities of nursing intervention are to:

- Reduce the patient's anxieties and recognise the risk of altered consciousness due to uraemia and electrolyte imbalance.
- Control fluid and electrolyte balance by:
  - monitoring cardiac status for signs of dysrhythmias
  - monitoring pulse, respiration and blood pressure for signs of overload and hypertension
  - restricting fluid intake and ensuring the accurate measuring and recording of urine output and other losses; daily weighing may be required
  - administering prescribed medication and carrying out urinary assays as required.
- Assess and maintain nutritional status within the necessary limitations by the oral, enteral or parenteral route and monitor the nutritional status of the patient.
- Prevent infection due to uraemia by strict asepsis with regard to infusion sites and catheter management and by close monitoring of temperature and the patient's reported symptoms.
- Manage anaemia by the safe administration of blood transfusions, if required.
- Promote comfort at all times.

The diuretic and recovery phases

The oliguric phase of renal failure may last 1–2 weeks and is followed by the diuretic phase, which indicates that renal function is returning. This is often a time of relief, but because the kidneys will not yet have regained their capacity for selective reabsorption, urine output can be as much as 4 L/day. This, in itself, could potentiate dehydration and electrolyte imbalances. Close monitoring must therefore continue. The recovery phase that follows can last several months and will require close medical follow-up of renal function. Convalescence in the form of rest, restricted activity, the avoidance of infections and alertness to any symptoms that might indicate renal problems may be a source of considerable stress to the patient, who may also be concerned about fulfilling family and work responsibilities.

Chronic renal failure

Chronic renal failure (CRF) is the gradual and progressive reduction in renal function. Failure may occur over weeks, months or even years. Each year, acceptance rates for renal replacement therapies are increasing, at a rate that exceeds death rates, and this is predicted to continue for the next 10 years (Department of Health 2004). The available treatments are dialysis – haemodialysis, peritoneal dialysis – or transplantation, which may be from cadaveric, living related donors or linked unrelated donors (i.e. a 'swop').

PATHOPHYSIOLOGY

Any disorder that damages kidney function can result in renal failure. Common causes are outlined in Box 8.5.

Clinical features

In the initial stages of CRF the patient may be asymptomatic. Proteinuria, hypertension, anaemia or an elevated blood urea are, however, common presenting features.

As renal failure progresses the GFR declines and the patient may complain of fatigue, lethargy, pruritus, nausea, vomiting

Box 8.5 Information

Common causes of chronic renal failure (adapted from Boon et al 2006 with permission)

Congenital and inherited: 5%, e.g. polycystic kidney disease

Renal artery stenosis: 5%

Hypertension: 5–25% (see Ch. 2)

Glomerular disease: 10–20%, IgA nephropathy is the most common

Interstitial diseases of the kidney: 5–15%, e.g. chronic interstitial nephritis caused by a variety of conditions that include analgesic nephropathy, systemic lupus erythematosus (SLE), amyloidosis, etc.

Systemic inflammatory disease: 5%, e.g. vasculitis, SLE

Diabetes mellitus: 20–40% (see Ch. 5)

Unknown: 5–20%

and indigestion. Breathlessness on exertion, headaches, visual disturbances, pallor and loss of libido may also be noted. A reduced immune response occurs, making the patient prone to infection, particularly of the urinary tract (see Ch. 16).

Metabolic bone disease, generalised myopathy, neuropathy and metabolic acidosis can occur in advanced stages of renal impairment. Atherosclerosis due to altered lipid and carbohydrate metabolism and hypertension may also occur. Vascular calcification and pericarditis may also be identified.

MEDICAL MANAGEMENT

Treatment

Treatment aims to identify the cause, extent and complications of the renal failure and to preserve useful renal function for as long as possible.

Where hypertension is evident, antihypertensive drugs may be used to reduce and control blood pressure gradually. Lifestyle advice should also be given to assist with reducing blood pressure, e.g. stopping smoking, losing weight or maintaining normal weight and regular exercise.

Fluid restriction may be required if the GFR is less than 5 mL/min as fluid overload can exacerbate problems with hypertension. Poor urine concentration can, however, result in a urine output of more than 2.5 L/24 h, in which case an intake of about 3 L/day is required.

Dietary measures are likely to include potassium and phosphate restrictions. Sodium restriction is not indicated unless there is evidence of oedema, hypertension or cardiac failure. In the case of sodium-losing conditions, sodium supplements may be required. A diet with no added salt may be appropriate in some cases.

Regular monitoring of biochemistry, GFR, creatinine clearance and assessment of symptoms allow treatment to be readjusted and progression of the disease to be assessed.

Renal replacement therapy, in the form of haemodialysis or peritoneal dialysis, is the treatment available to replace the excretory functions of the kidneys (Box 8.6, Figure 8.9). At present, transplantation (Figure 8.9D) is restricted by a

Box 8.6 Information

Renal replacement therapy: dialysis

Dialysis requires a semipermeable membrane to combine three principles – diffusion, osmosis and filtration – in order to permit the removal of solutes (metabolic wastes, excess electrolytes) and fluids from patients with renal failure. A favourable solute gradient is required.

Diffusion is the movement of molecules from an area of high concentration, across a semipermeable membrane, to an area of low concentration. This process continues until the concentrations in each compartment are the same.

Osmosis is the movement of a fluid or solvent from a lower concentration to a higher one.

Filtration is the movement of both solvent and solute across a semipermeable membrane under pressure.

Haemodialysis (Figure 8.9A)

Haemodialysis requires a means of vascular access, e.g.:

- *Percutaneous access* including subclavian, femoral and jugular lines which are either temporary or permanent.
- *Arteriovenous fistula and arteriovenous grafts (synthetic)*. Forming a fistula involves the anastomosis of an artery and a vein. The increased blood flow causes increased pressure on the vein walls which leads to thickening and dilatation (arterialisation); this allows the repeated insertion of needles for dialysis. This developmental stage takes about 12 weeks. The fistula can be seen as well as felt.

The blood is pumped from the patient to an artificial kidney (the dialyser – comprising blood and dialysate compartments separated by a semipermeable membrane) and back to the patient, having now been 'cleansed' as unwanted solutes and fluid pass through the membrane into the dialysate (fluid formulated to promote diffusion and removal of waste). The dialyser is normally a disposable hollow fibre or flat plate dialyser; different dialysers consist of different membranes. The type of membrane used is important as part of the patient's individualised dialysis prescription. Issues to consider are desired clearance, fluid removal and biocompatibility.

Peritoneal dialysis (Figure 8.9C)

The patient's peritoneal membrane serves as the semipermeable membrane for dialysis. A temporary or permanent Tenckhoff catheter is placed into the peritoneal cavity. The dialysate is instilled into the abdomen (usually 2 L at each session). A set time ('dwell time') elapses and the dialysate is drained out.

- Continuous ambulatory peritoneal dialysis (CAPD) – 2 L of dialysate are instilled into the peritoneal cavity and left in place, usually for 6 h, when the fluid is exchanged. Once patients have been instructed in and are competent in this method, they can be more independent, visiting the hospital only for clinic appointments or when any problems arise; the main potential problems are peritonitis, dehydration and constipation.

Continued

Box 8.6 Information – cont'd

Other methods

Other methods of renal replacement therapy are often used in intensive care, including:

- continuous arteriovenous haemofiltration (CAVH)
- continuous arteriovenous haemodiafiltration (CAVHD)
- continuous venovenous haemofiltration (CVVH)

📖 **See website Figure 8.4**

- continuous venovenous haemodiafiltration (CVVHD).

Note: In haemofiltration the person's blood is passed through a filter allowing separation of an ultrafiltrate containing fluid and solutes. The ultrafiltrate is discarded and replaced with an isotonic solution (Figure 8.9B). The process is usually continuous as in continuous venovenous haemofiltration. Haemodiafiltration is similar, but with the addition of dialysate. Diffusion occurs and the removal of unwanted solutes is enhanced (Brooker 2010).

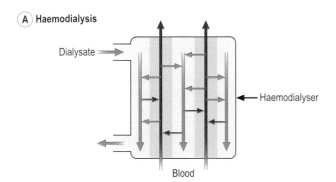

A Haemodialysis

Dialysate →

← Haemodialyser

Blood

- Typical small solute clearance 160 mL/min
- Used in both acute and chronic renal failure

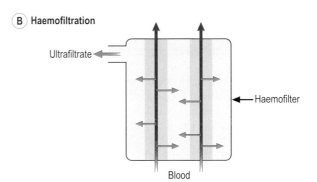

B Haemofiltration

Ultrafiltrate ←

← Haemofilter

Blood

- Typical small solute clearance (2 L/h exchanges) 33 mL/min
- ? Less circulatory instability than haemodialysis
- Used mostly in acute renal failure

- **Access to the circulation** for haemodialysis or filtration is required. Arteriovenous fistulae, temporary or semi-permanent tunnelled central venous lines or arteriovenous shunts (e.g. Scribner shunt) may be used. The extracorporeal circuit requires anticoagulation, typically with heparin

---

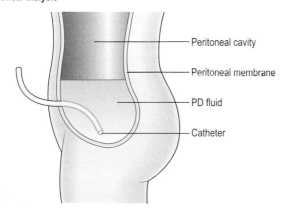

C Peritoneal dialysis

- Peritoneal cavity
- Peritoneal membrane
- PD fluid
- Catheter

- **Access to the peritoneal cavity** via 'Tenckhoff' catheter
- **Continuous ambulatory peritoneal dialysis** (CAPD): typically 4 exchanges of 2 L of fluid a day 4–6 h apart
- **Automated peritoneal dialysis** (APD): uses a machine to perform exchanges overnight (8–10 h). Used mostly in chronic renal failure

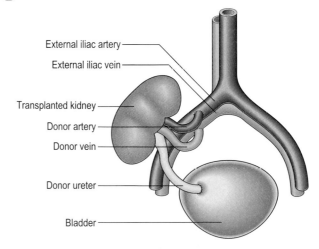

D Transplantation

- External iliac artery
- External iliac vein
- Transplanted kidney
- Donor artery
- Donor vein
- Donor ureter
- Bladder

- Successful transplantation extends the life expectancy of patients with end-stage CRF
- Requires long-term use of immunosuppressives with attendant risks

Figure 8.9 Renal replacement therapy. A. Haemodialysis. B. Haemofiltration. C. Peritoneal dialysis. D. Renal transplantation. (Reproduced from Boon et al 2006 with permission.)

lack of available cadaver donor kidneys. However, for some patients, it may be possible to consider a matched family member as a live donor. Recently there have been donations from live unrelated donors. Some are linked (two donors/ two recipients) in which the unrelated but matched donors donate a kidney to the unknown recipients (i.e. a 'swop').

 ## Nursing management and health promotion: chronic renal failure

Nursing management requires a strategy to help the patient and family come to terms with an illness for which there is no cure and in which sudden death can occur. Nursing intervention should aim to help the patient maintain a good quality of life by developing ways to cope with the constraints of the treatments and the possibility of complications occurring.

Adherence with treatment

Patient beliefs about the value and benefit of a treatment may differ markedly when compared with the priority given to the same treatment by the nurse. Failure to adhere to diet and fluid restrictions may indicate that the patient has an underlying problem, or is not coping with some aspect of the treatment; alternatively, there may be a lack of understanding of the importance of the treatment regimen. Knowing the patient and having an understanding of the patient's social and cultural background, especially their health beliefs, can give insight into behaviour with regard to a particular treatment.

Major problems experienced by patients

Fatigue and lethargy characteristic of CRF can reduce both ability and performance at work. Absence from work due to sickness or attendance at hospital may result in unemployment or reduction of income. Feelings of helplessness, hopelessness and depression are often expressed by patients with a long-term condition (see Ch. 32). Loss of control over many aspects of life and low self-esteem are likely to influence family relationships. Transplantation is acknowledged as the treatment of choice for a person with end-stage renal disease (ESRD). A successful transplant offers the patient freedom and independence as well as an enhanced quality of life.

Living with peritoneal dialysis

Peritoneal dialysis (PD) is performed either as continuous ambulatory peritoneal dialysis (CAPD) or automated peritoneal dialysis (APD) (Figure 8.9C). CAPD is a continuous treatment, generally performed four times a day; APD is achieved by machine, generally overnight in the patient's own home. PD offers patients a greater degree of control over their treatment and lifestyle. While the number of fluid exchanges per day will be prescribed by the doctor, the timing of each exchange can be decided by the patient, to fit in with family life or work commitments. In addition, freedom to be away from home for visits or holidays is possible. For travel abroad, the dialysate manufacturer may be able to deliver fluid requirements to the destination.

The need for regular fluid exchanges and aseptic technique can be limiting for some patients. Performing the exchange in a designated area at home can give confidence and reassure patients that they have done all they can to reduce the risk of peritonitis. There may be a reluctance to perform exchanges in the homes of friends and relatives, particularly if the patient's illness is poorly understood and a source of embarrassment.

The insertion of a tube and presence of fluid in the abdomen can alter body image and sexuality, thus discouraging those who are conscious of their appearance. A further disadvantage of CAPD is that it presents a constant reminder to the patient of their illness (for further information, see Thomas 2008 and in Further reading Levy et al 2009).

Nursing support during haemodialysis

Assessments to be performed before haemodialysis include:

* Weigh the patient – compare with weight after last dialysis and the patient's recognised dry weight, i.e. the weight at which there is no clinical evidence of oedema, increased jugular venous pressure (JVP), shortness of breath or hyper/hypotension.
* Record temperature, pulse and blood pressure – compare these with values after the last dialysis. Any temperature increase could indicate an infected dialysis site. Raised blood pressure may indicate fluid overloading.
* Enquire how the patient has been feeling, i.e. well or unwell.
* Assess any known specific medical problem, e.g. blood glucose in patients with diabetes mellitus.
* Once a month, take blood for urea and electrolyte levels pre- and post-dialysis; a full blood count should be checked every month.

During dialysis, the nurse should record the pulse and blood pressure. A drop in blood pressure may mean that the patient needs extra fluid. If necessary, the nurse should check the patient's weight halfway through the session.

At the end of dialysis, the patient's temperature, pulse, blood pressure and weight should be recorded in order to assess the effectiveness of the treatment. Any prescribed medications should be administered and the patient should be given the opportunity to raise any further concerns.

Disorders of the bladder

This section of the chapter deals with bladder cancer.

Bladder cancer

Tumours of the bladder, usually transitional cell carcinoma, occur more commonly in men than in women (M:F 4:1). The peak incidence of bladder cancer in the UK occurs at around 65 years of age. Bladder tumours are histologically similar to tumours of the renal pelvis and ureter. Approximately 95% are malignant, and benign tumours often recur after apparently successful treatment.

There are geographical variations in incidence: tumours are more common in industrialised regions than in underdeveloped regions. Possible causative agents or factors include:

- occupational exposure (industrial dyes, solvents)
- cigarette smoking
- calculi
- diverticula
- chronic inflammation due to indwelling catheterisation.

Screening of those in high-risk groups may help to reduce incidence and to monitor factors associated with bladder cancer, but as many years may elapse between exposure to a carcinogen and the development of cancer, direct connections are difficult to establish.

PATHOPHYSIOLOGY

Tumour growth usually commences in the transitional cell epithelium (urothelium) lining the bladder, often as a papillary growth (papillae are minute nipple-shaped projections). Benign growth will, without treatment, usually progress to malignancy and then, by stages, from superficial to deep muscle tissue involvement, eventually spreading locally into surrounding tissue and other parts of the urinary tract or organs.

Common presenting symptoms Approximately 80% of people with bladder cancer will notice haematuria (often painless). This may be the only presenting feature of the disease. Dysuria, frequency, symptoms of obstruction and cystitis may also be noticed, but embarrassment may prevent the individual from visiting their GP. Symptoms may not persist following initial presentation, e.g. if associated infection is resolved by a course of antibiotics. Investigations should, however, be undertaken if the cause of haematuria is unclear.

MEDICAL MANAGEMENT

Investigations

Diagnosis may be aided by physical examination, a full blood count, urea and electrolyte estimation and other biochemical assays. Examination of an MSU specimen will exclude evidence of infection. If the patient has microscopic or macroscopic haematuria and an infection has been excluded, the patient's upper urinary tract and bladder must be investigated. An IVU (p. 280) will be performed, which may exclude cancer of the renal pelvis. A cystoscopy is essential so that biopsies of suspicious lesions can be examined for abnormal cells. Computed tomography (CT) is performed if local spread of cancer is suspected. In situations where secondary (metastatic) spread of cancer is a possibility the patient will have a chest X-ray, a bone scan and liver function tests (LFTs).

The staging of bladder tumours is important for selecting the appropriate treatment modality (see Ch. 31).

Treatment

The choice of treatment will depend on the type of tumour and the degree of invasion of local tissue, as determined by cystoscopy. Superficial lesions without muscle invasion can be treated by:

- excision of the tumour through the urethra – transurethral resection (TUR) or cystodiathermy (using an electrocautery) during cystoscopy

- instillation of chemotherapy drugs or bacillus Calmette–Guérin vaccine (BCG) into the bladder.

Newer treatments for superficial bladder cancers include intravesical microwave hyperthermia with intravesical chemotherapy. This should, however, only be performed within a controlled clinical trial (National Institute for Health and Clinical Excellence 2007).

For invasive bladder tumours, a combination of surgery (i.e. total cystectomy), radiotherapy and chemotherapy may be used.

Total cystectomy involves removing the lower ureters, bladder, prostate, urethra and lymphatics in men, and also, in women, the reproductive organs. Urinary diversion is required, most commonly by ileal conduit and stoma formation. With this type of diversion, the ureters are anastomosed to an isolated section of the bowel, usually ileum with blood supply (in an operation known as ureteroileostomy or ileoureterostomy) and the loop brought to the abdominal surface as a stoma (Figure 8.10). This is a major procedure which will fundamentally affect the lifestyle of both the patient and family members. The complications (including those that occur later) must be discussed with the patient and their family to ensure that the patient is able to give fully informed consent for radical surgery (Box 8.7). Information about pre-operative and postoperative care, including a care plan for the first 24 h following surgery, is provided on the companion website.

See website for further content

Developments in reconstructive surgery have led to the use of bladder substitutes in place of urinary diversion, i.e. part of the intestine is anastomosed directly to the membranous urethra which provides a reservoir for urine; however, this technique is not appropriate for everyone as it requires major surgery (see Further reading, e.g. Pashos et al 2002).

Radiotherapy is normally given as an external treatment for bladder carcinoma over a 6-week period. It may be used as a palliative measure or in conjunction with surgery and/or chemotherapy, pre- or post-treatment. The age and general condition of the patient will determine whether treatment is given on an outpatient or inpatient basis. Sometimes the severity of the patient's symptoms leads to conversion from outpatient to inpatient care and a short period of respite from the treatment plan to allow the patient to recuperate before progressing to the next treatment.

Chemotherapy Treatment of invasive bladder cancer with systemic chemotherapy is under investigation. Regimens of treatment vary. Some patients receive care on a day-care basis, receiving i.v. injections, while others attend for inpatient hospital care involving 2–3 days in hospital for each cycle of treatment (see Ch. 31).

Intravesical chemotherapy may be offered in some cases. The recurrence of superficial bladder tumours resected endoscopically is approximately 65%. Recurrent tumours are usually of the same type and stage as those resected. Further endoscopic resection may be the treatment of choice, but intravesical chemotherapy is also given. A urethral catheter is inserted and the chosen medication is instilled via the catheter. Treatment may be weekly, monthly or bimonthly, depending upon the type of tumour and the medication used.

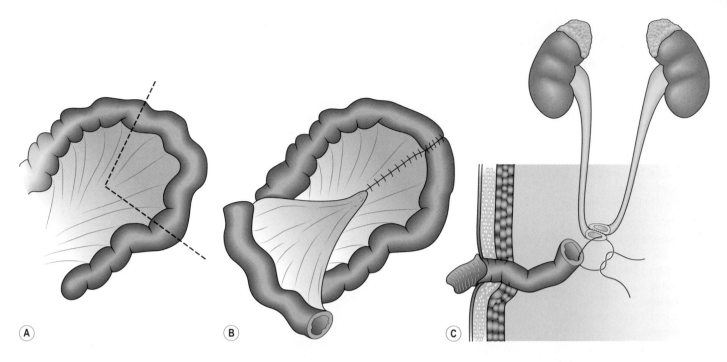

Figure 8.10 Ileal conduit urinary diversion. A, B. Isolation of segment of terminal ileum. C. Fashioning of the anastomosis between the ureters and ileum. The stoma is made to protrude from the skin to minimise skin contact with urine and so reduce irritation.

 Box 8.7 Information

Complications following total cystectomy

Specific complications post-cystectomy

- Breakdown of anastomosis
- Breakdown of blood supply to stoma leading to necrosis
- Pelvic abscess
- Urinary infection
- Poor wound healing post-radiotherapy
- Prolapse of stoma
- Retraction of stoma
- Renal failure

Later complications

- Depression
- Recurrence of tumour
- Prolapse of stoma
- Retraction of stoma
- Stenosis of stoma
- Stone formation
- Urinary infection
- Urinary reflux

Once the medication is instilled the catheter can be removed. The patient is asked to try to avoid passing urine for an hour and is asked to turn from back to front to sides every 15 min, in order to wash the medication around the bladder. The nurse administering the treatment should bear in mind that this patient may have difficulty in postponing the voiding of urine for up to 1 h because of frequency and bladder irritability. The patient should be reassured that an inability to comply with this request is not a sign of 'failure'.

After the treatment has been completed, the patient should be advised that urine passed will contain chemical substances that will irritate the skin and that leakages or dribbles should be washed off immediately.

The side-effects of the medications used in this treatment vary, but chemical cystitis leading to inflammation and bladder irritability, urgency and frequency is common. Sensitivity rashes are seen less commonly, as are more severe effects such as systemic toxicity and bone marrow suppression.

Effectiveness of treatment with intravesical chemotherapy varies considerably from individual to individual.

Disorders of the prostate

This section of the chapter outlines two important conditions affecting the prostate gland: benign enlargement and cancer.

Benign prostatic enlargement (BPE)

After the age of 40 years the prostate begins to enlarge and will gradually narrow the diameter of the urethra leading to urinary symptoms. The most bothersome symptom can be nocturia, (having to get up at night-time to empty the bladder). Fifty per cent of men over the age of 60 will have BPE, but not all will have symptoms (Thorpe & Neal 2003). Bladder outflow obstruction can occur for a number of reasons, but the most common cause is BPE (Box 8.8). Note: BPE is also known as benign prostatic hyperplasia (BPH).

PATHOPHYSIOLOGY

The precise cause of prostate enlargement has yet to be fully explained, but it is thought to be related to changes in androgen hormone (e.g. testosterone) levels.

Box 8.8 Information

Bladder outflow obstruction

Causes

- BPE (also known as benign prostatic hyperplasia)
- Bladder calculi
- Bladder tumour
- Phimosis
- Prostatic carcinoma
- Urethral strictures, stenosis, trauma
- Diuretic drugs
- Neurological disturbances

Common symptoms

- Diminished force of urine flow/stream
- Double voiding
- Dribbling post-voiding
- Dysuria
- Frequency
- Haematuria (occasional)
- Hesitancy
- Interrupted stream
- Loss of urinary continence
- Nocturia
- Urgency
- Urinary retention

Inadequate emptying of the bladder can result in an increased residual urine, increasing the risk of UTI and the incidence of bladder calculi formation.

Diagnosis

Diagnosis of bladder flow obstruction may be assisted by:

- History of symptoms
- Physical examination
- Routine urinalysis
- MSU for microscopy, culture and sensitivity
- Blood screen of urea, electrolytes and creatinine
- Urethroscopy and cystoscopy
- Ultrasound scan – residual urine volume and upper urinary tract
- Urodynamic evaluation
- Voiding cystometrogram (a record of the changes in pressure within the bladder during voiding)

Common presenting symptoms Symptoms of BPE include:

- urinary frequency
- hesitancy
- poor urinary flow
- incomplete bladder emptying, i.e. feeling the bladder retains urine
- having to strain to empty the bladder
- terminal dribbling
- urgency
- nocturia.

MEDICAL MANAGEMENT

Investigations

The diagnosis of prostate enlargement is made by digital rectal examination. However, more specific investigations are required to ascertain the nature of the enlargement and its effects:

- ultrasound scan
- urinary flow-rate test
- assessment of post-void residual urine
- blood for renal function tests
- full blood count
- symptom score to quantify symptoms and measure how 'bothersome' they are, for example, International Prostatic Symptom Score (IPSS)
- estimation of prostate-specific antigen (PSA) in the blood to eliminate diagnosis of cancer in selected men
- MSU.

Treatment

Treatment options include:

- watchful waiting
- medication – alpha blockers, e.g. alfuzosin, tamsulosin, or 5-alpha reductase inhibitors, e.g. dutasteride, finasteride, to reduce prostate size
- surgery, e.g. transurethral resection of the prostate (TURP), or variations of this (see Further reading, e.g. Garden et al 2007, Reynard et al 2008).

 See website for Critical thinking question 8.2

Transurethral resection of the prostate gland (TURP) is commonly used to treat prostate enlargement. A resectoscope is passed up the urethra to the prostate gland and small sections are chipped away from the prostatic lobes, removing the material that had been intruding into the urethra and bladder neck. Irrigation fluid (a non-electrolyte solution, glycine) constantly flushes out the bladder during the procedure. Most commonly, irrigation continues postoperatively, as the operative bed can give rise to considerable bleeding and clots could lead to obstruction. Box 8.9 outlines postoperative complications of TURP.

Box 8.9 Information

Postoperative complications of TURP

Potential postoperative complications

- Haemorrhage – evident as haematuria
- Clot retention
- Infection – UTI, epididymis or testis
- Extravasation – escape of urine into surrounding tissue due to bladder or urethral damage
- TUR syndrome – absorption of irrigant into the bloodstream, resulting in dilutional hyponatraemia (see Ch. 20)
- Venous thromboembolism – deep vein thrombosis and pulmonary embolism

Possible late complications

- Urethral stricture (see pp. 297–298)
- Loss of urinary continence
- Erectile dysfunction (ED)
- Retrograde ejaculation of semen into the bladder
- Bladder neck stenosis

Nursing management and health promotion: BPE

Caring for men with acute retention

Most men presenting with acute retention as a result of BPE will be discharged home with a catheter in situ and will return for planned surgery at a later date. Once the obstruction is relieved there is no urgency to perform surgery, which allows the treatment of any associated medical conditions and, when appropriate, the man can be admitted for surgery. However, the presence of a urinary catheter for any reason poses an infection risk.

Caring for men with chronic retention

Chronic urinary retention is usually the result of a crescendo of symptoms of 'prostatism'. These men do not always complain of symptoms of bladder outflow obstruction, but mainly of urge incontinence, dribbling urine or wet beds at night. They usually have no pain and, although they have a large amount of residual urine, their bladder distension is not always obvious to the eye or palpable on physical examination.

Because of the large volume of residual urine, these men are at risk of developing upper urinary tract dilatation and impaired renal function. It is urgent to make a diagnosis so that the level of hydration and renal function can be returned to normal. However, if there is no renal impairment, it is not essential that these individuals are catheterised.

Catheterisation will permit bladder drainage and allow renal function recovery. Once catheterised, the man may have a huge diuresis. His thirst mechanism will not allow adequate fluid replacement, making parenteral fluid replacement necessary. Large fluid replacement volumes put the man at risk of heart failure and it should be borne in mind that impaired renal function may have caused anaemia.

The use of urinary catheters is outlined in Box 8.10 and the principles of catheter management for both men and women are outlined in Box 8.11.

Once the man has been catheterised, his renal function restored and any anaemia corrected, there is no urgency to proceed to surgery. The individual may in fact benefit from a period of recuperation and bladder rest with the catheter in situ. Depending upon the ability of the individual to care for the catheter and upon community resources, ideally care will be given in the man's home.

A trial without the catheter should not be made, as this would again lead to chronic retention followed by renal failure.

For those with milder symptoms, it is a matter of discussion between the man and his doctor as to whether symptoms are interfering with the individual's lifestyle sufficiently to warrant an operation and whether he stands a good chance of improvement from surgery. In rare cases where there is poor life expectancy or the man is too unfit for surgery, operative treatment may not be offered and a permanent indwelling catheter may be considered the best management.

Caring for men undergoing TURP

The man must be given a clear explanation of the after-effects of TURP, so that he can give his informed consent prior to the procedure. The surgery and the complications

---

Box 8.10 Information

The use of catheters

Indications for catheterisation

- Acute or chronic retention of urine
- Diagnostic investigations of the bladder function
- Specific pre- and post-operative needs
- Following trauma, burns, road traffic accidents or any trauma to the lower urinary tract
- Therapeutic instillations of medication, e.g. chemotherapy
- Intractable incontinence where all other methods have failed
- Protracted loss of consciousness.

Choice of catheter

Points to consider when choosing a catheter include:

- Purpose of the catheterisation
- Length of time the catheter must remain in situ
- Whether a self-retaining catheter is necessary
- Presence of latex allergy
- Age and gender.

Features of the catheter

- The smallest catheter that will adequately drain the bladder should be used: size 12–16 FG for adults with clear urine; size 18–22 FG for adults with haematuria.
- The lumen of the catheter will vary depending on the material used. A latex catheter is made up of several layers of material, often coated inside with silicone, and its lumen will be smaller than that of a silicone catheter, which is extruded from one piece of material (Pomfret 2001).
- Balloon size: the larger the balloon, the higher the drainage eye lies in the bladder. This can impair drainage and cause more irritation to the sensitive trigone of the bladder (Figure 8.4, p. 276). The balloon should be just large enough to stop the catheter falling out or being pushed out if the patient bears down. The recommended balloon size for routine use is 5–10 mL. A 30 mL balloon should be used only following surgery on the prostate gland.

    Note that underinflation of a large-capacity balloon causes distortion of the tip of the catheter and occlusion of the drainage eye. Therefore a large balloon should be filled with at least 20 mL of water. A smaller-ballooned catheter, because the water must reach the balloon, should be filled with at least 10 mL.

- Catheters for short-term use are made of a latex material that can cause irritation of the urethra and build-up of crystals in the bladder. Therefore it is not recommended to use this type of catheter for longer than 2 or 3 weeks.
- Catheters for long-term use are made of 100% silicone material; they are less irritating, softer, and cause less build-up of crystals.

(outlined in Box 8.9 above) should be discussed with all men and their questions honestly answered. It should never be presumed that any specific groups of men are not sexually active. Apart from the general anxieties associated with the prospect of surgery and an anaesthetic (see Ch. 26), many men will worry about loss of continence, erectile dysfunction (ED) and a decrease in fertility (Box 8.12). Since many men have retrograde ejaculation (ejaculation of semen into the bladder) after prostate surgery, it is essential that they are counselled adequately beforehand. Retrograde

Box 8.11 Information

Principles of catheter management: for men and women

Performing catheterisation

The nurse performing catheterisation must introduce the catheter into the bladder using aseptic technique, without causing trauma and with minimum discomfort to the person. The following considerations are essential:

- Providing sufficient information to allow the person to give informed consent to the procedure.
- Positioning the person correctly.
- Adequate cleaning of the genital area.
- Working under good light, especially when catheterising women.
- Ensuring the person's privacy.
- Ensuring adequate anaesthesia of the urethra for both men and women. A local anaesthetic-containing antiseptic should be instilled and left to take effect for a minimum of 5 min.

Management of the indwelling catheter

The main priorities of catheter care are to prevent infection and to safeguard the person's dignity. To minimise the risk of infection the nurse should:

- Establish and maintain a closed system of drainage.
- Promote good personal hygiene – meatal hygiene can be achieved by washing with soap and water daily (National Institute for Health and Clinical Excellence 2003). More recently, evidence-based guidelines indicate that a daily bath or shower is sufficient (Pratt et al 2007).
- Encourage a fluid intake of 2–4 L daily, according to the individual's needs.
- Encourage maximum mobility.
- Avoid causing trauma to the urethra and bladder neck.
- Give bladder washouts only when absolutely necessary, i.e. when the catheter is blocked or when washouts have been prescribed as a treatment (Getliffe & Dolman 2003). Bladder washouts should not be employed as a prophylactic treatment for urine infections.

Maintaining the person's dignity

The following measures will help to preserve the person's dignity and self-esteem by:

- Providing education and promoting self-care where possible in meatal hygiene, emptying and changing bags.
- Using the correct length catheter for gender and the use of leg bags which allows people to conceal the bag more easily and have a choice of clothing, for example a woman may wish to wear a skirt.
- Encouraging maximum mobility to promote confidence and give better drainage.

Changes, problems and possible interventions

The nurse should be prepared for the following changes or potential problems:

An increase in urethral discharge

- Urethral secretion is increased with the presence of a foreign body, i.e. the catheter. To prevent this becoming troublesome the person is advised that daily meatal hygiene (see above) should be instituted from the first day of catheterisation.

Bypassing

- Check to see if the catheter or drainage tube is blocked, kinked or looped.
- Consider changing to a smaller gauge catheter. It is a misconception that if the catheter bypasses, a larger catheter is required.
- Check whether or not medication which can cause spasm has been prescribed.
- Exclude constipation – relieve constipation immediately and emphasise the importance of a high-fibre diet.
- Check with the doctor or other prescriber about the possibility of prescribing anticholinergic drugs if the bypassing still persists.

Balloon not deflating

- Attach a syringe to the valve in position without aspiration. It may self-deflate.
- The balloon may be burst by injecting 2–5 mL of dilute ether via the balloon inflating channel.
- A fine sterile wire may be passed up the inflating channel and the balloon burst.
- Never cut off the end of the inflation channel of the catheter.

Blockage

- May be caused by medication, e.g. aperients causing phosphate debris in the urine – change or stop the drug, encourage the person to take a high-fibre diet and encourage more exercise.
- Infection must be treated with the correct antibiotic. Check the amount of fluid intake and where possible try to increase this. Check the standard of personal hygiene.
- If clots occur, carry out a bladder washout with 0.9% sodium chloride solution.

---

ejaculation does not cause ED, but a man who has not been given adequate reassurance on this point could suffer psychological effects resulting in difficulty in achieving or maintaining an erection. Retrograde ejaculation will not render the man sterile, but neither will it necessarily permit him to father children easily.

Specific nursing considerations

Risk of haemorrhage Since haemorrhage is a major risk after prostate surgery, pre-operative care should involve determining baseline haematological values. Careful consideration must be given to those individuals receiving oral anticoagulants for any other disease, since the risk of haemorrhage is considerable. It may be necessary to discontinue oral therapy pre-operatively and to use heparin postoperatively until the oral regimen can be recommenced and stabilised. This may take some weeks to achieve and will require the patient to make additional visits to the hospital or GP surgery.

Fluid and electrolyte balance (see Ch. 20) Pre-operative determination of urea and electrolyte levels will provide baseline measurements and permit correction before surgery if required. This may involve urethral catheterisation to enable adequate bladder drainage and the use of i.v. fluids to achieve hydration.

During TURP, the bladder is irrigated with fluid to provide a clear view for the surgeon. Some of this fluid is

Box 8.12 Reflection

Providing information before TURP

Carlos, who is 63 years old, has been admitted for a TURP for BPE. He lives with his long-term partner and works as an electrician. When you and your mentor are checking his details and recording baseline vital signs he asks how often complications such as ED and urinary incontinence occur following TURP.

Activity

- Think about and reflect on how these potential problems could impact on his life.
- Search the literature to find out the level of risk of these problems occurring and discuss your findings with your mentor/lecturer.

Resource

British Urological Foundation http://www.buf.org.uk/

usually absorbed, and if there is an interruption in the venous system during the resection, the fluid absorbed can be excessive, leading to TUR syndrome. Excessive absorption of irrigant (usually glycine) will cause the patient to become hyponatraemic. This can lead to confusion, a restless mental state and, in some cases, altered consciousness. This imbalance can be corrected by restricting fluid intake and encouraging diuresis but medical assistance will be required in respect of the electrolyte balance (Steggall 1999).

Urinary infection The presence of an indwelling urethral catheter pre-operatively is associated with a high risk of infective complications. The effectiveness of prophylactic antibiotics is uncertain, but it would seem that those who do not receive systemic therapy at the time of operation, followed by a postoperative course, will be likely to develop bacteraemia and become unwell.

Management of irrigation

An irrigation set with a Y-connection will be used to allow two 3 L bags of 0.9% sodium chloride solution to be in place at any one time, with one bag running at a time. The irrigation runs into the bladder via the irrigating channel of the catheter, diluting the urine, which then drains out through the outlet channel of the catheter into a drainage bag. Irrigation prevents blood clots forming and obstructing the catheter. The irrigation is regulated, via a clamp, to run at a speed sufficient to keep the bladder clear of blood clots. The bags are numbered and the amount of irrigation fluid recorded on a fluid chart. The patient's total output, i.e. urine and irrigation fluid, should be measured and recorded. The amount of irrigation fluid used should be subtracted from the measured output to give an approximate urine output volume (note that the urine will initially contain blood).

The nurse should:

- Observe and palpate the man's lower abdomen. Abdominal distension may indicate clot retention or extravasation. Clot retention is a common complication in the first 12–24 h. Bladder washout or deflation and reinflation of the catheter balloon may be required.

- Note the colour of the irrigation fluid: a bright red colour may indicate fresh bleeding; a dark red colour would suggest old blood.
- In an uncircumcised man, check that the prepuce (foreskin) is over the glans penis to prevent paraphimosis (pp. 298–299).

The morning following surgery, the irrigation will be discontinued, provided the man is able to drink sufficient fluid to help flush the prostatic bed of any further bleeding or clots.

Pain relief should be adequate to allow the man to rest and feel comfortable.

Catheter care A common problem while the catheter is in situ is the bypassing of urine around it. This is sometimes difficult to resolve, and the nurse should take the following preventive measures:

- Check that the catheter is not blocked by clots or debris and that it is in the bladder.
- Check the amount of water in the balloon. If it is 30 mL, then reduce it to approximately 20 mL or so, but not less than 15 mL.
- Give anticholinergic medication as prescribed, e.g. oxybutynin.
- Encourage the man to continue to drink sufficient fluids.

The catheter will remain in situ for 2–3 days following surgery or until the urine output is clear. Before removing it, the nurse should ensure that the man has had a bowel movement, as straining following catheter removal can lead to further urethral bleeding. Following removal, the man may experience urgency and frequency as before. He should be reassured that this is normal and that it may take up to 8 weeks for a normal voiding pattern to be established. The man should be educated to tighten the sphincter muscle and to hold on as long as possible before passing urine.

Men who had chronic retention before surgery often fail to void postoperatively. A long-term catheter will normally be inserted in such cases, and the patient allowed home for several weeks (usually 6). This time period allows the bladder to rest and regain its elasticity.

Discharge

Once the man's urine is clear, the catheter can normally be removed. This is usually done in the morning to allow him to establish a normal voiding pattern before retiring to bed. Provided the man is able to pass urine without difficulty, he may be discharged from hospital the following day.

Many men feel, after the operation, that they have gained no relief from their problems. It must be understood that it will take about 6 weeks for the prostatic bed to heal, such that full urinary control is possible. During the early postoperative weeks, the man should refrain from vigorous exercise. He should drink sufficient fluids and avoid becoming constipated. The practice nurse or community nurse will give advice and support should urinary problems occur.

It should be noted that at about 14 days postoperatively, when desiccated tissue has sloughed off the prostatic bed, secondary haemorrhage can occur (see Ch. 26).

Occasionally, urethral stricture (see pp. 287–298) occurs as the urethral mucosa in the prostatic region heals.

Prostate cancer

Prostate cancer is the most commonly diagnosed malignancy in men. According to Cancer Research UK (2009) there were over 34 000 cases of prostate cancer diagnosed in the UK during 2005, and prostatic cancer accounted for 25% of new cancer diagnoses. The incidence of prostatic cancer increases with age and postmortem studies have shown that approximately 30% of asymptomatic men over the age of 50, and 90% over the age of 90, have microscopic foci, evident only on histological examination. About 10% of men thought to have benign prostate disease on examination are later found by histological examination to have prostatic cancer.

PATHOPHYSIOLOGY

The cause of prostate cancer is not clear, but there is some evidence to show that hormonal activity plays a part in the transformation of certain normal cells into cancerous ones. Benign enlargement (due to hyperplasia) and cancer arise in different parts of the gland. Cancer occurs in the peripheral gland. Metastases (secondary spread) often occur in bone, where they are associated with severe pain. In cases of extreme bony destruction, pathological fractures may occur. It has been known for vertebral destruction to cause spinal cord compression (SCC) which without urgent treatment can lead to paraplegia.

Common presenting symptoms The diagnosis of prostate cancer is difficult because the man is often asymptomatic. The GP is likely to see men who present with advanced disease which is already beyond cure. Men with locally advanced disease are likely to complain of symptoms associated with bladder outflow obstruction (see Box 8.8, p. 292), a sudden onset of urgency to void urine, and possibly haematuria or haematospermia (blood in semen).

Chronic urinary retention secondary to bladder outflow obstruction may cause renal damage by dilating the upper renal tracts. The man may present with a palpable bladder or with renal failure; he is likely to be generally unwell and losing weight. Renal failure may also be caused by ureteric infiltration of tumour or by para-aortic lymph node enlargement causing ureteric obstruction. Those who feel unwell and are anaemic are likely to have suffered bone marrow infiltration and/or renal failure. A complaint of persistent backache may suggest bone metastases.

An irregular, enlarged, hard prostate gland does not prove the diagnosis, although most advanced carcinomas will be felt as such on rectal examination. However, prostatitis or prostatic stone disease may feel similar on rectal examination. Moreover, if there is a cancer within the anterior part of the gland, rectal examination will reveal no abnormality.

MEDICAL MANAGEMENT

Investigations

The only certain means of making a diagnosis is by histological examination. Fine-needle transrectal prostatic biopsy can be done without anaesthetic for this purpose. Specimens (prostatic chips) resected at the time of transurethral or open prostatectomy should be sent for histological examination.

However, this may yield a false negative if the sample is not taken from the peripheral part of the gland. Prostatic cancer is graded histologically to assess malignant potential, such as by using the five-stage Gleason grading system.

Additional investigations to provide evidence of local and metastatic spread include IVU, CT scan, MRI scan, ultrasound scanning, bone scan and lymphangiography.

Treatment

The nature of the treatment offered and whether it is given on an outpatient or an inpatient basis will depend upon the extent of the disease and on how the man presents symptomatically and clinically.

Surgery TURP can be carried out to relieve urinary symptoms and retention. This does not, however, afford a cure. Radical prostatectomy and clearance of any pelvic lymphatic involvement are performed in the hope of achieving a cure. This treatment is restricted to those with disease localised to the prostate, a life expectancy of greater than 10 years and no significant co-morbidity. The man should be counselled pre-operatively about his disease and the almost certain complication of urinary incontinence and ED.

Radiotherapy This is given as either external beam or interstitial seed implantation (brachytherapy). For external beam radiotherapy, if the man is generally fit, he will probably attend for daily treatment as an outpatient. In some cases, the side-effects will necessitate hospitalisation, e.g. when nausea, vomiting and diarrhoea cause dehydration, or when urinary frequency or incontinence causes severe physical and psychological distress.

Cryotherapy Cryotherapy is being used more commonly to treat prostate cancer, but long-term data on its efficacy are currently unavailable. It is offered to men as a primary treatment or for recurrent prostate cancer following radiotherapy (salvage cryotherapy). The procedure involves freezing the prostate gland in order to destroy it, and is achieved by inserting probes into the prostate gland via the perineum.

Before treatment can be planned, a rectal ultrasound is required to ensure that the prostate gland is of small enough size. A staging biopsy may also be required to ensure that the man does have prostate cancer (in those men referred for salvage treatment) and that the PSA is not rising for some other reason.

This procedure is carried out under general or spinal anaesthetic and the man needs to remain in hospital for 24–48 hours. The man will be discharged with an indwelling urethral catheter in situ which is required to stay in for 2–3 weeks after the procedure.

The side-effects of cryotherapy are urinary incontinence (4–5%), ED (65% long-term ED in men having cryotherapy as a primary treatment, 100% in men having cryotherapy as a follow-up treatment to radiotherapy) and urethral–rectal fistula (1–2%).

Following cryotherapy, PSA levels and clinical signs will be monitored to determine whether the patient is deemed disease-free.

High-intensity focused ultrasound (HIFU) HIFU uses ultrasound energy to kill cancer cells in the prostate with minimal damage to the surrounding tissue. This technique has only been approved for use within the NHS for a short period of time, and therefore long-term data about its efficacy are not yet available.

Like cryotherapy, HIFU can be used as a primary treatment or for recurrent prostate cancer following radiotherapy (salvage treatment) and works by delivering a beam of high-intensity ultrasound to the prostate gland via a rectal probe. The ultrasound beam increases the temperature of the prostate gland and destroys the prostate cells.

This procedure is carried out under a general or spinal anaesthetic, and an indwelling urethral catheter needs to remain in situ for a few days after this procedure to allow the prostate to heal.

Potential side-effects of HIFU include ED, urinary tract infection, urethral stricture, stress incontinence and urethral–rectal fistula.

Treating advanced disease The aims of treatment in advanced disease are to provide symptomatic relief and to preserve an acceptable quality of life for the individual. There is no universally accepted definition of locally advanced prostate cancer. Current recommendations from NICE (2008) recommend treatment of locally advanced prostate cancer with luteinising hormone-releasing hormone agonists (LHRHa), but this may be in combination with radiotherapy. As testosterone can cause prostate cells to grow, removal of testosterone can help to prevent or limit cancer growth. To achieve this, there are three options to lower testosterone: bilateral orchidectomy (surgical removal of the testes), injections (LHRHa) or antiandrogen tablets (see NICE 2008, CG58).

Injection therapy is with goserelin or leuprorelin acetate. These need to be given every 3 months. A common side-effect of this medication is ED. Antiandrogens can also be given as a single therapy or in combination with LHRHa. Examples of antiandrogens include bicalutamide, flutamide and cyproterone acetate. Not all prostate cancers can be controlled by antiandrogens or LHRHa and for these men oestrogens (e.g. diethylstilbestrol) can be used. Unfortunately, treatment for prostate cancer invariably affects men's ability to gain or maintain erections, and therefore referral to a specialised clinic for ED is recommended (see Ch. 7).

Radiotherapy is sometimes beneficial in the relief of bony pain caused by metastases. Vertebral collapse caused by metastatic disease leading to spinal cord compression requires emergency radiotherapy or laminectomy and hormonal manipulation. If effective, these measures may prevent neurological manifestations including paraplegia from developing.

Pain control by means of opiate analgesics may cause constipation; this in turn can cause urinary retention. It may be more appropriate to administer non-steroidal anti-inflammatory drugs (NSAIDs) to avoid this side-effect. Should analgesics be required, they should be given in doses which prevent pain occurring (see Chs 19, 31). Sustained or slow-release medication is often very useful.

Nursing management and health promotion: prostate cancer

The nursing management of the man with prostatic cancer is very much influenced by the particular presentation and the stage of the disease in each individual. The nurse should take a problem-solving approach to care, and promote independence and self-care for as long as possible. The nurse should bear in mind that constipation and urinary retention or urinary incontinence are commonly encountered and can be very distressing both for the individual and for his family. Ongoing liaison between hospital and community teams will help to ensure that care is effective and genuinely responsive to the man's unique situation (see Chs 31, 33).

A range of medical interventions may be necessary at different stages in the disease process. Nursing involvement will then include assisting with procedures such as:

• correction of anaemia by blood transfusion
• TURP to relieve retention
• bilateral subcapsular orchidectomy to reduce the androgen hormone level, help prevent the spread of metastases and reduce pain.

In some cases, medical intervention can offer only temporary improvement, and the emphasis of care will turn to palliation. Treatment of advanced disease is usually shared between hospital and home, and the patient and his family will need a great deal of moral and practical support in both settings. It is important to convey a sense of optimism so that life can continue to be enjoyed to the fullest degree possible. Once the end-of-life stage of the illness has been reached, however, it should not be seen as a defeat or failure to help the man and his family to let go of life and face death with dignity (see Ch. 33).

Urethral stricture and disorders of the male urethra and penis

This section of the chapter outlines a range of conditions including urethral stricture and those affecting the male urethra and penis: phimosis, paraphimosis and congenital conditions.

Urethral stricture

A stricture is a narrowing within the lumen of the urethra which may be congenital or acquired.

PATHOPHYSIOLOGY

Urethral strictures can be congenital, caused by trauma (as in pelvic fracture), occur as a consequence of instrumentation of the urethra (e.g. cystoscopy) or result from the presence of an indwelling urethral catheter. Inflammation caused by infections such as non-gonococcal urethritis (previously known as non-specific urethritis) and gonorrhoea (see Ch. 35) may also result in stricture formation. It is a condition that more commonly affects men because of the length and structure of the male urethra. A stricture may also result from muscular spasm or from occlusion of the urethra by a cancerous growth.

Common presenting symptoms can prove to be both distressing and frustrating. They include poor urinary flow, a feeling of incomplete bladder emptying, frequency, dysuria or haematuria, and dribbling incontinence, secondary to chronic urinary retention.

MEDICAL MANAGEMENT

Tests and investigations required are flow-rate studies, retrograde urethrogram, urethroscopy, and full blood screening.

The treatment options include the following:

Urethrotomy The use of an optical urethrotome allows the surgeon, under direct vision, to divide the urethral stricture. A silicone catheter will normally be left in place for a specified period to allow healing. However, the length of time it will be left in situ is variable.

Self-dilatation This is often used in conjunction with urethrotomy. The technique involves the person using a self-lubricating urethral catheter on a regular basis to increase the urethral diameter and keep the urethral passage open.

Urethroplasty This reconstructive procedure is usually performed in two stages, involving excision of the stricture and anastomosis. In some cases a graft is required to replace the excised urethral tissue. This surgery requires a longer stay in hospital and is normally performed only after other treatments have failed.

Phimosis

In this condition, the foreskin or prepuce of the penis is too tight to be retracted over the glans penis. It may be caused by balanitis xerotica obliterans (BXO) (Csillag's disease), a group of chronic disorders that cause soreness and irritation (see Ch. 7). Other causes include infection, trauma as a result of early attempts to draw back the foreskin before it has naturally separated or developed fully in size, or a poorly performed circumcision operation.

PATHOPHYSIOLOGY

The natural separation of the two layers of skin from the glans penis normally occurs by about the age of 2 years. Following separation, daily bathing is necessary to ensure hygiene is maintained. Poor personal hygiene can give rise to inflammation and infection and has been implicated as a cause of penile cancer (Downey 2000).

Common presenting symptoms Phimosis often causes balanoposthitis (inflammation of glans penis [balanitis] and the prepuce [posthitis]). Presenting features include itching, a white discharge, pain, discomfort and bleeding during sexual intercourse, and sometimes urinary retention.

MEDICAL MANAGEMENT

The initial treatment may be with antibacterial or anti-candidal agents. If the individual is sexually active, he and his partner will both require treatment to prevent the infection being passed back and forth. Circumcision is the treatment of choice and may have to be performed as an emergency if urinary retention has occurred (Box 8.13).

Box 8.13 Information

Male circumcision

Circumcision, the surgical removal of the prepuce (foreskin), may be indicated for penile carcinoma, balanitis (inflammation of the glans penis), candidal infection, phimosis or adherent prepuce. These conditions generally affect adults. Circumcision may also be performed in accordance with religious practices, in which case the procedure is usually performed in infancy or childhood.

The main complications of circumcision are infection and bleeding. Painful erections in the immediate postoperative period can usually be relieved by the application of a local anaesthetic gel. Postoperative swelling or oedema may make micturition difficult. Dribbling or urinary leakage to the wound area can delay or prevent wound healing and cause secondary infection. The insertion of a urethral catheter may be necessary to relieve this problem in order that wound healing may take place.

Nursing management and health promotion: phimosis

Prevention

Health promotion is important for prevention, and information should be available to parents/carers in the early years. They should be advised that retraction of the foreskin for cleansing should not be attempted before natural separation around 2 years of age. During childhood older boys should be taught to retract the foreskin to wash the glans penis (during bathing or showering), dry the area and reposition the foreskin.

Promoting wound healing after circumcision

The nurse can promote wound healing by:

- teaching good personal hygiene to the newly circumcised man
- washing the wound area daily with soap and water and applying a protective, non-adherent dressing to prevent clothing disturbing wound healing
- providing more frequent washing and dressing changes should urine leakage occur onto the wound or dressing
- counselling the man to refrain from sexual intercourse until the wound is well healed.

Further information about phimosis and circumcision is provided in Chapter 7, Part 1.

Paraphimosis

Paraphimosis is a condition in which a foreskin that has been retracted over the glans penis cannot be returned to its usual position. The swollen band of foreskin obstructs the circulation to the glans, which in turn becomes swollen and painful. It is a medical emergency as delayed action may lead to gangrene of the glans.

Cold compresses applied to the penis may help to relieve the swelling and pain. The health professional may be able to manipulate the glans back under the foreskin with or without anaesthesia. Because of extreme pain, men may require a penile nerve block, topical analgesic or oral opioids. If manipulation is unsuccessful, a dorsal slit may be made in the foreskin. There remains a risk of recurrence of the paraphimosis and circumcision may be advisable at a later date. Further information about the prevention of paraphimosis is provided in Chapter 7, Part 1.

Congenital disorders of the urethra and penis

At birth, an infant is examined to confirm its sex and to make sure that expected bodily structures are present. In boys, the urethral meatus is normally seen at the anterior tip of the glans penis. Occasionally a malformation of the urethra is identified as a congenital defect.

Hypospadias

Hypospadias is a condition where the urethral meatus is positioned on the undersurface of the glans penis. It is the commonest congenital penile abnormality (Underwood et al 2003). The condition is usually treated quite effectively by enlargement of the meatus by plastic surgery. In some cases the urethral orifice is positioned further back on the lower surface of the penis, and this will complicate treatment. Surgical reconstruction should take place before the age of 2 years, as this avoids cosmetic and fertility problems in later life. The position of the meatus, distal urethra and presence or absence of chordee (downward curvature of the penis) will influence the surgical approach adopted.

Epispadias

In epispadias the urethra opens onto the upper surface, or dorsum, of the penis. The meatus of the urethra may be positioned anywhere along the length of the penile surface. Epispadias may coexist with other serious congenital abnormalities involving a poorly developed anterior section of the urinary bladder and abdominal wall. Surgical reconstruction is likely to be complex and may involve transplantation of ureters.

SUMMARY: KEY NURSING ISSUES

- Nursing people with disorders of the urinary system is a challenging and rapidly developing area of practice in which to work, one in which the role of the nurse is constantly developing.
- Caring for people who have problems within the urinary system is complex and demanding.
- Conditions that affect the urinary tract can be either acute or chronic and it is important that the nurse recognises that the person's needs are often multifactorial.
- In order to provide high quality nursing care, when caring for people with urinary problems the nurse must demonstrate not only a good understanding of anatomy and physiology, the disease process and the potential complications but also good interpersonal skills and sensitivity in the experience of illness.

REFLECTION AND LEARNING – WHAT NEXT?

- **Test** your knowledge by visiting the website 🐭 and answering the multiple choice questions and critical thinking questions.
- **Consolidate** your learning by looking at some of the further reading suggestions, references and specialist websites.
- **Revisit** some of the additional material on the website.
- **Consider** what you have learnt and how this will help your professional development.
- **Reflect** on how you can apply this knowledge to the care of your patients.
- **Discuss** your learning with your mentor/supervisor, lecturer and colleagues.

REFERENCES

Boon NA, Colledge NR, Walker BR, editors: *Davidson's Principles and Practice of Medicine*, ed 20, Edinburgh, 2006, Churchill Livingstone.

Brooker C, editor: *Mosby's Dictionary of Medicine, Nursing and Health Professions UK Edition*, Edinburgh, 2010, Mosby.

Cancer Research UK: *CancerStats Key Facts on Prostate Cancer*, 2009. Available online http://info.cancerresearchuk.org/cancerstats/types/prostate/?a=5441.

Department of Health: *The National Service Framework for Renal Services. Part One: Dialysis and Transplantation*, London, 2004, DH.

Downey P, editor: *Introduction to urological nursing*, London, 2000, Whurr.

Getliffe K, Dolman M: *Promoting continence. A clinical research resource*, ed 2, London, 2003, Baillière Tindall.

Goddard J, Turner AN, Cumming AD, et al: Kidney and urinary tract disease. In Boon NA, Colledge NR, Walker BR, editors: *Davidson's Principles and Practice of Medicine*, ed 20, Edinburgh, 2006, Churchill Livingstone, p 471.

Holdgate A, Pollock T: Systematic review of the relative efficacy of nonsteroidal anti-inflammatory drugs and opioids in the treatment of acute renal failure, *Br Med J* 328(7453):1407, 2004.

Jepson RG, Craig JC: Cranberries for preventing urinary tract infections, *Cochrane Database of Syst Rev* (1):CD001321, 2008.

National Institute for Health and Clinical Excellence (NICE): Infection Control, Prevention of Healthcare-associated Infection in Primary and Community Care, *Clinical guideline CG2* 2003. Available online http://www.nice.org.uk.

National Institute for Health and Clinical Excellence (NICE): Intravesical microwave hyperthermia with intravesical chemotherapy for superficial bladder cancer, *Interventional procedure guidance IPG235* 2007. Available online http://www.nice.org.uk.

National Institute for Health and Clinical Excellence (NICE): Prostate Cancer; diagnosis and treatment, *Clinical Guideline CG58* 2008. Available online http://www.nice.org.uk.

Pomfret I: Selecting the appropriate method of catheterization, *Journal of Community Nursing* 15(4):39–42, 2001.

Pratt RJ, Pellowe CM, Wilson JA, et al: epic2: National Evidence-Based Guidelines for Preventing Healthcare-Associated Infections in NHS Hospitals in England, *J Hosp Infect* 65(Suppl 1):S1–S64, 2007. Available online http://www.epic.tvu.ac.uk.

Steggall MJ: Transurethral Resection Syndrome: a risk after prostatic surgery, *Prof Nurse* 14(5):323–326, 1999.

Steggall MJ: Urine samples and Urinalysis, *Nurs Stand* 22(14):42–45, 2007.

Steggall MJ, O'Mara M: Urinary tract stones: types, nursing care and treatment options, *Br J Nurs (Continence Supplement)* 17(9):S20–S23, 2008.

Thomas N, editor: *Renal nursing*, ed 3, Edinburgh, 2008, Baillière Tindall.

Thorpe A, Neal D: Benign prostatic hyperplasia, *Lancet* 361(9366):1359–1367, 2003.

Underwood M, Alexander R, Gurun M, Jones G: *Key topics in urology*, Oxford, 2003, BIOS Scientific Publishers.

FURTHER READING

Colledge NR, Walker BR, Ralston SH, editors: *Davidson's principles and practice of medicine*, ed 21, Edinburgh, 2010, Churchill Livingstone.

Doherty W, Winder A: Indwelling catheters: practical guidelines for catheter blockage, *Br J Nurs* 9(18):2006–2014, 2000.

Donovan JL, Frankel SJ, Neal DE, Hamdy FC: Screening for prostate cancer in the UK, *Br Med J* 323(7361):763–764, 2001.

Evans A, Godfrey H: Bladder washouts in the management of long-term catheters, *Br J Nurs* 9(14):900–906, 2000.

Feehally J, Floege J, Johnson R: *Comprehensive Clinical Nephrology*, ed 4, Edinburgh, 2007, Mosby.

Garden JO, Bradbury AW, Forsythe J, Parks RW: *Principles and practice of surgery*, ed 5, Edinburgh, 2007, Churchill Livingstone.

Kirby R: Causes, risk factors and natural history of clinical BPH, *Trends in Urology, Gynaecology and Sexual Health* (July/Aug):19–23, 2003.

Kjellman A, Akre O, Norming U, et al: 15-Year Followup of a Population Based Prostate Cancer Screening Study, *J Urol* 181:1615–1621, 2009.

Levy J, Brown E, Daley C, Lawrence A: *Oxford handbook of dialysis*, ed 3, Oxford, 2009, Oxford University Press.

Pashos CL, Bottemann MF, Laskin BL, Redaelli A: Bladder cancer, epidemiology, diagnosis and management, *Cancer Pract* 10(6):311–322, 2002.

Reynard J, Mark S, Turner K, et al: *Urological surgery*, Oxford, 2008, Oxford University Press.

Reynard J, Brewster S, Biers S: *Oxford handbook of urology*, ed 2, Oxford, 2009, Oxford University Press.

Robinson J: Choosing a catheter, *Journal of Community Nursing* 17(3):37–42, 2003.

Thibodeau GA, Patton KT: *Anatomy and Physiology*, ed 6, St Louis, 2007, Mosby Elsevier.

USEFUL WEBSITES

British Association of Urological Nursing (links to other sites): www.baun.co.uk

British Urological Foundation: www.buf.org.uk

Evidence-based, Urinary: www.medicine.ox.ac.uk/bandolier/booth/booths/urine

Kidney patient guide: www.kidneypatientguide.org.uk

Kidney Research UK: www.kidneyresearchuk.org

National Institute for Health and Clinical Excellence (Improving outcomes in urological cancers): www.nice.org.uk/Guidance/CSGUC

Prostate Cancer Charity: www.prostate-cancer.org.uk

The Renal Association: www.renal.org/pages

UK Prostate Link: www.prostate-link.org.uk

Nursing patients with disorders of the nervous system

Sue Woodward

Introduction

Many nurses may have contact with patients suffering from neurological disorders. Community nursing staff are increasingly involved in the care of patients recovering at home following acute neurosurgical interventions or with long-term neurological conditions. The *National Service Framework for Long-Term (Neurological) Conditions* (Department of Health 2005) has highlighted the need for quality care of patients with neurological conditions, regardless of the setting in which they are cared for (Box 9.1 outlines the experiences of living with a lifelong illness).

This chapter considers the more common neurological and neurosurgical disorders and, where appropriate, makes reference to the less common disorders. The further reading suggestions at the end of the chapter provide more detailed information. It is hoped that the information contained here will raise awareness of this specialised field of nursing, and stimulate further discussion on how best to meet the needs of the patient with a neurological condition and of their family and/or significant others.

Anatomy and physiology

The nervous system is a complex, interrelated body system responsible for many functions including communication, coordination, behaviour and intelligence. It constantly receives data from the external and internal environments, interprets these, and then responds by adapting appropriately to demands.

The nervous system has two main divisions; the central nervous system (CNS), comprising the brain and spinal cord, and the peripheral nervous system (PNS), consisting of the cranial and spinal nerves. The PNS has two functional parts, the somatic (sensory and motor) and autonomic divisions (pp. 308–311).

Basic tissue structure

Nervous tissue consists of neuroglia (glial cells) and neurones (nerve cells). The neuroglia markedly outnumber the neurones and form a supportive, nutritive and protective network for the nervous system. In the PNS, supporting cells, called Schwann cells, form the myelin sheath as well as having a phagocytic role.

Box 9.1 Evidence-based practice

Living with a lifelong or long-term illness

'Idiopathic normal pressure hydrocephalus (iNPH) is a complex and multifaceted disorder of cerebrospinal fluid (CSF) circulation. This paper presents the findings of grounded theory research undertaken to explore the health and illness experiences of individuals diagnosed with iNPH. Purposive and theoretical sampling was used to recruit 26 participants who all had a confirmed diagnosis of iNPH for at least 6 months before data collection. Data were collected through in-depth semi-structured recorded interviews (n = 15) and written personal biographies (n = 11) and analysed using the Glaserian grounded theory method. Four themes emerged from the data: hope, frustration, isolation and life-long illness, and are used to explore and explain the experiences of those living with iNPH. Greater understanding of patients' experiences will help health professionals provide meaningful and effective care for patients and their families.'

> Gelling L, McVicar A: Living with idiopathic normal pressure hydrocephalus: A grounded theory study, *British Journal of Neuroscience Nursing* 5(4):173–178, 2009.

Activity

- Access the study by Gelling & McVicar (2009) and read about the four themes that emerged.
- Discuss with your mentor how you can use the experiences of people with lifelong or long-term illness to enhance the care you provide.

Myelin protects and electrically insulates nerve fibres from one another and speeds up nerve impulse transmission. Myelinated nerve impulses are transmitted by saltatory conduction, whereby the impulse jumps from one node of Ranvier to the next (Figure 9.1). Impulses in myelinated nerves are therefore transmitted very much faster than in unmyelinated nerves and require much less energy.

Neurones

Neurones are the structural and functional unit of the nervous system. They are capable of conducting impulses throughout the nervous system and to other excitable tissues, including muscles and glands. The structure of a typical multipolar neurone is shown in Figure 9.1.

The axons of sensory and motor neurones constitute the nerve fibres. They are bundled together in the peripheral nervous system by connective tissue to form the peripheral nerves.

🖱 **See website Figure 9.1**

Sensory (afferent) neurones transmit impulses from receptors in the skin, sense organs and viscera to the brain and spinal cord. These are usually unipolar (cells with processes projecting from one pole), or bipolar, (processes project from two poles at opposite ends of the cell body). Bipolar neurones are found only in special sense organs, e.g. the retina of the eye.

Motor (efferent) neurones transmit impulses from the brain and spinal cord to muscles and glands in the body (the effectors) (Figure 9.1).

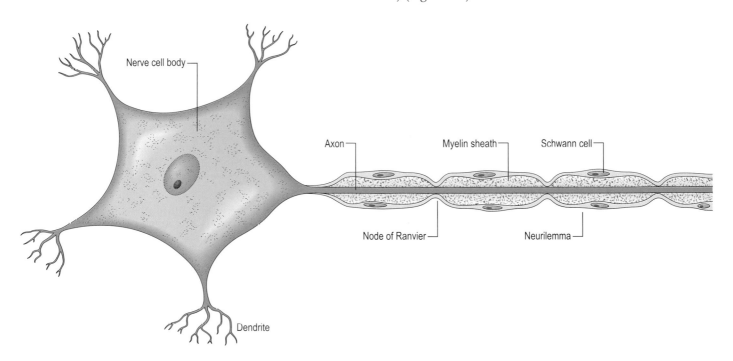

Figure 9.1 Structure of a multipolar neurone. It consists of three parts: (1) The nerve cell body, which is grey in colour. Each cell body is enclosed in a selectively permeable membrane, which also extends along the cell processes. The cell body contains a nucleus surrounded by cytoplasm which also contains other structures called organelles. (2) The dendrites are thread-like extensions of the cell body which increase the surface area available to receive signals from other neurones. (3) The axon is a single long process that conducts impulses away from the cell body. In many large peripheral axons, the axolemma is surrounded by another covering called the myelin sheath. This is a multiple-layered covering of fatty material which is white in colour. Its function is to insulate the neurone electrically and thus speed up the conduction of the nerve impulse, by segmentation. Each interruption of the sheath is known as a node of Ranvier and the speed of the impulse is increased by its 'jumping' from node to node. The axon and its collaterals branch into axon terminals, the ends of which form a bulb-like structure. These help to transmit an impulse from one neurone to another across the gap (synapse) between them or at the junctions with effector cells.

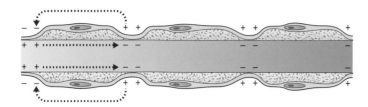

Figure 9.2 Saltatory conduction in a myelinated nerve.

Interneurones convey impulses from one neurone to another within the CNS.

The nerve impulse

A nerve impulse can be initiated by a stimulus such as a change in temperature, pressure or the chemical environment, or impulses can be generated spontaneously by pacemaker cells. The impulse is a self-propagating wave of electrical charge along the neuronal membrane.

At rest, the neurone has an unequal distribution of potassium and sodium ions on either side of the plasma membrane, which are necessary to maintain the chemical difference that produces an electrical difference: the inside of the cell is negatively charged in relation to the outside. This has been measured at $-70\,mV$ and is termed the resting membrane potential. This state is maintained by exchange of ions between the intracellular and extracellular fluids. A property of all neurones is their ability to produce an impulse when a stimulus is sufficient to initiate certain electrical and chemical changes within the cell membrane. These positive–negative changes occur in rapid succession, spreading to the end of the axon. (See Further reading, e.g. Marieb & Hoehn 2007.)

Generally, the larger the diameter of the axon, the quicker the nerve impulse travels, but the alternative device of saltatory conduction is found in myelinated neurones (Figure 9.2).

Neurotransmitters

The junctions between one neurone and another, and between neurones and muscles or glands, are known as synapses. Nerve impulses are transmitted across the gap at most synapses by chemical transmitters (neurotransmitters). The chemical is stored in vesicles in the expanded end of the axon and is released when the nerve impulse reaches this point. Several neurotransmitters have been identified, the most common ones being acetylcholine and noradrenaline. Many neurotransmitters are excitatory, resulting in the nerve impulse producing an effect such as contraction of muscle cells. Some, however, have an inhibiting effect and prevent the onward transmission of impulses, allowing, for example, muscle cells to relax. The effect of the neurotransmitter is terminated when it is destroyed by enzymes or reabsorbed into the neurone.

The central nervous system

The CNS consists of the brain and spinal cord.

The brain

The cerebrum

The cerebrum forms the bulk of the brain. The outer surface, the cortex (grey matter) consists of neuronal cell bodies. The surface area of the cerebral cortex is increased by folding into a series of grooves (sulci) and ridges (gyri). The deeper

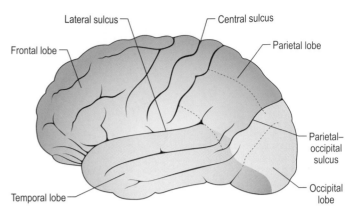

Figure 9.3 The lobes and sulci of the cerebrum. Each of the lobes is bounded by 'landmark' fissures: the frontal lobe is separated from the parietal lobe by the central sulcus; the temporal lobe is separated from the frontal and parietal lobes by the lateral sulcus; and the occipital lobe is separated from the temporal and parietal lobes by the parietal–occipital sulcus.

grooves are termed fissures and some form landmarks, e.g. the longitudinal fissure which almost splits the brain into left and right hemispheres (Figure 9.3).

Each hemisphere is subdivided into lobes, and each lobe is named according to the skull bones it underlies:

- frontal
- temporal
- parietal
- occipital.

The cerebral cortex is responsible for three main functions:

- receiving and interpreting sensory information from the internal and external environments
- initiating and controlling voluntary movement in response to the sensory information received
- integrating crucial functions such as memory and consciousness.

Certain areas of the cerebral cortex have been identified as being responsible for specific functions, and can be mapped (Figure 9.4).

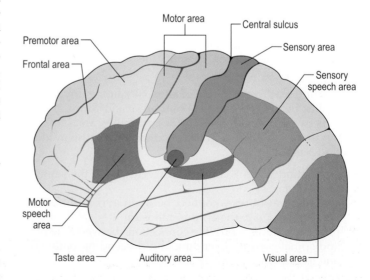

Figure 9.4 The cerebrum showing the functional areas.

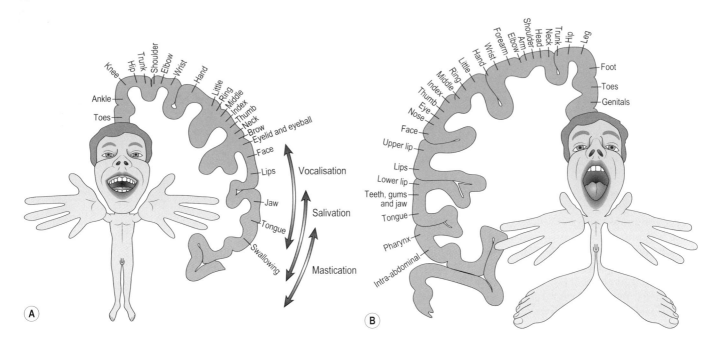

Figure 9.5 A. The motor homunculus showing how the body is represented in the motor area of the cerebrum. B. The sensory homunculus showing how the body is represented in the sensory area of the cerebrum. (Reproduced from Montague et al 2005 with permission.)

Relative size The thumbs, fingers, lips, tongue and vocal cords are more sensitive than the trunk, due to the greater number of receptors found in them. The homunculus (Figure 9.5) illustrates how the various parts of the body are represented in the corresponding motor and sensory areas of the cerebral hemispheres, i.e. representation is proportional not to the relative size of the body parts, but to each part's complexity of movement or the extent of its sensory innervation.

Cerebral dominance Some functions (e.g. speech) are found in only one hemisphere, i.e. they are lateralised. Motor control is usually more highly developed in one cerebral hemisphere than in the other. This is referred to as dominance. Approximately 95% of the population are dominant in the left hemisphere and are right-handed. If the dominant hemisphere is damaged, the opposite hemisphere is capable of taking over and assuming a dominant role.

Association areas Association areas are less well defined and are thought to be responsible for complex functions such as integration of the senses, memory, learning, thought processes, behaviour and emotion.

Connecting pathways White matter containing myelinated axons lies below the outer cortical layer and forms connections between the cerebral cortex and other areas of grey matter in the CNS. Three types of connecting pathways have been identified:

- association fibres – connect between gyri in the same hemisphere
- commissural fibres – connect between gyri in different hemispheres, e.g. the corpus callosum
- projection fibres – provide connections between the brain and spinal cord in ascending and descending pathways; one example is the internal capsule.

See website Figure 9.2

Basal nuclei (commonly called basal ganglia) Within the white matter of the cerebrum are paired islands of grey matter called the basal nuclei (N.B. 'ganglia' more properly describes structures in the PNS). They control subconscious movements, such as swinging the arms while walking, and regulating muscle tone for specific body movements, a function that is lost in Parkinson's disease.

Cerebellum

The cerebellum is located below the posterior part of the cerebrum and is separated from it by a fold of dura mater (p. 305). It consists of two hemispheres separated by a narrow strip called the vermis. The cortex of the cerebellum consists of grey matter, folded to increase its surface area. The interior comprises white matter presented in a branching configuration termed the arbor vitae (tree of life). Links to the rest of the brain and spinal cord allow the cerebellum to receive sensory information and thereby to maintain equilibrium and modify voluntary movement, making it smooth and coordinated.

Pituitary gland

The pituitary gland is situated at the base of the brain in a depression or fossa in the sphenoid bone called the 'sella turcica'. It is attached to the brain via a stalk which is continuous with the hypothalamus, and communication is by means of nerve fibres and blood vessels (see Ch. 5, Part 1).

Diencephalon

Three bilaterally symmetrical structures comprise the diencephalon:

- the thalamus
- the hypothalamus
- the epithalamus.

The thalamus consists of two oval-shaped masses, mainly consisting of grey matter, situated within the cerebral hemispheres just below the corpus callosum. Sensory impulses associated with pain, temperature, pressure and touch are conveyed to the thalamus, which acts as a 'gateway'. Chaos would reign if all sensory information were allowed to reach the sensory cortex.

The hypothalamus is situated below the thalamus and forms the walls and floor of the third ventricle. It controls the output of the hormones from the pituitary gland. Other functions include the regulation of hunger, thirst and body temperature (see Chs 20, 21, 22).

The epithalamus forms the roof of the third ventricle. Extending from its posterior border is the pineal gland that contains high concentrations of melatonin and is thought to influence circadian rhythms, e.g. the sleep/wake cycle (see Ch. 25).

Brain stem

This comprises three structures: the medulla, the pons and the midbrain. Inferiorly the medulla is continuous with the spinal cord and connects with the pons above. The pons is continuous with the midbrain, which connects with the lower portion of the diencephalon.

The medulla All the spinal pathways pass through the medulla. Descending motor pathways (corticospinal and corticobulbar) cross to the opposite side in triangular-shaped structures called the pyramids, a process known as decussation. The medulla:

- contains the reticular formation, a diffuse area of grey and white matter that connects with the rest of the brain stem and cerebral cortex, within which is the reticular activating system (RAS), responsible for consciousness and arousal
- accommodates the reflex centres that control vital functions:
  - the cardiac centre – regulates heartbeat and force of contraction
  - the medullary rhythmicity area – adjusts the rhythm of breathing
  - the vasomotor centre (VMC) – regulates the diameter of blood vessels
- contains other non-vital centres, including those responsible for coordinating swallowing, vomiting, coughing, sneezing and hiccupping
- contains the nuclei of cranial nerves VIII to XII (see Table 9.1, p. 309).

The pons The pons is a bridge between the medulla and the midbrain. It comprises fibres that connect with the cerebellum and fibres that link between the spinal cord and the brain. It contains the nuclei of cranial nerves V to VIII inclusive (see Table 9.1, p. 309). Other important nuclei also exert an influence on respiration.

The midbrain The midbrain contains the centres for visual, auditory and postural reflexes. It is located above the pons and contains the nuclei of cranial nerves III and IV (see Table 9.1, p. 309). Cranial nerves I and II originate in the cerebrum.

The limbic system

A diffuse collection of nuclei, the limbic system, comprises an interconnected complex of structures, with links to the hypothalamus, cerebral cortex and the olfactory system. These are thought to be responsible for behaviour associated with emotions, subconscious motor and sensory drives and feelings of pain and pleasure.

The meninges

The brain and spinal cord are surrounded and protected by three meninges. From inside working out they are:

- pia mater
- arachnoid mater
- dura mater.

Pia mater has its own blood supply and is a delicate layer that closely follows and adheres to the contours of the brain and spinal cord.

Arachnoid mater is a fibrous layer between the pia and dura maters. It is separated from the pia mater by the subarachnoid space which contains cerebrospinal fluid (CSF). The arachnoid mater projects villi into the venous sinuses, which are responsible for the absorption of CSF.

Dura mater is a double layer of dense fibrous tissue. It is separated from the arachnoid mater by the subdural space. The outer layer adheres closely to the underside of the cranial bones, whilst the inner, meningeal layer is much thinner. The spinal dura mater has only one layer, which corresponds to the meningeal layer of the cranium. The two layers of the dura mater separate at several locations and these spaces contain the venous sinuses, e.g. the falx cerebri and the tentorium cerebelli. The former forms an incomplete division dipping down between the two cerebral hemispheres (Figure 9.6). The tentorium cerebelli forms a division between the occipital lobes of the cerebrum and the cerebellum.

The ventricular system

The ventricular system of the brain comprises four fluid-filled irregular cavities (ventricles) interconnected by narrow pathways (Figure 9.7) and connected with the central canal of the spinal cord and the subarachnoid space. There are two lateral ventricles, one in each cerebral hemisphere, one ventricle (the third) located in the diencephalic region and the fourth located in the medulla.

Cerebrospinal fluid circulates within the closed ventricular system. The normal features of CSF are:

- colour – crystal clear
- cells – $<5 \times 10^6$/L (all mononuclear)
- protein (total) – 100–400 mg/L
- glucose – 2.5–4.0 mmol/L.

The CSF production–absorption cycle is continuous and a fairly constant volume of 120–150 mL is maintained. When this process is interrupted and the volume is increased beyond normal limits, hydrocephalus occurs.

Most CSF is produced by the choroid plexus, a collection of specialised capillaries located within the lining of the ventricles, the largest amount being produced in the lateral ventricles. From here, the CSF passes through two interventricular foramina (foramen of Monro) to the third ventricle, then via the single cerebral aqueduct (aqueduct of Sylvius)

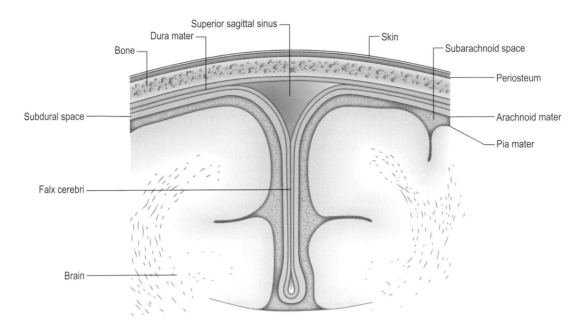

Figure 9.6 The meninges.

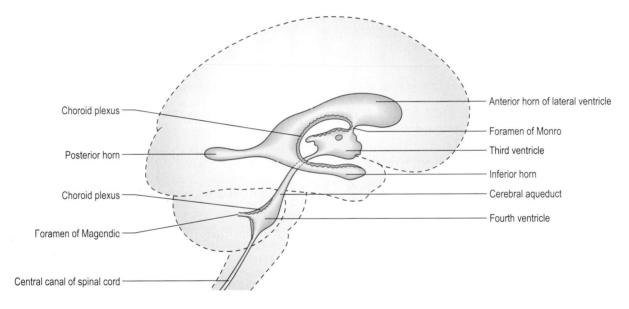

Figure 9.7 The ventricular system.

to the fourth ventricle. Some CSF passes down into the central canal of the spinal cord but most passes up through the two lateral and one medial foramina in the roof of the fourth ventricle, to circulate round the brain and spinal cord in the subarachnoid space before being reabsorbed into the blood via the arachnoid villi.

The functions of CSF are to:

- protect and cushion the brain and spinal cord
- provide nourishment
- maintain a uniform intracranial pressure
- remove waste products.

Blood supply and drainage

The brain cannot survive without a constant supply of oxygen and glucose and receives 850 mL of oxygenated blood

per minute. The blood supply to the head arises from the left and right common carotid arteries, which subdivide to form the internal and external carotid arteries. These supply blood to the anterior part of the brain, and the vertebral arteries supply the posterior part.

The greater part of the brain is supplied with blood by the arteries branching from the circulus arteriosus (circle of Willis), a ring of blood vessels located at the base of the brain (Figure 9.8).

Venous drainage is by small veins in the brain stem and cerebellum, and external and internal veins draining the cerebrum. Some of the external and internal veins empty into one large vein called the vein of Galen (great cerebral vein). Unlike other parts of the body, these veins do not correspond with their arterial supply. All these veins empty directly into a system of venous sinuses, including the

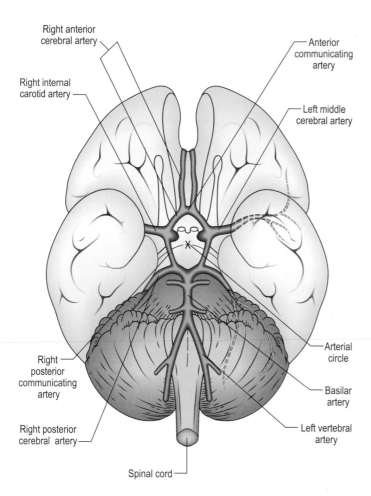

Figure 9.8 The blood supply to the brain.

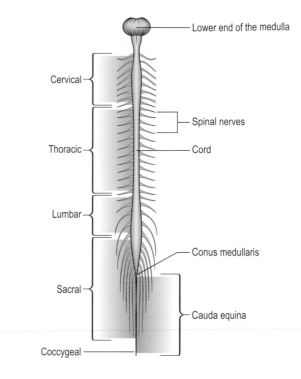

Figure 9.9 The spinal cord.

superior and inferior sagittal, the straight, transverse, sigmoid and cavernous sinuses.

🖰 See website Figure 9.3

The blood–brain barrier

This selective barrier normally prevents many harmful substances crossing from the blood to the brain, e.g. microorganisms. The blood–brain barrier (BBB) is formed by the capillary endothelial cells which have 'tight junctions' and are supported by astrocytes (a type of neuroglial cells) to ensure that the capillary wall is relatively impermeable. The barrier allows the passage of oxygen, nutrients and metabolic waste, and some drugs, alcohol and other toxic substances.

The spinal cord

The spinal cord is an oval cylinder that lies within the spinal cavity of the vertebral column. In adults, it is approximately 45 cm long and extends from the medulla to the first or second lumbar vertebrae. Beyond this, the spinal nerves from the lumbar and sacral segments of the cord form the cauda equina, or 'horse's tail'. The lower part of the cord is attached to the coccyx by the filum terminale and is tapered in shape (Figure 9.9).

The cord is segmented into five parts or regions, each corresponding to the specific vertebrae:

- cervical (C1–7)
- thoracic (T1–12)
- lumbar (L1–5)
- sacral (S1–5 fused bones)
- coccygeal (C1 fused bones).

A labelling system identifies different levels within the spinal cord and vertebrae; the third cervical vertebra becomes C3, the fourth lumbar vertebra becomes L4 and so on.

Two enlargements of the spinal cord are seen: (i) from C4 to T1 containing the nerve supply for the upper limbs; and (ii) from L2 to S3 which supplies innervation to the lower limbs. Paired spinal nerves, part of the PNS, are attached by two short roots to the cord (see pp. 308, 309).

The structure of the spinal cord is illustrated in cross-section in Figure 9.10.

The spinal pathways are described as:

- sensory – ascending from the body and transmitting impulses to the sensory cerebral cortex for interpretation
- motor – descending from the brain to skeletal muscles, where they initiate a motor response.

Each pathway has a name, derived from the spinal column in which it travels, the origin of the cell bodies and the termination of the axon.

Sensory pathways

These consist of the:

- posterior column pathway
- spinothalamic pathway
- cerebellar pathway.

Posterior column pathway Each pathway comprises a chain of three neurones which transmit information such as

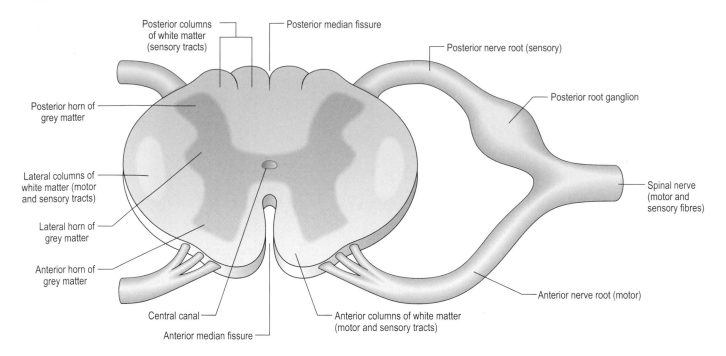

Figure 9.10 Cross-section of the spinal cord. The cord is incompletely divided into right and left halves by the posterior and anterior median fissures. In the centre is the central canal which contains CSF originating from the fourth ventricle. Extending the entire length of the cord, this is located within an H-shaped area of grey matter with posterior and anterior and, at some levels, lateral horns. The remainder of the cord is made up of white matter organised in columns in the posterior, lateral and anterior segments.

discriminative touch and vibration sense from the appropriate receptors to the sensory cortex.

See website Figure 9.4

Spinothalamic pathways are the lateral and anterior spinothalamic tracts. The first order neurone in both pathways connects the receptor with the spinal cord where it synapses with the second order neurone in the posterior grey horn. The pathway crosses over to the opposite side of the cord and ascends in either the lateral or anterior spinothalamic tract to the thalamus. The second order neurone synapses with the third order neurone, which then continues, terminating in the sensory cortex. Between them the spinothalamic tracts are responsible for conveying information about pain (see Ch. 19) and temperature, light touch and pressure.

Cerebellar pathways are the posterior spinocerebellar and anterior spinocerebellar tracts. Both tracts convey impulses about joint position sense (proprioception) from muscles and joints, terminating in the cerebellum instead of the cerebral cortex. This time there are only two neurones involved, synapsing in the posterior grey horn.

See website Figure 9.5

Motor pathways

Once a motor process is initiated within the cerebral cortex, the impulses descend via two main motor pathways:

- pyramidal tracts that pass through the internal capsule and form the main pathway for impulses to voluntary muscles
- extrapyramidal tracts consisting of all the descending motor pathways that do not pass through the pyramids; extrapyramidal tracts collectively assist in maintaining

muscle tone, posture and balance and gross automatic skeletal muscle movements.

See website for further content

Upper and lower motor neurones These are the functional units of the motor system and convey motor impulses. Damage to one or the other will result in very different functional impairment. Damage to an upper motor neurone results in spasticity, while damage to a lower motor neurone results in flaccid paralysis.

Upper motor neurones extend from the motor cortex to either the cranial nerve nuclei in the brain stem or the anterior horn of the spinal cord. The upper motor neurone is contained entirely within the CNS.

Lower motor neurones start within the brain stem or anterior horn of the spinal cord and pass via cranial or spinal nerves respectively to the motor end-plate of muscles.

The peripheral nervous system

The PNS has two functional parts:

- somatic nervous system, which is further subdivided into motor and sensory divisions
- autonomic nervous system (ANS), which conducts impulses from the CNS to smooth muscle, cardiac muscle and glands.

The cranial nerves

The 12 pairs of cranial nerves pass from their origin, principally within the brain stem, out via small openings in the skull to innervate structures around the head and neck, and beyond (Table 9.1). Cranial nerves were formerly described as either motor or sensory, or mixed nerves; however, most motor nerves are now considered to be mixed, but with a dominance of motor or sensory fibres. (See Further reading, e.g. Tortora & Derrickson 2009.)

Spinal nerves

There are 31 pairs of spinal nerves, named and grouped according to the vertebrae with which they are associated. There are:

- 8 cervical
- 12 thoracic
- 5 lumbar
- 5 sacral
- 1 coccygeal.

It should be noted that there is one more pair of cervical spinal nerves than there are vertebrae. This is because the first pair leave the vertebral canal between the occipital bone and the atlas, i.e. above C1, and the eighth pair leave below C7. Thereafter, the spinal nerves are named according to the vertebra immediately above.

Each spinal nerve has an anterior (motor nerve fibres) and a posterior root (sensory) (see Figure 9.10). The posterior root can be distinguished by its root ganglion, a cluster of nerve cell bodies.

Shortly after leaving the intervertebral foramina, both roots join together to form a mixed nerve. From here the spinal nerves continue to form a complex network all over the body, carrying motor signals to effectors such as the skeletal muscles and conveying sensory information such as touch to the CNS for interpretation. (See Further reading, e.g. Tortora & Derrickson 2009.)

Table 9.1 Outline of the cranial nerves (adapted from Bowie & Woodward 2003)		
CRANIAL NERVE NAME AND NUMBER	**TYPE**	**FUNCTIONS**
Olfactory (I)	Sensory	Smell (olfaction)
Optic (II)	Sensory	Vision
Oculomotor (III)	Motor Sensory	Controls four of the extrinsic (external) muscles that move the eyeball, and the muscle that raises the upper eyelid Some fibres control the iris muscle that constricts the pupil, and the ciliary muscle, which changes lens shape Proprioception
Trochlear (IV)	Motor Sensory	Controls the external muscle that moves the eyeball down and outwards Proprioception
Trigeminal (V) (three branches: ophthalmic, maxillary, mandibular)	Motor Sensory	Motor to the muscles of chewing (mastication) Sensory to the face, mouth, teeth and the nose
Abducens (VI)	Motor Sensory	Controls the extrinsic (external) muscle that moves the eyeball outwards Proprioception
Facial (VII)	Motor Sensory	Controls the facial, scalp and some neck muscles – facial expression. Autonomic fibres to the lacrimal (tear), nasal and some salivary glands – lacrimation and salivation Also controls the tiny stapedius muscle in the middle ear Taste
Vestibulocochlear (VIII)	Sensory	Hearing (audition) and balance
Glossopharyngeal (IX)	Motor Sensory	Controls the pharyngeal muscles involved in swallowing. Autonomic fibres to some salivary glands – salivation Taste Carotid sinus – regulation of blood pressure Proprioception
Vagus (X)	Motor Sensory	Supplies external ear, heart, larynx, trachea, bronchi, lungs, pharynx, oesophagus, stomach, small intestine and proximal part of large intestine, the liver, gallbladder and pancreas – swallowing, digestive secretions and movement, etc. Taste and other sensory inputs from structures innervated
Accessory (XI)	Motor Sensory	Controls muscles of the neck and shoulders – head movement, shoulder shrugging. The pharynx, soft palate and larynx – swallowing Proprioception
Hypoglossal (XII)	Motor Sensory	Tongue movements during speech and swallowing Proprioception

The autonomic nervous system

The ANS comprises the nerves carrying motor impulses to the internal organs; thus it is exclusively peripheral and motor. Its activity is influenced by many factors, including sensory information from the internal organs, numerous peptides and hormones, and signals from higher control centres such as the hypothalamus. It is described as having two divisions, the sympathetic and parasympathetic, each imposing different effects (Figures 9.11, 9.12). (See Further reading, e.g. Tortora & Derrickson 2009.)

Neurological investigations

Patients may undergo a range of neurological investigations depending on their condition. Pre-procedure preparation and post-procedure care is identified in Table 9.2. The specific investigations performed for each condition are detailed throughout the chapter.

Head injury and raised intracranial pressure

In 2006/2007 almost 156 000 people were admitted to hospital in England as a result of head injury, the majority of whom were young males. These figures have risen significantly since the implementation of the NICE head injury guidelines in 2003, which were updated in 2007 (Goodacre 2008). The majority of head injuries are mild (Glasgow coma scale [GCS] 13–15) but moderate (GCS 9–12) or severe injuries (GCS 3–8) are more likely to result in morbidity and mortality (see Ch. 28).

Falls (24–43%) and assaults (30–50%) are the most common causes of mild head injury in the UK, followed by road accidents (25%), although these account for a far greater proportion of moderate to severe head injuries. Alcohol may be implicated in up to 65% of all adult head injuries (NICE 2007a).

PATHOPHYSIOLOGY

The adult skull can be considered as a rigid box divided into two major compartments, containing non-compressible components. A uniform pressure, called intracranial pressure (ICP), is maintained, defined as the pressure exerted within the cerebral ventricular system. When an individual sustains a head injury or there is some abnormal pathology, e.g. a tumour, it can cause ICP to rise.

Three intracranial components contribute to maintaining ICP:

- brain tissue
- CSF
- blood.

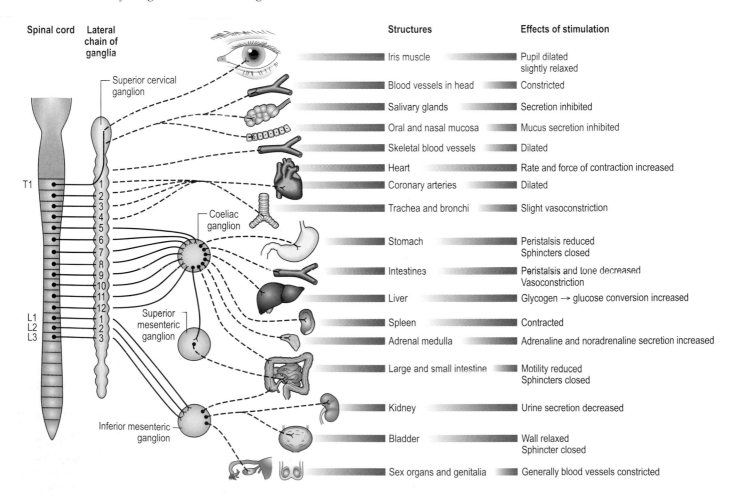

Figure 9.11 The sympathetic outflow, the main structures supplied and the effects of stimulation. Solid lines, preganglionic fibres; broken lines, postganglionic fibres.

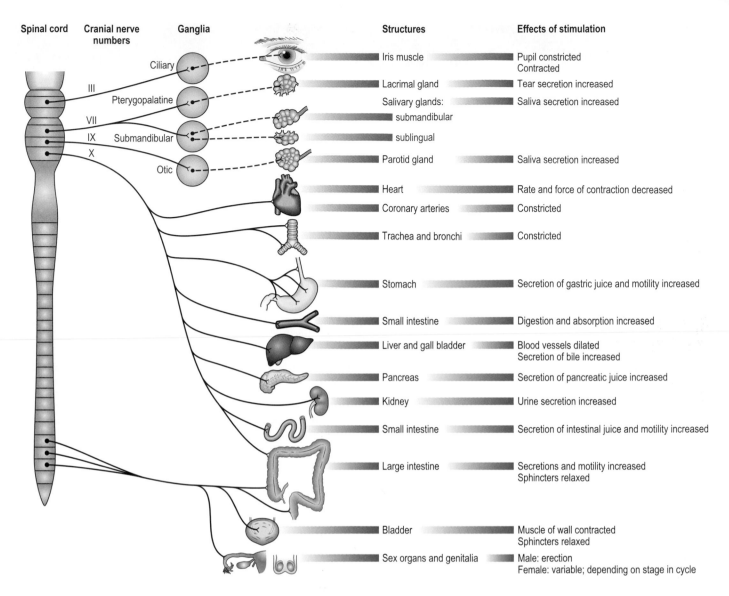

Figure 9.12 The parasympathetic outflow, the main structures supplied and the effects of stimulation. Solid lines, preganglionic fibres; broken lines, postganglionic fibres. Where there are no broken lines, the second neurone is in the wall of the structure.

The brain tissue contributes 80% of the content. The remaining 20% is taken up in equal proportion by the CSF and the blood. Under normal circumstances, ICP is maintained within normal limits (0–15 mmHg), but when there is an increase in the volume of one of these components within the confined space of the skull a rise in ICP may occur. Transient rises in pressure occur with activities such as coughing or sneezing and this is a normal physiological response.

Changes to the brain and its associated structures following trauma may cause ICP to rise to a dangerous level, resulting in coma and leading to permanent brain damage or even death.

The causes and presenting symptoms of raised ICP

A raised ICP can be due to intracerebral or extracerebral causes (Box 9.2).

A rise in ICP can develop over a number of months in a slow-growing brain tumour, with the patient hardly noticing any symptoms, or it can occur in a matter of minutes following severe head injury, when the patient becomes immediately unconscious. A distinct correlation exists between ICP and conscious level; as ICP rises, conscious level deteriorates.

A relationship exists between the volume of a lesion inside the head and ICP, represented by the pressure–volume curve (Figure 9.13).

During the initial rise in ICP, compensatory mechanisms come into play. The cerebral ventricular system can reduce the volume of CSF by displacing it into a distensible spinal dural sac. A reduction in cerebral blood volume also occurs as a result of autoregulation, the ability of blood vessels to constrict according to local conditions. This is represented by the flattened part of the curve. However, this is only a temporary measure and, as the volume of the expanding lesion increases, compensation is overcome and the steep part of the curve is entered. Then for every small increase in volume, the corresponding rise in ICP is dramatic. This process has four identifiable stages (Box 9.3).

Table 9.2 Neurological investigations (adapted from Woodward & Waterhouse 2009)

INVESTIGATION	DESCRIPTION	PRE-PROCEDURE CARE	POST-PROCEDURE CARE
Computed tomography (CT) scan	Specialised X-ray in which multiple X-rays are taken at different slices through the brain. These are then reconstructed by computer. The scan reveals different densities of tissue	No specific care is required. Any allergies, particularly to iodine-based contrast media, should be noted	No specific post-procedure care is required
Magnetic resonance imaging (MRI) scan	A patient is bombarded by radio waves as they lie inside a large magnet. This affects the atoms within the body and as the atoms move back to their original alignment, an energy signal is emitted. This is picked up by the scanner and a computer is then able to produce detailed images of body tissues	Completion of a checklist is vital as some patients are unable to enter an MRI scanner (e.g. those with pacemakers, metal fragments in the eye or some other metal prostheses) All jewellery and watches should be removed and no mobile phones, credit cards or other devices with magnetic information should be taken into the scan room Patients should be warned of possible claustrophobia and the need to lie still. Some patients may require mild sedation or a general anaesthetic	No specific post-procedure care is required, unless the patient has undergone a general anaesthetic
Lumbar puncture (LP)	A lumbar puncture involves passing a fine needle through the space between two vertebrae (normally L4/5 or L5/S1 in an adult) to obtain a specimen of CSF	Explain the procedure and the need to lie still in a 'fetal position' on their side. During the procedure the nurse should remain with the patient and reassure them throughout, but may also be required to assist the doctor to collect specimens of CSF	A small plaster will be placed over the puncture site. Check the wound site for signs of a CSF leak over the first few hours Encourage the patient to rest on their bed for a while and take oral fluids as they feel able Some patients will develop a post-LP headache. Administer simple analgesia if this occurs
Electroencephalogram (EEG)	An EEG involves placing small electrodes onto the patient's scalp in order to record the electrical activity within the brain	No specific pre-procedure care is required	The patient may require assistance to wash their hair and remove the electrode gel and glue that has been used
Angiography	Angiography involves the injection of contrast media into the arterial system and X-ray images are taken as the contrast media circulates round the cerebral circulation. This has been superseded by MR angiography in most cases as this is non-invasive	Patients normally undergo sedation or a general anaesthetic, so all the normal preparation for this is required	Half-hourly systemic and neurological observations are required – patients are at risk of neurological deterioration and developing signs of stroke, as well as bleeding from the puncture site Check the puncture site regularly for signs of bleeding or haematoma Report any haemorrhage immediately and apply pressure Ensure the patient remains on bed rest for at least 4 hours
Evoked potentials	Visual, auditory and somatosensory evoked potentials record the conduction velocities along nerve pathways	No specific pre-procedure preparation is required	No specific post-procedure care is required

Other factors which have an influence on this complex process include cerebral blood flow and cerebral oedema. (See Further reading, e.g. Woodward & Mestecky 2011.)

Herniation

The skull has two compartments:

- the supratentorial compartment above the tentorium
- the infratentorial compartment below the tentorium.

Herniation is the process by which tissue in a high-pressure compartment is compressed and forced through an available opening into an adjoining low-pressure compartment. Such a situation can exist in the patient with raised ICP.

The opening that permits trans-tentorial herniation is the tentorial notch, and that which permits tonsillar herniation is the foramen magnum.

Box 9.2 Information

Causes of raised intracranial pressure

Intracerebral causes

- Tumours
- Haematomas
- Cerebral oedema
- Cerebral abscess
- Hydrocephalus (due to increased production, decreased absorption or blockage to the flow of CSF)
- Idiopathic intracranial hypertension

Extracerebral causes

- Hepatic encephalopathy
- Hypercarbia (hypercapnia) – raised CO_2 tension in arterial blood
- Anoxia leading to cerebral oedema

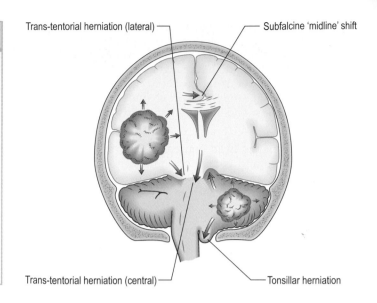

Figure 9.14 Types of herniation.

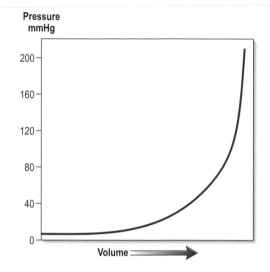

Figure 9.13 Volume–pressure curve.

Box 9.3 Information

Stages of volume–pressure relationship in raised intracranial pressure

Stage 1 Compensation phase: there is no rise in ICP and conscious level remains unaltered.

Stage 2 Early phase of reversible decompensation: a slight increase in ICP. Early signs of deterioration in conscious level are noted and focal neurological deficits.

Stage 3 Late phase of reversible decompensation: ICP is very high and conscious level deteriorates rapidly accompanied by pupil changes. Detrimental changes occur in the respiratory rate and pattern. ICP will soon equal mean arterial blood pressure (MABP) with, ultimately, cessation of cerebral blood flow.

Stage 4 Irreversible decompensation phase: brain herniation leads to 'coning' and death.

Subfalcine herniation involves the herniation of brain tissue across the midline from one side of the head to the other, under the falx cerebri.

Trans-tentorial herniation involves the downward displacement of the cerebral hemispheres, diencephalon and midbrain (central herniation). The nerves and posterior cerebral arteries are stretched and compression of the oculomotor nerve (IIIrd cranial nerve) occurs, resulting in a non-reactive pupil that may also be dilated. These and other structures are displaced into the posterior fossa.

Lateral trans-tentorial herniation occurs in the presence of an expanding lesion located close to the temporal lobe. The medial part of the temporal lobe (the uncus) is forced downwards and can subsequently develop into a central herniation (Figure 9.14).

Tonsillar herniation is the downward displacement of the lower part of the cerebellum (the cerebellar tonsils) through the foramen magnum, where compression of the medulla results.

MEDICAL/SURGICAL MANAGEMENT

Common presenting symptoms The head-injured patient with raised ICP may be fully alert and orientated, but consciousness is usually impaired. Neurological deficits can be found, e.g. limb weakness or occurrence of a seizure. Answers to the questions listed below should be obtained as they have an influence on the management and outcome:

- *How long has the patient been unconscious?* The period of unconsciousness relates to the severity of brain damage, i.e. the longer the patient is unconscious, the more severe the damage.
- *Does post-traumatic amnesia (PTA) exist and for how long?* The patient's memory for events following injury is an indicator of the severity of brain damage, i.e. the longer the period of PTA, the worse the brain damage.
- *What were the cause and circumstances of the injury?* This may indicate if other extracranial injuries exist.
- *Does the patient have any headache or vomiting?*

Early signs and symptoms of raised ICP include reduction in level of consciousness and focal neurological deficits (e.g. limb weakness or speech deficits), followed by pupil changes and finally systemic changes (Cushing's triad – bradycardia, hypertension and reduced/irregular respiratory rate). Hyperthermia may also occur due to compression of the hypothalamus and loss of the ability to autoregulate temperature.

Investigations In the head-injured patient, skull X-ray may reveal a fracture and computed tomography (CT) or magnetic resonance imaging (MRI) may demonstrate cerebral contusions or lacerations and/or an intracranial haematoma (Hickey 2002) (Box 9.4).

ICP monitoring One of the most important diagnostic measures is the monitoring of ICP. This is an invasive technique involving direct measurement of ICP. A typical system comprises a fibreoptic transducer-tipped catheter, which can be placed in the lateral ventricle, subdural or extradural space. The level of ICP is then transmitted to a digital data display as a waveform. A pulsatile waveform will be demonstrated along with a pressure level indicating if the patient's ICP is within normal limits ($\leq$15 mmHg) (Figure 9.15).

Treatment In the past, the treatment of head injury focused primarily on the interventions required to reduce ICP. However, greater emphasis is now placed on maintaining cerebral perfusion pressure (CPP) which is the pressure needed to perfuse the brain with blood, at more than 70 mmHg

Box 9.4 Information

Brain injuries

Contusions

Contusions are bruising of the cerebral tissue, most commonly affecting the frontal, occipital and undersurface of the temporal lobes.

There are two types:

- coup – indicates haemorrhage and oedema immediately under the injury site
- contrecoup – damage occurs directly opposite the injury site. This is caused by the rapid acceleration or deceleration movement of the brain within the skull following severe trauma, resulting in cerebral oedema and raised ICP.

Lacerations

Brain tissue is lacerated as a result of, for example, a skull fracture, resulting in disruption to cellular activity which will produce focal neurological deficits such as hemiparesis (weakness on one side of the body).

Contusions and cerebral oedema may also occur.

Haematoma

A localised collection of blood, named according to its location:

- extradural – between the skull and the dura mater
- subdural – between the dura mater and the arachnoid mater
- intracerebral – within the brain substance.

Diffuse brain injury

Here, there is no specific focal pathology. Shearing of the white matter occurs, causing disruption and tearing of the axons.

(Box 9.5). Those patients with a high ICP, low blood pressure and low CPP make a poorer recovery. The means by which this is achieved are varied according to circumstances.

Hyperosmolar agents An intravenous infusion of 100 mL of 20% mannitol over 15 min will reduce ICP by establishing an osmotic gradient between the plasma and brain tissue, thus removing water from the oedematous brain tissue to the blood. This will 'buy' time to allow the patient to be prepared for transfer to a specialist unit or for surgery. Repeated boluses may be administered over 24 hours, but may lead to a rebound increase in ICP.

Controlled ventilation In the past it was recommended that the reduction of $PaCO_2$ would reduce ICP. However, it also causes vasoconstriction, thus reducing cerebral blood volume. The resultant reduction in cerebral blood flow may itself cause ischaemic brain damage (Lindsay & Bone 2004) so patients are ventilated to keep $PaCO_2$ within normal limits. Maintaining the blood pressure and CPP appear to be as important, if not more important, than lowering ICP.

Fluid management Dextrose infusions should not be given to patients with head injuries. Due to disruption to the BBB, administration of dextrose could exacerbate cerebral oedema. 0.9% sodium chloride is the fluid of choice initially.

Sedatives If ICP fails to respond to standard measures then sedation, under carefully controlled conditions, may help by reducing cerebral metabolism and thus offering a degree of protection for the brain (Lindsay & Bone 2004).

Surgical intervention Surgery may be performed to remove a focal lesion such as an expanding haematoma and this may be combined with decompression. Withdrawal of small amounts of CSF via a ventricular catheter results in a reduction of ICP, but this provides only temporary relief. To be effective, drainage would require to be continuous, but this is often impractical.

 ## Nursing management and health promotion: head injury

Head injury is preventable. This is an area in which nurses should exercise their health promotion skills, e.g. by emphasising the dangers associated with head injury and its detrimental effects when communicating with patients who have experience of minor head injury with good recovery, and with their families. This may include consideration of driver behaviour or unsafe work practices. The use of seatbelts for the driver and all car passengers has led to a reduction in head injuries, as has the use of protective headgear for motorcyclists and horse riders (Headway 2004). Because a common contributing factor in head injury is alcohol intake, where appropriate, the patient can be encouraged to consider personal lifestyle and the consumption of alcohol.

Head-injured patients with raised ICP can present in different ways on admission to hospital. The person may initially appear not to have sustained an injury but can progress to become drowsy or confused, or develop speech problems or limb deficits. Seizures may occur.

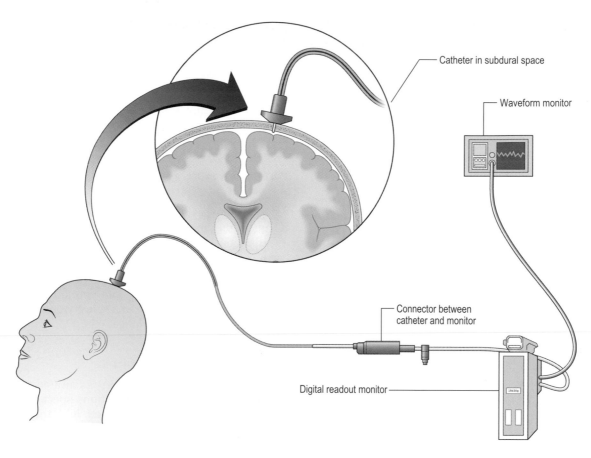

Catheter in subdural space

Waveform monitor

Connector between
catheter and monitor

Digital readout monitor

Figure 9.15 The fibreoptic transducer-tipped catheter system for monitoring intracranial pressure (Camino system). (Adapted from Hickey 2002.)

 Box 9.5 Reflection

Relationship between cerebral perfusion pressure (CPP), ICP and MABP

CPP is equal to the mean arterial blood pressure MABP − ICP (i.e. CPP = MABP − ICP)

Activity

- Reflect on what might happen to the CPP of a patient whose ICP rose significantly or who became hypotensive. What effects might these changes have on brain function? Discuss your conclusions with your mentor.

Box 9.6 Information

Respiratory care priorities in a patient with raised intracranial pressure

- Assess the rate, depth and pattern of respirations to indicate the patency of the airway. Report if the rate is less than 12 and more than 20, and any irregularities in rate or rhythm, as these may indicate a rise in ICP.
- Monitor O_2 saturations and assess the skin/mucosae for cyanosis, which would indicate inadequate respiration as a late sign.
- Apply oropharyngeal and tracheal suctioning only as required to remove secretions. Suction for no more than 15 s and consider preoxygenation prior to suctioning with 100% oxygen to prevent a build-up of carbon dioxide in the blood, resulting in further elevation of ICP.
- Institute measures to achieve optimal respiratory status including insertion of a Guedel airway, positioning the patient on their side with a 30 degree head-up tilt, and administer oxygen as prescribed.
- Assist with monitoring arterial blood gases and mechanical ventilation as required.

Immediate priorities

The immediate nursing aim is to prevent further damaging rises in ICP, and the first priority is to identify any alteration in respiratory function due to an inability to maintain an airway (Box 9.6). The nurse should be aware of the presence of other injuries, e.g. if the patient has been in a road traffic accident (see Chs 18, 27 for detail of assessment and interventions).

Assessment of neurological status

This is performed in order to:

- identify any immediate action that needs to be taken
- record a baseline to detect any changes in neurological condition.

Any deterioration in neurological status may be an early indication that ICP is rising further, thus increasing the likelihood of herniation (Mestecky 2007). Neurological assessment is important, as this may be the only indication that the patient's condition is deteriorating and a standardised method of monitoring neurological status enhances this process. The gold standard method is the Glasgow Coma Scale (NICE 2007a) (Ch. 28).

The frequency of observations is determined by the patient's condition, ranging from intervals of 15 min to 2 h. Conducting serial assessments is more important than a one-off set of observations. Medical staff should be promptly informed of any pertinent changes in the patient's neurological status.

The nurse, as the health care professional who normally spends most time with the patient, should learn to observe changes in the patient's behaviour which may herald an impending change in neurological status, e.g. the patient who does not answer questions so readily or who is becoming agitated and restless (Box 9.7).

The expert neurosurgical nurse will be alert to the early warning signs that must be reported so that treatment can be carried out as soon as possible (p. 314).

Cardiovascular assessment

The final life-threatening concern in a patient with a rising ICP is the effect of alterations to systemic and cerebral circulation, due to shock and cardiovascular instability. Unless requested by medical staff to do otherwise, the nurse should always report if:

- systolic pressure is less than 90 or more than 170 mmHg
- diastolic pressure is less than 50 or more than 100 mmHg
- the pulse rate is less than 50 or more than 100 beats/min.

Readings which are outwith these parameters will render the patient more susceptible to brain damage as a result of

raised ICP and lowered CPP. The recognition of the vulnerable patient has been greatly facilitated by the use of early warning system charts.

Surgery

Pre-operative care Urgent surgery (e.g. craniotomy) may be indicated on admission or in response to subsequent deterioration. The nurse may need to prepare the patient in a very short time and also provide adequate explanation and reassurance (see Ch. 26).

Postoperative care The overall priorities for patients following neurosurgery are:

- continuous assessment of neurological status (see Ch. 28)
- instituting measures to avoid secondary brain damage
- administration of appropriate therapies.

Table 9.3 outlines the main complications of neurosurgery.

As the patient progresses, their needs will require to be reassessed and the nursing interventions adjusted accordingly. The aim of care is to ensure optimal function and the early detection of complications.

Subsequent considerations

All of the nursing interventions identified in Chapter 26 will apply. Only those interventions specific to the patient who is unconscious due to raised ICP are included here. The main aim of care remains that of preventing further rises in ICP.

The patient care outlined in the following sections uses the Roper et al (1980) framework of the activities of living model.

Communicating

Unpleasant stimuli are known to increase ICP, so the nurse should take a calm, reassuring approach. Relatives should be encouraged to talk to the patient and, although they may feel rather foolish at first, they will be encouraged if they see the nurse doing this. They should, however, be warned to avoid discussing potentially upsetting topics as the unconscious patient may still be able to hear (Hickey 2002) and this may cause their ICP to rise.

Box 9.7 Reflection

Caring for a patient with raised ICP

A range of signs and symptoms may become apparent in a patient with raised ICP (see Box 9.3).

Activity

- Reflect on what sequence of events/changes in neurological observations might occur. Discuss these with your mentor.

Table 9.3 Complications of neurosurgery

COMPLICATIONS	CAUSE	INTERVENTIONS
Altered conscious level	Increased ICP due to cerebral haemorrhage/oedema	Frequent assessment of neurological status
Onset of seizures	Cerebral irritation	Observation of seizures. Appropriate interventions if they occur (see section on epilepsy)
Limb weakness	Increased ICP due to cerebral haemorrhage/oedema	Frequent assessment of limb movements
Speech problems	Increased ICP due to cerebral haemorrhage/oedema	Frequent assessment of verbal responses
Respiratory problems	Increased ICP due to cerebral haemorrhage/oedema	Frequent assessment of respiratory status
Loss of swallowing reflex	Increased ICP due to cerebral haemorrhage/oedema	Assessment of swallowing and keep nil by mouth
Loss of corneal reflex	Increased ICP due to cerebral haemorrhage/oedema	Eye care. Keep eyes closed to protect cornea
Periorbital oedema	Direct result of surgery	Observe for swollen/bruised periorbital tissues

Non-verbal communication, particularly touch, has been shown to decrease ICP, so relatives should be encouraged to touch the patient, e.g. holding hands, despite the extensive equipment which may surround them.

Any investigations or care to be performed should be explained to the patient and their family who will be anxious and distressed at this time, particularly as outcomes may be uncertain.

Breathing

Respiratory assessment and appropriate intervention will continue as long as the ICP remains elevated. The patient's position should be changed every two hours or as the need arises, and chest physiotherapy should be instituted to help prevent pooling of secretions in the lungs and atelectasis. The patient, if able, should be encouraged to undertake deep-breathing exercises. There is evidence to demonstrate the benefits of adopting the prone position to improve respiratory status and CPP in brain-injured patients in ITU, but it may lead to a further rise in ICP (Nekludov et al 2006) (see Ch. 29).

Maintaining a safe environment

The patient's bed should be positioned where they can be easily observed. If the patient is restless or agitated, the nurse should attempt to find out why. Adequate non-narcotic analgesics, such as codeine phosphate and tramadol, may relieve a headache, but patients suffer significant pain following craniotomy, which is often unrelieved by these analgesics, or patients experience side-effects (nausea and vomiting). Opioids have been avoided in these patients due to fears of masking neurological signs, but there is now mounting evidence that morphine is safe and effective following cranial surgery (Sudheer et al 2007). If the patient is confused, they may attempt to climb out of bed and may not appreciate their limb deficit and attempt to walk, thus endangering themselves. If appropriate, relatives can help persuade the patient to stay in bed. Any form of restraint (e.g. sedation, bed rails) should always be a last resort and only used following risk assessment, discussion with the family, in accordance with local policy and after all conservative methods of managing challenging behaviour have been exhausted. If the patient's behaviour proves very difficult to manage, it may be necessary to replace the bed with a mattress on the floor. (See Further reading, e.g. Braine [2005], Waterhouse [2007] and Useful websites, e.g. National Neuroscience Benchmarking Group.)

Controlling body temperature

Each 1°C rise in body temperature increases the metabolic demand of the brain by 10% (Hickey 2002). This increases blood pressure and encourages vasodilatation, which will increase ICP. Body temperature should be recorded at least 4-hourly (see Ch. 22), as an increase may indicate hypothalamic damage or infection. Any source of potential infection, such as leakage of CSF from the patient's ears (otorrhoea) or nose (rhinorrhoea) from a base-of-skull or anterior-fossa fracture, must be identified and reported. Confirmation of this is obtained by testing the fluid for the presence of glucose, using a reagent strip. A positive result, although not conclusive, is indicative of the presence of CSF.

Mobility

The patient will require frequent positional changes to avoid developing pressure ulcers. Semi-prone and lateral positions are both suitable. Moving the patient also encourages expansion of the lungs and prevents pooling of secretions. A head-up tilt of 30 degrees will reduce ICP, aid lung expansion and prevent chest infection. The patient's body should be maintained in neutral alignment, avoiding neck flexion and rotation. The hips should be carefully positioned, avoiding flexion over 90 degrees. These positions aid venous drainage as they minimise intra-abdominal and intrathoracic pressure, which will help to decrease ICP.

Passive exercises should be performed to prevent muscle wasting and limb contractures, but isometric exercising should be avoided as this raises ICP. Thromboembolism deterrent (TED) stockings or sequential compression devices should be used to minimise the risk of deep venous thrombosis, but anticoagulation should not be given or used with caution in neurosurgical patients (NICE 2007b).

As the patient's condition improves, further movement should be encouraged. Sitting out of bed in a chair will help to reduce respiratory complications and encourage limb movements. It may also act as an important psychological boost for the patient and their family as they will view this as progress and referral to physiotherapy is indicated.

Eating and drinking

As soon as the patient is able, oral food and fluid intake should be encouraged. Intravenous fluids may be required, however, and fluid restrictions should be carefully monitored and recorded to avoid inadvertent increases in ICP due to worsening cerebral oedema. Some patients may require enteral feeding, and the nurse should observe all the usual precautions (see Chs 4, 21). The patient with a basal skull fracture must not have the tube passed nasally as there is a danger of further damage and infection; the tube should be passed orally.

Eliminating

Observation of urinary output should be monitored and some patients require urinary catheterisation (see Ch. 8). As the level of consciousness improves, the patient may attempt to remove the catheter. Constipation should be avoided to minimise rises in ICP caused by straining at stool (see Ch. 4).

Rehabilitation

This forms a crucial part of the recovery process and the principles are outlined in Ch. 32. The aim is to maintain and promote function, and prevent further deterioration and occurrence of complications. The neurological deficits which can impede progress during rehabilitation include:

- motor impairment, e.g. spasticity or ataxia
- sensory impairment, e.g. loss of sense of pain or touch
- communication disability, e.g. dysphasia
- psychological disability:
  - cognitive impairment, e.g. memory loss
  - perceptual, e.g. eye–hand coordination
  - emotional, e.g. irritability
  - behaviour or personality, e.g. poor self-image
- social disability, e.g. social withdrawal
- educational or vocational disability.

All the above have an effect on the patient's ability to resume employment and educational or vocational activities.

The multidisciplinary team (MDT), in partnership with the patient and their family, should aim to assess the patient's needs and provide optimal care and support. Realistic goals should be set as rehabilitation may take months or years to achieve. Some patients may remain in a persistent vegetative state requiring constant nursing in a care facility (see Ch. 28).

In some circumstances, the patient's role within the family changes. They may previously have been the provider within a family and may now be dependent on others. Employment prospects may alter and, for some, a return to work is impossible. This can affect both the family's short- and long-term plans and may also have financial implications. An alteration to the patient's personality may affect relationships within a family, resulting in stress and discord. Indeed, some families will report that the person has completely changed and is now different from the person they knew before (see Ch. 32). Sinnakaruppan & Williams (2001) reviewed the perceived needs of family carers and identified that information giving and emotional support were the two most important, so resources of the voluntary sector and support groups may help.

Preparation for discharge

Many patients and their families will be particularly anxious as the time for discharge approaches. Much of this anxiety can be allayed by appropriate preparation and reassurance and an effective plan for discharge. The residual problems that may persist vary widely, ranging from headache to major behavioural changes. A home assessment may be performed jointly by the occupational therapist (OT) and community nurse. Pre-discharge visits home may be considered and will help to identify potential problems. If appropriate, referral to a community nurse and/or to the primary health care team should be made to enable optimal assessment and support within the community setting.

Despite these preparations, it is not usually until the patient is at home that the family members fully appreciate the difficulties that may be before them. Home routines may require to be adjusted, and whilst this may be easy in the early stages, it becomes more difficult to accept in the long term. Other members of the family will often view the disruption to their personal lives negatively and much of the early support gradually disappears. The patient's partner may be left to shoulder the burden alone, and in this situation a support group, e.g. Headway (see Useful websites), may help. Some families acknowledge a sense of failure should the patient require to be admitted for long-term care. They may feel that they have let their loved one down and do not like to admit that they are unable to cope.

Cerebrovascular disease

Cerebrovascular disease occurs as a result of a disorder of the blood vessels or the blood supply to the brain. This section considers:

- stroke – the most common cerebrovascular disorder
- subarachnoid haemorrhage – an uncommon but major life-threatening situation that demands acute neurosurgical intervention.

Stroke

A stroke can occur at any time during adult life. In the UK, 150 000 strokes occur annually, with someone having a stroke somewhere in the UK every five minutes. Age increases the risk. Most strokes occur in the 65–75 year age group and are more common in men. It is a leading cause of disability with over 250 000 people living in the UK with disability as a result of stroke. Stroke is the third most common cause of death in developed countries. The mortality rate rises in proportion to the length of time the patient is unconscious. Of patients unconscious for 48 h or more, 98% will die, compared with 12% where there is no loss of consciousness (Lindsay & Bone 2004).

Subarachnoid haemorrhage

Subarachnoid haemorrhage (SAH) is bleeding into the subarachnoid space, but is often wrongly referred to as 'cerebral' or 'brain haemorrhage'. It affects 10 000–15 000 people per year, with 15% dying before they reach hospital. It has a male bias in the under-40s, but this changes to a female bias in the over-40s (Lindsay & Bone 2004).

PATHOPHYSIOLOGY

The three main causes of stroke are:

- cerebral thrombosis
- cerebral embolus
- cerebral haemorrhage.

As a result of the rise in substance misuse, an increasing cause of stroke in the under-45s is the detrimental effects of illegal drugs such as crack cocaine.

Cerebral thrombosis This is the most common cause of stroke, in which atherosclerosis causes narrowing of the lumen of the affected blood vessels (Lindsay & Bone 2004) (see Ch. 2). As the atheroma builds up, it initially only partially occludes the blood vessel until the blood supply is suddenly disrupted. During the 24–48 h following this, neurological deficits frequently worsen.

Cerebral embolus An embolus may lodge in the narrowed lumen of a bifurcation in the cerebral circulation. The usual origin of the embolus is a cardiac thrombus, in the presence of cardiac disease such as myocardial infarction. Air or fat, the latter for example from a fractured femur (see Ch. 10), can also act as an embolus.

Cerebral haemorrhage Haemorrhage can occur into the cerebral tissues – intracerebral haemorrhage, or the subarachnoid space – SAH.

Approximately 85% of SAHs are caused by a weakness in the wall of a cerebral blood vessel, which causes a dilatation (aneurysm). Other causes include arteriovenous malformations (AVMs), but in some patients no cause is identified. Hypertension may be present, but damage caused by arteriosclerotic changes is common. Most aneurysms form on the anterior part of the circulus arteriosus (circle of Willis) and some patients have multiple aneurysms.

The exact cause of aneurysm formation remains unknown and some remain silent, causing no symptoms. Some bleeding can occur through the very thin aneurysmal wall and produce mild signs and symptoms of SAH without rupture occurring.

Risk factors

Certain predisposing factors increase the likelihood of cerebrovascular disease, such as raised serum cholesterol, hypertension and tobacco smoking (see Ch. 2).

Classification of stroke

A classification system for stroke is outlined in Box 9.8.

The effects of a stroke

A stroke results in an interruption to the cerebral blood supply, reducing the supply of oxygen and glucose reaching the brain. Within hours, oedema occurs at the site of the main lesion as a result of the changes to the cell membranes, allowing fluid to leak into the extracellular space. This gradually worsens, peaking between the fifth and seventh day and then gradually resolving.

The damage caused by a stroke is due largely to the extent of ischaemia that occurs. It has been established that there is a reduction in global cerebral blood flow following stroke. In and around the immediate area of the infarction, more subtle changes are detected in regional cerebral blood flow. Progression from reversible ischaemia to infarction depends on the degree and duration of the reduced blood flow (Lindsay & Bone 2004). The affected area of the brain loses its ability to carry out its function, e.g.:

- controlling movement in a specific part of the body
- controlling cognitive or emotional processes, speech or language.

Cerebral oedema also occurs and as the oedema subsides, cells begin to function again, explaining the rapid progress potentially made in the first 2–3 weeks.

After the initial period, recovery is slower, partly due to other cells taking over the functions of permanently damaged cells. At this stage, the patient begins to learn ways of handling their disability.

Generally speaking, if a patient shows a marked improvement within the first week, then minimal deficit will result. Conversely, if little or no improvement is made during this time, the outcome is likely to be poorer. Box 9.9 lists the most common types of residual disability.

Common presenting symptoms/signs The onset of cerebrovascular disease can be difficult to pinpoint. In thrombotic and embolic stroke, minor symptoms are often dismissed by patients and it is not until a significant symptom presents that the patient seeks medical help. Earlier symptoms, e.g. tingling and weakness of a limb, are the result of mild transient interruptions of neurological function. Major episodes requiring medical intervention include loss of consciousness, speech difficulties and hemiplegia, which may be accompanied by loss of vision on the affected side. Stroke needs to be recognised early and treated as a medical emergency because 'time is brain' (Department of Health 2007). The

---

Box 9.9 Information

Common types of disability caused by stroke
Motor deficits
- Movement deficits
  - loss of movement in the limbs on one side of the body (hemiplegia)
  - weakness in the arms and legs (hemiparesis)
- Speech difficulties
  - dysarthria, where the patient has distorted and indistinct speech but is able to understand what is said and can still read and write
  - dysphasia, i.e. loss of the ability to talk, read and write
- Facial paralysis on the affected side, causing drooling, indistinct speech and difficulty in chewing and swallowing

Sensory deficits
- Visual deficits
  - partial loss of the visual field
  - double vision (diplopia)
  - poorer vision than previously
- Poor response to superficial sensation, e.g. heat and cold
- Perceptual deficits, such as incorrect perception of the environment or loss of sense of smell
- Lack of awareness of the disabled part of the body

Loss of consciousness
- From mild impairment to coma
- Loss of memory or shortened attention span

Emotional deficits
- Emotional disturbances, e.g. change of personality, from quiet and pleasant to surly and aggressive, or vice versa
- Loss of self-control or inhibitions
- Confusion
- Depression

Bladder/bowel dysfunction
- Loss of bladder and/or bowel control (incontinence)
- Urinary frequency and urgency
- Constipation

Box 9.8 Information

Classification of stroke
Transient ischaemic attacks (TIA)
- Onset and disappearance of a neurological deficit within 24 h due to temporary disturbance of blood supply to the brain
- No residual neurological deficit
- Symptoms last from several minutes up to 24 h

Reversible ischaemic neurological deficit
- Neurological deficit persists longer than 12–24 h
- Symptoms may last days or weeks
- Minimal, partial or no residual neurological deficit

Stroke in evolution
- Symptoms persist beyond 24 h with an associated progressive deterioration of neurological status
- Residual neurological deficits
- Probably due to a failure of collateral circulation

Completed stroke
- Condition stabilises and neurological deficit remains

FAST test (**F**acial weakness, **A**rm and leg weakness, **S**peech problems, **T**ime to call 999) is used by paramedics and its wider use by GPs and the public is being encouraged by the Government and the Stroke Association.

SAH typically causes sudden, severe headache, often accompanied by vomiting. The patient may be alert and orientated and may feel intense fear at what they are experiencing. Alternatively, there may be loss of consciousness, seizures and evidence of neurological deficits such as IIIrd cranial nerve palsy, hemiplegia or hemiparesis (Lindsay & Bone 2004). Many of these symptoms/signs are related to the effects of raised ICP (see pp. 313–314).

The patient may still have a residual headache and neck stiffness which may be confirmed by passive neck flexion. This indicates meningism, caused by the presence of blood in the subarachnoid space irritating the meninges. Other findings may include hypertension and pyrexia. Signs and symptoms will depend on a variety of factors, including the area of the brain affected (see Figure 9.4, p. 303).

MEDICAL/SURGICAL MANAGEMENT

The Intercollegiate Stroke Working Party (Royal College of Physicians [RCP] 2008), the Scottish Intercollegiate Guidelines Network (SIGN 2002) and NICE (2008) have published guidelines for the management of stroke. These have now been complemented by a National Stroke Strategy (Department of Health 2007). Stroke patients should be managed in an acute stroke unit as there is clear evidence that patients cared for outside of such centres have worse clinical outcomes.

Investigations

CT scan must be performed within 24 h (RCP 2008) to determine the location and type of stroke and to ensure that there is no other lesion to account for the symptoms, although in practice stroke patients are often now fast-tracked for brain imaging so that thrombolysis may be considered within 3 h as part of hyperacute care. CT may also reveal subarachnoid or other haemorrhagic stroke.

Lumbar puncture If an SAH is suspected, but not evident on CT, and the patient is alert, obeying commands and has no focal neurological deficits, a lumbar puncture is indicated. Examination of the CSF reveals uniform bloodstaining or, if 6 h have elapsed since the original bleed, straw-coloured CSF (xanthochromia) is apparent due to the breakdown of haemoglobin.

If the patient is displaying signs of raised ICP, e.g. altered consciousness or has a neurological deficit, lumbar puncture is contraindicated because of the risk of brain herniation (see pp. 312–313).

Angiography/magnetic resonance angiography (MRA) If blood is detected, either by lumbar puncture or CT scan, angiography is indicated. The presence and location of aneurysms and other blood vessel anomalies such as stenosis will be demonstrated. Angiography is not without risk and MRA is more commonly used as this is non-invasive.

Treatment

Approaches to stroke management vary widely because of the variety of presentations. The aims are to prevent further brain damage, reduce the risk factors, provide supportive care and regain functional independence.

Hyperacute care and thrombolysis There is clear evidence to support the use of thrombolysis with recombinant tissue plasminogen activator (rTPA), alteplase, and this is recommended by NICE (2007c). Patients need to undergo CT scanning within 3 h to exclude haemorrhagic stroke.

Antiplatelet agents The use of aspirin as an antiplatelet agent in secondary prevention is now well-established practice, but there is no evidence that it can prevent stroke in patients who have never had a stroke or TIA.

Surgical management for stroke Carotid endarterectomy involves the removal of stenosing atheromatous lesions within the common carotid arteries.

Aims of treatment in SAH

The main aims of treatment are to avoid ischaemia and potentially fatal recurrence of bleeding. Of untreated patients, 30% will re-bleed within 28 days, and 70% of these will die.

Interventional radiology Most patients with SAH are treated with endovascular coiling by the insertion of helical platinum coils into the aneurysmal sac to induce thrombosis. There is now clear evidence supporting this technique over surgical interventions (Molyneux et al 2005).

Surgery An aneurysm may also be treated by placing a metal clip across the neck of the aneurysm via a craniotomy. This prevents blood flowing into the aneurysm and therefore prevents re-bleeding. Clipping may not be possible due to the size or location of the aneurysm; it may then be treated by wrapping in muslin gauze. The aim is to operate early so that vasospasm can be treated aggressively with Triple-H therapy (see below).

Pharmacological management Calcium antagonists, e.g. nimodipine, have been used in patients following SAH and reduce the incidence of cerebral infarction due to vasospasm following SAH. Triple-H therapy (hypervolaemia, hypertension and haemodilution) treats vasospasm aggressively with fluid administration (Mestecky 2005).

Other complications of SAH

Hydrocephalus The normal drainage of cerebrospinal fluid may be impaired by the presence of a haematoma pressing on the narrow pathways or by haemorrhage into the CSF impeding the flow and blocking the arachnoid villi (Box 9.10).

Intracerebral haematoma The haemorrhage may result in a haematoma, which will raise ICP.

Epilepsy Seizures may occur, necessitating treatment with anticonvulsants (see pp. 324, 325).

 ## Nursing management and health promotion: stroke

Prevention

One of the most important aspects of stroke management is prevention, by identifying at-risk individuals and dealing with early predisposing factors such as hypertension.

Box 9.10 Information

Hydrocephalus

Hydrocephalus is a progressive dilatation of the cerebral ventricular system due to a production of CSF which exceeds the absorption rate. This may be brought about by an obstruction to the flow of CSF, overproduction or reduced absorption. It can occur at all ages; it may be congenital in the newborn or secondary to some other intracranial pathology in the older child and adult.

Treatment is by insertion of a ventriculoperitoneal shunt. This is a long narrow plastic tubing, valve and reservoir device. One end is inserted into the lateral cerebral ventricle and the other end is sutured into the patient's peritoneal cavity via a subcutaneous route. The excess CSF is now 'shunted' from the ventricles into the peritoneal cavity, from where it then returns to the bloodstream. In the acute stages of hydrocephalus an external ventricular drain may be inserted (Woodward et al 2002).

Reference

Woodward S, Addison C, Shah S et al: Benchmarking best practice for external ventricular drainage. *Br J Nur* 11(1):47–53, 2002.

Transient ischaemic attack (TIA) and secondary prevention

A TIA is caused by insufficient blood reaching the brain, for a brief period (see Box 9.7, p. 316). If an individual or their relative notices the symptoms of a mild TIA, they should dial 999. Patients will often be seen in a nurse-led TIA clinic and secondary prevention to reduce risk factors (Table 9.4) will be instituted.

Nursing care following a stroke

Often the immediate priorities and follow-up care overlap, and they are separated here for the purposes of explanation only. An optimal outcome is more likely when appropriate techniques and resources are utilised, encompassing every member of the MDT, and when the rehabilitation process commences as soon as possible. NHS Education for Scotland (2005) provides a framework of core competencies for all

Table 9.4 Risk factors for stroke and TIA

FACTORS THAT CAN BE CHANGED (MODIFIABLE)	FACTORS THAT CANNOT BE CHANGED
• Hypertension	• Age
• Heart disease	• Sex
• Peripheral vascular disease	• Race
• Smoking	• Family history of TIA and stroke
• Obesity	• Past medical history of TIA and stroke
• Diabetes	
• Sedentary lifestyle	
• High cholesterol	
• Excess alcohol intake	
• Other rare factors e.g. clotting disorders, oral contraceptive pill	

health care professionals involved in the care of individuals with or at risk of a stroke, in acute and primary care settings.

Immediate priorities

Breathing Techniques for maintaining a patent airway and adequate ventilation (see Box 9.6, p. 315) are a priority (see Ch. 28). Patients are particularly at risk of aspiration (silent or otherwise) and may develop chest infections. Nurses need to be alert for wet, gurgly voice or respiratory difficulty.

Safety and comfort Hemiplegia often results from stroke, so the care of paralysed limbs and avoiding the hazards of immobility are vital. Similarly the patient with a decreased level of consciousness will require to have their safety needs met (see Ch. 28). ICP may be raised due to cerebral oedema (see interventions for care of a patient with a head injury, pp. 314–316).

The patient who has experienced a haemorrhage will be assessed for headache and an analgesic prescribed. An antiemetic may also be prescribed for nausea and vomiting.

Patient safety and comfort are greatly enhanced when consideration is given to the patient's ability to communicate and to their emotional well-being, as well as that of their family.

Communicating Speech impairment or loss can be a frightening experience for the patient and their family. Early referral to a speech and language therapist (SLT) is important, so that an expert assessment can be performed and an appropriate strategy identified. It is crucial to ascertain the type and nature of the speech deficit.

Powerful emotions are often apparent and patients may become emotionally labile due to the damage to the brain or become depressed (Dundas 2006). Patients who are unable to communicate their feelings verbally may feel trapped inside a body that refuses to do as they want. Some patients are convinced that their words are properly formed and fail to realise that what the nurse or family is hearing is indistinct or jumbled. Patients and their friends and family can become very distressed when they meet and this needs to be handled with sensitivity.

(See Further reading, e.g. Woodward & Mestecky 2011.)

Mobility The nurse should ensure that any obstacles are removed and that the patient is wearing appropriate clothing and footwear, i.e. outdoor shoes rather than loose-fitting slippers.

Visual impairment, such as diplopia, may also be dangerous for the patient. Simple interventions that may help include providing an eye patch to eliminate double vision and approaching the patient with homonymous hemianopia, i.e. loss of vision in the same half (right or left) of the visual field in both eyes, from the unaffected side. These interventions should also be explained to the patient's family, who should be advised about similar safety precautions at home following discharge. Patients should also be referred for physiotherapy and should be positioned to prevent spasticity and contractures (neutral alignment and support of affected limbs). The patient's affected shoulder is at risk of subluxation and should be moved carefully. Pressure area risk assessment and care is also vital (see Ch. 23).

Differences of opinion exist with regard to mobility following SAH. One approach advocates that patients should have strict bed rest and that their visitors should be restricted;

however, this can heighten the patient's anxiety, particularly when they feel well. An alternative approach is to allow the patient up to the toilet provided they are symptom-free. The patient with a neurological deficit or alteration in conscious level should be nursed in an easily observable bed.

Eating and drinking Fluid intake via an intravenous infusion may be required and the nurse will be responsible for maintaining this accurately. Oral diet may be introduced after detailed swallowing assessment (in conjunction with the SLT) has been performed and shown to be safe. The patient may need help with feeding, or can be given adapted eating utensils which allow them to feed themselves. Being fed can be embarrassing and sensitivity is required to preserve the patient's dignity and self-esteem. The nurse should determine the patient's capability; for example, hemiplegia may prevent them from cutting up their own food but, once this is done, they can feed themselves.

Dysphagia may put patients at risk of aspiration and they may need to be kept nil orally. Recommendations may include the use of nasogastric feeding with a prescribed proprietary liquid diet (see Ch. 21) and the use of specialised exercises and techniques to aid swallowing. Increased oral hygiene is important in both instances. The patient with dysphagia receiving nasogastric feeding will be more prone to a dry mouth and the patient who is managing to take an oral diet may leave food debris in the affected side of their mouth. Regular oral inspection and oral hygiene are essential (see Ch. 15).

Eliminating Incontinence of urine may occur due to the damage to the brain (urge urinary incontinence) or due to loss of consciousness and enforced immobility. Urge urinary incontinence can be treated by bladder retraining or administering anticholinergic drugs. Urinary incontinence may also be helped by using bedpans or urinals at specified intervals, rather than resorting to catheterisation. Urinary sheaths may be suitable for male patients, but these are not without practical problems. No successful female equivalent is yet available (see Ch. 24).

Constipation may also be a problem and bowel habit must be monitored and treated as necessary.

Rehabilitation

The overall aim of rehabilitation (see Ch. 32) is the active promotion and restoration of independence, and this applies equally to all patients following a stroke, whether they are at home, in hospital or in a rehabilitation centre (Box 9.11).

Therapy Clear evidence exists of the value of an MDT approach to managing the patient.

Physiotherapists can assist people with mobility and suggest suitable aids. They can also help the patient to regain movement in paralysed arms, improve balance and advise on managing spasticity.

OTs can help patients learn adaptive ways to dress and cook for themselves, and can suggest suitable home aids. They can also advise on emotional and cognitive care.

Box 9.11 Reflection

Individualised discharge advice

Farida had a stroke leaving her completely paralysed on the right side and unable to speak. A CT scan showed a large area of ischaemic damage on the left side. Within 12 days her speech was normal, but she still could not walk at all or use her right arm. She took her first steps after another 3 weeks, and 1 month later was walking alone using a tripod. A little movement returned in her right arm 6 weeks after her stroke. She was discharged 2 months after the stroke, and after 5 months she was walking to the local shops, talking normally and was able to use her right hand and arm for holding cans.

Activity

- Reflect on Farida's recovery and consider the specific advice she might need to be given prior to discharge.

SLTs help patients to overcome problems with speech and swallowing.

Nursing interventions identified during the acute period will be continued during rehabilitation. Attention to speech difficulties and sensory deficits and preparing the patient for discharge home with adequate support and advice within a well-constructed care package will be required. Involvement of the patient's family in the recovery phase is crucial as their cooperation can result in the increased likelihood of success (Boxes 9.12, 9.13).

The patient will have been referred to the local primary health care team for assessment and support. Once home, the patient's ability to live independently can be enhanced by aids such as hand rails in the bathroom and adapted cutlery. Information from the Stroke Association (see Useful websites) should be considered along with help and support from appropriate community groups.

 See website Critical thinking question 9.1

Box 9.12 Reflection

Advice for home carers of individuals recovering from stroke

- Do not overprotect the individual.
- Do encourage them to exercise.
- Do not accuse them of 'not trying'.
- Do not pull their weak arm.
- Do encourage friends to visit.
- Do not become gloomy and pessimistic.
- Do think twice before selling the double bed.
- Do continue a normal sex life.
- Do continue to position and support limbs as shown in hospital.

Activity

- Reflect on the points above and concentrate on two or three points.
- Discuss with your mentor how easy it will be for carers to follow the advice.

Box 9.13 Evidence-based practice

Long-term caregivers

'During the first few months after a stroke, family caregivers must learn how to care for the stroke survivor in the home setting. Although there are some studies that address the needs and concerns of stroke caregivers during the early post-stroke period, there are very few caregiver studies that report strategies used by caregivers to deal with their needs and concerns. Studies are also lacking that report the advice that caregivers would offer to others. The purpose of this study was to determine the self-reported needs, concerns, strategies and advice of family caregivers of stroke survivors during the first 6 months after hospital discharge. Using open-ended questions, 14 female family caregivers of stroke survivors were interviewed to identify their needs and concerns, strategies they used to deal with stroke and advice they would offer to other stroke caregivers. Findings revealed five major categories of caregiver needs and concerns: information, emotions and behaviours, physical care, instrumental care and personal responses to caregiving. Based on the findings, an initial needs and concerns checklist was developed. This checklist, as well as the list of strategies and advice, may help to identify relevant areas for caregiver intervention.'

Bakas T, Austin JK, Okonkwo KF, Lewis RR, Chadwick L: Needs, concerns, strategies and advice of stroke caregivers the first 6 months after discharge. *J Neurosci Nurs* 34(5):242–251, 2002.

Activities

- Access the study by Bakas et al (2002) and identify the items on the checklist.
- Consider how the experiences of longer-term caregivers could be used to assist family members caring for relatives with other chronic conditions.

Intracranial tumours

Approximately 3500 people in the UK die from a brain tumour (or other CNS tumour) every year (Cancer Research UK 2009). The cause of primary brain tumours is unknown. Astrocytoma, a malignant tumour of astrocytes (neuroglia), occurs twice as often in males as in females and is most common in the 40–60 year age group. There are two age peaks for intracranial tumours: the first decade of life, and the 50s and 60s.

PATHOPHYSIOLOGY

Intracranial tumours can be classified according to their pathology. Primary brain tumours arise from the neuroglial cells within the brain (glioma is the umbrella term), whereas secondary tumours metastasise to the brain from elsewhere in the body. Primary brain tumours are named after the cell from which they arise, e.g. astrocytomas from astrocytes, but this can only be determined when a biopsy is taken and examined.

See website for further content

Brain tumours may be benign or malignant, but even benign tumours (e.g. meningioma) can cause a life-threatening rise in ICP. Cerebral oedema is common due to disruption of the BBB.

Common presenting symptoms Presentation will be determined by the location, type, size and speed of growth of the tumour and its effect on surrounding structures.

The neurological symptoms of brain tumours include epilepsy, focal symptoms such as hemiparesis or cranial nerve deficits, and signs of raised ICP such as headache.

Patients with pituitary tumours will often present with visual field defects.

MEDICAL/SURGICAL MANAGEMENT

Investigations CT or MRI scanning are likely to be the investigations of choice. Additional investigations include measuring the ESR and taking a chest X-ray to establish the possible presence of metastases. If a pituitary tumour is suspected, endocrine studies and visual field testing will be performed. If acoustic neuroma is suspected, audiometric studies will be performed.

Exploratory surgical procedure Burr hole biopsy, in which a small piece of tissue is removed for pathological examination, may confirm the diagnosis.

Treatment

This may be with surgery, radiotherapy and/or chemotherapy. Patients are also usually prescribed dexamethasone (steroid) to reduce the cerebral oedema around the tumour.

Surgery The tumour is removed (if possible) using an approach that depends on the type and location of the tumour, e.g. craniotomy, posterior fossa craniectomy or transsphenoidal, and a combination of radiotherapy and surgery may be indicated where surgery alone cannot remove all of the tumour.

A tumour may be inoperable due to inaccessibility or because of its type and size. This situation poses a considerable challenge to all members of the MDT to be able to communicate effectively and offer adequate support (see Chs 31, 33). Sherwood et al (2004) highlight the needs of bereaved caregivers and identify the work of caring, informal and formal support, information and dealing with symptoms as key issues in achieving optimal end-of-life care.

Chemotherapy Use of chemotherapy is limited due to difficulty in getting the drugs across the BBB. Chemotherapy treatment is usually palliative, but some newer treatments are being developed (Woodward & Waterhouse 2009).

(See Further reading Woodward & Mestecky 2011.)

 ## Nursing management and health promotion: intracranial tumours

Assessment should be made of the patient's and family's understanding of the reason for admission. Someone with an intracranial tumour can usually carry out their normal daily activities, unless there is a rise in ICP caused by swelling or by tumour enlargement.

Immediate priorities

The patient should be assessed for increasing ICP, primarily through the use of neurological observations, and the nurse should observe for any deterioration in the patient's condition. If the patient has experienced seizures before admission, this should be carefully noted and the nurse should be prepared should a seizure occur.

If the patient has speech problems, e.g. dysphasia, time should be taken to ensure they have communicated their needs, possibly drawing on information from relatives.

Subsequent considerations

After physical and neurological assessment, the SLT, physiotherapist and OT should be involved in assessing the patient, offering advice and assistance.

Psychological support

The patient will be anxious to know the results of investigations and worried about the diagnosis. The investigations can confirm the diagnosis and/or identify the type of tumour, and the patient should be encouraged to discuss their fears and anxieties. An excellent account of the problems encountered by patients can be found at news.bbc.co.uk/1/hi/health/3636697.stm and news.bbc.co.uk/1/hi/health/4193093.stm. This diary was maintained by Ivan Noble, a BBC reporter who had a malignant tumour, and in it he spoke honestly of his feelings and concerns. He died, aged 37, early in 2005, but his account of his personal journey and comments from people worldwide who read the diary provide a remarkable insight into one person's experience of tumour and the impact his sharing of the experience has had for people in several countries. The nurse should be aware of the reality of a grieving process should the diagnosis be life limiting and accept the patient's reactions. Some fears and anxieties may be unfounded and can be alleviated by sensitive nursing interactions.

Ongoing care

Preparation for discharge

Many patients have a good neurological recovery, with no residual deficits and no recurrence of tumour growth. Others may have only slight deficits, such as limb weakness. If this is so, they should be encouraged to maintain their previous lifestyle.

If the patient has severe neurological deficits and requires considerable assistance with daily living, the situation should be discussed with both patient and family.

If the family members are anxious to have the patient at home, their wishes should be discussed with the ward team, community nurses and the patient's GP in order to ensure adequate support is available and in place prior to the patient's discharge. A home visit by the OT or physiotherapist may be advisable to assess the patient's requirements when at home.

It may be necessary to discuss issues around end of life and the patient's preferred place of care in accordance with the *End of Life Care Strategy...* (Department of Health 2008).

Epilepsy

Epilepsy affects 1 in 200 of the population and can be a symptom of an underlying pathology, but more commonly it is a disorder with no identifiable cause (idiopathic). Five per cent of the population will have a seizure in their lifetime, but with recurrence in only 0.5% (Lindsay & Bone 2004). The occurrence of an isolated seizure does not mean that the person has epilepsy. Epileptic seizures can occur at any age, although the age of onset can often provide a clue as to the cause, such as pyrexia in infants, trauma in adults or vascular disease in later life.

🖰 **See website for further content**

PATHOPHYSIOLOGY

An intermittent, uncontrolled discharge of neurones within the CNS results in a seizure. It can range from a major motor convulsion to a brief period of lack of awareness and can occur in any individual at any time.

Common presenting symptoms depend on when the person is examined. During certain types of seizure, the patient may be unconscious, apnoeic and incontinent of urine, whilst in others, changes are barely noticeable. Between seizures, the patient may show no neurological impairment or deficit. Seizures have been classified by the International League Against Epilepsy (ILAE) and are currently under review (see www.ilae.org).

MEDICAL/SURGICAL MANAGEMENT

Investigations Electroencephalography (EEG) will be performed. Other investigations such as CT and MRI may also be considered in order to identify possible organic causes.

The most dependable diagnostic tool is a reliable eyewitness account of the seizure.

Treatment The mainstay of therapy is medication, which is effective in keeping many people seizure free. A range of antiepileptic (anticonvulsant) medications is available (e.g. carbamazepine, lamotrigine, etc.) and guidance is provided by NICE (2004) on their use.

Epilepsy surgery For those patients who have intractable epilepsy with frequent seizures that impact on quality of life and an identifiable focus, surgery may be considered. This may involve resection of the specific cortical area, e.g. temporal resection, hemispherectomy, corpus callostomy, or more recently vagal nerve stimulation.

▷ **Nursing management and health promotion: epileptic seizures**

Most individuals with seizures live independently, with regular monitoring by the primary care team, but NICE recommends annual review by a specialist (NICE 2004).

Immediate priorities

Once notification is received that a patient is to be admitted with seizures, the following essential equipment should be readily available:

- oxygen and suction in working order
- a selection of various sizes of artificial airways
- charts for recording neurological status, vital signs and seizures

- side rails in place and possibly padded for additional safety
- anticonvulsant medication, particularly in parenteral preparations.

If the patient is having a seizure, the following actions must always be carried out:

- Ensure privacy for the patient if at all possible.
- Ensure side rails are in place, using pillows as padding if required.
- Ensure safety by removing any objects or furniture likely to cause harm.
- Loosen any restrictive clothing.
- Insert an airway *only* when teeth have unclenched (after the tonic stage); any attempts to insert objects into the patient's mouth prior to this serve no purpose and may cause harm to the nurse (bitten fingers) or to the patient (broken teeth).

Immediately following a seizure the nurse should:

- Place the patient in the recovery position, to facilitate the drainage of secretions.
- Use suction if necessary to prevent aspiration of secretions.
- Administer oxygen as prescribed.
- Allow the patient to recover with minimal disturbance.
- Allow time for the patient to wake up and provide gentle reassurance and assistance to encourage reorientation.
- Record a description of what happened on the seizure observation chart (Box 9.14).

Prescribed anticonvulsant medication should be administered and, where appropriate, medical staff informed. (See Further reading, e.g. Woodward & Mestecky 2011.)

Further considerations

The patient should be allowed to express their feelings and fears and they and their family should be given adequate explanations and support. Discussion about the medication, its effects and side-effects, will promote the patient's concordance with prescribed regimens. Monitoring of medication serum levels should be carried out, as this test will indicate if there is an adequate or inadequate dosage of the

medication, or if the blood levels are too high. If too high, the patient may experience side-effects; if too low, seizures may recur. Common side-effects of anticonvulsants are:

- drowsiness
- dizziness
- gastric upset
- diplopia
- ataxia.

Overdose or sudden withdrawal of medication can also lead to a rebound rise in seizure frequency.

The patient must be allowed time to come to terms with the diagnosis of epilepsy. They may experience feelings of anger, grief and/or disbelief, and the nurse should discuss with both the patient and family the realities of epilepsy, but encourage a positive outlook.

The patient may experience an aura (warning) prior to a seizure and the nurse can advise how to use the time available to ensure personal safety. Advice should be given prior to discharge about safety in the home and the involvement of the primary care team.

 See website Critical thinking question 9.2

Equally, 'triggers' that may induce a seizure should be discussed, such as:

- lack of food and sleep
- excessive heat
- constipation
- menstruation
- alcohol
- anxiety or stress.

Medical opinion varies as to whether someone with epilepsy should drink alcohol, as it can interact with antiepileptic medications, preventing them from achieving optimal seizure control. Large amounts of any liquid are known to trigger a seizure, but significant alcohol intake is also often associated with late-night, irregular eating habits and forgotten tablets. The decision to drink alcohol is an individual one, but patients should bear in mind the medical advice.

Patients may be encouraged to wear a MedicAlert® bracelet to inform others about their condition should a seizure occur.

Employment

Most people with epilepsy work, but the safety of the individual and others is paramount. Employment should be discussed, especially if it entails driving or operating machinery. The patient must be told that they have to inform the Driver and Vehicle Licensing Agency (DVLA) of their liability to have seizures and should be advised to stop driving in the meantime, otherwise their motor insurance will be invalid. The health care professional is responsible for telling the patient that informing the DVLA is their responsibility and this conversation must be documented in the medical records. This may present major problems to the patient, who may have to look for alternative employment; this may affect self-esteem or outlook for the future.

It is illegal not to employ someone simply because they have epilepsy; patients are protected by the Disability Discrimination Act (1995) and employers must make reasonable adjustments. Some careers are barred by law to people with

---

Box 9.14 Information

Documentation of seizure activity

- Time at which seizures occurred
- What the patient was doing at the time
- Any aura or crying out prior to the seizure
- Any loss of consciousness
- Which parts of the body were affected and any sequence to this
- Any stiffening or jerky movements
- Urinary or faecal incontinence
- The duration of the seizure (ictal phase)
- The duration of the (post-ictal) recovery period
- Patient's behaviour after the seizure
- Pupil reactions

epilepsy, however, e.g. pilot, diver, fire fighter, train driver, child minder.

Physical activity

The patient should be encouraged to continue normal physical activities, with some emphasis being placed on the need to take adequate precautions, e.g. when swimming the patient should let someone know or take a friend who could deal with a potential seizure.

Involving the patient's family

The patient's family should be given time and the opportunity to express their concerns, and the nurse should be prepared to provide advice and explanations. The nurse should explain about the type of seizure the patient is experiencing and family members should be told what to expect if a seizure occurs, e.g. that the patient will have sudden uncontrolled movements and will appear to be holding their breath. They should know exactly what to do and why they are doing it. Epilepsy Action provides helpful advice through their website (see Useful websites). Consideration must be given to meeting the needs of children whose parents have epilepsy. Advice should include the following:

- Ensure the safety of the individual, which can involve removing harmful objects and loosening all restrictive clothing.
- After the seizure, place them in the recovery position, and allow them to sleep, giving them adequate time to wake up and reorientate to time and place.
- Seek medical advice if a seizure lasts longer than usual or if seizures continue without the individual recovering in between.
- Ensure that the family is aware that the individual may have feelings of shock, anger and lack of self-esteem and that time should be allowed for them to come to terms with these feelings.

Women and epilepsy

Seizure frequency may increase during menstruation. Some anticonvulsants may reduce the effectiveness of the oral contraceptive pill.

Pre-conceptual counselling may be required as some anticonvulsants can lead to fetal abnormalities.

Multiple sclerosis

Multiple sclerosis (MS) is a chronic, progressive, demyelinating neurological disorder and is one of the most common neurological causes of long-term disability (Boon et al 2006). The age of onset is 20–50 years and it is slightly more common in females. The aetiology is considered to be an interaction between a number of environmental and genetic factors. MS typically follows a remitting and relapsing course, but the disease has several forms.

The prevalence of MS varies significantly in different parts of the world. It is described as a disorder of temperate climates. However, those who move from an area of high risk to one of low risk before the age of 7 reduce the chance of the disease occurring. MS is not hereditary, but the risk of a child developing MS where a parent is afflicted is approximately 15 times greater than in the unaffected population (Lindsay & Bone 2004).

A definitive diagnosis may be difficult initially, because demyelination develops over a varying period of time. To be conclusive, attacks must occur on multiple occasions and at multiple sites throughout the CNS. New MRI diagnostic criteria were developed and revised to be used with clinical examination (Polman et al 2005).

PATHOPHYSIOLOGY

MS is thought to be an autoimmune disorder, whereby the body's own myelin within the CNS is recognised as 'foreign' and attacked by the immune system, possibly as an abnormal response to a virus. The demyelination results in scarring or sclerotic patches, and the remission, typical in MS, is the result of healing of these areas. However, in time, these lesions degenerate to a point where recovery is unlikely and the resultant disruption of function becomes permanent.

Common presenting symptoms Clinical features vary considerably, depending on which nerves are affected, but may include:

- blurred or double vision – a common early symptom due to optic neuritis
- weakness and dragging of limbs
- slurred speech
- nystagmus – a disturbance in eye movement in which a slow drift in one direction is followed by a fast corrective movement
- loss of sensation in a specific area of the body or loss of proprioception
- extreme fatigue
- 'stiff limbs'
- intention tremor
- clumsiness/difficulty with movement
- urge urinary incontinence/retention of urine.

MEDICAL MANAGEMENT

Investigations

MRI identifies areas of demyelination, particularly in the white matter around the ventricles and within the brain stem, and is the primary investigation conducted.

Lumbar puncture Examination of the CSF may reveal changes in protein levels and the presence of oligoclonal bands.

Evoked potentials A delay in conduction velocity may be seen in visual, auditory or somatosensory pathways.

Treatment

There is no curative treatment. There is evidence that beta-interferons (disease-modifying drugs) can reduce the number of relapses and NICE recommends their use for patients with minimal disability and who have remitting–relapsing disease (Box 9.15).

Corticosteroid therapy may be helpful in acute exacerbations to manage symptoms and physiotherapy is helpful in the rehabilitation of numb, affected limbs. Many complementary therapies exist and are used with varying degrees of success, e.g. special diets, reflexology and hyperbaric oxygen. Patients will often use cannabis illegally for pain relief.

Box 9.15 Evidence-based practice

Experiences of patients treated with interferon-beta 1a

'The purpose of this study was to describe the experiences of patients with relapsing multiple sclerosis (MS) who are being treated with interferon beta-1a. MS patients often experience fear and uncertainty about their future and derive benefit from understanding their diagnosis, as well as learning about their anticipated disease course. Interferon beta-1a treatment can delay the accumulation of physical disability that naturally occurs over time in patients with untreated relapsing MS and thus offer hope for their future. However, patients may be afraid to start interferon beta-1a because they do not know what to expect.

The researchers undertook serial interviews of 15 patients with relapsing MS. The theme clusters that emerged were learning, feelings, adaptation and interferon beta-1a issues.

An exhaustive description of the phenomena that were derived illustrates the patients' process of learning about their illness and adapting to changes in their lives. Starting a new treatment requires coping and challenges use of resources. Social support is vital to patients, particularly those who have difficulty injecting themselves. Most of the patients expressed a sense of improvement in their condition since starting on interferon beta-1a treatment and considered it crucial to their hope for the future.'

Miller C, Jezewski MA: A phenomenologic assessment of relapsing MS patients' experiences during treatment with interferon beta-1a. *J Neurosci Nurs* 33(5):240–244, 2001.

Activity

- Access the study by Miller & Jezewski (2001) and identify the process patients go through as they adapt to life with MS and commencing beta-interferon.
- Consider with your mentor or colleagues how nurses can assist patients to adapt to the changing situation they find themselves in when commencing disease modifying therapy.

Essentially, care consists of supporting the patient and their family and alleviating symptoms.

Nursing management and health promotion: multiple sclerosis

Many patients with MS lead a normal life at home, requiring admission to hospital only if they experience deterioration in their condition. Comprehensive guidelines on the management of patients in both primary and secondary care have been issued by NICE (2003).

Williams (2004) reviews the evidence for current practice in the management of patients during a relapse or exacerbation of their condition and evaluates how the evidence can be incorporated into patient care.

Immediate priorities

Communicating

The patient undergoing investigations is likely to be anxious and will require adequate explanation about the procedures to be carried out. Frequently, the nurse is asked about these tests and should be prepared to answer questions or, if unable to do so, should find the answer for the patient (see Table 9.2, p. 312). It is important that there is an awareness of the patient's knowledge regarding the condition, as the patient will either fear the worst, often with only a partial understanding of what the diagnosis may be, or may not be aware of the possibility of having MS until the diagnosis is confirmed. Increasingly, patients are well informed from use of the internet.

It is advisable for the nurse to be present when the doctor is speaking to the patient, so that the nurse knows what information the patient has received. Often the patient wishes to discuss certain points and will find it reassuring to seek supporting advice and information from the nurse after the doctor has left.

The patient will need time to consider the condition and what effects it will have on their outlook for the future. Patients often experience a range of feelings and emotions related to the loss of self-esteem and body image and may worry about how the condition will eventually affect them. Normally, the patient's family will be included, with the patient's consent, and they will require explanations about their relative's condition. They too should be provided with opportunities to discuss their feelings and fears. Providing information about support groups, e.g. the MS Society (see Useful websites) is often helpful.

Admission to hospital during the course of the disease progression can cause considerable stress, especially for the patient who has a set routine at home that allows maintenance of independence. The nurse should encourage the patient to continue to be independent and to follow their daily routine as far as possible when in hospital.

Subsequent considerations

Communication

Communication impairment in the patient with MS can include difficulties in pronouncing words, slow and/or slurred speech and poor concentration.

The SLT should be involved and can give advice on how to improve the patient's ability to communicate. Useful techniques to help the patient include:

- ensuring that an erect posture is maintained, as this aids breathing and assists with speech
- reducing background noise as much as possible
- encouraging the patient to express the most important points at the beginning of a sentence, when energy and concentration are greatest
- using communication aids such as picture boards or computer.

Maintaining a safe environment

The patient with MS can experience difficulties with:

- movement, e.g. ataxia or spasticity
- vision, e.g. diplopia
- sensory disturbance, e.g. detection of pain and temperature.

When in hospital, an accurate assessment of the patient's condition, level of understanding and, if necessary, home conditions should be made. This will involve assessments by the community team as adaptations to the home may be required in order to maintain safety.

In hospital, the nurse should involve the patient in making any necessary changes to their new surroundings, as they will know best what suits them, e.g. the location and height of the bed, depending on their mobility. Ensure there is adequate space to manoeuvre a wheelchair properly. The nurse-call system should be within easy reach and the patient should be instructed in its use. The patient with clumsiness of movement or tremor may require assistance with some activities, e.g. at mealtimes.

Mobility

Maintaining mobility is vital for being independent. A problem for the patient with MS is the uncertainty of the rate at which deterioration in mobility will occur.

The attitude of the ward team is very important; the members should work together to encourage a positive outlook for the patient, while making time to understand the patient's and family's feelings and fears.

If the patient uses mobility aids at home, they should also be used when hospitalised. This enables the patient to maintain independence and also allows the physiotherapist to assess the effectiveness of any aids. Common problems may include ataxia, limb weakness and spasticity. Techniques which may be useful in helping these problems are:

- maintaining good posture
- making contact with the ground with the heel of the foot first
- taking care to place feet firmly in the direction of travel
- looking straight ahead rather than down at the ground
- relaxing and trying not to feel self-conscious.

The physiotherapist may suggest exercises to maintain a good functional position and range of limb movements. Rietberg et al (2005), in a systematic review of exercise therapy, concluded that exercise can be beneficial for those patients not experiencing a relapse.

Skin care

The patient and family should be taught the importance of regular skin inspection, e.g. to observe the sacrum and heels closely and to look for redness or blanching of the skin (see Ch. 23). If this occurs, the patient should be aware of the importance of relieving the pressure from the problem area, e.g. by lying on their side.

Using a wheelchair

The physiotherapist and OT may advise that the patient requires a wheelchair in order to maintain mobility. It can be very distressing for the patient to realise that this stage has been reached. It must be emphasised that this does not mean that the patient becomes totally reliant on the wheelchair and is unable to maintain independence.

If the patient requires physiotherapy when at home, advice and support can be obtained from the community physiotherapist. Some local MS societies also offer a physiotherapy service.

Advice should be given to the patient about when to use the wheelchair, in particular:

- The wheelchair should be used only when necessary.
- Emphasise the importance of relieving pressure.
- Careful positioning of limbs should be ensured.
- The footrest on the wheelchair should always be used.
- The legs should be placed in proper alignment and the patient should check regularly that the limbs are safely in position on the footrest.

Balance of rest and exercise

Fatigue is a common feature of MS. The patient should be advised about the importance of rest periods to avoid becoming overtired or overstressed, which will exacerbate the condition. Relaxation techniques and a specific rest/exercise programme may be beneficial and should be discussed with the patient and their family.

Although rest is very important, exercise is also vital to maintain muscle strength and help reduce the risk of spasticity. It will also improve circulation and prevent pressure ulcers and joint stiffness. Exercise will contribute to maintaining the patient's independence.

Temperature control

Fatigue and MS symptoms are also exacerbated by heat, which slows conduction velocities. Patients should be advised to avoid hot baths, hot climates and infections if at all possible.

Employment

If the patient's current employment involves physical exertion, this may prove problematic with regard to returning to work. The patient may have to consider how their disorder will affect current employment and think about finding alternative work, although in many cases this may prove impossible. Patients with MS are protected by the Disability Discrimination Act and employers have to make reasonable adjustments or consider redeployment.

Eliminating

The patient may experience bladder dysfunction, which can vary in severity and include incontinence, urinary frequency or urine retention. Problems with constipation are also of concern. The urinary problems are due to the reflex action of the bladder having been disturbed due to sites of demyelination in the lower spinal cord, particularly the sacral segments.

The social implications of incontinence can be enormous and some patients will avoid going out for fear of embarrassment (see Ch. 24). If a urine infection is suspected, a specimen should be sent to bacteriology for culture and sensitivity. Bladder retraining and antimuscarinic drugs (e.g. oxybutynin) may help, but it may be necessary to use aids such as protective clothing and pads (see Ch. 24).

Urinary catheterisation may be required if persistent urinary retention is experienced. Intermittent self-catheterisation is preferable and many become very competent at performing this procedure. Advice from a continence advisor may also be useful (see Ch. 24).

Some patients will require an indwelling catheter, and support should be provided to enable them to come to terms with this alteration to body image.

The importance of an adequate fluid intake of 2.5–3 L/day should be stressed. Many patients mistakenly think that if they stop drinking they will no longer be incontinent.

The immobile patient will be especially prone to constipation, which will aggravate coexisting urinary problems. The patient and the family should be advised as to how constipation can be avoided by taking an appropriate diet, an adequate fluid intake and maintaining as much mobility as possible. Regular oral laxatives may be required and the occasional use of enemas and suppositories may be indicated.

Expressing sexuality

The patient may experience a change in body image. Sexual counselling may be beneficial for both partners.

Men may experience erectile dysfunction and women diminished libido, due to neurological damage. The patient may be too embarrassed or worried to discuss such difficulties with a health professional, and support groups and relationship guidance services may be helpful. A free booklet published by the MS Society is available online (http://www.mssociety.org.uk/about_ms/symptoms/sex_relationships_and_intimacy/index.html).

Advice on contraception may be required, especially by women, as some oral contraceptives may interfere with existing medication. Pregnancy should be avoided during active stages of the disease as this may exacerbate the symptoms, although successful pregnancy may be achieved.

Eating and drinking

There has been some research into the link between diet and MS, and a number of specialised diets have been identified. It has been demonstrated that people with MS have higher levels of saturated fats and lower levels of polyunsaturated fats in the myelin sheath and the patient should take a healthy diet and reduce the intake of saturated fats (see Ch. 21).

The SLT and dietitian may be able to offer assistance and advice if the patient has swallowing difficulties. The nurse can assist by encouraging the patient to:

- Sit up straight with the head supported, if necessary.
- Eat in a quiet, relaxed atmosphere and not speak while eating.
- Take time when eating, to avoid choking.
- Eat foods that are easier to swallow, e.g. semi-solid or liquidised foods, following advice from SLT.

Personal cleansing and dressing

The patient should be encouraged to maintain independence with regard to washing and dressing. It may seem to the patient, and at times to the nurse or to the patient's family, that it would be quicker and easier for the nurse to perform these activities for the patient. The patient may feel under stress to hurry in order to release the nurse to go and attend to other patients. The nurse should explain that there is no hurry to have everything finished for a set time.

The OT can assess the patient and give advice regarding washing and dressing, offer a range of dressing aids and suggest specially adapted clothing, e.g. with Velcro instead of buttons and zips.

Education

The patient and the family should be as well informed as possible about the diagnosis of MS and should be aware of the most successful methods of maintaining independence. They should also be aware of the possibility of the occurrence of behavioural and mood changes. Euphoria, depression, apathy and emotional lability are common. Many MS nurse specialists run courses for newly diagnosed patients or an expert patient programme may be available.

Preparation for discharge

Episodic hospitalisation may become necessary as the disease progresses and the patient and family should be given the opportunity to voice any worries or fears to allow adequate preparation for discharge. Some adjustments may be required in the house, e.g. bath aids and rearrangement of furniture. If the patient depends on a wheelchair for mobility, the doorways may have to be widened, cupboards lowered, and a shower may be required instead of a bath.

Rehousing to ground floor accommodation may be needed to allow wheelchair access. This involves major changes not only for the patient but also for the family and can be very traumatic.

Advice regarding income and benefits available, e.g. Disability Living Allowance (DLA), can be given by the social worker. Outpatient appointments can be arranged for physiotherapy, occupational or speech therapy, if necessary.

Some doctors advocate discussing the possibility of relapse so that the patient is better prepared when it occurs. On the other hand, some patients may not have a period of relapse for up to 20 years and may worry unnecessarily if the subject is broached too soon. Some patients may benefit from being informed of the availability of support groups,

Parkinson's disease

Parkinson's disease (PD) is a chronic neurodegenerative disorder of the basal nuclei (see p. 304), with a slow onset that progresses gradually, often resulting in premature death (Woodward & Waterhouse 2009). It has an annual incidence of approximately 0.2/1000 and a prevalence of 1.5/1000 in the UK (Boon et al 2006). Both incidence and prevalence increase with age, with the majority of those diagnosed aged over 60, but one in 20 will be under 40 years.

Progressive supranuclear palsy and multisystem atrophy both present with parkinsonian features and patients are often misdiagnosed with PD.

PATHOPHYSIOLOGY

PD is characterised by degenerative changes in the substantia nigra within the basal nuclei. Depletion of the dopaminergic neurones in the substantia nigra results in a decrease in the levels of the neurotransmitter, dopamine, essential for the control of movement, coordination and posture. As a result, the balance between dopamine and acetylcholine is lost and the acetylcholine effects exaggerated. Parkinsonism may also be seen as a side-effect of some drugs. Although genetic and environmental factors have been implicated, the cause of the degenerative changes is unknown.

Common presenting signs/symptoms The diagnostic features of PD are a triad of features: tremor, muscle rigidity and bradykinesia (slowness in initiating or repeating movements) with impairment of fine movements.

Other clinical features include:

- expressionless face
- disturbance in free-flowing movement, stooped posture and festinating gait, recurrent falls
- micrographia (tiny handwriting)
- loss of postural reflexes
- autonomic manifestations, e.g. excessive perspiration, drooling and excess salivation
- constipation and urge urinary incontinence
- microphonia (weak voice).

(See Further reading, e.g. Woodward & Mestecky 2011.)

MEDICAL/SURGICAL MANAGEMENT

Investigations

Investigations such as CT scanning may be considered in order to eliminate other disorders. There is no specific diagnostic test for PD. Diagnosis is usually based on clinical presentation.

Treatment

Medication is the mainstay of treatment. Treatment is symptomatic, does not halt the pathological process and requires careful management and monitoring (see Further reading, e.g. British National Formulary).

Dopaminergic preparations such as levodopa are administered to replace the depleted dopamine. In older people, levodopa with a dopa-decarboxylase inhibitor is often used (e.g. co-beneldopa), but it is only used once the symptoms of the disease compromise the individual's normal functioning. In younger patients, dopamine agonists are given to stimulate the surviving dopamine receptors. The enzymes monoamine oxidase A and B play a key role in the breakdown of dopamine. Selegiline is a medication which inhibits this process and appears to have a symptomatic effect. Amantadine acts by allowing the dopamine to stay longer at its site of action without being used up by other cells. It may be useful in the control of tremor but helps only a small proportion of patients. Catechol-O-methyltransferase (COMT) inhibitors (e.g. entacapone) block the action of an enzyme that breaks down levodopa and, given in combination, may prolong the action of levodopa.

Patients who experience sudden fluctuations in their symptoms in spite of careful management of their medications may be prescribed apomorphine. This is a potent dopa agonist and is sometimes given as a 'rescue' medicine in advanced states. It produces a direct effect at the sites where dopamine is active in the brain.

Many of the medications have variable side-effects and accurate titration usually necessitates admission to hospital. Another drug effect is an 'on–off' phenomenon, whereby the patient loses the benefit of the dopamine and becomes rigid and immobile for a period of time. Surgery, e.g. deep brain stimulation (Breen & Heisters 2007) may be indicated for some patients.

▷ Nursing management and health promotion: Parkinson's disease

The support of the patient's family or carer and of the primary health care team is important. The family's/carer's ability to cope with the mobility and other problems associated with PD can make the difference between a level of independence, with the patient living in their own home, and total dependence in long-term care.

Immediate priorities

Many of the early symptoms of PD may be treated by the family doctor, with the patient and their family making necessary adjustments to their home, e.g. removal of rugs and other obstacles.

The progress of the disease can vary, but should the patient's condition worsen, admission to hospital may become necessary. This provides an opportunity for nursing staff, physiotherapist, SLT and OT, to advise the patient and the family on how to deal with the problems which are interfering with the patient's daily life.

The most important priority is to ensure medication is given on time, especially before meals, to promote maximal functional abilities and independence.

Mobility

Problems can include difficulty in starting to walk or stopping, shuffling, tottering, impaired balance when turning and ongoing stiffness, interrupted by a 'freezing' of movement. Falls are also common. Passive and active range of movement exercises are a good starting point. Relatives should be advised to continue this activity at home. Effort should also be directed towards improving the patient's gait, with the assistance of the physiotherapist. Useful tips are given in Box 9.16.

Moving and handling assessment is required. Some patients find a monkey pole or rope ladder attached to the foot of the bed helpful in hospital. If the patient experiences difficulty in rolling over in bed or getting in and out of bed, they can be advised to use a low bed with a firm mattress or to place a board under their existing mattress (Box 9.16). (See Useful websites, e.g. Parkinson's Disease Society, where additional suggestions inspired by patients themselves can be accessed.)

Exercise

Some patients may benefit from an exercise programme to assist mobility and improve posture. It is important that this programme is performed under supervision initially, until the patient and their helper are conversant with the techniques. Again, the importance of continuing these at home should be stressed to both patient and family.

Eating and drinking

The person with PD may have difficulty with eating and drinking due to abnormal posture, tremor, poor swallowing and excessive saliva, resulting in malnutrition. There may be embarrassment about their untidiness when eating, and the length of time it takes to eat often results in food going cold. People will often choose to eat alone rather than endure the social embarrassment of seeing others watching them eat. Nutrition risk assessment should be undertaken (see Ch. 21) and eating small amounts at frequent intervals is preferable.

The SLT may do a swallowing assessment and prepare a programme of swallowing management. This could include techniques to encourage swallowing, e.g. taking a sip of iced water to stimulate the swallowing reflex.

Box 9.16 Information

Useful tips for the nurse/carer to encourage a frail older person with Parkinson's disease to move

General tips

- Advise the person to consciously lift each foot as he is walking and to place his heel on the ground first. To encourage this, ask the person to think that he has a series of imaginary steps to climb.
- Teach the person to broaden his stance to provide a more stable base.
- Remind the person to think about his posture and to stand erect.
- If the person starts to shuffle, ask him to stop and start again.
- Ask the person to adopt the habit of taking small steps when he is turning and to turn only in a forward direction.

Rolling over in bed

- The person is advised to bend his knees so that his feet are flat on the mattress and then swing the knees in the direction that he wishes to turn.
- The person then clasps his hands and lifts them straight up, straightening the elbows, then turns the head and swings the arms in the same direction as the legs.
- The person then grips the edge of the mattress and adjusts his position until comfortable.

Getting into and out of bed independently

- To get into bed, the person sits on the edge of the bed near the pillow.
- The person then only has to lift his legs onto the bed and then adjust himself into a comfortable position.

N.B. Getting out of bed is more complicated and several techniques can be suggested by a physiotherapist.

Rising from a chair

- The person should avoid low chairs, choosing instead firm, high-backed chairs. In the home, the height of a low chair can be increased with blocks under the legs.
- Cushions or a spring-ejector seat will also help.

The dietitian's advice should also be sought. It is usual to establish what kind of foods the patient likes best. A review of their current dietary intake will alert the nurse to any deficiencies. If tremor is a problem, the patient can be taught to hold their arm close in to their body, using their elbow as a pivot. Bendable straws could be used and cups containing hot liquids should only be filled halfway to avoid spillage or scalding.

It is important for the patient's self-esteem to resist the temptation to feed them before this is absolutely necessary. Many patients may still be able to feed themselves if their food is cut up for them. Feeding the patient for the convenience of speed is unacceptable.

Some signs/symptoms of dysphagia are:

- coughing within a few seconds of swallowing
- food sticking in the throat
- nasal regurgitation
- fear of swallowing
- drooling
- food remaining in the mouth after the meal.

If the patient wears dentures, these should be checked frequently to ensure a proper fit. The importance of good oral hygiene should be emphasised. Patients should check and record their body weight weekly, as weight loss may occur. Some hospitalised patients need to have suctioning equipment readily available whilst eating, in case they choke.

Communication

The communication impairment seen in the patient with PD includes loss of facial expression, which may lead to the assumption that the patient is cognitively impaired. Loss of normal eye contact and body language may occur due to the stooping posture. Facial exercises encourage the patient to pronounce sounds more clearly, e.g. by mouthing words slowly and clearly. There are also exercises for breathing, strengthening the voice and controlling the speed of speech, many of which can be continued in the patient's home.

Eventually the voice may become so weak that meaningful communication is impossible and an alternative means of communication becomes necessary. Communication aids must be appropriate to the patient's needs, and advice regarding their use should be taken from the SLT.

It may be possible for the patient to write down messages using pen and paper. However, the ability to write also deteriorates progressively and the writing becomes smaller and smaller (micrographia) as muscle stiffness increases. The progressive difficulties with communications are frustrating for both patient and their family (Box 9.17).

Elimination

The impairment of mobility in conjunction with urinary frequency or hesitancy can lead to embarrassing episodes of incontinence and increases the risk of falls. Urge incontinence may occur and bladder retraining and continence aids may be indicated (see Ch. 24). It is important that patients are encouraged to maintain a fluid intake of 2.5–3 L/day. Eventually urinary catheterisation may be unavoidable.

Constipation is a common problem in PD, so the patient and family should be taught preventive action. A high-fibre diet and plenty of fluids will encourage regular bowel motions. Failing this, it will be necessary to administer oral faecal softeners or bulking agents regularly and, when required, an enema.

Box 9.17 Reflection

Parkinson's disease: the family's perspective

We are 7 years into living with Father's PD. There have been so many challenges for him and for us over the years, and the challenges keep changing as the disease progresses. With each new admission to care, we are having to work harder to make sure that staff understand that the painfully slow speech from an expressionless face still conveys humour, awareness of world events, kindness and insight.

Activity

- Reflect on how nurses can assist patients with progressive PD to communicate effectively.
- Discuss with your mentor how nurses and other members of the health care team could support the family in the scenario.

Personal cleansing and dressing

The oily skin and excessive perspiration seen in patients with PD demand more frequent washing and bathing. If tremor is present, men will find an electric or battery-operated shaver safer and easier to use.

Slowness in performing voluntary movement (bradykinesia) can make daily activities such as dressing difficult. Adaptations to clothing style or fastenings without loss of dignity, e.g. wearing tracksuit trousers or replacing buttons and zips with Velcro, and the use of appropriate aids will allow the patient to continue to dress independently for as long as possible.

Discharge

Every opportunity should be taken to advise the patient and family about the best way to manage the disorder at home. Each of the areas already outlined should be included in the discharge plan.

Additional points to consider following discharge from hospital are as follows:

- The names and times of the medicines to be taken should be written down. The importance of maintaining the correct dosage is emphasised and some indication of the medicine's action and possible side-effects should be given.
- A daily exercise programme should be devised for the patient.
- Contact should be established with the appropriate community services, who may be providing the patient and family with support at home.
- Advice on dietary intake along with sample menus should be provided.
- Advice on safety, e.g. removal of loose rugs and other obstacles, should be given.

The patient should be encouraged to remain as active as possible for as long as possible, but should also be warned to pace their activity. Each individual will approach this situation in their own unique way and this has to be taken into account when proffering advice. (See Further reading, e.g. Rudkins & Aird 2006.)

Infections of the central nervous system

This section outlines three infections of the CNS – meningitis, encephalitis and cerebral abscess.

Meningitis

Meningitis is inflammation of the meninges; it may be bacterial, viral, fungal or protozoal. The most serious infective organism that causes meningitis is the *Neisseria meningitidis* (meningococcus) bacterium (group B causes most cases in the UK as group C has declined since vaccination was introduced), which causes a characteristic non-blanching rash and can rapidly result in septicaemia and death. Other bacteria include:

- *Haemophilus influenzae* type B (Hib)
- *Streptococcus pneumoniae* (pneumococcus)
- and, less commonly, *Mycobacterium tuberculosis*.

Most victims of meningococcal meningitis are young children, teenagers and university students who work in close proximity. Meningitis and meningococcal septicaemia are notifiable in the UK. Vaccines against Hib (introduced 1992), group C meningococcal disease (1999) and pneumococcal disease (2007) are part of the routine immunisation programme in the UK (see Health Protection Agency www.hpa.org.uk/ for up-to-date epidemiological data on cases of meningococcal meningitis). Since these vaccines were introduced there has been a significant reduction in cases – Hib infection in general reduced by 99%, deaths from group C meningococcal disease have reduced from an average of 79 per year to less than 1 death on average, and it is estimated that the pneumococcal vaccine has prevented 900 serious cases (Department of Health 2009). At the time of writing, a vaccine against group B meningococcal disease is likely to be available within the next three years (Department of Health 2009).

Approximately 10 000 people contract viral meningitis annually (also known as aseptic/chemical meningitis) but rarely require hospitalisation. Patients present with headache, which resolves spontaneously. Fungal meningitis is rare and usually seen in immunosuppressed patients, e.g. in HIV disease, and may be caused by *Cryptococcus neoformans* or *Candida* infections.

Encephalitis

This much rarer infection affects 2–4 people per 100 000 per annum. The most common infective organism is the herpes simplex virus.

Cerebral abscess

Cerebral abscess is a focal collection of pus within the white/grey matter of the brain, caused by pyogenic bacteria such as staphylococci and streptococci (Hacking & Hunt 2007).

PATHOPHYSIOLOGY OF CNS INFECTIONS

Meningitis In bacterial meningitis, purulent exudate is found in the subarachnoid space. The most likely route of entry is via the bloodstream, which can carry microorganisms from, for example, an infected middle ear. Other routes of entry include direct extension from a skull or facial fracture, via the CSF, and extensions along cranial and spinal nerves. The circulating CSF acts as an effective means of spreading the microorganisms.

Encephalitis Herpes simplex encephalitis produces swelling and necrosis of the temporal lobes, accompanied by inflammation and haemorrhage.

Cerebral abscess most commonly occurs following middle ear and mastoid infections or dental abscess. Pus accumulates in the cerebral tissue and becomes encapsulated. Other related conditions are extradural abscess, where pus accumulates in the extradural space, and subdural empyema, where pus accumulates in the subdural space. Cerebral abscess is highly irritant with many patients developing epilepsy and/or raised ICP.

Common presenting symptoms Infections of the central nervous system affect all age groups. Common signs and symptoms are described in Box 9.18. Admission to hospital

Box 9.18 Information

Features in the presentation of CNS infections

Bacterial meningitis (abrupt onset; N.B. except in meningitis caused by *Mycobacterium tuberculosis* when it is insidious)

Non-specific:

- Vague 'flu-like' symptoms
- Vomiting
- Fever, although the person may have cold extremities
- Back, muscle or joint pains
- Headache
- Drowsiness

More specific:

- Neck stiffness
- Photophobia
- Phonophobia
- Confusion
- Altered consciousness
- Seizures
- Purpuric or petechial rash that does not blanch under pressure

N.B. Infants may exhibit some of the following:

- Pallor
- Irritability
- Decreased responses
- A high-pitched cry
- Refusing feeds
- Floppiness – reduced muscle tone
- Bulging fontanelle ('soft spot')

Late:

- Coma
- Neck retraction (in severe cases this, in combination with spasm, causing the heels to bend backwards, produces opisthotonos)
- Shock due to septicaemia
- Widespread haemorrhagic rash

Viral encephalitis (insidious onset)

- Headache
- Fever
- Conscious level deteriorates gradually
- Confusion is common
- Moderate neck stiffness
- Seizures can occur
- ICP may be elevated as a result of cerebral oedema
- Cranial nerve deficits and focal neurological signs may be present

Cerebral abscess (insidious onset, 2–3 weeks or more)

- Headache is recurrent
- Fever is usually present
- Confusion
- Drowsiness
- Neck stiffness (indicative of circulating CSF infection)
- Partial or generalised seizures may occur
- ICP is elevated as abscess expands
- Cranial nerve deficits occur and focal neurological signs include speech disorders, motor and sensory deficits and ataxia

will be necessary and, if the patient's condition is serious, referral to a neurosurgeon will be made as the condition can become fatal, especially in children. Complications include deafness, seizures, personality changes, fatigue and death.

MEDICAL/SURGICAL MANAGEMENT

Investigations

The patient with any focal neurological signs, or presenting with a Glasgow Coma Scale <7, should have a CT scan performed to exclude an intracranial mass, such as an abscess. A lumbar puncture is usually performed to identify the offending organism in meningitis. The changes seen in the CSF are outlined in Table 9.5.

Other investigations may include blood cultures and X-rays to detect the source of infection. Brain biopsy guided by CT scan may be helpful. When an abscess is suspected, the CT scan should be enhanced with contrast medium to highlight small lesions (daughter loculi) which may otherwise be missed. The abscess will enhance with a ring surrounding the pus-filled centre on CT scan.

Treatment

The patient with bacterial meningitis or a cerebral abscess should commence antibiotics as soon as possible (before admission to hospital in suspected bacterial meningitis). Penicillin is the antibiotic of choice and is usually given

Table 9.5 Cerebrospinal fluid in bacterial meningitis and viral encephalitis		
CSF PARAMETERS	ACUTE BACTERIAL MENINGITIS	VIRAL ENCEPHALITIS
Appearance	Yellow	Clear
Cells	Polymorphonuclear $1000-5000 \times 10^6$/L	Mononuclear $50-1500 \times 10^6$/L
Protein	Elevated	Mildly elevated
Glucose	Low	Normal
Organisms	Present on culture	Absent on culture. Require specialist virological testing to identify
Pressure	Increased	Increased

intravenously in high doses; alternative antibiotics are used if the person has an allergy to penicillin (see Ch. 6).

Surgery will be performed to drain a cerebral abscess and adequate explanations should be given to the patient and family of what is involved in this course of treatment. This may involve burr hole aspiration, primary excision of the whole abscess or evacuation of the abscess contents leaving the capsule intact. This avoids damaging the surrounding brain.

Patients with encephalitis will be prescribed intravenous aciclovir (antiviral) and anticonvulsants.

Nursing management and health promotion: CNS infections

For those patients who require surgery, the general pre- and postoperative care is as given in Chapter 26. The nurse should observe the patient for signs of raised ICP postoperatively (see p. 314). The patient's family will require explanations, support and comfort.

Immediate priorities

Neurological status and vital signs

The patient with an intracranial infection may have a decreased conscious level and may deteriorate rapidly, therefore observations should be recorded and any change in condition reported immediately. Vital signs are important as the patient may be pyrexial. Pulse, temperature, blood pressure and respirations may be high when recorded, owing to infection: any changes in these observations should be reported. There may be signs of raised ICP.

Breathing

The respiratory pattern should be observed for rate, depth and frequency. Any respiratory distress should be reported immediately. Oxygen may be prescribed and the nurse should encourage the patient to tolerate it, giving explanations when necessary. Nursing the patient with a head-up tilt of 30 degrees will not only help to decrease ICP, but also encourage lung expansion. The nurse should be aware of the risk of a chest infection developing.

Controlling body temperature

In order to detect and reduce pyrexia, the patient's temperature should be recorded frequently and any further rise reported immediately, as this may indicate that the antibiotics are not controlling the infection and that the patient's condition could deteriorate. Each 1°C increase in temperature increases the body's demand for oxygen by 10%, which encourages vasodilatation and increases ICP. Nursing measures to reduce pyrexia are discussed in Chapter 22.

Observe seizure activity

Seizures are common with abscess and encephalitis. Seizures should be recorded, noting the type of seizure, its duration and exactly what happened (see p. 325). An airway, oxygen and suction should be available.

Communication

Communication can be difficult, as the patient may be experiencing severe headache, nausea and vomiting, have photophobia and be disorientated and drowsy. A calm darkened environment will comfort the patient, who will be distressed about their condition and what is happening to them. Patients may become aggressive and behaviour becomes challenging (see Further reading, e.g. Woodward & Mestecky 2011).

Explanations should be given to the patient about what is happening and why, and the patient should be given time to ask questions and express their feelings.

The family will also require reassurance and explanations, but they should be advised not to overstimulate the patient.

Maintaining a safe environment

Side rails should be in position to prevent the patient falling out of bed due to restlessness or confusion following risk assessment. In extreme circumstances the patient may be nursed on a mattress on the floor.

Medication and fluid balance

Patients will have headache and analgesics should be administered.

The nurse should ensure that prescribed antibiotics are given or taken at the correct time by the patient, to ensure maintenance of the medication at a therapeutic level in the bloodstream. People who have been in close contact with patients with meningococcal meningitis will need to be traced and prescribed prophylactic antibiotics, e.g. rifampicin, ciprofloxacin or ceftriaxone.

An accurate fluid balance chart should be maintained as the patient can become dehydrated due to pyrexia, nausea and vomiting. Intravenous fluids will be prescribed until the patient is able to tolerate adequate oral fluids (see Ch. 20).

Personal cleansing and dressing

If the patient has a decreased conscious level, care should be exercised in meeting their needs and, as their condition improves, independence should be encouraged.

Mobility

Initially, bed rest may be necessary and all care should be taken to ensure that the patient's position is changed 2-hourly. Examination of the skin should be carried out at frequent intervals in order to detect signs of pressure, such as redness.

Preparation for discharge home

If the source of the infection has been treated successfully, e.g. in sinusitis or an ear infection, the patient should be advised to contact their GP if there is a recurrence of the infection. The need to continue medication on discharge should be fully explained, with emphasis on the importance of completion of the course of antibiotics.

While rehabilitating in the ward, the patient will have been assessed by the ward team. Maintenance of optimal function (both physically and mentally) is vital and outpatient appointments may be required, e.g. for physiotherapy. The patient's family should be involved in the patient's planned discharge and rehabilitation programme at home. Advice should also be given about employment, driving and other activities, especially if the patient has experienced seizures (see pp. 325–326).

Both the Meningitis Trust and the Encephalitis Society (see Useful websites) offer a comprehensive support system for those affected. Complete recovery takes time and they provide guidance on how to deal with a range of minor after-effects, e.g. general tiredness, headaches and difficulty in concentration.

Huntington's disease

Huntington's disease is an autosomal dominant inherited neurological condition, therefore affecting males and females equally. Signs and symptoms, which may vary, usually start during middle age but they can occur earlier. Signs and symptoms include:

- involuntary movements (chorea)
- poor concentration and memory problems
- mood changes, depression
- cognitive and behavioural changes
- later dementia
- weight loss
- dysarthria and dysphagia.

Patients progressively deteriorate until they are totally dependent and require full nursing care. They will eventually die from secondary infections, e.g. pneumonia. There is currently no cure and treatment is symptomatic only, such as drugs to control involuntary movements. Family members should be offered presymptomatic testing, genetic counselling and ongoing support. A detailed discussion of this and other inherited neurological diseases is beyond the scope of this book and readers can find information from the appropriate support group, e.g. Huntington's Disease Association (see Useful websites).

SUMMARY: KEY NURSING ISSUES

- Patients with neurological conditions have complex needs.
- Detailed assessment of consciousness, neurological function and other vital systems is essential.
- Treatment of patients with many long-term neurological conditions is often symptomatic and nurses play a vital role at the centre of a multidisciplinary team in helping patients maintain function and independence as far as possible.
- Nurses caring for such patients require excellent communication skills and to be able to provide psychological and emotional support to patients and their families.

REFLECTION AND LEARNING – WHAT NEXT?

- **Test** your knowledge by visiting the website 🖱 and answering the multiple choice questions and critical thinking questions.
- **Consolidate** your learning by looking at some of the further reading suggestions, references and specialist websites.
- **Revisit** some of the additional material on the website.
- **Consider** what you have learnt and how this will help your professional development.
- **Reflect** on how you can apply this knowledge to the care of your patients.
- **Discuss** your learning with your mentor/supervisor, lecturer and colleagues.

REFERENCES

Bakas T, Austin JK, Okonkwo KF, Lewis RR, Chadwick L: Needs, concerns, strategies and advice of stroke caregivers the first 6 months after discharge, *J Neurosci Nurs* 34(5):242–251, 2002.

Boon NA, Colledge NR, Walker BR: *Davidson's Principles and Practice of Medicine*, ed 20, Edinburgh, 2006, Churchill Livingstone.

Bowie I, Woodward S: Nursing patients with neurological problems. In Brooker C, Nicol M, editors: *Nursing Adults – The practice of caring*, Edinburgh, 2003, Mosby.

Breen K, Heisters D: A guide to deep brain stimulation surgery: A treatment for Parkinson's disease, *British Journal of Neuroscience Nursing* 3(12):554–559, 2007.

Cancer Research UK: *UK Brain and central nervous system cancer mortality statistics*, 2009. Available online http://info.cancerresearchuk.org/cancerstats/types/brain/mortality/.

Department of Health (DH): *National Service Framework for Long-Term (Neurological) Conditions*, 2005. Available online http://www.dh.gov.uk.

Department of Health (DH): *National Stroke Strategy*, 2007. Available online http://www.dh.gov.uk/en/Publicationsandstatistics/Publications/PublicationsPolicyAndGuidance/DH_081062.

Department of Health (DH): *End of life Care Strategy – promoting high quality care for all adults at the end of life*, 2008. Available online http://www.dh.gov.uk/en/Publicationsandstatistics/Publications/PublicationsPolicyAndGuidance/DH_086277.

Department of Health (DH): *Meningitis cases hit record low*, 2009. Available online http://www.dh.gov.uk/en/News/Recentstories/DH_098524.

Dundas J: An evaluation of use of the HADS scale to screen for post-stroke depression in practice, *British Journal of Neuroscience Nursing* 2(8):399–403, 2006.

Goodacre S: Hospital admissions with head injury following publication of NICE guidance, *Emergency Medical Journal* 25:556–557, 2008.

Hacking R, Hunt K: Cerebral abscess: A review of its pathophysiology, diagnosis and management, *British Journal of Neuroscience Nursing* 3(9):400–403, 2007.

Headway: *Prevention and safety (head injury)*, 2004. Available online http://www.headway.org.uk.

Hickey JV: *The clinical practice of neurological and neurosurgical nursing*, ed 5, Philadelphia, 2002, Lippincott.

Lindsay K, Bone I: *Neurology and neurosurgery illustrated*, ed 4, Edinburgh, 2004, Churchill Livingstone.

Mestecky AM: Modes of treatment for cerebral vasospasm following aneurysmal subarachnoid haemorrhage, *British Journal of Neuroscience Nursing* 1(1):20–27, 2005.

Mestecky AM: Management of severe traumatic brain injury: The need for the knowledgeable nurse, *British Journal of Neuroscience Nursing* 3(1):7–13, 2007.

Miller C, Jezewski MA: A phenomenologic assessment of relapsing MS patients' experiences during treatment with interferon beta-1a, *J Neurosci Nurs* 33(5):240–244, 2001.

Molyneux AJ, Kerr RSC, Yu LM: International Subarachnoid Aneurysm Trial (ISAT) of neurosurgical clipping versus endovascular coiling in 2143 patients with ruptured intracranial aneurysms: a randomised comparison of effects on survival, dependency, seizures, rebleeding, subgroups and aneurysm occlusion, *Lancet* 366:809–817, 2005.

Montague SE, Watson R, Herbert R: *Physiology for nursing practice*, ed 3, London, 2005, Baillière Tindall.

National Institute for Health and Clinical Excellence (NICE): Management of multiple sclerosis in primary and secondary care, *Clinical guideline CG8* 2003. Available online http://www.nice.org.uk/Guidance/CG8.

National Institute for Health and Clinical Excellence (NICE): Epilepsy (Adults) – Newer drugs, *Technical appraisal TA76* 2004. Available online http://www.nice.org.uk/Guidance/TA76.

National Institute for Health and Clinical Excellence (NICE): Head injury: triage, assessment, investigation and early management of head injury in infants, children and adults, *Clinical guideline CG 56* 2007a. Available online http://www.nice.org.uk/Guidance/CG56.

National Institute for Health and Clinical Excellence (NICE): Venous thromboembolism: reducing the risk of venous thromboembolism (deep vein thrombosis and pulmonary embolism) in inpatients undergoing surgery, *Clinical guideline CG 46* 2007b. Available online http://www.nice.org.uk/Guidance/CG46.

National Institute for Health and Clinical Excellence (NICE): Alteplase for the treatment of acute ischaemic stroke, *Technical appraisal TA122* 2007c. Available online http://www.nice.org.uk/Guidance/TA122.

National Institute for Health and Clinical Excellence (NICE): Diagnosis and initial management of acute stroke and transient ischaemic attack (TIA), *Clinical guideline CG 68* 2008. Available online http://www.nice.org.uk/Guidance/CG68.

Nekludov M, Bellander BM, Mure M: Oxygenation and cerebral perfusion pressure improved in the prone position, *Acta Anaesthesiol Scand* 50(8):932–936, 2006.

NHS Education for Scotland: Stroke: core competencies for healthcare staff, 2005: Available online http://www.nes.scot.nhs.uk.

Polman CH, Reingold SC, Edan G, et al: Diagnostic criteria for multiple sclerosis: 2005 revisions to the 'McDonald Criteria', *Ann Neurol* 58(6):840–846, 2005.

Rietberg MB, Brooks D, Uitdehaag BMJ, Kwakkel G: *Exercise therapy for multiple sclerosis*, Oxford, 2005, The Cochrane Library.

Roper N, Logan W, Tierney AJ: *The Roper–Logan–Tierney model of nursing, The activities of living model*, Edinburgh, 1980, Churchill Livingstone.

Royal College of Physicians (RCP): *National Clinical Guidelines for Stroke*, ed 3, London, 2008, RCP.

Scottish Intercollegiate Guidelines Network (SIGN): *Management of Patients with Stroke*, 2002. Available online http://www.sign.ac.uk.

Sherwood PR, Given BA, Doorenbos AZ, et al: Forgotten voices: lessons from bereaved caregivers of persons with a brain tumour, *Int J Palliat Nurs* 10(2):67–75, 2004.

Sinnakaruppan I, Williams DM: Family carers and the adult head injured: a critical review of carers' needs, *Brain Inj* 15(8):653–672, 2001.

Sudheer PS, Logan SW, Terblanche C, et al: Comparison of the analgesic efficacy and respiratory effects of morphine, tramadol and codeine after craniotomy, *Anaesthesia* 62:555–560, 2007.

Williams G: Management of patients who have relapses in multiple sclerosis, *Br J Nurs* 13(17):1012–1016, 2004.

Woodward S, Waterhouse C: *Oxford Handbook of Neuroscience Nursing*, Oxford, 2009, Oxford University Press.

FURTHER READING

Braine M: The minimal and appropriate use of physical restraint in neuroscience nursing, *British Journal of Neuroscience Nursing* 1(4):177–184, 2005.

British National Formulary (BNF): Updated twice yearly. Available online http://www.bnf.org/bnf/.

Cheung J, Hocking P: The experience of spousal carers of people with multiple sclerosis, *Qual Health Res* 14(2):153–166, 2004.

Colledge NR, Walker BR, Ralston SH, *Davidson's principles and practice of medicine*, ed 21, Edinburgh, 2010, Churchill Livingstone.

Finlayson M, Van Denend T, Hudson E: Aging with multiple sclerosis, *Journal of Neuroscience Nursing* 36(5):245–251, 259, 2004.

Gimenez R: My experience with a second brain aneurysm, *Clin Nurse Spec* 14(6):253–255, 2000.

Greenhill L, Betts T: The lifelong needs of women with epilepsy, *Practice Nursing* 14(7):302, 304–306, 308–309, 2003.

Marieb EN, Hoehn K: *Human Anatomy and Physiology*, ed 7, San Francisco, 2007, Benjamin Cummings.

Mhor DC, Hart SL, Julian L, et al: Association between stressful life events and exacerbation in multiple sclerosis: a meta-analysis, *Br Med J* 328(7442):731–733, 2004.

Price AM, Collins TJ, Gallacher A: Nursing care of the acute head injury: a review of the evidence, *Nurs Crit Care* 8(3):126–133, 2003.

Roberts I, Schierhout G: *Hyperventilation therapy for acute traumatic brain injury*, Oxford, 2004, Cochrane Library.

Rudkins H, Aird T: The importance of early consideration of palliative care in Parkinson's disease, *British Journal of Neuroscience Nursing* 2(1):10–16, 2006.

Sullivan J: Positioning of patients with severe traumatic brain injury: research-based practice, *J Neurosci Nurs* 32(4):204–209, 2000.

Tortora G, Derrickson B: *Principles of anatomy and physiology*, ed 12, New Jersey, 2009, Wiley.

Waterhouse C: Development of a tool for risk assessment to facilitate safety and appropriate restraint, *British Journal of Neuroscicence Nursing* 3(9):421–426, 2007.

Woodward S, Mestecky AM: *Neuroscience Nursing – Evidence based practice*, Oxford, 2011, Wiley-Blackwell.

Yang J, Wang K, Chiang Y, et al: Effects of head elevation on cerebral blood flow velocity in post-cerebral operation patients, *J Nurs Res* 11(2):129–136, 2003.

USEFUL WEBSITES

British Association of Neuroscience Nurses: www.bann.org.uk

Encephalitis Society: www.encephalitis.info

Epilepsy Action: www.epilepsy.org.uk

Headway – the brain injury association: www.headway.org.uk

Huntington's Disease Association: www.hda.org.uk

Meningitis Trust: www.meningitis-trust.org

MS Trust: www.mstrust.org.uk

Multiple Sclerosis Society: www.mssociety.org.uk

National Neuroscience Benchmarking Group: www.nnbg.org.uk

National Society for Epilepsy: www.epilepsynse.org.uk

Parkinson's Disease Society: www.parkinsons.org.uk

Scottish Huntington's Association: www.hdscotland.org

Stroke Association: www.stroke.org.uk

Nursing patients with musculoskeletal disorders

Brian Lucas

Introduction

A fully functioning musculoskeletal system is fundamental to optimal health in the normal active human being. Injury or disease involving this system can have a profound effect on an individual's ability to perform the activities of daily living and can result in either temporary or permanent disability, one of the main problems usually being the degree of decreased mobility.

This chapter outlines the relevant anatomy and physiology and describes some of the more common disorders of the musculoskeletal system caused by trauma or disease and the principles of nursing management and health promotion. The main causes of musculoskeletal trauma or disease in the UK include road traffic collisions (RTCs), industrial and other work-related accidents, sporting accidents and damage due to underlying disease such as osteoarthritis or osteoporosis. The overall aim of nursing care is to prevent further injury, reduce the risk of complications, promote healing, maximise independence and promote optimal rehabilitation.

Anatomy and physiology of the musculoskeletal system

This section gives a brief overview of the anatomy and physiology of the musculoskeletal system (see Further reading, e.g. Marieb & Hoehn 2007).

The skeletal system

The skeletal system consists of bones and the joints where they articulate and move.

The main functions of the skeleton are:

- support for the body
- protection for internal organs
- movement – bones and muscles act as levers to produce movement through joints
- mineral storage – minerals such as calcium and phosphorus
- blood cell formation – red bone marrow produces red and white blood cells and platelets.

Structurally, the skeletal system consists of two types of connective tissue: bone and cartilage.

Bone

Bone contains large amounts of calcium which provides its strength. There are two types of bone tissue: compact and cancellous.

The hard outer layer of a bone is compact bone tissue (cortical bone), while cancellous tissue fills the inside. Cancellous tissue is spongier in appearance and the larger spaces contain the highly vascular red bone marrow and the fatty yellow bone marrow. The thickness of each type of tissue varies, depending on the type and function of the particular bone. In long bones such as the femur, the shaft (diaphysis) is enclosed by a thick layer of cortical tissue which gives strength for weight-bearing, while at each end, the epiphyses, the cortical tissue is thinner and encloses a greater mass of cancellous tissue. Bone tissue is constantly being renewed due to the actions of three types of bone

cell: osteoblasts, osteocytes and osteoclasts. Osteoblasts are involved in bone production, osteoclasts in bone resorption and osteocytes maintain bone tissue structure.

Cartilage

This is another form of connective tissue; it is tough, flexible, avascular and devoid of nerve fibres. It forms part of the support mechanism of the body.

There are three types of cartilage:

- hyaline cartilage – firm yet pliable and forms the articular cartilage that covers the articulating surfaces of synovial joints
- fibrocartilage – strong, compressible and tension-resistant and is found in areas such as the intervertebral discs
- elastic cartilage – contains more elastin fibres than the others and therefore has a greater ability to stretch whilst retaining its strength; it is found in the external ear and the epiglottis.

The axial skeletal system

The skull, vertebral (spinal) column and the sternum/ribcage form the central axis of the skeletal system. The spinal column is a strong, flexible column of 33/34 bones, 24 of which are 'true' vertebrae – the 7 cervical (C), 12 thoracic (T) and 5 lumbar (L) vertebrae – the remainder being 9/10 fused bones that form the sacrum (S) and coccyx (C) (Figure 10.1). Between each of the vertebrae from C2 to S1

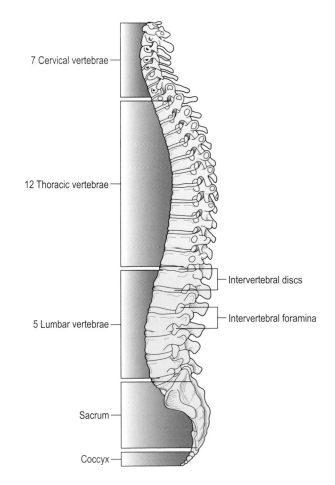

7 Cervical vertebrae

12 Thoracic vertebrae

Intervertebral discs

Intervertebral foramina

5 Lumbar vertebrae

Sacrum

Coccyx

Figure 10.1 The vertebral (spinal) column – lateral view.

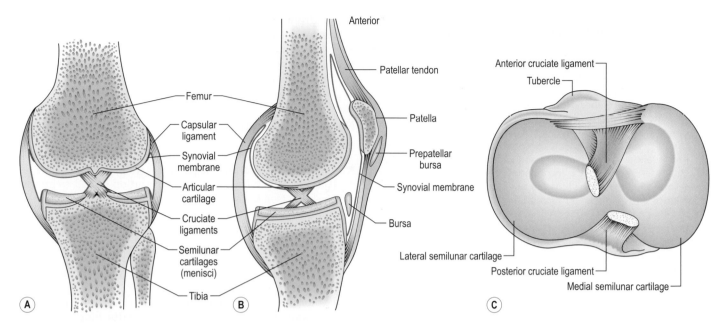

Figure 10.2 A synovial joint – the knee joint. A. Section viewed from front. B. Section viewed from side. C. Superior surface of the tibia showing the semilunar cartilages and cruciate ligaments.

is a strong joint created by the fibrocartilaginous intervertebral discs, which allow flexibility and act as shock absorbers when the spine is exposed to vertical forces.

The vertebral (spinal) column functions to protect the spinal cord, to support the skull and to act as a point of attachment for the ribs and muscles of the back.

The appendicular skeletal system

The bones of the upper and lower limbs and their girdles (the upper pectoral girdle and the lower pelvic girdle) are the main parts of the appendicular skeletal system. They are characterised by the presence of synovial joints which connect the articular surfaces of adjoining bones (Figure 10.2). The bones that make up the joint are held within a fibrous capsule, which consists of two layers:

- an outer layer of dense connective tissue which allows movement but resists dislocation
- an inner layer lined with synovial membrane which secretes synovial fluid; this provides nourishment and lubrication.

The articular surfaces of the bones involved are covered in hyaline cartilage – articular cartilage.

Ligaments

Ligaments attach bone to bone and are vital in maintaining the stability of a joint. They are made of dense connective tissue and have a relatively poor blood supply. A joint may have many ligaments, such as the knee which has the cruciate ligaments to prevent the femur and tibia moving forwards on each other and the medial and lateral collateral ligaments which prevent side to side movement (Figure 10.2). Damage to ligaments can result in an unstable and painful joint, common in football injuries.

The muscular system

Skeletal muscle (voluntary or striated muscle) tissue is composed of multinucleated muscle cells which are long and cylindrical in appearance. Each muscle is made up of muscle fibres and connective tissue. A good blood and nerve supply is essential for muscle function and the mechanics of movement.

Tendons

Tendons attach muscle to bone and allow movement of joints to take place. As with ligaments, tendons have a relatively poor blood supply. Damage to tendons can therefore be as serious as bony injury and prevent movement in an individual.

 ## Nursing management and health promotion: general principles of musculoskeletal disorders

Nursing assessment

This will involve a holistic assessment of the patient, as musculoskeletal disorders can have profound effects on a patient physically, psychologically and socially. In addition, visual inspection, palpation, measurement, and other investigations such as radiological/imaging studies (Box 10.1) and blood tests in rheumatoid arthritis, for example, are necessary.

In particular the nurse should assess for:

- the patient's perception of the cause of the primary problem
- the patient's knowledge and understanding of the condition
- the patient's description of pain and other symptoms

339

Box 10.1 Information

Investigations for musculoskeletal abnormalities

Radiological and imaging studies

- Radiograph (X-ray) – to detect abnormal position, fractures, arthritis and presence of fluid or abnormalities in joint capsules.
- Computed tomography scan (CT scan) – makes use of the fact that different tissues have varying radiodensities. A series of radiographs are made at different angles and planes and the computer integrates the information to produce pictorial slices (sometimes 3D) which can be used to detect soft tissue injuries or tumours and inflammatory or metastatic skeletal disease or fracture.
- Magnetic resonance imaging (MRI) – magnetic fields are used to show the difference in hydrogen density of various muscle and soft tissues, indicating the presence of abnormalities especially of the back and knee.
- Dual energy X-ray absorptiometry (DEXA) scan – scan for bone density, e.g. to detect osteoporosis.

Joint examination

- Arthroscopy – endoscopic visualisation of structures inside a joint undertaken under general or spinal anaesthetic. May also involve withdrawal of synovial fluid for analysis, and treatments such as washout of the joint to remove debris or the trimming of any damaged structures, e.g. the menisci in the knee joint.

Muscle and nerve studies

- Electromyography (EMG) – measures electrical potential of muscle during rest and activity.
- Nerve conduction velocities (NCVs) – measure speed of nerve impulse conduction.

Other tests

- These include bone biopsy, total body calcium and various blood tests (biochemical haematological studies) that include full blood count (FBC), erythrocyte sedimentation rate (ESR), rheumatoid factor, C-reactive protein (CRP), hormone and mineral levels, blood culture, etc.

syndrome, venous thromboembolism (VTE) and fat embolus (see below and p. 341)
- psychosocial consequences
- patient and family strengths – these should be defined and used constructively
- rehabilitation.

Nursing interventions

These will include:

- Treat life-threatening problems – ABC of resuscitation (see Chs 2, 27). Ensure early recognition of and treatment of shock (see Ch. 18).
- Relieve pain.
- Maintain an appropriate degree of therapeutic restriction and mobility.
- Constantly monitor and reduce the risk of neurovascular complications such as compartment syndrome and VTE.
- Maintain a safe environment.
- Explore the patient's and family's understanding of the condition and provide support and education based on individual needs.
- Coordinate multidisciplinary intervention for psychosocial problems.
- Facilitate rehabilitation.

 Nursing management and health promotion: core potential complications

The three potential complications – compartment syndrome, VTE and fat embolus – are common to many musculoskeletal injuries and can also occur after orthopaedic surgery. They are thus to be considered when caring for patients with any acute musculoskeletal injury or condition.

Compartment syndrome (CS)

Compartments within the body are areas where muscle, nerve and blood vessels are confined within inelastic boundaries of skin, fascia and/or bone. Compartment syndrome occurs when there is increased tissue pressure resulting in compromised circulation and function of tissues within a compartment (Lucas & Davis 2004). This results in tissue death (necrosis) and permanent loss of function, which can occur within 6–8 h. Increased pressure can result from direct trauma to the area, surgery or the application of a cast or other immobilisation aid. Nursing observations include examination of the colour, warmth, sensation and movement (CWSM) of the foot or hand distal to the injury, surgery site or constricting device such as a cast. The '5 Ps' that should be looked for are:

- pain (out of proportion to the injury and despite analgesia)
- paraesthesia – altered sensation such as 'pins and needles' or numbness
- paralysis
- pallor
- pulselessness (a late sign).

In order to reduce the risk of CS developing the affected limb should be elevated, unless CS is suspected to have

- abnormal position or appearance of limbs or affected part, with loss of function (compare with contralateral side)
- abnormal posture or gait
- use of walking aids or prostheses
- concurrent health problems, allergies and medications
- the impact on activities of living (ALs), especially relating to impaired mobility (see Further reading, e.g. Holland et al 2008)
- the patient's and the family's expectations and coping strategies.

Problems and strengths (actual and potential) are identified in the following categories:

- life-threatening problems such as shock
- pain
- impaired mobility
- knowledge deficit
- potential for further injury – physical safety and neurovascular complications, especially compartment

occurred, when elevation can exacerbate the condition and should be stopped (Lucas & Davis 2004). Compartment syndrome is an orthopaedic emergency and patients need to have surgery to relieve the pressure – a fasciotomy where the inelastic tissue surrounding the compartment is cut open.

Venous thromboembolism

Venous thromboembolism is a collective name for two conditions: deep vein thrombosis (DVT) and pulmonary embolism (PE). The risk factors for DVT are:

- venous stasis, such as when patients have reduced mobility after musculoskeletal trauma or surgery
- damage to veins after trauma
- hypercoagulability of the blood after injury.

It is usually a combination of these factors that causes a DVT. The result is a clot in the deep veins (of the leg or pelvis), most commonly of the lower leg. Signs and symptoms may include pain/tenderness, calf pain when the foot is dorsiflexed, redness, heat, swelling and hardness of the affected areas. Sometimes, however, there are no physical signs. Nursing management and health promotion includes educating vulnerable patients about the signs and symptoms so that they can inform staff if they occur, and the use of preventative measures to reduce the risk (see Ch. 26). These measures may be pharmacological, for example low molecular weight heparin injections, or non-pharmacological such as properly fitted antiembolism stockings, foot impulse device and early mobilisation (National Collaborating Centre for Acute Care 2007).

A DVT which breaks off and travels through the heart to the pulmonary circulation is known as a PE. This is an emergency as it can lead to respiratory arrest and death. The clinical presentation depends on severity but includes sudden sharp chest pain, tachycardia, dyspnoea, cough, cyanosis, fainting, sometimes haemoptysis, and restlessness/confusion in previously orientated patients. There will also be characteristic electrocardiogram changes. (See Further reading, e.g. Farley et al 2009, for details of PE.)

Fat embolus

Fat emboli can occur following fracture of any long bone or after orthopaedic surgery where a long bone is cut, such as a joint replacement. There are two theories relating to the cause: one is that fat cells from damaged tissue migrate into ruptured veins; the other is that catecholamines released through the stress of trauma mobilise lipids from fatty tissue. In the lung, these droplets are converted into free fatty acids which are toxic to lung tissue and disrupt alveolar function. Additionally, the droplets may become enmeshed in the capillary network of the alveoli and disrupt gas exchange. This can lead to cerebral hypoxia and, if large vessels in the pulmonary system are involved, to respiratory failure and death. Early signs of fat emboli are increased respiratory rate, anxiety, confusion, and transient petechial haemorrhage (tiny broken capillary blood vessels) on the head, neck and face.

The nurse must be alert for early signs of altered mental status – anxiety, irritability and especially confusion. Report

this immediately and be prepared to deal with respiratory failure and arrest and to transfer the patient to intensive care. Equipment should be ready for immediate blood gas analysis.

SKELETAL DISORDERS

This section of the chapter outlines a range of skeletal injuries and conditions, including fractures, spinal injury, osteoporosis, tumours and infections.

Fractures

A fracture or 'broken bone' is a break in the continuity of a bone (Langstaff 2000) as a result of direct or indirect trauma, underlying disease (pathological fracture) or repeated stress on a bone (stress fracture). It is described as a closed fracture when there is no communication between the external environment and the fracture site, and open when communication occurs. Stable fractures are those where the bone ends are lying in a position from which they are unlikely to move. In unstable fractures the bone ends are displaced or have the potential to be displaced. The edges of the broken bones may damage soft tissues or blood vessels/nerves at the time of the injury or later through poor handling of the limb.

MEDICAL/SURGICAL MANAGEMENT

All fractures, regardless of their position or the size of the bone involved, are managed according to three principles: reduction, maintenance of position and rehabilitation. The aim is to allow bone healing to take place. The stages of bone healing are demonstrated in Figure 10.3.

Reduction of fractures Fractures are said to be reduced when displaced bone fragments are pulled into their normal anatomical position. In many cases, a general anaesthetic will be necessary to overcome the protective muscle spasm and severe pain.

Maintenance of position The fracture needs to be held in the correct position until bony healing takes place, which can take from 6 to 12 weeks depending on the fracture site. Position can be maintained by external splintage using an orthosis, i.e. a removable splint, plaster of Paris (POP) or synthetic (resin/plastic based) casts, skin or skeletal traction, or an external fixator frame. Operative reduction with internal fixation by metal pins, plates, screws or nails may also be used to hold the bony fragments in position. When the blood supply is grossly affected, it may be necessary to implant a prosthesis to replace the affected bone, e.g. in some cases of fractured neck of femur. Without adequate maintenance of position the fracture may heal with the bone ends not properly aligned (malunion), take longer to heal (delayed union) or not unite at all (non-union).

Restoration of function Joints and muscles near to the fracture can become stiff and weak and physiotherapy and exercise is essential.

Patients require varying degrees of rehabilitation, involving a multidisciplinary team approach (see Ch. 32). It should

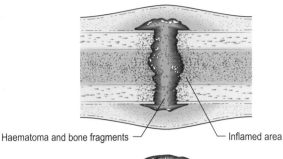

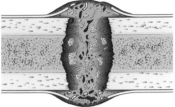

Haematoma and bone fragments — — Inflamed area

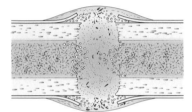

Phagocytosis of clot and debris.
Growth of granulation tissue begins

Osteoblasts begin to form new bone

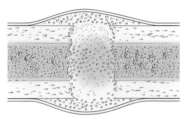

Gradual spread of new bone to bridge gap

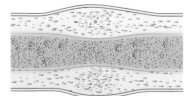

Bone healed. Osteoclasts reshape bone

Figure 10.3 Stages in bone healing.

be remembered that even when the physical damage is slight, the psychosocial impact may be considerable.

Traction

Orthopaedic traction occurs when a pulling force is applied to a part or parts of the body, and counter-traction, a pulling force in the opposite direction, is also applied (Lucas & Davis 2004). Counter-traction is usually supplied by the

body weight of the patient. It is used in the following circumstances:

- to reduce and immobilise fractures/dislocations and maintain normal alignment of all injured tissues
- to prevent and correct deformity
- to reduce muscle spasm
- to relieve pain
- to immobilise an injured or inflamed joint
- to keep joint surfaces apart.

Traction is less used than in the past as alternative methods, in particular internal fixation, enable patients to become mobile more quickly and therefore avoid the problems of bed rest. However, it still has its place in treatment and nurses must know the principles of its use.

Types of traction

Balanced or sliding traction This relies on the patient's own body weight to produce the necessary counter-traction, usually by tilting of the bed. Skeletal pins may be used to provide a firm point of attachment (Figure 10.4), but the most common type of balanced traction uses skin traction. This is Buck's traction which is used as a temporary measure for pain relief in patients with a fractured neck of femur (Figure 10.5). However, a Cochrane Review (Parker & Handoll 2006) could find no evidence which conclusively demonstrated the benefit of such traction for the outcome measures of pain relief or ease of fracture reduction at the time of surgery and its use has been discontinued in many orthopaedic centres.

Fixed traction This is the application of counter-traction acting through an appliance which obtains purchase on a part of the body (Figure 10.6). The most common is a Thomas' splint, used for restricting movement of a fractured shaft of femur when transferring a patient, e.g. between hospitals, or in the treatment of fractures of the shaft of femur in children (Lucas & Davis 2004).

 Nursing management and health promotion: traction

In addition to the general principles outlined earlier for management of musculoskeletal disorders (p. 339), the following are specific to a patient in traction.

Health promotion

Patients need to understand the reasons for their traction and how to move safely within the bed.

Management of equipment

All parts of frames, pulleys, ropes and slings should be inspected at regular intervals every day to ensure that they are correctly positioned and in good working order; this is especially important when the patient has been moved, e.g. after using a bedpan.

Reducing the risk of complications

- Observation of colour, warmth, sensation and movement (CWSM) of the injured limb must be carried out throughout

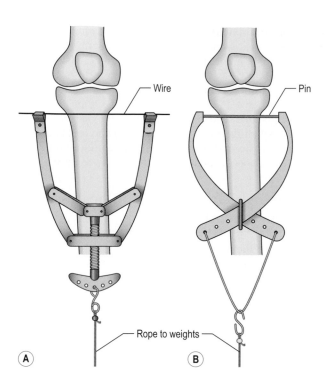

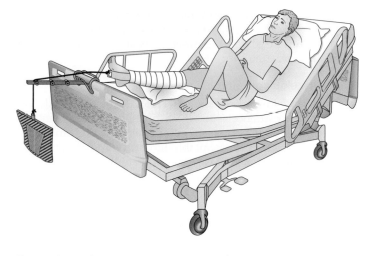

Figure 10.5 Buck's traction for femoral neck fractures.

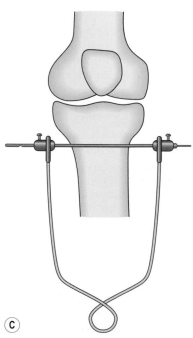

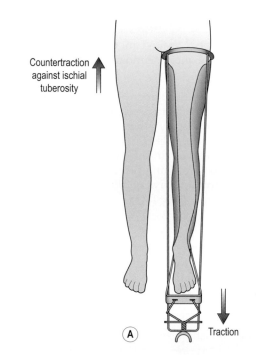

Figure 10.4 Skeletal traction may be applied by: A, a Kirschner wire and traction stirrup; B, a Steinmann pin and traction stirrup; or C, a Steinmann pin and Böhler stirrup.

the patient's stay in hospital for early detection of compartment syndrome (Lucas & Davis 2004).

- Potential skin breakdown around the traction and in vulnerable areas such as the sacrum should be monitored and appropriate pressure-relieving devices used.
- Observe for drop foot caused by excessive pressure on the common peroneal nerve located around the head of the fibula.

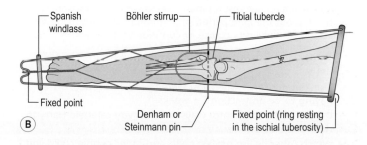

Figure 10.6 A. Fixed traction using skin traction and Thomas' splint. B. Fixed traction using skeletal pin and Thomas' splint.

- Work with the physiotherapists to ensure that patients are aware of the importance of deep breathing exercises and exercise of limbs to prevent chest infection, DVT and muscle wasting.

Care of skeletal pin sites

A Cochrane Review (Lethaby et al 2008) concluded that there is little evidence as to which pin site care regimen best reduces infection rates but there are best practice guidelines available based on the available literature and expert opinion (Lee-Smith et al 2001). These indicate that:

- Pin sites do not need to be cleaned if there is no exudate present. However, when necessary, cleaning should be done using 0.9% saline
- Pin site crusts should be removed as this allows visualisation of the wound and free drainage of exudate
- Pin sites may be left exposed if there is no exudate, otherwise woven gauze should be used.

Purulent discharge, redness or inflammation suggests infection and a wound swab should be taken to identify the causative organisms. The appropriate antibiotics should be commenced and the pin sites cleaned with 0.9% saline and dressed with woven gauze, changed as necessary (Lee-Smith et al 2001).

Fundamental aspects of care

Patients on traction have limited mobility and may be on bed rest for 6 weeks or more. Fundamental nursing issues to consider are:

- maintaining adequate fluid and dietary intake to prevent constipation and urinary tract infection
- maintaining patient dignity when meeting patient hygiene and toileting needs
- helping patients to maintain their contact with partners, family and friends, providing privacy as required
- helping patients to find ways of alleviating the boredom of prolonged bed rest (Box 10.2).

Casts

A cast is a splinting device comprising layers of bandages impregnated with POP, fibreglass or resin, some of which are applied wet and solidify as they dry out. Their main uses are

to immobilise and hold bone fragments in reduction and to support and stabilise weak joints. POP moulds more easily but it takes 48 h to dry and it is heavy. Synthetic casts set within 20 min and allow early weight-bearing but do not accommodate swelling and are not usually used in the initial stages of treatment, when a POP backslab is used. Other types of casts include adjustable focused rigidity primary casts which can be adjusted as swelling reduces (Large 2001) and cast braces which have hinges at the joints to allow restricted amounts of flexion or bend to stimulate cartilage nutrition (Dandy & Edwards 2009).

 ## Nursing management and health promotion: casts

In addition to the general principles of nursing management for musculoskeletal disorders (p. 339), the following will also apply.

Care of the cast

POP casts should be handled carefully when drying, using the palms of the hands rather than the fingers to prevent indentations which may cause pressure points. Patients should understand that a cast should not get wet and that synthetic protective covers can be used to permit them to take a shower. Patients should be taught how to protect the cast when washing and when using bedpans and urinals.

Many patients will go home wearing casts and need clear verbal and written instructions specific to their cast (Box 10.3 outlines advice for a patient with a hand to elbow plaster).

 Box 10.3 Information

Advice to a patient with a hand to elbow plaster

The plaster holds all the broken bones firmly in place to allow them to heal in the correct position. To prevent your fingers swelling, support your arm in the sling provided during the day and on pillows at night. It is important that you exercise the finger, elbow and shoulder joints of your injured arm at regular intervals, otherwise they will become stiff and painful to move.

The following exercises should be carried out at least four times each day:

- Make a firm fist then stretch the fingers as wide as possible.
- Try to touch each fingertip with the thumb of that hand.
- Bend and stretch the elbow joint.
- Lift your arm high above your head – use the other arm to help.
- Move your arm behind your back as if you wanted to scratch between your shoulder blades.

Do not wet, heat or otherwise interfere with the plaster and do not insert sharp objects between the plaster and the skin to scratch – this could cause skin damage and infection.

Report to the doctor or Emergency Department AT ONCE if:

- The plaster cracks, becomes loose or uncomfortable.
- There is pain.
- The fingers become numb or difficult to move.
- The fingers become more swollen, blue or very pale.
- There is discharge.
- You have any other problems.

 Box 10.2 Reflection

Dealing with boredom

Harry may be on bed rest for many weeks whilst on traction. He is worried about the long period of immobility and not being able to attend his university course or continue with his active social life.

Activity

- Think about times when you were bored and reflect on having to be on traction for weeks.
- Discuss with your mentor ways in which you can help Harry to relieve the boredom.
- Which other health professionals and other people could you call upon to help in this respect?

Potential for neurovascular impairment

Swelling or a too tight cast may lead to neurovascular impairment such as CS. CWSM observations should be carried out for early identification of problems. If CS or neurovascular impairment is suspected the cast needs to be split or bivalved down to the skin. If a local pressure ulcer develops beneath a cast, usually identifiable by specifically located pain, an inspection window can be cut and the ulcer dressed before the window is taped or bandaged back into place.

Removal of a cast

Removal of a cast is a skilled activity and should only be carried out by nurses who have been deemed competent in this role. Removal can be achieved using plaster shears for POPs or an electric oscillating saw for POPs and synthetic casts.

External fixation

Bone fragments are held in position by skeletal pins inserted into the bone on either side of the fracture and held in alignment by a scaffold or a ring fixator (Figure 10.7). They are used for the treatment of some closed fractures, e.g. the pelvis, to stabilise open fractures with extensive soft tissue loss until the soft tissue has healed, for fractures that have not united by other methods, and for reconstructive surgery such as leg lengthening. Depending on the reason for their use they can be in place for as little as 6 weeks, e.g. for treatment of a closed fracture, or up to 1 year, e.g. in non-union of a tibial fracture.

 ## Nursing management and health promotion: external fixation

The general principles relating to potential neurovascular impairment, positioning and potential for pin site infection that have already been discussed are important in the care of patients with an external fixator. In addition it is important that the patient, carers and community staff are confident in caring for the external fixator when the patient is

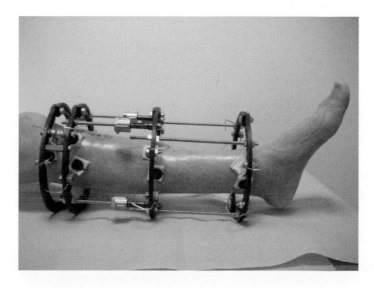

Figure 10.7 An example of external fixation – Ilizarov frame. (Courtesy of Barts and the London NHS Trust.)

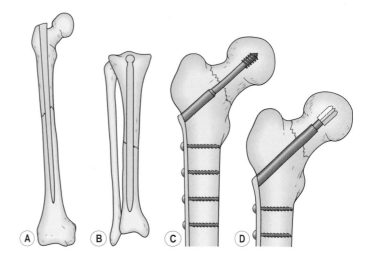

Figure 10.8 Types of internal fixation. A, B. Intramedullary nails. C. Compression nail for fixation of femoral neck. D. Sliding nail fixation of the femoral neck.

discharged from hospital, including managing issues related to altered body image (Limb 2004). (See Further reading, e.g. Dandy & Edwards 2009.)

Internal fixation

Fractures may also be stabilised by surgical intervention where nails, plates, wires, screws or rods hold the bone fragments in place (Figure 10.8). Again this permits earlier mobilisation and reduces the potential for complications. The general principles of nursing management and health promotion of musculoskeletal disorders and of core potential complications (pp. 339–341) apply. In addition the perioperative principles of nursing management are also relevant (see Ch. 26).

Fractures of specific sites – lower limb

Any of the bones in the lower limb can be fractured due to trauma, and the principles of reduction, maintenance of position and restoration of function apply to all. The specific treatment and associated nursing care and health promotion depend on the exact nature of the fracture and the patient involved. Two of the commonest fractures are those of the femoral neck and the tibia/fibula, and these are discussed in more detail.

Fracture of neck of femur

There are approximately 70 000 fractures of the femoral neck, commonly known as a hip fracture or fractured neck of femur (and abbreviated as #NOF), in the UK each year (British Orthopaedic Association [BOA] 2007). They are most common in older people, particularly women who may have osteoporosis. There is much evidence that a coordinated approach to care of this patient group can improve patient outcomes (Box 10.4).

MEDICAL/SURGICAL MANAGEMENT
History and examination

The patient will complain of severe pain in the hip or knee and there may be visible shortening and external rotation of

Box 10.4 Evidence-based practice

Hip fracture: the care of patients with fragility fracture: the 'Blue Book' guidelines

The British Orthopaedic Association and the British Geriatrics Society, together with other organisations including the Royal College of Nursing, has examined the evidence for the care of patients with a hip fracture and published good practice guidelines. The *six standards* are:

1. All patients with hip fracture should be admitted to an acute orthopaedic ward within 4 hours of presentation.

2. All patients with hip fracture who are medically fit should have surgery within 48 hours of admission, and during normal working hours.

3. All patients with hip fracture should be assessed and cared for with a view to minimising their risk of developing a pressure ulcer.

4. All patients presenting with a fragility fracture should be managed on an orthopaedic ward with routine access to acute orthogeriatric medical support from the time of admission.

5. All patients presenting with fragility fracture should be assessed to determine their need for antiresorptive therapy to prevent future osteoporotic fractures.

6. All patients presenting with a fragility fracture following a fall should be offered multidisciplinary assessment and intervention to prevent future falls.

(The British Orthopaedic Association, 2007.)

Activities

- Access *Care of Patients with Fragility Fractures* at www.nhfd.co.uk and identify which team members it considers to be essential for the multidisciplinary care of patients with a hip fracture.

- What is the role of the 'Hip Fracture' nurse specialist, according to the document?

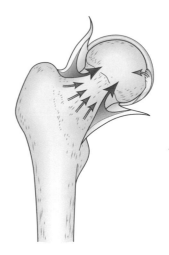

Figure 10.9 Blood supply of the femoral head via the capsule, intramedullary vessels and ligamentum teres.

the affected leg. Diagnosis will be confirmed by X-ray. A history of the fall is important as it may identify underlying conditions such as hypotension and indicate how long the patient may have been lying on the floor before receiving help.

Treatment

Depending on the site of the fracture, and the age and condition of the patient, the treatment will be either internal fixation with a plate and screws or replacement of the head of femur with a metal prosthesis if the fracture is inside the joint capsule and there is a risk of damage to the blood supply of the femoral head (Figure 10.9). The underlying osteoporosis needs to be treated (see p. 351).

▷ ## Nursing management and health promotion: fracture of neck of femur

In addition to the general principles relating to musculoskeletal injury and fractures, the following priorities need to be addressed.

Potential complications As a result of age and general physical condition when found, the patient may be confused and fearful and need a great deal of comfort and reassurance. Measures

will be taken to reverse any hypothermia and dehydration (see Chs 20, 22). Risk assessment of the patient for skin breakdown using an approved scale such as the Waterlow scale (see Ch. 23) should be recorded and the patient may be nursed on a therapeutic bed. Vital signs will be monitored at least 4-hourly intervals to detect early signs of complications.

Pain With an extracapsular fracture there is often extensive bruising which adds to the severe pain. Pain assessment and pain relief measures should be implemented (see Ch. 19) including repositioning and supporting the limb, and administering prescribed analgesics.

Increased risk of multisystem complications For an older patient, such acute trauma and associated surgery may lead to multisystem failure (see Ch. 18).

Rehabilitation Discharge planning should commence within 48 h of admission (Scottish Intercollegiate Guidelines Network [SIGN] 2002). The use of an integrated care pathway (ICP) can help to improve the standard of overall care by ensuring that each member of the multidisciplinary team knows the best available evidence for care and when that care should be carried out (Tarling et al 2002) (Table 10.1, Box 10.5). Early supported discharge schemes, often led by nurses, can help to ensure that patients are discharged rapidly but safely to their home environment (British Orthopaedic Association 2007).

Fracture of the tibia and fibula

Fracture of the tibia and fibula is one of the most common injuries dealt with by orthopaedic surgeons. These fractures usually result from direct impact to the limb, and extensive skin and soft tissue damage may be present. RTCs and sports injuries are common causes.

MEDICAL/SURGICAL MANAGEMENT

Treatment

There are three choices of treatment.

- *Cast immobilisation.* This is the treatment of choice for closed, stable injuries and the patient may remain in a cast for 12–16 weeks.

Table 10.1 Extract from the integrated care pathway of a patient with a fractured neck of femur – postoperative day 1 (nursing part only)

PATIENT PROBLEM/ NEED	NURSING INTERVENTION	EXPECTED OUTCOME
Recovery from anaesthetic	At least 4-hourly monitoring of vital signs	Vital signs within patient's normal limits
Wound care	Check wound site dressing Check and record wound drainage	Dressing dry and intact Drain to be removed at 24 h after surgery as further drainage minimal
Neurovascular status of limb	Monitor neurovascular status of affected limb	No neurovascular deficit
Relief of pain	Use pain score with patient at least 4-hourly Administer analgesics as prescribed	Pain relief at level acceptable to patient
Risk of deep vein thrombosis (DVT)	Ensure antiembolism stocking in situ Thromboprophylaxis injection as prescribed Monitor for signs of DVT	Reduction in risk and early detection of problem
Reduced mobility	Ensure patient understands correct way to transfer and mobilise	Patient to sit in chair Patient to walk to end of bed with aid of Zimmer frame

Box 10.5 Reflection

Integrated care pathways (ICP)

An ICP is different from traditional medical and nursing notes in many ways.

Activities

- Think about the material in Table 10.1, Tarling et al (2002) and, if possible, an ICP in use in your placement.
- Discuss with your mentor the differences between 'traditional' medical and nursing notes and ICPs and the relative advantages and disadvantages of each.

- *Internal fixation.* Fractures which are closed but unstable will be internally fixed with a nail. Routine postoperative care will be required (see Ch. 26). The patient will be able to use crutches once fully recovered from the effects of surgery. Information about the correct use of crutches/sticks is provided on the companion website.

 See website for further content

- *External fixation.* If there is skin loss or a contaminated wound at the fracture site, the choice of treatment is

Box 10.6 Reflection

Ken

Ken is a 40-year-old man who lives alone. He sustained an open fracture to his left tibia and fibula while skiing with friends.

Confirmation of the diagnosis was made by radiography and it was decided to take Ken to the operating theatre for application of an external fixator to his left leg. This was explained to him and a picture of an external fixator in position was shown to him and the two friends who had accompanied him.

After an uneventful postoperative period, Ken was allowed to sit in an armchair on day 1 with his leg elevated on a stool to reduce the swelling. The wound had been dressed in theatre following the local dressing policy of the institution. The physiotherapist gradually assisted Ken to walk with the help of crutches, and showed him how to manage the awkward appliance to avoid injuring himself. He was helped to widen two pairs of trousers below the knee so that he could cover the external fixator.

Ken was discharged home 6 days after his accident with a return appointment for 2 weeks later.

Activity

- Reflect on the discharge needs of Ken. Discuss with your mentor how these can be managed.

more commonly an external fixator which is applied under a general anaesthetic in an operating theatre. The patient may be weight bearing or not, depending on the stability of the fixation (Box 10.6).

▷ **Nursing management and health promotion: fracture of the tibia and fibula**

The principles of nursing management for each type of treatment are given on the following pages: casts (p. 344), internal fixation (p. 345) and external fixation (p. 345).

Fractures of specific sites – upper limb

As with the lower limb there are many different fractures of the upper limb. The two commonest are those of the neck of the humerus (the upper arm) and a Colles' fracture (the wrist).

Fracture of neck of humerus

A fracture of the neck of the humerus commonly occurs in older adults with osteoporosis after a fall on an outstretched hand.

MEDICAL MANAGEMENT

Treatment

This injury can usually be treated at home following the initial visit to the Emergency Department, providing there is no gross displacement or neurovascular complications (when internal fixation is required). The arm is supported in a shoulder immobiliser, broad arm sling or collar and cuff for approximately 2 weeks. Movement is gradually introduced, followed by outpatient physiotherapy, in order to avoid the major complication – development of a stiff shoulder joint. If the fracture does not heal, internal fixation may be required.

▷ Nursing management and health promotion: fracture of neck of humerus

In addition to the general principles of nursing management, including core potential complications (pp. 339–341), the following also apply.

Assessment of ability to carry out normal activities of daily living This is done before the patient is discharged home from the Emergency Department. Home nursing and home help are arranged accordingly, or a supported discharge scheme may be in place (Renton & Brown 2001) (Boxes 10.7, 10.8).

Skin care of injured arm If a supported discharge scheme is not available, it is necessary to arrange for the community nursing service to attend to wash the injured arm two or three times a week, taking particular care of the axilla. The sling is reapplied and neurovascular status and degree of mobility monitored.

Colles' fracture

This is one of the most common fractures seen at the Emergency Department and usually involves the lower end of the radius within 2.5 cm of the wrist joint, with a classic 'dinner fork' deformity (see Figure 10.10). It is commonly found in middle-aged and older women after a fall on an outstretched hand.

MEDICAL MANAGEMENT

Examination

Diagnosis will be confirmed by the appearance of the patient's wrist and by plain X-rays.

Box 10.7 Reflection

Shoulder immobilisation

Support for a humeral or other arm fracture can be achieved by a broad arm sling, a high arm sling or a collar and cuff.

Activities

- Think about the appropriate choice of sling for patients and discuss it with your tutor or mentor.
- After initial instruction from your tutor or mentor and with a fellow student, practise applying a broad arm sling, a high sling and a collar and cuff. Put the sling on your dominant arm and attempt to carry out an ordinary task, such as combing your hair or cutting up food.
- How difficult was it to undertake the task? Reflect on the potential difficulties for patients who may well be considerably older than yourself.

Box 10.8 Reflection

Mrs Linda Browne

Mrs Browne is a 70-year-old lady living alone in sheltered housing. She was admitted to the Emergency Department following a fractured neck of humerus after a fall, which was treated with a sling. The supported discharge scheme sister undertook a multidisciplinary assessment of Mrs Browne, who was discharged home after a stay of 2 h in the Emergency Department. The social worker within the supported discharge team arranged a suitable social care package to provide the support Mrs Browne would require.

The supported discharge scheme staff nurse visited Mrs Browne at home to wash and dry the skin around her injured shoulder, inspecting it for any signs of friction or pressure. Extensive bruising was noted over the shoulder region. The sling was reapplied. The nurse checked that Mrs Browne was moving her joints as advised and that no joint stiffness was present. It was established that no neurovascular deficit was present and Mrs Browne was educated to look for any developing signs of tingling or numbness of the fingers, change in finger colour or warmth, and/or reduced ability to move the arm.

The team's occupational therapist carried out an assessment and suggested changes to the environment, such as removing the bath mat on which Mrs Browne had slipped and replacing it with a non-slip one. Mrs Browne attended the hospital outpatient department 10 days later where she was seen by an orthopaedic specialist. The supported discharge team completed their package of care at this point, but social services continued to provide social care, including help with hygiene needs.

Activity

- Think about the psychological needs Mrs Browne might have after her fall and fracture, and how the primary care nursing staff might help her to meet these needs.

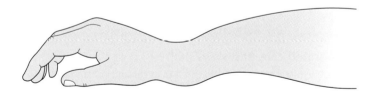

Figure 10.10 The 'dinner fork' deformity of Colles' fracture.

Treatment

The fracture usually requires reduction under local or general anaesthesia followed by application of a backslab (a half POP cast) until any swelling has reduced and then a full below elbow cast for 6 weeks. Internal or external fixation may be necessary if closed reduction is unsuccessful.

▷ Nursing management and health promotion: Colles' fracture

In addition to the management principles already discussed which relate to musculoskeletal trauma, fractures and plaster casts, the following priorities should be noted.

Health promotion A Colles' fracture is often the first sign of osteoporosis and patients should be investigated and treated as appropriate (p. 351). Advice should be given on how to prevent future falls and referral may be made to a falls clinic.

Removal of rings Marked swelling of the fingers is likely to occur and it is important to remove all rings and bracelets from the injured hand as soon as possible.

Prevention of complications of fractures – summary

The prevention of some general complications of fractures, such as neurovascular compromise, malunion, infection, etc., is summarised in Table 10.2.

Spinal injuries

Injury or damage to the vertebral (spinal) column which protects the spinal cord may be confined to bony and/or ligament injury or may be accompanied by damage to the cord itself. This spinal cord damage can happen at the time of injury or be the result of poor handling of the patient by health care professionals. It is estimated that 500–700 people per year in the UK sustain traumatic injury to the spinal cord (Harrison 2000) but many more sustain vertebral fractures or ligament damage with no spinal cord damage. Common reasons for spinal cord injury (Smith 2004a) are:

- road traffic collisions
- falls, such as falling downstairs
- industrial injuries, mainly building site falls
- sports injuries, e.g. rugby, skiing and diving.

PATHOPHYSIOLOGY

The resultant damage can involve transection, compression, contusion or interference to the spinal cord, accompanied by varying degrees of paralysis and sensory deficit below the level of the lesion (Figure 10.11).

MEDICAL/SURGICAL MANAGEMENT

The three principles of management (Smith 2004a) are:

- *Preserving existing neurological function*, which includes correct moving and handling of the patient. Every patient with spinal trauma should be treated as having a potential spinal cord injury until investigations such as magnetic resonance imaging (MRI) or X-rays have provided a clear diagnosis. Vertebral fractures may be stabilised by surgery or with halo vest traction (Figure 10.12) which facilitates early mobilisation in patients with intact neurological function. Some stable fractures, especially lower thoracic and lumbar fractures, can be treated by bed rest on a firm base. Patients who have damaged the ligaments supporting the vertebral (spinal) column may have a potentially dangerous unstable spine.
- *Physiological resuscitation*, i.e. attending to the potential life-threatening respiratory and cardiovascular effects related to spinal cord injury, which include:

Table 10.2 Prevention of complications of fractures

COMPLICATION	CAUSE	PREVENTION
Damage to soft tissue – neurovascular compromise	Trauma Sharp fragments/edge of bone	Monitor neurovascular function regularly – report abnormalities
Complications associated with immobility: Diminished function of all body systems Muscle atrophy – decreased range of movement – contractures	Decreased physical stimulation Lack of normal exercise	Encourage active and passive exercise Coordinate physiotherapy programme
Altered psychological processes	Decreased social stimulation	Provide social and mental stimulation
Pressure ulcers	Casts – prolonged pressure	Regular pressure area care and position change
Infection	Open wound postoperatively Skeletal pin sites	Apply principles of infection prevention and control
Malunion	Mal-apposition of bony fragments. Inadequate cast fit (e.g. when swelling subsides – cast becomes loose)	Meticulous and regular monitoring of cast fit and traction alignment
Delayed union	Unstable fracture Poor blood supply	Maintain adequate circulation and splintage
Non-union	Infection Soft tissue intrusion	Infection prevention and control
Fat embolus – emergency	Fat globules released into circulation from bone marrow at fracture site – usually associated with fractured femur or multiple fractures	Early reduction and splintage Ensure early diagnosis and treatment by reporting confusion, petechial haemorrhages, chest pain, dyspnoea immediately (see p. 341)

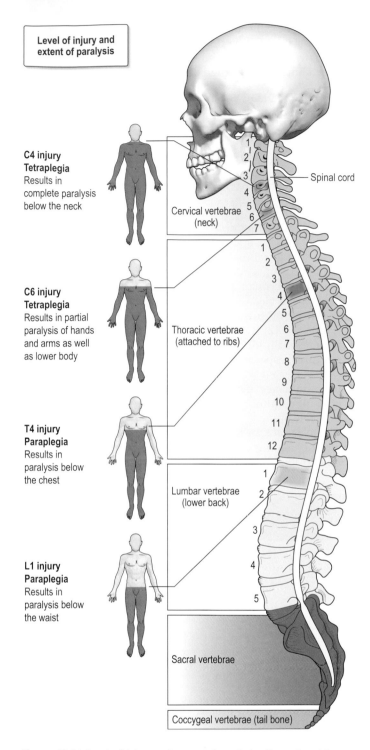

| Level of injury and extent of paralysis |

C4 injury
Tetraplegia
Results in complete paralysis below the neck

C6 injury
Tetraplegia
Results in partial paralysis of hands and arms as well as lower body

T4 injury
Paraplegia
Results in paralysis below the chest

L1 injury
Paraplegia
Results in paralysis below the waist

Spinal cord

Cervical vertebrae (neck)

Thoracic vertebrae (attached to ribs)

Lumbar vertebrae (lower back)

Sacral vertebrae

Coccygeal vertebrae (tail bone)

Figure 10.11 Level of injury and extent of paralysis. (Reproduced from Harrison 2000 with permission from the Spinal Injuries Association and Claire MacDonald.)

- ineffective airway clearance
- ineffective breathing pattern
- hypotension
- bradycardia
- hypothermia.

The last three are caused by spinal shock, i.e. the cessation of conduction within the spinal cord neurones.

This results in a loss of voluntary movement and sensation below the level of the injury and progressive

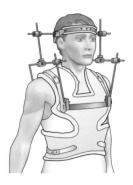

Figure 10.12 'Halo-vest' traction. A halo fixed to the skull – attached to bars mounted on the chest.

loss of sympathetic and parasympathetic activity which can last for up to 6 weeks.

- *Prevention of secondary complications*, which may be physical or psychological (see p. 351). Patients will usually be transferred to a spinal injuries unit (SIU) but this may not happen for a few days due to bed availability, and patients may initially be treated in a general hospital.

▷ Nursing management and health promotion: spinal injuries

Basic principles of positioning and moving patients with spinal injury

All nurses should be aware of the importance of maintaining anatomical alignment of the vertebral (spinal) column in patients with suspected and actual spinal cord injury both before patients reach hospital and once they are admitted, to avoid scenarios such as that outlined in Box 10.9. Manoeuvres such as log rolling the patient (see Ch. 27) (for thoracolumbar injuries), pelvic twists (for cervical injuries) and

---

Box 10.9 Reflection

First aid for accident victims: the effect on outcome

Two 18-year-old men were brought into the Emergency Department on the same night. They had both sustained multiple injuries to the head and body in similar road traffic collisions – the first (Pete) had been moved from his overturned vehicle by well-meaning people at the scene of the accident whilst waiting for the ambulance to arrive, whereas the second (Wayne) was supported in the position in which he was found until the ambulance team arrived. They applied a neck collar and maintained skeletal alignment whilst transferring him to the ambulance and at all times subsequently. Spinal X-rays showed that the men had identical injuries to the cervical spine.

Two months later, Wayne walked out of the spinal injuries unit; many months later, Pete was wheeled out of the same unit with quadriplegia.

Activity
- Think about the two scenarios and discuss with your mentor the main reasons for such different outcomes of the two accident victims.

using special beds (e.g. an electric turning bed) are carried out under the guidance of an experienced nurse.

Respiratory and cardiovascular monitoring

This is a vital nursing responsibility, to detect any deterioration in the functioning of these systems. Depending on the level of injury patients may be ventilated. VTE is a potential complication and prophylaxis should be carried out according to local policy.

Additional physical care

Patients with a spinal cord injury have the potential to develop additional physical problems, in particular paralytic ileus, gastric ulceration and pressure ulcers. During the acute stage of spinal cord injury the patient will have a flaccid bowel and bladder, and therefore urinary catheterisation will be necessary and manual evacuation of faeces will be undertaken by a suitably qualified practitioner.

Psychological care

Spinal cord injury is a life-changing event, not only for the patient but also for the family. The experience of SIU staff is that two of the most important interventions nurses can perform are to be truthful at all times, ensuring all staff are providing the same information, and to reduce the effects of sensory deprivation through the use of therapeutic touch and aids such as mirrors (Harrison 2000). Long-term support and adaptation will be necessary and organisations such as the Spinal Injuries Association are vital in this (see Useful websites).

 See website Critical thinking question 10.1

Osteoporosis

Osteoporosis is a 'progressive, systemic skeletal disorder characterised by low bone mass and micro-architectural deterioration of bone tissue, with a consequent increase in bone fragility and susceptibility to fracture' (NICE 2008a). It is estimated that 1 in 3 women and 1 in 12 men in the UK will develop clinically significant osteoporosis (Allsworth 2004).

PATHOPHYSIOLOGY

The characteristic overall reduction in bone mineral density (BMD) is caused by both uncontrollable and modifiable factors (Howard 2001). Eighty per cent of BMD is determined by genetically determined risk factors such as race, gender and stature. The remaining 20% is influenced by non-genetic factors which can be modified to enhance BMD (see below). Patients become susceptible to fractures, with the wrist, e.g. Colles' fracture, vertebrae and neck of femur as the most common sites.

MEDICAL MANAGEMENT

Prevention is aimed at ensuring that patients have as high a BMD as possible. Modifications to diet such as increased calcium and ensuring sufficient weight-bearing exercise are key in this. Peak BMD is reached by a person's early 30s and therefore such modifications should ideally be made before this, although there are benefits in all age groups.

Early identification is also key. It has long been recognised that a low-impact or fragility fracture, i.e. one sustained by falling from standing height or less, especially a distal radial fracture, is suggestive of osteoporosis and merits further investigation and patient education (BOA 2007). All patients over 50 with a fragility fracture should have their bone density measured (by dual-energy X-ray absorptiometry [DEXA] scan) and appropriate treatment initiated by their GP or local osteoporosis unit (BOA 2007).

In the presence of osteoporosis, medication therapy is instituted to inhibit bone resorption by osteoclasts and therefore slow down the rate of bone loss. A group of drugs known as the bisphosphonates are widely prescribed and are designed to bind calcium to bone; in the UK, alendronate, etidronate and risedronate are amongst those licensed for use (NICE 2008a). Vitamin D and calcium supplements are also prescribed, as vitamin D is required for the absorption of calcium, and calcium supplementation is vital in the prevention and treatment of postmenopausal osteoporosis (James 2000).

 See website Critical thinking question 10.2

Hormone replacement therapy (HRT) was widely prescribed for the prevention and treatment of osteoporosis but questions about long-term safety, in particular the increased risk of breast cancer, have led to a change in thinking. A review of the evidence (Lookinland & Beckstrand 2003) concludes that HRT should not be used for the primary prevention of chronic diseases such as osteoporosis, and if it is used to control menopausal symptoms it should be limited to 2–3 years at the lowest dose (see Ch. 7).

▷ Nursing management and health promotion: osteoporosis

Prevention

Nurses can play a key role in education of the population about the importance of diet and exercise in the prevention of bone problems later in life. Community nurses, school nurses and health visitors are specific groups that can contribute, but all nurses can use time spent with patients as a health promotion opportunity.

Early detection and treatment

A number of hospitals are developing schemes whereby patients identified as at risk of osteoporosis, especially patients who have had a Colles' or femoral neck fracture, are screened for osteoporosis and treated appropriately. Many of these schemes are nurse led (Content et al 2003).

Bone tumours

Primary bone tumours can be benign or malignant, although some benign tumours may become malignant. Bone tumours are usually classified according to the cell type from which they originate (Table 10.3).

Metastatic bone disease is malignant bone disease due to secondary deposits in bone tissue from a primary cancer elsewhere, such as those in the breast (see Chs 7, 31). Their

Table 10.3 A classification of bone tumours

TISSUE OF ORIGIN	BENIGN TUMOUR	MALIGNANT TUMOUR
Bone	Osteoid osteoma Osteoblastoma Aneurysmal bone cysts	Osteosarcoma
Cartilage	Osteochondroma Chondroma Enchondroma	Chondrosarcoma
Fibrous marrow	Fibroma	Fibrosarcoma Myeloma
Uncertain	Giant cell tumour Benign fibrous histiocytoma	Ewing's sarcoma Malignant fibrous histiocytoma

Reproduced with permission from Henry (2004).

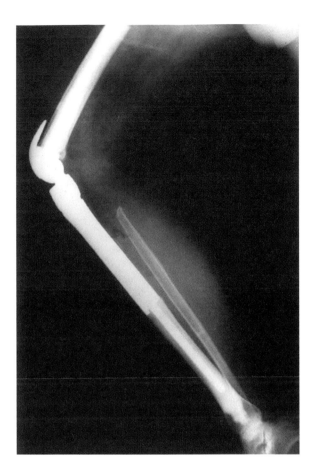

Figure 10.13 Endoprosthetic replacement of the proximal tibia (lateral view) with distal femoral component and excision of head of fibula.

treatment requires multidisciplinary care and nursing plays a key role in coordination of this care and supporting the patient through their journey.

PATHOPHYSIOLOGY

As a bone tumour grows, eruption into the surrounding tissues can occur and may be noted as a warm swelling of the affected area. The tumour will originate from a specific cell type within the bone tissue, but may then involve a variety of bone cells.

Skeletal metastases occur in approximately 30–70% of all new cancers; of these, 80% are cancers of the breast, prostate and lung, with those of the kidney and thyroid being a less common source (Dupuy & Goldberg 2001). Bony metastases are usually transmitted by the blood and tend to occur in sites where red bone marrow is present, the commonest sites being the femur, humerus and acetabulum.

MEDICAL/SURGICAL MANAGEMENT

History

Patients most commonly present with pain, due to stretching of the surrounding tissue by the tumour and/or its impingement on nerves and blood vessels. Pain at night and pain not relieved by rest are indications of malignant tumours. Other symptoms include swelling, reduction in movement of the affected limb and reduced sensation (Henry 2004).

Investigations

Diagnosis is confirmed by:

- blood tests
- X-rays and other imaging techniques such as MRI or CT scan
- biopsy to determine histopathology and microbiology.

Treatment

This is usually dependent on the type of bone tumour.

Benign bone tumours Osteochondroma, the most common type, is managed by wide excision. Osteoclastoma, common

in the femur and tibia, may require excision and insertion of an endoprosthesis (Figure 10.13). Prostheses are now being used which are extendable, allowing for growth in skeletally immature patients.

Malignant bone tumours The most common type, osteosarcoma, which affects young people up to 30 years of age, is usually treated with chemotherapy followed by surgery, either limb sparing, with endoprosthesis, or amputation. The second most common, chondrosarcoma, occurs in people aged 40–60 and is usually treated by wide excision (with endoprosthesis) or amputation.

Metastatic bone disease The treatment of a patient with metastatic bone disease tends to be symptomatic and in particular the management of pain by analgesics, radiotherapy, chemotherapy and/or surgery (see Ch. 31).

 Nursing management and health promotion: primary bone tumours

Once the patient has seen their GP, immediate hospitalisation will ensue. The care of a patient undergoing chemotherapy and/or radiotherapy is described in Chapter 31.

The care of a patient who has a custom-built prosthetic implant will be specific to the implant but the principles of postoperative care are similar to the care of a patient following joint arthroplasty (see pp. 358–359).

Psychological care is paramount for patients with bone tumours, as treatment can last for several months and be very debilitating, e.g. chemotherapy followed by major surgery. Concerns about body image may arise and there will be many fears, including fear of the unknown and of dependence (Henry 2004).

Amputation of a limb

With the development of new treatments amputation is becoming less common, but it can still be necessary in some instances. The most common reasons are bone tumour, crushing injury, peripheral vascular disease (see Ch. 2), congenital anomaly and severe osteomyelitis with systemic complications.

 ## Nursing management and health promotion: amputation of a limb

Coping with loss Loss of a limb through amputation is like any other major loss. As the majority of amputations are carried out as elective procedures, the nurse will be able to make physiological, psychological and social assessments of the patient, and therefore plan care which will assist in the adjustment and adaptation process for the patient (Ellis 2002). This may include arranging for the patient to visit the local prosthetic department or to meet a patient who has had an amputation and is coping successfully.

Occasionally a patient may undergo an amputation as an emergency procedure following a severe crushing injury. In this case, the psychological preparation of the patient and family can only be very limited. They are very likely to require extra support and understanding during the postoperative period.

Wound dressing A stump bandage is used for the first few days and then replaced with a special shrinker sock, which has better elastic properties and is lighter than a crepe bandage. It maintains uniform compression on the wound, thereby reducing oedema, promoting wound healing and beginning to shape the stump, which eases the fitting of the prosthesis.

Phantom sensation (phantom limb) describes the painful sensation experienced by some patients following an amputation (see Ch. 19). If it becomes a chronic problem, treatment in the form of transcutaneous electrical nerve stimulation (TENS), ultrasound, local nerve blocks, relaxation therapy or medication, such as the adjuvant analgesic carbamazepine, may be effective (Ellis 2002).

Pneumatic post-amputation mobility aid Some centres use a prosthesis known as a pneumatic post-amputation mobility (PPAM) aid to help the patient regain balance, reduce oedema of the stump and encourage early walking after lower limb amputation. The aid consists of an inflatable plastic tube which is placed around the patient's stump. The tube is encased in a metal frame with a rocker foot. The use of the PPAM aid can help the patient adjust to the change in body image as the time without an artificial limb is reduced.

Bone infections

Antibiotic resistance, the re-emergence of tuberculosis (TB) in Western countries, and the increased use of metallic implants in orthopaedic surgery all mean that the potential for orthopaedic infections is ever present. This section will outline the three most common types: osteomyelitis, septic arthritis and TB.

Osteomyelitis

Osteomyelitis is a local or generalised infection affecting bone tissue and bone marrow.

PATHOPHYSIOLOGY

Acute osteomyelitis is most commonly caused by *Staphylococcus aureus* and the bacteria usually accumulate in the metaphyseal plate where they proliferate (Burden & Kneale 2004). The microorganisms usually gain entry during surgery or trauma, but spread from existing infection or via the bloodstream also occurs. As the infection spreads, the patient develops pyrexia and severe pain and the affected part is hot and swollen (Dandy & Edwards 2009). If untreated, the infection spreads through the marrow and erodes the cortex and the periosteum. An abscess forms, which will eventually discharge through the skin. By this stage it has become chronic osteomyelitis. If the infection is close to a joint it may track into the joint, causing septic arthritis; this most commonly occurs at the hip, knee, shoulder, elbow and wrist joints (Dandy & Edwards 2009).

MEDICAL/SURGICAL MANAGEMENT
History

Patients may have had recent trauma affecting the bone or an infection elsewhere in the body. Local signs of infection will be pain, heat and redness, and systemic symptoms of pyrexia, nausea, sweating and malaise may also be present.

Investigations

Blood cultures, wound swabs or needle biopsy samples are taken to identify the causative organism and thus ensure the appropriate antibiotic(s) is prescribed. Blood tests will show raised inflammatory markers: white blood cell (WBC) count, erythrocyte sedimentation rate (ESR) and C-reactive protein (CRP).

A plain X-ray will exclude any other causes for the symptoms, and a CT scan will highlight bony abscesses or sinus tracks. An MRI scan may also be carried out to detect any soft tissue or bone marrow involvement.

Treatment

Antibiotic therapy is the first line of treatment. If this is not successful surgical intervention, involving removal of infected material and bone grafting or external fixation, may be carried out. In severe cases amputation may be necessary.

Nursing management and health promotion: osteomyelitis

Early detection Patients and nurses need to be alert to the condition so that early referral and treatment can be instituted to prevent progression.

Elevation of the affected part This will reduce pain and may be accompanied by the use of traction, splints or casts to rest the affected area.

Pain relief and comfort Rest, gentle handling, use of bed cradles to relieve pressure of bedclothes, prompt administration of analgesics and antipyretics, reassurance and distracting activity will all help to relieve pain to some extent.

Antibiotic therapy Initially, antibiotics will be administered intravenously. Increasingly this is being carried out in the community by appropriately skilled nurses, thereby reducing the need for prolonged inpatient stay. If antibiotics are instilled directly into the bone the patient will remain in hospital (Sims et al 2001).

Managing chronic osteomyelitis Patients with chronic infection may have many hospital admissions and treatments and be anxious about the long-term prognosis. Nurses can help by ensuring patients are kept fully informed of their condition and its treatments, and by referring them to appropriate agencies such as social services or occupational therapy.

Joint infection – septic arthritis

Septic arthritis is an acute bacterial inflammation of a joint.

PATHOPHYSIOLOGY

Septic arthritis can be caused by osteomyelitis, infection from a penetrating wound or bacteraemia from a distant focus of infection.

MEDICAL MANAGEMENT

History Septic arthritis usually presents as a hot, swollen, red and painful joint which the patient is reluctant to move.

Investigations Blood cultures, blood tests and aspiration of the joint will confirm the presence of infection and identify the causative organism. Imaging, such as X-rays, CT and MRI, will help to identify the extent of the problem.

Treatment The joint is drained by needle aspiration, arthroscopic washout or open surgery, depending on the joint involved. Antibiotic therapy is instituted, usually intravenously at first. If treatment is not successful, patients may be left with long-term arthritic changes and reduced mobility.

 Nursing management and health promotion: septic arthritis

The priorities are similar to those for patients with osteomyelitis.

Tuberculosis and bone infection

Rates of tuberculosis (TB) have increased recently for a number of reasons, including movement of unvaccinated people between countries and susceptibility to infection of immunosuppressed patients such as those with HIV (see Chs 3, 6, 35). The emergence of strains of multidrug resistant-tuberculosis (MDR-TB) and extensively drug-resistant tuberculosis (XDR-TB) limits treatment options and is cause for great concern.

PATHOPHYSIOLOGY

TB usually occurs in the lungs and may spread to the skeletal system, especially the vertebral (spinal) column, where half of all cases of skeletal infection occur (Burden & Kneale 2004). The course of the disease is similar to that of osteomyelitis, although the pace is much slower. It can cause vertebral fractures and in some cases paraplegia. Surgical treatment may be necessary once the active disease has been controlled, including vertebral fusion to prevent further collapse of vertebrae, or joint replacement.

MEDICAL MANAGEMENT
History

Symptoms usually develop slowly with little redness or heat initially. Localised tenderness sometimes occurs.

Investigations

Blood tests, sputum/urine tests, X-rays and MRI are all used to aid diagnosis.

Treatment

This involves a combination of antitubercular drugs, e.g. rifampicin, for a long period (sometimes years) and addressing the symptoms.

 Nursing management and health promotion: tuberculosis and bone infection

Nursing management involves implementation of the principles of infection prevention and control (see Ch. 16), health promotion and comfort measures to alleviate symptoms. It may take up to 2 years to successfully treat skeletal TB and patients require support, for example, regular supervision and monitoring of medication regimen for side-effects to ensure completion of the treatment. In some areas specialist TB teams have been set up for this reason.

DISORDERS OF JOINTS

This section outlines the management of disorders of the lumbar spine, osteoarthritis (OA) and rheumatoid arthritis (RA).

Disorders of the lumbar spine – back pain

Lumbar spine disorders or 'back pain' account for more lost working hours than any other medical condition and up to 25% of referrals to some orthopaedic clinics are for this condition (Dandy & Edwards 2009). This part of the chapter will focus on management of acute back strain, recurrent back strain and prolapsed intervertebral disc (PID).

PATHOPHYSIOLOGY

Damage or trauma to the vertebrae, ligaments or intervertebral discs can result in instability and potential impingement on the spinal cord and nerves. Figure 10.14 illustrates the major causes of low back pain. In the lumbar spine mechanical causes are the most common, i.e. abuse, overuse or underuse of the back (Smith 2004b).

Acute back pain/strain

This is associated with a sudden sharp movement or an attempt to lift a heavy object from an extended position, or it may occur when people with sedentary occupations indulge in bursts of excessive exercise. It may be manifest by sudden severe pain in the lumbar region, due to an acute muscle or ligament strain in the lumbar spine.

MEDICAL MANAGEMENT

Management includes:

- rest for 24 h maximum in the most comfortable position and then resumption of activity
- analgesics, non-steroidal anti-inflammatory drugs (NSAIDs) and/or antispasmodic medication (Krismer & van Tulder 2007).

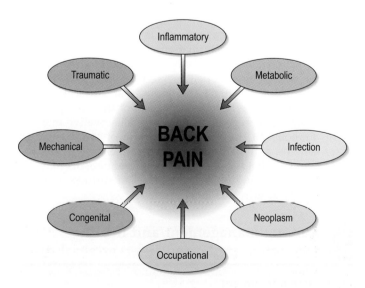

Figure 10.14 Causes of back pain.

▷ Nursing management and health promotion: acute back pain/strain

Nurses have many opportunities in the workplace, community and hospital to teach people how to organise their environment and activities in order to avoid acute back strain. Relevant health promotion is vital in prevention. Much research has gone into the ergonomics of correct lifting techniques and many teaching aids such as videos and leaflets are available (see Further reading and Useful websites, e.g. Disabled Living Foundation, Health and Safety Executive).

Nurses are themselves a high-risk group for back injury and a code of practice has been published by the Royal College of Nursing (RCN) Advisory Panel for Back Pain in Nurses (2002). Both employer and employee responsibilities are set out and there are specific guidelines for assessment and planning of patient care (Box 10.10).

 Box 10.10 Reflection

Moving and handling of patients/clients

Assessment and planning

Particularly heavy patients, or helpless patients with no ability to assist nurses, need to be individually assessed by a competent patient handling team. Student nurses and support workers should not be expected to undertake these assessments without competent supervision.

The care plan or profile should include the following information:

- The current weight of the patient.
- The extent of the patient's ability to assist and weight-bear, and any other relevant information.
- The technique to be employed to handle that particular patient which should be consistent with the activity undertaken. This should be based upon:
  - the task
  - the individual
  - the load
  - the environment.

Manual Handling Operations Regulations 1992 (Health and Safety Executive 2004) do not contain any weight limits and state that there is no threshold below which handling may be regarded as safe. All patient handling should be assessed looking at all risk factors, not just weight.

Mechanical handling devices or equipment should be used for moving totally dependent patients from bed to chair, trolley, toilet, etc. Sliding equipment should be used for moving totally dependent patients in bed.

(From the RCN Advisory Panel for Back Pain in Nurses, 2002.)

Activities

- Find out which moving and handling aids are available in the clinical area to which you are currently attached. How often are they used?
- Reflect on the different techniques for moving and handling patients you have seen or used. Discuss the safety, suitability and effectiveness of each technique with your mentor.

Recurrent back pain/strain

A patient who suffers recurrent back pain or strain should be fully investigated to rule out any other causes, such as a spinal tumour or a prolapsed intervertebral disc.

MEDICAL MANAGEMENT

Physiotherapy, medication and strategies for dealing with chronic pain are the mainstays of treatment. Specific medication may include tricyclic antidepressants and gabapentin (see Ch. 19). Patients are often referred to a chronic pain clinic where an interprofessional team aims both to relieve pain and to enable patients to live with their pain (Hansson et al 2001). This is achieved by helping patients to understand the reason for their pain, and by teaching behavioural techniques that can help to reduce it, such as pacing activities over time and learning to use relaxation techniques (Oliver & Ryan 2004).

 ## Nursing management and health promotion: recurrent back pain/strain

The nursing role within a chronic back pain management programme can encompass case management, administration and monitoring of analgesics, education and, with an appropriate qualification, counselling (Smith 2004b).

Prolapsed intervertebral disc

A prolapsed intervertebral disc (PID) is the protrusion of the disc nucleus into the spinal canal.

PATHOPHYSIOLOGY

The intervertebral discs consist of a firm nucleus pulposus surrounded by a ring of fibrocartilage and fibrous tissue which links two vertebrae together. Age-related loss of water content and an increase in collagen content leads to stiffening of the discs (Smith 2004b). The disc space becomes narrowed and distorted, leading to increased stress on the spine and intervertebral discs. Eventually the disc may rupture and the soft contents, the pulposus, will prolapse, causing compression and stretching of nerve roots or fibres. Ninety per cent of lumbar disc protrusions involve L4–5 or L5–S1 (Dandy & Edwards 2009) (Figure 10.15).

MEDICAL/SURGICAL MANAGEMENT
History

Patients classically present with acute lumbar pain radiating down the thigh and lower leg.

Examination

Muscle spasm and an intense focal area of pain may be identified. The straight leg raising test will indicate restriction of movement well below 90 degrees of hip flexion and there may be neurological signs such as numbness, tingling or diminished motor function. If necessary, an MRI scan will confirm the diagnosis.

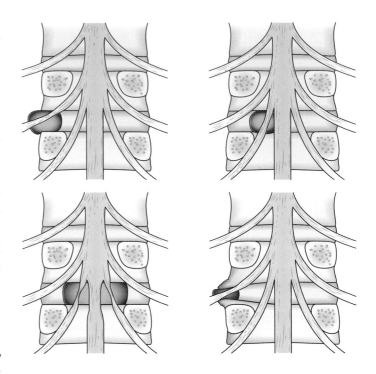

Figure 10.15 Disc prolapse and root compression in the lumbar spine. A laterally placed prolapse may compress the L4 root, a more central prolapse will compress L5, and a central prolapse will compress the cauda equina. Osteophytes in the lateral canal will also produce root compression.

Treatment

A patient who presents with a central disc prolapse is an orthopaedic emergency as the prolapsed disc causes pressure directly on the spinal cord and prompt surgical decompression is required. For other prolapses conservative treatment for acute back pain as outlined above should be tried first, although manipulation of a spine with acute disc prolapse is said to be dangerous as it could lead to a spinal cord injury (Dandy & Edwards 2009). Localised epidural steroid injections may prove beneficial (Smith 2004b).

The indication for disc excision is when there is proven disc protrusion with accompanying neurological signs and no improvement after 6 weeks of conservative treatment, or if any neurological deficit worsens. A Cochrane Review (Gibson & Waddell 2007) concludes that surgical discectomy, removal of the herniated portion of the disc, provides faster relief from an acute attack than conservative management. Removal of the herniated portion of the disc means there will be a reduction in its shock-absorbing function with the result that between 30 and 60% of patients may suffer permanent, though varying, degrees of stiffness and back pain (Dandy & Edwards 2009).

 ## Nursing management and health promotion: prolapsed intervertebral disc

Conservative treatment

As most of the conservative treatment can be carried out at home, it is the primary care nurse who will have responsibility for advising and supporting the patient and family in all comfort measures.

🖱 **See website Critical thinking question 10.3**

Operative treatment

In addition to the general principles for perioperative care and for musculoskeletal care, the following points are specific to postoperative management of patients having disc excision.

Pain The use of patient controlled analgesia (PCA) or of epidural analgesia following spinal surgery will help to ensure that the patient's pain is well controlled.

Positioning and mobilising Spinal alignment should be maintained after surgery. Normal movements can be gradually resumed as soon as the patient's general condition permits. A supportive brace may need to be worn before mobilisation can begin. Minimal flexion of the knees, using a knee rest or a pillow for support while in the supine position, will allow spinal muscles to relax. A pillow between the knees will provide comfortable alignment when in the lateral position.

Early mobilisation is usually prescribed. The bed should be lowered and the patient taught to roll to the edge, swing the legs to the floor and stand up in one smooth movement.

Degenerative and inflammatory joint disorders

There are over 200 conditions that can affect synovial joints and tissues. This section focuses on two common joint diseases: osteoarthritis and rheumatoid arthritis (Figure 10.16).

Osteoarthritis

Osteoarthritis (OA) is by far the most prevalent joint disorder with up to 8.5 million people in the UK affected by it (NICE 2008b).

PATHOPHYSIOLOGY

OA is characterised by a relatively slow deterioration of the articular cartilage that covers the bone ends in a synovial joint. Although not primarily an inflammatory disease, there is some inflammation in the joint due to the presence of cartilage debris and some synovitis (Maher et al 2002). The disease may be classified as primary or secondary, the former being a progressive condition of unknown origin, more common in the older person, especially females. Secondary OA can affect people of any age or gender and is usually associated with a previous injury/condition of the joint, such as a previous fracture or a childhood hip condition such as Perthes' disease. It can also develop following repeated high-impact joint movements in sport or occupation, e.g. professional footballers are particularly prone to hip and knee OA.

MEDICAL/SURGICAL MANAGEMENT

History and examination

Pain on movement, stiffness at rest and reduced joint function are the most common symptoms. The joint will have a

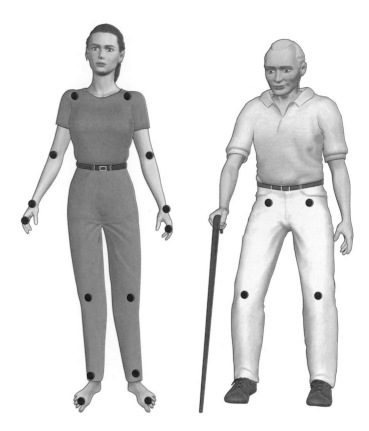

Figure 10.16 Some differences between rheumatoid arthritis and osteoarthritis. Rheumatoid arthritis affects small joints, is symmetrical and is more common in young women. Osteoarthritis mainly affects the weight-bearing joints and is more common in older people.

reduced range of movement on examination and this may be accompanied by pain.

Investigations and diagnosis

There are no specific diagnostic tests for OA, and diagnosis is usually made on history and examination. X-ray of an osteoarthritic joint will show loss of joint space and bony outgrowths, known as osteophytes. However, the degree of destruction of the joint space does not always correlate to the degree of pain and disability a patient is experiencing, and thus X-ray is usually reserved for patients where joint replacement is being considered or to rule out other disease such as a tumour. Blood tests are not necessary unless infection or inflammatory disease is suspected.

Treatment

The National Institute for Health and Clinical Excellence (NICE) has reviewed the evidence for effectiveness of treatments and provided good practice guidelines (NICE 2008b) (Box 10.11).

Surgery is considered when conservative methods are no longer effective in relieving the pain of OA. For hip and knee OA in younger people consideration may be given to osteotomy, the correction of malalignment through cutting a wedge of bone out of the distal or proximal bone (Zhang et al 2008). The surgical treatment of choice for hip and knee OA is joint replacement, i.e. the removal of the damaged ends of the bones and their replacement with a combination

Box 10.11 Evidence-based practice

The care and management of osteoarthritis in adults

The National Institute for Health and Clinical Excellence (NICE 2008b) has examined the evidence for osteoarthritis care in adults and produced evidence-based guidelines on which to base practice.

The three core treatments which should be considered initially are:

- education and advice
- strengthening and aerobic exercises
- weight loss if overweight or obese.

Relatively safe pharmacological treatments which should be considered when further treatment is required are:

- paracetamol
- topical non-steroidal anti-inflammatory drugs (NSAIDs) – creams applied to the skin for superficial joints.

Adjunctive treatments – those with less evidence of their efficacy or those with increased risk to the patient:

- oral opioids such as co-dydramol
- NSAIDs
- intra-articular injections
- transcutaneous electrical nerve stimulation (TENS)
- shock-absorbing shoes or insoles
- supports/braces
- local heat or cold
- walking sticks or assistive devices
- joint arthroplasty (joint replacement).

Activities

- Access the guidelines (http://www.nice.org.uk/Guidance/CG59) and read the section covering the three core treatments.
- Reflect on the role of the nurse in the three core treatments and discuss your conclusions with your mentor.

(National Institute for Health and Clinical Excellence [NICE] 2008b Osteoarthritis: the care and management of osteoarthritis in adults. Clinical guideline CG59.)

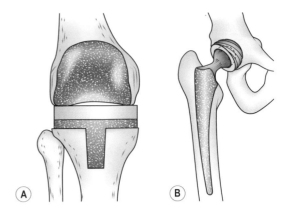

Figure 10.17 Examples of a total knee replacement (A) and a total hip replacement (B).

are generic and some disease specific, with organisations such as Arthritis Care running specific programmes for people with OA. The evidence from these programmes indicates that they can increase patient self-efficacy, the belief in the ability to change behaviour and manage disease, and that this can lead to better symptom management and enhanced quality of life (Coulter & Ellins 2006).

▷ Nursing management and health promotion: joint replacement

Pre-operative care

Preparation should begin as soon as a patient's name is added to the waiting list, with provision of written information and the opportunity to attend an assessment and information session, often known as a hip or knee clinic. These are usually multidisciplinary but coordinated and led by orthopaedic nurse practitioners.

Postoperative care

Postoperative care will follow the basic principles (see Ch. 26) and the general principles of care for musculoskeletal disorders outlined earlier (pp. 339–341), in particular regarding VTE as hip and knee replacement surgery have the highest reported rate of DVT if prophylaxis is not used, at 44% and 27% respectively (National Collaborating Centre for Acute Care 2007).

Mobility and rehabilitation The patient may begin to mobilise as soon as their condition permits, which is usually on the first day postoperatively. This will be supervised by the physiotherapist and the nurse. After a hip replacement there is a risk of dislocation of the prosthesis and it is important that the knee is not raised higher than the hip; a raised bed, chair and toilet seat are usually necessary. A walking frame may be used at first and the physiotherapist will re-educate the patient to use a normal walking gait. Depending on progress, the patient should practise using crutches or walking sticks before discharge.

See website for further content

Aids to living The occupational therapist will provide aids for dressing, such as a stocking applicator, and any other

of metal (cobalt chromium or titanium) and plastic (polyethylene) components (Maher et al 2002) (Figure 10.17). Total hip replacement (THR) and total knee replacement (TKR) prostheses are long lasting and studies show that at 10 years after surgery 90–95% of THRs (Berry et al 2002) and TKRs (Johnson et al 2003) are still functioning well. For hand OA arthrodesis (fusing of the joint) or joint replacement may be considered if all other treatments have been ineffective.

▷ Nursing management and health promotion: conservative treatments for osteoarthritis

The key to OA treatment is patient self-management and nurses can play a leading role in helping patients to develop the necessary skills and knowledge to do this. Nurses can provide the education and support themselves or refer patients to a self-management programme. Within the UK the Expert Patients Programme uses peer educators to help patients to manage their disease. Some of these programmes aids found to be necessary after an assessment of the home environment and the patient's capabilities.

Discharge planning Discharge planning should begin pre-operatively and in some centres patients will be identified as suitable for an early supported discharge scheme where a hospital at home environment is provided. Where such services do not exist, the community nurse will provide care, such as wound suture removal, and will liaise with the hospital team as necessary (Box 10.12).

Box 10.12 Reflection

A patient's reflection on having a total hip replacement

Two months after an operation for hip replacement I am trying to record my experiences, but one thought predominates to such an extent that everything else fades into insignificance. I can think of nothing other than the fact that I have no pain: no pain walking, no pain sitting, no pain lying in bed, no pain at all. Two ideas arise from this: one, that it does not seem at all healthy to be so conscious of the absence of pain. The hope must be that sooner or later being pain-free will become the normal unobserved fact of life. The other is a retrospective awareness of the debilitating effect of continuous chronic pain, the insidious way in which everything developed. People now keep exclaiming that I look so well, that my colour has improved so much. They never in the past told me that I looked old and grey. This must have been as unremarkable to others as the experience of continuous pain was to me.

There were many different kinds of pain. The worst in intensity was probably the pain on weight-bearing, but somehow it did not bother me so very much. I felt I could anticipate it, control it by leaning on a stick or furniture, or by refraining from walking altogether. There were sudden and very acute bouts of pain, sharp like toothache, on sudden movements or jolts, but these passed and did not matter much. There was the impossibility of ever sitting or lying in comfort – much less severe pain, but the most difficult to bear. It was when that particular pain suddenly got much worse that I first told the GP how I felt. When, in spite of anti-inflammatory painkillers, even the weight of the sheet became intolerable and lack of sleep became difficult to cope with, an appointment was made with the orthopaedic specialist services. I saw an orthopaedic nurse practitioner in the outpatient clinic and she asked me about my symptoms, examined me and talked through the X-ray with me. My hip joint was almost completely worn out and we agreed that it was time for a total hip replacement.

I was very apprehensive as I did not know a great deal about the operation. However I was given a comprehensive information booklet and invited to the 'Hip Clinic'. At this session I met other people waiting for their operation and we had the opportunity to talk with two people who had already had theirs. It was very reassuring to hear about their experiences. The orthopaedic nurse practitioner answered any questions we had and showed us a hip replacement. There was also an occupational therapist there who explained what adaptations we would need to our home, such as a raised toilet seat, and a physiotherapist taught us the exercises we would have to do after our operation so that we could practise them before we came into hospital. At the end of this I felt I knew what was going to happen, though I was still a little apprehensive.

Now, after the operation, I have joined the ranks of those who extol its virtue, but even the most enthusiastic supporters had not prepared me for the speed with which it would be possible to lead a normal life: walking within 24 h, discharged from hospital within 5 days, fully independent by the time of the follow-up outpatient appointment 6 weeks after operation. Here, in summary, are the events which I now believe made the whole experience entirely positive: on first appointment at the orthopaedic outpatient clinic the thorough examination, the fact that the nurse practitioner appeared to understand how much pain I had – perhaps even better than I did – and did not belittle what I was saying. The fact that I attended the Hip Clinic and that I was only on the waiting list for 12 weeks. Two weeks before the operation there was a day of tests and examinations in the ward to which I was to be admitted, giving a good opportunity to allay anxiety.

On admission I was immediately aware of the cordiality and friendliness of the nursing staff and of the community spirit of the patients who made me feel welcome and who augmented the very adequate information given to me by the staff, both in print and in discussion.

Pre-operative relief of anxiety and postoperative pain control were superb; after the initial intravenous analgesic cover, painkillers were offered every 4 h, but not really needed, except before physiotherapy, after the first few days. It was interesting to observe that all patients who had hip operations went through the same progression of skill acquisition and setbacks, learning how to get in and out of bed, how to turn in bed, how to walk, first with a Zimmer frame, then with two sticks, and later one stick, how to pick things up off the floor, to put on stockings and shoes, to shower independently, to dress and undress, to climb stairs and to get in and out of a car. It was evident that all the nurses knew exactly what each patient was capable of doing. All were willing to help but clearly expected and encouraged independence. The nurses' awareness of patients' progress and the supervision of the activities of less highly qualified staff were always in evidence. It was reassuring to notice that there was vigilance in case deep vein thrombosis arose. With the emphasis throughout on what one can do by oneself and encouragement to get moving, it was a boost to self-confidence to know that nurses were vigilant for complications and setbacks. I found it helpful to have been shown the X-ray of the new hip as it makes it possible to visualise what the joint is doing during various activities, and to understand why one is advised never to cross the legs, to get on all fours or to pick things up off the floor from the sitting position. A pillow between the legs during sleep helps prevent crossing the legs accidentally.

There were 12 women in the ward, most of them in for hip or knee operations. The impression gained on admission of a friendly, supportive group spirit was reinforced throughout. What a wealth of experience, what a reservoir of knowledge, what abundance of empathy, goodwill and helpfulness. There was also a tremendous amount of fun and humour, perhaps enhanced by the experience all had of being pain-free all of a sudden. On discharge I was part of a supported discharge scheme, which meant that a physiotherapist and nurses visited me during my first few weeks at home to check that I was continuing to make progress. It was reassuring to have this support when I got home.

I learned a lot, not only about health and illness, but also about emotional, social and economic stress, and about coping strategies. The importance of the patient community and its therapeutic potential is seldom recognised in general nursing but it should never be underestimated.

Activity

- Using information from the chapter and the patient's reflection, write a concise discharge plan for a patient who has undergone an uncomplicated total hip replacement. Discuss the plan with your mentor.

Rheumatoid arthritis

Rheumatoid arthritis (RA) is a systemic disease of connective tissue which affects approximately one million people in the UK (Hill & Ryan 2000).

PATHOPHYSIOLOGY

RA is an autoimmune disease, i.e. the body's immune system attacks its own tissues and becomes self-destructive (see Ch. 6). The cause of this is not yet known and research continues. The joints are acutely inflamed due to inflammatory changes in the synovial membrane. The synovium becomes thicker, very vascular and the site of increased cell infiltration which may cause an effusion within the joint that manifests as a swollen joint. As the proliferative tissue spreads as a 'pannus' over the articular cartilage, the cartilage is slowly eroded.

Systemic inflammatory changes can affect many of the body's organs and lead to pericarditis, pleuritis and bowel vasculitis, as well as general malaise and anaemia. It is therefore potentially a very debilitating chronic disease. Life expectancy is reduced by approximately 7 years in men and 3 years in women, mainly due to infections, renal or respiratory disease, or the RA itself (Hakim et al 2006). However, there is no one path of RA progression and some patients have permanent remission whilst others have severe relentless deterioration in symptoms; each patient must therefore be assessed individually.

MEDICAL/SURGICAL MANAGEMENT

History

The disease most commonly starts when a person is in their 30s or 40s with a gradual onset of pain and stiffness, particularly in the morning, affecting the small joints of the hands and feet. The person may also present to their GP complaining of loss of appetite and weight, mild pyrexia, and characteristics of anaemia. As the RA progresses, other joints may become involved, with inflammation, swelling and progressive loss of function. Commonly the wrists, elbows, shoulders, cervical spine, temporomandibular joints, knees and ankles are affected.

For some patients the onset of RA is acute, with multiple joint involvement from the onset, with rapid progress to loss of function.

Examination

The affected joints will appear swollen and be warm to the touch. The patient will complain of pain when the normal range of movement is attempted.

Investigations

X-rays of both hands and feet will usually confirm erosions. A blood specimen will be taken for assessment of the level of haemoglobin, number of white blood cells, ESR, CRP and the presence of rheumatoid factor.

Diagnosis

The American Rheumatism Association criteria for classification of RA provide a diagnostic guideline (Arnett et al 1988). The seven criteria are:

- morning stiffness
- arthritis in three or more joints with swelling
- arthritis of the hand joints
- symmetrical arthritis
- subcutaneous nodules
- presence of rheumatoid factor
- joint changes on X-ray.

The first four criteria must have been present for at least 6 weeks and a patient must have four or more of the seven criteria to be diagnosed as having RA.

Treatment

There is no known cure for RA, and therefore intervention is directed towards relieving pain, modifying the level of disease activity and maintaining optimal functional ability for each individual (Ryan & Oliver 2002).

The aims of medical treatment are to:

- Reduce the patient's pain with the use of analgesics, e.g. NSAIDs.
- Reduce joint destruction with the use of disease-modifying anti-rheumatic drugs (DMARDs) such as methotrexate, and/or early short-term use of local or systemic corticosteroid therapy. Newer treatments, biological agents such as infliximab, etanercept and adalimumab are also being used (Lorenzi & Kelly 2008). These alter the normal immune response by blocking the normal inflammatory process.
- Prevent or minimise deformity of a joint by splinting damaged or painful joints.
- Assist the patient to adapt their lifestyle.
- Correct anaemia.

The main surgical treatments are:

- synovectomy (removal of excess synovial membrane from within the joint capsule)
- osteotomy
- joint replacement or arthrodesis (most commonly of the ankle).

 Nursing management and health promotion: rheumatoid arthritis

The aim of care is to relieve symptoms and to maintain and, if possible, improve quality of life. A multidisciplinary approach is essential, but coordination of care and therapeutic interventions such as joint injections often fall within the remit of rheumatology nurse specialists.

Patient involvement/empowerment

As with OA the current emphasis for RA management is on patient involvement and self-management through Expert Patient programmes.

Controlling pain

A range of analgesics may need to be considered, from paracetamol/aspirin to compound analgesics, such as co-codamol, to NSAIDs. Corticosteroids are usually used in the short term in acute episodes of pain/inflammation. When they are used for long-term therapy, abrupt withdrawal must be avoided as the body may not have sufficient glucocorticoids to deal with stress (see Ch. 5). Herbal therapy is tried by many patients but there is often little evidence for its effectiveness and some herbal medication can interact with prescribed drugs, for example Devil's Claw can increase the effects of warfarin (Vitetta et al 2008). However, some patients do gain benefit from such herbal remedies and nurses play an important role in ensuring that patients are aware of any potential side-effects.

Local pain control can be achieved in some joints by other methods, such as splints for the hand and wrist joints.

Maintaining independence and fostering well-being

Exercise and mobility The principles of joint protection should be explained to the patient, such as respecting pain and not being fearful or ignoring it, balancing work and rest, using the larger or stronger joints rather than small ones, and reducing the effort to a joint (Maher et al 2002).

Adaptation of living space The muscle power of the patient with RA is reduced, and therefore the use of aids such as a variable-height bed, raised or ejector chair and raised toilet seat may be of assistance.

Walking aids, such as a stick or elbow crutches, may help to retain the patient's level of mobility by reducing the weight load placed on specific joints. The hand pieces of the aids may need to be adapted to accommodate the finger and wrist deformities that are common features of the disease.

Diet The patient with RA may require assistance in maintaining nutritional status due to anorexia and/or difficulty in using eating and drinking utensils. Frequent, light, appetising meals should be served. The occupational therapist can supply a variety of utensils, such as large-handled cutlery and a tilting kettle stand, which will help the patient to retain independence. A patient with RA is likely to develop anaemia due to the chronic inflammatory process of the disease and/or from gastrointestinal bleeding caused by non-steroidal anti-inflammatory medication therapy, and iron supplements may be prescribed.

Sexual activity Counselling regarding sexual activity may be required. The Arthritis Research Campaign has produced booklets containing useful information for RA patients and their partners (see Useful websites).

SOFT TISSUE INJURIES

This section of the chapter outlines a range of soft tissue injuries, including those affecting ligaments, muscles and tendons and peripheral nerves.

Ligament injuries

Injuries to ligaments may involve a partial or complete rupture of the ligament.

PATHOPHYSIOLOGY

Injuries are caused by excessive extension, flexion and/or rotation of a joint. 'Whiplash injury' is the term used to describe a ligamentous injury to the cervical spine area often occurring after an RTC. This injury is due to excessive flexion and extension movements to the neck. The knee is heavily dependent on its ligaments for stability and they are susceptible to injury, particularly the anterior cruciate ligament which limits forward movement of the tibia on the femur. Injured ligaments never heal soundly or regain their former strength as the scar tissue that forms at the site is never as strong as the original tissue (Dandy & Edwards 2009).

MEDICAL MANAGEMENT

History and examination

People who suffer these injuries are often young and will complain of severe pain around the injured area after feeling or hearing something snap or tear. Limitation of normal joint movement may be found with swelling of the injured part and joint instability may be noted during the physical examination.

Investigations

Plain radiographs are taken to rule out a bony injury to the area. An MRI scan or examination of the joint under general anaesthesia may be undertaken.

Treatment

The injured area will be supported, e.g. using a cervical collar for a whiplash injury (Figure 10.18) or a POP cylinder/knee brace for a knee injury. Physiotherapy is instituted in order to build up muscle groups that surround the joint which the injured ligament normally supports. Surgical intervention is usually needed only when the injury affects the knee joint or where there is damage to more than one ligament and/or gross instability of the joint. Repairing ruptured ligaments is generally not successful, because the repaired ligament will not have the same 'stretchiness' as the original, and therefore they are usually replaced with a length of tendon or prosthetic material (Dandy & Edwards 2009).

▷ **Nursing management and health promotion: ligament injuries**

If no other injury has been sustained, the patient may be treated and discharged from the Emergency Department to attend as an outpatient.

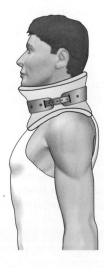

Figure 10.18 Cervical collar.

Pain relief This will be the major patient problem on presentation at hospital. Such pain should be assessed (see Ch. 19) and an effective analgesic prescribed. As ligamentous injuries are sustained following severe trauma to the body part, the surrounding soft tissues will also be involved, causing further bleeding which will increase the swelling and irritate the surrounding tissues, thus increasing the patient's pain. The use of NSAIDs will be of value to reduce the inflammatory process.

Muscle spasm This is a common sign of soft tissue irritation and, if severe, the patient may need to be prescribed a mild antispasmodic as well as an analgesic.

Support/immobilisation Refer to priorities and management of patients in casts (p. 344). When a cervical collar is worn, it can usually be removed to allow daily skin care. Following anterior cruciate ligament repair a patient may wear a knee brace for the first 6–8 weeks, which prevents flexion greater than 90 degrees, and nurses should ensure that the patient can correctly apply the device.

Psychosocial care Ligamentous injury may take up to a year to heal completely, and work and financial status, as well as social interaction, can be affected (Smith 2004c).

Muscle and tendon injuries

PATHOPHYSIOLOGY

These injuries are most often caused either by direct trauma at the site of the injury or by a sudden sharp movement of the joint associated with sports such as tennis and squash. The large tendons and muscles of the lower limbs, such as the Achilles tendon that inserts the gastrocnemius and soleus muscles into the heel bone, are the most common sites of injury.

MEDICAL MANAGEMENT

History and examination

The patient will experience a distressing tearing sensation or a kick at the site of the injury and possibly an inability to put the foot down. Swelling and tenderness will develop within a few hours following the injury. Bruising will appear later and may be extensive and alarming for the patient. On examination, a gap between the ends of the muscle or tendon may be felt in superficial muscle injuries. MRI or ultrasound may be used to determine the extent of the injury.

Treatment

For muscle injuries the principles of RICE – Rest, Ice, Compression and Elevation – should be followed in order to control haemorrhage and limit haematoma formation. Early mobilisation within pain limits is important, as muscle healing occurs through aerobic metabolic pathways and therefore needs adequate circulation. Surgery may be necessary if there is a large intramuscular haematoma or if there is a large muscle tear affecting movement of a joint.

Tendon injuries are usually treated conservatively, with a cast or splint holding the ends together until healed. Surgery may be required for a complete tendon rupture, particularly of the Achilles tendon. A systematic review of surgical versus conservative treatment of Achilles tendon injury concluded that whilst surgery reduced the risk of re-rupture, it significantly increases the risk of other complications such as infection (Khan et al 2004).

 ## Nursing management and health promotion: muscle and tendon injuries

Comfort The nurse has a key role in helping the patient to institute and maintain RICE.

Mobility Once activity is commenced, the physiotherapist will teach the patient to use the most appropriate walking aid, usually a pair of crutches, and nurses should ensure that the patients use these correctly.

See website for further content

Assessment of the patient's home circumstances with regard to mobility will be required and referral to an occupational therapist may be necessary.

Following surgery, routine postoperative care will be necessary (see Ch. 26). The use of a cast or brace will necessitate education of the patient in its care and management.

Peripheral nerve injuries

Nerves can be damaged due to underlying disease or following trauma. In this section, the focus will be on nerve injuries following trauma.

PATHOPHYSIOLOGY

A single nerve or group of nerves may be damaged depending on the site of injury. Nerve injuries can be due to either direct or indirect force and can be divided into three types (Wellington 2004):

- neuropraxia – intact nerves with temporary damage usually due to compression
- axonotmesis – divided axons with maintenance of the endoneural tubes, usually due to severe blow or traction, a pulling injury; prognosis is good
- neurotmesis – the whole nerve is divided, usually from a penetrating wound such as a stabbing; no recovery is possible without surgical repair.

MEDICAL MANAGEMENT

History and examination

Following an accident, a patient may become aware of tingling (paraesthesia), numbness and/or loss of movement of the affected part. Examination of the distribution of the loss of sensation and movement will aid diagnosis as to the extent of the injury.

Investigations

Plain radiographs are useful to assess bony injury and for the presence of any foreign material, such as glass fragments, which may have caused the injury.

Diagnosis

This is confirmed by the absence or alteration of neurological function and sensation of the affected part. Nerve conduction studies, which involve stimulating a nerve with a wave pulse to evaluate the sensory and motor responses along the course of the peripheral nerve, may be carried out (Dandy & Edwards 2009). Electromyography (EMG), which records motor activity at rest and on attempted muscle contraction, may also be used (Wellington 2004).

Treatment

Non-operative management involves immobilisation of the affected part in the anatomical position, using a lightweight cast or splint. Peripheral nerves are capable of regenerating at a rate of 1–2 mm/day (Wellington 2004). It is possible to calculate roughly the length of time to recovery although there is no guarantee that each nerve cell will heal. Primary surgical repair is indicated only when a nerve has been cleanly divided. Secondary repair may include suturing and grafting of nerve tissue from a less important nerve within the patient's body.

Nursing management and health promotion: peripheral nerve injuries

Complete recovery may occur but can take a few weeks, months or years. However, the patient may need to adapt to permanent and severely disabling physical, psychological and social changes (Wellington 2004).

In the short term, as the patient will have been involved in some form of trauma, nursing care as outlined in Chapter 27 will apply. Should the patient require surgery, general perioperative care will be needed (see Ch. 26).

Health promotion – preventing further injury

The patient will have partial or complete loss of the protective mechanisms of touch and pain, and care must be taken to prevent further injury to the affected part. Movement of the injured limb must be through the normal range of passive joint movements, otherwise joints, muscles, tendons, ligaments and other nerves could be damaged further. To prevent the development of joint contracture and deformity, the patient may be fitted with a lightweight splint which holds the joints in their anatomical position. This may be needed for a long period. Exposure to extremes of temperature should be avoided, to prevent a skin burn.

Other considerations

Pain Sharp shooting pain and a constant tingling sensation can be very troublesome and the patient may need prolonged use of analgesics. Antidepressant medication, such as amitriptyline, and adjuvant analgesics are known to be beneficial as a supplementary medication in the relief of neuropathic pain (see Ch. 19).

Washing and dressing The patient will need advice and information to assist in adapting their usual mode of personal cleansing and dressing. For example, a patient with a median nerve injury due to a laceration of the wrist of the dominant hand may have difficulty in brushing their teeth or combing their hair. The occupational therapist can provide advice and appropriate aids.

Splints If a splint is used, the patient will need information and advice about the correct method of application and removal.

Support As recovery from a peripheral nerve injury may be prolonged, the patient will require support and understanding from family, friends and the members of the health care team to relieve boredom and prevent the development of depression. Group sessions for patients with similar injuries who are receiving physiotherapy, occupational therapy and/or diversional therapy can be an excellent psychological support mechanism. The social worker can assist with social and/or financial problems which may develop due to the possible lengthy absence from employment.

Permanent disability If the nerve injury prevents return to the previous occupation, it will be necessary to ensure that the patient has access to specialist advice about retraining and new employment opportunities. In some instances, alteration to body image could have a severe psychological effect. Nurses should be aware of this and provide support and counselling as needed by the patient.

SUMMARY: KEY NURSING ISSUES

- The overall aims of nursing care of patients with musculoskeletal injury or disorder are to prevent further injury, reduce the risk of complications, promote healing, maximise independence and promote optimal rehabilitation.
- Three key potential complications which must be considered with musculoskeletal injury or the treatment of musculoskeletal disorders are compartment syndrome, venous thromboembolism (VTE) and fat embolus. Nurses play a key role in reducing the risk of these complications and their early identification.
- Fracture treatment consists of reducing the fracture, maintaining its position whilst it heals, and restoring function. Nurses caring for patients with fractures need an understanding of the various methods used to achieve fracture healing, including casts, traction and internal or external fixation.
- The management of joint disorders such as osteoarthritis and rheumatoid arthritis requires patients to play a central role in the management of their condition. Nurses can help to ensure that patients have the necessary knowledge and self-management skills to achieve this.
- Patients with musculoskeletal injury or disorder will be cared for in a wide variety of settings and not just an orthopaedic ward. All nurses need some understanding of the common conditions such as osteoporosis and osteoarthritis and their attendant treatments such as medication and joint replacement.

REFLECTION AND LEARNING – WHAT NEXT?

- **Test** your knowledge by visiting the website and answering the multiple choice questions and critical thinking questions.
- **Consolidate** your learning by looking at some of the further reading suggestions, references and specialist websites.
- **Revisit** some of the additional material on the website.
- **Consider** what you have learnt and how this will help your professional development.

- **Reflect** on how you can apply this knowledge to the care of your patients.
- **Discuss** your learning with your mentor/supervisor, lecturer and colleagues.

REFERENCES

Allsworth A: Osteoporosis: nursing implications. In Kneale J, Davis P, editors: *Orthopaedic and trauma nursing*, ed 2, Edinburgh, 2004, Churchill Livingstone, pp 380–389.

Arnett FC, Edsworth SM, Block DA: The American Rheumatism Association 1987 revised criteria for the classification of rheumatoid arthritis, *Arthritis Rheum* 31(3):315–324, 1988.

Berry D, Harmsen S, Cabanela M, et al: 25-year survivorship of 2000 consecutive primary Charnley total hip replacements, *J Bone Joint Surg* 84A(2):171–177, 2002.

British Orthopaedic Association (BOA): *The care of patients with fragility fracture*, ed 2, 2007. Available online http://www.nhfd.co.uk.

Burden J, Kneale JD: Orthopaedic infections. In Kneale J, Davis P, editors: *Orthopaedic and trauma nursing*, ed 2, Edinburgh, 2004, Churchill Livingstone, pp 215–236.

Content G, Hajela V, Lucas B: Osteoporosis screening and education following distal radial fracture: an expanding role for fracture clinic nurses, *J Orthop Nurs* 7(3):137–140, 2003.

Coulter A, Ellins J: *Patient focus interventions: a review of the evidence*, London, 2006, The Health Foundation.

Dandy DJ, Edwards DJ: *Essential orthopaedics and trauma*, ed 5, Edinburgh, 2009, Churchill Livingstone.

Dupuy D, Goldberg N: Image-guided radiofrequency tumour ablation: challenges and opportunities – part II, *J Vasc Interv Radiol* 12(10): 1135–1148, 2001.

Ellis K: A review of amputation, phantom pain and nursing responsibilities, *Br J Nurs* 11(3):155–163, 2002.

Gibson JNA, Waddell G: Surgical interventions for lumbar disc prolapse, *Cochrane Database Syst Rev* (2):CD001350, 2007.

Hakim A, Clunie G, Haq I: *The essential pocket guide to rheumatology: Oxford Handbook of rheumatology*, Oxford, 2006, Oxford University Press.

Hansson M, Bostrom C, Harms-Ringdahl K: Living with spine-related pain in a changing society: a qualitative study, *Disabil Rehabil* 23(7): 286–295, 2001.

Harrison P: *Managing spinal injury: critical care*, London, 2000, Spinal Injuries Association.

Health and Safety Executive: *Manual Handling Operations Regulations 1992 (as amended). Guidance on Regulations L23*, ed 3, London, 2004, HSE Books.

Henry C: Care of patients with bone tumours. In Kneale J, Davis P, editors: *Orthopaedic and trauma nursing*, ed 2, Edinburgh, 2004, Churchill Livingstone, pp 265–285.

Hill J, Ryan S, editors: *Rheumatology: a handbook for community nurses*, London, 2000, Whurr.

Howard WJ: A critical review of the role of targeted education for osteoporosis prevention, *J Orthop Nurs* 5(3):131–135, 2001.

James A: Osteoporosis: cause and treatment, *Nurs Times* 96(22):36–37, 2000.

Johnson GV-V, Worland RL, Keenan J, et al: Patient demographics as a predictor of the ten-year survival rate in primary total knee replacement, *J Bone Joint Surg* 85-B(1):52–56, 2003.

Khan RJK, Fick D, Brammar TJ, et al: Surgical interventions for treating acute Achilles tendon ruptures, *Cochrane Database Syst Rev 2004* (3): CD003674, 2004.

Kneale J, Davis P, editors: *Nursing the orthopaedic patient*, ed 2, Edinburgh, 2004, Churchill Livingstone.

Krismer M, van Tulder M: Low back pain (non-specific), *Best Pract Res Clin Rheumatol* 21(1):77–91, 2007.

Langstaff R: Fracture healing and principles of fracture management. In Langstaff D, Christie J, editors: *Trauma care: a team approach* Oxford, 2000, Butterworth-Heinemann, pp 13–25.

Large P: A 'new focus' in casting – an introduction to the concepts of focus rigidity casting, *J Orthop Nurs* 5:176–179, 2001.

Lee-Smith J, Santy J, Davis P, et al: Pin site management. Towards a consensus: part 1, *J Orthop Nurs* 5:37–42, 2001.

Lethaby A, Temple J, Santy J: Pin site care for preventing infections associated with external bone fixators and pins, *Cochrane Database Syst Rev* (4):CD004551, 2008.

Limb MK: An evaluation survey of self-concept issue in adult patients undergoing limb reconstruction procedures, *J Orthop Nurs* 8(1):34–40, 2004.

Lookinland S, Beckstrand RL: HRT: decide based on the evidence, *Nurse Pract* 28(9):46–54, 2003.

Lorenzi A, Kelly C: What's new in rheumatology, *Medicine* 36(8):442–446, 2008.

Lucas B, Davis PS: Why restricting movement is important. In Kneale J, Davis P, editors: *Orthopaedic and trauma nursing*, ed 2, Edinburgh, 2004, Churchill Livingstone, pp 105–139.

Maher AB, Salmond SW, Pelino TA: *Orthopaedic nursing*, ed 3, Philadelphia, 2002, Saunders.

National Collaborating Centre for Acute Care: *Reducing the risk of venous thromboembolism (deep vein thrombosis and pulmonary embolism) in inpatients undergoing surgery*, London, 2007, National Collaborating Centre for Acute Care.

National Institute for Health and Clinical Excellence (NICE): *Osteoporosis – primary prevention. Technology appraisal TA 160*, 2008a. Available online http://www.nice.org.uk/Guidance/TA160.

National Institute for Health and Clinical Excellence (NICE): *Osteoarthritis: the care and management of osteoarthritis in adults. Clinical guideline CG59*, 2008b. Available online http://www.nice.org.uk/Guidance/CG59.

Oliver S, Ryan S: Effective pain management for patients with arthritis, *Nurs Stand* 18(50):43–52, 2004.

Parker MJ, Handoll HHG: Pre-operative traction for fractures of the proximal femur in adults, *Cochrane Database Syst Rev* (3): CD000168, 2006.

Renton S, Brown J: An evaluation of an orthopaedic supported discharge service, *J Orthop Nurs* 5(3):120–124, 2001.

Royal College of Nursing (RCN) Advisory Panel for Back Pain in Nurses: *Code of practice for patient handling*, London, 2002, RCN.

Ryan S, Oliver S: Rheumatoid arthritis, *Nurs Stand* 16(20):45–52, 2002.

Scottish Intercollegiate Guidelines Network (SIGN): *Prevention and management of hip fractures in older people No. 56*, 2002. Available online http://www.sign.ac.uk.

Sims M, Trent J-C, Lake S, et al: The Lautenbach method for chronic osteomyelitis: nursing roles, responsibilities and challenges, *J Orthop Nurs* 5(4):198–205, 2001.

Smith M: Care of patients with acute spinal cord injuries. In Kneale J, Davis P, editors: *Orthopaedic and trauma nursing*, ed 2, Edinburgh, 2004a, Churchill Livingstone, pp 390–410.

Smith M: Care of patients with spinal conditions and injuries. In Kneale J, Davis P, editors: *Orthopaedic and trauma nursing*, ed 2, Edinburgh, 2004b, Churchill Livingstone, pp 359–379.

Smith M: Sports injuries. In Kneale J, Davis P, editors: *Orthopaedic and trauma nursing*, ed 2, Edinburgh, 2004c, Churchill Livingstone, pp 495–512.

Tarling M, Aitken E, Lahoti O, et al: Closing the audit loop: the role of a pilot in the development of a fractured neck of femur integrated care pathway, *J Orthop Nurs* 6(3):130–134, 2002.

Vitetta L, Cicuttini F, Sali A: Alternative therapies for musculoskeletal conditions, *Best Pract Res Clin Rheumatol* 22(3):499–522, 2008.

Wellington B: Peripheral nerve injuries. In Kneale J, Davis P, editors: *Orthopaedic and trauma nursing*, ed 2, Edinburgh, 2004, Churchill Livingstone, pp 436–449.

Zhang W, Moskowitz RW, Nuki G, et al: OARSI recommendations for the management of hip and knee osteoarthritis, Part II: OARSI evidence-based, expert consensus guideline, *Osteoarthritis Cartilage* 16(2): 137–162, 2008.

FURTHER READING

Dandy DJ, Edwards DJ: *Essential orthopaedics and trauma*, ed 5, Edinburgh, 2009, Churchill Livingstone.

Farley A, McLafferty E, Hendry C: Pulmonary embolism: identification, clinical features and management, *Nurs Stand* 23(28):49–56, 2009.

Health and Safety Executive: *Musculoskeletal disorders in health and social care*, 2009. Available online http://www.hse.gov.uk/healthservices/msd/index.htm.

Holland K, Jenkins J, Solomon J, Whittam S, editors: *Applying the Roper–Logan–Tierney Model in Practice*, ed 2, Edinburgh, 2008, Churchill Livingstone.

Kneale J, Davis P, editors: *Orthopaedic and trauma nursing*, ed 2, Edinburgh, 2004, Churchill Livingstone.

Knight C, Mathew A, Muir JK: The locomotor system. In Kneale J, Davis P, editors: *Orthopaedic and trauma nursing*, ed 2, Edinburgh, 2004, Churchill Livingstone, pp 47–75.

Langstaff D, Christie J: *Trauma care: a team approach*, Oxford, 2000, Butterworth-Heinemann.

Maher AB, Salmond SW, Pellino TA: *Orthopaedic nursing*, ed 3, Philadelphia, 2002, Saunders.

Marieb EN, Hoehn K: *Human Anatomy and Physiology*, ed 7, San Francisco, 2007, Benjamin Cummings.

Ramachandran VS, Hirsten W: The perception of phantom limbs: the D.O. Hebb lecture, *Brain* 121(9):1603–1630, 1998.

Santy J, Vincent M, Duffield B: The principles of caring for patients with Ilizarov external fixation, *Nurs Stand* 23(26):50–55, 2009.

Scottish Intercollegiate Guidelines Network (SIGN): *Prophylaxis of venous thromboembolism*, No. 62, 2002. Available online http://www.sign.ac.uk.

USEFUL WEBSITES

Arthritis Care: www.arthritiscare.org.uk
Arthritis Research Campaign: www.arthritisresearchuk.org
Disabled Living Foundation: www.dlf.org.uk
Health and Safety Executive: www.hse.gov.uk
National Osteoporosis Society: www.nos.org.uk
RCN Society of Orthopaedic and Trauma Nursing: www.rcn.org.uk/development/communities/specialisms/orthopaedic_and_trauma
Spinal Injuries Association: www.spinal.co.uk.

CHAPTER 11

Nursing patients with blood disorders

Jacqueline Bloomfield

Introduction

Disorders of the blood are diverse and the nursing care of a patient with a blood disorder will depend on the type and nature of the condition. They can be acute or chronic and can affect all age groups. Some blood disorders, such as haemophilia, are sex-linked. Others, such as the hereditary haemoglobinopathies sickle cell disease and thalassaemia, are more prevalent among certain groups whereas others, such as iron-deficiency anaemia, occur generally. Some blood disorders, such as acute leukaemia, are life-threatening and require urgent treatment. Nursing patients with a blood disorder is challenging and requires expert knowledge and skills in order to ensure individualised, holistic care. This chapter provides a brief overview of the anatomy and physiology of blood and haematopoiesis (blood cell production) (see Further reading, e.g. Tortora & Derrickson 2009).

Disorders of blood, investigations and treatments are also described with a focus on nursing management and health promotion.

Anatomy and physiology

The haematological system comprises the blood, bone marrow and lymphoid tissue. The three primary functions of blood include:

- Transportation of oxygen, carbon dioxide, essential nutrients, enzymes and hormones. Blood also carries waste products to the excretory organs.
- Regulation of water, electrolyte and acid–base balance and body temperature.
- Protection against infection. As blood contains coagulation factors, it also protects the body from excessive blood loss.

367

All blood cells originate from pluripotent haematopoietic stem cells. Stem cells are capable of self-renewal, proliferation and differentiation into separate cell lineages, which give rise to distinct blood cell populations. This multistep process, known as haematopoiesis, is stimulated and regulated by a range of cytokines, hormones and growth factors including erythropoietin, thrombopoietin, colony-stimulating factors (CSFs) and interleukins (Hoffbrand et al 2006).

Blood cells have a limited lifespan and an estimated 100 billion new blood cells are required daily in order to maintain a healthy, steady state (Huether & McCance 2008). Consequently, haematopoiesis is a continual process which takes place in different anatomical sites throughout the lifespan. These include the embryonic yolk sac, the fetal liver and spleen, and in all bone marrow during infancy. From childhood onwards, red bone marrow is progressively replaced with fat. In adults haematopoiesis occurs primarily in the medullary cavity of flat bones. Sites include the:

- ends of the humerus and femur
- pelvis
- vertebrae
- ribs
- sternum
- skull.

Additional sites may be recruited when there is an increased demand for blood cells such as in the case of illness.

Blood constantly circulates around the body and the normal total blood volume depends on the size of the individual, e.g. 5–6 L in an average adult male. Blood is composed of both cellular and fluid elements.

Cellular components of blood

The three main cellular components of blood are:

- erythrocytes (red blood cells)
- leucocytes (white blood cells)
- thrombocytes (platelets).

Erythrocytes (red blood cells)

Erythrocytes, the most numerous of all blood cell types in the blood, constitute approximately 40% of total blood volume. Biconcave in shape, erythrocytes are responsible for the transportation of oxygen to the tissues and some carbon dioxide to the lungs. Haemoglobin, the oxygen-carrying molecule contained within the cell, contributes to a third of its weight and gives blood its characteristic red colour. Iron is an essential component of haemoglobin. Erythrocytes are soft and pliable, allowing them to travel easily through capillaries, and their thin cellular membrane facilitates gaseous exchange between the cell and surrounding tissues.

The total number of circulating erythrocytes remains fairly stable at 3.8–6.5×10^{12} cells/L, with women having less than men. Erythropoietin has a vital role in the regulation of red cell production (erythropoiesis) and is produced mainly by the kidneys in response to tissue hypoxia. During maturation, the erythrocyte synthesises haemoglobin and extrudes its nucleus, thereby rendering the mature cell incapable of reproduction, repair, growth or haemoglobin production (Figure 11.1). The average lifespan of a red blood cell

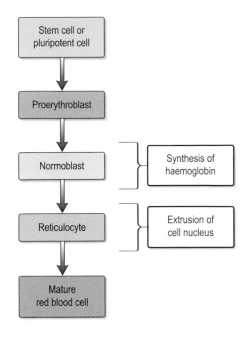

Figure 11.1 Maturation of red blood cells.

(RBC) is 120 days, after which it is sequestered in the spleen where it is destroyed by the phagocytic cells of the reticuloendothelial system (also known as mononuclear–phagocytic system).

Leucocytes (white blood cells)

Leucocytes or white blood cells (WBCs), of which there are several distinct types, make up approximately 1% of blood volume and are instrumental in defending the body against infection. The total number of WBCs is between 4.0 and 11.0×10^9 cells/L. Leucocyte maturation is regulated by specific haematopoietic growth factors such as granulocyte colony stimulating factor (G-CSF), and their lifespan will vary according to type (Figure 11.2). For example, neutrophils circulate for about 7–8 hours in the blood before migrating into the tissues, where they die after a few days. Lymphocytes may live from 100 days to several years, whereas macrophages can survive for many years.

Leucocytes are classified according to their structure as either granulocytes or non-granulocytes or in relation to their function (phagocytes or immunocytes).

Granulocytes These cells contain enzyme-rich granules within their cytoplasm, which assist with phagocytosis and inflammatory and immune functions. Subtypes of granulocytes include neutrophils, eosinophils and basophils (the polymorphonuclear cells). (See Appendix for the normal numbers of each type.)

Neutrophils are the largest component of the WBC population, and the primary phagocytes of infection control. These cells spend 8–10 hours in circulation before migrating to the tissues where they are responsible for non-specific defence against bacterial and fungal infections.

Eosinophils circulate in the peripheral blood for approximately 5 hours. Phagocytic eosinophils exit to the tissues where they are responsible for defence against infestation

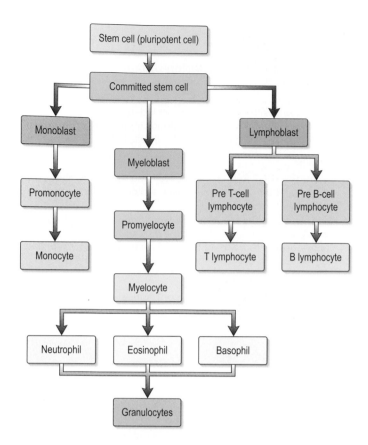

Figure 11.2 Development of different types of leucocyte.

by parasites. Eosinophils also have a role in allergic responses (see Ch. 6).

Basophils comprise the smallest number of WBCs. Basophils and mast cells contain heparin and histamine and are involved in anaphylactic, hypersensitivity and inflammatory responses (see Ch. 6).

Agranulocytes These WBCs have a large nucleus and, as their name suggests, do not contain granules in their cytoplasm. They include monocytes and lymphocytes, both of which perform a range of protective functions. (See Appendix for the normal numbers of each type.)

Monocytes The largest of the WBCs, monocytes start as immature macrophages which are present in the blood for 20–40 hours before travelling to tissue sites where they mature into powerful phagocytes. Tissue macrophages also process and present antigens to lymphoid cells and play a role in the production of cytokines and growth factors important for haematopoiesis, inflammation and cellular responses (Mehta & Hoffbrand 2009).

Lymphocytes are the chief cells of the immune response and make up approximately 36% of total leucocyte count. Lymphocytes mature in either bone marrow (B lymphocytes or B cells) or the thymus gland (T lymphocytes or T cells). B lymphocytes are responsible for antibody-mediated (humoral) immunity while T lymphocytes play an integral role in specific cell-mediated (cellular) immunity (see Ch. 6). Natural killer (NK) cells are a subset of lymphocytes which share many features of cytotoxic T cells, a type of T lymphocytes.

Thrombocytes (platelets)

Platelets are very small, non-nucleated cell fragments that play a vital role in haemostasis (arrest of bleeding). The normal platelet count is $140–400 \times 10^9/L$.

Originating from the pluripotent stem cell, these cells differentiate and mature into megakaryocytes, which then fragment to form platelets. Platelets are involved in the first three phases of haemostasis, but not the final phase:

- vasoconstriction of the injured vessel
- formation of a platelet plug
- coagulation – formation of a fibrin clot
- fibrinolysis – dissolution of the fibrin clot.

Information about blood coagulation factors and haemostasis is available on the companion website.

See website for further content

About one third of platelets are stored in the spleen, from which they are released in response to cellular damage or injury. Platelets survive for about 10 days before being destroyed by macrophages.

Plasma

Plasma comprises 50–55% of total blood volume and is a straw-coloured aqueous solution containing plasma proteins, i.e. albumin, globulins and fibrinogen. It also contains inorganic ions that regulate cell function, blood pH and osmotic pressure. These ions include sodium, potassium, chloride, phosphate, magnesium and calcium. Small amounts of nutrients, waste products, drugs, hormones and gases are also present in plasma.

Blood groups

ABO blood groups

Red blood cells have specific inherited antigens (also known as agglutinogens) on their membrane. These are important in terms of defining the ABO blood group classification system and a person can possess the A or B antigen, neither, or both. As such there are four main blood groups: A, B, AB and O.

A person with the antigen A (blood group A) has anti-B antibodies (also called agglutinins) in the plasma whereas a person with antigen B (blood group B) has the anti-A antibodies. A person with both antigens A and B (blood group AB) has no antibodies in the plasma, whilst a person with neither A nor B antigens (blood group O) has both anti-A and anti-B antibodies in the plasma (Table 11.1).

Table 11.1 Antigens and antibodies present in ABO blood groups		
ABO BLOOD GROUP	**ANTIGEN ON RED BLOOD CELL MEMBRANE**	**ANTIBODIES PRESENT IN THE PLASMA**
A	A	Anti-B
B	B	Anti-A
AB	A and B	None
O	None	Anti-A and anti-B

The importance of the A and B antigens is evident when one person receives blood from another. If a person receives a transfusion of ABO incompatible blood, the transfused red cells will clump together (agglutinate) and break down (haemolyse), which may be fatal. Thus, if the recipient's plasma contains anti-B antibody, they must only receive blood from a group A or O donor.

WBCs and platelets also possess ABO antigens. Therefore, if a patient is to receive a transfusion of other cellular components, the correct blood group must also be used.

The Rhesus D factor

In the UK, 85% of the population have a second important class of antigen present on their red cells: the Rhesus (Rh) D factor. Thus a person may be either RhD-positive or RhD-negative.

The antibody, anti-D, does not occur naturally in the plasma of RhD-negative blood, but stimulation to produce it can occur if a RhD-negative person receives a RhD-positive blood transfusion or if, during pregnancy or childbirth, red blood cells from a RhD-positive fetus cross the placental barrier into the circulation of a RhD-negative woman. In these circumstances later exposure to RhD-positive red blood cells will result in agglutination and haemolysis. Blood products to be transfused must therefore be carefully cross-matched for the RhD factor as well as ABO groups.

Other blood groups

In addition to the ABO and RhD factor blood groupings there are several further blood classification systems, e.g. Duffy, Kell and other Rhesus antigens. These do not usually cause agglutination unless multiple blood transfusions are required, in which cases it would be essential to check that donor blood is compatible with the recipient's blood serum antibodies.

(See Further reading, e.g. Daniels & Bromilow 2007.)

Blood transfusion

Blood transfusion, the administration of whole blood or blood products donated by one person to another, makes it possible to save lives. Transfusion does, however, expose patients to the risk of potentially fatal complications, e.g. infection, haemolytic reactions or receiving an incompatible unit of blood (Box 11.1). Box 11.2 provides an opportunity for you to consider how nurses can improve safety during transfusion.

 See website Critical thinking question 11.1

Many people who require blood transfusions fear being infected with a transmittable disease, such as HIV, hepatitis or variant Creutzfeldt–Jakob disease (vCJD). It is therefore necessary that the screening procedures undertaken on all blood donors and the testing and processing of donated blood are explained. For instance, in the UK, white cells are routinely removed from donated blood to minimise the risk of transmitting vCJD. Some religious groups such as Jehovah's Witnesses may refuse blood transfusions while some others may wish to consult family and religious leaders before giving consent. The blood transfusion products readily available are listed in Table 11.2.

 Box 11.1 Reflection

Serious hazards of transfusion of blood and blood products

The SHOT (Serious Hazards of Transfusion) Annual Report 2007 analysed 332 adverse events. These included 46 'wrong blood' events where a patient received a blood component intended for a different patient or of an incorrect group (SHOT 2007).

Activities

- Access the SHOT Annual Report 2007 and read more about the episodes where people were given a blood component of an incorrect group.
- Find out about the checks used when a sample of blood is taken for group and cross-match, and the tests and checks taken in the laboratory to ensure that blood of the correct group is supplied for the patient. Discuss these measures with your mentor.

Resource

SHOT (Serious Hazards of Transfusion) Annual Report 2007. Available online http:// www.shotuk.org.

Box 11.2 Evidence-based practice

Promoting safer blood transfusion

Results from a national audit of bedside transfusion practice revealed that patients in the UK are at risk of misidentification and poor monitoring when undergoing a blood transfusion. Parris & Grant-Casey (2007) identify the implications of the audit findings and explore initiatives to improve blood transfusion safety.

Activities

- Access the article by Parris & Grant-Casey (2007) and list the key recommendations for improving safety during blood transfusion.
- Consider your own practice area. What could be done to ensure that all staff members involved in the administration of blood products comply with these guidelines?

Before a patient receives a transfusion of a blood product their blood is grouped. The donated blood is then tested for compatibility with that of the recipient. The donor's blood should be of the same ABO blood group and a RhD-negative recipient should receive RhD-negative blood products. Details of the cross-matching are recorded along with the blood unit number on the documentation sent with the unit of blood. After the transfusion, this documentation is retained in case of a transfusion reaction. Patients may be able to donate their own red cells prior to elective surgery. This is known as an autologous transfusion and avoids the risks associated with allogeneic blood transfusions.

(See Further reading, e.g. Gray & Illingworth 2005.)

DISORDERS OF THE BLOOD

The following sections address a range of blood disorders affecting RBCs, WBCs and platelets. Although the specific responsibilities of nurses caring for patients with blood disorders will depend on their particular role and workplace setting, key elements will include:

Table 11.2 Blood transfusion products available

PRODUCT	INDICATIONS FOR USE	SPECIAL POINTS
Whole blood (infrequently given)	Acute, severe bleeding requiring replacement of red blood cells and plasma and coagulation factors	Stored at 4°C for up to 35 days Platelets and coagulation factors have much reduced viability
Fresh whole blood (infrequently given)	As above	Blood <24 h old, therefore more likely to contain viable coagulation factors
Red cell concentrate	Replacement of red blood cells only. Therefore used when haemoglobin level is low	Up to 200 mL plasma removed per 500 mL blood
Washed red cells	As for red cell concentrate Specially prepared to remove antigens	Prevents anaphylactic transfusion reactions
Frozen red cells	As for red cell concentrate	Storage lifespan lengthened, therefore useful for rare blood groups
Platelet concentrate	Patients with platelet count <20 × 10^{9}cells/L but not actively bleeding	Platelet units from blood banks contain platelets from many units of blood, therefore there are frequent reactions. Patient may require i.v. hydrocortisone plus i.v. chlorphenamine prior to transfusion. Stored at 20°C. Viability of platelet concentrate only 24 h. Never place in fridge
Other blood components		
Fresh frozen plasma	Hereditary or acquired bleeding disorder Volume replacement Liver disease Disseminated intravascular coagulation (DIC)	Frozen within 6 h of cell separation and viable for 1 year. Once thawed, use within 30 min
Cryoprecipitate (factor VIII, fibrinogen)	Haemophilia	From fresh frozen plasma Last part to thaw is cryoprecipitate
Factor VIII	Haemophilia A	From fresh frozen powder (half-life 12 h)
Factor IX	Haemophilia B (Christmas disease)	
Human immunoglobulin	Passive immunity, especially immunosuppressed patients	
Albumin solution	Hypoproteinaemic oedema, ascites, acute volume replacement	

- detecting and monitoring signs of illness and response to treatment
- assisting with medical investigations
- administering treatment and supportive therapies
- providing information and patient education
- health promotion regarding nutrition, lifestyle and the prevention of complications
- assessment and management of pain
- implementing strategies aimed at infection prevention and control
- providing emotional support and reassurance
- liaising with and making referrals to multidisciplinary health team members.

Investigations used in the diagnosis of blood disorders

A range of investigations are used for the diagnosis of blood disorders, Specific tests will depend on the nature of the suspected disorder but may include:

Blood tests

- Full blood count (FBC) – to establish the total number of red cells, white cells and platelets.
- Haemoglobin concentration – a level 10% below normal is considered indicative of anaemia.
- Packed cell volume (PCV) or haematocrit – the volume of red blood cells expressed as a percentage of the total volume of blood.
- Reticulocyte (immature RBCs) count – a small percentage are normally present in the blood, but a larger percentage may indicate increased bone marrow activity if the red cell count is low.
- Mean cell volume (MCV) – measures the average red cell volume.
- Mean cell haemoglobin (MCH) – measures the average haemoglobin concentration.
- Erythrocyte sedimentation rate (ESR) – measures the rate of fall of red cells in plasma left standing for an hour.

Box 11.3 Information

Bone marrow aspiration

Purposes

- Diagnosis – to examine cell populations and thus determine type of anaemia, leukaemia or lymphoma.
- Monitoring – to assess progress of disease and response to treatment.

Sites

Red bone marrow is found in the cavities of the flat bones of the adult, e.g. skull, clavicle, scapula and iliac crest. The site usually chosen (for ease of access to minimise trauma to nearby structures) is the iliac crest – left and right, anterior and posterior.

The nurse's role

The patient may be anxious about this investigation, especially if there is awareness that the results may show a malignant condition. This anxiety may be heightened if the patient has been talking with others who have undergone the procedure.

Providing the patient with information on all aspects of the test – the use of premedication and local anaesthetic, the site to be used, the degree of discomfort to be expected, the time that it will take, and when the results will be reported – will help to reduce anxiety.

It is the policy of some doctors, especially where repeated aspiration will be required, to give a sedative such as lorazepam or a light general anaesthetic. The individual may undergo the procedure as an outpatient, inpatient or as a day case. Whatever the setting, the nurse's role will include:

- assessing the patient's understanding of the test and providing more information if necessary
- ensuring that the patient's platelet count has been checked prior to the procedure and that the results are available
- preparing the equipment
- ensuring that the patient is comfortable and is positioned correctly
- observing the patient throughout the procedure and drawing attention to any change in condition
- assisting the doctor
- applying a pressure dressing and making the patient comfortable after the procedure
- inspecting the aspiration site frequently for signs of haemorrhage or haematoma formation
- documenting the patient's response to the procedure
- preparing the patient for discharge by explaining care of puncture site, what discomfort may be expected, who to contact if ill-effects arise, when results will be available and timing of the next appointment.

Possible complications

- Haemorrhage – the patient's platelet count should be checked before aspiration.
- Infection.

- Ferritin (an iron storage protein) – measures the amount of iron stores.
- Vitamin B_{12} and folate.

Blood film

This is the examination of blood cells under a microscope to examine cell morphology in order to detect abnormalities in their size, structure or shape.

Bone marrow aspiration and trephine biopsy

This involves the removal of a small amount of bone marrow from the posterior iliac crest or sternum. This is mounted on slides and stained for microscopic examination. This test is not done routinely but is indicated if there is evidence of severe anaemia or of another blood disorder such as aplastic anaemia or leukaemia (Box 11.3).

Other investigative techniques

These include cytogenetic studies, immunophenotyping and molecular studies which assist in the detection of chromosomal and genetic abnormalities and are important prognostic indicators for many haematological malignancies.

Disorders of red blood cells – anaemias (general aspects)

Anaemias are a complex group of blood disorders found in all age groups resulting from a reduction in the number of RBCs and/or haemoglobin concentration in the blood (Figure 11.3). Defined by the World Health Organization (WHO et al 2001) as haemoglobin level less than 13.0 g/dL in males over 15 years of age, less than 12 g/dL in non-pregnant females over 15 years and children aged 12–14 years, and less than 11 g/dL in pregnancy, anaemia may be caused by:

- decreased red cell production
- excessive destruction of red cells
- chronic or acute blood loss.

Anaemia may be the primary presenting illness or may occur secondary to another condition such as cancer, chronic renal failure or an inherited disorder of haemoglobin synthesis. Anaemia may also be acquired due to environmental, iatrogenic or nutritional factors.

Interestingly, many people are diagnosed with anaemia by chance when they seek medical advice for an unrelated symptom or during a routine medical examination.

PATHOPHYSIOLOGY

Anaemia arises when the oxygen-carrying capacity of the red blood cells is reduced. Symptoms stem from a lack of oxygen in the tissues and are primarily due to compensatory mechanisms which occur in response to hypoxia (reduced levels of oxygen in the tissues). The severity of symptoms will depend on the haemoglobin concentration of the red blood cell and the ability of the person to adapt to a lower oxygen concentration.

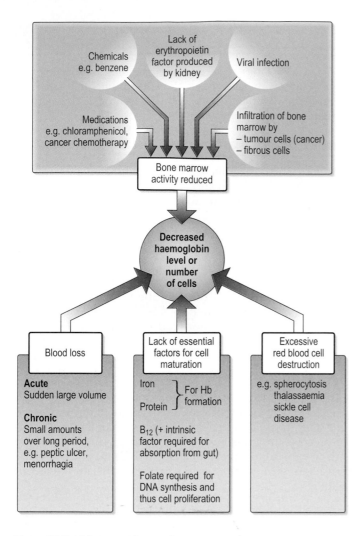

Figure 11.3 Main types of anaemia.

Clinical presentation

The clinical presentation of anaemia is diverse and each type of anaemia has specific attributes. However, features common to all types include:

- tiredness and lethargy
- pallor
- breathlessness
- palpitations
- tachycardia
- dizziness, fainting and dimness of vision
- headache and lack of concentration
- angina and/or intermittent claudication.

MEDICAL MANAGEMENT

History and examination

A diagnosis of anaemia requires a thorough patient assessment. A detailed history, looking at the patient's past and present health and lifestyle, should be undertaken. The use of medications such as aspirin or phenytoin should be identified as these may contribute to anaemia. Assessing the person's social circumstances and nutritional intake is also important.

Physical examination may reveal:

- pallor of the skin and mucous membranes
- signs of complications of anaemia such as jaundice, dyspnoea and cardiac failure
- bleeding
- changes to hair and skin texture or pigmentation
- signs of underlying disease or conditions such as cancer or pregnancy.

Investigations

Blood samples will be taken for FBC, haemoglobin level, MCV, MCH, ESR, PCV, serum iron and blood film. Bone marrow aspiration is not undertaken routinely but is indicated if the anaemia is severe.

Treatment

Treatment will depend on the cause, type and severity of anaemia. Some patients may need to be hospitalised but most can be treated in the community with medication, lifestyle changes and health education. The underlying cause of the anaemia must also be treated. Blood transfusions may be needed either initially or repeatedly over a period of time. Follow-up care for all anaemic patients is important to encourage and monitor compliance with medication and to prevent recurrence and long-term adverse effects.

 ## Nursing management and health promotion: anaemia

Patients may experience some general problems common to most anaemias in addition to those specific to their type of anaemia. This section outlines the nursing management of general problems. The specific problems and nursing management are discussed in subsequent sections. It is vital that the patient is treated as an individual and that care is holistic. A nursing assessment of the patient's background, lifestyle, illness, needs and goals should be undertaken, after which a care plan will be agreed.

General problems associated with anaemia

Tiredness

Patients may tire easily because of hypoxia. It is important that their daily routine in hospital or at home includes periods of rest. If cardiac failure is evident, the patient may need to be nursed in bed or in a chair. The nurse should be aware of the potential problems of immobility, paying particular attention to pressure areas and the prevention of venous thromboembolism (VTE). Assistance with personal hygiene and dressing may also be needed. Patients should be reassured that their tiredness is not imaginary but is part of the anaemia and that it will lessen as treatment progresses.

Breathlessness

Breathlessness may be mild, occurring only on exertion, or it may be a major problem causing considerable distress and debility. Nursing priorities will focus on ensuring maximum perfusion of oxygen to the tissues and reducing the patient's distress. These can be achieved by nursing the patient in an upright position, administering oxygen as prescribed, explaining to the patient the reason for the breathlessness and giving reassurance that it will lessen as the anaemia improves.

Nutrition

The anaemic patient will require a high-protein diet which includes all the nutrients necessary for red cell production (p. 368). Breathlessness, a lack of energy to shop and prepare food, a sore mouth and dysphagia may all contribute to anorexia. A sore mouth can be especially distressing and the nurse will need to carry out an oral assessment using an appropriate assessment tool. Care should include not only that which will improve and heal the mouth but also relevant health education about oral hygiene including teeth cleaning and/or care of dentures, mouth washes and lip care.

Patients who have a low income and/or a poor understanding of nutrition may need referral to a dietitian or specialist nutritional nurse for specific guidance about nutrition and diet. A social worker referral may also be needed for advice about budgeting and social security benefits.

Safety

Faintness, light-headedness and sensitivity to cold make the anaemic patient prone to injury. As the body responds to poor oxygenation by preserving the blood supply to the essential organs, anaemic patients will have poor peripheral circulation and, consequently, fragile skin. The reduced attention span typical of anaemic patients will also make them vulnerable to falls, minor injuries and hypothermia. Anaemic patients should be warned against changing position suddenly, especially from lying to standing, and should be given instruction on first aid for minor injuries and on the prevention of hypothermia (see Ch. 22).

Skin integrity

The anaemic patient's reduced oxygen and nutrient supply to the skin increases the risk of pressure ulcers. Hypoxic skin will not necessarily break down quickly, but if damaged it will take longer than usual to heal. An initial and continuing assessment of all pressure areas should be made using appropriate risk assessment tools (see Ch. 23).

Once the patient's level of risk of developing pressure ulcers has been determined, appropriate interventions should be instigated. These will include ensuring that the patient's position is changed 2 hourly, the use of appropriate pressure-relieving devices and instructing the patient about the importance of regular re-positioning (European Pressure Ulcer Advisory Panel [EPUAP] 2008).

Anxiety and communication

Prior to diagnosis, the anaemic patient may fear the presence of a life-threatening illness, particularly if frightening symptoms such as breathlessness, palpitations and chronic headaches have been experienced. The disorientation and confusion arising from cerebral hypoxia can be distressing. Explanation of the causes of these symptoms and reassurance that they should improve as the anaemia responds to treatment may help to reduce the anxiety suffered by both the patient and the family.

Specific anaemias

The section outlines some specific anaemias: iron deficiency, megaloblastic, aplastic, haemolytic including the inherited haemoglobinopathies (sickle cell disease and thalassaemia), and anaemia caused by blood loss.

Iron deficiency anaemia

Iron deficiency anaemia affects an estimated 600 million people (Craig et al 2006) and is recognised as one of the most common types of anaemia worldwide.

PATHOPHYSIOLOGY

Iron is a constituent of haemoglobin and is essential for cellular function and erythropoiesis. Iron deficiency anaemia arises when absorption of iron from food does not meet the daily requirements. This may be due to chronic blood loss (discussed more fully on pp. 375–376) or malabsorption, although the most common cause is inadequate dietary intake (Mehta & Hoffbrand 2009).

Clinical presentation

As the onset of iron deficiency anaemia is usually very gradual, the patient may not seek medical attention until some time after symptoms appear. The most common presenting features are tiredness and pallor, although any of the other general symptoms of anaemia (see p. 373) may be apparent. Signs and symptoms specific to iron deficiency anaemia include:

- glossitis – a smooth, sore tongue
- hair thinning
- angular cheilosis – maceration at the angles of the mouth
- koilonychia – spoon-shaped (concave) and brittle nails
- pica – a strong desire to eat unusual substances such as ice or coal.

MEDICAL MANAGEMENT

History and examination

The patient may give a history suggestive of inadequate iron intake or chronic blood loss, e.g. menorrhagia or bleeding from the gastrointestinal tract. Examination may reveal general signs of anaemia.

Investigations

Blood samples will be taken for tests, such as FBC, haemoglobin level, MCV, MCH, ESR, blood film, serum iron and total iron-binding capacity (TIBC). Estimates of ferritin (an iron storage protein) measure iron stores and a subnormal level is caused by iron deficiency (Craig et al 2006). Other investigations such as faecal occult blood testing (FOB), endoscopy or barium studies may be undertaken to establish the cause of the deficiency.

Treatment

If dietary changes are insufficient to correct the anaemia, oral iron (ferrous salts) supplements, usually ferrous sulphate, will be prescribed. Medication should be continued for 3–6 months after the haemoglobin level has returned to normal to replenish iron stores. Side-effects, which include constipation, nausea, abdominal pain and diarrhoea, often lead to poor compliance with medication and these should be explained to the patient. Intramuscular iron injections are usually given only where there is proven malabsorption syndrome or poor compliance. If the anaemia is very severe (less than 7 g/dL) blood transfusions may be required.

 ## Nursing management and health promotion: iron deficiency anaemia

Many of the nursing considerations for the general care of anaemic patients (see pp. 373–374) are relevant for iron deficiency anaemia. Other nursing management strategies will focus on patient education and discharge planning with an emphasis on health promotion.

Patient education and health promotion

Helping the patient to understand the disorder will assist in promoting compliance with treatment. Information about foods that are rich in available iron should be given and advice on selecting and budgeting for a well-balanced diet may also be needed (Box 11.4). Assessing the patient's perception of the problem, level of knowledge and sociocultural background can help to ensure that the advice offered is relevant and comprehensible. Referral to a social worker may also be appropriate.

Clear instructions should be given to reinforce the prescriber's directions regarding medication. Patients should also be made aware that ferrous salts of iron cause blackened stools and discolouration of the urine.

If inpatient treatment has been required the following should be discussed with the patient and family/carers before discharge:

- conditions at home and the availability of support services if family or friends are unable to help
- the importance of follow-up appointments with health professionals
- the importance of taking prescribed medication.

In older people, there is often a link between recent bereavement and the onset of iron deficiency anaemia, as loneliness, grief and depression may lead to self-neglect. Such patients should have the necessary follow-up and support by the health visitor, social worker or bereavement support counsellor.

Anaemia resulting from chronic blood loss

Iron deficiency anaemia may result from blood loss. This may either be:

- acute – the loss of a large volume of blood over a short period of time, as in haemorrhage (Chs 18, 27), or
- chronic – the loss of small amounts of blood over an extended period of time.

Chronic blood loss, which will be addressed in this section, is not uncommon and may present secondary to a number of other disorders. Frequently, it is only when a diagnosis of iron deficiency anaemia has been established that the underlying cause is suspected. The most common causes of chronic blood loss are listed in Box 11.5.

 Box 11.4 Reflection

Nutrition and the prevention of iron-deficiency anaemia

Tom is 45 years old and has been diagnosed with iron deficiency anaemia. He tells you that he works as a long-distance lorry driver and is often away from home for long periods of time. Subsequently he does not eat regular meals and most of his diet comprises chips, sweets and take-away meals.

You have been asked to provide Tom with advice about his diet and improving his intake of iron-rich foods.

Activity

- Access the *Iron deficiency* page on the Food Standards Agency website (see below) and consider the following issues:
  - foods rich in iron
  - absorption of iron
  - the role of vitamin C in iron absorption
  - foods and beverages that inhibit iron absorption
  - suggestions for meals and snacks.
- Consider the advice that you would give to Tom about his diet. Plan some iron-rich meals and snacks that fit into Tom's work pattern.

Resource

Food Standards Agency *Iron deficiency*. Available online (June 2009): http://www.eatwell.gov.uk/healthissues/irondeficiency/?lang=en.

 Box 11.5 Information

Common causes of chronic blood loss

Gastrointestinal blood loss is the commonest cause in men and postmenopausal women (Craig et al 2006).

Gastrointestinal bleeding (see Ch. 4)

- Gastritis – excessive alcohol intake, drugs such as NSAIDs and aspirin.
- Peptic ulceration – infection with the bacterium *Helicobacter pylori*, corticosteroid therapy.
- Oesophageal varices (blood loss may be acute).
- Inflammatory bowel disease.
- Diverticulitis.
- Gastric or colorectal cancer.
- Intestinal parasites such as hookworm infestations are important causes worldwide.

Genitourinary bleeding (see Chs 7, 8)

- Menorrhagia (heavy regular menstrual flow) – a common cause.
- Haematuria – bladder cancer.

Respiratory bleeding (see Ch. 3)

- Chronic haemoptysis – lung cancer, tuberculosis, bronchiectasis, pulmonary infarction.

PATHOPHYSIOLOGY

It is unlikely that ill-effects of chronic blood loss will be noticed until it has caused depletion of the body's iron stores. The pathophysiology is similar to that of iron deficiency anaemia caused by poor dietary intake of iron (see p. 374).

Clinical presentation

In addition to those of iron deficiency anaemia, clinical features of anaemia occurring as a result of blood loss occur in accordance with the underlying disorder. Examples include indigestion, abdominal pain, menorrhagia, weight loss, blood in stools or haematuria.

MEDICAL MANAGEMENT

History and examination

These are similar to those used for the diagnosis of iron deficiency anaemia (see p. 374).

Investigations

These are as for the diagnosis of iron deficiency anaemia (see p. 374).

Treatment

Treatment will depend on the specific cause of the blood loss; however, treatment options include oral iron preparations to replenish iron stores and possibly blood transfusion.

Nursing management and health promotion: anaemia due to chronic blood loss

The patient may be feeling apprehensive and frightened, and providing clear information about investigations, especially invasive procedures such as endoscopy (see Ch. 4), may help to alleviate anxiety. Information should address any pre-investigative preparation such as fasting, approximate durations of tests and what they will involve. It is also important to discuss whether the patient will be fit to return home unaccompanied after investigative procedures and when the results can be expected.

When planning care, the nurse must prioritise the patient's needs and be sensitive to their individual values and perceptions. Comprehensive assessment will help to establish the cause of bleeding and this will incorporate sensitive questioning, observation, monitoring of vital signs and discussion with the patient's family and friends as appropriate.

Megaloblastic anaemias

Megaloblastic anaemias are characterised by large, immature and dysfunctional RBCs (megaloblasts) in the bone marrow.

PATHOPHYSIOLOGY

Megaloblastic anaemias are due to defective DNA synthesis, commonly caused by a deficiency of either:

- vitamin B_{12} (cobalamins), or
- folates (group of B vitamins).

Although in these conditions the haemoglobin content of the cells is typically normal, the defective cells have a considerably reduced lifespan, which decreases their numbers in the bloodstream resulting in anaemia.

Vitamin B_{12} deficiency

As vitamin B_{12} is found predominantly in meat, eggs and dairy products, vegans are at particular risk; however, the most common cause of vitamin B_{12} deficiency is malabsorption due to pernicious anaemia. This condition, caused by autoimmune gastritis, affects 1 in 100 people of all races over the age of 60 (Hoffbrand & Provan 2007). It occurs when the gastric mucosa atrophies, resulting in a failure to produce intrinsic factor required for vitamin B_{12} absorption. Table 11.3 outlines other causes.

Folate deficiency

Folates are found in green leafy vegetables, potatoes, fruits, fortified breakfast cereals and bread, liver, milk and dairy products, and yeast extract. Deficiency is commonly due to an inadequate dietary intake of folic acid. (See Table 11.3 for other causes.) This may occur either alone or in conjunction with a condition such as pregnancy, in which folate utilisation is increased. Fetal abnormalities, e.g. neural tube

Table 11.3 Causes of the megaloblastic anaemias	
TYPE	**CAUSES**
Folate deficiency	Inadequate dietary intake Malabsorption: • disease of small bowel, e.g. coeliac disease, extensive surgical resection of small bowel • alcohol misuse Increased demands: • very active cell proliferation, e.g. in haemolytic anaemia or leukaemia • pregnancy Excessive loss: • heart failure • long-term dialysis Drugs: • the cytotoxic drug methotrexate • antiepileptic medications, e.g. phenytoin • oral contraceptive
Vitamin B_{12} deficiency	Inadequate vitamin B_{12} in diet (especially vegans) Malabsorption: • reduced gastric acid (hypochlorhydria) • gastric surgery • pernicious anaemia caused by autoimmune gastritis that leads to gastric atrophy and intrinsic factor deficiency • pancreatic insufficiency • inflammatory disease of terminal ileum where vitamin B_{12} is absorbed, e.g. Crohn's disease • small bowel resection involving the ileum

defects (NTDs), are associated with inadequate folate intake around the time of conception and during the first few weeks of pregnancy.

Clinical presentation

As vitamin B_{12} and folic acid are essential for all dividing cells, a deficiency of these not only affects RBCs but also the gastrointestinal epithelium, leading to glossitis, anorexia, diarrhoea and malabsorption. In addition to these and other general signs of anaemia, megaloblastic anaemia may cause mild jaundice and skin pigmentation.

Pernicious anaemia develops gradually so the condition may be very advanced when treatment is sought. Because vitamin B_{12} is important for myelin production, up to 40% of people with this deficiency may develop spinal cord damage or peripheral nerve problems causing:

- paraesthesia
- coldness or numbness in limbs
- ataxia
- atrophy of optic nerve
- dementia.

MEDICAL MANAGEMENT

History and examination

History and examination is similar to that for anaemia (see p. 373). However, if megaloblastic anaemia is suspected the doctor will be alert to a history of gastrointestinal surgery, alcohol misuse or epilepsy and to the following specific features identified above.

Investigations

Blood tests will be similar to those for the diagnosis of iron deficiency anaemia (see p. 374) Additional specific diagnostic blood tests for megaloblastic anaemia include serum B_{12} levels and folate assays. Other investigations may include:

- gastric parietal cell antibodies
- Schilling test (to determine cobalamin absorption)
- endoscopy
- bone marrow aspiration (see Box 11.3)
- neurological examination (see Ch. 9).

Treatment

Vitamin B_{12} deficiency is usually treated with injections of hydroxycobalamin until blood count improves. Maintenance doses of hydroxycobalamin are usually required every 3 months for life.

Folate deficiency is conventionally treated with oral folic acid, for several weeks. This is usually continued as a weekly maintenance dose if the underlying cause cannot be rectified.

Nursing management and health promotion: megaloblastic anaemias

Patients with vitamin B_{12} and intrinsic factor deficiency may need to be admitted to hospital for diagnosis and treatment in the initial stages, but most will be diagnosed by their GP. If the anaemia is not yet advanced, treatment can be started immediately by a community or practice nurse, who will administer prescribed vitamin B_{12} injections. Assistance with personal care and other activities of daily living may be needed if the patient is experiencing breathlessness or fatigue.

The patient and family should be encouraged to participate in their management, possibly by learning how to administer the hydroxycobalamin injections themselves.

Advanced stages of pernicious anaemia are rarely seen today; however, if cardiac failure and severe neurological problems develop, specific nursing and medical interventions will be required (see Chs 2, 9).

Health promotion and education regarding a healthy diet and compliance with medication is a nursing priority when managing patients with folate deficiency anaemia. Patients will need to know which foods contain folic acid, how to shop and budget for these and how to avoid destroying folic acid during food preparation and cooking (see Useful websites, e.g. British Nutrition Foundation). An understanding of how to take folic acid supplements correctly is also essential. The importance of follow-up checks should also be emphasised.

Aplastic anaemia

Aplastic anaemia is a rare and life-threatening condition. It manifests when haematopoietic stem cells in the bone marrow fail to mature and proliferate and are replaced by fat cells. This results in pancytopenia – lack of RBCs (anaemia), WBCs (leucopenia) and platelets (thrombocytopenia).

PATHOPHYSIOLOGY

Aplastic anaemia may be due to an inherited condition such as the rare Fanconi anaemia. However, it may also be acquired, and in 20–50% of all cases onset is thought to be associated with exposure to one of the following:

- chemicals, especially benzene, coal tar derivatives and petroleum products
- drugs, including chloramphenicol, certain cytotoxic chemotherapeutic agents, phenothiazines and anticonvulsants
- ionising radiation (see Ch. 31)
- viral infection, notably hepatitis viruses and Epstein–Barr virus (EBV).

The remaining 50–80% of cases have no detectable cause. In North America and Europe acquired aplastic anaemia affects 2 per million population per year (Montané et al 2008). There is a 2–3 times higher incidence in East Asia (British Committee for Standards in Haematology [BCSH] 2009).

Clinical presentation

The onset of aplastic anaemia is usually insidious and months may elapse between exposure to the causal agent and the development of symptoms. It can occur at any age and the presenting symptoms will vary relative to the extent of the pancytopenia. These may include:

- general symptoms of anaemia
- infections
- bleeding – especially from the nose, gums or gastrointestinal tract.

MEDICAL MANAGEMENT

History and examination

Initial examination may detect no abnormality other than the presenting symptoms. However, further assessment may reveal exposure to chemicals or the use of over-the-counter medication and a thorough drug history is essential.

Investigations

Investigations undertaken to provide a definitive diagnosis include among others:

- full blood count including a reticulocyte count
- blood film
- bone marrow aspiration and trephine biopsy.

Treatment

Immediate admission to hospital may be required once a diagnosis of aplastic anaemia is made, particularly if the condition is advanced. Supportive therapy with blood and platelet transfusion will be given based on clinical need. Broad spectrum antibiotic therapy and antifungal drugs may be needed to treat any infections. Other medications that may be prescribed include antithymocyte globulin, ciclosporin and haematopoietic growth factors (BCSH 2009).

Allogeneic haematopoietic stem cell transplantation (HSCT) has become the treatment of choice for younger patients with severe or very severe aplastic anaemia when an appropriate donor is available (Grundy 2006). Immunosuppressive therapy is recommended for patients with non-severe aplastic anaemia who are transfusion dependent, patients with severe or very severe disease who are over 40 years old and for younger patients with severe or very severe disease who do not have an appropriate donor (BCSH 2009). (See also Box 11.10, p. 383, and Table 11.4, p. 384, in the section covering leukaemia.)

 Nursing management and health promotion: aplastic anaemia

Nursing management of patients with aplastic anaemia requires expert skills and knowledge to prevent the development of serious life-threatening complications. Nursing care will include the:

- prevention and early detection of infections (Chs 16, 31)
- initiation of immediate treatment for septic patients
- prevention and early treatment of haemorrhage.

The nurse will play an important role in the coordination of the numerous tests necessary for diagnosis and will be instrumental in the care of the patient if HSCT is undertaken. Further details regarding transplantation and the care of profoundly pancytopenic patients are included in the subsequent section on leukaemia.

Communication and psychological support

Supporting the patient and their family psychologically is an important aspect of care and sensitivity is required as the patient comes to terms with their diagnosis, prognosis and effects of treatment.

Education

Patients and their family need information about how to prevent fatigue, infection and haemorrhage and to identify signs of these should they occur. The nurse should also assess the patient's understanding of the need for medication, what action to take if medication is inadvertently missed and how to obtain new supplies. The patient should also be advised to inform any doctor or dentist about prescribed corticosteroids and always to carry information with details of their medication.

Rehabilitation and health promotion

Patient rehabilitation will involve the multidisciplinary team and must be planned before discharge in response to the patient's specific needs and potential for recovery. Realistic goals should be set in partnership with the patient as it may be necessary to make lifestyle or career changes. Before discharge it is important to discuss with the patient, family and carers any fears or apprehensions and to clarify details of who to contact if there are any further episodes of illness. Information about support outside the hospital including support groups should also be provided.

Haemolytic anaemias

Haemolytic anaemias are rare and result from the premature destruction of RBCs in response to an inherited or an acquired defect. The most common inherited anaemias are the haemoglobinopathies – sickle cell disease and thalassaemia. These are outlined in this section. The most common acquired forms result from direct cell injury following infection or medical treatment (Box 11.6).

 Box 11.6 Information

Causes of haemolytic anaemia

Inherited

- RBC membrane fragility
  - spherocytosis (RBCs round in shape)
  - elliptocytosis (RBCs elliptical in shape)
- Haemoglobinopathies (haemoglobin defects: structure or synthesis)
  - sickle cell disease
  - thalassaemia
- RBC enzyme defects
  - glucose-6-phosphate dehydrogenase (G6PD) deficiency
  - pyruvate kinase deficiency

Acquired

- Antibody attack, e.g. mismatched blood transfusion
- Autoimmune haemolytic anaemia (warm or cold antibodies)
- Non-immune haemolytic anaemia
  - traumatic (disruption of RBCs), e.g. prosthetic heart valve, burns injury, intense exercise
  - chemical or drug induced, e.g. sodium chlorate, dapsone, sulfasalazine, nitrites
  - infection, e.g. malaria (*Plasmodium falciparum*), etc.

PATHOPHYSIOLOGY

Haemolytic anaemia is characterised by a reduced lifespan of the RBCs, due to fragility and excessive breakdown (haemolysis). This results in a reduced oxygen-carrying capacity and tissue hypoxia. The production of erythropoietin, a growth factor which stimulates erythropoiesis, is increased; however, if the RBC lifespan is greatly reduced (<15 days) the bone marrow will not be able to compensate adequately and the person will experience symptoms of anaemia. Because the products of RBC breakdown are retained in the body, signs of increased bilirubin and urobilinogen may be evident.

Thalassaemia

The thalassaemias are a group of inherited autosomal recessive disorders that cause an impaired rate of synthesis of one of the two globin chains (alpha α or beta β) of adult haemoglobin (Huether & McCance 2008). The resultant imbalance leads to ineffective erythropoiesis and a reduced RBC lifespan. Thalassaemias are among the most common genetic disorders in the world. Cases occur sporadically in the general population; however, they are more common in people who originate from around the Mediterranean, the Middle East, South and East Asia. In the UK the condition occurs most often among people of Cypriot, Italian, Greek, Indian, Pakistani, Bangladeshi and Chinese descent. This is because the mutations that cause thalassaemia originally occurred in countries in which *falciparum* malaria was common (Hoffbrand et al 2006).

PATHOPHYSIOLOGY

A haemoglobin molecule comprises four ferrous iron-containing haem groups and four matching globin (protein) chains. To function effectively haemoglobin requires two α globin chains and two β globin chains. There are two forms of thalassaemia – α thalassaemia and β thalassaemia. Both types have major or minor subtypes, depending on how many genes are defective and whether the defects are inherited homozygously (thalassaemia major) or heterozygously (thalassaemia minor).

Clinical presentation

There are a number of clinical syndromes associated with thalassaemia and clinical presentation will depend on mode of inheritance. β thalassaemias occur more frequently than α thalassaemias.

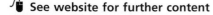 **See website for further content**

MEDICAL MANAGEMENT

Treatment

Blood transfusion is the mainstay treatment for thalassaemia and a patient typically requires 3 units of blood every 3–4 weeks. This carries an increased risk of transfusion-related reactions due to the development of antibodies against donor blood. Excessive accumulation of iron can also be problematic, particularly if it affects the heart, liver and endocrine organs. This risk can be minimised by the regular administration of an iron chelating drug, e.g. desferrioxamine, which is usually administered overnight via subcutaneous infusion (Hoffbrand et al 2006).

 Nursing management and health promotion: thalassaemia

Thalassaemia and its treatment can have a disruptive impact on the individual's life and requires expert, supportive nursing care. In many areas this will be provided by specialist nurses and will involve:

- the safe administration of blood and vigilant monitoring for transfusion reactions in accordance with national and local policy
- sensitivity to the patient's fears or concerns regarding the transmission of infections during blood transfusions
- educating the patient and their family/carers how to administer drugs safely and the provision of support to encourage compliance
- referral to relevant support groups (see Useful websites)
- health promotion and advice regarding nutrition, lifestyle and compliance with medication and treatments.

Sickle cell disorders

Sickle cell disorders (SCDs) comprise a group of disorders caused by an inherited structural abnormality in the haemoglobin molecule. The abnormal haemoglobin (HbS) causes a characteristic sickle shape of the red blood cell when it is deoxygenated (Figure 11.4).

It is inherited as a recessive, autosomal disorder of which there are two types. In the heterozygous variant, the person inherits the abnormal haemoglobin gene (HbS) from one parent and the normal (HbA) gene from the other parent. This person has sickle cell trait (HbSA) and usually is unaware of the abnormality unless tested for the trait or if they develop symptoms when exposed to hypoxic conditions, such as during an anaesthetic. In the homozygous type, the abnormal gene is inherited from both parents and the person will have sickle cell anaemia.

A crucial factor in diagnosing this haemoglobinopathy is knowledge of the family's genetic history. Sickle cell disorder occurs more commonly among people of African, Caribbean, Eastern Mediterranean, Middle Eastern, Indian and

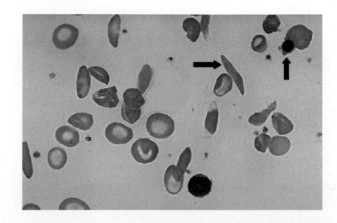

Figure 11.4 Blood film showing a sickle cell. (Reproduced from Craig et al 2006 with permission.)

Pakistani origin. In the UK, it affects 1 in 2400 live births and there are currently estimated to be 12 500 people living with sickle cell disease in England, making it the most common genetic disorder (Sickle Cell Society 2008).

PATHOPHYSIOLOGY

The amino acid sequence in the beta globin chains of haemoglobin is altered in HbS by a substitution of one amino acid for another. HbS has certain properties which distinguish it from normal HbA haemoglobin. When it becomes deoxygenated, crystals are formed within the RBC making it more rigid and distorting it into a sickle shape (Hoffbrand et al 2006). Affected RBCs are destroyed prematurely and have a lifespan of between 5 and 30 days (normally 120 days).

Clinical presentation

Sickle cell disease normally presents in childhood. It is characterised by chronic haemolytic anaemia in which mild jaundice and splenomegaly may be evident and intermittent painful crises in response to a triggering factor (Box 11.7). People with sickle cell anaemia have an increased risk of infection, tissue necrosis and renal insufficiency.

During a sickle cell crisis large numbers of RBCs become sickle-shaped, causing subsequent blood vessel occlusion and tissue ischaemia. Pain is caused by the obstruction of small blood vessels in the tissues and is typically characterised by the acuteness of its onset and unresponsiveness to mild analgesics. The location of the pain depends on the location of the obstruction.

Acute chest syndrome (ACS), a common form of acute lung injury that may lead to acute/adult respiratory distress syndrome (ARDS), is a leading cause of death in people with sickle cell disease (Box 11.8). Central to its effective management is an awareness of its clinical presentation, anticipation of its development and prompt intervention. Nurses and medical teams should be educated to recognise and manage acute chest syndrome, and patients and their carers should be taught about it and to seek urgent medical attention should symptoms arise (Sickle Cell Society 2008).

Box 11.7 Information

Trigger factors in sickle cell anaemia

- Reduced oxygen, e.g. during strenuous exercise
- Anaesthesia
- Dehydration
- Infection
- Fever
- Pregnancy
- Sudden change in temperature
- Alcohol – possibly because of dehydration
- Emotional stress
- Extreme fatigue

Box 11.8 Information

Acute chest syndrome (ACS) in sickle cell disease

The characteristic presentation includes:

- tachypnoea
- chest pain
- cough
- dyspnoea
- fever
- hypoxia.

Early recognition is vital and all patients admitted to hospital should be assessed for these signs and symptoms and a chest X-ray performed if chest pain, respiratory symptoms or reduced oxygen saturations are found. All patients should be monitored for the development of ACS using regular pulse oximetry and observation of pulse and respiratory rates throughout admission, especially if they are having opiate analgesia.

Protocols should be in place for the management of ACS and will include:

- analgesia
- measurement of arterial blood gases (ABGs)
- nursing observations (respiratory rate and effort, colour, temperature, pulse, blood pressure, oxygen saturations, level of reported pain, fluid balance, etc.)
- fluid management
- oxygen and respiratory support (see Chs 3, 29)
- incentive spirometry
- bronchodilator therapy for patients with evidence of wheeze, reversible airway disease or a history of asthma, antibiotics and indications for blood transfusion.

See Further reading suggestions, e.g. Sickle Cell Society 2008.

MEDICAL MANAGEMENT

Investigations

Investigations for diagnosis include FBC, blood film and reticulocyte count. The presence of HbS can be demonstrated when the RBCs are mixed with a solution of sodium metabisulphite. The screening test for sickle cell anaemia and sickle cell trait uses electrophoretic analysis to measure the rates of movement of the different haemoglobins in an electrical field.

Treatment

Currently there is no cure for sickle cell disease. Management is based on alleviation of symptoms, the prevention of complications and the promotion of a lifestyle that minimises crisis events. This includes:

- avoiding situations that may trigger a crisis (see Box 11.7)
- prompt treatment of any infections, even minor ones
- prophylactic penicillin and pneumococcal vaccination
- education on general health and nutrition and prophylactic use of folic acid 5 mg daily
- recognising complications of sickle cell disease including: bone and joint pains, leg ulcers, priapism (prolonged penile erection without sexual stimulation), gallstones, blurred vision, kidney disease in patients over 50 years of age, and peptic ulceration

- frequent follow-up in special clinics to monitor disease
- genetic counselling and vigilant antenatal care
- alerting other relevant health professionals to the condition
- obtaining support from sickle cell centres and support groups.

Patients experiencing a severe sickle cell crisis will need hospitalisation and should be managed with adequate analgesics, antibiotics, oxygen therapy, rehydration and close observation. An exchange blood transfusion may be needed if the crisis does not resolve or if there is continued hypoxia. Some patients are prescribed hydroxycarbamine in an attempt to reduce the frequency and severity of crises. Allogeneic HSCT is currently being investigated as a possible curative treatment strategy.

 ## Nursing management and health promotion: sickle cell disease

A patient or the parents of a child newly diagnosed with sickle cell disease will require comprehensive education about the disorder, addressing ways to minimise complications and necessary lifestyle changes.

All family members should be offered screening if this has not been done previously and genetic counselling should be available. Some areas with a high incidence of sickle cell disease employ specialist nurses and nurse counsellors to carry out these roles. The emphasis for care is on promoting health and minimising ill health.

Sickle cell crisis is an emergency and must be treated as such. Accordingly, nurses must act promptly to manage symptoms and initiate treatment in order to prevent complications. This will involve:

- vigilant observation and monitoring
- assessing the severity of the pain and likely need for opiates, and administering these regularly as prescribed
- commencing an intravenous infusion to rehydrate the patient to aid the reduction of blood viscosity
- administering antibiotics and other prescribed medications
- administering oxygen therapy to alleviate hypoxia.

Patients experiencing a sickle cell crisis are often frightened and require considerable emotional support. Some patients may have had several previous episodes and may know the best way that they should be treated when in a crisis and nurses should be mindful of this.

Males may be admitted with priapism due to thrombosis in the corpora cavernosa (two lateral columns of spongy erectile tissue in the penis). This requires both the administration of analgesics and intravenous hydration as well as possibly exchange blood transfusion to reduce the percentage of sickle cells. Chronic priapism can occur and the man's sexual function may be impaired.

Before discharge, patients should be made aware of the importance of recognising and avoiding situations that may trigger a sickle cell crisis and of the need to seek medical advice at the onset of further painful episodes (Box 11.9).

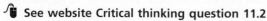 **See website Critical thinking question 11.2**

 Box 11.9 Reflection

Minimising the risk of a sickle cell crisis

Josh, a 16-year-old male with sickle cell disease, is studying for school exams which start next month. He is worried that he might experience a sickle cell crisis in the lead-up to his exams.

Activity

- Reflect on the trigger factors for sickle cell crisis (see Box 11.7). What advice can you give Josh?

See Sickle Cell Society 2008 for information about the care of patients with sickle cell disease.

Disorders of red blood cells – overproduction

Excessive RBC production is referred to as polycythaemia (or erythrocytosis). Relative polycythaemia occurs when there is an increased concentration of blood cells due to dehydration. Absolute polycythaemia occurs as a physiological response to hypoxia such as in people living at high altitudes, those with congenital heart disease or those with chronic pulmonary disease, and is referred to as secondary polycythaemia. It may also be caused by an inappropriate production of erythropoietin or similar substances in certain conditions such as cancer. The over-production of erythrocytes with no erythropoietin stimulus is called polycythaemia vera (or primary proliferative polycythaemia).

Polycythaemia vera

This is a myeloproliferative disorder (a condition characterised by the proliferation of one or more of the cellular components of the bone marrow) which originates from a neoplastic haematopoietic stem cell. This disease is distinguished by hypercellularity of the bone marrow and an overproduction of erythrocytes. Increased WBC (leucocytosis) and platelet counts (thrombocythaemia) are not uncommon and the spleen is often enlarged (splenomegaly). The condition occurs most frequently in Caucasian males aged between 55 and 80 years (Huether & McCance 2008).

PATHOPHYSIOLOGY

The raised RBC, WBC, platelet count and haemoglobin level have a number of implications. These include hyperviscosity of the blood, thrombosis and hypertension, all of which could precipitate cardiac failure or peripheral vascular disease.

Clinical presentation

Often characterised by a ruddy appearance and suffused conjunctiva, hyperviscosity of the blood can also give rise to symptoms associated with a sluggish circulation and arterial and venous thrombosis. The patient may therefore present with symptoms of:

- cerebral vascular disease, e.g. headaches, dizziness, blackouts, visual disturbances

- peripheral vascular disease, e.g. intermittent claudication
- hypertension, e.g. headaches, epistaxis, dyspnoea
- angina and cardiac failure.

Gout may also arise due to the increased cell turnover and raised uric acid levels. Excess histamine production released from basophils can cause gastric ulceration and pruritus, especially on exposure to temperature extremes.

MEDICAL MANAGEMENT

History and examination

The patient may be found to have hypertension during a routine check-up. A ruddy complexion may be evident and the palms of the hands and the oral mucosal membrane may be deep red. Splenomegaly may also be detected.

Investigations

These will include FBC, haemoglobin level, PCV and blood viscosity. Estimation of the red blood cell mass will be made. Bone marrow aspiration will also be performed.

Treatment

Venesection is the simplest form of treatment and involves the drainage of 300–500 mL of whole blood, usually via a needle in the arm. This procedure is normally carried out in the outpatient setting and will typically be repeated regularly until the PCV drops sufficiently and there is an alleviation of symptoms. Thereafter, less frequent but regular venesection will maintain this level.

Once the diagnosis is established, the underlying myeloproliferation can be controlled with treatments such as interferon, hydroxycarbamine or alkylating agents such as chlorambucil to suppress bone marrow function (Craig et al 2006). Aspirin may be prescribed to reduce platelet activity and prevent clot formation.

All patients will require frequent monitoring to minimise the effects of the disorder.

 Nursing management and health promotion: polycythaemia vera

Psychological support may be needed as the patient and their family come to terms with the diagnosis of chronic disorder that may impact on lifestyle and longevity. Clear information regarding investigations, treatment and monitoring should be provided to the patient and their family. It is important to teach the patient how to monitor for signs and symptoms of thrombosis, such as pain or swelling. If medication has been prescribed detailed instructions about taking this should be provided. The necessity of continued monitoring, via blood tests and outpatient appointments, should also be emphasised.

While undergoing venesection, the patient must be monitored closely for signs and symptoms of shock (see Ch. 18). If prescribed radioactive phosphorus, the patient must be given clear instructions regarding limitations of activities or contact with people, in view of radioactivity. If admission to hospital is required, the need for isolation to protect other patients, visitors and staff must be tactfully explained to the patient.

Disorders of white blood cells and lymphoid tissue

Disorders of the WBCs and lymphoid tissue are highly diverse and specific nursing management will vary as discussed in subsequent sections. However, nurses have an essential role throughout the disease trajectory and are central to providing the continuity and coordination essential for efficient patient care. The prevention and management of specific disease- and treatment-related complications is also of utmost importance.

This section of the chapter provides an outline of:

- leukaemia
- lymphoma
- multiple myeloma
- myelodysplastic syndrome.

Leukaemia

The leukaemias are a group of blood disorders in which there is an abnormal and excessive proliferation of malignant WBCs. Leukaemia is typically divided into acute and chronic types. These are then further subdivided into myeloid or lymphoid classifications depending on the type of WBC affected. Leukaemia is uncommon, representing less than 3% of cancers in the UK (Cancer Research UK 2009a) but it occurs in all ages, in both sexes and in all races.

Aetiology

The aetiology of leukaemia is not fully understood but, like other cancers, appears to be a multistep process involving accumulated genetic mutations which disrupt normal cellular functions controlling proliferation and differentiation (Howard & Hamilton 2008). Exposure to factors such as ionising radiation, viruses, petroleum-based chemicals and some cytotoxic medications has been associated with increased incidence. Congenital factors or genetic disorders such as Down's syndrome are also implicated in the development of leukaemia.

Acute leukaemia

Acute leukaemia is subdivided into acute myeloid (myelogenous) leukaemia (AML), originating in the myeloid stem cell, and acute lymphoblastic leukaemia (ALL), arising from the lymphoid stem cell. In adults, AML is more common than ALL with an annual UK incidence of 10 per 100 000 population (Leukaemia and Lymphoma Research 2009a), while in children ALL accounts for most cases (Howard & Hamilton 2008). The internationally recognised WHO classification system categorises acute leukaemia into subgroups according to morphological, cytogenetic and molecular characteristics, which have gained recognition as significant prognostic factors (Craig et al 2006).

PATHOPHYSIOLOGY

Acute leukaemia is characterised by uncontrolled malignant proliferation occurring at the blast level of cell maturity and is defined as the presence of over 20% of blast (immature) cells in the blood or bone marrow (Hoffbrand et al 2006).

It is thought to arise from a genetic alteration in a stem cell which proliferates to produce a clone of identical cells. As these abnormal cells proliferate, they gradually crowd out the bone marrow, affecting the production of normal blood cells. This leads to anaemia, thrombocytopenia and neutropenia (reduction in the number of neutrophils).

Clinical features

There is little uniformity in the presentation of acute leukaemia; however, clinical features, which derive from the effects of the disease on the bone marrow, include:

* acute infection, associated with fever
* bleeding of the gums, epistaxis or bruising
* anaemia – pallor, breathlessness and lethargy.

Other signs and symptoms may occur if leukaemic cells infiltrate tissues and organs leading to:

* bone pain
* hepatosplenomegaly (enlargement of liver and spleen) causing abdominal pain
* hypertrophy or swelling of the gums
* skin lesions.

MEDICAL MANAGEMENT

History and examination During a detailed medical history the patient may describe either:

* an acute onset of symptoms occurring over the previous 72 hours with pallor, pyrexia and tachycardia and exhibiting other signs and symptoms of acute infection, or
* a 2–3 month history of minor recurrent infections.

Physical examination may reveal pallor, lymphadenopathy (enlargement of the lymph nodes), splenomegaly, gum bleeding, petechiae, purpura and bruising.

Investigations Typically, a diagnosis of leukaemia will be established through a series of investigations including blood count, biochemistry and microscopic examination of a blood film.

This diagnosis will be confirmed by examination of a bone marrow aspirate and biopsy (see Box 11.3, p. 372).

🖱 **See website Critical thinking question 11.3**

Further laboratory testing of the marrow using cytochemistry, immunophenotyping, cytogenetic analysis and molecular studies will lead to a precise diagnosis of a particular subtype of acute leukaemia.

Further aspirations of bone marrow are taken and examined during and after treatment to assess the response of the disease and help to indicate the prognosis.

If the patient has ALL, further diagnostic investigations will be carried out. These include:

* lumbar puncture, as there is a high risk of central nervous system involvement, especially in the cerebrospinal fluid
* examination of the testes, as this is a region to which leukaemia may spread.

Treatment Acute leukaemia is a life-threatening condition and such a diagnosis requires urgent treatment. The aim is elimination of the disease and involves hospitalisation, intensive chemotherapy and, in some cases, HSCT (Box 11.10, Table 11.4). Research into the use of novel therapies, such as monoclonal antibodies, is currently ongoing.

Cytotoxic chemotherapy is the mainstay treatment in the management of acute leukaemia. Chemotherapeutic agents act on the cell cycle disrupting cell growth and replication. As many chemotherapy agents are non-selective, normal cells undergoing cell division are also damaged, giving rise to potentially life-threatening complications. These include infection and haemorrhage caused by bone marrow suppression and side-effects such as nausea and vomiting, mucositis, alopecia and infertility (see pp. 384–386 and Ch. 31).

Box 11.10 Information

Haematopoietic stem cell transplant

In some cases, HSCT may be considered the sole chance of a cure for a number of haematological conditions including acute leukaemia. It involves the transplantation of healthy haematopoietic progenitor cells to re-establish healthy bone marrow function in someone whose bone marrow has been destroyed or depleted as a result of a disease or its treatment. Prior to receiving the stem cells, a preparatory regimen, known as conditioning, is administered. This typically consists of high-dose chemotherapy and/or total body irradiation. Consequently, myeloid and lymphoid blood cells are destroyed leaving the patient extremely vulnerable to infection. Administered in a similar way to blood transfusion, the stem cells are then given with the goal of repopulating the patient's marrow to restore normal haemopoietic function.

The type of transplant is defined according to the donor and source of stem cells. Stem cells may be donated from a related or unrelated HLA (human leucocyte antigen) compatible donor (allogeneic) or they may be obtained from the patient (autologous). Haematopoietic stem cells can be harvested from the peripheral blood following mobilisation using growth factor injections. They can also be obtained from the bone marrow or umbilical cord blood.

There are many potential life-threatening complications associated with stem cell transplantation which are largely due to the myeloablative (describes the therapy used intentionally to 'knock out' the patient's bone marrow) effects of conventional conditioning regimens. As such, guidelines identify which patients are most likely to benefit from this procedure. Although these are constantly being refined, they typically exclude older patients and those with co-morbidities. Recently, reduced intensity transplants, also known as 'mini transplants', which are less toxic than standard full intensity transplants have emerged as a potential treatment strategy. This approach has potentially extended the chance of cure to patients with acute leukaemia and other blood disorders who are ineligible for transplant due to age or co-morbidity (Provan 2007). Reduced intensity transplants attempt to utilise an immunological 'graft versus leukaemia' effect to eradicate the malignant cell clone and have resulted in a reduction in transplant-related mortality, although they are still undergoing investigation (Craig et al 2006).

For different types of transplant see Table 11.4.

See Further reading, e.g. Ezzone & Schmit-Pokorny 2007, Grundy 2006.

Table 11.4 Transplantation for malignant haematological disease

TYPE OF TRANSPLANT	EXPLANATION
Bone marrow transplantation	A term to describe the transplantation of bone marrow, which contains haematopoietic progenitor cells, to re-establish haematopoiesis in someone whose bone marrow has been destroyed or damaged by high-dose therapy. Donor marrow is usually harvested from the posterior iliac crests in the pelvis under general anaesthetic and infused intravenously to the recipient
Haematopoietic stem cell transplantation	The transplantation of haematopoietic stem cells to re-establish haematopoiesis in someone whose bone marrow function has been destroyed or damaged by high-dose therapy. Stem cells may be obtained from peripheral blood or the umbilical cord and are infused intravenously
Syngeneic transplant	Transplantation of bone marrow or haematopoietic stem cells between identical twins
Allogeneic sibling transplant	The use of bone marrow or haematopoietic stem cells from a matched sibling donor obtained from a bone marrow harvest or peripheral blood stem cell collection
Matched unrelated donor transplant (MUD)	Where a matched related donor is not available, a volunteer donor of bone marrow or stem cells may be found from national or international donor registries
Autologous transplant (rescue)	The use of a patient's own bone marrow or blood stem cells following high-dose therapy to reduce the period of pancytopenia. The cells are usually harvested during a period of remission, preserved and returned at a later date

Before treatment commences, several issues need to be considered including:

- a detailed, holistic assessment to determine the patient's general state of health and organ function
- the insertion of a long-term central venous access device (CVAD) such as a Hickman catheter
- referral for a wig fitting due to the likelihood of alopecia
- fertility issues must be discussed with patients of child-bearing age; male patients should be offered sperm banking facilities and female patients the opportunity to review the strategies available to them to maintain the possibility of future fertility (Foster 2002).

The chemotherapy regimens used to treat acute leukaemia are based on national protocols of treatment devised by the Medical Research Council (MRC) and change over time in the light of ongoing research and drug development. At the time of diagnosis most patients will be entered into a clinical trial. Typically, several cycles of treatment, each lasting several days, are required using a combination of agents that induce cell death by different means.

Initial treatment for AML, known as the induction phase, is aimed at achieving a disease remission indicated by a reduction of blast cells to <5% of the total WBC in the bone marrow (Cook & Craddock 2007). This is followed by further chemotherapy (the consolidation phase) which aims to eliminate any remaining leukaemic cells. However, some patients may undergo HSCT once induction is complete. Examples of chemotherapies used in the treatment of AML include daunorubicin, idarubicin, cytosine arabinoside, thioguanine, amsacrine and etoposide. Newer agents including gemtuzumab ozogamicin, tipifarnib and CEP701 are currently being investigated in the UK in relation to their role in the treatment of AML.

Treatment regimens for ALL are principally the same as for AML but may include an intensification phase, after the induction phase. This is then followed by consolidation therapy. Drug regimens will vary but may conventionally include vincristine, asparaginase and daunorubicin during induction with the addition of methotrexate and cytosine arabinoside during consolidation therapy. Maintenance therapy is administered to patients with ALL for a further one to two years after the completion of consolidation chemotherapy (Howard & Hamilton 2008). Additionally, regular doses of chemotherapy via the intrathecal (within the subarachnoid space) route are given prophylactically with the aim of treating or preventing the spread of leukaemia to the central nervous system (CNS) (Cook & Craddock 2007). Cranial irradiation may also be used.

Tumour lysis syndrome

Acute tumour lysis syndrome (TLS) is more likely in patients presenting with a high WBC and results from the rapid lysis (breakdown) of tumour cells during chemotherapy, leading to metabolic disturbances (including hyperkalaemia, hypocalcaemia and hyperphosphataemia) caused by the excessive production of uric acid and high levels in the blood (hyperuricaemia) (BCSH 2005). To slow uric acid production and prevent renal failure oral allopurinol and intravenous hydration are administered from the commencement of treatment. Some patients may also require apheresis prior to treatment to avoid this.

Supportive therapy

Leukaemic disease and aggressive treatment result in the suppression of normal blood cell production and, as outlined earlier, the patient will be predisposed to bleeding caused by thrombocytopenia, anaemia and infection. Supportive interventions will be required as detailed below.

Bleeding caused by thrombocytopenia Platelet transfusion will be required if the platelet count falls below 10×10^9cells/L (BCSH 2005). Platelets will also be required with higher counts in other specific instances, such as bleeding gums or epistaxis.

Anaemia caused by reduced numbers of RBCs RBC transfusions are used to minimise the effects of anaemia by maintaining the haemoglobin level above 10 g/dL (Craig et al 2006). As for platelet transfusions, some patients may require cytomegalovirus (CMV) negative and/or irradiated blood products.

Infection caused by neutropenia To reduce the incidence of infection, prophylactic antibiotics are often administered from the start of chemotherapy and for some time after the completion of treatment. Prophylactic antifungal and antiviral agents are also typically prescribed.

Neutropenic patients are extremely vulnerable to infection and once an infection develops, the lack of normal defence mechanisms means that the patient's condition can rapidly deteriorate, leading to septic shock. A temperature of >38°C for more than 1 hour may indicate sepsis and requires urgent intervention. Treatment protocols for the management of neutropenic sepsis are specific to individual haematology units; however, these typically involve blood cultures and swabs, urine and faecal specimens, medical examination, chest X-ray and the prompt administration of broad spectrum intravenous antibiotics. To reduce the period of neutropenia for select patients, granulocyte colony stimulating factor (GCSF) may be administered by subcutaneous injection.

Nursing management and health promotion: acute leukaemia

Nursing care for the patient with acute leukaemia must meet their individual physical and psychological needs throughout the disease trajectory. Treatment is intensive and has potentially life-threatening side-effects, thereby requiring expert care. Nurses are instrumental in administering treatments and supportive therapies, monitoring condition and providing appropriate information, emotional support and reassurance to the patient and their family.

Prevention of infection

An essential aspect of nursing patients undergoing treatment for acute leukaemia is to minimise the risk of infection. Some patients may require protective isolation in a single room to reduce contact with environmental microorganisms, while others will be nursed in general areas away from infectious patients. Other interventions to reduce the risk of infection include:

- Meticulous hand hygiene and decontamination using bactericidal solutions prior to patient contact and between tasks performed for the same patient.
- Use of protective clothing such as disposable plastic aprons and gloves during close contact with the patient or when blood and body fluid are present.
- Use of sterile gloves and aseptic technique for invasive procedures.
- Restricting visitor numbers.
- Encouraging compliance with a diet recommended for neutropenic patients. For patients with a neutrophil count between 0.5 and 2.0×10^9/L, for example, avoiding soft cheeses, such as brie, live yoghurts and foods containing raw or undercooked eggs. For patients with a neutrophil count below 0.5×10^9/L there are more restrictions such as avoiding raw fruit and vegetables (Leukaemia and Lymphoma Research 2007) (Box 11.11).
- Removal of flowers and pot plants which may harbour fungal spores and infection.

As the patient's own microflora will also pose a threat to the immunosuppressed patient, the risk of infection can be reduced by:

- regular and vigilant observation of the patient, e.g. 4-hourly recordings of temperature, pulse, respirations and blood pressure

> **Box 11.11 Reflection**

Dietary restrictions for patients with neutropenia

Dietary restrictions are required for neutropenic patients as part of the measures put in place to minimise the risk of infection.

Activities

- Access *Dietary advice for patients with neutropenia* (Leukaemia and Lymphoma Research 2007) and consider the following:
  - the general type of foods/beverages that are excluded
  - the differences in the foods excluded for a patient with neutropenia and one with severe neutropenia
  - the alternatives and other food suggestions provided.
- Reflect on having to exclude so many food items from the diet – how would you feel and what would you most miss?

Resources

Leukaemia and Lymphoma Research 2007 Dietary advice for patients with neutropenia. Available online http://www.beatbloodcancers.org/sites/default/files/Dietary%20advice%20for%20patients%20with%20neutropenia%20booklet.pdf

- management of CVADs according to local protocol
- encouraging attention to personal hygiene including daily showers and regular handwashing
- regular assessment and care of the oral cavity using appropriate solutions (see p. 386 and Ch. 15).

Prevention of haemorrhage

The patient should be closely monitored for bleeding and any indication of this must be acted on promptly. Such actions will include:

- immediately reporting signs and symptoms of bleeding to medical staff
- administering prescribed platelet transfusions promptly in accordance with national and local policy
- monitoring pulse and blood pressure readings at least 4-hourly
- undertaking daily urinalysis for blood
- testing stools for occult blood
- observing for changes in levels of consciousness or development of headaches which may indicate cerebral haemorrhage
- inspecting sputum and vomit for blood
- assessing the skin daily for purpura and bruising
- monitoring pain, especially in the abdomen, as this may be an indication of haemorrhage
- avoiding intramuscular injections and the use of aspirin-based medications
- advising the patient against the use of wet razors or harsh toothbrushes.

Communication and psychological support

The nature of acute leukaemia means that chemotherapy is often started before the patient has had time to fully assimilate their diagnosis and its associated implications. Treatment typically lasts several months and the impact of this on the patient and their family can be devastating and should never be underestimated. Treatment usually involves repeated admission to hospital and patients may find this difficult to cope with. Periods of social isolation and lengthy disruptions to normal life may promote anxiety and this may be coupled with feelings of uncertainty about the future or a fear of death. Helping the patient to understand their illness and its treatment may help them to retain a sense of control, even when very ill. This can be achieved through effective communication and the provision of support and reassurance. Providing patients and their families with information relevant to their needs in relation to investigations, treatment strategies and expected side-effects is also essential.

Minimising the side-effects of chemotherapy

General side-effects of chemotherapy are discussed in Chapter 31. Common short-term side-effects experienced by patients receiving chemotherapy for leukaemia are outlined here.

Nausea and vomiting If left untreated, nausea and vomiting may lead to fluid and electrolyte imbalance (see Ch. 20), malnutrition (see Ch. 21) and a possible reluctance by the patient to accept further treatment. However, control is possible through the use of antiemetic medications given prior to, during and after the administration of treatment. A wide range of antiemetics are currently available and alternatives can be used if first-line medications are ineffective. The use of relaxation techniques or distraction therapies may also help.

Compromised nutritional intake Loss of appetite is common during and after chemotherapy and may be influenced by factors such as nausea and vomiting, stomatitis and anxiety. Advice should be sought from the dietitian about appropriate food and drinks and nutritional supplements. Occasionally it may be necessary for the patient to receive enteral or parenteral nutrition for a short period of time (see Ch. 21). In such circumstances the patient will require careful assessment and monitoring to ensure fluid and electrolyte balance. Daily or weekly weight monitoring may also be indicated.

Mucositis/stomatitis Chemotherapy inhibits cell replication of the mucosa lining the oral cavity and may lead to inflammation known as stomatitis. The production of saliva is also reduced leading to changes in the normal microflora of the mouth, thus increasing the possibility of infection. Ulcers, which often develop within the oral cavity, increase the risk of microorganisms entering the circulation. Mouth ulcers may also compromise nutrition and cause considerable pain which is sometimes severe enough to merit the administration of opioid analgesia. Baseline and daily oral assessment using a specialist tool will help to ensure that changes are detected promptly and that appropriate management strategies are implemented. Patients may be required to use a bactericidal mouthwash several times a day, often in conjunction with an antifungal agent.

Patient education

Providing clear, accurate information about treatment, procedures and expected side-effects is essential. The active involvement of the family should be encouraged as the patient is given guidance in the following areas:

- monitoring body temperature
- recognising and responding to the symptoms of infection and haemorrhage

- maintaining a high standard of personal hygiene and oral care
- recognising and responding to complications associated with a CVAD
- adhering to the oral medication regimen.

Discharge planning

On discharge patients should receive a date for an outpatient appointment. The patient's GP and community nurse will be informed of discharge and arrangements made regarding continuing care. It is also important that patients receive information about who to contact in the event of an emergency.

Chronic leukaemia

Unlike acute leukaemia, the onset of chronic leukaemia is insidious and the disease may be present for some time before medical attention is sought. Diagnosis may result from incidental blood testing for other conditions. Chronic leukaemia is subdivided into chronic myeloid leukaemia (CML) and chronic lymphocytic leukaemia (CLL).

PATHOPHYSIOLOGY

CML is a disease of the pluripotent stem cells leading to an overproduction of granulocytes and their precursors in the peripheral blood. The annual UK incidence is about 1.8/100 000 (Craig et al 2006). Presentation is most likely in people aged 50–60 years. Over 95% of the leukaemic cells have an abnormal chromosome known as the Philadelphia (Ph) chromosome (a shortened chromosome 22) (Mehta & Hoffbrand 2009). CML is characterised by three stages. After a chronic phase, which may last 2–3 years, the disease enters an accelerated stage and finally transforms into acute leukaemia which is often the main cause of death.

CLL is a malignant disorder of the mature B lymphocytes which proliferate and accumulate in the blood, bone marrow, lymph nodes and spleen. The aetiology of CLL is unknown and most cases occur in adults aged over 50 years. CLL is the most common type of leukaemia in Western countries. The incidence in the UK is approximately 2750 annually (Leukaemia and Lymphoma Research 2009b).

Clinical presentation

Presentation of chronic leukaemia is extremely variable. Presentation may be similar to that of acute leukaemia and include:

- fatigue
- anaemia
- weight loss
- infection, sweats and fevers
- painless lymphadenopathy (in CLL)
- abdominal discomfort due to splenomegaly.

MEDICAL MANAGEMENT

History and examination Of patients with suspected CML, 90% will have splenomegaly and 50% will have hepatomegaly. Of patients with suspected CLL, more than 66% will present with painless lymphadenopathy, infection and symptoms derived from bone marrow failure, e.g. anaemia, thrombocytopenia (BCSH 2004).

Investigations A diagnosis of chronic leukaemia will be confirmed by further investigations including peripheral blood count, reticulocyte count, examination of bone marrow aspirate and trephine biopsy, biochemical tests, computed tomography (CT) scans and chest radiography. Lymph node biopsy may also be needed in some cases (BCSH 2004). Staging is important in CLL as it assists with prognostic information and treatment decisions (Howard & Hamilton 2008).

Treatment of chronic myeloid leukaemia Imatinib is now recommended by the National Institute for Health and Clinical Excellence (NICE) (2003) as the first treatment for adults with the Ph-chromosome type of CML in the chronic phase.

It is also recommended as treatment for adults diagnosed with Ph-chromosome type CML in the accelerated or blast crisis phase and for those patients whose disease has been resistant to other therapies such as interferon (Craig et al 2006). Other treatment options include oral hydroxycarbamide, and interferon alfa, which may be used alone or in combination with cytarabine.

For patients in the accelerated phase, treatment is highly problematic. Patients in blast crisis may be treated with chemotherapy suitable for treating acute leukaemia; however, response is usually short-lived.

Allogeneic HSCT is a potentially curative option and may be used for younger patients who have a matched sibling donor. Best results have been seen when transplant has been performed during the early chronic phase within one year of diagnosis (Howard & Hamilton 2008). For those who do not have a sibling donor, matched unrelated donor HSCT may offer the possibility of a cure.

Treatment of chronic lymphocytic leukaemia Although there is no curative treatment for CLL, evidence suggests that there is no advantage from early treatment of asymptomatic patients. Hence, current practice follows a 'wait and watch' approach during which the patient is monitored regularly for signs of disease progression.

In accordance with the BCSH CLL guidelines (2004), patient follow-up may be undertaken in primary care with detailed guidelines as when to refer to the haematologist.

Chemotherapy can be used to control the disease and should be started when the patient develops advancing disease manifested by progressive bone marrow failure, enlarged spleen and lymph nodes, increasing lymphocyte counts and systemic symptoms such as weight loss, fatigue, fever and night sweats (Bishop & Pearce 2007). Splenectomy, leucopheresis and supportive care may be used alongside chemotherapy.

Chlorambucil (an alkylating agent) has conventionally been the mainstay treatment for CLL and is generally well tolerated by patients. Fludarabine, used either alone or in conjunction with other agents such as cyclophosphamide, is now favoured over oral chlorambucil as first-line treatment due to its higher clinical response and remission rates (Howard & Hamilton 2008). The use of monoclonal antibodies, such as rituximab and alemtuzumab, as supplements to first-line treatment, is also attracting interest and studies of autologous and allogeneic stem cell (particularly reduced intensity allogeneic) transplantation are also in progress.

Supportive care may include the administration of intravenous immunoglobulin and antibiotics for patients experiencing recurrent infections, allopurinol to control hyperuricaemia, and radiotherapy to relieve local obstruction.

Nursing management and health promotion: chronic leukaemia

A diagnosis of chronic leukaemia is a significant, life-changing event. Unless intensive treatment is required many patients remain at home but they require regular monitoring. Hospital-based nurses may be involved in assisting with diagnostic procedures and the administration of supportive therapies. However, if more intensive treatment or transplantation is pursued the nursing responsibilities will include:

- providing information about tests, diagnosis and treatment options
- administering treatment such as chemotherapy
- providing psychological support to help the patient come to terms with a chronic and potentially life-threatening illness
- educating the patient about medication, including the importance of continuing with intermittent courses of chemotherapy
- assisting with activities of daily living
- giving advice about the level of work and activity that can realistically be attempted
- reinforcing the importance of follow-up in outpatient clinics.

Lymphoma

The lymphomas are a group of malignant disorders characterised by a proliferation of lymphoid cells originating in the lymph nodes or lymphoid tissue. Most often the disease is of B-cell origin. Traditionally, lymphomas are divided into two groups:

- Hodgkin's lymphoma (HL) (previously called Hodgkin's disease)
- non-Hodgkin lymphoma (NHL).

HL is uncommon and accounts for 0.5% of all cancers (Cancer Research UK 2009b).The incidence of HL is approximately 2.7/100 000 of the population per year with an annual incidence in the UK of around 1600 cases, and causing 311 deaths in 2007 (Cancer Research UK 2009b). It is more common among men than women and among people aged between 20 and 30 years, peaking again after 50 years of age.

NHL is the fifth most common cancer in the UK, representing 4% of all cancers and causing over 4500 deaths in 2007 (Cancer Research UK 2009c). Incidence increases with age and, as with HL, it seems to be more common in males than in females.

PATHOPHYSIOLOGY

Lymphomas arise from the uncontrolled growth of lymphocytes and in both HL and NHL, cells in the affected lymph tissue (usually lymph nodes) reveal a disruption of normal structure. HL is characterised by the presence of large, malignant, multinucleated cells of B-cell origin known as

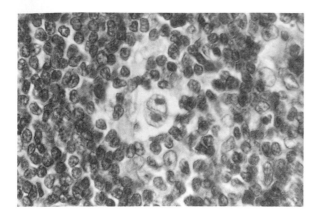

Figure 11.5 Hodgkin's lymphoma showing a typical Reed–Sternberg cell. (Reproduced from Craig et al 2006 with permission.)

Reed–Sternberg cells within the lymphoma tumour mass (Figure 11.5). HL has two main types:

- classical Hodgkin's lymphoma, of which there are four subtypes
- nodular lymphocyte-predominant lymphoma.

NHL is more difficult to classify as it encompasses a wide range of diseases. The recent WHO classification system is based on the Revised European–American Lymphoma classification (REAL) and attempts to group lymphomas by cell type. The most commonly occurring NHLs are:

- diffuse large B-cell lymphoma
- follicular lymphoma.

Lymphoma spreads via the blood and lymphatic systems and can infiltrate tissue and organs.

Clinical presentation

Hodgkin's lymphoma

For 80–90% of patients with HL, the most common manifestation is a painless enlarged lymph node, often described as 'rubbery'. Such nodes are found in the neck and supraclavicular fossae, axillae or inguinal regions. These may grow slowly or rapidly and compromise other organs by compression or obstruction. Other symptoms include infection, pruritus and pain in the diseased lymph nodes on consuming alcohol. The reasons for this are unclear (Hoffbrand et al 2006).

Non-Hodgkin lymphoma

Patients with NHL may present similarly to those with HL with painless lymphadenopathy. However, NHL is often widely disseminated at presentation and a wider range of symptoms can occur and will depend on the extent and site of the diseased nodes. Examples include:

- breathlessness due to enlarged mediastinal lymph nodes or obstruction of the superior vena cava
- lymphoedema in the arms or legs due to obstructed lymph drainage in the axillary or inguinal node
- anaemia or pancytopenia due to bone marrow involvement
- infection caused by defective humoral and/or cell-mediated immunity (see Ch. 6).

Some patients also present with systemic symptoms, which are medically known as B symptoms. These may include one or more of the following:

- persistent unexplained fever of 38°C
- drenching night sweats requiring the patient to change bed linen and night clothes
- weight loss >10% of body weight.

These symptoms are important when staging the disease and give some indication of prognosis.

MEDICAL MANAGEMENT

Investigations

Diagnosis of lymphoma is generally made by means of:

- lymph node biopsy
- blood tests including FBC, ESR, renal function tests
- bone marrow aspiration (see p. 372)
- chest X-ray
- CT scan of chest, abdomen and pelvis
- magnetic resonance imaging (MRI) or positron emission tomography (PET) scan.

After clinical examination and once results of the investigations are known, the disease is staged. For HL this is now typically based on the modified Ann Arbor system (the Cotswold Classification) (Box 11.12). This important prognostic indicator determines the extent of the disease by examining the number and location of involved lymph nodes or extralymphatic sites and takes into account the presence or absence of B symptoms.

An international prognostic index (IPI) based on age, stage, bulk of disease, performance status and the serum lactate dehydrogenase (LDH) level is used as a predictor of adverse outcome in NHL (Howard & Hamilton 2008).

Treatment

Hodgkin's lymphoma Treatment depends on the stage of the disease. For early stage disease a short course (2–3 cycles) of combination chemotherapy is usually given and is followed by reduced-dose localised radiotherapy. Doxorubicin (previously the proprietary name Adriamycin® was used), bleomycin, vinblastine and dacarbazine (ABVD) is now considered standard treatment.

> **Box 11.12 Information**
>
> **Staging of lymphomas: the Cotswold Classification**
>
> | | |
> |---|---|
> | Stage I | One lymph node region involved or one extralymphatic site, e.g. stomach, Peyer's patches, thyroid |
> | Stage II | Two or more lymph node regions involved but on the same side of the diaphragm or an extralymphatic site plus lymph nodes on the same side |
> | Stage III | Lymph node involvement on both sides of the diaphragm with or without extralymphatic sites |
> | Stage IV | Diffuse involvement of extralymphatic sites, e.g. bone marrow, liver |
>
> Associated with each stage will be either A (no symptoms) or B (fever, night sweats, >10% weight loss in preceding 6 months).

Advanced stage disease is typically treated with 6–8 cycles of combination chemotherapy. Again, the most common ABVD combination is used, although alternate chemotherapy regimens are also in use. If there is no response or the patient relapses, the combination of medications is changed. Patients with 'bulky' (i.e. large diseased lymph nodes) mediastinal disease may be given chemotherapy followed by radiotherapy.

Patients who relapse post radiotherapy will be offered chemotherapy. Those who relapse post chemotherapy for advanced disease may be offered high-dose chemotherapy with HSCT.

Non-Hodgkin's lymphoma Specific chemotherapy regimens are prescribed according to the type of lymphoma and the stage of the disease. Regimens are continually being refined as clinical understanding improves.

'Low-grade' NHL Patients who are asymptomatic with 'low-grade' NHL are generally monitored closely without treatment until symptoms indicate the need. Local disease may be treated with radiotherapy. When required, chemotherapy will be administered either as single agents, e.g. chlorambucil, cyclophosphamide, fludarabine, or in combination, e.g. cyclophosphamide, doxorubicin, vincristine and prednisolone. Relapsed patients may respond to the same treatment that induced remission

'High grade' NHL (diffuse large B-cell lymphoma) In the UK the gold standard treatment to date is CHOP (cyclophosphamide, doxorubicin hydrochloride [previously called Adriamycin®], vincristine [Oncovin®] and prednisolone). For patients who relapse, further chemotherapy followed by autologous stem cell rescue or allogeneic HSCT may be offered. Current research involving the use of monoclonal antibodies which target specific cells is being evaluated (Provan 2007); however, rituximab is now widely used in conjunction with the CHOP protocol.

 Nursing management and health promotion: lymphoma

As lymphoma comprises such a diverse group of disorders and treatment is so varied, nursing care cannot be prescriptive. Some patients will be treated as outpatients, whereas others will be hospitalised throughout the course of treatment. Regardless of the setting in which the patient is treated, nursing interventions will include:

- explanation of diagnostic and staging investigations
- information about the disease
- administering specific treatment and managing side-effects with care and skill
- offering psychological support to patients and their families who may be shocked by the possibility of serious illness.

After the course of treatment patients should be given detailed information about post-radiotherapy/chemotherapy care (see Ch. 31). This should include:

- a contact number for help or advice
- the signs of infection or bleeding and who to contact should either of these occur

- medication and details about how and when to take it, and potential side-effects
- dietary advice
- advice regarding skin care
- recommended level of activity and when to return to employment
- the importance of attendance at follow-up clinics
- appropriate self-help and support groups
- sexual counselling as appropriate
- referral to community nurse, social worker and GP.

Whatever the outcome of treatment, patients with HL or NHL require high-quality physical and psychological care from nursing staff who are able to recognise and meet their individual needs, and concerns.

Myeloma

Myeloma, also referred to as multiple myeloma, is an uncommon malignant disorder characterised by an abnormal and unregulated proliferation of plasma cells which develop from mature B lymphocytes. Myeloma accounts for 1% of all cancers in the UK, with 3970 new cases diagnosed in 2005 (Cancer Research UK 2009d). There were 2695 deaths in 2007 (Cancer Research UK 2009d). The disease is rare in young people and primarily occurs over the age of 40. It is a disease that is twice as common in people of African Caribbean descent, and is more prevalent in men than in women (Singer 2007).

PATHOPHYSIOLOGY

Normal plasma cells develop from B lymphocytes following antigen stimulation. Each plasma cell produces a specific immunoglobulin, which contains a variety of heavy and light chains. In myeloma there is a malignant proliferation of one clone of plasma cells, which produce a single heavy or light chain known as a paraprotein. Depending on the type secreted, the abnormal paraprotein may be detected in the serum. It may also be present in the urine where it is referred to as Bence Jones protein. Measurement of paraprotein is commonly used to monitor the course of the disease.

The majority of malignant plasma cells exist in the bone marrow. Here they produce cytokines which stimulate osteoclasts, which normally regulate bone resorption and formation at a constant rate. Myeloma cells disrupt this process by promoting osteoclast activity. This results in increased bone resorption and a reduction in bone formation. Multiple lytic bone lesions, hence the term 'multiple myeloma', also occur due to the secretion of bone-damaging cytokines by the myeloma cells.

Although the cause of myeloma is unknown there appears to be some connection with occupational exposure to certain products such as pesticides, radiation and benzene.

Clinical features

The onset of myeloma is often insidious and it is not uncommon for the disease to be advanced at time of presentation. Some patients may experience a sudden onset of bone pain caused by pathological fracture or severe bone tenderness throughout the body. Others present with pneumonia due to neutropenia and lowered immunoglobulin levels, and yet others may present with clinical features of renal failure and/or hypercalcaemia.

The most common presenting features associated with multiple myeloma are:

- bone pain, especially in the lower back region, and pathological fractures
- spinal cord compression (SCC) due to vertebral collapse
- anaemia, mediated by cytokines rather than by marrow replacement
- renal failure
- hypercalcaemia
- infection
- amyloidosis (deposition of the abnormal protein, amyloid, in organ systems) affecting the kidney and leading to proteinuria and nephrotic syndrome.

MEDICAL MANAGEMENT

Investigations

Investigations undertaken to diagnose myeloma include:

- the presence of paraproteins in blood or urine – electrophoresis and immunoelectrophoresis
- X-ray skeletal survey, isotope bone scan, MRI
- bone marrow aspiration and trephine biopsy
- blood tests – FBC, urea and electrolytes, calcium, albumin, alkaline phosphatase, coagulation tests, creatinine, uric acid, immunoglobulins.

To confirm the diagnosis of myeloma and determine its stage, evidence of two of the following is required:

- the presence of paraprotein
- lytic bone lesions
- infiltration of the bone marrow by excess plasma cells.

Treatment

Myeloma is currently an incurable disease. Patients with minimal symptoms may not require intervention. In more advanced disease, treatment is aimed at controlling symptoms of the disease, particularly pain. High fluid intake of 3–4 L of fluid a day is recommended to prevent and treat renal impairment and hypercalcaemia, and in some cases intravenous fluids may be needed.

Chemotherapy Standard first-line treatment is dexamethasone, either used alone or in combination with vincristine and doxorubicin (VAD) or with lenalidomide, an analogue of thalidomide. Lenalidomide may be used for people with multiple myeloma who have received at least one prior therapy (NICE 2009).

Haematopoietic stem cell harvesting and more intensive treatment using high-dose melphalan and autologous stem cell rescue may then follow. Allogeneic transplantation may cure some patients and should be considered (Howard & Hamilton 2008).

In older patients, where transplantation is not appropriate, a combination of low-dose oral melphalan and prednisolone may be prescribed. Bortezomib is recommended by NICE (2007) as a possible treatment for people with relapsed multiple myeloma, and who have had a bone marrow transplant, unless it is not suitable for them.

Bisphosphonates have been shown to substantially reduce bone destruction by inhibiting osteoclast activity and are recommended for all patients requiring treatment.

Radiotherapy is useful in the treatment of myeloma. Specific bony lesions can be targeted, thus preventing fractures and reducing pain.

Surgery Internal fixation of fractured bones or areas of lytic lesions that are liable to fracture may be necessary to stabilise bones which are diseased (see Ch. 10).

Plasmapheresis may be used to reduce a high blood viscosity, as the removal of the patient's plasma will also reduce the paraprotein level. This is done only as a temporary measure whilst other treatment is given.

Nursing management and health promotion: myeloma

Myeloma is a very complex disorder with multisystem effects, some of which are potentially life-threatening. In order to plan and implement care, it is important that the nurse has a thorough knowledge of the disease and its effects on the patient.

Pain management

Often the most distressing and debilitating symptom for the patient is pain. Assessment should take into account the multidimensional effects of pain and that the pain may have been present for some time. Pain management strategies will depend on the cause and severity of the pain but may include the use of analgesia including opioids and NSAIDs, and non-pharmaceutical methods such as relaxation, massage and the application of hot or cold packs. Palliative chemotherapy and/or radiotherapy may be used to reduce pain.

Maintaining mobility whilst preventing fractures

Whilst prolonged periods of bed rest should be avoided to decrease the risk of hypercalcaemia and pulmonary embolism, so too should activity which increases the risk of fracturing weak bones. Management strategies include:

- ensuring pain is controlled prior to exercise and being aware that increased activity may increase the level of pain and the need for analgesics
- working with the physiotherapist and occupational therapist to help the patient attain an optimal level of activity
- provision of lightweight braces which provide support for the spine for patients with multiple lytic lesions
- maintaining a safe environment
- ensuring that a home assessment has been carried out prior to discharge to identify any modifications that may be needed within the patient's home.

Prevention of infection

Preventative strategies include:

- monitoring the patient for signs and symptoms of infection and treating these promptly with prescribed antibiotics
- ensuring maintanance of adequate hydration

- avoiding urinary catheterisation to prevent the possibility of infection
- maintaining a diet high in calories and essential nutrients to support the immune system.

Fatigue due to anaemia

Anaemia causing fatigue will be corrected by regular blood transfusion. Patients may need reassurance about the frequency of transfusion and to be assisted in establishing strategies to maximise their energy by ensuring a balance between rest and activity.

Prevention of spinal cord compression

SCC is an oncological emergency which can occur in patients who have myeloma. Nurses need to know the presentation of SCC, which includes pain or impaired sensation and paralysis, and must recognise the importance of urgent reporting to medical staff and immediate interventions.

Communication and psychological support

In addition to coping with distressing and debilitating symptoms, the patient faces a diagnosis of a malignant disease which is probably incurable. Nursing management strategies include listening to the patient's anxieties and answering questions honestly, in a way that is appropriate for the patient.

Patient education

Acquiring knowledge about the disease and its management may help the patient to feel more in control. The patient should receive information about:

- side-effects of treatment and self-monitoring
- preventing or minimising complications, e.g. sufficient oral fluids
- safe techniques for moving and handling
- reducing muscle weakness
- the importance of follow-up with the GP and hospital outpatient clinics and relevant support groups (see Useful websites).

Discharge planning

This will depend on the patient's physical and psychological state, the type of treatment received and the availability of carers at home or in the community. Planning needs to address the following:

- the patient's level of dependency
- the availability of home carers – the type and degree of support needed
- the skills needed by carers, e.g. safe moving and handling of the patient.

(See Further reading, e.g. Smith et al 2007.)

Myelodysplastic syndrome

Myelodysplastic syndrome (MDS) is a group of disorders derived from an abnormal stem cell which retains the capacity to differentiate into end-stage cells. However, this differentiation is disordered and ineffective and leads to peripheral blood cytopenias of RBCs, WBCs and platelets (Hoffbrand et al 2006). Morphological abnormalities and impaired maturation of RBCs, WBCs and platelets are common and these form the basis for diagnosis. Disease progression is extremely variable but during the course of MDS the abnormal clone is prone to lose its ability to differentiate, with some cases transforming into acute leukaemia.

MDS is more common in men than women, and although it can affect all ages tends to be a disease affecting older people. The annual incidence in the UK has been reported as 1 new case per 100 000 population (Leukaemia and Lymphoma Research 2009c), but as many cases remain undiagnosed, the true incidence is probably higher.

It occurs most often as a primary condition with an unknown cause, but may also develop secondary to exposure to cytotoxic medications (e.g. alkylating agents), chemicals (e.g. benzene) and radiation.

PATHOPHYSIOLOGY

MDS occurs as a result of DNA damage to a pluripotent stem cell leading to more rapid cell division in the abnormal clone of cells when compared to normal cells. The disease is classified into five subgroups according to the widely used French–American–British (FAB) system. However, the newer WHO classification system is based on the combination of bone marrow and peripheral blood morphology and also divides MDS into different subgroups (Cahalin & Liu Yin 2007). (See Further reading, e.g. Green 2006.)

Clinical presentation

The clinical presentation of MDS is highly variable. Some patients may have symptoms of bone marrow failure such as fatigue caused by anaemia, infection caused by neutropenia, or bruising due to thrombocytopenia. Others may be diagnosed through unrelated routine blood tests. In some cases hepatosplenomegaly may be present and occasionally gum hypertrophy, pleural and pericardial effusion, and painful, swollen joints.

The course and prognosis of MDS is variable and unpredictable. Some patients remain stable for many years, whilst others experience rapid progression to AML.

MEDICAL MANAGEMENT

Investigations

After a thorough history, diagnosis is made on findings from the following investigations:

- bone marrow aspiration and trephine biopsy
- FBC and film
- cytogenetic analysis.

Vitamin B_{12} and folate levels are usually checked to eliminate any deficiency that would affect the blood results.

Treatment

Treatment of MDS depends on the patient's health status, co-morbidities and severity of the myelodysplasia. Treatment is most often aimed at supportive care in order to prolong survival and delay transformation to acute leukaemia. Interventions include:

- regular blood transfusion
- platelet transfusion administered prophylactically and when spontaneous bleeding occurs

- infection prevention strategies and swift treatment in the event of detection
- immunosuppression with antithymocyte globulin
- colony stimulating factors such as GCSF and erythropoietin
- low-dose or intensive chemotherapy.

Other potential treatments include lenalidomide, arsenic trioxide and farnesyl transferase inhibitors.

Allogeneic bone marrow transplantation is the only curative treatment and may be considered for patients with a suitable donor.

 ## Nursing management and health promotion: myelodysplastic syndrome

Nursing a patient with MDS requires specific skills and expert knowledge in relation to the disease process, treatment options and side-effects. Due to the unpredictability of the disease and the seriousness of its effects, MDS may have significant psychological and social implications and the effect of these on the patient and their family should not be underestimated. Strategies aimed at promoting health and minimising the risk of complications should be provided to the patient with an emphasis on maintaining quality of life. As such, nursing priorities will include:

- monitoring the patient for signs of anaemia, infection and bleeding and acting promptly if these are detected
- educating the patient and their family about the disease, treatment and associated risks and what to do if complications arise
- administering prescribed treatment and supportive therapies such as blood transfusion in line with national and local policy guidance
- demonstrating flexibility when planning hospital appointments and treatment in order to minimise disruption to daily life
- referral to a social worker or counsellor for psychological support and assistance with financial issues if required.

Disorders of coagulation

Disorders of coagulation can be subdivided into three types:

- disorders due to lack of coagulation (clotting) factors
- platelet disorders
- disorders due to other causes such as lack of vitamin K or liver disease (see Ch. 4).

These disorders may be inherited or acquired and all age groups are affected. Some problems with coagulation are caused by genetic disorders, for example haemophilia. Coagulation factor disorders involve a deficiency in one or more of the blood factors required for haemostasis. Inherited coagulation disorders result from the lack of specific coagulation factors. The acquired disorders involve the failure of certain coagulation factors to be activated, usually as a result of vitamin K deficiency or liver disease.

This section provides an outline of haemophilia and thrombocytopenia (deficiency of platelets).

Haemophilia

The haemophilias are a group of inherited disorders in which an essential coagulation factor is either partly or completely missing. This causes a person with haemophilia to bleed for longer than normal. A rare acquired autoimmune haemophilia also occurs in older people (Haemophilia Society 2008). Haemophilia is evident worldwide and occurs in all racial groups.

PATHOPHYSIOLOGY

Haemophilia is a recessive X-linked condition (sex-linked inheritance) which nearly always affects males while females carry the defective gene (Box 11.13). Notably, it is possible for a female to have haemophilia or a tendency to bleed (Haemophilia Society 2008). There are two types of haemophilia, the most common being haemophilia A (classical haemophilia), in which factor VIII is lacking. This type affects approximately 1/10 000 people (Craig et al 2006). In haemophilia B, also known as Christmas disease, factor IX is lacking. Both types of the disorder share similar symptoms.

Clinical presentation

Despite haemophilia being an inherited disorder, it is unusual for excessive bleeding to occur before 6 months of age, when superficial bleeding or bruising may occur (Craig et al 2006). A full blood count and coagulation assays will be required for diagnosis and a family history must be taken to ascertain whether the condition is inherited.

Haemophilia is classified as mild, moderate or severe and clinical presentation will vary accordingly. In mild cases, superficial bruising and excessive bleeding after minor injuries or procedures may be evident, while if haemophilia is severe, spontaneous recurrent bleeding in major joints and muscles is common. Serious long-term effects of this include pain, arthritic changes and mobility problems.

MEDICAL MANAGEMENT

There is no cure for haemophilia, and people with haemophilia may be managed in specialist units. Treatment involves replacing the deficient coagulation factors and is

---

 Box 11.13 Reflection

Haemophilia and health promotion

Belinda and Marvin are expecting their first baby. One of Belinda's brothers has haemophilia A, as do several other male relatives. She has been tested and knows that she is a genetic carrier of the disorder. Belinda and Marvin are worried that their baby will be affected and that, if this is the case, he or she will not be able to have a fulfilling life.

Activity

- Access *Introduction to haemophilia* (Haemophilia Society 2008) and find out (a) how likely it is that their baby will be affected, (b) information about the management of haemophilia and lifestyle if they have a son who has haemophilia.
- Reflect on Belinda and Marvin's situation. Are their concerns valid and what information and advice should they be given?

dependent on the degree of factor deficiency and severity of the bleed. People with mild haemophilia A may be prescribed desmopressin (DDAVP), a synthetic hormone which stimulates factor XIII release and may be given in combination with tranexamic acid. More severe cases will require regular intravenous infusions of factor VIII concentrate. This may be derived from human blood plasma and is also available in recombinant form which is considerably safer in terms of reducing viral contamination. Since the risk of transmitting variant Creutzfeldt–Jakob Disease (vCJD) through blood was first considered, a number of precautionary measures have been introduced to minimise the risk from the UK blood supply. UK plasma has not been used for the manufacture of coagulation factors since 1999 and synthetic coagulation factors are provided for all patients for whom they are suitable (Health Protection Agency 2009).

A serious consequence of regular factor VIII replacement therapy is the development of antibodies to factors which may render treatment ineffective. In such cases higher doses may be required or factor from other sources such as pigs (porcine). Alternatively immune tolerance therapy (ITT) may be required (Haemophilia Society 2008).

Thrombocytopenia

Any disturbance in the number or function of circulating platelets will affect the normal coagulation process. Thrombocytopenia implies a reduction in the number of platelets and may be inherited or acquired.

PATHOPHYSIOLOGY

Inherited thrombocytopenia is fortunately rare. Acquired thrombocytopenia may occur as a result of factors which either decrease normal platelet production or increase platelet consumption/destruction (Box 11.14).

Decreased production is usually caused by drugs or some other agent whereby the bone marrow is suppressed. The most common cause of increased platelet consumption/destruction is idiopathic thrombocytopenic purpura (ITP). This commonly affects individuals in their teens or early 20s and is thought to be autoimmune in origin. Whatever the cause, ITP will result in a prolonged bleeding time, giving rise to bruising, purpura or petechiae and, more seriously, gastrointestinal, retinal or intracranial bleeding.

Common presenting symptoms

These may include a history of bleeding gums, epistaxis, melaena and haematuria. In contrast to haemophilia, if pressure is applied to the bleeding point, bleeding will stop and not recur unless further trauma occurs.

MEDICAL MANAGEMENT

History and examination

A thorough clinical history is required to identify any recent minor illness or drug therapy, including over-the-counter medicines. Clinical examination is carried out to detect any signs of bruising, petechiae, purpura or any underlying disorder.

Box 11.14 Information

Causes of acquired thrombocytopenia (adapted from Craig et al 2006 with permission)

Decrease in platelet production

- Idiopathic
- Drug induced, e.g. cytotoxic chemotherapy (note: drugs such as NSAIDs, penicillin and β-blockers can inhibit platelet function)
- Aplastic anaemia
- Vitamin B_{12}, folate deficiency
- Bone marrow infiltration:
  - leukaemia
  - myeloma
  - lymphoma
  - carcinoma
  - myelofibrosis (formation of fibrous tissue within the bone marrow cavity)

Excess consumption/destruction of platelets

- Viral infection, e.g. EBV, HIV
- Bacterial infection, e.g. Gram-negative septicaemia
- Liver disease
- Hypersplenism
- Connective tissue disease, e.g. systemic lupus erythematosus
- Idiopathic thrombocytopenic purpura (ITP)
- Disseminated intravascular coagulation (DIC) (see Ch. 29)

Note: Due to the short lifespan of platelets, there may be no viable platelets in blood transfusion units, and a patient requiring a large volume of blood may have insufficient platelets.

Investigations

These will include:

- FBC and blood film
- bone marrow aspiration
- coagulation screen
- biochemical screen.

Treatment

Some cases of ITP resolve spontaneously; however, it usually becomes a chronic condition. In cases where an exacerbating factor such as a medication is withdrawn, spontaneous remission may also occur.

Corticosteroids improve platelet survival and these may be given until resolution occurs. However, thrombocytopenia may recur when the corticosteroids are withdrawn. Intravenous immunoglobulin (IVIg) may be given. Splenectomy may also be required in some cases, as the spleen is a major site of platelet destruction. Platelet transfusions are given if bleeding is severe.

Nursing management and health promotion: thrombocytopenia

Nursing priorities for the hospitalised patient with platelet disorders include:

- controlling any superficial bleeding by the application of external pressure

- ensuring that the patient is protected from injury by advising on environmental safety and that feeling faint may indicate anaemia or low blood pressure
- providing explanations and support during tests and treatment
- observing the patient for evidence of bleeding by:
  - regular monitoring of patient's pulse (note: caution should be used if blood pressure measurement is required as this may cause bruising and petechiae)
  - inspection of the skin for petechiae, purpura and bruises, and of the mouth for bleeding and infection
  - regular testing of urine, stools and vomit for blood
  - being alert to complaints of headaches and drowsiness, as these may indicate intracranial bleeding.

Health promotion is of utmost importance and the importance of monitoring all episodes of bleeding must be stressed, along with the need for regular follow-up.

Specific points that the patient should be advised about include:

- taking medicines as prescribed
- avoiding aspirin preparations
- avoiding intramuscular injections
- carrying identification such as a Medic-Alert® card
- minimising potential for soft tissue injury
- avoiding contact sports.

The family should be included in the education programme to ensure that all members understand the necessity of certain restrictions upon lifestyle. However, it should also be stressed that it is important for the patient to maintain a balance between being overcautious and taking unnecessary risks.

SUMMARY: KEY NURSING ISSUES

- Haematology is a challenging and constantly developing area of practice in which ongoing research continues to improve patient outcomes.
- Nurses are instrumental in the planning, delivery and evaluation of care of people with blood disorders and require a range of skills underpinned by a sound knowledge of blood and haematopoiesis as well as an understanding of disorders, treatment and potential complications.
- Anaemia is a common blood disorder. It is associated with various factors including diet and disease and can impact on physical and psychological well-being.
- An understanding of infection prevention and control by nurses is vital when caring for patients with WBC disorders. Signs of infection require prompt action.
- The nature of acute leukaemia means that chemotherapy is often started before the patient has had time to fully assimilate the diagnosis and its implications. Nurses can assist by providing accurate information and ongoing psychosocial support in response to the needs of the patient and their family.
- HSCT or bone marrow transplantation may be the only curative treatment for a number of blood conditions. It typically involves preparatory regimens which render the patient extremely vulnerable to infection and other complications.

- Some blood disorders are inherited and this may have implications for the family members.
- Many blood disorders are incurable and in such cases effective symptom control and maintaining quality of life should be a priority.

REFLECTION AND LEARNING – WHAT NEXT?

- **Test** your knowledge by visiting the website 🖱 and answering the multiple choice questions and critical thinking questions.
- **Consolidate** your learning by looking at some of the further reading suggestions, references and specialist websites.
- **Revisit** some of the additional material on the website.
- **Consider** what you have learnt and how this will help your professional development.
- **Reflect** on how you can apply this knowledge to the care of your patients.
- **Discuss** your learning with your mentor/supervisor, lecturer and colleagues.

REFERENCES

Bishop L, Pearce H: Chronic lymphocytic leukaemia: a common but overlooked cancer, *Cancer Nursing Practice* 6(9):29–35, 2007.

British Committee for Standards in Haematology (BCSH): Guidelines for diagnosis and management of chronic lymphocytic leukaemia, *Br J Haematol* 125:294–317, 2004.

British Committee for Standards in Haematology (BCSH): *Guidelines on the management of acute myeloid leukaemia in adults*, 2005. Available online http://www.bcshguidelines.com/pdf/AML_230505.pdf.

British Committee for Standards in Haematology (BCSH): *Guidelines for diagnosis and management of acquired aplastic anaemia*, 2009. Available online http://www.bcshguidelines.com/pdf/published_AA_june10.pdf.

Cahalin PA, Liu Yin JA: The myelodysplastic syndromes. In Provan D, editor: *ABC of clinical haematology*, Oxford, 2007, Blackwell, pp 40–44.

Cancer Research UK: *UK Leukaemia incidence statistics*, 2009a. Available online http://info.cancerresearchuk.org/cancerstats/types/leukaemia/incidence/.

Cancer Research UK: *UK Hodgkin's lymphoma incidence statistics*, 2009b. Available online http://info.cancerresearchuk.org/cancerstats/types/hodgkinslymphoma/incidence/.

Cancer Research UK: *UK Cancer incidence statistics for common cancers*, 2009c. Available online http://info.cancerresearchuk.org/cancerstats/incidence/commoncancers/.

Cancer Research UK: *UK Multiple myeloma statistics*, 2009d. Available online http://info.cancerresearchuk.org/cancerstats/types/multiplemyeloma/?a=5441.

Cook M, Craddock C: The acute leukaemias. In Provan D, editor: *ABC of clinical haematology*, Oxford, 2007, Blackwell Publishing, pp 27–32.

Craig JIO, McClelland DBL, Ludlam CA: Blood disorders. In Boon NA, et al, editor: *Davidson's Principles and practice of medicine*, ed 20, Edinburgh, 2006, Churchill Livingstone, pp 999–1064.

European Pressure Ulcer Advisory Panel (EPUAP): *Pressure ulcer prevention guidelines*, 2008. Available online http://www.epuap.org/glprevention.html.

Foster R: Fertility issues in patients with cancer, *Cancer Nursing Practice* 1(1):26–30, 2002.

Grundy M, editor: *Nursing in Haematological Oncology*, ed 2, Edinburgh, 2006, Baillière Tindall.

Haemophilia Society: *An Introduction to Haemophilia*, 2008. Available online http://www.haemophilia.org.uk.

Health Protection Agency: *vCJD abnormal prion protein found in a patient with haemophilia at post mortem*, 2009. Available online http://www.hpa.org.uk/webw/HPAweb&HPAwebStandard/HPAweb_C/1234859690542?.

Hoffbrand AV, Moss PAH, Pettit JE: *Essential Haematology*, ed 5, Oxford, 2006, Blackwell Publishing.

Hoffbrand V, Provan D: Macrocytic anaemias. In Provan D, editor: *ABC of clinical haematology*, ed 3, Oxford, 2007, Blackwell, pp 6–10.

Howard MR, Hamilton PJ: *Haematology: An Illustrated Colour Text*, ed 3, Edinburgh, 2008, Churchill Livingstone.

Huether SE, McCance KL: *Understanding Pathophysiology*, ed 4, St Louis, 2008, Mosby.

Leukaemia and Lymphoma Research: *Dietary advice for patients with neutropaenia*, 2007. Available online http://www.beatbloodcancers.org/sites/default/files/Dietary%20advice%20for%20patients%20with%20neutropenia%20booklet.pdf.

Leukaemia and Lymphoma Research: *Adult acute myeloid leukaemia*, 2009a. Available online http://www.beatbloodcancers.org/.

Leukaemia and Lymphoma Research: *Chronic lymphocytic leukaemia*, 2009b. Available online http://www.beatbloodcancers.org/.

Leukaemia and Lymphoma Research: *Myelodysplastic syndromes (MDS)*, 2009c. Available online http://www.beatbloodcancers.org/.

Mehta A, Hoffbrand V: *Haematology at a Glance*, ed 3, Oxford, 2009, Blackwell Science.

Montané E, Ibáñez L, Vidal X, et al: for the Catalan Group for the Study of Agranulocytosis and Aplastic Anemia: Epidemiology of aplastic anemia: a prospective multicenter study, *Haematologica* 93:518–523, 2008.

National Institute for Health and Clinical Excellence (NICE): *Guidance on use of imatinib for chronic myeloid leukaemia. Technology Appraisal 70*, 2003. Available online http://www.nice.org.uk/nicemedia/pdf/TA70_Imatinib_fullguidance.pdf.

National Institute for Health and Clinical Excellence (NICE): *Bortezomid monotherapy for relapsed multiple myeloma. Technical appraisal 129*, 2007. Available online http://www.nice.org.uk/nicemedia/pdf/TA129Guidance.pdf.

National Institute for Health and Clinical Excellence (NICE): *Lenalidomide for the treatment of multiple myeloma in people who have received at least one prior therapy. Technical appraisal 171*, 2009. Available online http://www.nice.org.uk/nicemedia/pdf/TA171GuidanceWord.doc.

Parris E, Grant-Casey J: Promoting safer blood transfusion practice in hospital, *Nurs Stand* 21(41):35–38, 2007.

Provan D, editor: *ABC of clinical haematology*, Oxford, 2007, Blackwell Publishing.

SHOT (Serious Hazards of Transfusion): *Annual report 2007*, 2007. Available online http://www.shotuk.org/shot-reports/reports-and-summaries-2007/.

Sickle Cell Society: *Standards for the Clinical Care of Adults with Sickle Cell Disease in the UK*, 2008. Available online http://www.sicklecellsociety.org/pdf/CareBook.pdf.

Singer CRJ: Multiple myeloma and related conditions. In Provan D, editor: *ABC of clinical haematology*, Oxford, 2007, Blackwell Publishing, pp 45–51.

World Health Organization, UN Children's Fund and UN University: *Iron deficiency anaemia: assessment, prevention, and control. A guide for programme managers*, Geneva, 2001, WHO/NHD/01.3 WHO.

FURTHER READING

Daniels G, Bromilow I: *Essential guide to blood groups*, Oxford, 2007, Blackwell Publishing.

Dougherty L, Lister S, editors: *The Royal Marsden Hospital Manual of Clinical Nursing Procedures*, ed 7, Oxford, 2008, Wiley-Blackwell.

Ezzone S, Schmit-Pokorny K: *Blood and Marrow Stem Cell Transplantation*, ed 3, Boston, 2007, Jones and Bartlett Publishers.

Gray A, Illingworth J: *Right blood, right patient, right time. RCN guidance for improving transfusion practice*, London, 2005, Royal College of Nursing. Available online http://www.rcn.org.uk/__data/assets/pdf_file/0009/78615/002306.pdf.

Green J: Myelodysplastic syndromes. In Grundy M, editor: *Nursing in Haematological Oncology*, ed 2, Edinburgh, 2006, Baillière Tindall, pp 29–41.

Grundy M, editor: *Nursing in Haematological Oncology*, ed 2, Edinburgh, 2006, Baillière Tindall.

Liptrott S: Quality of life in stem cell transplant patients – a literature review, *Cancer Nursing Practice* 6(10):29–33, 2007.

Newcomb P: Pathophysiology of sickle cell disease crisis, *Emerg Nurse* 9(9):19–22, 2002.

Sickle Cell Society: *Standards for the Clinical Care of Adults with Sickle Cell Disease in the UK*, 2008. Available online http://www.sicklecellsociety.org/pdf/CareBook.pdf.

Smith PJ, Cox CL, Kelly D: Multiple myeloma: understanding the impact of the disease, *Cancer Nursing Practice* 6(1):25–28, 2007.

Tortora GJ, Derrickson B: *Principles of anatomy and physiology*, ed 12, New Jersey, 2009, John Wiley.

USEFUL WEBSITES

British Nutrition Foundation (BNF): www.nutrition.org.uk
Cancer Research UK: www.cancerresearchuk.org
Haemophilia Society: www.haemophilia.org.uk
Leukaemia and Lymphoma Research: www.beatbloodcancer.org
Lymphoma Association: www.lymphomas.org.uk
Myeloma UK: www.myelomaonline.org.uk
National Institute for Health and Clinical Excellence: www.nice.org.uk
NHS National Blood Service: www.blood.co.uk/index.html
SHOT Serious Hazards of Transfusion: www.shotuk.org
Sickle Cell Society: www.sicklecellsociety.org
UK Thalassaemia Society: www.ukts.org

Nursing patients with skin disorders

Jill Peters

Introduction

This chapter introduces dermatology nursing and the most common conditions encountered. Skin disorders range from minor conditions, resolved with over-the-counter (OTC) preparations, to potentially life-threatening skin conditions requiring intensive care and treatment (Skin failure p. 415). Many conditions are of a cyclical long-term nature with patients requiring care in different settings: inpatient, outpatient and community. Dermatology is a visual specialty and readers can access colour images in Further reading, e.g. Buxton 2003, the companion website and Useful websites.

Skin disorders are encountered in all fields of nursing. A good knowledge base helps the nurse to dispel myths about the contagious nature of skin disorders, as the psychosocial implications of skin disease should not be dismissed lightly. Success, power and achievement are often dependent on 'image'. The media support images of the soft-skinned baby, blemish-free teenager and smooth sophisticated adult, and such images are reflected in money spent by both genders who aspire to cosmetic perfection.

Various research-based tools, e.g. Dermatology Life Quality Index (DLQI) (Finlay & Khan 1994) are used to investigate the quality of life (QoL) of patients with skin disorders and how skin disease impacts on their life.

🖰 **See website for further content**

The experience of skin disease may restrict social, professional and personal activities and impact on careers and relationships. Problems with sexuality and relationships can be linked to low self-esteem and the self-concept of an altered body image associated with having a skin condition (Marks 2003). The psychological morbidity of skin disease is often unrecognised by professionals (Lewis-Jones 1999) despite patients reporting their experiences of ostracism, stigmatisation and isolation – the 'unclean leper' status of having a skin disorder (Box 12.1).

Epidemiology of skin diseases

Skin disease is common. Approximately 20% of the UK population have a skin disorder meriting medical management. The type, incidence and prevalence of skin disorders depend on social, economic, geographical, racial and cultural factors (Gawkrodger 2008). Internal and external factors contribute to skin disorders (Table 12.1). The economic implications of skin disease can be considerable for individuals, families and employers. Skin diseases are the most common group of occupational health problems leading to absence from work. Work-induced dermatoses (skin disease) leads to lost working time and often to compensation claims.

Age is an important factor in diagnosing disorders, some conditions being exclusive to a particular age group, and others persisting throughout life. Atopic eczema, for example, is most common in infancy, while acne develops in adolescence and normally wanes by the late 30s. Older people show expected degenerative skin changes, with 27% having malignant skin lesions. Psoriasis and eczema occur in all age groups and can be cyclical in nature throughout life.

Malignant melanoma, the deadliest form of skin cancer, is the second most common cancer in young adults (aged 15–34) (Cancer Research UK 2009a). It is largely preventable and may be curable if diagnosed and treated early (All Party Parliamentary Group [APPG] 2008). Non-melanoma skin cancer is also increasing with estimates suggesting doubling of rates every 10–20 years (APPG 2008). Current UK campaigns aim to change behaviour in relation to sunlight

exposure and to UVL during sunbed use by educating people that a suntan is a sign of damaged skin rather than a desirable fashion statement. People should be alert for specific changes, a vital factor in early detection of melanoma.

Genetic or hereditary factors can be relevant to the diagnosis, and a family history should be part of the assessment. Psychological stress (exams, divorce, etc.) is common as a trigger, but most skin disorders are stressful conditions in their own right. Certain skin disorders are recognised as being entirely of psychogenic origin, e.g. trichotillomania (breaking of hair).

Social factors impact on skin disorders, and improvements in standards of living, personal hygiene and nutrition have reduced the rate of certain skin disorders (Gawkrodger 2008). The current rise in the number of patients with asthma and eczema appears to be associated with environment changes of the home, e.g. central heating, carpeting, etc. Unemployment and low wages restrict job mobility and people with industrial skin diseases may have difficulty in changing jobs to alleviate the condition. Homelessness and poor housing create problems in maintaining skin care, the former often resulting in limited access to medical care.

The nurse's role

Patients with skin disorders and support groups have asserted their right to access specialist staff and be nursed in specialist areas (Department of Health [DH] 2004). If nurses can spend time talking with the patient, educating and demonstrating skin care techniques, it increases their confidence and potentially the patient becomes the 'expert' and the burden of skin care can be alleviated by supported self management (Dermatology Workforce Group 2007), a strategy that fits with Government position on long-term conditions (DH 2006).

Cure is not a word widely used in dermatology given the cyclical nature of many conditions, so nurses involved often forge long-term relationships with patients. Nurses with experience of chronic skin disease can help patients who require empathy and guidance from specialist practitioners who have the time, knowledge and willingness to share clinical skills with this motivated client group. Kurwa & Finlay (1995) reported inpatient management as improving QoL for dermatology patients, while peer group interaction between patients in dermatology wards is recognised as beneficial.

It is important to share this specialist knowledge with primary care nurses as 'care moves closer to the patient' with dermatology being one of the specialisms moving into the community from secondary care (DH 2006). The supportive role of nurses in primary care is vital. Only a small minority of patients are referred to dermatologists. Self-medication, OTC therapies and nurse prescribing mean that, for many, pharmacists and community teams are the first contact for most patients. The dermatology nurse specialist/practitioner/liaison uses educational input to support the primary care team in providing information and therapies that are valid, accurate and up-to-date and, in an advisory and consultative capacity, helps sustain continuity of care (Stone 1997). Dermatology nurse practitioners/specialists have introduced initiatives in many areas of practice such as nurse-led clinics for chronic disease management (eczema,

Table 12.1 External and internal factors causing skin disease	
EXTERNAL	**INTERNAL**
Ultraviolet light (UVL)/sunshine	Psychological factors/stress
Extremes of temperature – heat and cold	Genetic factors
Allergens	Systemic disease
Chemicals	Prescribed medications
Irritants	Herbal or over-the-counter products
Infections	Infections
Skin trauma/friction	Behavioural – scratching/picking

psoriasis, acne) utilising non-medical prescribing and managing patients with skin cancer. Nurses are therefore an important group within the dermatology team, playing a vital role in the provision of direct specialised care.

Anatomy and physiology

A brief outline of the structure and functions of the skin is provided. For further information readers should consult their own anatomy and physiology book.

Structure of the skin

The skin is composed of two layers: epidermis and dermis. Beneath these layers, a layer of subcutaneous fat protects and insulates the underlying structures.

Epidermis

The epidermis is composed of stratified epithelium and varies in thickness between different parts of the body; skin on the palms and soles is thicker than that on the face or back. The epidermis is avascular, the cells being nourished by means of diffusion of materials. Structures passing through the epidermis include hair follicles and sebaceous and sweat glands (Figure 12.1A). The epidermis has several layers, its health depending on three factors:

- regular division and migration of epidermal cells to the skin surface
- gradual keratinisation of these cells
- desquamation or rubbing away of these cells.

The layers of the epidermis are (Figure 12.1B):

Basal layer (stratum basale) The cells lying nearest the dermis form the germinative layer where cell division occurs. Cells migrate upwards from this layer, becoming keratinised over a period of 21–28 days before being shed.

Prickle cell layer (stratum spinosum) Cells in this layer have intercellular connections that protect against shearing forces or trauma to the skin.

Granular layer (stratum granulosum) This layer contains keratohyalin, a precursor of keratin, which gradually replaces the cytoplasm of the cells.

Clear cell layer (stratum lucidum) Present only where the skin is thickened, e.g. the soles of feet. The cells exhibit nuclear degeneration and contain large amounts of keratin. Skin injury or friction increases cell production, resulting in a callus or corn.

Cornified, horny layer (stratum corneum) Comprises thin, flat, non-nucleated cells, the cytoplasm of which has been totally replaced by keratin.

The epidermal/dermal junction is convoluted into dips and ridges which help to prevent damage to the skin from shearing forces. The configuration of these ridges is visible at the epidermal surface as corresponding characteristic, individualised patterns, e.g. at the fingertips.

Dermis

The dermis is composed of fibrous connective tissue providing a supportive meshwork for the structures and organs within. The papillary layer has many capillaries and lies next to the basal layer of the epidermis. The reticular layer, lying above the subcutaneous fat layer, has fewer blood vessels and is less reactive.

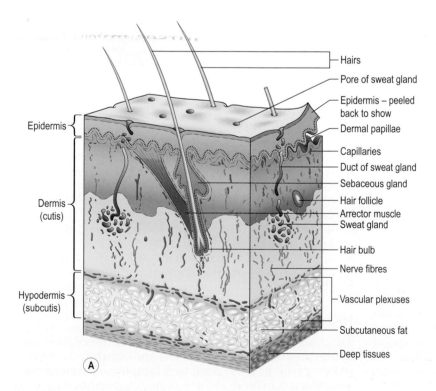

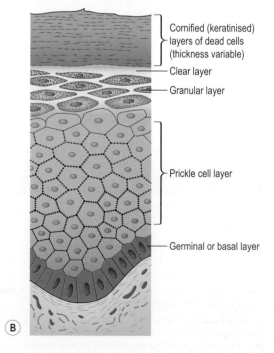

Figure 12.1 A. The structure of the skin. B. The layers of the epidermis.

The ground substance of the dermis is a jelly-like material acting as a support and a transport medium. Tissue mast cells are often found near hair follicles and blood vessels, producing heparin and histamine when damaged. Tissue macrophages engulf foreign particles within the dermis.

Fibroblasts generate collagen fibres, a process requiring vitamin C. These strong fibres bind with water molecules to give skin its tight, 'plump' appearance. Elastin fibres are also formed by fibroblasts. They are bound loosely around bundles of collagen and, in combination with the ground substance and collagen, help the dermis to maintain its characteristic properties.

Lymph vessels drain excess tissue fluid and plasma proteins from the dermis, thereby maintaining correct volume and composition of tissue fluids.

Specialised nerve endings (sensory receptors) present in the dermis and basal layer of the epidermis detect mechanical and thermal changes (see Ch. 22).

Glands

Sweat glands are coiled tubes of epithelial tissue opening as pores onto the skin surface. They have individual nerve and blood supplies and secrete a slightly acid fluid containing excess excretory products (water, salts). Sweat glands are of two types: eccrine and apocrine. Eccrine glands are controlled by the sympathetic nervous system, producing secretions in response to temperature elevation or fear. Apocrine glands in the pubic and axillary areas are not functional until puberty. They are thought to secrete pheromones, chemical signals released into the external environment.

Sebaceous glands are lined with epidermal tissue, secreting sebum, a greasy, slightly acid substance which helps to form a waterproof covering over the skin and, like sweat, to keep the keratin supple. The acid sebum has antibacterial and antifungal properties. Most sebaceous glands open into hair follicles (collectively a pilosebaceous unit). Sebum production is influenced by sex hormone levels.

Functions of the skin

Intact skin is vital to health and well-being. As the largest organ in the body, weighing approximately 4 kg, and having a surface area of $2\ m^2$, the skin has many vital functions (Hughes 2001):

- protection
- sensation
- vitamin D synthesis
- temperature regulation
- insulation and protection of internal organs
- a barrier to harmful external factors.

Protection

The horny layer forms a waterproof seal against undue entry or loss of water. The skin surface protects against microorganisms (through its acidity) and acts as a barrier to chemicals, gases and gamma and beta radiation. Internal structures are shielded by the skin from minor mechanical trauma, and repeated pressure or friction stimulates an increase in cell division, producing thickened areas of skin, e.g. corns and calluses. Melanin produced in the basal layer of the epidermis screens the dermis from UVL.

Sensation

Nerve endings continually monitor the environment and are most highly concentrated in areas such as the fingertips and lips. Innervated hair follicles help the individual to avoid injury by stimulating reflex action in response to touch.

Vitamin D synthesis

Epidermal cells produce 7-dehydrocholesterol, which is slowly converted to vitamin D when skin is exposed to UVL (see Chs 10, 21).

Temperature regulation

The skin is vital in temperature regulation (see Ch. 22). In cold conditions heat is conserved by vasoconstriction and generated by the involuntary muscular action of shivering. Body hair becomes erect to trap warm air on the skin. During overheating, sweating is induced and vasodilatation occurs. As sweat evaporates from the skin, latent heat is lost from the skin surface, causing it to cool. Vasodilatation allows large quantities of blood to circulate in the uppermost layers of the dermis. Heat is then lost through convection, radiation and conduction. Blood flow is controlled to direct blood either to the capillary bed closer to the skin surface (maximum heat loss) or to the deeper tissues of the skin (minimising heat loss).

Other functions

During starvation, subcutaneous fat is utilised both as an energy source and as a water reserve. The dermis functions as a water reservoir which may also be utilised by the body in an emergency, e.g. haemorrhage. The skin is able to absorb various substances, a property utilised for the administration of various drugs. The skin also has an excretory function, with urea and salts being excreted in small amounts through sweat.

Skin assessment

In completing a comprehensive skin assessment, it is important to obtain a full history, which should include:

- onset, initial site and duration of the condition
- associated symptoms, e.g. itch, redness
- actions that worsen the condition, e.g. sunlight exposure
- family history, e.g. genetic predisposition, allergies
- associated systemic disorders, e.g. asthma, hay fever
- current medication – oral and topical therapies, prescribed, OTC or illegal
- social history – occupation, hobbies, housing, alcohol/ drug intake
- impact of the disorder on daily life – personal coping strategies, self-esteem and self image
- allergies.

History taking

The history should reveal the person's description and understanding of the disorder as well as their perception of living with it. It can often be a symptom of systemic disease or a condition in its own right, e.g. pruritus may indicate liver disease/low ferritin or dry skin. An effective assessment should determine the impact of the skin disorder on those around the patient. Skin disease, with all its social implications, has a major cultural impact that varies within a multicultural society. Cultural beliefs need to be identified if treatment programmes are to be adapted to acknowledge such issues. It is important to ask patients what they have already used to treat their skin disorder. Many OTC preparations or treatments, borrowed from well-meaning friends, can exacerbate an existing skin condition. When examining skin, the nurse must have knowledge of 'normal' skin to be able to identify the abnormal at any age.

Physical examination

The entire skin surface is examined to determine the extent of the disorder. Touch is very important – lightly run the tips of the fingers over the skin surface. Palpation of skin lesions will determine changes in skin texture with associated crusting or scaling. In skin disorders, the term 'lesion' describes a small area of disease, while an 'eruption' or 'rash' describes widespread skin involvement.

See website for further content

Skin assessment includes routine examination of the hair and nails as changes can aid diagnosis, e.g. nail changes in psoriasis or fungal infection. The distribution of lesions can vary. Psoriasis tends to localise on the outer aspects of elbows and knees, while eczema is most common in the skin flexures.

During assessment, the nurse should recognise that skin changes can be a manifestation of systemic disorders, e.g. liver disease. Peters (2001) reminds the nurse to recognise the wide diversity of skin colour and pigmentation in society. The pathophysiology of the disorder will be unchanged, but skin pigmentation can influence skin changes during illness.

See website for further content

Communication with patients is important for accurate assessment, as a patient's description of symptoms is relevant to diagnosis and management. Initial nursing management involves alleviation of distressing symptoms while awaiting diagnosis.

The nurse should also recognise that the effect of the physical appearance of a skin disorder on quality of life is often viewed by the patient as being of greater importance than the discomfort of having abnormal skin (Lewis-Jones 1999).

Investigations

Investigations assist with the process of elimination or act as supporting evidence to develop a working diagnosis. Interpretation of the result is important, while identifying the relevance to the current clinical picture and the patient.

Common investigations include:

- skin swabs (bacterial or viral)
- skin scraping/nail clippings/hair debris (mycology)
- skin biopsy (histopathology)
- blood tests, e.g. full blood count, immunoglobulin E (IgE), etc.
- patch testing
- prick testing.

See website for further content and website
Figures 12.1–12.5

Principles of therapy in skin disorders

This section outlines the range of treatments used to treat skin disorders. They are often used in combinations of topical and systemic treatments.

Topical therapies

Topical therapies are usually known as first-line treatments and are applied directly on the skin which is the target organ and readily accessible. Various classes of topical preparations are used (Box 12.2).

Ongoing commitment is needed to maintain treatment as topical therapies can be messy, time-consuming and smelly (Box 12.3). Treatment programmes often have to be customised because therapeutic responses can differ with each patient.

Box 12.2 Information

Classification of topical preparations

- Creams – have a light effect due to high water content. They rub in easily and cool the skin.
- Lotions – used if skin is 'weeping'. Good for scalp treatment as they are not greasy to apply.
- Ointments – greasy preparations used as a base for the drug being applied. They last for 6–8 h on the skin, encouraging absorption by a barrier effect.
- Pastes – ointments applied to medicated bandages for occlusive use or used in combination as a stiffer paste to apply treatment directly to lesions. This permits a slower, more effective absorption on the target sites.

Box 12.3 Reflection

Advantages and disadvantages of topical therapy
Advantages
- Drug delivered directly to target area
- Reduces systemic absorption
- Patient can view improvement
- Side-effects easily identified

Disadvantages
- Time-consuming
- Messy and potential to stain clothing
- Preparations smell or stain the skin
- Patient can see deterioration or lack of improvement
- Inability to apply to oneself due to lack of dexterity

Activities
- Reflect on the advantages that would motivate you to persevere with topical therapy, and the disadvantages most likely to stop you using the treatment.
- Discuss with your mentor how you would deal with the disadvantages while teaching a patient how to use their medication.

Regular nursing assessment will identify improvements or deterioration and allow treatment to be amended appropriately. A maintenance programme is needed as well as the treatment response for a flare. The patient needs to have the therapies at home so they can also use them immediately a flare occurs – step-up step-down. In order to achieve the desired outcome, the skilled practitioner needs a sound knowledge of dermatology therapies balanced with abilities to educate, support and motivate the patient to complete lengthy treatment programmes.

A fire hazard is associated with the use of paraffin-based skin products (National Patient Safety Agency 2007) and nurses must alert patients to this danger.

Emollients

Agents which moisturise and lubricate the skin are the mainstay of dermatological treatment. They are used in different forms such as soap substitute/bath additives or leave-on preparations. They can be used in skin maintenance programmes and are vital in preparing the skin for the specific therapies available for different disorders, e.g. tar, corticosteroids. The choice of emollient depends on the disorder:

- Dry, hyperkeratotic skin – use oily occlusive ointments.
- Flaky, rough, excoriated skin – use grease-based preparations.
- Erythematous, inflamed skin – benefits from the cooling effect of water-soluble creams.

Patients may use a combination of emollients for different areas of the body. Taking time to demonstrate application technique and trial different moisturisers so the patient is involved in choice (Peters et al 2008) is key to compliance. For further information see Ersser et al (2007) and Useful websites, e.g. Dermatology UK.

Topical corticosteroids

Topical corticosteroids should be applied after the topical emollient or bathing with a bath oil or soap substitute to the affected areas only. Advice given about the use of topical corticosteroids should be balanced: they are safe to use but often patients are anxious because there is emphasis on thinning of the skin

The potential side-effects, such as skin thinning, bruising/purpura, hirsutism, systemic effects, etc., depend on the age, site and frequency of the product used. A recent review stated that 'the intermittent use of topical corticosteroids is highly effective; bears little risk, and is relatively inexpensive' (Hengge et al 2006, p. 12).

A concern with children is that they are more prone to the development of systemic reactions based on their higher ratio of total body surface area to body weight. Epidermal thinning does occur within 1–3 weeks of treatment with potent or very potent topical steroids on normal skin but reverses within 4 weeks of stopping (O'Donoghue 2005). It is now recognised that emollient therapy is potentially steroid sparing (Grimalt et al 2007) and this potentially corrects the defect in the skin barrier, so using emollient therapy for washing, bathing and as a leave-on preparation is key to the day to day management with intermittent use of topical corticosteroids.

Other topical therapies

Other topical therapies used include:

- vitamin D analogues or dithranol for psoriasis
- cleansers, vitamin A analogues or antibiotics for acne
- fluorouracil, diclofenac sodium, imiquimod for sun-damaged skin or basal cell carcinoma (BCC).

Each therapy has to be applied in a different manner and nurses advising the patient must know the difference and the potential effect it has on the skin in order to advise the patient. See Useful websites, e.g. British Dermatological Nursing Group (BDNG).

Systemic therapies

A range of oral medication, from antibiotics to immunosuppressant to biological drugs, is used to treat long-term inflammatory conditions as well as acute inflammatory or bullous conditions. Monitoring of patients on oral medication is often undertaken by dermatology nurses who work as non-medical prescribers: they interpret blood results and alter doses or initiate alternative therapies used in conjunction with topical therapies (see Useful websites, e.g. The British Association of Dermatologists). Nurses must know the potential side-effects of topical and systemic therapies in order to provide safe care and when necessary be able to adjust therapy accordingly.

Phototherapy (ultraviolet light B)

Certain skin disorders, most commonly psoriasis and eczema, can be treated with ultraviolet light B (UVB) in measured doses. UVB is the wavelength in natural sunlight responsible for sunburn. Treatment requires outpatient attendance two to three times weekly over a period of weeks. Phototherapy is given in a cabinet with fluorescent lamps emitting UVB.

🖱 **See website Figure 12.6**

A test dose administered to the patient's back determines a safe starting dose. This dose is gradually increased over the treatment period.

Photochemotherapy (psoralen and ultraviolet light A)

The treatment combination of psoralen and ultraviolet light A (PUVA) requires the patient to take oral psoralen (a natural plant extract) 2 h before exposure to UVA. Photochemotherapy is given in a cabinet with fluorescent lamps emitting UVA.

🖱 **See website Figure 12.7**

Bath PUVA (methoxypsoralen lotion) is a treatment in which a measured amount of psoralen is added to 150 L of bath water. Patients soak for a specific time, pat the skin dry and then treatment is given in a UVA light cabinet. Again, psoriasis and eczema can both be treated with PUVA. A test dose is administered to determine a safe starting dose and treatment is given in twice weekly sessions.

Patients having light therapy wear protective goggles during UVB/PUVA exposure. After PUVA they must also wear dark glasses for 24 h to protect the eye if psoralen is taken orally. UVB/PUVA is administered in specialist units to ensure accurate recording of the amount of light therapy given, as guidelines exist that restrict the amount a patient may receive.

Complementary therapies

The increasing interest in complementary therapies to treat skin disorders reflects a rise in public awareness of non-traditional approaches to treatment, perhaps stimulated by the failure of orthodox medicine to provide 'cures'. The nurse is ideally placed to discuss both the orthodox and complementary options available. Discussion should focus on the safe use of complementary therapies initiated by referral to a practitioner who has undergone accredited training and is a licensed practitioner with insurance. Complementary therapy should be considered as an adjunct and not as an alternative to routine therapies.

DISORDERS OF THE SKIN

Psoriasis

Psoriasis is a chronic, non-infectious inflammatory skin disorder characterised by well-demarcated erythematous plaques with adherent silver scales. The epidermal cell proliferation rate increases greatly, while epidermal turnover time is reduced. Psoriasis is prevalent in 2% of the UK population, yet the cause remains unknown. It can occur in any age group and is characterised by exacerbations and remissions. Genetic influences predispose to the condition, with 35% of patients showing a family history.

Precipitating/aggravating factors include:

- infection – streptococcal throat infection
- medications – can exacerbate or trigger psoriasis
- sunlight – in some patients, psoriasis improves during the summer and relapses during the winter; however, others report that sunlight aggravates the condition
- hormonal change – psoriasis can get better or worse during pregnancy or during the climacteric
- alcohol – can exacerbate the condition
- psychological stress – can exacerbate psoriasis, but the condition itself is recognised as stressful
- trauma – creates the 'Köebner effect' where psoriasis is triggered in damaged skin, e.g. the site of an injury or surgical scar.

Psoriasis varies from mild forms, with plaques localised to the knees and elbows, to severe forms which are potentially life threatening. Classification of psoriasis is made on clinical presentation or location (Weller et al 2008).

Guttate presents as drop-like symmetrical lesions on the trunk and limbs. It is most common in adolescents and young adults and is often triggered by a streptococcal throat infection.

Plaque presents as well-demarcated, erythematous plaques covered in dry, white waxy scale often localised to the knees and elbows (Figure 12.2). Plaques vary in size and extend to cover the trunk and scalp. Plaque psoriasis tends to be chronic, with exacerbations and periods of remission.

Flexural affects the axillae, submammary and anogenital areas. Plaques are sharply defined but the skin has a thin glistening redness, often with painful fissures in the skin folds.

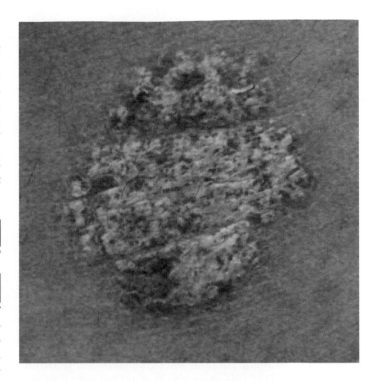

Figure 12.2 Plaque psoriasis – erythema with silvery scale and a well-demarcated edge.

Pustular is a localised form affecting the hands and feet. It is characterised by yellow/brown pustules which dry into brown scaly macules (Figure 12.3). It is a painful condition, difficult to treat and linked to smoking and very debilitating.

Generalised pustular is a rare yet serious form of the disease. Sheets of sterile pustules develop, merging on an

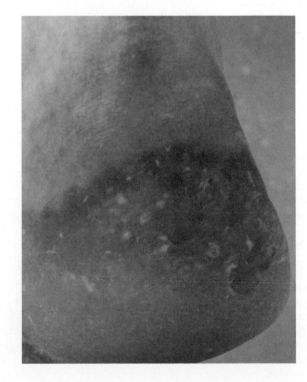

Figure 12.3 Pustular psoriasis – sterile pustules along the demarcated edge.

erythematous background. These areas of skin shear and the patient will present with pyrexia and malaise and require hospital admission. It is often triggered when attempts are made to withdraw oral or topical corticosteroids, or may just reflect the instability of the condition.

Scalp can often be the sole manifestation of the disorder. Thick scale adheres to the scalp and can extend to the scalp margin and behind the ears.

Nail changes Psoriasis can involve pitting of nails and onycholysis, where the distal edge of the nail separates from the nail bed. There is no effective topical treatment for psoriatic nail changes.

Erythrodermic is a rare but severe form of skin failure that can be life threatening and warrants hospital admission. The skin becomes uniformly red due to high blood flow volume. The patient feels unwell and maintaining body temperature is difficult. It can be triggered by the irritant effects of therapies, or by withdrawal of oral/systemic corticosteroids or by a medication reaction. The condition can progress to a generalised pustular psoriasis.

Psoriatic arthropathy is a rheumatoid-like arthritis affecting about 5% of psoriatic patients. Joint changes occur in hands, feet, spine and sacroiliac joints. This arthropathy mimics rheumatoid disease but notably the rheumatoid factor test is negative (see Ch. 10). Psoriatic arthropathy is difficult to treat, meriting the combined expertise of a rheumatologist and a dermatologist.

PATHOPHYSIOLOGY

The epidermis thickens, with an associated increased blood flow to the skin, and becomes raised to accommodate skin changes (parakeratosis) (Figure 12.4). Epidermal cell proliferation rate increases. The transit time of epidermal cells maturing through normal skin is approximately 21–28 days, whereas in psoriasis it is 4 days. The increased cell production and transit time mean that cells do not keratinise completely and so cannot be shed. This causes the build-up of a white, waxy silver scale as immature skin cells remain adherent to the skin. Psoriasis results from an increase in activity of dividing cells associated with an increase in their rate of reproduction. The cause is not fully understood but is interlinked with the immune system.

Common presenting signs/symptoms include:

- *Pain.* Fissures form, particularly on hands and feet, because of loss of flexibility in the thickened epidermis.
- *Erythema.* Generalised redness and heat loss.
- *Scaling.* A build-up of cells creates the silver-scale appearance diagnostic of psoriasis.
- *Pustules.* In inflammatory conditions, an infiltration of white blood cells is normal. Increased infiltration in pustular psoriasis accumulates as microabscesses in the outer layer of the skin.
- *Pruritus (itch).* Many textbooks describe psoriasis as non-itchy, but patients often report itch to be troublesome.
- *Sore throat.* In guttate psoriasis.

MEDICAL MANAGEMENT

Where possible, psoriasis is managed on an outpatient basis, but the severity of activity in erythrodermic/pustular psoriasis will result in hospital admission to prevent potential life-threatening complications of an unstable psoriatic state and to move the patient into remission.

Investigations

Diagnosis can be made from the clinical picture and relevant history:

- skin biopsy
- throat swab
- Auspitz sign – gentle removal of the silvery scale from a plaque reveals pinpoint bleeding from the dilated superficial capillaries
- blood tests – if considering systemic therapy.

Treatment

This may involve topical and systemic medication and phototherapy. PUVA and UVB are effective therapies for psoriasis (see p. 402). The combination of therapies chosen depends on diagnosis and severity of the disorder, topical prescribed therapies being the mainstay of psoriasis treatment (see Nursing management and health promotion section pp. 405–406).

Medication Combined systemic and topical medication is useful in the management of psoriasis. Systemic medications used include:

- antihistamines – alleviate itch and promote sleep and rest

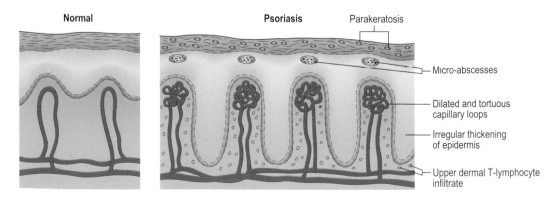

Figure 12.4 Histology of psoriasis. (Reproduced from Boon et al 2006 with permission.)

- analgesics – reduce the pain and discomfort of inflamed skin
- antibiotics – for streptococcal throat infections.

The majority of patients with psoriasis respond to topical therapies, but the more extensive forms of psoriasis may require a systemic approach (Weller et al 2008). Medications that are particularly important in this regard are methotrexate, ciclosporin, retinoids (e.g. acitretin) and biologics (e.g. etanercept).

 See website for further content

Nursing management and health promotion: psoriasis

The goals of nursing management will vary depending on the type and severity of the person's psoriasis. If the epidermal barrier is breached as in severe erythroderma leading to acute skin failure, measures are needed to support the epidermal barrier (see Skin failure, p. 415). Generalised pustular psoriasis and erythrodermic psoriasis can be life-threatening conditions requiring skilled nursing.

 See website Critical thinking question 12.1

Intensive nursing care is essential for comfort, preventing infection, and monitoring and acting on the early signs or noting change in general health status.

However, the majority of people manage their condition at home by themselves or by family members. Applying topical therapies can be time consuming and messy with the need to carry out additional washing and vacuuming to remove shed skin scale. The role of the nurse is to:

- support self care, exchanging explanations on techniques of application of the different therapies
- discuss life activities/style to reduce potential causes of exacerbations while promoting confidence and reducing stress
- work in collaboration with patient/family to achieve the maximum benefit for the minimal risk of the therapy (topical or systemic).

Many patients who have a long-term skin disorder such as psoriasis may wish to use a complementary treatment (see p. 403). Acupuncture, hypnotherapy and aromatherapy have all been used with varying degrees of success.

Psychological support

People react to events differently and so it is important to ask the patient about how the psoriasis affects their everyday life. This sometimes can be obvious in that they are too self-conscious to expose their skin to go to the gym or swimming. Use of excessive clothing hides their skin from public view or even from their partners through embarrassment. A referral to a clinical psychologist may be needed to work with the patient on areas of body image, sexuality, quality of life and personal coping strategies. These are all management considerations, and effective counselling can enhance the therapeutic effect.

Management of topical therapy

A range of topical therapies are used for outpatient management of psoriasis. By talking together, the patient and nurse can choose the therapies that fit into the patient's lifestyle and if necessary ensure that there is someone at home to assist. It is important to review the patient once therapies are commenced and to adjust accordingly. Of course, all therapies take some weeks to cause improvement so a realistic timeframe is essential. The nurse should also explain the different preparations used, giving advice on correct application/location of use on the body and potential side-effects. By providing clear information and ongoing psychological support, the nurse can help to ensure the patient perseveres with treatment. Specific considerations in using topical preparations are as follows:

Emollients Bland emollients (e.g. emulsifying ointment) moisturise and lubricate the skin, helping to ease scaling and promote comfort. Regular applications seal the stratum cornum, thus reducing transdermal heat and fluid loss, which is particularly relevant in erythrodermic psoriasis. Erythrodermic or generalised pustular psoriasis is often treated with emollients initially to allow fiery skin to 'settle' before other treatments. Emollient bath additives, e.g. Oilatum®, and soap substitutes, such as aqueous cream, are available.

Coal tar ointments are usually blended with white soft paraffin and have an anti-pruritic, anti-inflammatory and keratolytic effect. Low concentrations are used initially and gradually increased according to the tolerance of the skin. Tar applications are messy and smelly and they stain, so tend to be used for inpatient treatment. Proprietary blends of cleaner tar creams are available for outpatient therapy; some may be more appropriate for the face/hairline and skin folds than crude coal tar.

Patients must be advised that if ointment irritates or burns the skin, it should be removed immediately in an emollient bath and advice sought.

Dithranol suppresses cell proliferation. It is available in many forms, but patients must be informed that it can stain skin and clothes; staining can last for 10–14 days after treatment has finished. If the patient is attending daily to a day unit then dithranol is applied by spatula to affected skin and powdered or covered with stockinette gauze to prevent the ointment spreading to surrounding skin. It then stays on the skin between 1 and 12 hours before being cleaned off. This procedure is time consuming and messy but effective. For outpatient therapy, short-contact treatment is available. Cream is applied to the plaque and removed 30–60 minutes later.

Vitamin D analogues such as calcipotriol are applied as a cream or ointment directly to plaques. They are non-messy, non-staining and well tolerated. Calcipotriol inhibits cell proliferation and stimulates epidermal cell differentiation, correcting the increased cell turnover time associated with psoriasis. It can be combined with corticosteroids. Due to potential systemic absorption, there is a restriction on the quantities (100 g) to be applied over 1 week. This restriction will relate to the extent and severity of the psoriasis and it is important that patients are aware of the prescriptive guidelines.

Corticosteroids Immunosuppressants can be useful to reduce itch on body or scalp. Newer combinations of corticosteroids and vitamin D analogues can be useful in chronic plaque psoriasis but should be pulsed, e.g. 4 weeks daily then take a break, or if psoriasis is still present switch to plain vitamin D analogues.

PUVA/UVB (see p. 402). The treatment programme varies for each individual depending on identification of skin type and tolerance of sunlight. Koek et al (2009) found that UVB phototherapy administered at home is as safe and effective as that given in outpatient departments. Moreover, using the treatment at home reduced the burden of treatment and increased patient satisfaction. Retinoids can be given with PUVA to stimulate more rapid skin clearance at lower total doses of UVL.

🖱 See website for further content

Goeckerman regimen An effective combination treatment comprising a tar bath prior to exposure to UVL.

Ingram regimen A combination therapy involving tar baths, UVL and dithranol applications.

Cocois ointment A blend of tar, emulsifying ointment and salicylic acid used to treat scalp psoriasis. It is gently massaged into the scalp, left overnight/occluded overnight with a showercap and removed with shampoo of the patient's choice.

Olive oil (warmed) reduces the build-up of scale on the scalp.

Eczema

Eczema describes a range of inflammatory skin disorders. The aetiology of eczema is unknown. Most classifications of eczematous skin disorders use the term 'eczema' synonymously with 'dermatitis', as both terms apply to the inflammatory skin changes provoked by either internal (endogenous) or external (exogenous) factors. Eczema may result from one or both types of factor (Gawrodger 2008).

Priorities of medical and nursing management are similar for all classifications of eczema. In common with other skin conditions some types of eczema can lead to life-threatening skin failure (see p. 415).

Endogenous eczema

Atopic eczema

Atopic eczema is a common inflammatory skin disorder affecting 20% of infants in the UK; there are associated genetic and environmental factors. Atopy covers the classification of related disorders, e.g. asthma, eczema and hay fever. Atopic eczema can be a chronic itchy distressing disorder, having a major impact on a child's behaviour and quality of life and causing severe disruption to family life. Strict diagnostic criteria are followed (National Institute for Health and Clinical Excellence [NICE] 2007). Infantile eczema can resolve spontaneously but sometimes progresses to a chronic pattern of episodic exacerbations. Commonly affected sites are the flexural aspects of knees and elbows with involvement of the face and wrists. The pattern of distribution can alter into adulthood and late onset can be very distressing to the older person. (Figure 12.5). See Further reading, e.g. Royal College of Nursing (2008).

Pompholyx eczema

This is a 'blistering' eczema localised to palms and soles. It develops rapidly, causes acute discomfort and can become secondarily infected. The cause is unknown and outbreaks

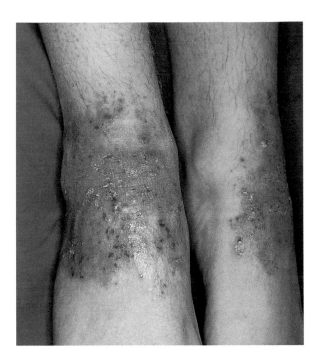

Figure 12.5 Atopic (subacute) eczema on the fronts of the ankle in a teenager. These are sites of predilection, along with the cubital and popliteal fossae, in atopic eczema. (Reproduced from Boon et al 2006 with permission.)

can be linked to heat/humidity or reaction of contact dermatitis or fungal infections.

Discoid eczema

Characteristic symmetrical coin-shaped lesions affect the limbs and can be intensely itchy. It is more common in middle-aged and older people and may only last for a few weeks.

Asteatotic eczema

This mainly affects older people, commonly on the lower legs. It appears to be associated with a deficiency of sebaceous secreting glands, resulting in excessive dryness and scaling of the skin. Central heating, diuretic therapy and over-frequent washing are also implicated as possible causes.

Varicose eczema

Chronic patchy eczema of the legs occurs, with or without the presence of a venous ulcer (see Ch. 23). It is associated with chronic venous stasis, and there may be varicose veins, oedema and pigmentation of the skin (due to haemosiderin from the blood leaking through capillary walls) (Gawrodger 2008). The area involved may become itchy and hot to touch and a secondary response may produce associated eczematous areas on other parts of the body.

Exogenous eczema

Irritant contact dermatitis

This is very common, especially in industrial/work settings. It usually erupts at the maximum point of contact, but presentation varies according to the nature of the irritant contact. The epidermis may be damaged by water or abrasion, and the effect of the irritant, e.g. cement, is exacerbated by rubbing against clothing. Epidermal necrosis may occur within hours of contact with strong chemicals, while eczema triggered by milder substances, e.g. detergents, may take longer to evolve. Many patients with atopic eczema appear prone to irritant contact dermatitis and should be advised to avoid work where exposure to irritants could occur.

Allergic contact dermatitis

In this condition the skin develops a specific immunological hypersensitivity. The most common allergy is to nickel (found in inexpensive jewellery/body piercing). Continued exposure to the allergen results in an eczematous response, ranging from mild to severe. Allergy patch testing may identify the allergen; in many cases a change of job or avoidance of the allergen may be necessary (Weller et al 2008). The most difficult cases to treat are those in which allergic contact dermatitis is suspected but no definitive triggering factor is found.

PATHOPHYSIOLOGY

The skin generally becomes drier to the touch and then erythema and swelling caused by vasodilatation and oedema occur. The erythema may be generalised or limited to localised areas. It can be exacerbated by scratching extending to an exudative, scaling and crusting phase. Blistering can occur as part of the inflammatory process.

In chronic conditions involving recurrent exacerbations, the skin is scaly, excoriated, thickened and pigmented. The eczematous areas will be localised to more defined parts of the body and lichenification will be apparent (Figure 12.6). Lichenification is the skin's response to mechanical damage (rubbing/scratching) in which the affected areas become thickened, toughened and show a marked exaggeration of normal skin markings. Painful fissuring of the skin occurs as normal elasticity is lost.

Common presenting symptoms

- *Itch (pruritus)* accompanies most eczematous conditions and can be acute and distressing. The itch–scratch–itch cycle quickly becomes established. The skin is well supplied with sensory nerves that respond quickly to the mechanical stimulation of scratching or any external stimulation.

- *Redness.* Inflammatory skin diseases cause vasodilatation of blood vessels feeding the skin, leading to generalised total body redness (erythroderma) (see p. 415). In atopic eczema, white dermographism can be evoked – firm strokes of the skin normally produce a 'weal and flare' response, a pink raised weal lasting about 30 min, but in atopic patients a simple white line arises, with no erythema.
- *Fissures/lichenification.* In the chronic stages there is also a generalised thickening of some layers of the skin over flexures or any area traumatised by scratching. Open fissures are painful and slow to heal.
- *Infections.* Primary or secondary bacterial infections (e.g. *Staphylococcus* or *Streptococcus*) can exacerbate eczema. Patients with atopic eczema tend to be more susceptible to viral infections, e.g. eczema herpeticum (see p. 412).

MEDICAL MANAGEMENT

Diagnosis is made from the presentation and the patient's history. Many of the exogenous conditions are managed in an outpatient setting; however, severe exacerbations warrant hospital admission.

Investigations

Precise diagnosis may require all or a combination of the following.

Laboratory investigations may include:

- skin swabs – excoriated lesions may result in secondary infection
- skin scrapings – to exclude fungal infection
- skin biopsy – for immunohistological examination when the diagnosis is in doubt
- blood test – to ascertain the level of IgE or the presence of specific antibodies to external factors, e.g. house dust mite, pollen, cat/dog or food proteins
- prick tests – to ascertain type 1 reaction to specific allergens, e.g. house dust mite (see Ch. 3).

Patch testing may be carried out to confirm allergic contact dermatitis. A range of patch tests is available in which suspected allergens, e.g. nickel, fragrance, hairdressing products, plant material and rubber, are made up in a concentration which would normally produce no reaction unless the patient was sensitive to them.

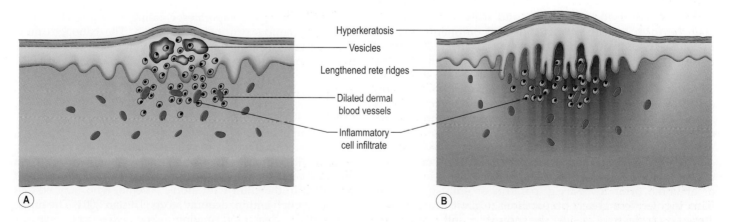

Hyperkeratosis

Vesicles

Lengthened rete ridges

Dilated dermal blood vessels

Inflammatory cell infiltrate

(A)   (B)

Figure 12.6 The histology of acute (A) and chronic (B) dermatitis.

Treatment

This is topical, systemic or both.

Topical therapies (see Nursing management and health promotion section below)

- First line treatment for dry skin is emollient therapy and the avoidance of products, e.g. soap, that remove the skin's natural moisturising factor (NMF).
- Soap substitutes or bath additives cleanse the skin without removing the NMF. 'Leave-on' skin preparations help restore the epidermal barrier.
- Second line treatment is the use of corticosteroids to suppress the inflammation and reduce itch. Sometimes combined with an antibiotic for local infection.
- Bandaging.

Systemic medication therapy

- Antihistamines – to reduce itch; the side-effect of drowsiness may aid sleep and rest.
- Antibiotics – to treat bacterial infection, specifically *Staphylococcus aureus*, for generalised infection.
- Analgesics – to ease heat, tenderness and localised pain. (Further information about drugs used is available on the companion website.)

  See website for further content

▷ Nursing management and health promotion: eczema

The immediate priority is to alleviate discomfort. A tired, hot, itchy patient is not in an ideal state to absorb information and learn self-care techniques, and therefore an immediate and sympathetic approach to care is important. Ongoing support and reassurance are fundamental to achieving long-term goals. Informing the patient about eczema, triggers, treatments and techniques of applications creates greater understanding of the condition and its outlook.

Substantial time and effort can be required to motivate, educate and empower the patient to share condition management. Patients and families should be informed of relevant support groups (see Useful websites, e.g. National Eczema Society).

Nursing considerations in topical therapy

Emollients

Emollients are used to make dry and scaly skin smoother, take the form of bath oils, creams and ointments and are the mainstay of treatment. Itch, heat and dryness all respond promptly to lubrication. Many emollients create a barrier for inflamed skin, preventing further fluid/heat loss. Eczema is a condition in which the skin is chronically dry, so long-term use of emollients maintains good skin moisture. Patients should be advised to avoid perfumed products and use prescribed bath additives and soap substitutes. When bathing, water temperature, length of immersion and the hardness of water can affect eczema (McNally et al 1998). Very greasy preparations are used when the skin is very dry in hospital or at home prior to bed e.g. paraffin or emulsifying wax base. Lighter/less greasy preparations, e.g. oil/water based, are used for daytime or over the summer months. Many are available in a pump dispenser to encourage use.

Emollient preparations should be applied lightly, with smooth downward strokes in the direction of hair growth to prevent follicle blockage, inflammation and infection. Rubbing creates heat in the skin causing itch, and if emollient is applied thickly it traps body heat causing itching. Frequent applications are needed throughout the day.

Corticosteroids

Topical corticosteroid therapy will have a major impact on the eczematous skin, therefore it is important that the patient understands the correct methods of application. Absorption of topical corticosteroid and the volume of cream used will be greater if the skin is dry and excoriated (Morris 1998), thus the skin must be regularly moisturised with emollient during corticosteroid therapy. Corticosteroids should be applied to freshly bathed skin (if using emollient) or at least 60 min after the application of an emollient. Using the 'fingertip unit of approximately 0.5 g', measured amounts of cream are gently massaged into the affected areas for maximum effect (Weller et al 2008) but not rubbed to irritate and cause itch.

The best treatment advice is to be proactive and use the correct potency to match the location and extent of inflammation; however, many eczematous conditions require a potent corticosteroid to inhibit the inflammatory process. Treatment programmes start with a potent corticosteroid (moderate potent to face) applied twice daily, gradually reducing the strength as the condition improves. The 'step-up step-down' approach is recommended by NICE (2007). Many patients are aware of the side-effects of topical corticosteroids, e.g. systemic absorption, skin thinning. The nurse must emphasise that it is prolonged use of potent corticosteroids with inadequate use of emollients that potentially produces side-effects. In eczema, secondary bacterial infection may be present and treatment may include a combined corticosteroid and antibiotic cream.

Bandaging

A variety of occlusive, medicated bandages is available. Applied overnight, occlusive bandaging creates a moist environment which aids the absorption of medication. Bandaging is a mechanical barrier, preventing skin damage from scratching. The use of wet wrap dressings should only be used under close supervision. The technique involves the initial application of emollient, or corticosteroid and emollient, followed by covering with, first, a wet layer of elasticated viscose stockinette, a tubular conforming bandage/or clothing, and then a second dry layer of the same product. Water in the moist bandages evaporates, creating a cooling effect that markedly reduces pruritus (Page 2003). The bandages need to be kept moist and not allowed to dry out. This is used short term and only after assessment of previously used treatments.

Other considerations

Rest

Rest is imperative for recovery in more severe eczematous conditions. This involves hospitalisation or taking home sick leave to allow the skin to heal by having time to concentrate on skin care. Disruptive, manipulative behaviour is often described in the child with atopic eczema, who may be distraught by itch and inadequate sleep (Titman 2003). The nurse must give clear information about the safe use of antihistamine medication in children. Many parents avoid giving their child medicines, but the judicious use of antihistamines will provide rest for the eczema sufferer and the family.

Diet

Diet is implicated in some forms of infantile eczema when the history strongly suggests the infant is allergic or intolerant to milk or milk products. The best advice is to maintain a well-balanced diet while avoiding foods known to cause irritation. Exclusion diets to identify food allergy are difficult and should be attempted only under the supervision of a dietitian (Lawton 2001).

Complementary therapies

When conventional medicine cannot offer a cure, parents or adults with atopic eczema may turn to alternative therapies, e.g. homeopathy, herbal medicine, aromatherapy.

Traditional Chinese medicine using self-help tools from energy-based therapies, e.g. Shiatsu, can blend with Western techniques to reduce stress and boost the body's natural healing capacity.

Behaviour modification for eczema is based on habit reversal (scratching/picking), creating awareness of the attitudes and circumstances that lead to scratching. Treatment methods vary for each age group so specialist help must be sought.

The contribution of the nurse

In detailing the provision of more care closer to home the Department of Health (DH 2006) places the primary care team at the forefront of skin care, and therefore their clinical skills and educational abilities must address the identified need. A multidisciplinary team approach ensures that care is coordinated and holistic and that people with eczema and their families are supported.

School nurses can support and motivate the child to maintain skin care at school while educating teachers about the physical and psychosocial impact of eczema (National Eczema Society 2003). Health visitors should be involved in regular monitoring to ensure therapies are not inhibiting the child's development.

Occupational health nurses advise on changes in work practice to reduce risk factors and the incidence of industrial-acquired skin disorders. In every setting, the nurse practitioner should utilise all available resources and refer patients appropriately to the relevant agencies and support groups.

Skin infections and infestations

Many skin infections and infestations cause anxiety among sufferers because of their real or perceived social implications.

Fungal skin infections

These are a group of infections caused by fungi that include dermatophytes (*Trichophyton* [ringworm]), non-dermatophyte moulds (*Aspergillus, Scopulariopsis*) and yeasts (*Candida albicans, Pityrosporum* [*Malassezia*]).

Dermatophyte infections

Dermatophytes are fungi responsible for superficial fungal infection occurring in keratin (i.e. stratum corneum, hair and nails). Some dermatophyte infections are confined to humans, while others principally affect animals and can transfer from animal to human, causing severe inflammatory skin reactions. The term 'tinea' is the generic description given to these fungal infections. Fungal infections are usually unilateral. A dermatophyte can be identified by scaly erythema-defined edge plaques with central clearing, excessive scaling in the skin creases or, if by stretching the skin between two fingers (5 cm apart), fine scaling is seen. Superficial fungal infections are very common in small children and can be hard to eradicate but rarely compromise a child's life.

Tinea pedis or athlete's foot. The patient complains of itchy, scaling skin between the toe webs.

Tinea capitis affecting the scalp, can result in loss of hair and scarring.

Tinea cruris affects young males, presenting as scaly erythematous lesions on the inner thighs and spreading to the perineum and buttocks. The source of infection is usually athlete's foot and the fungus is transferred to the groins on fingers or towels.

Tinea unguium is a fungal dystrophy of the toenails in which the nail thickens, discolours and becomes very friable.

Cattle ringworm (tinea corporis) is common amongst farm workers or visitors to farms. The fungus is picked up from gates or fences where cattle have left keratin debris containing the organism. The face and forearm tend to be affected and the fungus provokes a severe inflammatory reaction.

MEDICAL MANAGEMENT

Topical treatments (e.g. clotrimazole, miconazole creams) are usually first line for all, but for multiple nails or hair infection then systemic therapy is effective with confirmation of mycology results, especially if considering treatment in children.

Investigations Skin scraping/nail clipping/hair debris are sent for mycology to confirm dermatophyte infection.

🖱 **See website Figure 12.2**

A specimen of blood may be needed for liver and renal function tests to monitor for adverse effects of 'azole' drugs.

▷ Nursing management and health promotion: dermatophyte infection

Nursing management focuses on containment of infection and promotion of basic hygiene. Avoidance of shared face cloths/towels prevents further spread. The nurse can advise on prescribed and OTC therapies and their correct method of application. Treatment programmes may involve combined oral and topical therapies, and patients should be advised to persevere where therapies take time to resolve the condition. Conditions can recur, so educating the patient in management of the condition is beneficial in preventing this.

Candida infection

Candidiasis (thrush) is a yeast infection of the skin and mucous membranes caused by *Candida albicans*. The microorganism is a normal commensal of the human digestive system, only becoming pathogenic if the opportunity presents itself. Immunosuppressed patients, people with diabetes, and patients having broad-spectrum antibiotics or topical and systemic corticosteroid therapies are all at risk from this opportunistic infection. Yeast infections are often moist with pustules along the periphery and on nearby healthy skin or macerated in between skin webs. Yeast infections can be intensely itchy – scratching can cause secondary bacterial infection and spread.

Buccal mucosal candidiasis Oral thrush presents as milky curd-like spots on the tongue and inner cheeks. It often affects babies, older people and patients having broad-spectrum antibiotics (see Ch. 15).

Candida vulvovaginitis presents with a creamy vaginal discharge and itchy erythema of the vulva. It tends to be associated with pregnancy, use of oral contraceptives, antibiotics and diabetes.

Candida balanitis is a thrush infection of the foreskin and glans. It tends to be more common in uncircumcised males and may be associated with poor hygiene or diabetes. It can recur if a sexual partner also has candidiasis.

Chronic paronychia is a candidal infection of the nail plate which is common in people whose occupation involves repeated immersion of the hands in water, e.g. hairdressers, nurses, bartenders. The nails become distorted and the nail base is painful, red and swollen.

Intertrigo Candidal infection is common where two skin folds are in contact and there is increased heat and humidity, such as the groins (nappy rash), axillae and beneath the breasts or pendulous abdomen. Obesity and poor hygiene exacerbate the problem. The skin displays erythematous, well-demarcated erosive lesions and is tender, moist and painful in these areas.

Angular cheilitis is a common condition of older people where the deep grooves at the side of the mouth tend to be moist with saliva; a *Candida* infection exacerbates the problem. It is common in denture wearers but can also be a feature of vitamin B$_2$ deficiency.

MEDICAL MANAGEMENT

The diagnosis is confirmed from the clinical picture and skin swab results. The use of topical preparations can be effective.

Investigations
- Skin swabs.

 See website Figure 12.1

- Urinalysis and fasting blood sugar to exclude diabetes.
- A full blood count must be carried out in older people with angular cheilitis.

Treatment is specific to the area affected. Antifungals in the form of creams, ointments and pessaries are very effective. A combined moderate corticosteroid/antifungal, e.g. Trimovate®, is appropriate to treat intertrigo, reducing both inflammation and infection. Combination packs of vaginal pessary and cream are available for vaginal thrush, e.g. clotrimazole, and these are usually single applications, depending on the dose/strength of the preparation. Newer OTC preparations include a single dose of the antifungal drug fluconazole.

 Nursing management and health promotion: candidiasis

The nurse must be able to identify those at risk of opportunistic infection, e.g. older people, babies and patients having chemotherapy. The nurse's role as counsellor is vital in the treatment of genital candidiasis and confidential information should be respected when sexual partners are treated concurrently to prevent reinfection.

Bacterial skin infections

Cellulitis

Cellulitis is an acute, spreading and potentially serious infection of dermal and subcutaneous tissue, characterised by red, oedematous, tender skin that is hot and painful. Patients feel unwell with rigors and fever and local lymph nodes may be enlarged. Microorganisms implicated in cellulitis include *Staphylococcus aureus* and *Streptococcus pyogenes* (Group A β-haemolytic streptococcus). In adults, the most common presentation is cellulitis affecting the lower limbs, with the point of entry of infection usually being a fissure between the toes which may be secondary to tinea pedis. Cellulitis is common in older people who have lower limb oedema. Infection enters the skin in a variety of ways, including surgical wounds, stasis eczema or leg ulcers, insect bites, minor abrasions and intravenous drug injection sites. A superficial streptococcal infection of the skin is called erysipelas.

MEDICAL MANAGEMENT

Management involves the prompt administration of appropriate oral or intravenous antibiotic therapy (sometimes involving several different antibiotics). Analgesics reduce the pain of inflammation.

Investigations Where appropriate:

- blood culture – bacterial growth
- Doppler – to rule out deep vein thrombosis (see Chs 2, 10).

 Nursing management and health promotion: cellulitis

Initial care includes bed rest, monitoring of temperature and dealing with rigors (see Ch. 22). Pain assessment and administration of regular analgesics will ease discomfort. Early intervention teams often initiate intravenous antibiotics in the patient's own home to prevent admission into hospital. A limb affected by cellulitis requires elevation to reduce oedema. Exercising reduces the complications of bed rest but mobilisation should occur as soon as possible. Once the condition resolves, general advice on basic skin care and avoidance of predisposing factors is helpful. Patients can have recurrent cellulitis and may be prescribed prophylactic antibiotic therapy to prevent future episodes.

Other staphylococcal skin infections

Impetigo is a superficial skin infection caused by *Staphylococcus aureus*, sometimes with *Streptococcus pyogenes*. The head and neck are the most common sites. The condition starts as a small but gradually enlarging pustule that ruptures to leave a raw exuding surface. The exudate dries and forms the yellow golden crust typical of impetigo. It is common amongst children as it spreads very quickly within a nursery/school environment. It can also occur as a secondary infection, e.g. associated with eczema and scabies.

Folliculitis Infection of superficial hair follicles by *Staphylococcus aureus* presents as a small pustule on an erythematous base centred around the follicle. Folliculitis may be exacerbated by the use of greasy ointments, occlusive bandages and tar therapies. This is why technique of application is important, i.e. application in the direction of hair growth.

MEDICAL MANAGEMENT

Treatment involves the use of topical and/or oral antibiotics depending on whether the bacterial infection is localised or generalised. Careful selection of antibiotics (see local policies) reduces antibiotic resistance and healthcare-associated infection (HCAI).

Viral skin infections

Warts

Infection by the human papilloma virus (HPV) affects the DNA in epidermal cells, creating warts. Warts are benign, highly contagious and can be unsightly or catch on clothing.

 See website Figure 12.8

Some are self-limiting (between 6 months and 2 years) and are non-scarring. Transmission occurs during direct contact, e.g. in gyms, swimming baths or schools. The classification of warts is outlined in Box 12.4.

MEDICAL MANAGEMENT

Diagnosis is based on history and clinical appearance. Treatment may involve topical application of ointments or premedicated plasters containing salicylic acid to soften and remove the wart, or cryosurgery (effective for palmar warts)

▷ **Nursing management and health promotion: warts**

The nurse should explain virus transmission and encourage the meticulous continuation of treatment. Many patients become disheartened by the slow resolution of the problem and discontinue treatment. Regular assessment by the

---

Box 12.4 Information

Classification of warts

- Common warts – hyperkeratotic nodules occurring on the hands and feet of children. These often resolve spontaneously.
- Plane warts – smooth flat-topped warts appearing on the face and hands.
- Plantar warts (verrucae) – the HPV is pressured into the dermis, creating a callus. The most common site is the feet.
- Genital warts – a mass of warts with a cauliflower-like appearance present on the perianal and genital areas.

---

practice nurse may encourage adherence to treatment. If warts occur on hands, especially of people in the catering trade, then the use of liquid nitrogen is viable but can cause scarring.

 See website Figures 12.9, 12.10

Molluscum contagiosum

A pox virus produces solid, skin-coloured or pearly-white papules on the skin. It affects adults but is more common in children, arising over a period of 2–3 months. The lesions may be single or multiple, occurring on the neck and trunk.

MEDICAL MANAGEMENT

Initial diagnosis is based on history and clinical appearance. The condition should resolve spontaneously and patients or parents can be reassured that it tends to be self-limiting. Normal basic hygiene rules prevent further spread. Treat any local infection if the lesions are traumatised.

Herpes simplex virus (HSV)

There are two types of HSV – HSV-1 associated with orolabial herpes (cold sores) and HSV-2 associated with genital herpes – but either can cause genital herpes. Initial contact with the herpes simplex virus is usually in childhood and often goes unnoticed. However, development of primary cutaneous herpes simplex can occur and, in a patient with atopic eczema, it can be a severe life-threatening condition. Following primary infection, HSV-1 can establish itself in sensory ganglia (trigeminal) and be reactivated by, for example, sunlight, stress and colds. Reactivation of the virus is preceded by a tingling sensation before a cluster of small vesicles develops. The vesicles burst and lesions then crust, usually resolving in 10–14 days. Genital herpes is a sexually transmitted infection affecting the penis, vulva, perianal area and rectum. Following the primary episode, HSV-2 persists in the presacral ganglion and can recur. This can be serious in pregnant women because of the risk of transmitting the virus to the fetus during labour and delivery.

MEDICAL MANAGEMENT

Recurrent herpes simplex is treated with topical aciclovir which is now available OTC. It must be used immediately on awareness of the tingling sensation, and applied five times daily for 5 days to inhibit vesicle eruption. Patients with genital herpes should be referred to a sexual health clinic for investigations, management and expert counselling.

▷ **Nursing management and health promotion: herpes simplex**

The nurse can advise patients at risk of recurrent episodes of herpes simplex on the use of topical aciclovir and should recommend completing the course. The patient should be reminded of basic hygiene standards to avoid further transmission of the virus during the active phase. Patients with genital herpes should be encouraged to access specialist support and counselling at the sexual health clinic. A pregnant woman with genital herpes requires effective liaison between herself, the midwife and obstetrician, to acknowledge the condition and its potential complications and to initiate appropriate action to minimise virus transfer during delivery (Gawkrodger 2008).

Eczema herpeticum

Eczema herpeticum is a widespread cutaneous HSV infection occurring in patients with atopic eczema. In children it can be life threatening, and any patient can be systemically unwell and febrile. Vesicles erupt rapidly over the face and neck and can extend over the rest of the body. The skin is taut, red and painful. As vesicles erupt and rupture, the patient becomes susceptible to secondary bacterial infection.

MEDICAL MANAGEMENT

Treatment depends on the severity of illness and is a combination of antiviral drugs and antibiotics. The patient who is pyrexial and systemically unwell should be hospitalised. A side room is ideal, but effective standard (universal) precautions are required to minimise the infection risk to other susceptible patients (see Ch. 16). Oral aciclovir is adequate in minor cases, but if the patient is unwell aciclovir is given by the intravenous route. Prompt referral to an ophthalmologist is vital for the patient with any eye involvement (see Ch. 13). Patients with eczema discontinue topical corticosteroids until the virus resolves. Secondary bacterial infection should be treated with topical antibiotic cream and/or oral antibiotics. Appropriate analgesics may be required.

Nursing management and health promotion: eczema herpeticum

The nurse's role is to maintain effective infection prevention and control procedures in order to reduce the transmission of infection. The patient who is systemically unwell requires regular observations of temperature, fluid intake and rest until infection resolves. The nurse should assist in topical applications of prescribed creams as the patient may feel too unwell or too distressed by pain to manage this independently. Once the infection resolves, the nurse can advise the patient on restarting topical corticosteroids for the eczema. Patients who have had HSV previously and are at risk of cold sores should keep aciclovir in reserve to use promptly if a cold sore develops and avoid contact with people who have them. Aciclovir is available OTC so effective treatment is easier to achieve. Delay in seeing the GP can be detrimental as this condition erupts quickly.

Herpes zoster (shingles)

Herpes zoster is caused by the varicella-zoster virus (VZV). After an attack of childhood chickenpox, the virus remains dormant in the dorsal root ganglia of the spinal cord but can be reactivated later in life to cause shingles. The trigger factor is unknown, but the condition occurs in immunosuppressed people, stress and serious illness, and commonly affects middle-aged and older people.

Once reactivated, VZV multiplies within host cells. The cells lyse and virus particles are released to invade other cells. The virus particles migrate along the sensory nerve fibres causing nerve damage and pain. Fluid-filled vesicles erupt along a thoracic and/or cranial dermatome with a characteristic unilateral band-like distribution of the sensory nerve. Pain and tenderness often precede the vesicular erosions, and patients may have fever and feel unwell. As the vesicles crust over, the infective risk resolves over a period of 2–3 weeks.

MEDICAL MANAGEMENT

Early treatment with antivirals such as topical aciclovir, ideally 72 h before the development of the vesicles, can reduce the intensity. Diagnosis is confirmed by clinical history and viral culture. Oral or intravenous aciclovir is essential management in immunosuppressed patients. The potential complications of herpes zoster are:

- herpes zoster ophthalmicus (causing corneal vesicles, ulceration and scarring)
- postherpetic neuralgia (requiring input from the specialist pain team).

Nursing management and health promotion: herpes zoster (shingles)

In an acute attack of shingles, the patient may require hospitalisation. Standard (universal) precautions and isolation are required until the infectious stage resolves. The patient should be nursed by staff who have had chickenpox, as non-immune people can develop chickenpox following contact with a patient with shingles. Nurses should encourage people to seek early treatment before the vesicles erupt (see above).

Certain groups of people are particularly susceptible to the transmission of herpes zoster, e.g. patients having radiotherapy and/or chemotherapy, and immunocompromised patients on oral or topical corticosteroids. Community nurses should be aware of the long-term problems associated with shingles. A small proportion of patients report persistent pain (postherpetic neuralgia) continuing for many years. Chronic pain has a major impact on daily living and requires full assessment (see Ch. 19). Treatment options available for postherpetic neuralgia include transcutaneous electrical nerve stimulation (TENS), topical capsaicin, ultrasound, antidepressants and/or anticonvulsant therapy. Referral to a pain control clinic is advisable for intractable pain.

Infestations

Scabies

Scabies is a skin infestation caused by the itch mite *Sarcoptes scabiei* and acquired by prolonged close physical contact with the mite. The female scabies mite burrows into the stratum corneum, and after fertilisation begins to lay eggs along the burrow. For the first 4–6 weeks after infestation there may be no itching, but thereafter pruritus is intense, especially at night. This is thought to be due to a hypersensitive response to the mite. Skin examination usually reveals burrows, principally on the hands and feet, the sides of fingers/toes, between finger and toe webs, the wrists and the insteps. Burrows can also present on the male genitalia.

A scabies 'rash' may be present in the axillae, umbilicus and thighs. Excoriation can cause burrows to become eczematised and infected, which can often confuse diagnosis.

 See website Figure 12.11

Crusty scabies is the form of scabies presenting in patients who have sensory deficits where the sensation of itch is absent, e.g. in spinal injuries, or in patients who are immunosuppressed either because of disease or treatment, e.g. HIV disease, lymphoma, systemic corticosteroids or transplantation. Absence of scratching leads to large numbers of mites remaining on the skin in crusted lesions.

During skin shedding, mites are shed into the environment, and therefore any person in contact is at considerable risk of developing scabies from the patient.

MEDICAL MANAGEMENT

Diagnosis can be confirmed by using a needle to remove a mite from a burrow and examining it microscopically, or a burrow can be visualised with a dermoscopy. Current topical therapies are permethrin and malathion. Once the infestation is treated, further therapy with a combined corticosteroid/antibiotic cream may be necessary to reduce itch and treat excoriated lesions until the skin is healed. Antihistamine tablets are appropriate if itch disturbs sleep. Soothing topical preparations, e.g. Eurax® cream, can be useful until residual itch disappears.

 ## ▷ Nursing management and health promotion: scabies

The priority is to treat the patient and identify close contacts requiring treatment. The nurse combines practical advice with psychological support, recognising the social embarrassment associated with scabies. The nurse must identify current treatments and their correct method of application (Box 12.5). As recurrent scabies is often due to poorly applied treatments, both patient and nurse should read carefully the advice leaflets provided with topical scabicides,

 Box 12.5 Reflection

Treating scabies

Rosa, Carlos and their three children (aged 15, 6 and 3 years) need to use a topical preparation for a scabies infestation.

Activities

- Think about how you would guide the family in obtaining information from the worldwide web.
- Reflect on any potential problems with treating the whole family.
- Access some professional health websites to download the information (see below) and discuss their suitability with your mentor.

Resources

New Zealand Dermatological Society Inc – www.dermnetnz. org/arthropods/scabies.html
The British Association of Dermatologists (BAD) – www.bad. org.uk/site/871/default.aspx

always remembering to leave some preparation to reapply to the hands if they are washed after initial application. Treatments are usually repeated after 7 days. Transient contact with the patient is unlikely to cause transmission. However, the patient with crusty scabies is highly contagious and should avoid contact with others while treatment is ongoing. Normal washing of linen and clothes is adequate.

Head lice (pediculosis capitis)

Head lice are transmitted by close contact. The adult female louse lays eggs which are cemented to the hair approximately 0.5 cm from the root. Scalp irritation and itch are due to the saliva produced as the louse bites the scalp. The 'nit' is the empty case left once the larva has hatched — the case becomes white and is more easily detected.

 See website Figure 12.12

Head lice is an emotive topic, as infestation continues to be endemic amongst schoolchildren.

▷ Nursing management and health promotion: head lice

The priority is to treat the patient and appropriate contacts. Treatment usually consists of an insecticide lotion applied to the scalp, e.g. malathion or pyrethroid (phenothrin), which is left on for a number of hours and then shampooed out. Treatment is repeated after 7 days to destroy newly hatched lice. Combing with a fine-tooth comb assists in the final removal of nits. The practice of rotating products to prevent the development of resistance is no longer advocated: current advice is that if an insecticide does not destroy the lice, use a different one for the next course (British National Formulary [BNF] 2009). Education of parents regarding the guidelines for each product is essential as the burden of treatment falls on them. Some will opt to use nightly wet combing after conditioning, rather than use chemicals.

Bullous disorders

Bullous disorders are characterised by large watery blisters (bullae) arising within or immediately under the epidermis (Weller et al 2008). The aetiology of autoimmune bullous diseases remains unknown – genetic factors may have a role – and histological location influences the classification of the disorder. Early detection and treatment are essential, as many of the bullous conditions are severe and potentially life threatening.

Pemphigus (intraepidermal bullae)

PATHOPHYSIOLOGY

This autoimmune disease occurs in adults. It is characterised by the development of autoantibodies against epidermal cell surface molecules creating superficial erosions and blisters on epidermal and mucosal surfaces.

Common presenting symptoms Superficial fluid-filled blisters are present within the epidermis. These blisters are flaccid, thin-roofed and offer little resistance; consequently they shear, leaving raw, denuded skin. Pain from the exposed sites is a major factor. Oral lesions are common affecting nutrition and hydration. Diagnosis is confirmed by a positive Nikolsky's sign – when lateral pressure is applied to the skin surface with a thumb, the epidermis shears and appears to slide over the dermis.

Pemphigoid (subepidermal bullae)

PATHOPHYSIOLOGY

This is more common in older people: 80% of patients are aged 60 and over (Marks 2003). Like pemphigus, pemphigoid is an autoimmune disease and can be triggered by certain drugs (Denyer & Hughes 2001). Antibodies bind to the junction between dermis and epidermis, and blisters are formed in response to enzymes released from inflammatory cells (Figure 12.7).

Common presenting symptoms include generalised intense itch, followed by erythematous plaques on the skin (pre-pemphigoid stage), followed by the development of tense intact blisters affecting any area of the body. Nikolsky's sign is negative.

Toxic epidermal/epidermolytic necrolysis (TEN) (subepidermal)

PATHOPHYSIOLOGY

TEN presents as a dermatological emergency and is often precipitated by drug hypersensitivity (severe form of Stevens–Johnson syndrome). The skin split is subepidermal and the entire epidermis shears off in layers, leaving raw, denuded areas. A review of the patient's medication and removal of the causative factor(s) are essential.

Common presenting symptoms The skin is erythrodermic and painful, with the skin shearing off in sheets.

🖱 See website Figure 12.13

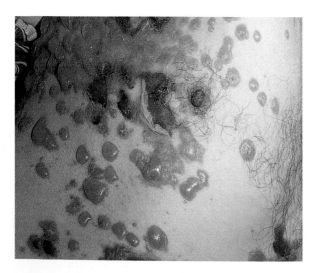

Figure 12.7 Bullous pemphigoid. Large tense and unilocular blisters clustered in and around the axilla. (Reproduced from Boon et al 2006 with permission.)

Nikolsky's sign is positive. There is pain and erosions may be present in the mouth, oesophagus and bronchus.

MEDICAL MANAGEMENT OF BULLOUS DISORDERS

Early diagnosis and hospitalisation is imperative due to the life-threatening potential of bullous disorders.

Investigations include:

- skin biopsy – to identify the type of skin split
- blood tests – full blood count, urea and electrolytes to monitor fluid loss from eroded skin; presence of antibodies in pemphigus
- skin swab – to diagnose secondary bacterial infection.

Treatment might involve the following:

- Antibiotics – for secondary infection.
- Corticosteroids – in pemphigus and pemphigoid, high-dose oral corticosteroids, e.g. prednisolone, are the first line of management and are maintained until blistering stops. The dose is gradually reduced, aiming for low-dose maintenance therapy.
- Analgesics – to control pain from eroded skin lesions.
- Antihistamines – to reduce itch and aid rest.
- Immunosuppressants, e.g. cyclophosphamide, azathioprine, are used in combination with oral corticosteroids to control the disease process of pemphigus and pemphigoid.
- Plasmapheresis to remove antibodies is considered in severe cases; it also allows monitoring of circulating pemphigus antibodies.

▷ Nursing management and health promotion: bullous disorders

The general nursing care of bullous disorders is outlined. Although rare, they are more commonly seen in dermatology units. The nursing priorities are similar to those needed by patients with severe burn injuries (see Ch. 30).

Major nursing considerations

Analgesia

Analgesia must be effective and consistent. Pemphigus and TEN are distressing, painful conditions when shearing of the skin is active. Pain assessment tools (see Ch. 19) permit the nurse and patient to determine pain control needs, ensure accurate delivery of analgesics, and evaluate their efficacy, which is particularly relevant prior to dressing changes.

Bed rest, special beds/pressure-relieving equipment

Facilitating rest and comfort is a primary aim to avoid further trauma to the skin. The use of low-pressure, air-fluidised beds enhances comfort and reduces the need for positional changes which contribute to shearing forces on the skin. The temperature regulator in these beds maintains an appropriately warm environment, helping the patient to maintain body temperature. This warm environment also increases the amount of insensible fluid loss, so the patient's fluid intake must be increased to compensate. Dressings remain moist with the use of these beds, and are usually easily removed.

Hygiene

The maintenance of good personal hygiene and the prevention of infection are extremely important. Gentle washing or the application of soaks, i.e. potassium permanganate, for their mild antiseptic/antipruritic effect can be soothing and help to minimise further trauma.

Infection prevention (see Ch. 16)

Isolation may be necessary due to skin loss. The patient will be susceptible to infection and the use of immunosuppressants will increase this susceptibility. Patients with TEN are often cared for in burns units (see Ch. 30).

Diet

Approximately 20% of an adult's dietary protein is used for skin repair and growth in normal health. Therefore, an increased intake of protein is advisable in bullous conditions. Referral to a dietitian will ensure the prescription of any necessary supplements. Constipation induced by fluid loss, or as a side-effect of analgesics, is an associated problem. Mild laxatives may be indicated to prevent discomfort.

Monitoring vital signs

Regular measurement of body temperature is required, as fluctuations may occur due to fluid and heat loss from the skin. Variations in environmental temperature can be reduced by nursing the patient in a side room.

Blood pressure is checked regularly if there is associated fluid loss, corticosteroid-induced hypertension or hydration by intravenous fluids.

Monitoring electrolyte and fluid balance

This is imperative in any condition associated with skin loss. Rehydration may initially be achievable by increasing the patient's oral intake and monitoring output. An intravenous infusion may be necessary in severe cases. If skin loss presents problems in siting a peripheral infusion, a central line may be required, with monitoring of central venous pressure providing an accurate assessment of fluid requirements.

Urine should be tested for glycosuria in order to detect a potential diabetic state induced by oral corticosteroid therapy.

Dressings and topical therapy

A dressing procedure provides the best opportunity to complete a skin assessment and evaluate disease activity. In pemphigus and TEN, raw areas are recorded and dressed. The tense bullae of pemphigoid are identified and left intact to permit reabsorption of blister fluid, thereby minimising trauma and infection risk. Blisters restricting movement are uncomfortable for the patient and can be aspirated using a sterile syringe and needle, leaving the blister roof intact (Deyner & Hughes 2001). Administration of analgesics prior to the application of topical therapy is important to reduce the patient's apprehension about dressing changes. Individual needs and disease severity determine dressing requirements, but the aims are to:

- keep dressing changes to a minimum
- maximise comfort
- ensure dressings are removable without traumatising the skin.

Meeting these aims ensures that further trauma is minimised and healing is promoted. Simple applications of soothing emollients or a non-adherent dressing secured by gauze stockinette will possibly be all that is tolerated. Heavier pads and bandaging create constriction and pain. Dressing choices should be guided by the patient's comments and nurses will adjust dressings appropriately.

Care in the community

Although these conditions are rare, as numbers of older people increase, the incidence will rise. The community nurse has a dual role: firstly, in identifying disorders and coordinating referral for specialist help; and secondly, after discharge from hospital, in ensuring the patient understands the rationale behind long-term maintenance medication, encouraging adherence to and monitoring side-effects of systemic therapies.

Acute skin failure

This life-threatening condition is associated with a number of serious skin disorders, for example erythrodermic psoriasis, eczema, bullous diseases, etc.

 ## Nursing management and health promotion: acute skin failure

The nursing goals will vary depending on the type and severity of the presenting condition. If the epidermal barrier is breached, as it is in severe erythroderma associated with types of psoriasis and eczema or autoimmune blistering conditions, the nursing interventions need to support the epidermal barrier:

- loss of body temperature control – bed rest, use of warmth, management of rigors
- loss of water through the skin surface – increase oral fluid
- loss of protein – high-protein diet
- discomfort and pain – analgesia, emollient therapy hourly and antihistamines if itchy.

Intensive nursing care is essential for the safety and comfort of the patient including infection prevention and monitoring and acting on early signs of deterioration in the patient's condition. (Box 12.6)

 See website for further content

Acne

Acne is a disorder of the pilosebaceous units. It is a common condition, usually developing during adolescence, between 11 and 14 years. It reaches a peak between 17 and 21 years, gradually improving and disappearing. However, 6% of adults between 25 and 40 years still experience acne (Cunliffe & Gollnick 2001). The psychosocial impact of acne should not be underestimated, as its onset during the years when visual appearance is important to developing new relationships can have a devastating effect on the young adult. Dermatologists are very aware of the impact that acne can have on quality of life.

Box 12.6 Information

Monitoring patients with acute skin disorders/failure

The type and frequency of observations and investigations depend on the severity of the person's condition.

- Level of consciousness
- Temperature and shivering
- Heart rate
- Respiratory rate
- Blood pressure
- Gastric emptying
- Fluid balance
- Urinary volume may be measured hourly
- Urinary osmolality

- Extent of skin lesions
- Body weight
- Calculation of fluid loss
- Arterial blood gases
- Chest X-ray
- Blood tests
  - full blood count
  - urea and electrolytes
  - glucose
  - serum proteins
  - liver enzymes
- Urine tested for glucose (glycosuria)

PATHOPHYSIOLOGY

During puberty, circulating androgen hormones stimulate sebum production. Hyperkeratosis occurs at the mouth of the hair follicle and the dilated chamber fills with sebum. The organism *Propionibacterium acnes* grows in large numbers, creating the comedone. *P. acnes* acts on sebum to produce inflammatory chemicals which leak into the surrounding dermis or out through a rupture in the follicle wall (Gawkrodger 2008) (Figure 12.8).

Common presenting symptoms Acne affects the face, neck, upper back and front of the chest. In more severe cases, these lesions may spread further. Lesions can include comedones, papules, pustules, nodules, cysts and residual scars.

 See website Figures 12.14–12.16

MEDICAL MANAGEMENT

Mild acne is managed with topical therapies, antiseptic washes and antibiotic preparations, whereas moderate/severe acne requires both topical and systemic therapies.

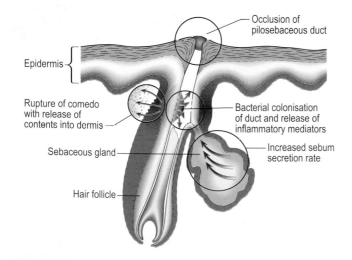

Figure 12.8 The pathogenesis of acne. (Reproduced from Boon et al 2006 with permission.)

Antibiotics Oral tetracyclines given over a 6-month period reduce the inflammatory process. Side-effects of and contra-indications to tetracycline should be noted (see BNF 2009). If patients are intolerant of tetracycline, erythromycin can be prescribed.

Isotretinoin (a retinoid) reduces sebum production. Its side-effects necessitate regular monitoring of liver function and blood lipids levels. The medication is teratogenic: pregnancy must be ruled out before starting treatment and female patients must use reliable contraception (see BNF 2009). Isotretinoin clears acne in most patients with no recurrence.

▷ Nursing management and health promotion: acne

Nurses are key to educating patients and dispelling misinformation about acne. The patient should be reassured that acne is not linked to poor diet, an excess of sweets or chocolate (per se) or poor hygiene. Indeed, most acne sufferers are overzealous in personal hygiene. The nurse should encourage continuation of therapies for the full treatment course. Nurses must ensure that females starting a course of isotretinoin understand that they must not become pregnant and that they are enrolled into the pregnancy prevention programme prior to commencing treatment. The nurse must respond empathetically to the acne sufferer. The degree of distress may not always equate with the severity of disease, and care must address the psychosocial impact of acne. Skin disease has provoked suicide, and the nurse working with acne patients should recognise that individuals can become so disturbed that they are pushed to this extreme (Cotterill & Cunliffe 1997). Part of the monitoring of isotretinoin is around the emotional impact that the drug has in magnifying moods and could lead to sadness and potential self harm. It is imperative that the impact of acne is not underestimated, and prompt referral to a dermatologist will initiate effective treatment.

Photodermatoses

Photodermatoses are skin disorders induced or aggravated by sunlight. They are relatively common and can impose severe limitations on daily life. Nursing management focuses on assisting the patient to maintain independent living within the limitations imposed by photosensitivity.

Sunlight

Sunlight is composed of different wavelengths of UVL, divided into UVA, UVB and visible light. UVA in larger doses can produce erythema, passes through window glass and is less variable in intensity. UVB causes sunburn. Visible light easily penetrates the epidermis, usually with minimal significance. Some conditions, however, demonstrate an abnormal sensitivity to visible light. Factors affecting the intensity of sunlight include:

- time of day – strongest between 11.00 and 15.00 h
- geography – weaker in northern latitudes
- season – UVB less intensive in winter months
- reflective effect of snow, water and sand.

Note that clouds do not protect against sunburn as UVB penetrates cloud cover.

Types of photodermatosis

Polymorphic light eruption (PLE) is very common, with women being affected twice as frequently as men (Gawkrodger 2008). It affects patients in early spring, disappearing in autumn. Several hours after exposure to sunlight, the patient develops an itchy papular rash, which persists for 7–10 days. The rash is provoked by UVB or UVA wavelengths, and it should be remembered that UVA also penetrates window glass and thin clothing.

Photo-aggravated dermatoses Some pre-existing skin conditions, e.g. atopic eczema, psoriasis, herpes simplex, can be exacerbated by sunlight.

Photo-contact dermatitis In these disorders direct contact of the skin with a substance, e.g. tars, sunscreens, followed by exposure to UVL provokes dermatitis. Certain genetic disorders, e.g. xeroderma pigmentosum, also produce a photosensitive reaction.

Chronic actinic dermatitis usually affects men over 50 years of age but can also occur in women (Gawkrodger 2008). Patients are sensitive to sunlight (all components) and artificial light and have allergies to substances in direct contact with their skin, e.g. plants, wood, perfumes, sunscreens and rubber. Sparing of the shaded skin can be present, e.g. behind ears, under a watch strap. The condition presents with marked erythema, eczema and thickening of the skin of the face, neck and hands. Skin changes may be less evident in areas covered by clothing.

MEDICAL MANAGEMENT

A full history is required and assessment of related factors, such as skin type, sites involved, drugs, hobbies, occupation, etc.

Signs and symptoms include eczema, erythema, heat, itch, oedema, pain and urticaria.

Investigations:
- *Phototesting* – available in specialist photobiology/dermatology units. Phototesting involves the use of a monochromator (Ferguson 2004) to identify if abnormal light sensitivity is present and establish which wavelengths are responsible, i.e. UVA, UVB or visible light. Varying doses at different wavelengths are irradiated to small areas on the back and delayed erythema is noted at 7 and 24 h. Responses are compared with those of a control group, to determine the degree of photosensitivity and wavelengths responsible.
- *Patch testing* (p. 401).

Treatment involves:
- systemic and topical therapy and/or phototherapy
- antihistamines, immunosuppressants, oral and/or topical corticosteroids
- sunscreens – offer a sun protection factor (SPF) either chemically (absorbing/filtering UVL) or physically (reflecting/scattering UVL) to protect the skin. A combination sunscreen creates a more effective sun block.

Some light-sensitive conditions, e.g. PLE, can be treated with a course of phototherapy desensitisation and patients should be encouraged to continue exposure to maintain their new tolerance level. Unfortunately, this is lost during winter and repeat phototherapy is needed the following spring.

 ## Nursing management and health promotion: photodermatoses

Patients require practical help and support from nurses trained in the management of photodermatology. Many patients are relieved that investigations have produced a diagnosis rather than a dismissal of symptoms as merely 'a bit of sunburn'. Information from nursing staff is vital if the patient is to cope with lifestyle changes imposed by the diagnosis. Advice includes:

- regular use of emollients
- meticulous, regular (every 2 h) application of prescribed sunscreens to exposed sites
- treatment with topical corticosteroid if the condition flares
- sun avoidance between 11.00 and 15.00 h
- wear closely woven clothing as an effective barrier; a wide-brimmed hat, scarf and gloves may prove helpful
- apply clear museum film (blocks UVL) to windows (home, workplace and car).

Psychological support

Social isolation is a major problem for individuals with severe photosensitive disorders. Many patients, distressed by their diagnosis and the restrictions it entails, reject management regimens which would lead to a life indoors or only leaving home after sundown. Others accept the limitations and persevere with the use of sunscreens to permit them some freedom, albeit restricted daily living.

The nurse must display a sympathetic understanding of the psychological impact of the diagnosis and restrictions. Nursing support should aim for the patient to control skin management in an informed way, with easy access to professional help as needed.

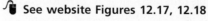 ## Urticaria

Urticaria is a common condition. Lesions are described as 'hives' or nettle rash. The skin feels irritable with white raised weals that turn pink with a bordered edge.

✍ **See website Figures 12.17, 12.18**

There are many causes, and it often resolves spontaneously. Severe cases may lead to swelling around the eyes, mouth and throat known as angioedema (see Ch. 6). In severe attacks, the airway is compromised, so immediate emergency treatment is needed. Urticaria may also be associated with anaphylaxis (see Ch. 6).

PATHOPHYSIOLOGY

In response to the initial trigger factor, the dermis becomes oedematous, blood vessels dilate and mast cells release histamine. The weal of urticaria is oedema of the dermis and can extend rapidly into the subcutaneous tissues causing angioedema.

Classification of urticaria (Box 12.7) Acute contact urticaria is related to contact factors, e.g. animal fur, plants, insect stings. Extensive urticaria associated with angioedema is usually idiopathic but can be related to the ingestion of food or drugs (strawberries, nuts, penicillin, etc.). Urticaria is more common in individuals with atopic eczema. Cold, heat, sun, pressure and water can all induce physical urticaria. Sweating after physical exercise or eating spicy food may also induce urticaria with isolated facial swelling.

MEDICAL MANAGEMENT

History and skin examination assist in determining the provoking factors. Antihistamines are essential, they block histamine release and some, e.g. desloratadine, are non-sedating. In acute attacks, the patient requires oral antihistamines until the condition resolves, usually in a few days. In chronic urticaria, maintenance antihistamines may be needed for several months. Severe urticaria may also require short-term use of systemic corticosteroids. The management of angioedema, anaphylaxis and training patients to self-administer adrenaline is outlined in Chapter 6.

Nursing management and health promotion: urticaria

The nurse in every setting will encounter the patient with allergies. Angioedema and anaphylaxis can prove fatal, so professionals must recognise the urgency of the situation and be trained and competent in emergency procedures. On a day-to-day basis the nursing role is to provide factual information and manage the condition.

Dietitians provide dietary advice about avoiding foods that trigger urticaria. Dietary exclusion is difficult, as food labelling is not always helpful. Public pressure has persuaded food companies and supermarkets to provide accurate food labelling, for example to protect those with nut allergy. Nut allergy and sensitisation can lead to anaphylaxis and death, so accurate food labelling is vital. In cases of severe allergic reactions the patient/parents should be trained to use adrenaline pens. The nurse can help the patient and family in relation to all aspects of the allergy, in particular to recognise warning symptoms and to use the adrenaline promptly whilst seeking medical assistance (see Ch. 6).

Skin tumours

The skin can develop a wide diversity of tumours, both benign and malignant, within the epidermis and dermis (e.g. seborrhoeic warts, actinic keratoses, basal cell carcinoma [BCC], squamous cell carcinoma [SCC], malignant melanoma, etc.). Skin biopsy for histology is necessary in the diagnosis, prognosis and management of skin tumours (NICE 2006) involving multidisciplinary teams and skin cancer nurse specialists.

 See website Figures 12.19–12.23

Malignant melanoma

Malignant melanoma is the most serious of the skin tumours and its incidence is rising. Melanoma is responsible for most skin cancer deaths – over 2000 per annum in the UK (Cancer Research UK 2009a). UK survival figures indicate that 78% of men and 91% of women with melanoma are alive 5 years following diagnosis (Cancer Research UK 2009a). Melanoma commonly arises in a naevus (mole) (Figure 12.9), involves the pigment-producing melanocytes and can metastasise rapidly via the blood and lymph (unlike other skin tumours). Early detection and excision of thin tumours (less than 1 mm thick) carries an excellent prognosis and potential cure. Late-stage untreated melanoma with metastases has a poorer outcome and treatment is often palliative, e.g. radiotherapy (Figure 12.10).

Health promotion

Research suggests that excessive childhood sun exposure is an important factor in the aetiology of melanoma. Current campaigns such as *SunSmart* (Cancer Research UK 2009b) encourage people to protect themselves and their children from the sun's harmful rays and so reduce their risk of skin cancer. However, it is important to recognise the importance of safe

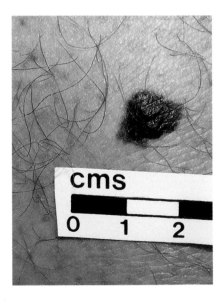

Figure 12.9 Malignant melanoma. A changing mole which fails the ABCDE test (**A**symmetry, **B**order irregular, **C**olour irregular, **D**iameter often greater than 0.5 cm and **E**levation irregular). (Reproduced from Boon et al 2006 with permission.)

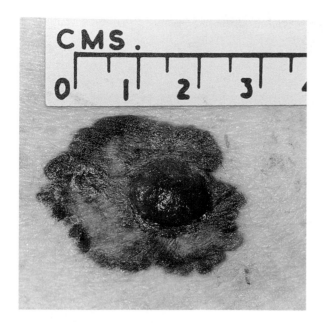

Figure 12.10 Superficial spreading melanoma. Note the irregular, asymmetrical shape and different hues, including depigmented areas signifying spontaneous regression. (Reproduced from Boon et al 2006 with permission.)

exposure to UVL and adequate vitamin D in older people at risk of osteoporosis and falls (see Chs 7, 10, 34). Campaigns stress the importance of the individual being aware of the appearance of their own moles, emphasising the fact that all moles change slowly over the years (Figures 12.9, 12.10) and promote 'safe sun' and encourage behavioural and social changes that might prevent or reduce the incidence of melanoma.

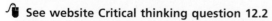 **See website for further content**

Advice includes:

- avoidance of direct sun between 11.00 and 15.00 h
- use of high SPF sun creams
- use of T-shirts/sun hats.

Nurses can encourage regular checking of moles as a preventive strategy, which could have a profound impact on the early detection, incidence and mortality rates of malignant melanoma. Nurses also should raise awareness of skin cancers that occur without there first being a mole present and advise patients to seek medical advice if they develop a non-healing lesion or lesions that are red and get very scaly rather than ignoring them.

See website Critical thinking question 12.2

SUMMARY: KEY NURSING ISSUES

- This chapter focuses on some of the more common skin disorders.
- Dermatology is a major specialty and all nurses will encounter people with skin conditions.
- When assessing and managing skin conditions it is important to consider the psychosocial and economic impact on patients and families.
- A sound knowledge and skills in dermatology are important for all nurses, particularly so for nurses who are non-medical prescribers.

- Publication of competency frameworks to underpin clinical development (Further reading, e.g. NHS Education for Scotland 2003) aims to open up this specialty, so increasing access for patients.

REFLECTION AND LEARNING – WHAT NEXT?

- **Test** your knowledge by visiting the website and answering the multiple choice questions and critical thinking questions.
- **Consolidate** your learning by looking at some of the further reading suggestions, references and specialist websites.
- **Revisit** some of the additional material on the website.
- **Consider** what you have learnt and how this will help your professional development.
- **Reflect** on how you can apply this knowledge to the care of your patients.
- **Discuss** your learning with your mentor/supervisor, lecturer and colleagues.

REFERENCES

All Party Parliamentary Group (APPG): *Skin cancer – improving prevention, treatment and care*, London, 2004, APPG.

Boon NA, Colledge NR, Walker BR: *Davidson's Principles and Practice of Medicine*, ed 20, Edinburgh, 2006, Churchill Livingstone.

British National Formulary (BNF): 2009. Available online http://www.bnf.org.uk.

Cancer Research UK: *CancerStats Key Facts on Skin Cancer*, 2009a. Available online http://info.cancerresearchuk.org/cancerstats/types/skin/.

Cancer Research UK: *SunSmart*, 2009b. Available online http://info.cancerresearchuk.org/healthyliving/sunsmart/about-sunsmart/.

Cotterill JA, Cunliffe WJ: Suicide in dermatology patients, *Br J Dermatol* 137:246–250, 1997.

Cunliffe WJ, Gollnick HPM: *Acne diagnosis and management*, London, 2001, Martin Dunitz.

Denyer J, Hughes E: Epidermolysis bullosa and bullous diseases. In Hughes E, Van Onselen J, editors: *Dermatology nursing: a practical guide*, Edinburgh, 2001, Churchill Livingstone, pp 221–234.

Department of Health: *The NHS improvement plan. Putting people at the heart of public services (Section 2)*, 2004. Available online http://www.dh.gov.uk/en/Publicationsandstatistics/Publications/PublicationsPolicyAndGuidance/Browsable/DH_4097241.

Department of Health: *Our health, Our care, Our say*, 2006. Available online http://www.dh.gov.uk/en/Healthcare/Ourhealthourcareoursay/index.htm.

Dermatology Workforce Group: *Models of integrated service delivery in dermatology*, 2007. Available online http://www.skincarecampaign.org/.

Ersser S, Maguire S, Nicol N, Penzer R, Peters J: *Best practice in emollient therapy. A statement for health professionals*, Aberdeen, 2007, Dermatological Nursing.

Ferguson J: Chronic actinic dermatitis, *J Eur Acad Dermatol Venereol* 18(Suppl 1), 2004.

Finlay AY, Khan GK: Dermatology Life Quality Index: A simple practical measure for routine clinical use, *Clin Exp Dermatol* 19:210–216, 1994.

Gawkrodger DJ: *Dermatology: an illustrated colour text*, ed 4, Edinburgh, 2008, Churchill Livingstone.

Grimalt R, Mangeaud U, Cambazard F: The steroid sparing effect of emollient therapy in infants with atopic dermatitis: A randomised controlled study, *Dermatology* 214(1):61–67, 2007.

Hengge UR, Ruzicka T, Schwartz RA, et al: Adverse effects of topical glucocorticosteroids, *J Am Acad Dermatol* 54(1):1–15, 2006.

Hughes E: Skin: its structure, function and related pathology. In Hughes E, Van Onselen J, editors: *Dermatology nursing: a practical guide*, Edinburgh, 2001, Churchill Livingstone, pp 1–18.

Koek MB, Buskens E, van Weelden H, et al: Home versus outpatient ultraviolet B phototherapy for mild to severe psoriasis: pragmatic multicentre randomised non-inferiority trial (PLUTO) study, *BMJ* 338:b1542, 2009.

Kurwa HA, Finlay AY: Dermatology inpatient management greatly improves life quality, *Br J Dermatol* 113:575–578, 1995.

Lawton S: Eczema. In Hughes E, Van Onselen J, editors: *Dermatology nursing: a practical guide*, Edinburgh, 2001, Churchill Livingstone, pp 151–169.

Lewis-Jones S: Quality of life – skin disease and disability, *Dermatology in Practice* 7(3):8–10, 1999.

Marks R: *Roxburgh's Common skin diseases*, London, 2003, Arnold.

McNally NJ, Williams HC, Phillips DR, et al: Atopic eczema and domestic water hardness, *Lancet* 352(15):527–531, 1998.

Morris A: Effects of long-term topical corticosteroids, *Dermatology in Practice* 6(3):5–8, 1998.

National Eczema Society: *Schools packs*, London, 2003, NES.

National Institute for Health and Clinical Excellence (NICE): *Improving outcomes for patients with skin tumours including melanoma*, 2006. Available online http://www.nice.org.uk/nicemedia/pdf/CSG_Skin_EvidenceReview.pdf.

National Institute for Health and Clinical Excellence (NICE): *Atopic eczema in children; Management of atopic eczema in children from birth up to the age of 12 years clinical guidelines. In collaboration with National Collaborating Centre for Women's and children's Health*, 2007. Available online http://www.nice.org.uk/CG57.

National Patient Safety Agency: *Potential hazard with paraffin based skin products on dressings and clothing*, 2007. Available online http://www.npsa.nhs.uk/.

O'Donoghue N: Corticosteroids in dermatology, *Dermatological Nursing* 4(1):11–13, 2005.

Page BE: Wet wraps, *Nursing Scotland* (March/April):22, 2003.

Peters J: Assessment of the dermatology patient. In Hughes E, Van Onselen J, editors: *Dermatology nursing: a practical guide*, Edinburgh, 2001, Churchill Livingstone, pp 19–39.

Peters J, Sterling A, Robertson S: Knowledge and application of topical emollients: an audit, *Dermatological Nursing* 7(2):30–35, 2008.

Stone L: Dermatology nursing: planning for the future, *Nurs Stand* 11(49):39–41, 1997.

Titman P: *Understanding childhood eczema*, Chichester, 2003, Wiley.

Weller R, Hunter J, Savin J, Dahl M: *Clinical dermatology*, ed 4, Oxford, 2008, Wiley-Blackwell.

FURTHER READING

Buxton P: *ABC Dermatology*, London, 2003, British Medical Journal.

Gawkrodger DJ: *Dermatology: an illustrated colour text*, ed 4, Edinburgh, 2008, Churchill Livingstone.

Lawton S, Gill M: Contact dermatitis: types, triggers and treatment strategies, *Nurs Stand* 23(34):40–46, 2009.

McWilliam J: Acne vulgaris: clinical features, assessment and treatment, *Nurs Stand* 23(34):49–56, 2009.

NHS Education for Scotland: *Caring for people with dermatological conditions: a core curriculum*, Edinburgh, 2003, NHS Education for Scotland.

Penzer R, Ersser S: *Principles of Skin Care: A Guide for Nurses and Health Care Practitioners*, Oxford, 2010, Wiley-Blackwell.

Peters J: Adult eczema and behaviour modification, *Dermatological Nursing* 3(2):8–10, 2004.

Peters J: Dermatology. In Cross S, Rimmer V, editors: *Nurse Practitioner Manual of Clinical Skills*, ed 2, London, 2007, Saunders, pp 27–62.

Royal College of Nursing (RCN): *Caring for children and young people with atopic eczema: guidance for nurses*, London, 2008, RCN.

White G: *Color atlas of dermatology*, ed 3, London, 2004, Mosby.

USEFUL WEBSITES

British Dermatological Nursing Group: www.bdng.org.uk

National Eczema Society: www.eczema.org

New Zealand Dermatological Society Inc: www.dermnetnz.org

Nottingham University Hospitals: www.nottingham.ac.uk/dermatology

Psoriasis Association: www.psoriasis-association.org.uk

Skin Care Campaign: www.skincarecampaign.org

The British Association of Dermatologists (BAD): www.bad.org.uk

Wessex Cancer service sponsoring MARC's Line: www.wessexcancer.org

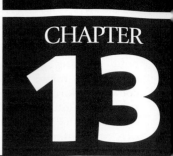

Nursing patients with disorders of the eye and vision

Christine Thom, Allyson Sanderson

Introduction

The aims of this chapter are to present the knowledge and specialised care required for the ophthalmic patient, to raise awareness pertaining to visual impairment (VI) and how VI impacts upon all aspects of daily living, and to consider the implications for practice relating to the Disability Discrimination Act (DDA) in 2005 (http://www.direct.gov.uk). It is estimated that 100 people a day lose their vision, and sight loss is feared more than AIDS, stroke, cancer, heart disease and diabetes (http://www.vision2020uk.org.uk). As life expectancy increases in the UK, there is a higher incidence of cataract, age-related maculopathy and diabetic eye disease and, therefore, it is increasingly important for health care professionals to recognise adverse ocular signs and symptoms and ensure prompt referral for specialised care.

It is predicted that by 2020 many specialised nurses will be retiring (http://www.rcn.org.uk) at a time when a large percentage of the population will be over 60 years of age and by association there will be a higher incidence of VI/eye disease. The need for service modernisation which would improve efficiency and delivery of care (Cuber-Dochan et al 2006) and the reduction in junior doctors' hours (Calpin-Davies 2001) have served as catalysts for developing the role of the health care professional in this dynamic field of health care. As the professional need and desire to develop ophthalmic knowledge (Marsden & Shaw 2007) continues, the nursing roles are evolving in response to the influence of technological, statutory and organisational change. These roles, which have increased both nursing autonomy and responsibility, include performing minor lid surgery, emergency eye care, glaucoma monitoring and cataract care among a variety of other nurse-led initiatives. The health care professional in all environments has a duty of care to be up-to-date in practice, to facilitate health promotion, screening, primary and secondary care (Nursing and Midwifery Council [NMC] 2008). The ocular conditions and diseases presented in this chapter will provide the reader with a sound knowledge base related to causes, diagnoses, management and related nursing care. Not all ocular conditions cause VI; many clinical conditions are successfully treated with medical and surgical interventions. The main causes of VI in the UK are cataract (p. 431) and glaucoma (p. 432), age-related macular degeneration (p. 443) and diabetic eye disease (p. 444).

The term 'visually impaired' will be used throughout this chapter as an alternative term for people who do not wish to be labelled as 'blind' or 'partially sighted', as they can feel that these terms are negative and misleading (http://www.afbp.org/). It is estimated, globally, that 135 million people are visually impaired (VI) with 80% having eye disease that is believed to be treatable or preventable (http://www.who.int). The risk of blindness in developing countries is 10–14 times higher than in developed countries and it is predicted that the incidence of VI will double by 2020, due to an increase in the population and longer life expectancy (Bunce & Wormald 2006).

The World Health Organization is at the forefront of *Vision 2020 – The Right to Sight: A Global Initiative for the Elimination of Avoidable Blindness* (http://www.vision2020uk.org.uk). The aim is to eliminate avoidable blindness as a public health problem by the year 2020 (http://www.who.int). The Royal College of Ophthalmologists (http://www.rcopht.ac.uk) estimates

that 4.3 million people over 65 years of age in the UK have a VI in one or both eyes (http://www.guidedogs.org.uk).

Anatomy and physiology

It is important to understand that the structures that compose the eyeball do not themselves produce sight but serve as a gateway for visual impulses which are then processed via the optic nerves and tracts, the visual cortex and associated areas of the brain. Accessory structures play a vital role in enabling the eyes to scan and focus on objects in the environment and in protecting and maintaining the optical properties of the eyes.

The eye

The eyeball

The eyeball is generally spherical in shape and approximately 24 mm in length. It is sited for protection within the bony structures of the orbit and behind the eyelids. It receives light stimuli through the clear anterior structures of the cornea and lens which refract or bend the light in such a way as to direct the light stimuli through the clear posterior structure of the vitreous. In this way the light is focused on to the photoreceptor cells of the retina and more particularly on to the macula, which is responsible for detailed vision.

The eyeball or globe is a structure composed of three main layers of tissue (Figure 13.1):

1   The outer layer of the globe consists of the fibrous white sclera posteriorly and the transparent cornea anteriorly. The junction of the two is called the limbus. The cornea is transparent due to its avascularity and is supplied with nerve endings from the trigeminal nerve.

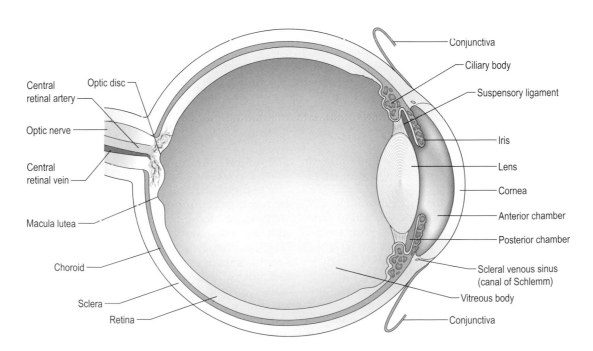

Figure 13.1 Section of the eye. (Adapted from Waugh & Grant 2006.)

2 The middle vascular layer, known as the uveal tract, consists of the choroid, the ciliary body and the iris. The choroid lines the sclera in the posterior compartment of the eye and continues into the muscular ciliary body, into which are inserted the suspensory ligaments. These ligaments, known as the zonules, extend to the lens and hold it in position. The contraction or relaxation of the ciliary body changes the shape of the lens and controls its refractive and focusing power. The iris is the pigmented anterior portion of the uveal tract. It contains circular and radial muscle fibres which control the size of the pupil.

3 The inner layer of the eyeball is the retina. It contains several million photoreceptive cells that are responsible for converting light into electrical impulses. The retina arises just behind the equator of the eyeball in an area known as the ora serrata. This leaves a small anterior section of the choroid – the pars plana – exposed, which allows surgical access without retinal damage.

The retina consists of two layers: the pigmented outer layer, which lines the choroid, and the innermost neural layer, which is in contact with the vitreous humor. Rod cells predominate in the periphery and function best in dim light. Cone cells predominate near the centre of the retina and are adapted for bright light and colour vision. These photoreceptor cells are linked through a series of synapses to ganglion cells whose axons run together to form the optic nerve. For further anatomy and physiology see Waugh & Grant (2006) or Field & Tillotson (2008).

The two segments of the eye

Inside the globe, the lens acts to divide the eye into two main segments:

* The anterior segment, which is divided into two chambers: the anterior chamber in front of the iris and the posterior chamber behind the iris.
* The posterior segment behind the lens, which contains the clear jelly-like substance called the vitreous humor. In conjunction with the aqueous this exerts sufficient pressure to maintain the shape of the eye.

Internal environment and intraocular pressure (IOP)

The anterior compartment is bathed in a clear aqueous fluid (humor) that is produced by the ciliary body and provides nutrients to the lens and cornea. Aqueous flows from the posterior chamber through the pupil to the anterior chamber and drains away through the sieve-like fibrous trabecular meshwork located in the angle between the iris and cornea around the circumference of the eye. This then drains into the vascular canal of Schlemm and into the systemic venous circulation. The production and drainage of aqueous must be constant in order to maintain a normal IOP within the range of 10–20 mmHg (Waugh & Grant 2006).

The depth of the anterior chamber and thus the angle between the cornea and iris, affects the functioning of the drainage system. The larger, elongated eye of the myope (short-sighted person) has a naturally occurring deep anterior chamber with an open angle, whilst the small eye of the hypermetrope (long-sighted person) has a shallow anterior chamber with a narrow angle (Box 13.1). Any interference with

Box 13.1 Information

Terms associated with visual acuity and refractive errors

* Emmetropia – normal sight; light rays focus on the retina
* Ametropia – defective sight due to refractive error
* Myopia – short-sightedness; light rays focus in front of the retina
* Hypermetropia – long-sightedness; light rays focus behind the retina
* Presbyopia – loss of focused reading/near-vision capacity, resulting from loss of lens elasticity due to ageing
* Astigmatism – irregular curvature of the cornea which prevents light rays from focusing at a single point

normal drainage of the aqueous humor raises the IOP, leading to the decreased blood supply, pain and impaired vision associated with conditions such as glaucoma.

The visual pathways and interpretative centres

The optic nerve runs from the posterior aspect of the globe and enters the cranial cavity via the optic foramen. The medial nerve fibres cross over to the opposite side at the optic chiasma (Figure 13.2) to join with the lateral fibres and form the optic tract before synapsing in the lateral geniculate body of the thalamus. The fibres then run in the optic radiations to the occipital cerebral cortex of the brain. The main blood supply to the eye is via the ophthalmic artery, a branch of the internal carotid artery.

Accessory structures

The exposed anterior aspect of the eyeball is protected by the eyebrow, eyelids and eyelashes. The conjunctiva, a mucous membrane, lines the eyelids (palpebral conjunctiva) and reflects back on itself (bulbar conjunctiva) to cover the sclera. This fold forms the conjunctival sac or fornix and is an ideal site for the instillation of topical drugs. At the limbus, the conjunctiva is modified to form the epithelial layer of the cornea. The conjunctiva facilitates free movement of the eyelids over the globe.

The exposed surface of the eye is covered by a three-layered film of tear fluid. Mucous secretion from conjunctival goblet cells forms the first layer of the tear film and ensures an even spread of tears over the cornea. The middle layer is the watery fluid secreted by the lacrimal glands (situated under the upper orbital rim) and by the accessory glands in the conjunctiva. The outer lipid layer of tear film is secreted by the meibomian glands of the lids. This is thought to reduce the evaporation rate of tears and to prevent the lids sticking together during sleep. The main functions of tear fluid are to lubricate the eye, to facilitate O_2 and CO_2 exchange, to provide an optically smooth corneal surface and to cleanse the eye with a bacteriostatic enzyme called lysozyme. Excess tears are drained from the eye via the lacrimal punctum and apparatus at the inner canthus (nasal end of the lid margins) into the lacrimal sac and thence into the nose through the nasolacrimal duct (Figure 13.3).

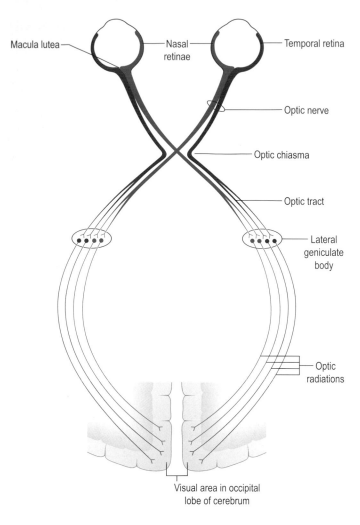

Figure 13.2 The optic nerves and their pathways. (Reproduced with kind permission from Waugh & Grant 2006.)

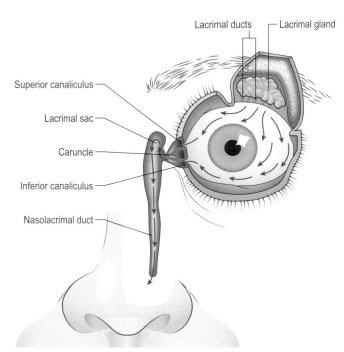

Figure 13.3 The lacrimal apparatus. Arrows show the direction of the flow of tears. (Reproduced with kind permission of Waugh & Grant 2006.)

Posteriorly and laterally the globe is protected by the bony orbit, the extraocular recti and oblique muscles (responsible for tracking movements) and by orbital fat.

The physiology of vision

Light rays are bent (refracted) as they pass through the varying densities of the clear media of the cornea, aqueous, lens and vitreous to focus on the retina. The cornea is relatively constant in shape and is responsible for about two thirds of the refractive power of the eye. The zonules extend from the ciliary body into the lens through 360 degrees so that any contraction or relaxation of the body will change the shape of the lens and affect its focusing (refractive) power. The normal eye in its relaxed state brings rays of light from distant objects into sharp focus. However, for clear focusing on near objects, an autonomic reflex known as the synkinetic near reflex comes into play. This reflex involves accommodation, miosis and convergence, as follows:

- Accommodation – the ciliary body contracts and changes shape, thus releasing tension on the zonular fibres and allowing the lens to thicken and increase its refractive power. This allows objects at different distances to be visualised with equal clarity.
- Miosis, or constriction of the pupil, accompanies accommodation and ensures that light rays are concentrated to pass through the centre of the lens and focus on the macula.
- Convergence, or in-turning of the eyes, seeks out the object to be focused on.

Failure to focus may be described as ametropia, or refractive error (see Box 13.1).

Once the rays of light are focused on the retina, their energy is converted into neuroelectrical energy by the photoreceptor cells. These nerve impulses are transmitted via the visual pathway to the visual cortex. Here, they are interpreted as sensations of light, form and colour and are processed into images of objects that are given meaning by other cerebral areas (see Ch. 9).

🖰 See website for Multiple choice questions

Assessing the eye and visual function

Examination of structure

It is necessary to know what a normal eye looks like and the normal expectations for an eye recovering from surgery or disease. It is vital for nurses working with ophthalmic patients to examine the eye in a systematic way and to be able to recognise significant abnormalities. It is recommended the nurse works in good light using a well-charged pen torch and examines all ocular structures from outermost to innermost. The possible implications of clinical features

Table 13.1 Significance of clinical features found on eye examination

STRUCTURE	CLINICAL FEATURES	POSSIBLE SIGNIFICANCE
Lids	Bruising (ecchymosis) Swelling Drooping Increased lacrimation Discharge	Surgical handling Trauma Infection
Conjunctiva	Redness (injection) Swelling (chemosis)	Surgical handling Trauma Allergy Infection
Cornea	Cloudy Crinkled Fluorescein staining Suture line not intact Penetrating injury	Increased IOP Infection Loss of AC Ulceration
Anterior chamber (AC)	Hyphaema (blood in AC) Hypopyon (pus in AC) Shallow AC	Hyphaema due to surgery should gradually resolve Increasing IOP = bleeding/inflammation Hypopyon = infection Shallow = ? aqueous loss
Iris	Muddy	Inflammation
Pupil	Irregular shape	Iris prolapse Adhesions Trauma

that may be found in the course of an eye examination are listed in Table 13.1. For further information on initial visual assessment see Field & Tillotson (2008).

Testing visual function

Visual acuity

Obtaining an accurate visual acuity (VA) assessment is vital in order to assist the clinician in the choice of treatment options. Visual acuity is the mathematical estimation of visual function for different distances.

Distance vision This is tested using Snellen test-type charts, which display letters or pictures arranged in rows of precise and diminishing size (Figure 13.4A). Each eye should be tested separately, with the benefit, if worn, of any spectacles or contact lenses, to ensure that 'best corrected vision' is being checked. The eye not being tested must be completely occluded. In normal testing, patients are positioned 6 m away from the chart and asked to read each line aloud until they can no longer make out the letters. The result is recorded as a fraction of the distance from the chart in metres over the normal reading distance of the last complete line read, plus the number of extra letters read from the line below or minus the number of letters read incorrectly, e.g. 6/9 − 2 (Figure 13.4). If glasses or contact lenses are worn this is also recorded.

Normal distance acuity is accepted as 6/6, although what the patient is likely to achieve will vary with their age.

If the patient sees less than 6/12 or 6/9 (there may be variations from one eye unit to another), they may be asked to read the chart again, looking through a pinhole (PH). A pure refractive error should improve with this simple method of sharpening focus by cutting out peripheral light stimulation.

If the patient cannot read the top letter (6/60) then ability to count fingers (CF) at 1 metre, detect hand movements (HM) or perceive light (PL) is tested. Testing when the patient does not read or understand English can be facilitated by using a Snellen 'E' chart (Figure 13.4B). If the patient has learning difficulties, poor concentration or expressive dysphasia then VA testing can be done by using a Sheridan-Gardiner singles booklet in which single letters or pictures of varying size are presented one at a time and the patient is asked match them on a card with a limited choice of symbols. When increased sensitivity of testing is required the LogMAR system may be used at a distance of 4 m. It is conducted in a similar fashion to the Snellen test, but the scoring system for every letter missed is more rigorous (Marsden 2008).

Near vision is tested in good illumination and the patient is asked to read text in various sizes of standard print that are prefixed with the letter N. N5 is accepted as normal reading acuity.

Binocular vision involves simultaneous perception of an image by both eyes and fusion of the two images in the visual cortex to form a single image. Binocular vision is thought to play a role in depth perception. Having two eyes also widens the field of vision and counters gaps in the visual field caused by natural blind spots (Box 13.2).

The visual field refers to what the eye can see with respect to angle of view (rather than distance). Normally this is about 60 degrees nasally, 90 degrees temporally, 50 degrees superiorly and 70 degrees inferiorly. Assessment of the integrity of the visual field is essential in the management of glaucoma and an important aid to diagnosis of neurological disease and retinal detachment. In the primary care environment and in the absence of automated equipment visual field testing can be carried out by means of a simple confrontation test, whereby the examiner sits directly in front and approximately one metre from the patient and compares the patient's field of vision with their own (Douglas et al 2005). In the ophthalmic setting it is performed by means of perimetry using field analyser systems to gain accurate measurements of visual field defects known as scotomas (Khaw et al 2004).

Colour-blindness

Colour vision depends on the normal functioning of the retinal cones. A colour-blind person is unable to distinguish between some colours – usually red and green. While approximately 8% of the male population is born with defective colour vision, this problem is estimated at only 1% in females. Colour-blindness can be congenital or acquired through certain conditions such as optic neuritis or drug dependency. For further information on colour vision deficiency see http://www.healthinfoplus.scot.nhs.uk.

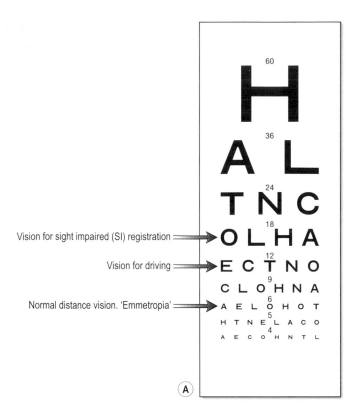
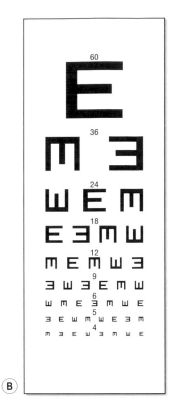

Vision for sight impaired (SI) registration ——➤

Vision for driving ——➤

Normal distance vision. 'Emmetropia' ——➤

(A)   (B)

Figure 13.4 Eye testing charts. A. Snellen test-type chart; the standard method for testing visual acuity in the UK. B. 'E' chart for non-English speakers. The patient is given a wooden or plastic E, which they move to indicate the positions in which they see it on the chart.

 Box 13.2 Reflection

Binocular vision

Look carefully straight ahead and note what you see. Now close one eye. What do you not see? Now repeat with the other eye. What do you no longer see?

The most common method of testing for colour blindness is by means of a series of Ishihara colour-dotted plates. A person with defective colour vision would be unable to distinguish the numbers from the surrounding background. Some occupations, such as pilots and electricians, require normal colour vision, usually for reasons of safety but there are no restrictions on driving cars, lorries or buses, as traffic lights have a fixed sequence and can be recognised by position rather than colour.

Eye changes with ageing

By age 70, most people will need some form of visual aid because the elasticity of the lens decreases with age. Focusing is affected as the cornea flattens, causing astigmatism (see Box 13.1). Retinal cells become less efficient due to deposits laid down by ageing pigment epithelial cells. Tear film is reduced in volume and altered in structure, with the result that tears evaporate more quickly, leading to dryness and irritation of the eye. Conversely, some elderly patients complain of watering eyes due to muscle laxity and malposition of eyelids (see Entropion and Ectropion, p. 444).

 Nursing management and health promotion: preservation of vision

Health care professionals can do a great deal through health education and active intervention to help people preserve their vision by observing individual behaviour and general appearance; missed appointments, unkempt clothes and a reluctance to go out may suggest ocular problems (http://www.rnib.org.uk) (Box 13.3). Should any changes be noted, prompt action and referral to an optician to ensure early screening and accurate diagnosis are vital.

The following will contribute to health education and promotion.

- Promote the maintenance of good health through a balanced diet, regular exercise and avoidance of smoking (Khan et al 2006). It is believed, although not proven, that this will reduce the risk of ocular degeneration.
- Encourage regular eye examinations, especially in people over 40 years of age and individuals in high-risk groups (e.g. those with diabetes or hypertension). In the UK free sight testing is available for those over 60 years as well as

 Box 13.3 Reflection

Visual impairment recognition

Consider the changes in behaviour or appearance that may be indicative of deteriorating vision. Check your ideas with information on the RNIB website – http://www.rnib.org.uk

for those in high-risk groups, lower income groups and people over 40 years old who have a family history of glaucoma.

- Provide advice and ensure the correct use, storage and cleaning of glasses and contact lenses. It is vital that contact lenses are properly maintained and used according to optometrists' and manufacturers' guidance. If guidance is not followed, there is a risk of long-term, possibly permanent damage to the cornea, due to infection, ulceration or abrasion (Jackson 2008).
- Encourage the prompt treatment of eye infections and ailments to prevent long-term ocular damage.
- Both work and leisure-related eye injuries can be prevented by wearing eye protection; 85% of ocular injuries occur in males aged 20–40 with approximately 70% being the result of industrial accidents (http://www.rnib.org.uk). While statutory health and safety regulations and better supervision by occupational health nurses have helped to reduce the number of industrial eye injuries, lack of eye protection remains a problem (http://www.dh.org.uk). The wearing of eye protection is mandatory in certain work environments, e.g. chemical laboratories and any area where grinding of metal occurs (Health and Safety at Work Act [1974] and Personal Protective Equipment Work Regulations [1992]). The health care professional must be aware that education is vital as the lack of use of eye protection may be associated with poor reliability as well as an uncomfortable design which deters, rather than promotes wear (Box 13.4).
- Advocate the correct and safe labelling of chemical products, and ensure first aid (e.g. eye irrigation) is available for emergency use. Individuals in the workplace and at home should be urged to heed the labels on chemical products indicating whether they are harmful to the eyes and make a careful note of first aid instructions in case of accidental splashing.
- Ensure that visual display units (VDUs) are used in accordance with the Health and Safety Executive (2003) recommendations for short, frequent rest periods to prevent eye fatigue. Employers must provide an annual sight test for all VDU users.
- Promote the wearing of sunglasses. It is not known exactly what type of ocular damage exposure to sunlight can cause, but it is believed to contribute to long-term ocular changes, i.e. cataract, macular degeneration (http://www.abfp.org).

Box 13.4 Reflection

Concordance and compliance

If we accept that concordance is not necessarily the same concept as compliance or adherence (consult the *Phamaceutical Journal Online* – http://www.pharmj.com/ – and type in 'concordance' in the search box), how do you as a nurse see your role with a patient who is prescribed topical anti-glaucoma treatment?

The visually impaired person (VIP)

Good vision is generally taken for granted and therefore it can be difficult to appreciate fully the value and importance of vision in everyday life. For example, when blindfolded it is difficult to accomplish the most simple task, such as making a sandwich, even when in a familiar environment.

Certification of vision impairment (CVI)

Most visually impaired people have some residual sight and there are few VIPs with a visual acuity of no perception of light (NPL). An ophthalmologist is required to certify the degree of impairment (Table 13.2) and certify that the patient is either Severely Sight Impaired (SSI, previously known as blind) or Sight Impaired (SI, previously known as partially sighted). In England a 'certificate of vision impairment' form (http://www.dh.gov.uk) is used and in Scotland it is a 'blind person' form. For information regarding registration in Wales and Northern Ireland see http:www.rnib.org.uk.

Registration is completely voluntary and entitles the individual to many local and national benefits; however, rehabilitation support can be obtained without registration. The social worker visiting individuals in their homes and helping to arrange the appropriate support will explain these issues. Some areas also have the benefit of a mobility or rehabilitation officer who is specially trained to help newly registered individuals to relearn certain daily living skills, and to move about safely in their own environment. This may involve the use of special canes or guide dogs. Rehabilitation officers also teach communication and information technology skills and advise on retraining for employment. Their overall aim is to enable the visually impaired person to function as independently as possible.

People with impaired vision may be referred to a low-vision clinic and assessed by an optometrist or specialist nurse to determine the need for low visual aids (LVAs) in the form of a monocular telescope, for reading bus numbers at a distance, or a magnifying glass for near vision tasks such as reading newspapers. Closed circuit television (CCTV) allows the VIP to comfortably view a magnified image of material such as photographs or objects such as pill boxes with added clarity and so can help individuals to make best use of their residual sight. These professionals may also provide information and advice on adaptation or retraining for employment. Employers can also be advised by various agencies, including the Royal National Institute of Blind People (http://www.rnib.org.uk) and Action for

Table 13.2 Defining visual impairment (adapted from the Royal National Institute of Blind People)	
TYPE OF VI	**DEFINITION/ STANDARDS FOR CVI**
SSI	VA less than 3/60 with full visual field (VF) VA between 3/60 and 6/60 with reduced VF VA 6/60 or above with reduced VF
SI	VA 3/60 to 6/60 with full VF VA up to 6/24 with altered VF VA up to 6/18 with large VF defect

Blind People (http://www.afbp.org) about the sophisticated electronic equipment now available for VI employees. The introduction of the Disability Discrimination Act (DDA) in 1995 made it unlawful to treat disabled individuals in a discriminatory way, stating that employers and service providers, including the NHS and Primary Care Trusts (PCTs), must make reasonable adjustments to their services, ensuring for example equal access for disabled persons (http://www.direct.gov.uk).

Considering the needs of the visually impaired person

All client care should be planned using a structured approach to assessment and implemented with an ongoing recognition of the degree of assistance the VIP actually wants. The principles for care listed below echo the tenets of the Roper, Logan and Tierney (1990) model for nursing which is based on activities of living; it is a nursing model in which care is orientated to the patient and provided in a way that enables or supports the patient.

 See website Critical thinking question 13.1

Some general principles of care for the visually impaired person are outlined below:

- *Communication.* Approximately 80% of sensory information is obtained visually (http://www.guidedogs.org.uk). Perception through focused use of other senses, especially hearing and touch, will be therefore heightened (http://www.rnib.org.uk). Ensure the person has access to radio, talking books/newspapers, information in large print or Braille or on audiotape and other more sophisticated means of communication as required.
- When approaching the individual, address them by name and identify yourself. Describe what you are doing so that they feel involved. Remember also to inform the VIP when you leave, as otherwise they may not be aware of this.
- *Orientation to place.* If the person is at home the environment is familiar and it is therefore important to keep things in their usual place. Assistance should be given to help VIPs move around the community and workplace until they are confident to do so independently. Appropriate visual aids such as magnifiers should be used. If the person is admitted to hospital, it is the duty of the health care professional to orientate them (http://www.nmc.org.uk). Older people can become confused in this situation and need constant reassurance and support.
- *Mobility.* Early mobilisation should be encouraged in the home and hospital with appropriate assistance given. The preferred method of guiding a person with visual impairment is illustrated in Figure 13.5.
- *Maintaining a safe environment.* It is essential to remove any hazardous objects in the person's environment. Doors should be fully open or properly closed. Fires should have guards. Loose flooring must be secured.
- *Eating and drinking.* Bearing in mind the patient's functioning visual field, food should be placed close to the patient and the content and position of food on the

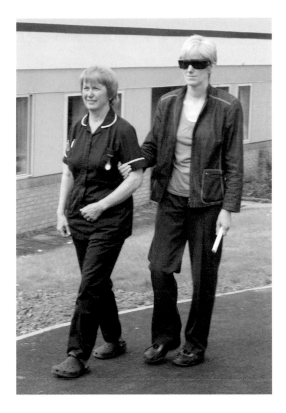

Figure 13.5 Guiding a VIP. Before you set off, offer your arm to the VIP. Ask which side they prefer. They should hold your arm just above the elbow. Check that the VIP is ready to go. Always walk one pace in front and at the same pace as the person. Describe the environment and warn the VIP of any obstacles or changes in the journey, i.e. stairs – up or down, doors, kerbs. In this way, the VIP can sense any turning of the guide's body and can walk more confidently. The long cane or guide dog is in the VIP's 'free' hand. (Reproduced with permission from the Medical Photography Department, St John's Hospital.)

plate should be described using a clock-face analogy. Plate guards, non-slip mats and using crockery that contrasts with the food colour can be helpful for those with severe visual impairment. Many safety devices are available for use in the home to help with cooking (http://www.rnib.org.uk).
- *Personal hygiene and grooming.* After initial orientation and help, the VIP should be encouraged to be as independent as possible.

With good rehabilitation training and family support, the visually impaired person should be able to get around in their environment safely and effectively. It will take confidence, time and patience to achieve this level of ability, and the VIP will require understanding and ongoing support.

▷ Nursing management and health promotion: ophthalmic care

The following principles must be followed when carrying out ophthalmic nursing procedures, not only in the perioperative period but also in the context of emergency care and the clinic setting. The reader is urged to consult specialist ophthalmic nursing texts listed in the references section.

General principles for ophthalmic care

In relation to those conditions that require surgical intervention the term 'intraocular surgery' describes procedures that are performed inside the globe of the eye involving structures in the anterior and/or posterior segments. This chapter will focus on cataract, retinal detachment, glaucoma and corneal transplant. These conditions share common certain general priorities for ophthalmic nursing management but specific priorities relating to each condition are outlined below.

Alleviating stress and giving information

Anxiety levels for ophthalmic patients attending or admitted to hospital may be exacerbated by fear of blindness and loss of independence. It is important to anticipate and dispel any misconceptions that the patient may have about eye surgery. The patient should be given the opportunity to discuss particular fears and should be provided with realistic information that does not raise false expectations about operative results. The patient's concerns about managing practical activities following ophthalmic treatment or surgery should be addressed and the individual should be reassured with information regarding what guidance and support will be available from the acute and primary health care team and from local organisations with a role in supporting the VIP.

If a local anaesthetic is to be used, the person may be concerned about their level of awareness during the procedure and about whether they will be able to cooperate. Depending on the patient's visual acuity, it is often helpful to discuss the operation using a model of the eye. Some patients will want only the minimum details and so the nurse should provide the appropriate amount and depth of information for each individual in order that the patient's wishes are respected. See Chapter 26 for further discussion of the principles of peri-operative nursing, anxiety, informed consent and information giving.

Asepsis and infection control issues

Although asepsis and infection control measures must be observed by the nurse and the underlying principles taught to patients and relatives, the nurse must be realistic about what the patient and relatives will manage in the home. Education and planning regarding self-care on discharge should be tailored to individual need and capability.

Each eye should be treated separately. Drops and ointments should only be used in the eye for which they are prescribed. In hospital, topical medication should be dated upon opening and discarded after one week (after 4 weeks in the community). These precautions and simple handwashing measures (see Ch. 16) will reduce the risk of eye infection, which can pose a threat to vision.

Instilling eye drops and ointments

If the patient is able to carry out self-medication, instruction in the instillation of drops can provide a good opportunity to begin a teaching programme for postoperative self-care. Eye drops are inserted into the middle to outer third of the lower conjunctival sac. To facilitate this, the patient is asked to tilt the head back and look up while the lower lid is gently pulled down (Figure 13.6). Dropping the solution onto the sensitive cornea will cause discomfort and trigger a reflexive squeezing

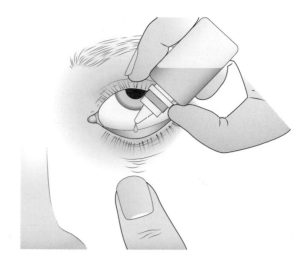

Figure 13.6 Instilling eye drops into the lower central fornix.

shut of the eye. After drop instillation the patient is asked to close their eyes gently for 30 s to maximise absorption.

Eye ointment is instilled into the lower conjunctival sac with the patient's head tilted back as described above. Contact of the tube with the eye should be avoided. For information about topical and systemic drugs and other ophthalmic preparations see http://www.bnf.org/bnf/.

Managing eye dressings

Pressure on the eyeball must be avoided. This applies particularly when cleansing the upper eyelids. A sterile, moist, dental roll is used to wipe from inner to outer canthus along the eyelash line and is discarded after a single use. Cotton wool balls can be used only if they have been thoroughly soaked and squeezed out to ensure that no dry fibres are protruding. Patients should be cautioned against rubbing their eyes. The cornea is vulnerable to abrasion injuries, particularly after the instillation of local anaesthetic.

Eye pads are used to apply pressure to the eye and occasionally for comfort when photophobia or lacrimation (tear production) is excessive. The term 'double padding' means that two pads are applied to the treated eye; padding both eyes at the same time is generally avoided to prevent the disorientation and distress that this sudden visual deficit will incur. Eye pads are applied after eyes have been cleansed (if required), examined and treatment instilled. Ensure that the eye is closed underneath the pad at all times to prevent corneal damage.

The eye pad is held in position and tape is applied by first attaching one end to the forehead, then stretching diagonally across the eye pad towards the lateral aspect of the cheek, where it is secured. The downward movement facilitates lid closure and the diagonal position of the tape permits facial muscle movement. To aid removal a tab should be made by turning under the top of the tape. The skin on the forehead and cheek are supported during removal of the tape to reduce any dragging movement on the eyeball. The eye is examined when a pad is removed and the pad must be inspected for signs of infection or haemorrhage before discarding.

When the eye cannot be closed voluntarily, e.g. in the unconscious patient, care should be taken to avoid corneal abrasion from bedclothes or other articles when attending to the patient. The cornea can be kept moist by the instillation of lubricants and lid closure can sometimes be improved with the application of paraffin gauze, as in the case of a sedated and ventilated patient.

Postoperatively the eye is protected by a plastic shield at night for up to a week. Dark glasses may be worn during the day to reduce the discomfort of glare; patients should be taught to put the glasses on over their forehead to avoid accidentally pushing the earpieces into the eye.

Irrigation

This is a procedure that is generally confined to the emergency or occupation health setting. When irrigating the eye, the warmed solution of sodium chloride 0.9% should be directed across the skin of the lateral cheek so as to prepare the patient for the solution coming into contact with the eye. After this the irrigating motion should be directed away from the nasal side of the sclera. This will wash harmful foreign material away from the lacrimal duct to the side of the cheek, where it can be received in a kidney dish (Box 13.5).

Patient positioning and activity

As a general rule, any position or activity that markedly increases venous pressure in the head should be avoided in ophthalmic surgical patients. In most situations an upright head position is recommended except in cases of retinal detachment, macular hole surgery and following vitrectomy (removal of some of the gel-like substance in the posterior segment of the eye) when the surgeon's instructions for positioning must be followed precisely.

Nausea and vomiting

Postoperative vomiting should be prevented by ensuring that an antiemetic is prescribed and given promptly if the patient complains of nausea. Increased blood flow caused by a head-down position when vomiting or retching will

raise intraocular pressure and can result in damage to optical structures or suture lines. The majority of patients go home shortly after surgery and therefore explanation of any restrictions on activity and positioning and the duration of the restrictions must be clear and concise. This information must be explained to the patient as early as possible to allow time to consider the ramifications, which might include taking time off work or being unable to provide care for a relative.

Assessing visual status

It is important to establish a baseline visual status so that the patient is not demeaned by inappropriate restrictions. It is equally important to identify any risks, in order to ensure that a safe environment is maintained. Any significant change in visual acuity must be reported. Patients should be oriented to the clinical area with a view to maintaining their normal degree of independence as far as possible. The dependency level will fluctuate during the perioperative period due to anaesthesia, treatment and/or padding of the eye. The potential difficulties should be discussed fully with the patient.

Examining the eye

Providing there is no underlying pathology it is often helpful to use the non-affected eye as a baseline against which to compare the operated or injured eye and also because the unaffected eye may react in sympathy with the affected eye (sympathetic ophthalmitis). The patient should be asked to describe how each eye feels. As eye complications can develop rapidly, early recognition and reporting of abnormalities and increasing pain is vital in reducing the risk of potential permanent loss of sight.

The examination using a pen torch should be systematic and allow the nurse to check for signs of infection and evidence of healing. Subconjunctival haemorrhage is not abnormal, particularly in patients who have had cataract surgery under local anaesthetic. Often a localised subconjunctival bleed may be noted in the area of the anaesthetic infiltration or in the postoperative antibiotic injection site, if the needle or cannula has disrupted a small blood vessel. If bleeding into the anterior chamber (hyphaema) is present, it should be recorded and a diagram indicating size relative to the anterior chamber entered in the medical and nursing notes. Some degree of lid bruising and swelling may be seen postoperatively, especially following local anaesthesia. Conjunctival redness (injection) and oedema (chemosis) is sometimes noted to spread out from the postoperative antibiotic injection site. The cornea and anterior chamber (AC) should be clear. A fine suture line may be evident, although cataract wound size is often so small and the wound tunnelled in such a self-sealing way that sutures are not required. Glaucoma and cataract surgery wounds are concealed under the top lid and examined by asking the patient look downwards and the gently retracting the top lid. The depth and shape of the AC should be noted, as a shallow AC (one in which there appears to be a decreased space between the cornea and the iris) may indicate that aqueous from the AC is leaking from the site of the wound. Photophobia (sensitivity to light) is to be expected postoperatively and following trauma.

Box 13.5 Information

Irrigation of an eye

Copiously irrigate the affected eye(s), preferably with 1 litre of sodium chloride 0.9% via an i.v. giving set or ideally a Morgan lens (http://www.morganlens.com). Ensure the patient is comfortable, reclining with their head and neck supported. Clothing should be protected by waterproof cape and towels. Ask the patient to hold the receiver dish and to turn their head slightly to the affected side. Instill topical anaesthetic drops, e.g. proxymetacaine 1 to 2 drops. Pull down the lower eyelid and irrigate with a steady flow of fluid, while asking the patient to move their eye around and to evert the upper lid to ensure thorough irrigation. Continue irrigation for at least 15 minutes, re-instilling local anaesthetic drops as required. Remove particles or foreign bodies with moistened cotton bud or forceps. Wait 5 minutes prior to checking pH levels of the tear film, which should be 7.5 or below. Continue irrigation until this neutral pH is indicated when reading the colour reaction of a strip of universal pH paper when it touches the tear film in the lower fornix of the eye (Marsden 2008).

Conditions requiring surgical intervention

Cataract

Any opacity of the lens can be defined as a cataract. Cataracts can develop as part of the ageing process. They can also be congenital or develop following trauma, as sequelae to inflammatory and degenerative disease, or as a result of the prolonged use of some systemic drugs such as corticosteroids.

The lens of the eye is normally transparent due to the regular arrangement of its crystalline fibres and the nature of the proteins inside them. These fibres, which originate in the epithelium of the lens capsule, continue to be laid down throughout life. This results in thickening and a loss of elasticity. Opacity will eventually develop with ageing.

Clinical features The main feature of a mature cataract is that it reflects as a grey or milky white lens behind the pupil, which normally appears black.

Common presenting symptoms of age-related cataract are as follows:

- gradually decreasing acuity affecting distance vision more than near vision
- general dimming of vision because of the reduction of light reaching the retina
- more frequent refractive errors because of reduced lens elasticity
- increased dazzle and glare in bright light and appearance of haloes around lights at night
- monocular diplopia (double vision or a 'ghosting' effect in one eye)
- alteration in colour and depth perception.

MEDICAL MANAGEMENT

During the developmental stages of cataract spectacles may provide a degree of improvement in visual acuity but, as it is impossible to reverse the opacification process, surgical removal of the cataract will ultimately be the only effective treatment (Riaz et al 2006). Local anaesthetic day care is likely to remain popular as it offers the least disruption to the patient's daily routine and makes effective economic use of health resources. For the most recent UK guidelines on cataract surgery by the Royal College of Ophthalmologists see http://www.rcoph.ac.uk.

Cataract removal and lens implantation is performed when the cataract interferes with activities of daily living. Cataract removal and lens implantation will still be considered in the presence of co-existing ocular pathology such as age-related maculopathy or glaucoma (see pp. 432, 443), even though the visual outcome may be poor (guarded prognosis). Before the operation, the pupil is dilated to facilitate access to the lens and to reduce the risk of damage to the iris. An incision is then made into the globe at the limbus in the 12 o'clock section of the eye. The two principal methods of lens removal are:

- Phaco-emulsification – ultrasonic fragmentation to break up the nucleus and aspirate soft lens material, leaving the posterior capsule intact.

- Extracapsular extraction – removal of the entire nucleus and cortex through a large incision, leaving the posterior capsule intact. This is carried out more often in developing countries as it is not dependent on the availability and sophisticated, technical maintenance of phacoemulsification equipment

Intraocular lens implantation

The best visual correction is achieved by the insertion of an intraocular lens (IOL) positioned in front of the posterior capsule at the time of cataract removal. Unforeseen surgical complication, such as severe posterior capsular rupture with the release of a large amount of vitreous into the anterior chamber, is the main contraindication to non-insertion of an IOL. The strength of lens is calculated for each patient based on a combination of biometry (measurement of the axial length of the eye along the visual axis), keratometry (measurement of the corneal curvature) and their previous optical history. The nurse must not only be able to carry out the tests, but also understand the underlying principles and pro-actively interpret the results with a view to obtaining the best postoperative vision.

An intraocular lens may be inserted as a secondary procedure. In the rare situation when no IOL is inserted, a contact lens or corrective spectacle may be issued.

 ## Nursing management and health promotion: cataract extraction and implantation of intraocular lens

Day case cataract surgery has become routine and ophthalmic units have developed care pathways on the basis of local or national clinical guidelines such as those of the Scottish Intercollegiate Guidelines Network (SIGN 2001) and the Department of Health (DH 2000). The principles of care relating to intraocular surgery are detailed in the Nursing care plan on the website.

See website for Nursing care plan 13.1

The following points are specific to cataract extraction and IOL implantation.

Intraocular lens management

It is important for the nurse to know which method of local anaesthetic has been used – topical or peribulbar (injection around the eye) – as this will affect the length of time the patient has an anaesthetic and akinetic (temporary paralysis of movement of the eye) effect on the operated eye. The nurse must also be aware if surgery has deviated from the routine course, in which case the IOL may not have been implanted and the postoperative drop and medication regimen will be different from the normal pathway.

Problems that may arise following IOL implantation include:

- a secondary rise in intraocular pressure, usually accompanied by severe one-sided headache above the brow of the operated eye
- cystoid macular oedema which results in the patient noting reduction and distortion of vision
- infection with the rare, but sight-threatening possibility of endophthalmitis (severe infection inside the eye).

Patients and relatives need to know who to contact promptly should any of these signs and symptoms occur so that action can be taken to prevent permanent eye damage. It should be explained that during the healing process there will be a period of adaptation as the brain adjusts to changes in visual perception. Although there are generally no restrictions on mobility the patient should take care during this period if they have any pre-existing conditions that affect their balance.

Postoperative medication The inflammatory response that accompanies healing within the eye is controlled by a combination of topical steroids and antibiotics. There has been a concerted drive to shorten and normalise this surgical event to a 2–3 hour visit, with no fasting requirements (for local anaesthesia) or need to remove patient clothing, This may lead patients to misinterpret the situation and equate what appears to be 'low care' with 'no care'. As a result they may view the postoperative eye drop administration as an optional extra rather than a necessary part of the total care package. It is part of the nurse's role to ensure that patients and their relatives/carers understand the importance of completing the prescribed course of postoperative drops.

Refractive laser treatments

Individuals with myopia, hypermetropia or astigmatism (see Box 13.1) have become dissatisfied with the inability to obtain their best vision with either glasses or contact lens, resulting in the practice of laser surgery to correct refractive errors. Current laser techniques, whereby laser energy is used to reshape the cornea, include photorefractive keratectomy (PRK), which alters corneal curvature by ablating surface corneal tissue and results in a reduction of refractive power. Laser in situ keratomileusis (LASIK) consists of cutting a hinged flap of cornea under very precise conditions, performing the laser ablation in the corneal bed and then replacing the flap.

Before considering treatment, it is essential to seek advice from an ophthalmologist, as complications can occur, including over-correction, under-correction and loss of best corrected VA. The National Institute for Health and Clinical Excellence (NICE) offers interventional procedure guidance for these treatments at http://www.nice.org.uk/IPG164.

Glaucoma

Glaucoma is a disease process with a characteristic pattern of cupping of the optic disc and permanent field loss. The IOP may be raised or normal. The condition may be acquired or genetic in origin. Acquired glaucoma can be further classified as primary open-angle glaucoma (POAG), primary closed-angle glaucoma (PCAG – both acute and chronic) and glaucoma secondary to pathological processes (secondary glaucoma).

Primary open-angle glaucoma

This type of glaucoma (also known as chronic simple glaucoma) causes progressive and irreversible loss of the peripheral visual field, with the central 10% being spared until a later stage. The normal range of IOP is 12–20 mmHg and this varies throughout the 24-hour period. In POAG, the pressure is generally elevated and the diurnal variation may show considerable fluctuation (Kanski 2007).

Raised IOP decreases the blood flow in the optic disc capillaries with resultant excavation and atrophy of the optic nerve head and subsequent loss of nerve fibres passing through it (cupping). A progressive loss of the visual field results from damage to nerve fibre bundles as they enter the optic disc.

Clinical features The outward appearance of the eye is normal. On examination, if there is cupping of the optic disc, peripheral visual field loss and possible raised IOP, a diagnosis of glaucoma may be made.

Common presenting symptoms There is usually a gradual and painless loss of peripheral vision. The patient rarely notices this deterioration until considerable damage has been done. This loss of vision is irreversible. The glaucoma is often detected by an optometrist during a routine eye examination.

MEDICAL MANAGEMENT

The main aim of treatment is to reduce IOP to allow better capillary perfusion at the optic nerve head. This involves improving the aqueous drainage system or decreasing the production of aqueous, or a combination of both. Medical treatment is the mainstay in the majority of cases (European Glaucoma Society 2008) although there is a growing trend towards early surgical or laser intervention.

Tests and investigations

Diagnosis and medical assessment of the nature and severity of the condition will rely on the following:

- tonometry – measurement of IOP with instruments that allow for corneal contact
- visual field analysis (perimetry)
- ophthalmoscopy to examine the optic nerve head and estimate the degree of cupping
- gonioscopy – examination of the state and depth of the angle of the anterior chamber
- phasing – measurement of IOP by tonometry at different times of the day.

Treatment

Whether the medical regimen is implemented alone or in combination with a surgical procedure, it is important to maintain monitoring of the efficiency of treatment indefinitely. The regimen may include the administration of some combination of the following medications (for more information see Chapter 11 of the British National Formulary):

- Topical beta blockers, and systemic carbonic anhydrase inhibitors to reduce aqueous production. Topical regimens may be prescribed for long-term continuous use; systemic drugs such as acetazolamide are generally prescribed for short-term or intermittent use.
- Topical prostaglandin analogues to increase uveoscleral outflow are also used in the initial treatment of POAG.
- Topical sympathomimetics in the form of alpha-2 adrenergic agonist which have a dual mechanism to reduce aqueous production and increase uveoscleral outflow.

- Topical miotic drops to constrict the pupil and stretch open the trabecular meshwork, thus facilitating aqueous drainage.

Surgical treatment for POAG is usually performed when conservative management has failed, which is indicated by progression of visual field loss and persistent elevation of IOP, or when the patient's social situation or health prevents them from adhering to the recommended treatment regimen.

The most commonly used procedure is trabeculectomy, which involves creating a fistula between the anterior chamber and the subconjunctival space in order to bypass the existing drainage system and increase the outflow of aqueous. Postoperatively a small blister-like bleb under the conjunctival flap will be visible if the top lid is retracted. The success of surgery is evaluated by whether the IOP remains within normal limits, however there is no actual improvement in visual acuity (VA); the aim is prevention of further deterioration in the VA. If a trabeculectomy drains well, topical treatment may be discontinued.

Laser treatment involves applying short bursts of a laser beam through a special lens, targeting selected areas of the trabecular meshwork. Application of argon laser burns to the trabecular meshwork (argon laser trabeculoplasty) has been found to be effective in selected cases in reducing IOP. The scarring caused by the laser appears to stretch the tissues between the burns, thus opening up spaces in the trabecular meshwork and facilitating drainage of aqueous. This is a very precise procedure and the patient must therefore maintain a steady head position during treatment. A nurse may need to hold the patient's head in situations such as a head tremor or laboured breathing when it is difficult for the patient to do this alone. All attending staff must wear appropriate goggles for protection. After the treatment the patient should be advised of follow-up arrangements and time allowed for explaining any changes in topical or systemic medication.

Nursing management and health promotion: primary open-angle glaucoma (POAG)

There are three major nursing considerations for patients with POAG: screening, concordance with treatment recommendations and postoperative observation and monitoring.

Screening

Measurement of IOP and visual field testing (see p. 423) may be carried out in the community by the optometry service as part of a 'shared care' scheme or in hospital-based screening clinics.

Patient concordance with treatment recommendations

Concordance is a major concern as patients are generally unaware of any positive physiological changes that derive from treatment. It is the nurse's responsibility to assess the patient's understanding of their condition and treatment and their ability to instill the eye drops and continue with aspects of treatment such as occlusion of lid puncta after beta blocker eye drops are instilled to reduce the risk of the drug being absorbed into the body (systemic absorption) (see Box 13.4). Self-administration of eye drops requires arm

and neck flexibility and hand dexterity to successfully manage the bottle. Administration aids are available to help with the procedure but it requires skilful demonstration and encouragement to patients and carers with low confidence to improve their chances of success.

Postoperative observation and monitoring

Depth of the anterior chamber (AC) The depth of the AC in the operated eye should be compared to that of the unoperated eye and variations must be reported. It is possible for over-drainage to result in a shallow AC or for under-drainage to result in a deeper AC.

Signs of raised IOP Severe postoperative pain, accompanied by a cloudy cornea and flat AC, is abnormal and must be investigated.

Retinal detachment

Retinal detachment describes a separation between the neural and pigmented layers of the retina.

The light-sensitive cells in the neural layer are detached from the essential pigments in the pigment layer as fluid effusion between the layers gradually causes more separation. Retinal detachments are most frequently associated with holes or tears in the retina. These occur as a consequence of vitreous traction, degenerative disease or vitreous loss, which may be traumatic or postoperative. Predisposing factors include myopia, aphakia (without a natural lens), blunt trauma or retinal/choroidal tumour. If one eye is affected, the other is also at risk.

Common presenting symptoms The patient may present at various stages with painless visual disturbances or loss of vision. The external appearance of the eye is unchanged, unless recent traumatic injury or surgery has occurred. During the early stages, the rods and cones are falsely activated, causing sensations of flashing light. As flakes of pigment are shed into the vitreous, the patient may see showers of floating shapes and strands in the vitreous field and in later stages may describe an impression of a curtain coming down or across their line of vision.

MEDICAL MANAGEMENT

The exact nature and extent of the retinal detachment and the presence of retinal fluid will dictate the specific procedure for repair that is used (Ehlers & Shah 2008). External cryotherapy in the form of a CO_2 freezing probe can be applied to the sclera behind the detached retina or internal laser can be targeted at the appropriate area of the retina to induce adhesion of the detached neurosensory and pigment epithelium layers. An internal approach using a vitrectomy (removal of some of the vitreous humour) and volume replacement with expansile gas or silicone oil will almost inevitably induce a cataract within a 1–2-year period and the patient should be made aware of this. Depending on the precise location of the detachment, an external surgical approach with the use of an explant such as a scleral band and buckle may be more appropriate to repair the detachment by means of inducing a compressive effect on the exterior surface of the retina (Khaw et al 2004).

Surgical procedures

The aim of surgery is to produce a controlled inflammatory response to seal the detachment, release the subretinal fluid and bring the retinal layers into normal apposition. Control of the postoperative inflammatory response is achieved by mydriatic and steroid eye drops. Surgery should be undertaken at the earliest opportunity to give the best possible visual outcome, especially in those situations where the macula is still attached or has been detached for less than 1 week. Patients may have concerns about sutures being left in place, but they should be advised that non-absorbable sutures are used and left in place in order to sustain their compressive effect over time.

Nursing management and health promotion: retinal detachment

There are four major nursing considerations for patients with retinal detachment: positioning, education and counselling, pain management and observation of the eye.

Patient positioning

Individualised head positioning regimens determined by the surgeon must be strictly observed in order to improve the success of surgery. The prescribed positioning will depend on the site and the nature of the surgical repair procedure and whether intravitreal air or gas is used. Patients must be fully informed of the reasons for positioning as their adherence to the regimen is very important to the success of the treatment. If the outcome of the surgery is simply re-attachment with no predicted improvement in vision, the patient may decide against surgery and the associated positioning, which can prove arduous for those with musculoskeletal and respiratory conditions. Normal functional positions are usually allowed at mealtimes and for toilet purposes. Complete bed rest is seldom necessary for longer than 24 h postoperatively but head-down positioning may be necessary for 2–6 weeks postoperatively. The aim is to enable the detached area to move back into position preoperatively and to maintain normal apposition postoperatively. This surgery is more likely to be performed under general anaesthetic. The same positioning rules are likely to apply to patients who have had surgical macular hole repair. See Box 13.6 for research into head-down posturing by Waterman et al (2005).

Patient education and counselling

Patients should be warned that the vision may be temporarily poorer than before surgery and will improve only gradually. This is because of the manipulation of the eye, the postoperative mydriatic drops and the alterations to the focusing power of the eye resulting from any compressive explant in the form of a surgical band or buckle, which might be sutured onto the sclera.

Postoperative pain

Postoperative pain can be expected to be fairly severe, depending on the complexity and the duration of the surgery. If severe pain persists despite the use of narcotic analgesics, an acute rise in IOP, possibly precipitated by

---

Box 13.6 Evidence-based practice

Advancing ophthalmic nursing practice through action research

Surgical repair of macular hole is a retinal procedure after which patients are sometimes required to adopt a face-down posture for several weeks. There is anecdotal evidence that patients find this difficult to achieve. An action research project was initiated with the aim of promoting face-down posturing following macular hole surgery in order that patient outcomes might be enhanced. The methodology was participative and cyclical and started with qualitative interviews of 18 members of staff to elicit views on posturing. Seven action objectives were set and three further projects were identified and undertaken. The findings revealed that education of staff and patients, appropriately timed services, clear lines of responsibility for patient care, good communication and availability of equipment were the factors that influenced whether patients adopted a face-down posture after surgery.

Waterman H, Harker H, MacDonald H, et al: Advancing ophthalmic nursing practice through action research. Journal of Advanced Nursing 52(3):281–290, 2005.

Activities

- Access the Waterman et al study (2005) and read the 'methods' section to identify the authors' justification for adopting an action research approach in this instance. Consider other areas in which an action research approach might be appropriate.
- Consider the project's limitations regarding change and evaluation processes in light of your experience of working within the hospital context.

retinal surgery, should be suspected and reported. If severe pain persists and the IOP is within normal limits, some problem with the explant must be suspected.

Postoperative appearance of the eye

In retinal surgery, the conjunctival incision is encircling, there is extensive handling of the globe and, if vitrectomy instruments have been used, there may be considerable trauma to the conjunctiva. Marked chemosis with bruising and swelling of the eyelids, described as a 'meaty' appearance, is therefore expected. The eye must be monitored to ensure that the conjunctival incision heals cleanly and that there is no evidence of rejection or extrusion of the silicone explant.

Corneal transplant (keratoplasty)

Indications for corneal transplant include destruction of the cornea by injury or disease, some cases of advanced keratoconus (conical cornea) and corneal opacity. Transplants may be full thickness or partial thickness. Keratoplasty is primarily an elective procedure with 90% of donor material in the UK supplied by the Corneal Transplant Service Eye Banks in Bristol and Manchester. In 2006/2007 2403 people had their sight restored by corneal transplant in the UK, but there is still a shortage of donor material (http://www.uktransplant.org.uk). The donor material has to be harvested within 24 h of death and is screened to ensure that no infection or corneal disorder is present.

Nursing management and health promotion: corneal transplant

The peri-operative period is managed as for other intraocular surgery but there are some special considerations following keratoplasty.

The use of donated tissue

Recipients rarely ask questions regarding the source of a donated cornea, but nurses must be ready to give reassurance and support, as the use of donor corneas can be an emotive issue. The website http://www.uktransplant.org.uk offers a good resource to direct patients or potential donors who want more information.

Postoperative examination

The peri-operative period is managed as for any other intraocular surgery. Following the procedure, any conjunctival redness (injection) should gradually lessen. If the conjunctiva does not soon return to the 'white eye' state and if the cornea reveals a loss of clarity the cause may be raised IOP or transplant rejection. The wound should be examined to ensure the suture line remains intact and the corneal disc (transplant) has stayed in position, as disruption of either may affect the optical power of the transplant.

Patient involvement and cooperation

Patients and their relatives/carers should be made aware that corneal transplant requires a lengthy follow-up period. The cornea is an avascular structure, and therefore healing will be slow. The corneal sutures will remain in situ for several months or, if a good optical result has been obtained, it may be decided to leave the sutures in indefinitely rather than risk disturbing the transplant.

It must also be emphasised that it is vital to continue any topical medication prescribed to avoid rejection of the transplant and to prevent infection. Some may be disappointed by the initial outcome, when vision may seem poorer than before transplant. Patients should be warned that optimal visual recovery cannot be expected until some months, or even up to two years after surgery.

Patient education should stress the need for attending review appointments, and being aware of the importance of early recognition of symptoms of transplant rejection which include:

- increased redness of the conjunctiva
- cloudiness of the cornea
- reduction of visual function
- discomfort in the operated eye.

Red eye

This section focuses on the acute aspects of eye care, and the most common presentation is the 'red eye'. For any eye injury or ailment there are core areas that can affect all individuals regardless of severity of the ocular condition.

Triage

Utilising the Manchester triage system is essential (Marsden 2008) to ensure accurate and prompt assessment and the intervention of required care.

Anxiety

Suffering eye injuries can cause high levels of anxiety, and the role of the health care professional is to provide reassurance and emotional support by explaining the procedures, answering questions, ensuring adequate pain control and contacting the patient's family. It is essential to acknowledge that the patient may experience severe pain and fear at the potential loss of vision. Reassurance and support are vital at this time through effective communication. Liaison with support groups and counselling options should be discussed.

Education and safe environment

Some conditions will require the patient to have their eye padded and have dilated pupils, the latter of which causes photophobia (sensitivity to light) and dazzle/glare especially when driving. It is a medicolegal requirement to avoid driving and operating heavy machinery during this treatment regimen (http://www.dvla.gov.uk).

Prevention of cross-infection and hospital-acquired infection (HAI) is a priority. The practice of handwashing, wearing gloves, proper storage and instillation of eye drops and correct aseptic technique are essential. Please refer to Chapter 16 for further information.

Return to the community

It is necessary, in cases of sight loss, to ensure that the patient and carers are fully supported and are offered appropriate advice by special community services for the visually impaired person.

It is also essential for the patient, despite their shocked and confused state, to understand the need to maintain prescribed treatment and to attend follow-up outpatient appointments

Primary acute closed-angle glaucoma (PCAG/ACAG)

This presents as an acute episode of severe raised IOP, usually unilateral. It is an ophthalmic emergency and requires immediate intervention as permanent ocular damage occurs if treated incorrectly. Prophylactic treatment is also given for the unaffected eye.

Raised IOP develops as a result of disruption of the circulation of aqueous humor in the anterior chamber, which can be associated with hypermetropia. Pupil dilatation is accompanied by forward displacement of the iris, which blocks the trabecular meshwork, reducing or stopping the flow of aqueous to the canal of Schlemm. The pupillary margin of the iris also comes into contact with the lens, causing the pupil to become semi-dilated and fixed, further impeding the flow of aqueous and increasing forward displacement of the iris. Aqueous build-up results in corneal oedema and disturbance of sensory nerve fibres. The symptoms are as follows:

- red eye, especially around the limbal area (due to marked ciliary injection)
- nausea and possible vomiting; these symptoms can sometimes lead to a misdiagnosis of gastric or abdominal problems
- severe pain in one eye accompanied by fronto-temporal headache on the affected side
- photophobia and increased lacrimation
- blurred, reduced vision
- corneal haze due to oedema
- semi-dilated pupil, unreactive to light
- poorly defined iris details (muddy in appearance)
- on palpation over a closed lid, the eye feels hard because of raised IOP.

MANAGEMENT

Tests and investigations include the following:

- a full history (Table 13.3)
- systematic ocular examination using a slit lamp, which is a binocular microscope that illuminates and magnifies the ocular structures with a narrow band of light, facilitating examination for accurate diagnosis
- gonioscopy (examination of the angle of the eye)
- measurement of IOP.

Acute signs and symptoms should be managed as follows:

- Pain relief by analgesics, including intramuscular opiates.
- Control of nausea and vomiting with intramuscular antiemetics.
- Increase in outflow of aqueous humor by freeing the iris angle. To achieve this, a regimen of intensive topical miotic therapy is commenced to constrict the pupil rapidly and draw the iris away from the angle.

Prophylactic therapy is prescribed for the other eye to prevent an acute attack.

- Reduction in production of aqueous by administration of carbonic anhydrase inhibitors such as acetazolamide (Diamox) either orally or intravenously. If the reduction in IOP is poor, osmotic diuretics such as oral glycerol or intravenous mannitol can be used (Kanski 2007).

Surgical intervention This will be decided upon once the acute signs and symptoms have been managed. Further tests, for example of visual fields and of IOP, should be delayed until acute signs and symptoms have resolved (Kanski 2007). The method depends on the appearance of clinical presentation and may incorporate the following:

- argon laser trabeculoplasty (ALT) – small holes are created in the peripheral iris of the affected eye
- surgical procedures, including trabeculectomy (see Glaucoma, p. 432) or iridectomy whereby a small triangular area is excised from the peripheral iris to improve aqueous circulation
- post ALT, topical steroid treatment and possible long-term anti-glaucoma therapy (see http://www.bnf.org.uk) to reduce inflammation and stabilise IOP.

See website for Nursing care plan 13.1

Uveitis

Uveitis is inflammation of the uveal tract, incorporating the iris and/or the ciliary body, (anterior uveitis or iritis) or the choroid (choroiditis/posterior uveitis). It is an acute condition, which should be seen urgently. The exact cause may be unknown, although it is often associated with the HLA-B27

Table 13.3 Systematic approach to history-taking		
ASSESSMENT	**QUESTION**	**RATIONALE**
History of injury	How did the accident occur? When did the accident occur? Where did the accident occur? Which eye is affected? Is the injury unilateral/bilateral? Were safety goggles worn?	To aid diagnosis For medicolegal reasons
Ophthalmic history	Are glasses or contact lenses worn? Has a similar accident occurred before? Has patient had a previous eye injury or operation?	To ascertain if preventive lessons are learnt To aid clinical examination and diagnosis
Medical history	Does patient have any general health problems? Has patient had previous surgery?	Some systemic disorders may affect the eye, e.g. diabetes mellitus, hypertension, altered thyroid activity Patient may require surgery and may have had a reaction to an anaesthetic previously
Medications	Is patient taking medication at present?	Some medications may affect the eye, e.g. aspirin and the contraceptive pill Patient may have an allergy to a medication To ensure safe prescribing and avoidance of any contraindications to use
Allergies	Is patient allergic to any substance, e.g. medications, Sellotape, Elastoplast?	A substance may inadvertently be given to which the patient is allergic, complicating the condition

histocompatibility antigen (used to detect gene/antigen compatibility and autoimmune disease), rheumatoid conditions, irritable bowel syndrome (IBS), ankylosing spondylitis and sarcoidosis (Denniston & Murray 2008). The prevalence is greater in males than females with a 1.5:1 ratio (Di Lorenzo 2006).

Recurrent episodes are expected but they usually respond to prompt treatment with a good prognosis. Secondary uveitis may accompany other eye infections or trauma.

Clinical features are as follows:

- mild to severe pain, due to ciliary body spasm
- red eye due to vascular congestion in the conjunctival vessels at the limbus
- photophobia
- cloudy aqueous due to the increase in aqueous protein content and presence of white blood cells (the debris floating in the aqueous is known as 'flare and cells')
- reduced vision, dependent on the severity of the attack and degree of inflammation
- cellular exudates (keratic precipitates or KPs) may be present on the posterior endothelial surface of the cornea
- loss of iris details (muddy iris)
- inflammation of the iris may cause it to adhere to the anterior surface of the lens (synechiae formation); this will interfere with aqueous flow
- possible raised IOP which, if untreated, may progress to secondary glaucoma.

MANAGEMENT

- Blood tests will be used to determine the cause in patients with recurrent uveitis: the most commonly used tests are HLA-B27 and erythrocyte sedimentation rate (ESR) (Blann 2008). The aetiology is most commonly idiopathic or autoimmune.
- Outpatient review is usual, but in severe cases hospital admission may be required.
- Usual treatment is with topical steroids and cycloplegics (Hopkins & Pearson 2007); however, in severe cases, these may be given via subconjunctival injection.
- Raised IOP must be treated, as described in the PCAG section (see p. 435).
- Treatment will be long-term if attacks are frequent with acute flare-ups.

Keratitis

Keratitis refers to inflammatory conditions of the cornea, associated with trauma, external eye disease, dry eye and extensive contact lens wear (Jackson 2008). The main causes are certain bacteria, viruses or fungi. If the superficial layer (epithelium) alone is affected, there is minimal damage with little visual loss. If the middle portion (stroma) is involved, loss of transparency and altered corneal curvature may lead to significant loss of vision. Severe inflammation may result in inflammatory debris being shed into the anterior chamber and settling as a collection of cells (hypopyon).

Clinical features are as follows (severity of signs and symptoms will vary depending upon actual cause):

- red, injected eye
- photophobia with spasm of the eyelid (blepharospasm)
- lacrimation/profuse tearing in most cases, although there are some instances of dry eye presentation

- reduced vision
- possible discharge and 'sticky' eye.

Bacterial keratitis

The most common causative agents are *Pneumococcus*, *Streptococcus* and *Pseudomonas*, which invade the cornea, resulting in an inflammatory reaction. The condition tends to recur, may range from superficial to severe and may result in corneal thinning and, in rare cases, perforation.

Viral keratitis

The most common form is dendritic (herpetic) ulcer, which is caused by the herpes simplex virus. Its distinguishing feature is the branching, tree-like pattern it forms on the cornea, which is visible on corneal staining with fluorescein (http://www.revoptom.com).

Fungal keratitis

Fungal infections of the eye are an increasing problem. The damage they cause is severe, and specific antifungal treatment agents are limited, making clinical management complex. Complications can develop rapidly. The distinguishing feature of this kind of ulceration is that it appears as fluffy, feathery extensions over the cornea. Often it can be associated with minor trauma from vegetation or with contact lenses.

Acanthamoeba

This organism inhabits polluted water and swimming pools. Although rare, it is serious and is linked with certain features of contact lens wear: use of soft, disposable lenses, poor hygiene levels and excessive contact lens wear which breaches the manufacturer's guidance (Kanski 2007). Clinical features include ring abscess formation and corneal melt (also known as corneal thinning resulting from inflammation, infection or degeneration) as well as typical signs and symptoms of keratitis listed above. Treatment is medical with an intensive eye drop regimen, but poor response to this treatment can result in severe visual impairment.

MANAGEMENT

Patients should be managed, wherever possible, by an ophthalmic corneal consultant. Conjunctival and corneal swabs and fluorescein staining can confirm diagnosis. The fluorescein fixes to damaged corneal tissue and turns the affected area a bright fluorescent green, indicating the extent of the damage. Topical antibiotic, antiviral or antifungal therapy is usually commenced immediately to avoid rapid development of complications (Hopkins & Pearson 2007). Differential diagnosis must be sought by the following:

- obtaining a thorough patient history
- taking of corneal scrapings
- slit lamp examination
- sending away contact lens for culture and sensitivity.

Possible secondary ocular complications of raised IOP or uveitis must be treated as necessary. It is important to note that steroids are contraindicated, as they suppress the response to infection (Dale & Haylett 2005).

Nursing management and health promotion: keratitis

Patients are generally managed on an outpatient basis, unless they present in an acute state and require intensive topical treatment day and night – this can be as frequent as drops every quarter of an hour. The care and education for patients with keratitis should be as follows:

- The patient should be taught not to touch or rub the eye as this may extend the ulceration.
- Careful hygiene is essential to prevent cross-infection. Tears should be wiped from the cheek only, with a clean disposable tissue on each occasion. Principles of isolation and infection control will be observed in the hospital situation (see Ch. 16) with correct handwashing techniques (http://www.npsa.nhs.uk).
- With dendritic ulcers, it is important to note that anyone who has an outbreak of herpes simplex – commonly known as 'cold sores' – should be advised to guard against touching the sores and then rubbing their eyes. Nursing staff with active sores should not have contact with ophthalmic patients.
- Re-education regarding contact lens wear. Long-term use may be contraindicated. Contact lens care is of vital importance and must incorporate the following (Marsden 2008):
  - maintaining strict hygienic practice
  - not exceeding the recommended wearing time
  - cleaning with sterile water or lens cleaning products, not with saliva or tap water
  - removing lenses if the eyes become inflamed or sore, and not reinserting until advised by a specialist
  - removing soft lenses before administering drops containing preservatives.

Conjunctivitis

Inflammation of the conjunctiva is a common condition, which may be acute, subacute or chronic. It can be unilateral or bilateral in presentation, the latter form often being due to cross-infection. Causative agents are bacteria, viruses, chlamydia, fungi, parasites, toxins, chemicals, foreign bodies and allergies, which cause vascular dilatation of the palpebral and bulbar conjunctiva, cellular infiltration leading to formation of papillae and follicles, and serous exudation. In severe cases, oedema of the conjunctiva (chemosis) may occur.

Clinical features include:

- a brick-red appearance
- a gritty feeling as if there is a foreign body in the eye
- mucopurulent discharge (common with bacterial conjunctivitis), with eyelids sticking together at night
- varying degrees of pain.

The eye may be photophobic, but the visual acuity is not necessarily affected. Eversion (Box 13.7) of the lids may reveal follicle formation, which is the cause of the gritty sensation (Marsden 2008).

 Box 13.7 Information

Eversion of an eyelid

This should be done if a foreign body (FB) is suspected or a gritty sensation reported under the upper eyelid. With the patient's eyes open and looking down, the upper lid lashes are grasped. At the same time, the upper edge of the tarsal plate (at the crease of the eyelid) is depressed, using a glass rod or cotton bud. This allows the lid to be turned over to expose the subtarsal conjunctiva and facilitates inspection, irrigation and foreign body removal (Marsden 2008).

▷ Nursing management and health promotion: conjunctivitis

This includes diagnosis through history taking, slit lamp examination, and conjunctival swabs or scrapings, if clinically indicated, then treating the cause. As well as educating the patient in eye hygiene and self-medication, the nurse must monitor for complications such as secondary corneal inflammation (kerato-conjunctivitis), which would cause visual reduction. Conjunctivitis is highly infectious and family members, peers and other patients should be advised about the prevention of cross-infection by strict handwashing and the use of individual towels and face cloths (Kanski 2007).

Herpes zoster ophthalmicus (ophthalmic shingles)

This is an acute unilateral infection of the trigeminal ganglion, which extends from the scalp to the nose and includes the eye. It is caused by the chickenpox virus and is relatively common in people over 50 years of age (Simon et al 2005).

Common presenting symptoms and signs, all on the affected side, are:

- Regional adenopathy and general malaise of the patient.
- Pain and tingling sensation.
- Skin rash of the forehead and around the eye.
- Swollen eyelids.
- Characteristic vesicular eruptions over the course of the nerve.
- There may be serious ocular complications, including uveitis, keratitis and conjunctivitis.

MANAGEMENT

- Treatment with systemic antiviral agents should begin immediately, as it is only effective if initiated within 48 h after onset, is expensive and has limited benefits especially in immunocompetent patients (Simon et al 2005).
- Treatment with topical antiviral agents, usually commenced by the ophthalmologist.
- Analgesia for post-herpetic pain.
- Possibly ocular lubricants to relieve ocular discomfort.
- Regular eye-bathing if there is ocular discharge.

Allergy to topical medication

This presents as chemosis (swelling of the conjunctiva) and inflammation of the eyelids extending to the cheeks. Common causative agents are atropine, neomycin and preservatives in eye drops.

Clinical signs are:

- red and oedematous eyelids
- epiphora (excessive watering) and intense itching in the acute stage.

MANAGEMENT

- Review and suspend all medication for 24 h if clinically indicated.
- Substitute an alternative agent.
- Systemic antihistamines to relieve itching.
- Cortisone lotion may be prescribed for the affected skin area to relieve itching and oedema.
- Cool eye-bathing may be used as a therapeutic measure.

External eye conditions

These are common and easily treated, once accurately diagnosed (Khaw et al 2004). Nurse specialists in many ophthalmic units now manage patients with such diseases.

Blepharitis

This is a chronic inflammatory condition of the eyelids and eyelashes, resulting in redness, crusting and itchiness. This condition may predispose the patient to stye or chalazion (see below) and may recur, requiring long-term management using:

- lid hygiene and application of warm flannel compresses to remove crusting and excess oily secretions from the eyelids (http://www.patient.co.uk/blepharitis)
- topical antibiotics
- ocular lubricants, if associated with dry eye (refer to Age-related conditions, p. 443)
- systemic antibiotics.

If there is acne rosacea, psoriasis or eczema and if treatment is ineffective, referral to a dermatologist should be considered (Jackson 2008).

Stye

This is an infection of an eyelash follicle, which should be treated with warm compresses and topical antibiotics.

Chalazion or meibomian cyst

This is a blocked duct from the meibomian 'lipid secreting' glands. Treatment is as for blepharitis in the first instance, progressing to 'incision and curettage' if the condition persists (http://www.revoptom.co.uk). This procedure is performed under a local anaesthetic in the outpatient department. Biopsy of the cyst contents is necessary should the cyst reoccur as cysts and lesions of the eyelids can have a similar clinical appearance. Therefore careful history of the duration and pathology is essential, and referral to an ophthalmic consultant is advised if possible malignancies are suspected (Collins 2006).

Diplopia (double vision)

This is defined as 'seeing separate or overlapping images instead of one single one' (Field & Tillotson 2008). It can be either monocular, affecting one eye only, associated with cataract, refractive error, macular disease and retinal detachment, or binocular, present with both eyes, usually associated with nerve palsies, squint, trauma or myasthenia gravis.

▷ **Nursing management and health promotion: diplopia**

The exact cause of diplopia must be investigated and established, prior to any intervention or long-term treatment to alleviate symptoms. Binocular diplopia that is of sudden onset must be referred promptly to rule out any underlying life-threatening cause such a space-occupying lesion or tumour.

MANAGEMENT

Following diagnosis, treatment is specific and ongoing and may include:

- Occlusion of one eye after assessment by an orthoptist and ophthalmologist.
- Use of prisms on the patient's glasses.
- Injection of botulinum toxin into overactive muscle. This results in temporary paralysis (approximately 3 months) and encourages increased function of the underactive muscle. The botulinum blocks the transmission of the nerve impulses at the neuromuscular junction by interfering with release of the neurotransmitter acetylcholine (see Ch. 9).
- Surgical intervention to correct squint. This is either 'recession' or 'resection', the weakening or strengthening of extraocular muscles, by moving their attachment to the sclera backwards or forwards.

Eye injuries

It is vital to record an accurate history (Table 13.3) to rule out any non-visible injury such as intraocular foreign body (IOFB). The VA must be measured and a systematic eye examination made to establish a diagnosis and for medico-legal reasons. The Manchester triage system is used in clinical practice (Mackway-Jones et al 2005) to support the health care professional's judgement, in order to facilitate the preservation of vision (Box 13.8). Some of the more prevalent eye injuries are described below.

Hyphaema

This refers to a haemorrhage in the anterior chamber (AC) of the eye. Most commonly it is a primary hyphaema, which is due to a direct blow to the eye, causing rupture of the small iris blood vessels. It may be microscopic, with diffuse red

Box 13.8 Reflection

Triage exercise

Using the Manchester triage system (Marsden 2008) list the following ophthalmic conditions in order of priority for emergency treatment: conjunctivitis; uveitis; retinal detachment; entropion; perforating eye injury; chemical injury.

Answers

Red = chemical injury; orange = perforating eye injury; yellow = retinal detachment, uveitis; green = conjunctivitis, entropion.

cells visible only with the aid of a slit lamp, or severe with a level of blood seen in the anterior chamber of the eye (Field & Tillotson 2008). Occasionally the blood can completely fill the AC. The degree of pain and reduction in vision depend upon the severity of the bleeding. A secondary hyphaema may occur after intraocular surgery.

MANAGEMENT

A patient with a microscopic or moderate hyphaema will not be admitted to hospital but advised to rest at home for several days. These hyphaemas rarely re-bleed. A patient with a severe hyphaema may be admitted for observation, as there could be an associated rise in IOP or further bleeding. Investigations will include B-scan (an ultrasound technique in which a probe which is used to detect vitreal or retinal haemorrhages), fundal examination, blood tests to estimate clotting time, and possibly CT scan to determine cause. Topical drops will be prescribed including antibiotics, cycloplegics and steroids (Hopkins & Pearson 2007).

▷ Nursing management and health promotion: hyphaema

Ocular observation of the level of hyphaema is made according to the ophthalmologist's instruction. Gentle activity such as listening to radio, music or audio books will be encouraged. The patient is advised to bend at the knees to reach things from below waist height and not to bend over, lift or strain. On discharge, the patient will be advised to avoid active or contact sports until the first follow-up appointment and to assess visual function in the injured eye daily, to detect possible complications such as retinal detachment (p. 433). Protective eyewear will be necessary in the future, e.g. whilst playing squash.

Penetrating injuries

Depending on the results following history-taking and examination, a penetrating injury must always be treated as an emergency and thoroughly investigated with X-rays and ultrasound scanning to confirm the presence, location and type of any foreign body.

MANAGEMENT

Treatment is dependent on the cause and extent of the injury. It may include the administration of mydriatic (dilating), steroid or antibiotic eye drops, and possibly systemic antibiotics to reduce the risk of complications from inflammation and infection (Ehlers & Shah 2008). In addition, the measures described below will be taken.

Perforating injuries The patient will be admitted to hospital for surgical repair of the wound and possible excision of iris prolapse. If the lens is damaged it may be removed at the same time. If facial or other injuries are present, these will be reviewed then treated by the appropriate specialists.

Small puncture wounds These may seal themselves, but the patient is admitted to ensure that the wound stays closed and that intraocular infection does not develop. If the wound is not completely sealed, acrylic glue may be instilled onto the affected cornea and a 'bandage' contact lens placed over this site to seal the wound and hold the lens in place until the wound has healed. The glue gradually dissolves to allow for removal of the lens (Marsden 2008).

Intraocular foreign bodies Admission is essential for surgical removal of the foreign body, which could be embedded in the iris, vitreous or lens. If it is found in the lens, a lens extraction is carried out (see p. 431). Vitrectomy may be necessary if there has been vitreous haemorrhage.

Complications following penetrating injury The most common complications are corneal scarring, raised IOP, cataract formation, haemorrhage, hypopyon, iris prolapse and retinal detachments (see relevant sections for further detail).

Severe infections can occur following any injury, making intensive treatment with antibiotic eye drops and systemic antibiotics necessary.

It is always very important to examine the uninjured eye for signs of 'sympathetic ophthalmitis', a rare complication that presents as a low-grade uveitis. The cause of the sympathetic inflammatory process is thought to involve an immune response to damaged uveal tissue. The use of topical steroids has reduced the occurrence of this potentially sight-threatening condition, which was formerly managed by enucleating the injured eye (Jackson 2008).

A severely damaged eye with no prospect of useful vision may become very painful and unresponsive to analgesics, in which case it may be necessary to enucleate the eye to give relief to the patient.

Following repair of large penetrating injuries (or severe infections), the eye may collapse entirely and become a shrunken mass (phthisis bulbi) in the orbit. This can be unsightly and the patient may wish the eye to be enucleated for cosmetic reasons (see p. 442).

▷ Nursing management and health promotion: penetrating injuries

The patient's main concern is the degree of visual impairment, as well as altered body image (http://www.changingfaces.org.uk/home) and changes in working life and everyday lifestyle. Discussion and effective communication among staff are vital to prevent any misunderstandings. Any questions and concerns must be answered honestly. A process of grieving is normal when any degree of vision is lost.

The community nurse should be advised of the immediate practical measures regarding dressings and wound care and also how they can access further support information on behalf of the patient, such as from a psychologist if the patient is psychologically unable to comes to terms with their altered appearance or from an orbital prosthetist if they have queries about cosmetic results.

Ocular burns

These must be treated as emergencies and if chemicals (acids, alkalis, solvents or detergents) are splashed into the eye, irrigation (see Box 13.5) must be started immediately (Field & Tillotson 2008), prior to prompt referral to an ophthalmic emergency department. Many chemical substances have antidotes, so the chemical label or details on the container should be taken to the emergency department along with the patient (http://www.toxbase.org).

A burn may be caused by either acid or alkali. In general, acids cause only superficial burns because coagulation of the tissues prevents further penetration. The structures involved are usually the palpebral (lining the eyelids) and bulbar (covering the eyeball) conjunctivae and the cornea. Alkalis penetrate the conjunctivae, cornea, sclera and eyelids more deeply and can cause severe damage. Other substances that cause burns include antifreeze, car battery acid, household cleaning agents, cement and superglue.

Clinical signs/symptoms

- Severe, burning pain due to the exposure of the pain receptors of the trigeminal nerve.
- Extreme watering of the eyes due to reflex action.
- Lids will be very swollen and red.
- Burns to the surrounding skin may also be evident.

Absence of pain or a white eye, 'blanching', does not mean the burn is mild: it may be so severe that it has compromised conjunctival circulation and destroyed the nerve endings.

MANAGEMENT

The eye must be irrigated immediately (see Box 13.5) as this is the one time when visual acuity is not assessed before treatment (Marsden 2008). Once the nurse is sure that all traces of the chemical have been removed, a full history can be taken and visual acuity assessed. Post irrigation, ocular examination will be done using a slit lamp to assess the extent of the injury. Chemical injuries are usually successfully treated without causing any long-term damage. Occasionally, however, the burn can cause extensive damage to the cornea and conjunctiva.

Treatment for minor burns An antibiotic ointment is prescribed and possibly cycloplegics (http://www.bnf.org) to relieve iris spasm, prior to an eye pad being applied for 6 h. The topical treatment is prescribed for several days and the patient is often given a follow-up appointment for the next one to two days.

Treatment for severe burns Admission to the ward for intensive treatment and observation is usual. Depending on the severity of the pain, intramuscular analgesics are given for at least the first 24 h. An antibiotic ointment is applied at least four times daily to lubricate the inner eyelids and reduce the risk of secondary infection, and mydriatic eye drops are instilled to relieve accompanying iris spasm and iritis. Topical steroids are often administered in addition to vitamin C eye drops, which are thought to aid collagen remodelling and speed healing time to promote better visual outcome in severe burns (Ehlers & Shah 2008). Monitoring of IOP using a slit lamp by the specialised nurse or doctor is required in the event that uveitis occurs and leads to a secondary glaucoma. If there is permanent damage to one or both corneas, a keratoplasty may be carried out (see p. 434).

Radiation injuries

Irradiation from ultraviolet, infrared or laser light can cause eye damage.

Ultraviolet radiation causes corneal epithelial damage (arc eye, welders' flash) and most commonly occurs when approved eye goggles with protective sides are not worn during welding or when the individual is using a sun bed. Usually the signs and symptoms do not appear until several hours after exposure, when the patient presents with photophobia, pain and excessive lacrimation. Fluorescein drops show dot-like staining of the cornea. Treatment is with topical antibiotics and includes pain relief and the use of eye pads or dark glasses. The corneal healing is variable but there should be no long-term effects.

In environments where workers are exposed to hot material such as molten glass or metal infrared radiation may penetrate the eye through the cornea and can cause cataract.

Sunbeds emit both UVA and UVB rays, which according to the WHO (2010) can damage the DNA of the cells. This can cause irreversible damage to the retina and so the safe use of appropriate eye protection for sun beds should always be encouraged.

Central retinal artery occlusion (CRAO)

This condition is an ophthalmic emergency, recognized as 'orange' in the Manchester triage system (see p. 439). The patient will experience sudden, complete and painless loss of vision in one eye, due to an obstruction of the central retinal artery. It is associated with emboli, thrombosis, diabetes mellitus, hypertension, giant cell arteritis and trauma (Kanski 2007). The retinal artery and some of its branches may be obliterated. The damage to retinal cells is irreparable.

MANAGEMENT

Treatment must begin within minutes if any degree of visual recovery is to be achieved. Valuable time is often lost as the patient may think that the visual loss is transitory and therefore may not seek help immediately. The aim is to reduce IOP rapidly by massage of the globe and administration of osmotic medication such as intravenous mannitol to draw fluid from the eye by osmosis to release aqueous from the anterior chamber. This will further reduce the IOP and should allow the retinal artery to dilate so that the clot may be flushed along to a peripheral branch.

Once the emergency stage has passed the patient is given a full examination. Any underlying medical condition such as hypertension should be referred to, and treated in, primary care.

Minor eye injuries

Corneal foreign body

There is usually a history of something entering the eye. The eye will be extremely painful, especially on blinking. On examination, a foreign body (FB) or rust ring (oxidisation if the object is a long-standing metal FB) will be visible on the anterior surface of the cornea. Anaesthetic eye drops are instilled and the foreign body is removed with a moistened cotton bud or a 10 G needle, dependent on the depth and location of the FB. This can be carried out by an experienced practitioner.

Subtarsal foreign body

The nurse should suspect the presence of a FB when, despite the patient's complaint of something entering his eye, nothing can be seen on normal inspection. There will be discomfort, especially on blinking. The upper lid should be everted (see Box 13.7) and the foreign body, if present, removed with a moistened cotton bud. It is necessary to check for possible corneal abrasion.

Corneal abrasion

This can be caused by a fingernail, a twig or other sharp object. It is an extremely painful condition with profuse lacrimation. Fluorescein eye drops should be instilled in order to determine the extent of the abrasion. An eye pad is not always required after treatment for abrasion or FB removal (Marsden 2008). The need depends upon the severity and location, i.e. if the abrasion is central and large. If the patient feels more comfortable with the eye closed, a pad may be worn for about 6 h. Antibiotic ointment may be prescribed to prevent infection, as well as mydriatics (Field & Tillotson 2008) if pain from ciliary spasm is severe. A follow-up appointment may be given depending on the severity of the abrasion or the depth at which the foreign body was embedded.

Surgical removal of an eye

There are three methods of removing an eye:

- *Enucleation.* This is surgical removal of the globe. The extraocular muscles are cut at their insertion and the optic nerve severed.
- *Evisceration.* This is the removal of the contents of the globe, leaving the scleral shell.
- *Exenteration.* This is a more extensive operation which involves removing the eye and surrounding tissues.

Special considerations

The choice of operation is dependent upon the diagnosis that has necessitated the removal of an eye. A badly injured eye may be enucleated whilst a blind infected eye may require to be eviscerated. Exenteration would be required when a malignant tumour extended beyond the globe. The need for good cosmetic appearance post surgery has led to the development of a range of socket and orbital implants, which may reduce psychological trauma.

Management is as for extensive penetrating injuries. The nurse may find that if patients have suffered severe pain and blindness in an eye, the relief from pain after surgical removal may help them to cope with the loss. Contact through support groups with others who have had a similar experience may help to reassure the patient that it is possible to adapt to the changes.

Artificial eye fitting

The National Artificial Eye Service (NAES) in Blackpool in the UK provides training to enable personnel to make and fit artificial eyes. Patient education, support and follow-up services are also provided by technicians in local ocular prosthetic departments. See http://www.naes.nhs.uk.

An artificial eye is individually designed to fit the socket and implant exactly and is painted by an ocular artist to match the patient's other eye. The prosthesis is shell-like in shape and form and not, as one would imagine, ball-shaped. If an orbital implant has been inserted, the artificial eye will move in unison with the natural eye because the extraocular muscles have been preserved and attached to the implant.

Lack of information about artificial eyes can cause a great deal of anxiety and a degree of revulsion. This may be dispelled by explaining that the appearance of the socket is similar to the inside of the mouth. Anxiety is further reduced by the opportunity to speak to an orbital prosthetist and handle an artificial eye before surgery and thereby gain reassurance that it looks quite natural.

Principles of artificial eye care

Nurses should be prepared to assist in or advise on the care of an artificial eye. Principles of daily management are as follows.

Removal of an artificial eye

A special extractor is provided by the ocular prosthesis department. The eyelids are opened with the thumb and forefinger, and the lower edge of the eye is gently levered out with the aid of the extractor. If an extractor is not available, then a finger will suffice (see Figure 13.7A).

Insertion of an artificial eye

The eyelids are opened with the thumb and forefinger. The eye is inserted under the upper lid with the curve of the eye towards the nose. The lower lid is depressed slightly. The eye can then be slipped into position (see Figure 13.7B).

Care of the artificial eye

An artificial eye should be cleaned at least once a day with ordinary soap in cold or lukewarm water. It should be thoroughly rinsed afterwards under running water. Chemical cleansers or disinfectants must not be used. Patients are encouraged to wear the eye both day and night. If they prefer not to, the eye should be placed in cold water or a saline solution in a clean, labelled container. When not in regular use, the eye should be stored in cotton wool or tissue to prevent scratching.

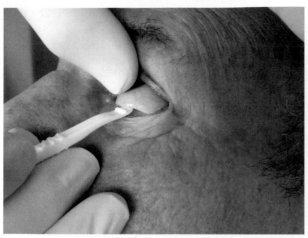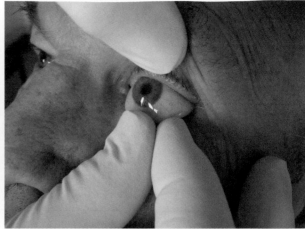

Figure 13.7 A. Removing an artificial eye. B. Inserting an artificial eye. (Reproduced with kind permission of the National Artificial Eye Service [NAES 1998].)

Through normal wear the eye may lose its high polish. In this case it can be sent to the nearest ocular prosthetic department for polishing. Replacements can be obtained cost-free from the same department. The community nurse may need to prompt elderly patients to take advantage of this service or may need to approach their GP for initial referral to a consultant.

Care of the socket

The socket should remain healthy if the artificial eye is kept clean using procedures recommended by the NAES. Infection or irritation of the socket may result from scratches on the eye and lead to ulceration.

The socket can be irrigated with normal saline and treated with an antibiotic ointment for a short period. The artificial eye should not be inserted until the infection or irritation has cleared up. It is not advisable to leave the eye out for long periods as shrinkage of the socket can occur, causing difficulty and discomfort on reinsertion of the eye.

Age-related conditions

Age-related macular degeneration (AMD)

Macular degeneration is the major cause of blindness in the elderly in developed countries. It is accountable for 50% of individuals on the blind (severely sight impaired) or partially sighted (sight impaired) register and the incidence is increasing. It affects detailed central and colour vision primarily and the patient notices difficulty with activities such as reading and sewing, and problems in identifying faces and coins. In some cases, a new blood vessel membrane may develop and cause lifting of the central retina, which results in distorted and blurred central vision, but peripheral vision is maintained. AMD can occur in wet and dry form, as shown below, and in the presence of other eye conditions such as cataract and glaucoma, complicating the diagnosis and treatment. The website http://www.maculardisease.org is a patient information site that covers aspects of both clinical and psychosocial support and encourages discussion between members.

Dry AMD
- AMD usually begins as the dry type and will remain so in the majority of people.
- Dry AMD develops slowly and in most cases causes mild symptoms. However, advanced dry AMD can cause marked visual loss.
- With dry AMD in one eye, there is an increased risk of developing it in the other.

Wet AMD
- Wet AMD can rapidly damage the macula and can result in a fast and severe vision loss.
- Wet AMD accounts for 10–15% of all cases of AMD, but is responsible for 80% of the cases of severe AMD-associated vision loss.

Retinal pigment epithelial cells (RPEs) wear out with age and are never replaced. As they degenerate they deposit material on the underlying membrane, which accumulates to form yellowish white spots on the retina. Initially this process does not affect vision, but eventually the cell loss will result in atrophy of the RPE layer, which may then disperse pigment into the macula.

MANAGEMENT

Before treatment the specific type of AMD should be accurately diagnosed through assessment of visual acuity (reading and distance), Amsler grid – which is a grid pattern which allows the patient to recognise small changes in central vision (http://www.maculardisease.org), colour vision, clinical examination and possible fundal fluorescein angiogram (FFA) (see Diabetic retinopathy, p. 445). No treatment is currently available for the dry form of the disease which accounts for the majority of cases, but laboratory research on stem cell and gene therapy may offer the possibility of viable treatment in the future.

Developments for treatment and care include:

- Recent NICE guidance from 2008 recommends options for treatment of wet AMD including ranibizumab and pegaptanib (http://www.nice.org.uk/TA155), which are classified as vascular endothelial growth factor inhibitors or anti-VEGF therapy. These medications are given directly into the eye by intravitreal injection.

- *Argon laser treatment* – may be beneficial if there are early symptoms of new blood vessel membrane formation. In some cases a degree of vision can be regained following this, although if there is foveal (central area of the macula) damage there will be a persistent central scotoma (blind spot)
- *Photodynamic therapy (PDT)* – this treatment is the process of intravenous injection of verteporfin, 'a light sensitive drug', circulated into the retinal vessels to allow photodynamic laser treatment of the degenerated tissue (Marsden 2008).
- *High-dose vitamin and mineral supplements* – are believed to reduce the progression in advanced AMD, and are recommended for use by those with intermediate AMD in one or both eyes, and those with advanced disease in one eye but not the other eye but not in early AMD (AREDS 2001) (see the commercial site http://www. viteyes.com for an example of one supplier and their advertising). Discussion with the GP is essential prior to starting treatment, as the AREDS-recommended vitamins have been linked with certain systemic side-effects. For example, high-dose beta carotene has been linked with an increased risk of lung cancer and is contraindicated in smokers.
- *Low visual aids (LVA) and referral to a welfare advisor* – to discuss registration as visually impaired (p. 427), available support, local and national organisations.

Nurses play a supportive and educational role, especially at the point of diagnosis and possible registration, as grief, fear and depression are common (http://www.vision2020uk.org.uk). Liaison with the multidisciplinary team and social services is essential to ensure that the VIP is fully supported and empowered to live as independently as possible.

 See website Critical thinking question 13.2

Entropion

Defined as a malposition of the eyelid with the lid margin turned towards the globe, this condition most commonly affects the lower lid and is caused by reduced elasticity of the connective tissue, which may be a result of the ageing process, of trauma or of a badly applied eye pad. The inturned eyelashes irritate the cornea and can cause discomfort and ulceration (Jackson 2008).

MANAGEMENT

Discomfort can be relieved in the following ways (Marsden 2008):

- short-term intervention by the application of tape to the affected lid margin, usually the lower one, to retract it in such a way that downward traction of the tape, when applied to the cheek, restores the normal position
- ocular lubricants, either ointment or drops to lubricate the eye
- topical antibiotics if the cornea is damaged by infection or abrasion
- botulinum toxin injection, as a short-term measure and alternative to taping
- repositioning of the lid by either a simple surgical procedure or eversion sutures.

Ectropion

Ectropion is malposition of the eyelid when the lid margin is turned away from the globe, mainly affecting the lower lid. This condition is associated with atonic tissue around the eyes. Due to malposition of the lid and punctum, tears overflow and run down the cheeks. The individual constantly wipes their eyes, drawing the lid even further down and exacerbating the condition.

MANAGEMENT

The use of ocular lubricants may be required if the eye is infected or sore. Topical cream to the skin is soothing if excessive watering (epiphora) is causing excoriation. Cautery to the inner eyelid contracts the tarsal conjunctiva and inverts the lid. Minor oculoplastic surgery may be required to reposition the eyelid (Collins 2006).

Dry eye syndrome (keratitis sicca)

This is a common, chronic and bilateral condition, requiring prompt assessment, diagnosis and management. Either a reduced quantity of tear production, poor quality of tear film, or both, results in symptoms of dry, burning and gritty eyes, occasionally with excessive epiphora, exacerbated by humidity, wind and smoke. The diagnosis can be complex as the condition is associated with systemic disease such as rheumatoid arthritis and Sjögren's syndrome, which is an autoimmune disease that attacks and destroys the body's own moisture-producing glands. The main symptoms are dry eyes and mouth, as well as dryness of joints and major organs (Kanski 2007).

MANAGEMENT

This is dependent upon the severity and actual cause of the condition, but consists of one or more of the following:

- Instillation of ocular lubricants instilled 4 times a day or as required and at night – the ophthalmologist may recommend a preservative-free preparation as some types of artificial tears contain preservatives such as benzalkonium hexachloride. If drops containing benzalkonium chloride are used for long periods, they may cause a toxicity reaction within the cornea.
- Punctal occlusion, inserting collagen or silicone plugs into the upper and lower punctum, preventing drainage of tears.
- Punctal cautery to seal the puncta.
- Corrective surgery, e.g. tarsorrhaphy, which involves partial closure of the lids, thereby decreasing the surface area of the cornea from which the tear film evaporates (Collins 2006).

Entropion, ectropion and dry eyes are common conditions in the elderly, who may not realise that a simple treatment such as the instillation of lubricants or minor lid surgery is often effective in treating the discomfort associated with the conditions (Denniston & Murray 2008).

Systemic disease and disorders of the eye

The eye is a sensitive indicator of systemic disease. Visual disturbance or abnormal appearance of the retina or optic disc may be the first manifestation of health breakdown.

In this section, ophthalmic conditions associated with some of the more common systemic diseases will be described. Other conditions are described in Table 13.4. The reader should refer to relevant chapters in the present text for further information on the underlying systemic disease.

Diabetes mellitus

Diabetic retinopathy represents the major cause of sight-threatening disease in the developed world. The incidence of diabetes is increasing markedly in developed and developing countries as diets include more processed foods and refined sugars (see Ch. 5, Part 2). Poorly controlled diabetes can lead to retinopathy, early cataract development, vascularisation of the iris (rubeosis) and a high incidence of minor eye conditions such as chalazion.

Diabetic retinopathy

Elevated blood sugar levels, associated with prolonged poor diabetic control, damage the blood vessel basement membrane. In the retina, this leads to leakage and the formation of fatty and haemorrhagic lesions. These changes are termed 'retinopathy'. The patient will usually complain of gradual and painless loss of vision – unless there is bleeding into the vitreous, in which case loss of vision may be sudden and frightening. The diagnosis and progression of the disease can be confirmed by fluorescein angiography, whereby photos of the retinal blood vessels are taken immediately after intravenous injection of fluorescein dye. Diabetic retinopathy is the leading cause of preventable blindness in the working population in developed countries. See http://www.rcophth.ac.uk or http://www.patient.co.uk for the 2005 Diabetic Retinopathy guidelines.

Table 13.4 Further eye problems secondary to systemic diseases

DISORDER	MAIN OPHTHALMIC CLINICAL FEATURES	CAUSE	TREATMENT
Thyroid function imbalance (Graves' disease)	Upper lid retraction Exposure keratitis Swelling of lids and conjunctiva Exophthalmos Compression of optic nerve Diplopia	Sympathetic nerve innervation Exposure of eyeball Infiltration of lymphocytes in orbital tissue and associated oedema Infiltration of lymphocytes in muscle tissue leading to fibrosis	Lubricating drops during day and antibiotic ointment nightly As above Partial tarsorrhaphy Systemic steroids Surgical decompression Prism spectacles Botulinum A neurotoxin injection into the appropriate lid muscle Strabismus surgery
Nephritis	Blurred vision Papilloedema Retinal haemorrhage Retinal detachment	Hypertension	Reduce hypertension Laser treatment Vitrectomy Surgical repair of detachment
Multiple sclerosis	Uniocular Small unequal pupils: do not react to light but do with accommodation, unable to dilate with atropine Optic neuritis Rapid reduction of central vision Sudden onset of pain especially when looking upwards Central scotoma Diplopia	Localised demyelinating lesion to the cranial nerves III IV VI	Symptoms may recover spontaneously but will always recur Systemic painkillers Prism spectacles Botulinum A neurotoxin injection Strabismus surgery
Intracranial aneurysm	Uniocular/binocular diplopia Blurred vision Ptosis Visual field defects	Pressure on visual pathway Pressure on cranial nerves III IV VI	Detection and clipping of aneurysm Botulinum A neurotoxin injection Strabismus surgery
Migraine	Headache with visual disturbances Characteristic aura: multicoloured, jagged shape, firework-like	Idiopathic; possibly chemical changes in the brain caused by various triggers, e.g. stress, or dietary, e.g. eating oranges or chocolate	Feverfew herbal remedy Ergotamine Rest

Classification of the condition as introduced by the Early Treatment Diabetic Retinopathy Study (ETDRS 1987) is as follows:

Background or non-proliferative diabetic retinopathy (NPDR) The small retinal vessels become fragile, microaneurysms form and leakage occurs, causing localised oedema and haemorrhages. If these changes are in the periphery they may not have much visual effect. Moderate to severe NPDR can have ischaemic features that can cause changes to the fovea and macula.

Proliferative retinopathy In this condition there is further deterioration as new blood vessels and fibrous bands form in response to breakdown and occlusion of the normal circulation. The main complications that arise from this are bleeding into the vitreous and tractional retinal detachment as a result of scar tissue formation from the bleeding. Eventually, proliferative vascularisation can affect the angle of the eye by blocking the trabecular meshwork and causing secondary glaucoma.

Maculopathy This is the commonest cause of blindness in type 2 diabetes. The leakage round the macula will result in the subsequent deposit of hard exudates within the macula, thereby reducing central visual function (Khaw et al 2004).

MANAGEMENT

Early diagnosis is critical, as is good control of blood sugar levels and regular monitoring of ophthalmic status. Laser treatment may be used to delay the progress of proliferative retinopathy. This involves treating the peripheral retina with multiple laser burns (panretinal ablation) so that the oxygen requirement of retinal tissue is reduced. This in turn reduces the stimulus for new vessel formation. Focal burns may also be used to seal off leaking blood vessels. Small 'grid' pattern burns may be used to aid the absorption of the fluid from vessel leakage around the macula.

Severe vitreous haemorrhage with subsequent scar formation and tractional retinal detachment may be treated by removing the vitreous (vitrectomy) and replacing it with clear fluid, gas or silicone oil. See Kanski & Milewski (2002) for retinal photography of diabetic eye complications and surgical diagrams.

 Nursing management and health promotion: diabetic retinopathy

Patient education

Ongoing education and encouragement to adhere to diabetic regimens are important in the attempt to delay the onset or progression of complications and to encourage early awareness of visual changes. The nurse has a key role in reinforcing the connection between maintaining good blood sugar levels and reducing the risk of ophthalmic complications. Explanation and support during laser treatment is important to maximise the patient's cooperation to prevent accidental burns.

Vitrectomy management

Peri-operative care for patients undergoing vitrectomy is the same as for other retinal detachment surgery (see p. 434), with a particular emphasis on ensuring that any prescribed head-down or head-tilt postoperative posturing is maintained, as with retinal detachment described on page 434. Outpatient care and education is aimed at encouraging active patient participation and attendance for review.

Cerebrovascular accident (CVA)

A CVA involves an interruption of the blood supply to a part of the brain and may be caused by blockage or rupture of a blood vessel. CVA results in ischaemia (deficient blood supply) of the affected part and development of neurological defects. If the visual pathways are involved, vision will be affected and the damage may be permanent. When a patient suffers a transient ischaemic attack (TIA), vision may be temporarily affected but will usually be restored when the attack subsides (see Ch. 9).

 Nursing management and health promotion: cerebrovascular accident (CVA)

The extent of the visual deficit must be assessed to facilitate rehabilitation and maintain patient safety. This may be difficult if the patient's ability to communicate has been affected by the CVA. The accuracy of the assessment is dependent upon the nurse's skilled observation and on the patient's health status at the time of assessment. If the CVA has occurred very recently, you may observe that the patient's concentration and ability to express themselves or process information may be compromised; this will make it more difficult to test visual acuity. This will be observed if there has been damage to the occipital lobe or orbital pathways, as the patient may not recognise letters or may see only part of them due to hemianopia.

🖰 **See website Critical thinking question 13.3**

Temporal arteritis (giant cell arteritis, cranial arteritis)

This is a progressive disease process affecting the over-60 age group in which the middle layer of medium-sized arteries becomes inflamed. When the external carotid system is involved, ocular damage results with sudden loss of vision, which may be preceded by, or accompany, polymyalgia rheumatica (stiff aching muscles, especially around the shoulders) (Ehlers & Shah 2008).

There is degeneration of the retina, which results from thrombosis or occlusion of the ophthalmic artery, secondary to necrotic inflammatory changes in the middle layer of the temporal and cranial arteries. The cells in the destroyed middle layer are replaced by collagen. During the active phase of this process, there is a raised erythrocyte sedimentation rate (ESR) (Blann 2008).

Clinical features Patients often complain of general malaise, loss of weight and lethargy, or a 'flu-like' illness which may last for a few days or weeks and which precedes a sustained visual disturbance. This is in contrast to the prodromal phase during which there are symptoms which signal the impending onset of the condition: in this case fleeting episodes of blurred vision may occur, accompanied by unilateral temporal or occipital headache. On presentation the patient may complain of scalp tenderness and jaw claudication whereby pain is experienced on chewing due to insufficient blood supply to the muscles of the jaw. The loss of vision is sudden in onset, usually affecting one eye before the other. The length of time between both eyes being affected is extremely variable, ranging from several hours to several days (Simon et al 2005).

MEDICAL MANAGEMENT

Diagnosis is made following fundoscopy, examination of the retina with an ophthalmoscope, and the discovery of a raised ESR. The ESR may not be high in the early stages of the disease and repeat tests may be necessary. The diagnosis may be confirmed by carrying out a temporal artery biopsy. Treatment may be instigated in the community or in hospital and consists of systemic corticosteroid therapy, which reduces the ESR to within normal limits and may be administered for up to 2 years (Jackson 2008). Topical treatment is not usually prescribed unless a secondary condition, e.g. iritis, develops.

 ## Nursing management and health promotion: temporal arteritis

Nursing care is directed towards supporting the patient undergoing corticosteroid therapy. In particular, monitoring and recording regimens, e.g. of blood pressure, urinalysis and body weight, will be required to give warning of any complication arising from the therapy. If vision impairment is severe, then help and support will be necessary, with registration being required.

Hypertension

The condition of the retina and optic disc are used to aid the diagnosis of hypertension; fundal examination of the eye is in fact part of the screening process for hypertension (see Ch. 2).

Hypertensive retinopathy in a young adult appears as widespread narrowing of the arteries caused by spasm of the arterial walls. In an older person with arteriosclerosis, the arteries are narrow and rigid. As hypertension increases in severity, haemorrhages and exudates are visible. The haemorrhages are flame-like in appearance and are found close to the optic disc. The exudates are due to lipid deposits and occur around the macula. Oedema of the retina occurs in malignant hypertension and may also be present in some cases of mild hypertension. The optic disc is swollen and hyperaemic. The patient will complain of varying degrees of visual disturbance. The condition is painless. The outward appearance of the eye remains normal. The eye condition improves as hypertension is brought under control by appropriate treatment (see Ch. 2).

Acquired immune deficiency syndrome (AIDS)

Ophthalmic complications affecting both the anterior segment of the eye and the retina develop in about 30% of patients with AIDS. They are caused by HIV infection, opportunistic infections and AIDS-related neoplasms, and may affect any part of the eye.

HIV retinopathy

Clinical signs are yellowish-grey, cotton wool-like spots, dot-like haemorrhages and micro-aneurysms over the retina. Vision remains normal unless the macula is involved. Some patients respond to antiviral agents.

HIV encephalopathy nystagmus

In central nervous system involvement, nystagmus, gaze palsies and visual field defects may occur. No treatment is available at present.

Opportunistic infections

HIV/AIDS patients are prone to all types of eye infections. The most common infections include severe herpes zoster ophthalmicus, herpes simplex, Candida retinitis, Toxoplasma choroidoretinitis and cytomegalovirus (CMV) retinitis. CMV retinitis, the most common retinal infection in AIDS, is seen in 15–46% of patients, in particular when the CD4 count is <50 cells/mm^3 (see Ch. 35) (Kaiser et al 2004).

Fear of blindness is often more distressing for the patient than fear of dying. CMV retinitis, with intraretinal haemorrhages and retinal necrosis, leads to retinal detachments and progressive loss of vision, but the use of highly active antiretroviral therapy (HAART) has dramatically reduced the incidence of this infection in developed countries (Khaw et al 2004). Palliative treatment by intravitreal or intravenous antiviral agents such as ganciclovir may be offered in an attempt to prevent blindness in the last few months of life.

AIDS-related neoplasms

Kaposi's sarcoma may involve any of the ocular structures. Treatment may include cryotherapy, radiotherapy or the administration of cytotoxic drugs.

 ## Nursing management and health promotion: AIDS-related eye diseases

The general principles of nursing a patient with AIDS (see Ch. 35), together with the principles of nursing a patient with eye infections, apply in all of the above. Full care and support should be mobilised for the patients and their family/partners.

🖰 **See website Critical thinking question 13.4**

SUMMARY: KEY NURSING ISSUES

- Specialised care is required for ophthalmic patients and the visually impaired. It is necessary for general and community health care professionals to have a sound knowledge base pertaining to ophthalmic nursing care, so that they too can prepare and support the individual and their family and/or carers, as well as working in partnership with the ophthalmic unit.

- Ophthalmic nurses are available to their hospital and community colleagues as a local resource for technical and practical information relating to the care of the ophthalmic patient and the visually impaired.

- The impact of visual impairment on everyday life must never be underestimated. Visually impaired patients who require to be hospitalised for whatever reason (e.g. cardiac, ophthalmic, obstetric, respiratory) are likely to need extra consideration with regard to the practical and communication issues that arise from sensory deficit.

- It is important to recognise the significance of adverse signs and symptoms and the fact that delay can result in irreparable damage and permanent loss of sight.
- Ophthalmic nursing has been shown to be a leader in role development, especially within the realm of technical expertise, but the emphasis is that ophthalmic care should be 'seamless' and seek to address both the clinical and psychosocial aspects of patient need, especially for those whose sight loss cannot be remedied by medicine or surgery.

REFLECTION AND LEARNING – WHAT NEXT?

- **Test** your knowledge by visiting the website 🖱 and answering the multiple choice questions and critical thinking questions.
- **Consolidate** your learning by looking at some of the further reading suggestions, references and specialist websites.
- **Revisit** some of the additional material on the website.
- **Consider** what you have learnt and how this will help your professional development.
- **Reflect** on how you can apply this knowledge to the care of your patients.
- **Discuss** your learning with your mentor/supervisor, lecturer and colleagues.

REFERENCES

Age-Related Eye Disease Study (AREDS) Research Group: A randomized, placebo controlled clinical trial of high dose supplements with vitamin c and e, beta carotene, and zinc for age-related macular degeneration and vision loss, *Arch Ophthal* 119:1417–1436, 2001. Report no 8.

Blann A: *Routine Blood Results Explained*, ed 2, Keswick, 2008, M&K Publishing.

Bunce C, Wormald R: *Leading causes of certification for blindness and partial sight in England and Wales*, 2006. Available online http://www.biomedcentral.com/bmcpublichealth/.

Calpin-Davies PJ: Doctor–nurse substitution: the workforce equation, *J Nurs Manag* 7(1):71–79, 2001.

Collins JRO: *A manual of systematic eyelid surgery*, ed 3, Edinburgh, 2006, Butterworth-Heinemann.

Cuber-Dochan WJ, Waterman CG, Waterman HA: Atrophy and anarchy: the third national survey of nursing skill-mix and advanced nursing practice in ophthalmology, *J Adv Nurs* 15:1480–1488, 2006.

Dale MM, Haylett DG: *Pharmacology condensed*, Edinburgh, 2005, Churchill Livingstone.

Denniston AKO, Murray PI: *Oxford Handbook of Ophthalmology*, Oxford, 2008, Oxford University Press.

Department of Health: *Action on cataracts: good practice guidance HMSO Online*, 2000. Available online http://www.dh.gov.uk/en/Publicationsandstatistics/Publications/PublicationsPolicyAndGuidance/DH_4005637.

Di Lorenzo A: HLA-B27 Syndromes. Ophthalmology, genetic disorders, *Emedicine* 2006. Available online http://emedicine.com/oph/topicc721.htm.

Disability Discrimination Act: 1995. Available online http://www.opsi.gov.uk/acts/acts1995/1995050.htm.

Disability Discrimination Act: 2005. Available online http://www.opsi.gov.uk/ACTS/acts2005/20050013.htm.

Douglas G, Nicol F, Robertson C: *Macleod's Clinical Examination*, ed 11, Edinburgh, 2005, Elsevier.

Early Treatment Diabetic Retinopathy Study Group (EDTRS): Treatment techniques and clinical guidelines for photocoagulation of diabetic macular edema, EDTRS Report Number 2. *Ophthalmology* 94:761–774, 1987.

Ehlers JP, Shah CP: *The Wills Eye manual: Office and emergency room diagnosis and treatment of eye disease*, ed 5, Philadelphia, 2008, Lippincott Williams and Wilkins.

European Glaucoma Society: *Terminology and Guidelines for the treatment of glaucoma*, ed 3, Italy, 2008, EGS.

Field D, Tillotson J: *Eye Emergencies: The practitioner's guide*, Keswick, 2008, M&K Publishing.

Health and Safety at Work Act: London, 1974, HMSO.

Health and Safety Executive: *The law on VDUs: An easy guide*, Suffolk, 2003, Health and Safety Executive Books.

Hopkins G, Pearson R: *Ophthalmic drugs; Diagnostic and therapeutic uses*, ed 5, Edinburgh, 2007, Butterworth-Heinemann.

Jackson TL: *Moorfields Manual of Ophthalmology*, Edinburgh, 2008, Mosby.

Kaiser PK, Freidman NJ, Pineda R: *The Massachusetts Eye and Ear Infirmary illustrated manual of ophthalmology*, ed 2, Philadelphia, 2004, Elsevier Science.

Kanski JJ: *Clinical Ophthalmology: A synopsis*, Edinburgh, 2007, Butterworth-Heinemann.

Kanski JJ, Milewski SA: *Diseases of the macula: a practical approach*, Edinburgh, 2002, Mosby.

Khan JC, Thurlby DA, Shahid H, et al: Smoking and age related macular degeneration; the number of pack years of cigarette smoking is a major determinant of risk for both geographic atrophy and choroidal neovascularisation, *Br J Ophthalmol* 90:75–80, 2006.

Khaw PT, Shah P, Elkington AR: *ABC of Eyes*, ed 4, London, 2004, BMJ Books.

Mackway-Jones K, Marsden J, Windle J: *Emergency Triage*, ed 2, London, 2005, BMJ Publishing Group.

Marsden J: *An Evidence base for ophthalmic nursing practice*, Chichester, 2008, Wiley.

Marsden J, Shaw M: The development of advanced practice in ophthalmic nursing, *Practice Development in Health Care* 6(2):119–130, 2007.

Nursing and Midwifery Council (NMC): *Code of professional conduct*, London, 2008, NMC.

Personal Protective and Equipment Work Regulations: London, 1992, HMSO.

Riaz Y, Mehta JS, Wormald R, et al: Surgical interventions for age-related cataract, *Cochrane Database Syst Rev* (4), 2006.

Roper N, Logan W, Tierney A: *The Elements of Nursing*, ed 3, London, 1990, Churchill Livingstone.

Scottish Intercollegiate Guidelines Network: *Day Case Cataract Surgery Guideline No. 53. A national clinical guideline*, Edinburgh, 2001, SIGN.

Simon C, Everitt H, Kendrick T: *Oxford handbook of general practice*, ed 2, Oxford, 2005, Oxford University Press.

Waterman HA, Harker R, McLauchlan R, et al: Advancing ophthalmic nursing practice though action research, *J Adv Nurs* 52(3):281–290, 2005.

Waugh A, Grant A: *Ross and Wilson's Anatomy and physiology in health and illness*, ed 10, Edinburgh, 2006, Churchill Livingstone.

World Health Organization (WHO): *Sunbeds, tanning and UV exposure*, 2010. Available online http://www.whoint/mediacentre/factsheets/fs287.

USEFUL WEBSITES

Action for Blind People: www.afbp.org

British National Formulary: www.bnf.org

Guide Dogs: www.guidedogs.org.uk

Macular Disease Society: www.maculardisease.org

National Artificial Eye Service (NAES): www.naes.nhs.uk

National Institute for Health and Clinical Excellence (NICE): www.nice.org.uk

NHS Blood and Transplant: www.uktransplant.org.uk

Patient UK: www.patient.co.uk

Royal College of Ophthalmologists: www.rcopht.ac.uk

Royal National Institute of Blind People (RNIB): www.rnib.org.uk

Vision 2020 UK: www.vision2020uk.org.uk

World Health Organization: www.who.int

Nursing patients with disorders of the ear, nose and throat

Hilary Harkin

Introduction

Some problems of the ear, nose and throat (ENT) are very common; most people at some time in their lives suffer from nosebleeds, sore throats or earache. Many of these problems will be dealt with successfully at home, often with the advice of a pharmacist or general practitioner (GP). Some ENT problems, however, can be life threatening, requiring an immediate visit to an emergency department (ED), surgery and, in some cases, a period of nursing care at home following discharge.

To nurse ENT patients effectively in a home or hospital setting, a basic knowledge of the anatomy and physiology of the relevant structures, along with a thorough understanding of the clinical features of common disorders, is essential. The health visitor, community nurse, school nurse or occupational health nurse is often in a position to detect problems before the medical practitioner or even the patient is aware of them.

This chapter will outline the basic structure and functioning of the ear, nose and throat, describing the most commonly encountered disorders of each, and outlining appropriate medical and nursing interventions. As in every area of nursing care, one of the most important contributions that nurses can make is in the area of communication and education as they provide support and reassurance to the patient and family, and convey information about the causes of the patient's condition, its treatment and measures to prevent its recurrence.

THE EAR

Anatomy and physiology of the ear

The ear can be divided into three sections: the external ear, the middle ear and the inner ear. The external and middle ears are primarily involved with the transmission of sound. The inner ear contains the organ of hearing as well as structures concerned with body balance (Figure 14.1).

The external ear comprises the cartilaginous pinna and the external auditory canal/meatus (EAM), the inner two thirds of which is composed of bone rather than cartilage. The purpose of the pinna and canal is to capture sound waves and funnel them to the tympanic membrane, which is located at the end of the external canal and divides the external from the middle ear.

The middle ear is ventilated by the eustachian tube, which communicates with the nasopharynx. Three small bones, called the auditory ossicles, pass on sound vibrations received by the tympanic membrane to the inner ear. The first of these, the malleus, is attached to the tympanic membrane and articulates with the incus, which in turn articulates with the stapes. The 'footplate' of the stapes lies against the membranous oval window or fenestra of the inner ear.

The inner ear houses the cochlea, which is shaped like a snail shell and is the organ of hearing. The cochlea contains the organ of Corti, which consists of cells with hair-like projections on a membranous layer and connects with the terminal ends of the auditory nerve. The canals of the cochlea and the organ of Corti are bathed in endolymph. Perilymph is the fluid contained within the bony (osseous) cavities of the inner ear, whereas endolymph is the fluid within membranous cavities. As sound waves are transmitted by the ossicles they travel along this fluid and disturb the hair cells. This disturbance changes to impulses, which travel along the auditory nerve to the brain stem and cortex, where they are interpreted as meaningful sound.

The posterior part of the inner ear is formed by three semicircular canals and by the vestibular apparatus. These assist in the perception of body position against gravity and in the maintenance of balance. The vestibular apparatus consists of the utricle and saccule and is sensitive to linear acceleration. The semicircular canals are sensitive to rotatory acceleration. Balance is maintained by the adjustment of muscles, joints, tendons and ligaments in response to information gathered by the vestibular apparatus and the canals as well as that received by the eyes. For further information, see Tortora (2009).

Disorders of the external ear

Otitis externa

The most common causes of otitis externa, inflammation of the external ear, are infection and allergy. Infection may be caused by excess wax trapping water in the EAM or scratching the ear with contaminated fingernails, cotton buds or other sharp objects. Itching is an early symptom of allergy and is more common in dry skin and dermatological conditions. In otitis externa, multiple bacteriological flora are usually present. The condition most commonly occurs in hot, humid climates, where it tends to be recurrent and may be severe. Patients usually present with a sensation of a blocked ear and a history of localised pain and itching and a burning sensation followed by a discharge, which initially may be watery and then becomes thicker. If there is gross oedema of the meatus and a large amount of debris is present, the patient may suffer from conductive deafness (see p. 452).

▷ ### Nursing management and health promotion: otitis externa

The first priority of the nursing staff is to clean the EAM so that an examination can be carried out and any prescribed treatment administered effectively. This procedure is called aural toilet and should only be carried out by an appropriately qualified ENT nurse. Cotton wool can be tightly applied to an instrument specifically designed for aural toilet (Figure 14.2). This looks similar to a cotton bud, however

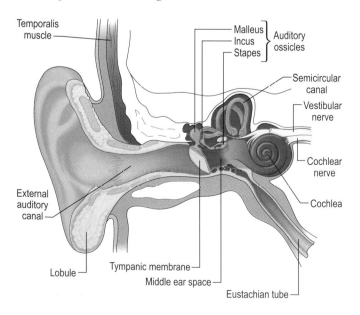

Figure 14.1 Sagittal section of the ear.

Temporalis muscle
Malleus
Incus — Auditory ossicles
Stapes
Semicircular canal
Vestibular nerve
Cochlear nerve
Cochlea
External auditory canal
Lobule
Tympanic membrane
Middle ear space
Eustachian tube

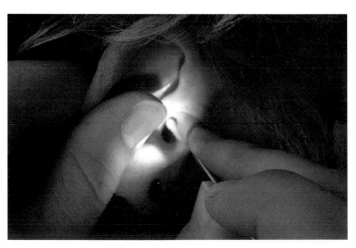

Figure 14.2 Aural toilet using cotton wool.

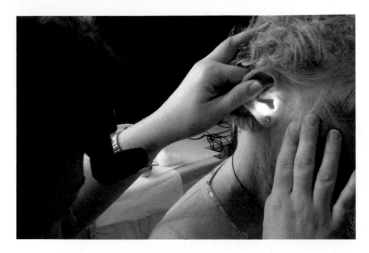

Figure 14.3 Straightening the ear canal.

the area of cotton is designed to be narrower to ensure the ear canal is not occluded once the cotton-tipped instrument is inserted into the canal. Care must be taken not to damage the skin. Gentle pulling of the pinna will straighten the canal and allow easier access (as demonstrated in Figure 14.3). A good light source should be used or an operating microscope. Gentle irrigation with water can clean the EAM but large amounts of discharge and debris are best removed by an appropriately qualified nurse or doctor using microsuction via a fine-bore tube under an operating microscope in the outpatient department.

It may be necessary to administer an oral analgesic before the external auditory canal can be properly examined, as often any movement of the pinna is painful, see Box 14.1.

Since the vast majority of patients are seen in the community or outpatient department, the nurse's involvement will range from the total management of ear conditions in a nurse-led clinic to demonstrating how to administer topical preparations effectively. The nurse should also teach the patient to keep the ear dry from water entry and not to insert implements into the ear and stress the importance of frequent, thorough cleansing of any appliances, including hearing aids, that are put in the ear.

Cerumen excess

Cerumen is the normal waxy secretion of special glands in the external auditory canal. Along with shed skin scales and hair, the cerumen normally migrates naturally out of the EAM but can be hindered by coarse hair, narrow canals or by the person impacting the material by attempting to clean the ears with cotton wool buds or other instruments. Nurses should provide patients with health education information regarding the normal cleansing mechanism and avoiding the use of cotton buds and other foreign bodies (Reynolds 2004). The patient usually presents with a blocked feeling in the ear. Tinnitus may develop, causing the patient distress (see p. 458), and disturbance of balance may result from pressure of the hard material on the tympanic membrane.

MEDICAL MANAGEMENT

If there is an excessive amount of wax, or the patient needs to have a hearing test or hearing aid review, the doctor, community nurse or outpatient nurse will need to clear the EAM. The wax can be removed manually with instruments, by irrigation with water using an electronic irrigator or by microscope and suction. If the wax is too hard and compacted for this to be carried out, water can be inserted into the EAM for 15 minutes to soften the wax (Roland et al 2008). To improve patient comfort, written information can be given at the time of booking recommending they use olive oil for a few days before the procedure. An advice sheet regarding ear care and how to insert ear drops is available on the website.

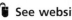 **See website for further content**

 Box 14.1 Reflection

History of a patient with otitis externa

At the end of August Mr Smith had just returned from a short break in Cornwall. He had been swimming in the sea in the warm weather. His right ear felt blocked as if he had some water left in it, so he tried to dry his ear with a cotton bud. The ear continued to feel blocked and also became very itchy. On the Monday night Mr Smith woke up in the early hours of the morning with severe earache and a ringing noise on the same side of his head. He was finding it painful to talk as jaw movement hurt his ear and paracetemol had not relieved the discomfort. There was a small amount of dried liquid on the outside of the ear and it was uncomfortable to touch the ear itself. He was worried that there was something dreadfully wrong as he had never had any problems with his ear before.

Mr Smith attended the minor injuries department and the triage nurse examined his ear. The nurse said that there was debris present and the ear canal was mildly swollen. She explained it would be necessary to clean the ear canal to optimise the chance of clearing the infection. The nurse gently irrigated Mr Smith's ear with water to remove the debris. Mr Smith found this quite relieving and the ear felt better once the nurse dried the canal with a cotton-tipped carrier. He was diagnosed with otitis externa and the nurse prescribed an ear spray with combined steroid and antibiotic. The nurse advised Mr Smith to be careful not to allow water enter the ear and to stop using the cotton buds. The nurse warned that he was to follow this advice forever or the ear infection might re-occur. The pain in the ear subsided very quickly and within 3 days Mr Smith's ear was better; however, he continued to use the drops for the full week of the prescription.

Activities

Look at the website (irrigation guidelines and ear care advice) before attempting to answer the following questions and think about what questions the nurse will have asked Mr Smith about his ear prior to carrying out irrigation with water.

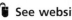 **See website for further content**

- How would you have advised Mr Smith to keep his ears dry from any entry of water?
- Is there any further advice you would give Mr Smith about taking care of his ears?

Nursing management and health promotion: cerumen excess

Individuals with cerumen excess are usually seen in the doctor's surgery or, more rarely, in the outpatient department, for removal of the impacted wax. Ear syringing with a metal syringe is now obsolete and impacted wax is removed by instrumentation, ear irrigation with water, or microsuction.

The doctor or nurse who performs the irrigation should first take a full history to ensure there are no contraindications to irrigation with water. In order to protect against the transmission of infection, gloves and disposable aprons should be worn and a disposable cape/apron placed over the patient's shoulders to keep them dry. The nurse should obtain valid consent and should be seated at the same level as the patient. The contraindications to irrigation with water and full guidelines for the procedure are available on the website.

 See website for further content

Patients should also be advised that, following effective wax removal, they should prevent water entry to the EAM for approximately 4–5 days and may be hypersensitive to even quite normal sounds for a short time.

Foreign bodies in the ear

Small objects may become lodged in the ear by some mishap or, as frequently occurs among children, by accident during play (Reynolds 2004). Such objects may lie undetected for years unless they have damaged the tympanic membrane. Sometimes gentle irrigation with water or microsuction will remove the foreign body, but if it has become impacted it may be necessary for the patient to be admitted to hospital as a day case and for the object to be removed under general anaesthetic. Only objects that will not expand when in contact with water should be irrigated. Hydroscopic matter such as peas and lentils will absorb the water and become enlarged and often impacted in the canal; as a result removal from the EAM will be through microsuction and/or instrumentation.

Deafness and hearing loss

Although total deafness is comparatively rare, many people suffer hearing loss to varying degrees. Deafness can affect both adults and children. There are 840 babies born each year in the UK with significant deafness. Many children who are deaf continue to be so for all of their lives, but some can be helped to maximise auditory function. This section will concentrate on hearing problems among adults. There are estimated to be 9 million deaf and hard of hearing adults in the UK. This figure is rising as the number of those over 60 increases, with 698 000 of this age group being severely or profoundly deaf (RNID 2008a). A high proportion of severely or profoundly deaf people have other disabilities as well. Among those under 60, 45% have additional disabilities, which are more likely to be physical disabilities. Among severely or profoundly deaf people over 60 years of age, 77% have some additional disability. For 45%, this means significant dexterity or sight difficulties, or both.

PATHOPHYSIOLOGY AND MEDICAL MANAGEMENT

Deafness is usually classified into conductive and sensorineural disorders. Conductive deafness can often be helped by removing any obstruction (cerumen or a foreign body, see above) or by amplifying sounds by means of a hearing aid. Because the external and middle ear are fairly accessible, surgical intervention may also be an option. By contrast, in sensorineural deafness, where the damage is to the organ of Corti or the cochlear portion of the VIIIth cranial nerve, surgery does not usually have much effect. Diagnosis of the type of hearing loss will be by examination and audiometry.

Hearing tests

Voice tests are a simple method of establishing if the patient has a degree of hearing impairment. The RNID offers free simple hearing checks on their website for people to complete while they are online.

Tuning fork tests

These tests are a simple means of determining a patient's basic auditory status. They may be performed in a clinical or home environment. Nurses and doctors can perform these tests, however an audiometric assessment of hearing is generally carried out by the audiologist.

Rinne test Air conduction is tested by holding a vibrating 512 Hz tuning fork first to the front of the ear and then by placing the base of the tuning fork against the mastoid bone, which is located behind the ear. Patients should hear sound louder to the front of the ear. A Rinne positive result indicates normal hearing.

Weber test Bone conduction is tested by placing the base of a vibrating 512 Hz tuning fork to the middle of the forehead. This sound should be heard centrally within the head. A conductive hearing loss is indicated if the sound is lateralised to the ear that has reduced hearing. If sensorineural hearing loss is present, sound will be localised to the better hearing ear.

Audiometry

Audiometric tests measure hearing acuity. These tests, which include delivering tones of variable frequency and intensity, the spoken word and measuring middle ear pressures, are amongst the methods used to determine the type and source of any hearing loss. Electric response audiometry measures the patient's response to an acoustic stimulus by way of an electroencephalogram and can provide reliable and exact information on the site of a disorder, e.g. the cochlea, auditory nerve tract or brain stem. Detailed descriptions of these tests can be found in Maltby (2002).

Conductive deafness

This results from a reduced ability of the sound waves to reach the fluid in the cochlea. The sound is quieter but not distorted. This can be due to:

- congenital abnormality
- otitis externa
- foreign bodies
- excessive cerumen
- otitis media (secretory and suppurative)
- damage to the tympanic membrane, incus, malleus or stapes.

Sensorineural deafness

This is caused by a defect of the cochlea or its connecting nerves. The sound heard is quieter and is also distorted. This is a result of the loss of the high frequencies, which register consonant sounds. In severe cases, patients may not be able to hear the sound of their own voice. This can be due to:

- ageing
- medication
- trauma, including head injury and noise
- infection
- Ménière's disease
- congenital malformation.

Presbycusis the most common type of sensorineural deafness, develops as a consequence of ageing and is becoming increasingly prevalent in Western society. In the UK, 71.1% of people over 70 and 41.7% of people over the age of 50 years will have some kind of hearing loss (RNID 2008a). Audiometry initially shows loss of ability to hear high tones, but there is gradual deterioration of lower tone hearing as well. Degeneration of the nervous tissue leads to loss of intelligibility in the sounds that are heard. Hearing loss in this disorder is symmetrical, i.e. it affects both ears. A hearing aid may be of slight advantage, but distortion and poor discrimination may cancel out any benefit from amplification. When communicating with these patients, it is important to speak a little slower and more distinctly and to try to eliminate any background noise. Because the high tones are affected first, the individual may have trouble hearing consonants, as these are usually of higher tone than vowels. Durga et al (2007) has found that taking a daily folic acid supplement (800 µg) may be helpful in slowing down the progression of presbycusis.

Medication It has been recognised for some time that salicylates and quinine can cause deafness, but this can be reversed by discontinuing these medications. Other drugs, such as antibiotics of the aminoglycoside group, some diuretics, such as intravenous furosemide, and cytotoxic agents of the nitrogen mustard group, are ototoxic and can cause irreparable damage.

Trauma Noise-induced hearing loss is well documented and has become recognised as an industrial disease. Socioacusis, the term used to describe the hearing loss caused by sources of noise outside work (loud music, traffic), can be as great a risk as loud noise in the workplace (RNID 2008b). A single exposure to a loud noise such as an explosion or gunshot can cause permanent deafness, or the injury may be temporary. Tinnitus usually accompanies this injury and often takes longer to resolve than any deafness (see p. 458). Exposure to loud noise over a period of time leads to destruction of the hair cells in the organ of Corti. The Noise at Work Regulations (HMSO 1989) laid down strict standards of noise control and protection for employers in the UK, who are liable to be prosecuted if they do not comply (see Useful websites for more information). Occupational health nurses have a role to play in monitoring noise levels and encouraging auditory health through education. On audiometry, early changes in hearing caused by exposure to noise are seen as a dip that gradually deepens and involves adjacent frequencies.

Head injuries or other trauma resulting in deafness usually involve fractures or penetrating injuries of the temporal bone. Occasionally, concussion (see Ch. 9) can cause deafness due to haemorrhage into the middle ear or cochlea. These injuries are often accompanied by severe vertigo, nausea and vomiting.

Infection leading to deafness is usually viral in origin. The causative viruses are those associated with mumps, measles, meningitis, chickenpox and rubella.

Ménière's disease See page 458.

▷ Nursing management and health promotion: deafness and hearing loss

In the case of conductive deafness, the nurse's role may be to prepare the patient for surgery and facilitate postoperative recovery. Some of the surgical procedures that may benefit patients are myringoplasty (repair of the tympanic membrane), ossiculoplasty (repair to the ossicular chain in the middle ear) and stapedectomy (a prosthetic stapes is inserted to replace the damaged bone). A patient for whom surgery is not feasible may be fitted with a hearing aid and educated in its use by members of the audiology department, including the hearing therapist. In this case the nurse, as a member of the multiprofessional team, should also explain how to obtain the greatest benefit from the aid (see guide to looking after hearing aids on the website).

♫ **See website for further content**

Most patients in this situation also benefit from learning how to lip-read. Lip-reading sessions are usually available as a day or evening class at audiology departments or a local college. It can take many months to become proficient at lip-reading, so the earlier the patient starts the better. Slow progress, combined with deteriorating hearing, can be very demotivating.

Communicating effectively with a hearing-impaired patient is a very important nursing priority (Box 14.2). In the assessment, the nurse should obtain and record information about the patient's preferred method of communicating, e.g. lip-reading, finger-spelling or sign language. A study by the RNID (2008a) suggested that deaf adults who used sign language were dissatisfied with and disadvantaged in their communication with health care staff, including nurses. According to Ratna (1994), the problems deaf clients bring to counselling include isolation, frustration, discrimination and physical and sexual abuse.

It is now recognised that deafness can have a profound psychological impact and that hearing-impaired individuals may require support to help resolve problems. Many deaf people would prefer to have counselling from a counsellor who is deaf, and attempts should be made to find such a professional if preferred (via the British Association for Counselling and Psychotherapy [BACP] if necessary, see Useful websites). Older adults and their carers have complained of symptoms such as depression, anxiety, decreased social activity and emotional turmoil (Berry et al 2004).

Box 14.2 Information

Talking with someone who has a hearing deficit

- Do not speak until you have the person's attention and they can see your full face.
- Never turn your back on the person when you are speaking or cover your mouth.
- Ask the person if they can lip-read.
- Do not exaggerate your lip movements.
- Direct your voice to one ear if it has better hearing than the other.
- Speak slowly, enunciate clearly and do not shout.
- Remember that vowels are heard more easily than consonants.
- Check that the person has understood what you have said.
- If the person has difficulty in understanding, try rephrasing the sentence.
- Do not laugh at misinterpretations.
- Have patience. Give the person time to adjust their hearing aid if necessary.
- Encourage the person to participate in group conversations when the occasion arises.
- If verbal communication is impossible, explore alternative means, e.g. sign language.

Community nurses can provide tremendous help and support for patients and their relatives when sensorineural deafness is a problem. They should be able to assist their patients to obtain many of the aids available, including a hearing dog for the deaf, which can help to overcome communication difficulties in everyday life. There are many associations, both voluntary and professional, which can provide support and help. The nurse working in the community should be a resource person for patients and guide them to the support that is available (see Useful websites and Box 14.3).

Hearing aids

About 2 million people in the UK have hearing aids, but only 1.4 million use them regularly. There are at least another 4 million people who do not have hearing aids but experience significant hearing difficulties in everyday life. They would be likely to benefit from hearing aids. All electronic hearing aids have a microphone, which picks up the sound; the sound is processed electronically either by analogue or digital circuits to make it more audible. This is then delivered to the receiver, converted back to sound and reaches the ear via an ear mould. For further information on hearing aids see the website.

 See website for further content

Box 14.3 Evidence-based practice

Are we being heard?

- The RNID decided to commission this report because of the frequency with which it received examples of poor communication experienced by deaf and hard of hearing people when attempting to use the NHS. The study took place within the context of the Disability Discrimination Act (1995), which came into force in 2004 and places a legal obligation on the NHS to meet the needs of disabled people. The NHS in England, Wales and Scotland has acknowledged defects in services which affect disabled people, including difficulties in communication with staff and in finding their way around premises. There are thought to be approximately 9 million deaf and hard of hearing people in the UK. As one in every seven people in the UK has some level of hearing loss, and it is known that the average GP will have up to four patients with hearing loss in their surgery daily, it is important that health care professionals in all care settings are aware of the particular needs for effective communication of those who have reduced hearing.
- The RNID and the UK Council on Deafness conducted this research in collaboration with 21 UK-based deaf and hard of hearing groups and charities; a total of 866 participants completed the survey.
- The main findings reported by deaf and hard of hearing people when using GP services were that 35% had experienced difficulty communicating with their GP or practice nurse and 15% avoided going to see their GP because of communication problems. Making and keeping appointments was another problematic area, with 28% reporting that they found their hearing loss made it difficult for them to make an appointment: of 24% who stated they had missed an appointment, 19% had missed more than five. Of those who did see their GP or nurse, 35% reported being unclear about their condition because of communication problems. Of those who used British Sign Language (BSL), 33% were either unsure about medication instructions or had taken inaccurate doses.

- The situation in NHS hospitals is equally disturbing, as 42% of the deaf and hard of hearing who had visited a hospital for non-emergency treatment found it difficult to communicate with staff. BSL users experienced even more difficulties, with 77% of this group reporting communication problems for emergency and non-emergency overnight stays and 70% of those admitted to emergency departments were not provided with a BSL/English interpreter to facilitate effective communication.
- Overall, the picture is one of poor communication, resulting in people having inadequate access to health care and insufficient information about their health condition and treatment, thus limiting their ability to make informed choices, and being placed in higher risk situations than their hearing counterparts. It is also unacceptable that family, including young children, and friends have to act as interpreters and on occasion convey critical health information. The financial cost to the NHS of missed appointments is put at approximately £20 million a year. The financial and non-financial costs to the patient, family and friends will never be known.
- The report notes that NHS staff do wish to deliver a better and more equitable service to the deaf and hard of hearing but that often the necessary resources and infrastructure are not available. Solutions recommended include increasing the number of BSL/English interpreters, using video phones, providing improved written information, installing loop systems to allow better use of hearing aids in noisy environments, providing visual displays in appointment areas and clear lighting, and providing deaf awareness education, including communication skills, for all health care staff, whether working in hospital or community settings. Deaf awareness seminars should be provided for appropriate hospital departments and GP surgery staff, so that these areas have at least one formally trained 'front line' staff member.

RNID 2004 A simple cure. A national report into deaf and hard of hearing people's experiences of the National Health Service. RNID, London. (See also Useful websites.)

Disorders of the middle ear

Secretory otitis media (glue ear)

Glue ear is the most common cause of hearing impairment and the most common reason for elective surgery in children. Approximately 80% of children will suffer from glue ear before they are 4 years old (Scottish Intercollegiate Guidelines Network [SIGN] 2003). This disorder is known as glue ear because it is characterised by a thick, tenacious fluid that collects in the middle ear. Normally, the mucosal secretions of the middle ear drain down the eustachian tube into the naso-pharynx (see Figure 14.1). It is not certain whether the abnormal accumulation of this fluid is caused by the viscosity of the fluid, congestion of the eustachian tubes or obstruction caused by enlarged adenoids or a tumour.

Common presenting symptoms Pain is rarely associated with this condition. The adult patient usually comes to the medical practitioner complaining of hearing loss. A child might never complain, and their condition might be discovered only upon investigation into poor performance at school or during routine screening of hearing at school.

MEDICAL MANAGEMENT

Examination of the tympanic membrane by auriscope usually confirms the diagnosis, as in this disorder the membrane has a characteristic dull grey or orange appearance. It will also lose its normal translucence and become retracted.

Conservative treatment is to prescribe a decongestant, or antihistamines, to reduce oedema of the nasal mucosa. Mucolytics, which liquefy the mucus, have been shown to have no effect on the condition (SIGN 2003).

Surgical intervention involves performing a myringotomy (incising the tympanic membrane) and suctioning of the glue. If a grommet is not inserted, the delicate tympanic membrane heals within a few days. The fluid may, of course, accumulate again. The insertion of a grommet (Figure 14.4) is sometimes considered appropriate, although some specialists think this can lead to scar formation in later years which will impair hearing. If a grommet is inserted, it usually is extruded from the tympanic membrane at 9–12 months; patients sometimes find it on their pillow when they waken one morning. A grommet allows aeration of the middle ear, thus restoring middle ear air pressure. There is usually a marked improvement in hearing after this procedure which is maintained in about 75% of patients.

 ## Nursing management and health promotion: secretory otitis media (glue ear)

Only care specific to ENT patients is outlined in this chapter. The reader is referred to Chapter 26 for details of routine peri-operative care.

Pre-operative care

Most of this surgery is carried out on a day case basis, and the nurse must ensure that the patient and family are adequately informed about what the surgical procedure will entail. This may involve the use of diagrams and it may be helpful to

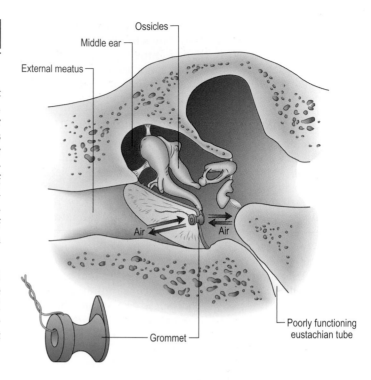

Figure 14.4 Grommet and grommet in situ.

show them a grommet if one is to be inserted. When communicating with the patient pre-operatively, the nurse should make allowances for hearing loss (see Box 14.2).

Postoperative care

The anaesthetic for this operation is very light. Measures to prevent the spread of infection, e.g. washing the hands before and after touching the affected ear, how to change and dispose of cotton wool plugs in the external auditory canal, and specific instructions about whether and when it is safe to allow water to enter the ear must be discussed with the patient. When a grommet is in place, most surgeons allow swimming, as long as the patient does not dive or swim underwater. Usually, a cotton wool plug moistened with petroleum jelly is inserted in the external canal when the hair is being washed or when taking a shower. The nurse must ensure that the patient and family understand this advice and are given information booklets or advice sheets. Patients should be told to see their GP if they experience any pain or if there is a bloodstained discharge from the ear. Most of these precautions apply to all patients who have undergone aural surgery. The patient may be asked to see their GP for regular checks of the position of the grommet rather than requiring them to attend the outpatient department.

Otosclerosis

Otosclerosis is a condition in which the ossicles in the middle ear, along with the temporal bone (see Figure 14.1), begin to soften. This spongy bone gradually becomes a dense sclerotic mass; the ossicles may become fixed and less effective in passing on auditory vibrations. The individual with this condition will complain of increasing hearing loss. While this loss is conductive in origin, if the damage extends to the cochlea, sensorineural loss of hearing will also occur.

Mild tinnitus (see p. 458) may also be experienced, in which case some people find that they can actually hear better in a noisy environment where their tinnitus is masked.

This disorder commonly begins in adolescence and its cause is as yet unknown. Heredity, vitamin deficiency and otitis media have all been cited as significant factors.

MEDICAL MANAGEMENT AND NURSING PRIORITIES

Although no cure for otosclerosis is known, surgery can often dramatically improve hearing. The surgery of choice, stapedectomy, involves freeing the stapes and replacing it with a prosthesis. This restores the vibration necessary to permit the transmission of sound waves. Surgery may be performed under local anaesthetic, and hospital admission may be no more than 24 h.

Great care must be taken in the early postoperative period, as the patient may take a little while to regain their sense of balance. This short-term vertigo, if discussed and explained in the pre-operative period, should cause minimal distress to the patient. Prior to discharge, advice should be given on the prevention of aural infection (keep the ears dry from water entry, do not insert implements into the ear) and the need to guard against blowing the nose until the operative site is completely healed. Violent nose blowing can force air up the eustachian tube, increasing middle ear pressure, which can affect the operated area and prosthesis. Patients should be advised to keep their mouth open when sneezing to reduce middle ear pressure, and also to avoid flight and Eurotunnel travel until they have discussed this at their outpatient follow-up appointment.

Acute suppurative otitis media (ASOM)

This is an acute bacterial infection of the middle ear which is especially common in childhood. The most common causative organisms are *Streptococcus pneumoniae, Haemophilus influenzae, Streptococcus pyogenes* and *Staphylococcus aureus*. Onset usually follows acute tonsillitis, the common cold or influenza, when infection travels up the eustachian tube to the middle ear. The whole middle ear may be affected, including the mastoid air cells, small air spaces in the posterior portion of the temporal bone, behind the middle ear (see Figure 14.1).

Common presenting symptoms The patient usually presents with acute ear pain. There may be deafness, general malaise and pyrexia. On examination, the eardrum is red and bulging due to the collection of pus in the middle ear. The tympanic membrane may rupture, releasing the discharge and dramatically and instantaneously relieving the pain.

MEDICAL MANAGEMENT AND TREATMENT

The patient with ASOM is usually seen and treated by a GP. The exact treatment given will depend on the stage of the infection, as follows.

Early stage The eardrum may appear red with no light being reflected. Analgesics such as paracetamol alternated with ibuprofen will be necessary to relieve pain and reduce fever. Vasoconstricting nasal sprays may also be helpful in keeping the eustachian tubes patent, thereby allowing escape of fluid from the middle ear. In severe cases, admission for intravenous antibiotics and pain control may be necessary (SIGN 2003).

Bulging eardrum If the infection has reached this stage, a myringotomy may be performed. This involves applying a local anaesthetic before making an incision in the tympanic membrane to allow the pus to escape. If a myringotomy is performed in preference to allowing the eardrum to rupture, the membrane will heal with less scarring and hearing should not be impaired. During this procedure a swab of the discharge will be taken for culture and sensitivity so that the appropriate antibiotic can be prescribed.

Discharging ear By this stage the tympanic membrane will already have ruptured. A swab of the discharge will be taken and the ear carefully mopped out and then dressed with a small plug of cotton wool. Broad-spectrum antibiotics will be prescribed in the first instance while the results of bacteriology are awaited.

The patient will have to visit the GP regularly so that healing of the membrane can be monitored. If the perforation does not heal the patient will suffer with intermittent discharge from the ear which would be unpleasant. If water enters the ear, this discharge usually will increase, making bathing and swimming difficult. If necessary, a myringoplasty (repair of the eardrum) will be performed.

Nursing management and health promotion: acute suppurative otitis media (ASOM)

Early stage

If at this stage a nurse, possibly a practice nurse, is involved, their role will be to ensure that the prescribed course of antibiotics is completed in order to eradicate all the organisms. It may be necessary to teach the patient or a relative/carer how to administer a nasal spray.

Discharging ear

If the disease has reached this stage, the nurse's role will include mopping out the external ear as often as required and carrying out microsuction clearance of the debris. Microsuction is performed using the same equipment and suction pressure as for tracheal suctioning. Looking down the microscope, the specialist nurse uses disposable thin suckers to remove any debris or wax from the ear canal. The benefit of the microscope is that it offers magnification and binocular vision and depth of field. If appropriate treatment is given early enough, ASOM should resolve and hearing return to normal. Occasionally, complications do occur, including chronic suppurative otitis media and acute mastoiditis, which are described below.

Chronic suppurative otitis media (CSOM)

PATHOPHYSIOLOGY

This condition follows unresolved ASOM. The patient will present with a perforated tympanic membrane, a discharging ear and some degree of conductive deafness. Pain is not usually a complaint. The discharge may be intermittent and is mucoid, becoming purulent in the presence of secondary infection.

MEDICAL MANAGEMENT

The recommended treatment is to keep the ear dry by the use of topical medication before correcting the hearing loss by performing a tympanoplasty.

Tympanoplasty Following removal of diseased tissue, an attempt may be made to re-establish the sound transmission mechanism in the middle ear by reconstructing the tympanic membrane (myringoplasty) using a connective tissue graft taken from the fascia covering the temporal bone and reconstructing the ossicular chain (ossiculoplasty). This combined reconstruction is known as a tympanoplasty. For further information on middle ear surgery see Ludman (2007).

 Nursing management and health promotion: tympanoplasty

Pre-operative care

The patient is usually admitted on the day of surgery. In view of their obvious hearing deficit, the establishment of good communication is very important. To help avoid complications, the ear must be dry and free from infection. Hearing tests will be carried out to confirm the degree of hearing loss. To help alleviate anxiety, the nurse should give the patient information about the procedure and warn about sensations that may be experienced afterwards, such as dizziness and tinnitus (see p. 458). It is also important to describe the very bulky bandage that will be present around the head and affected ear so that this does not alarm the patient and family. Hearing aids should be worn to the operating theatre. The theatre nurse should remove the hearing aid as the patient is anaesthetised and place it in the patient's notes. If the hearing aid was worn in the ear that was not operated on, it should be reinserted by the recovery nurse before the patient is extubated.

Postoperative care

General postoperative care is as described in Chapter 26. The majority of patients undergoing ear surgery are given a hypotensive anaesthetic in order to reduce bleeding and thereby allow the surgeon a clearer view of the tiny operative field. This involves the intravenous administration of a hypotensive agent. Frequent blood pressure readings are therefore required until the pre-operative baseline levels are regained.

Following the operation, the patient should be encouraged to lie with the affected area uppermost and should be observed for nausea, vomiting and vertigo, all of which might be present due to possible interference with the semicircular canals during surgery. The aim of the pressure dressing and bandage is to prevent bleeding and haematoma formation, but the nurse should always observe the patient's bandages and pillows for bloodstains.

Because of its location, the VIIth cranial (facial) nerve is at risk of damage during surgery to the middle or inner ear. Following this type of surgery, patients should be asked to smile, wrinkle their nose and shut their eyes tightly. The ability to perform these movements indicates that there has been no damage to the facial nerve. A record of the time of checking and level of function of the nerve should always be documented for medical and legal reasons.

Most patients are able to be up on the evening of surgery and return home the next day. The surgeon usually requests the nurse to remove the head bandage the morning after surgery. The patient should be advised that they may experience dizziness during the following 2 or 3 weeks and should avoid sudden movements such as quickly turning the head. Sutures should be removed in 5–7 days, either at the GP's surgery or on the ward. Packing usually remains in the EAM for between 1 and 3 weeks following surgery. The patient will be shown how to change the piece of cotton wool at the entrance to the meatus as required, without disturbing the packing. The packing is removed by the surgeon in the outpatients department and the patient should be recommended to take a mild analgesic such as paracetamol before their appointment as this will be slightly uncomfortable.

CSOM with cholesteatoma

This potentially dangerous condition is sometimes called attico-antral disease, because it is found in the attic (upper) area of the middle ear. Cholesteatoma is an ingrowth of keratinising squamous epithelium from the external ear into the middle ear, usually from the site of a previous perforation. It may be possible to see this on examination. The squamous epithelium growing within the middle ear produces keratin, which has the ability to erode the bony ossicles and may even spread into the inner ear.

Common presenting symptoms The patient will complain of a foul-smelling discharge from the ear and of deafness.

MEDICAL MANAGEMENT

The treatment of choice is mastoidectomy (see below).

Acute mastoiditis

This condition arises from acute otitis media and is caused by the infection spreading to the bony walls of the cells of the mastoid process.

MEDICAL MANAGEMENT

Conservative management is by administration of antibiotics; surgical management is a cortical mastoidectomy.

Mastoidectomy A cortical mastoidectomy is so called because the surgeon removes the superficial cortex of bone overlying the mastoid air cells. Surgery involves incision, drainage and removal of unhealthy mucosa and bone cells from the mastoid process of the temporal bone, leaving the middle ear structures intact. A modified mastoidectomy may be performed if the disease is confined to the upper area and the patient has good hearing. This is currently the most common surgical procedure for middle ear infection. The procedure involves clearing out the mastoid cells and removing the outer attic and posterior wall, thus leaving a large cavity to allow air from the ear canal to circulate and dry up secretions.

Nursing care is as for patients undergoing tympanoplasty (see p. 457).

Other complications of middle ear infection

Less common complications of middle ear infection are facial nerve paralysis, meningitis, extradural or subdural abscess, labyrinthitis, lateral sinus thrombosis and brain abscess.

Disorders of the inner ear

Tinnitus

Tinnitus is a little understood but most distressing feature of some ear diseases and disorders. It may also occur spontaneously or as a postoperative complication. Possibly because it is so puzzling, has no known cause and is not a visible symptom, sufferers often feel that they receive very little sympathy and understanding.

Tinnitus is usually a subjective sensation of sound in the ear. It is a relatively common complaint that may arise in association with a wide range of conditions, including inner and middle ear disease, overuse of medications such as aspirin and quinine, abnormalities of the auditory nerve, renal problems, cardiac problems and anaemia. It is often accompanied by vertigo and/or deafness. The Tinnitus Association helps sufferers and produces an excellent range of factsheets and a free newsletter for interested professionals (see Useful websites).

Common presenting symptoms Tinnitus can vary in severity from an intermittent mild ringing sensation in the ear to an incessant noise, loud enough to make life unbearable. The perceived sound varies in volume and character from one individual to another. Some patients are aware of the sound only during their waking hours, while others are aware of it mainly at night or when they are somewhere very quiet. Tinnitus may cause difficulty in sleeping, with irritability, tiredness and lack of concentration following restless nights. The persistent symptoms cause many tinnitus sufferers to feel anxious and depressed (Box 14.4). The feelings are exacerbated in some by fears that the tinnitus is an indication of a more serious underlying disease or that it will cause an increase in hearing loss. In the worst cases, individuals with tinnitus may suffer total deafness because the noise in their ear eliminates all other sounds.

MEDICAL MANAGEMENT

To aid diagnosis, a careful history must be taken, including information about all other symptoms and any medications. This should be done in a tinnitus clinic within an ENT department. A hearing test and careful examination of the ear (including radiography) may help determine the cause. Unfortunately, in many instances, no treatable cause will be found. For further information, read Anderson (2005).

Nursing management and health promotion: tinnitus

Very few tinnitus sufferers will be patients in hospital, unless their condition has arisen as an early postoperative complication. The majority will attend their GP's surgery or their nearest ENT outpatient department. Wherever nursing staff encounter these patients, high priority should be given to allowing them to express their fears and to recognising and relieving their anxiety and possible depression. Once an ENT specialist has carried out all the tests required to determine a diagnosis, any prescribed treatment and training can be commenced. Where there is no medical treatment, a planned programme of care, including tinnitus

Box 14.4 Reflection

An experience of tinnitus

I shall never forget the first time I experienced tinnitus. It was in the dead of night when I heard a high-pitched whine in my left ear. I was so taken aback that I got up out of bed and went in search of the source of the noise. Before long, however, I realised that the noise was being carried with me.

The tinnitus had been preceded about a month beforehand by nausea and severe vertigo which I had accepted as transitory. To find that I was left with this noise made me feel very anxious indeed. I had difficulty in coming to terms with the fact that it might always be present. My reaction was 'It can't be! There must be something to combat it and make the noise go away!'.

When it became clear to me that I was now a 'tinnitus sufferer' I experienced a phase of reactive depression and felt that life was not worthwhile. Naturally, I searched for a cure and eventually joined the local branch of the Tinnitus Association. This was a move which I made by myself, but the Association proved to be an invaluable source of emotional and practical support and information. A hearing therapist and a clinic psychologist have now joined the team at my audiology clinic and they are giving tinnitus sufferers like me a great deal of help in many ways.

Activities

- Reflect on the support you would offer the patient with tinnitus.
- How would you explain what tinnitus is to the patient's relatives?
- If the patient does not have a computer at home, how would you recommend they gain access to the internet?

retraining therapy, counselling, explanations and information giving, such as details of support groups, will be necessary to help the patient adapt and to relieve any worries. There are more than 100 tinnitus support groups in the UK (see Useful websites) and they can be of enormous help to sufferers by providing ongoing emotional support (see Box 14.4). For further information about tinnitus and health anxiety, see Anderson (2005).

Vertigo

Vertigo is a disturbance of equilibrium, in the absence of an external cause, which creates a sensation of rotating motion of oneself or one's surroundings. It is usually caused by irritation of the vestibular apparatus and is most frequently associated with disorders of the bony labyrinth and with Ménière's disease. Cardiac, neurological or viral infections and therapeutic medications such as streptomycin can also cause vertigo.

Common presenting symptoms Vertigo is a disabling and often frightening sensation that may be transient or recurring. It is not the same as dizziness and may be relatively mild or quite severe. The motion perceived is often described as a whirling sensation, but rocking and swaying sensations are also reported. Severe attacks of vertigo may be sudden and dramatic, accompanied by pallor, nausea and vomiting. For more information about vertigo management, see Luxon & Davies (1997).

MEDICAL MANAGEMENT

A careful history is required from the patient and must include any precipitating factors such as head and neck movements. Any other symptoms such as tinnitus or deafness should be ascertained. It is also helpful to know how long the periods of vertigo last. Details of medication and any recent trauma can also aid diagnosis. A neurological and cardiovascular examination and perhaps radiography, hearing tests and blood tests may be advisable.

Occasionally, surgery will be required to treat the particular disorder of which vertigo is a symptom, but treatment is more commonly pharmacological or uses the Epley manoeuvre or Cooksey Cawthorne head and neck exercises, which are taught by a physiotherapist (for more information on these exercises see Luxon & Davies 1997). An occupational therapy assessment of home safety may also be beneficial.

Nursing management and health promotion: vertigo

As is the case with tinnitus sufferers, the majority of individuals who suffer from vertigo will be distressed and incapacitated by their condition. They will usually be seen in their homes, as they are likely to feel unsafe venturing out. The first nursing priority for these patients is safety. The attacks of vertigo may be unpredictable, or may be associated with a particular head movement. For example, for one individual, a precipitating circumstance might be standing on a stepladder with their head back and to one side in order to change a light bulb; for another, it may be simply a quick movement to bend down and pick up a baby from its cot. The nurse should discuss with the patient and family how to avoid the particular head and/or other movements in order to eliminate attacks, if this is possible.

Ménière's disease

In Ménière's disease, the membranous labyrinth is distended by an increase in the endolymph, at the expense of the perilymph, and the organ of Corti degenerates. The most widely held theory of its cause is that it arises as a result of local ischaemia, although it has been suggested that it may be due to viral infection, biochemical disturbance, vitamin deficiency or local physiological faults (Luxon & Davies 1997). It may arise at any age but is most common among individuals aged 30–50.

Common presenting symptoms Ménière's disease is characterised by four disabling features:

- vertigo
- tinnitus
- sensorineural hearing loss
- nausea and vomiting.

As it runs its course over a period of many years, deafness increases. Although this hearing loss may initially affect only one ear, it will, in 10% of patients, eventually affect the other as well (McAllen 1996). Many patients have a warning that an attack is imminent, e.g. there is a feeling of fullness in the ear or the character of the tinnitus changes.

During an attack the patient will have vertigo, nausea and vomiting and will want to lie down and remain as still as possible, in order to relieve these distressing symptoms. Nystagmus (involuntary, rhythmic eyeball rolling) may be present and sweating, bradycardia and diarrhoea may occur.

MEDICAL MANAGEMENT

It may be difficult to arrive at a conclusive diagnosis of Ménière's disease, as many other disorders, e.g. labyrinthitis, intracranial disease and acoustic neuroma, display similar symptoms (see Ch. 9). Given that, between attacks, clinical examination may prove negative, diagnosis will rely heavily on careful history taking and audiological investigations (see p. 452).

Treatment The most common treatment for the symptoms of Ménière's disease is the prescription of medication, e.g. a labyrinthine sedative (medication to dampen the sensation of unsteadiness) such as cinnarizine, and diuretics. A vasodilator such as nicotinic acid or moxisylyte may be prescribed to alleviate local ischaemia. The majority of patients respond well to medication therapy and may have long periods of respite from severe symptoms. Adherence to a low-salt diet may be advised to reduce the volume of endolymph.

Surgery may occasionally help to relieve symptoms. This may take the form of decompression of the endolymphatic sac, the creation of a fistula between the endolymph and perilymph reservoirs, or a vestibular neurectomy.

Nursing management and health promotion: Ménière's disease

The main nursing priority in case of an attack of Ménière's disease is to ensure the patient's safety. Attacks are often so severe that the patient needs to lie as still as possible, and, if in hospital, may gain a sense of security if the side rails on the bed are raised. Vomiting can be so severe as to cause dehydration. If the patient cannot take fluids orally, intravenous fluids and antiemetic drugs will be necessary until oral medication and feeding can be tolerated.

Patients suffering from Ménière's disease often have to make lifestyle changes in order to cope with some of the symptoms of the disorder. The nurse should be prepared to offer advice on lifestyle adaptations. As an individual faced with the problems associated with Ménière's disease is likely to feel anxiety, it is vital that the nurse provides clear information and explanations, particularly with regard to prognosis.

THE NOSE

Anatomy and physiology of the nose

The principal function of the nose is to provide a passageway for air entering and leaving the respiratory tract (Figure 14.5). In so doing, it acts as an 'air conditioner', ensuring that inspired air is humidified, sufficiently warm and free from particulate matter.

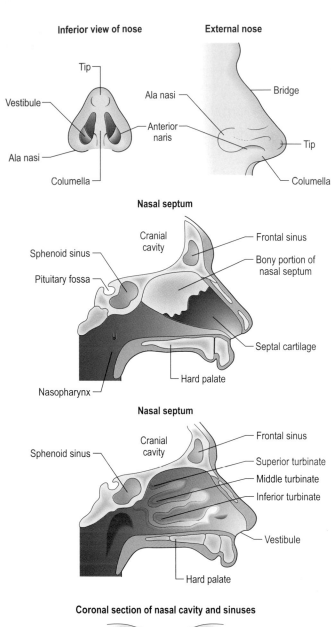

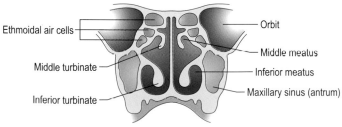

Figure 14.5 The nose and paranasal sinuses.

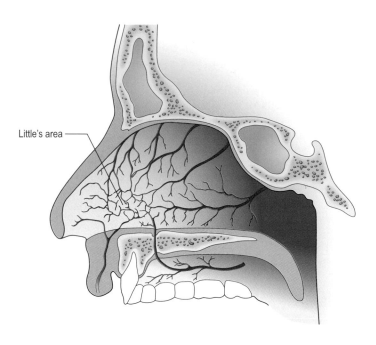

Figure 14.6 Blood supply to the nose (sagittal section).

The terminal fibres of the olfactory nerve are located in the roof of the nasal cavity. The lower two thirds of the nose are supported by cartilage and the upper third is enclosed by bone. The cavity is divided in half by the septum which consists of cartilage anteriorly and bone posteriorly. The entrance is lined with stratified squamous epithelium and coarse hairs (termed vibrissae) and the passages are lined with a mucous membrane of ciliated columnar epithelium.

These passages are highly vascularised. A branch of the maxillary artery supplies the lower posterior section of the cavity, and the anterior and posterior ethmoidal arteries supply the mucous membrane. All these vessels join at Little's area on each side of the septum (see Figure 14.6).

Disorders of the nose

Epistaxis

Epistaxis is bleeding from the nose. It is not a disease in itself but a symptom of some other disorder, which may be of a local or general nature. Local causative disorders include idiopathic, trauma caused by nose-picking, foreign bodies, a blow to the nose or surgery. More generalised disorders that sometimes give rise to nosebleeds can be:

- vascular, e.g. hypertension and cardiac failure
- congenital, e.g. haemophilia and hereditary haemorrhagic telangiectasia
- neoplastic, e.g. leukaemia
- medication-induced, e.g. a side-effect of anticoagulant therapy
- infections, e.g. influenza, rhinitis, sinusitis and the common cold.

Common presenting symptoms Epistaxis can affect males and females equally and can occur at any age but is most common in childhood and early adolescence, when it usually occurs in Little's area (Figure 14.6) and is often the result of trauma or infection. In middle-aged or older individuals, the bleeding is more likely to occur in the posterior part of the nose and may be associated with hypertension. This form of epistaxis may be very frightening and can be life threatening if it proves difficult to control. See Box 14.5 for the management of epistaxis.

Box 14.5 Information

Management of a patient with epistaxis

- Provide reassurance to the patient. Guide them to a bed and recommend they sit down, leaning slightly forwards so the blood drains out of the nose rather than the back of the throat. Swallowing the blood will make the patient feel nauseous and they may vomit. Encourage the patient to breathe through their mouth and spit out the blood so the amount of blood loss can be monitored.

- Pinch all the soft parts of the nose (located below the nasal bones) between your thumb and forefinger. If the bleeding continues, apply ice to the forehead and back of the neck to constrict the blood supply to the nose. Monitor the patient's vital signs, ensuring they remain cardiovascularly stable. Speak gently with the patient, question them as to what the cause of the bleeding may be, what medication they take and if there is a history of nose bleeds or other medical issues.

Bleeding from nose → apply pressure to soft area towards the front of the nose for 10 minutes

Bleeding stops; vital signs normal, patient can go home with antibiotic nasal ointment and the following advice:

- Rest, and do not pick your nose.
- Do not blow your nose. If you have to sneeze, open your mouth to reduce the pressure of air in your nose.
- Do not strain or bend down to lift anything heavy.
- No hot liquids for 24 h.
- Do not strain during bowel movements; use a stool softener if necessary.
- If you take blood thinning medication, ensure you have weekly blood monitoring until your blood levels have stabilised.
- If you are spending a lot of time in air conditioned or heated environments, ensure your nose is well moistened or use a saline nasal spray.

Bleeding continues despite compression of soft area of nose:

- Continue monitoring vital signs and take bloods.
- If the bleeding point is seen on examination of the nose, nasal cautery will be carried out.
- Bleeding stops; patient can go home if blood results are normal. Patient will require antibiotic nasal ointment and advice as above.

Bleeding continues despite compression and no bleeding is point visible in the nose:

- Continue monitoring vital signs and take bloods.
- Nasal packing inserted into each nostril, apply bolster dressing under nose.
- Oral antibiotics and mild sedation prescribed.
- Encourage good oral hygiene and plenty of cold fluids.
- Packing removed after 24 h. If no further bleeding the patient can go home with advice.
- Outpatient appointment to ensure underlying cause of epistaxis treated.

Profuse bleeding from further back in nose:

- Continue monitoring vital signs and take bloods.
- Nasal packing and nasal catheter inserted with air used to inflate balloon, bolster dressing applied under nose.
- Encourage good oral hygiene and plenty of cold fluids.
- Oral antibiotics and mild sedation.
- Packing and catheter removed in 24–48 h.
- If no further bleeding patient can go home with advice as above and an outpatient's appointment.

Profuse bleeding continues despite packing:

- Ensure patient's cardiovascular system remains stable.
- Prepare patient for theatre to undergo ligation of nasal arteries (refer to Ch. 26 for details of routine peri-operative care).
- Specific nasal postoperative care as above.

Patients often present at clinics with a history of recurrent epistaxis, but are rarely actually bleeding at that time. On examination, dilated blood vessels may be apparent. The best treatment to prevent the bleeding recurring is cautery by the use of a chemical, such as silver nitrate, electrocautery or diathermy.

MEDICAL MANAGEMENT

The management of epistaxis can be divided into resuscitation of the patient, arrest of the haemorrhage and diagnosis and treatment of any underlying cause (Ludman 2007). A patient with severe active epistaxis is usually admitted to hospital as an emergency. Vital signs are recorded to monitor for shock, as bleeding may be severe enough to necessitate blood transfusion. Treatment is by insertion of a nasal pack. This usually takes the form of a nasal tampon or pneumatic packing with an inflatable balloon. Nasal packs are usually left in place for 24–72 h. Antibiotics are given if the packs are in longer than 24 h, to prevent any risk of infection developing and spreading to the middle ear. Occasionally, when these measures fail to control the bleeding, arterial ligation is necessary. If the bleed is the result of some underlying medical condition, this will need to be investigated and treated at the same time.

 ## Nursing management and health promotion: epistaxis

Nursing intervention will vary depending on the site, severity and cause of the epistaxis, and the patient's age. Most patients with anterior nosebleeds (bleeding from the front of the nose) are children or adolescents and will be treated as outpatients in their GP's surgery or at the hospital.

The first priority of nursing intervention is to stop the bleeding, whilst providing psychological support. The patient should be helped to sit upright with the head slightly forward and asked to mouth breathe and spit out all blood. This helps to estimate the blood loss and prevents the blood from being swallowed and causing nausea. Digital pressure with the thumb and forefinger should be applied to the cartilaginous part of the nose and ice packs to the area above it, i.e. Little's area (see Figure 14.6). This area has many surface arterioles which may have weakened walls. Ten continuous minutes of this pressure is usually sufficient to control an anterior nosebleed. If these first aid measures fail, or if there are recurrent nosebleeds, the patient will probably be transferred to hospital for insertion of a nasal pack or cautery of the area.

Once the bleeding is under control, the nurse should explain to the patient and, where appropriate, to the parents, how to prevent nosebleeds from recurring. Advice should be given about blowing the nose gently, avoiding picking the nose and trying to keep the nasal mucosa slightly moist by using soft petroleum jelly. An explanation of how to cope with and control a nosebleed should also be given (Box 14.5).

Hospital treatment

This will be necessary for severe epistaxis that cannot be controlled by the above measures. By providing clear and concise information, the nurse can help alleviate the patient's anxiety and aid recovery. Some patients admitted as emergencies with uncontrollable nosebleeds will be in hypovolaemic shock (see Ch. 18, p. 538).

A specialist nurse can pack the nasal cavity or assist the medical practitioner to do so. When a nasal pack is in place, the patient will only be able to breathe through the mouth and may be afraid of suffocation. Frequent oral hygiene and plenty of cold oral fluids should be offered to prevent the oral mucosa becoming dry. These drinks must not be hot, as this can cause local dilatation of blood vessels and exacerbate the problem. Eye care may be necessary as the packing may obstruct the nasolacrimal duct, causing tears to overflow (see Ch. 13). Nasal packing can also cause hypoxia, leading to disorientation as well as alterations to vital signs. Oxygen therapy and blood gas monitoring with appropriate monitoring of O_2 saturation will be needed in this situation. Areas that have been cauterised may become encrusted. Soft petroleum jelly should be applied to such areas twice a day for a few weeks until the mucosa has healed.

Although anxieties can be reduced by answering the patient's questions and giving information, sedatives may also be prescribed. Following an epistaxis, patients are usually nursed propped up in bed to aid venous return from the area and to make it easier for them to spit out any blood. Ice packs may be applied to the nose to help constrict the vessels and control bleeding. The nurse should explain to the patient how to breathe through the mouth and a vomit bowl or sputum carton should be to hand. Again, it is important to offer frequent oral hygiene, plenty of cool drinks and eye care as necessary. As these patients often have dysphagia because of the pressure of the nasal pack on the soft palate, a nutritious soft or even liquid diet may be appropriate. Bed rest is usually advised, although patients should be allowed to use the commode at the side of the bed rather than a bedpan to ease the strain of elimination.

Packing is usually removed in 2 or 3 days. If the bleeding has not been controlled, the patient will have the appropriate arteries ligated in theatre. If a deviated nasal septum (see p. 464) has been a contributory cause, corrective surgery may be performed.

If hypertension or another medical disorder has caused the nosebleed, an appropriate specialist medical opinion is sought and treatment commenced. The nurse may, in the meantime, obtain appropriate patient education booklets or information sheets in relation to the relevant disorder from colleagues working in the ward(s) specialising in the care of such patients, so that the patient can be given appropriate advice (see Ch. 2).

Community care

To prevent the recurrence of epistaxis, support should continue after the patient has returned home and resumed normal activities. If the patient is at home, the GP and practice nurse will be informed of their condition so that they can encourage the patient to implement the advice received in hospital and can monitor hypertension if present. Refer to Box 14.6.

Disorders of the paranasal sinuses

The paranasal sinuses are a group of air spaces surrounding the nose which, it is said, make the skull lighter and add resonance to the voice. They consist of two frontal, two maxillary

---

Box 14.6 Reflection

An experience of epistaxis

It first started on a Saturday morning. I bent down to pick up my bag from the floor and realised my nose was running. On wiping it, I saw fresh blood. Going into the bathroom, I could still feel it running and the tissue was getting soggy with blood. Remembering some first aid, I squeezed the soft front of my nose, sat down and leaned forward. At least it stopped the blood coming out of my nose, although I could taste some in my mouth now. After 10 min I stopped squeezing and the bleeding stopped. I cleaned around the front of my nose, but spent the rest of the day not daring to blow my nose in case the bleeding started again.

All was well until Wednesday evening. I'd just had a bath and was watching TV, when I felt my nose running. Again, there was blood on the tissue and dripping from my nose. Like the previous time, I squeezed my nose, but after 10 min, when I released the pressure, the blood started dripping and I squeezed again. Again, on releasing the pressure, the blood continued to drip and I now had a pile of bloodstained tissues in the bin and patches of blood all over the bathroom floor as I tried stuffing tissues up my nose as well. By now an hour had passed and still the blood dripped. I didn't think it was ever going to stop and wasn't sure what to do.

My flatmate suggested contacting NHS Direct. She phoned and we were advised to go to the emergency department of our local hospital. So my flatmate drove me to the hospital and I took the washing up bowl to catch the blood, as I didn't want to mess up the car!

On arriving at the emergency department, my flatmate booked me in and I was seen very quickly by a nurse. On releasing the squeeze on my nose, the blood still continued to drip out and the nurse said I would see a doctor. The nurse then squeezed my nose for me. I was glad as my arms were aching from all the squeezing I had done. My blood pressure was taken and the doctor saw me.

Despite all the blood coming out of my nose the doctor sprayed it with a local anaesthetic and had a look inside. They could see a blood vessel at the front of my nose that was bleeding, so they put a stick on it to cauterise the vessel and the bleeding stopped. It was a great relief and after an hour of no further bleeding I was allowed to go home with some nasal ointment and an outpatient's appointment for 4 weeks' time.

Activity

- Reflect on what advice you would give the patient with an active nosebleed if you had answered the telephone to them.

and two ethmoid sinuses and a single sphenoid sinus divided by a septum. These sinuses all drain into the nose (see Figure 14.5).

Acute sinusitis

Acute sinusitis is the inflammation of one or more of the paranasal sinuses. It usually develops as an infection secondary to an upper respiratory tract infection or dental disease. Because of the close anatomical connection of the sinuses with the nose, sinus infection is common. It may be acute or chronic.

Common presenting symptoms Pain is a symptom, and it may be facial, supraorbital (above the eye) or intraocular (within the globe of the eye), depending on the sinus involved. Tenderness in the area of pain and nasal obstruction may also be features, and nasal discharge may be present. The patient usually complains of general malaise and has a raised temperature (pyrexia).

MEDICAL MANAGEMENT

A nasal swab may be taken for culture and sensitivity. Sinus radiography may also be performed to determine which sinuses are affected. Medical treatment usually consists of the prescription of mild analgesics, antibiotics and nasal decongestant drops.

Nursing management and health promotion: acute sinusitis

The patient with acute sinusitis is usually nursed at home, and will be advised to rest in bed, to drink plenty of fluids, to take mild analgesics such as paracetamol and to self-administer any prescribed nasal drops. Oral hygiene is also important as the individual will probably be mouth breathing because of the nasal obstruction. Moist steam inhalations can also bring some relief and help to loosen crusting in the nasal cavities. Many sufferers find inhalations very soothing first thing in the morning and last thing at night. The patient can cover their head with a towel and leaning over a basin of hot water they should try and breathe the steam in through their nose and out through their mouth. They should blow their nose when necessary to release mucus rather than sniffing and swallowing. Patients need to take care that the hot water is placed on a stable surface to minimise the risk of burning themselves. Eucalyptus oil can be added to the water but there is no reliable research demonstrating that this is of benefit. After 2 or 3 days the person should have improved sufficiently to be fully active again.

Chronic sinusitis

Chronic sinusitis is common and can be quite debilitating. It can develop for several reasons, including:

- inadequate treatment of an acute episode
- septal deviation or nasal polyps preventing adequate drainage of the sinuses
- pollution, e.g. cigarette smoke
- allergic nasal disease.

Common presenting symptoms The main symptoms of chronic sinusitis are purulent nasal discharge, postnasal drip (mucus draining from the nose down to the back of the throat), facial pain, headache and recurrent throat infections.

MEDICAL MANAGEMENT

Treatment is initially conservative, consisting of treating any infection with prescribed antibiotics and nasal decongestant sprays. Surgery may be necessary to remove all of the diseased mucosal lining and widen the opening to the nasal passage to allow more effective drainage. This is functional endoscopic sinus surgery (FESS). CT and/or MRI scans are vital for both diagnostic and intraoperative use. For further information see Ludman (2007).

Nursing management and health promotion: chronic sinusitis

Nursing priorities when caring for these patients are:

- to prepare the patient for surgery and to observe for any possible complications, including haemorrhage and infection
- removal of nasal packing as per the surgeon's instructions
- administration of prescribed analgesics and antibiotics.

On discharge, the patient must be advised on the correct method for instillation of nasal drops and the importance of steam inhalations. See website for the procedures for aural toilet and insertion of ear drops.

 See website for further content

Nasal injury

Injuries to the nose are fairly common and usually occur in sporting activities, falls, accidents and assaults. A blow to one side of the nose may fracture and displace the bone, causing deviation on the other side. A direct blow to the front of the nose can splay out the nasal bones, resulting in a depressed bridge. An injury that is sufficiently severe to fracture the nasal bones will also cause soft tissue swelling and may cause epistaxis.

MEDICAL MANAGEMENT

Investigations will involve a radiographic examination, although this does not always reveal the fracture or may simply reveal a previously undetected fracture. An examination of the nose using a nasal speculum will allow the practitioner to see if the airways are patent and if there is any damage to the septum. Palpation of the nasal bones must be carried out very gently, as they will be very tender and painful for up to 3 weeks following a fracture.

Treatment of a broken nose involves manipulating the fractured bones. Occasionally this can be done at the time of the accident, but more commonly it is done a few days later, when the oedema has subsided, usually as a day case procedure. The manipulation must be performed within 10 days of injury to prevent calcification of the nasal bones. If the corrected fracture is unstable, a plaster of Paris cast is usually taped in position over the nose for about 10 days to allow the fracture to set correctly.

Nursing management and health promotion: nasal injury

First aid treatment of a fractured nose will involve measures to stop any epistaxis and to limit the oedema. This involves compressing the end of the nostrils gently between the thumb and forefinger, which unfortunately will be painful for the patient, and encouraging the patient to sit with the head slightly forwards and to spit out any blood. If ice is available, an ice pack applied to the bridge of the nose can help to control bleeding and swelling. Any epistaxis which results from a blow to the nose is usually short lived.

Disorders of the nasal septum

Deviation of the nasal septum

The nasal septum separates the nostrils. It is usually thin and quite straight. The upper part is composed of bone and the lower part of cartilage. Deviations of the nasal septum can range from a simple bulge to a marked S-shaped deformity. Most people have some degree of deviation; hence, when introducing a nasogastric tube, the patient should always be asked which nostril is easier to breathe through.

Developmental problems or trauma may result in a deviated nasal septum. Patients usually complain of nasal obstruction, infection of the sinuses or chronic otitis media due to the inability of the eustachian tubes to function properly (see p. 450). Any combination of these symptoms may be present, or there may be no symptoms; simply having a septal deviation is not a reason to operate on it.

MEDICAL MANAGEMENT

An assessment by the medical practitioner of the symptoms, correlated with the degree of the deformity, should be carried out before a treatment plan is agreed. Inspection of the nose with a nasal speculum should reveal the extent of the deviation. If surgery is the chosen treatment, this is likely to be either a submucous resection or a septoplasty. For further details of these procedures see Roland (2001)

 Nursing management and health promotion: deviation of the nasal septum

Septal surgery is often carried out as a day case and packs can be in place from 4 to 24 h. Nursing care in hospital will be similar to that given for epistaxis (see p. 461). Patients are usually discharged 2–4 h after the nasal packing has been removed. There will be a degree of nasal obstruction for 2 or 3 weeks after surgery, until the post-surgical swelling has subsided. Patients are usually advised to stay away from work or crowded places for 10–14 days after surgery to minimise the risk of infection. They are also advised to follow the surgeon's instructions with regard to steam inhalations, nasal douches (sniffing up a solution, usually water based, into each nostril) or decongestant sprays.

Septal haematoma

This usually results from trauma or surgery, and is a collection of blood beneath the mucoperichondrium of the septum. The patient complains of nasal obstruction and pain. Examination usually reveals a bilateral swelling in the nasal cavities. Antibiotics are given to prevent infection and it is often necessary to incise and drain the haematoma.

Septal perforation

Trauma or snorting illegal drugs is usually the cause of a hole in the septum. Although the patient is often symptom-free, excessive crusting or epistaxis may occur. Occasionally the patient complains of whistling on inspiration. If symptoms are troublesome, surgical closure may be attempted.

Nasal obstruction

Obstruction of the nasal cavities can result from a number of causes but patients usually present with similar symptoms, the most common being obstructed breathing and increased nasal discharge. Some of the most common causes are:

- infection
- allergy
- deviated nasal septum (see p. 464)
- foreign bodies
- polyps
- neoplasms.

Infection and allergy

Infection and allergy can cause an inflammatory reaction in the mucosa of the nose resulting in a sensation of blockage. This is one of the reasons that patients are often prescribed topical steroids and antihistamines in the form of intranasal sprays to reduce the swelling in the nose.

Foreign bodies in the nose

It is usually very young children, aged 2–4 years, or those with learning difficulties who insert foreign bodies into the nasal cavity. These objects may be organic or inorganic. Inorganic objects include buttons, beads and small plastic or metal objects which may lie undetected for a long time, only to be found during a routine examination, sometimes as late as when the child reaches adolescence or adulthood. Organic bodies such as peas, wood, paper, cotton wool or sweets cause a local inflammatory reaction which will eventually lead to the formation of granulation tissue. The resulting nasal discharge will eventually become purulent, foul-smelling and bloodstained. Characteristically, the discharge is from only one cavity.

MEDICAL MANAGEMENT

Following a thorough examination, the foreign body is usually removed in the outpatient department. Occasionally it has been in place for such a long time that a general anaesthetic is needed for smooth and safe removal.

Nursing management and health promotion: foreign body

Support will be given to both the patient and the family as removal can be frightening. Epistaxis is a possible complication following removal, irrespective of the type of anaesthetic used.

Nasal polyps

Nasal polyps are projections of oedematous mucous membrane and may look like bunches of grapes. They result from prolonged infection or allergy and are usually bilateral and multiple. They occur more commonly in adult males than in females.

Common presenting symptoms Patients usually complain of nasal obstruction and discharge. Occasionally the size of the polyps may cause broadening of the external nose. The patient may complain of headaches if there is sinus involvement and there may be loss of smell and taste.

MEDICAL MANAGEMENT

On examination, a characteristic glossy, greyish swelling will be visible. If probed, it will be found to be soft, insensitive and mobile. Surgical removal is the treatment of choice. This may be carried out under local or general anaesthetic. The patient who is given a local anaesthetic will require less time in hospital, but the decongestant that the local anaesthetic contains shrinks the polyps and makes them more difficult to identify and remove. With a general anaesthetic, the polyps can be removed at a less hurried pace but bleeding may be more profuse and might therefore obscure some of the smaller polyps. Recurrences are common and an attempt should be made to treat any underlying infection or allergy.

Nursing management and health promotion: nasal polyps

Nursing staff should be alert to epistaxis, which is the main postoperative complication of polyp removal. Given that polyps can be associated with allergies, many patients may also suffer from asthma and should be closely observed in this regard. A nasal pack is usually inserted after the procedure. Appropriate nursing care is detailed on page 461. As it is fairly common for polyps to recur, the importance of attending the outpatient department for follow-up should be emphasised.

Neoplasms

Nasal and sinus tumours are rare. When they occur, they are usually unilateral. Malignant tumours are often infected and ulcerated, in which case they usually produce epistaxis or a profuse purulent discharge. Headache may also be a feature if there is sinus involvement.

Treatment may consist of surgery, radiotherapy, chemotherapy or a combination of these. Patients receiving radiotherapy or chemotherapy are usually treated as outpatients and may be visited by community nurses, including Macmillan nurses, if they experience any side-effects of treatment requiring nursing intervention. For further information on nasal and sinus neoplasms and treatments, see Roland (2001).

Common problems during nasal surgery

- *Bleeding* – this occurs because the nasal mucosa has such a rich blood supply. It can be controlled by the use of ice packs. If the surgeon suspects that the bleeding might be severe, a nasal pack may be inserted.
- *Oedema* – oedema of the mucosa is likely to occur as a consequence of manipulation. Ice packs may help to minimise swelling.
- *Watery discharge* – the irritation of the mucosa, which results from surgery, will cause the production of an excessive amount of watery discharge known as rhinorrhoea. The nurse should provide an adequate supply of tissues or apply a nasal bolster made of gauze to absorb discharge. This helps to make the problem more manageable.
- *Pain* – as the nose is blocked after surgery, the patient may experience frontal headaches, which should be alleviated with prescribed analgesics, e.g. paracetamol.

THE THROAT

Anatomy and physiology of the throat

The throat is usually considered to consist of the pharynx and the larynx. The pharynx may be divided into the nasopharynx and the oropharynx. The nasopharynx extends from the nasal septum to the eustachian tubes and rests behind and above the soft palate. The oropharynx extends from the posterior boundary of the hard palate to the hyoid bone; it contains the uvula and the tonsils and is surrounded by lymphoid tissue (Figure 14.7).

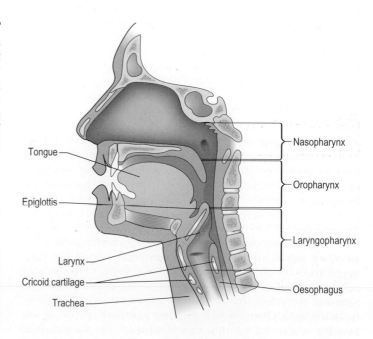

Figure 14.7 Sagittal section of the pharynx and larynx.

The larynx is the organ of voice production and airway protection. It is composed mainly of cartilage and muscle and is lined with a mucosa of stratified squamous epithelium (upper part) and ciliated pseudostratified columnar epithelium (lower part).

Disorders of the throat

Benign tumours

These generally arise as a result of voice overuse and the patient usually presents with continued hoarseness. The tumours are usually attached to the vocal cords and vary greatly in size.

Resolution of small nodules may be achieved by voice rest and appropriate speech therapy. Larger nodules may require surgical removal. For further information on benign and malignant tumours, see Roland (2001).

Carcinoma of the larynx

Carcinoma of the larynx is classified according to its location and extent, i.e. supraglottic (above the vocal cords), glottic (confined to the vocal cords) or subglottic (below the vocal cords) (see Figure 14.7). It accounts for 1% of all malignant disease and is more common in males than in females. The majority of patients have a history of heavy smoking, although the disorder does occasionally occur in non-smokers. High levels of alcohol consumption can be an influencing factor. The most common form of the disease is squamous cell carcinoma. About 10% of all patients with carcinoma of the larynx have a coexisting carcinoma of the bronchus.

Common presenting symptoms Some patients with laryngeal carcinoma do not seek medical help until the disease is advanced, having ignored the symptom of hoarseness for some time. Occasionally patients are treated initially for laryngitis, and by the time a tumour has been diagnosed it is advanced. Otalgia (earache), dyspnoea (shortness of breath), dysphagia (difficulty swallowing), neck lumps and weight loss are all symptoms of advanced laryngeal carcinoma. The impact of the diagnosis and the community care needs of a patient newly diagnosed with cancer are discussed by Glover & Cameron (2004).

MEDICAL MANAGEMENT

Carcinoma of the larynx has a high rate of cure if detected early. The form of treatment offered will depend on the site of the tumour and how early it has been detected. If the tumour is confined to the vocal cords it is usually diagnosed as a result of the patient consulting their GP with a history of hoarseness. Patients who have suffered from hoarseness for more than 3 weeks should have a mirror examination of their larynx (indirect laryngoscopy) to investigate the possibility of carcinoma. Diagnosis is confirmed by an examination of the patient's larynx under general anaesthesia (direct laryngoscopy) and a histological examination of a biopsy of the tumour.

If the patient has a positive biopsy result, depending on the size and spread of the tumour they may undergo CO_2 laser, radiotherapy, chemoradiation (chemotherapy given at certain points during a course of radiotherapy) or surgery with a total laryngectomy (see website). Laryngeal surgery may

also have to be performed on patients who have a residual or recurrent tumour following radiotherapy. Nursing interventions following laryngectomy are outlined on the website.

See website for further content

Very advanced tumours of the larynx may be considered inoperable, in which case the patient may be given palliative radiotherapy and/or chemotherapy to relieve some of the more distressing symptoms (see Ch. 31). A study by Forbes (1997) found that the most frequent symptoms and problems experienced by patients with head and neck cancer, in a palliative care situation, are pain, weight loss, feeding difficulties, respiratory problems and communication difficulties. A tracheostomy is sometimes performed (see p. 466) to relieve any respiratory obstruction and a percutaneous endoscopic gastrostomy (PEG) tube inserted to aid nutrition, hydration, administration of medications and patient comfort (see Ch. 21). For detailed information regarding the care of the patient with head and neck cancer and laryngectomy please see the website.

See website for further content

Tracheostomy

The surgical procedure of tracheostomy involves making an opening through the skin and structures of the neck into the trachea. It is one of the earliest operations described; there is evidence that it was performed by the Egyptians in biblical times. A tracheostomy may be short or long term and may be planned as elective surgery or performed as an emergency procedure.

Indications

The indications for a tracheostomy are as follows:

- *Airway obstruction* – this may be caused by the inhalation and impaction of a foreign body in the larynx. Severe inflammation may also cause obstruction, as might laryngeal cancer which is being treated by radiotherapy.
- *Bronchial toilet* – after head injury, drug overdose, cerebrovascular accident, coma or certain neurological disorders, the patient may require assistance with respiration and removal of bronchial secretions.
- *Need to improve respiratory efficiency* – when patients with impaired respiration are relying on their own efforts rather than assisted ventilation, the performance of a tracheostomy cuts down dead space and improves respiratory efficiency by 30–50% (Serra 2000).
- *Artificial ventilation* – if artificial ventilation is required for more than 72 h, a tracheostomy may be indicated, as it has been shown that endotracheal intubation for 72 h or longer can cause laryngotracheal damage.
- *Major head and neck surgery* – a tracheostomy will maintain the airway and protect it from haemorrhage and obstruction due to oedema both during and after surgery (see also Ch. 28). Box 14.7 lists some indications for short- and long-term tracheostomy

MEDICAL MANAGEMENT

Prior to performing a tracheostomy, the medical staff must explain to the conscious patient what is involved and the effect the procedure will have. In an emergency situation,

Box 14.7 Information

Indications for tracheostomy

Short-term tracheostomy

- Assisted ventilation
- Burns and scalds
- Foreign body lodged in trachea
- Major head and neck surgery
- Severe infection
- Trauma to larynx, face, mouth or oropharynx
- Vocal cord paralysis

Long-term tracheostomy

- Congenital deformity
- Trauma causing permanent damage
- Untreatable tumours, causing airway obstruction
- Vocal cord paralysis

such as when the patient presents with stridor or is unconscious, when there is minimal opportunity or time to prepare the patient pre-operatively, a planned programme of support and explanation will be required afterwards.

Tracheostomy is usually carried out with the patient under a general anaesthetic, but in emergencies a local anaesthetic may be used. Tracheostomy involves making an incision into the trachea through the third and fourth tracheal rings. An appropriately sized tracheostomy tube is inserted. For the first 24–48 h, a cuffed tracheostomy tube (Figure 14.8) is

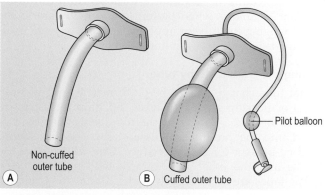

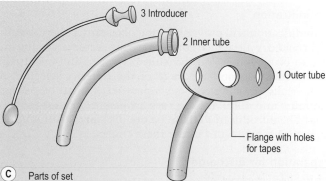

Figure 14.8 Tracheostomy tubes in common use. A. Non-cuffed tube. B. Cuffed outer tube. C. Parts of tracheostomy tube set.

normally used to prevent blood from the wound being aspirated into the lungs and aspiration pneumonia developing (see Ch. 26). A permanent tract usually forms 2–3 days postoperatively, at which time it is possible to change the tube. Tracheal dilators must always be to hand to keep the stoma open in case the tube is expelled accidentally. Most hospitals have a policy regarding the first tube change, which is likely to be performed by medical staff or experienced nursing staff with medical back-up.

There are several types of tracheostomy tube available, and the most appropriate one will be chosen for each patient. As discussed above, a cuffed tube, preferably with a low-pressure cuff, may be inserted during the operation. Single-use disposable tubes are usually employed and may be cuffed or plain. All tubes have an introducer, which is removed immediately on insertion, and an inner tube, which can be removed for cleaning without necessitating removal of the whole tube. Most tubes are made of polyvinyl chloride (PVC) and silicone, although silver tubes are occasionally used.

Nursing management and health promotion: tracheostomy

Pre-operative priorities

Physical and psychological preparation of the individual for a tracheostomy is a priority of pre-operative nursing care as the procedure can cause many difficulties. If the tracheostomy is short term, these problems will be of limited duration, but if it is to be long term, the patient and family will require additional information and education. They may need help in coming to terms not only with the problems presented by the stoma but also with the diagnosis, e.g. cancer, that necessitated surgery. Patients who have been well prepared for a tracheostomy tend to cope better than those who have not. Unprepared patients may become insecure, withdrawn and depressed. Ideally, a patient undergoing tracheostomy should be nursed in a single room initially and care assigned to one nurse who can gain the confidence of the patient and family. The main problems in the immediate postoperative period, for which the patient has to be prepared prior to surgery, are as follows:

Temporary loss of voice Air will bypass the vocal cords following the tracheostomy, making speech impossible unless a tube with a speaking valve is inserted. A system of communication whereby the patient can make themselves understood by staff and family members should be worked out beforehand.

Altered body image Body image is concerned with the control and function as well as physical appearance of the body. The very thought of coughing out sputum, which most people usually go to great lengths to hide, but which in the case of the patient who has a tracheostomy must be done through an open hole and tube in their neck, as well as their need for suction, is not easy to understand and accept. High-quality information and education must be offered to help the patient and family adjust to the presence of a tube in the neck. A visit from a patient who has adjusted well to having a tracheostomy may help.

Increased secretions These are produced because of the irritation caused by the tube and air bypassing the nose. This should be explained to the patient along with the need for suction. It is helpful, if possible, to show the equipment required for this prior to surgery.

Postoperative priorities

Maintenance of the airway

On return to the ward the patient should be nursed in a sitting position with the neck well supported; the tapes around the neck, which are fixed to the flange of the tracheostomy tube, must be tied securely in position.

Tracheal suction should be carried out regularly to clear secretions from the tube. To prevent infection, it is necessary to perform this procedure with a clean technique, according to Harris (1984) and Harris & Hyman (1984), whose research has not yet been superseded (see also Ch. 28). A sterile catheter should be used each time and should touch only the inside of the tracheostomy tube. A study on tracheal suction by Day et al (2002) indicated poor levels of knowledge and potentially unsafe practice among the nurses studied. The catheter diameter should be no more than half that of the tube to allow adequate flow of gases around it. If it is too wide, it will draw air out of the lungs more quickly than it can be replaced, which can cause atelectasis. Russell & Matta (2004) give a formula and chart to allow calculation of the correct catheter size.

Suction should be applied only as the catheter is being removed. Thumb-control catheters are ideal for this. Since the patient is unable to breathe during suction, it should be performed for no longer than 10–15 s; the patient should be allowed enough time to recover before it is repeated. The amount and type of secretions should be observed and recorded.

The physiotherapist will teach the patient how to cough into a tissue; as the patient becomes competent at this, the need for suction will gradually be eliminated.

Continuous humidification is given immediately postoperatively via a mechanical humidifier. When the patient begins to mobilise, a protector over the stoma will humidify inhaled air, act as a filter and have a cosmetic effect by covering the tube.

Care of the wound

The stoma (the surgically created opening into the trachea from the neck) into which the tube is inserted will require regular cleansing to prevent crusting and infection. A dressing beneath the tracheostomy tube can aid comfort and help to prevent sores caused by the tube and hard flanges as well as excoriation of the skin from tracheal secretions. However, these dressings can be a source of infection (Bond et al 2003). Skin can be protected with a barrier cream or film. If sutures are present, these will be removed according to local policy (see Ch. 23). For further information on adult tracheostomy care, see Russell & Matta (2004); for a pictorial guide, see Harkin & Russell (2001).

Complications

Blockage of tracheostomy tube Tracheal dilators and a spare cuffed tracheostomy tube must always be kept to hand in case this problem arises. Sometimes the blockage can be relieved by suction or by changing the inner tube. At other times it will be necessary to change the whole tube.

Displacement of the tube The tube can become displaced into the pre-tracheal tissue or completely out of the stoma if the tapes holding it in place have not been secured adequately. Dilators should be used to keep the stoma open until the tube can be replaced. Tapes should be checked for correct fit at least twice daily. Assessment and management of a patient in this situation are described by Russell & Matta (2004).

Surgical emphysema Emphysema is the abnormal presence of air in the tissues. Surgical emphysema is iatrogenic in origin, being a result of faulty suturing, and can be corrected by releasing the sutures.

Haemorrhage The insertion of a cuffed tracheostomy tube can help to control bleeding and prevent aspiration of blood. It is possible, however, for a major blood vessel to be eroded by a badly placed or poorly managed tube, causing a massive haemorrhage.

Dysphagia, nausea, vomiting If the tracheostomy tube is the wrong shape for the type of tracheostomy and the size of the patient, it may also tether the larynx and exert excess pressure on the posterior wall of the trachea and oesophagus, resulting in nausea, dysphagia and vomiting. These effects can be relieved by the insertion of a different type of tube.

Damage to the tracheal mucosa This can result from poor suctioning technique, badly chosen or improperly inserted tubes, or prolonged and/or over-inflation of the tube cuff. Ulceration of the anterior wall or a tracheo-oesophageal fistula may result and can lead to tracheal stenosis.

Infection A wound or respiratory tract infection can result from poor technique when performing wound care to the stoma, changing the tube or applying suction, or from inadequate management of respiratory problems.

Changing the tracheostomy tube

The first tube change should be performed by experienced medical or nursing staff, as it takes 2–3 days for a tract to form and there is a danger of the tube being displaced or inserted into the pre-tracheal tissues. Two people should always be present for this procedure. One will remove the old tube and the other will immediately insert the new one. The tapes are then securely tied.

Humidification

Humidification will prevent the tracheostomy patient breathing in cold dry air, which could cause the secretions of the trachea to become dry and difficult to remove and eventually lead to infection and blockage of the tube. A selection of aesthetically pleasing covers shaped like a small bib, which humidify and filter the air, are available and the patient should be introduced to these before discharge. A humidifying device can be worn under these covers.

Preparation for discharge

Before discharge can take place, the patient and family must be well prepared for all foreseeable difficulties and should be proficient in total care of the tracheostomy tube. The teaching of self-care techniques can begin with the nurse demonstrating procedures while the patient watches in a mirror. Rudy & McCullagh (2001) describe a nurse teaching programme initiated in order to help non-specialist nurses develop skills and confidence in identifying barriers to learning and motivation when teaching tracheostomy care to their patients. It is wise to teach not only the patient but also the family how to care for the tracheostomy in case the occasion arises when the patient is unable to do this themselves. However, some surgeons do prefer their patients to report to the ward or unit for a weekly tube change. For an outline of outpatient nursing care, see Russell & Matta (2004).

The community nurse will be actively involved in the patient's discharge into the community. Ideally, they will visit the patient in hospital and arrange for suction apparatus to be installed in the home if necessary. After discharge, they should visit regularly to ensure that the patient is coping with the stoma and altered body image.

Decannulation or removal of the tube

The tube can be removed without any preliminaries, but usually the patient is gradually reintroduced to breathing through the nose and mouth prior to removal of the tube. A tube with a speaking valve allows the patient to breathe in through the tube and out through the larynx. Once the patient has become accustomed to this, the tube can be replaced by a 'blocker' so that the patient has to breathe in through the nose and mouth. Once the patient is able to tolerate this continuously for 24 h and oxygen saturation levels are satisfactory day and night, the tracheostomy tube can be removed. Another method of achieving decannulation is to insert a smaller tube each time it is changed.

Whichever method is used, after removal of the tube a dressing must be applied to allow the tracheostomy site to heal. This can be a very anxious time for patients, and support and encouragement are necessary. The stoma should shrink rapidly and close off in a short time.

Tonsillitis

The tonsils are composed of lymphoid tissue and lie between the faucial pillars (Figure 14.9). During early childhood they enlarge in response to upper respiratory tract

infections and in adulthood should become reduced in size. In old age they normally atrophy. It is generally agreed that tonsils have a role to play in the body's defence system against infection.

Common presenting symptoms Patients usually present with a sore throat. Tonsil pain increases with swallowing and is often referred to the ear because of the involvement of the trigeminal nerve, which supplies both sites. They may also present with pyrexia, inflamed tonsils with exudate, lethargy and the absence of a cough (SIGN 1999). Recurrent bouts of infection are the most common reason for the removal of tonsils. Infection may take the form of acute tonsillitis, acute otitis media (see p. 456) or a peritonsillar abscess (see p. 470). Streptococci, staphylococci and *Haemophilus influenzae* are the organisms most commonly present.

Patients with tonsillar tumours normally present with dysphagia. These patients usually also complain of weight loss and may have speech problems. They may also suffer from facial pain and deafness because of the involvement of cranial nerves. Tonsillar tumours are rare.

MEDICAL MANAGEMENT

There is some controversy among medical practitioners about when tonsil infections should be treated conservatively and when tonsillectomy, with or without adenoidectomy, should be performed. The size of the tonsils is not usually the main criterion, but rather the history of the effect of repeated infections on the general health of the patient. Consideration is also given to absence from school or work, loss of appetite, speech defects, nasal catarrh or colds, hearing loss, breathing problems and abdominal pain, the last a sign of mesenteric adenitis, which occurs because of transmission of infection through the lymphatic system (SIGN 1999).

Tonsillectomy is an elective operation and is not considered in the presence of respiratory tract infections, during the incubation period after contact with an infectious disease, or if there is tonsillar inflammation. Tonsils are removed by dissection and any bleeding vessels are ligated or diathermy is applied.

> ### Nursing management and health promotion: post tonsillectomy

Airway

On returning from theatre, patients should be positioned in the post-tonsillectomy position, i.e. semi-prone, as this allows any blood or saliva to flow out of the mouth and helps keep the airway clear.

Haemorrhage

Half-hourly recordings of pulse and blood pressure and observations of breathing, pallor, restlessness and frequent swallowing are carried out to ensure early diagnosis of haemorrhage. Frequent swallowing is one of the first signs of tonsil haemorrhage and can go unnoticed unless the patient is closely observed. Particular attention must be paid to the sleeping patient.

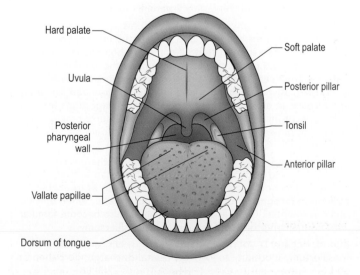

Figure 14.9 Tonsils and surrounding area.

Hard palate
Uvula
Posterior pharyngeal wall
Vallate papillae
Dorsum of tongue
Soft palate
Posterior pillar
Tonsil
Anterior pillar

Chewing and swallowing

Encouraging the patient to eat regularly and to swallow is important, as the exercising of the throat muscles seems to help keep the tonsil bed free from infection and to prevent the occurrence of secondary haemorrhage (Roland 2001).

Infection

Pyrexia is not uncommon on the first postoperative day, as part of the general metabolic response to the trauma of surgery, but if it continues, antibiotics should be prescribed and the source of infection sought.

Analgesics

Prescribed analgesics should be administered and their effectiveness observed. They should be administered before meals, before going to sleep and first thing in the morning. Good pain management is vital in ensuring the patient has a comfortable and uncomplicated postoperative recovery.

Preparation for discharge

Patients are usually discharged from hospital within 24 h. They are advised to avoid dirty, dusty atmospheres for approximately 2 weeks and to take a similar amount of time away from work or school/college. An advice sheet should be given on discharge with a contact number should any difficulties be experienced at home, including bleeding, pyrexia and otalgia (earache) (Box 14.8).

Peritonsillar abscess (quinsy)

This is a very painful condition and can be life threatening. It usually occurs as a complication of acute tonsillitis. Pus forms in the space behind the capsule of the tonsil. The abscess is usually unilateral and affects males more than females.

The patient presents with a pyrexia high enough to cause a rigor (see Ch. 22). There is usually a history of an episode of acute tonsillitis that has subsided, only to return on one side.

There is acute pain radiating to the ear on the affected side, trismus (spasm of the jaw muscles) is present and swallowing is so difficult that saliva dribbles out of the mouth. The voice becomes muffled because of the large swelling that affects the function of the palate. The neck glands on the affected side will be enlarged and tender.

MEDICAL MANAGEMENT

Antibiotic cover must be prescribed and the abscess may need to be incised and drained. Usually it is necessary to administer intravenous fluids, and antibiotics are always given parenterally for the first 24 h. Analgesics will be required when the pain is severe. Very rarely the swelling will be so severe that it will obstruct the airway; it may then be necessary to perform a tracheostomy to enable the patient to breathe.

 ## Nursing management and health promotion: peritonsillar abscess

Nursing care of the patient with peritonsillar abscess will include:

- physical and psychological support of the patient
- administration of analgesics, antipyretics and antibiotics
- administration of prescribed intravenous fluids
- good oral hygiene
- observation and recording of the patient's airway, temperature, pulse, blood pressure, fluid intake and output
- care of the tracheostomy if this has been performed (see p. 466).

Patients who require admission to hospital will be very anxious, agitated and in pain. They will require explanations, reassurance and swift administration of analgesics. As many will be unable to swallow, observations must be made for signs of dehydration; if dehydration is present, it

---

 Box 14.8 Evidence-based practice

Early post-tonsillectomy morbidity

This prospective study was undertaken to assess the amount and nature of post-tonsillectomy morbidity within 2 weeks of discharge from hospital. Complete follow up data were obtained from 149 patients (103 children under 16 years and 46 adults) when they attended a follow-up review with one of the authors. All patients were admitted on the day of surgery, had their tonsils removed by dissection and, with two exceptions, were discharged within 24 h. The two exceptions were discharged within 36 h when pyrexia had subsided and oral antibiotics had been commenced.

Following verbal advice from medical and nursing staff, all patients were discharged with oral analgesics and a written information sheet, which advised different actions for specific problems. In spite of this, a surprisingly large number of patients contacted their GP. Whether these patients were adults or children is not stated. Forty patients (27%) were responsible for a total of 53 GP consultations: 23 were prescribed antibiotics and 2 were prescribed mouthwashes. Throat pain was the commonest reason for consultation. Two out of 5 patients who consulted for otalgia were inappropriately prescribed a topical steroid and antibiotic. The responses to secondary haemorrhage were particularly worrying.

Nineteen patients had this potentially fatal complication. Despite clear advice to the contrary, only 7 patients sought advice or care.

The inability to recognise expected symptoms, such as throat pain, or to seek advice for haemorrhage, despite the information given, led the authors to suggest that all patients who experienced any operation-related problems should telephone the ward in the first instance. The need to improve or reinforce information was recognised, as well as the very real increase in workload for GPs and increase in antibiotic prescriptions. Other suggestions for improvement included routine assessment by a nurse practitioner and giving patients a review appointment that could be cancelled if all was well.

As the number of day case patients and early discharges continues to rise, the need to provide patients with information that can be clearly understood, remembered and accepted, so as to enable patients to recognise problems and act appropriately when they do occur, is essential. General practitioners must also become familiar with normal symptoms and responses to tonsillectomy.

Kuo M, Hegarty D, Johnson A, Stevenson S 1995 Early post-tonsillectomy morbidity following hospital discharge: do patients and GPs know what to expect? Health Trends 27(3):98–100.

will be necessary to administer intravenous fluids as prescribed by medical staff.

Good oral hygiene is important, especially once the abscess has been drained, as the patient will have had to spit out pus and will have a foul taste in the mouth. Once the pain has been relieved by analgesics and drainage of the abscess, the patient will be able to commence oral fluids and gradually begin taking a normal diet. Oral antibiotics will be substituted for intravenous administration.

The patient is usually discharged once apyrexial for 24 h and able to eat and drink normally. If the abscess was severe enough to require a tracheostomy, this would be removed (see p. 469) and the patient discharged only when the wound had healed. Patients are often sent home before they have finished their course of antibiotics; the importance of completing the course must therefore be clearly explained to them. Most patients who have a previous history of tonsillitis are re-admitted in 6–8 weeks to have a tonsillectomy performed as peritonsillar abscesses have a habit of recurring. For further details of the management and care of a patient with a peritonsillar abscess, see Ludman (2007).

Snoring/obstructive sleep apnoea (OSA)

Over the last few years, the issue of snoring in association with OSA has been addressed as it has been recognised that these individuals may have a contributing anatomical defect. The patient may show signs of chronic sleep deprivation. The patient's partner and/or family may complain of loud snoring and periods of breath-holding when the patient is asleep. This may be as a result of the tissues of the soft palate and pharynx collapsing and causing a temporary obstruction of the oropharynx. When the patient breathes, this tissue, including the uvula and possibly large tonsils, may vibrate, resulting in loud snoring. Patients may hold their breath due to this obstructing tissue. This condition can be dangerous, due to the possible development of severe hypoxaemia and systemic and pulmonary hypertension.

MEDICAL MANAGEMENT

Investigations Admission to hospital for a sedation nasendoscopy will be necessary. By means of a nasendoscope the medical staff can view the oropharynx of the sleeping patient and observe the activity and position of the tissues and structures. At this time monitoring of oxygen saturation levels is also possible.

Many centres now carry out sleep studies, which record the patient's breathing, snoring and pattern of electrical activity during overnight sleep.

Treatment A variety of treatments is available. These include weight loss in overweight people, change of sleeping position, mandibular advancement splints and the use of nasal decongestants. Continuous positive airway pressure may also be used (see below).

If it is obvious that there is collapse of excess tissues in the oropharynx, then the surgical technique of uvulopalatopharyngoplasty, with or without tonsillectomy, may be performed at a later date. This involves tightening of the soft palate and pharyngeal tissue, removal of the uvula and possible tonsillectomy. Correction using a laser or punctate diathermy is an alternative procedure.

 ## Nursing management and health promotion: uvulopalatopharyngoplasty

The priorities and management are the same as for tonsillectomy (see p. 469). Patients may experience nasal regurgitation on swallowing. This will usually resolve over a short period of time.

Continuous positive airway pressure (CPAP)

This treatment avoids surgery and can be carried out by the patient at home each night. The patient requires a considerable amount of education and supervision during the initial stages and continuous ongoing support. This education and support are usually provided by a specialist nurse who plays a key role in coordinating and implementing continuity of care from the initial sleep investigation stage and throughout.

Nasal CPAP works as a pneumatic splint, as the continuous positive pressure stops the pharynx collapsing and vibrating. At night the patient wears a well-fitting nasal mask which is connected via tubing to a small machine which delivers the positive pressure airflow. The mouth is left uncovered. The nasal cavity needs to be free of obstruction.

Most patients tolerate CPAP well, despite occasional problems with nasal and face irritation. It is most commonly used for moderate to severe OSA.

SUMMARY: KEY NURSING ISSUES

- The speciality of ENT care is continually evolving and presents many challenges to the nurse, who will encounter patients of various ages and backgrounds, each with specific needs in regard to the intensity, duration and setting of treatment.
- The ENT nurse is likely to encounter a wide range of disorders, some of which will have profound implications for the patient's ability to function within family, work and social spheres and which will require thorough assessment and individualised care planning.
- The nurse's ability as communicator will do much to determine the effectiveness of interventions; the need for skill and inventiveness in communication is especially important.
- In order to successfully educate the patient about their ENT condition a good knowledge of anatomy and physiology is required.
- The acoustics of the hospital and ward often make it difficult for older adults to hear. Turn off televisions and radios, shut the door and, facing the patient with a positive attitude, repeat yourself as necessary.
- All older adults should have their ears examined on an annual basis. Patients who wear hearing aids or who have a history of wax build-up should have their ears checked on a more regular basis and wax or debris removed as necessary.
- All hearing aid users and their families/carers should understand the basic care of the hearing aid and what to do if they encounter the common problems.

See website for further content

- Personal stereos are capable of producing the same volume of sound as a pneumatic drill, and thus present a serious risk of hearing impairment.

- Many ENT conditions are successfully managed within the primary setting. Health education and promotion are vital to maintain the patient's ability to function within the community.
- Most large ENT units also care for patients suffering from head and neck cancer. *Cancer – Implementation of Cancer Improving Guidelines* (Department of Health 2000) has implications not only for where these patients should receive their care but also for the education and training needs of the nurses who care for them.
- As the causes of certain ENT disorders become better understood, and as pharmacological and surgical treatments make further strides forward, ENT nursing will continue to offer challenges and rewards for nurses in a variety of care settings.

➡ REFLECTION AND LEARNING – WHAT NEXT?

- **Test** your knowledge by visiting the website 🖱 and answering the multiple choice questions and critical thinking questions.
- **Consolidate** your learning by looking at some of the further reading suggestions, references and specialist websites.
- **Revisit** some of the additional material on the website.
- **Consider** what you have learnt and how this will help your professional development.
- **Reflect** on how you can apply this knowledge to the care of your patients.
- **Discuss** your learning with your mentor/supervisor, lecturer and colleagues.

REFERENCES

Anderson G: *Tinnitus: a multi-disciplinary approach*, London, 2005, Whurr.

Berry P, Mascia J, Steinman BA: Vision and hearing loss in older adults: double trouble, *Care Manag J* 5(1):35–40, 2004.

Bond P, Grant F, Coltart L, et al: Best practice in the care of patients with a tracheostomy, *Nurs Times* 99(30):24–25, 2003.

Day T, Farnell S, Haynes S, et al: Tracheal suctioning: an exploration of nurses' knowledge and competence in acute and high dependency ward areas, *J Adv Nurs* 39(11):35–45, 2002.

Department of Health: *The NHS cancer plan*, London, 2000, TSO.

Durga J, Verhoef P, Anteunis JCL, et al: The effects of folic acid supplementation on hearing in older adults (randomized controlled trial), *Ann Intern Med* 146:1–9, 2007.

Glover E, Cameron S: Support in the community, *Cancer Nursing Practice* 3(10):34–39, 2004.

Harkin H, Russell C: Tracheostomy patient care: step-by-step pictorial guide, *Nurs Times* 97(25):34–37, 2001.

Harris RB: National survey of aseptic tracheostomy care techniques in hospitals with head and neck/ENT surgical departments, *Cancer Nurs* 7(1):23–32, 1984.

Harris RH, Hyman RB: Clean vs. sterile tracheostomy care and level of pulmonary infection, *Nurs Res* 33(2):80–85, 1984.

HMSO: *The Noise at Work Regulations*, Statutory Instrument 1989 No 790. London, 1989, HMSO.

Ludman H: *ABC of ear nose and throat*, ed 5, London, 2007, Blackwell Publishing.

Luxon LM, Davies RA: *Handbook of vestibular rehabilitation*, London, 1997, Whurr.

Maltby MT: *Principles of hearing aid audiology*, ed 2, London, 2002, Whurr.

McAllen PA: Managing Ménière's disease, *Am J Nurs* 96(6):16E–16H, 1996.

Ratna H: Counselling deaf and hard of hearing clients, *Counselling* 5(2):128–131, 1994.

Reynolds T: Ear, nose and throat problems in Accident & Emergency, *Nurs Stand* 18(26):47–53, 2004 55.

RNID: *Noise exposure and hearing loss*, London, 2008a, Royal National Institute for Deaf People, Policy Division.

RNID: *How many people use hearing aids?*, London, 2008b, Royal National Institute for Deaf People.

Roland NJ: *Key topics in otolaryngology and head and neck surgery*, ed 2, London, 2001, BIOS.

Roland PS, Smith TL, Schwartz SR, et al: Clinical practice guideline: cerumen impaction, *Otolaryngol Head Neck Surg* 139:S1–S21, 2008.

Rudy SF, McCullagh L: Overcoming the top 10 tracheostomy self-care learning barriers, *ORL Head Neck Nurs* 19(2):8–14, 2001.

Russell C, Matta A: *Tracheostomy: a multiprofessional handbook*, Cambridge, 2004, Cambridge University Press.

Scottish Intercollegiate Guidelines Network (SIGN): *Management of sore throat and indications for tonsillectomy*, Publication No 34, Edinburgh, 1999, SIGN.

Scottish Intercollegiate Guidelines Network (SIGN): *Diagnosis and management of childhood otitis media in primary care*, Publication No 66, Edinburgh, 2003, SIGN.

Serra A: Tracheostomy care, *Nurs Stand* 14(42):45–52, 2000.

Tortora G: *Principles of Human Anatomy*, ed 11, London, 2009, John Wiley.

FURTHER READING

Cochrane MA: Establishment of a nurse-run acupuncture treatment for hayfever, *Complement Ther Nurs Midwifery* 8:17–20, 2002.

Davis R, Roberts D: Nursing care of the patient with head and neck cancer, *Oncology Nurses Today* 4(1):9–15, 1999.

Dixson RK: The why, what, and how of endoscopic sinus surgery, *Semin Perioper Nurs* 9(4):163–167, 2000.

Dobbins M, Gunson J, Bale S, et al: Improving patient care and quality of life after laryngectomy/glossectomy, *Br J Nurs* 14(12):634–640, 2005.

Edwards M, Feber T: Working with anxiety in cancer: psychooncological care, *Cancer Nursing Practice* 2(1):19–26, 2003.

Ell SR, Parker AJ: A study of epistaxis in the elderly, *Care of the Elderly* 4(2):80–83, 1992.

Forbes K: Palliative care in patients with cancer of the head and neck, *Clin Otolaryngol Allied Sci* 22:117–122, 1997.

Harkin H: *Action on ENT: ear care guidance*, London, 2002, NHS Modernisation Agency.

Harkin H, Russell C: A guide to tracheostomy patient care, *Nurs Times* 97(25):34–36, 2001a.

Harkin H, Russell C: Preparing the patient for tracheostomy tube removal, *Nurs Times* 97(26):34–36, 2001b.

Haw S: Providing support to stop smoking, *Prof Nurse* 17(8):458–459, 2002.

Jamieson EM, McCall JM, Whyte L: *Guidelines for clinical nursing practices*, ed 4, Edinburgh, 2003, Churchill Livingstone.

Kendrick AH: Sleep apnoea, *Prof Nurse* 10(10):624–628, 1995.

Macdougald I: Laser therapy for OSAS, *Nurs Times* 90(19):32–34, 1994.

Malem F, Butler K: Nurse-aid management of ear and nose emergencies 2, *Br J Nurs* 2(18):926–928, 1993.

NHS Quality Improvement Scotland. *Caring for the patient with a tracheostomy. Best Practice Statement*, Edinburgh, 2003, NHS Quality Improvement Scotland. Available online http://www.nhshealthquality.org.

Semple CJ: The role of the CNS in head and neck oncology, *Nurs Stand* 15(23):39–42, 2002.

Semple CJ, McGowan B: Need for appropriate written information for patients with particular reference to head and neck cancer, *J Clin Nurs* 11:585–593, 2002.

Wright D: Swallowing difficulties protocol: medication administration, *Nurs Stand* 17(14–15):43–45, 2002.

Zeitoun H, Demajunder R, Hemmings C, et al: Developing a nurse-led aural care clinic, *Nurs Times* 93(45):45–46, 1997.

USEFUL WEBSITES

Association of Teachers of Lip reading to Adults (ATLA): www.lipreading.org.uk

British Association for Counselling and Psychotherapy (BACP): www.bacp.co.uk

British Association of Head and Neck Oncology Nurses: www.bahnon.co.uk

British Deaf Association: www.britishdeafassociation.org.uk

Hearing Concern: www.hearingconcern.org.uk

Hearing Dogs for Deaf People: www.hearing-dogs.co.uk

Information for ENT Nurses: www.entnursing.com

Let's Face It (a national and international group for the facially disfigured, including cancer sufferers): www.letsfaceit.force9.co.uk

National Association of Laryngectomee Clubs (NALC) (for laryngectomy patients, but tracheostomy and head and neck cancer patients are also welcome): www.nalc.ik.com

National Deaf Children's Society: www.ndcs.org.uk

Royal College of Nursing ENT/Maxillofacial Nursing Forum: www.rcn.org.uk/ent

Royal National Institute for Deaf People (RNID): www.rnid.org.uk

Scottish Council on Deafness: www.scod.org.uk

Tinnitus Helpline (contact via the RNID): www.rnid.org.uk

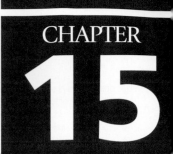

Nursing patients with disorders of the mouth

Susan Stringer

Introduction

The mouth is central to many activities of daily living that we take for granted until some minor but painful problem reminds us of the importance of the condition of the mouth to our feeling of well-being. The mouth is the source of the infant's first pleasurable activity, the sucking reflex being present at birth, and, perhaps, during teething, of the first experience of *dis*-ease. For individuals approaching the end of life, or for anyone who is acutely ill, good mouth care can give much comfort and relief and help to preserve dignity. Although this book addresses adult health, it is important to realise that good oral health practices laid down in childhood can influence adult health in a positive way.

Nurses remain the 'key personnel' in the multidisciplinary team (MDT) in the early detection of oral symptoms and potential problems patients may encounter with performing oral hygiene procedures (Murphy 2005). However, McGuire (2002) notes that: '...there are a number of barriers that prevent patients from receiving needed care. These barriers range from a lack of knowledge, to inconsistent practice, to administrative and environmental issues' and oral care remains an often neglected aspect of nursing care. It has been recognised that many nurses feel uncomfortable about raising the topic of oral hygiene with their patients, and may consider an oral examination to be an 'infringement of patients' integrity' (Murphy 2005). Miller & Kearney (2001, p. 241) suggest that 'mouth care has become a ritualistic and banal activity, a topic of conflicting advice and subjective conclusions from sporadic research'. McAuliffe (2007)

reports similar experiences, adding that oral hygiene practice is also carried out 'without reference to patients' individual needs', and is a task delegated to junior nurses or auxiliary staff, who may have received little educational preparation. Mouth care should not be regarded as a standard procedure, but must be adapted to meet the needs of individuals in various care settings throughout life, and at various points on the health–illness continuum.

Oral diseases are generally not given priority over other complex medical problems despite the often profound effects of oral problems on a person's quality of life (Doyle & Dalton 2008). The mouth is often the first indicator of generalised systemic disease or disease in adjacent structures and its immediate visibility gives any dysfunction a particular significance for the individual, who may be acutely aware of any disfigurement (cosmetic or functional). This can give rise to many difficulties affecting the person's self-perception and quality of life.

Anatomy and physiology

The oral cavity has evolved as a 'workshop', where much activity associated with chewing (mastication), drinking and speaking takes place (Figure 15.1):

- The mouth is the first portion of the alimentary canal. It is lined with a mucous membrane with the lips marking the transition from mucous membrane to skin. It is bounded laterally and in front by the alveolar arches, which contain the teeth.

1(A) Oral stage: preparatory phase
(Time taken varies)

Lips open; saliva is stimulated
Liquid or portion of food is taken
↓
Solid material is broken down by
teeth, moistened by saliva
↓
Strenuous movements of jaw and
cheek muscles and mobile tongue
against the hard palate, teeth
and alveolar ridges form food
into bolus
↓
Tongue tip gathers stray food
particles from between lips and
teeth and from the floor of the
mouth and incorporates them
into bolus
↓
The lips must be closed. The soft
palate is lowered and bolus or
liquid is propelled backwards by
strong humping movements and
funnelling of the tongue

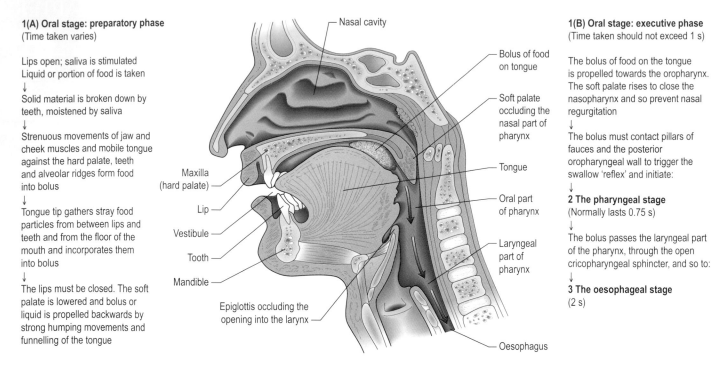

1(B) Oral stage: executive phase
(Time taken should not exceed 1 s)

The bolus of food on the tongue
is propelled towards the oropharynx.
The soft palate rises to close the
nasopharynx and so prevent nasal
regurgitation
↓
The bolus must contact pillars of
fauces and the posterior
oropharyngeal wall to trigger the
swallow 'reflex' and initiate:
↓
2 The pharyngeal stage
(Normally lasts 0.75 s)
↓
The bolus passes the laryngeal part
of the pharynx, through the open
cricopharyngeal sphincter, and so to:
↓
3 The oesophageal stage
(2 s)

Labels on figure:
Nasal cavity
Bolus of food on tongue
Soft palate occluding the nasal part of pharynx
Tongue
Oral part of pharynx
Laryngeal part of pharynx
Oesophagus
Maxilla (hard palate)
Lip
Vestibule
Tooth
Mandible
Epiglottis occluding the opening into the larynx

Figure 15.1 The importance of oral competence to the process of feeding, chewing and swallowing.

- The roof of the mouth is formed by the bony hard palate and muscular soft palate.
- Lateral walls are formed by the muscles of the cheeks (buccal region). The parotid duct drains into the cheeks at the level adjacent to the upper second molar.
- The floor of the oral cavity is almost entirely filled by the muscular tongue, which is very mobile and sensitive. Tiny projections on it, called papillae, contain nerve endings which include taste buds. In the floor of the mouth under the tongue there are also openings from two pairs of salivary glands: submandibular and sublingual.
- The rear exit to the oral cavity is under the border of the soft palate, through two archways (palatoglossal and palatopharyngeal) which enclose the palatine tonsil. This area is known as the oropharynx. The area posterior to the molar teeth is known as the retromolar trigone.
- The entire oral cavity is lined with mucous membrane, much of which is stratified squamous epithelium to cope with the daily trauma of eating, drinking and talking.
- It has a rich blood supply and lymphatic system.

The mouth is situated close to many other structures (the eye, ear, nose, maxillary sinuses, pharynx, larynx and neck) and disease or injury of the mouth may also affect these areas. A thorough knowledge of the anatomy is important to understand the relationship between the blood supply and lymphatic drainage. This will affect the way certain infections and diseases will present and is important in the management of patients with these conditions.

The stages of swallowing

Swallowing (deglutition) is a complex mechanism using both skeletal muscle (tongue) and smooth muscles of the pharynx and oesophagus. Only in the mouth is there any voluntary

control over the process of swallowing. The first stage (oral or buccal) must be accomplished so that the swallowing reflex is triggered when the bolus reaches the posterior pharyngeal wall, and the second stage (pharyngeal) then commences. During this stage and the third (oesophageal stage), swallowing is involuntary and is coordinated by the autonomic nervous system. Any problem in the oral phase can affect the patient's ability to swallow normally. Several cranial nerves are involved in the acts of swallowing and voice production.

 See website Table 15.1

A means of communication

The oral structures, together with throat and facial muscles, manipulate sound to give quality and resonance to speech. Thus any disturbance to the norm can cause diminution or failure of these very basic functions and so reduce quality of life. The psychosocial impact of poor oral health may be far reaching, as the mouth plays an integral role in communication through both speech and physical expression.

Saliva

This is formed by a combination of secretions from the parotid, submandibular and sublingual glands and from the numerous minor glands in the mucous membrane. Saliva plays an essential role in lubrication and protection of the oral mucous membranes (Xavier 2000), and salivary amylase is the enzyme that begins starch digestion whilst the food is still in the mouth. For more information about the physiology of salivation, see Holmes (1998).

Teeth

Teeth are important structures for biting and chewing food. Children have 20 temporary (deciduous) teeth, which are

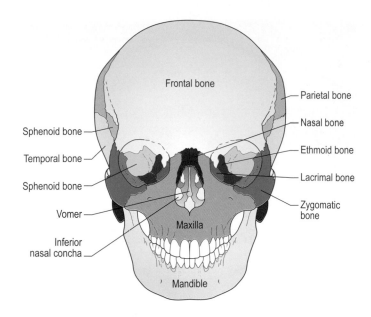

Figure 15.2 The bones of the face.

gradually replaced by 32 permanent teeth between the ages of 6 and 16 years. The dental age can be estimated in children depending on which teeth have erupted but there can be considerable individual variation. Overcrowding of teeth may necessitate extractions and orthodontic treatment in children. Impacted third molars (wisdom teeth) are removed if they cause problems themselves or with adjacent teeth.

Bones of the face (Figure 15.2)

Many of these bones are complex and fragile, and hence trauma to the mouth may result in a complicated injury.

DISORDERS OF THE MOUTH

Disorders of the mouth can be broadly classified into five categories:

- congenital orofacial deformity
- oro-dental disease
- infections
- traumatic injuries
- tumours (benign or malignant).

Congenital orofacial deformity

Defects involving the mouth may require a series of corrective procedures and may present the individual with physical, social and emotional problems in childhood, young adulthood and maturity. The most commonly occurring congenital malformations of the mouth are dental and jaw disproportion. Cleft lip (cheiloschisis) and cleft palate (palatoschisis) (the most widely recognised orofacial congenital defects) have an incidence of approximately 1 in 700–1000 live births. Of this number, roughly one third are isolated cleft lip, one third isolated cleft palate, and the remaining third cleft lip and palate. Other deformities of the face and mouth are comparatively rare, but can be devastating for both child and

parents, and may involve dilemmas for parents if diagnosed prenatally. These can involve defects of not only the mouth and face but the entire skull, so-called 'craniofacial defects'.

Problems associated with such facial deformities may include:

- appearance
- dentition/occlusion
- eating and drinking
- speech (e.g. speech articulation errors, hypernasal voice resonance and nasal emissions)
- hearing/increased incidence of ear infections
- facial growth (maxillary hypoplasia in cleft lip and palate for example)
- psychosocial adjustment/social alienation
- significant financial and emotional burden.

Cleft lip and palate

A cleft lip and palate is a congenital deformity in the body's natural structure caused by an embryonic developmental failure 6–12 weeks after conception. Cleft lip may be unilateral or bilateral and can vary in severity from a slight notch to complete division of lip and gum which presents the child with significant functional and aesthetic implications (Zuk 2008). Cleft palate can result in inability of the soft palate to meet the posterior pharyngeal wall and close off the nasopharynx. If uncorrected, speech is affected, producing a typically 'nasal' delivery in which certain consonants, particularly C, D, K, P, S and T, cannot be properly enunciated. For further information on rarer deformities of the mouth and face, see Wray et al (2003).

MEDICAL MANAGEMENT

Treatment

The medical management of oral defects requires a multidisciplinary approach extending from infancy to adulthood. Treatment protocol will depend on the extent of the deformity and the age of the child, but typically the patient will endure numerous procedures over the course of at least a decade. The aim of cleft surgery is timely reconstruction of the functional units that have been disrupted by the cleft (lip/nose and palate), so that normal facial development can be achieved (Oxley 2001). For management of cleft lip/palate, see Zuk (2008) and Table 15.1.

Orthognathic surgery (surgery to correct facial deformities) is an important area of maxillofacial surgery and is carried out in most maxillofacial units in collaboration with orthodontists (dentists specialising in moving teeth with braces). Craniofacial surgery, on the other hand, is only performed in designated craniofacial centres.

 Nursing management and health promotion: congenital orofacial deformity

Nursing considerations

Although deformities may be discovered by prenatal screening, the experience for parents of such a newborn child may be very traumatic, and the provision of sensitive and

Table 15.1 Treatment of cleft lip and palate

PROCEDURE	TIMING/PATIENT'S AGE
Lip repair	0–6 months
Palate repair	4–24 months
Bone graft to alveolus	9–11 years
Osteotomy (for correction of defect of hard palate) Rhinoplasty (for nasal defect)	Around 18 years
Pharyngoplasty (to correct the pharynx) Myringotomy revision procedures	As and when necessary
Orthodontic treatment	Throughout childhood and into adulthood
Speech therapy	As and when necessary

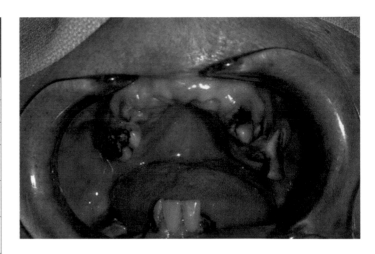

Figure 15.3 Periodontal disease with loss of teeth.

supportive counselling is vital. The way in which nurses care for and support the parents can aid their adjustment to the situation (Hodgkinson et al 2005). Parents should be given a clear and accurate account of the expected management plan for their baby at the earliest opportunity (Filies et al 2007).

The currently accepted model of care for the management of patients with a cleft lip/plate is a multidisciplinary team approach and they should be referred to the relevant professionals, e.g. specialist nurse, orofacial consultant, orthodontist, speech therapist, genetic specialist. With the increase in antenatal diagnosis, contact with the specialist team often happens before the birth. Information on local support groups or other appropriate self-help groups should also be provided. Professional psychological support may also be required and it is recommended that the team should include a mental health professional (De Sousa 2008).

Oral hygiene Nurses should emphasise to parents the importance of good dental hygiene. Parents may mistakenly feel that, compared with gross abnormality, the loss of a few teeth due to dental caries is inconsequential but dental health education, fluoride supplementation and dental attendance must be maintained throughout childhood.

Pre- and postoperative nursing care of patients undergoing major corrective surgery will take into account the general considerations discussed in Chapter 26, incorporating the specialised skills and techniques demanded by each procedure.

Oral health and orodental disease

Dental and periodontal disease (Figure 15.3) continue to pose an important public health problem (Jones et al 2005), affecting about 95% of the population of the UK in varying degrees and accounting for the largest proportion of mouth disorders. Although loss of teeth is not a lethal disease, the burden of oral disease in terms of financial, social and personal impacts is considerable (Kwan et al 2005).

Changing patterns of dental health

From the early 1970s, there was a substantial improvement in dental health in the UK. More people retained their natural teeth into later life, and there was a marked decrease in dental caries in children. Dental caries, also known as tooth decay, is a disease where bacterial processes dissolve the tooth structure, causing the progressive breakdown of the hard structures of the tooth, and producing holes (cavities) in the teeth. By 1998, dentate adults had fewer missing teeth and greater numbers of sound, untreated teeth on average than in 1978. However, improvement in children's dental health appears to be reversing and there was no improvement in 2001/2002 compared to the two previous years. Furthermore, the 2003 Children's Dental Health Survey reported that since the previous survey in 1993, the proportion of children with plaque and gum disease had risen in 5, 8, 12 and 15 year olds (White & Lader 2004). In the UK, 40% of children have dental decay (Morgan et al 2008), but there is wide regional variation. Most epidemiological studies conclude a direct correlation between socioeconomic status and periodontal disease (Peterson & Ogawa 2005). The most recent survey into children's dental health in the UK (Lader et al 2005) confirmed this relationship, with the average number of teeth showing obvious decay being lower among children from professional and managerial backgrounds compared with those from routine and manual families. There are serious implications for health in later years if dental disease remains untreated in childhood.

Promoting oral health

As illustrated by Box 15.1, nurses in all spheres of practice can help with early education in the simple preventative measures that are key to oral health.

A nurse-led initiative described by Black (2000) is aimed at educating children and their parents to improve their diet and dental health, and to identify orodental problems early. Such health promotion messages can be reinforced throughout the most influential stages of children's lives, enabling them to develop lifelong sustainable attitudes and skills (Kwan et al 2005).

Box 15.1 Information

Contribution of nurses and midwives to orodental health

Health visitors and public health nurses

Encourage oral hygiene in childhood and visits to dentist and orthodontist. This is a primary preventive function of the health visitor, school nurse and public health nurse. Educate on oral cancer prevention (smoking, alcohol and other substance abuse). Demonstrate dental hygiene. Alert parents to the need for children's visits to the dentist. Encourage healthy eating principles.

Occupational health nurses and practice nurses

Educate on adverse effects of smoking and excessive alcohol. Raise awareness of symptoms of intraoral cancer. Advise on good handwashing practices and healthy eating.

District nurses

Identify potential problems in older people. Advise on continued dental examination. Raise awareness of oral cancer.

Nurses caring for older people

As above. Increase mouth comfort and self-esteem.

Nurses working with those with learning disability

Supervise early and continued dental care and thus minimise need for restorative dentistry.

Midwives

Give dental care advice in pregnancy.

All nurses

Encourage and/or assist with oral hygiene for patients' comfort and health. Have dental/oral health literature available.

Oral hygiene

Parents should introduce a dental hygiene routine as soon as their child's first teeth appear, using a soft, baby toothbrush. Most children will require supervision until they are 7 or 8 years old.

The teeth should be brushed last thing at night and, ideally, after every meal. The toothbrush should be held at an angle of 45 degrees and the teeth brushed horizontally to avoid damage to the gums. All exposed surfaces of the teeth should be brushed.

Toothbrushes should be renewed every 3 months, and certainly when the bristles start to bend outwards. Hard brushes and traumatic technique should be avoided as these can cause abrasion of the teeth and gums.

Toothpaste with added fluoride is recommended, except in areas with fluoridated water, as the adverse effects of fluoride (see below) depend on total fluoride dosage from all sources. Current advice is that it is unnecessary to rinse, thus leaving a film of fluoride toothpaste. It should be emphasised that 'topical' fluorides such as toothpaste can have a 'systemic' effect when they are inadvertently ingested by young children. Studies have shown that 47–72% of dental fluorosis in children can be attributed to the systemic effect of fluoride toothpaste (Jones et al 2005). Ingestion of fluoride

before 3–4 years (i.e. pre-eruptive fluoride exposure) is critical to the probability of fluorosis, as this is when the formation of the permanent teeth occurs.

Fluoride is a substance naturally present in water in some areas. It is taken up by growing teeth and makes enamel harder and more resistant to the development of caries. There is strong evidence that the incidence of caries is considerably reduced in areas of naturally occurring fluoridated water (Stephen et al 2002). However, much controversy surrounds water fluoridation (Cross & Carton 2003). Excessive intake of fluoride, either through fluoride in the water supply, naturally occurring or added to it, or through other sources, causes fluorosis. This can appear as faint white 'mottling'; but in its severe form it is characterised by black and brown stains and pitting of the teeth. This pitting and loss of enamel in the more severe form of fluorosis increases the risk of dental caries (Levy 2003).

Dental floss with or without added fluoride should be used to remove food and dental plaque from between the teeth and at the gumline, where periodontal disease and gingivitis often begins. Overzealous use can damage the gums and it is best not used by children.

Disclosing tablets can be useful to demonstrate how plaque is left after inadequate brushing. Chewed after cleansing, the tablet produces a stain on any teeth still covered with plaque. Correct brushing should then remove the plaque.

Common misconceptions Chewing gum after meals to increase saliva is of limited value in reducing decay. To be of any benefit, sugar-free gum must be chewed for 20 min and be backed up by other forms of dental care. Chewing an apple after a meal does not clean the teeth. Rather, it is acidic and can cause erosion of the enamel.

Diet There is a direct correlation between the incidence of dental caries and availability of sucrose, with poor diet predisposing to dental decay in children. Children are particularly vulnerable to sophisticated TV advertising promoting high fat, sugar and salt containing foods, such as confectionery (Morgan et al 2008). Nurses can contribute to health education in this area, and emphasise the damaging effects of non-milk sugars, which include fruit juices, honey and sugar, especially when consumed by young children last thing at night.

Access to dental care The dental surgery is often the first remembered clinical setting for health care. If these first visits are pleasant, a positive attitude may be created towards future regular dental check-ups, and subsequent disease can then be diagnosed early. In the adult population with learning difficulties, changes from institutional living to community-based housing may be associated with reduction in dental attendance and treatment (Stanfield et al 2003). Older housebound people face similar problems.

The future dental health of the nation may be affected by factors including regional variation in accessibility of NHS dentistry, increased treatment charges and changes in funding of dental services. Although 75% of British adults consider oral health to be important to quality of life (McGrath & Bedi 2002), only 59% of adults were likely to attend for regular dental check-ups, and younger adults (16–24 years) were less likely to do so than when they were 5 years younger (Nuttall et al 2001).

Dental and periodontal disease

PATHOPHYSIOLOGY

Plaque is a firmly adherent, non-calcified deposit of bacteria, mucus, food particles and cellular debris which accumulates on the surface of a tooth, particularly at the base. The microorganisms present in dental plaque are all naturally present in the oral cavity, and are normally harmless. However, in the absence of good oral hygiene plaque builds up into a thick layer and reacts with sugar to form an acid which can attack and erode tooth enamel. Saliva is also unable to penetrate the build-up of plaque and thus cannot act to neutralise the acid produced by the bacteria and remineralise the tooth surface.

Calculus (tartar) is hard mineralised plaque which requires removal by a dental surgeon or dental hygienist.

Caries is progressive, localised decay of teeth caused by bacterial action. It is characterised by demineralisation of the inorganic portion and destruction of the organic substance of the tooth.

Gingivitis – inflammation of the gums Normal gums are pink (in Caucasians) or brown (in Asian and African people) and are firm with no bleeding when touched by a toothbrush. In gingivitis, the gums are inflamed and can be red to purple and often look swollen and puffy. They may be tender and may bleed easily on tooth brushing. The early stages are reversible with effective oral hygiene and dental care. Untreated, gingivitis can lead to gum recession and the formation of pockets (periodontal disease) (found in 75% of dentate adults) around the base of teeth, in which plaque and calculus can collect. Further infection from bacteria in plaque may lead to periodontitis.

Periodontitis is characterised by gradual loss of the supporting periodontal membrane of the teeth and erosion of supporting alveolar bone (Figure 15.4). Once the periodontal membrane and bone have been destroyed they cannot be replaced and subsequent loosening of teeth occurs.

Acute ulcerative gingivitis is caused by a mixed infection of a bacillus and spirochaetes. This is associated with poor oral hygiene and smoking, but can be associated with HIV infection and immunosuppression due to other causes. The gums are sore and bleed very easily and ulcers develop on the

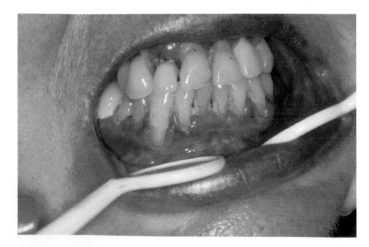

Figure 15.4 Periodontitis.

inderdental papillae (the cone-shaped pad of gingiva filling the space between the teeth) which may spread more deeply. There is foul-smelling halitosis, and cervical or neck lymph glands may be enlarged.

Halitosis, commonly known as bad breath, is very common, and in most cases originates in the mouth itself (although there are other possible sources such as the airways, oesophagus and stomach). It usually results from the anaerobic breakdown of proteins by bacteria somewhere in the mouth, with the most common part of the mouth for halitosis to originate being the back of the tongue. Here, large quantities of bacteria can remain relatively undisturbed by normal activity, and the continually-forming coating of food debris, dead cells and post-nasal drip allows these bacteria to flourish.

Common presenting symptoms

The patient commonly presents to the general practitioner (GP) or dentist with a combination of symptoms which may include toothache, bleeding gums and emission of pus from the gums (pyorrhoea). If oral hygiene has been habitually poor, the patient is more likely to wait until pain is severe before visiting the GP.

MEDICAL MANAGEMENT

Investigations include dental X-rays and relevant blood tests and a thorough clinical examination.

Dental surgery or outpatient procedures Most orodental problems are treated in dental surgeries. Standard dental treatments such as extractions, fillings, etc., are carried out with the patient under a local anaesthetic administered by the dentist. More complex procedures necessitate general anaesthesia, which is administered by an anaesthetist. This is not performed in a dental surgery setting and the patient is usually referred to a specialist department in hospital. Treatment of gingivitis is called scaling (removal of the plaque and calculus), and is more easily carried out when any swelling has subsided. Mouthwashes and systemic oral antibiotics are also helpful.

Inpatient or day-case procedures Procedures that can be classed as minor oral surgery but which may require hospital treatment in a dental hospital or oral and maxillofacial unit include:

- removal of impacted teeth, including wisdom teeth
- removal of cysts of the jaws
- minor soft tissue surgery (e.g. excision of oral polyps, frenulectomy, excision of mucoceles)
- apicectomy – excision of apex of tooth root following root canal therapy (often associated with cyst removal as well)
- pre-prosthetic surgery
- placement of dental implants.

Patients taking certain types of medication and those with the following medical conditions may require hospital treatment (Wray et al 2003):

- Diabetes mellitus – insulin dosage needs to be monitored according to blood sugar levels. There is a risk of infection in these patients (see Ch. 5).
- Heart valve disease – NICE guidelines (2000) state that the vast majority of these patients do not require any special treatment. They used to be given prophylactic antibiotics to prevent the development of infective endocarditis (see Ch. 2).

- Corticosteroid medication – must be monitored. Healing may be delayed.
- Anticoagulants – must be monitored and if necessary stopped pre-operatively or changed. There is increased risk of haemorrhage.

 ## Nursing management and health promotion: orodental disease

Nursing considerations

Outpatient care Individuals treated in dental surgeries or as hospital outpatients will require reassurance and advice on aftercare at home (Box 15.2).

Inpatient care Many patients are treated as day cases. However, stay may be longer if the patient has any relevant medical conditions (see above). Because of 'dentist phobia',

patients undergoing dental surgery often experience anxiety which may seem disproportionate to the size of the procedure, and need much reassurance. Postoperatively, the patient may experience pain, swelling and bruising. The nursing care plan on the website provides an example of the care that is required following a wisdom tooth extraction.

 See website Nursing care plan 15.1

On discharge, the patient should be given clear, adequate information on self-care and a number to call should further advice be needed (see Box 15.2).

Promoting oral health and comfort in special client groups

Most people are able to maintain good oral hygiene independently throughout much of their lives. Others, for reasons of

---

Box 15.2 Information

Information for patients having minor oral surgery

Following surgery to your mouth, you can expect some swelling and discomfort. This may last for some days. The following information will help you in the postoperative period.

On the day of treatment

1 Rest for a few hours. For the first night following surgery, when you lie down, elevate your head with pillows if possible to prevent any bleeding.

2 Avoid strenuous exercise for 24 h, and do not bend or do any heavy lifting for 2–3 days.

3 Avoid rinsing your mouth for 24 h, even if it tastes unpleasant. It is important to allow the socket to heal, and disturbing the clot by rinsing may cause bleeding and can allow infection into the socket and delay healing. Similarly, try to avoid disturbing the clot with tongue movements, eating on that side or brushing near the extraction site for 3–4 days. You can carefully wipe the area with a clean, wet gauze pad. Chlorhexidine mouthwash is also a useful adjunct.

4 Avoid sucking (e.g. through a straw), spitting and blowing your nose, as increased positive or negative pressure could dislodge the blood clot.

5 Your lips and/or tongue may be numb. Be careful not to bite or burn them inadvertently.

6 Avoid hot food and fluids until the anaesthetic wears off. This is important as you cannot feel pain properly and may burn or scald your mouth.

7 Avoid alcohol for at least 24 h, as this can encourage bleeding and delay the healing process.

8 Try to avoid smoking for as long as possible, but at the very least for the rest of the day.

9 Stick to a liquid or soft food diet for a day or two.

10 Pain or soreness can be relieved with a mild painkiller, e.g. co-codamol or paracetamol (no more than eight tablets in 24 h for an adult). Avoid aspirin-containing medications, as this can thin the blood slightly and may lead to bleeding. Check with your chemist or dentist if you are concerned or feel that you need something stronger.

11 There may be some slight bleeding for the first day or two. If you do notice bleeding, do not rinse out, but apply firm pressure to the socket. Bite firmly on a folded piece of gauze or

clean cotton material such as a handkerchief for at least 15 minutes. Make sure that the pad is placed directly over the extraction site, and replace the pad as necessary. If the bleeding has not stopped after an hour or two, contact your dentist.

12 If you are at all worried, or if anything untoward occurs, such as prolonged bleeding, excessive pain or swelling, please telephone the oral surgery department where you received treatment.

After the first 24 hours

It is important to keep your mouth and the extraction site as clean as possible, ensuring that the socket is kept clear of all food and debris. A mouthwash can now be used to cleanse the mouth. It is not necessary to purchase a proprietary mouthwash, although you can if you wish. It is the mechanical action of washing out the mouth which is of importance, rather than the substance used.

Warm salty water is very effective to cleanse and freshen the mouth. Dissolve one teaspoon of salt in a tumbler of warm water. Hold a mouthful of the solution in the mouth for a minute or two and then spit it out (but not forcefully). Finish the tumbler in the same way. Repeat the procedure several times a day for at least 5 days.

Pain that lasts up to a week or so but gradually gets better is normal. Pain that starts to get worse after 2 days is considered abnormal, and you may want to see your dentist. This may be a sign of a 'dry socket'. This occurs when the blood clot for healing becomes dislodged or does not form. In that case, the bone and fine nerve endings are not protected and are exposed to air, food and liquids. This delays the healing process and can be painful. If you suspect dry socket, see your dentist. He/she will place a medicated dressing into the socket, which will almost instantly relieve pain. A course of antibiotics may also be prescribed if the area is infected.

Follow-up

You will have been given another appointment if further treatment is necessary. If you have any problems please contact the oral surgery department for advice.

Sources

What to do following an extraction. British Dental Health Foundation. www.dentalhealth.org.uk Accessed 13th September 2009.

Healing after extractions and oral surgery. www.dentalfearcentral. org/healing.html Accessed 13th September 2009.

physical or cognitive disability, or infirmity due to illness or advanced age, will need supervision and assistance in carrying out dental and periodontal care routines. The importance of this aspect of daily care must not be minimised, as poor orodental health can seriously compromise the individual's well-being, both functionally and socially.

Physically disadvantaged and those with learning difficulties

Individuals with limited motor control or manual dexterity may require help with brushing teeth. Toothbrushes with adapted handles are available to aid gripping and the nurse should be aware of how these can be obtained (often from an occupational therapist). Electric toothbrushes often make tooth brushing more effective and easier to perform. Many people with limited movement depend on the mouth and teeth to hold or control equipment; it is thus especially important that their teeth are kept in good condition. Occasionally, it is difficult to gain the cooperation of a disadvantaged person who needs dental treatment; in such cases, general anaesthesia may be required even for a simple procedure. In the case of patients who have suffered a stroke, mouth care is particularly important. As recognised by Brady et al (2007), a stroke may result in physical weakness, lack of coordination and cognitive problems, all which may impact on the ability to maintain effective oral hygiene.

The older person

Effective dental care for older people can greatly enhance quality of life with regard to comfort, self-image and social interaction. Much of the care is not supported by research, and oral care practices have remained unchanged for many years.

See website Table 15.2

More people now retain their natural teeth into later life, and dentures are no longer an inevitable consequence of old age (Holman et al 2005). Good oral hygiene and regular assessment of oral/dental health for older people in hospital should form part of any nursing care plan (Box 15.3). However, Samaranayake et al (1995) found considerable unmet dental need among a group of 147 older people in five long-stay wards. Oral diseases are usually progressive and cumulative, and older people in general have a high prevalence of co-morbidities, health care challenges, and barriers to care, such as:

- Gum retraction/resorption – this occurs naturally (becoming 'long in the tooth'), causing root surfaces to be exposed, and with abrasive wear of the teeth can necessitate restorative treatment. The tooth root is exposed, and the tooth may be sensitive due to the exposed dentin.

Box 15.3 Reflection

Oral care for older patients

Consider the nursing care of older patients. Is the same quality of care given to teeth as to washing face and hands and combing hair?

Holman et al (2005) describe mouth care in detail. See also the website and Langlais et al (2009) for illustrations of oral disease that nurses might encounter during routine oral inspection and which would warrant seeking specialist advice.

- Dry mouth (xerostomia) – increases the risk of tooth decay. Older people are more likely to take medications that cause xerostomia (Holman et al 2005), and may have a host of medical disorders that cause salivary dysfunction (Russell & Ship 2008, p. 237). It is difficult to estimate the prevalence of xerostomia due to the limited number of epidemiological studies available; however, it is estimated that approximately 30% of the elderly population experience this (Turner & Ship 2007). Xerostomia may predispose the patient to microbial infections, altered taste, diminished food enjoyment and impaired denture use (as retention of dentures may be difficult if the salivary film is inadequate) (Russell & Ship 2008, p. 237). Many may also complain of a coated tongue.
- Ill-fitting dentures – as a result of the natural resorption of the alveolar bone the mouth continues to change when teeth are lost. After a few years dentures will not fit effectively and should be renewed every 5–7 years. Continuous wearing of dentures can lead to the development of *Candida*-associated denture stomatitis (inflammation of the mouth). Dentures should therefore be removed at night, cleaned and kept in water or a weak solution of Milton or other proprietary cleanser. Dentures left dry for any length of time can shrink.
- Angular cheilitis – this often develops because of old dentures and loss of lower facial height. It is characterised by irritation and fissuring (inflammation, deep ulceration and breaks in the tissue) in the corners of the mouth.
- Loss of appetite – older people who have lost interest in meals should be examined for any of the above and for early indications of intraoral cancer. Specialist opinion should always be sought for any mouth ulcer that does not heal within 2–3 weeks.
- Reduced manual dexterity and general weakness. Becoming accustomed to new dentures, or managing brushing and flossing techniques may be extremely difficult if an older person has one of the common diseases of later life such as Parkinson's disease, Alzheimer's disease or stroke (Holman et al 2005).
- Risk of developing oral cancer. The three greatest risk factors for developing oral cancer are age, tobacco use and alcohol. Almost 50% of oral cancers occur in people over the age of 65 years (Russell & Ship 2008, p. 236).

The acutely ill patient

During the acute phase of any illness, the patient may require assistance or supervision in carrying out oral hygiene, but the objective should be to encourage optimal independence as far as possible. Many acutely ill patients suffer from stomatitis and/or candidiasis and will require special measures (see below). These can give rise to considerable pain and discomfort.

Oral infections/inflammation

The mouth may be affected by the following:

- local and systemic infections

See website Table 15.3

- oral manifestations of a generalised systemic disease:
  - gastrointestinal and nutritional disorders (see Chs 4, 20, 21)

⌗ See website Table 15.4
- blood and endocrine disorders (see Chs 5, 11)
- dermatological disorders (see Ch. 12).

Stomatitis (oral mucositis)

Stomatitis means inflammation of the mouth (stoma) and can be caused by the following:

- vitamin deficiency (B_{12}, folic acid)
- viral infections (e.g. herpes infection and HIV)
- medical treatments:
  - radiotherapy to head and neck
  - chemotherapy
  - bone marrow transplantation (BMT) and graft-versus-host disease (GVHD)
  - liver failure
  - renal failure.

Common presenting symptoms This is an ulcerative inflammatory condition, where cell regeneration in the epithelium of the mucous membrane cannot keep pace with the rate of destruction that occurs as a result of any of the above. The mucosa becomes thin and there is erythema and loss of taste. Later, oedema develops and the mucosa breaks down at the slightest trauma, giving rise to haemorrhage and ulceration (Wells 2003).

The pain caused by stomatitis can be excruciating, and can considerably impact patient morbidity (Murphy 2005). A sore mouth is one of the side-effects that makes chemotherapy, radiotherapy to the head and neck area or preparation for bone marrow transplantation (BMT) an unhappy experience for many people (see Ch. 31). In health, saliva helps to clear the mouth of harmful pathogens; however, in these patients saliva becomes increasingly viscoid, resulting in xerostomia (dry mouth) which upsets the normal pH balance (Holmes 1998), creating an ideal environment for invasion by *Candida albicans*.

In addition to the effect on the quality of life and daily activities including nutrition, stomatitis also impacts in other ways. These include disruption to therapies, social isolation and distress, and systemic infections in immunocompromised patients (Wood 2004, Murphy 2005).

Candidiasis (thrush)

Candidosis, candidiasis or moniliasis is caused by infection with *Candida (Monilia) albicans*, a yeast-like fungus normally found in the respiratory, alimentary and (in females) genital tracts of healthy people. Oral candidiasis is very common in people who are ill, debilitated, older or terminally ill (Figure 15.5). Its presentation and predisposing factors are summarised in website Table 15.3. Most cases of oral candidiasis may be treated with locally applied antifungal drugs in the form of drops, lozenges or gel. For more severe cases, or for candidiasis persisting after first-line treatment, antifungal medication may be given systemically.

Aphthous ulcers

These are painful open sores inside the mouth, caused by a break in the mucous membrane. Recurrent aphthous ulceration is one of the most common oral conditions, and is classified according to the diameter of the lesion. Lesions between 3 and 10 mm are classed as minor ulceration, those greater than

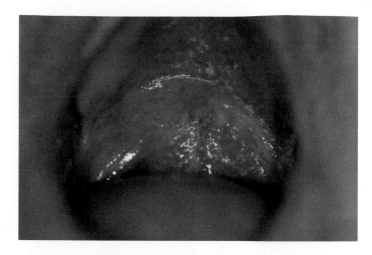

Figure 15.5 Oral candidiasis.

10 mm are classed as major ulceration, and clusters of numerous 1–3 mm ulcers are known as herpetiform ulceration.

Systemic diseases with oral manifestations

These include blood disorders such as leukaemia (bleeding gums), polycythaemia vera (bright red oral mucosa) and thrombocytopenic purpura (petechiae on the tongue) (see Ch. 11). In dermatological conditions examples of oral symptoms are Koplik's spots in measles and oral vesicles in chickenpox (varicella) (see Ch. 12).

Burning mouth syndrome (glossodynia)

This is a relatively common condition, particularly among older women. It is characterised by burning sensations within the oral cavity (particularly the tongue), with no detectable abnormalities of the mucous membranes. Frequently, patients also complain of xerostomia and dysgeusia (altered perception of taste) (Meiss et al 2004).

Aetiological factors include nutritional deficiencies, allergies, side-effects of some drugs, haematological disorders, undiagnosed diabetes, oral disorders such as thrush or xerostomia and cancer phobia (the latter causing much anxiety). Antidepressants have previously been the therapy of choice for burning mouth syndrome, but these often result in dry mouth and aggravation of symptoms due to their anticholinergic side-effects. Gabapentin has been used in the treatment of neuropathic pain for some time, and studies have proven this to be superior to antidepressants in the treatment of glossodynia (Meiss et al 2004).

Other inflammatory or infective conditions of the mouth include lichen planus and black hairy tongue (caused by too much bacteria or fungus growth in the mouth).

⌗ See website Figures 15.1, 15.2

MEDICAL MANAGEMENT OF INFECTIONS AND INFLAMMATORY CONDITIONS

Treatment begins with identification of the pathogen by culture swab or saliva washings. An appropriate antibiotic or antifungal agent is prescribed. All patients having radiotherapy, chemotherapy or preparation for bone marrow transplant should be referred for dental assessment before treatment. If being treated for a systemic disease, the patient's medication should be reviewed, with appropriate consideration of drug interactions. Appropriate mouthwashes may be prescribed (such as saline mouthwashes, antiseptic or antibacterial mouthwashes, locally acting analgesic and anti-inflammatory mouthwashes, or topical corticosteroids) depending on the underlying cause.

Nursing management and health promotion: oral infections/inflammation

Many patients with these conditions are already ill and to have to cope with an excruciatingly painful mouth can often overwhelm them and lead to total demoralisation. Nurses may help in this situation by carrying out and documenting a full oral hygiene assessment, (preferably using a valid assessment tool) and planning care using effective evidence-based interventions.

Nursing responsibilities for oral care

Much of the traditional ritual of oral care is unsuited to a sick person with xerostomia, acute stomatitis (oral mucositis) and/or candidiasis. It is difficult to encompass the many aspects of care in a single chapter, but nurses should consider the following when caring for patients and should challenge inappropriate practice:

Self-care should be encouraged whenever possible as patients know what their own mouths will tolerate and are more likely to cooperate.

Assessment The condition of the oral cavity may change from day to day. Frequent assessment is vital, using an oral assessment tool (to identify problems and initiate appropriate interventions) and a chart (to evaluate progress and document changes). Thorough examination is necessary and although the patient may find this intrusive, it can be used as an opportunity to supervise and offer encouragement. As recognised by Malkin (2009), a number of assessment tools have been proposed but evidence remains limited on the effectiveness of these. Holmes & Mountain (1993) and Wells (2003) evaluate oral assessment tools which have benefits in different care settings and Lockwood (2000) describes the development, piloting and evaluation of a new oral hygiene assessment tool, which includes quite specific details, with grading on many of the risk factors.

Frequency There is general agreement that care should be regular, but opinions vary as to frequency. Four times daily may be adequate for some patients, but those able to tolerate only rinsing or even just moistening, may benefit from half-hourly care. This may be an opportunity for the patient's family/carers to contribute to care.

Regimen A simple regimen is advocated. If possible, dentate patients should continue using toothbrush and toothpaste (a soft brush and toothpaste with added fluoride are recommended). If there is fragile mucosa, foam sticks may remove debris but will not remove plaque. Gauze swabs held in forceps or wrapped around a finger are too rough and may remove a layer of regenerating epithelium. Irrigation with a syringe may be appropriate in some circumstances, but

forceful use may damage mucosa. Following intraoral surgery, a patient may find it difficult to adapt to the changes inside the mouth because of alteration to contour and presence of insensate (lacking sensation) flaps, so supervision may be necessary to ensure removal of debris.

Oral care preparations A mouth with acute stomatitis can be regarded as an open wound, and the nurse must consider whether or not some traditionally used oral care products are appropriate treatment. Evidence for and against the use of a range of oral care equipment and preparations is summarised on the website.

See website Table 15.2

From the information available, it is clear that there is considerable variation in the opinions of practitioners and researchers. In the absence of compelling evidence, current opinion considers best practice to include brushing with fluoride toothpaste for natural teeth, use of chlorhexidine mouthwash to prevent plaque, and mouth moisturising systems for xerostomia.

Temperature is important. Ice cubes may seem soothing if a mouth feels inflamed, but may delay the healing process. Warm saline solution is recommended for wound irrigation; it should assist in healing a damaged mouth and is often preferred by patients. Hot salt mouthwashes are very simple and easily self-administered. Most patients find these helpful in most post-surgical and sore mouth situations (approximately one teaspoon per tumbler of water).

Analgesics must be adequate and timed appropriately, for example to give maximum benefit at mealtimes and to cover periods away from the ward or home when receiving treatment. Opioids may be appropriate; topical anaesthetic agents including benzydamine mouthwash, Mucaine® or lozenges containing local anaesthetic may be used (Wells 2003). Topically active anaesthetic agents, such as lidocaine gel, are also effective in particularly uncomfortable cases.

Dignity and self-esteem Consideration should be given at all times to the importance to the patient of maintaining dignity and self-esteem. All nursing care plans for oral care must form part of holistic care and must consider any therapeutic measures being implemented by other members of the multidisciplinary team.

Orofacial trauma

Traumatic injury to the mouth or face typically gives rise to much anxiety concerning disfigurement. Because of the high vascularity of this area, blood loss at the time of injury may be considerable and the patient, together with companions or relatives, is likely to be very alarmed.

Causes

Causes of maxillofacial trauma are multifaceted (Laski et al 2004), and the types of injuries produced are varied.

See website Figures 15.3, 15.4

Soft tissue injuries to the face range from simple lacerations, knife wounds and bites (Figure 15.6), to multiple injuries

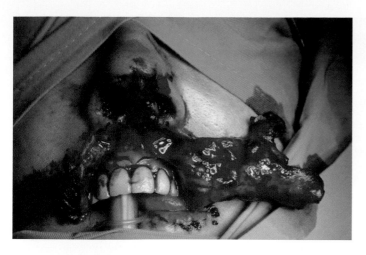

Figure 15.6 Dog bite.

resulting in tissue loss. Bone injuries include fracture of the mandible,

 See website Figure 15.5

the zygomatic complex (malar fractures) and the maxilla and nasal complex.

Violence

Assault is the most common reason for maxillofacial trauma. Many of these patients are young adults and alcohol is often associated with either victim or assailant. Zazzali et al (2007) assert that as with all violence-related injury, orofacial injury disproportionately affects socioeconomically disadvantaged minority populations. Domestic violence is another factor, and is often unreported by the victim. Lydon (1996) comments that domestic violence is often trivialised and challenges nurses to be proactive in bringing this serious issue in our society to the fore (Box 15.4).

Road traffic collisions (RTCs)

The incidence of facial injuries was reduced following the introduction of seat belt legislation (Department of Health

---

Box 15.4 Reflection

Domestic violence

Ms Y, aged 23, was brought to the Emergency Department by a neighbour who heard a disturbance and found her dazed. She was found to be suffering from concussion, a fractured malar bone and facial lacerations, and was admitted. Ms Y explained that she received these injuries when she tripped and fell against a door. While she was on the ward, Ms Y began to disclose some of her domestic problems and indicated that she would consider accepting assistance from a women's support group. A social worker arranged for Ms Y's children to be cared for until she was ready for discharge. Ms Y's discharge was planned well in advance. Through liaison with women's support agencies, she was assisted in reviewing her home circumstances and was offered alternative accommodation with her children.

Activity

- Think about what factors may make women scared to report domestic violence.

---

and Social Security 1978), and the more recent introduction of airbags has reduced fatalities and severity of injuries to the head.

Industrial injuries

Accidents in the workplace involving machinery or equipment are often followed by claims for compensation. Nurses should therefore not comment on the circumstances of any incident, either in person or by telephone, other than by using standard statements agreed by hospital policy (Nursing and Midwifery Council 2008).

Sports injuries are usually the result of a collision or fall and are commonly soft tissue injuries. Wearing helmets and gum shields may reduce the severity of injury.

Accidents

Accidental falls are common among older people, often resulting in facial injury. The underlying cause of the fall may require investigation. As recognised by NICE (2004a), older people who present for medical attention as a result of a fall should be offered a multifactorial risk assessment.

Burns

The treatment of burn injuries is discussed in Chapter 30. In order to assist in the prevention of contractures of the mouth and subsequent difficulty in function, patients with burns should be encouraged to drink from a cup as early as possible and to avoid the use of straws.

MEDICAL MANAGEMENT

Immediate intervention

Emergency treatment will involve whatever resuscitative measures are required to maintain the patient's airway, breathing and circulation and to prevent the development of shock (see Chs 18, 27). Priorities for intervention will have to be set, as cerebral and pulmonary injuries are often associated with maxillofacial injuries in severely injured trauma patients (NICE 2004a). A full physical examination will involve neurological observations and X-rays as appropriate, and will be followed by referral to the appropriate specialists, e.g. maxillofacial, orthopaedic or ophthalmic surgeons. Cannell et al (1996) state that, in using an injury assessment tool (Ali & Shepherd 1994) when assessing multiply injured patients, maxillofacial injuries often tend to be scored too low and that a maxillofacial surgeon should be involved as soon as possible to minimise facial deformity. However, the person with a maxillofacial injury with minimal displacement of bone and no symptoms of head injury may delay attending for treatment.

Treatment of maxillofacial injuries

The signs and symptoms of maxillofacial injuries, together with appropriate treatments, are summarised in Table 15.2.

Soft tissue injuries require thorough cleansing. This may entail scrubbing of the wound under general anaesthesia, to remove glass, debris, gravel or dirt. Failure to clean the injury adequately will lead to 'tattoo scarring', i.e. a permanent blue-grey scar. Facial suturing should adhere to plastic surgery techniques (McGregor & McGregor 2000).

Table 15.2 Characteristics and management of maxillofacial fractures

FRACTURE	SIGNS AND SYMPTOMS	MANAGEMENT
Fractured nasal bones	Nasal deviation or flattening; bruising Septal haematoma causing obstructed breathing	Manipulation of nasal bones and septum; nasal pack and plaster of Paris for 1–2 weeks Drainage of haematoma
Fractured malar bone	Black eye; swelling over cheek, sometimes flattening; anaesthesia of areas supplied by injured nerves (infraorbital and superior dental); inability to open mouth; diplopia	Elevation of malar bone through incision in temporal region May require fixation by wiring of bone
'Blow-out' fracture of malar	Periorbital haematoma; diplopia	Insertion of implant to orbital floor to stop eye dropping
Fractured maxilla/ middle third fracture	Grossly swollen face; failure of teeth to occlude properly; bilateral periorbital haematoma; fractured nasal bones; teeth may be loosened; CSF rhinorrhoea	Intermaxillary fixation (IMF) eyelet wires, Gunning splints, etc. Open reduction and internal fixation (ORIF) using wires, screws, plates
Fractured mandible with/without other fractured facial bones	Displaced or undisplaced; local pain and swelling; severe pain on opening mouth, sublingual haematoma	Undisplaced: usually no treatment Displaced: reduction with wires, splints or plate depending on site of fracture

NB: There will be considerable variation in presentation and in the timing of manipulative procedures, in accordance with the exact site and combination of fractures.

Bone injuries The objectives of treatment are to restore pre-existing anatomy, functional occlusion of teeth and facial appearance. Undisplaced fractures of the mandible generally require no active surgical treatment. The most common method of immobilisation now employed in the treatment of displaced fractures of the mandible is open reduction and internal fixation (ORIF). The fracture is exposed, reduced (repositioned) and fixed with plates and screws (Figure 15.7). The metalwork may be left in situ permanently or removed after several months.

Other methods of indirect fixation using the patient's teeth, known as intermaxillary fixation (IMF), may still be used successfully, for example:

- *Eyelet wiring* – wires are twisted around the upper and lower teeth, leaving a loop (eyelet). The teeth are then brought into proper occlusion and wired together.

- *Arch bar wiring* – a metal bar is wired to the teeth in each jaw and then, using cleats on the bar, the jaws are wired together (Figure 15.8).
- Gunning splint and cast cap splints are largely historical methods of IMF.

A fractured maxilla can be treated by open reduction and internal fixation or closed reduction with fixation applied externally using IMF and external frames or suspension wires.

External fixation is now less commonly seen but may still be effective in some cases.

Treatment of a fractured zygoma (malar) may take the following forms:

- Closed reduction, via an incision in the temporal region and elevation of the fractured bone.

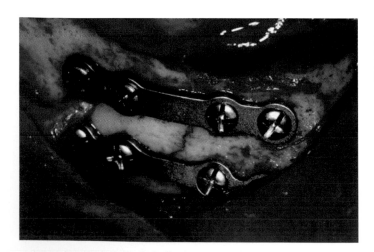

Figure 15.7 Open reduction and internal fixation of fractured mandible.

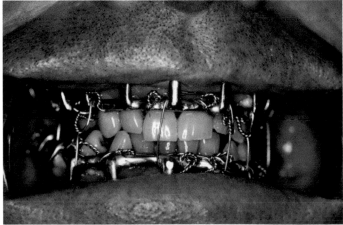

Figure 15.8 Intermaxillary fixation.

- Open reduction and internal fixation with plates and screws applied to some or all of the fracture sites (wires were used in the past).
- Kirschner wires (K-wires) – rigid wires which may be inserted into the bone in one or more directions, and the ends cut just clear of the skin. They then require removal 3 weeks later.
- Orbital floor fractures are commonly associated with this type of injury. An implant may be required to reconstruct the floor but sometimes this is achieved with adequate bony reduction alone.

Fractured nasal bones may also form part of a compound facial injury. Here, the fracture is reduced by manipulation of the nasal bones and may be immobilised by a splint.

Nursing management and health promotion: orofacial trauma

Orofacial injuries vary widely both in presentation and in their impact upon the individual's lifestyle and psychological well-being. While the treatment of individuals who have suffered orofacial trauma must take into account a range of physical and emotional considerations, only that care which is specific to the mouth and face will be described here.

Life-threatening concerns

For patients who have suffered maxillofacial injury, the immediate concern is to preserve the airway (Roberts et al 2000). Respiratory difficulty and haemorrhage require immediate care.

Respiratory difficulty

This can vary in severity and may be due to swelling of the tongue caused by oedema or haematoma, or to the patient's inability to control the tongue because of disturbance of the muscle attachments. If conscious and if other injuries allow, the patient should be sitting up and propped forward as soon as possible. The airway must be kept clear. If the maxilla is fractured, it may be necessary to insert two fingers into the patient's mouth and hook behind the hard palate and pull forwards to re-establish the airway by disimpacting the maxilla from the skull base. The use of an airway adjunct, usually an oropharyngeal or nasopharyngeal airway, is common in the Accident and Emergency department in some patients for short-term use. However, nasopharyngeal airways should be used cautiously in patients with severe craniofacial injuries, and similarly an oropharyngeal airway should not be used in patients with loose or avulsed teeth (Springhouse 2006, p. 328). In severe cases, early intubation or tracheostomy may be necessary.

Haemorrhage

There may be significant haemorrhage from middle third of the face fractures, with exsanguination and surgical shock a real possibility in some cases. Such bleeding may also further compromise the airway. Anterior nasal packing and the insertion of posterior nasal packs may be required to stem the bleeding (see Ch. 14). Bleeding may also be profuse when soft tissue injury alone has occurred, and immediate measures such as applying pressure on a bleeding point or pressure point may be necessary until ligation of the damaged vessel can be performed.

Shock

Nursing and medical staff must be alert to the warning signs of shock and should be prepared to take urgent action (see Ch. 18).

Observation and monitoring

Vital signs Temperature, pulse, pulse oximetry, respiration, blood pressure and pain should be monitored at regular intervals. Neurological observations will be appropriate (see Ch. 9).

Rhinorrhoea The nurse should also watch for the presence of rhinorrhoea (nasal discharge) caused by leakage of cerebrospinal fluid (CSF). This can occur in fracture of the maxilla if the cribriform plate of the ethmoid bone is disturbed. CSF contains glucose and therefore gives a positive reaction to glucose if tested with a urine testing strip.

Eye integrity/vision The nurse should check for abnormal pupil reactions, proptosis (forward projection or displacement of the eyeball) and acute pain. Vision should be checked hourly at first, especially if the patient cannot open the eyes because of oedema; the nurse should gently open the eyes and check pupil reaction (see Ch. 13). Any rapid decrease in visual acuity can indicate retrobulbar haemorrhage (bleeding from the back of the eyeball), which can lead to blindness and requires urgent action. Double vision can indicate a fracture of the orbital floor.

Other concerns

Pain management

Pain must be assessed (see Ch. 19). It is important not to underestimate the patient's pain, and to explain why analgesics may have to be withheld initially while investigations are carried out. Administration of strong systemic analgesics should be avoided until after a full assessment, as opiates may impair consciousness and mask symptoms of intracranial injury (see Ch. 27).

Anxiety

Anxiety caused by fear of disfigurement and scarring may be the first concern of many patients and relatives. Patients and relatives should be given the opportunity to talk about their fears. Nurses should offer the reassurance that healing is usually rapid and that as much as possible will be done to minimise scarring. However, it is equally important not to raise expectations unduly. Some people have unrealistic ideas about the results that surgery can produce, and it is unfair to allow them to imagine that what existed before can always be fully restored. Scars can fade and may be camouflaged, but it is not always possible to disguise the disfigurement caused by major tissue loss or bone displacement and it may be appropriate to introduce psychological support at an early stage.

Oral hygiene

Every effort should be made to clean blood and debris from the patient before relatives arrive, in order to avoid unnecessary distress. Oral hygiene should be carried out within the limitations of the patient's condition. For example, a blood clot should be left undisturbed as far as possible to minimise further bleeding, but broken teeth, debris and so on should be removed.

Nursing care in surgical interventions

Many patients with maxillofacial fractures will require surgical intervention to reduce and stabilise the fracture. The timing of this surgery will vary according to the patient's overall condition, and may not be an immediate priority (Roberts et al 2000). Localised swelling may also make assessment of the fracture difficult, and in some cases, fixation is best left for a few days. If the general condition permits, the patient may be discharged home for the interim. Alternatively, direct transfer to a specialised unit may be arranged or more complex surgery planned and executed when the appropriate surgical teams are available.

POSTOPERATIVE MANAGEMENT

The aim of postoperative management is to assist as necessary with the activities of daily living and to help the patient achieve independence in these activities as soon as possible.

Monitoring vital signs In the initial postoperative period, the patient's vital signs should be recorded every 15 min. As the condition stabilises, the patient can gradually be raised to a sitting position to aid respiration, help drainage and minimise oedema.

Respiration Many patients will have fractures fixed with internal metal plates. However, if the jaw is immobilised by other means, appropriate instruments for releasing the fixation, i.e. wire cutters, or scissors for elastic bands, must always be available at the patient's bedside for immediate use should any danger of airway obstruction arise.

The patient may have a nasal airway in situ to assist breathing and this will need occasional suction to ensure it remains patent. The mouth may also need gentle suction using a Yankauer sucker if the patient is afraid to swallow saliva for fear of choking. The patient should be encouraged to relax and to practise gentle swallowing movements.

Oral hygiene It is very important to help the patient maintain good oral hygiene. If the jaws have been wired, a soft toothbrush can be used to keep the anterior surface of the teeth and splints clean. The inside of the mouth can be cleansed with mouthwash taken through a straw (or a feeding cup with a spout) and squeezed out between the teeth. An alternative method is to have the patient lean forward and to irrigate the mouth through gaps between the teeth, using an oral irrigating syringe, letting the fluid run out. Chlorhexidine is an effective 'chemical toothbrush'.

Preventing wound infection The skin entry points of external fixation should be kept free of crusting by cleaning with normal saline. An ointment such as sterile petroleum jelly may be applied.

Sutures to facial lacerations can be kept clean with normal saline and removed in 3–4 days to minimise scarring. Supporting Steri-strips® may then be applied over the wound for a further 3–4 days. Wound care advice should be given, including sunlight avoidance for a few months, use of moisturising creams, etc. Any intraoral lacerations are usually repaired using a resorbable material that will gradually dissolve and does not require removal but the mouth should be checked in case any non-absorbent sutures have been used.

Maintenance of fixation The guiding principle of the treatment of maxillofacial fractures is, as for any other type of fracture, to obtain healing in the optimal position. Instruments for tightening screws on external fixators should be at hand, and the fixation checked at regular intervals. Most patients will be aware if it becomes loose, but older people or those with head injury may not be.

Nutrition (see also Ch. 21). A nasogastric tube may be inserted to allow for postoperative aspiration and/or drainage of old blood. Oral feeding should be encouraged as soon as possible, and there are particular problems if the jaws must be kept wired for several weeks. A liquid diet must be taken, which may make it difficult for the patient to consume sufficient calories to maintain body weight. All food must be liquidised and supplemented with 'sip feeds'. Frequent, small meals should be taken throughout the day.

The dietitian should be consulted, ideally before the surgery takes place, to assess the patient's dietary requirements. Older patients with a low body mass index will require special monitoring and encouragement. This is especially important if food is served by non-nursing personnel who may not appreciate the significance of unfinished meals.

Allaying fears The patient is likely to be very alarmed on recovery from anaesthesia to find that interdental or external fixation is in place, even if pre-warned. It is important that the patient is given some means of expressing feelings and concerns (see below) and is briefed fully on how to manage basic functions such as eating and how to avoid choking if coughing up sputum or vomiting. The patient may require help as they sip fluids through a straw or from a spoon, and nasogastric feeding may be necessary. Antiemetic drugs should be administered for the first few days after the injury, and in the event of choking or vomiting, the wires must be cut. Therefore, a wire cutter must be kept near the patient at all times.

Communication will be frustrating for the patient initially if the jaws have been wired together. Writing pads, 'magic' slates, picture cards and other aids may be used to facilitate communication. Special care will be needed for patients with learning difficulties.

Mobility When and how well the patient will be able to return to normal activity will depend on the nature of any other injuries incurred. Patients with facial injuries can be up on the day following surgery, but there are obvious restrictions if a cranio-maxillary frame is in place.

Body image Disfigurement caused by facial injuries is of great concern to most patients, and for the majority scarring will be a source of continuing anxiety. De Sousa (2008) suggests that people disfigured as a result of injury may have many problems in common with those disfigured by facial cancer.

Discharge planning

Patients who are fit and who can maintain adequate self-care can be discharged when postoperative swelling has subsided. They should be provided with written instructions on diet and oral hygiene, and given a telephone number to call in case of emergency. Referral to the community nurse should be made for care of wounds if appropriate. A follow-up appointment should be made for the patient to return to the outpatient department, usually within 1–2 weeks.

Alcohol Smith et al (2003) showed the benefit of a nurse-led psychological intervention on alcohol consumption and misuse in young males following alcohol-related facial injury.

Post-traumatic stress disorder (PTSD)

There is growing awareness of the psychological impact of a traumatic event, and of the need to address the long-term psychological problems that many trauma patients experience. Zazzali et al (2007, p. 5814) highlight the growing evidence which suggests that assaultive injuries in particular are associated with 'short and long-term psychological morbidity, impaired social and role functioning, and a degraded quality of life'. They go on to suggest that an aftercare programme to address the psychosocial issues that these patients face is paramount. Furthermore, it has been suggested that the degree of social anxiety is directly proportional to the size of the injury and the scar it leaves (De Sousa 2008).

Older patients who are already frail may never recover fully from maxillofacial injury and surgery. Some who are fit to go home may be too afraid or self-conscious to go out of their house. The community nurse is in an ideal position to encourage such individuals to venture into the outside world again. Some may require long-term care, whether within the family, in sheltered housing or in an appropriate care home.

Tumours of the mouth

Oral cancer is more common than is often realised. However, public awareness of oral cancer is low, probably due to its *relative* rarity (NICE 2004b), and attempts are being made to raise awareness (www.mouthcancerawareness.org.uk). Despite current progress in treatments, the mortality rates for oral cancer have not improved dramatically (Sargeran et al 2008). This reflects the large proportion of patients who have advanced disease by the time they are referred for specialist treatment. The 5-year survival rate for early stage localised disease is 80% (NICE 2004b), therefore mortality rates could be much reduced. It is recognised that at least three quarters of all oral cancers could be prevented by the elimination of tobacco smoking, and a reduction in alcohol consumption. In both high-risk groups and the general population neither the symptoms of oral cancer nor the main risk factors are well understood. It is clear that public education is

urgently required, and nurses in their role as health educators can make a significant contribution to this reduction (see Box 15.1, p. 479).

Treatment of intraoral tumours is generally carried out in specialised units. As patients are discharged into the community at an earlier stage, nurses in more general areas of practice are likely to encounter these patients. To help to ensure continuity of care from hospital to the community, it is important for general nurses to have an understanding of the long-term problems faced by these patients (Rogers et al 2005).

Treatment plans vary from centre to centre and there are different schools of thought within the medical profession as to which treatment schedule best promotes survival and a good quality of life. However treated, it is likely that many patients will suffer some disruption of several basic mechanisms which control the functions of eating and speaking. Patients may be left with short-term, long-term or permanent malfunction, which will vary greatly from patient to patient and is dependent on many factors.

It must be stressed that each patient is very much an individual whose needs and priorities will differ significantly from those of another seemingly similar patient. There can therefore be no set plan of care, and nurses must be ready and equipped to modify their ideas, working in conjunction with the other members of the multidisciplinary team and with the patient, to meet that individual's needs. As rehabilitation may take many months or years, it is often necessary for this multidisciplinary liaison to continue for some considerable time to ensure the best possible quality of care.

The pathophysiology and common presenting symptoms of tumours of the mouth are described under the following headings:

- tumours of the lips
- tumours of the tongue and floor of the mouth
- tumours of the palate and maxilla

🖱 **See website Figure 15.6**

- tumours of the salivary glands.

Because the separate functions of the mouth (speaking, chewing and swallowing) are frequently interdependent, medical and nursing management will be discussed with reference to the whole mouth.

Tumours of the lips

Malignant disease may take the form of basal cell carcinoma (BCC, often called 'rodent ulcer' because of its pattern of 'gnawing' into tissue) or squamous cell carcinoma (SCC).

🖱 **See website Figure 15.7**

Malignant melanomas may also rarely occur on the lips (see Ch. 12). Predisposing factors include prolonged, unprotected exposure to sunlight, e.g. among outdoor workers, people with fair skin and pipe smokers. The lower incidence of lip cancers among women may possibly be due to the barrier effect of cosmetics.

Common presenting symptoms Basal cell carcinoma may appear as a nodule or as a small, unstable ulcerating area with persistent crusting. However, it may also be diffuse and invasive. The ulcer may have 'pearlised' rolled edges. These tumours are generally slow growing and do not metastasise.

Squamous cell carcinoma is more aggressive and usually presents as a non-healing ulcer or a nodule. This can be painful, and if untreated, may assume the 'cauliflower' look of a malignant ulcer and will eventually fungate and cause severe pain.

Tumours of the tongue and floor of the mouth

Cancers of the tongue (Figure 15.9) account for approximately one third of all intraoral tumours in the UK. Others included in the category of the floor of the mouth are found on the lower alveolus, tonsillar fossae and retromolar trigones, and about 90% are of the SCC type (NICE 2004b). Fifty years ago the male to female ratio was 5:1; it is now 2:1 and incidence and mortality are also rising in almost all EU countries. Registration rates for oral cancer have risen by 20% in the last three decades, particularly in people under 65 years of age (NICE 2004b). Spread usually involves the local lymph nodes; distant metastases occur rarely at presentation but are usually in the lung.

Predisposing factors Heavy smoking combined with excessive alcohol consumption is associated with these cancers. However, there is an increase in younger people with no history of smoking or excess alcohol consumption, and it is now accepted that oral cancer may occur in any age group. Other risk factors are deprivation, diets poor in fruit and vegetables and chewing betel nut. There are also connections with anaemia, vitamin deficiencies and chronic oral infections, e.g. syphilis, herpes simplex virus, human papillomavirus and HIV.

🖰 See website Figure 15.8

The role of viruses remains unclear, but evidence is perhaps strongest for infection with high-risk human papillomavirus (HPV); transmission of HPV via oral sex is one possibility (D'Souza et al 2007).

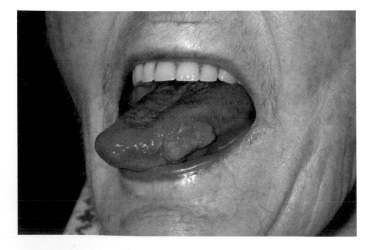

Figure 15.9 Squamous cell carcinoma of the tongue.

Common presenting symptoms In the early stages, intraoral SCC is easily mistaken for infection, irritation from dentures or a simple aphthous ulcer.

🖰 See website Figures 15.9, 15.10

Benign lesions may also occur and may be mistaken for a malignant tumour.

🖰 See website Figures 15.11, 15.12

Dysplasia, i.e. abnormal mucosa which presents as white patches (leucoplakia) or red patches (erythroplakia), is a precancerous condition that can revert to normal if the individual reduces risk factors such as stopping smoking.

🖰 See website Figure 15.13

Unchecked, this condition may become malignant. More advanced tumours are usually unmistakable but many patients present late for various reasons, including fear, misdiagnosis and self-neglect.

🖰 See website Figures 15.14, 15.15, 15.16

Tumours of the hard and soft palate

These tumours may arise from the epithelium of the mucous membrane (SCC), in the maxillary sinuses, in the maxilla or in the minor salivary glands in the palate. They are less common than tumours of the floor of the mouth, but spread may occur locally to involve the floor of the orbit or even the eye.

Common presenting symptoms Onset may be insidious. The patient may notice a dull ache for some time and may complain of sinusitis. The pain will eventually increase and swelling may develop over the cheek. There may be some displacement of the eye (proptosis) in advanced cases. Rarely, a malignant melanoma appears as a pigmented lesion of the palate and goes unnoticed until the individual presents with a secondary tumour of the cheek or neck.

Tumours of the salivary glands

The most common cause of swelling of the parotid gland is mumps (acute parotitis), an infectious, inflammatory condition that usually resolves without treatment. Mumps may, however, be relatively severe in adults and lead to pancreatitis or orchitis (a painful acute inflammatory reaction of the testicle secondary to infection, see Ch. 7, Part 1).

Benign or malignant tumours may develop in any salivary gland such as the parotid, submandibular, sublingual and other minor salivary glands.

🖰 See website Figure 15.17

Benign disease is more commonly the cause of a parotid lump and malignant disease is more often the cause of a submandibular lump.

Common presenting symptoms The patient presents with a swelling, which is often asymptomatic, and therefore sometimes long-standing, in the area of the affected gland. A malignant parotid gland tumour may involve the facial nerve (cranial nerve VII), resulting in facial palsy. Sometimes this is a presenting feature depending on the location of the tumour.

Medical management of tumours of the mouth

Tests and investigations

A treatment plan for malignant tumours will be devised on the basis of careful staging of the cancer (see website Table 15.5 and Ch. 31) and the patient's age, general physical condition and mental outlook.

🖰 **See website Table 15.5**

Management may include the following:

- history and physical examination
- blood tests
- diagnostic X-rays
- orthopantomogram (OPT or OPG) (a panoramic X-ray, providing a two-dimensional view of the upper and lower jaw)
- computed tomography (CT) scan
- magnetic resonance imaging (MRI)
- positron emission tomography (PET) scan
- examination under anaesthetic
- fine needle aspiration or biopsy
- sentinel node biopsy (SNB) to evaluate spread of cancer to the neck (Ross et al 2002); this may be a useful technique in the future.

Treatment

Patients are generally seen at a combined clinic, where many medical and other professional personnel are present. At this clinic different specialist consultants, e.g. surgeons and oncologists, liaise to plan treatment, which may be radical, i.e. intended to effect a cure, or conservative, i.e. intended to alleviate pain and prevent fungating tumours and subsequent haemorrhage. Radical treatment may involve extremely difficult adjustments for patients and, for some, a significant reduction in the quality of life.

The main forms of curative treatments for oral tumours are radiotherapy, surgery and chemotherapy, although this is less common as first-line treatment. These treatment modalities may be used singly or in combination. Choice of treatment depends on a number of factors, including the patient's wishes, site of the primary tumour, risk of hidden disease, need to preserve function, side-effects and medical resources.

Chemotherapy was previously reserved for palliation but is now usually given concurrently with other treatment (for example, to enhance the effects of radiation). It may be used to reduce the bulk of some tumours prior to surgery or in cases of recurrent tumours.

Radiotherapy can be given as the sole treatment, or pre- or postoperatively. It may take either of the following forms (see Ch. 31):

- external beam radiation
- brachytherapy (a radioactive source is placed in or near the tumour, e.g. interstitial needles to tumours of the lip or oral cavity); this treatment can be used in tongue cancer to try to maximise quality of life.

Many tumours, e.g. SCC, are highly curable by radiotherapy. Sarcoma and malignant melanoma, on the other hand, are less radiosensitive (see Ch. 31).

Surgical excision Treatment by this method ranges from small local excisions with direct closure, to major operations with full reconstruction. Benign tumours are usually excised but may still require the full range of resection and reconstructive options to be available. Table 15.3 summarises current surgical procedures. Microvascular transfer of free tissue (free flaps) has revolutionised reconstruction after radical excisions of oral cancers (Smith et al 2006). However, an effective monitoring protocol is essential in order to ensure early detection of vessel thrombosis and therefore ensure survival of the flap. The role of nursing staff is essential in the safe and effective monitoring of free flaps (Jackson et al 2009) (Figure 15.10).

Both radiotherapy and surgery treat SCC successfully, either independently or in combination. Gene, viral oncolytic and antibody therapies are being researched (Ganly 2003).

External beam radiotherapy can potentially cause skin damage, and nurses should be aware of the effects of radiation on the epithelium (Wells 2003). Prophylactic skincare procedures are necessary, and where skin damage does occur, appropriate interventions to promote healing will be necessary (see Ch. 31). Following radical radiotherapy, healing after surgery may be delayed; occasionally, orocutaneous (between mouth and skin) fistulae may develop. A late effect may be bone necrosis (osteoradionecrosis).

Table 15.3 Surgery for tumours of the mouth		
SITE	**EXCISION**	**RECONSTRUCTION**
Superficial lesion of lip, leucoplakia	Shaving	None
Lip, parotid gland, T1 tumour of mouth	Simple excision	None: direct (primary) closure
Lip	Wedge excision	Direct closure
Tongue	Local excision	Split-skin graft
Lip, alveolus, tongue	Local excision	Local flap: many varieties – Abbe, tongue, buccal, nasolabial, etc. (see Soutar & Tiwari 1996)
Mouth/pharynx (all sites), cheek, neck	Local/wide excision ± neck dissection	Free flap common in many centres
As above (especially for recurrent tumour as palliative procedure)	As above	Pedicled flap (deltopectoral, pectoralis major)

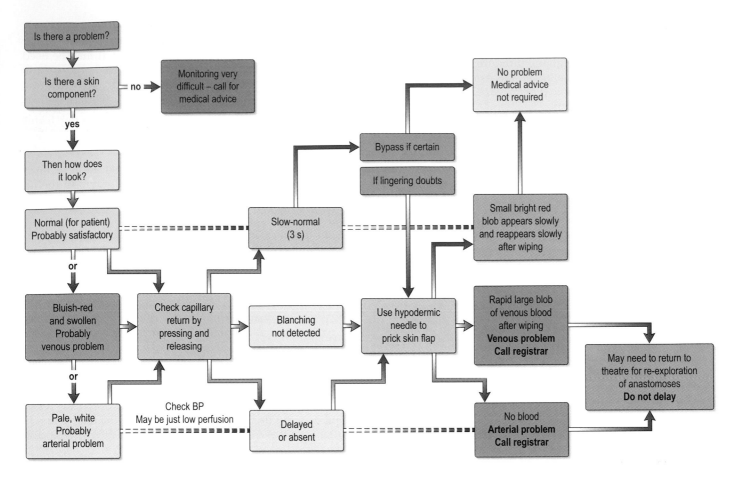

Figure 15.10 An algorithm for monitoring free flaps.

Follow-up and aftercare will require regular outpatient appointments for at least 5 years. Dental and/or prosthetic provision may include dentures, obturators (prostheses designed to fill a defect in the palate after maxillectomy) and other prostheses. Referral to other consultants, e.g. ENT, ophthalmic, thoracic and neurological specialists, will be made as appropriate. Speech therapy and dietary advice will be essential for many patients.

 Nursing management and health promotion: tumours of the mouth

The presence of an oral tumour may not give rise to immediate life-threatening concerns, except where a long-neglected tumour causes respiratory distress or haemorrhage. Patients vary widely in the symptoms with which they present, and usually require much reassurance when a biopsy confirms the diagnosis. A gastrostomy (see Ch. 21) may be planned if swallowing difficulties are anticipated. The nurse's role as the patient's advocate, to ensure adequate understanding before consent to treatment, will be important (Box 15.5).

 Box 15.5 Reflection

Support for patients with oral cancer

Mrs C, a 45-year-old housewife with two teenage children, was referred to an oncology unit from a dental hospital after she reported that she had had a lump in her mouth for some weeks. No lymphatic nodes were palpable in her neck and Mrs C was not too concerned that she might have cancer because she had never smoked and rarely took alcohol. She and her husband were consequently very shocked when they were given the result of a biopsy which showed squamous cell carcinoma. Mrs C was assured that the disease was treatable and was advised to have surgical excision in the first instance, possibly followed by radiotherapy.

Activity

- Reflect on Mrs C's situation and consider what measures could be put into place to support her and her family, and allay her fears.
- Consider the ways in which other members of the MDT (see p. 493) would be able to contribute to Mrs C's care while in hospital and when at home.

Immediate nursing priorities

This chapter will focus on specific care for patients undergoing surgery for oral tumours (for general perioperative care see Ch. 26). Nursing intervention in the early stages of treatment will focus on controlling pain (see Ch. 19), relieving anxiety, encouraging self-care in oral hygiene, and nutritional assessment (see Ch. 21). Supplementary feeding may be necessary, as weight loss is common among this group of patients. Existing physical conditions must be taken into account in any nursing plan. An additional concern may be the assessment and control of alcoholism. Excessive consumption of alcohol is a causative factor in many cases of oral cancer, and advice and information on limiting the intake of alcohol may be given by nurses (see Ch. 4).

Pre-operative preparation

Giving information

Patients will require adequate and honest information about the proposed treatment and its implications in order to give informed consent. In view of the many variations in procedures, and the diverse presentations and responses to treatment that are possible, nurses should be wary of giving information based on limited knowledge of apparently similar cases. What is feasible for one person may not be possible for another. The patient must be given the opportunity to voice any concerns about the disease and its implications for normal functioning and for appearance. It is important for their needs to be recognised and any unfounded anxiety relieved.

A multidisciplinary approach

A successful outcome will depend partly on the continuity of care provided by the multidisciplinary team. Treatment planning is often complex, due to the anatomical position of the disease and the long-term effects of subsequent treatment. Along with medical staff, the nursing team will include ward, theatre and high-dependency unit nurses, specialist nurses, community nurses and possibly Macmillan and Marie Curie nurses. The following professionals also contribute to care, and the nurse must be aware of each team member's role and facilitate liaison wherever appropriate:

- Dietitian – assesses dietary intake and advises staff and patient on maintaining adequate nutrition; liaises with the nutritional support person in the commercial companies and the community dietitian for provision of enteral feeding equipment.
- Speech and language therapist – advises the patient on pre- and postoperative exercises to assist with speech and swallowing difficulties; advises on alternative means of communicating if loss of voice is permanent.
- Physiotherapist – gives instruction and assistance with pre- and postoperative exercises to assist breathing, expectoration, limb and shoulder movements.
- Dentist (restorative) – assesses need for ongoing dental care, and provides the prosthetic rehabilitation including implant-borne restorations and obturators.

See website Box 15.1 and Figure 15.18

Pre-operative assessment prior to radiotherapy is important in minimising the development of radiation caries and osteoradionecrosis.

- Dental hygienist – advises the patient on care of teeth and oral hygiene, especially during radiotherapy and/or chemotherapy and after-treatment maintenance.
- Maxillofacial technician – advises on whether provision of a prosthesis is realistically possible; designs, constructs and fits this when appropriate for each individual patient.
- Medical social worker – gives information and advice on availability of grants for special needs; arranges home help, day care.
- Hospital chaplain or other religious counseller – gives spiritual comfort and practical help.
- Voluntary support agencies – provide emotional and practical support for patient and family.

Postoperative care

The postoperative nursing care of individuals who have undergone major surgery for intraoral cancer is highly specialised and combines the skills of many specialties. There will be variations in procedures and approaches among centres, and each patient will require a highly individualised plan for care. Many centres reconstruct facial defects using free tissue transfer. Figure 15.10 outlines nursing procedures for the monitoring of free flaps. See Jackson et al (2009), Marsh et al (2009) and Devine et al (2001) for information about nursing responsibility for monitoring free flaps.

Support for family/carers

Oral tumours and the effects of treatment may have far-reaching consequences not only for the patients, but also their families. Relatives must often provide care for the patient after discharge and are likely to experience much anxiety. They will need constant reassurance, especially during the early postoperative days, and should be counselled before the first postoperative visit, which is often very stressful. It is advisable to reinforce and supplement verbal advice with written information, particularly with regard to oral hygiene, diet, radiotherapy/chemotherapy and local support groups. Written information is now often available locally and general information booklets are also available from various websites and organisations (such as www.Macmillan.org.uk).

Altered body image

The impact of surgery to the face and mouth is visible to everyone. Basic activities such as breathing, eating and drinking may have to be performed with some loss of dignity.

See website Table 15.6

This, together with the disfiguring effects of the surgery, will require the patient to accept an altered body image, which can be a very difficult adjustment to make. Many patients, e.g. those who have had a tracheostomy, will be temporarily unable to speak following their surgery. It is important for nurses to bear in mind that it may be difficult for these individuals to convey their emotions in writing.

Discharge planning

Prior to the patient's discharge, liaison should be established with the GP and community nurse and appropriate appointments and home visits arranged. In most centres a specialist nurse will visit the patient in the ward and will continue to give support at home. Each of these professionals will coordinate subsequent visits through the local health centre according to assessment of the patient's needs and should be encouraged to contact any member of the hospital team for help and support at any time.

Particular advance planning will be required if the patient's social circumstances are less than optimal; for example, many patients live alone, and early liaison with social workers will ensure that the best possible social support is provided.

Rehabilitation

Despite technical advances in treatments, patients still have many difficulties, particularly with speech, chewing, swallowing, oral rehabilitation, nutrition, shoulder function and appearance. Cure is only one aspect of the effective management of such patients (Smith et al 2006). Covert alterations in body structure, loss of function and its implications for social interaction have been linked to depression. These problems are augmented by the additional burdens of difficulty with communication and social rejection (Millsopp et al 2005). Women experiencing facial cancers often have higher levels of depression and may take longer to adjust to their disfigurement.

Following discharge after major oral surgery and radiotherapy, the process of rehabilitation may not be complete for a period of some months or even years. Patients will need ongoing support as they learn to cope with changes in lifestyle and in the activities of daily living. Support is a vital component of the healing process, and websites such as that of The Mouth Cancer Foundation Charity (www.mouthcancerfoundation.org) provide an important source of information for patients trying to gain a better understanding of their illness.

Planning for rehabilitation should start from the day of admission and must take into account the following considerations:

- *Living arrangements* – the patient may need to live with relatives temporarily or permanently, or may need rehousing if they are to live alone. Long-term nursing support, e.g. from Macmillan and Marie Curie nurses, and community-based services, e.g. Meals-on-Wheels, may need to be arranged.
- *Breathing* – patients with a tracheal stoma will need to be instructed in its management and will need support in adjusting to their altered appearance (Ch. 14).
- *Oral hygiene; eating and drinking* – the patient (or carer) will need to be proficient in maintaining oral hygiene and, if necessary, giving enteral feeds (Ch. 21).
- *Communication* – training in alternative forms of communication will be needed if there is loss of speech.
- *Psychological support* – the patient should receive pre-discharge counselling to help in adjusting to an altered body image. Ongoing professional support may be needed for some time after discharge as the patient readjusts to life in the community (Robinson et al 1996), and both the patient and family should be able to contact members of the hospital team for support and advice. The patient and family should also be informed about local self-help groups where they can obtain practical and psychological support.

- *Work* – the patient will need help in adjusting to new employment circumstances, whether changing jobs, stopping working or returning to a previous job, and in learning to cope with a changed appearance and function and with the reactions of colleagues.
- *Education* – the patient may need information on such matters as nutrition, giving up smoking and reducing alcohol intake (Scottish Intercollegiate Guidelines Network 2003).

Nursing and stress

Caring for patients with intraoral tumours can give rise to considerable stress and nurses may find this area of care quite harrowing. Unfortunately, ward nurses frequently see patients return with a recurrence of the cancer, and some may question whether radical treatment has in fact been justified. However, many patients do in fact survive to lead fulfilling lives for many years after treatment. For information about staff support in cancer nursing see Chapters 17 and 31.

Palliative care

Only approximately 10% of patients with oral cancer survive over 5 years in cases of advanced disease. There is therefore a need to address issues of palliation, often from time of diagnosis (see Ch. 33).

SUMMARY: KEY NURSING ISSUES

- Oral health problems need to be given the same priority as other medical problems as they can have a profound effect on the individual.
- Poor orodental health can not only precipitate distress and discomfort for patients, it may also result in a decline in general health, dignity, self-esteem, social integration and overall quality of life.
- Oral care is a quality of life issue that must be a fundamental priority for nurses in any health care setting.
- Many medical conditions and treatments have an enormous adverse impact on oral health; unfortunately such problems are often not recognised, or are under-reported. As a result, many oral problems are inadequately assessed or treated, with often devastating consequences for the patient.
- Optimal assessment using a mouth care assessment tool is a necessity in order to make an initial assessment. Use of such tools also prevents the use of mouth care practices that are historical, rather than research-based, and promotes a high standard of evidence-based oral care via a coordinated approach.
- Nurses remain the key personnel within the multidisciplinary team in the early detection of oral symptoms and potential problems that patients may encounter. Nurse-led initiatives are also vital; for example, in improving children's diet and oral health, and identifying oro-dental problems at an early stage.
- Given the importance of good oral care, it is hoped that this chapter will stimulate the reader to consider the causes of oral health problems for patients encountered in their own area of practice, and reflect on their personal practice of oral care assessment and management.
- Nurses should consider what oral assessment is currently used in their clinical area, and whether any training programme and evaluation is in place to ensure that the tool is being utilised correctly.

REFLECTION AND LEARNING – WHAT NEXT?

- **Test** your knowledge by visiting the website 🖱 and answering the multiple choice questions and critical thinking questions.

- **Consolidate** your learning by looking at some of the further reading suggestions, references and specialist websites.

- **Revisit** some of the additional material on the website.

- **Consider** what you have learnt and how this will help your professional development.

- **Reflect** on how you can apply this knowledge to the care of your patients.

- **Discuss** your learning with your mentor/supervisor, lecturer and colleagues.

REFERENCES

Ali T, Shepherd JP: The measurement of injury severity, *Br J Oral Maxillofac Surg* 32(1):13–18, 1994.

Black S: Teething troubles, *Nurs Stand* 15(1):22–23, 2000.

Brady MC, Furlanetto DLC, Hunter RV, et al: Improving oral hygiene in patients after stroke, *Stroke* 38:1115–1116, 2007.

Cannell H, Paterson A, Loukota R: Maxillofacial injuries in multiply injured patients, *Br J Oral Maxillofac Surg* 34:303–308, 1996.

Cross DN, Carton RJ: Fluoridation: a violation of medical ethics and human rights, *Int J Occup Environ Health* 9(1):24–29, 2003.

Department of Health and Social Security: *Road accident statistics*, London, 1978, HMSO.

De Sousa A: Psychological issues in oral and maxillofacial reconstructive surgery, *Br J Oral Maxillofac Surg* 192:1–4, 2008.

Devine JC, Potter LA, Magennis JS, et al: Flap monitoring after head and neck reconstruction: evaluating an observation protocol, *J Wound Care* 10(1):525–529, 2001.

Doyle S, Dalton C: Developing clinical guidelines on promoting oral health: an action research approach, *Learning Disability Practice* 11(2):12–15, 2008.

D'Souza D, Kreimer A, Viscidi R, et al: Case control study of human papilloma virus and oropharyngeal cancer, *N Engl J Med* 356:1944–1956, 2007.

Filies T, Homann C, Meyer U, et al: Perioperative complications in infant cleft repair, *Head and Face Medicine* 3(9):1–5, 2007.

Ganly I: Novel and experimental treatments, 2003: In Bagg J, McFarlane TW, McCann M, Soutar DS, editors: *The A–Z of oral cancer – an holistic route*, Edinburgh, 2003, The Royal Society of Edinburgh, pp 17–20. Available online http://www.royalsoced.org.uk/events/reports/oral_health2002.pdf.

Hodgkinson PD, Brown S, Duncan D, et al: Management of children with cleft lip and palate: A review describing the application of multidisciplinary team working in this condition based upon the experiences of a regional cleft lip and palate centre in the UK, *Fetal and Maternal Medicine Review* 16:11–27, 2005.

Holman C, Roberts S, Nicol M: Promoting oral hygiene, *Nurs Older People* 16(10):37–38, 2005.

Holmes S: Xerostomia: aetiology and management in cancer patients, *Support Care Cancer* 6:348 355, 1998.

Holmes S, Mountain E: Assessment of oral status: evaluation of three oral assessment guides, *J Clin Nurs* 2(1):35–40, 1993.

Jackson RS, Walker RJ, Varvares MA, et al: Postoperative monitoring in free tissue transfer patients: Effective use of nursing and resident staff, *Otolaryngol Head Neck Surg* 1:1–5, 2009.

Jones S, Burt BA, Petersen PE, et al: The effective use of fluorides in public health, *Bull World Health Organ* 83(9):670–676, 2005.

Kwan SYL, Peterson PE, Pine C, et al: Health-promoting schools: an opportunity for oral health promotion, *Bull World Health Organ* 83(9):677–685, 2005.

Lader D, Chadwick B, Chestnutt I, et al: *Children's dental health in the UK 2003: Summary Report*, London, 2005, Office for National Statistics, p 2.

Langlais RP, Nield-Gehrig JS, Miller CS: *Colour atlas of common oral diseases*, ed 4, 2009, Lippincott Williams and Wilkins.

Laski R, Ziccardi VB, Broder HL, et al: Facial Trauma: a recurrent disease? The potential role of disease prevention, *J Oral Maxillofac Surg* 62:685–688, 2004.

Levy SM: An update of fluoride and fluorosis, *J Can Dent Assoc (Tor)* 69(5):286–291, 2003.

Lockwood A: Implementing an oral hygiene assessment tool on an acute medical ward for older people, *Nurs Older People* 12(7):18–19, 2000.

Lydon C: Too slap happy? *Nurs Times* 92(45):48–49, 1996.

Malkin B: The importance of patients' oral health and nurses' role in assessing and maintaining it, *Nurs Times* 105(17):11, 2009.

Marsh M, Elliott S, Anand R: Early postoperative care for free flap head and neck reconstructive surgery – a national survey of practice, *Br J Oral Maxillofac Surg* 47:182–185, 2009.

McAuliffe A: Nursing students' practice in providing oral hygiene for patients, *Nurs Stand* 21(33):35–39, 2007.

McGrath C, Bedi R: Understanding the value of oral health to people in Britain – importance to life quality, *Community Dent Health* 19(4):211–214, 2002.

McGregor AD, McGregor IA: *Fundamental techniques of plastic surgery and their surgical applications*, ed 10, Edinburgh, 2000, Churchill Livingstone.

McGuire DB: Mucosal tissue injury in cancer therapy: more than mucositis and mouthwash, *Cancer Pract* 10(4):179–191, 2002.

Meiss F, Fielder E, Taube, et al: Gabapentin in the treatment of glossodynia, *Dermatology and Psychosomatics* 5(1):17–21, 2004.

Miller M, Kearney N: Oral care for patients with cancer: a review of the literature, *Cancer Nurs* 24(4):241–254, 2001.

Millsopp L, Brandom L, Humphris G, et al: Facial appearance after operations for oral and oropharyngeal cancer: A comparison of casenotes and patient-completed questionnaire, *Br J Oral Maxillofac Surg* 44:358–363, 2005.

Morgan M, Fairchild R, Phillips A, et al: A content analysis of children's television advertising: focus on food and oral health, *Public Health Nutr* 2008:1–8, 2008.

Murphy L: Oral mucositis: a challenge for nurses, *Cancer Nursing Practice* 4(6):21–24, 2005.

National Institute for Health and Clinical Excellence (NICE): *Guidance on the extraction of wisdom teeth*, London, 2000, NICE.

National Institute for Health and Clinical Excellence (NICE): *Clinical Practice Guideline for the assessment and prevention of falls in older people*, London, 2004a, NICE.

National Institute for Health and Clinical Excellence (NICE): *Improving Outcomes in Head and Neck Cancers*, London, 2004b, NICE.

Nursing and Midwifery Council (NMC): *The Code – Standards of conduct, performance and ethics for nurses and midwives*, London, 2008, NMC.

Nuttall NM, Bradnock G, White D, et al: Dental attendance in 1998 and implications for the future, *Br Dent J* 190(4):177–182, 2001.

Oxley J: Are arm splints required following cleft lip/palate repair? *Paediatr Nurs* 13(1):27–30, 2001.

Peterson PE, Ogawa: Strengthening the prevention of periodontal disease: The WHO approach, *J Periodontol* 76:2187–2193, 2005.

Roberts G, Scully C, Shotts R: ABC of oral health: Dental emergencies, *Br Med J* 321:559–562, 2000.

Robinson E, Rumsey N, Partridge J: An evaluation of the impact of social interaction skills for facially disfigured people, *Br J Plast Surg* 49(5):281–289, 1996.

Rogers SN, Panasar J, Pritchard K, et al: Survey of oral rehabilitation in a consecutive series of 130 patients treated by primary resection for oral and oropharyngeal squamous cell carcinoma, *Br J Oral Maxillofac Surg* 43:23–30, 2005.

Ross G, Soutar DS, Shoaib T, et al: The ability of lymphoscintigraphy to direct sentinel node biopsy in the clinically N0 (node-negative) neck for patients with head and neck squamous cell carcinoma, *Br J Radiol* 75(900):950–958, 2002.

Russell SL, Ship JA: Normal oral mucosal, dental, periodontal and alveolar bone changes associated with aging. In Lamster IB, Northridge ME, Takamura JC, editors: *Improving oral health for the elderly: An interdisciplinary approach*, New York, 2008, Springer, pp 233–246.

Samaranayake LP, Wilkieson CA, Lamey P-J, et al: Oral disease in the elderly in long-term hospital care, *Oral Dis* 1(3):147–151, 1995.

Sargeran K, Murtomaa H, Safavi SMR, et al: Survival after diagnosis of cancer of the oral cavity, *Br J Oral Maxillofac Surg* 46:187–191, 2008.

Scottish Intercollegiate Guidelines Network (SIGN): *Guideline 74. Management of harmful drinking and alcohol dependence in primary care*, Edinburgh, 2003, SIGN.

Smith AJ, Hodgson RJ, Bridgman K, et al: A randomized controlled trial of a brief intervention after alcohol-related facial injury, *Addiction* 98(1):43–52, 2003.

Smith GI, Yeo D, Clark J, et al: Measures of health-related quality of life and functional status in survivors of oral cavity cancer who have had defects reconstructed with radial forearm free flaps, *Br J Oral Maxillofac Surg* 44:187–192, 2006.

Soutar DS, Tiwari R, editors: *Excision and reconstruction in head and neck cancer*, Edinburgh, 1996, Churchill Livingstone.

Springhouse: Respiratory care (Ch 6). In *Best Practices: Evidence-based nursing procedures*, ed 2, Philadelphia, 2006, Lippincott Williams and Wilkins, pp 282–365.

Stanfield M, Stanfield M, Scully C, et al: Oral healthcare of clients with learning disability: changes following relocation from hospital to community, *Br Dent J* 194(5):271–277, 2003.

Stephen K, Macpherson L, Gilmour W, et al: A blind caries and fluorosis prevalence study of school-children in naturally fluoridated and nonfluoridated townships of Morayshire, Scotland, *Community Dent Oral Epidemiol* 30(1):70–79, 2002.

Turner MD, Ship JA: Dry mouth and its effects on the oral health of elderly people, *J Am Dent Assoc* 138(Suppl 1):15S–20S, 2007.

Wells M: Oropharyngeal effects of radiotherapy. In Faithfull S, Wells M, editors: *Supportive care in radiotherapy*, Edinburgh, 2003, Churchill Livingstone, pp 182–212.

White D, Lader D: *Periodontal condition, hygiene behaviour and attitudes to oral health: Children's dental health in the UK 2003*, London, 2004, Office for National Statistics, p 8.

Wood A: Mouth care and ritualistic practice, *Cancer Nursing Practice* 3(4):34–39, 2004.

Wray D, Stenhouse D, Lee D, Clark A, editors: *Textbook of general and oral surgery*, Edinburgh, 2003, Churchill Livingstone.

Xavier G: The importance of mouth care in preventing infection, *Nurs Stand* 14(18):47–52, 2000.

Zazzali JL, Marshall GN, Shetty V, et al: Provider perceptions of patient psychosocial needs after orofacial injury, *J Oral Maxillofac Surg* 65:1584–1589, 2007.

Zuk PA: Tissue engineering craniofacial defects with adult stem cells: Are we ready yet? *Pediatr Res* 63(5):478–486, 2008.

FURTHER READING

Newcastle University School of Dental Sciences, Nutrition and Oral Health Group. Available online http://www.ncl.ac.uk/dental/research/diet.

Sweeney MP, Bagg J: *Making sense of the mouth (video and CD-ROM)*, Glasgow, 1997, Partnership in Oral Care.

USEFUL WEBSITES

British Dental Health Foundation: www.dentalhealth.org.uk

Changing Faces: www.changingfaces.org.uk

CLAPA (Cleft Lip and Palate Association): www.clapa.com

Craniofacial Support Group: headlines.org.uk

Let's Face It: www.letsfaceit.force9.co.uk

Macmillan Cancerline: www.macmillan.org.uk

Mouth Cancer Foundation: www.mouthcancerawareness.org.uk

Core nursing issues

Infection prevention and control

Jacqui Prieto, Claire Kilpatrick

Introduction

Infection prevention measures are essential in everyday clinical practice to minimise the risk of infection to patients, their relatives/carers and health care staff. Patients receiving health care, either in a health care facility or at home, may be at increased risk of infection due to their underlying illness or need for treatment. Those being cared for in close proximity to other patients, for example in a hospital ward, are more likely to be exposed to infections harboured by others, particularly given the frequency of contact with health care staff and the sharing of equipment and the environment. In all settings where health care is delivered, it is important for nurses and other health care staff to understand the ways in which infection is spread and the precautions necessary to minimise the risk of spread in order to protect patients, themselves and others from infection. The nurse, along with all other members of the multi-professional team, is responsible for ensuring that infection prevention measures are implemented correctly as part of routine patient care and safety. In this rapidly changing area of practice it is essential for health professionals to keep up to date with the latest evidence and recommended best practice. Throughout the chapter, reference is made to websites that provide current information, evidence-based guidance and other resources for use by health care professionals.

An overview of the problems with and management of health care associated infection and infectious diseases

Health care associated infection (HCAI), previously known as hospital-acquired infection (HAI) and in some countries as nosocomial infection, is the term used to refer to infection acquired during receipt of some form of health care. This updated terminology more accurately reflects the diverse range of settings in which health care is delivered and where infection may arise. There is ongoing concern and activity in the UK, and globally, in relation both to HCAI and the prevention and control of all infectious diseases.

Infectious agents, including different bacteria and viruses capable of rapid spread within health care environments, cause major disruption and impact significantly on the provision of high-quality health care. Currently, these include *Clostridium difficile*, influenza, norovirus (known as winter vomiting diarrhoeal disease) and respiratory syncytial virus (RSV, in paediatric wards). The occurrence of antimicrobial-resistant microorganisms, such as meticillin-resistant *Staphylococcus aureus* (MRSA) and glycopeptide-resistant enterococci (GRE), attributed in part to many years of use and misuse of antimicrobial agents, has also risen over the last two decades, causing significant patient safety concerns in

UK health care. Common microorganisms, including *Staphylococcus aureus,* continue to genetically mutate, developing resistance to antimicrobial agents in order to ensure their survival in a changing environment.

The latest HCAI prevalence surveys in adult patients were conducted in 2006 in acute hospitals across England, Wales, Northern Ireland and the Republic of Ireland (Smyth et al 2008) and in 2005–2006 in both acute and non-acute hospitals in Scotland (Reilly et al 2008). The results estimate the prevalence of HCAI to be between 7.3 and 9.5%, which means that at any one time approximately one in eight patients could have an HCAI. Infections associated with invasive procedures and the use of medical devices such as intravascular devices and urinary catheters account for a high proportion of HCAI. Prevalence and incidence results in the UK also reiterate the fact that common microorganisms like those that have already been mentioned continue to cause problems.

It had been thought that up to one third of all HCAIs would be preventable by better application of proven methods of prevention (Haley et al 1985, Harbarth et al 2003). However, more recently it has been claimed that certain HCAIs, in particular central venous catheter-related bloodstream infections, could potentially be eliminated (Pronovost et al 2006). The nurse has a crucial role in achieving this, as described in this chapter.

Emerging infections such as Legionnaire's disease, human immunodeficiency virus (HIV), severe acute respiratory syndrome (SARS) and pandemic influenza also continually pose challenges to public health as well as to health care settings. This necessitates contingency planning both at population level and within organisations, including health care systems. For example, during the 2009 influenza A (H1N1), or 'swine flu' pandemic, the extensive planning that had taken place across many parts of the world and within health care systems in the preceding years enabled a rapid response to the situation as it evolved over time. The tremendous increase in world travel over recent years has added to concerns about the threat posed by infectious diseases, many of which can spread rapidly around the world affecting large numbers of people. Whilst in the UK, the long-standing, vaccine-preventable infectious diseases including measles, mumps and rubella (MMR) affect only a small number of people compared to the past, reduced uptake of childhood immunisations such as the MMR vaccine has in recent years resulted in lowered 'herd' immunity (immunity across an entire population) and, consequently, an increase in these diseases. Infections familiar only to older generations, for example smallpox, have caused recent concern in an age when there is heightened awareness of the risks from bioterrorism. Governments internationally are preparing both for the re-emergence of diseases that have previously been eradicated or controlled and for the emergence of new diseases, at the same time as attempting to control the common HCAIs occurring in our health care settings.

Less common in the UK, but often with drastic outcomes, are infections spread via the food-borne route. In the past these have had a major impact on both hospital settings and the community. The outbreak of *Escherichia coli* O157 infection, spread through meat in a butcher's shop in Wishaw, Lanarkshire, in 1996, resulted in the death of many people within that community and attracted much media interest over hygiene controls in food premises. In hospitals and care facilities, guidance on effective food preparation, production and distribution techniques is vital for effective infection control. The nurse's role in food hygiene often involves basic measures such as ensuring patients' own food is in date, stored and reheated correctly. It may also include maintaining correct hygiene procedures relating to enteral feeding systems. Awareness of the importance of food hygiene overall is essential.

Infection prevention and control measures aim to reduce the burden of HCAI and other infectious or communicable diseases, on individuals, health care organisations, and within the National Health Service as a whole. The Health Protection Agency, Health Protection Scotland and Departments of Health in all UK countries coordinate many activities, such as national surveillance and control programmes, in order to highlight and act upon the actual burden in specific settings (see Useful websites, p. 515). Nurses are well placed to contribute to the prevention, control and management of infection within health care settings and beyond. Indeed, nurses occupy a wide diversity of roles, including those concerned with public health, providing ever-increasing opportunities to influence the health protection and patient safety agendas.

For further information about the national burden of HCAI and spread of other infectious diseases, see the recent national prevalence surveys (Reilly et al 2008, Smyth et al 2008), National Audit Office reports (2000, 2004, 2009), the Care Quality Commission's work, the UK Health Department websites, the Health Protection Agency and Health Protection Scotland websites (see Useful websites, p. 516).

How infection spreads

The terms 'infection process', 'cycle of infection' and 'chain of infection' are often used to describe the circumstances that can lead to patients or others developing an HCAI or any infectious disease. The rationale for applying infection prevention measures is based on this chain of events. It is crucial to understand how microorganisms spread and infection occurs. The infection process involves:

- The presence of *an infectious agent*, i.e. microorganisms that are capable of causing infection.
- *A reservoir or source* where microorganisms can be found. Within health care settings, this includes people (i.e. patients, staff and visitors) and also the environment, e.g. dust, bedding, equipment, furniture, sinks, washbowls, commode chairs and surfaces.
- The potential for microorganisms to be transmitted from sources. This is often called a *'portal of exit'* and is the means by which microorganisms are expelled from the body, such as exhalation, aerosolisation (when liquid droplets are dispersed into the air, e.g. when coughing or sneezing), secretion and excretion.
- *A means or route of transmission* of microorganisms, categorised as contact, droplet, air-borne, blood-borne, food- and water-borne (common vehicle) and vector-borne.
- The potential for microorganisms to enter the body through a susceptible site. This is often called a *'portal of entry'* and includes a breach in skin integrity such as a wound or open skin lesion, mucous membranes,

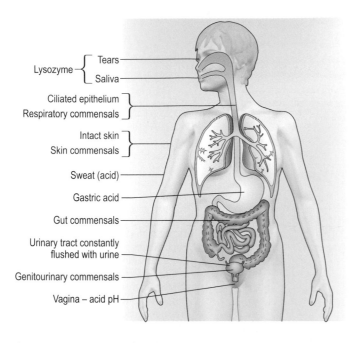

Lysozyme — Tears
Lysozyme — Saliva
Ciliated epithelium
Respiratory commensals
Intact skin
Skin commensals
Sweat (acid)
Gastric acid
Gut commensals
Urinary tract constantly flushed with urine
Genitourinary commensals
Vagina – acid pH

Figure 16.1 Barriers to infection.

ingestion and any breach in normal immune defences (Figure 16.1), commonly through a variety of invasive devices, e.g. intravascular catheters, urinary catheters, respiratory devices.

- *A susceptible host* – anyone who, for whatever reason, is at risk of infection by microorganisms, including those that

would not normally cause them harm. Factors that affect the body's natural ability to fight infection include:
- the presence of underlying disease, e.g. diabetes mellitus
- being immunocompromised, e.g. HIV infection, chemotherapy treatment
- poor nutritional status
- extremes of age, i.e. the very young and the very old.

The principles relating to all infection prevention measures are based on the interruption of this process. If these measures are not taken, a cycle will continue whereby patients, and possibly staff and others, may be exposed to potentially pathogenic (disease-causing) microorganisms that can cause harm.

Microbiology

Microbiology is the study of microorganisms and other causes of infection, including bacteria, viruses, fungi, protozoa, prions and helminths.

Bacteria

Bacteria, including variations of the microscopic beings such as mycoplasmas, rickettsiae and chlamydiae, are small microorganisms of simple primitive form. Bacteria are commonly found living within the human body and in the environment, for example in soil and water. Those species of bacteria capable of causing disease in humans are known as 'pathogens'. Some are more 'pathogenic' than others. Most are acquired though contact with other people or the environment (i.e. 'exogenous' sources). Table 16.1 gives some examples of

Table 16.1 Examples of common bacteria encountered while providing health care			
ORGANISM	**MAIN SOURCES**	**MAIN MODE OF SPREAD AND MEANS OF ENTRY**	**EXAMPLES OF RESULTING DISEASE/CONDITIONS**
Staphylococcus aureus including MRSA	Found in people, in skin, wounds, and at times in sputum and urine Environmental dust	Direct and indirect contact with persons carrying the organism or from the environment. Entry through susceptible sites, e.g. open wounds, invasive devices	Wound and skin infection, bacteraemia, endocarditis, osteomyelitis and septic arthritis
Clostridium difficile	Found in people, in the lower bowel, therefore faeces and any faecally contaminated areas. Especially found in hospitalised patients who have received antibiotic therapy that has disturbed their normal bowel flora	Direct and indirect contact with persons carrying the organism or from the environment, especially as it forms spores that survive for long periods in the environment. Often also called faecal–oral spread if ingestion occurs resulting in further gastrointestinal (GI) upset/infection	GI infection, characterised by loose, foul-smelling green stools and abdominal pain. The most common diarrhoeal cause of HCAI. Can lead to pseudomembranous colitis
Streptococci	Found in people, at various sites, and in the environment	Direct and indirect contact with persons carrying the organism or from the environment. Through droplets from infected respiratory tract	Pharyngitis, wound infection, rarely necrotising fasciitis, septicaemia toxin-mediated disease, e.g. scarlet fever, toxic shock syndrome, pneumonia and associated bacteraemia
Escherichia coli	Found in humans, particularly the GI tract, and in the environment	Direct and indirect contact with persons carrying the organism or from the environment	Urinary tract infection; bacteraemia; GI infection (uncommon in the health care environment)

Continued

501

Table 16.1 Examples of common bacteria encountered while providing health care – cont'd

ORGANISM	MAIN SOURCES	MAIN MODE OF SPREAD AND MEANS OF ENTRY	EXAMPLES OF RESULTING DISEASE/CONDITIONS
Enterococci, including glycopeptide-resistant enterococci (VRE)	Mainly environmental sources but also in the human GI tract. In the lower bowel of animals and humans, most commonly in hospitalised patients who have received antibiotic therapy. Moist sites in the environment, but especially poorly draining shower areas and open fluid containers	Direct and indirect contact with persons carrying the organism or from the environment	Urinary tract infection Wound infection Endocarditis Eye and ear infections Wound infections, e.g. in burns Septicaemia Respiratory infections, especially in the immunocompromised, e.g. cystic fibrosis patients
Pseudomonas aeruginosa	Mainly environmental sources (soil and ground water). Contaminates moist/wet reservoirs in hospitals such as respiratory equipment and indwelling catheters	Direct and indirect contact with persons carrying the organism or from the environment	Urinary tract infection Wound infection Endocarditis Eye and ear infections Wound infections, e.g. in burns Septicaemia Respiratory infections, especially in the immunocompromised, e.g. cystic fibrosis patients
Mycobacterium tuberculosis (TB)	Found in humans, animals and in the environment	Through the air-borne route when respiratory infection is present. Through direct contact when other systems are infected	Respiratory or pulmonary TB; can be termed as open TB. Closed TB, where another system or site of the body is infected. It can infect any organ in the body (see Ch. 3)

pathogenic bacteria commonly encountered while providing health care. Bacteria that constitute the normal commensal flora within the body are not normally pathogenic (Table 16.2). However, in certain situations, such as when these bacteria gain access to a different anatomical location within the body,

Table 16.2 Normal commensal microorganisms

SITE	ORGANISM
Skin	*Staphylococcus epidermidis* Diphtheroids *Corynebacterium* sp.
Mouth and throat	Staphylococci Streptococci Anaerobes *Neisseria* sp.
Nose	Staphylococci Diphtheroids
Gut	*Escherichia coli* *Klebsiella* sp. *Proteus* sp. *Streptococcus faecalis* *Clostridium perfringens* Yeasts (*Candida*)
Kidneys and bladder	Normally sterile
Vagina	Lactobacilli Streptococci Staphylococci Anaerobes

they can cause disease. This is known as 'endogenous' infection. It is not always clear when infections are exogenous or endogenous.

Viruses

Viruses are a group of parasitic infective agents so small that they are visible only through electron microscopy. Viruses have no independent metabolic activity and may replicate only within the cell of a living plant, animal or human. Viruses in humans therefore tend to spread due to close human contact, although some can also survive and be spread through environmental contamination.

Fungi

Fungi are simple plants that are parasitic on other plants, animals and humans. A few can cause fatal disease and illness in humans. Fungi can cause 'opportunistic' infection in people with increased susceptibility to infection. For example, in a postoperative patient, where antibiotic therapy may not only eradicate the infective organism but also protective normal flora, fungi such as *Candida albicans* can proliferate and cause infection.

Protozoa

Protozoa are single-cell microbes, which are the smallest organism in the animal kingdom. Some species can cause human disease, particularly in hot climates. Examples include *Plasmodium*, the protozoan that causes malaria, and *Entamoeba histolytica*, which causes amoebic dysentery. Protozoal infections do not pose a risk of person-to-person spread within health care settings, as depending on the type, they are spread via contaminated water or food, insect bites or sexual intercourse.

Prions

Prions are minute protein particles that cause transmissible spongiform encephalopathies (TSEs) in humans and animals. Creutzfeldt–Jakob disease (CJD) is a human TSE which is fatal. It causes the destruction of neural tissue, leading to progressive brain damage. Variant CJD (vCJD) has been associated with cases in young people.

Helminths

Helminths are worms, some of which can be a major cause of morbidity in humans, mainly in developing countries. In the Western world, many species of helminths can infest humans. These are most frequently spread within a household or shared living space and are not commonly encountered in the context of health care.

For further information on all microorganisms, see Gould & Brooker (2008) and Wilson (2000).

Routes of transmission

Clear understanding of the most common routes or means of transmission of microorganisms can ensure that appropriate precautions are taken to minimise the risk of spread of infection in all situations.

- *Contact* – direct or indirect. This is regarded as the most common route of transmission related to HCAI. Direct contact is the transfer of microorganisms from one person to another, through direct body contact without the involvement of an object or a third person, e.g. direct contact between the colonised skin of one individual and the mucous membranes of another. Indirect contact means the transfer of microorganisms via items within the environment, known as 'fomites' (any inanimate object that can carry pathogenic organisms, such as a contaminated commode chair or a reusable washbowl), or via another person, e.g. the hands of health care workers.
- *Air-borne* – air-borne transmission is by small particles within the respirable size range (less than or equal to 5 µm). They can remain infectious in the air for long periods of time and can be widely dispersed by air currents and cause infection by entering the respiratory tract of susceptible individuals.
- *Droplet* – droplet transmission differs from air-borne transmission as the particles are larger (greater than 5 µm) and therefore do not remain suspended in the air and only travel short distances, i.e. less than 1 metre. Spread is therefore through close contact with infected persons who may be sneezing, coughing, talking or undergoing airway procedures such as intubation or bronchoscopy. The droplets can also settle in the environment close to where they have originated, e.g. within 1 metre of an infected coughing person.
- *Blood-borne* – through sexual transmission, injury or inoculation (penetration through the skin). The main concern within health care settings or for health care workers in the community is the transmission of hepatitis

B, hepatitis C and HIV through sharps injuries or blood splashes.
- *Food- and water-borne* (also known as common vehicle) – food and water can be common reservoirs for microorganisms, but the term 'common vehicle' also includes transmission through medication, blood or other solutions, such as parenteral feeds (given into a vein) and enteral feeds (used for nasogastric or percutaneous endoscopic gastrostomy [PEG] feeding).
- *Vector-borne* – usually spread via insects such as mosquitoes and ticks, but cockroaches, ants and flies can also transmit infection. This mode of transmission is not common in the UK but should be considered in pest control policies.

Certain organisms can be transmitted through more than one of these routes and all modes of spread must be considered when carrying out risk assessments and providing safe care.

The infection prevention team

Health care workers, patients, relatives and carers together have a contribution to make in the prevention, control and management of the spread of infection. Those involved include nurses, doctors and dentists, allied health professionals, microbiology laboratory scientists, health care assistants, domestic and catering services, estates management, sterile services staff, administrative and management staff, education and training staff.

The role of the infection prevention team (IPT) has been defined and includes the utilisation of the risk management approach (see p. 505), provision of relevant specialist advice, ensuring appropriate measures and action plans are in place and supporting sustained improvement through a change of culture throughout their health care organisation. The team has clear accountability for reporting infection prevention and control progress and issues through relevant management structures, such as clinical governance and patient safety committees and, at times, directly to chief executives. The infection prevention doctor (IPD) and infection prevention nurse (IPN) have clear responsibilities within the health care organisation. More recently, leadership and management roles, including the Nurse Consultant, Director of Infection Prevention and Control (in England and Wales) and Infection Control Manager (in Scotland) have added to the structure.

Other recent additions to the IPT include audit and surveillance staff amongst other invaluable support staff. Whilst in secondary care settings this arrangement is generally well established, this is not always so within primary care, where the community-based IPT may be a relatively new addition, yet provide a vital service, both for commissioning and provision of specialist services. The role of the health protection nurse working at regional or national level may also be a relatively new contact for infection prevention and control teams, but provides an important link as part of the strategic infection prevention work within a locality and nationally.

Many settings also have infection prevention link personnel to enhance the effectiveness of the work of the team. The link person in a ward, department or community team receives additional education to improve the communication between infection prevention and control teams and the clinical setting and may assist with clinical audit and awareness of clinical staff in relation to Standard Precautions (see p. 507).

The work of the infection prevention team is guided by the Control of Infection Committee, which is responsible for strategic and operational decisions about infection prevention and control within a given organisation or, in the case of the community, across a locality. However, the IPT also reports to clinical governance, risk management and patient safety committees to ensure action and effective cross-facility outcomes. The outcomes for infection prevention programmes of work at organisation level, as led by teams, are guided by national and local requirements and needs.

The nurse's role in infection prevention

Nurses can contribute to all aspects of infection prevention in clinical practice, acting as role models and educating others. Nurses have a pivotal role in managing infection in acute and primary care settings by:

- maintaining up-to-date knowledge and high standards of clinical practice based on best available evidence, including training and educating clinical colleagues
- reporting and acting upon incidents when it has not been possible to implement best practice
- assessing infection risks to patients, staff and others and identifying the actions required to minimise them
- promptly identifying signs and symptoms of infection and taking the appropriate actions (e.g. referral to a medical practitioner, collection of a clinical specimen)
- seeking specialist advice for support with risk assessment when required
- involvement in the promotion of messages about best practice and monitoring standards of infection prevention
- educating patients and their carers about infection prevention measures.

Nurses in the UK have a duty of care as stated in the Health and Safety at Work Act (1974) to prevent, control and manage infection. Nurses, as the largest staff group in health care, have a responsibility to deliver care based on the best available evidence or best practice (Nursing and Midwifery Council [NMC] 2008). This includes preventing the spread of infection, ensuring they do not put themselves and others at unnecessary risk from infection. In England and Wales, The Health and Social Care Act (DH 2008, p. 2) requires health care professionals to 'demonstrate good infection control and hygiene practice'.

Nursing assessment is vital to health and infection prevention, whether the health care setting is the home, the hospital, the clinic or the care home, as it can reveal crucial information about patients, their surroundings and their behaviours. Nursing models and processes must incorporate approaches to prevention, control and management of infection, for example, within care plans and pathways.

The health of nurses while at work is also important. Nurses should:

- stay away from work if unwell, particularly if the illness could be communicated to others, e.g. influenza, infection with the Group A streptococcus, or *Streptococcus pyogenes* (particularly in the throat)

- be aware of their own immunity to infectious diseases such as rubella, chickenpox, measles, tetanus and hepatitis B; nurses can obtain advice from their general practitioner (GP) or from their employer's occupational health department
- discuss other health concerns that may have an impact upon the ability to work, or upon others, with the Occupational Health Department, e.g. allergies that may be caused by supplies used during work and skin conditions that may harbour and spread microorganisms.

Diagnostic sampling

The collection of specimens for microbiological examination is an important element of a nurse's role. It enables identification of microorganisms to aid diagnosis and ensure appropriate treatment. In the case of bacterial infection, accurate diagnosis enables the use of narrow-spectrum rather than broad-spectrum antimicrobial agents, which optimises treatment and reduces problems associated with antimicrobial use. A sample may also be taken for screening purposes, e.g. to exclude previous known infections or as part of contact tracing. The UK countries currently have a range of policies on screening for antimicrobial-resistant organisms and, in particular, MRSA (see Useful websites p. 516).

Samples may be taken from various sources according to the person's presenting symptoms or, in the case of screening, the most likely sites of colonisation. These include swabs from sites such as the ear, nose, throat, eye, vagina, skin or wound. A fluid specimen or, in some instances, a sample of tissue, may be taken from the respiratory tract (e.g. nasopharyngeal aspirate, sputum), the gastrointestinal tract and biliary system (e.g. faeces), the genitourinary tract (e.g. urine) and the circulatory system (e.g. blood). Samples of vomit are not normally sent for testing as the results are of limited analytical value. In order to avoid false positive and false negative results, it is important to ensure that there is no contamination from other microorganisms while obtaining samples, that an adequate amount of a sample is taken and that it is sent promptly to the laboratory or stored appropriately until it is sent. The storage requirement for different samples varies, so it is important to ensure the correct procedure is followed. For example, a sputum specimen must be sent to the laboratory immediately, as respiratory pathogens do not survive for long periods. Although urine ideally should be examined in the laboratory within 2 hours, it can be stored in a specimen fridge for up to 24 hours to prevent bacteria multiplying and giving misleading results. Likewise, a wound or MRSA swab can be stored overnight in a specimen fridge. Blood cultures differ, as they must be sent to the laboratory immediately or stored at room temperature, but must not be refrigerated.

The value of swab sampling is frequently questioned, but it is a common, convenient and inexpensive option in clinical practice. If contamination occurs, for example, from intact skin surrounding a suspected infected surgical wound (false positive), or not enough sample is sent to the laboratory, for example a dry swab is used to sample a small patch of dry skin for microbiological screening purposes (false negative), analysis will be limited and results will not be meaningful. Accurate completion of laboratory forms is also essential to provide laboratory staff with the information needed to select appropriate diagnostic tests. Whilst demographic information about the patient is often computer generated nowadays, relevant information about the patient's condition, current medication or treatments (e.g. antibiotics), the source of the specimen and its purpose (e.g. screening or confirming the diagnosis of infection) is important to include.

Epidemiology

Epidemiology is the study of disease in relation to populations, e.g. who is being affected by MRSA or influenza, and when and where they are being affected. Epidemiological data are crucial in guiding actions and therefore all staff should support and become involved in collecting data and taking on board feedback in order to enhance targeted patient care and treatment. A population considered at risk, for example from *Clostridium difficile*, could be monitored using epidemiological methods to gather information which relates the disease to the population by studying both ill and healthy individuals. Epidemiology is closely linked with risk assessment and management. Results of epidemiological monitoring help to affect outcomes, for example reductions in infection rates by influencing infection prevention and control measures featured in, for example, action plans and care plans.

In order to identify infectious diseases including HCAI, methods must be in place to gather the appropriate information to inform knowledge of the distribution of such diseases. There are various ways to monitor disease.

- *Incidence* is the number of new cases in a defined period within a specific population, e.g. incidence of wound infections postoperatively in all patients undergoing surgery in the next financial year.
- *Prevalence* is the number of cases that occur either at a particular time (point prevalence) or over a defined period of time (period prevalence), e.g. the number of patients with urinary tract infection at any one time within a hospital.
- *Surveillance* is the ongoing systematic collection and analysis of data about an infectious disease that is essential to the planning, implementation and evaluation of public health practice and can lead to action being taken to control or prevent the disease.

Data collected over time show the changing patterns of infectious diseases in our society, providing information about newly emerging diseases and identifying specific problem areas, e.g. outbreaks and seasonality of diseases. This informs the risk management process, which contributes to the prevention of infections and the control of outbreaks of infection.

Mandatory surveillance systems are in place throughout the UK and tools are provided to support the collection and collation of data. It is important that principles, including definitions, for epidemiological monitoring are followed to allow for reliable and comparable data in order to show improvement or deterioration over time.

The risk management approach

The risk to health from infection is one of many risks to be managed in health care settings. The risk management approach to HCAI was developed during the 1970s as part of the growing health and safety agenda around the developed world. The World Health Organization (WHO 2008) definitions provide a basis for the risk management approach in relation to infection prevention and control:

- *hazard* – a biological, chemical or physical agent with the potential to cause an adverse health effect
- *risk* – a function of the probability of an adverse health effect and the severity of that effect associated with exposure to a hazard.

Hazards and risks from microorganisms are present in our environment at all times. Once they are identified, appropriate control measures and action plans must be adopted to ensure that the greatest time and resource is spent in the areas with the greatest risks of infection. For example, the approach to the management of MRSA within the health care environment varies according to the risk to patients. In the hospital environment and, in particular, wards and units where patients are deemed to be at high risk of infection with MRSA, such as intensive care units and orthopaedic surgical wards, a more stringent approach to screening, decolonisation treatment and the isolation of patients colonised or infected with MRSA may be taken, as compared with community settings such as care homes and the patient's own home (Box 16.1). As hazards and risks may change over time, up-to-date guidance on infection prevention and control measures is required for the health and safety of patients and staff.

The correct systems, management and culture must be in place to ensure that actions are effective in preventing, controlling and managing the risks that present from HCAI:

- *Systems* include structures and processes at national, organisational and individual practitioner level, e.g. guidance given through policies and procedures, education and training, and frequent planned monitoring of outcome through audit, surveillance and research.
- *Management* includes the appropriate support being available and a clear commitment towards addressing the risks of infection, considering these alongside the many other pressures faced within health care. Ensuring that the correct processes are in place to achieve this must be a management priority. This includes the provision of training and education of health care staff, which is mandatory in many health care organisations.
- *Culture* includes the continuous improvement of quality through individual behaviour, whereby nurses, for example, can be seen as role models, aware of the systems and processes to manage hazards and risks from infection. Good infection prevention and control practice by health care and associated staff helps maintain an overall culture of good practice, making it easier for all to comply, especially during periods of stress.

There are many approaches and tools used for supporting risk management, available locally, nationally and internationally.

Root cause analysis

Root cause analysis is one way to identify the cause of infection-related problems and to support all staff in finding

Box 16.1 Reflection

Mr Brown's journey

The following scenario concerns an infectious condition that is commonly encountered, both in community and hospital settings. From the information provided, consider: (i) Mr Brown's susceptibility to infection before admission to hospital; (ii) how Mr Brown's susceptibility to infection will be affected by his hospital admission and need for surgery; (iii) the ways in which infection risks can be minimised both to Mr Brown and other patients on the ward.

Mr Brown is due to be admitted to hospital for total hip replacement surgery. He is assessed in the outpatients' clinic 2 weeks before his operation is due. He is 62 years old with type 2 diabetes, treated by hypoglycaemics. On assessment, the significant factors noted are: he is overweight and is a smoker, he states that he eats well and controls his diabetes, his skin is dry in places and he is a social drinker.

His wife is with him and is recovering from a hysterectomy, for which she was discharged from hospital 4 weeks ago. It later transpires that she is continuing to see the practice nurse for an ongoing postoperative wound problem.

Mr Brown is found to have a foot ulcer. During examination of the foot ulcer, signs and symptoms of infection are present, i.e. erythema (redness), swelling and heat, with evidence of scanty serous exudate. Samples are taken and sent to the microbiology laboratory. Also, a nose swab is taken to screen for MRSA. The multidisciplinary team are eager to manage and treat the ulcer appropriately in order to progress with Mr Brown's proposed hip surgery and are considering antibiotic therapy on results of the samples taken.

The results from Mr Brown's MRSA screen and foot ulcer yielded MRSA.

Activities

- What further information do you think the team should collect to try to ascertain the epidemiology of the MRSA infection?
- Reflect on how you would manage discussions that might take place with Mrs Brown.

NB: Further critical thinking questions relating to this scenario are available on the website.

 See website Critical thinking question 16.1

---

solutions to managing the associated risks. The National Patient Safety Agency for England and Wales, among others, has developed toolkits to support clinical staff in identifying causes of problems and taking action to ensure patient safety. They provide step-by-step guidance on how to perform analysis and how to direct action in relation to preventing future avoidable HCAI. Nurses have a pivotal role in supporting root cause analysis as their presence within clinical settings allows them to have an understanding of what works well and what does not work in relation to patient care on a day-to-day basis. For further information, the National Patient Safety Agency website contains a range of resources, including a specific tool relating to the reduction of infection, which is promoted for use in England and Wales (http://www.npsa.nhs.uk).

Policies and procedures, training and education

Underpinning much of the work undertaken in clinical practice are the policies and procedures that guide best practice related to hand hygiene, isolation of infectious patients, aseptic technique and insertion and maintenance of medical devices, including urinary and intravascular catheters. These must be current and must have planned timescales for review. Many nurses are involved in policy writing, including those at management, specialist and general level. However, it is not enough to have infection control policy documents; the recommended practices must be learned, applied and monitored, with feedback given to ensure continuous quality improvement for up-to-date patient care (Box 16.2). It is part of being professionally accountable that each member of the multidisciplinary team adheres to policies and procedures; failure to do so may be considered a breach of the Health and Safety at Work Act (1974) and, in England and Wales, the Health and Social Care Act (2008).

It is also part of the nurse's role both to attend and provide education and training. This can take many different forms including face-to-face lecture style sessions, online programmes and shorter, interactive sessions within clinical settings to overcome the difficulties with time for attending formal sessions. The principles contained within infection prevention and control education and training sessions range from specific measures to be taken to broad principles of risk management and quality improvement.

Quality improvement

The correct and reliable implementation of evidence-based policies and procedures by all health care staff on a routine basis is a cornerstone of high-quality patient care and safety. Despite an increasingly robust body of evidence, it is widely known that the measures within policies and procedures are often not fully implemented in practice and can be ineffective in changing the behaviours of health care staff. For

Box 16.2 Reflection

Infection prevention and control policies

- Locate the infection prevention and control policy in your area of work and familiarise yourself with the guidance it provides, related to your nursing duties.
- How do you contact the local infection prevention team for further guidance if needed?
- How would you monitor the standards set within the guidance against what is actually happening in your practice?
- How might you update your knowledge if you were not sure how to apply the guidance?

example, adherence to hand hygiene policies is notoriously problematic and average compliance with hand hygiene recommendations is usually estimated as below 50% with baseline rates ranging from 5 to 89% (WHO 2009).

Quality improvement strategies aim to change behaviours and create and sustain reliable systems of care. In order to be effective, such strategies must be aimed not only at individual level, but also at group and institutional levels, including the commitment of senior management. There are many models, one of which is the approach used by the Institute for Healthcare Improvement (IHI). The IHI Model for Improvement features key questions that must be asked in order to frame the overall improvement process, along with the use of rapid 'plan, do, study, act' (PDSA) cycles. This approach has been considered and adapted for use throughout the UK in recent times. Nurses play an important role in the multidisciplinary team approach to implementing and evaluating quality improvement strategies, in order to constantly improve patient safety. Other strategies also ensure improvement, including the use of care bundles and checklists. For further information on quality improvement approaches as applied to the prevention and control of infection, see the following websites: http://www.npsa.nhs.uk/nrls/improvingpatientsafety; http://www.nhshealthquality.org/nhsqis; http://www.patientsafetyalliance.scot.nhs.uk/programme; http://www.wales.nhs.uk (1000 Lives Campaign); http://www.health.org.uk/news/northern_ireland.html.

Valid and reliable tools for collecting and collating data in relation to all of these monitoring and reporting aspects are essential. Tools for audit and quality improvement are available under the auspices of the Infection Prevention Society in the UK and Ireland. These have been commissioned and are provided to support infection control specialists and clinical staff in their work to prevent and control infections.

Specific infection prevention measures

In everyday clinical practice, specific infection prevention measures are required routinely in order to minimise the risk of infection to patients, their relatives/carers and health care staff. This includes the use of: standard precautions, decontamination of reusable medical devices, transmission-based precautions, aseptic and clean techniques, use of evidence-based practice guidelines, antimicrobial stewardship and outbreak management. All the following points must be considered in both the hospital and the community setting, although the focus for infection rate reduction programmes is frequently on acute critical care and other high-risk settings. There are also other specific targeted measures pertaining to key areas of concern related to HCAI incidence and prevalence, and their prevention.

Standard Precautions

Standard Precautions are the measures applied at all times when performing health care activities in order to minimise the risk of spreading microorganisms to patients, health care staff and others. They should be applied routinely in all situations, whether or not an infection has been identified, to ensure a safe and effective approach to infection prevention (Box 16.3).

Box 16.3 Reflection

Assessing infection risks and applying standard precautions during nursing care

- Think about a patient you have cared for recently. Bearing in mind the steps in the infection process (p. 500), how did you consider the risks for potentially spreading infection to the patient and to others during provision of nursing care?
- Which Standard Precautions did you apply, or should you have applied, and why did you/did you not apply them?

Standard Precautions incorporate previously recommended measures known as 'Universal Precautions', which were first introduced during the initial HIV epidemic in the 1980s to protect against exposure to blood and body fluids whether or not the patient's infection status with regard to blood-borne pathogens was known. These precautions appeared to motivate and greatly improve compliance with general infection control measures and ultimately had a major impact on health care, for example the increased use of gloves for clinical procedures. Standard Precautions take account of the many microorganisms that can be spread while providing care and not only blood-borne viruses such as HIV. There are nine elements to Standard Precautions. Some of these will now be covered in detail (see also Table 16.3).

Hand hygiene

People's hands are considered the most common way in which microorganisms might be transported and cause infection to those who are susceptible. Therefore, hand hygiene is considered to be the most important step in preventing HCAI. All of the steps that lead to adequate hand decontamination must be considered and applied in practice in all settings. In the community setting, there is at times a need to adapt the approach according to the equipment available for use but hand hygiene is equally important wherever care is being delivered.

Recognising the times when hand hygiene is required is crucially important, yet the problem of poor adherence to recommended practice is well known. The World Health Organization's first Global Patient Safety Challenge *Clean Care is Safer Care* has identified 'My 5 moments for hand hygiene' to highlight the most fundamental times when hands should be cleansed during care delivery and daily routines (Sax et al 2007). These moments are: before touching a patient, before invasive procedures including aseptic tasks, after body fluid exposure risk, after touching a patient and touching patient surroundings. For more information on the 'Your 5 moments for hand hygiene', the technique for performing adequate hand hygiene and hand hygiene campaigns going on throughout the UK, see the following websites: http://www.who.int/gpsc/en/; http://www.washyourhandsofthem.com; http://www.npsa.nhs.uk/cleanyourhands/.

In most situations, plain liquid soap is the cleansing agent of choice to physically remove visible soiling and the 'transient' microorganisms acquired temporarily on the skin. Alcohol-based hand rubs have become common in recent times due to their effectiveness and ease of use. They are a convenient

Table 16.3 Standard Precautions

ELEMENT	ACTION/TIMING	RATIONALE
1. Hand hygiene	At the point of care (see WHO 'My 5 moments for hand hygiene', http://www.who.int/gpsc/en) in the most appropriate way for the situation. Alcohol-based hand rubs are recommended for ensuring effective hand hygiene in all patient care situations except when: • hands are visibly soiled with blood or other body fluids or after using the toilet • the patient is experiencing vomiting and/or diarrhoea • there is an outbreak of norovirus, *Clostridium difficile* or other diarrhoeal illnesses In these instances hands should always be cleaned with liquid soap and water of a comfortable temperature	Frequently referred to as the single most important action to prevent, control and manage infection
2. Personal protective equipment (PPE)*	Gloves (powder-free): • non-latex alternatives should be available and their use is being increasingly encouraged due to the adverse affects of latex Aprons, gowns Eye and mouth protection, for example masks, goggles, face shields • Use when exposure to blood or other body fluids might occur	To protect mouth and eyes in particular, and the skin of the face, hands and the rest of the body with the use of clothing and equipment in order to avoid contamination/soiling/splashing and potential exposure to harmful microorganisms, originating from patients, the environment or even live vaccinations. The use of gloves does not negate the need for hand decontamination and all PPE must be disposed of safely and properly immediately after being removed; often this is into clinical waste
3. Prevention of occupational exposure to infection	Cover all breaks in skin Avoid sharps injuries: • never re-sheathe sharps such as needles • utilise sharps receptacles close to the point of use • never try to retrieve any items from sharps receptacles Avoid splashes with blood or body fluids by using PPE when exposure is anticipated Report any exposure incidents immediately following local policies (see http://www.riddor.gov.uk/info.html)	To additionally protect health care workers, carers and others from exposure to microorganisms that cause infection, e.g. hepatitis B and C, HIV, MRSA
4. Management of blood and body fluid spillages	Utilise cleaning products and disinfectants (often found in 'spillage kits') immediately spillages occur, following local policies	To protect all of those in the surrounding area from exposure to microorganisms found within spillages that could cause harm and to protect the environment from contamination
5. Management of equipment utilised during care	Prevent reuse of single-use devices Prevent single-patient use devices being used on other patients Ensure reusable devices are handled safely and decontaminated between use on the same patient and before use on others, following local policies: • basic cleaning measures are a vital part of health care and should also be performed before any required disinfection processes	To ensure that items used during care are not a factor in the spread of potentially infectious microorganisms directly to patients or a factor in the contamination of patients' environment leading to indirect spread of infection
6. Environment control	Cleanliness and maintenance of the environment must be kept at an optimum level. Maintenance and audit schedules are required as per local policies, and must be applied routinely and in the case of outbreaks/incidents	To ensure that the care setting, its fixtures and fittings and other items within it are adequately decontaminated and maintained to prevent cross-infection occurring through this route
7. Safe disposal of waste, including sharps	Waste is categorised by regulations so that it will be segregated and subsequently destroyed safely and effectively: • clinical waste generated in the home and community is often dealt with differently from that generated in hospital settings; local policies reflecting current regulations must be followed • the area around the opening of clinical waste bags and sharps containers is often the most contaminated in	To prevent the risk of inappropriate, avoidable exposure to the microorganisms found contaminating clinical waste in particular, thus protecting all health care workers and others The use of PPE when handling waste is essential

Continued

Table 16.3 Standard Precautions – cont'd

ELEMENT	ACTION/TIMING	RATIONALE
	health care settings and should never be touched; 'hands-free' waste sack holders, e.g. foot-operated, must always be in place Attaching waste bags to other pieces of furniture, e.g. trolleys, is not generally acceptable, nor is overfilling of bags	
8. Linen	Safe handling, transport and processing of bags: • linen should never be held against the body or shaken, even if protective clothing is worn • linen should always be disposed of into appropriate receptacles immediately after being removed and never placed on the floor/other surfaces	To prevent the risk of inappropriate, avoidable exposure to microorganisms when linen is being handled or reused, thus protecting health care workers and others and preventing contamination of the environment. Linen can be heavily contaminated with potentially pathogenic microorganisms; items such as urinary catheters, needles, etc. are often found in linen by laundry staff, putting them at unnecessary risk. Use of PPE when handling used linen is essential
9. Appropriate patient placement	Choosing the most appropriate site/area to care for a patient must be considered using a risk management approach at all times, e.g. consider the route of transmission of any known or suspected infections/colonisation, how these might then spread to others, the potential outcomes of this spread, the availability of resources to site patients in the best place	To prevent exposure of others and the environment to potentially infectious microorganisms and to protect the patient as far as possible

*Also known as protective clothing.

alternative to handwashing with soap and water in the majority of situations including the 'My 5 moments for hand hygiene' (see Table 16.3). However, since alcohol-based hand rubs are not reliable against the spore-forming bacterium *C. difficile*, they are not recommended for use when caring for patients strongly suspected to have *C. difficile* infection or for any patient with diarrhoeal illness that may be infectious. It should be noted however that the use of intact gloves also plays a part in protecting hands from contamination. Therefore, if hands have been protected by intact gloves in any situation and there is no concern of contamination with body fluids, e.g. faeces, alcohol-based hand rubs are still acceptable and consideration should be given to the importance of some form of hand hygiene rather than none at all when sinks are not readily available.

An effective hand hygiene technique is important in ensuring adequate hand hygiene standards, as detailed in Table 16.4. This includes ensuring thorough cleansing and drying of all areas of the hands (palms, fingers including tips, thumbs, backs of hands and wrists) and avoiding re-contamination when closing taps and disposing of paper towels.

Being a role model by setting a good example and encouraging others to perform hand hygiene, including making facilities available to patients as appropriate, is an important part of the nurse's role, as are supporting strategies for ensuring hand hygiene is performed reliably over time. This includes ensuring facilities and guidelines are in place, supporting and adhering to social marketing messages, such as hand hygiene poster displays, performing and taking part in education training programmes and monitoring hand hygiene compliance, for example through taking part in compliance monitoring. It must also always be remembered that the use of gloves does not negate the need for hand hygiene.

Personal protective equipment

Personal protective equipment (PPE) is the disposable, single use clothing and equipment available to health care workers, and at times visitors, to protect them from exposure to microorganisms no matter in which setting they are working. PPE includes disposable gloves, aprons/gowns, goggles/visors and masks/respirators (Box 16.4). As well as protecting the health care worker, use of PPE also minimises microbial contamination of hands and clothing. Therefore it plays a key part in preventing the spread of microorganisms to patients and others.

The use of PPE is based on a risk assessment, depending on the task in hand and according to the likelihood of exposure to body fluids or other infectious substances. It is important to select the most appropriate PPE for each procedure/situation, ensuring it fits closely and securely, so as to provide adequate protection. For example, a visor or a well-fitting surgical mask worn in conjunction with goggles provides protection from splashing of blood and body fluids. The type of PPE most appropriate for the activity being undertaken should be donned at the start of a patient care procedure, in order to protect against exposure to microorganisms. It is important to ensure prompt removal of PPE between tasks on the same patient and between different patients. When this is overlooked it can lead to cross-contamination and, potentially, infection. It is also essential to change PPE when damaged, torn or soiled, e.g. if a surgical mask is clearly wet with moisture, including from breath, it should be changed. Hand hygiene should always be performed following removal of PPE.

Environmental control and care of equipment

A clean environment contributes to the prevention and control of infection. It is common sense and good practice to ensure that the environment and all equipment in it is clean so that patients are reassured that standards of cleanliness and hygiene are high and every effort is being made to prevent infections as far as possible.

The responsibilities for ensuring the patient's environment is clean must be made clear to all. Assigning the specific

Table 16.4 Steps involved in performing effective hand hygiene

PREPARATION FOR HAND HYGIENE

- Ensure all equipment is available and the handwash basin is free from extraneous items, e.g. medicine cups, utensils
- Remove or adjust long-sleeved clothing so that wrists and forearms are exposed below the elbows
- Remove all jewellery including stoned rings and wrist watch
- Ensure nails are short (artificial nails must not be worn)

PROCEDURE FOR HANDWASHING WITH SOAP AND WATER

- Turn on tap(s) and adjust to a comfortable temperature (warm)
- Wet hands and wrists
- Apply cleansing agent
- Vigorously rub hands together, generating a good lather
- Wash all surfaces of the hands (front and back) for 15 seconds, paying particular attention to finger tips and thumbs
- Rinse well under running water
- Turn off taps using a 'hands-free technique' (elbows or disposable paper towel)
- Dry thoroughly all parts of the hands and wrists, paying particular attention to interdigital surfaces of the fingers and thumbs
- Dispose of paper towel in a bin without re-contaminating hands

PROCEDURE FOR HAND HYGIENE WITH ALCOHOL-BASED HAND RUB

- Ensure hands are visibly clean
- Apply hand rub to all surfaces of the hands in the same way as described above
- Allow to dry naturally
- Alcohol-based hand rubs are not reliable against spore-forming organisms (e.g. *Clostridium difficile*) and viral causes of gastroenteritis (e.g. norovirus)

APPLICATION IN COMMUNITY SETTINGS

- Carry a supply of alcohol-based hand rub at all times, as in some situations, this may be the only available option for hand hygiene
- In a patient's/client's home, whenever possible, request a freshly laundered hand towel and liquid soap for use during your visit

---

 Box 16.4 Reflection

Selection of face, eye and nose/mouth protection

There are various forms of PPE to protect the face, eyes and nose/mouth. These include surgical masks, particulate respirators (often referred to as FFP3 respirator masks and most commonly used to protect from pathogenic microorganisms spread via the air-borne route), goggles and visors.

Activities

- Locate the infection prevention and control policy in your area of work and familiarise yourself with the guidance relating to the use of PPE to protect the face, eyes and nose/mouth.
- In which situations might you need to wear a FFP3 respirator mask?
- Which forms of PPE for the face, eyes, nose/mouth are available in your area of work and how can you access those that are not supplied there?

The use of alcohol wipes is commonplace in health care environments. This is acceptable, in keeping with local policy, as long as the wipes are used for hard surface disinfection where the surface is physically clean and wipes are moist throughout use.

If any visible contamination of the environment or equipment is observed, decontamination must take place immediately. Particular attention must be given to frequently touched horizontal surfaces, e.g. bedrails, commodes, bedside cabinets, chair arms and tables, as well as other equipment at the point of care, such as infusion pumps. While recent media headlines have implicated items such as lift buttons and computer keyboards, those items closer to patient care are probably most important with regard to environment control and protection of patients.

Cleaning and decontamination schedules must reflect specific risks, e.g. the volume of activity, the patient's infectious condition and the procedures being undertaken. This applies to clinical areas as well as local or central storage

---

 Box 16.5 Reflection

The use of nebulisers and associated risks

A newspaper article revealed that a patient had acquired *Legionella* following a hospital stay. Following investigation of the source of this infection, an alert was distributed from the Medicines and Healthcare Products Regulatory Agency in England and Wales and Scottish Healthcare Supplies in Scotland, stating the importance of the care of nebulisers, in particular cleaning them after use. Manufacturers' instructions should be followed and recent reviews have highlighted sufficient evidence to recommend cleaning them with sterile water rather than tap water to avoid contamination from microorganisms such as *Legionella*. *Legionella* can cause disease in humans following inhalation from contaminated water vapour. If water sources are adequately treated and managed for home and health care setting consumption, *Legionella* should be avoided. Immediate drying and storage of nebulisers are equally as important so that they do not become a source of infection between uses on the same patient; nebulisers are considered single-patient use items.

---

responsibilities of health care organisation and cleanliness to domestic services staff and other clinical staff including nurses is important in order to avoid confusion about whose role it is to clean what. Cleaning is usually conducted using a general purpose detergent, warm water in a clean receptacle and clean or disposable cloths or mops. Disposable wipes impregnated with detergent offer a convenient alternative, although owing to the wide variety of wipes now available, care should be taken to select a suitable product for use. Drying is an important part of the cleaning process when using the detergent and water method, although large surfaces, e.g. floors, may have to be 'air-dried'. Stagnant moisture or fluid can be a focus for microorganisms and could potentially lead to HCAI (see example in Box 16.5). Disinfectants in addition to general purpose detergents may be used when particular risks are known, under guidance from the infection prevention and control team and from local policies and procedures.

areas for supplies such as personal protective equipment (PPE), waste and linen. Cleaning of soft furnishings such as curtains, chairs and carpets should include vacuuming and/or laundering as appropriate. Increasing the frequency of cleaning and reviewing methods of cleaning is essential during outbreaks or when there is increased risk of cross-infection, e.g. from incontinent patients or the presence of antimicrobial-resistant microorganisms. Schedules for the collection of linen and waste bags are also important and must be agreed, recorded and monitored.

Many disciplines are involved in environment control and 'service level agreements' for example can ensure that all are aware of the standards to be achieved and tasks to be undertaken. Many reports, including findings of audits, have been published about the lack of cleanliness and hygiene in health care premises, particularly NHS hospitals, often focusing on the potential effects of the reduced numbers of dedicated cleaning staff. Roles such as the modern matron, director of infection prevention and control, nurse consultant in infection prevention and infection control manager, as well as the infection prevention team, should help to create a positive culture towards cleaning as one part of the broad range of infection prevention and control measures.

Standard Precautions for control of respiratory infections

The spread of respiratory infections, e.g. influenza, has put respiratory hygiene and cough etiquette on the health agenda. These precautions have been incorporated into the latest revision of the guidelines on Standard Precautions (Siegel et al 2007) and apply to all persons with signs and symptoms of respiratory tract infection (cough, congestion, runny nose, increased production of respiratory secretions), including patients/clients, health care staff and visitors. Suggested preventative measures include:

- covering the mouth and nose when coughing or sneezing
- using disposable tissues and disposing of them directly into bins
- performing hand hygiene after any contact with respiratory secretions, used tissues and/or potentially contaminated surfaces.

The proximity of patients to one another in areas such as waiting rooms is also a consideration for the spread of respiratory infections and regularly updated guidance will be made available to address such ongoing concerns, particularly from the Health Protection Agency and Health Protection Scotland. Key Standard Precautions points representing good practice in preventing infection are shown in Table 16.3.

Decontamination of reusable medical devices

Decontamination means the removal of unwanted substances, including dust, dirt and microorganisms, from an item or surface, rendering it safe for reuse. Health care workers require specific guidance on the processes involved in decontamination of reusable medical devices, such as surgical instruments (Figure 16.2). Decontamination encompasses cleaning,

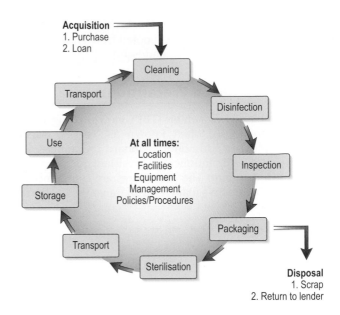

Figure 16.2 Decontamination cycle.

disinfection and sterilisation. The main areas to consider when undertaking decontamination include:

- The risk of HCAI from a reusable device and the most appropriate technique to protect patients from infection. Transmissible spongiform encephalopathies (TSEs), including Creutzfeldt–Jakob Disease (CJD) and variant CJD (vCJD), present a serious risk and need particular guidance, which can be obtained from the infection prevention and control team.
- General patient and staff safety to protect them from potentially infective microorganisms where devices are in use and to ensure that devices are safe to be handled and only used following decontamination.
- Recognition of the symbols that guide health care workers in relation to handling and reprocessing medical devices, e.g. the symbols for 'do not reuse', 'single use only' and 'sterile', which can be found on the packaging of all items.

Many health care workers, including nurses, are responsible for handling and packaging items before sending them to a reprocessing department, e.g. central sterilising unit, returning them to stores for redistribution or sending them for repair. Training on central sterilising unit policies is essential for those responsible for reprocessing surgical instruments to avoid decontamination failures that can lead to HCAI. Automatic washer disinfectors and ultrasonic cleaners should be used. If cleaning is not carried out correctly, failures will occur, even in sterilised items. Cleaning prior to sterilisation is as important as sterilisation itself. Manual cleaning is discouraged, both to protect the health care worker from cross-infection and also because the automated process is often more efficient. Where manual cleaning of instruments is essential, guidance must be sought from the infection prevention team and from the most up-to-date policies, including the use of appropriate PPE. Items with hollow bores and areas that are hard to reach are particular harbours of microorganisms, and clear guidance on their decontamination must be available and followed to avoid incidents that can lead to potentially serious infections in patients where the same device has been used for invasive procedures. Outbreaks have been noted from reuse of poorly decontaminated items such as endoscopes.

Transmission-based Precautions

Transmission-based Precautions (TBP), incorporating isolation procedures, previously often known as 'barrier nursing', should be applied in addition to Standard Precautions when highly transmissible or antimicrobial-resistant microorganisms are present in a patient. The procedures are commonly categorised by the organism's main route of transmission, the most common being:

- contact
- droplet
- air-borne.

Knowledge of the route of transmission will make the precautions to be taken clear and easy to understand without the need for more in-depth knowledge of the specific microorganism or infection. However, it is important to remember that some microorganisms are spread by more than one route and may therefore require a combination of precautions. For example, respiratory viruses spread via the airborne or droplet route may also arrive at susceptible portals of entry (i.e. nasal mucosa, conjunctivae and less frequently, the mouth) by the contact route, via hands that have become contaminated by the virus. Noroviruses are transmitted by contact, food- and water-borne routes, but may also be spread through aerosolisation of infectious particles from vomitus or faecal material.

Full details of the measures to be adopted in addition to Standard Precautions should be available within local infection prevention and control policies and from the infection prevention team. Although internationally accepted recommendations are specific with regards to measures to prevent and control the spread of infection through identified routes of transmission, slight variations may occur due to local situations and facilities.

Contact precautions are the measures directed towards prevention of spread via the contact route of transmission. They are particularly important, as it has been found that 'contact', particularly via contaminated hands, is the most common route of spread in relation to HCAI (Pittet et al 2006). If contact precautions are applied, infections such as MRSA and *Clostridium difficile* can be prevented and controlled. Measures to control diarrhoea are extremely important due to the number of infections presenting that are spread through this route. Steps such as appropriate single room isolation as well as targeted hand hygiene, use of appropriate PPE, decontamination of equipment and the environment and prompt treatment for patients are crucial.

For further information, see Siegel et al (2007) and Health Protection Scotland model infection control policies, which include particularly useful summary pages at the end of each Transmission-based Precaution policy and procedure (http://www.hps. scot.nhs.uk/haiic/ic/modelinfectioncontrolpolicies. aspx#devtbp). For information about those infectious diseases that require to be 'notified' for monitoring purposes, whether an isolated case or during an outbreak situation, see http:// www.hpa.org.uk/infections and http://www.isdscotland.org.

People being cared for under TBPs, whether in hospital or in the home, may be embarrassed or depressed because they feel that they are in some way 'dirty'. They may require increased psychological support, including more regular 'social' visits by nursing staff, particularly when nursed in single room isolation (see below). Nurses are legally responsible for keeping patient information confidential and may divulge such information only if it is essential for the benefit of the patient or the safety of others. Nurses should explain this to patients to minimise embarrassment or unease. Avoiding unnecessary use of PPE, positioning the call bell within easy reach and involving visitors in helping find ways to relieve boredom may all help to minimise the adverse effects of single room isolation and should be part of the routine care of the isolated patient (Madeo 2001).

Nursing a patient in single room isolation

The use of single room isolation for a patient who poses a risk of infection to others is an important part of TBPs. However, it can lead to anxiety in the patient and also their visitors. The nurse's role in providing accurate information, support and reassurance is vital. It is important to explain to the patient and their visitors the infection prevention and control procedures being used.

Isolation procedures can cause confusion amongst health care staff regarding rationales for best practice and this can lead to inconsistent implementation (Prieto & Macleod Clark 2005). In particular, there can be a tendency to introduce unnecessary practices, such as the overuse of PPE, double-bagging of clinical waste and the use of disposable crockery and cutlery, out of concern to minimise the risk of infection transmission. Other health care workers and visitors to the patient in isolation look towards nurses to guide them in the correct use of isolation procedures. It is therefore especially important for nurses to understand the rationale underpinning isolation procedures in order to promote their correct and consistent use, thereby reducing anxiety amongst colleagues, visitors and the patient and minimising the risk of spread of infection. Ensuring that all staff have access to readily available information on the steps to be taken is important.

Aseptic technique

Aseptic technique is designed to prevent the entry of pathogenic microorganisms into susceptible sites, for example surgical sites and insertion sites of invasive devices. The appropriate use of dressings and effective maintenance and care of invasive lines and tubes also prevents microbial invasion. Dressings when applied should keep a wound or insertion site free from potential contamination and infection and be impermeable to bacteria. For surgical wounds healing by primary intention, it is particularly important not to disturb the wound dressing for the first 48 hours after surgery when the fibrin layer is developing. Variations in the use of terminology, techniques and practice have led to calls to standardise the practice of aseptic technique (Aziz 2009, Rowley et al 2010) in order to minimise confusion and promote best practice. The term aseptic non touch technique (ANTT) has been proposed as an umbrella term that can be applied to all aseptic procedures (Rowley et al 2010).

Aseptic non touch technique (ANTT)

The term 'asepsis' means being free from living, foreign pathogenic microorganisms. Maintaining asepsis involves the application of targeted hand hygiene and at times a surgical scrub technique, sterile gloves and a sterile dressing pack/towel plus non-touch methods.

It may also be achieved by using sterile products, but not necessarily a sterile dressing pack, sterile towel or sterile gloves by preventing direct or indirect contact with sterile or 'key' parts of equipment by a non-touch method and other appropriate precautions including hand hygiene. ANTT was first described in relation to intravascular therapy (Rowley 2001) and the term has since been applied more widely (Rowley & Sinclair 2004), hence recognition of the need to standardise terminology, techniques and practice (Aziz 2009, Rowley et al 2010).

Dougherty & Lister (2008) identify that aseptic technique should be employed for the following invasive procedures:

- care of wounds healing by primary intention, e.g. surgical incisions, fresh breaks in the skin or burns
- suturing of wounds
- insertion of intravascular devices, e.g. central venous catheters, peripheral venous catheters
- insertion of indwelling urinary catheters
- insertion of percutaneous endoscopic gastrostomy and jejunostomy tubes
- insertion of tracheostomy tubes or chest drains
- vaginal examination using instruments
- assisted delivery, e.g. forceps and ventouse
- biopsies.

It is important to ensure that:

- all equipment and fluids used are sterile and in date, with packaging intact
- the surface used, e.g. the dressing trolley, is prepared by washing it with detergent and water and drying it
- Standard Precautions are adopted by personnel involved, including the use of alcohol-based hand rub or antiseptic scrub, sterile gloves and a disposable plastic apron
- the patient is prepared for the procedure and has given consent and analgesia is used if needed
- only sterile items and fluids come into contact with the wound surface/susceptible body site
- items are disposed of or reprocessed appropriately following the procedure
- appropriate documentation is completed to describe the procedure and any findings.

A risk assessment approach, based on assessment of the immediate physical and air environment, the complexity of the procedure and the competency and expertise of the health care professional undertaking it, will determine the appropriateness of glove selection and choice of aseptic field equipment (Rowley et al 2010). Before proceeding, liaison with the infection prevention team or other nurse specialist, for example the tissue viability nurse, may be advisable. For further information see Dougherty & Lister (2008).

Use of evidence-based practice guidelines to ensure targeted measures to prevent HCAI

The evidence base to support best practice in relation to HCAI prevention has become increasingly well defined in recent years. Procedures associated with a high risk of infection have become a focus for the production of guidelines, applicable in all settings. These include the prevention of urinary tract infection (UTI), surgical site infection (SSI) and bloodstream infection. Care bundles have been defined as 'a structured way of improving the processes of care and patient outcomes: a small, straightforward set of practices – generally three to five – that, when performed collectively and reliably, have been proven to improve patient outcomes' (Haradon 2006). The use of care bundles that feature evidence-based criteria is one way in which to implement improvement aimed at minimising or eliminating specific HCAI.

The prevention of urinary tract infections, surgical site infections, skin and soft tissue infections, respiratory tract infections, particularly those associated with mechanical ventilation, and intravascular line infections are all of current concern and clear plans of action are required to ensure these infections are minimised as far as possible.

- Urinary tract infections are known to account for approximately 20% of all HCAIs and most of these (80–95%) originate from indwelling urinary catheters. For further information, see Chapter 8 and the UK prevalence surveys (Reilly et al 2008, Smyth et al 2008). It is important to use a urinary catheter only when necessary and remove it as soon as it is no longer needed. Selection of the most suitable catheter for the patient is essential. Both insertion and ongoing maintenance of the urinary catheter system must be conducted using aseptic technique (Pratt et al 2007).
- Surgical site infections account for at least 15% of all HCAIs, although this is an underestimate, because many of these infections occur after the patient has been discharged from hospital. There is much that nurses can do to minimise infection risks before, during and after surgery. For further information see Owens & Stoessel (2008) and Chapters 23 and 26.
- Mild to severe skin and soft tissue infections, such as abscesses, cellulitis and impetigo, have more recently been noted as causing a significant HCAI burden, accounting for approximately 10% of all HCAIs. The increasing prevalence of skin and soft tissue infections caused by antimicrobial-resistant microorganisms such as community-associated MRSA is of concern and it is recognised that further work in both the acute and community settings is needed to better understand the contribution these emerging infections may make to the problem of HCAI (Skov & Jensen 2009).
- Lower respiratory tract infections, including pneumonias, account for approximately 20% of all HCAIs. Ventilator-associated pneumonia accounts for almost one fifth of all health care-associated pneumonias (see Ch. 29). Nurses have a key role in minimising the risk of lower respiratory tract infection, for example encouraging all postoperative patients to take deep breaths, move about the bed and ambulate unless medically contraindicated. For mechanically ventilated

patients, the nurse must ensure the patient is positioned correctly (elevating the head of bed to 30–45 degrees) and must adhere to Standard Precautions during care of the patient and their breathing apparatus, changing ventilator breathing circuits when soiled. For further information see Resar et al (2005) and Tablan et al (2003).

- Bloodstream infection accounts for approximately 7% of all HCAIs and is associated with a higher mortality rate than most other HCAIs. A significant proportion of bloodstream infections are related to the use of an intravascular device (for further information see the UK prevalence surveys and HPA and HPS websites featuring routine *Staphylococcus aureus* bacteraemia reports). As with urinary catheters, a peripheral or central intravascular device should be inserted only when necessary and removed as soon as no longer needed. Aseptic technique and thorough disinfection of the skin around the insertion site is essential. Care should be taken to avoid contamination of the dressing used to cover the device and of all other equipment (e.g. during attachment of the administration set and infusion fluid). The nurse has a vital role in regularly assessing the insertion site for signs of phlebitis and infection, recording the visual infusion phlebitis or 'VIP' score and taking the appropriate actions promptly when signs first appear. Routine replacement of an intravascular device should be conducted in accordance with agreed protocols, and clear documentation to support this, including documenting the date of insertion, is crucial. The role of catheter-associated bloodstream infection (CLABSI) prevention programmes is a high priority in many countries. For further information, see Sawyer et al (2010).

Infection prevention and control is a rapidly changing area of practice. For the most recent advice and further information on the use of care bundles in the UK visit http://www.hps.scot.nhs.uk/haiic/ic/index.aspx; http://www.dh.gov.uk (go to public health, health protection, then healthcare associated infection); http://www.clean-safe-care.nhs.uk; or http://www.devices.mhra.gov.uk. See also Chapters 3 and 29.

Other areas of practice that relate to infection prevention and control

Antimicrobial stewardship

Another important area of practice in which policy should be available to guide health care practitioners is antimicrobial prescribing and use. This is a topic of worldwide concern and now of particular concern to those nurses who have a role in prescribing, as antimicrobial resistance (Box 16.6) is increasing and strategies and recommendations have been published by the WHO and in UK countries to combat the problem. There have recently been cases in the developed world where patients have died from infections that could not be treated, as the causative microorganism was resistant to all the available antimicrobial agents. This is of great concern in a world that has relied heavily upon the benefits of antimicrobial agents. Recently, recommendations have been made and steps have been taken to establish antimicrobial pharmacists/teams to work alongside or as part of IPTs to give clear direction

Box 16.6 Reflection

Antimicrobial use and resistance

- Antimicrobials can work in different ways to treat infections. They can be bacteriostatic – stopping bacteria from multiplying, or they can be bactericidal – interfering with the cell wall of bacteria, thus killing them.
- Bacteria mutate and change to protect their cell structure against antimicrobials, thus becoming resistant. Drug-resistant organisms can not only spread and cause further harm but can also transfer their resistance to other organisms. Even as new antimicrobials are introduced it is anticipated that bacteria will continue to protect themselves by mutating and again become resistant.
- Misuse and overuse of antimicrobials are thought to have contributed to the problem. Pressure from patients to be given antimicrobials, the contribution of topical antimicrobials to antimicrobial resistance and over-the-counter availability of antimicrobials in many countries outside the UK are all considerations. Some resistance, however, will be inevitable.
- Policies should include guidance on the appropriate use of antimicrobials for treatment in all clinical eventualities, including the use of 'broad spectrum' and 'narrow spectrum' antimicrobials, and the length of time antimicrobials should be taken. Guidance on use of antimicrobials for prophylaxis is equally important, e.g. the use of antimicrobials before, during and after surgery to prevent rather than treat infection.
- Nurse prescribing and its role in antimicrobial resistance is important at this time when nurse prescribing is being extended. Points for consideration include the difficulties associated with diagnosing infection accurately, awareness of allergies to and toxic effects of antimicrobials, the potential side-effects and the reduction in effectiveness of other medications when taking antimicrobials, e.g. the oral contraceptive pill. Patient education is also important, e.g. there is often no point in taking antimicrobials for viral complaints such as a sore throat, and completing an entire course of antimicrobials as prescribed is essential.

on appropriate prescribing. They also have a key responsibility to report antimicrobial prescribing through to senior management, including chief executives. For further information, see Department of Health (2000), HPS web pages, HPA web pages, http://www.advisorybodies.doh.gov.uk/arhai/, http://www.who.int/patientsafety/amr/en/.

Outbreak management

When an outbreak of infectious disease occurs, a prompt, well-coordinated, multidisciplinary response will help to minimise its impact. An outbreak may have minimal impact or major, widespread implications, including death or serious illness. Local infection prevention and control policies state the response that will be mounted when an outbreak is suspected or confirmed, including the definition of what is considered an outbreak, as this can vary between settings.

The factors that constitute an outbreak depend upon a number of considerations including the number of people involved, the pathogenicity of the organism and its potential for spread. Some infections should be automatically regarded as outbreaks, for example suspected food poisoning related to food supplied or serious communicable disease such as influenza or *Legionella*. Other examples include organisms with a higher antimicrobial resistance profile (e.g. epidemic strains of MRSA) or an increase in infectious conditions that may be caused by different organisms (e.g. wound infections).

Policies on outbreak management should include details of the personnel involved and their roles during the incident, the communication processes and the actions to be taken, including risk assessments. Communication is crucial in these situations, as it is within all health care provision. Meetings are convened during an outbreak to facilitate the response and this might include extraordinary meetings of the Control of Infection Committee. Involvement of staff from the local health protection unit is especially important for outbreaks affecting primary care settings and the wider community. Similarly, outbreaks in the community often spread to health care settings, where patients may be more susceptible to infection, in an environment already conducive to the spread of infection.

As described earlier, the nurse's role in supporting infection prevention and control includes taking corrective action when outbreaks are suspected or proven. This entails alerting the infection prevention and control team to any concerns over increasing numbers of infections and following the specific direction given on the care and treatment of patients involved in an outbreak.

Infection prevention and control measures at home

In the home environment, risk assessments must be carried out and the most appropriate and common-sense approach used when applying Standard Precautions. For example, asking a patient's partner to wear full PPE when cleaning up a urine or vomit spillage may be unrealistic. Education and support from the community nurse is essential to provide people at home with the information necessary to prevent the spread of infection, while ensuring a clean and safe environment for those who are vulnerable. The use of Standard Precautions by health care workers in order to minimise the risk of spread of infection to patients, carers and themselves remains essential (Box 16.7).

Transition from home to hospital and hospital to home

Effective communication between staff working within primary and acute care settings is vital if infections that might be introduced to the home from hospital or to the hospital

from home are to be prevented or controlled and managed appropriately. Nurses should liaise between settings, disciplines and agencies to influence and inform decision-making in relation to infection prevention and control. Whether working in the NHS, in education as a school nurse or lecturer, in the prison service, general practice, independent hospitals or care homes, or with commercial companies providing health care products, nurses must consider ways in which the potential for infection can be managed across the spectrum of health care services. Communication in all its forms is core to this.

SUMMARY: KEY NURSING ISSUES

- The prevention and control of all infectious diseases and, in particular, health care associated infection (HCAI), is an essential part of safe, high-quality patient care.
- Standard Precautions form a cornerstone of safe and effective infection prevention practice and are used in combination with risk management strategies to ensure the safety of patients, health care workers and visitors/family.
- Hand hygiene is part of Standard Precautions and is widely regarded to be the most important step in preventing HCAI.
- Nurses, along with other members of the multi-professional team, have a key role to play in ensuring that infection prevention measures are implemented consistently and reliably in whatever setting care is being delivered and that they are practising in accordance with the latest evidence and best practice recommendations.
- Nurses should feel confident to challenge their own practices and the behaviours of others to ensure recommended infection prevention measures are embedded into day-to-day routines. Education, training and communication are key to achieving this.
- By working closely with infection prevention teams and specialists, nurses can enhance their understanding of prevalent hazards and risks which must be considered and addressed in order to adapt to the ever-changing challenges and threats posed by infectious diseases and HCAI.

REFLECTION AND LEARNING – WHAT NEXT?

- **Test** your knowledge by visiting the website and answering the multiple choice questions and critical thinking questions.
- **Consolidate** your learning by looking at some of the further reading suggestions, references and specialist websites.
- **Revisit** some of the additional material on the website.
- **Consider** what you have learnt and how this will help your professional development.
- **Reflect** on how you can apply this knowledge to the care of your patients.
- **Discuss** your learning with your mentor/supervisor, lecturer and colleagues.

Box 16.7 Reflection

Applying infection prevention measures in the community

- Discuss with a community nurse how infection prevention measures such as hand hygiene, use of protective clothing, aseptic techniques and disinfection of equipment can be achieved in the patient's home.

REFERENCES

Aziz A: Variations in aseptic technique and implications for infection control, *Br J Nurs* 8(28):26–31, 2009.

Department of Health (DH): *UK Antimicrobial resistance strategy and action plan*, London, 2000, DH.

Department of Health (DH): *The Health and Social Care Act 2008 Code of Practice for the NHS on the Prevention and Control of Healthcare Associated Infections and Related Guidance*, London, 2008, DH.

Dougherty L, Lister S, editors: *The Royal Marsden Manual of Clinical Nursing Procedures*, ed 7, Oxford, 2008, Wiley-Blackwell.

Gould D, Brooker C: *Infection Prevention and Control, Applied microbiology for healthcare*, ed 2, London, 2008, Palgrave.

Haley RW, Culver DH, White JW, et al: The efficacy of infection surveillance and control programs in preventing nosocomial infections in US hospitals, *Am J Epidemiol* 121:182–205, 1985.

Haradon C: *What Is a Bundle?*, vol 2007, Boston MA, 2006, Institute for Healthcare Improvement.

Harbarth S, Sax H, Gastmeier P: The preventable proportion of nosocomial infections: an overview of published reports, *J Hosp Infect* 54(4):258–266, 2003.

Health and Safety at Work Act: *(Application outside Great Britain Order) 2001*, London, 1974, The Stationery Office.

Madeo M: Understanding the MRSA experience, *Nurs Times* 97(30):36–37, 2001.

National Audit Office: *Report by the Comptroller and Auditor General: The management and control of hospital acquired infection in acute NHS trusts in England*, London, 2000, NAO.

National Audit Office: *Report by the Comptroller and Auditor General: Improving patient care by reducing the risk of hospital acquired infection: a progress report*, London, 2004, NAO.

National Audit Office: *Report by the Comptroller and Auditor General: Reducing healthcare associated infection in hospitals in England*, London, 2009, NAO.

Nursing and Midwifery Council (NMC): *The Code: Standards of Conduct, Performance and Ethics for Nurses and Midwives*, London, 2008, NMC.

Owens CD, Stoessel K: Surgical site infections: epidemiology, microbiology and prevention, *J Hosp Infect* 70(S2):3–10, 2008.

Pittet D, Allegranzi B, Sax H, et al: on behalf of the WHO: Evidence-based model for hand transmission during patient care and the role of improved practices, *Lancet Infect Dis* 6(10):641–652, 2006.

Pratt RJ, Pellowe CM, Wilson JA, et al: Epic2: National evidence-based guidelines for preventing healthcare associated infections in NHS hospitals in England, *J Hosp Infect* 65(Suppl 1):S1–S64, 2007.

Prieto J, Macleod Clark J: Contact precautions for *Clostridium difficile* and methicillin-resistant *Staphylococcus aureus* (MRSA): Assessing the impact of a supportive intervention, *Journal of Research in Nursing* 10(5):511–526, 2005.

Pronovost P, Needham D, Berenholtz S, et al: An intervention to prevent catheter-related bloodstream infections in the ICU, *N Engl J Med* 355(26):2725–2732, 2006.

Reilly J, Stewart S, Allardice GA, et al: Results from the Scottish national HAI prevalence survey, *J Hosp Infect* 69:62–68, 2008.

Resar R, Pronovost P, Haraden C, et al: Using a bundle approach to improve ventilator care processes and reduce ventilator associated pneumonia, *Jt Comm J Qual Patient Saf* 31(5):243–248, 2005.

Rowley S: Aseptic non-touch technique, *Nursing Times Plus* 97(7):6–8, 2001.

Rowley S, Sinclair S: Working towards an NHS standard for aseptic non-touch technique, *Nurs Times* 100(8):50–52, 2004.

Rowley S, Clare S, Macqueen S, Molyneux R: ANTT v2: An updated practice framework for aseptic technique, *Br J Nurs (Intravenous Supplement)* 19(5):S5–S11, 2010.

Sawyer M, Weeks K, Goeschel C, et al: Using evidence, rigorous measurement, and collaboration to eliminate central catheter-associated bloodstream infections, *Crit Care Med* 38:S292–298, 2010.

Sax H, Allegranzi B, Uçkay I, et al: 'My five moments for hand hygiene': a user-centred design approach to understand, train, monitor and report hand hygiene, *J Hosp Infect* 67(1):9–21, 2007.

Siegel J, Rhinehart E, Jackson M, et al: and the Healthcare Infection Control Practices Advisory Committee 2007 Guideline for Isolation Precautions: *Preventing Transmission of Infectious Agents In Healthcare Settings*, Atlanta GA, 2007, Centers for Disease Control and Prevention.

Available online http://www.cdc.gov/ncidod/dhqp/pdf/isolation 2007.pdf.

Skov RL, Jensen KS: Community-associated meticillin-resistant *Staphylococcus aureus* as a cause of hospital-acquired infections, *J Hosp Infect* 73:364–370, 2009.

Smyth ETM, McIlvenny G, Enstone JE, et al: on behalf of the Hospital Infection Society Prevalence Survey Steering Group: Four country healthcare associated infection prevalence survey 2006: overview of the results, *J Hosp Infect* 69(3):230–248, 2008.

Tablan O, Anderson L, Besser R, et al: Guidelines for preventing health-care associated pneumonia. Recommendations of CDC and the Health care Infection Control Practices Advisory Committee, *Morb Mortal Weekly Rep* 53(RR03):1–36, 2003.

Wilson J: *Clinical Microbiology: An Introduction for Healthcare Professionals*, ed 8, Edinburgh, 2000, Baillière Tindall.

World Health Organization: *Definitions of risk analysis terms related to food safety*, 2008. Available online http://www.who.int/foodsafety/publications/micro/riskanalysis_definitions/en/.

World Health Organization: *WHO Guidelines on Hand Hygiene in Health Care*, Geneva, 2009, WHO.

FURTHER READING

Gould D, Brooker C: *Infection Prevention and Control*, ed 2, Basingstoke, 2008, Palgrave Macmillan.

Mangram A, Horan T, Pearson M, et al: Guideline for prevention of surgical site infection, *Am J Infect Control* 27(2):96–134, 1999.

Wilson J: *Infection Control in Clinical Practice*, ed 3, Edinburgh, 2006, Baillière Tindall.

USEFUL WEBSITES

Advisory Committee on Antimicrobial Resistance and Healthcare Associated Infection: www.dh.gov.uk/ab/ARHAI

Advisory Committee on Dangerous Pathogens: www.dh.gov.uk/ab/ACDP

Association of Medical Microbiologists: www.amm.co.uk

British Society of Antimicrobial Chemotherapy: www.bsac.org.uk

British Thoracic Society: www.brit-thoracic.org.uk

Care Commission: www.carecommission.com

Care Quality Commission: www.cqc.org.uk

Centers for Disease Control and Prevention (USA): www.cdc.gov

Department for Environment, Food and Rural Affairs: www.defra.gov.uk/environment/waste/topics/clinical.htm

Department of Health: www.dh.gov.uk

Department of Health – Saving Lives Delivery Programme: www.dh.gov.uk/prod_consum_dh/groups/dh_digitalassets/@dh/@en/documents/digitalasset/dh_4113480.pdf

Department of Health, Social Services and Public Safety in Northern Ireland: www.dhsspsni.gov.uk

Department of Health Wales: wales.gov.uk/topics/health/protection/communicabledisease/?lang=en

The Green Book (for up-to-date information on immunisation against infectious disease): www.dh.gov.uk/publicationsandstatistics

Health Protection Agency: www.hpa.org.uk
(for notification of infectious diseases in England: www.hpa.org.uk/infections)

Health Protection Scotland (formerly Scottish Centre for Infection and Environmental Health): www.hps.scot.nhs.uk

Health and Safety Executive (including Care of Substances Hazardous to Health Regulations): www.hse.gov.uk/coshh

Healthcare A–Z: www.healthcarea2z.org

Hospital Infection Society: www.his.org.uk

Infection Prevention Society (incorporating the ICNA): www.ips.uk.net

Institute for Healthcare Improvement: www.ihi.org

ISD Scotland (for notification of infectious diseases in Scotland): www.isdscotland.org

Medicines and Healthcare products Regulatory Agency: www.mhra.gov.uk

National Institute for Health and Clinical Excellence (NICE): www.nice.org.uk

National Patient Safety Agency: www.npsa.nhs.uk

National Resource for Infection Control: www.nric.org.uk

NHS Health Facilities Scotland: www.hfs.scot.nhs.uk

NHS Institute for Innovation and Improvement: www.institute.nhs.uk

NHS Purchasing and Supply Agency (PASA): www.pasa.nhs.uk

NHS Quality Improvement Scotland: www.nhshealthquality.org

NHS Scotland (Fit for Travel – travel advice for the public on infectious diseases around the world, maintained and updated by Health Protection Scotland): www.fitfortravel.nhs.uk

Scottish Government Health Department: www.sehd.scot.nhs.uk

World Health Organization (including WHO Guidelines on Hand Hygiene in Health Care): www.who.int

Stress and anxiety

Graeme D. Smith, Tonks N. Fawcett

Introduction

Most people would probably describe themselves as being 'stressed' from time to time, but what does this really mean? Is stress something that resides within the environment, in situations that are threatening, harmful or unpleasant, or is it essentially an internal state, an effect of the individual's perception of what is happening to them? Benner & Wrubel (1989), in their seminal text, defined stress as 'the disruption of meanings, understanding and smooth functioning so that harm, loss or challenge is experienced and sorrow, interpretation or new skill acquisition is required'.

Stress may have physiological or psychosocial origins and research into stress is a highly complex field involving a number of sciences, including biology, physiology, psychology and sociology. When biologists and physiologists talk of sources of stress, they are referring to empirical phenomena. Their interest is in examining identifiable events and their measurable effects upon the organism or system under stress. Anything which affects the equilibrium of the organism may be described as a stressor; this would include bacterial infections, dehydration, extremes of temperature, inadequate food, and so on. Therefore stress can be viewed as a disturbed homeostasis that manifests itself via certain physiological and psychological imbalances (Watson & Fawcett 2003). The impact of stress occurs only when the cumulative effects of stressors surpass the individual's ability easily to return to equilibrium. However, despite the popular connotations, not all stress is a bad thing. Having the optimal amount of stress to keep us performing at our best, adapting to life's daily challenges, is called eustress, good stress. Distress means that our functional adaptability is impaired in some way; this can take many forms, such as anxiety, low mood or physical illness. Commonly associated triggers related to stress are outlined in Box 17.1.

Social scientists view stress in terms of the pressures upon the individual to conform (or not) to societal norms. The inherent values expressed in a society's organisation and functioning may themselves be a source of stress to the individual. Modern industrial society, for example, provides food, safety and shelter for its members in return for a commitment to work, often at some sacrifice to personal interests, leisure and family life.

Psychologists view stress from the perspective of the interaction of individuals and groups with the environment, describing the effects of stress on cognition, emotional well-being and behaviour.

It is important for nurses to have a clear understanding of the concept of stress as they endeavour to provide the best possible care for their patients/clients and to appreciate why patients/clients might be feeling stressed and how this might be alleviated. In relation to the nurse's own well-being, an understanding of stress and its effects is equally important. Nursing is physically and emotionally demanding work, and nurses need to recognise signs of stress in themselves, its meaning and management.

Box 17.1 Reflection

Common triggers of stress (adapted from the Stress Management Society)

- Bereavement
- Illness, injury or trauma
- Interpersonal conflict
- Environmental factors
- Financial issues
- Uncertainty/change
- Work overload

Activity

Since starting your nursing course it is possible that you have been affected by one or more of the stress triggers listed above, for example work overload (with assignments), financial issues and uncertainty/change.

- Take some time to reflect on how you felt – were there physical effects or did it affect your mood?
- How did you cope with the stress and the trigger? If appropriate, discuss coping strategies with other students in your group.

This chapter begins by looking at the physiological consequences of a stressor, identifying some of the more influential models that seek to explain the phenomenon of stress, before examining the relationship between stress and disease. The concept of 'coping' and various therapeutic strategies available to assist the individual in managing stress are then explored.

Physiological responses to stress

The physiological response to stress seeks to enable the individual to meet the challenges set by whatever is perceived as a stressor, by:

- the activation of the sympathetic nervous system (see Ch. 9)
- the increased secretion of several hormones from the endocrine system (see Ch. 5, Part 1).

The stress response

In 1935, Cannon summarised the response of an individual, or animal, to external threat as the 'flight, fight or fright' reaction, often referred to as the 'acute stress response'. Real and imagined psychosocial stressors are an essential component of living and, when present to a moderate degree, have been described as 'eustress' since they optimise performance and improve learning. It is when a threat is perceived to be of an order which endangers either a person's sense of self-worth or even life itself, that the full manifestations of the acute stress response are seen. After events such as a car crash, bomb explosion or unexpected physical attack, rapid physiological adaptations of the acute stress response are activated. This can, in some circumstances, be life saving. Consider, for example, the situation in which smoke suddenly appears in a room and, all too soon, the first flames begin to spread; a person will often find a sudden unexpected ability for rapid action to deal with such an emergency. Along with a surge of physical strength, there will be an increased ability to tackle the flames and a marked enhancement in the ability to run and thereby escape the danger. Such a response is enabled by a release of hormones brought about by activation of the sympathetic nervous system and the adrenal medulla (see Ch. 5, Part 1).

An alarm reaction of lesser magnitude is a common occurrence in the more ordinary trials of life. This occurs, for example, in such circumstances as running out of petrol on the motorway en route to an important engagement, losing one's front door keys, or being with someone who unexpectedly becomes acutely ill. The severity of the alarm reaction varies considerably between different individuals and also between different occurrences of a similar situation. Thus, when a person's car breaks down on the motorway for a second time, they may feel even more distressed than on the first occasion. Alternatively, they may be more confident in their ability to deal with the event and consequently be less 'stressed'.

The manifestation of stress is derived not merely from external problems or dangers but from the way in which people attempt to manage these problems. Stress is described as the state of affairs that exists when the way in which people attempt to manage problems taxes or exceeds their coping resources. When the response to a stressor is severe, normal social relationships can be affected, as aspects of the 'flight, fight or fright' response potentially impinge upon rational behaviour.

As indicated, aversive physical stimuli that provoke stress events include excessive noise, cold or heat, and physiological imbalances such as those associated with sleep deprivation, lack of food or chronic pain. Such stressors not only act to bring about hormonal changes associated with the acute stress response, but also have their own selective effects on physiological functioning.

An example of such a selective effect can be seen in the body's response to cold, as it strives to maintain homeostasis. In cold conditions, the blood supply is redistributed to less exposed areas in order to limit heat loss and, via the mechanical act of shivering, the body temperature can be increased (see Ch. 22). In addition, the secretion of thyrotrophin-releasing hormone from the hypothalamus is increased, thereby stimulating the anterior pituitary gland to secrete thyroid-stimulating hormone (TSH). This in turn causes enhanced release of the thyroid hormones thyroxine and triiodothyronine, which raise basal metabolic rate and hence increase heat production and core temperature.

To maintain homeostasis when threatened by a stressor, the body employs a range of physiological mechanisms. Some stressors are short lived, in which case the body may be able to react to the situation and quickly resolve the disturbance evoked by the stressor. Other stressors may last for days, months or even years. There are many examples of this chronic form of stress, for example when people must live with chronic disease or social disharmony. Where there has been repeated exposure to a particularly stressful or aversive event, there can be a further reaction, characterised by a conditioned fear response to any neutral stimulus experienced at the same time as the previous stressor. This effect is responsible for many of the anxiety reactions or acts of avoidance some people show in response to specific harmless objects.

The general adaptation syndrome (GAS)

Hans Selye, in his seminal work on the response-based model of stress, noted that the diverse noxious stimuli which challenged the ability of the body to maintain homeostasis induced a common pattern of effects (Selye 1936, 1976).

Selye deduced that, whatever the nature of the stressor, it resulted in a pattern of non-specific responses that formed part of what he described as a general adaptation syndrome (GAS). These responses, providing they were not over-whelming, enabled a physiological adaptation to take place (Selye 1976).

The syndrome is considered to have three phases:

- first phase – 'alarm reaction'
- second phase – 'resistance'
- third phase – 'exhaustion'.

In the 'alarm reaction', the sympathetic nervous system and the adrenal glands are activated. Together they prepare the body for flight or fight. If the stressor continues, the triggering of neural and endocrine responses in the alarm reaction is followed by 'resistance' phase. Stimulation of the hypothalamo–pituitary–adrenal axis results in increased secretion of corticosteroids, the endocrine response. In this phase, the internal responses of the body mobilise resources and enable tissue defences to achieve the maximum adaptation possible. The final phase of the GAS is 'exhaustion', in which the body may succumb to the stressor.

The GAS is criticised for providing a somewhat simplistic, stereotypical model of the responses of the body and failing to take full account of the individual variations of psychological and physiological responses. Lazarus (1966) argued that there is a circularity about Selye's model, in so far as something about the stimulus elicits a particular stress response while something about the response indicates the presence of a stressor.

The acute stress response

During the alarm reaction to stress, a series of physiological responses involving limbic and brain stem structures are triggered (Fox 2004). Neural pathways from nuclei in the limbic system mediate responses to emotional stress, and pathways from the reticular formation in the brain stem mediate responses to physiological stressors such as pain and injury. This activates the hypothalamo–pituitary–adrenal axis and results in the secretion of a range of hormones.

An immediate response to threat or stress involves the neural connections from the hypothalamus to the sympathetic outflow, activating both postganglionic and preganglionic sympathetic nerves passing to the adrenal medulla. This is the emergency reaction which was first described by Cannon (1935). In the adrenal medulla, acetylcholine released at preganglionic sympathetic nerve terminals activates the chromaffin cells to secrete the catecholamines adrenaline and noradrenaline. In humans, adrenaline is secreted in greater amounts than noradrenaline. The release of these hormones takes place in a matter of seconds or minutes.

The hormones liberated from the adrenal medulla have many effects which facilitate emergency reactions. For example, adrenaline and noradrenaline improve cardiac and respiratory function. Heart rate and force of contraction are increased. Bronchioles are dilated and the depth and rate of respiration are increased. Blood flow is redistributed to areas of need, i.e. the heart and skeletal muscles. Blood glucose and basal metabolism are raised and blood clotting facilitated. The increase of blood glucose is due mainly to the actions of adrenaline on the liver to promote glycogen breakdown and enhance gluconeogenesis (production of glucose from non-carbohydrate substances) from fatty acids and proteins. Adrenaline also acts on the pancreas to inhibit insulin secretion. Piloerection and pupillary dilatation, so characteristic of the behaviour of fighting cats, represent yet another physiological consequence of hormone release from the adrenal medulla. Sweating by the eccrine glands (the most abundant sweat glands) is increased. In the meantime, functioning of the digestive tract is reduced and urinary sphincters are closed.

The physiological effects of adrenaline and noradrenaline are explained in Chapter 5 (Part 1).

In the more long-term responses to stress described by Selye, the centre of activity passes from the adrenal medulla to the adrenal cortex, and to the hypothalamus and pituitary, which are responsible for activating the adrenal cortex. Corticotrophin-releasing hormone (CRH) is secreted by the hypothalamus as well as other sites in the brain. CRH acts on the anterior pituitary gland, stimulating the secretion of adrenocorticotrophic hormone (ACTH) and beta-endorphin.

Beta-endorphin reduces susceptibility to pain and is probably one of the means by which stress and the stimuli of conditioned fear give rise to endogenous analgesia. Opiates act in a similar way to endorphins, but are not rapidly degraded by the body, as natural endorphins are, and thus have a long-lasting effect on pain perception and mood (Pert 1997).

Other factors influence the release of ACTH, including antidiuretic hormone (ADH) and hypothalamic vasoactive intestinal peptide (VIP). The ACTH liberated by the anterior pituitary acts to stimulate cells in the adrenal cortex to secrete corticosteroids.

Glucocorticoids, mostly cortisol (hydrocortisone), secreted by the adrenal cortex play a key role in adaptation to stress. Glucocorticoids modify metabolism so as to increase blood glucose concentrations. They do this by mobilising tissue protein and amino acids and by these actions may induce a negative nitrogen balance (see Ch. 21). Glucocorticoids are needed to enable other hormones to bring about the mobilisation and metabolism of fat. These metabolic effects of glucocorticoids ensure the supply of adequate fuel to the cells when the body is under stress, and in this respect the adrenal cortex provides an important back-up system for the adrenal medulla. In addition, glucocorticoids play important roles in the proper functioning of many organ systems and tissues in the body, including the cardiovascular system, the nervous system, lymphoid tissue and skeletal muscle.

Glucocorticoids, such as cortisol, possess appreciable mineralocorticoid activity, retaining sodium chloride and indirectly increasing extracellular fluid (ECF) volume, although they are much less potent in this respect than aldosterone (see Ch. 20). The secretion of aldosterone is not regulated by ACTH, and so its release is independent of the stress response. Mineralocorticoid activity by hormones such as cortisol may in part underlie important, though poorly understood, actions on the cardiovascular system. An increase of ECF volume can be of great importance under circumstances when stressors induce shock or when there is loss of body fluids after haemorrhage or burn injury (see Chs 18, 29, 30).

Additionally, glucocorticoids can decrease the number of some types of circulating white blood cells and, at pharmacological concentrations, suppress the immune response. In addition to their direct effects, the corticosteroids exert an enabling influence on the actions of several other hormones and are necessary for the body to show a full response to the adrenaline and noradrenaline released from the adrenal medulla. It can be seen that due to its wide-ranging functions, especially in the maintenance of fluid and electrolyte balance, the adrenal gland is essential to life and the maintenance of physiological homeostasis and psychological equilibrium (Box 17.2).

The chronic stress response

Clearly, as Selye (1976) established, there are limits to the body's ability to maintain its phase of resistance and adaptation in the face of excessive or continuing stress; environmental stressors can be toxic and physiologically overwhelming. As Selye noted as long ago as the 1950s, when an individual

Box 17.2 Information

Hormones and effects of short- and long-term stress

Short-term stress
Mediated by the release of the catecholamines adrenaline and noradrenaline from the adrenal medulla, short-term stress leads to:

- increased heart rate
- bronchodilatation
- increased blood pressure
- liver conversion of glycogen stores to glucose for release into the bloodstream
- altered blood flow patterns to increase arousal and decrease digestive and urinary activity via selective vasoconstriction
- increased platelet aggregation
- pupil dilatation and piloerection
- increased metabolic rate
- sweating from eccrine glands.

Long-term stress
Mediated by the release of glucocorticoids and mineralocorticoids from the adrenal cortex, long-term stress leads to:

- gluconeogenesis whereby proteins and fats are broken down to form glucose
- increased blood glucose levels
- retention of sodium and water by the kidneys (aldosterone effect)
- increased blood volume and blood pressure via the above plus vasoconstriction and reduced fluid shift
- increased coagulability and viscosity of the blood
- suppression of the immune system and inflammatory response
- altered blood biochemistry, e.g. in 5-hydroxytryptamine (serotonin), endorphin and dopamine levels.

is physiologically challenged but not overwhelmed, as in conditions of prolonged, chronic stress, enlargement of the adrenal glands and atrophy of the thymus and lymphatic structures (thymicolymphatic atrophy) will occur. When stress persists beyond a certain period of time, disturbances occur in the homeostatic balance of the body and there is an ever-increasing danger that disease processes will be precipitated.

An important part of the body's defence mechanism in the phase of resistance is the pituitary secretion of ACTH, which in turn stimulates the adrenal cortex to release corticosteroids. One of the early signs of the body's inability to meet the demands of unremitting stress is a blunting of the amounts of ACTH released by the anterior pituitary in response to that stress. Under these circumstances, the adrenal cortex frequently shows hyperplasia, which persists despite the reduced secretion of ACTH. This blunting of the ACTH response to stress also occurs in long-standing timidity, which is possibly due to high arousal together with slow habituation to the stressors. This is coupled with an associated enlargement of the adrenal glands and hypersecretion of corticosteroids under comparatively non-threatening circumstances. Likewise, blunting of the ACTH responses to stressors is seen in depressive illness and in many forms of anxiety. In individuals experiencing low mood, there is frequently a high corticosteroid excretion associated with enlargement of the adrenal glands and an increase in the concentrations of CRH in cerebrospinal fluid.

Emotional as well as hormonal changes characterise chronic stress. These include emotional exhaustion, a decreased sensitivity to rewards and a withdrawal from decision making, which is characteristic of fatigue. This can progress to the condition known as 'burnout', a complex phenomenon involving extreme physical and emotional distress which, for the individual, is often linked to organisational factors (Hall 2004). In burnout, the physical and emotional fatigue may be manifest as a lack of involvement with, or sympathy or respect for, colleagues and clients. At its final stage, chronic stress may result in total collapse. Long-lasting stress in which there is a poor coping strategy is correlated with increased occurrence of a variety of diseases (Levi 1971, Cooper 2004, Hesselink et al 2004). These may be described as diseases of adaptation and are related to deranged secretion of adaptive hormones in the phase of resistance. These conditions include digestive disturbances, hypertension, myocardial infarction, allergies and sleep disturbances (see Chs 2, 4, 6, 25). Such chronic stress may also lead to anxiety, low mood or behavioural disturbances, such as appetite disorders or increased usage of alcohol, tobacco, caffeine or even illegal substances. Clearly, in such situations, physiological homeostasis and psychological equilibrium are under threat.

From homeostasis to allostasis

The concept of allostasis, as opposed to homeostasis, refers to the maintenance of stability through change. It is seen as a fundamental process by which organisms actively adjust to both predictable and unpredictable events. This theoretical development suggests that both homeostasis and allostasis are endogenous systems responsible for maintaining the internal stability of an organism. However, homeostasis means remaining stable by staying the same. Allostasis comes from the Greek allo, which means 'variable', thus remaining stable by being variable. Thus the allostatic state refers to the altered physiological and emotional activity in response to changing environments and challenges, e.g. an excessive or inadequate production of, for example, cortisol or cytokines (McEwan & Wingfield 2003). Cytokines are a group of intercellular signalling molecules, e.g. interleukins, interferons, which act on immune cells.

The allostatic load refers to excessive or prolonged alteration in allostatic state that is outwith the individual's ability to cope and which arguably leads to detrimental health outcomes. The perception of stress is influenced by the individual's unique makeup, their genetics, experiences and behaviour (Lazarus 1966). From the theoretical stance of allostasis, when a source is perceived as stressful, physiological and behavioural responses are initiated leading to an altered allostatic state and, ideally, adaptation. However if the source of stress does not resolve, over time the allostatic load can accumulate and the overexposure to neural, endocrine and immune stress mediators can begin to have adverse effects on organs and systems of the body, leading to disease.

There are considered to be four types of allostatic load:

- Simply too much 'stress' in the form of repeated, novel events that cause repeated elevations of stress mediators over a long period, e.g. economic hardship.
- A failure to habituate or adapt to the same stressor. This leads to the overexposure to stress mediators because of the failure of the body to dampen or eliminate the hormonal stress response to a repeated event.
- A failure to switch off either the hormonal stress response or to display the normal diurnal pattern of the glucocorticoid production in the body.
- Inadequate hormonal stress response which allows other systems, such as the inflammatory cytokines, to become overactive (McEwan & Wingfield 2003, Wingfield 2003).

Models of stress

The physicist Robert Hooke (1635–1703) used the word 'stress' in the 17th century to refer to the ratio of an external force (created by a load) to the area over which that force was exerted. The resultant strain created a deformation or distortion of the object by what became known as Hooke's Law.

There is an interesting similarity between this use of the word stress and its modern application in the realm of human emotion and behaviour; indeed, people frequently use words such as 'weight' and 'strain' when describing their feelings of anxiety and stress.

During the 20th century, the adoption of the concept of stress by the biological and behavioural sciences resulted in the formulation of a number of models to describe stress and its effects, including the:

- stimulus-based model
- response-based model
- general adaptation syndrome
- transactional model
- phenomenological model or approach.

The stimulus-based model

In this model the person is viewed as being constantly exposed to general or specific 'stressors' in their daily life, e.g. the demands of work, family responsibilities, illness, accidents, bereavement or disability. These stressors have the potential, however, to cause both physical symptoms and distressing feelings that will undermine well-being.

In the stimulus-based model, stress is a state that can generally be empirically observed, measured and evaluated, and which can potentially be removed or altered to reduce the individual's stress: it is possible, in theory, to persuade noisy neighbours to be quieter, for traumatic wounds to heal, or to make a cold working environment warmer. However, in many situations, such as a bereavement or disablement, the original stressor cannot be changed or adapted to reduce distressing feelings. Even in relatively simple situations, removing the stressor is not necessarily a straightforward matter (Box 17.3). It quickly becomes apparent that the stimulus-based model has substantial shortcomings when considered in relation to the breadth of human experience (Sutherland & Cooper 2000) and has difficulty explaining why some people experience stress in certain situations while others, in similar circumstances, do not, or explain why a given situation may be stressful at one time but not at another. The model offers no explanation as to why a person may be stressed in response to apparently neutral stimuli such as birds, spiders or aeroplanes. Lazarus (1966), in his seminal text, argued that it is not possible to evaluate the human experience of stress objectively; only a personal account of feelings and experiences can adequately convey the nature of an individual's stress.

Box 17.3 Reflection

Janice

A health visitor could not understand initially why her client, Janice, an unsupported mother of two, appeared to be tense and unhappy when they met at the child health clinic. She asked how Janice was feeling, and Janice described how she had new neighbours in the flat above her who played loud music until early in the morning, preventing her and her two children from getting enough sleep. She had tried to talk with them but they had been hostile towards her and made her feel apprehensive. She didn't dare complain to them again. The lack of sleep was affecting Janice and her children. Janice had difficulty concentrating at work and felt like crying frequently during the day; the children were overtired and generally irritable, making it even more difficult for her to cope. The health visitor asked Janice if she could intervene by contacting the environmental health department of the local council on her behalf, but Janice said that she was afraid that this would make matters worse.

Activities

- Reflect on Janice's situation and consider how else the health visitor could support her.
- Read the chapter material covering other models of stress and discuss with your lecturer or mentor the relative advantages and limitations of each in Janice's situation.

The response-based model

In this model, the word 'stress' is used to describe the response of a person who feels they are in a threatening or difficult situation. Stress is thus a person's response to threat which, as in the stimulus-based model, is not necessarily inherent in the environment or situation. By using the response-based model, it is possible to make sense of an individual's unique stress responses and even of responses that might seem, within the stimulus-based model, to be irrational, such as a fear of birds, spiders or of flying. Hans Selye's extensive physiological research as an endocrinologist (Selye 1936, 1946a,b, 1976) was largely based upon the response-based model of stress.

The transactional model

A behavioural model of stress that incorporates a dynamic view of the individual and their interaction with the stress in their environment is called a transactional model. As discussed above, the person appraises, or seeks meaning in, what is perceived to be a potentially threatening situation in an attempt to respond in a way that minimises the distress. The process of appraisal is highly individual; each person will perceive a threatening situation differently and attach their own meanings to it (Lazarus & Folkman 1984). Moreover, the relationship between the individual and their environment is a dynamic one which constantly changes as the process of appraisal, coping and adaptation takes place.

The role of appraisal

How individuals appraise, or find meaning in, adversity is crucial to how they withstand it. The concept of resilience may explain why some people, e.g. patients with cancer or AIDS (Polk 1997), can withstand and survive the adversity whilst others cannot. Appraisal is crucial to the individual's ability to continue a healthy life after catastrophe or illness, and, as with resilience, the personal traits of the individual will influence their ability to find meaning in what is happening to them. It should be recognised, however, that the process of appraisal may be a spontaneous emotional reaction rather than a well thought-out process.

The phenomenological model or approach

Phenomenological models and approaches rest largely upon the description given by the individual of their own experience of stress. The writings of phenomenological philosophers such as Merleau-Ponty and Heidegger describe human experience as 'being in the world' whereby each person is defined by their own thoughts, feelings, memories, relationships and social settings. Mind and body are described not as separate but as one integral whole (Benner & Wrubel 1989). This topic is further examined under 'psychosomatic' problems (p. 525). The body is the physical means of knowing and sensing the world and, with disability or disease, the experience of the person will be impaired (Benner & Wrubel 1989).

This view of human experience invites the nurse to use an intuitive approach when working with people who are distressed, because it acknowledges the complexity of individual responses, and recognises that providing the right kind of help is, similarly, a complex and subtle task. The description of human experience from a phenomenological viewpoint attributes to the person a wisdom about themselves and their problems that cannot easily be gained from an 'objective' position (Benner & Wrubel 1989). However, does this mean that the nurse is merely a passive observer when working with distressed people? If suggestions and advice cannot be offered in any but the most uncomplicated situations, then what help can be offered? The most effective help that can be given by the clinical nurse is support in enabling the person to identify what is causing their stress and to deal with it in their own way. This does not entail the nurse, however subtly, suggesting what they think the patient should do. Rather, it involves being aware and respectful of the person's right to choose what they feel is appropriate for them. This is not a passive position for the nurse to take but is a highly interactive and enabling one (Rogers 1974, Egan 1997, Kennedy & Charles 2002).

Phenomenology, appraisal and the role of stress

In a sense, all appraisal is phenomenological, because it rests upon the individual's own attribution of meaning to a situation (Lazarus & Folkman 1984). Personality factors play a large part in determining to what features of their environment an individual attends, and what they attend to is a feature of the meaning that a situation has for them (Lazarus & Folkman 1984, Benner & Wrubel 1989). Rather than describing the individual as 'appraising' a situation, however, Benner and Wrubel (1989) prefer to speak of the person 'being in' a situation. They emphasise that the attribution of meaning to a situation is unique for every individual, even though many people's interpretations appear to coincide. Taking this further, they argue that there are no situations with an objective reality beyond the highly individual interpretations that are put upon them.

For Benner and Wrubel (1989), stress is woven into the fabric of our 'being in the world' and is not 'out there' to be dealt with and it would be seen as harmful to suppress painful emotions, as these assist us in our interpretations of the world. Emotions such as anger or guilt give guidance to people about what is happening to them in the world. To teach people to relax may give them some short respite from painful tension until they are ready to confront their problems again but to teach relaxation as a way of *dealing* with problems may be misguided. Stress is part of the person's self, their concerns, thoughts, feelings about the past and future, memories and relationships to others and to objects.

The concept of resilience

An interesting and developing concept is that of resilience in individuals, which enables them to 'spring back' following distressing events (Jacelon 1997). The research indicates that people who can spring back have a constellation of personality traits such as above-average intelligence, interest in life, a positive outlook and flexibility. Those who can visualise their own future are also more likely to be resilient.

The notion of resilience as a process is less well researched, although nurses will recognise the individual learning and change described by Polk (1997) as 'survival, recovery and rehabilitation'. Gillespie et al (2007) argue that resilience as a process can be developed at any time during a lifespan and can be gained by transforming stressful experiences using constructs such as self-efficacy, hope and coping.

Stress and disease

It is well established that stress can be a contributory factor in disease presentation. There are several physical and psychological factors which are commonly associated with stress (Box 17.4).

See website Critical thinking question 17.1

A relatively new area of behavioural medicine, psychoimmunology, looks at how the body's immune system is affected by psychological factors, such as stress. Psychoimmunologists believe that many stress-related diseases may result from the immune system's inability to deal with stress. These include inflammatory bowel disease, cancer, allergies and arthritic disorders, all of which may be related in some way to the body's inability to defend itself from stress.

In the following section the role of stress in several common disorders is examined.

Psychosomatic problems

The term 'psychosomatic' means mind ('psyche') and body ('soma'). Such a disorder is one which therefore involves both mind and body. Of course our very existence involves the inseparability of the mind and the body. However, the term 'psychosomatic disorder' specifically refers to a physical disease which is thought to be caused, or made worse, by psychological factors. Some physical diseases are thought to be particularly prone to be worsened by factors such as psychological stress, e.g. irritable bowel syndrome (IBS), psoriasis, eczema, peptic ulcer, hypertension and heart disease (see Chs 2, 4, 12). It is thought that the physical element of the illness, e.g. the extent of a rash, the level of the blood pressure, can be affected by psychological factors.

Biologically, this is entirely reasonable as part of the stress response causes such things as a faster heart rate, tremor, fast breathing, sweating, dry mouth, headache and a 'knot

in the stomach'. When these physical symptoms persist and are caused by mental or emotional stress it is called somatisation. For example, many people have occasional headaches caused by mental stress. The tension headache is due to increased tone of muscles of the neck and the scalp. However, stress can cause many other physical symptoms such as tiredness, dizziness, back pain, diarrhoea and, in women, dysmenorrhoea. The somatic symptoms due to anxiety result from enhanced activity of the autonomic nervous system. Psychogenic factors may produce muscle tension and pain. This autonomic nervous overactivity may manifest itself in several bodily systems, including, as illustrated below, the gastrointestinal system.

Anxiety attacks

As previously noted, a certain amount of anxiety and stress is a vital and healthy adaptation mechanism. In a moderate and appropriate degree, stress arouses and alerts us, improving mental and physical activity and helping us to perform better, for example in interviews, or enabling us to avoid dangerous situations.

Anxiety or panic attacks are characterised by severe sympathetic arousal, often in the absence of any immediately obvious stressor. Panic attacks are a common presenting problem in those visiting their general practitioner (GP) with feelings of stress. During an attack, the person often experiences intense fear, accompanied by physiological signs such as palpitations, sweating, trembling, rapid respiration and pallor. The fear may be associated with a fear of collapse, death or a need to escape. Sufferers often explain they feel that their heart might burst.

By explaining the nature of these attacks, the doctor, counsellor or nurse can sometimes bring an element of relief to the sufferer. It is true that the circularity of being afraid of the fear often intensifies the symptoms. Practical advice on the management of attacks is also helpful. Anxiety attacks are symptomatic of underlying distress. They can be acute and of rapid onset, occurring perhaps only once or twice, or can develop into a chronic symptom. Attacks may occur at any time, causing intense feelings of fear where there is no obvious cause, such as fear or discomfort in a centre seat at the cinema or on a bus. The stressor causing the attack may only become apparent, if at all, upon later therapeutic introspection.

There is increasing evidence that complementary and alternative medicine (CAM) can be helpful for stress-related symptoms and anxiety and depression and may used either alongside, or instead of, conventional medication-based treatment. Many of these therapies arguably have fewer side-effects than medication (Kessler et al 2001).

Post-traumatic stress disorder (PTSD)

This condition, recognised for many years, can affect people who have experienced any serious accident or trauma outside the range of their normal experience, such as a serious road traffic accident, rape, physical attack, plane crash, bomb blast, war or terrorist attack. The disorder can follow one or more of such events and can occur not only in those directly involved but also in those called to assist, such as emergency workers or onlookers. The greater the scale of

---

Box 17.4 Information

Physical and psychological factors associated with stress

- Headaches
- Altered bowel function
- Insomnia
- Recurrent fatigue
- Depression
- Anxiety
- Reduced self-esteem
- Poor concentration

the incident, the more likely it is for post-traumatic stress disorder to arise.

The person, having escaped adversity and perhaps having a sense of relief at having escaped relatively unharmed, can be very perplexed at the occurrence of distressing symptoms, sometimes a considerable time after the event. There may be a loss of memory and total amnesia and sufferers often report feeling mentally numbed (Fagan & Freme 2004, Rhoads et al 2008). Symptoms may include:

- mood swings and feelings of aggression
- feelings of alarm, anxiety and irritability
- feeling jumpy
- flashbacks to the original trauma that leave the person feeling as though they were back in the traumatic situation
- loss of interest in pleasurable events
- phobic and depressed feelings, panic
- sleep disturbances, e.g.
  - waking in alarm and unable to return to sleep
  - difficulty in getting to sleep
  - early morning waking
  - distressing nightmares
  - night sweats.

Migraine/headache

Migraine headaches are common and among the most disabling non-fatal conditions of humankind (Jung 2007). Changes in the size of blood vessels and the levels of neurotransmitter substances are thought to be responsible for migraine headaches. It is recognised that they are not caused solely by stress but have a number of precipitating factors such as menstrual cycle, diet, dehydration and certain sounds and smells which, in conjunction with a feeling of stress, may trigger an attack. Many people report that the attack paradoxically occurs after the cessation of the stressful event.

Migraine has been likened to a storm building up and causing, instead of lightning, wind and rain, intense pain, nausea and vomiting, often lasting for several hours. The person is often prevented from continuing normal activities. The phases of an attack are outlined in Box 17.5.

The understanding of migraine pathophysiology has evolved from the belief that migraine is a vascular disorder, to evidence that better defines migraine as a neurogenic disorder associated with secondary changes in brain perfusion (Biondi 2006) and that stress precipitates this pathology through increased activity in catecholamine (adrenaline, noradrenaline, dopamine) pathways, thereby increasing the risk of migraine.

Interventions

The person should, if possible, identify any trigger factors of their migraine attacks and avoid them (Jung 2007). The pain can, in some cases, be treated with simple analgesics in conjunction with antiemetic medication for associated nausea and vomiting. A specific group of drugs – the 5-hydroxytryptamine ($5HT_1$) agonists (triptans), such as sumatriptan – are used to treat acute migraine. CAM, including acupuncture, osteopathy, relaxation therapy and homeopathy, is commonly used for the management of migraine/headache. However, Griggs & Jenson (2006) caution that the evidence base, for example for acupuncture, is still conflicting and lacking robust research trials.

Box 17.5 Information

Migraine phases

Migraine attacks usually follow a pattern consisting of the five phases described below (Blau 1987). The third and fourth phases are prerequisites of a diagnosis of classical migraine.

Phase 1 Prodrome
- Subtle symptoms; may not be noticed
- Craving to eat sweet food
- Mood variations
- Tiredness
- Mild photophobia
- Heightened visual perception

Phase 2 Aura
- Multicoloured visual disturbances
- Scotoma with flickering, scintillating edge
- Tingling of face, sometimes one sided
- Numbness of face

Phase 3 Headache
- Slowly developing throbbing pain
- Lasts 2–72 h

Phase 4 Resolution
- Sleep is major resolving mechanism
- Vomiting

Phase 5 Postdromal
- 'Washed-out' or drained feeling
- Euphoria
- Impaired concentration
- Irritability
- Cerebral blood flow observations indicate that anomalies can outlast the headache by 24 h

Chronic fatigue syndrome (myalgic encephalomyelitis [ME])

Chronic fatigue syndrome (CFS) is characterised by protracted periods of fatigue associated with a wide range of accompanying symptoms (Box 17.6).

The symptoms of this perplexing illness, known also as myalgic encephalomyelitis (ME), include extreme muscle fatigue, poor memory and concentration and slips of the tongue (Aylett & Fawcett 2003). This condition can cause considerable distress and disability over a period of months and sometimes years. The individual may, with devastating consequences, be unable to continue full or even part-time work or be forced to take frequent periods of sick leave. This, and other implications of the illness, can cause stress to loved ones and adversely affect the well-being of the family as a whole.

Fatigue and depression as sequelae to infections have long been recognised, particularly in relation to Epstein–Barr, Coxsackie and other enteroviruses. It is important, however, that postviral fatigue syndrome is not mistaken for mental illness (Sharpe & Wilks 2002).

Some health professionals advise rest, while others, recognising the adverse effects of long-term inactivity, advise

Box 17.6 Reflection

Chronic fatigue syndrome (CFS/ME)

CFS can present with a wide range of symptoms:

- Substantial impairment in short-term memory or concentration
- Sore throat
- Tender lymph nodes
- Muscle pain
- Multi-joint pain without swelling or redness
- Headaches of a new type, pattern or severity
- Poor sleep
- Post-exertional malaise lasting more than 24 h

Based on data from Sharpe & Wilks (2002) and Aylett & Fawcett (2003).

Activities

- Reflect on the difficulties that people may have in obtaining a diagnosis of CFS/ME given the varied presentation.
- Some health care professionals advise rest, whereas others advise limited exercise. Consider how patients and their families may feel about receiving conflicting advice.
- Access the NICE guidance (http://guidance.nice.org.uk/CG053). How will this guidance help to standardise the management of CFS/ME?

exercise. Good emotional support is vital, and it is most important that depression, where present, is treated. Other treatments are aimed at the detection of possible intercurrent disorder and at maintaining a good diet.

Many patients who are able to undertake a modest amount of exercise report some improvement in symptoms. Conventional treatment approaches to CFS/ME include the prescription of antidepressant medication to promote sleep, and anti-inflammatory medication, i.e. aspirin and ibuprofen, may be prescribed to reduce muscular aches and pains. CAM therapies are sought by many patients who do not find improvement or look to enhance the improvement from conventional medicines. Despite limited scientific evidence, herbal remedies, acupuncture, osteopathy and aromatherapy are widely used for the management of CFS/ME. Recommendations from NICE (2007) have gone some way in recognising the reality and management of this disorder which may be both a cause and consequence of stress.

Irritable bowel syndrome (IBS)

Stressful life events have long been associated with the development of IBS. IBS is a common functional disorder characterised by abdominal pain and altered bowel function. Although IBS is not life threatening, for many patients it can have a serious impact on their daily activities and health-related quality of life. There are several factors which can trigger attacks of IBS in some people, e.g. work stress and examinations.

People with anxious personality traits may find symptoms difficult to control. The relationship between the mind, brain, nervous impulses and overactivity of internal organs such as the gut is complex (Lea & Whorwell 2003). Some patients have reported relaxation techniques, stress counselling, cognitive therapy and psychotherapy useful in controlling symptoms. CAM therapies are also commonly employed in the management of IBS, for example gut-directed hypnotherapy, acupuncture and homeopathy are all used with good effect. Reducing chronic stress is an appropriate and highly achievable therapeutic goal in the management of IBS (Smith 2006).

Depression

Depression is a psychological state of melancholy and dejection that can have physical symptoms. It is not the case that everyone who feels stressed also has depression, but the illness can be the outcome of feelings of stress; conversely, people experiencing depression can also become stressed. An interesting debate in relation to the stress vulnerability model of depression is given by Taylor & Ashelford (2008). The link between stress and depression and other mood disorders is explored in the field of psychoneuroimmunology (Starkweather et al 2005).

The experience of depression seems to range from unpleasant but normal feelings of being 'fed up' to severe states of mental ill-health requiring psychiatric intervention. It is important to recognise that clinical depression, which is a serious mental illness, can be life threatening, as suicide and self-harm are frequent outcomes in severe depression. All health professionals need to be alert to this possibility. Houston et al (2003) argued that the GP, in particular, can play a major role in the detection and management of depression and in the after-care of patients who deliberately self-harm, along with the community psychiatric nurse (CPN).

Symptoms of depression

The presence of depression is often not obvious to the nurse, as observable signs do not always reflect the unpleasantness of the feelings experienced. However, certain symptoms occurring in combination strongly indicate the presence of depression, for example early morning wakening, a feeling of grinding tiredness and loss of energy, of interest in sexual relationships and appetite alongside feeling 'down' and bad tempered. The link between anxiety and depression is debatable, but if this division is dispensed with, the list of potential symptoms of depression might arguably be expanded to include panic or anxiety attacks.

Feelings associated with depression

People experiencing depression often describe their circumstances in terms that denote an ongoing feeling of oppression, as of being under a cloud, of everything looking black or grey, or of being in a tunnel without an end. Feelings of hope diminish, replaced by feelings of helplessness and hopelessness. They often feel uncared for and alone even when this is not the case. Inertia takes the place of activity. Depressed individuals often blame themselves for problems in their relationships or daily lives, where others who are not depressed might show anger. This leads to the hypothesis that depression is anger turned in on itself when for some reason it cannot be expressed openly (Freud 1917, Worden 2002).

Causes of depression

Depression can occur at any time in life and may follow on from any painful event or loss, such as the death of a loved one or the loss of a job. Depression which, when it occurs in adulthood, does not have an obvious cause, may be the result

Box 17.7 Information

Complementary and alternative medicine used in depression

- *Psychological therapies* – cognitive behavioural therapy and relaxation training.
- *Acupuncture* – traditional acupuncture treatment or electroacupuncture can ease depression. Some studies found this to be superior to antidepressant medication and with fewer side-effects.
- *Homeopathy* – various remedies may help. The remedy ignatia is often used to ease grief, pulsatilla may relieve tearfulness, sulphur is often indicated for despair and aurum metallicum, a natural mineral derived from gold, is used for suicidal feelings.
- *Herbal medicine* – the herb St John's wort (*Hypericum perforatum*) has been clinically proven to relieve mild or moderate depression.
- *Reflexology, meditation and yoga* – these have also been used in the treatment of depression but have not yet been tested by research.
- *Light therapy* – exposure to bright light and the use of light boxes can help people suffering from seasonal affective disorder (SAD).

of early childhood loss or distress. Individuals who have been the victims of sexual, physical or emotional abuse as children may suffer depression as adults in a delayed response to the loss associated with abuse, which is triggered by a more recent experience of distress. Early unresolved loss has been suggested as a possible explanation for the distressing symptoms of depression following childbirth. Depression may also be triggered by the lack of light and sunlight exposure during the winter months, known as seasonal affective disorder (SAD). Conventional medical approaches for moderate to severe depression often require antidepressant medication. In milder cases of depression, counselling and psychotherapy may be helpful, in conjunction with lifestyle, exercise and dietary advice. CAM can be used in the treatment and prevention of depression (Box 17.7).

Coping

The concept of coping

Used in a neutral sense, the term 'coping' refers to the way in which the individual responds to a stressful situation or to the perception of threat, by attempting consciously and unconsciously to maintain equilibrium. It is revealing, however, to reflect upon everyday usage of the word, as it can be a value-laden term, used in intrinsically judgemental descriptions of an individual's degree of mastery over a situation or environment. Consider the degree of approval or disapproval that might be implied in the following statements:

- 'She coped well in her first managerial position.'
- 'She cannot cope.'
- 'He finds it difficult to cope with exams.'
- 'He couldn't cope with the patient's relatives.'

The association of 'coping' with mastery and of 'failure to cope' with weakness should not be automatic. It may be the

case that the individual who succumbs to feelings of stress is better able to sense tension in a situation than the person who gives the appearance of coping well. The person who effects their removal from a situation may in fact be 'coping' with it, by acknowledging that distancing or disengagement is the best way, in the circumstances, to preserve emotional health or physical safety. In some situations, the determination to persevere or to achieve mastery may be a damaging choice, ending in disease.

Different situations demand different strategies for coping. In some cases the individual may need to confront a difficulty or overcome an obstacle. In other circumstances, the person must learn how to carry on with their life in the face of an ongoing situation such as bereavement, disability or unemployment. What 'coping' entails will depend upon the individual's unique circumstances and needs, and various models such as resilience and hardiness have been put forward in an attempt to identify the factors that contribute to an individual's style of coping (Klag & Bradley 2004).

Management of stress

Effective stress management techniques can prevent stress-related ailments, boost vitality and improve quality of life. The management of stress can be approached in a number of ways (Box 17.8).

One stress management technique often employed is to offer the individual the opportunity to examine the sources of their stress in present or past experience and to consider ways of modifying their responses to that stress. This therapy can be provided by a psychotherapist, clinical psychologist or qualified counsellor who may also be a nurse.

Some individuals suffering from acute anxiety or depression may find it impossible to confront the source of their difficulty and to make constructive changes without

Box 17.8 Information

Stress management techniques

- *Deep breathing* – this means taking a long, slow breath in, and very slowly breathing out. If you do this a few times, and concentrate fully on breathing, you may find it quite relaxing.
- *Muscular tensing and stretching* – try twisting your neck around each way as far as is comfortable, and then relax. Try fully tensing your shoulder and back muscles for several seconds, and then relax completely.
- *Improve your diet* – reduce caffeine, nicotine, junk foods and sugar, and increase whole grains, vegetables, fruit and water.
- *Vitamins and minerals* – stress puts added strain on the liver and nervous system. To strengthen these, boost intake of B vitamins, vitamin C, zinc and magnesium.
- *List major stresses* and consider solutions or lifestyle changes for each. Prioritise, practise time management and learn to delegate and say, 'No'.
- *Make time for rest and relaxation* and time for yourself on a regular basis.
- *Take regular exercise* to relieve stress and stimulate endorphin production, which has a relaxing effect.

Adapted from the Stress Management Society.

first being given some relief from their distressing feelings. Here, the carefully monitored use of appropriate medication (see below and p. 530) can facilitate recovery and change. The individual suffering from stress can also learn a number of techniques that will assist them to reduce or manage their stress in day-to-day life. The role of CAM in stress management is examined in the next section.

Techniques such as relaxation, yoga, biofeedback, visualisation and meditation have all gained in credibility and popularity in recent years (Thomas et al 2001). When taught effectively and followed up with continuing support, courses in such techniques can help people to adopt a new approach to the problem of stress. Moreover, learning a new skill such as deep relaxation can impart to the individual a feeling of well-being which may facilitate positive change in other areas of their life. However, if stress lies in the interaction between the person and their environment, or in the meaning they attribute to their situation, then clearly a short course on relaxation, for example, cannot hope to address in depth the source of their stress. Indeed, it should be borne in mind that there is a potential for courses in stress reduction to exacerbate the problem, if the individual is made to feel that any stress that is not helped by such techniques offered is intractable or somehow abnormal.

🖰 See website Critical thinking question 17.2

Counselling in stress

Counselling and psychotherapy aim to assist people to overcome the emotional barriers or psychological problems caused by stress and enable them to address their problems and make the life changes needed to improve their health and well-being.

Finding and choosing therapeutic help

There are a number of ways to find therapeutic help and various professional bodies for counselling and psychotherapy will give suggestions, although the availability of some types of psychotherapy will depend upon where in the UK the person seeking help lives. Whilst many people travel long distances to see a counsellor or psychotherapist, the regular nature of the consultations, which may be weekly, may cause an added burden if extensive travel is required.

If psychotherapeutic help is sought through the NHS, a referral can be made by the GP. Many departments of clinical psychology will accept self-referrals, but will ask the person if they may contact their GP. Where the therapy being sought is through the private sector, the person pays a fee for each consultation.

For therapy to be effective, it must respond to the person within their own frame of reference and be relevant to their own life from their own unique perspective. Finding an appropriate form of therapy may be very difficult for the individual, and many people are reluctant to approach a professional agency or voluntary organisation for assistance with personal problems. Many wait for long periods before finding the courage to seek help, and often their first point of contact is with the primary care team at their local surgery; this may be the GP, the practice nurse or another member of the team, such as the health visitor or community psychiatric nurse. The practice nurse, or nurse practitioner undertaking screening programmes, is well placed to be able to listen to patients who are distressed (Cunningham 1996).

Often, just discussing the problem with a member of the practice team can provide considerable relief. However, when further help is required, the patient can be referred to the community mental health team.

The GP may also wish to discuss with the patient the possibility of prescribing antidepressants, whilst also ensuring that a physical illness such as hypothyroidism or anaemia, which can cause symptoms similar to depression, has been excluded. Reassurance can be given that panic attacks are not life threatening and advice given on how to deal with them. The GP can also authorise sick leave to enable the patient to focus on rest and restorative interventions.

The therapist–client relationship

People are highly individual in their feelings, experiences, backgrounds and personalities. A form of therapy which is helpful to one person may not suit another, and a therapist who is helpful to one person may fail to establish a rapport with another. For this reason it is important for therapists to be clear with their clients about the way in which they work, what the work involves, its likely duration and, if private consultation is sought, its cost. It is possible for the client to change therapists if the therapy does not seem to be helpful, although there is one major proviso to this. For personal change to take place, therapist and client must work closely in a relationship of trust. This will enable the therapist to reflect and challenge the behaviour that is causing the client distress. The fact that this can be an unsettling experience for the client may not be the right reason for them to abandon therapy. Nevertheless, the therapist should be willing to discuss any feeling on the client's part that the therapy is proving detrimental or unhelpful and, if appropriate, to give guidance on finding an alternative therapist.

To become a therapist involves undertaking appropriate theoretical education and supervised work with clients. Nurses working in clinical settings may undertake shortened courses which will help them to develop the necessary skills to listen in a therapeutic way to people in their daily work.

Medication

The personal experience of stress can be so severe and overwhelming that the individual becomes unable to take any action to alleviate their feelings. Severe anxiety or depression, perhaps in combination with an overpowering feeling that a serious physical illness is lurking, can have an immobilising effect on the person so that even the prospect of action to alleviate symptoms is daunting. When people feel as severely distressed as this, they may begin to entertain thoughts of suicide.

Medication can help to alleviate severe distress by relieving its most acute symptoms and thus enabling emotional rest to take place. Some medications are intended to help with sleeplessness (see Ch. 25), while others which do not have a tranquillising effect will permit those taking them to continue to work, to problem-solve, to drive, and so on. Medication should always be supplemented by continued monitoring and support by the medical practitioner. The following provides a brief overview of the main types of medication used in the treatment of stress-related conditions.

Tricyclic and related antidepressants

The most common antidepressant medications used in severe stress and depression are the tricyclic and related groups.

The group, which includes amitriptyline, imipramine and related drugs such as trazodone, blocks the reuptake of serotonin (5-hydroxytryptamine) and noradrenaline. Some drugs such as trazodone and clomipramine cause more sedation. Tricyclic antidepressants are usually prescribed to people suffering from moderate to severe depression, although it is important to realise that they work by alleviating symptoms. This can be useful; for instance, the person who is debilitated by anxiety might be able to find ways of living that are more constructive once their feelings of anxiety are lifted. These medications may not be helpful, however, when the depression is related to bereavement, an unhappy working environment, overwhelming family responsibilities or disturbing memories of abuse or neglect, for it is only when the underlying cause of depression can be understood, and appropriately treated, that the person is likely to obtain any lasting benefit.

Management The person prescribed tricyclic antidepressants must be seen frequently following prescription as they may take 2–4 weeks before having a therapeutic effect; during this time the patient may feel isolated and helpless. Side-effects include the following:

- constipation
- sleepiness
- dry mouth
- blurred vision
- urinary retention
- sweating.

Tolerance seems to develop over time and some of the side-effects become less apparent.

If the individual's depression is severe, careful support and perhaps hospitalisation may be essential. Treatment with this group of medications should be continued for at least 1 month (BNF 2008). Reduction or withdrawal should be carried out very slowly to avoid symptoms such as strange and fragmented dreams, headaches, recurrence of anxiety, depression or restlessness.

Selective serotonin reuptake inhibitors (SSRIs)

Serotonin, also known as 5-hydroxytryptamine, is a substance widely distributed in body tissue. Serotonin participates in the transmission of nerve impulses and has a function in controlling mood. SSRIs block the reuptake of serotonin, producing an increase in the amount of the neurotransmitter at central synapses. Examples of commonly prescribed SSRIs for stress-related conditions are citalopram, fluoxetine and paroxetine. In contrast to the tricyclic antidepressants, SSRIs have few antimuscarinic and anticholinergic effects, and cause little sedation or weight gain. They may, however, cause nausea, diarrhoea, insomnia and anorexia.

Benzodiazepines

Drugs belonging to the benzodiazepine class include diazepam, flurazepam, temazepam, etc.; they have different durations of action. They are used as anxiolytics or as hypnotics. They act at a specific central nervous system receptor or by potentiating the action of inhibitory neurotransmitters to help calm patients and promote rest and sleep. They are therefore used to help treat, but not cure, the symptoms of anxiety, such as tension, tremor, sweating and disturbed thought processes.

However, this class of medication fell into disrepute when individuals who were taking the medication for extended periods of time found that their original symptoms were intensified and that the medication was addictive. It is now recommended that benzodiazepines are prescribed for periods not exceeding 2 or 3 weeks and under careful supervision (BNF 2008).

Monoamine oxidase inhibitors

Monoamine oxidase inhibitors (MAOIs) prevent the breakdown of monoamine neurotransmitters, thereby prolonging their action. Monoamines, which include noradrenaline, dopamine and tyramine, play an important role in the metabolism of the brain. MAOIs are recommended for people with depression, anxiety and somatic complaints, for patients who do not respond to tricyclics and patients with agoraphobia. They are used less commonly than tricyclic antidepressants or SSRIs because of dangers of dietary and medication interactions.

Beta-adrenoceptor-blocking drugs

Beta-adrenoceptor-blocking drugs, also called beta-blockers, act by blocking the stimulation of beta-adrenergic receptors by the neurotransmitters adrenaline and noradrenaline. These are produced at the nerve endings of that part of the sympathetic nervous system which facilitates the body's reaction to anxiety, stress and exercise. Beta-blockers act to reduce anxiety and some physical symptoms, such as trembling, which are caused by a stress reaction. They are particularly useful for situational anxiety. For example, some musicians who become stressed take a beta-blocker to ease their shakiness before a concert performance.

Alcohol and stress

It is commonly believed that a way to cope with stress is to use alcohol. However, although alcohol may give short-term relief of stress, in the long run it does not, and drinking alcohol to 'calm nerves' is often a slippery slope to heavier and problem drinking. For most people who stay within the recommended drinking levels, alcohol can be an enjoyable part of relaxation and socialising. However, the more an individual uses alcohol to relieve stress, the less effective it becomes. Eventually, more and more alcohol is required to achieve the desired effect of relaxation. The after-effects of alcohol may also increase feelings of anxiety and depression.

Other means of stress reduction

The other stress-reducing methods discussed here are CAM, exercise and relaxation.

Complementary and alternative medicine

There is an increasing interest in the use of CAM in stress management. Examples of CAM therapies are:

- osteopathy
- chiropractice
- herbal medicine
- acupuncture
- homeopathy.

Other well-known therapies include hypnotherapy, aromatherapy and massage, all of which are increasingly used in stress management. CAM focuses on the whole person, with lifestyle, environment, diet, mental, emotional and spiritual health being considered alongside physical symptoms. Many CAM therapies are based on the belief that the body naturally strives to maintain emotional equilibrium. Interventions aim to stimulate this natural propensity. Taking responsibility for one's own health is regarded as an important part of healing, so clients are often actively involved in their own therapy. For example, self-hypnosis techniques are employed in hypnotherapy (Gonsalkorale et al 2002).

Exercise

Although there is both research-based and anecdotal evidence that regular physical exercise has a positive effect upon the individual's ability to deal with feelings of depression and stress, the effects of exercise are not generally accepted or understood (Ströhle 2009). For instance, those taking physical exercise may have considerable exposure to light and this, in itself, may have a therapeutic effect upon feelings of depression (Groom & O'Connor 1996). Proponents of exercise as a means of stress reduction argue that exercise may be essential for psychological, physiological and social development, having a direct effect upon feelings of self-esteem (Segar et al 1998). Exercise works in a paradoxical manner in reducing stress. It is itself a physical stressor causing an acute stress response but nonetheless functions as a relaxant. The physiological effects of exercise include increased blood flow and oxygen consumption, as well as changes in blood pressure, heart rate, respiration and metabolic rate.

Physical exercise acts as a relaxant for a number of reasons:

- Most exercise involves effort and concentration and thus it can be difficult to sustain anxious thoughts whilst engaged in physical exercise.
- Meeting a physical challenge can give the individual a sense of achievement.

- During strenuous exercise the body produces noradrenaline and endorphins; these substances help to alleviate depression and arguably bring about feelings of happiness and tranquillity (Pert 1997).
- Exercise can be taken in the company of other people and so can diminish feelings of social isolation.

Relaxation

Relaxation has long been known to help alleviate feelings of stress and to enhance health-seeking behaviour (Vines 1994). Relaxation may take various forms, including relieving muscle tension, e.g. through exercise, taking time off, either on a daily or weekly basis or as a scheduled holiday, and meditation. Everly & Benson (1989), Knight (1995) and Nyklicek & Kuijpers (2008) have discussed the response elicited physiologically and psychologically by certain types of meditative relaxation, identifying components of these meditation techniques which cause the relaxation response and a reduction in feelings of stress.

There are six types of activity which specifically foster this type of meditative relaxation:

- meditation/mindfulness-based stress reduction (MBSR)
- autogenic training
- pre-suggestion hypnosis
- prayer (repetitive or liturgical)
- yoga exercises
- t'ai chi chu'an.

For many people, these techniques produce a sense of well-being as well as an increase in concentration and energy.

It is argued that, during relaxation, there are physiological alterations consistent with a decrease in central and peripheral adrenergic excitation, and a reduction in stress-induced psychological or physiological responses and proinflammatory cytokines (Koh et al 2008). Those who undertake regular meditative relaxation (Box 17.9) appear to recover faster from stressful events than those who do not relax in this way.

 Box 17.9 Information

Guidelines for meditative relaxation

Setting the scene

- Find a quiet, warm, comfortable room where you are unlikely to be disturbed (try to exclude children, pets, ticking clocks or telephones).
- Meditate sitting upright and well supported in a comfortable chair. Rest the feet flat on the floor and the hands loosely in your lap.
- Have a watch or clock in clear view. The session lasts 20 minutes. If you feel that you are likely to fall asleep, set an alarm.
- Loosen any tight clothing; slip off your shoes if this makes you more comfortable.
- Meditate whilst neither too hungry nor too full.
- Try to meditate twice each day for 20 minutes. Because you may feel deeply relaxed, it is better not to meditate close to bedtime, as this might interfere with your sleep patterns.

The process

During the process of meditation you will remain completely conscious.

- You may prefer to meditate with your eyes closed. Begin the process by taking one or two deep, relaxing breaths.
- Gently begin to count, either on each inhalation or exhalation, with the number one, then two, then three… Every time you become aware of a thought, any thought, calmly return to number one. It is unlikely, though, that after a number of years of regular meditating you will go beyond the number one; indeed, the principle of this sort of meditation is not one of mastery, but of the gentle pushing aside of thoughts to enable the body and the mind to achieve complete rest.
- You may find that you have spent the whole session thinking over a problem. If so, do not worry; before you finish the session gently return to the counting, for 1 or 2 minutes.
- If you find that you have fallen asleep, do not worry about this. It may be that you are very tired and your body needs sleep. Before finishing the relaxation, gently return to the counting for 1 or 2 minutes. If you find that during the meditation you have solved a major problem, written a poem or worked out a solution, before finishing the session, gently return to your counting.

At the end of the session, before moving, stretch gently and sit with the eyes closed for a few moments.

SUMMARY: KEY NURSING ISSUES

- Stress is not in itself a pathological or abnormal phenomenon. Having the optimal amount of stress to keep us performing at our best, adapting to life's daily challenges, is called eustress, good stress.

- Stress (distress) means that our functional adaptability to the daily challenges is impaired in some way, the stressor exceeding the ability to cope.

- Stress can be closely associated with serious physical, emotional or mental health problems, including heart disease and depression.

- Stress can also give rise to detrimental coping behaviours such as drug, alcohol and other forms of substance misuse.

- For this reason it is vital that stress is taken seriously by health professionals and that its mechanisms and effects are clearly understood.

- From the nurse's perspective, the most important aspect of the experience of stress is its uniqueness for each individual. The experience of stress, like the experience of pain, must be assessed in each person, and approaches to stress management must be congruent with the individual's personality, experiences and values.

- Nurses need to acquire both a theoretical and a practical understanding of stress and its effects, whereby they are equipped to provide a positive contribution to the therapeutic management of stress and stress-related disorders in their patients.

- In addition such knowledge and understanding will also allow the nurse to recognise and rise to the challenge of stress in their own professional and personal life.

REFLECTION AND LEARNING – WHAT NEXT?

- **Test** your knowledge by visiting the website 🖱 and answering the multiple choice questions and critical thinking questions.

- **Consolidate** your learning by looking at some of the further reading suggestions, references and specialist websites.

- **Revisit** some of the additional material on the website.

- **Consider** what you have learnt and how this will help your professional development.

- **Reflect** on how you can apply this knowledge to the care of your patients.

- **Discuss** your learning with your mentor/supervisor, lecturer and colleagues.

REFERENCES

Aylett E, Fawcett TN: Chronic fatigue syndrome: the nurse's role, *Nursing Standard* 17(35):33–37, 2003.

Benner P, Wrubel J: *The primacy of caring*, London, 1989, Addison Wesley.

Biondi DM: Is migraine a neuropathic syndrome? *Curr Pain Headache Rep* 10(3):167–178, 2006.

Blau JN, editor: *Migraine: clinical, therapeutic, conceptual and research aspects*, London, 1987, Chapman and Hall, Ch 11, pp 185–204.

British National Formulary, 2008. (No 56). Available online http://www. bnf.org/.

Cannon WB: Stresses and strains of homeostasis, *American Journal of Medical Science* 189:1, 1935.

Cooper CL: *Handbook of stress, medicine and health*, ed 2, London, 2004, CRC Press.

Cunningham J: For better or for worse, *Practice Nurse* 12(10):624–627, 1996.

Egan G: *The skilled helper: a systematic approach to effective helping*, Pacific Grove, CA, 1997, Brooks/Cole.

Everly GS, Benson H: Disorders of arousal and the relaxation response: speculations on the nature and treatment of stress related diseases, *Int J Psychosom* 36(1–4):15–21, 1989.

Fagan N, Freme K: Confronting post traumatic stress disorder, *Nursing* 34(2):52–53, 2004.

Fox SI: *Human physiology*, ed 8, Boston, 2004, McGraw-Hill.

Freud S: *Mourning and melancholia. Standard edition* (vol XIV), London, 1917, Hogarth Press.

Gillespie BM, Chaboyer W, Wallis M: Development of a theoretically derived model of resilience through concept analysis, *Contemp Nurse* 25(1–2):124–125, 2007.

Gonsalkorale WM, Houghton LA, Whorwell PJ: Hypnotherapy in irritable bowel syndrome: a large scale audit of a clinical service with examination of factors influencing responsiveness, *Am J Gastroenterol* 94:954–961, 2002.

Griggs C, Jenson J: Effectiveness of acupuncture for migraine: critical literature review, *J Adv Nurs* 54(4):491–501, 2006.

Groom KN, O'Connor ME: Relation of light and exercise to seasonal depressive symptoms: preliminary development of a scale, *Percept Mot Skills* 83(2):379–383, 1996.

Hall DS: Work-related stress of registered nurses in a hospital setting, *J Nurses Staff Dev* 20(1):6–14, 2004.

Hesselink AE, Penninx BW, Schlosser MA, Wijnhoven HA: The role of coping resources and coping style in quality of life of patients with asthma and COPD, *Qual Life Res* 13(2):509–518, 2004.

Houston K, Haw D, Townsend E, Hawton K: General practitioner contacts with patients before and after deliberate self harm, *British Journal of General Practitioners* 53(490):365–370, 2003.

Jacelon CS: The trait and process of resilience, *J Adv Nurs* 25(1):123–129, 1997.

Jung S: The impact of migraine: a case study, *J Neurosci Nurs* 39(4):213–216, 2007.

Kennedy E, Charles SC: *On becoming a counsellor: the basic guide for non-professional counsellors*, London, 2002, Newleaf Publications.

Kessler RC, Soukup J, Davis RB, et al: The use of complementary and alternative therapies to treat anxiety and depression in the United States, *Am J Psychiatry* 158(2):289–294, 2001.

Klag S, Bradley G: The role of hardiness in stress and illness: an exploration of the effect of negativity, affectivity and gender, *Br J Health Psychol* 9(Pt 20):137–161, 2004.

Knight S: Use of transcendental meditation to relieve stress and promote health, *Br J Nurs* 4(6):315–318, 1995.

Koh KB, Lee YJ, Beyn KM, et al: Counter-stress effects of relaxation on proinflammatory and antiinflammatory cytokines, *Brain Behav Immun* 22(8):1130–1137, 2008.

Lazarus RS: *Psychological stress and the coping process*, New York, 1966, McGraw-Hill.

Lazarus RS, Folkman S: *Stress, appraisal, and coping*, New York, 1984, Springer.

Lea R, Whorwell PJ: New insights into the psychosocial aspects of irritable bowel syndrome, *Curr Gastroenterol Rep* 5:343–350, 2003.

Levi L, editor: *Society, stress and disease*, vol 1, Oxford, 1971, Oxford University Press, pp 280–366.

McEwan BS, Wingfield JC: The concept of allostasis in biology and biomedicine, *Horm Behav* 43(1):2–15, 2003.

National Institute for Health and Clinical Excellence (NICE): *Chronic fatigue syndrome/myalgic encephalomyelitis (or encephalopathy): diagnosis and management of CFS/ME in adults and children*, 2007. Available online http://guidance.nice.org.uk/CG053.

Nyklicek I, Kuijpers KF: Effects of mindfulness-based stress reduction intervention on psychological well-being and quality of life: is increased mindfulness indeed the mechanism? *Ann Behav Med* 35(3):331–340, 2008.

Pert C: *Molecules of emotion*, London, 1997, Simon and Schuster.

Polk LV: Towards a middle-range theory of resilience, *Advanced Nursing Science* 19(3):1–13, 1997.

Rhoads L, Pearman T, Rick S: PTSD: therapeutic interventions post Katrina, *Crit Care Nurs Clin North Am* 20(1):73–81, 2008.

Rogers CR: *On becoming a person*, London, 1974, Constable.

Segar ML, Katch VL, Roth RS, et al: The effect of aerobic exercise on self-esteem and depressive and anxiety symptoms among breast cancer survivors, *Oncol Nurs Forum* 25(1):107–113, 1998.

Selye H: Syndrome produced by diverse nocuous agents, *Nature (London)* 138:32, 1936.

Selye H: The general adaptation syndrome and the diseases of adaptation, *Journal of Clinical Endocrinology* 6:117, 1946a.

Selye H: What is stress? *Metabolism* 5:525, 1946b.

Selye H: *The stress of life*, New York, 1976, McGraw-Hill.

Sharpe M, Wilks D: ABC of psychological medicine: fatigue, *Br Med J* 325(7362):480–483, 2002.

Smith GD: Irritable bowel syndrome: Quality of life and nursing interventions, *Br J Nurs* 15(21):1152–1156, 2006.

Starkweather A, Witek-Janusek L, Matthews HL: Applying the psychoneuroimmunology framework to nursing research, *J Neurosci Nurs* 7(1):56–62, 2005.

Ströhle A: Physical activity, exercise, depression and anxiety disorders, *J Neural Transm* 116:777–784, 2009.

Sutherland VJ, Cooper CL: *Strategic stress management*, London, 2000, Macmillan.

Taylor V, Ashelford S: Understanding depression in palliative and end-of-life care, *Nurs Stand* 23(12):48–57, 2008.

Thomas KJ, Coleman P, Nichol JP: Use and expenditure on complementary medicine in England: a population based survey, *Complement Ther Med* 9:2–11, 2001.

Vines SW: Relaxation with guided imagery: effects on employees' psychological distress and health seeking behaviors, *American Association of Occupational Health Nursing Journal* 42(5):206–213, 1994.

Watson R, Fawcett TN: *Pathophysiology, homeostasis and nursing*, London, 2003, Routledge.

Wingfield JC: Anniversary Essay: Control of behavioural strategies for capricious environments, *Anim Behav* 66(5):807–816, 2003.

Worden JW: *Grief counselling and grief therapy: a handbook for the mental health practitioner*, ed 3, London, 2002, Routledge.

FURTHER READING

Bowlby J: *Attachment and loss: loss, sadness and depression* (vol 3), London, 1980, Tavistock.

Cunningham SM: Migraine: helping clients choose the right treatment and identify triggers, *Br J Nurs* 8(22):1515–1523, 1999.

Diamond S, Franklin MA: *Conquering your migraine*, London, 2001, Simon and Schuster.

Dryden W: *Individual therapy*, Milton Keynes, 1990, Open University Press.

Healy D: *Psychiatric drugs explained*, ed 5, Edinburgh, 2009, Churchill Livingstone.

Palmer JA, Palmer LK, Michiels K, Thigpen B: Effects of type of exercise on depression in recovering substance abusers, *Percept Mot Skills* 80(2):523–530, 1995.

Parkes CM: *Bereavement*, London, 1972, Tavistock.

Parkes CM: Determinants of outcome following bereavement, *Omega* 6:303–323, 1972.

Payne RA: *Relaxation techniques*, ed 3, Edinburgh, 2005, Churchill Livingstone.

Segar ML, Katch V, L Roth RS, et al: The effect of aerobic exercise on self-esteem and depressive and anxiety symptoms among breast cancer survivors, *Oncol Nurs Forum* 25(1):107–113, 1998.

USEFUL WEBSITES

International Stress Management Association (UK): www.isma.org.uk

Migraines.net: http://migraines.net

Mind Tools: www.mindtools.com

Stress Coping (Counselling, Strategies & Management Advice): www.stress-counselling.co.uk

Stress Management Society: www.stress.org.uk

Stressbusting.co.uk: www.stressbusting.co.uk

The National Center for Complementary and Alternative Medicine (NCCAM), part of the US National Institutes of Health: nccam.nih.gov

UK National Work-Stress Network: www.workstress.net

Recognising and managing shock

Carol Ball

Introduction

Despite advances in diagnosis, treatment and management, shock remains one of the leading causes of death in the acutely ill patient (Dellinger et al 2008). It is important that nurses from all areas of clinical practice have the knowledge required to identify patients at risk and ensure timely and appropriate intervention is carried out. Identification of the acutely deteriorating patient is a key function of the nurse. The timely and accurate recording of vital signs is an essential part of this identification. Allied to this is the appropriate escalation of management to the appropriate personnel (NICE 2007). The aim of this chapter is to help you understand the pathophysiology of shock and the associated care as this is the responsibility of all nurses.

In any clinical environment, awareness of the predisposing factors which may lead to shock, early detection and prompt action are vital for a good prognosis. Caring for patients who are suffering from shock requires not only an understanding of the pathophysiology of shock and the principles of its treatment and management, but also an awareness of the devastating psychological and social impact such a sudden change from health to illness can have on patients and their families.

The pathophysiology of shock

Circulatory homeostasis exists when the circulating blood volume and the vascular tone of blood vessels are in dynamic equilibrium (Marieb & Hoehn 2007, pp. 733–742). Shock is a state in which tissue perfusion is inadequate to maintain the supply of oxygen and nutrients necessary for normal cellular function and disequilibrium ensues. If there is an inadequate supply of oxygen and nutrients to two or more organs this is known as multi-organ dysfunction and indicates that the patient is at significant risk of becoming critically ill if appropriate treatment is not given immediately (Richards & Edwards 2003).

Tissue perfusion is reflected by the arterial blood pressure (Marieb & Hoehn 2007, pp. 723–733). Hypotension (systolic blood pressure below 90 mmHg or a mean arterial pressure of below 70 mmHg) is a result of either inadequate cardiac output or low systemic vascular resistance. Glomerular filtration (see Ch. 8) is dependent on an adequate blood pressure and in the presence of hypotension the urine output will drop (Marieb & Hoehn 2007, pp. 1007–1011). Inadequate perfusion to the brain may induce a change in behaviour which could be manifested through decreased arousal or agitation. Decreased arousal can be assessed using a simple mnemonic, AVPU – **A**lert; responds to **V**oice; responds to **P**ain; **U**nconscious (McNarry & Goldhill 2004). In order to maintain cardiac output, in the presence of hypotension, the heart rate will rise (Marieb & Hoehn 2007, pp. 698–705). To maintain adequate oxygenation it is likely that the respiratory rate will also increase. Thus shock is evident in the presence of:

- a systolic blood pressure below 90 mmHg (or 40 mmHg below the usual systolic pressure)
- a rising heart rate (particularly if this is over 100 beats per minute) and respiratory rate (over 25 breaths per minute)
- a lowered urine output (below 0.5 mL/kg/h or less than 30 mL/h)
- an altered level of consciousness.

Of these the most important observation is a fall in blood pressure, which will require immediate attention.

Shock may be the result of a reduced amount of blood returning to the heart (inadequate ventricular filling), an inability of the heart to contract with sufficient strength (reduced ventricular contractility) or a decrease in the resistance to blood flow caused by dilation of the blood vessels (decreased systemic vascular resistance). Shock may be classified as follows (Bridges & Dukes 2005):

- hypovolaemic – a reduction in circulating blood volume (e.g. haemorrhage, burns, diarrhoea, inadequate fluid intake, excessive urine output)
- cardiogenic – a decrease in myocardial contractility (e.g. myocardial ischaemia, myocardial infarction)
- obstructive – an obstruction to blood flow in the circulation (e.g. pulmonary embolus, cardiac tamponade)
- distributive – a decrease in systemic vascular resistance (e.g. septic, neurogenic, spinal or anaphylactic shock).

The stages of shock

Shock represents a complex set of physiological reactions which comprise activation of the sympathetic nervous and immune systems, hormonal response and metabolic derangement (Marieb & Hoehn 2007, pp. 740–742). To interpret the signs and symptoms that present and the appropriate management of shock it is necessary to understand these underlying physiological reactions. These can be divided into four stages:

1 initial stage
2 compensatory stage
3 progressive stage
4 refractory stage.

It is important to understand that the stages of shock comprise continuous and complex processes. There is usually no sudden transition from one stage to the next, although some individuals may progress rapidly through the four stages.

The initial stage

At this point there are no signs and symptoms but cellular changes begin to occur in response to a disturbance in cell perfusion and oxygenation.

The compensatory stage

In this stage physiological adaptations occur in an attempt to overcome the original problem, e.g. hypovolaemia. The

compensatory stage strives to maintain cardiac output, which comprises stroke volume and heart rate (CO = SV × HR, see Ch. 2). In the absence of direct measurement of cardiac output, blood pressure and central venous pressure are used as surrogates in the assessment of cardiac output. The normal cardiac output is approximately 5 L, as is circulating volume. When circulation becomes inadequate due to a reduction in circulating volume, diminished myocardial contractility or massive vasodilatation, various mechanisms are activated in response to hypotension, hypoxaemia, acidosis or a combination of these.

Sympathetic nervous system Hypotension leads to decreased stimulation of the aortic and carotid sinus baroreceptors (Marieb & Hoehn 2007, pp. 727–732). This reduces impulses to the vasomotor centre and thus activates vasoconstriction. Stimulation of the sympathetic nervous system occurs, resulting in activation of the stress response. Catecholamines, namely adrenaline and noradrenaline, are released from the adrenal medulla (Marieb & Hoehn 2007, pp. 631). The stimulation of alpha-adrenergic receptors by the catecholamines results in vasoconstriction of the skin, kidneys, gastrointestinal tract and other organs together with a rise in heart rate (Marieb & Hoehn 2007, pp. 543). This demonstrates an attempt to preserve the blood supply to the heart and brain. Conversely, beta-adrenergic receptors stimulate vasodilation in the lungs and skeletal muscle. Vasoconstriction may initially restore the arterial blood pressure to normal, but peripheral resistance will be raised, making the myocardium work harder to maintain cardiac output. Urine output and peristalsis will decrease, and the individual's skin will become pale and cool. Sympathetic nervous system stimulation will also result in increased respiratory rate and depth, dilated pupils and increased sweat gland activity, causing the 'clammy' skin typically found in all forms of shock, other than early septic and anaphylactic shock.

Immune response The disorder to blood flow caused by generalised vasoconstriction results in the production of proinflammatory mediators by neutrophils and macrophages (Marieb & Hoehn 2007, pp. 657–660). These include interleukins 1, 6 and 8, TNFα and prostaglandins (Greenwood & Murgo 2007). They are designed to fight foreign antigens and promote wound healing (Marieb & Hoehn 2007, pp. 790–798). At the same time anti-inflammatory mediators are produced to ameliorate the effect of these. If homeostasis is not regained then the proinflammatory mediators proliferate and damage to the endothelium occurs (Marieb & Hoehn 2007, p. 120). Neutrophils adhere to the damaged endothelium and produce more proinflammatory mediators which in turn activate the clotting cascade through the production of platelet activating factor. Small clots form which, in addition to vasoconstriction, disrupt blood flow through the organs resulting in reduced delivery of oxygen and glucose to the cells. The composition of endothelial cells is also disrupted by proinflammatory mediators and the movement of water and plasma proteins from the intravascular to the extravascular space becomes apparent in the formation of oedema.

Hormonal response Adrenaline (epinephrine) stimulates the anterior pituitary gland to release adrenocorticotrophic hormone (ACTH), which causes the adrenal cortex to release glucocorticoids such as hydrocortisone and mineralocorticoids such as aldosterone (Marieb & Hoehn 2007, pp. 616, 626–629).

Glucocorticoids raise blood sugar by increasing gluconeogenesis and thereby the availability of glucose for energy. In addition, the glucocorticoids mobilise amino acids from the tissues and decrease protein synthesis. They also reduce glucose uptake by the cells and mobilise fatty acids from the adipose tissue into the plasma. Cortisol shifts cell metabolism from glucose to fatty acids for energy, enhancing fatty acid oxidation, and also reduces tissue destruction by stabilising lysosomal membranes.

Aldosterone increases reabsorption of sodium and chloride by the kidney. To maintain electrolyte balance at the renal tubular level, the excretion of potassium and hydrogen ions is increased. Thus hypokalaemia can occur. A higher concentration of sodium chloride raises the serum osmolality stimulating the hypothalamic osmoreceptors. In turn this leads to the release of antidiuretic hormone (ADH) from the posterior pituitary gland (Marieb & Hoehn 2007, pp. 627–628).

ADH stimulates an increase in renal tubular water reabsorption, in an attempt to augment circulating volume and blood pressure whilst restoring normal serum osmolality (Marieb & Hoehn 2007, pp. 617–619). Urine output is diminished.

Renin is secreted by the kidney in response to secretion of noradrenaline by the adrenal medulla, which results in renal artery vasoconstriction. In the circulation, renin reacts with angiotensinogen, producing angiotensin I. This is converted by an enzyme in the lungs to angiotensin II, which causes venous constriction and increases aldosterone release, thus leading to increased fluid and sodium retention, increased blood volume and therefore increased venous return, blood pressure and renal perfusion (Marieb & Hoehn 2007, p. 628).

Thyroxine secreted by the thyroid gland sensitises the beta-receptors in the heart to noradrenaline and so increases heart rate, systolic pressure, stroke volume and cardiac output (Marieb & Hoehn 2007, p. 620).

The classic clinical picture at this stage of shock is cool, pale, clammy skin, decreased urinary output and increased heart rate. However, this is not the case in septic, anaphylactic and neurogenic shock, which present with vasodilatation and the skin appears warm and pink. This can be misleading but the disorder to blood flow through the organs, due to a relative reduction in blood volume caused by the vasodilatation, is such that a decreased urine output and tachycardia will still be apparent. The patient may be anxious, restless or confused due to the cerebral effects of hypoxia and sympathetic nervous system stimulation. Anxiety will intensify the physiological responses to stress and thus it is very important for the nurse to provide much needed reassurance to both the patient and any relatives during this major life crisis.

The progressive stage

Now the compensatory mechanisms begin to fail and produce adverse effects. This disturbance progresses to a change from aerobic to anaerobic cellular metabolism, in which production of lactic acid and pyruvic acid leads to metabolic acidosis. Although the compensatory mechanisms may appear at first to reverse the effects of shock, if the cause is not treated appropriately then the next stage of shock soon becomes evident.

If tissue perfusion is not restored and blood flow through the organs remains erratic then the supply of oxygen and glucose to the cells will be inadequate to produce sufficient adenosine triphosphate (ATP) (Marieb & Hoehn 2007, p. 57). The sodium pump will fail and the amount of intracellular calcium increase. Anaerobic metabolism by the cell, which results from an inadequate oxygen supply, will increase the production of lactic acid resulting in a metabolic acidosis (pH <7.35) (Edwards 2008).

Prolonged disruption to the supply of oxygen and glucose and the consequent impact on cell function will soon compromise the functioning of the vital organs, as follows:

- The lungs will become less compliant as fluid and plasma proteins leak from the pulmonary capillaries into the alveoli, leading to pulmonary oedema and acute lung injury. This in turn affects gaseous exchange reducing the diffusion of oxygen into the blood. Thus, hypoxaemia is evident in a reduced peripheral oxygen saturation (SpO_2) and partial pressure of oxygen (PaO_2). In the early stages a higher respiratory rate will demonstrate an attempt to increase oxygen supplies, and a corresponding drop in carbon dioxide levels will be apparent. However, in the later stages of shock carbon dioxide levels may increase, even though it is a more soluble gas, if the pulmonary oedema intensifies and the acute lung injury deteriorates to acute respiratory distress syndrome (ARDS, see Ch. 3). Hypercapnia is demonstrated through a rising partial pressure of carbon dioxide ($PaCO_2$).
- Myocardial workload will be increased due to the increased heart rate caused by stimulation of the sympathetic nervous system and the effort made to eject blood from the left ventricle (stroke volume) against the high peripheral resistance caused by vasoconstriction. Even if vasodilatation is evident the heart rate will still be raised due to the relative drop in the amount of blood returning to the heart. The heart will eventually fail as coronary perfusion and oxygen supply become inadequate to meet the demands of the myocardium.
- The kidneys will be unable to filter, reabsorb and excrete fluid normally. Urine will become concentrated in appearance, osmolality will increase and output will be reduced to below 0.5 mL/kg/h. Acute tubular necrosis may occur (see Ch. 8), causing a marked rise in blood creatinine and urea.
- Alteration in cerebral function may have a number of effects, ranging from a dulling of responses to major behavioural changes.
- Ischaemic damage to the intestinal mucosa will potentially result in the release of bacteria and toxins from the gut into the circulation.
- Pancreatic cells will release the enzymes amylase and lipase into the circulation, contributing to the formation of myocardial depressant factor (MDF), which decreases myocardial contractility.

The refractory stage

In this stage pathophysiological processes are set in motion that cannot be arrested or reversed. Death is imminent.

Continuing circulatory collapse, an inability to restore circulating blood volume, increasing metabolic acidosis and the formation of micro-emboli will all contribute to decreased tissue perfusion (Marieb & Hoehn 2007). Inadequate ventilation will lead to increasingly inadequate oxygenation. Renal failure will contribute to increasing metabolic abnormalities, and vital centres in the brain will eventually cease to function due to ischaemia and hypoxia. If the refractory stage is reached, shock is irreversible and death will occur.

Types of shock

The following sections describe the distinguishing features of hypovolaemic shock, cardiogenic shock, obstructive shock and the different forms of distributive shock (Skinner & Jonas 2007). It is essential that deterioration in the patient's condition is communicated effectively and escalated to experienced staff. This is addressed in a later section of this chapter. (See Boxes 18.1, 18.2.)

Hypovolaemic shock

This is the most common type of shock. Its primary cause is loss of fluid from the circulation, which may be described as:

Box 18.1 Reflection

Prevention is better than cure

Two days ago Mrs R underwent a hysterectomy with bilateral salpingo-oophorectomy to remove a dermoid cyst. She required blood and crystalloid replacement following surgery but is now eating and drinking. The area around her intravenous cannula is now looking red and swollen, her blood pressure is 80/50 mmHg, pulse rate 110 and temperature 39°C.

Activity:
• What might have been done to avoid this problem?
Answer: remove the intravenous cannula when no longer required.

Box 18.2 Reflection

What type of shock are you observing?

Mr W is obese and has type 2 diabetes. Recently he fell at home, following a non-ST elevation myocardial infarction, and sustained a subdural haematoma. This afternoon he has complained of an ache on the left side of his chest, affecting his arm and jaw. This was thought to be related to his recent fall. You have just taken his observations and note he is very drowsy, temperature 36.5°C, blood pressure 80/60 mmHg, heart rate 80 and the pulse feels 'thready'; skin is cold to touch and appears cyanosed.

Activity
• What type of shock are you observing?
Answer: cardiogenic shock.

• *External fluid loss* – due to external bleeding, vomiting, diarrhoea, overuse of diuretics or burns.
• *Internal fluid loss* – due to internal bleeding such as haemothorax or bleeding into tissues at fracture sites after injuries, paralytic ileus, intestinal obstruction or acute dilatation of the stomach. Although hidden, the effects of internal fluid loss can be very serious. For example, 1 litre (approximately 20% of the blood volume of an average person) or more of fluid may be sequestered (i.e. lost from the circulation) in the gastrointestinal tract during paralytic ileus and/or acute dilatation of the stomach, and the same volume or more of blood may escape into the tissues and/or thorax as a result of multiple injuries.

The physiological implications of hypovolaemia are:

• reduced blood volume
↓
• decreased venous return
↓
• decreased cardiac output
↓
• reduced tissue perfusion.

In early hypovolaemic shock, the compensatory mechanisms described (see above) are activated when the blood pressure starts to fall. These mechanisms will compensate for up to 10% reduction of the circulating volume of a healthy person without the development of marked symptoms. However, if a greater volume of fluid is lost and is not replaced quickly, the compensatory mechanisms may fail quite suddenly, in which case the patient's condition will deteriorate rapidly. It should be recognised that, in older people, the cardiovascular system is often less able to cope with haemodynamic changes, and the heart may be less able to pump faster and harder in order to maintain cardiac output against high peripheral resistance.

Recognising hypovolaemic shock

The following signs and symptoms of hypovolaemic shock are reliable only if they are considered in relation to one another and the patient's previous, stable condition. Nevertheless, when several of these indicators occur together the possibility of shock should be considered as a successful outcome depends upon early intervention. It is essential that the measurement of vital signs is done manually as it is impossible to ascertain respiratory rate and the characteristics of a pulse when using electronic machines. The nurse should be alert to the following:

• rapid and deep respirations, in response to sympathetic nervous system stimulation, hypoxia and acidosis
• a rapid, weak, thready pulse, due to low blood flow despite a rapid heart rate
• systolic blood pressure below 90 mmHg
• narrowing of the pulse pressure, i.e. a reduced difference between systolic and diastolic pressures due to decreased stroke volume and increased peripheral resistance indicating vasoconstriction of the skin and viscera, reflecting decreased blood flow

- anxiety, restlessness and confusion, which may indicate decreased cerebral perfusion and oxygenation
- cool, clammy skin and cold peripheries, due to vasoconstriction and sympathetic stimulation of sweat glands
- decreased urinary output, due to renal artery vasoconstriction and endocrine compensatory mechanisms
- lowered body temperature, which may be related to altered metabolism, perfusion and oxygenation and, possibly, heat loss caused by evaporation of sweat from the skin
- thirst and a dry mouth related to fluid depletion and possibly to sympathetic nervous system stimulation
- fatigue, probably related to inadequate perfusion and oxygenation of the tissues and vital organs.

It is relatively easy to diagnose hypovolaemic shock when a patient is bleeding externally. Diagnosis is more difficult when hypovolaemia is developing as a consequence of an internal crisis. Nurses must be alert to recognise the above signs and context of the crisis and to ensure that prompt action is taken and/or help is sought.

Cardiogenic shock

Primary angioplasty and progress in the prevention, detection and treatment of coronary heart disease over the past eight years has led to a 40% reduction in cardiovascular disease related deaths (Department of Health [DH] 2008). Cardiogenic shock is far less prevalent than in the previous decade; however, coronary heart disease is still responsible for death in 1 in 5 men and 1 in 6 women (DH 2008).

The clinical definition of cardiogenic shock is hypotension with evidence of impaired perfusion of the coronary arteries, in the presence of acute myocardial infarction (see Ch. 2). A variety of other causes such as myocardial contusion, myocarditis and cardiomyopathy can produce cardiogenic shock, but the majority of cases result from atherosclerosis and the resulting myocardial necrosis (cell death due to interruption of the blood supply) (Jowett & Thompson 2007). Ischaemic muscle is deprived of adequate oxygen and substrates for effective contraction, and infarcted muscle or scar tissue is unable to contract. When more than approximately 40% of the left ventricle is infarcted the ability to maintain the systemic circulation is significantly impaired.

The compensatory mechanisms that normally act to prevent hypotension can worsen the situation. The catecholamine release produces tachycardia, vasoconstriction and increased cardiac contractility. All these increase myocardial oxygen demand and the workload of the left ventricle, potentially causing extension of the infarct and further compromising left ventricular function.

In addition, because the left ventricle cannot contract sufficiently to eject its contents, the left ventricle does not empty effectively. As a result pressure rises in the left atrium, the pulmonary circulation and the right side of the heart. Pulmonary oedema ensues, reducing oxygenation (see Ch. 3). Thus, not only will the tissues be poorly perfused, but the blood which does reach the tissues will carry less oxygen.

Signs of cardiogenic shock

The signs of cardiogenic shock include:

- systolic pressure <80 mmHg
- tachycardia and a weak, thready pulse
- dyspnoea
- cold, clammy skin
- oliguria – urine output <0.5 mL/kg/h
- confusion
- mottling of the extremities, particularly the legs
- raised jugular venous pressure.

Management of cardiogenic shock will require the use of vasoactive drugs (e.g. glyceryl trinitrate), pulmonary artery catheterisation and advanced therapies such as the intra-aortic balloon pump (IABP) (Gowda et al 2008). The patient should therefore be transferred to a coronary or intensive care unit immediately.

Obstructive shock

This type of shock is caused by obstruction to blood flow in the circulation (Skinner & Jonas 2007). Causes of obstructive shock include pulmonary embolus, pericardial tamponade, tension pneumothorax and lung hyperinflation. Clinical signs of obstructive shock are similar to hypovolaemic and cardiogenic shock, i.e. cold peripheries, cyanosis, weak central pulses and low cardiac output.

Distributive shock

Distributive shock can be divided into three different types: septic, neurogenic and anaphylactic. All are characterised by a loss of blood vessel tone, enlargement of the vascular compartment and displacement of the vascular volume away from the heart. In contrast to hypovolaemic, cardiogenic and obstructive shock, due to vasodilatation patients are warm and pink rather than cold and cyanosed. Although the blood volume remains the same, due to vasodilatation the vascular compartment has expanded, resulting in a reduction in cardiac output. Normally the circulating volume of blood in the body is approximately 5 litres flowing around a circuit that has the same capacity. In distributive shock the capacity of the circuit increases, and although the physiological mechanisms described earlier will come in to play, these are usually insufficient and hypotension ensues due to the drop in cardiac output.

Septic shock

Septic shock is the most common type of distributive shock. It affects millions of people each year and is increasing in incidence, to the extent that international guidelines have been published as part of the Surviving Sepsis campaign (Dellinger et al 2008). It is a medical emergency and full assessment of the patient may need to wait until fluid resuscitation and antimicrobial drugs have commenced (Figure 18.1). It is a major cause of admission to intensive care and mortality.

Sepsis represents the systemic response to infection, known as the systemic inflammatory response (SIRS) (Bone et al 1992). It is characterised by a temperature above 38°C or lower than 36°C, a heart rate above 90 beats per minute

Patient ID sticker	*Organ dysfunction/hypoperfusion care pathway*	Date: Initial ward/area:

EWS Triggered: PARRT Team called: PARRT Team arrived:

1. Assess for evidence of organ dysfunction/hypoperfusion. Is there one or more of:

SBP <90 mmHg or MAP <70 mmHg for >1 hour	☐		
Urine output <0.5 mL/kg/h for >1 hour	☐	Y N	HH : MM
Unexplained confusion/deterioration in conscious level	☐		
Arterial pH <7.3 and base deficit >5 mmol/L	☐		
Lactate >4 mmol/L on arterial blood gas	☐		

THIS IS A MEDICAL EMERGENCY

Begin resuscitation immediately and notify responsible SPR and consultant

TO BE COMPLETED IN FIRST HOUR

2. Initial Resuscitation

Action	Done?	Time	If omitted give reason:
100% Oxygen via non-rebreathing face mask	Y N	HH : MM	
Large bore IV access (ideally grey or brown venflon)	Y N	HH : MM	
Fluid bolus: 10–20 mL/kg Gelofusine over 20 minutes	Y N	HH : MM	
Urinary catheter inserted	Y N	HH : MM	
Arterial blood sample for blood gas and lactate	Y N	HH : MM	
Check for haemorrhage and treat if found	Y N	HH : MM	
Check for hypoglycaemia and administer glucose if required	Y N	HH : MM	

3. Assess for evidence of sepsis. Is there:

Known or suspected infection?	☐		
AND any two of:			
Temperature >38°C or <36°C?	☐		
Heart Rate >90 beats per minute?	☐	Y N	HH : MM
Resp Rate >20 or PaCO$_2$ <4.3 kPa?	☐		
White Cell Count >12.0 or <4.0?	☐		
C Reactive Protein >20 mmol/L?	☐		

IF SEPSIS SUSPECTED THEN BEGIN TREATMENT IF NOT GO TO STEP 5

4. Management of sepsis

Action	Done?	Time	If omitted give reason
Blood cultures (also consider sputum, urine, line tips & HVS)	Y N	HH : MM	
Prescribe IV broad spectrum antibiotics	Y N	HH : MM	
Administer IV broad spectrum antibiotics	Y N	HH : MM	

ONE HOUR CHECK :   HH : MM   ALL ACTIONS COMPLETE?   Y   N

5. Consider the need for:

	Need?	Decided	Done	Comments
Infection source control	Y N	HH : MM	HH : MM	
Further fluid bolus(es) 10–20 mL/kg over 20 mins	Y N	HH : MM	HH : MM	
CVP insertion	Y N	HH : MM	HH : MM	
Repeat arterial blood gas and lactate	Y N	HH : MM	HH : MM	
Hb check and transfusion to maintain Hb >7 g/dL	Y N	HH : MM	HH : MM	

SIX HOUR CHECK :   HH : MM   **6. Persistent problems? Any one of:**

SBP <90 mmHg or MAP <70 mmHg for >1 hour	☐		
Urine output <0.5 mL/kg/h for >1 hour	☐		
Unexplained confusion/deterioration in conscious level	☐	Y N	HH : MM
Arterial pH <7.3 and base deficit >5 mmol/L	☐		
Lactate >4 mmol/L on arterial blood gas			
If not already refer to ICU SpR Bleep 71-1030	☐		

IF PROBLEMS PERSIST SEEK ADVICE AT ANY STAGE FROM THE INTENSIVE CARE REGISTRAR – BLEEP 71-1030

Form to be completed by parent medical team and filed in the patient's notes.

Signed: Dr..Date....................Time....................

Figure 18.1 Hypoperfusion pathway.

and a respiratory rate above 20 breaths per minute, which may be reflected in a lower carbon dioxide level in the blood. The patient may also demonstrate an altered mental status, significant peripheral oedema and hyperglycaemia in the absence of diabetes (Levy et al 2003). Therefore blood sugar measurement and arterial blood gas analysis are essential to the diagnosis of sepsis. Sepsis-induced hypotension is defined as a systolic blood pressure less than 90 mmHg or mean arterial pressure less than 70 mmHg, or a fall of more than 40 mmHg below the patient's normal blood pressure. Thus septic shock is described as sepsis-induced hypotension which persists despite initial fluid resuscitation or blood lactate >4 mmol/L. The judgement as to whether fluid resuscitation is adequate can be complex, especially in the presence of peripheral oedema. However, it is important to remember that the oedema reflects the movement of water and plasma proteins from the intravascular space to the extravascular space. Thus a significant amount of fluid will have been lost from the circulation. This requires replacement in an attempt to restore circulating volume and consequently blood pressure. In order to assess the circulating volume more accurately a central venous line may be sited to evaluate central venous pressure (see p. 547). Tissue hypoperfusion will be represented by oliguria and a raised lactate. Lactate is produced by the cell as a result of anaerobic metabolism, due to the tissue hypoperfusion and reduced oxygen supply to the cell.

Septic shock is often related to pneumonia, surgical wound sites, indwelling catheters and intravenous devices (O'Brien et al 2007), all of which demonstrate that septic shock is preventable. Those particularly at risk are the elderly, the obese, the immunocompromised and those in whom there is significant co-morbidity, e.g. diabetes, heart disease. To avoid pneumonia patients should be in a sitting position and mobilised frequently. Peripheral and central venous cannulae can cause bacteraemia. Thus the date on which indwelling catheters have to be changed should be prominent in the patient's records and intravenous devices should be in place for no longer than the period they are required for treatment. They should also be reviewed daily for signs of inflammation and must be removed as soon as any signs of inflammation become apparent. Strict asepsis should be used in the management of wounds. Should any pus, sputum or exudate become apparent, specimens should be taken and sent immediately for culture.

Neurogenic shock

This type of distributive shock is associated with the central nervous system. It can occur when a disease process, drug or traumatic injury blocks sympathetic nerve impulses from the brain's vasomotor centre and thus increases parasympathetic activity. Neurogenic shock produces a picture of vasodilatation with loss of vascular tone. Venous return is reduced, cardiac output falls and hypotension rapidly follows.

There are a number of preconditions which may, over the course of several hours, or even a few weeks or months, lead to the development of neurogenic shock. One of the most common causes is spinal anaesthesia especially that which extends up the length of the spinal cord and results in a blockage of sympathetic impulses. Cerebral trauma such as contusions or concussion, particularly to the brain stem or medulla oblongata, may also produce severe neurogenic shock. Another potential cause is spinal cord trauma in which all reflex activity below the level of the lesion is lost.

Spinal shock

Trauma to the head, neck, back or shoulders resulting from an accident may cause injury to the vertebral column and/or spinal cord. Spinal injuries are most prevalent among young men who have been previously healthy and for whom the injury is a catastrophic event necessitating major changes in lifestyle.

The degree and type of force exerted on the spine at the time of injury will determine the nature and severity of the injury. The most frequently seen and, unfortunately, the most damaging type of spinal injury as a result of a road traffic accident is a sudden hyperflexion and rotation with fracture-dislocation of the vertebral column at C5 and C6, and T12 to L1. Within 30–60 min of the trauma, autonomic and motor reflexes below the level of the injury are suppressed. This state is known as spinal shock and it may last hours or even weeks.

Anaphylactic shock

If not dealt with immediately, this type of shock is life threatening. It arises when the individual develops hypersensitivity in response to an antigen, drug or foreign protein in which the release of histamine causes widespread vasodilatation resulting in hypotension and increased capillary permeability causing loss of fluid from the intravascular to the extravascular space and the formation of oedema. Laryngeal oedema is particularly evident and the airway may become compromised. Endotracheal intubation may be required to secure the airway and this is an emergency situation.

The main causes of systemic anaphylaxis are insect bites and stings, particularly from bees and wasps; drugs, notably penicillin; and food such as peanuts, eggs or shellfish. Occasionally, diagnostic contrast media used by radiographers may also precipitate anaphylactic reactions. The individual developing anaphylactic shock presents with some, or all, of the following symptoms:

- laryngeal stridor, dyspnoea, cough and, occasionally, cyanosis
- local oedema, particularly around the face
- a weak and rapid pulse
- skin eruptions, large weals.

Treatment will be needed urgently because of the respiratory problems caused by local tissue swelling, laryngeal oedema and/or bronchospasm in addition to circulatory insufficiency.

General principles of the management and treatment of shock (Box 18.3)

The early recognition of shock is vital (Nolan et al 2005). In order to make the signs of deterioration more widely known, it is recommended that physiological track and

Identifying patients at risk of experiencing shock

- Has the patient experienced multiple trauma?
- Has the patient had surgery recently?
- Has the patient suffered severe burns?
- Is the patient postpartum?
- Does the patient have a history of oesophageal varices or peptic ulceration?
- Is the patient taking anticoagulant therapy?

The above factors put the patient at risk of *hypovolaemic* shock

- Has the patient experienced chest pain recently or suffered a myocardial infarction – especially in vessels supplying the anterior wall of the left ventricle?
- Does the patient have a history of cardiac failure or cardiac dysrhythmias?

The above factors put the patient at risk of *cardiogenic* shock

- Does the patient have impaired immunity, e.g. are they suffering from HIV or cancer, or undergoing chemotherapy?
- Does the patient have a resistant deep-seated infection?
- Is the patient seriously ill and requiring multiple invasive catheters and devices?

The above factors put the patient at risk of *septic* shock

- Does the patient suffer from any disordered state resulting in impaired nervous stimuli to vascular smooth muscle?
- Has the patient experienced recent spinal anaesthesia?
- Has the patient experienced trauma to the brain and/or spinal cord?

The above factors put the patient at risk of experiencing *neurogenic* or *spinal* shock

- Does the patient have significant allergies or sensitivities?
- Is the patient undergoing tests requiring contrast media?

The above factors put the patient at risk of experiencing *anaphylactic* shock

---

trigger systems should be in place to alert all health care practitioners to deterioration in the patient's condition (NICE 2007). Physiological observations should be taken at least 12-hourly or as requested in the patient's management plan. This forms the 'track' part of the system, where patients' normal physiological parameters are documented on the observation chart (Figure 18.2). The 'trigger' denotes the alteration from normal to abnormal physiological signs. These usually involve blood pressure, heart and respiratory rate, coupled with oxygen saturation and urine output. These are combined to form an early warning score (EWS). No one type of scoring system has demonstrated superiority (Gao et al 2007), but all will combine blood pressure, heart and respiratory rate, oxygen saturation and urine output (Table 18.1). A graded response should then be in place, which escalates the management of the patient to appropriate personnel (Figure 18.2). Frequency of observations should be automatically increased to quarter hourly.

The track and trigger mechanism is only part of the story, however. Key to the appropriate management of a deteriorating patient is communication. In these acute circumstances it is vital that the correct information is imparted in an effective manner. Vague, unstructured communication leads to delay and the increased possibility of death.

One such example is the use of SBAR (situation, background, assessment, recommendation) (Pope et al 2008). An example could be as follows:

- **Situation**: Mrs X has just lost 1 litre of sero-sanguineous fluid into her Robinson drain.
- **Background**: She returned from the operating theatre one hour ago, following hemi-colectomy.
- **Assessment**: On assessment her blood pressure is 80 mmHg systolic compared to a pre-operative systolic of 130 mmHg, heart rate is 115, respiratory rate 22, oxygen saturation 93% on 2 L oxygen via nasal 'specs'; she is cold peripherally and rousable to voice.
- **Recommendation**: Please will you come and see her immediately?

In its early stages, shock demands immediate intervention. The initial treatment priority is the control of life-threatening abnormalities through assessment of airway, breathing and circulation and assessment of disability (reduced consciousness) (Nolan et al 2005). When obtaining a patient's initial history the nurse should take note of the risk factors listed in Box 18.3. Thereafter, the management of shock includes treatment of the underlying cause, restoration of tissue perfusion and patient support. The purpose of oxygen support is to restore and help maintain adequate tissue oxygenation. The goals of haemodynamic support are to restore an effective blood pressure, ensure tissue perfusion and normalise cellular metabolism.

Management and treatment of hypovolaemic shock (Box 18.4)

Regardless of what may have triggered the patient's hypovolaemia, the restoration of circulating fluid volume is the key to management. As soon as the patient's airway has been secured and oxygen therapy instituted, the next priority is to assess circulatory status and commence replacement intravenous fluids via two large-bore cannulae. Fluid therapy remains the cornerstone for almost every form of shock, although the original insult must also be identified and resolved where possible. Fluid replacement must be accurately recorded on a fluid balance chart and observations taken regularly to assess the patient's response. The desired outcome is restoration of the patient's physiological observations such that they no longer trigger early warning signs (EWS) (Table 18.1). The best choice of fluid replacement (crystalloids, colloids or blood) has been the subject of some debate (Finfer et al 2004).

Crystalloids

A crystalloid is water containing other molecules such as glucose or salt (sodium chloride).

Normal saline solution (sodium chloride 0.9%) is often the first replacement fluid administered to the shocked patient, although its large concentration of chloride ions could be

continued

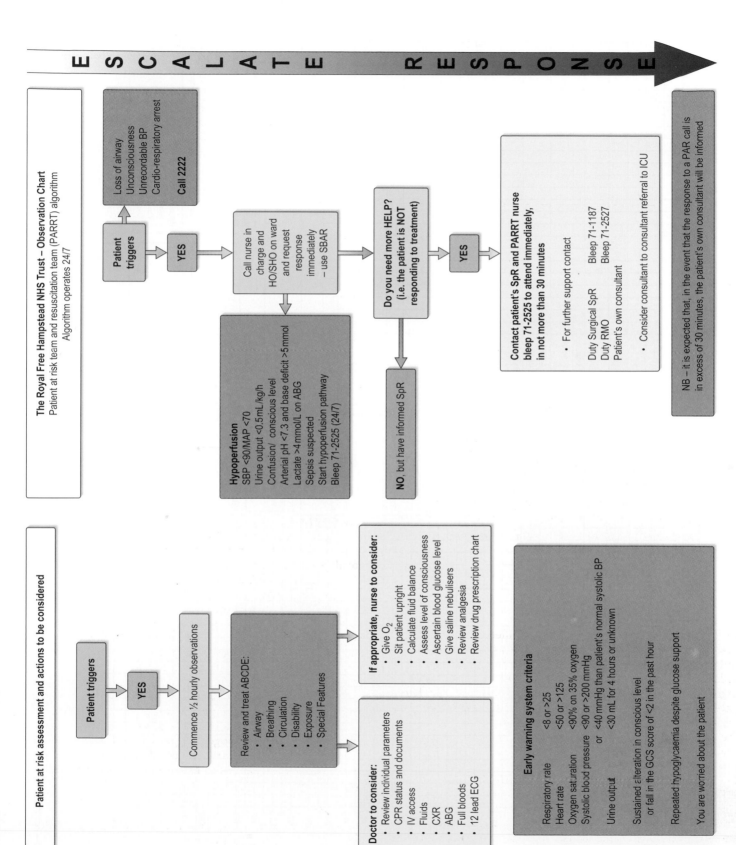

E S C A L A T E   R E S P O N S E

The Royal Free Hampstead NHS Trust – Observation Chart
Patient at risk team and resuscitation team (PARRT) algorithm
Algorithm operates 24/7

Loss of airway
Unconsciousness
Unrecordable BP
Cardio-respiratory arrest

Call 2222

Patient triggers

YES

Call nurse in charge and HO/SHO on ward and request response immediately – use SBAR

Hypoperfusion
SBP <90/MAP <70
Urine output <0.5mL/kg/h
Confusion/ conscious level
Arterial pH <7.3 and base deficit >5mmol
Lactate >4mmol/L on ABG
Sepsis suspected
Start hypoperfusion pathway
Bleep 71-2525 (24/7)

Do you need more HELP?
(i.e. the patient is NOT responding to treatment)

YES

NO, but have informed SpR

Contact patient's SpR and PARRT nurse bleep 71-2525 to attend immediately, in not more than 30 minutes

- For further support contact

Duty Surgical SpR   Bleep 71-1187
Duty RMO   Bleep 71-2527
Patient's own consultant

- Consider consultant to consultant referral to ICU

NB – it is expected that, in the event that the response to a PAR call is in excess of 30 minutes, the patient's own consultant will be informed

Patient at risk assessment and actions to be considered

Patient triggers

YES

Commence ½ hourly observations

Review and treat ABCDE:
- Airway
- Breathing
- Circulation
- Disability
- Exposure
- Special Features

If appropriate, nurse to consider:
- Give O$_2$
- Sit patient upright
- Calculate fluid balance
- Assess level of consciousness
- Ascertain blood glucose level
- Give saline nebulisers
- Review analgesia
- Review drug prescription chart

Doctor to consider:
- Review individual parameters
- CPR status and documents
- IV access
- Fluids
- CXR
- ABG
- Full bloods
- 12 lead ECG

Early warning system criteria

Respiratory rate   <8 or >25
Heart rate   <50 or >125
Oxygen saturation   <90% on 35% oxygen
Systolic blood pressure <90 or >200 mmHg
                        or <40 mmHg than patient's normal systolic BP
Urine output   <30 mL for 4 hours or unknown

Sustained alteration in conscious level or fall in the GCS score of <2 in the past hour

Repeated hypoglycaemia despite glucose support

You are worried about the patient

Figure 18.2 Escalating patient management.

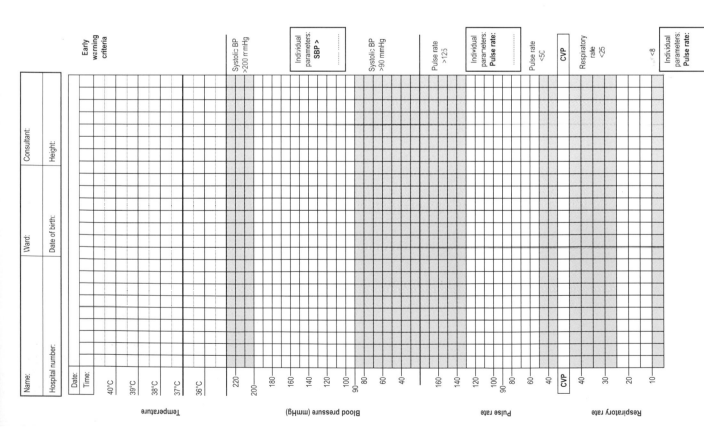

Glasgow Coma Score

Eyes open	Spontaneously	4
	To speech	3
	To pain	2
	None	1

Best verbal response	Orientated	5
	Confused	4
	Words	3
	Sounds	2
	None	1

Best motor response	Obey commands	6
	Localise to pain	5
	Flexion to pain	4
	Abnormal flexion to pain	3
	Extension to pain	2
	None	1

Pain score

Assess pain on movements, deep breathing or coughing
- No pain at rest or on movement — 0
- No pain at rest, slight pain on movement — 1
- Intermittent pain at rest, moderate pain on movement — 2
- Continuous pain at rest, severe pain on movement — 3

Nausea score
- None — 0
- Nausea — 1
- Vomiting — 2

Sedation score
- Sleep — S
- None, patient alert — 0
- Mild, occasionally drowsy, easy to rouse — 1
- Moderate, often drowsy, easy to rouse — 2
- Severe, somnolent, difficult to rouse — 3

Figure 18.2—cont'd

Table 18.1 Track and trigger system	
PHYSIOLOGICAL TRIGGER	**CRITERIA**
Respiratory rate	<8 or >25
Systolic blood pressure	<90 mmHg or >200 mmHg (or 40 mmHg less than the patient's normal BP)
O_2 saturation	<90% on 35% oxygen or more
Urine output	<30 mL/h for 4 h or unknown

disadvantageous to the patient whose renal function is already impaired.

Colloids

A colloid is a solution containing medium to large particles, such as protein, which help to restore the interstitial osmotic pressure. Examples of colloids are albumin and fresh frozen plasma. However, synthetic solutions such as succinylated gelatin (Gelofusine) are commonly used as they are relatively inexpensive and reduce the risks associated with the use of human products. Colloids stay in the circulation for a longer period than crystalloid, but the amount of time varies between individuals.

Blood

After initial resuscitation with crystalloids, colloids or a blood transfusion may be required to improve the oxygen-carrying capacity of the circulation. It may be necessary to use a pressure infuser to increase the rate of delivery and a blood warmer to bring the blood up to body temperature in order to avoid excessive cooling of the patient. Initially packed cells will be used, followed by other blood products such as platelets or clotting factors if blood loss has been profound. A haemoglobin level of 8–9 g/dL is considered acceptable as this combines adequate oxygen-carrying capacity without compromising blood flow through the tissues, thereby improving tissue oxygenation (Babb & Farmery 2003).

Management and treatment of cardiogenic shock (see Box 18.4)

The main goals of therapy in cardiogenic shock are:

* to re-establish circulation to the myocardium
* to minimise heart muscle damage
* to improve the effectiveness of the heart as a pump.

Damage to cardiac muscle can be minimised by improving myocardial oxygen supply and, at the same time, reducing its oxygen demand. Oxygen supply can be increased by the administration of high percentage O_2. The effective delivery of oxygen should be monitored using pulse oximetry and blood gas analysis. Dobutamine may be used, via continuous infusion, as this has both inotropic properties (can increase strength of myocardial contractility and therefore blood pressure) and vasodilatory effects. Vasodilatation decreases the resistance against which the left ventricle has

Box 18.4 Information

Definitive and supportive therapy in clinical shock

For all patients the nurse must be confident the airway is secure and that oxygen is delivered to the patient by a fixed performance mask. If the SpO_2 is <93% deliver 60% oxygen via the fixed performance mask.

Hypovolaemic shock

* Restore intravascular volume with crystalloid or colloid.
* If possible, apply pressure to reduce blood loss.
* Maintain Hb 9–10 g/dL.
* Accurately document fluid balance.

Cardiogenic shock

* Control pain with morphine.
* Increase effectiveness of the heart as a pump via inotropic medication and vasodilatation with nitrates.

Septic shock

* Restore adequate intravascular volume with crystalloid or colloid.
* Achieve CVP 8–10, mean arterial blood pressure >65 mmHg, urine output >0.5 mL/kg/h.
* Identify and control the source of infection via bacterial screening.
* Administer appropriate antibiotics.
* Remove the cause of infection if possible.

Anaphylactic shock

* Identify and remove the causative antigen.
* Reduce effects of mediator substances that have caused massive vasodilatation, e.g. give adrenaline to restore vascular tone, antihistamines to reverse histamine effects, bronchodilators to oppose bronchial constriction.
* Restore adequate intravascular volume with crystalloid or colloid.

to pump, thus reducing myocardial workload and oxygen demand. However, due to the vasodilatory properties of dobutamine, the heart rate can increase. This increases myocardial workload and oxygen demand and therefore adrenaline may be the inotrope of choice. Glyceryl trinitrate may also be prescribed as it will dilate the coronary arteries, thus increasing oxygen supply, and through peripheral vasodilation reduce workload and therefore oxygen demand.

An essential part of management is the control of pain. The administration of intravenous morphine is ideal as it also dilates the blood vessels and reduces peripheral resistance, which in turn will further reduce oxygen demand.

Management and treatment of septic shock (see Box 18.4)

International guidelines recommend the use of protocols to guide the management of septic shock (Figure 18.1) (Dellinger et al 2008). Resuscitation should be commenced immediately. The goals of resuscitation are to achieve:

* central venous pressure (CVP) 8–12 mmHg
* mean arterial pressure above 65 mmHg
* urine output greater than 0.5 mL/kg/h

- central venous oxygen saturation greater than 70% or mixed venous oxygen saturation greater than 65%.

Both central venous oxygen saturation and mixed venous oxygen saturation represent percentage saturation of oxygen on the haemoglobin once it has returned from the capillaries. It indicates the amount of oxygen which has been utilised by the cells. Goal-directed therapy has been demonstrated to improve survival, in an extremely influential single centre randomised controlled study (Rivers et al 2001). As with hypovolaemic shock, fluid resuscitation may be with crystalloid or colloid. Fluid challenges (the administration of 1 litre of normal saline or 300–500 mL of colloid over 30 minutes) should be used to evaluate the effectiveness or otherwise of fluid resuscitation. These challenges should be repeated until the CVP is 8–12 mmHg. It should be noted that even when this is achieved continued vasodilatation and capillary leak may prevent a sustained effect and further fluid resuscitation will be required. If fluid resuscitation fails to improve the blood pressure then inotropes will be required. These should only be delivered through a central intravenous line, and the blood pressure should be monitored via an arterial line, requiring management in an intensive care or high-dependency unit. Noradrenaline is the primary inotrope of choice, followed by adrenaline if response to noradrenaline is poor (Dellinger et al 2008). Use of hydrocortisone is only recommended when the blood pressure responds poorly to fluid resuscitation and inotropic therapy. Recombinant protein C, a drug which acts on the microthrombi produced in sepsis and has the potential to restore blood flow to the tissues, can be used patients who are in multiple organ failure (Dellinger et al 2008). Again, its use would be restricted to the intensive care or high-dependency unit. Once tissue perfusion has been re-established packed cells should be administered to restore the haemoglobin level to 7–9 g/dL.

Central venous or mixed venous oxygen saturation measure the amount of oxygen extracted from the haemoglobin and can be seen to reflect tissue hypoxia. However, this can be misleading. If flow through the capillary bed is reduced due to the formation of microthrombi then blood flow is disrupted and tissues are unable to extract oxygen. In such a situation venous oxygenation could be more than 70% but despite this tissues are engaged in anaerobic metabolism due to hypoxia. Thus blood lactate concentration is an extremely useful measurement in assessing cellular metabolism and the effectiveness of goal-directed therapy because it represents the degree of anaerobic metabolism undertaken by the cells.

Establishing the cause

Two or more blood cultures should be taken, one of which should be percutaneous and one from each vascular access site. Other sites should be cultured also, e.g. wounds, sputum, urine. Following this, broad spectrum antibiotics should be administered intravenously within one hour of sepsis being suspected. The source of the infection should be established as soon as possible and if amenable to drainage or debridement this should be undertaken as a matter of urgency with the exception of infected pancreatic necrosis where surgical intervention is best delayed (Mier et al 1997). Where intravascular access is implicated all devices should be re-sited according to EPIC2 guidelines (Pratt et al 2007).

It is essential that the patient with septic shock is transferred to a high-dependency or intensive care unit where mechanical ventilation and advanced monitoring can be established and support provided for sequential organ failure.

Management and treatment of anaphylactic shock (see Box 18.4)

Swift recognition of anaphylactic shock, which results from a severe allergic reaction to a specific antigen, is vital to the individual's survival. Intervention should aim first at identifying and, if possible, removing the cause. If this is not possible, the effects of the reaction must be reversed.

Immediate assessment should be made of the adequacy of the patient's airway, breathing circulation and conscious level. If swelling around the throat or face, hoarseness or stridor, rapid breathing, a wheeze, hypotension or confusion is apparent the patient's management should be immediately escalated to experienced staff using an effective form of communication such as the SBAR approach described above (p. 542) and immediate resuscitation should commence. The patient should be laid flat with the legs raised. High-flow oxygen via a non-rebreathe mask should be commenced and intravenous access established with large-bore cannulae. Adrenaline 1:1000 500 µg should be given intramuscularly, and repeated after 5 minutes if there is no improvement. Crystalloid is usually the resuscitation fluid of choice as this is less allergenic than colloid. However, if hypotension is profound then colloids may be used. Any colloid infusion running at the time anaphylaxis occurs should be discontinued.

Monitoring the patient in shock

Monitoring and observation of the patient's ever-changing condition will facilitate the prompt correction of deficits. The following are the most important indicators of tissue perfusion and are discussed in the following sections:

- cardiac status
- respiratory status
- haemodynamic status
- level of consciousness
- renal function
- body temperature
- skin condition.

Monitoring cardiac status

The manual assessment of an arterial pulse, usually the radial artery, is the most fundamental and vital form of cardiac monitoring. It can demonstrate not only the rate but the rhythm of the heart together with an impression of blood pressure and whether this is 'bounding' (strong) or 'thready' (weak). A bounding pulse represents a raised blood pressure, whereas a 'thready' one denotes a low blood pressure.

Electrocardiography

An electrocardiogram (ECG) is a recording of the electrical activity of the myocardium and indicates the changes which occur as a result of contraction. The contraction of any heart muscle is associated with electrical changes called depolarisation and these can be detected by electrodes attached to the surface of the body (see Ch. 2). An ECG can be obtained quickly in an emergency department or with a portable electrocardiograph at the patient's bedside. It can provide further useful information about the rate and rhythm of the heart. Thus, if arrhythmias arise, they can be detected and treated immediately. However, electrocardiographs should only be used by specialist staff who can interpret waveforms accurately. Thus, ECG monitoring is usually only performed in coronary, high-dependency or intensive care units.

Monitoring respiratory status

Respiratory rate is an extremely sensitive indicator of deterioration and should *always* be monitored together with haemodynamic observations. Sadly, if automated devices are used respiratory rate is often omitted because it is not measured by the device. The nurse should always be alert to hypo- or hyperventilation. Hyperventilation will result in fatigue of the respiratory muscles. This may lead to shallow breathing and the risk of respiratory distress, necessitating mechanical ventilation. Hypoventilation may be a very late sign of shock, as the patient begins to tire and has insufficient reserve to maintain ventilation. It may also be associated with the administration of opiates, such as morphine, often administered in cardiogenic shock.

Monitoring oxygen saturation

The level of O_2 saturation in the patient's blood (SpO_2) will give some indication of respiratory status. Continuous monitoring will provide valuable information related to the individual's response to interventions and can provide early warning of hypoxaemia. However, poor oxygen delivery to the tissues may also occur in the presence of a normal SpO_2. It is, therefore, also important to know the patient's haemoglobin level in order to assess whether the oxygen-carrying capacity of the blood is adequate (Hb 9–10 g/dL).

Pulse oximetry

Arterial O_2 saturation along with pulse rate can be monitored continuously by means of a non-invasive electronic device called a pulse oximeter. This functions by measuring the absorption of red and infrared light passed through living tissue, usually a finger, toe or ear lobe. Results usually correspond closely to arterial blood gas values and this instrument reduces the need for blood samples. Vasoconstriction can impair SpO_2 readings and if this is the case then arterial blood gases should be taken. Readings are not affected by skin colour but can be distorted by high blood bilirubin levels, as in jaundice, and in cases of carbon monoxide poisoning and smoke inhalation. Results for very heavy smokers may also be difficult to interpret.

Monitoring haemodynamic status

The importance of monitoring the blood pressure has already been established through its use not only to recognise deterioration, but also to evaluate the effectiveness of fluid resuscitation. Pulse pressure is also a very useful determinant of haemodynamic status. The pulse pressure is the difference between the systolic and diastolic pressure. Thus if the BP is 110/80 the pulse pressure will be 30. If this narrows it indicates the activation of the sympathetic nervous system and vasoconstriction. If it widens it can denote vasodilatation, indicating a reduction in circulating volume and the need for fluid resuscitation. The absolute values of the pulse pressure are of less significance than the trend. Therefore, in documenting the blood pressure it is important to establish the status of the pulse pressure. The importance of accurate monitoring of these two physiological observations cannot be overemphasised. In addition to BP and pulse pressure, CVP and cardiac output measures are also useful in the management of shock. These are outlined below.

Central venous pressure (CVP) monitoring

CVP is the pressure within the right atrium and superior vena cava. Its measurement can give information about circulating blood volume. It can also give an indication of vascular tone and pulmonary vascular resistance, as well as the effectiveness of the right myocardium. However, it does not measure left ventricular function and it can be unreliable in the critically ill patient with chronic lung disease, right and left heart failure or valve disease.

CVP monitoring reflects the rate of blood return to the right side of the heart and can be an accurate guide for fluid replacement. A CVP of approximately $2 \, cmH_2O$ in the presence of a low arterial blood pressure usually indicates hypovolaemia, whereas a CVP above $14 \, cmH_2O$ in the presence of a low arterial blood pressure indicates cardiogenic shock.

Technique A large-bore catheter is inserted under strict aseptic conditions into the internal or external jugular, or subclavian vein, using ultrasound techniques to correctly site the catheter. In wards the CVP can be measured as shown in Figure 18.3. In the intensive care or high-dependency unit, a transducer can be attached to the central line in order to obtain a waveform and digital display of the CVP reading in mmHg. Continuous monitoring will indicate the effectiveness of treatment.

Central venous lines, although extremely important for a critically ill patient, present a danger of bacterial infection. Nurses can make an important contribution to care by ensuring that aseptic techniques are adhered to when the line is inserted and that the insertion site is kept clean and dry. Once it is no longer needed, the line should be removed as quickly as possible to reduce the risk of infection (Pratt et al 2007).

Non-invasive methods of measuring cardiac output

Cardiac output measurements can be very useful as they provide information concerning left ventricular filling and resistance to blood flow from the left ventricle (systemic vascular resistance). This can be performed using either Doppler or bioimpedance measurements (Albert 2006). Doppler involves the placing of a probe in the patient's oesophagus adjacent to the descending aorta. Bioimpedance cardiography involves the measurement of impedance (or resistance) to transmission of a small electrical current though the chest

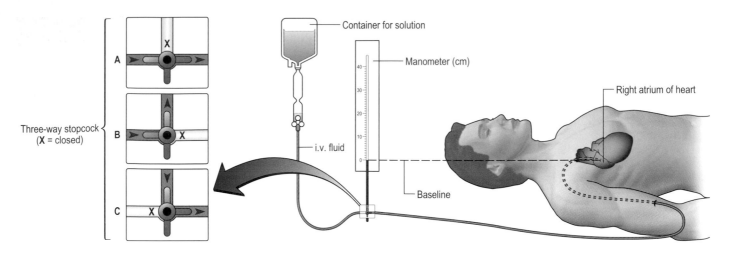

Figure 18.3 Diagram of a CVP water manometer. A. Before measuring central venous pressure (CVP), the infusion flow is to the patient and the three-way stopcock is closed to the manometer. B. To measure CVP, the stopcock is turned so that it is closed to the patient. This allows the manometer to be refilled with fluid. C. The stopcock is turned so that it is closed to the infusion fluid. This allows a free flow of fluid from the manometer to the intravenous catheter. The fluid level will fall until the level corresponds with the pressure in the right atrium or superior vena cava. (Adapted from Jamieson et al 2003.)

area (thoracic bioimpedance) or the whole body (whole body impedance). These measurements are useful because they provide information regarding stroke volume, a prerequisite of cardiac output. They are more accurate in assessing cardiac status than central venous pressure measurements as they measure volume and not pressure. In health, pressure and volume are contiguous, e.g. if the blood volume rises then the pressure increases (Starling's law); however, in shock states this is not always the case and therefore blood pressure may not always accurately reflect blood volume. Also, the central venous pressure reading can reflect high pulmonary pressures rather than those of the left ventricle. Currently, Doppler and bioimpedance are not widely used but are likely to become so in the near future (Ahrens 2008).

Monitoring level of consciousness

In the early stages of shock, the patient may still be quite alert and anxious. They may complain of pain and may be able to give a history, which will help the clinician to establish a diagnosis. However, if cerebral perfusion pressure falls, with resulting cerebral hypoxia, the patient will gradually become less coherent and may eventually become comatose. The nurse should observe the patient carefully to ensure changes in the state of consciousness are noted as they occur, and management escalated to the appropriate personnel (e.g. senior ward nurse, specialist registrar, critical care outreach team, anaesthetist). There is a danger that if a patient has been agitated, due to hypoxia, and then becomes quiet the nurse may consider the patient is responding to treatment, whereas the opposite may be the case. Once the conscious level drops it is vital to ensure that the airway is maintained and a Guedel airway or intubation may be required. It may be advisable to place the patient in the left lateral position. The Glasgow Coma Scale (GCS, see Ch. 28) is a useful tool with which to assess the patient's cerebral function. The mnemonic AVPU is also now widely used because it is easier to calculate than the GCS. AVPU refers to an assessment of consciousness in which the patient is **A**lert, alert to **V**oice only, roused by **P**ain, **U**nconscious.

For a detailed discussion of consciousness levels, see Chapter 28.

Monitoring renal function

Renal function is a very good indicator of tissue perfusion and should therefore be monitored carefully in patients suffering from shock. A urinary catheter and accurate fluid balance chart are therefore vital to the patient's management. Since the kidneys are dependent on adequate tissue perfusion, a drop in urinary output indicates poor perfusion. The urinary output should be 0.5–1.0 mL per kg per hour or not less than 200 mL in the last 6 hours. A lower figure may represent dehydration, as well as shock; however, both conditions require fluid resuscitation and dehydration may lead to hypovolaemic shock. Urinary catheterisation and hourly urine measurement greatly assist the early detection of decreasing renal perfusion.

Measurement of specific gravity (SG) reflects the concentration of the urine. The normal urinary specific gravity is between 1.002 and 1.028. In the early stages of shock, when urine volume falls, the concentration of excreted waste products rises. This is reflected in a raised SG and osmolality. However, if the shocked state progresses and urine volumes remain low, the ability of the kidneys to concentrate the urine is fixed or low (Ch. 8). Levels of creatinine and urea in the blood will also rise in the presence of decreased renal perfusion and function.

Monitoring body temperature

The importance of obtaining accurate body temperature measurements should not be underestimated, as many clinical interventions are based on these readings. These factors, as well as procedures for obtaining accurate core temperature readings, are described in detail in Chapter 22.

Observing skin condition

Direct observation of the skin colour, temperature and condition will reflect the stage of shock that the patient is in. Intense activation of the sympathetic nervous system will result in pale, clammy skin and a dry mouth. Capillary refill is a common measure of peripheral perfusion. It is the rate at which blood refills the empty capillaries. It is measured by pressing on the fingernail bed until it turns white and noting the time it takes for the colour to return. Refill should occur within 2 seconds once the nail bed is released. Failure of capillary refill indicates sustained and prolonged vasoconstriction. If oxygen delivery is severely impaired, the skin will become cold, mottled and cyanosed. However, it should be noted that the clinical picture in septic, neurogenic and anaphylactic shock is different. In these types of shock, the skin is warm, dry and flushed due to vasodilatation.

Laboratory and diagnostic tests

Arterial blood gas (ABG) analysis provides a guide to oxygenation, tissue perfusion and aerobic or anaerobic respiration by the cells (Coombs 2001). In all types of shock, it is not uncommon to find a fall in the partial pressure of oxygen (PaO_2) and a rise in the partial pressure of carbon dioxide ($PaCO_2$). However, $PaCO_2$ may fall due to hyperventilation (Woodrow 2004). With an increase in anaerobic metabolism resulting in the production of lactic acid, metabolic acidosis is frequently seen in the severely shocked patient (Edwards 2008).

Information on a range of diagnostic tests including ABGs is given in the Appendix.

SUMMARY – KEY NURSING ISSUES

- Fundamental to the recognition and effective management of shock is the accurate recording and documentation of physiological parameters and fluid balance.
- In assessing the patient, continual review of the airway, breathing, circulation and disability (conscious level) is vital, together with the exposure of the patient to ascertain alteration in skin colour, or the presence of oedema, urticaria (rash) or inflammation.
- If shock is established then treatment must be swift as this is a medical emergency and effective communication is imperative.
- Use of the SBAR system enables complex information to be escalated efficiently.
- Once management is instigated the nurse again plays a crucial role in monitoring the effectiveness of treatment. Successful resuscitation of the patient relies, almost uniquely, on the vigilance of the nurse.

REFLECTION AND LEARNING – WHAT NEXT?

- **Test** your knowledge by visiting the website 🖰 and answering the multiple choice questions and critical thinking questions.
- **Consolidate** your learning by looking at some of the further reading suggestions, references and specialist websites.
- **Revisit** some of the additional material on the website.
- **Consider** what you have learnt and how this will help your professional development.
- **Reflect** on how you can apply this knowledge to the care of your patients.
- **Discuss** your learning with your mentor/supervisor, lecturer and colleagues.

REFERENCES

Ahrens T: The most important vital signs are not being measured, *Aust Crit Care* 21:3–5, 2008.

Albert NM: Bioimpedance cardiography measurements of cardiac output and other cardiovascular parameters, *Crit Care Nurs Clin North Am* 18:195–202, 2006.

Babb MA, Farmery AD: Haemorrhagic shock, *Surgery* 8:208A–208E, 2003.

Bone RC, Balk RA, Cerra FB, et al: Definitions for sepsis and organ failure and guidelines for the use of innovative therapies in sepsis, *Chest* 101:1644–1655, 1992.

Bridges EJ, Dukes S: Cardiovascular aspects of septic shock: pathophysiology, monitoring and treatment, *Critical Care Nursing* 25:14–24, 2005.

Coombs M: Making sense of arterial blood gases, *Nurs Times* 97:36–38, 2001.

Dellinger RP, Levy MM, Carlet JM, Bion J, Parker MM, Jaeschke R, et al: Surviving Sepsis campaign: international guidelines for management of severe sepsis and septic shock: 2008, *Intensive Care Med* 34:17–60, 2008.

Department of Health: *The coronary heart disease national service framework: building for the future progress report for 2007*, 2008, DH. Available online http://www.dh.gov.uk/publications.

Edwards SL: Pathophysiology of acid base balance: the theory practice relationship, *Intensive Crit Care Nurs* 24:28–40, 2008.

Finfer S, Bellomo R, Boyce N, French J, Myburgh J, Norton R: A comparison of albumin and saline for fluid resuscitation in the intensive care unit, *N Engl J Med* 350:2247–2256, 2004.

Gao H, McDonnell A, Harrison DA, Moore T, Adam S, Esmonde L, Goldhill DR, Parry GJ, Rashidian A, Subbe CP, Harvey S: Systematic review and evaluation of physiological track and trigger warning systems for identifying at-risk patients on the ward, *Intensive Care Med* 33:667–679, 2007.

Gowda RM, Fox JT, Khan IA: Cardiogenic shock: basics and clinical considerations, *Int J Cardiol* 123:221–228, 2008.

Greenwood M, Murgo M: Management of multi-organ dysfunctions. In Elliott D, Aitken L, Chaboyer W, editors: *ACCCN's Critical Care Nursing*, Sydney, 2007, Mosby Elsevier, pp 435–461.

Jamieson EM, McCall JM, Blythe R, White LA: *Guidelines for clinical nursing practices*, ed 4, Edinburgh, 2004, Churchill Livingstone.

Jowett NI, Thompson DR: *Comprehensive Coronary Care*, ed 4, Baillière Tindall, 2007, Edinburgh, pp 239–242.

Levy MM, Fink MP, Marshall JC, Abraham E, Angus D, Cook D, Cohen J, Opal SM, Vincent JL, Ramsey G, et al: International sepsis definitions conference, *Crit Care Med* 31:1250–1256, 2003.

Marieb EN, Hoehn K: *Human anatomy and physiology*, ed 7, San Francisco, 2007, Pearson Benjamin.

Mcnarry AF, Goldhill DR: Simple bedside assessment of level of consciousness: comparison of two simple scales with Glasgow coma scale, *Anaesthesia* 59:34–37, 2004.

Mier J, Leon EL, Castillo A, Robledo F, Blanco R: Early versus late necrosectomy in severe necrotising pancreatitis, *Am J Surg* 173:71–75, 1997.

National Institute for Health and Clinical Excellence (NICE): Acutely ill patients in hospital: recognition of and response to acute illness in adults in hospital, *NICE Clinical Guideline 50*, July 2007.

Nolan JP, Deakin CD, Soar J, Bottiger BW, Smith G: European Resuscitation Council guidelines for resuscitation 2005. Section 4 Adult advanced life support, *Resuscitation* 67(Suppl 1):s39–s86, 2005.

O'Brien JM, Ali NA, Aberegg SK, Abraham E: Sepsis, *Am J Med* 120:1012–1022, 2007.

Pope BB, Rodzen L, Spross G: Raising the SBAR: how better communication improves patient outcomes, *Nursing* 38:41–43, 2008.

Pratt RJ, Pellowe CM, Wilson JA, Loveday HP, Harper PJ, Jones SRLJ, Mcdougall C, Wilcox MH: EPIC2: National evidence-based guidelines for preventing healthcare-associated infections in NHS hospitals in England, *J Hosp Infect* 655:s1–s64, 2007.

Richards A, Edwards S: *A nurse's survival guide to the ward*, Churchill Livingstone, 2003, Edinburgh.

Rivers E, Nguyen B, Havstad S, Ressler J, Muzzin A, Knoblich B, Peterson E, Tomlanovitch M. Early Goal Directed Therapy Collaborative Group: Early goal directed therapy in the treatment of severe sepsis and septic shock, *N Engl J Med* 345:1368–1377, 2001.

Skinner B, Jonas M: Causes and management of shock, *Anaesthesia and Intensive Care Medicine* 8:520–524, 2007.

Woodrow P: Arterial blood gas analysis, *Nurs Stand* 18:45–52, 2004.

FURTHER READING

Adam S, Osborne S: *Oxford Handbook of critical care nursing*, ed 2, Oxford, 2009, OUP.

Moore T, Woodrow P: *High Dependency nursing care*, ed 2, London, 2004, Routledge.

Sheppard M, Wright M: *High dependency nursing*, ed 2, Edinburgh, 2006, Elsevier.

Pain management

Carol Chamley

Introduction

Acute pain has been described as a worldwide phenomenon, and the belief that pain is an inevitable part of the human condition is widespread (Brennan et al 2007). The pain and suffering endured by people commands universal interest, and as knowledge and research develops exponentially, science and technology continues to support our understanding of pain treatment and management. Throughout the world it is estimated that tens of millions of people are affected by life-threatening diseases, such as cancer, HIV/AIDS disease, etc., coupled with episodes of acute and chronic enduring pain (Sepúlveda et al 2002). Furthermore, it is estimated that 10 million new cases of cancer are diagnosed annually, and by 2020 this figure will double, with approximately 70% of incidences occurring in the developing nations (Selva 1997), with huge implications for the delivery of safe and ethical pain management.

Pain is an important component, and at times the only element, of disease processes. Pain management and subsequent nursing interventions entail a moral, humanitarian, ethical and legal obligation to ensure that people in our care have their pain relieved. This requires competent and knowledgeable practitioners who are 'fit for purpose'. The Nursing and Midwifery Council (NMC) has identified *Essential Skills Clusters* (NMC 2007); several subsections within the clusters relate to pain including: *Care, Compassion,* and *Organisational Aspects of Care and Medicines Management* (Ellson 2008).

> *...pain is a critical ethical issue because it has the capacity to dehumanize the human person (Lisson 1987)*

Effective pain management as a fundamental human right is a moral imperative that is universally acknowledged, but pain on a global scale remains inadequately treated because of cultural, attitudinal, educational, legal and system-related ideologies (Brennan et al 2007, Fisherman 2007). Today the best available evidence indicates a gap between an increasingly sophisticated understanding of the pathophysiology of pain, and the widespread inadequacy in its treatment. In the poorest and most socially deprived nations, this is exacerbated by the huge numbers affected by HIV/AIDS disease coupled with poverty, war, oppression and violence (Brennan et al 2007). However, pain-related activities in medicine, law and ethics have reached a critical point – it is accepted that pain is ubiquitous and complex, yet often under-treated and at best manageable. The global pain community has now declared that pain management is a human right and that unreasonable failure to treat an individual's pain is unethical and a breach of human rights (Brennan et al 2007). Furthermore, adequate pain management is founded upon the duty of health practitioners to act ethically. Values and ethics embraced within *The Code: Standards of Conduct, Performance and Ethics for Nurses and Midwives* (NMC 2008) reflect the duty of care that nurses have towards those in their care.

Every person, irrespective of age, deserves to be pain free. The particular rights of children are recognised in the *National Service Framework for Children, Young People, and Maternity Services* (NSF) (Department of Health [DH] 2004), and enshrined in the *Declaration of the Rights of the Child* (United Nations 1989).

It is accepted that pain is an international problem requiring international solutions. The World Health Organization (WHO) undertakes a critical role in solutions through:

- promoting and disseminating guidelines relating to pain management
- advocacy for improved access to opioid analgesics (pain killers)
- national programmes of palliative care and pain relief.

Worldwide, there are some outstanding examples of public health programmes for pain management and palliative care. The best have combined policy with an integrated approach and commitment to education. Brennan et al (2007) conclude that pain management is an issue of central importance related to disciplines such as medicine, law and ethics, where they are at an *'inflection point'*. Unreasonable failure to treat an individual's pain is viewed globally as poor medicine, unethical practice and an abrogation of a fundamental human right (Brennan et al 2007, p. 205).

Nurses working within a multidisciplinary team (MDT) need up-to-date evidence-based knowledge and understanding of pain in order to competently prevent and minimise pain. Davies & Taylor (2003) summarise the information needed by health care staff as:

- the causes of pain and major influences on the perception of pain
- the effects of unrelieved pain on the individual
- appropriate methods of pain assessment
- pharmacological interventions according to the needs of the person
- complications of pharmacological interventions
- the use of appropriate non-pharmacological interventions (Davies & Taylor 2003, p. 118).

This chapter outlines some of the central issues relating to pain – the difficulty in defining and describing pain due to its elusive, complex and subjective nature and how historical perspectives, including myths and misconceptions, have helped to shape contemporary practice and policy. Tools for the assessment of pain and the subjects of pharmacological and non-pharmacological pain management are described. The chapter provides interactive boxes, cross-references to relevant chapters (e.g. Chs 9, 26, 31, 33) and suggestions for further reading.

Defining pain: competing perspectives

Historically pain has often been attributed, in some cultures, to wrong doing, suffering and punishment. Pain is described as being multidimensional, embracing physical, psychosocial emotional and spiritual components (Chamley & James 2007, p. 653). Furthermore, the multidimensional nature of pain makes it possible to be with an individual who is in pain and be unaware of their pain. It is therefore increasingly recognised that pain is a complex phenomenon and it is difficult to assign a simple single definition. The International Association for the Study of Pain (IASP) describes pain as:

> . . . *an unpleasant sensory and emotional experience associated with actual or potential tissue damage or described in terms of such damage (IASP 1994)*

Whilst this definition describes both the sensory and emotional aspects of pain it has limitations because it fails to account for other peripheral nervous system (PNS) activity and stimuli within the central nervous system (CNS), and the variable way in which the nervous system can respond to injury. Moreover, this definition disregards the sociocultural aspects of an individual's life, as pain is influenced by body, mind and culture. Over forty years ago McCaffery (1968) proposed a simple definition which has been widely accepted within nursing and has encouraged nurses to focus upon the patient/client's pain perspective.

> *Pain is whatever the patient says it is and exists when he says it does.*

This definition embraces the subjective nature of pain and has encouraged nurses and others to value the person's reporting of their pain. Despite a lack of consensus on the definition of pain, ongoing research has expanded our understanding of the pain experience. Therefore, health care professionals must be aware of and responsive to an individual's pain, taking account of many variables which influence the individual's lived-in experience of pain (Box 19.1).

Historical perspectives and contemporary thinking about pain

The history of pain treatment is extensive: ample literature and documentary evidence describes the pervasive influence and intrusive nature of pain on every facet of life since the

---

 Box 19.1 Reflection

Factors influencing the pain experience

Think about your own pain experiences, for example with a headache, and how the intensity of pain may have been influenced by other factors. These factors may include position, noise, stress, tiredness, hunger, frustration, a row, a fast-approaching assignment deadline, not having enough information, a big occasion such as a wedding, etc.

Activity

Discuss your thoughts with colleagues and list the factors that reduce pain intensity, and what increases pain intensity.

earliest human experience (Brennan et al 2007, p. 207). The treatment and management of pain has evolved over the centuries from early treatments with herbs to modern day pain management with drugs and non-pharmacological methods. The antecedents of pain theories and treatments can be traced back to early civilisations which had very different views of pain; often the commonly held belief was that pain was the consequence of, or the punishment for sins committed, or the magical influence of spirits of the dead. Nearly every religion has addressed the issue of pain, and religion, philosophy and folklore have saturated pain with meaning (Brennan et al 2007).

As long as 4500 years ago the Chinese had a well-developed system of pain management based upon acupuncture. They also used herbal remedies, and evidence from very early in their history suggests that they used opioids or other narcotics. The Egyptians appear to have believed that pain was inflicted by either a god or disincarnate spirit, and as in India the Egyptians believed the heart to be at the centre of sensation.

The Indian culture attached much more significance to the emotional roots of pain. It was the ancient Greeks who introduced the concept of the brain as the main organ in which pain was raised to the level of consciousness. However, this was refuted by Aristotle who also considered the heart as the main organ for pain sensation. Hippocrates (the 'father of medicine') held a view which was closely aligned to the Chinese theory of the 'elements' or 'humors': blood, phlegm, yellow bile and black bile. The humors were traditionally associated with the causation of disease, whereby disease was caused by an imbalance of the humors, or excess or deficiency of these humors caused pain.

Eventually the reality that the brain was the centre for the recognition and sensation of pain was gradually accepted. The ancient Greeks established that the brain and peripheral nerves were intimately connected. Galen demonstrated that both CNS and PNS components were collectively involved in pain sensation. Even so, Galen continued to hold the view that pain was a 'passion of the soul'. Pain is the oldest medical problem, yet its pathophysiology has been poorly understood until fairly recently.

Pain theories have developed from the best available scientific literature yet none of them has been able to completely explain the phenomenon of pain and all have shortcomings. Wall (2007) asserts that over the last three decades there has been sustained scientific development and refinement of pain theories and science now rejects the model of a pain mechanism, which has a dedicated action, and 'fixed rigid modality'. The process which produces pain is described as plastic and changing sequentially over time. The essential mobility of the pain mechanism exists in damaged tissue in the PNS. The movement of pathology from the periphery to the centre triggers reactive processes in the brain. Ultimately this presents the practitioner with a scattered and potentially migrating target (Wall 2007).

Theories of pain

This section of the chapter outlines three theories: the specificity theory, the pattern or summation theory and the gate control theory.

Specificity theory

Descartes (1596–1650) proposed what is described as the classic specificity theory. This traditionally held theory proposed a direct channel for pain from the periphery of the body to the brain, proposing that when the body was exposed to a painful stimulus, this was relayed to the brain by a specific pain pathway. The historical importance of this theory should not be underestimated, and it is only relatively recently that more refined theories have been proposed and accepted, thus demonstrating the inherent inadequacies of specificity theory (Latham 1991). According to Melzack & Wall (1999) its biggest flaw is that it cannot account for how a single stimulus can create different responses including emotional and cognitive.

Pattern or summation theory

According to Field & Smith (2008) the pattern theory was dominant from the end of the nineteenth century until the early 1960s. Goldscheider, at the end of the nineteenth century, proposed the pattern or summation theory which was based upon the excitatory effects of converging stimuli. He claimed that the summation of the skin impulses had a sensory input at the dorsal horn cells and produced particular patterns of nerve impulses that produced pain. When receptors normally activated by non-noxious heat or touch were subject to excessive stimulation or pathological conditions these would enhance the summation of impulses and eventually produce acute pain, and abnormally long periods of summation would produce chronic pain (Latham 1991). In 1943, Livingstone first proposed a central summation theory asserting that a central neural mechanism was responsible for pain syndromes such as phantom limb pain. However, this was strongly counter-argued because when surgical lesions of the spinal cord are performed, in the majority of cases this does not eliminate pain for any sustained length of time, indicating that a mechanism operates at a higher level than the dorsal horns.

Gate control theory

Gate control theory was developed by Melzack & Wall (1965). According to this theory, the transmission of information from a potentially painful stimulus can be modified by a gating mechanism situated in the cells (substantia gelatinosa) of the dorsal horn of the spinal cord. This mechanism can increase or decrease the flow of nerve impulses from the periphery to the CNS. If the gate is open, impulses pass through; if it is partially open, some pass through; and if shut, no impulses get through and pain is not experienced.

Melzack & Wall (1965), in their seminal text, argued that whether the gate is open or closed is determined by:

- activity in small-diameter fibres (A-δ and C fibres, which transmit pain)
- activity in large-diameter fibres (A-β fibres, which transmit touch)
- descending influences from higher centres, including those concerned with motivational and cognitive processes.

Melzack & Wall (1965) proposed that the substantia gelatinosa is activated by large A-β fibres that shut the gate and inhibited by small A-δ and C fibres that open the gate. This activity then influences the information sent to the brain, which in turn initiates descending inhibitory controls depending on the information from other areas such as the cortex (Figure 19.1)

Understanding of the physiology of pain has developed since the gate control theory was first proposed, such as the discovery of endogenous opioid neurotransmitters (e.g. endorphins). Chemicals, such as prostaglandins, released in response to a painful stimulus also influence whether the gate is closed or open. However, the inherent fundamental principles have stood the test of time and influenced pain management. The principles of gate control theory are used in nursing care, such as the application of heat/cold, massage, etc. The use of touch and massage stimulates the skin, increasing large fibre (A-β) activity and thereby closing the gate at the spinal cord level and relieving pain. This rationale also explains the benefit of advice to 'rub it better'.

Closing the gate at the brain stem level can sometimes be achieved by ensuring sufficient sensory input, e.g. by using distraction (see p. 570). Similarly, at the level of the cortex/thalamus, the gate can be closed by reducing anxiety, e.g. by providing accurate information about the cause, likely course and relief of pain and thereby increasing the person's confidence and sense of control.

Factors that may exacerbate pain (i.e. opening the gate) may include injury, anxiety, low mood, fatigue or boredom and focusing too much upon the pain (Chamley & James 2007).

Interestingly, Descartes had earlier made the observation for which Melzack, Wall and others such as Beecher take credit: that the nervous system has the ability to regulate the intensity of the pain experience (Grady et al 2007).

Pain physiology and functional anatomy – an overview

A basic overview of pain physiology and functional anatomy is provided. Readers requiring more information should consult their own anatomy and physiology books, or Further reading (e.g. Clancy & McVicar 2009). The structures and substances involved in the pain sensation include:

- Nociceptors (noxious sensation receptors) – specialised neurones found throughout the body, especially in the skin. They are classified according to the speed at which they can conduct nerve impulses, which is dependent upon the diameter of the axon and whether or not it is myelinated. Therefore, larger axons would conduct faster than smaller axons. The myelin acts as an electrical insulator to enhance the speed of transmission. Nociceptors may be mechanoceptors or polymodal nociceptors which are responsible for different types of impulses and have different characteristics. For example, mechanoceptors respond to strong pressure over a wide skin area, whereas polymodal receptors respond to tissue damage caused by mechanical stimuli, chemicals released in response to damaged tissue, e.g. kinins, histamine, 5-hydroxytryptamine (5-HT, serotonin), substance P and prostaglandins, or thermal insults (Carter 1994).

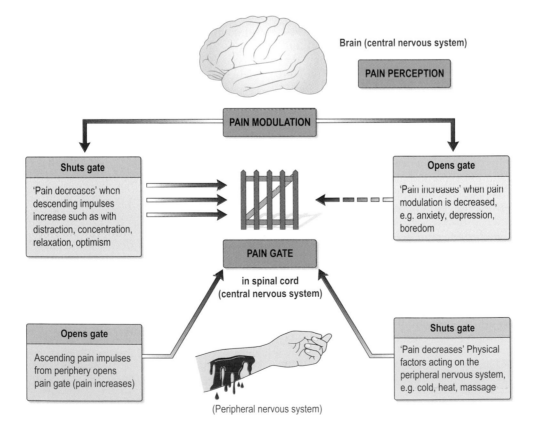

Figure 19.1 Gate-control theory. (Reproduced from Brooker & Waugh 2007 with permission.)

Silent nociceptors which are inactive or in a resting state, refractory to mechanical or electrical stimuli. However, in the presence of tissue damage or inflammation the nociceptors 'switch on' and become active. It is believed that although these are described as silent from the point of nerve impulse propagation, they do provide the sensory system with continuous data from the tissue environment, which is signalled to the spinal cord via microtubular mechanisms in the axon of nerve cells (Grady et al 2007).

- Peripheral nerve pathways – once a nociceptor is activated, an electrical impulse is conducted along an afferent (sensory) neurone.
- The impulse travels in the dorsal columns of the spinal cord to the brain. The impulse may be modified by the gate control mechanism within the spinal cord (see pp. 553–554). Impulses can also be modified by descending control from the brain (Davies & Taylor 2003). Further modification in the spinal cord and brain stem prevent many pain impulses ever reaching consciousness.
- The brain stem processes and integrates pain sensations. According to Melzack & Wall (1999) there is extensive evidence to suggest that a mechanism, operating in the brain stem, leads to reduced pain perception. Endogenous opioid neurotransmitters capable of reducing pain perception are released from brain tissue, e.g. endorphins and enkephalins (Davies & Taylor 2003).

CLASSIFICATION OF TYPES OF PAIN

In order for nurses to provide evidence-based care it is crucial to understand the person's pain experience, which in its broadest sense is classified according to timescale (Chamley & James 2007) (Figure 19.2). However, timescale may be too simplistic for the complex spectrum of the pain experience.

Pain may be classified according to factors such as the presumed origin that may include related pathology and type of pain or clinical speciality and client group. Historically pain was distinguished as being either acute or chronic, but clear distinctions between the two are not easily discernable (McCaffery & Pasero 1999). Horn & Munafo (1997) propose that acute and chronic pain may be usefully regarded as being at the ends of a spectrum rather than being fundamentally separate conditions.

Acute pain

This is often described as being short lived, that is less than 6 weeks, and is commonly nociceptive pain associated with surgery, trauma or acute disease. Acute pain will usually diminish as healing occurs before ceasing completely. Acute pain may occur suddenly or the onset may be slower. It can be of any intensity ranging from a mild headache to agonising chest pain with a major heart attack (see Ch. 2). Ongoing time-limited pain (chronic–acute) may last for a prolonged period but usually it will cease once the cause is removed or treated such as with burns pain. Four processes are involved in acute nociceptive pain: transduction, transmission, modulation and perception (McCaffery & Pasero 1999):

Transduction occurs when nociceptors of C fibres and A-δ fibres of afferent neurones respond to painful stimuli causing the release of inflammatory chemicals including prostaglandins, kinins, histamine, 5-HT, etc., forming an 'algesic (*pain causing*) soup'. The categories of noxious stimuli include:

- mechanical – pressure, swelling, abscess, incision and tumours
- thermal – burns and scalds
- chemical – including inflammation/infection, ischaemia and toxins.

The effects of inflammatory chemicals released from damaged tissue can be modified by non-steroidal anti-inflammatory drugs (NSAIDs), e.g. ibuprofen.

Figure 19.2 Types of pain. (Reproduced from Brooker & Waugh 2007 with permission.)

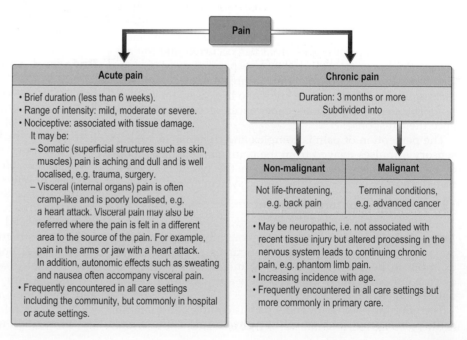

Transmission The pain impulse is transmitted from the site of transduction along the nociceptor fibre to the dorsal horn of the spinal cord and onwards to the brain stem, thalamus, the cerebral cortex and higher centres. As there is no dedicated pain centre, impulses that arrive in the thalamus are directed to multiple areas within the brain for processing. Many pharmacological treatments for pain interfere with the transmission of pain impulses along the pathway between the site of tissue injury and the cerebral cortex, for example topical anaesthetic and analgesic (against pain) products.

Modulation This occurs when the pain impulse is inhibited or changed (modulated) by chemical or neural influences on the 'pain gate'. The complex and multiple pathways involved in pain modulation are described as the descending modulatory pain pathways, and activities within these pathways can either increase transmission of pain impulses (excitatory) or inhibit or decrease transmission.

Nerves descending from the brain stem to the spinal cord close the gate by releasing endogenous opioids, and this may be the reason why nociceptive pain is responsive to opioids and accounts for the variation in pain perception seen in clinical practice. That is, some patients have more effective modulation than others (McCaffery & Pasero 1999). Chamley & James (2007) draw our attention to the 'placebo effect' which has been identified in individuals who have an analgesic response to a masked inert substance (such as a sugar pill) in a double-blind trial of inert substance versus an active drug. Some individuals respond to the placebo whilst others have a poor or no response. Placebo responders may be those with a well-developed endogenous opioid system (Chamley & James 2007).

Perception is the end result of neural activity where pain becomes a conscious multidimensional experience. As there is no 'pain centre' in the brain, pain perception occurs through an 'action system'. Opioid-binding sites have been identified in several parts of the brain, indicating that they have a role in pain perception. When painful stimuli are transmitted to the brain stem and thalamus, multiple cortical areas are activated and a response is elicited. The first aspect of pain perception is warning and protection and the individual would rapidly assess what has occurred and initiate action (Melzack & Wall 1988), but psychological factors also have an important role, for example anxiety, emotional distress and helplessness are known to increase pain perception. The person's previous experiences of pain will influence their response.

The perception of pain is complex and dynamic involving sensory impulses relayed from the pain gates and activation of pain responses mediated through the reticular system, somatosensory cortex and the limbic system (Wood 2008).

🖱 **See website for further content**

Acute episodes of pain occur throughout life. These episodes are usually self-contained and sometimes predictable, for example in people who experience migraine or sickle cell disease episodes, but in between these episodes the individual is pain free.

The neurophysiology of acute pain is complex and intense acute pain is often accompanied by physiological effects, e.g.

Box 19.2 Information

Physiological and behavioural responses to pain (adapted from Chamley & James 2007)

Physiological responses include:

- Sweating
- Increased heart rate, respiratory rate and blood pressure
- Vomiting due to gastric stasis

Behavioural responses include:

- Anxiety
- Withdrawal and lack of cooperation
- Aggression, abusiveness, swearing, agitation
- Attention seeking
- Quietness
- Poor concentration (focused on pain)
- Grimacing, frowning
- Rubbing or holding the painful part
- Thrashing about, pacing, adopting a particular position, keeping very still
- Moaning, shouting, screaming, crying
- (In children) fractiousness, food refusal, withdrawal

People who have learning disabilities may exhibit changes in their behaviour but it is important that the pain is recognised and changes in behaviour are not just attributed to personality/disability.

tachycardia, sweating, as the body responds to the potent stressor (see Ch. 17). Initially these are activated by the sympathetic division of the autonomic nervous system and are referred to as 'flight or fight' responses which are automatic, primitive survival mechanisms. It is important for nurses to understand the physiological and behavioural effects of pain (Box 19.2). This is crucial when caring for people who have difficulties in communication or are unable to articulate their pain such as pre-verbal children, some individuals who have learning disabilities and associated communication problems or people with dementia.

Referred pain

Referred pain occurs when acute nociceptive pain originates in an internal organ such as the heart and the pain is experienced some distance away from the chest, i.e. in the arms (particularly the left arm) or the back, neck and jaw. This is due to sensory impulses from the left arm and the heart entering the spinal cord at the same level. Normally, few sensory impulses are processed from the heart so when more impulses than normal are received to be processed this results in the perception of pain in the arm. The pain is usually referred to a structure developed from the same embryonic structure or sclerotome.

Stannard & Booth (2004) describe *trigger points* which are also associated with referred pain. These are small areas of hypersensitivity located in muscles or connective tissue, and when they are triggered the pain is felt at a distance. This type of referred pain is not aligned to a dermatome but stimulation will produce pain in a predictable location.

Chronic pain

When acute pain has not resolved after 3 months it is termed chronic (British Pain Society & Royal College of Anaesthetists 2003). However, increased knowledge of the pathophysiology of disorders that were traditionally associated with chronic pain has made the classification by time potentially redundant (IASP 1994). Increasingly, the term 'persistent pain' is used to describe chronic pain, and to classify pain by pathophysiological mechanisms including nociceptive and neuropathic pain (see below). Nociceptive pain is caused by tissue damage, whereas neuropathic pain describes pain that persists beyond the original cause, such as a nerve injury or infective cause. These pain types are defined as non-life threatening (benign) or non-malignant. Pain may be intermittent, for example irritable bowel syndrome (IBS), rheumatoid arthritis or back pain. The pain has not responded to conventional treatment and may last for life. Low back pain currently accounts for over 50% of all musculoskeletal disabilities; work loss due to back pain in the UK is approximately 52 million days per year (Box 19.3). Disability due to low back pain has reached epidemic proportions and treatment costs amount to 1% of the total NHS budget (Grady et al 2007).

The exact mechanisms involved in the pathophysiology of chronic persistent pain are complex and to date remain unclear. Even after the original acute painful episode has healed, chronic pain may manifest, and in some instances presents with no initial physiological assault. Ko & Zhou (2004) suggest that chronic pain may follow injury or disease with rapid long-term changes occurring within the CNS, particularly if the acute episode was not effectively managed. Within the spinal cord a central mechanism exists known as 'wind-up', which has links to physiological hypersensitivity and hyperexcitability. Wind-up occurs when there are repeated, prolonged and sustained noxious stimuli which cause the dorsal horn cells to fire and transmit progressively increasing numbers of pain impulses (Wood 2008). More recently, it was considered that spinal cord glial (supportive) cells are involved in chronic persistent pain; glial cells regulate extracellular ions and neurotransmitters, and clear away debris. Therefore, the suggestion is that glial cells are potentially responsible for amplifying pain by releasing substances that stimulate the pain response.

During episodes of chronic pain sensitisation can occur; there is amplification and distortion of pain messages and the painful condition is out of proportion to the original injury (Field & Smith 2008). Furthermore, spinal cord sensitisation can result from chemical reactions which increase pain messages being forwarded to the brain. PNS sensitisation can result from inflammation which causes nociceptors to fire with greater intensity.

Chronic pain is generally subdivided into:

- chronic non-malignant pain (nociceptive and neuropathic pain); NB, both types may coexist
- malignant (life-threatening) pain.

Chronic non-malignant pain

There is persuasive evidence, mainly from developed countries, which suggests that chronic pain is a widespread public health issue. Some community-based studies have found that between 15 and 25% of adults suffer from chronic pain at any given time, and this figure can increase to 50% in populations over 65 years of age (Brennan et al 2007). Chronic non-malignant pain can be caused by persistent tissue injury where a degenerative condition exists: 46.5% of the population have conditions which result in chronic pain (Elliot et al 1999). It is thought that chronic non-malignant pain involves physiological changes to pain processing in the CNS which results in pain memories and leads to conditions such as phantom pain following amputation.

See website Critical thinking question 19.1

Chronic non-malignant pain can be as destructive as malignant pain, as eventually it impacts on the individual's family and social life and employment (McCaffery & Beebe 1989). Furthermore, it leads to isolation, relationship difficulties and mental health problems including suicidal ideation.

Chronic malignant pain

Chronic malignant pain is associated with life-threatening conditions and most frequently with cancer in which there may be progressive spread of the disease which contributes to the chronicity of pain.

Pain associated with cancer is rarely a presenting feature, but the person's 'cancer journey' may begin with acute pain (nociceptive) resulting from diagnostic procedures, including surgery. If the cancer metastasises, the pain becomes chronic, involving nociceptive and neuropathic elements but also psychoemotional ones. There needs to be regular assessment and readjustment of treatment to meet the needs of the individual; this requires the skills of an MDT (see Chs 31, 33). The prevalence of cancer increases with age, and pain is one of the most distressing symptoms. Unfortunately, for many older people it is more likely that pain will be under-reported and undertreated.

Chronic pain and depression may occur concomitantly as chronic pain may exacerbate depression and vice versa. A study by Gureje et al (1998) revealed that people living with chronic pain are four times more likely than those

Box 19.3 Reflection

Chronic pain (persistent pain)

The National Institute for Health and Clinical Excellence (NICE) has published guidance relating to persistent low back pain.

Activity

- Access the NICE guidance and review the recommendations.
- Consider how the specific recommendations for persistent non-specific low back pain could be used to inform your nursing practice when caring for a person with persistent pain.

Resource

National Institute for Health and Clinical Excellence 2009 Early management of persistent non-specific low back pain. Clinical guidance 88. Available online http://guidance.nice.org.uk/CG88

Box 19.4 Evidence-based practice

Chronic pain and depressive illness

Pain syndrome is thought to play a role in depression. This study assesses the prevalence of chronic (≥6 months' duration) painful physical conditions (CPPCs) (joint/articular, limb, or back pain, headaches, or gastrointestinal diseases) and their relationship with major depressive disorder...

Of all subjects interviewed, 17.1% reported having at least 1 CPPC (95% confidence interval [CI], 16.5%–17.6%). At least 1 depressive symptom (sadness, depression, hopelessness, loss of interest, or lack of pleasure) was present in 16.5% of subjects (95% CI, 16.0%–17.1%); 27.6% of these subjects had at least 1 CPPC. Major depressive disorder was diagnosed in 4.0% of subjects; 43.4% of these subjects had at least 1 CPPC, which was 4 times more often than in subjects without major depressive disorder (odds ratio [OR], 4.0; 95% CI, 3.5–4.7). In a logistic regression model, CPPC was strongly associated with major depressive disorder (OR: CPPC alone, 3.6; CPPC + nonpainful medical condition, 5.2); 24-hour presence of pain made an independent contribution to major depressive disorder diagnosis (OR, 1.6)...

The presence of CPPCs increases the duration of depressive mood. Patients seeking consultation for a CPPC should be systematically evaluated for depression. (Ohayon & Schatzberg [2003] from the Abstract)

Activity

- Access the full article by Ohayon & Schatzberg (2003) and consider the link between chronic pain and depression.
- Think about the implications of the study findings for your care of people with chronic pain and discuss the issues with your mentor.

Resource

Ohayon M M, Schatzberg A F 2003 Using chronic pain to predict depressive morbidity in the general population. Archives of General Psychiatry 60(1): 39–47. Available online http://archpsyc.ama-assn.org/cgi/content/full/60/1/39

---

without to suffer from depression and anxiety, which is consistent with other statistics on pain as a risk factor for both conditions (Fishbain 1999) (Box 19.4). It is estimated that 28% of people attending pain clinics (see p. 569) have a well-defined affective illness and people may manifest depression during the course of a painful illness without having being depressed previously (Grady et al 2007). However, approximately half of all depressed people have pain. Atypical facial pain was a common presenting feature in 66% of a series of depressed women, and in a smaller proportion of both sexes tension headaches were the most common presenting feature of depression.

Pain disorder or the chronic pain syndrome is a specific syndrome characterised by:

- pain as the predominant presenting complaint
- pain causing significant distress or impairment in social, occupational or other aspects of life
- psychological factors that are considered to play a significant role in the onset, severity exacerbation and/or maintenance of pain
- no malingering
- no alternative explanation such as depressive disorder, including anxiety or mood disorders.

There are advantages in the recognition and acceptance of pain disorder – there is the recognition that affective factors need to be addressed in order for there to be a chance of improvement for the person. There is the need to acknowledge that chronic pain is an illness and that it warrants holistic management embracing the wholeness of the individual.

Nociceptive pain

Nociceptive pain is the most common type of pain seen in clinical settings and may be somatic or visceral (see Figure 19.2, p. 555). Pain results from stimulation of nociceptors following tissue damage or inflammation, e.g. surgery, infection or trauma. Intense and ongoing stimulation of nociceptors increases the excitability of neurones in the spinal cord leading to central sensitisation.

Neuropathic pain

Neuropathic pain is initiated or caused by a primary lesion or dysfunction of the PNS or CNS (IASP 1994). The damage to the PNS and CNS can be due to stroke, spinal cord injury, brachial plexus avulsion, herpes zoster (shingles) leading to post-herpetic neuralgia, or follow amputation.

Damage leads to the development of central sensitisation causing reorganisation of synapses in the spinal cord and hyperexcitability in the peripheral nerves, and as a result the individual experiences symptoms that are characteristic of neuropathic pain. This definition has attracted some criticism, being described as vague, particularly in relation to the term 'dysfunction' which blurs the distinction between neuropathic pain and other possible pain types that may arise from different underlying mechanisms (Backonja 2003). It has been observed that pain and other neurological symptoms due to PNS or CNS disease/injury present in very similar ways, and this observation has led to a group designation of neuropathic pain. This definition is based upon the presence of neurological disease; however, it is important to note that most disorders that involve the nociceptors responsive to thermal stimuli do not present with pain and would suggest that these people have conditions that are genetic in origin (Backonja 2003).

Affected individuals can experience increased sympathetic activity including sweating and changes to skin colour, texture and temperature. Pain in an area of sensory loss may be described as spontaneous, paroxysmal, sharp, shooting or stabbing.

Depending on the exact cause it may manifest as:

- Phantom (limb) pain/syndrome – feeling that a limb is still part of the body following amputation. The pain felt appears to originate from the amputated limb. It is caused by altered pain processing in the CNS, possibly due to earlier nerve or tissue damage. Effective pain relief before amputation can minimise the risk of this occurring. If phantom pain does become chronic, treatment with nerve blocks and adjuvant drugs, and/or various non-pharmacological therapies such as ultrasound, relaxation or transcutaneous electrical nerve stimulation (TENS), may be helpful (see pp. 569–570).

See website Critical thinking question 19.1

- Allodynia – sensation of pain in response to a non-noxious stimulus, such as touch.
- Hyperalgesia – extreme sensitivity to a stimulus that is normally painful.
- Dysaesthesia – abnormal sensations, e.g. tingling, burning or numbness.

Neuropathic pain may respond poorly to opioids.

KEY CONCEPTS

This section of the chapter outlines the concepts of pain threshold and pain tolerance – terms often confused and used erroneously. Pain myths/misconceptions and individual differences in pain tolerance (mainly related to gender and cultural influences) are discussed.

Pain threshold

The pain threshold is 'the least experience of pain which a subject can recognize' (IASP 1994). Laboratory studies of pain have demonstrated that pain thresholds are fairly constant across the population. In other words, the vast majority of people agree on the point at which a sensation becomes painful.

Pain tolerance

Pain tolerance is 'the greatest level of pain which a subject is prepared to tolerate' (IASP 1994). Pain tolerance must be distinguished from drug threshold.

Pain tolerance differs widely amongst people and is a far more important concept than pain threshold in medicine and nursing, as it usually means that the pain has gone beyond an acceptable tolerance level and at this point the individual will seek professional help (Field & Smith 2008).

Advancing age is known to be associated with a greater prevalence of pain, ranging from 25 to 65% in older people living at home and upwards of 80% in older adults requiring residential/nursing home care (Helme & Gibson 2001). It has been suggested by Briggs (2003) that older people have lower pain tolerances and experience pain at a greater intensity. The experimental evidence would assert that this may result from the ageing process and associated physiological and neurological changes. Moreover, older adults are more likely to have co-morbidities and polypharmacy. There is little evidence to suggest that neonates, infants and children have a different pain tolerance from adults and the previously held belief that infants were incapable of experiencing pain is now completely accepted to be a myth (Carter 1994).

Pain myths

Pain management may be subject to traditional and ill-informed prejudice which sometimes holds sway over evidence and a common sense approach to pain management (McQuay et al 1997). There are enduring myths, misconceptions, false judgements, mistaken beliefs and misunderstandings which reflect outmoded beliefs and lack of knowledge and understanding in relation to the pain experience of another (Box 19.5). Children in particular have been disadvantaged over time, as it has only been since the 1970s that child pain assessment and management has

---

i | **Box 19.5 Information**

Pain myths: explained

- Pain is the earliest symptom of cancer – except in cancers involving nerve tissue or bone. Pain is usually a late symptom of advanced cancer.
- Older adults and health professionals may believe that chronic pain is inevitable during ageing – this myth is firmly embedded in sociocultural beliefs and poses significant barriers to pain relief for older people. Pain may be overlooked as part of the ageing process. It is a common symptom associated with co-morbidities of old age. The ability of the older person to withstand chronic illness and pain may also depend upon their circumstances and coping mechanisms.
- Pain medication always causes heavy sedation – people with chronic and enduring pain will have had problems sleeping. Therefore, opioid analgesics may produce some initial sedation for 24 hours which allows them some rest and sleep.
- Infants cannot feel pain due to their immature nervous system – complete development of nerves is not required for pain perception, and neonates exhibit both behavioural and physiological responses to pain.
- Infants and children experience less pain than adults – younger children may perceive a greater intensity of pain than older children and adults.

- A person's behaviour accurately reflects their level of pain – children and adults who are sleeping, or who are active, playing, reading, etc., may still be experiencing pain but are coping with it.
- Psychological dependence and respiratory depression are common side-effects of opioid analgesics – these are uncommon but fear of them can hamper effective pain management.
- There are some types of pain that cannot be treated – some types of pain require combined approaches (multimodality) for effective pain relief. The recent advances in pain management ensure that all types of pain can be controlled.
- People have to be in hospital to receive effective pain management – it is easier to provide safe and effective pain relief at home than it is in the average hospital.
- Treating depression in older people with chronic illness has little effect on coping with pain – treating depression in older people enhances coping with the pain associated with chronic illnesses and improves quality of life.
- Complementary and alternative therapies do not have an important role in pain management – various techniques can be used by people as coping strategies for managing pain.

attracted any interest. The lack of scientific evidence encouraged poor practice: children, in particular infants, were operated upon, sutured, injected and subjected to intense levels of procedural pain. Advances in science and technology have provided evidence which refutes many of these myths and increasingly evidence-based practice is used to provide effective pain management across the lifespan.

A barrier to effective pain relief was linked to misconceptions relating to medications, particularly opioids, among health care professionals. There was concern regarding opioid addiction, tolerance and hyperalgesia, including correct dosage, escalation and physical dependence. Fear of opioids among health care professionals is compounded by their ignorance of opioids (Brennan et al 2007). At the heart of these concerns are inadequate education and training among health care professionals and patients who express high levels of concern about opioids, particularly with advancing age. Results of countless surveys over the last 20 years provide incontrovertible proof that many nurses still lack adequate information about pain management and there remain concerns regarding determination of effective opioid dose and exaggerated fear of addiction (McCaffery & Ferrell 1997). Opioids remain the drug of choice for the treatment of moderate to severe pain regardless of aetiology, but fear of opioid misuse and addiction continue to shape policy and prescription of these drugs.

Individual differences in pain perception

The way in which an individual perceives and responds to pain is unique to the individual and is the culmination of many variables that include gender, past pain experiences, social and cultural factors. Furthermore, it is recognised that pain experiences very early in life can influence pain processing over the rest of the lifespan, as is illustrated in children who remember their early pain experiences but can learn to modify their responses. The inter-relationship between pain, anxiety and fear has been extensively investigated and the evidence would suggest that anxiety and fear magnify pain, particularly in children. Therefore, the person's emotional state is important and various factors contribute to that state including diagnosis, prognosis, coping ability and their social support networks coupled with their own beliefs and meanings they assign to pain (Field & Smith 2008).

Locus of control testing indicates how people will respond and adapt to pain. People with an internal locus of control believe that through their own behaviour they more readily exert control over their own health; the perception of lack of control can result in increased anxiety. Those with an external locus of control believe that they have little or no influence over the outcomes of their pain experience and that their health is in the 'hands of others', fate or chance. They may therefore appear to be very dependent upon others.

Contemporary thinking has moved away from the idea that personality and overt pain behaviours are inter-related and places greater emphasis upon the mental processes such as memory, locus of control, self-efficacy and comprehension that help to mediate individual pain behaviour (Chamley & James 2007).

Gender

It has been suggested that men are better able to tolerate pain than women, but the evidence for this is inconclusive and mostly taken from data reporting the incidence of pain. A population prevalence study found women reported significantly more incidence of pain than men (Müllersdorf & Söderback 2000). Similar findings were reported from an epidemiological study of pain (Elliott et al 1999) and from a population-based telephone survey by Portenoy et al (2004). These findings may be explained by the different ways in which men and women are socialised (Bendelow 1993). In some societies men are expected to be 'brave', and tend not to report pain, whereas women are expected to be expressive or 'emotional', and tend to report pain. Another possibility is that gender differences can be explained in terms of coping style. Rollnick et al (2003) found that women were more likely to adopt passive coping strategies, whereas men were more likely to adopt active coping strategies. Passive coping strategies are more likely to result in disability as a consequence of pain.

Coping is also influenced by socioeconomic factors. Portenoy et al (2004) argue that women are more likely to have poorer socioeconomic conditions than men, which may provide an alternative explanation for gender differences in the pain experience and behavioural response.

Cultural influences on pain expression

Few studies have been undertaken to understand the way in which society shapes the meaning and treatment of pain (Lasch 2002), although Carr & Mann (2000) and Portenoy et al (2004) suggest that people from minority cultural groups are more likely to experience poor pain management. However, more research has been undertaken about cultural perception and expression of pain. Each cultural group has its own behaviours, beliefs, values and meaning 'scripts' that shape responses to pain, as well as help-seeking activities and receptivity to health care interventions. For example, many British people traditionally value control over the display of emotions – maintaining a 'stiff upper lip' – which has the effect of discouraging people from reporting pain. Kikuya and Masai tribesmen are expected to respond to pain with dignity and composure, whereas it is acceptable for the women to cry and wail, except during labour when stoicism is required (Carter 1994).

A classic study by Zborowski (1952) illustrates the link between culture and pain. Men from three groups were compared: 'old Americans' (i.e. their grandparents or earlier forebears were born in the USA and they did not identify with a particular cultural group), Italian Americans and Jewish Americans. The 'old Americans' attempted to avoid showing any pain, tended to withdraw and preferred to be alone when in severe pain. The Italian and Jewish Americans, however, openly expressed their pain and did not want to be alone. The Italian Americans were concerned with relief of their pain, while the Jewish Americans were concerned about the implications of their pain for the future. This study has been criticised for selecting people whose culture, and consequently their responses, may have been 'diluted' by living in the USA; nevertheless, the study points to the influence of culture on expression and experience.

The influence of culture on the experience and expression of pain has more recently been explored through narrative research. This approach to understanding the influence of culture on the experience of pain enables the beliefs and values that shape this experience to be understood.

MANAGEMENT OF PAIN

Pain assessment and measurement are critical to the holistic care and management of the individual's pain: one of the most challenging and commonly undertaken tasks for nurses. Pain assessment is complex and depends upon the interaction of a number of variables, not least the therapeutic relationship between the nurse and the person with pain. Objective and systematic assessment of pain is a fundamental right of everyone and Article 3 of the Human Rights Act (1998) states that 'No one shall be subject to torture or to inhumane or degrading treatment or punishment'.

The NMC states that in order to provide optimal care nurses require appropriate knowledge, skills and attitudes towards pain, and the associated assessment and management of patients' pain journey. This must be based upon the best available evidence to prevent patients from suffering (NMC 2008). It is unacceptable for people to experience unmanaged pain, or for nurses to have inadequate knowledge about pain and poor understanding of their professional accountability in this aspect of care (Dimond 2002). Furthermore, pain has been identified as the fifth vital sign in an attempt to facilitate and engender greater accountability for pain assessment and management (Chronic Pain Coalition 2007). The 'gold standard' is to ask and believe the person about their pain experience and assessment should not be based upon, for instance, the expected pain associated with a particular surgical procedure or a medical condition, which will underestimate the pain (Sjöström et al 2000).

There is no single test for pain, and to date there is no single evidence-based document for pain management. However, the DH in England has recently published completely new *Essence of Care Benchmarks for the Prevention and Management of Pain* (DH 2010). There are a variety of measures which can inform the overall pain assessment, including biomedical, psychosocial and behavioural responses.

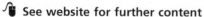 **See website for further content**

Pain assessment

Pain assessment also encompasses pain measurement (see below). Assessment is the overall appraisal of the factors which are influencing the experience and expression of pain (McCaffery & Pasero 1999). This is the comprehensive process of describing the pain and its effect upon the person's function based upon a systematic process of assessment, measurement and reassessment or evaluation. Melzack & Katz (1994) outline the aims of assessment, including to:

- determine the intensity, quality and duration of pain
- aid diagnosis
- determine the most appropriate therapy

- evaluate the relative effectiveness of different treatment modalities
- monitor the standards of clinical practice.

Field & Smith (2008) suggest four main approaches to pain assessment:

- Talk to the person.
- Observe the person's behaviour.
- Record physiological signs.
- Utilise appropriate pain assessment tools.

Talking with the person and discussing their pain is the most fundamental way to assess the pain – after all, only the person with the pain knows how much it hurts. This aspect of pain assessment is often undervalued and studies report that few patients were asked about their pain and as a consequence experienced unnecessary pain (Carr & Thomas 1997). However, in studies where the person or carers were asked by nurses how they could help to relieve the person's pain, this reinforced the importance and central role of the nurse in listening and being sensitive to the needs of the patient (Manias et al 2002). The interplay of many variables can influence this process. In the first instance the person may be reluctant to report pain because they do not want to worry family or interrupt the work of busy nursing staff. Children may lack either the language or cognitive ability, and adults with learning disabilities or cognitive impairment such as dementia may not be able to articulate their pain. Furthermore, personal biases, myths and prejudices of the nurses may influence the assessment, who may believe that pain should be managed according to their own views of pain.

Pain measurement

Measuring pain enables the nurse to assess the amount of pain the person is experiencing. Where possible the person's self-report of their pain is regarded as the highest standard of pain assessment-measures by providing the most valid pain measurement (Peter & Watt-Watson 2002). Pain measurement enables appropriate intervention, evaluation and understanding of the individual's pain. Measurement refers to pain on a scale, that is the application of some metric to a specific element, usually pain intensity. Therefore, pain should be measured using an appropriate pain assessment tool that identifies both quantitative and/or qualitative dimensions of the person's pain. However, an assumption may be made that pain measurement is subjective and therefore will be of little value. Furthermore, some nursing staff appear to distrust patients' self-reporting of pain, which suggests that some nurses may have their own personal benchmarks of what is deemed acceptable as to when and how people should express their pain (Watt-Watson 2001). The reality is that if measurements are carried out properly, sensitive and consistent results can be obtained. However, there are some circumstances when it may not be possible to measure pain or when reports are likely to be unreliable. Most acute pain analgesic studies include measurements of pain intensity and/or pain relief and the commonest tools are categorical and visual analogue scales (see below).

Nursing management and health promotion: assessing and measuring pain

Pain assessment, which includes pain measurement, is the responsibility of every nurse – not just those nurse specialists working within pain teams (see p. 569).

Pain is generally measured on a scale without taking into consideration any other component related to pain, such as mood (Chamley & James 2007). A valid pain assessment is one that involves the person in pain, meaning that the nurse should not assess the patient's pain in isolation from the patient (Field & Smith 2008). Always asking the person about their pain ensures that they can verbalise (if able) their unique pain experience (Davies & Taylor 2003).

Therefore communication skills are essential for effective pain assessment and the nurse must consider how she/he frames questions. Some questions that may help to understand and characterise the person's pain include:

- When did your pain start?
- How long does it usually last?
- Is there anything which makes the pain worse (such as movement or eating/drinking)?
- Where does it hurt?
- Does the pain stop you from doing anything?
- What do you do to relieve your pain?
- Does the pain occur at certain times of the day or night?
- Does the pain stop you from sleeping?

Nurses need to be aware of potential barriers and individual differences in the expression of pain, such as age, cognitive ability, gender and culture (see pp. 559–561). Also nurses should not be influenced by their own beliefs, prejudices, personal experiences, attitudes and values (Field & Smith 2008). Equally it is crucial to acknowledge that for some people verbal communication may be absent or difficult because of coexisting pathology, e.g. after a stroke, or other language difficulties, or when the language is not understood or fully developed. This is because during assessment of the individual's pain the nurse is not only measuring pain intensity but asking what this experience means to the person and how it affects their activities of living. As already mentioned, Carr & Thomas (1997) report that this aspect of pain assessment is undervalued in some studies where people were not questioned about their pain.

McCaffery & Pasero (1999) outline the essential issues of pain assessment:

- Ask about the pain, but appreciate that people may not use traditional descriptors for their pain (see below).
- Accept and respect what they have to say about their pain – they know it best.
- Intervene appropriately to relieve the pain.
- Ask them after intervention about their pain.

The words often used to describe pain include: aching, agonising, biting, boring, burning, bursting, colicky, cramping, crushing, cutting, discomfort, dragging, drawing, dull, exhausting, gnawing, grinding, gripping, heavy, hurting, irritation, lancing, penetrating, piercing, pinching, pins and needles, pounding, pressing, punishing, scalding, sharp, shooting, smarting, soreness, spasms, stabbing, stinging, takes my breath away, tearing, tender, throbbing, tingle, twinge, torture, wearing.

Pain assessment is cyclical (assess–plan–intervention–evaluation) involving the MDT working inter-professionally to secure positive outcomes for the person.

Observation alone is difficult and unreliable but should not be dismissed. People who are in pain may articulate this in their behavioural responses, especially infants and children who do not have the language skills and people with cognitive impairment.

Pain maps

Pain maps are increasingly used during assessment to help identify or locate the person's pain. These comprise a picture of a body outline (anterior and posterior) combined with other forms of evaluation; the person marks or identifies the areas of pain and records other information, such as intensity, nature of the pain(s) and what makes it worse or better.

🖱 **See website Figure 19.1**

The maps are an important way for the person to retain 'ownership' of their pain management, empowering carers and patients particularly those with chronic pain. Pain maps are useful tools for evaluating pain.

Pain diaries

Keeping a pain diary can be an effective means of identifying patterns of pain and this can be useful especially for people who experience chronic pain. Pain diaries can also inform the assessment and management process because people may document some of the complex components associated with the pain experience, such as the emotional, social and financial effects as well as the physical.

🖱 **See website for further content**

Pain assessment tools

A pain assessment tool must be reliable and valid. Reliability refers to consistency, stability and the reproducibility of measurements made by different nurses. Validity refers to the appropriateness, applicability and the representativeness of measurements which reflect the true findings of an individual's pain at any given time. Selecting an appropriate pain assessment tool is important. Coll et al (2004) suggest utilising a framework developed by Fitzpatrick et al (1998). The framework was formulated from a comprehensive review of 5621 abstracts and articles that focused upon methodological perspectives of patient-based outcome measures including eight criteria:

- appropriate – for the purpose and setting
- reliable – in terms of internal consistency and reproducibility
- valid – it should measure the person's perception of pain
- responsive – it should capture changes that are important to the person
- precise – accurate and discriminating
- interpretable – meaningful information is produced
- acceptable – to those using the tool
- feasible – in relation to the burden of effort.

A further consideration is that assessing different pain types requires different pain assessment tools that are appropriate for the age and cognitive ability of the individual. To assess acute pain the nurse may utilise a tool that is quick and easy to use, for example a visual analogue scale, numerical rating scale or a verbal/descriptive scale. However, the assessment of types of chronic pain, including pain associated with cancer, may require a more detailed assessment tool that can be used to provide a more comprehensive analysis of the person's pain and how it might be relieved (Field & Smith 2008).

Pain assessment tools may be unidimensional or multidimensional. Unidimensional tools collect and measure one dimension of the pain experience, e.g. pain intensity. They are accurate, quick and easy to use and understand, e.g. body map, numerical scales, picture scales or verbal rating scales. Multidimensional tools capture both qualitative and quantitative pain data. They are useful for neuropathic pain, but they do require that the person is able to communicate effectively and they take longer to complete. Examples include the hospital anxiety and depression questionnaire (HAD), brief pain inventory, McGill pain questionnaire (MPQ), Pain Disability Index, cognitively impaired/dementia pain scales and multidimensional pain inventory.

Observational tools are useful for people with altered consciousness or who are sedated or cognitively impaired. These tools assess physiological responses and behavioural responses, such as grimace, restlessness, etc. Global scales are useful to rate the effectiveness of patient-controlled analgesia (PCA) for acute pain management, or transcutaneous electrical nerve stimulation (TENS) in chronic pain management. Pain assessment tools are classified as:

- self-report
- observational
- physiological measurement.

Self-report pain assessment tools

Self-report scales include a variety of simple methods to collect data relating to the person's pain (Box 19.6). These include visual analogue scale (VAS), numerical rating scale (NRS) and verbal rating scale (VRS). Other scales in this category may also include questionnaires and interviews. Self-reporting can be adapted for children by modifying the scale, for example using a 'pain thermometer' scale, or children can use their own words on a scale of no pain to worst hurt. Moreover, Chamley & James (2007) suggest that the

pain thermometer with a scale of 0–10/100 has been well received by older people (see Further reading, e.g. Royal College of Physicians 2007). However, patient preference is all important with acceptability and engagement with a tool.

Visual analogue scale (VAS) is usually a 10 cm line (usually horizontal but can be vertical) with 'no pain' at one end and 'worst pain possible' at the other end (Figure 19.3A). The person marks the position on the scale which best reflects their pain. The assessor measures the mark in cm from the left-hand side or the foot of a vertical scale to obtain the 'score'. The advantages of this scale include the absence of numbers or words; the person in pain is not required to assign a precise numerical value to the pain or to choose a word that may not exactly represent their pain. Furthermore, these tools can be modified to use with children (9–10 years) who have the cognitive ability to understand proportions and translate their experience into an analogue format (Chamley & James 2007).

Numerical rating scale (NRS) is similar to the VAS but is calibrated with the numbers 0–10 (Figure 19.3B). The person selects a number on the scale which best describes their pain intensity.

Verbal rating scale (VRS) According to Closs et al (2004), the VRS provides a more reliable guide to the person's pain intensity than other tools. This tool provides graded categories: 'no pain', 'slight pain', 'moderate pain', 'very bad pain' and 'agonising pain' (Figure 19.3C). Many people find this scale easy to use although it has the disadvantage of fewer assessment points compared to a 0–10 scale and therefore is not as sensitive.

The visual, numerical and verbal pain scales rate pain intensity, which is only one aspect of pain experience. These tools also encourage a linear assessment of pain intensity. Turk (1989) noted that pain intensity may not be perceived in a linear fashion, and that linear scales may constrain and distort the person's experience. This was borne out by a participant in Whelan's (2003) study who commented on the difficulty of expressing the meaning of the pain when using

Box 19.6 Reflection

Pain assessment tools

With your mentor discuss the pain assessment tools used in your practice area and consider the rationale for choice.

Activities

- Have there been any problems with implementation of the tools? If so, what were the main reasons for this?
- Reflect on how existing pain assessment tools could be adapted further to capture pain assessment data more effectively.
- Consider your patient group. Are there any barriers such as sociocultural or language barriers which could interfere with using self-report tools?

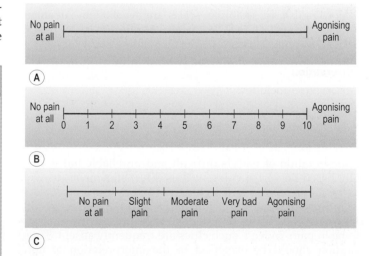

Figure 19.3 Self-report pain scales. A. Visual analogue scale. B. Numerical rating scale. C. Verbal rating scale.

a numerical scale: 'I wanted to put a meaning next to those numbers, so that if I said to my doctor "I'm having pain that's about a seven" what I mean is, it's really bad, it's incapacitating enough that I'm not able to do my daily duties, but it's not so bad that I'm not able to get out of bed.'

Although people find these scales easy to use and understand, the effectiveness may be distorted if the person inadvertently or deliberately denies or minimises their pain (McCaffery & Pasero 1999).

Detailed coverage of assessing children's pain is not within the scope of this chapter; however, all nurses will have some contact with children, such as in emergency departments or health centres.

Children have the right to feel secure and to be nursed in an atmosphere where compassion, trust and caring are at the heart of all decisions (DH 2004, Royal College of Nursing [RCN] 2009). Accurate pain assessment in children and young people is complex and challenging and despite the huge impact of pain on the child it is still reported as inadequately assessed and managed (Simons & MacDonald 2004).

Children and young people need careful consideration because of age, cognitive and developmental ability. However, a number of self-report scales are available and in current use for children, e.g. Faces Scale, Pain Thermometer, Colour Scale used together with a body map.

Groups with special needs

Whilst the assessment of pain is recognised as an essential component of quality care, the assessment and management of pain for certain groups needs special consideration. Visually impaired individuals may not be able to use a VAS and may benefit from using a verbal rating scale which is adapted to their individual needs. Older adults may use a range of words other than pain to describe their pain, and cognitively impaired individuals may have problems using a range of pain measurement tools, but self-report tools have been reported as more effective. For people with marked cognitive impairment it may be more appropriate to use an observational rating scale (see Further reading, e.g. Bjoro & Herr 2008, Flaherty 2008).

The British Pain Society has produced a series of pain scales to assist in the assessment of individuals whose first language is not English; for example, scales are available in Albanian, Arabic, Bengali, Greek, Gujarati, Hindi, Polish, Punjabi, Somali, Swahili, Turkish, Urdu, Vietnamese and Welsh.

Observation

Observation includes:

- pain behaviours
- verbal and motor responses
- sleep and rest patterns.

Observation of pain is difficult and unreliable but is usually based on verbal clues such as direct statements, as well as moaning, crying and sighing, and non-verbal clues such as grimacing, guarding, bracing and lying perfectly still. However, these clues do not have to be present for someone to be in pain. Indeed, such clues are frequently absent. Thus, caution should be exercised in the interpretation of non-verbal signals. However, they remain an important source of assessment for people who cannot respond verbally, such

as those who have altered consciousness or are disorientated and confused.

Herr et al (2010) stress the importance of selecting the best available pain-behaviour assessment tool for use in nursing home residents who have dementia.

Physiological measurements

The usefulness and reliability of physiological measurements continue to be debated and in part the difficulty is due to the fact that physiological responses can be also attributed to competing stressors. It is also important to note that ongoing pain leads to adaptation, which may result in pain not presenting through physiological assessment. Physiological measurements relate to the objective measurement of pain. The parameters that are usually measured are vital signs such as heart rate, respiratory rate and oxygen saturation, and endocrine and metabolic responses. Although these measures have their limitations they have been utilised in the assessment of neonatal pain as there are few reliable measures for this group. See the website for more information on biomedical, psychosocial and behavioural responses.

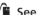 **See website for further content**

 # Nursing management and health promotion: pain

Nurses have a very significant role to play in pain management. Effective pain management depends upon the therapeutic relationship developed between the nurse and the person and, in part, this is why pain assessment is so important, as it sets the 'spirit' of that relationship, whether the person's concerns will be taken seriously and how they will be responded to. The importance of this kind of therapeutic relationship, and of the nature of the characteristics required to achieve it, can be drawn from several studies that represent the 'patient view'. A respondent in Carr & Thomas's (1997) study emphasised the importance of this relationship: 'If she [the acute pain nurse] had just walked away I don't know what I would have done. Her being with me enabled her to understand what I was going through. I didn't feel alone. I felt that I had someone who was helping... you know. She was sort of experiencing it with me. Really, it was a wonderful feeling in that way... that she was with me'.

The respondents in Madjar's (1998) research identified particular qualities that they valued in the ways that nurses responded to their pain. These included:

- gentleness – a softness and tenderness in the way a nurse saw to their comfort
- trustworthiness – a combination of characteristics such as calmness and ability to inspire confidence
- sensitivity – responding through appropriate use of talk and silence and pacing nursing care according to the person's ability to tolerate it
- technical competence – being organised and efficient and able to perform technical tasks with skill and agility
- knowledge and skilful communication – being able to judge what information would be important at a particular time and the ability to communicate it in a way that fostered reassurance and encouragement.

Manias et al (2002) point to another nursing skill in pain management. This study highlighted that nurses are regularly interrupted in their work and needed skill in managing frequent interruptions and the competing demands placed on their time, since these qualities influenced pain management, e.g. how long a person waits for analgesics.

Information and explanation are important aspects of support and therefore crucial to the nurse's role. The purpose of these activities is to ensure the person has realistic expectations and that the nurse works towards achieving these. The aim is to achieve congruence between a person's expectations and their experience, since this has been shown by studies to reduce distress (Carr & Thomas 1997, Boström et al 2004).

Congruence between expectation and experience will also depend on the type of pain. In neuropathic pain it may take time to reduce pain, although much can be done to help people cope. On the other hand, nociceptive pain can be relieved in nearly everyone and it is realistic to work towards considerable pain relief. However, despite advances in pain management, some health care professionals still believe that pain is an unavoidable outcome of treatment and care (Carr & Mann 2000) and overestimate people's ability to cope with pain (Madjar 1998). This is compounded by people not understanding that they can ask for pain relief (McCaffery & Pasero 1999) or waiting until they are in severe pain before asking for an analgesic (Carr & Mann 2000). Carr & Thomas (1997) suggest that this is due both to the lack of information and to the fact that people see that nurses are busy.

The nurse's role in pain management extends to the family. Part of the nurse–family relationship is to recognise that family members have information needs of their own, particularly if they are the key carers. The carers in Oldham & Kristjanson's (2004) study of cancer pain identified the need to have the following concerns addressed: the nature of pain, concerns about medication and how to provide comfort.

This section of the chapter discusses the strategies for managing pain: pharmacological and non-pharmacological modalities. However, we should remember that relieving pain and enhancing the patient's experience can also depend upon the simplest of nursing measures. These might include ensuring analgesia is given before movement; skillful positioning with use of pillows, wedges or bed cage/cradle; a warm bath; and many more initiatives that give comfort. Nurses should ensure that people have sufficient rest and sleep, as this too will enhance coping abilities.

Pharmacological pain management

Most pain can be managed with drugs, and effective relief can be achieved using non-opioids (e.g. paracetamol) including the NSAIDs (e.g. ibuprofen), or opioids (e.g. codeine, morphine) and sometimes with adjuvants for certain types of pain. Problems can be overcome with most standard interventions and protocols but there are certain groups that will require special consideration to prevent predictable problems including:

- older people with co-morbidities
- some people with learning disabilities
- people unable to speak and/or understand English

- patients with:
  - chronic respiratory disease
  - renal failure
  - speech problems, e.g. following a stroke
  - brain injury or impaired consciousness
  - drug misuse, or patients already prescribed opioids
  - sickle cell disease
- infants and pre-verbal children.

Patient understanding of the pain experience is important as some may feel reluctant to request pain relief, seeing it as a sign of weakness, or not wanting to bother busy nursing staff (Field & Smith 2008). Furthermore, people may be reluctant to take 'strong' medication because of the myths and misconceptions relating to opioid addiction. It is important that people are given the information needed to empower them to make informed decisions about their pain relief in partnership with the medical and nursing staff, i.e. concordance.

Pain algorithms, e.g. for postoperative pain relief, are increasingly being developed and utilised in clinical practice. These are based upon the best available evidence and aim to expedite recovery and enhance the quality of the patient's pain journey. An algorithm is any set of detailed instructions that results in a predictable end state, for example in assembling flatpack furniture. Applied to the management of pain it is regarded as a recommended patient management strategy that has been developed to direct decision-making, such as a flow chart, decision grid or a decision tree.

Drug groups used in pain management

Analgesics are a large and diverse group of drugs that act upon the CNS and PNS to relieve pain. They can be divided into non-opioids (including the NSAIDs) and opioids. Non-opioids include over-the-counter (OTC) medications such as paracetamol and ibuprofen. Opioids range from mild drugs such as codeine which are available OTC and strong morphine. In addition, a variety of adjuvant drugs such as amitriptyline are used with analgesics to relieve some types of pain.

Readers should always consult their national formulary, e.g. the British National Formulary (BNF), for authoritative information relating to analgesics (see Useful websites).

The person's age, pain type and intensity, health problems and the setting are important considerations when determining the appropriate type of analgesic. It is especially important to be aware that the action of analgesic drugs may be affected by individual pharmacokinetics and metabolism, e.g. in older people or those with renal or hepatic dysfunction.

Non-opioid analgesics

Non-opioid analgesic drugs include:

Paracetamol This has both analgesic and antipyretic properties, but has no anti-inflammatory action. Paracetamol is commonly used for mild pain and is thought to work centrally (in the CNS) and peripherally at the point of the pain by inhibiting the production of pain mediators such as kinins, histamine, etc. (Field & Smith 2008). Paracetamol can cause liver and less commonly kidney damage in quite moderate overdose.

Aspirin (acetylsalicylic acid) is commonly used for mild to moderate pain and to relieve inflammation. Aspirin acts by inhibiting prostaglandin production. Aspirin must be used with caution as it can cause gastrointestinal bleeding. It should not be given to children under the age of 16 years, except in certain conditions, as there is a link between aspirin and Reye's syndrome. Reye's syndrome is most likely to affect children under 5 years but can also in rare cases affect older children and can be fatal (see Useful websites, e.g. BNF).

NB: Aspirin is also used as an antiplatelet drug (see Ch. 2).

NSAIDs include a wide range of drugs, e.g. ibuprofen, diclofenac, naproxen, some of which can be bought OTC, for example ibuprofen. They are used to relieve mild to moderate pain and inflammation. Most NSAIDs are absorbed quickly and act at the point of pain. They too inhibit the production of inflammatory chemicals such as prostaglandins. Gastrointestinal side-effects include discomfort and possible bleeding and ulceration.

In terms of differences in pain relief between mild analgesics, such as aspirin and paracetamol, Edwards et al 2000 conclude that pain relief attained with aspirin was very similar milligram for milligram to that attained with paracetamol.

Opioid analgesics

Opioid analgesics may be derived from the opium poppy or synthetic analgesics which mimic the action of the natural substance. They act upon the opioid receptors in the CNS to block pain transmission by mimicking the effects of naturally occurring endorphins at the receptor sites, thereby minimising pain. Opioids include codeine, buprenorphine, diamorphine, dihydrocodeine, fentanyl, pethidine, methadone, morphine, oxycodone, tramadol, etc. They vary in efficacy and strength, ranging from codeine (a mild opioid used for moderate pain) to morphine (a strong opioid used for severe pain). Opioids cause constipation, may cause nausea, vomiting and sleepiness, and can depress respiration (see Ch. 33).

Misuse of opioid drugs can lead to physical dependence and addiction. Recently the NHS Central Alerting System (DH 2009) issued new warnings and tighter controls over the sales of OTC medicines containing codeine or dihydrocodeine. These initiatives were introduced to minimise the risk of overuse and addiction of these drugs in line with advice from the Commission on Human Medicines (CHM). For example, pharmacists should offer safety advice to the public regarding short-term use and avoidance of the risk of addiction by taking codeine for no more than 3 days as recommended.

Adjuvants

Adjuvant agents or drugs act to modify or enhance the effects of pharmacological agents or other treatments. They may be needed in the management of neuropathic pain. Examples include:

- Antidepressants, e.g. amitriptyline, prevent the reuptake of noradrenaline (norepinephrine) from the synaptic cleft after its release by the neurone to transfer chemically an action potential, thus depleting available neurotransmitters.
- Corticosteroids, e.g. dexamethasone, are used to reduce swelling. They are used in nerve compression and to reduce cerebral oedema.

- Antiepileptics (anticonvulsants), e.g. gabapentin, carbamazepine, sodium valproate, act in a variety of ways to decrease the effects of neuropathic pain.
- Antispasmodics, e.g. hyoscine butylbromide.
- Capsaicin, an irritant chemical present in sweet peppers, is used topically for postherpetic neuralgia.

Frameworks for the use of analgesics

Two frameworks can guide the use of analgesics: the World Health Organization pain relief ladder (http://www.who.int/cancer/palliative/painladder/en/) and systematic reviews of analgesic effectiveness. These frameworks have in common the principle that safe and effective analgesia can be provided by titrating the dose of analgesics to gain a balance between therapeutic effect and side-effect.

The World Health Organization pain relief ladder

The World Health Organization (WHO) pain relief ladder, first proposed in the 1980s and developed in 1996, is a three-step ladder that guides analgesic decision making. In clinical studies assessing the effectiveness of this framework, pain relief was attained in 80–90% of cases (WHO 2004). The underpinning principle of this framework is that the right drug should be given, at the right dose, at the right time. In persistent pain, titration should be done by moving from non-opioids, e.g. paracetamol, and NSAIDs through to mild opioids, e.g. codeine, and then to strong opioids, e.g. morphine, i.e. moving up the ladder. In surgical or trauma pain, titration will move in reverse order, from strong opioids to weak opioids to non-opioids and NSAIDs (Figure 19.4). In both cases analgesics should be given regularly to maintain a constant analgesic plasma concentration (Figure 19.5).

See website Critical thinking question 19.2

For example, if a patient needs morphine, this will require to be given 4-hourly unless given as a modified-release preparation such as MST continus® 12-hourly or MXL® 24-hourly.

The right dose of analgesic is that which provides pain relief with the lowest side-effect profile. When moving from strong opioids to weak opioids, or vice versa, it is important to take into account the equipotency of the drugs involved. If the person has been having 60 mg oral codeine 6-hourly and still has pain, the starting dose of oral morphine needs to be equivalent to more than this dose, in order to increase analgesia.

Opioids are central to cancer pain management, either used alone or in combination with other medication. Chapter 33 provides detailed information regarding the use of the WHO pain relief ladder in palliative care.

Some people will require more intensive measures and/or mixed modalities of treatment. Other treatments may include some type of nerve block or spinal analgesia (epidural or intrathecal). Associated neuropathic pain may be opioid responsive but may require specific antineuropathic medication, and pain can also be treated using drugs that specifically target the pathological processes responsible for cancer pain (Grady et al 2007).

Opioids are often the first-line treatment for severe acute pain, including postoperatively, and there is no compelling evidence that one opioid is better than another. The key message for safe and effective use of opioids is to titrate the dose

Figure 19.4 Pain relief (analgesic) ladder (based on WHO 2005). (Reproduced from Brooker & Waugh 2007 with permission.)

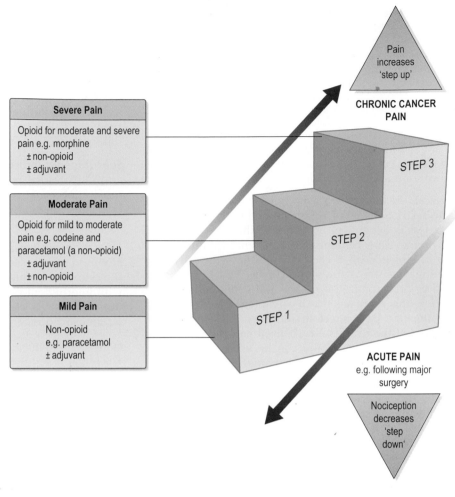

Severe Pain

Opioid for moderate and severe pain e.g. morphine
± non-opioid
± adjuvant

Moderate Pain

Opioid for mild to moderate pain e.g. codeine and paracetamol (a non-opioid)
± adjuvant
± non-opioid

Mild Pain

Non-opioid
e.g. paracetamol
± adjuvant

Pain increases 'step up'

CHRONIC CANCER PAIN

STEP 3

STEP 2

STEP 1

ACUTE PAIN
e.g. following major surgery

Nociception decreases 'step down'

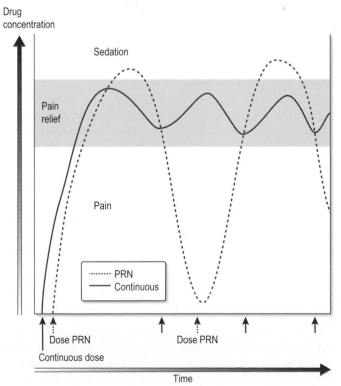

Figure 19.5 PRN versus around-the-clock administration of analgesics.

against the desired effect (pain relief) and minimise the unwanted side-effects. If the person is asking for more pain relief then it is usually a sign of inadequate pain control which may be due to:

- too little drug administered
- too long between doses
- poor pain assessment
- too rigid application of protocols.

Routes and modes of delivery

The age of the person is an important consideration when analgesic drugs are prescribed: infants, young children, adults and older people all have different body composition and the metabolism and elimination of drugs are influenced by their life stage. Also, a child's age, weight and height are important in calculating doses. In older people reduced metabolism and drug excretion can result in an accumulative effect and polypharmacy may cause drug interactions.

There is a general saying that if the person is cooperative and can swallow it is best to give the drug orally, but this is not always possible or desirable. Routes of administration include:

- oral
- sublingual or buccal
- intranasal
- inhalation

- subcutaneous
- intramuscular
- epidermal
- intravenous
- intrapleural
- transdermal
- rectal
- intraspinal.

It is important that nurses are familiar with the advantages, disadvantages and effectiveness of each route, and this been greatly improved by the availability and use of algorithms. The more commonly used routes are outlined below.

Oral Tablets or liquids are usually easy to administer and place no restrictions on a person's mobility. However, their effectiveness is dependent on patient adherence. Sustained-release preparations can enhance adherence by limiting the number of tablets needed each day and have the advantage of attaining consistent drug plasma levels. However, absorption will be compromised if nausea and vomiting is present. In addition, this route has the disadvantage that it is susceptible to the first-pass effect in the liver and intestine, by which some of the drug is metabolised and thus less enters the circulation. The oral route can be used for both mild non-opioids and oral opioids such as morphine.

Intramuscular This route was often used to relieve postoperative pain, but has mostly been superseded by some type of PCA. It has the advantage that it enables the rapid absorption of drugs, although morphine may be more slowly and erratically absorbed than water-based drugs such as diamorphine. Intramuscular injections can be painful, particularly so if the volume of drug exceeds 4 mL. Moreover, people may have to move to expose an injection site, thus causing additional pain.

Intravenous The action of analgesics administered by this route is rapid in onset but of short duration, and therefore a continuous infusion rather than bolus injection may be more effective in maintaining the level of analgesic in the bloodstream.

Rectal Analgesics, e.g. diclofenac, morphine, given as a suppository are absorbed across the rectal mucosa, and generally opioid availability when given rectally is at least equivalent to oral administration. However, absorption is affected in the presence of hard faeces in the rectum. The rectal route is useful for people who have nausea and vomiting or dysphagia. Rectal preparations may not be suitable for people who are neutropenic or in danger of being so. Minor trauma from insertion of the drug may allow entry of gastrointestinal commensals into the bloodstream resulting in septicaemia. Rectal administration can be used at home and is useful in palliative care. However, some people find rectal administration unacceptable (Stannard & Booth 2004).

Sublingual and buccal Medication is placed under the tongue or between the upper lip and gum or between the cheek and gum. These routes may avoid the first-pass effect and are rapid in onset of action. However, there is the disadvantage that the person may inadvertently swallow the drug, and buccal administration may be difficult for people with upper dentures. An example of an analgesic drug administered by this route is buprenorphine.

Transdermal A drug-containing patch is placed directly onto the skin, where absorption occurs. The opioid fentanyl provides effective pain relief by this route. Patches need to be changed, usually every 3 days, and have the advantage of continuous pain relief without the need to remember to take tablets throughout the 24 hours. This route is dependent on the patch being in contact with the skin and on the availability of oral morphine to control 'breakthrough' pain. NSAIDs such as diclofenac are available as gels/creams OTC for mild pain.

Subcutaneous infusion is used for administration of opioids and NSAIDs for people with chronic disorders when oral medication is not possible. It offers a simple, safe and effective alternative to intravenous or intramuscular injections and can be used safely at home.

Inhalation enables rapid absorption of gaseous, volatile and atomised substances. For example, nitrous oxide and oxygen (Entonox®) administered via mask or mouthpiece can help with intermittent pain, as in labour, or during minor procedures, dressings, etc. However, it can be difficult to administer an exact dose and there may be airway irritation.

Spinal Medications given directly into the epidural or subarachnoid space have rapid onset of effect and can provide effective pain relief in a variety of situations (Stannard & Booth 2004). Typically opioids and anaesthetic agents are given by this route. The direct access to the CNS means that much smaller doses are required. Whilst this route has many advantages, including a reduction in postoperative complications (Buggy & Smith 1999) and neuromodulation of persistent pain, using opioids to reduce wind-up in neuropathic pain, it has important and potentially serious complications – respiratory depression and sudden dramatic hypotension. Despite the need for caution, many people with persistent pain are managed at home for long periods of time, with spinal analgesics administered via a small portable syringe pump or through a medication pump implanted under the skin.

Patient controlled analgesia (PCA)

PCA refers to the administration of analgesics by any appropriate and safe route over which the person has control. When they feel pain, pressing a button delivers a prescribed dose of medication, usually an opioid. Usual routes include intravenous, subcutaneous or epidural (see also inhaled Entonox® above). Regular assessment of the patient is important, as is monitoring for nausea and vomiting which are common side-effects of opioids (see Ch. 26).

The pump is set with 'lock-out' intervals and doses to regulate the amount of drug administered. This method is typically used postoperatively, but can be used in other painful situations. The person must be able and willing to use it and therefore meeting the person's information needs is important, for example explaining potential side-effects and reassurance that it is safe, and that overdose and addiction are not possible.

There is evidence that PCA offers improved pain relief and quicker recovery following surgery, resulting in earlier discharge (Chang et al 2004). The most frequently purported psychological benefit of PCA is the person's specific control over pain, PCA eliminating the need to wait for nurse-administered analgesia. To test the influence of this on pain experience, Shiloh et al (2003) undertook a randomised quasi-experimental design trial in which 120 postoperative patients were assigned to one of three groups, each receiving different pain management regimens. The authors suggest that the main effect of PCA is increased pain tolerance and that this may be due to the person's control over their pain and thus a decrease in uncertainty about the availability and effectiveness of pain relief. This may in turn lead to an increase in the use of strategies such as diversion to help the pain.

Other medical interventions

Local anaesthesia and regional nerve blocks are achieved with the injection of local anaesthetic, sometimes together with a corticosteroid, near to or in a peripheral nerve or major nerve plexus or into the spine. Although there can be adverse reactions and complications, the pain-relieving effects often outlast the duration of the local anaesthetic.

Surgery Nerve transection can reduce or eliminate intractable pain. Although this may work initially, pain often returns and may be worse than it was pre-surgery (Stannard & Booth 2004). For this reason, other techniques, such as spinal cord stimulation, are more common. Implanted epidural electrodes are controlled either via an external radiofrequency transmitter or an implanted pulse generator. Pulse generators implanted subcutaneously are used to stimulate the brain.

Radiotherapy, chemotherapy and specific drug therapy Radiotherapy and chemotherapy may be used to relieve pain, for example in metastatic cancer. Bisphosphonates such as pamidronate are effective in relieving pain from bone metastases (see Chs 31, 33).

Specialised pain services

Acute pain services

In response to evidence of inadequate postoperative pain relief and a recommendation by the British Pain Society in collaboration with the Royal College of Anaesthetists (2003), multiprofessional acute pain services are now well established in many hospitals in the UK. Davies & Taylor (2003) summarise the overall functions of such teams:

The multiprofessional team can assist in:

- formalising staff and patient education
- organising and monitoring acute pain management
- safely introducing new techniques and maximising the potential of existing ones
- standardising pain assessment
- formulating and introducing practice guidelines
- auditing service efficacy (Davies & Taylor 2003, p. 121).

The British Pain Society (2003) in *Pain Management Services. Good Practice* include all of the above plus further provisions for acute pain services:

- provision of specialist care and advice for difficult acute pain problems such as occur in people who misuse opioids
- seamless liaison with other health care teams responsible for the shared care of people with acute pain

- back-up arrangements, education programmes and appropriate guidelines or protocols to ensure that there is continuous cover for acute pain management around the clock, 7 days a week.

There is emerging evidence of the impact of specialist acute pain teams on nurses' knowledge and attitudes towards pain management. Mackintosh et al (2000) found a consistent positive trend in improved knowledge and attitudes in pain management following the development of a pain service, and Barton et al (2004) found that nurses who were unaware of an acute pain service in their organisation had less knowledge about pain than nurses who were aware of the service.

Hospice/palliative care teams have a wealth of expertise in pain and symptom control and can be a valuable resource (see Ch. 33). Such teams are usually multidisciplinary and situated in a variety of care settings. The key functions of such teams are to provide support to other professionals in caring for people with life-threatening illness.

Chronic or 'persistent' pain services

These offer a service to people with persistent pain. Clinics are usually multidisciplinary and may be staffed by anaesthetists, nurses, psychologists, physiotherapists, occupational therapists and pharmacists with the aim of increasing the person's ability to function and lead a more fulfilled life. This aim incorporates the belief that persistent pain is the result of multiple interrelating physical, psychological and social or occupational factors.

Non-pharmacological pain management

Over recent years the use of non-pharmacological methods of pain control has received greater acceptance in conventional health care systems. Although there is still a paucity of robust evidence, they have become more acceptable and more widely available. Non-pharmacological methods include complementary and alternative medicine (CAM) therapies, which many nurses have incorporated into their practice. Nursing staff who provide CAM therapies are subject to *The Code: Standards of Conduct, Performance and Ethics for Nurses and Midwives* (NMC 2008). The nurse must have undertaken an approved course or programme of study that deems the practitioner competent to administer such treatments. Furthermore, the nurse must work within the framework of clinical governance which aims for continuous quality improvement in order to provide safe and effective patient care (see pp. 570–571). An employed nurse must first have authority from the NHS Trust or other employer to practise CAM and must ascertain that the employer's vicarious liability covers such activity. Self-employed nurses should have professional indemnity insurance that includes CAM, such as the schemes offered by professional organisations.

This section of the chapter outlines non-pharmacological methods, including some CAM therapies used in pain management. Non-pharmacological methods can be classified into two broad types: physical (counter-irritation) and psychological. However, some methods such as massage have both physical and psychological benefits.

Physical methods:

- acupuncture
- aromatherapy

- chiropractic
- herbal medicine
- homeopathy
- hot/cold
- low-level laser therapy (LLLT) photobiomodulation
- massage
- osteopathy
- reflexology
- therapeutic touch
- transcutaneous electrical nerve stimulation (TENS)
- ultrasound
- yoga.

Psychological methods:

- art therapy
- behavioural therapy
- biofeedback
- distraction
- drama therapy
- hypnosis
- imagery
- music therapy
- relaxation.

Hot or cold therapy The application of superficial heat promotes vasodilation, thereby increasing blood flow to an area, and pain-inducing chemical mediators are 'diluted'. Equally the application of cooling measures reduces the metabolic rate and lowers cellular activity and the consumption of oxygen. If the cooling is sufficiently intense, pain and cold sensations are suppressed. Caution must be exercised in using these therapies if there is existing reduction in skin sensation or if this therapy is contraindicated by the patient's condition, for example impaired blood supply to an area.

Massage is an ancient form of pain relief often used in conjunction with oils or creams. The evidence for the effectiveness of massage is sparse. It is thought that massage activates certain elements of the gate-control mechanisms and releases endorphins. The pain relief achieved when rubbing an area after a knock or a bump is an example of this and massage not only provides healing but relaxes tight muscles that may be associated with stress.

Acupuncture treats the person and not the disease. It is based upon a technique whereby fine needles are inserted and manipulated in specific points (approximately 365) along meridians. The meridians are channels through which energy known as *Qi* is said to flow. The effects of such treatment are still subject to scientific scrutiny. A similar technique using pressure without needles can be used on the acupuncture points, which may be more acceptable to some people who are needle-phobic.

Distraction relies on distracting attention away from the painful stimulus. This may involve asking the person to breathe deeply, the aim of which is to shield the sensation of pain by increasing sensation via another sensory route (Field & Smith 2008). The list of distracters includes those for adults and children. They include:

- company and conversation
- humour and laughter
- reading

- television
- listening to music
- hobbies
- companion animals
- exercise, activity and sport if applicable
- e-mailing friends and 'surfing' the internet
- computer games
- blowing bubbles
- storytelling, reading to children
- music and singing, shouting and yelling
- visits by well-known people and role models.

Transcutaneous electrical nerve stimulation (TENS) is a method of pain relief in which a controlled level of low-voltage electricity is applied to the body via electrodes. This is understood to relieve pain by stimulating the release of endorphins. It may be useful during labour and for chronic pain.

See website Figure 19.2

Low-level laser therapy (LLLT) or photobiomodulation used in pain management utilises a different type of laser from the heat-generating lasers used in surgery (Grady et al 2007). The non-thermal application of red and infrared laser light has selective stimulatory effects at cellular level. According to the evidence (Grady et al 2007) the laser light action in managing pain is multifaceted. It includes a reduction in inflammatory and pain chemicals and normalisation of nerve outputs and their membrane function which reduces pain transmission at the spinal gate. Adrenocorticotrophic hormone (ACTH) and endorphins are released as a secondary response. LLLT has been used in the treatment of conditions such as failed back surgery, musculoskeletal pain, chronic post-surgical pain and post-traumatic pain of the spine and limbs. LLLT is not associated with serious adverse reactions and has a high benefit to risk ratio.

A detailed account of CAM therapies is beyond the scope of this book; readers requiring more information are directed to Further reading (e.g. Plant 2007, Zollman et al 2008).

Support and self-help groups

Pain is isolating, particularly so in chronic pain where the person and their carers may withdraw from social interactions. Contact with appropriate self-help and support groups can help to reduce the isolation of pain. The chance to share experiences and feelings provides emotional support, encourages hope and promotes empowerment and control. Sharing information about coping strategies can be especially useful. Nurses can discuss the potential benefits of self-help groups (see Useful websites) with the person, but the importance of close family support, emphasised in some cultures, should be respected.

Clinical governance in pain management

Standards set through the National Service Frameworks (NSFs) (e.g. DH 2005), National Institute for Health and Clinical Excellence (NICE) guidance (e.g. NICE 2009) and the Scottish Intercollegiate Guidelines Network (SIGN) (e.g. SIGN 2008) ensure that services and clinical standards are delivered through local systems of clinical governance. Clinical governance is a systematic approach to maintaining and improving the quality of care within health systems. It is also a doctrine whereby the practitioner is responsible to the employing authority as well as their professional body for aspects of professional and ethical conduct. Scally & Donaldson (1998) define clinical governance as 'a framework through which the NHS organisations are accountable for continuously improving the quality of their services and safeguarding high standards of care by creating an environment in which excellence in clinical care will flourish'.

Clinical governance involves at least the following elements:

- risk assessment
- risk management
- clinical audit
- clinical effectiveness
- transparency and openness
- education and training
- research and development.

It can be argued that all these elements are applicable to pain management.

Role of guidelines and policies in pain management

Despite the increasing numbers of initiatives to improve pain management, powerful myths can cloud rational actions, and entrenched perceptions can spread with ease independent of logic and professional acumen. Combating these myths and outmoded ideals has been made easier by the availability of government-endorsed clinical practice guidelines and local initiatives (Brennan et al 2007). Many professional bodies have issued guidelines, recommendations, etc., relating to pain management (British Pain Society 2003, RCN 2009). Common to all is a clear commitment to quality pain management achieved through the highest professional standards. The best not only state that the person has the right to pain management, but that the person has the right to be believed in their expression of pain and the right to appropriate pain assessment and management strategies that take account of individual differences. However, it is worth mentioning that recommendations alone do not change professional attitudes or behaviour but collectively they provide professionals with the clarity, structure and rationale of pain management that has been sadly lacking in previous decades (Brennan et al 2007).

Practice guidelines are systematically developed recommendations that assist practitioners and those in their care in making informed decisions about health care. In turn recommendations can be adopted, modified or rejected according to the needs of the client population and clinicians' needs and constraints (American Society of Anesthesiologists 2004). However, practice guidelines cannot guarantee specific outcomes, or revision subject to advances in professional knowledge, technology and practice – only people can do that.

SUMMARY: KEY NURSING ISSUES

- 'Pain is whatever the patient says it is and exists when he says it does' (McCaffery 1968).
- Nurses are part of the MDT who use up-to-date evidence-based knowledge and understanding of pain in order to competently prevent and minimise pain.
- Pain is a complex, subjective and multidimensional experience that has physical, psychosocial, emotional, cultural and spiritual influences.
- Pain assessment and measurement are critical to the holistic care of a person with pain.
- Relieving pain and enhancing the patient's experience can also depend upon the simplest of nursing measures.
- Holistic pain management involves both pharmacological and non-pharmacological approaches.
- Nurses empower people with chronic pain by encouraging independence and coping skills.
- Ineffective pain management impedes recovery after surgery/trauma and may lead to unrelieved chronic pain.
- Effective pain management is a quality issue for all nurses.

REFLECTION AND LEARNING – WHAT NEXT?

- **Test** your knowledge by visiting the website and answering the multiple choice questions and critical thinking questions.
- **Consolidate** your learning by looking at some of the further reading suggestions, references and specialist websites.
- **Revisit** some of the additional material on the website.
- **Consider** what you have learnt and how this will help your professional development.
- **Reflect** on how you can apply this knowledge to the care of your patients.
- **Discuss** your learning with your mentor/supervisor, lecturer and colleagues.

REFERENCES

American Society of Anesthesiologists Task Force on Acute Pain Management: Practice guidelines for acute pain management in the perioperative setting, *Anesthesiology* 100(6):1573–1581, 2004.

Backonja MM: Defining neuropathic pain, *Anesthetic Analgesia* 97:785–790, 2003.

Barton J, Don M, Foureur M: Nurses' and midwives' pain knowledge improves under the influence of an acute pain service, *Acute Pain* 6(2):47–51, 2004.

Bendelow GA: Pain perceptions, emotions and gender, *Sociol Health Illn* 15(3):273–294, 1993.

Boström B, Sandh M, Lundberg D, et al: Cancer-related pain in palliative care: patients' perceptions of pain management, *J Adv Nurs* 45(4):410–419, 2004.

Brennan F, Carr D, Cousins M: Pain management: a fundamental human right, *International Anesthesia Research Society* 105(1):205–221, 2007.

Briggs E: The nursing management of pain in older people, *Nurs Stand* 17:47–53, 2003.

British Pain Society in collaboration with Royal College of Anaesthetists: *Pain management services. Good practice*, 2003. (Updated 3-yearly). Available online http://www.britishpainsociety.org/pub_professional.htm#pmp2.

Brooker C, Waugh A, editors: *Foundations of Nursing Practice. Fundamentals of holistic care*, Edinburgh, 2007, Mosby.

Buggy DJ, Smith G: Epidural anaesthesia and analgesia: better outcome after major surgery? *Br Med J* 319:530–531, 1999.

Carr EC, Mann E: *Pain: Creative approaches to effective pain management*, Basingstoke, 2000, Palgrave.

Carr EC, Thomas V: Anticipating and experiencing post-operative pain: the patient's experience, *J Clin Nurs* 6(3):191–201, 1997.

Carter B: *Child and infant pain: principles of nursing care and management*, London, 1994, Chapman & Hall.

Chamley C, James G: Pain management – minimizing the pain experience. In Brooker C, Waugh A, editors: *Foundations of Nursing Practice: Fundamentals of Holistic Care*, Edinburgh, 2007, Mosby, pp 653–679.

Chang AM, Ip WY, Cheung TH: Patient controlled analgesia versus conventional intramuscular injection: a cost effectiveness analysis, *J Adv Nurs* 46(5):531–541, 2004.

Chronic Pain Coalition: *A new pain manifesto*, 2007. Available online http://www.paincoalition.org.uk/.

Closs S, Barr B, Briggs M: Cognitive status and analgesic provision in nursing home residents, *Br J Gen Pract* 54(509):919–921, 2004.

Coll AM, Ameen J, Mead D: Postoperative pain assessment tools in day surgery: Literature review, *J Adv Nurs* 46(1):124–133, 2004.

Davies K, Taylor A: Pain. In Brooker C, Nicol M, editors: *Nursing Adults: The Practice of Caring*, Edinburgh, 2003, Mosby, pp 113–119, 118–121.

Department of Health (DH): *National Service Framework for Children, Young People, and Maternity Services – Core Standards*, 2004. Available online http://www.dh.gov.uk/en/Publicationsandstatistics/Publications/PublicationsPolicyAndGuidance/Browsable/DH_4094329.

Department of Health (DH): *National Service Framework for long-term conditions*, 2005. (See Ch. 2 Quality requirement, quality requirement 9: palliative care pdf.) Available online http://www.dh.gov.uk/en/Publicationsandstatistics/Publications/PublicationsPolicyAndGuidance/DH_4105361.

Department of Health (DH): *Central Alerting System: Updated advice on non-prescription medicines containing codeine or dihydrocodeine*, London, 2009, DH.

Department of Health (DH): *Essence of Care Benchmarks for the Prevention and Management of Pain*, 2010. Available online http://www.dh.gov.uk/

Dimond B: *Legal aspects of pain management*, Salisbury, 2002, Quay Books.

Edwards JE, Oldman A, Smith L, et al: Single dose oral aspirin for acute pain, *Cochrane Database Syst Rev* (2):2000, CD002067.

Elliot AM, Smith BH, Penny KI, et al: The epidemiology of chronic pain in the community, *Lancet* 354:1248–1252, 1999.

Ellson R: Pain management. In Richardson, editor: *Clinical skills for student nurses. Theory, practice and reflection*, Devon, 2008, Reflect Press Ltd, pp 84–114.

Field L, Smith B: Pain management. In Field L, Smith B, editors: *Nursing care: an essential guide*, Harlow, 2008, Pearson Education Limited, pp 193–233.

Fishbain D: Approaches to treatment decisions for psychiatric co-morbidity in management of the chronic pain patient, *Med Clin North Am* 83:737–760, 1999.

Fisherman S: Recognizing pain management as a human right: A first step, *International Anesthesia Research Society* 105(1):205–221, 2007.

Fitzpatrick R, Davey C, Buxton MJ, et al: Evaluating patient-based outcome measures for use in clinical trials, *Health Technol Assess* 2:1–4, 1998.

Grady K, Severn A, Eldridge P: *Key topics in pain medicine*, ed 3, Hampshire, 2007, Thompson Publishing Services.

Gureje O, Von Korff M, Simon GE, et al: Persistent pain and well being: a World Health Organization study in primary care, *JAMA* 280:147–151, 1998.

Helme RD, Gibson SJ: The epidemiology of pain in elderly people, *Geriatric Medicine* 7:417–431, 2001.

Herr K, Bursch H, Ersek M, et al: Use of pain-behavioral assessment tools in nursing homes, *J Gerontol Nurs* 36(3):18–29, 2010, quiz 30–1.

Horn S, Munafo M: *Pain theory, research and intervention*, Buckingham, 1997, Open University Press.

Human Rights Act: London, 1998, TSO. Available online http://www.opsi.gov.uk/.

International Association for the Study of Pain (IASP) Task Force on Taxonomy: IASP pain terminology. In Merskey N, Bogduk N, editors: *Classification of chronic pain*, ed 2, Seattle, 1994, IASP Press, pp 209–214.

Ko SM, Zhou M: Central plasticity and persistent pain. Drug discovery today: disease models, *Pain and Anaesthesia* 1(2):101–106, 2004.

Lasch KE: Culture and pain, *Pain Clinical Updates* X(5):1–10, 2002.

Latham J: *Pain control*, ed 2, London, 1991, Mosby.

Lisson EL: Ethical issues related to pain control, *Nurs Clin North Am* 22(3):649–659, 1987.

Mackintosh C, Bowles S, Mackintosh S: The effect of an acute pain service on nurses' knowledge and beliefs about postoperative pain, *J Clin Nurs* 9(1):119–126, 2000.

Madjar I: *Giving comfort and inflicting pain*, Edmonton, 1998, Qualitative Institute Press.

Manias E, Botti M, Bucknell T: Observation of pain assessment and management: the complexities of clinical practice, *J Clin Nurs* 11:724–733, 2002.

McCaffery M: *Nursing practice theories related to cognition, bodily pain and man–environmental interactions*, California, 1968, UCLA Students Store.

McCaffery M, Beebe A: *Pain Clinical Manual for Nursing Practice*, St Louis, 1989, Mosby.

McCaffery M, Ferrell B: Nurses' knowledge of pain assessment and management: How much progress have we made? *Journal of Pain Management* 14(3):175–186, 1997.

McCaffery M, Pasero C: *Pain clinical manual*, ed 2, St Louis, 1999, Mosby.

McQuay H, Moore A, Justins D: Treating acute pain in hospital, *Br Med J* 314(7093):1531–1535, 1997.

Melzack R, Katz J: Measurement in persons in pain. In Wall P, Melzack R, editors: *Textbook of pain*, ed 3, Edinburgh, 1994, Churchill Livingstone, p 672.

Melzeck R, Wall P: Pain mechanisms: A new theory, *Science* 150:971–979, 1965.

Melzack R, Wall PD: *The challenge of pain*, ed 2, London, 1988, Penguin Books.

Melzack R, Wall P: *Textbook of pain*, ed 4, Edinburgh, 1999, Churchill Livingstone.

Müllersdorf M, Söderback I: The actual state of the effects, treatment and incidence of disabling pain in a gender perspective – a Swedish study, *Disabil Rehabil* 22(18):840–854, 2000.

National Institute for Health and Clinical Excellence (NICE): Early management of persistent non-specific low back pain, *Clinical guidance* 88, 2009. Available online http://guidance.nice.org.uk/CG88.

Nursing and Midwifery Council (NMC): *Essential Skills Clusters*, 2007. Available online http://www.nmc-uk.org.

Nursing and Midwifery Council (NMC): *The Code: Standards of Conduct, Performance and Ethics for Nurses and Midwives*, 2008. Available online http://www.nmc-uk.org.

Oldham L, Kristjanson LJ: Development of a pain management programme for family carers of advanced cancer patients, *International Journal of Palliative Care* 10(2):91–98, 2004.

Peter E, Watt-Watson J: Unrelieved pain: an ethical and epistemological analysis of distrust in patients, *Can J Res* 34(2):65–80, 2002.

Portenoy RK, Ugarte C, Fuller I, et al: Population-based survey of pain in the United States: differences amongst White, African, American and Hispanic subjects, *J Pain* 5(6):317–328, 2004.

Rollnick JD, Karst M, Pieoenbrock S, et al: Gender differences in coping with tension-type headaches, *Eur Neurol* 50(2):73–78, 2003.

Royal College of Nursing (RCN): *Clinical practice guidelines: The recognition and assessment of acute pain in children*, 2009. Available online http://www.rcn.org.uk/__data/assets/pdf_file/0004/269185/003542.pdf.

Scally G, Donaldson LJ: The NHS's 50th anniversary, Clinical governance and the drive for quality improvement in the new NHS in England, *Br Med J* 317(7150):61–65, 1998.

Scottish Intercollegiate Guidelines Network (SIGN): *Control of pain in adults with cancer*, 2008. Guideline No 106. Available online http://www.sign.ac.uk/guidelines/fulltext/106/index.html.

Selva C: International control of opioids for medical use, *European Journal of Palliative Care* 4:194–198, 1997.

Sepúlveda C, Marlin M, Yoshida T: Palliative care: The World Health Organization's global perspective, *Journal of Pain Management* 24(2):91–96, 2002.

Shiloh S, Zukerman G, Butin B, et al: Postoperative patient-controlled analgesia (PCA): how much control and how much analgesia? *Psychology and Health* 18(6):753–770, 2003.

Simons JM, MacDonald LM: Pain assessment tools: Children's nurses' views, *J Child Health Care* 8(4):264–278, 2004.

Sjöström D, Dahlgren LO, Heljamáe H: Strategies used in post-operative pain assessment and their clinical accuracy, *J Clin Nurs* 9:111–118, 2000.

Stannard C, Booth S: *Pain*, ed 2, Edinburgh, 2004, Churchill Livingstone.

Turk DC: Assessment of pain: the elusiveness of latent constructs. In Chapman CR, Loeser JD, editors: *Issues in pain measurement. Advances in pain research and therapy*, Vol 12, New York, 1989, Raven Press, pp 267–279.

United Nations: *Declaration of the Rights of the Child*, 1989. Available online http://www.dcsf.gov.uk/everychildmatters/strategy/strategyandgovernance/uncrc/unitednationsarticles/uncrcarticles/.

Wall P: Preface. In Grady K, Severn A, Eldridge P, editors: *Key topics in pain medicine*, ed 3, Hampshire, 2007, Thompson Publishing Services, pp 69–71.

Watt-Watson JB: Relationships between nurses' knowledge and pain management outcomes for their postoperative cardiac patients, *J Adv Nurs* 36(4):535–545, 2001.

Whelan E: Putting pain to paper: Endometriosis and the documentation of suffering, *Health* 7(4):463–482, 2003.

Wood S: *Anatomy and Physiology of Pain*, 2008. Available online http://www.nursingtimes.net/nursing-practice-clinical-research/anatomy-and-physiology-of-pain/1860931.article.

World Health Organization: *WHO's Pain Relief Ladder*, 2005. Available online http://www.who.int/cancer/palliative/painladder/en/.

Zborowski M: Cultural components in response to pain, *Journal of Social Issues* 8(4):16–30, 1952.

FURTHER READING

Bjoro K, Herr K: Assessment of pain in the nonverbal or cognitively impaired older adult, *Clin Geriatr Med* 24(2):237–262, 2008.

Clancy J, McVicar A: *Physiology and Anatomy for Nurses and Healthcare Practitioners*, ed 3, London, 2009, Hodder Education (Ch. 20), pp 971–974.

Field L, Adams N: Pain management 2: Use of psychological approaches to pain, *Br J Nurs* 10(5):971–974, 2001.

Flaherty E: Using pain scales with older adults, *Am J Nurs* 108(6):40–47, 2008.

Kaasalainen S: Pain assessment in older adults with dementia: Using behavioural observational methods in clinical practice, *J Gerontol Nurs* 33(6):6–10, 2007.

Plant AN: Sleep, rest, relaxation, complementary and alternative therapies. In Brooker C, Waugh A, editors: *Foundations of Nursing Practice: Fundamentals of Holistic Care*, Edinburgh, 2007, Mosby, pp 251–275.

Royal College of Physicians: *Concise guidance to good practice series, No 8. The Assessment of Pain in Older People: National Guidelines*, 2007. Available online http://www.rcplondon.ac.uk/.

Smith HS: *Current therapy in pain*, St Louis, 2010, WB Saunders.

Stannard C, Kalso E, Ballantyne J: *Evidence-based Chronic Pain Management*, Oxford, 2010, Wiley-Blackwell.

Wood S: *Investigations and Pain Management Guidelines*, 2008. Available online http://www.nursingtimes.net/nursing-practice-clinical-research/investigations-and-pain-management-guidelines/1861192.article.

Zollman C, Vickers A, Richardson J: *ABC of Complementary Medicine*, ed 2, Oxford, 2008, Wiley-Blackwell.

USEFUL WEBSITES

Bandolier Oxford Pain Internet Site: www.medicine.ox.ac.uk/bandolier/booth/painpag/index2.html

British National Formulary: www.bnf.org

British Pain Society: www.britishpainsociety.org

Chronic Pain Coalition: www.paincoalition.org.uk

International Association for the Study of Pain: www.iasp-pain.org

Migraine Action: www.migraine.org.uk

Pain-talk (UK discussion forum for health care professionals): www.pain-talk.co.uk

Maintaining fluid, electrolyte and acid–base balance

Michelle Cowen, Debra Ugboma

Introduction

Monitoring and manipulating body fluid and electrolytes form a crucial aspect of nursing care. For a lean adult male, about 18% of the body weight is protein, 15% fat and 7% minerals; 60% is water. For health, body water and electrolytes must be maintained within a limited range. Homeostatic mechanisms regulate parameters such as body fluid volume, acid–base balance (pH) and electrolyte concentrations, maintaining a delicate, dynamic balance which can be destabilised during illness. In extreme cases, the fluid or electrolyte deficit or excess can lead to death. Consequently, nurses must have a clear understanding of fluid and electrolyte homeostasis (autoregulatory processes that maintain fluid and electrolyte levels, pH, blood glucose, etc. within set parameters) so that they can assess fluid and electrolyte status, anticipate and recognise deterioration and implement corrective interventions.

Nursing interventions in relation to fluid therapy may range from encouraging the patient to drink an afternoon cup of tea to managing a complicated intravenous fluid regimen. Ill-defined terms, such as 'encourage fluids', and instructions to record fluid intake/output or daily weight, are commonly encountered. However, without a knowledgeable appreciation of the physiology and pathophysiology of fluid and electrolyte balance there is a real risk that these activities will be performed in a somewhat mechanistic fashion, without sufficient thought or understanding.

This chapter reviews the normal mechanisms which regulate body fluid and electrolytes and outlines some of the basic adaptive responses to imbalances. The regulation of acid–base balance is also considered, along with basic principles in the management of fluid and electrolyte disorders. Within the chapter, typical clinical situations where fluid and electrolyte control may be compromised are identified. Students who are unfamiliar with the physiology of fluid, electrolyte and acid–base balance or need to refresh their understanding are advised to read this chapter in conjunction with their physiology textbooks.

Nursing goals in the care of patients with existing or potential fluid and electrolyte problems include:

- the promotion and maintenance of a healthy pattern of fluid intake/output appropriate to the patient's lifestyle and wishes
- the detection of existing or potential fluid and electrolyte imbalances
- the re-establishment of fluid and electrolyte balance when homeostasis is disturbed
- the development of educational programmes for the maintenance of fluid and electrolyte balance.

This chapter will provide some of the essential knowledge necessary to achieving these goals.

Fluid in the body

Water is essential to life and has a range of functions within the body including giving form to body structures and acting as a transport medium for nutrients, electrolytes, blood gases, metabolic wastes, heat and electrical currents. Water makes up nearly three quarters of the body's active tissues and homeostatic regulation of body fluids is essential to normal function and health.

An average young adult man has a total body water (TBW) of about 60% of his body weight, or approximately 40 L in a 70 kg man. The percentage of body weight represented by the TBW varies from one individual to another depending on factors such as age, gender and build. Most of this variation is due to fat (adipose tissue). Adipose tissue contains only about 10% of water and so contributes little towards TBW. A 70 kg woman of average build would have a TBW of about 52% (36 L) due to the greater proportion of adipose (fatty) tissue. In both genders, the percentage of body water decreases with age.

Fluid compartments

Body water is distributed between two major compartments: approximately two thirds as intracellular fluid (ICF) and one third extracellular fluid (ECF) (Figure 20.1). The volume of ICF is around 28 L in a 70 kg male. The ECF has a volume of approximately 12 L. It comprises the *intravascular fluid* (about 2.5 L within the heart and vessels) and the *interstitial fluid* (about 9.5 L) surrounding the cells and forming a relatively constant environment. In addition, there are very small quantities of transcellular fluid (e.g. within the eye, cerebrospinal fluid, glandular secretions) and water in bone.

In infants and children, although the actual ECF volume is much smaller than in adults, the ECF:ICF ratio is larger, i.e. the ECF represents a greater percentage of the TBW. Fluid loss in children can rapidly lead to dehydration and is potentially more serious in the infant than in the adult.

The distinction between the different fluid compartments is maintained by the selective permeability of cell membranes. The membrane is freely permeable to water and the movement of other solutes is influenced by amongst other things the size of molecule, concentration gradient and electrical charge. Large proteins which are synthesised by the cell remain inside as they are too big to pass through the membrane. Distribution of electrolytes and water is influenced by selective membrane transport processes.

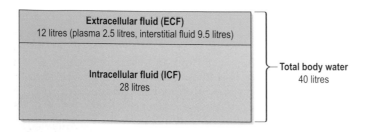

Figure 20.1 Distribution of body water in a 70 kg person. (Reproduced from Waugh & Grant 2006 with permission.)

Electrolytes in the body

Fluid in the body cannot be equated simply with water, as it also contains dissolved substances or solutes as well as larger particles in suspension (colloids). Solutes may be complete molecules (non-electrolytes) or parts of molecules (electrolytes). An electrolyte is a chemical compound that, when in solution, dissociates into electrically charged particles called *ions*. These ions can be positively charged (cation) or negatively charged (anion). The main electrolytes found within the body are sodium (Na^+), chloride (Cl^-), potassium (K^+), magnesium (Mg^{2+}), calcium (Ca^{2+}), phosphorus as phosphates ($H_2PO_4^-$ and HPO_4^{2-}) and bicarbonate (HCO_3^-). In solution, a molecule of sodium chloride dissociates into a positively charged sodium ion Na^+ (cation) and a negatively charged chloride ion Cl^- (anion). Sodium is the dominant cation in the ECF. Chloride and bicarbonate (HCO_3^-) are the major extracellular anions. Inside the cell, potassium (K^+) is the dominant cation. Glucose is a good example of a non-electrolyte in that it dissolves in body water but does not dissociate into ions.

Electrolytes are essential for cellular activity and need to remain within a specific range for optimal function. In clinical practice, serum electrolytes are measured by a simple blood test, urea and electrolytes, often known as 'U&Es'. Nurses should be aware of normal ranges and factors which may cause electrolyte imbalances in patients for whom they are caring, for example patients with cardiovascular disease or renal disease or those receiving diuretic medication. This knowledge will assist nurses and other health professionals to respond with appropriate care interventions. Box 20.1 provides a more detailed description of the common electrolytes.

Box 20.1 Information

Common electrolytes: functions and features (adapted from Waugh 2003 with permission)

Sodium (Na^+) – normal range 135–143 mmol/L

- Most abundant cation in ECF
- Provides plasma with up to half its osmotic pressure
- Required for action potential in neurones and muscle
- Levels regulated by the hormones aldosterone, antidiuretic hormone and atrial natriuretic peptide (ANP)
- Exchanged for K^+ ions when Na^+ crosses cell membrane
- Average dietary intake usually exceeds daily requirements
- Kidney can conserve sodium if necessary
- Sweating increases loss of sodium

Potassium (K^+) – normal range 3.3–4.7 mmol/L

- Most abundant cation in ICF
- As the majority of K^+ is intracellular, serum levels do not accurately reflect total K^+ in the body
- Plays a key role in resting membrane potential, repolarisation of neurones and muscle cells
- Maintains ICF volume
- Exchanged for Na^+ ions when K^+ crosses cell membrane
- Levels regulated by the hormone aldosterone
- K^+ mainly lost in urine with small amount in faeces and sweat

Continued

Box 20.1 Information – cont'd

- Kidneys cannot conserve K^+ in the same way as they conserve Na^+

Calcium (Ca^{2+}) – normal range 2.1–2.6 mmol/L

- Most abundant mineral in the body
- Majority combined with phosphate as salts
- Essential for blood clotting
- Controls release of neurotransmitters
- Essential for excitability of nerves and muscles
- In its ionised form (Ca^{2+}) is mainly extracellular
- Levels in the blood are controlled by parathyroid hormone and calcitonin

Magnesium (Mg^{2+}) – normal range 0.75–1.0 mmol/L

- Magnesium is a co-factor required for enzyme action
- Required for the sodium–potassium pump
- Half of body magnesium found in bone matrix as magnesium salts
- Remainder is ionised (Mg^{2+}) and found mainly in ICF

Chloride (Cl^-) – normal range 97–106 mmol/L

- Most common extracellular anion (Cl^-)
- Crosses cell membrane freely in exchange for bicarbonate

Phosphate – normal range 0.8–1.4 mmol/L

- Ionic forms of phosphate ($H_2PO_4^-$ and HPO_4^{2-}) have a role in phosphate buffer system
- Found as a salt in bones and teeth
- Present in nucleic acids and adenosine triphosphate (ATP)
- Principally found in ICF
- Levels controlled by parathyroid hormone and calcitonin

Bicarbonate (HCO_3^-) – normal range 22–28 mmol/L

- Essential for homeostasis of blood pH through the bicarbonate buffer system
- Second most abundant extracellular anion
- Levels regulated by kidneys in response to pH of blood

Water and electrolyte homeostasis

Maintaining fluid and electrolyte balance

Maintaining normal, healthy fluid intake and the constancy of the internal environment is essential for efficient cell function. Fluid balance in the body is maintained by a number of physiological mechanisms. These mechanisms help to ensure that water gain and water loss are balanced (Table 20.1) and prevent the consequences of imbalances such as dehydration

Table 20.1 Water balance – water gain and water loss (adult)	
INPUT – WATER GAIN	**OUTPUT – WATER LOSS**
Beverages 1500 mL Food 750 mL Water produced during metabolism 250 mL	Urine 1500 mL Faeces 100 mL Sweat 200 mL Skin and respiration 700 mL (insensible loss)
Total 2500 mL	Total 2500 mL

and possible death. The main stimulus for increasing intake of fluid is the thirst mechanism.

Fluid and electrolyte balance is inextricably linked and in health the volume and composition of the different fluid compartments are finely regulated, with daily fluctuations in TBW of less than 0.2%. Water and electrolytes are ingested and absorbed through the gastrointestinal (GI) tract, although a small volume of water is produced through the oxidation of hydrogen in food. Excess water, electrolytes and waste products are excreted via the kidneys and in faeces. Additional water and salt loss occurs via the skin and respiratory tract, known as insensible loss. Since losses from the gastrointestinal and respiratory tract are not subject to fine regulation, the kidney is the main regulator of fluid and electrolyte balance (see Ch. 8). The flow of blood through the kidney is known as the glomerular filtration rate (GFR) and a normal GFR is 125 mL/min. In 24 hours, the total blood flow through the kidneys is approximately 180 L; this means that the plasma contained within the body is filtered and reabsorbed about 60 times a day. The kidney regulates not only fluid volume, but also electrolyte composition, pH and osmolality. Central to the renal regulation of body fluid osmolality and volume is the kidney's role in the handling of sodium and water.

The osmotic pressure of a solution is expressed as the osmolality (the number of particles present per kilogram of solvent). Osmolality is a standard measure used in medicine and in the very simplest of terms could be considered a measure of the concentration of a solution. Each of the constituents within the ECF and plasma, e.g. the principal ions (sodium, potassium, chloride, etc.) and other non-ionic substances such as glucose and amino acids, exerts a different osmotic pressure. The total sum of these is the measure of the osmolality of the ECF and plasma within 1 kg of the principal solvent within the body, water. The ECF and plasma are said to have an osmolality of around 300 mOsm/kg. The osmotic pressure produced by the proteins, although small, plays an important role in the exchange of fluid between body compartments (Pocock & Richards 2006).

Fluid exchange between the intracellular and extracellular compartments

The movement of body fluids and their constituents between the different compartments is dynamic and involves the processes:

- diffusion
- osmosis
- facilitated diffusion
- active transport
- filtration.

These processes take place through the selectively permeable membrane separating the different fluid compartments, that is, the cell membrane and the capillary wall (single-cell layer of endothelium). The cell membrane separates the ICF from the ECF, and the capillary wall represents the boundary between the intravascular and interstitial compartments of the ECF.

Diffusion is the movement of solutes from an area of higher concentration to an area of lower concentration, which results in an equal concentration in both areas. Diffusion is a form of passive transport because no energy is required and the solutes just move or flow across the membrane.

Osmosis is the passive movement of fluid from an area of lower concentration (of solutes) to an area of higher concentration, in an attempt to dilute the 'stronger' solution and achieve an equal balance on both sides of the membrane. The capillary wall is selectively permeable to substances of a molecular weight less than 69 000 Daltons (69.0 kDa) and to lipid-soluble molecules. Lipid-soluble substances diffuse directly through the cell membrane, while water and electrolytes utilise channels formed by membrane proteins. The membrane is freely permeable to water but is only selectively permeable to electrolytes. Permeability is affected by the size and charge of the hydrated ion; for example, the membrane is 50–100 times more permeable to potassium than to sodium.

Some substances move through *facilitated diffusion* or *active transport*, for example, glucose moves under the influence of insulin. The most important example of active transport is the sodium–potassium pump. This pump is a membrane protein that couples the active transport of sodium out of the cell with the active transport of potassium inwards. It requires energy derived from the hydrolysis of adenosine triphosphate (ATP) to function.

The exchange of water, electrolytes, metabolites and waste products between the plasma and interstitial fluid occurs in the capillary bed. The capillary endothelium is freely permeable to water and solutes but the larger plasma proteins are retained. The movement of fluid through the capillaries relies on a process called capillary filtration. At the arterial end, fluid is forced out of the capillary by hydrostatic pressure. As water is lost from the capillary, the plasma proteins become more concentrated and the colloid osmotic or oncotic pressure exerted by the plasma proteins increases. At the venous end, the hydrostatic pressure, now lower than the rising osmotic pressure, results in fluid being drawn back into the capillary.

The lymphatic system is central to maintaining interstitial fluid volume. Blind-ended lymphatic capillaries in the interstitium are more permeable than the capillaries and easily take up and remove any plasma proteins that have leaked out and fluid from the interstitial space. The fluid formed in these vessels – lymph – is carried through the lymphatic system, eventually returning to the circulation via the central lymphatic and the thoracic duct.

Disturbances in fluid exchange

As approximately 20% of body fluid is found in the interstitial or tissue spaces, the maintenance of fluid volume in this compartment plays a key role in homeostasis. Normally, a dynamic equilibrium exists which maintains the extracellular fluid content of both the plasma and the tissue spaces. However, this delicate balance can easily be disturbed by the following factors and the resulting clinical picture for many of them will be oedema (Box 20.2). Further information about oedema is available on the website.

See website for further content

- *Alterations in capillary pressure* – changes in pressure at either end of the capillary bed will alter net movement of fluid. Increased arterial pressure or venous congestion

Box 20.2 Reflection

Oedema

Think back to a patient you have cared for who had peripheral oedema.

Activity

- What had caused their oedema? What clinical manifestations did they have?
- How was their oedema being managed and what nursing care did they require?
- Reflect upon the effectiveness of the care given in terms of patient comfort.

both tend to favour the loss of fluid to the interstitial space. Examples include hypertension, hypotension, heart failure, and arterial or venous obstruction.
- *Alterations in the plasma proteins* – a reduction in plasma proteins due to malnutrition, liver or renal disease, loss of circulating plasma or leakage of proteins into the tissue fluids will alter the osmotic pressure gradient and prevent fluid being reclaimed from the tissue spaces. Failure of the lymphatics to remove this fluid will increase the osmotic pressure of the interstitial fluid and favour fluid retention.
- *Changes in the integrity of the capillary endothelium* – factors which alter the normal mechanisms regulating the permeability/pore size of the capillary endothelium also change the osmotic or hydrostatic pressures. These effects may be local or systemic. Examples include membrane damage from burns, anoxia, pressure, septicaemia and the presence of inflammatory mediators such as bradykinin or histamine.
- *Accumulation of metabolites* – an accumulation of metabolites within the tissue fluid can alter the hydrostatic and colloidal osmotic pressures with consequent changes in fluid movement. For example, in some states of shock or tissue hypoxia, the cumulative effects of lactic acid and carbon dioxide when combined with vasoactive substances may result in oedema.

Regulation and adjustments of ECF volume, osmolality and sodium

The circulatory system comprises the arterial system of high pressure and low volume and the venous system which operates with a lower pressure and higher volume. Approximately 55% of the plasma volume is in the venous system, 10% in the arterial system and the remaining 35% distributed in the heart, lungs and capillaries (see Ch. 2). Thus changes in volume are usually accommodated by the venous system. The effect of gravity upon fluid in the circulatory system is marked, causing pooling of blood in the venous system with a consequent reduction in the arterial blood volume. If an individual stands for a prolonged period, particularly in a warm environment, there is a reduction in arterial flow to the cells; inadequate venous return then leads to a fall in end-diastolic volume and hence cardiac output. Inadequate perfusion of the brain can then lead to fainting.

The tissue spaces can accommodate large volumes of fluid, but the process is slow and causes fewer disturbances to the ICF or plasma. Adults can usually tolerate changes of about 2 L in the tissue spaces before there are noticeable signs of a volume shift. This 'hidden' accumulation of fluid may, however, be noticed by changes in body weight, 1 L of water (pure) being equivalent to 1 kg.

Volume and osmolality regulation of the ECF involves a series of homeostatic mechanisms. Although the plasma compartment is small, it is dynamic, with shifts in volume and pressure occurring in response to internal and external stimuli. Sodium is also a major factor in the regulation of ECF. The kidney regulates sodium and water ingestion/excretion under the influence of two hormones, aldosterone and antidiuretic hormone (ADH; also known as arginine vasopressin [AVP] or vasopressin).

Influence of antidiuretic hormone

Within the hypothalamus are specialised cells called osmoreceptors which monitor and respond to changes in plasma osmolality (see above). They are very sensitive and respond to changes of as little as ± 3 milliosmoles (mOsm). Plasma osmolality is normally in the range of 300 mOsmL/kg water. The osmoreceptors respond to variations in plasma osmolality by stimulating two mechanisms: thirst and ADH release.

The stimulation of the thirst centre will make the active, independent individual seek fluid to drink, thus attempting to correct any dehydration or shortage of water. ADH will act on the epithelial cells of the nephron collecting ducts to increase/decrease tubular permeability to water. If there is fluid loss, or excess ingestion of salt, plasma osmolality is increased and registered by the osmoreceptors and the individual should begin to feel thirsty. The release of ADH (from the posterior pituitary gland) affects the permeability of the nephron collecting ducts, and water will be reabsorbed into the blood to dilute the hypertonic plasma. This will result in a decrease in urine volume and increase in urine osmolality – urine produced will have a darker, more concentrated appearance. Conversely, if a large volume of water is ingested, the plasma sodium is diluted, causing a fall in the plasma osmolality. This fall is registered by the osmoreceptors, with a resultant decrease in ADH release. Lowered plasma ADH then results in decreased tubular permeability, less water is reabsorbed and water is excreted in the form of a more dilute urine.

The presence of a non-absorbable solute in the renal tubular lumen will also increase water loss. For example, when plasma glucose levels are raised, as in poorly controlled diabetes mellitus (see Ch. 5), and filtered glucose exceeds the ability of the nephrons to reabsorb it, urine production is increased. The glucose exerts an osmotic force, keeping water in the tubule. Osmotic diuresis can also be induced therapeutically by the i.v. administration of a non-absorbable molecule such as the sugar mannitol.

Other factors affecting ADH regulation of osmolality

ADH release may be altered by some drugs, including nicotine and alcohol. Alcohol inhibits the release of ADH, with a resulting diuresis. Nicotine, morphine and barbiturates (which are rarely used) are drugs which increase ADH release. Adrenal insufficiency alters the renal response to water loading. Deficiency in adrenal glucocorticoids (e.g. cortisol) causes an increase in distal tubular permeability to water. Water reabsorption is increased and dilute urine cannot be produced. Tubular response to ADH is decreased and, even in the absence of ADH, permeability to water remains high.

Influence of aldosterone

ECF volume is principally determined by sodium, and body sodium is regulated by the kidney, mainly under the influence of aldosterone. Aldosterone is a mineralocorticoid, released from the adrenal cortex, and is essential for sodium (with associated water) reabsorption. Aldosterone release is stimulated by changes in ECF volume, plasma sodium concentration and plasma potassium concentration. Increases in serum potassium levels of as little as 0.2 mmol/L can cause a marked increase in aldosterone release.

The release of aldosterone is part of a physiological mechanism often known as the *renin–angiotensin–aldosterone* system. Renin is a proteolytic enzyme released from the kidney; more specifically from the juxtaglomerular apparatus (JGA) situated near the afferent arteriole of the glomerulus. It is released in response to changes in plasma sodium and effective circulating volume. Renin acts on a circulating plasma protein (angiotensinogen) to form angiotensin I. Angiotensin I is in turn altered by a converting enzyme found in the lungs to its active form angiotensin II. Angiotensin II has several actions: it is a potent vasoconstrictor and it stimulates the release of aldosterone. This release of aldosterone will then result in an increase in sodium (and water) reabsorption within the distal tubule of the nephron. The increase in sodium reabsorption is in direct exchange for potassium. A rising serum potassium will directly stimulate the production of aldosterone, which in turn will increase sodium reabsorption from the kidney tubule in exchange for potassium which will be lost in the urine.

Hypovolaemia (reduced volume of blood circulating), which reflects a fall in sodium content (as opposed to concentration), will increase aldosterone secretion via the renin–angiotensin system. The resulting vasoconstriction and reabsorption of sodium and water reflects the body's attempt to correct the intravascular volume and thereby maintain blood pressure.

In certain types of hypertension, this mechanism malfunctions and is managed by medication such as angiotensin converting enzyme inhibitors (ACE inhibitors) and angiotensin II receptor blockers (ARBs).

Fluid and electrolyte disturbances

Water volume and sodium imbalances frequently occur in combination with other electrolyte problems, although occasionally they occur alone. Principal causes of disturbance can be related to:

- insufficient or excessive intake or output
- problems in the regulation of intake and output which may be associated with disease states, e.g. heart failure or renal disorders
- problems related to fluid shifts within the body.

Assessment of fluid and electrolyte balance is covered later (pp. 585–589 including Tables 20.4 and 20.5 that outline some of the signs associated with fluid and electrolyte disturbances and measurable parameters and their significance).

Fluid imbalances

Fluid imbalances may be *isotonic* or *osmolar* in nature depending upon the composition of the fluid lost and the resulting balance of water and electrolytes in relation to the ECF. Isotonic imbalances result from the loss of water and electrolytes in proportion to their normal levels in the ECF. Osmolar imbalances are the result of water loss (hyperosmolar) or water gain (hypo-osmolar) which affects the concentration of electrolytes in the ECF and changes the serum osmolarity. Most fluid imbalances are often a combination of both isotonic and osmolar disturbances. This next section considers the effects of fluid imbalances such as dehydration (fluid deficit) or overhydration (water intoxication) of the body and tissues.

Fluid deficits

An ECF volume deficit will arise when fluid loss exceeds fluid intake. Insufficient intake may be related to a number of factors.

Hyperosmolar losses

Dehydration

Strictly speaking, dehydration refers only to water losses from the body that exceed intake, leaving the person with a corresponding accumulation of sodium (a hyperosmolar state). This might be seen for example in a confused, disoriented person who does not drink adequately and over a period of days becomes dehydrated. This shortage of water results in a rise in sodium and an increase in serum osmolality. Water will then shift from the cells (ICF) into the ECF and vascular compartment to try to correct the imbalance, although this will result in the cells themselves becoming dehydrated.

Pure water losses are unusual and it is more common for water to be lost in conjunction with sodium (and other electrolytes) as is seen in vomiting and diarrhoea.

Initially, compensatory mechanisms will maintain blood pressure and heart rate and the kidneys will reduce output, but as the dehydration continues, blood pressure falls, pulse volume weakens, and heart rate and packed cell volume (PCV) (also known as haematocrit) rise. Haemoconcentration (relative increase in the volume of red blood cells to that of plasma) also causes apparent rises in haemoglobin and albumin levels. Eventually the person will be unable to meet the obligatory volume necessary to excrete waste products in the urine. The sequelae of this – metabolite accumulation, acidosis (the processes that result in the build-up of excess acid in the body), renal failure and toxaemia – may lead to death.

Dehydration can be categorised according to the approximate percentage of body water that is lost; in the adult this may be defined as follows:

- mild: 4% (3 L)
- moderate: 5–8% (4–6 L)
- severe: 8–10% (7 L).

The management of dehydration is often complex, especially in severe states where there is gross derangement of body chemistry. In mild to moderate dehydration, fluid losses should be replaced slowly to prevent sudden shifts of water and/or electrolytes between fluid compartments, which would aggravate ionic balance. However, in cases of severe dehydration, as seen in diabetes insipidus or severe heat exhaustion, this may lead to fatal hypovolaemia and so aggressive therapy is required (see Chs 5, 22). The effects of hyponatraemia (decreased sodium concentration in the blood) and hypernatraemia (increased sodium concentration in the blood) which may accompany dehydration are summarised in Table 20.2.

Urinary loss

A number of disease states may result in an excessive production of urine. Patients who have incurred head injury, have undergone hypophysectomy (removal of the pituitary gland),

Table 20.2 Common electrolyte disturbances – deficits and excesses of sodium, potassium and calcium (see Further reading, e.g. Chernecky et al 2006, for information on disturbances affecting other electrolytes, such as magnesium, phosphate, chloride, bicarbonate)

ELECTROLYTE DISTURBANCE	REASONS	CLINICAL EXAMPLES	TYPICAL SIGNS AND SYMPTOMS
Hyponatraemia (serum sodium <135 mmol/L)	a. Excess sodium loss b. Sodium dilution c. Hormone-induced water gains	a. GI losses, exercise b. Excessive fluid intake c. Renal tubule dysfunction, increased ADH secretion	Muscle cramps, weakness, headache, mood changes, depression, lethargy, altered consciousness, tachycardia, hypotension, oedema
Hypernatraemia (serum sodium >143 mmol/L)	a. Excess sodium intake b. Decreased extracellular water c. Water deprivation and decreased water intake d. Hormone related	a. Diet, near drowning, excessive i.v. administration of solutions containing sodium b. Dehydration c. Confusion, impaired thirst sensation, communication difficulties d. Diabetes insipidus	Confusion, lethargy, twitching, convulsions, polydipsia (excessive thirst), hypertension, weight gain

Continued

Table 20.2 Common electrolyte disturbances – deficits and excesses of sodium, potassium and calcium (see Further reading, e.g. Chernecky et al 2006, for information on disturbances affecting other electrolytes, such as magnesium, phosphate, chloride, bicarbonate) – cont'd

ELECTROLYTE DISTURBANCE	REASONS	CLINICAL EXAMPLES	TYPICAL SIGNS AND SYMPTOMS
Hypokalaemia (serum potassium <3.3 mmol/L)	a. Inadequate intake b. Excessive GI losses c. Excessive renal losses d. Intercellular movement	a. Starvation, anorexia b. Diarrhoea, vomiting, excessive nasogastric tube aspiration c. Diuretic therapy, hyperaldosteronism d. Side-effect of some beta blockers, insulin therapy, e.g. diabetic ketoacidosis	Muscular weakness, cardiac dysrhythmias and cardiac arrest, alkalosis, mental confusion, fatigue and hypoventilation
Hyperkalaemia (serum potassium >4.7 mmol/L)	a. Excessive intake or gain b. Inadequate renal losses c. Release from cells (intracellular compartment)	a. Oral or i.v. potassium b. Renal failure, renal tubule dysfunction, side-effects of ACE inhibitors c. Tissue trauma, burns, crush injuries	Anxiety, confusion, cardiac dysrhythmias, bradycardia and cardiac arrest, twitching, muscle weakness, nausea, vomiting and other gastrointestinal disturbances
Hypocalcaemia (serum calcium <2.1 mmol/L)	a. Impaired ability to mobilise calcium from bone b. Abnormal calcium binding c. Abnormal losses d. Renal failure, liver disease	a. Hypoparathyroidism b. Increase in blood pH (more alkaline), such as with hyperventilation, rapid transfusion of citrated blood c. Pancreatitis d. Reduced absorption or intake	Paraesthesia, spasms, cramp, tetany, hypotension, ventricular dysrhythmias, bone pain
Hypercalcaemia (serum calcium >2.6 mmol/L)	a. Excessive gains b. Increased bone resorption c. Increased level of parathyroid hormone d. Inadequate losses e. Renal insufficiency	a. Increased vitamin D or calcium in the diet, excessive use of calcium-containing medicines, or nutritional supplements b. Metastatic tumours of bone, paraneoplastic syndrome, Paget's disease c. Hyperparathyroidism d. Thiazide diuretics, lithium therapy e. Altered calcium and phosphate absorption or binding	Polyuria, polydipsia. Vague symptoms of anorexia, abdominal pain, nausea, vomiting, constipation, muscle weakness/pain and lethargy. Cardiac disturbances

or who have a primary diagnosis of diabetes insipidus may excrete excessive volumes of water and electrolytes due to a disruption in the release of ADH from the pituitary gland. Diabetes insipidus occurs when there is either a deficiency in the manufacture and release of ADH, or an inability of the kidney tubules to respond to ADH (see Ch. 5, Part 1).

Isotonic losses

Gastrointestinal losses

Within the GI tract there is a continuous exchange of fluids, with most of the fluid produced being absorbed. Illnesses which present with diarrhoea or vomiting, or conditions in which fistulae, drainage tubes or GI suction are present, can result in excessive fluid and electrolyte losses, potentially up to 8–9 L/day. Continuous GI or fistula drainage will have the same consequences for a patient as severe diarrhoea and vomiting.

 See website Critical thinking question 20.1

Third space losses

The concept of the *third space* is used to describe the presence of fluids in areas of the body where they are usually absent, or present only in small quantities. This may occur in patients with sepsis, burns or major trauma. Although not lost from the body, the fluid is physiologically unavailable and thus the patient presents as if they are deficient in fluid.

Skin losses

The loss of sodium and water from the skin increases dramatically during excessive sweating or if large areas of the skin have been damaged. For example, in extreme hot weather as much as 1.5–2.0 L/h can be lost through sweat. In the patient with fever, water loss may be up to 3 L/24 h. Burns patients suffer excessive fluid losses; evaporation losses can increase ten times with severe burns (Porth & Matfin 2008) and total loss of fluid from severe burns can be as much as 6–8 L/24 h (see Ch. 30).

Osmotic diuresis

In osmotic diuresis, polyuria (excretion of excessive volume of urine) results from the presence of large quantities of solutes in the blood which enter the glomerular filtrate and are not reabsorbed. The high osmolality of the filtrate in the renal tubules inhibits the action of ADH and prevents reabsorption of water. This principle can be used to produce an osmotic diuresis therapeutically, for example when mannitol is administered to reduce intracranial pressure. In people with diabetes mellitus, an excess of glucose, leading to hyperglycaemia (too much glucose in the blood) or diabetic ketoacidosis, results in a level of glucose that exceeds the kidney's ability to reabsorb it. This causes polyuria, a common presenting symptom of diabetes mellitus.

Fluid volume excess

The retention of fluid and electrolytes results in a fluid volume excess. Such an imbalance can be caused by overloading with fluids or by reduced functioning of the body's homeostatic mechanisms responsible for maintaining fluid and electrolyte balance. The most likely scenario is retention of sodium accompanied by the retention of water as seen in congestive heart failure, renal disease and inappropriate administration of i.v. fluids containing sodium. Isotonic fluids such as 0.9% sodium chloride (physiological saline) or sodium lactate compound (Hartmann's solution) contain large amounts of sodium. With some patients, e.g. older people or those who have a history of heart or renal disease, careful attention must be given to i.v. fluid therapy. Other sources of sodium gain include some over-the-counter (OTC) drugs that contain significant amounts of sodium salts.

Hypo-osmolar imbalance or water excess

When a large volume of water is ingested, it begins to be absorbed within about 15 minutes, in consequence of which the osmolality of the blood decreases. This causes an inhibition of the production and secretion of ADH. Absence of ADH makes the distal convoluted tubule and collecting duct impermeable to water and so more urine is excreted by the kidney, thus producing a more dilute urine and a water diuresis. Following a single large intake of oral fluid, the maximum effect upon diuresis will be noticed about 40 minutes later. A similar effect is achieved if a bolus or fluid challenge of i.v. fluid is administered.

Water intoxication

The kidney has a maximum rate at which it can excrete fluid. If water ingestion, or a hypotonic i.v. fluid administration, exceeds this capacity, then the ECF remains hypotonic. The hypotonic ECF results in fluid moving into the ICF, with a subsequent swelling and bursting of cells. This is most serious in the brain, causing raised intracranial pressure (RIP), convulsions and death. Another significant cause of death from water intoxication occurs as a consequence of the use of the illegal drug ecstasy. Ecstasy reduces or suppresses the thirst sensation with a resultant risk of dehydration. To minimise harm and prevent the likelihood of dehydration, ecstasy users are advised to drink approximately a litre of water an hour if they become hot and/or expend energy, e.g. while dancing.

The danger is that the person misjudges how they should compensate their fluid intake while using ecstasy.

Risk factors and disorders associated with fluid and electrolyte imbalance

This section outlines some areas in which patients commonly experience difficulties with fluid and electrolyte control. Some patients may be at risk for a number of reasons and older people in particular are at increased risk. Nurses in many areas of practice will encounter patients whose fluid and electrolyte balance has been challenged, with potentially dire consequences, e.g. patients with burns, cardiac failure or respiratory problems. Some important risk factors associated with fluid and electrolyte imbalances include:

- *Shortage of water* – in developing countries, water is often in short supply or involves long journeys to obtain it. Drinking the required daily amount to maintain hydration (especially in hot climates) may be very difficult for some to achieve.
- *Fasting or restricted intake* – many medical procedures or the need for surgery require a period of 'nil by mouth' and it is important that this be no longer than necessary. For patients who are repeatedly starved it may be necessary to commence i.v. fluids. Some religious practices involve fasting and may put some members of the population, e.g. older people or those with renal impairment, at risk.
- *Inability to respond to thirst* – people who are confused, depressed, frail or debilitated may not be able to obtain their own fluid/drinks independently. It is important to identify such patients and ensure appropriate measures are taken for them to obtain adequate fluid.
- *Vomiting or loss of gastrointestinal fluid,* e.g. via nasogastric aspirate, if not replaced with appropriate fluid can cause dehydration. If prolonged or severe, it may also lead to metabolic alkalosis (see p. 584) and malnutrition (see Ch. 21). The loss of gastric juices, which contain hydrochloric acid and potassium ions, initially leads to metabolic alkalosis due to a surplus of bicarbonate ions. In severe, prolonged vomiting without adequate nutritional replacement, the body begins to metabolise fats as an energy source, producing ketone bodies and the potential for further acid–base disturbance (see pp. 583–584). Patients who have had abdominal surgery may develop paralytic ileus and the gastric fluid produced is drained via a nasogastric tube rather than being reabsorbed. This will result in a fluid deficit if not appropriately replaced by i.v. fluids.

🖱 **See website Critical thinking question 20.1**

- *Diarrhoea* – worldwide, diarrhoea is a serious problem and the most important indication for fluid and electrolyte replacement. It occurs when the body is unable to reclaim/absorb the fluids in the intestinal tract and the peristaltic contractions of the gut expel the intestinal contents. Generally, intestinal fluids are isotonic with the ECF until the colon is reached, at which point the contents gradually become hypotonic due to the colon's role in water reabsorption. Severe and prolonged diarrhoea, as seen in cholera or in some forms of infant gastroenteritis, can lead to severe electrolyte imbalance, dehydration and, ultimately, death if treatment is unsuccessful or delayed. Fluid and electrolyte replacement is an essential component in the management of the effects of diarrhoea, with accompanying management of the causative agent. Oral rehydration solution is frequently employed in cases of gastroenteritis and dehydration, providing the gut is able to absorb ingested fluids.

See website Critical thinking question 20.1

- *Problems associated with the mouth and throat* – patients who have had a stroke (cerebrovascular accident – CVA) and have dysphagia (difficulty in swallowing) will find taking oral fluids and food difficult and sometimes distressing. Full assessment by the speech and language therapist (SLT) will be essential before oral fluids are given to assess their ability to swallow without choking or risk aspirating fluid into the lungs. Other patients at risk include those who have facial trauma, or have had extensive oral or dental surgery.
- *Reduced mobility and dexterity* – many people will fit into this category. It may be a patient who has undergone a hip replacement; it could be someone who has a new disability such as following stroke, or someone with severe rheumatoid arthritis. For these patients, it is important to ensure that they can reach and easily access fluid so that they can drink independently, or the nurse should ensure that the patient is given fluids at regular intervals.
- *Cardiovascular and renal problems* – people with these problems often present with retention of sodium and water. This is the result of physiological mechanisms not functioning correctly, e.g. the renin–angiotensin–aldosterone mechanism. It is often necessary to restrict fluid intake to prevent fluid overload, and restriction of salt and potassium is also required for some patients.
- *Diuretic therapy* – diuretic medication increases urine output, and therefore influences fluid and electrolyte loss. It is important to monitor that the diuresis is not too far in excess of the patient's intake so that they risk becoming dehydrated. Patients who are required to take this medication may choose to omit it if they find they have to make repeated trips to the lavatory in the night (hence it is often prescribed first thing in the morning) or if they are afraid of falling whilst hurrying to the lavatory.
- *Loss of continence* – people with continence problems may sometimes restrict their fluid intake in a hope that it will reduce their need to pass urine or soil their underwear. This situation may also arise in hospital when patients may similarly reduce their fluid intake so that they do not have to ask for the commode/bedpan or ask to be taken to the lavatory too frequently.

Disorders of electrolyte balance

As stated earlier (p. 576), electrolytes are essential for cellular activity and their concentration in the blood must remain within a specific range for optimal function. There are many clinical situations which may result in disorders of electrolyte balance, some of which are life-threatening. Nurses should be aware of the normal biochemical ranges (Box 20.1, p. 576) and factors which may cause electrolyte imbalances in patients they are caring for (see above). Table 20.2 outlines a range of commonly encountered electrolyte disorders, including possible causes and the effects on bodily function. By fully understanding the implications of electrolyte disturbances, the nurse can respond with appropriate care interventions.

Maintaining acid–base balance

Body fluids are normally slightly alkaline (basic), within a pH range of 7.36–7.44 (hydrogen ion concentration ($[H^+]$) 35–45 nmol/L). Blood has an H^+ concentration of 40 nmol/L, or a pH of 7.4. Acidaemia occurs when the arterial blood pH is less than 7.36 (greater than 44 nmol/L H^+). An arterial pH greater than 7.44 (or less than 36 nmol/L H^+) is alkalaemia. The body enzymes which control most physiological processes are optimally active within the normal pH range, and variations from this range can rapidly result in severe physiological dysfunction or death. It is therefore essential to understand the basis of acid–base balance in health and the effects of disease on this balance. A pH outside the range 6.9–7.7 is incompatible with life; variations outside 7.36–7.44 are serious and may be difficult to rectify. Whilst the blood pH is maintained at a slightly alkaline level, the pH of urine is frequently acidic as the body seeks to excrete surplus acids which have been produced by both metabolic and respiratory processes.

The medium and long-term regulation of pH occurs through the lungs and kidneys, whilst chemical buffers in the blood provide an immediate response to changes in pH. With adjustments in respiratory rate, carbon dioxide levels, and hence pH, can also change. The response, involving the kidney, is slower and sometimes referred to as the 'renal lag'. The kidney's ability to regenerate bicarbonate ions whilst excreting hydrogen ions enables it to aid the regulation of pH. Crucial to the management of acid–base problems is the reversal or removal of the causative factor.

Disorders of acid–base balance

Homeostatic mechanisms within the body ensure that the environment for cellular activity is maintained within some important limits to allow them to function effectively. One of these mechanisms is regulation and balance of acids and bases (see above). Slight imbalances in the pH of body fluids can result in significant effects on body metabolism and essential functions. There are many potential causes of acid–base imbalances, for example infection, respiratory disease, renal disease or dysfunction and some medications. The resulting states may be:

- Acidosis – the process that results in the build-up of excess acid (hydrogen ions) in the body. It leads to acidaemia in which the pH of the blood is below normal (i.e. the pH shifts further towards the neutral point).
- Alkalosis – the process that results in low levels of acid (excess of alkali) in the body. It leads to alkalaemia in which there is a low level of acid (hydrogen ions) and an above normal pH.

Box 20.3 Information

Acid–base disturbances

Respiratory acidosis

- Respiratory acidosis is caused by an excess of carbon dioxide due to hypoventilation.
- It is most frequently caused by primary disorders of the respiratory tract, or by conditions which affect the respiratory centre, e.g. drugs overdose and central nervous system problems.
- Faults in the management of mechanical ventilation may also lead to respiratory acidosis.
- Compensation is through the renal system which retains bicarbonate ions to counter the high level of $PaCO_2$ (the partial pressure of carbon dioxide in arterial blood).
- People with chronic respiratory problems such as chronic obstructive pulmonary disease (COPD) may have well-established compensatory mechanisms.

Respiratory alkalosis

- The most common cause of respiratory alkalosis is hyperventilation, which may occur in a panic/anxiety attack (see also hypocalcaemia, p. 581).
- The subsequent removal of carbon dioxide leads to a raised pH and eventually a fall in the bicarbonate level when renal compensation has occurred.

Metabolic acidosis

- Common causes include renal failure, lactic acidosis (occurring in severe shock with poor tissue perfusion causing hypoxia, sepsis, cardiac and respiratory dysfunction), diabetic ketoacidosis, diuretic therapy with carbonic anhydrase inhibitors, excessive loss of GI fluid such as through a fistula or diarrhoea.
- Characterised by a low pH and low levels of bicarbonate ions.
- The lowered pH leads to a compensatory respiratory drive to hyperventilate, thus causing a transitory fall in the $PaCO_2$.
- Renal compensation is made through the excretion of excess hydrogen ions.
- If the acidosis is severe, cardiac contractility may be affected resulting in bradycardia with a consequent reduction in cardiac output.

Metabolic alkalosis

- Caused by a loss of hydrogen ions, e.g. through vomiting, gastric aspiration or a gain of alkali, as in excess intake of sodium bicarbonate. It may also be caused by some diuretic therapy, or excessive secretion of adrenal cortical hormones – Cushing's syndrome or hyperaldosteronism (see Ch. 5, Part 1).
- Characterised by high pH and a high concentration of bicarbonate ions.
- Respiratory response seeks to compensate by raising the $PaCO_2$ through a decreased respiratory effort.
- Renal compensation can occur through the conservation of hydrogen ions.

Because the lungs and the kidneys are ultimately responsible for the maintenance of acid–base balance, imbalances are categorised as having a respiratory or metabolic cause, i.e. respiratory or metabolic acidosis and respiratory or metabolic alkalosis. The four key disturbances of acid–base balance are outlined in Box 20.3. Sometimes, however, patients have a mixed disorder of acid–base balance. Any of these states may be life threatening. In the acute or critically unwell patient, the pH of the blood and other parameters are assessed via arterial blood gas measurements. The normal values of arterial blood gases are outlined in Table 20.3.

Table 20.3 Normal arterial blood gases (ABGs) (note: slight variations occur between laboratories)	
PARAMETER	**NORMAL RANGE**
pH	7.36–7.44
$[H^+]$	35–45 nmol/L
$PaCO_2$	4.6–5.6 kPa (35–42 mmHg)
PaO_2	11.3–14 kPa (90–105 mmHg)
HCO_3	23–31 mmol/L
Standard HCO_3^-	22–28 mmol/L
Base excess	−2 to 2 mmol/L
Saturation O_2	97%

▷ Nursing management and health promotion: fluid and electrolyte balance

Water is essential for life, and healthy living messages constantly advise people to drink 'plenty' – a minimum of 1200 mL (6–8 glasses) of fluid throughout the day (Food Standards Agency 2010). Despite this clear need for an adequate fluid intake, there is evidence to suggest that patients in hospital are not always being helped to meet this requirement (National Patient Safety Agency [NPSA] 2002). Indeed the situation was becoming so serious that the Nursing and Midwifery Council (NMC) identified *Nutrition and Fluid Management* as one of its Essential Skills Clusters for preregistration nursing programmes (NMC 2007). Every nursing student training within the UK is required to demonstrate competence in helping their patients to meet their fluid needs, whether it be orally or by other routes of administration in order to enter the branch programme. Competence in further skills is required for entry to the register.

One of the main reasons for an inadequate fluid intake is the lack of access to a drink when desired (Box 20.4). Whilst this is unlikely to be a problem for fit healthy adults, for those with reduced cognitive ability, mobility and/or dexterity it may be a significant obstacle. This may be as a result of age, illness or other mobility difficulties. The thirst sensation is diminished in older people and so they are less likely to seek hydration. Also, older adults living alone may be unable to prepare a drink for themselves, or carry it to where they wish to sit. The same could apply to individuals convalescing after surgery or debilitated by ill health. Therefore a fundamental role of the nurse is to ensure that whoever is caring for the individual is aware of the need for fluids to be always both available and accessible. This may include pouring a drink for someone who is unable to do so and making sure that it is within reach and in a suitable drinking vessel. Safety is paramount and the use of specialised cups and/or straws may mean that an individual is able to maintain their independence without the risk of injury. For those for whom help is only available at certain times of the day, equipment such as an insulated jug, preferably with a push-button dispenser, will allow the person easy access to hot or cold drinks for several hours.

A poor fluid intake may also be a result of a reduced desire to drink. Lukewarm water which has sat in a jug all day is unlikely to encourage anyone to drink. It is important that the nurse identifies what types of drink the individual likes and, unless medically contraindicated, tries to make these available. Simple measures such as providing cold, fresh water, perhaps with the addition of ice, if available, will make drinks much more palatable than lukewarm stale water.

Failure to meet a patient's need for adequate fluid can have catastrophic effects on their health and well-being. In two reports, the early signs of potential deterioration, often linked to inadequate fluid intake, were not being recognised and subsequently patients experienced delays in receiving appropriate treatment (National Confidential Enquiry into Patient Outcome and Death [NCEPOD] 2005 and NPSA 2007). In the NPSA report, out of the 576 deaths reported to them, 11% or 66 deaths were attributed to signs of deterioration not being recognised or acted upon. The need for comprehensive assessment is therefore paramount.

Assessment – fluid and electrolyte status

The effects of a fluid/electrolyte loss or gain depend to a large extent on the volume of the loss or gain and the rate at which it occurs. Effects are more acute when loss or gain develops rapidly, when the person is at the extremes of age and when the person is debilitated. Signs and symptoms observed by the nurse will depend upon the effects of the fluid loss or gain on the serum osmolality. A major problem in the assessment of fluid and electrolyte imbalance is that significant changes occur before they can be detected by clinical measurements such as blood pressure or central venous pressure. The nurse therefore needs to be able to use a wide range of skills to detect early changes. These include the following:

- *Knowing what to look for* – using a sound knowledge of physiology, the nurse will know what early and late clinical signs may be present, including signs of compensation by the body in its attempt to maintain homeostasis.
- *Knowing how often to look* – the nurse will be able to assess the severity of the situation and assess/monitor the patient accordingly.
- *Knowing what the anticipated effects of a variety of medical interventions are* – in order to assess effectiveness of treatment and plan further care.

Changes in tissue fluid volume are noticed mainly through observation of mucous membranes and skin elasticity, the latter being more easily observed over bony prominences. Skin turgor is a less reliable indicator of dehydration in an older person, due to the natural loss of elasticity of the skin. With an infant, the anterior fontanelle provides a good indication of hydration status.

The nurse's frequent contact with the patient should enable detection of any disturbances of features which may be related to fluid and electrolyte status. Unfortunately, nursing management of patients' needs for food and fluid is often neglected and notoriously full of errors and confusion. In illness, certain groups, such as older people, infants/children and pregnant women, are particularly susceptible to fluid and electrolyte problems. Others are at risk by virtue of an underlying pathological problem and/or as a result of nursing or medical interventions.

A number of parameters may indicate changes in fluid or electrolyte status, but minor changes are often recognised only by those familiar with the person. Thus effective communication is crucial between nurses, e.g. at handover reports, and with relatives and carers who may notice changes. The rapid detection of patterns and trends can be important in identifying deterioration or improvement in the patient's condition.

A structured approach to nursing assessment should facilitate the identification of actual and potential patient problems. Indeed, the initial assessment may not be completed until a 24-hour observation of the patient has been undertaken. Assessment of the patient's fluid and electrolyte status involves a four-stage process, some of which may run concurrently:

- Stage 1: Consider observable and reported parameters.
- Stage 2: Consider measurable parameters.
- Stage 3: Consider the underlying pathophysiology.
- Stage 4: Consider the effects of medications.

Many changes in tissue volume can be noticed through sensory observation or by the patient reporting symptoms. When this information is combined with the measurable data, it can give a reliable indicator of the patient's fluid status (Tables 20.4, 20.5). For further details of the physiological processes which influence fluid and electrolyte status (see Further reading suggestions, e.g. Porth & Matfin 2008). Underlying pathological processes and the effect of medications frequently distort clinical signs and therefore must also be considered.

Table 20.4 Observable/reportable signs of fluid and electrolyte disturbance and their possible significance

CLINICAL SIGNS/SYMPTOMS	CLINICAL SIGNIFICANCE	CAUTIONS IN INTERPRETATION
Mucous membranes will appear dry and the patient will complain of thirst	Decreased saliva production will result in a dry mouth and sensation of thirst. Osmoreceptors detecting hypovolaemia will also trigger a feeling of thirst. This acts as a useful backup, as effective oral hygiene often disguises the decreased saliva production	Mouth breathing Oxygen administration Anticholinergic drugs, e.g. dicycloverine hydrochloride
Tongue furrows	A normal tongue has one long longitudinal furrow, but in dehydration additional furrows will be present and the tongue will appear smaller due to fluid loss (Lapides et al 1965)	–
Sunken eyes	The result of decreased intraocular pressure	–
Increased jugular venous pressure (JVP). With a patient positioned at 45 degrees, venous distension should not exceed 2 cm above the sternal angle	Distended veins indicate fluid overload; flat veins indicate decreased plasma volume	Assessing the right internal jugular vein gives a more reliable reading than on the left as it is the most anatomically direct route to the right atrium
Reduced capillary refill time	Capillary refill taking 2–3 s indicates a mild fluid deficit Refill times in excess of 3 s signify severe fluid deficits	Peripheral shutdown due to cold will slow capillary refill irrespective of fluid status
Reduced skin turgor	Reduction in interstitial and intracellular fluid will reduce skin elasticity	In an older person it is difficult to detect changes in skin turgor due to the gradual loss of skin elasticity with age
Cool peripheral temperature and pale skin colour	As a result of the renin–angiotensin cycle, hypovolaemia will result in peripheral vasoconstriction and therefore reduced temperature and colour	Patients with poor circulation, e.g. peripheral vascular disease or Raynaud's disease, will normally have cool peripheries Certain antihypertensives including vasodilators and ACE inhibitors will disguise the body's normal compensatory mechanism
Dark urine	Hypovolaemia will trigger release of ADH, leading to more concentrated urine	Patients with liver disease may have bilirubin present in their urine giving it a very dark colour. Diuretic therapy will override the body's production of ADH
Peripheral oedema	Oedema occurs with the movement of fluid into interstitial spaces as a result of fluid excess and/or reduced levels of plasma proteins A consequent decrease in intravascular fluid may lead to a reduction in blood pressure	–
Pulmonary oedema (fluid within the lung alveoli), observable through frothy, pink-stained sputum and/or dyspnoea (shortness of breath)	Pulmonary oedema will result in decreased gaseous exchange, with a reduction in oxygen saturation and arterial oxygen levels	–

Monitoring fluid balance

The two most important components of monitoring a patient's fluid balance are measurements or estimations of fluid intake/output and weight. Insensible fluid losses are estimated according to standard norms and often account for a much larger volume than is usually estimated in clinical practice (Marieb & Hoehn 2007). It is therefore important to make adjustments for the following factors:

- body temperature
- ambient temperature
- basal metabolic rate (BMR)

- respiratory rate
- respiratory assistance, e.g. use of oxygen, humidification
- other pathologies
- fluid content in stools
- internal losses due to fluid movement
- losses through skin trauma.

Whilst some losses and gains have to be estimated, in appropriate circumstances others can be measured, for example:

- volume of oral fluid intake and fluid in foods
- i.v. fluids

Table 20.5 Measurable parameters and their significance in fluid and electrolyte imbalance

CLINICAL PARAMETERS/ MEASUREMENTS	CLINICAL SIGNIFICANCE	CAUTIONS IN INTERPRETATION
Pulse	If there is a reduction in circulating volume and therefore stroke volume, the heart rate will increase to compensate and maintain cardiac output (see Ch. 2) Initial assessment of rhythm, based on the regularity of the pulse, may be useful and indicate a need for an ECG recording	Cardiac drugs, e.g. beta-blockers, such as atenolol, celiprolol, will inhibit the body's compensatory mechanism and therefore block an increase in heart rate
Blood pressure	Measurement of blood pressure will give an indication of circulating volume. Pulse pressure, the difference between systolic and diastolic pressure, will give an indication of vasoconstriction, i.e. compensation by the body	As a result of numerous compensatory mechanisms, blood pressure is maintained by the body for as long as possible. A 'normal' blood pressure in the presence of compensation must be acted upon immediately
Central venous pressure (CVP)	Will be reduced as a result of hypovolaemia and/or vasodilatation An increase in CVP does not necessarily indicate fluid overload as CVP is influenced by numerous other factors including cardiac competence, systemic vascular resistance (SVR), intrathoracic and intra-abdominal pressure	For further information, see Chapter 18
Urine volume	In health, the body produces 1 mL urine/kg of body weight per h Acceptable urine output in the critically ill patient is equal to 0.5 mL urine/kg per h	A knowledge of the patient's weight and calculation of desired urine output based upon that is essential Administration of diuretics will override normal physiological processes. Their use must be noted when assessing volume of urine produced
Specific gravity (SG) of urine	Demonstrates the body's ability to concentrate urine as an indicator of kidney function and/or response to ADH production	Administration of diuretics will override normal physiological processes. Their use must be noted when assessing urinary SG

- GI gains through enteral feeding
- GI losses from gastric aspiration, fistulae and drains
- urine: volume and concentration, i.e. an output <0.5 mL/ kg body weight per h
- fluid pressures through observing the jugular venous pressure or measuring central venous pressure.

Unfortunately, the volume of oral fluid intake or fluid in food is usually estimated rather than measured. Indeed, some fluid-containing foods such as soups and custards are not necessarily included in fluid recording. This is particularly important in patients who are restricted to a liquid diet or whose fluid intake is restricted, as in renal failure.

Fluid balance charting: possible sources of error

Nurses should be aware of the many ways in which the accuracy of fluid intake/output calculations may be compromised. Examples include:

- duplication or omission of items
- use of estimations rather than measurements
- arithmetical errors
- i.v. fluids administered in theatre and not correctly accounted for
- staff shift change errors, i.e. in carrying forward from the previous shift
- not specifying whether fluid is colloid or crystalloid in calculations
- recording wrong i.v. bag – confusion between treatment chart and fluid chart

- failure to observe patterns in consecutive daily balance
- the patient is unable to accurately recall events and forgets their fluid or food intake
- unmeasurable loss, e.g. vomit over the floor.

Measurement errors also arise when inappropriate utensils are used (Box 20.5). To reduce the margin of error, low volumes of urine should be measured in containers with

Box 20.5 Reflection

Reducing errors in recording fluid balance

Reflect on your experience of recording fluid balance in practice and identify potential sources of error.

Activities

- Measure out 100 mL quantities of water using an accurate measure (e.g. a syringe) and transfer them into the following containers, observing the water levels: urinal, catheter drainage bag, a measuring jug and a standard glass, cup and cereal/soup bowl used in your placement.
- Determine how much liquid is contained in the standard glass, cup and bowl used, when full to the brim, about half full or filled to the level usually served by the catering staff.
- Consider the implications of your findings with regard to a patient's/client's hydration status and discuss them with your mentor or lecturer.
- Think about how the ward/unit team could reach a consensus about recording the exact volume of oral fluids.

gradations designed for low volumes. Large volumes measured from catheter drainage bags may prove to be different if the bag is emptied and then measured in a rigid measuring jug. Similarly, i.v. fluid bags may contain more than the actual amount specified. In the clinical setting it is possible to use scales to measure body fluids; subtracting the weight of the empty receptacle, e.g. vomit bowl or urinal, from the total weight. A very approximate conversion of weight to volume is straightforward, e.g. 250 g = 250 mL, but this simple conversion relates to pure water and further allowances must be made, for instance when vomit contains undigested food.

Understanding the relative acceptable margins of error is an essential but neglected aspect of fluid monitoring. In a fit, healthy person, small errors may not be significant, but in a vulnerable person they can lead to inappropriate treatment regimens with consequent problems. Due to the problems associated with estimating and measuring fluid intake and output volumes, many view the use of daily weight recordings as a more reliable indicator of fluid status. However, for these measurements to be accurate and meaningful, the weight should be taken at the same time each day and with the patient wearing the same clothes and shoes. Lean body mass changes do not occur quickly and the measurement of daily weight is particularly useful when assessing the older person and those with renal or cardiac impairment.

Finally, measurement of bioelectrical impedence may be a way forward in the assessment of fluid volumes within the body (Metheny 2000). This involves attaching a surface electrode to the patient's hand and foot before passing an imperceptible electrical current through their body fluids. The extent to which the body conducts electricity can be used to estimate fluid volumes and a study by Mequid et al (1992) suggested that bioelectrical impedance analysis provides a better correlation with fluid balance charts than daily weight measurement. They suggest that the speed and simplicity of this technique make it a valuable assessment tool. However, despite these findings it is not commonly seen in practice and further studies into its value may be beneficial to assess if it could help overcome the problems associated with inaccurate fluid balance charts.

Managing fluid and electrolyte therapy

The aims of all fluid and electrolyte therapy are to:

- Regulate, where possible, the patient's fluid and electrolyte balance by controlling the content and volume of fluids taken by the oral/enteral route. When the oral/enteral route is inadequate, venous access is required.
- Control excessive losses and gains, such as by means of surgical intervention to prevent blood loss or by the use of diuretics to regulate fluid balance.

Both the medical and nursing management of the patient's fluid and electrolyte status will be derived from the initial assessment. The patient may require one or more of the following interventions:

- assistance with the maintenance of normal fluid and electrolyte requirements; this usually occurs for a short period of time in a previously well-nourished person, e.g. following surgery or during a brief period of altered consciousness

- correction of fluid/electrolyte imbalances
- parenteral nutrition (PN) (see Chs 21, 28).

Occasionally, a person will require all three measures simultaneously; for example, someone with a major abdominal injury may need immediate correction of fluid loss (including blood loss) and electrolyte disturbances, followed by a need to ensure that normal fluid and electrolyte requirements are met, with consideration being given to changes in demand due to the injury. If oral/enteral feeding is unlikely to be resumed, then the introduction of parenteral feeding will be urgently considered by the multidisciplinary team (MDT).

In deciding on the most appropriate plan for a patient, consideration is given not only to the content of the therapy, but also to the resources available, the patient's coexisting problems, e.g. diabetes mellitus, and the particular hazards associated with the respective methods of administration. The timing, rate and duration of the therapy can also determine which route will be most effective.

Determining the volume and content of the therapy

The regimen prescribed for the patient will be based on the following essential considerations of what needs to be:

- replaced – measured and insensible or hidden losses from the body
- removed – where there is excess production or excretory failure
- adjusted – where there is translocation of fluids or electrolytes
- resolved – the cause of the problem, e.g. vomiting, haemorrhage.

The identification of these requirements will be based on nursing observation, medical assessment and laboratory analysis of specimens. However, the method of administration will influence the nature of the fluid regimen.

Routes for fluid and electrolyte therapy

The routes discussed include oral, parenteral, enteral, rectal and subcutaneous.

Oral route

Replacing fluids via the oral route is without doubt the safest method and one that maintains normality. In a healthy adult who has no circulatory or renal insufficiency, the need for fluid is 1500–3000 mL/24 h. Replacing fluids orally will involve identifying the person's preferred drinks and then making these available, where reasonable, in the desirable quantity.

In some situations the patient may be prescribed 'restricted fluids', the amount usually being stated. For example, a person with renal failure may have a restricted fluid intake of 1000 mL/24 h (usually based on the previous day's urine output plus an amount for insensible loss). In other circumstances the nurse may be instructed to 'encourage fluids', especially when the goal is to prevent urinary stasis in the catheterised patient.

Two key points for the nurse to bear in mind when caring for patients requiring replacement of fluid and electrolytes by the oral route are:

- Ascertain the exact meaning of vague orders (verbal or written) concerning fluid replacement, e.g. 'push fluids', 'encourage fluids', 'taking sips'. Remember that fluid and electrolyte balance is vital and that the nurse has a key role to play in preventing further problems.
- If at all possible, know exactly how much fluid a person is required to have over a 24-hour period. Medical orders can easily be written to identify appropriate daily fluid intake targets, e.g. 2000–2500 mL/24 h.

Sometimes patients having fluid replacement therapy still complain of thirst. Whilst the thirst response will be permanently relieved if the receptors in the hypothalamus are no longer stimulated, a temporary depression of the thirst mechanism has been associated with interventions related to the oropharyngeal region (Anderson & Rundgren 1982). The patient troubled by thirst may appreciate the nurse:

- providing frequent oral hygiene
- applying lubricant to lips
- giving mouth rinses with fresh water
- choosing carefully the type and temperature of fluids
- offering ice for the patient to suck.

Parenteral route

For a number of patients, fluid and electrolyte therapy must be administered via the parenteral route (a route other than the alimentary tract). Most commonly this is administered intravenously (i.v.). Parenteral fluid administration enables solutions to enter the extracellular compartment directly, enabling a rapid and controlled method of delivery. Managing an i.v. therapy regimen has become a common nursing responsibility, with some practitioners being qualified to initiate specified therapies under specified authority or using Patient Group Directions. Before commencing an i.v. therapy regimen, assessment should consider the adequacy of the patient's renal/cardiac function and current fluid/electrolyte status, referring to such objective measures as laboratory results, body surface area and intake/output.

Enteral route

A tube may be inserted into the stomach (nasogastric) or the small intestine (nasoenteral) to administer fluids and electrolytes; this may be as part of nutritional support (see Ch. 21). A nasogastric tube is used short-term, but for long-term therapy a percutaneous endoscopic gastrostomy (PEG) tube is inserted, or a jejunostomy is performed.

Rectal route

Fluids can be administered through the rectum (proctoclysis) and through ostomies, although these routes are not always effective. However, Bruera et al (1998) concluded that rectal fluid replacement can be effective for patients with terminal cancer and that it is a safe and inexpensive method of providing fluids and electrolytes.

Subcutaneous route

Subcutaneous fluid replacement is known as hypodermoclysis. In older patients in whom venous access may be difficult, in patients who are confused or find it difficult to tolerate an alternative route, or in the terminally ill patient, the use of subcutaneous fluid administration can be both appropriate and preferred (Mansfield & Monaghan Hall 1998). The sites of choice include the anterior or lateral aspects of the chest wall, the abdominal wall, the anterolateral aspects of the thigh and the scapula. The site of the subcutaneous administration should be regularly inspected and changed every 24 hours.

Major complications of i.v. therapy

Due to advances in technology, i.v. therapy is now relatively safe; however, it is still possible for serious complications to arise. Unfortunately, as noted in a classic study by Speechley & Toovey (1987), complications are sometimes regarded as routine occurrences or merely a 'nuisance'. Despite the age of this work the situation remains largely unchanged and to overlook or underestimate the potential risks of i.v. therapy is to lose sight of the aim of therapy, which is to effectively replace fluid and electrolytes without causing the patient discomfort or further injury. The most common complications are:

- occlusion
- infiltration, i.e. leakage of non-irritant or vesicant fluid into the tissues surrounding the vein
- extravasation, i.e. infiltration of irritants or vesicants that cause tissue damage
- phlebitis.

Factors associated with an increased incidence of phlebitis include:

- cannula location – lower extremities or proximity to joints presents an increased risk
- duration of therapy – increasing time raises the incidence, especially over 24 hours
- blood flow problems in the region of the cannula site
- inadequate cleaning of the cannula site
- pre-existent infection
- pH and osmolality of the fluid – acidic infusates in particular
- particulate matter which may contaminate the delivery system.

Selecting the site

Patients who are particularly vulnerable to complications are those with existing infections or immune suppression and those whose restlessness or mental state may lead them to traumatise the cannula site. In their seminal work, Maki et al (1973) pointed out that the cannula site is similar to an open surgical wound containing a foreign body and should be treated as such (see Further reading suggestions, e.g. Dougherty & Lamb 1999, Finlay 2004).

Some practical considerations are involved in site selection, namely:

- the nature and anticipated duration of the therapy
- situational and environmental factors
- patient and safety factors
- availability of products
- staff expertise.

Insertion of i.v. cannulae is often undertaken by medical staff but is now more commonly undertaken by a competent registered nurse who has undertaken appropriate training.

Some suggested competencies for i.v. drug administration are outlined by Finlay (2004) and are the subject of ongoing development by the Royal College of Nursing IV Therapy Forum. Effective communication between patient, nurse and doctor may enable a more effective and safe selection of site, materials and insertion technique. Tackling the reduction of infection associated with peripheral venous cannulae is now addressed as part of the *Saving Lives* initiative and more directly through the high-impact intervention 2 – peripheral venous cannula care bundle (Department of Health [DH] 2007). In life-threatening circumstances, the selection of the i.v. site is largely dependent upon the expertise of the staff available, the products to hand and the purpose of the i.v. line. Whilst infection control measures are important, at the scene of a disaster or accident environmental contaminants may be inevitable and speed may take priority. The more invasive the procedure, the greater is the importance of environmental control. Central venous catheters must also be inserted under strict aseptic conditions, and the Department of Health (DH) high-impact intervention 1 – central venous catheter care bundle (DH 2007) provides further guidance for appropriate care and management. Local factors which may be controlled during the time of insertion include the elimination of airborne contaminants and the avoidance of debris or bacteria entering via the insertion site.

Patient factors Patient mobility and comfort may be enhanced or hindered by site selection. It is wiser, and causes less discomfort, to site the i.v. cannula away from joints or sites where clothes may rub. Skin areas which are vulnerable to breakdown should also be avoided, including areas which are burned, oedematous, otherwise traumatised, inflamed or affected by conditions such as eczema or psoriasis. The integrity and state of the veins themselves should also influence selection.

The safety of i.v. lines in patients who are restless often poses a practical problem for nurses. Stability of the line may be enhanced by the method of attachment to the patient, and applying principles of countertraction, through the use of loops, may prevent unnecessary trauma. Modern dressings may also help tackle this problem.

Central lines (central venous catheters)

Central lines are used to measure central venous pressure (see Ch. 18) and for the long-term administration of infusates, e.g. PN and chemotherapy (cytotoxic and antibiotic) (see Chs 7, 11, 21, 31). However, the greatly increased incidence of complications associated with the use of central lines necessitates a very cautious and competent approach to their management. Finlay (2004) reminds nurses of the dangers associated with central line insertion and maintenance, namely pneumo- or haemothorax, arterial puncture, atrial fibrillation, venous embolism on insertion, during maintenance or upon withdrawal, infection and thrombosis.

Types of parenteral fluids

The nature of the products to be infused determines both the number and location of the lines. Some infusates cannot be mixed, and if concurrent administration is required, two or more lines may be needed. Infusates which increase the likelihood of microbial contamination include those used in PN, especially those containing high concentrations of glucose. Each infusate carries with it particular risks, and nurses should familiarise themselves with the specific potential side-effects associated with different infusates.

Broadly speaking, the infusates commonly used in i.v. therapy, as opposed to PN, may be categorised as:

- crystalloids – those containing water, electrolytes, glucose
- colloids – blood and blood products, plasma and plasma substitutes (Table 20.6).

Clinicians continue to debate which type of i.v. fluid is preferable in the resuscitation of the acutely ill. Research has provided mixed evidence, and several Cochrane Reviews have added to the debate but have not drawn firm conclusions (Alderson et al 2003, Bunn et al 2003).

Infusates can also be categorised with respect to their tonicity.

Isotonic solutions have the same osmolarity (tonicity) as serum or other body fluids and expand the intravascular compartment without affecting the intracellular and interstitial compartments; 0.9% saline is an isotonic fluid with respect to plasma.

Hypotonic solutions have a lower osmolarity than serum and cause body fluids to shift away from the intravascular compartment and into the intracellular and interstitial spaces to areas of higher osmolarity. Hypotonic solutions may be used in the case of cellular dehydration due to diabetic ketoacidosis.

Hypertonic solutions have a higher osmolarity than serum and cause fluid to move from the interstitial and intracellular compartments towards the intravascular compartments (see Ch. 18).

Problems associated with fluid and electrolyte imbalance

This section outlines some areas in which patients/clients experience difficulties with fluid and electrolyte balance – dehydration and hydration at the end of life, vomiting, diarrhoea and the special needs of the person undergoing surgery. This information is supported by additional material on the website and the opportunity to complete Critical thinking questions.

Dehydration and hydration in end-of-life care

The debate continues as to whether, and when, to withhold or withdraw intravenous, subcutaneous or nasogastric hydration in the days or hours before an expected death. Nurses may well be presented with situations where a decision regarding hydration of their patients must be made. Nurses need to be knowledgeable of the benefits and disadvantages of both terminal dehydration and the rationale for hydration (Salt 2007). Decisions made must be individualised and based on careful assessment that considers the clinical and ethical problems related to dehydration, the potential risks and benefits of fluid replacement and the patient's wishes at the time (or in the form of an Advance Directive), and those of the family. If individuals do not have the capacity to make decisions for

Table 20.6 Commonly used intravenous fluids – crystalloids and colloids		
INTRAVENOUS FLUID	**TYPE**	**FEATURES**
Glucose 5% contains glucose 50 mg/mL	Crystalloid	Frequently used as a maintenance fluid Used to replace minor fluid losses Provides some calorific value (small)
Sodium chloride 0.9% (physiological saline) contains 150 mmol/L of both sodium and chloride Note: it should not be referred to as *normal saline*	Crystalloid	Frequently used as a maintenance fluid Used to replace minor fluid losses Used to correct hyponatraemia
Sodium lactate compound (Hartmann's solution) contains sodium 131 mmol/L, potassium 5 mmol/L, chloride 111 mmol/L, calcium 2 mmol/L, lactate 29 mmol/L	Crystalloid	Can be used instead of sodium chloride 0.9% Contraindicated in renal or hepatic disease
Sodium bicarbonate 1.26% contains 150 mmol/L of both sodium and bicarbonate	Crystalloid	Used to treat metabolic acidosis
Blood – plasma depleted (packed cells)	Colloid	Used to replace red blood cells such as in severe anaemia or blood loss
Fresh frozen plasma	Colloid	Used to correct coagulation deficits
Gelatin solutions (a plasma substitute) examples include Gelofusine®, Haemaccel®	Colloid	Used in hypovolaemia to restore and/or maintain the intravascular fluid volume Hypersensitivity reactions can occur, rarely anaphylaxis
Etherified starch (a plasma substitute) Examples include hetastarch (non-proprietary), HAES-steril®	Colloid	Used in hypovolaemia to restore and/or maintain the intravascular fluid volume Extremely long half life
Albumin solutions (isotonic 4–5% or concentrated 15–25%)	Colloid	Used to restore and/or maintain intravascular fluid volume

Based on a table from Cowen MD 2009 Fluid management. In Childs L, Coles L, Marjoram BA, eds. Essential skills clusters for nurses: theory for practice. Oxford, Wiley-Blackwell.

themselves, procedures must be guided by the Mental Capacity Act 2005 (Ministry of Justice 2005) and there is also ongoing guidance from the General Medical Council (see Further reading).

Vomiting

Fluid loss caused by vomiting can rapidly cause dehydration and electrolyte imbalance; if prolonged or severe, it may lead to metabolic alkalosis and further acid–base disturbance (see pp. 583–584). The fluid and electrolyte losses caused by vomiting may be summarised as follows:

- depletion of the ECF volume
- hypochloraemia (low serum chloride level caused by loss of Cl⁻)
- alkalosis
- hypokalemia
- possible acidosis.

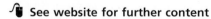 **See website Critical thinking question 20.1**

The nursing care required for a person who is vomiting is outlined on the website.

🖱 **See website for further content**

Diarrhoea

Worldwide, diarrhoea is a serious problem and the most important indication for fluid and electrolyte replacement (see pp. 588–590). The fluid losses from diarrhoea may cause:

- depletion of ECF volume
- hyponatraemia
- hypokalaemia
- metabolic acidosis (loss of bicarbonate in the digestive juices)
- severe water dehydration (if the colon is involved).

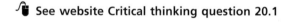 **See website Critical thinking question 20.1**

Special needs of the person undergoing surgery

The person undergoing surgery, whether elective or emergency, is particularly vulnerable to several disturbances of fluid and electrolyte balance. Disturbances in the composition and placement of the body fluids and electrolytes accompany many procedures and include blood loss, dehydration from pre-operative fasting, bowel preparation and surgical exposure (see Ch. 26).

🖱 **See website Critical thinking question 20.2**

SUMMARY: KEY NURSING ISSUES

- Homeostasis of water, electrolytes and acid–base balance is vital to cellular function.
- Fluid and electrolyte imbalance is associated with too little (caused by reduced intake and/or increased loss), or too much (caused by increased intake and/or decreased loss).
- Disturbances of fluid balance may be isotonic or osmolar.

- Nurses need a clear understanding of fluid, electrolyte and acid–base balance, and the common disorders in order to assess fluid and electrolyte status, anticipate and recognise deterioration and implement corrective interventions.
- Awareness of potential risk factors for fluid and electrolyte imbalance is vital.
- Nurses are key to the early recognition of disturbances and therefore need to be able to use a wide range of skills to detect early changes, such as monitoring fluid balance.
- Nursing interventions in relation to fluid therapy range from providing appropriate oral fluids to managing a complicated i.v. fluid regimen.
- Safe management of the person with a fluid, electrolyte or acid–base disturbance is complex and requires skilful and knowledgeable nursing practice.

REFLECTION AND LEARNING – WHAT NEXT?

- **Test** your knowledge by visiting the website 🖱 and answering the multiple choice questions and critical thinking questions.
- **Consolidate** your learning by looking at some of the further reading suggestions, references and specialist websites.
- **Revisit** some of the additional material on the website.
- **Consider** what you have learnt and how this will help your professional development.
- **Reflect** on how you can apply this knowledge to the care of your patients.
- **Discuss** your learning with your mentor/supervisor, lecturer and colleagues.

REFERENCES

Alderson P, Schierhout G, Roberts I, Bunn F: Colloids versus crystalloids for fluid resuscitation in critically ill patients (Cochrane Review). In *The Cochrane Library*, Issue 4, Chichester, 2003, Wiley.

Anderson B, Rundgren M: Thirst and its disorders, *Annu Rev Med* 33:231–239, 1982.

Bruera E, Pruvost M, Schoeller T, et al: Proctoclycis for hydration in terminally ill cancer patients, *J Pain Symptom Manage* 15(4):216–219, 1998.

Bunn F, Roberts I, Tasker R, Akpa E: Hypertonic versus crystalloids for fluid resuscitation in critically ill patients (Cochrane Review). In *The Cochrane Library*, Issue 4, Chichester, 2003, Wiley.

Cowen MD: Fluid management. In Childs L, Coles L, Marjoram BA, editors: *Essential skills clusters for nurses: theory for practice*, Oxford, 2009, Wiley-Blackwell, pp 185–197.

Department of Health: *Saving Lives: Reducing infection, delivering clean and safe care*, 2007. Available online http://www.dh.gov.uk.

Finlay T: *Intravenous therapy*, Oxford, 2004, Blackwell Science.

Food Standards Agency: *Healthy diet*, 2010. Available online http://www.eatwell.gov.uk/healthydiet/nutritionessentials/drinks/drinkingenough/.

Lapides J, Bourne R, Maclean L: Clinical signs of dehydration and extracellular fluid loss, *J Am Med Assoc* 191:413, 1965.

Maki DG, Goldman D, Rhame S: Infection control in IV therapy, *Ann Intern Med* 79(6):867–887, 1973.

Mansfield S, Monaghan Hall J: Subcutaneous administration and site maintenance, *Nurs Stand* 13(12):56–62, 1998.

Marieb EN, Hoehn K: *Human Anatomy and Physiology*, ed 7, San Francisco, 2007, Benjamin Cummings.

Mequid M, Lukaski H, Tripp M, et al: Rapid bedside method to assess changes in postoperative fluid status with bioelectrical impedance analysis, *Surgery* 112:502, 1992.

Metheny N: *Fluid and electrolyte balance: nursing considerations*, ed 4, Philadelphia, 2005, Lippincott.

Ministry of Justice: *Mental Capacity Act*, 2005. Available online http://www.justice.gov.uk/guidance/mental-capacity.htm.

National Confidential Enquiry into Patient Outcome and Death (NCEPOD): *An acute problem?*, 2005. Available online http://www.ncepod.org.uk/2005aap.htm.

National Patient Safety Agency (NPSA): *National reporting goes live*, 2002. Available online: http://www.npsa.nhs.uk.

National Patient Safety Agency (NPSA): *Safer care for the acutely ill patient: learning from serious incidents*, 2007. Available online http://www.npsa.nhs.uk/nrls/alerts-and-directives/directives-guidance/acutely-ill-patient/.

Nursing and Midwifery Council (NMC): *NMC Circular 07/2007 Annexe 2 Essential Skills Clusters (ESCs) for Pre-registration Nursing Programmes*, 2007. Available online http://www.nmc-uk.org.

Pocock G, Richards CD: *Human Physiology – The basis of Medicine*, ed 3, Oxford, 2006, Oxford University Press.

Porth CM, Matfin G: *Pathophysiology: concepts of altered health state*, ed 8, Philadelphia, 2008, Lippincott Williams and Wilkins.

Salt S: When a terminal patient is no longer able to eat or drink, *End of Life Care* 1(3):34–39, 2007.

Speechley V, Toovey J: Problems in i.v therapy, *Prof Nurse* 2(8):240–242, 1987.

Waugh A: Problems associated with fluid, electrolyte and acid-base balance. In Brooker C, Nicol M, editors: *Nursing Adults: The Practice of caring*, Edinburgh, 2003, Mosby, pp 135–136.

Waugh A, Grant A: *Ross and Wilson Anatomy and Physiology in Health and Illness*, ed 10, Edinburgh, 2006, Churchill Livingstone.

FURTHER READING

British National Formulary: 2010 (No. 59). Available online www.bnf.org.

Chernecky C, Macklin D, Murphy-Ende K: *Saunders Nursing Survival Guide: Fluid and Electrolytes*, ed 2, Philadelphia, 2006, Saunders.

Department of Health: *Benchmarks for the Fundamental Aspects of Care*, 2010. Available online http://www.dh.gov.uk.

Dougherty L, Lamb J, editors: *Intravenous therapy in nursing practice*, Edinburgh, 1999, Churchill Livingstone.

Dougherty L, Lister S: *The Royal Marsden Hospital Manual of Clinical Nursing Procedures*, ed 7, Oxford, 2008, Wiley-Blackwell.

Finlay T: *Intravenous therapy*, Oxford, 2004, Blackwell Science.

General Medical Council: *Withholding and withdrawing life-prolonging treatments: Good practice in decision-making*, 2002 (paragraphs 22–24, pp 12–13). Available online http://www.gmc-uk.org.

Neno R: Nurses confront the challenge of delivering dignified care, *Nurs Older People* 20(5):9–10, 2008.

Nursing and Midwifery Council (NMC): *Record Keeping*, 2007. Available online http://www.nmc-uk.org.

Nursing and Midwifery Council (NMC): *Standards for Medicines Management*, 2008. Available online http://www.nmc-uk.org.

Porth CM, Matfin G: *Pathophysiology: concepts of altered health state*, ed 8, Philadelphia, 2008, Lippincott Williams and Wilkins.

Pratt RJ, Pellowe CM, Wilson JA, et al: epic2: National Evidence-Based Guidelines for Preventing Healthcare-Associated Infections in NHS Hospitals in England, *J Hosp Infect* 65(Suppl 1):S1–S64, 2007. Available online www.epic.tvu.ac.uk.

Rochon PA, Gill SS, Litner J, et al: A systematic review of the evidence for hypodermoclysis to treat dehydration in older people, *Journal of Gerontology: Medical Sciences* 52A(3):M169–M176, 1997.

Woodrow P: Assessing fluid balance in older people: fluid needs, *Nurs Older People* 14(9):31–32, 2002.

Weinstein S: *Plumer's Principles and practice of intravenous therapy*, ed 8, Philadelphia, 2005, Lippincott Williams and Wilkins.

USEFUL WEBSITES

Food Standards Agency: www.eatwell.gov.uk

National Institute for Health and Clinical Excellence: www.nice.org.uk

National Library of Medicine (US) MedlinePlus: www.nlm.nih.gov/medlineplus/fluidandelectrolytebalance.html

National Patient Safety Agency: www.npsa.nhs.uk

NHS National Library for Health: www.library.nhs.uk/

Scottish Intercollegiate Guidelines Network (SIGN): www.sign.ac.uk

Nutrition and health

Sue Green

Introduction

Nutrients and water are essential for existence. An adequate intake of nutrients and water is required to maintain physiological function, to allow for growth and maintenance of tissues, and to provide energy to meet the demands of daily living (see Ch. 20). Although a biological necessity, eating and drinking have significance beyond the merely physiological, forming an important part of social and psychological well-being. Meals are used as a time for people to come together, food or drink may be offered to make a guest feel welcome, and formal meals are a feature of many family, religious or national ceremonies.

The importance of the role of the nurse in ensuring nutritional needs are met is well recognised. The Nursing and Midwifery Council (NMC) identifies nutrition as a component of the Essential Skills Clusters for pre-registration nursing programmes (NMC 2007). The responsibilities of the nurse concerning nutritional care are extremely varied and range from preventing malnutrition to caring for the malnourished. Nurses play a more minor role in the preparation and serving of food to individuals in their care than they have done in previous years. Changes in food delivery and serving methods have acted to reduce the nursing input required at mealtimes. In many areas there is a necessary delegation of responsibility concerning mealtime care to health care assistants or other staff. However, it must be remembered that it is the qualified nurse who is responsible for ensuring food is provided, as appropriate, to the patient in their care.

This chapter will consider principles of nutritional science, public health nutrition and the nutritional care of individuals by nurses. The principles of nutritional science are only briefly considered in this chapter and the reader is advised to obtain a good understanding of the form and function of macronutrients and micronutrients (see Further reading, e.g. Geissler & Powers 2009).

Principles of nutritional science

To maintain health, an adequate supply of nutrients is required. The foods that make up the diet can vary considerably but the nutritive constituents of the diet fall into two main groups: the energy-yielding macronutrients (carbohydrates, protein and fat) and micronutrients (vitamins and minerals).

🖰 **See website for further content**

Table 21.1 outlines the vitamins required by the body, and gives details of rich food sources, at-risk groups and symptoms of deficiency and Table 21.2 provides similar information about some of the minerals.

Alcohol, usually in the form of ethanol, may also be considered a form of macronutrient in that it is energy-yielding.

Some components of foods, such as non-starch polysaccharides (NSP) (or fibre) and water, provide few if any nutrients but are important for physiological function. The diet may also contain other substances such as food colourings, food preservatives and caffeine which have little or no nutritional value but can enhance the quality of the diet.

Nutrients have a complex role in physiological function and most nutrients have a number of roles in the body. Nutrients are required to form the structural components of the body, for example, protein is the major constituent of muscles. Nutrients are also important in metabolic pathways and enzyme systems that enable the body to function appropriately. They can either form a part of the pathway or assist in the enzymatic reactions in that pathway (a co-factor). For example, vitamin C is required in the pathway that forms collagen. Nutrients also provide energy for metabolism. Metabolic demand needs to be met by an effective supply of nutrients.

These come from two sources: the food eaten and the breakdown of body tissues. There is a dynamic process between food eaten, body tissues and metabolism. Carbohydrate and fat are the body's predominant energy sources but protein may be used if these are not readily available.

If food intake is inadequate, fat and muscle tissues will be used to supply the energy needed for metabolic demand.

In the UK, estimated nutritional requirements (EARs) for different groups of people within the population have been established (Department of Health [DH] 1991) and are termed dietary reference values (DRVs). Nutritional requirements vary across the lifespan. Infants and children require sufficient nutrients to grow and develop. Requirements for some nutrients are increased pre-conception (folic acid), during pregnancy (folic acid in the first 12 weeks) and whilst breast feeding, and also change with ageing (e.g. vitamin D and calcium). It is important to recognise that dietary reference values are not recommendations for intake by individuals but are estimates for healthy populations only; within a clinical setting the advice of a dietitian must be sought.

Table 21.1 Vitamins: rich food sources, at-risk groups and signs and symptoms of deficiency

NUTRIENT	RICH FOOD SOURCES	GROUPS AT RISK OF DEFICIENCY OR EXCESSIVE INTAKE AFFECTING HEALTH	SIGNS AND SYMPTOMS OF DEFICIENCY
Vitamin A (retinol)	Liver, fish oils, dairy products, fortified margarine, some green, yellow and orange fruits and vegetables	*Deficiency associated with:* fat malabsorption *Excessive intake affecting health:* pregnant women should avoid supplements containing vitamin A (unless advised otherwise at antenatal clinic) and liver and liver products. Postmenopausal women and older men who are more at risk of osteoporosis should not eat liver or liver products more than once a week and not take supplements if liver is eaten once a week (Food Standards Agency [FSA] 2010)	Dryness of the conjunctiva and cornea, impaired adaptation to dim light (night blindness), skin changes, impaired immune function, growth retardation
Vitamin B$_1$ (thiamin)	Found in most foods, particularly unrefined cereal grains, fortified flour, some breakfast cereals, meat, dairy products and legumes	*Deficiency associated with:* alcohol dependency	Headaches, tiredness, anorexia, muscle wasting. Deficiency disease (beriberi) affects the cardiovascular and nervous systems Wernicke–Korsakoff syndrome can develop in alcohol dependency
Vitamin B$_2$ (riboflavin)	Found in many foods, particularly dairy products, eggs, fortified cereals, ice cream, liver	*Deficiency associated with:* intestinal malabsorption, biliary atresia, older people with poor dietary intake, regular use of fibre-based laxatives, women who exercise excessively, alcohol dependency	Lesions of the mucocutaneous surfaces of the mouth, seborrhoeic skin lesions, vascularisation of the cornea, anaemia, retarded growth in childhood
Vitamin B$_3$ (niacin: generic term for nicotinic acid and nicotinamide)	Red meat, wheat flour, maize, eggs, milk	*Deficiency associated with:* alcohol dependency, long-term use of isoniazid medication	Changes in skin, oral mucosa, GI tract and nervous system. Deficiency disease (pellagra) is characterised by skin lesions in areas exposed to sun and pressure, and by diarrhoea and dementia

Continued

Table 21.1 Vitamins: rich food sources, at-risk groups and signs and symptoms of deficiency – cont'd

NUTRIENT	RICH FOOD SOURCES	GROUPS AT RISK OF DEFICIENCY OR EXCESSIVE INTAKE AFFECTING HEALTH	SIGNS AND SYMPTOMS OF DEFICIENCY
Vitamin B_6 (pyridoxine)	Meat, fish, eggs, milk, wheatgerm, brewer's yeast, brown rice, soybeans, unrefined wheat grains, some nuts	*Deficiency associated with:* use of drugs which cause depletion (e.g. isoniazid), intestinal malabsorption, renal dialysis, alcohol dependency. *Excessive intake affecting health:* women may take large amounts (without medical advice) to relieve premenstrual syndrome symptoms. The Food Standards Agency (2003) advises against taking more than 10 mg/day to avoid the development of neuropathy. Supplements may reduce therapeutic effects of levodopa. Pyridoxine interacts with some drugs, e.g. phenytoin and phenobarbitone	Severe deficiency rare. Inflammation and skin changes around the mouth, weakness, irritability
Vitamin B_{12} (cobalamins)	Made by microorganisms and incorporated into the food chain by animals. Appears in meats or foods of animal origin	*Deficiency associated with:* lack of gastric intrinsic factor, strict vegetarians and vegans, malabsorption syndrome, older people in institutional environments	Neuropathy (subacute combined degeneration of the spinal cord), megaloblastic anaemia
Folate (folic acid)	Widely distributed in foods, particularly liver, yeast extract, leafy green vegetables, fortified grains and breakfast cereals	*Deficiency associated with:* malabsorption, alcohol dependency, some anticonvulsant drugs, older people on restricted diets. Women in the first trimester of pregnancy or those thinking of becoming pregnant should take a daily supplement of 400 µg (FSA 2003). A higher dose may be recommended by the doctor or midwife if there is a history of neural tube defect	Effect on cell division leading to megaloblastic and macrocytic anaemia, elevation of plasma homocysteine, association with neural tube defect in pregnancy
Pantothenic acid	Widely distributed in foods, particularly animal products, whole grains, potatoes and tomato products	–	Rare and only demonstrated in those eating a very restricted diet
Biotin	Widely distributed in foods, particularly liver, egg yolk, soy flour, cereals and yeast	–	Rare and only demonstrated in those receiving parenteral nutrition or eating a very restricted diet
Vitamin C (ascorbic acid)	Fresh vegetables and fruit, particularly spinach, tomatoes, broccoli, strawberries and citrus fruits	*Deficiency associated with:* smokers, an absence of fruit and vegetables in the diet	Hair follicle eruption, petechial haemorrhage on limbs, bleeding gums, impairment of connective tissue formation in wound repair, joint pains, fatigue. Symptoms of deficiency disease (scurvy) result from the failure of the body to synthesise collagen
Vitamin D (calciferols)	Major source is exposure to sunlight. Found in fatty fish, liver, milk, eggs, fortified food such as margarine, breakfast cereals	*Deficiency associated with:* inadequate exposure to sunlight (e.g. nursing home residents, dark-skinned people who habitually cover their skin), malabsorption. Pregnant or breastfeeding women should take 10 µg of vitamin D a day (FSA 2010). *Excessive intake affecting health:* people with sarcoidosis should not take vitamin D supplements	Rickets in children, osteomalacia, muscle weakness, bone tenderness
Vitamin E (tocopherols)	Synthesised by plants. Plant oils, nuts and seeds are a rich source	–	Deficiency only demonstrated in preterm infants and those unable to absorb or utilise vitamin E. Deficiency results in cell membrane dysfunction
Vitamin K (phylloquinone and menaquinones)	Green leafy vegetables and vegetable oils. Also produced by bacteria in intestine	*Deficiency associated with:* malabsorption or impaired gut synthesis. Vitamin K supplement given prophylactically to prevent haemorrhagic disease of the newborn in many countries due to vitamin K deficiency in the newborn	Deficiency very rare in adults and results in bleeding disorder

Table 21.2 Minerals: rich food sources, at-risk groups and signs and symptoms of deficiency

NUTRIENT	RICH FOOD SOURCES	GROUPS AT RISK OF DEFICIENCY OR EXCESSIVE INTAKE AFFECTING HEALTH	SIGNS AND SYMPTOMS OF DEFICIENCY
Calcium	Milk, cheese, small fish, e.g. sardines, some green leafy vegetables, soybean products, fortified wheat flour and breakfast cereals, some nuts	*Deficiency associated with:* fat malabsorption, consumption of large amounts of phytates *Excessive intake affecting health:* excessive intake of calcium (e.g. antacids) and those with renal failure may be susceptible	Widespread effects of deficiency Stunted growth and bone malformation in children, skeletal and tooth changes in adults
Magnesium	Found widely in foods, particularly green leafy vegetables, grains, nuts	*Deficiency associated with:* malabsorption, excessive renal loss (e.g. diuretic use) *Excessive intake affecting health:* those with renal failure susceptible	Widespread effects including cardiovascular and skeletal system disorders. Severe deficiency of magnesium may be associated with hypocalcaemia and hypokalaemia
Phosphorus	Found widely in foods, particularly fish, poultry, red meat, dairy products, cereal grains	*Deficiency associated with:* some forms of rickets, excessive intakes of aluminium-containing antacids, vitamin D deficiency, alcohol dependency, diabetic ketoacidosis *Excessive intake affecting health:* those with renal failure susceptible	Widespread effects including osteomalacia, myopathy, growth failure
Sodium chloride	Salt and salty foods	*Excessive intake affecting health:* infants and young children should not have salt added to food as renal excretion is limited. In adults intake of no more than 6 g/day recommended to promote health	Rare except following excessive loss of body fluids, e.g. sweating. Leads to low blood pressure, dehydration and muscle cramps
Potassium	Milk, fruit, e.g. bananas, and vegetables, shellfish, red meat, white meat, liver	*Deficiency associated with:* use of some diuretics, very low energy diets *Excessive intake affecting health:* those taking potassium-sparing diuretics and some other types of drug. Those with renal disease, adrenal insufficiency and insulin deficiency susceptible	Rare except following excessive loss of body fluids, e.g. diarrhoea. Muscle weakness, arrhythmias, irritability, cardiac arrest
Iron (haem and non-haem form)	Liver, meat, beans, nuts, dried fruit, fish, enriched cereals, soybean flour, dark leafy green vegetables. Dietary factors influencing uptake include: form of iron ingested, presence of vitamin C, phytates, calcium, soy protein	*Deficiency associated with:* infants over 6 months, toddlers, adolescents, pregnant women, menstruating women, older people, people with parasitic infestations, high intake of inhibitors of absorption, e.g. tea *Excessive intake affecting health:* frequent blood transfusion recipients susceptible	Normocytic anaemia, microcytic anaemia, reduced work capacity, reduced intellectual performance, impaired resistance to infection, impaired thermoregulation
Zinc	Meat, unrefined cereals, fortified cereal products	–	Growth retardation, defects of rapidly dividing tissues, e.g. skin, intestinal mucosa, immune system
Selenium	Fish, offal, brazil nuts, cereals	Dietary deficiency endemic in some areas of the world, e.g. China	Deficiency associated with Keshan disease, a form of cardiomyopathy; inflammatory joint disease
Iodine	Marine fish, shellfish, sea salt, supplemented salt	Dietary deficiency endemic in some areas of the world (landlocked mountainous regions)	Goitre, hypothyroidism including the congenital form where fetal and infant growth and development is affected
Fluoride	Generally obtained from drinking water and dental products. Rich food sources include tea and fish	–	Fluoride is implicated in the development of tooth health

Molybdenum, manganese, copper, chromium are also required but these are widespread in foods and deficiency is only demonstrated in very restricted diets or certain medical conditions.

Nutritional requirements of individuals will vary depending on a person's basal metabolic rate (BMR), activity level and response to certain factors such as cold exposure and ingestion of food. BMR is the metabolic rate of the body at rest and is influenced by several factors, including genetic makeup, gender and body mass. Illness can increase the requirement for nutrients, but this may be counteracted by a reduction in physical activity level during the period of illness. If an individual has an inadequate intake of energy for a period of time, the body can adapt by reducing BMR.

If intake of a particular nutrient or range of nutrients affects physiological function adversely, then the person can be said to be malnourished. Malnutrition can refer to both overnutrition, i.e. intake of energy and nutrients in excess of requirements, and undernutrition, i.e. intake of insufficient energy and nutrients to meet requirements. Malnutrition may jeopardise health status in general and can affect morbidity and mortality.

It is important to understand the different nutrients required by the body, what the nutrients are used for and the consequence of a poor nutritional intake and use this understanding when working with people to enable them to achieve appropriate nutritional care.

Public health nutrition

Public health nutrition refers to the promotion of good nutritional health and the prevention of diet-related illness in groups of people, rather than the nutritional care of individuals. Public health nutrition can be an important aspect of the nurse's role, for example school nurses may work to improve the nutritional health of a group of school children. It is important to consider the wider aspects of nutritional care, for example, why people choose to eat certain foods.

The diet

The diet consists of the foods people eat from day to day. Although foods containing all known nutrients can be formulated, no single naturally occurring food can meet all the daily nutritional demands. Different types of food contain different proportions of macro- and micronutrients and, therefore, a range of foods is necessary to provide the daily requirement of individual nutrients. The diet should supply all the necessary nutrients in sufficient quantity, whilst avoiding excessive intake. There is considerable debate about the safety of some vitamin and mineral supplements that are not medically prescribed (Food Standards Agency [FSA] 2003). For up-to-date recommendations on the intake of particular nutrients see Useful websites (e.g. FSA www.food.gov.uk and www.eatwell.gov.uk). Government guidelines on dietary intake recommend an intake thought to promote maximum health for the population. For the UK these recommendations include a fat intake of less than 35% of dietary energy intake, of which no more than one third should be in the form of saturated fats, and a carbohydrate intake of approximately 50% of dietary energy intake (DH 1994). A salt intake of less than 6 g/day for adults is also recommended (FSA 2009a).

It is important to consider factors which influence food intake of populations and individuals. At a global level, government policies influence what a population eats because food supply and legislation is essentially determined by government policy. For example, the fortification of foods or water with particular nutrients is a feature in many countries and is usually managed at a central government level, e.g. fortification of flour with calcium. The policy for food labelling which can influence individuals' choice is determined centrally. Within a country, there are generally regional and socioeconomic differences in dietary intake which can influence what individuals eat, for example,

women with low incomes in the UK are more likely to eat low amounts of fruits and vegetables, whole grains and fish, and higher amounts of sugar and sweetened drinks compared with more affluent women (Anderson 2007).

At an individual level, people choose to eat a particular type of diet for a variety of reasons which include sociological, psychological, economic and behavioural factors. Sociological factors include age, culture, religion, income, food availability and cooking facilities. Psychological factors encompass a variety of factors ranging from aversions to particular foods, to overeating particular food types. Economic factors influence both the quality and quantity of dietary intake. If a type of food, such as fruit, is not available to buy or if there is insufficient money to buy a range of foods in appropriate amounts, dietary intake will be reduced in quality and quantity. Behavioural elements of food choice can also influence dietary intake. For example, toddlers can be very particular about the type of food that they will eat.

When food is available, the amount eaten is determined by appetite. Appetite is controlled by many factors, including the presence of nutrients in the gastrointestinal (GI) tract, levels of GI hormones, levels of nutrients in the blood and the response of the central nervous system to hunger signals from the rest of the body. Emotional factors may also influence what is eaten, for example, some people eat particular foods to 'cheer themselves up' or a celebratory meal may be eaten. The environment also affects appetite, for example, the smell of freshly baked bread when passing a bakery may instigate feelings of hunger. Conversely, smelling a very unpleasant odour when eating tends to diminish appetite. People tend to eat more when eating with other people in a social setting, although this is not always the case.

As outlined above there are many factors to consider when developing strategies to improve the diet of a group of people. In addition to the nutritional value to foods, the quality of foods is also an important factor and issues of food safety need to be considered.

Food safety

Food safety is a topic encompassing a wide range of factors which influence the quality of the foods that we eat. These include the use of aluminium foil and plastic to wrap food, pesticide residues in foods, natural toxins in foods and food-borne illness. Food-borne illnesses are a particular topic of nursing concern due to their impact on the health of individuals. Food-borne illnesses can be caused by improperly prepared or stored food.

Older people and children are particularly susceptible as they are less able to withstand the consequences of food-borne illness, such as prolonged nausea and vomiting. The Food Standards Agency (2009b) outlines that five food-borne bacteria account for the majority of cases of food-borne illness. These are salmonella, campylobacter, E. coli O157, Listeria monocytogenes and Clostridium perfringens. Viruses may cause food-borne disease but they are more likely to be spread from person to person.

Nurses must ensure that Food Hygiene Regulations are adhered to in areas where the RN is responsible for care delivered at both a group and individual level by following guidelines on storing and serving food and drink (Box 21.1).

Box 21.1 Reflection

Food Hygiene Regulations

You are on an acute hospital ward placement when a patient's relative asks you to store some takeaway meals (intended for several patients) in the ward fridge.

Activities

- Reflect on what your response to this request should be.
- Find out about the food hygiene regulations that apply to the ward kitchen and discuss the scenario with your mentor or lecturer.

Resource

Food Standards Agency – www.food.gov.uk/safereating/

Drug–nutrient interactions

Some medications may influence food intake, absorption and metabolism. In addition, some nutrients may influence medication absorption and metabolism. The interaction may potentiate or inhibit the activity of the medication or result in side-effects. The type of interaction will vary depending on the medication and the nutrient. This is an important issue for the nurse to consider when involved in the administration of medications and providing advice to patients, clients or carers about medication use. The nurse should be aware of the potential of commonly prescribed medications to interact with food. The hospital or community pharmacist can provide advice on this issue.

▷ Nursing management and health promotion: nutritional care

Nutritional care by nurses in the context of this chapter refers to the nutritional care given to individuals. It involves screening, assessment, planning, intervention and evaluation (Figure 21.1).

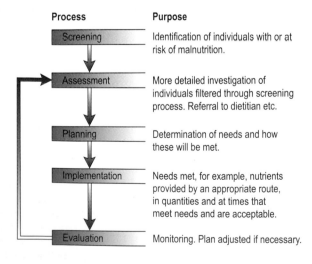

Figure 21.1 Process of nutritional care of individuals by nurses. (Adapted from McLaren & Green 1998 by permission of *Nursing Times*.)

Nutritional screening and assessment

A number of national publications (Nursing and Midwifery Practice Development Unit 2002, DH 2010, National Institute for Health and Clinical Excellence [NICE] 2006a) have highlighted the need for nutritional screening and assessment, and local guidelines for nursing practice have been developed from these. Nutritional screening aims to identify those with, or at risk of, malnutrition and can highlight potential causes. If an individual is considered to be at risk of or to have malnutrition, then a more detailed assessment must be undertaken. A variety of health care professionals may undertake this assessment depending on the type of problem identified at screening. The majority of patients will be referred to the dietitian if malnutrition is suspected. However, referral to another health care professional may also be appropriate; for example, referral to the speech and language therapist (SLT) if a swallowing deficit (dysphagia) is identified.

NICE (2006a) outlines that hospital inpatients, outpatients, people in care homes and people attending GP surgeries should be screened for malnutrition (guidelines for those >18 years). They should be screened on admission and subsequently assessed weekly for inpatients or more frequently if there is clinical concern (NICE 2006a).

 See website Critical thinking question 21.1

Specific guidelines concerning screening and assessing for eating disorders (NICE 2004) and obesity (NICE 2006b) are also available.

Screening and assessment allow identification of needs, planning of interventions and setting of goals (McLaren & Green 1998). Following this, interventions can be implemented. As always, interventions should be recorded and regularly evaluated and modified as required. Screening and assessment can also establish a baseline from which to monitor changes in status. There are five principal methods of screening or assessing for nutritional status:

- dietary history and intake
- clinical examination
- functional tests
- anthropometric measures
- biochemical tests.

Dietary history and intake

Elementary assessment by nurses of dietary history and intake is essential to determine the risk of malnutrition as well as to examine other factors, such as dietary habits, food preferences and economic factors affecting food intake. Changes in appetite, reduced food intake and absorption, the use of supplements and other issues, e.g. dietary adherence, can also be considered. The type of diet a person consumes is influenced by many factors, particularly in a home environment. In care environments, food charts can be used to record food intake over a period of time to assess whether dietary needs are being met. Asking a person to recall what they have eaten over the previous day or to describe what they generally eat, are also useful ways of assessing dietary intake. These methods can also be used to identify food that may have caused a reaction.

Assessment of food intake over a longer period of time, e.g. 7 days, by the use of a food diary can be useful in some circumstances, for example when working to promote dietary change in a person with obesity. Assessment of habitual intake will increase a person's awareness of their dietary intake and can highlight aspects that can be modified to help achieve an intake that follows the 'healthy eating guidelines'. The nurse is able to carry out an elementary assessment of food intake but more comprehensive dietary analyses should be undertaken by a dietitian as assessment of any individual's specific intake is a complex process.

Clinical examination

A clinical examination can identify medical conditions and treatment that may influence intake, digestion and absorption of nutrients. Drug and alcohol use can adversely affect nutritional status and should be considered in assessment. Changes in appetite, taste or smell, dental problems or ill-fitting dentures should be investigated. The person's usual activity level should also be considered, as well as general appearance and fit of clothes, condition of the hair, skin, eyes and mouth, and neurological and musculoskeletal systems. It is also important to assess a person's functional ability to eat; for example, are there physical or mental factors that might impair the process of eating? In addition, assessment of whether a person is able to read the language in which any dietary advice is written is essential. Issues such as literacy and visual impairment need to be considered if written dietary advice is to be given.

Functional tests

Functional tests of nutritional status are usually performed by the doctor or dietitian and include tests such as handgrip strength (using a dynamometer) and respiratory muscle strength.

Anthropometric tests

Simple anthropometric measures can be used by nurses to screen and assess nutritional status. Anthropometry refers to the measurement of the human body. It is important to weigh individuals on admission to care and periodically thereafter to identify any subsequent losses or gains. To ensure accuracy, the person should, if possible, be weighed on the same scales at the same time each day, preferably in the same clothes, and after emptying their bladder and bowel. Single measurements of weight are of limited value, but serial measurements permit trends in weight loss or gain to be identified.

Percentage weight change can be calculated using the equation:

$$\% \text{ weight loss/gain} = \frac{\text{usual weight} - \text{current weight (kg)} \times 100}{\text{usual weight (kg)}}$$

A loss of 10% in the previous 3 months is suggestive of malnutrition. However, caution is required when interpreting weight changes as factors such as dehydration, oedema or tumour growth can complicate the picture.

Weight considered in relation to height gives a more accurate assessment of the degree to which a person is under- or overweight than weight alone. Body mass index (BMI) is commonly used to assess weight in relation to height. This is simply the body weight in kilograms (kg) divided by the height in metres squared (m^2). For example, someone with a body weight of 57 kg and a height of 1.62 m has a BMI of $57/1.62^2 = 21.7 \text{ kg/m}^2$. Height can be difficult to determine, due to factors such as spine curvature and inability to stand. An estimation of height can be made, for example by using ulna length (Elia 2003).

The International Obesity Task Force (2003) has defined the following BMI categories:

- <18.5 underweight
- 18.5–24.9 normal range
- 25.0–29.9 overweight
- 30.0–34.9 obese (class 1)
- 35.0–39.9 obese (class 2)
- >40.0 obese (class 3).

When using BMI with older people the resulting plan and intervention need to be carefully considered as the usefulness of BMI as a predictor of risk of morbidity and mortality in the very old has been questioned (British Dietetic Association 2003).

Waist circumference can be used to assess the amount of fat located in the abdominal region. This measure is increasingly being used to screen for cardiovascular risk in primary care. Men with a waist circumference >102 cm and women with a waist circumference >88 cm should be advised that weight reduction would be beneficial (Lean 2000).

Anthropometric measures that assess fat levels or muscle mass (lean tissue) of the body can be used by dietitians or doctors in clinical environments. Nurses may use these measures in specialist units following training in their use. These measures include skin fold measures to estimate body fat, and mid-arm muscle circumference to estimate skeletal muscle mass. Electrical bioimpedance is a method of assessing the fat mass of the body which is being used increasingly in some environments such as health clubs.

Regular checks of accuracy and, if necessary, recalibration are essential for all equipment used to measure individuals, including weighing scales.

Biochemical tests

Biochemical measures to assess nutritional status include a number of parameters, obtained from investigation of plasma, urine and body tissues.

Measurement of proteins present in the blood, such as albumin and retinol-binding protein, can be useful in some clinical situations but the interpretation of what the level means needs to be considered carefully. Serum protein levels are usually more an indicator of clinical state than nutritional status in the acutely ill, as protein levels in the blood change in response to the trauma the body is experiencing. In addition, treatments such as administration of blood products will change serum protein levels. The clinical biochemist, doctor and dietitian are key members of the multidisciplinary team when considering the relationship between a patient's nutritional status and serum protein level. Biochemical investigations can also assess circulating lipoprotein levels to give an indication of cardiovascular risk. In addition, specific vitamin, e.g. vitamin C, or mineral, e.g. iron and selenium, levels can be evaluated.

Nitrogen balance studies provide an index of protein status. Nitrogen balance is determined by estimating protein intake and subtracting urinary nitrogen excretion with an allowance for nitrogen loss via hair, skin and faeces. Additionally, losses from wound drainage or GI fistulae must be considered. A positive nitrogen balance indicates that the patient is in an anabolic state, whereas a negative balance indicates catabolism.

Nutritional screening tools

Nutritional screening tools use risk factors that may lead to or be associated with malnourishment and are similar in format to a pressure ulcer risk assessment tool (see Ch. 23). They are typically in questionnaire format and are useful as an aide-mémoire for screening and as a record of information. An appropriate plan of action is identified by some. Of the many nutritional screening tools published, only a few have undergone rigorous testing of reliability and validity (Green & Watson 2005). The British Association of Parenteral and Enteral Nutrition (BAPEN) has introduced a valid and reliable screening tool for use by nurses in all areas of clinical practice (Elia 2003): the Malnutrition Universal Screening Tool (MUST). NICE (2006a) has endorsed the use of this tool. Accurate nutritional assessment relies on utilisation of data from a number of sources. Data from only one source can be open to misinterpretation due to the many factors, such as disease processes, that can influence individual parameters. A combination of two or more measures obtained from dietary history and intake, clinical examination, functional tests, anthropometric measures and biochemical tests is required to gain an accurate picture of an individual's nutritional status. The methods described above may be used by nurses in the context of a busy clinical environment. Other methods can be employed by dietitians and other health care professionals in the clinical environment and research settings (Geissler & Powers 2005).

Refeeding syndrome

If the patient is very malnourished problems can arise from sudden feeding, known as refeeding syndrome. This is caused by a rapid shift of electrolytes, glucose and water from extracellular to intracellular compartments, and can cause deficits in the extracellular fluid. As the syndrome can be life threatening it is crucial that anyone at risk of refeeding syndrome is identified before nutritional intervention is given so that appropriate intervention can be planned. A person who has had very little food intake for more than 5 days is at some risk. NICE (2006a) recommends that people who have eaten little or nothing for more than 5 days should have nutritional support at no more than 50% of requirements for the first 2 days. Following this the nutritional support can be increased if clinical and biochemical monitoring reveals no refeeding syndrome. See Further reading, e.g. Mehanna et al 2008.

NUTRITIONAL INTERVENTION

Following screening and assessment of an individual, the nurse will plan appropriate interventions. The following sections outline interventions that may be planned by the nurse, usually in association with other health care

professionals such as the dietitian. These include advising on a 'healthy diet', promoting oral intake and enteral and parenteral nutrition. Obesity and undernutrition are also discussed. In many situations referral to the dietitian is a necessary part of the nutritional plan of care. However, in some circumstances, for example, giving advice concerning healthy eating to an individual who is overweight, this can be given by the nurse.

Local guidelines should outline when referral to a dietitian is appropriate. Individuals who require therapeutic diets, e.g. those with diabetes mellitus, renal disease, coeliac disease (gluten sensitive enteropathy), hyperlipidaemia and food allergy, should always be referred to the dietitian. Nurses may then follow through a plan of care prescribed by the dietitian.

A healthy diet

The diet which is currently recommended to promote the health of the general population in the UK is shown in Figure 21.2.

The pictorial representation is termed the 'plate model'. It illustrates five food groups, and the proportion in which each group should be consumed can be used as a health promotion tool. Such a diet is sometimes termed a 'balanced diet', i.e. it provides the appropriate amounts of all nutrients in the correct proportions to meet the requirements of the body. This diet consists of 33% vegetables and fruit, 33% complex carbohydrate, 12% protein-containing foods, 15% dairy products or similar foods and 8% fat- and sugar-containing foods. Current recommendations suggest that individuals eat at least five or more portions of a variety of fruit and vegetables a day (FSA 2009c). The type of diet outlined above is not suitable for those under 5 years of age or those following a diet prescribed by the dietitian.

The Food Standards Agency provides *Eight Tips for Eating Well*:

- 'Base your meals on starchy foods.
- Eat lots of fruit and veg.

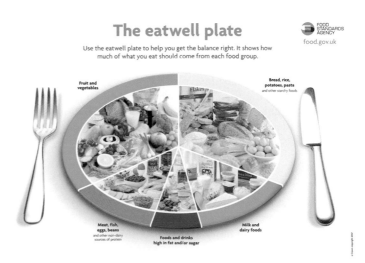

The eatwell plate

Use the eatwell plate to help you get the balance right. It shows how much of what you eat should come from each food group.

Fruit and vegetables

Bread, rice, potatoes, pasta and other starchy foods

Meat, fish, eggs, beans and other non-dairy sources of protein

Foods and drinks high in fat and/or sugar

Milk and dairy foods

Figure 21.2 The plate model based on the Government's Eight Guidelines for a Healthy Diet. © Crown copyright material is reproduced with the permission of the Controller of HMSO and Queen's Printer for Scotland.

- Eat more fish.
- Cut down on saturated fat and sugar.
- Try to eat less salt – no more than 6 g a day.
- Get active and try to be a healthy weight.
- Drink plenty of water.
- Don't skip breakfast.'

(Reproduced from the Food Standards Agency 2009d with permission.)

Obesity

Obesity is the condition of excessive accumulation of fat in the body, leading to an increase in weight beyond that considered desirable. Obesity quite simply results when intake of energy is greater than energy usage. However, the reasons why this happens are complex. Although many people have the genetic propensity to develop obesity, the propensity does not mean the person will become obese; customary diet and lifestyle play a major role (Ulijaszek & Lofink 2006). Rarely, obesity may result from a medical condition, such as hypothyroidism (see Ch. 5, Part 1).

Obesity is considered a major world health problem as the number of people who are obese is rapidly escalating (World Health Organization 2006). Obesity is associated with many common disorders such as coronary heart disease, hypertension, and type 2 diabetes mellitus (NICE 2006b). Individuals with obesity may also be subject to psychological distress and social penalties.

Treatment of obesity

There are a number of approaches to the treatment of obesity. Currently, few specialist obesity clinics exist and most people with obesity who seek help from health care professionals are assessed and managed by the primary care team. NICE (2006b) recommends multicomponent interventions for individuals which involve behaviour change to increase physical activity level, improvement of eating behaviour and quality of diet, and reduction in energy intake. Treatment programmes within the primary care setting should be individualised and involve assessment and goal setting. The Department of Health in London has produced a comprehensive package of material for health professionals as well as information for patients and clients concerning the management of obesity (DH 2009a). The package includes obesity care pathways for adults and children. Assessment of the patient or client by the nurse should follow the guidelines outlined by NICE (2006b) and include assessment of readiness to change.

Dietary change

NICE (2006b) outlines that a diet containing 600 kilocalories less than the person needs to stay the same weight or a diet that reduces energy intake by lowering the fat content should be recommended. Low energy (1000–1600 kcal) and very low energy diets (less than 1000 kcal/day) may be used in the short term. In the longer term a diet consistent with other healthy eating advice is recommended.

There are many types of diet published, advocating various types and combinations of foods.

NICE (2006b) does not recommend the use of very restrictive and nutritionally incomplete diets because they may be harmful and ineffective in the long term.

Physical activity

Increased physical activity can facilitate weight management (Mulvihill & Quigley 2003). Some individuals may be unable to increase their physical activity levels due to their medical condition, and the advice of the doctor should be sought. Adults should undertake 30 minutes (or more) of moderate-intensity physical activity on five or more days of the week. This can be as one session or several sessions of ten minutes or more (NICE 2006b). NICE (2006b) suggests that people who have been obese and lost weight may need to do 60–90 minutes of moderate activity a day. Activity within the daily routine, e.g. walking rather than driving, should be encouraged. Resistance training can also help, as it will conserve muscle mass and maintain resting metabolic rate as weight is lost (Hunter et al 2008). Exercise on prescription may also be a useful way of promoting activity level (DH 2001).

Behaviour

Changing behaviour underlies obesity management. Individuals with obesity need to change or modify their behaviour in order to change their diet and activity level. NICE (2006b) outlines that behavioural interventions for adults can include the following strategies: self monitoring of behaviour and progress, stimulus control, goal setting, slowing rate of eating, ensuring social support, problem solving, assertiveness, cognitive restructuring (modifying thoughts), reinforcement of changes and strategies for dealing with weight regain. Some people may find that they benefit from the support they gain from attending a reputable 'slimming club'.

Medication

Drug therapy may be indicated when a person who is obese has co-morbidities and has been unable to lose weight by dietary change (NICE 2006b). In the UK there is currently one type of medication that may be prescribed for the treatment of obesity. It inhibits the actions of lipases in the GI tract, thus limiting the absorption of fat, which is consequently excreted in the stools. It has been shown to be useful in promoting weight loss but there are side-effects associated with their use.

Surgery (see Ch. 26)

Obesity can be treated by surgical means if other methods of obesity management have failed (NICE 2006b), although currently in the UK only a select number of NHS hospitals offer this kind of surgery. The decision to undertake surgical treatment is not taken lightly as there are risks involved and eating patterns following surgery are vastly different from those before.

Surgical treatments involve reducing the size of the stomach ('stomach stapling' or gastric banding) or bypassing sections of the upper GI tract. Reducing the size of the stomach restricts the amount of food a person can eat, and bypassing sections of the GI tract results in fewer kilocalories being absorbed by the body. It is important that anyone undergoing surgical treatment for obesity is referred to the dietitian. Surgical treatment for obesity will not automatically result in the consumption of a healthier diet, and may actually lead to a poorer quality of diet being consumed. The nurse must be aware that, following surgery, whilst the patient may be pleased with a very fast weight loss, a poor diet may be the cause, which can lead to a risk of malnutrition. As with any method of weight loss, weight loss maintenance is important and diet and lifestyle changes are essential factors in this.

Prevention of obesity

Many European countries are developing strategies to promote activity level and healthy eating with the aim of both reducing and preventing obesity. For example, the Scottish Government published a national plan (The Scottish Government 2008), and in England the Department of Health published *Healthy Weight, Healthy Lives: A cross-government research and surveillance plan for England* (DH 2008) and launched the *Change4Life – Eat Well, Move More, Live Longer* campaign (DH 2009b). Prevention of obesity is an important issue as obesity levels, particularly in children, continue to escalate. Where appropriate, health promotion and education strategies by nurses should promote adherence to healthy eating guidelines and increased activity levels, not only for individuals but also for their families. Nurses who work with communities, such as school nurses and occupational health nurses, usually work to prevent obesity in their communities as well as working with individuals who are obese.

Undernutrition

Protein-energy malnutrition (PEM) affects large numbers of the world's population and contributes significantly to mortality and morbidity. Certain groups are at particular risk, including older adults, people with a low income, institutionalised people, people with acute or chronic conditions affecting nutrient intake, etc. (Box 21.2).

Undernutrition can occur as a result of reduced food intake or increased nutritional requirements as well as an impaired ability to digest, absorb or metabolise nutrients. Illness and long-term conditions can reduce food intake by causing anorexia (loss of appetite), pain, nausea, dysphagia,

Box 21.2 Reflection

Malnutrition in the UK

'Malnutrition is an under-recognised and under-treated problem facing the UK... At any given point in time, more than three million people in the UK are either malnourished or at risk of malnutrition. The vast majority of these (c. 93%) are living in the community...'

(Elia & Russell 2009)

Activities

- Reflect on the enormity of the statements from the report by Elia & Russell 2009.
- Discuss with your mentor or lecturer how this can happen in a developed country.

dyspnoea, fatigue and a reduction in the ability to obtain and eat food. Illness can increase the need for nutrients, for example pyrexia results in an increased metabolic rate and, therefore, increased energy demands. Infection and the process of tissue repair can increase the need for specific nutrients. However, some conditions can also result in a reduction in the need for some nutrients as physical activity level may be reduced. Some illnesses and conditions can cause changes in the function of the gastrointestinal tract resulting in altered digestive and absorptive processes and can also affect the body's ability to metabolise nutrients.

There is evidence of significant undernutrition in hospitalised patients (NICE 2006a) and concerns have been raised about the incidence of malnutrition in the community. Hospitalisation may predispose to undernutrition for a variety of reasons. Hospital admission can cause anxiety which reduces food intake and the condition the patient has been admitted for may make them unable to eat well. Hospitals may serve food and fluids that are unfamiliar to individuals and may not serve it at a time at which they are used to eating and drinking. The environment in hospitals may not be conducive to eating and investigations and treatments may interrupt normal eating patterns.

Enhancing nutritional intake

Nurses are ideally placed to help individuals, whether at home or in hospital, to meet their nutritional needs. In addition to meeting nutritional needs it is important for the nurse to acknowledge that food has a number of other roles, such as expressing beliefs and culture. Following screening and assessment the nurse should identify with the patient ways in which nutritional intake can be improved considering all the factors which affect their intake and produce a plan of care. The plan of care should include appropriate interventions and be evaluated at regular intervals. The next section discusses factors which can be assessed when planning care.

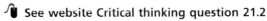 **See website Critical thinking question 21.2**

Factors influencing food acquisition

For an individual to eat an adequate oral diet at home, a number of activities are required and need to be considered:

- Is the person able to go shopping and to choose and purchase appropriate foods?
- Is the person's nutritional knowledge adequate for informed choice and have they the financial resources to purchase the required foods?
- Once purchased, can food be transported home or is a delivery service available?
- Are there adequate facilities for storing food at home e.g. refrigerator/freezer?
- Are adequate cooking facilities available and can the person use them safely?

If there are issues of concern in any of these areas, ways to address them need to be outlined in the plan of care. Ordering shopping using the internet, mobile shops and delivery services may help some individuals to cope with shopping for food. However, these services may not be available or appropriate for some and assistance will be required from family, informal carers, volunteer services or social services as appropriate. The home environment may need to be modified to enable independent food storage and preparation. If this is considered necessary the person should be referred to the occupational therapist (OT) for assessment.

Factors influencing eating

To eat and drink normally requires the ability to transfer food and fluids to the mouth, the ability to retain food in the mouth, to chew and to swallow. Sensory function is also important as appetite is improved if a person can see, smell and taste their food. As people age, the ability to detect sweetness and saltiness generally diminishes and more highly seasoned and sweeter food may be preferred by older adults. Some illnesses, conditions and treatment cause taste and smell changes resulting in a change in the types of foods liked by an individual or a reduction in appetite. Conditions such as upper respiratory tract infections can cause a temporary reduction in the sense of smell, which makes food less appealing. Reduced oral sensitivity or confusion may cause the temperature of food to be misjudged, resulting in a greater risk of burn injury from hot food and drinks.

Reduced mobility may cause problems in attaining a comfortable eating position. Some patients or clients are required to maintain a supine or prone position for eating. Individuals may have difficulty with arm or hand movement or hand–eye coordination making transferring food to their mouth difficult. The person may need to be offered specific food textures to enable eating, for example, soup or food that can be transferred to the mouth with fingers. Referral to the OT is required when it is considered that eating is restricted by reduced dexterity. The OT will be able to identify which eating aids, such as modified cutlery and plate guards, are appropriate for the person.

The state of the teeth and mouth is important. Teeth are needed for effective chewing; edentulous (without natural teeth) people may require food of a softer texture or food cut into smaller pieces. Such people are likely to eat fewer vegetables, less dietary fibre and be deficient in vitamins such as D (Finch et al 1998). Poor oral health can alter the taste and consequently enjoyment of a meal. If oral tissues are dry, inflamed or painful, a person may be reluctant to eat (see Ch. 15).

Visual appearance and texture of food

Meals that look unappetising or are poorly presented can reduce appetite and enjoyment of a meal. People with visual impairment may appreciate knowing where different foods are positioned on the plate by the server advising them when the food is served. People who have experienced a stroke or other brain injury may only perceive a portion of the plate and, therefore, need to be reminded about the remainder (see Chs 9, 27).

The texture of food is important. The person who has no natural teeth may choose not to eat particular food types. Some medical conditions cause difficulty chewing, closing the mouth or swallowing resulting in food dribbling from the mouth. This can cause the person to feel very self conscious and result in them avoiding eating.

Food texture may need to be modified for individuals who have dysphagia. Dysphagia can be caused by a number of conditions such as neurological injury (as in stroke), mechanical or motor obstruction of the oesophagus, oesophagitis and oesophageal cancer. The degree of dysphagia must be assessed by the SLT and local guidelines for the management of patients with swallowing difficulties followed. It may be that no oral intake or only soft foods or thickened fluids can be tolerated. If oral intake is problematic or impossible, then enteral feeding must be considered.

Organising effective mealtimes

Mealtimes are often the focal point of the day for patients or clients. Ensuring a supply of nutritious food, at the right temperature and in an attractive and hygienic manner, is the responsibility of both nursing and catering services. Food preparation is not usually a nursing task, but the nurse is responsible for ensuring that food is ordered and should act as advocate between the patient/client and the centralised catering services. Mealtime activity should be planned by the RN and delegated appropriately so the responsibilities of each member of the team are clear. Although RNs remain responsible for ensuring adequate nutrition, their role in the preparation and distribution of food has reduced in recent years. Meals are often delivered to patients or clients pre-plated in heated trolleys at fixed times. Some patients or clients may need or prefer more frequent and smaller amounts of food so snacks should be offered between meals. When a patient or client does miss a meal it is the nurse's responsibility to ensure an alternative is offered. In NHS hospitals (DH 2007) the *24 Catering Initiative* states that food is available at any time of day. In the past, reports have suggested that patients in hospitals have often missed a meal or had their meal interrupted due to ward and treatment activities. Recently the concept of *protected mealtimes* has been introduced to prevent this (DH 2007). Mealtimes should not coincide with other structured ward activities such as medication administration, shift handovers or staff breaks.

In continuing care settings some flexibility over meal timing is preferable and it is important that an effort is made to enable people to follow their normal pattern of eating. In a continuing care environment there is often a dining room or large table for people to sit at to eat meals. Eating with others in a dining room or at a table can encourage food intake, although it must be recognised that some individuals may prefer to eat alone. If a dining room is available for residents or patients it should be pleasantly decorated and provided with small tables to allow people to eat in their natural groupings. If a person has visitors during meals, this can be helpful, as relatives can be involved in assisting with eating or enjoy a meal with them.

Food selection and presentation

Although RNs do not always serve meals, it is important for them to make sure that each person receives the right food in sufficient quantities. Patients and clients need to be active in food selection where possible by filling in a menu card or choosing from a bulk trolley. Foods should be attractively served. Small portions should be offered to those with a small appetite as large portions can be daunting. For those requiring a pureed diet, food moulds can enhance the presentation of a meal.

The temperature of food is another factor that affects appetite; care should be taken to ensure hot foods are served hot and cold foods are served cold. It is also important that food is served using a no-touch technique. Chipped or cracked crockery should not be used as it will not clean properly and can become a source of cross infection.

Assisting a person to eat

When someone has difficulty eating, it becomes the RN's responsibility to assist with this activity of living. Before preparing for the meal, the person should be offered toilet facilities, followed by the opportunity to wash their hands. It is generally easier to eat sitting in a chair, but the person confined to bed can be assisted to sit upright (if this is not contraindicated). An appropriate table is required so that the food can be set out, allowing the person to see the food and indicate preferences. The patient or client should be offered protection for their clothing. Where possible, independence should be promoted by preparing food and drink for an individual so it is ready to eat. Sitting with a person and using verbal and non-verbal prompts as required may enable them to eat the meal independently. Where a person is unable to transfer food or drink into their mouths it is necessary to do this for them. This requires considerable skill and the consent of the patient or client is required. It should be recognised that having to be fed by someone can be a threat to the individual's integrity and self-esteem, so every effort should be made to minimise the negative aspects. The nurse should sit level with the person and encourage a relaxed social atmosphere. The rate and manner of assistance with eating and drinking should be at the person's normal pace and pattern. The pace of eating can be controlled by the person if their hand is placed on the nurse's forearm during assistance with feeding and drinking. Plenty of time is essential to allow the person to chew, to pause between mouthfuls and to have a drink when desired. The nurse should check that plates and food are at an appropriate temperature and ensure that any bones or fruit pips are removed. Fluid should be offered periodically as this will facilitate swallowing. Mouth care should be offered when the meal is finished and the person should remain sitting for a period of time after the meal to promote digestion. It is important to stop giving food and fluid to a patient/client if their voice sounds gurgly, they show signs of choking or food is pocketing in their mouth as this suggests that the swallow reflex is compromised and referral to the SLT may be appropriate. (See Further reading, e.g. Brooker & Waugh 2007, for information about mealtime environment and feeding patients/clients.)

Between meals a drink should be within the patient's/client's reach. If appropriate, snacks can also be positioned so the person can help themselves as required.

Supplementing the diet

If an individual's intake is poor, it is important to 'make every mouthful count'. This can be achieved through strategies such as encouraging the person to choose high-energy foods to eat and increasing the nutritional value of foods by adding butter or cheese to vegetables and ice cream to puddings and milk drinks.

People with a poor appetite or dysphagia may not be able to ingest enough food to meet nutritional needs, and oral nutritional supplements between meals may be prescribed. These consist of drinks, puddings, or powders that are mixed with milk or water that have added kilocalories and other nutrients. Supplements can be presented in a range of ways: frozen to the consistency of a mousse or ice cream or warmed to resemble soup. They should be served at the temperature recommended by the manufacturers. Once opened, they should be considered to be similar to a glass of milk and discarded promptly if not consumed. Patients/clients may prefer them served in a glass or cup rather than the container in which they are packaged. The short-term use of oral nutritional supplements has been shown to be a cost effective way of improving nutritional intake (Elia et al 2005).

In addition to oral nutritional supplement drink and puddings, a prescription for vitamin and mineral supplements may be required to correct specific micronutrient deficiencies or generally increase the intake of micronutrients.

Enteral feeding by tube

Enteral feeding by tube refers to the delivery of nutrients directly to the patient's stomach or small intestine via a tube. If a patient is not able to eat or drink sufficiently adequately to maintain nutritional status, enteral feeding should be considered and can be used as the sole form of nutrition or as a supplement to oral intake. There are several indications for enteral feeding (Box 21.3).

Box 21.3 Information

Indications for enteral feeding

Increased nutritional needs

- Hypercatabolic states, e.g. following extensive burns, major sepsis or severe trauma
- Major surgery – enteral feeding may be commenced pre-operatively to improve nutritional status

Compromised access to GI tract

- Head and neck surgery
- Obstruction due to tumour, e.g. cancer of the mouth or oesophagus
- Oesophageal stricture
- Oesophageal fistula

Inability to eat

- Altered consciousness
- Confusion
- Unwillingness to eat, e.g. persistent anorexia due to chemotherapy
- Persistent nausea and vomiting
- Dysphagia, e.g. following stroke

GI disorders

- Fistula
- Reduced absorption in GI tract, e.g. short bowel syndrome, inflammatory bowel disease, gastrectomy

---

If a person has a functioning gut, enteral nutrition should always be considered before parenteral nutrition (NICE 2006a). Enteral nutrition is less costly, safer and easier to manage and has fewer side-effects than parenteral nutrition. Compared to parenteral nutrition it is thought to preserve intestinal mucosal structure and function and allow for the absorption and utilisation of nutrients in a more physiologically normal way.

Enteral nutrition is contraindicated in some conditions, e.g. obstruction or incompleteness of the GI tract. The decision as to whether a person is enterally or parenterally fed should be informed by the Nutrition Support Team if present in the clinical setting, or made with the input of a dietitian and pharmacist if not. When deciding whether enteral nutrition is appropriate for an individual, ethical and legal issues need to be considered. For further information on this complex and important area of clinical practice, see NICE (2006a) and Körner et al (2006).

It is essential that a person receiving enteral feeding has a written plan of care so that all involved with the care of that person are aware of the goals of care, interventions planned and the evaluation strategies. It is also important that the plan of care is made in partnership with the patient/client where possible and that carers are informed where appropriate. Often it seems there is a lack of clarity in care settings as to what the overall plan of care is for an individual, for example why a particular type of tube is used, when it has been placed and the duration of any side-effects.

The major enteral route via the nose is to the stomach (nasogastric tube [NG]), although a tube may also be inserted from the nose to the duodenum (nasoduodenal tube) or jejunum (nasojejunal tube). Post-pyloric placement is indicated when the risk of aspiration (into the respiratory tract) is considered high or when the patient's medical condition, e.g. obstruction by tumour, or treatment, e.g. oesophageal surgery, indicates this. Less commonly a tube may be passed via the mouth to the stomach (orogastric tube). Tubes may also be inserted through the abdominal wall into the stomach (gastrostomy) or jejunum (jejunostomy). For short-term feeding, enteral feeding tubes are usually inserted via the nose, but if a tube is required in the longer term, a gastrostomy is the preferred route of choice. As nasogastric and gastrostomy tubes represent the most common approaches to tube feeding, they will be the focus of the rest of this section.

Nasogastric tube insertion and care

Nasogastric tube feeding is indicated when short-term nutritional support is required. As the nasogastric route interferes minimally with oral function, it can be used to supplement oral intake. The tube used should be narrow in diameter and flexible. Tubes that have a wide diameter are poorly tolerated as they are uncomfortable, can cause pressure necrosis in the nose and oropharynx and may encourage gastro-oesophageal (cardiac) sphincter/valve incompetence, thus increasing the risk of gastro-oesophageal reflux and aspiration. As fine-bore tubes are flexible, a wire introducer may be required when the nurse is inserting the tube. Fine-bore (6–8 FG) feeding tubes of PVC, silicone or polyurethane are available. PVC tubes degrade quite quickly and are less flexible but can be useful for feeding in the short term as they are less expensive. Polyurethane or silicone tubes are for longer-term use and can be left in position for up to a month. The exact length of time is detailed in the manufacturer's guidelines. Some of those with a guide wire (single-patient use) may also be reused on the same patient if they are displaced, although the guide wire must only be reinserted into the tube if the tube has been removed from the patient.

Insertion of the tube must follow guidelines approved by the clinical setting (see Further reading, e.g. Dougherty & Lister 2008, for information on how to insert tubes with and without guide wires). Nurses may insert tubes safely and effectively in most individuals; however, the insertion of fine-bore tubes following maxillofacial surgery and laryngectomy, or in those individuals with maxillofacial or oesophageal disorders, is not straightforward and in these situations either a doctor (BAPEN 1996) or a nurse with advanced clinical skills in this procedure should place the tube. Local guidelines on which patients/clients RNs may insert a nasogastric tube should be followed.

Once the tube is in place, its position may be checked by pH testing of aspirate using the appropriate pH range indicator strips or X-ray (National Patient Safety Agency [NPSA] 2005). Air auscultation – the 'whoosh' test – involving the rapid injection of 20–30 mL of air down the tube while listening over the stomach with a stethoscope, is no longer recommended (NPSA 2005). However, no method is foolproof; gastric aspirate may be obtained from the trachea if the person has aspirated, and an X-ray is only accurate at the time it was taken. Guidelines approved by the clinical setting must be followed when ascertaining the placement of a tube and the patient carefully observed for signs of respiratory distress or general discomfort once feeding has commenced.

Following insertion, the position of the tube should be checked before administration of any solution or medication, if the patient complains that the tube feels uncomfortable, if feed is seen in the mouth and following episodes of vomiting, coughing or suctioning. Regular flushing of the tube with water is essential to reduce the chance of blockage. A 50 mL syringe is considered to be the most appropriate size of syringe to use for flushing or aspirating, as use of a smaller syringe is thought to generate a higher pressure within the tube (BAPEN 2004). Excessive pressure should not be used to force fluids down the tube as this may split the tube wall. It has been suggested that the tube should be flushed with 30 mL of water at the beginning and end of each feed and before and after giving medication (BAPEN 2004). For some patients, fluid intake may be limited due to their medical condition, in which case advice from the Nutrition Nurse Specialist or pharmacist should be sought. Guidelines from the Infection Control Nurses Association (Skipper et al 2003) suggest that sterile water should be used to flush tubes in acute health care settings and all tubes which terminate in the jejunum. In the community setting, guidelines suggest that cooled, freshly boiled water or sterile water from a newly opened container should be used if the patient is immunosuppressed (NICE 2003). A 50 mL catheter-tipped syringe or syringe specifically designed for enteral tube use should be used to administer fluids.

Syringes intended for i.v. use should not be used due to the risk of accidental parenteral administration (BAPEN

2004). Syringes used for the administration of medication or flushing should be discarded after use (Skipper et al 2003). Premature removal of nasogastric tubes by patients is common (Pancorbo-Hidalgo et al 2001). A nasogastric tube should be secured to the nose and side of the face to prevent the tube from being displaced.

The act of eating and drinking cleanses and hydrates the oral mucosa. For patients/clients who are tube fed, frequent mouth care is a priority to keep the mouth in a clean and comfortable condition (Box 21.4).

Gastrostomy tube insertion and care

Gastrostomy feeding is used if enteral feeding is likely to continue for longer than a month (NICE 2006a). This has become a relatively common nutritional intervention. The procedures most commonly used to place a gastrostomy tube are termed 'percutaneous endoscopic gastrostomy' (PEG) and 'radiologically inserted gastrostomy' (RIG) although tubes may also be inserted surgically. Prior to the procedure the patient will require pre-operative preparation (see Ch. 26).

Gastrostomy placement is contraindicated in some medical conditions such as ascites. The doctor in charge of the patient's medical care or the Nutrition Support Team will assess the patient's suitability for gastrostomy placement prior to the procedure and obtain the patient's written consent. A gastrostomy is normally performed after the patient has received a sedative medication, therefore postoperative care should follow the general guidelines following an operative procedure under sedation (see Ch. 26). Complications of gastrostomy insertion can occur, such as bleeding and pneumoperitoneum (air/gas in the peritoneal cavity)

Box 21.4 Reflection

Oral and nasal care during enteral feeding

Krystyna has been nil by mouth for 4 days and is receiving an enteral feed via a nasogastric tube. She confides to you that her mouth feels dry and tastes unpleasant, and that her nose feels sore.

Activities

- Reflect on Krystyna's situation and why it has occurred. Think about how you would feel in similar circumstances.
- Look at the relevant guidelines used in your placement and Further reading suggestions, e.g Dougherty & Lister 2008, and note the main points pertaining to mouth and nasal care required during enteral feeding with a nasogastric tube.
- You will probably have a list that includes: regular teeth or denture brushing; frequent mouthwashes; possibly ice to suck; sugar-free chewing gum to minimise dryness; ensuring that the enteral feed regimen meets the patient's fluid needs; asking if the patient is allowed sips of water; checking the oral mucosa for signs of infection. Check that the nasogastric tube is not causing pressure within the nasal passages or where it is secured to the face; ensure that the skin around the nose is clean and dry and that the nostrils are clean and clear.
- Prepare a care plan for Krystyna that addresses her problems and discuss it with your mentor or lecturer.

(Schrag et al 2007) and the nurse should carefully observe the patient's condition in the postoperative period.

Following the procedure, tube feeding can usually commence within 4 hours of insertion of a PEG (NICE 2006a). Local guidelines should be followed after insertion of one of the other types of gastrostomy tube. Until the gastrostomy tract has granulated the site can be dressed with a dry dressing which is changed daily using an aseptic technique (see Further reading, e.g. Dougherty & Lister 2008). Once the tract has healed and the stoma formed, the site should be washed daily with water and dried thoroughly (NICE 2003). Some types of gastrostomy tube need to be rotated regularly once the tract is healed to prevent skin from growing around the tube. The frequency with which this should be carried out is variable, therefore local clinical guidelines must be followed. It is suggested that the tube should be gently pushed in by 1 cm and then returned to its original position whilst rotating it through 360 degrees. The fixation plate should be approximately 5 mm distance from the abdomen and should be undone and pulled back to facilitate cleaning. The patient with a gastrostomy tube can swim or bathe once the tract has healed.

If the gastrostomy tube is removed accidentally, then immediate action must be taken as the tract will close over within a matter of hours. If the tube cannot be reinserted by the Nutrition Nurse Specialist or doctor within a short period of time, then a replacement may be inserted to keep the stoma patent; fluid should never be infused until the position of the tube has been confirmed by a health care professional experienced in the care of gastrostomy tubes.

Complications as a result of gastrostomy formation are not uncommon and may include infection and leakage (Schrag et al 2007). Overgranulation of the stoma may also occur; advice on this may be sought from the Nutrition Nurse Specialist or in some situations from the Tissue Viability Nurse (see Ch. 23).

The procedure for the removal of a gastrostomy tube varies according to the type of tube placed. Some tubes can be withdrawn through the stoma, following deflation of the retainer in the stomach; some tubes may be cut and the portion remaining in the stomach removed endoscopically or allowed to pass through the GI tract. If a tube is to be removed, local guidelines should be followed or the advice of the Nutrition Nurse Specialist or unit personnel who have placed the tube should be obtained.

Administration of medications via enteral tube

The pharmacist should be consulted if medication is to be given via an enteral tube as there are risks associated with this route of administration such as tube blockage, drug toxicity and a reduction in drug efficacy. The pharmacist is able to advise on the appropriate route, formulation, timing and monitoring. Nurses must be aware that administration of a licensed medicine via an enteral tube is an unlicensed use and that they are professionally accountable for any adverse effects experienced as a result of using this route (Bowling 2004).

The location of the enteral tube needs to be considered before medication is given as some drugs are not absorbed effectively when delivered directly into the small intestine rather than to the stomach. Medications in the form of oral liquid and dispersible tablets are most easily administered via an enteral tube. However, some liquids may be hyperosmolar and cause diarrhoea, especially if directly administered further down the small intestine. Some viscous oral liquids may be diluted with water to ease administration. Tablets may be crushed, but the advice of the pharmacist must be sought. Medication which is coated (film or enteric) is rarely suitable for administration via an enteral tube. Tablets or capsules of cytotoxic, hormonal, steroidal or antibiotic medications should not be crushed or opened because of the potential risk of exposure to staff and others. (See Further reading, e.g. Dougherty & Lister 2008 for guidelines for the administration of medication via enteral feeding tubes.)

The pharmacist is also able to advise on the potential for drug–nutrient interactions; for example, the drugs phenytoin, carbamazepine and tetracycline should not be administered with feed as this can affect the amount of drug absorbed from the GI tract. If several medications are to be given at one time, the tube should be flushed with at least 10 mL of water between each medication (BAPEN 2004) or advice on the suitability of mixing medications sought from the pharmacist. Two drugs may interact with each other and their effects may change as a result.

Selection of enteral solution

There is a wide range of commercially prepared enteral solutions ('feeds') that may be prescribed. Commercially prepared feeds are of a known nutritional content, are sterile and are designed for ease of administration. The dietitian will choose the most appropriate feeding regimen for the patient, basing such choice on assessment of the patient's needs and medical condition. Generally, the dietitian will also order the feed and ensure it is available for the nurses to administer. Feeds may cause GI disturbances when feeding is being initiated or if they are infused too rapidly. Enteral solutions should be administered at room temperature, as administration of a cold feed can cause the patient to experience abdominal discomfort. Enteral solution should be stored according to the manufacturer's instructions and usually requires shaking prior to administration to disperse any sediment formed. 'Use by' dates should always be checked prior to administration.

Method of administration of enteral solution

The equipment for feeding consists of a reservoir, the nasogastric tube, and usually a giving set that connects to the reservoir and a pump. The reservoir may be a bottle or soft pack and may require filling or may be filled with feed at the manufacturing stage. Nasogastric feeds can be delivered intermittently or continuously. Intermittent feeding is the administration of a 'bolus' of feed periodically. Continuous feeding involves the delivery of a feed over a period of many hours. In clinical settings, enteral feeding pumps are commonly used to deliver a steady flow of solution over a period of time. Feeding intermittently reflects more closely the normal eating pattern and permits free movement between feeds; however, it may be more likely to result in feelings of nausea, intestinal distension, cramps and diarrhoea. There

may also be an increased risk of reflux and aspiration. The dietitian will prescribe the rate at which a solution should be administered following assessment of the individual. During feeding and for 1 h after, unless contraindicated, the patient should sit up at 30 degrees or higher to reduce the risk of aspiration (BAPEN 1999). The amount of feed remaining in the stomach (gastric residue) can be checked if the individual complains of nausea or gastric distension. In some clinical settings, e.g. intensive care units, checking the amount of feed in the stomach should be carried out periodically; local guidelines should be consulted on this issue.

Monitoring and complications of enteral feeding

Monitoring of a patient on enteral feeding is essential to observe for signs of complications and to ensure nutritional goals are being met. Monitoring should include assessment of fluid and food intake, vital signs, weight, gastrointestinal function, stool frequency, tube position and leakage and general clinical condition. Biochemical monitoring is carried out, the frequency determined by the patient's condition. For further details see the NICE guidelines on nutrition support for adults (NICE 2006a).

Complications of enteral feeding can be categorised into three broad groups: mechanical, biochemical and gastrointestinal/infectious (Table 21.3). The serious complication of refeeding syndrome is discussed earlier (p. 602).

The psychological effects of tube feeding should also be considered, since food has a profound influence on psychosocial well-being. One study highlighted that the placement of a gastrostomy has a major impact on the lifestyle of patients and their carers (Brotherton & Judd 2007). Effective symptom management and support are identified as important factors in enabling patients to cope (Brotherton & Judd 2007). The nurse should ensure that the nursing care recognises and meets the patient's and carer's needs.

If a patient is likely to be discharged from hospital with an enteral feeding tube in situ, then it is essential that appropriate discharge arrangements are made for the continuation of nutritional care (NICE 2006a). Patients and carers should receive training and education concerning their enteral feeding regimen before discharge and appropriate support by community services following discharge. NICE (2006a) outlines that the patient should have the support of a coordinated multidisciplinary team and an individualised care plan and that the patient and their carers should receive training and relevant information.

Parenteral nutrition

In parenteral feeding, nutrients in solution are infused directly into the venous system. Parenteral nutrition (PN) may be used as a supplement to oral or enteral feeding or it can be the sole form of feeding. Appropriate early intervention by PN can prevent or reduce the likelihood of malnutrition developing. This invasive technique is associated with several hazards and problems and should be used only when other methods of nutritional support have been excluded. The term 'TPN' (total parenteral nutrition) is commonly used, but 'PN' is preferred.

Table 21.3 Complications associated with enteral feeding

POTENTIAL COMPLICATION	PREVENTION/MANAGEMENT
A. Mechanical complications of enteral feeding	
Tube blockage	Flush tube with water regularly according to local guidelines Maintain continuous flow of feed according to feed prescription Replace tube as required Consult pharmacist concerning appropriate medications Clear tube blockage using solution detailed in local guidelines; these may include carbonated drinks or enzymes
Knotted tubes	Note any pain on tube withdrawal Consult Nutrition Nurse Specialist or doctor if pain is present
Tube displacement	Use correct procedure to insert tube Use appropriate type and length of tube Secure tube firmly Explain need for tube to patient
Aspiration of feed	Elevate head and shoulders by 30 degrees or more whilst feeding and for 1 h after Confirm position of tube prior to use Check gastric residual volume as indicated by local guidelines
Discomfort	Give mouth care regularly Lubricate lips Use smallest appropriate bore of tube Use alternate nostril for tube insertion
Excessive or inadequate feed flow	Use an enteral feeding pump and appropriate giving set and reservoir to administer feeds or follow dietitian's instruction concerning bolus feed administration Give feed at rate indicated by feed prescription. Do not interrupt feed unless clinically indicated and do not increase the feed rate beyond the prescribed amount
B. Biochemical complications of enteral feeding	
Changes in electrolyte levels	Monitor electrolyte levels in blood according to NICE (2006a) guidelines and act promptly if changes detected
Changes in hydration status	Record fluid input and output daily and weigh at least weekly
Refeeding syndrome	Follow dietitian's instructions concerning rate and type of feed Monitor electrolyte levels in blood according to NICE guidelines (2006a) Monitor clinical condition (e.g. temperature, blood pressure, pulse and respiration) daily initially or more frequently if clinical condition unstable Record fluid input and output daily
C. Gastrointestinal and infectious complications of enteral feeding	
Nausea and vomiting	Avoid administering high-osmolality fluids by ensuring medications are given in appropriate forms Avoid rapid infusion rates by adhering to prescribed feed rate Administer fluids at room temperature Check residual gastric volume if nausea is experienced and consult dietitian and doctor Stop feed if vomiting is experienced and consult dietitian Consider antiemetic administration Review procedures used to administer feeds and ensure giving set is changed according to local guidelines
Diarrhoea	Establish cause of diarrhoea: consider medications used, e.g. antibiotic therapy, laxatives and high-osmolality fluids, and medical diagnosis Consult dietitian as feed type and rate may need reviewing Administer feed at room temperature If diarrhoea persists, send a stool sample for culture Review procedures used to administer feeds and ensure giving set is changed according to clinical setting guidelines

Continued

Table 21.3 Complications associated with enteral feeding – cont'd

POTENTIAL COMPLICATION	PREVENTION/MANAGEMENT
Constipation	Monitor frequency and consistency of stool Contact dietitian, as feed type may need reviewing Encourage mobility Give laxatives as prescribed Ensure adequate fluid intake
Distension/cramps	Check gastric residual volume of feed Follow dietitian's instructions concerning rate and type of feed Consider antiemetic or antispasmodic use
Stoma site inflammation	Clean site daily Ensure fixation device is in the appropriate position to avoid external pressure at stoma site Avoid the use of a dressing around the site Rotate tube according to local guidelines Consult Nutrition Nurse Specialist or Tissue Viability Nurse Specialist for advice if inflammation persists or is severe Send swab from site for microbiological examination Observe for signs of systemic infection

Indications for PN

The risks and expense associated with PN are significant and the key factor to consider when deciding to use this form of feeding is the availability of the GI system. PN will be the method of choice if the GI system is unavailable. In addition patients may not be able to tolerate the oral or enteral intake required to rectify their nutrition deficits, and supplementary parenteral feeding may be considered. Conditions in which PN may be indicated include:

- trauma to the GI system resulting in an inability to ingest or absorb nutrients, e.g. perforated bowel
- postoperative complications delaying enteral feeding, e.g. paralytic ileus, obstruction, acute or chronic gastrointestinal inflammation which is not responding to treatment, e.g. Crohn's disease, ulcerative colitis
- malabsorption, e.g. in cancer and cancer chemotherapy or radiotherapy, where there is mucosal inflammation
- pancreatitis
- severe nausea and vomiting.

Many people will require only short-term PN (less than 2 weeks) until GI function has improved sufficiently. Some, however, with prolonged GI failure, will need long-term PN. Whilst there may be 'typical' indications for PN, each patient will have individual needs. In order to support and maintain a patient with PN successfully, a team approach is needed, involving not only the nursing and medical staff, but also the biochemist, pharmacist and dietitian, and the primary care team if the patient is to receive PN at home. Specialist nutrition teams assist patients and their carers to manage PN successfully at home, giving advice on such things as storage of PN bags, management of the regimen and equipment use.

Venous access for PN

PN can be administered through a peripheral or central vein. Central venous catheterisation is currently the route of choice for long-term PN and for those with inaccessible peripheral veins.

Infusion into the superior vena cava (SVC) promotes rapid dilution of the hypertonic fluid infused which avoids irritation of the veins by the PN. The SVC can be accessed by direct cannulation via the subclavian, external jugular, internal jugular or brachiocephalic veins. Central venous catheterisation can also be carried out through a peripheral vein in the antecubital fossa, using a long catheter that is threaded up to the SVC (peripherally inserted central catheter, or PICC line). PICC lines are suitable for medium- to long-term PN. For long-term PN (greater than 30 days) it is recommended that the catheter is a tunnelled subclavian catheter (NICE 2006a). With tunnelling, there is some distance between where the catheter enters the skin and the point at which it enters the vein, which may facilitate better positioning of the catheter and reduce the risk of infection.

Administration of PN via a peripheral venous catheter can be considered for patients who are receiving PN for less than 14 days and who do not require a central venous catheter for another reason (NICE 2006a). The route is not suitable for longer-term infusion of PN as the infused solution can irritate peripheral veins. Peripheral lines are often referred to as peripherally inserted catheters (PIC lines) and include both peripheral cannulae and midline catheters. Peripheral midline catheters are typically 20 cm, 22 FG catheters, which are sited in the antecubital fossa and stretch along the vein toward the SVC. These catheters are suitable for short- to medium-term use. Peripheral cannulas should be re-sited every 24–48 hours in the opposite arm but local policy should be consulted. The leg veins are not generally used for PN because of the risk of deep vein thrombosis and phlebitis.

Regardless of the approach adopted, an aseptic insertion technique and careful insertion site management are essential (see Ch. 20). The central venous line should be inserted either in the operating theatre, where maximum control of the environment is possible, or on the ward, using appropriate infection control measures (see Ch. 16). After insertion of a central catheter, an X-ray should be performed to ensure that the line is in the correct position and complications have not occurred.

Administration equipment

All nutrient solutions should be administered through a dedicated feeding line, using volumetric pump/controllers with occlusion and air in line alarms (NICE 2006a). This is important and will help to avoid complications associated with PN such as air embolism, catheter occlusion, and metabolic and fluid complications as a result of a rapid infusion rate. A large variety of i.v. catheters are available for parenteral feeding. A flexible, strong catheter made from an inert, soft material is ideal. It should also be detectable by X-ray, so that the tip position can be checked prior to PN commencing. In-line filters can be used to reduce particulate matter and may help to reduce bacterial contamination, depending on the type of filter employed.

Solutions for PN

Parenteral nutrition, if used exclusively, must meet as closely as possible all of a patient's requirements for water, energy, macro- and micronutrients. The fluid and electrolyte intake should cover loss via urine, faeces (especially if diarrhoea occurs or a fistula is present), respiration, perspiration and any abnormal losses via wounds or drains. All nutrient solutions should be compounded, under aseptic conditions, by the pharmacy department or a licensed manufacturer. This will ensure stability of solutions and minimise the risk of microbial contamination. Energy is provided by glucose and lipid solutions. Lipid solutions also provide essential fatty acids. Protein needs are met by the use of amino acid solutions with varying proportions of essential and non-essential amino acids. Micronutrients are added to the protein, fat and glucose solution to provide all the patient's nutritional requirements in a single bag of fluid.

Complications of PN

General complications associated with PN can be classed as catheter-related complications and metabolic and fluid related complications (NICE 2006a). The psychosocial impact of parenteral nutrition should also be considered.

Catheter-related complications

The general complications of i.v. therapy are discussed elsewhere, e.g. Ch. 20. The particular risks of i.v. therapy that involve parenteral nutrition are those related to the administration of large quantities of fluid rich in nutrients which increases the risk for catheter blockage, tissue damage in extravasation and microbial growth.

The catheters should be flushed regularly according to local policy and the flow rate should not be intermittent to prevent blockage. Strict asepsis should be followed when dressings and PN bags are changed. Disruption to the 'closed' infusion system should be minimised as this increases the risk of microorganisms entering the system. The insertion site should be observed for any signs of infection and the patient's general condition should be monitored carefully for signs of infection or PN leaking into the tissues. Feeding lines should be dedicated and not be used for the administration of medications or the withdrawal of blood.

Management of patients by Nutrition Support Teams or Nutrition Nurse Specialists has been suggested to reduce the complications experienced with PN (NICE 2006a). In order to reduce the risk of infection associated with PN bag changes and catheters, in some clinical areas this is considered an extended role of the nurse. Nurses in many clinical areas, therefore, need to undergo specific training in changing PN infusion bags and caring for catheters through which PN is being infused.

Metabolic and fluid related complications

Fluid related complications are related to the fluid being administered or the speed of administration. To avoid complications with the speed of infusion all PN should be commenced at the prescribed rate and the patient's clinical condition carefully monitored and appropriate action taken if overhydration or dehydration is suspected. Metabolic complications can arise because the infused nutrients may cause changes in the way carbohydrate and fat is used by the body and may affect intracellular electrolyte levels. As with other forms of nutritional support, malnourished patients are at risk of refeeding syndrome when PN is commenced (see p. 602). NICE (2006a) recommends that nutritional support should start at no more than 50% of the estimated energy and protein needs and be increased to meet full needs over the first 24–48 hours if clinical and biochemical monitoring indicate this is acceptable. As full requirements of fluid and electrolytes may be given from the start, the PN formulation may change over the first few days. Patients with diabetes mellitus who are controlled by insulin are generally prescribed a sliding scale of insulin to ensure blood glucose remains within the normal range (see Ch. 5, Part 2).

Monitoring of people receiving PN

People receiving PN need careful monitoring whether they are at home or in hospital. This includes monitoring of fluid and nutrient intake, weight, gastrointestinal functioning, the catheter entry site, and clinical condition. Monitoring of a patient's clinical condition includes basic clinical observations (such as temperature, pulse, respiration, blood pressure, blood glucose), and laboratory tests to measure micronutrient levels (including electrolytes), renal function, liver function, level of lipids in the blood (lipidaemia), urea and blood cell counts (NICE 2006a). People receiving PN over a long period of time will need monitoring for the whole time they are receiving PN nutrition and this will include looking at factors which can be affected by long-term nutritional support, such as bone density.

The psychosocial impact of PN

People who receive PN are usually either not able to eat or can eat but what they can eat is limited. The impact on normal daily life of drastically changing eating habits should not be underestimated. Eating and drinking is part of our everyday life and enables us to express our cultural and religious beliefs. Removing or reducing the ability to eat and drink normally will have a psychological and social impact on the person and the people with which they share their life. In addition a person who is receiving PN at home will have to adapt their home and lifestyle to deal with bag changes and PN infusion. Their work and social life will also be affected. The psychosocial impact will depend on the length of time nutritional support is given and a person's cognitive ability to appraise the situation. For example, if a person receives PN for 14 days when acutely ill, the psychosocial impact is likely to be much less than for a person who is informed that they will require PN for the rest of their life. It is important to support the patient and their family by providing appropriate information and enabling them to express their concerns. It is very difficult for health care professionals to really understand what people and their carers experience when they are prescribed long-term PN. They can be informed about the registered charity Patients on Intravenous and Nasogastric Nutrition Therapy (PINNT). This charity aims to support both adults and children who require nutrition therapy, to provide understanding and contact between patients and to eliminate some of the problems which come with treatment (PINNT 2008).

EVALUATION

The final stage of the process of nutritional care of individuals is evaluation. Nutritional plans of care must be evaluated to ensure that the nutritional plan is effective. The evaluation process should use the screening and assessment methods outlined above. If the patient's plan of care is not effectively improving their nutritional status or other identified goal then the plan of care needs to be reviewed. It is vital that interventions are evaluated to ensure that they are effective and that the evaluation process is appropriately recorded.

The Nutrition Support Team and the Nutrition Nurse Specialist

The establishment of an expert, multidisciplinary nutrition team within care settings to coordinate nutritional care has been recommended for a number of years (Silk 1994). Such a team is usually termed a Nutrition Support Team. Membership of a Nutrition Support Team varies between practice settings, but at a minimum usually includes a senior medical doctor, a Nutrition Nurse Specialist, a dietitian and a pharmacist. The team may also include biochemistry and microbiology laboratory staff members. The responsibilities of a team vary according to the practice setting but usually include ensuring enteral and parenteral nutrition is administered appropriately, providing nutritional education and training, conducting audit and setting standards of clinical practice in nutritional support through the development of policies and procedures. It has been suggested that the presence of a Nutrition Support Team leads to a reduction in complications and costs associated with enteral and parenteral feeding (NICE 2006a). The team can also ensure that the nutritional care of patients within each care setting is standard and follows local and national policy and guidelines.

The Nutrition Nurse Specialist (NNS) is a clinical nurse specialist who works with the Nutrition Support Team. NICE (2006a) recommends that all acute Trusts should employ at least one specialist nutrition support nurse. The NNS acts to ensure nursing practice concerning nutritional care is appropriate, follows policy and guidelines and is patient/client-centred. The role of the NNS varies according to the practice setting but generally includes clinical practice, education and training, management, audit and provision of advice and guidance. Research activity may also form part of the role of the NNS.

Future directions in nutritional care

Currently the nutritional care of patients in care settings varies, both at a regional and a national level. In 2002 The Council of Europe published national guidelines for food provision and nutritional care in hospitals and has recently highlighted malnutrition within the community as an issue of concern across Europe (Council of Europe 2007), aiming to encourage action to tackle malnutrition through a series of recommendations. In 2007 the Council of Europe also published a paper entitled *A Strategy for Europe on Nutrition, Overweight and Obesity related health issues* which sets out an integrated approach to reducing ill health due to overweight and obesity. In the UK, NICE has recently produced clinical guidelines concerning the management of obesity and nutrition support (NICE 2006a, b). The Nursing and Midwifery Council has outlined the skills required by nurses in relation to nutritional care in the Essential Skills Clusters (NMC 2007) for pre-registration nursing programmes. This will ensure that all nurses have the skills required to give appropriate nutritional care on entry to the register.

SUMMARY: KEY NURSING ISSUES

- Nurses are involved in aspects of public health nutrition by enabling groups of individuals to achieve a diet that meets their nutritional requirements.
- The nutritional care of individuals is a fundamental part of good nursing practice.
- The role of the nurse is to ensure nutritional care is carried out appropriately and in accordance with the patient's wishes.
- However, the nurse does not act independently to ensure nutritional needs are met – the involvement of the entire health care team is crucial.

REFLECTION AND LEARNING – WHAT NEXT?

- **Test** your knowledge by visiting the website 🖱 and answering the multiple choice questions and critical thinking questions.
- **Consolidate** your learning by looking at some of the further reading suggestions, references and specialist websites.
- **Revisit** some of the additional material on the website.
- **Consider** what you have learnt and how this will help your professional development.
- **Reflect** on how you can apply this knowledge to the care of your patients.
- **Discuss** your learning with your mentor/supervisor, lecturer and colleagues.

REFERENCES

Anderson A: Nutrition interventions in women in low-income groups in the UK, *Proc Nutr Soc* 66:25–32, 2007.

Bowling T: *Nutritional support for adults and children*, Abingdon, 2004, Radcliffe Medical Press.

British Association for Parenteral and Enteral Nutrition (BAPEN): *Standards and guidelines for nutritional support of patients in hospitals*, Maidenhead, 1996, BAPEN.

British Association for Parenteral and Enteral Nutrition (BAPEN): *Current perspectives on enteral nutrition in adults*, Maidenhead, 1999, BAPEN.

British Association for Parenteral and Enteral Nutrition (BAPEN): *Drug administration via enteral feeding tubes*, 2004. Available online http://www.nnng.org/Newsletters/NNNG_Iss2.pdf.

British Dietetic Association: Effective Practice Bulletin, issue 32: Challenging the use of body mass index (BMI) to assess under-nutrition in older people, *Dietetics Today* 38(3):15–19, 2003.

Brotherton AM, Judd PA: Quality of life in adult enteral tube feeding patients, *J Hum Nutr Diet* 20(6):513–522, 2007.

Council of Europe: *From Malnutrition to Wellnutrition: policy to practice*, 2007. Available online http://www.european-nutrition.org/files/pdf_pdf_38.pdf.

Department of Health (DH): *Dietary reference values for food energy and nutrients for the United Kingdom*, London, 1991, HMSO.

Department of Health (DH): *Nutritional aspects of cardiovascular disease*, Report on health and social subjects No. 46, London, 1994, HMSO.

Department of Health (DH): *Exercise referral systems: A national quality assurance framework*, London, 2001, Department of Health.

Department of Health (DH): *Hospital food*, 2007. Available online http://www.dh.gov.uk/en/Managingyourorganisation/Leadershipandmanagement/Healthcareenvironment/DH_4116450.

Department of Health (DH): *Healthy Weight, Healthy Lives: A cross government research and surveillance plan for England*, 2008. Available online http://www.dh.gov.uk/en/Publicationsandstatistics/Publications/DH_091964.

Department of Health (DH): *Obesity publications for health professionals*, 2009a. Available online http://www.dh.gov.uk/en/Publichealth/Healthimprovement/Obesity/DH_078102.

Department of Health (DH): *Change4Life – Eat Well, Move More, Live Longer*, 2009b. Available online http://www.dh.gov.uk/en/News/Currentcampaigns/Change4Life/index.htm.

Department of Health (DH): *Essence of Care: Benchmarks for the Fundamental Aspects of Care*, 2010. Available online http://www.dh.gov.uk/.

Elia M: *The 'MUST' report*, Redditch, 2003, BAPEN.

Elia M, Stratton R, Russell C, et al: *The cost of disease-related malnutrition in the UK and economic considerations for the use of oral nutritional supplements (ONS) in adults: executive summary*, 2005, BAPEN. Available online http://www.bapen.org.uk/pdfs/health_econ_exec_sum.pdf.

Elia M, Russell C: *Report of the Advisory Group on Malnutrition, led by BAPEN. Combating Malnutrition: Recommendations for Action*, 2009, BAPEN. Executive summary. Available online http://www.bapen.org.uk/pdfs/reports/advisory_group_report.pdf.

Finch S, Doyle W, Lowe C, et al: *National diet and nutrition survey: people aged 65 years and older. Volume 1: Report of the diet and nutrition survey*, London, 1998, TSO.

Food Standards Agency (FSA): *Safe upper levels for vitamins and minerals*, 2003. Available online http://www.eatwell.gov.uk/.

Food Standards Agency (FSA): *Healthy diet, Salt*, 2009a. Available online http://www.eatwell.gov.uk/healthydiet/fss/salt/.

Food Standards Agency (FSA): *Health issues, Food Poisoning*, 2009b. Available online http://www.eatwell.gov.uk/healthissues/foodpoisoning/.

Food Standards Agency (FSA): *Healthy diet, Nutrition Essentials, Fruit & vegetables*, 2009c. Available online http://www.eatwell.gov.uk/healthydiet/nutritionessentials/fruitandveg/.

Food Standards Agency (FSA): *Healthy diet, 8 tips for eating well*, 2009d. Available online http://www.eatwell.gov.uk/healthydiet/eighttipssection/8tips/.

Food Standards Agency (FSA): *Healthy diet, Vitamin A*, 2010. Available online http://www.eatwell.gov.uk/healthydiet/nutritionessentials/vitaminsandminerals/.

Geissler C, Powers H: *Human Nutrition*, Edinburgh, 2005, Churchill Livingstone.

Green SM, Watson R: Nutritional screening and assessment tools for use by nurses: literature review, *J Adv Nurs* 50(1):69–83, 2005.

Hunter GR, Byrne NM, Sirikul B, et al: Resistance training conserves fat-free mass and resting energy expenditure following weight loss, *Obesity* 16(5):1045–1051, 2008.

International Obesity Task Force: *About obesity*, Quebec, 2003, International Obesity Taskforce. Available online http://www.iotf.org.

Körner U, Bondolfi A, Bühler E, et al: Ethical and legal aspects of enteral nutrition, *Clin Nutr* 35:196–202, 2006.

Lean MEJ: Pathophysiology of obesity, *Proc Nutr Soc* 59:331–336, 2000.

McLaren S, Green S: Nutritional screening and assessment, *Prof Nurse* 13(6): S9–S14, 1998.

Mulvihill C, Quigley R: *The management of obesity and overweight: an analysis of reviews of diet, physical activity and behavioural approaches. Evidence briefing*, London, 2003, Health Development Agency.

National Institute for Health and Clinical Excellence (NICE): Infection control, prevention of healthcare-associated infections in primary and community care, *Clinical Guideline CG2*, 2003. Available online http://www.nice.org.uk/Guidance/CG2.

National Institute for Health and Clinical Excellence (NICE): Eating disorders, *Clinical Guideline CG9*, 2004. Available online http://www.nice.org.uk/Guidance/CG9.

National Institute for Health and Clinical Excellence (NICE): Nutrition support in adults, *Clinical Guideline CG32*, 2006a. Available online http://www.nice.org.uk/Guidance/CG32.

National Institute for Health and Clinical Excellence (NICE): Obesity, *Clinical guideline CG43*, 2006b. Available online http://www.nice.org.uk/Guidance/CG43.

National Patient Safety Agency (NPSA): *How to confirm the correct position of nasogastric feeding tubes in infants, children and adults*, 2005. Available online http://www.npsa.nhs.uk/patientsafety/alerts-and-directives/alerts/nasogastric-feeding-tubes/.

Nursing and Midwifery Council: *Essential Skills Clusters, Circular 07/2007 Annexe 2*, London, 2007, NMC.

Nursing and Midwifery Practice Development Unit: *Best practice statement: nutrition assessment and referral in the care of adults in hospital*, Edinburgh, 2002, Nursing and Midwifery Practice Development Unit.

Pancorbo-Hidalgo PL, Garcia-Fernandez FP, Ramirez-Pérez C: Complications associated with enteral nutrition by nasogastric tube in an internal medicine unit, *J Clin Nurs* 10:482–490, 2001.

PINNT: *Welcome to the PINNT website*, 2008. Available online http://www.pinnt.co.uk.

Schrag SP, Sharma R, Jaik NP, et al: Complications related to percutaneous endoscopic gastrostomy (PEG) tubes. A comprehensive clinical review, *J Gastrointestin Liver Dis* 16(4):407–418, 2007.

Scottish Government: *Healthy Eating, Active Living: An action plan to improve diet, increase physical activity and tackle obesity (2008–2011)*, 2008. Available online http://www.scotland.gov.uk/Publications/2008/06/20155902/0.

Silk DBA, editor: *Organisation of nutritional support in hospitals*, Maidenhead, 1994, BAPEN.

Skipper L, Cuffling J, Pratelli N: *Enteral feeding infection control guidelines*, Bathgate, 2003, Infection Control Nurses Association.

Ulijaszek SJ, Lofink H: Obesity in Biocultural Perspective, *Annual Review of Anthropology* 35:337–360, 2006.

World Health Organization (WHO): *Obesity and overweight*, 2006, Fact sheet No 311. Available online http://www.who.int/mediacentre/factsheets/fs311/en/.

FURTHER READING

Barasi ME: *Human nutrition. A health perspective*, London, 2003, Arnold.

Bowling T: *Nutritional support for adults and children*, Abingdon, 2004, Radcliffe Medical Press.

Brooker C, Waugh A: *Foundations of Nursing Practice. Fundamentals of Holistic care*, Edinburgh, 2007, Mosby.

Dougherty L, Lister S: *The Royal Marsden Hospital Manual of Clinical Nursing Procedures*, ed 7, Oxford, 2008, Wiley-Blackwell.

Geissler C, Powers H: *Fundamentals of Human Nutrition for Students and Practitioners in Health Sciences*, Edinburgh, 2009, Churchill Livingstone.

Jordan S, Griffiths H, Griffith R: Administration of medicines part 2: pharmacology, *Nurs Stand* 18(3):45–54, 2003.

Mehanna H, Moledina J, Travis J: Refeeding syndrome: what is it, and how to prevent and treat it, *Br Med J* 336:1495–1498, 2008.

Stratton RJ, Hackston A, Longmore D et al: Malnutrition in hospital outpatients and inpatients: prevalence, concurrent validity and ease of use of the 'malnutrition universal screening tool' ('MUST') for adults, *Br J Nutr* 92(5):799–808, 2004.

USEFUL WEBSITES

British Association for Parenteral and Enteral Nutrition (BAPEN): www.bapen.org.uk

British Nutrition Foundation: www.nutrition.org.uk

Food Standards Agency (FSA): www.food.gov.uk

Food Standards Agency (FSA), Eat well, be well: www.eatwell.gov.uk

Guidelines and Implementation Network: www.gain-ni.org

Health Protection Agency: www.hpa.org.uk

International Association for the Study of Obesity: www.iotf.org

National Institute for Health and Clinical Excellence (NICE): www.nice.org.uk

National Patient Safety Agency (NPSA): www.npsa.nhs.uk

Patients on Intravenous and Nasogastric Nutrition Therapy: www.pinnt.co.uk

World Health Organization (WHO): www.who.int/en

Maintaining body temperature

Charmaine Childs

Introduction

The aim of this chapter is to provide an understanding of the factors and processes involved in thermoregulation, i.e. the maintenance of body temperature at a near-constant level. An understanding of the physical, physiological and behavioural mechanisms will allow for a more rational approach to treatment for patients whose thermoregulatory system is disturbed. There are a number of reasons why body temperature might rise or fall from the 'normal' range, but before any decisions are made about treatment, the first step is to ensure that measurement is accurate.

The remarkably narrow range of normal temperature, together with the fact that infections cause body temperature to rise, allows us to use temperature as a measure of disease. However, the practice of temperature measurement and monitoring is often based on ritual rather than on rational decision-making. The responsibility of the nurse is to:

- understand the mechanisms for 'normal' control of body temperature at approximately 37°C
- ensure that temperature measurements are accurate and that the body site used for temperature measurement is appropriate
- monitor and evaluate the impact of any treatments used to regulate body temperature.

It is for the above reasons that patients should have their temperature measured and assessed by a registered nurse or nursing student under supervision.

Normal body temperature

'Body temperature' can be a misleading term because the body is not at a uniform temperature. For example, skin temperature varies considerably. The skin has been described as a mosaic of temperatures and even 'core' (deep body) temperature can vary slightly. For this reason it is good practice to use the same body site for each temperature measurement and to report the temperature of the site used, e.g. 'Axilla temperature of Mr A on admission to hospital was 36.9°C' or 'Oral temperature of Mrs B was 37.1°C'.

The temperature of the tissues of the body

Surface temperature

Under most circumstances, the skin surface or 'body shell' is the coolest part of the body. The organs, blood and deeper tissues are described as the body 'core' (Tortora & Derrickson 2006). Because the temperature of the skin is influenced by the temperature and humidity of the air (Figure 22.1), measurement of skin temperature is not a reliable method to detect temperature changes of the organs and deep body tissue (Box 22.1). This may be most important

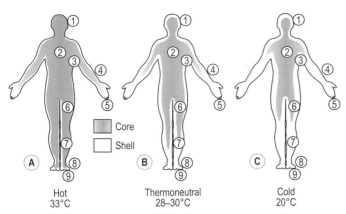

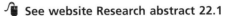

Site	A (°C)	B (°C)	C (°C)
1 Scalp	36.0	34.8	32.8
2 Chest	35.8	34.5	31.3
3 Axilla	36.5	36.4	36.4
4 Arm	35.9	33.5	27.6
5 Finger	35.9	33.2	21.0
6 Thigh	35.2	33.4	27.8
7 Leg	35.3	30.1	25.2
8 Foot	35.5	29.7	22.7
9 Toe	36.2	29.1	21.4

Figure 22.1 Core temperature and temperature of the skin surface at various sites in a hot, a thermoneutral and a cold environment. (Based on an original figure by Aschoff & Wever, cited in Stainer et al 1984, with additional data from Childs C.)

Box 22.1 Reflection

Differences in temperature between the surface and internal organs

The brain controls the temperature of the body so that it remains close to 37°C. The temperature of the skin, however, can vary.

Activity

Look at the manikins (A, B, C) in Figure 22.1. In each example body temperature (oral) is 36.8°C.

- What is the explanation for the higher skin temperatures at the extremities in A compared with C?
- What do you notice about the skin temperatures measured over the thigh, leg, foot and toe in A?
- Why is the pattern of skin temperature in these sites in A different from the patterns in B and C?

---

when caring for patients with critical illness where accurate temperature measurement is likely to be of importance in the diagnosis of infection.

Deep body (core) temperature

The organs of the head and thorax (the main components of core tissues), e.g. heart, liver and brain, are 'insulated' from environmental conditions by bone, fat and skin. The liver,

kidneys, brain and myocardium have a high metabolic rate and consequently a higher temperature than tissues with a lower rate of metabolic activity such as smooth muscle and skin (Houdas & Ring 1982).

In a recent publication by Moran et al (2007) the authors undertook a prospective observational cohort study to investigate whether tympanic measurements were a reliable measurement technique in the critically ill patient. Different conventional methods for body temperature measurement were compared. Access the paper by Moran and colleagues on the website to find out whether the authors considered tympanic membrane temperature to be a valuable measurement method in critically ill patients.

🖱 **See website Box 22.1**

See website Research abstract 22.1 for information about a study by LeFrant et al (2003) that demonstrated the variation in core temperatures in the different organs, muscles, etc.

🖱 **See website Research abstract 22.1**

Regulation of body temperature

Mammalian thermoregulation is controlled by the brain, specifically the pre-optic region within the anterior portion of the hypothalamus (POAH) (see website Figure 22.1 for anatomy of the hypothalamus). Incoming (afferent) signals to the hypothalamus from thermoreceptors in skin and organs are transmitted to and integrated within the POAH, which then responds by transmitting outgoing (efferent) signals to the body so that heat can be either generated/conserved or lost.

🖱 **See website Figure 22.1**

For example, if the temperature of the blood bathing the cells of the hypothalamus starts to rise above 'normal' (37°C), as in a fever, the outgoing, or efferent, signals stimulate 'effector' mechanisms so that heat is lost from the body. Conversely, if the incoming blood is at a lower temperature than the reference (set-point) temperature (i.e. <37°C), mechanisms to conserve or produce heat will be activated. In this way, deep body temperature is prevented from rising or falling from the biological set-point of 37°C. The pathways that help to maintain body temperature at a constant level are shown in Figure 22.2.

Mechanisms of heat conservation and heat production

Heat conservation

If skin or blood temperature falls, signals from peripheral thermoreceptors in skin are interpreted at the POAH and the heat-promoting centre stimulates mechanisms to retain heat as well as to increase the amount of heat produced within the body (endogenous heat production).

Behavioural thermoregulation The ability of humans to conserve heat by putting on more clothes or seeking shelter from the cold is often overlooked or forgotten, but such behaviours are the most fundamental of the protective

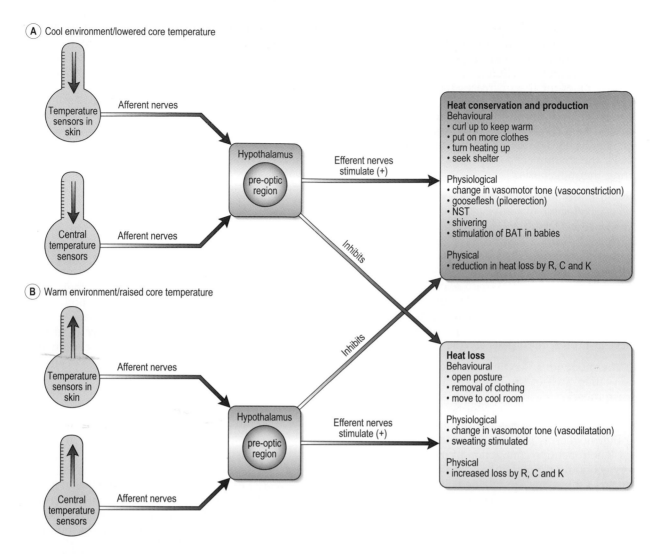

Figure 22.2 Control of body temperature. A. Responses to a cool environment or lowered core temperature. B. Responses to a warm environment or raised core temperature. BAT, brown adipose tissue; C, convection; K, conduction; NST, non-shivering thermogenesis; R, radiation.

thermoregulatory activities and are the 'first line' of defence against extreme heat or cold. Very young and very old people, as well as those who are immobile due to illness or who are sedated, are unable to protect themselves from heat or cold and so are more vulnerable to environmental temperature changes. It then becomes the responsibility of the nurse to place the patient in a comfortable environment to ensure that they are not at risk of hyper- or hypothermia.

Peripheral vasoconstriction As the person begins to feel cold, changes in the flow of blood to the skin also occur. Nerve impulses from the POAH, concerned with heat conservation, cause blood vessels, particularly in the hands, feet, ears and nose, to constrict. Sympathetic stimulation to nerves supplying the blood vessels in these regions results in peripheral vasoconstriction which leads to a reduction in the flow of warm blood from internal organs to the skin. This has the effect of retaining body heat, keeping the core tissues at or close to 37°C.

If body temperature continues to fall despite the above measures, body heat will be produced by a rise in the rate of metabolic heat production (see non-shivering and shivering thermogenesis below).

Heat production

In a healthy young adult, metabolic rate is between 35 and 39 kcal/m^2 body surface/h whereas in an infant, metabolic rate is 53 kcal/m^2 body surface/h. The fact that an infant has a higher metabolic rate than an adult can be explained by the rapid synthesis of cells in the growing body. However, in both adults and children, metabolic rate may rise well above the normal limit for a given age if the person is sick or injured. The most well recognised explanation for a rise in metabolic heat production is the onset of a fever (Childs & Little 1994, Jenney et al 1995) after an injury such as a burn.

In early studies, patients suffering from serious burns (see Ch. 30) were found to have a very high metabolic rate and also a very high body temperature (Childs 1994). Wilmore (1977) reported that metabolic heat production in severe burns was almost double that of a healthy person of the same age. Later, it was found that improvements in surgical management, wound care and analgesia ameliorated the enormous increases in metabolic rate and demand for energy (Childs 1994) although patients remained febrile. Part of the high metabolic 'cost' of burn injury could be reduced by early surgery (to promote healing of the burn wound) and pain management but fever can persist and is a cause of raised metabolic rate, especially if the patient develops a burn wound infection.

Any activity or event that increases the rate of chemical reactions in cells and the rate of oxygen uptake by the cell increases metabolic rate and thus the amount of metabolically produced heat (Frayn 1997). Body heat is produced in two ways: chemically by non-shivering thermogenesis, and physically by the rhythmical contractions of skeletal muscle, i.e. shivering thermogenesis.

Non-shivering thermogenesis Although peripheral vasoconstriction is very effective in conserving body heat, additional sources of heat may need to be generated to restore body temperature to 'normal'. This can be achieved by non-shivering thermogenesis (NST). As its name implies, NST does not involve muscular contraction to stimulate endogenous heat production, but relies upon release of the thermogenic hormone, noradrenaline, under the control of the sympathetic nervous system. Although muscle tissue is the most important source of chemically produced heat, other important heat-producing organs are the brain and liver.

Shivering thermogenesis People who are cold shiver. The heat conservation area of the brain stimulates mechanisms that increase muscle tone, i.e. shivering, such that heat production increases to five times the basal rate. Shivering occurs in most skeletal muscles but the greatest intensity of shivering thermogenesis is in the jaw and neck and is least in the legs. The repetitive contraction of muscle is not, however, a very economical process, as only 40% of the heat generated during shivering is retained by the body and shivering does not continue indefinitely (see Hypothermia, p. 627).

Mechanisms of heat loss

High air temperature and strenuous exercise will raise the temperature of the blood. If the heat gained during the exercise is not matched by an equivalent rate of heat loss, heat-losing mechanisms are initiated and heat-conserving mechanisms are inhibited (Figure 22.2). The series of events that protects the brain and core tissues from reaching dangerously high temperatures is as follows:

- A high air temperature warms the skin. The rise in skin temperature is detected by skin thermoreceptors which send afferent signals to the thermoregulatory centre in the POAH.
- The first reaction of the person is to reduce body insulation by removing some clothing.
- At the same time, blood vessels in acral regions (hands, feet, ear lobes and nose) dilate so that more blood is brought to the surface of the skin. Areas of the body such as the face and ears will then appear 'flushed', pink and warm.
- Providing the air temperature is lower than the skin temperature, heat will be lost by radiation and convection (Table 22.1). If, however, the air temperature is higher than skin temperature, the person will gain heat from the environment. This is why evaporative heat loss becomes so important when the temperature gradient

between skin and air is narrow, i.e. when skin temperature is close to air temperature.
- Stimulation of sweat glands in hot conditions is controlled by the sympathetic nervous system. Production of a fluid consisting mostly of water, but also containing salt, urea, lactic acid and potassium ions, onto the skin causes cooling when the thermal energy needed to transfer the fluid to a gas is removed from the body, i.e. from the skin surface to the air. This transfer of energy from a fluid to a gaseous state is called vaporisational heat loss and occurs during heat loss by sweating.

Fluctuations in a healthy person's temperature

Humans are able to make both physiological and behavioural adjustments to maintain deep body temperature close to 37°C. Like many mammals, humans have the ability to increase the amount of heat in the body as air temperature falls, or to increase heat loss when conditions become uncomfortably hot. It is for this reason that humans are able to live successfully in most climates on Earth.

Normal temperature range

Although central or hypothalamic temperature is 'set' at a relatively constant level, fluctuations do occur in healthy people, e.g. following exercise. No harm is done to the cells of the body by a change in temperature, providing core temperature does not rise above or fall below critical limits. Indeed, the ability of the thermoregulatory system to stimulate changes in heat production or heat loss indicates that the system is operating efficiently.

Website Figure 22.2 illustrates the range of 'normal' temperature in health.

🖱 **See website Figure 22.2**

In the early morning or during cold weather, body temperature may fall to 35–36°C. After moderate exercise, and also, for example, in crying babies, core temperature may rise to approximately 38°C; after hard exercise, body temperature can reach 40°C without causing harm. However, an increase of approximately 5°C above 37°C indicates a serious disruption of thermoregulation and a person's life may be at risk if deep body temperature rises above 43°C or falls below 24°C.

Circadian rhythm

Body temperature fluctuates in a characteristic pattern over a 24-h period. It is thought that this pattern is a result of regular, but normal, deviations of the body's own thermostat or hypothalamic set-point temperature. As with many other physiological functions, thermoregulation displays a circadian rhythm (diurnal variation). This rhythm persists during short periods of night work. Eventually, however, regular night work will reverse the normal pattern so that lower temperatures occur during the day and higher temperatures at night.

Table 22.1 Principles of heat transfer

ROUTE FOR HEAT LOSS	PRINCIPLE	RELEVANCE TO CLINICAL PRACTICE
Radiation (R)	Transfer of energy in the form of electromagnetic waves. The human body emits heat as infrared radiation. At the same time all dense objects (furniture, buildings, other people) are also radiating heat. The rate at which heat is emitted from the human body is dependent upon the temperature difference (gradient) between the skin and other objects and surfaces in the room. If the skin is hotter than the average temperature of objects in the room, heat will be lost. If the objects in the room are hotter, the body will gain heat	A person, naked, sitting quietly in a room at 25°C loses between 50 and 70% of heat by R, the major route for heat loss under such conditions. As air temperature increases, the temperature gradient between skin and air falls such that less heat is lost by this route. As air temperature rises towards skin temperature (35°C), the gradient will be so small that very little heat loss can take place by this route. Evaporative heat loss then becomes an important route for heat loss
Convection (C)	Air (or water) next to the body warms and moves slowly away because warm air is less dense and rises. As it moves away from the body, cooler air replaces it. This process can be speeded up if a strong draught (e.g. electric fan) is used to force the air away and cause a rapid replacement of warmed air with cool air	Nurses frequently increase the rate of heat loss by convection by placing electric fans close to their patients. This can be a very efficient way to lower skin temperature, but frequently the cool stimulus results in an inappropriate response, i.e. peripheral vasoconstriction. Heat retention within core tissues can cause core temperature to rise rather than fall. In febrile patients who have an elevated set-point, the use of electric fans is likely to cool the skin and return heat to the tissue
Conduction (K)	Heat loss by K involves transfer of thermal energy from atom to atom. The skin must be in contact with cooler or hotter objects for heat exchange to take place by K	Critically ill patients are often nursed on special beds designed to reduce the incidence of pressure ulcers. These beds are often maintained at a constant temperature to help prevent heat loss from the body. Sometimes the thermostat can fail and patients have been known to overheat or to cool because the temperature of the bed is too high or too low. Patients must be protected from body temperature disturbances of such an iatrogenic nature
Evaporation (E)	Evaporation of water from the skin and respiratory passages is the most important route for heat loss in hot conditions. The evaporation of water occurs when energy transforms water and sweat droplets to a gas. The heat (or thermal energy) needed to drive this process is taken from the body. Thus the more water there is on the skin, the more heat is taken from the body to turn it into a gas (vaporisation). The more heat removed from the body in the process of E, the more the body cools. The function of sweat (produced under the control of the sympathetic nervous system) as an agent for vaporisational heat loss can be enhanced by spraying the body with a fine mist of warm water	Patients with a high core temperature may not always sweat. During a rise in rectal temperature the body responds as though it were too cold and if patients are observed carefully it will be seen that their skin is dry. At this stage the hypothalamic set-point is above normal but the body continues to activate heat-conserving mechanisms to achieve the new set-point temperature. Only when the patient has reached the new central temperature set-point will heat loss by all routes (E included) be activated. Thus when nurses notice that patients with a high core temperature are sweating, it is more likely to indicate that core temperature has reached the new set-point. A fall in body temperature may then follow

In general, the lowest temperatures recorded over a 24-h cycle will be approximately 0.5°C lower than the afternoon temperature. By the evening, body temperature may be as much as 1.0°C above the early morning temperature. In the newborn, a circadian rhythm of core temperature is not fully developed (Waterhouse et al 2000).

An awareness of the normal changes in deep body temperature in health is necessary if nurses are to interpret temperature measurements correctly. For example, a moderately elevated axilla temperature recorded during the afternoon should be monitored closely before any action to lower the temperature is taken because of the cyclical nature of body temperature, otherwise treatment for pyrexia could be instigated unnecessarily.

Other factors affecting a healthy person's temperature
Babies and young children As long ago as 1937, Bayley & Stolz showed that rectal temperature begins to rise during the first 7 months of life, remaining fairly constant until the age of 2 years, after which it begins to fall. Average rectal temperature at age 1 month was reported to be 37.1–37.2°C, at 8 months 37.6–37.7°C, and at 18 months 37.7°C. By the time the children in the Bayley & Stolz study approached their third birthday, rectal temperature had settled to 37.1°C.

Higher temperatures in early childhood are thought to be a result of increased cellular and metabolic activity. The young of most mammals have a large body surface area relative to their body weight. As a result, babies have a higher risk of hypothermia because they cannot shiver and cannot increase their body insulation, as can adults, by putting on more clothes. This means that a naked baby will lose relatively more heat than an adult for every square metre of their body surface. Babies are therefore reliant on parents and carers to protect them from extremes of environmental temperature.

To counteract increased heat loss, babies have an important source of body heat: brown adipose tissue (BAT), a specialised type of fat cell (Cannon & Nedergaard 2004). BAT is a unique type of adipose tissue, shown by Hull (1976) to be an important source for heat production in small hibernating mammals, and has been described as the 'hibernating gland'. BAT is also stimulated in the human newborn infant after birth. Under the control of the sympathetic nervous system, the function of BAT is to transfer energy from food into heat (Cannon & Nedergaard 2004) and probably plays a role in the evolutionary success of mammals. BAT can be found around the kidneys, between the shoulder blades, around the great vessels and deep within the axillae (Frayn 1997). BAT is richly supplied with blood and oxygen and this dense blood supply is responsible for its brown colour. It becomes much less important in maintaining the temperature of the body as a baby gets older. In adults, BAT is scarce and probably not functional (Klaus 2004).

Adults and older people Unlike small infants, who rely principally on 'switching on' heat production to maintain a stable deep body temperature, adults are more efficient at conserving body heat. In other words, they rely on preventing body heat from being lost, either by putting on more clothes (behavioural thermoregulation) or by vasoconstriction at the extremities (physiological thermoregulation).

Older people, however, often have a lower body temperature than children or younger adults, for which there are a number of reasons:

- After the age of about 50 years, the metabolic rate starts to decline and, correspondingly, metabolic heat production also falls. Consequently, deep body temperature tends to be lower.
- Social and economic factors contribute to the inability of some older people to keep warm, particularly in winter, because, as people grow older, it is more difficult for them to detect extremes in temperature (see Ch. 34). This puts them at risk of hypothermia (Box 22.2 and see website Box 22.2).

 See website Box 22.2

- In warm conditions, deep body temperature in older people may rise slightly because the ability to sweat is reduced. Evaporative heat loss is therefore less efficient at a time when increased heat loss is needed to keep the temperature within the normal range.

Exercise Vigorous exercise can raise core body temperature by several degrees. Temperatures above 40°C have been recorded in marathon runners and, after a game of rugby,

---

Box 22.2 Reflection

Avoiding unnecessary heat loss

After a bath, patients often feel cold and uncomfortable if the nurse is slow in helping them to dry themselves. What is the cause of this feeling of discomfort when the body is wet and the room temperature is low? Why would leaving the bathroom door open make the patient feel cold? How can the nurse improve the patient's comfort when preparing them for a bath?

---

rectal temperatures over 39°C can occur. This rise in temperature can persist for many hours and represents an imbalance between heat production and heat loss (see pp. 618–620).

The menstrual cycle It is now well recognised that 80% of healthy women have higher oral temperatures at the time of ovulation, and a record of early morning oral temperature is used to reflect this. A slight drop in temperature occurs 24–36 h after ovulation. Temperature then rises abruptly by 0.3–0.4°C and continues at this slightly higher level for the rest of the cycle. Three days after the onset of the higher temperature is generally thought to coincide with the end of the fertile phase. The 'hot flushes' associated with the menopause are discussed on the website.

 See website Box 22.3

Eating a meal Mastication (chewing), digestion, absorption and assimilation of nutrients produce body heat. This metabolic heat production was originally described as the specific dynamic action (SDA) of food but now the term 'diet-induced thermogenesis' (DIT) is more often used (Frayn 1997). Metabolism of protein has a greater effect in generating heat than the metabolism of carbohydrate or fat.

The source of body heat – chemical thermogenesis

Heat is expressed in 'energy units' called calories (cal), or more usually in larger units, kilocalories (1 kcal = 1000 cal). The SI unit for energy is the kilojoule (1 kJ = 4.18 kcal).

Since nurses are involved in measuring body temperature, it is important for them to understand how body heat is generated. Most of the energy needed for growth and repair of tissues, for work and for body warmth comes from the food we eat. Most packaged foods have a label which lists the amount of energy (in kcal or kJ) contained in an average serving (or per 100 g) when oxidised or burned by the body. Heat is a by-product of oxidation and the process by which it is produced is called chemical thermogenesis. The rate at which heat is produced in the body is referred to as the metabolic rate.

Metabolic rate

If an awake, resting, lightly clothed man fasts overnight for 12 h in a warm (28–30°C) room, his metabolic rate, and thus his energy expenditure, will be at a minimal or basal level (basal metabolic rate, BMR). During sleep, metabolic rate will be close to basal level. If the man increases his activity, by walking, exercising or even shivering, metabolic rate will rise because more oxygen is being utilised. When this happens, some of the additional energy will be used in order to perform the exercise, i.e. to move from sitting to walking (between 2 and 25%, depending on the activity), but most will be lost as heat.

Business men and women spending most of the day at the office and taking little exercise have a relatively sedentary lifestyle. They can expect to increase their energy requirements by 25–40% above the basal rate during the course of a day. Assuming that 100% of their energy requirements were provided from the food they ate on that day and no energy was stored, approximately 10% would be lost as heat, as a by-product of the work involved in processing their food, 50% would be lost as heat in the conversion of potential energy in food to high-energy biochemical bonds, and 20% would be lost as heat as a result of internal work, e.g. respiration, cell pumps, glandular activity. In this example, the remainder (20%) of energy intake would be used for external work, e.g. muscular contraction for walking. Thus 80% of energy intake is lost as heat and only 20% is used for energy to do work (Wilmore 1977). It is clear that utilisation of food energy is a very inefficient process because most of the energy intake is lost as heat. However, the rate at which heat is produced does not necessarily reflect the rate at which it is lost from the body, because heat can be retained and stored. One of the most important stimuli for body heat storage is a slight fall in core temperature, particularly if the person is in a cool environment. Although a large amount of the energy from food is lost from the body as heat, it is known that many people eat more than is required. Thus, if the amount of calories ingested in food is in excess of the amount of calories used, then energy is stored and the person gains weight. If this is the case, the person is said to be in positive energy balance (see Ch. 21).

The measurement of body temperature

Thermometers

The clinical thermometer

The development of a reliable thermometer was made possible only after scientists came to an agreement about the meaning of temperature and devised a scale to measure it. The scale with which most nurses will be familiar in clinical practice is the Celsius or centigrade scale determined by Anders Celsius (1701–1744). The mercury-in-glass thermometer was the standard temperature-taking instrument for the last century. With modern instruments and techniques the mercury-in-glass thermometer is now rarely used in clinical practice.

Infrared radiation thermometers

Radiation from the sun travels through space mostly in the form of visible light and infrared rays. On striking a body, these waves are partly reflected and partly absorbed and can cause a rise in temperature. The skin absorbs as well as radiates infrared waves (infrared radiation). These waves are part of a 'family' of waves called the electromagnetic spectrum and can be detected with the aid of a special lens (detector) incorporated into a hand-held infrared thermometer. The most commonly used 'infrared' thermometers in hospital are tympanic thermometers.

The tympanic thermometer

The tympanic (ear) thermometer detects radiant heat emitted from the tympanic membrane. Since the tympanum (ear drum) shares a blood supply with deep parts of the brain, tympanic temperature is considered to be a very good substitute for deep body, even brain temperature.

The key point in this measurement technique is to ensure that the 'lens' is inserted correctly so that it can 'see' the tympanum; if the lens is facing the skin of the ear canal, the measurement will not be accurate. Tympanic thermometers are safe for use even in babies, do not present any risk of perforation to the ear drum, and a recording is available in 1–2 s. However, the accuracy of tympanic measurement has been questioned. When comparisons were made of results from three different brands of tympanic thermometer with results from rectal thermometers, differences as great as 2°C between tympanic and rectal temperature were found (Hoffman et al 1999). These data support the results of earlier studies (Talo et al 1991, Brogan et al 1993, Childs et al 1999, Craig et al 2002) and a more recent investigation (Childs 2008) confirming that tympanic thermometers are not a reliable surrogate for deep body (or brain) temperature (see website Figure 22.3).

See website Figure 22.3

Temporal artery thermometers

New methods of infrared thermometry have become available using a small scanner that can be passed over the forehead. The TemporalScanner™ TAT-5000 is manufactured by Exergen (Boston, MA) and the manufacturers claim that it provides a measure of core body temperature. A study by Kimberger et al (2007) compared the accuracy of the temporal artery scanner against tympanic thermometers. More recently, Kirk et al (2009) have shown that temporal artery thermometers perform better as a 'surrogate' for changes in brain temperature than tympanic readings.

Skin surface thermometers

Small infrared thermometers have also been developed to measure surface temperature. The benefit of these instruments is that they can be held in the nurse's hand just a few centimetres from the skin surface and a measurement can be made in seconds. In plastic surgery, surface temperature measurements are a useful and often important way of diagnosing burn depth (Cole et al 1991, Wyllie & Sutherland 1991), the deeper burn being colder than surrounding tissue (see Ch. 30). After transplantation of skin flaps, a reduction in temperature of a flap could indicate poor blood supply; a rise in temperature of a flap could indicate infection.

Electronic thermometers

Electronic thermometers have improved both safety and speed of measurement and revolutionised temperature monitoring for nurses in the UK over the last 20 years. For a single 'spot' measurement, electronic thermometers are quick and simple to use.

Disposable chemical thermometers

In 1999 a new 'generation' of single-use disposable chemical thermometers (e.g. Temp.a.Dot), became available. This type of thermometer is convenient and hygienic and useful in frail older patients, as well as those patients with stroke, where keeping the electronic thermometer in the mouth can be difficult and uncomfortable. Each thermometer has a series, or matrix, of temperature-indicating dots at the tip. Within each dot, a different combination of chemicals melts and changes colour from beige to blue at intervals of 0.1°C. The temperature is read by observing the number of dots that have changed colour. The range of temperature that can be measured with the disposable chemical thermometers is 35.5–40.4°C.

Whilst disposable chemical thermometers have some advantages over other methods, nurses should be aware that temperatures below 35.5°C or above 40.4°C will not be detected. These thermometers are therefore not suitable for temperature measurement when hypo- or hyperthermia is suspected but are considered useful in paediatrics (Macqueen 2001), correctly identifying fever in children with a sensitivity of 92% (Morley et al 1998).

Temperature recording

Recording an accurate body temperature depends not only on the reliability of the instrument, but also on the clinical skill of the nurse. Even the most accurate of instruments will give an incorrect reading if the nurse has a poor temperature-taking technique.

In the conscious patient, the options for deep body temperature measurement are limited to conventional sites such as the axillae, mouth and tympanum (auditory canal). However, when patients are critically ill, accurate temperature measurement becomes a priority (Table 22.2). The patient's temperature may need to be measured at a site which allows the thermometer to remain in situ for many hours, i.e. for continuous monitoring. This is common in the intensive care unit. In such cases, body core temperature can be measured using indwelling thermometers (thermistors) placed in the rectum, oesophagus, nasopharynx or urinary bladder. Continuous temperature measurements are displayed on bedside monitoring systems.

Brain-injured patients

In the brain-injured patient, a rise in temperature of 1–2°C above normal is linked to a poor neurological outcome (Natale et al 2000, Greer et al 2008). However, the evidence for an adverse neurological outcome due to raised temperature remains unproven (for reviews see Childs 2008, Sacho & Childs 2008). For many years it was not possible to measure temperature deep inside the head but today brain temperature monitoring can be performed at the bedside in

Table 22.2 Sites for body temperature measurement: advantages and disadvantages

SITE	NURSING PRACTICE	ADVANTAGES	DISADVANTAGES
Axilla	Place in centre of armpit, hold arm against chest. Leave in position for 9 min	Ideal for temperature measurement in babies and toddlers	Less accurate than oral or rectal measurements but can be a reasonable indicator of core temperature if thermometer is left in situ for the required length of time. Since measurement is not taken in a body cavity, there is more chance of external influences affecting the result
Mouth	Place chemical thermometer under the tongue close to the sublingual artery	Quick and easy to use. Note that there are no 'dots' below 35°C	Accurate readings cannot be expected if the patient has had a hot drink or has smoked a cigarette within the previous 20 min. Chemical thermometers are not suitable for patients where hypothermia is suspected
Ear (auditory canal) (e.g. using the Core Check thermometer, Ivac, Basingstoke, UK)	Ensure the 'lens' of the thermometer is clean (free from cerumen or ear wax). Apply lens cover. Gently hold the pinna and insert probe into the auditory canal. In small children it is important to pull the pinna gently backwards to straighten the ear canal (refer to manufacturer's instructions). Ensure lens is directed towards the tympanum and not to the skin inside the ear canal. After pressing the thermometer 'start' button, a bleep will be heard. It is advisable to repeat the measurement in the opposite ear to ensure parity of measurements in both ears. However, there is sometimes a difference between the temperature of the ears. This is particularly true in hospital where measurements are made on patients who have recently been lying on their side, with their ear on a pillow	Quick and easy to use, with little danger of ear perforation, even in babies. Always remember that thermometers must be calibrated regularly (6-monthly) by the hospital technical department	Unreliable measurements can occur if the ear is inadvertently cooled or warmed, either naturally or by recent local heating/cooling; e.g. if a tympanic temperature measurement is taken in patients who have recently been in a cold environment, or if patients are receiving body cooling treatment for a high temperature, especially where the scalp is involved. Where repeat measurements are made in the same ear, repeated placement of the thermometer in the same ear may cause the measurement to be lower each time it is made, because the instrument casing may slightly lower the temperature inside the ear canal

patients admitted to a neurocritical care unit. Brain temperature measurement, typically performed alongside intracranial pressure monitoring (see Ch. 9), can be made within brain tissue (parenchyma) as well as in the ventricles (Childs et al 2005).

Disturbances in temperature regulation

The causes of increased body temperature can be divided into two categories:

- a rise due to fever (pyrexia)
- an increase as a result of heat illness (due to too much stored body heat).

🖱 **See website Table 22.1**

It is important to recognise the fundamental differences between the causes of raised body temperature and to appreciate their implications for treatment.

Fever

The high 'core' or deep body temperature associated with fever is due to an upward re-set in the central hypothalamic set-point temperature. See website Figure 22.4 to understand the way in which the body thermostat is adjusted during and after fever onset.

🖱 **See website Figure 22.4**

If the set-point is shifted, for example from 37° to 39°C, thermoreceptors in the brain detect a discrepancy between the set-point temperature and the temperature of the blood circulating (37°C) through the hypothalamus. This is the error signal described on page 618. Since blood temperature is lower than the new, raised set-point temperature, heat gain mechanisms will be stimulated to achieve an increase in the temperature of the 'core'. This can be observed when

the febrile patient complains of being cold and pulls on more bedclothes or turns the heating up. Patients do this even when their core temperature has started to rise. They complain that their hands and feet feel cold. This is due to the blood in the skin being diverted away from the 'shell' to the central 'core'. The patient may also start to shiver. Very vigorous shivering is called a rigor. The occurrence of febrile convulsions in young children and the related nursing care are discussed in website Box 22.4.

🖱 **See website Box 22.4**

As body temperature rises, heat loss mechanisms are inhibited or 'switched off'. These thermoregulatory changes help the temperature to reach the new set-point level. At this stage, the nurse should not try to lower the patient's temperature by cooling, either by tepid sponging or with electric fans, because by doing so the stimulated heat conservation mechanisms already in operation will be counteracted. However, once the temperature of the blood and deep body tissues are at the new 'set-point' level and sufficient heat has been stored within the body to sustain the new set-point temperature, the patient will become more comfortable despite the higher (febrile) temperature.

The set-point will not remain at the higher level. Eventually, the biological effects of the pyrogen (see below) will wear off and the thermoregulatory 'set-point' will abruptly return to normal. When this happens, the patient will feel uncomfortable and hot (Table 22.3). Hands, face and feet will become red as peripheral vasodilatation replaces vasoconstriction. Vasodilatation allows skin blood flow to reach the most superficial layers of skin so that heat exchange from core tissues to the skin surface and from the skin to the environment can take place.

At this stage the patient should be put in the best position to allow natural dissipation of body heat. Forcing heat loss from the body by using a fan or allowing the temperature of the room to fall so low that the patient quickly becomes cold and uncomfortable will induce peripheral vasoconstriction again. If this happens, heat loss by radiation and

Table 22.3 Clinical appearance and observations of an apyrexial patient who complains of feeling hot: evidence for behavioural and physiological thermoregulation

OBSERVATION	RESPONSE
The bedclothes have been pushed to the bottom of the bed by the patient	This is a behavioural response to the sensation of feeling too warm. Removal of bedclothes/clothing exposes a larger area of the body surface for heat exchange by radiation and convection. If bedclothes/clothing are removed then sweat can freely evaporate to the room and so facilitate evaporative heat loss
Close inspection of the patient shows that the skin of the hands and feet is red and the veins in these areas dilated	Under control of the sympathetic nervous system, veins of the feet and hands vasodilate due to a reduction in vasomotor tone. Blood is therefore directed to the skin surface, resulting in the core tissues extending to the shell and the skin appearing flushed. The skin is now at a higher temperature, thus creating a wider temperature gradient between the body and the environment. The greater the temperature difference between the body surface and its surroundings, the greater the heat loss by dry routes
Small droplets of sweat appear on the forehead and trunk	Sweating is stimulated in response to either an increase in skin temperature or a rise in core temperature (note the exception to this described in Table 22.1). Sweating occurs first on the forehead, followed by the upper arms, hands, thighs, feet and, finally, the abdomen. Sweating has been shown to start when the average skin temperature is 34°C; as skin temperature increases so does the sweat rate

Box 22.3 Information

Non-steroidal anti-inflammatory drugs (NSAIDs)

In addition to their anti-inflammatory effects, NSAIDs are antipyretics. They act by inhibiting the production of prostaglandins from arachidonic acid in the cyclo-oxygenase pathway.

Since 1986, the NSAID aspirin (acetylsalicylic acid) has been withdrawn from general use in children under the age of 12 years because of the association between this drug and a serious condition called Reye's syndrome.*

Paracetamol (acetaminophen) is now the most commonly used antipyretic in children. Although not an NSAID, its antipyretic properties are thought to lie in its ability to prevent the synthesis of prostaglandins, which are thought to affect the temperature set-point when released into the brain (see p. 618).

Antipyretic drugs are not effective in conditions where high core temperatures are caused by heat illness; neither are they effective in lowering normal body temperature.

*Reye's syndrome is a rare illness that occurs typically in children and teenagers. The onset is usually during a viral illness such as influenza or chickenpox. This is then followed by protracted vomiting and neurological changes at just about the time when the child is beginning to recover from the original illness (Ward 1997). The use of aspirin during the illness has been identified as a factor contributing to the very serious metabolic disorders associated with it, i.e. encephalopathy and fatty degeneration of organs. Unexpected vomiting and disturbed brain function after a viral illness are symptoms of Reye's syndrome in children and teenagers, but in infants the symptoms may be slightly different and include diarrhoea, breathing difficulties and fits. The number of cases reported has fallen in countries where aspirin has been withdrawn from use in children (Larsen 1997).

convection will be prevented. Patients often have a drenching sweat when their set-point returns to normal. It is, however, possible to encourage heat loss by evaporation by spraying the patient with a fine mist of warm water. The use of non-steroidal anti-inflammatory drugs (NSAIDs) in the treatment of fever is discussed in Box 22.3.

How fever develops

Fever is caused by the action of pro-inflammatory cytokines acting within the brain. Cytokines are peptide molecules released from a variety of cells, including those of the immune system (see Ch. 16). In health, cytokines are essential for cell–cell communication. During episodes of disease, such as inflammation and injury, they are responsible for many of the exaggerated inflammatory changes that can lead to sepsis and multiple organ failure. However, cytokines are not always harmful in disease, because these molecules also have beneficial effects for the host. The anti-inflammatory cytokines such as interleukin-10 (IL-10) and transforming growth factor beta (TGFβ), for example, are important for healing and repair. Cytokines therefore have harmful as well as beneficial effects upon the patient.

For many years, the substances thought to be responsible for the fever associated with infection, tissue breakdown and necrosis, e.g. after traumatic injury or myocardial infarction, were a group of peptides called endogenous pyrogens (EPs). The endogenous pyrogens have now been shown to

include specific molecules and are collectively called interleukins. Interleukin-1 (IL-1) is generally believed to be the centrally acting pyrogen which acts in the brain to raise the set-point temperature to a higher level. IL-1 can be detected in the circulation in some but not all diseases. For example, after severe acute respiratory syndrome in children, patients have markedly elevated levels of IL-1 (Ng et al 2004). High levels of circulating IL-1 are also reported after acute myocardial infarction (Francis et al 2004) and stroke (Lucas et al 2006).

Release of IL-1 into the circulation is probably stimulated by other interleukins produced outside the brain. Interleukin-6 (IL-6), for example, is a cytokine produced by a number of different cells such as activated macrophages, monocytes, keratinocytes, fibroblasts and others. It is thought that IL-6 released at the site of inflammation or injury triggers the production of IL-1 in the brain. In the brain, IL-1 probably stimulates production of a group of substances called prostaglandins. These substances are thought ultimately to be responsible for elevating the thermoregulatory set-point (Ranels & Griffin 2003).

Chills and rigors

A sudden onset of fever with a 'chill' or 'rigor' is characteristic of some diseases. For example, the rigors associated with malaria are diagnostic of the infection and are often portrayed in novels and films as a serious symptom of tropical disease. Repeated rigors are typical not only of pyrogenic infections and bacteraemia but are now also recognised as a symptom of viral as well as bacterial infections. Rigors and chills also occur in other febrile illnesses and can be demonstrated experimentally. For example, fever can be induced in human volunteers by safe, intravenous administration of a pyrogen called endotoxin. Endotoxin is a lipopolysaccharide molecule produced by Gram-negative bacteria. In human volunteer studies of thermoregulation and metabolism, endotoxin administration produces a 1–1.5°C rise in body temperature, accompanied by chills, shivering, myalgia and flu-like symptoms. These symptoms begin approximately 90 min after the endotoxin is administered. All the symptoms disappear after 5–6 h (Soop et al 2002).

A chill or rigor is accompanied by intense feelings of cold. The patient's skin will be white or blue and cold and they will probably pull their bedclothes tightly around themselves and curl their body. Their teeth may chatter and they will feel very uncomfortable. Intense shivering and violent jerking movements will be uncontrollable.

Fever in myocardial infarction

Myocardial infarction is an example of a condition in which there is an acute rise in deep body temperature, probably due to release of pro-inflammatory cytokines from the injured myocardium (Francis et al 2004). Typically, body temperature rises after the first 24 h to 37.8–39.9°C and remains elevated for 2–3 days. By day 5, however, deep body temperature returns to normal. It is thought that the pattern of elevated body temperature reflects necrosis of myocardial tissue (see Ch. 2). If fever persists after the fifth day, the nurse should consider infection such as pneumonia, thrombophlebitis or a systemic infection as a possible cause.

How heat illness develops

Unlike fever, where the rise in temperature is part of an orchestrated and biological response to infection, inflammation or injury, heat illness and the more serious condition of heat stroke is due to an excessive, and often accidental overexposure to heat. This frequently can occur during hard exercise of endurance athletes (Lim et al 2006). Heat illness is a term which includes the following three clinical conditions:

- heat illness
- heat exhaustion
- heat stroke.

An elevated body temperature is not usually diagnostic of heat illness (or even of fever) but a rather non-specific signature of an underlying disturbance in homeostasis. In heat illness it indicates an increase in the heat content of cells and tissues. If extreme, this increase in tissue temperature can damage cell structures leading to a loss of function.

Heat illness can be a minor medical problem or so severe that it poses a threat to life. Its primary cause is not an inflammatory process (although this may develop if heat illness is not abated) but a variety of factors which can result in excessive heat storage. Similarly, overwrapping an infant by putting on too many clothes or leaving them in a closed space (such as a car with the windows closed) on a sunny day could lead to a mild form of heat illness. If exposure to a hot environment persists, dehydration could mark the onset of a fatal case of heat stroke. Another situation that can cause heat stroke is use of the 'recreational' drug MDMA, also known as ecstasy. This drug can lead to excessive heat production and a sudden and serious rise in body temperature (see website Box 22.5).

 See website Box 22.5

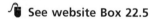

▷ Nursing management and health promotion: fever

Nursing the patient with fever is a skill. It demands knowledge of the mechanisms of thermoregulatory disturbance as well as good clinical practice. It is important for the nurse to appreciate the difference in the management of a patient with fever compared to hyperthermia due to heat stroke.

Fever may start abruptly with a shaking chill, or it can develop with little more than a sense of malaise and discomfort. When measured, core temperature may remain high or it may fluctuate (Edwards 1998). A fluctuating temperature with peaks and troughs can occur naturally as discussed on page 620, but in hospital, a peak followed by a trough is more likely to be due to the effects of administration of an antipyretic, such as paracetamol, or vigorous, often inappropriate, use of body surface cooling. A care plan for observation of a patient you suspect is developing a high temperature and the care you might consider can be found on the website.

 See website Table 22.2

In heat stress or heat stroke the primary problem is one of heat imbalance: too much heat stored, not enough body heat

lost. This can occur in elite athletes after a marathon or after too much sunbathing. In both situations the problem for the person is the same. Antipyretics are ineffective because the set-point remains unchanged. The first line of treatment is to aid the dissipation of heat from the body and to rehydrate the body. Mild cases of 'sunstroke' can be corrected by moving out of the sun and in to a cool environment so that heat can be lost from the body by radiation and convection: the dry heat loss routes. Cold drinks will also be helpful and comforting. In extreme situations, heat exhaustion may occur. The person is unable to lose heat by sweating because the sweat glands fail to produce sweat. The most effective treatment is to expose the body and spray the skin with warm (not cold) water to promote vaporisational heat loss, whilst taking care not to cause peripheral vasoconstriction. Heat exhaustion is a major risk for soldiers during combat in a hot climate.

Hypothermia

Hypothermia is a state in which the temperature of the body is lower than the thermoregulatory set-point. This situation can occur accidentally, i.e. spontaneous or accidental hypothermia, or it can be induced deliberately, i.e. therapeutic hypothermia. Nurses may encounter patients who have had a prolonged period of cold exposure due to an accident either inside or outside the home. In hospital, a subnormal temperature may occur in a patient who has undergone a prolonged surgical procedure. Nurses also now encounter therapies employing techniques specifically to lower the temperature of the body below normal to achieve hypothermia.

 See website Box 22.6

Causes of accidental hypothermia

Although accidental hypothermia does occur in fit young people, it is more often seen in neonates shortly after birth or in older people living at home. The young and the old are the most vulnerable to the effects of cold, particularly during the winter months. Resistance to cold in the fit and healthy person depends upon an efficient thermoregulatory system

Some impairment of thermoregulation may play a role in the predisposition of older people to the adverse effects of cold. Perception of cold may be impaired and the individual may therefore not respond to falling temperatures appropriately, for example by putting on extra clothing. Many older people become confined to a chair or their bed, so it is difficult for them to get up to put on extra clothes even when they do begin to feel the cold. Those caring for older people at home can help by leaving extra warm clothing close at hand to be used when needed. Wearing a hat at home may be useful to reduce heat loss from the head by convection. This is because a hat insulates the large surface area of the head and to some extent the face, thus reducing the transfer of heat from the body (especially if seated in a draft) to the room. Ensuring the older person has warm drinks close by, perhaps in a flask, and encouraging them to drink these, will help to warm the body.

Older people do not have the same ability as young adults to generate heat within the body because the metabolic rate for heat production is reduced with age. Other factors that may reduce the ability of the body to produce heat are:

- malnutrition
- hypothyroidism (see Ch. 5)
- hypoglycaemia, which may be a particular problem in older adults with diabetes, as it lowers the threshold for the onset of shivering (Passias et al 1996); this means that a much greater fall in body temperature can occur before a hypoglycaemic patient starts to shiver
- intoxication with alcohol, because it limits the availability of glucose; the resulting hypoglycaemia inhibits shivering thermogenesis.

In the UK, accidental hypothermia in older people is a real hazard (Ranhoff 2000). Sadly, each winter, there are newspaper reports of older people who have died of hypothermia – deaths that are preventable. The British media (BBC News Online 2001) reported that millions of older people lived in a cold home and could not afford to pay their fuel bills. With an estimated 30 000 deaths each year in cold weather, it is hoped that schemes to improve home insulation and winter fuel allowances will make a positive impact in reducing accidental hypothermia in the older population.

Donaldson et al (1998) found that even in the coldest regions of the earth, such as Eastern Siberia, mortality from hypothermia is not as high as it is during winter in regions where the climate is more temperate. This is thought to be because the population in extremely cold regions is better at using simple precautions to prevent themselves becoming cold. For example, they wear very warm clothing in several layers and stay as much as possible in their houses, which they keep warm.

When community nurses visit older people during the winter months, some assessment of their environment and of their thermoregulatory system should be made. If the nurse thinks that the patient's house is too cold, assessment of the risk of hypothermia should be carried out. The nurse should ensure that the thermometer selected is adequate for use with patients who may have a temperature well below normal (see p. 617).

Nursing management and health promotion: hypothermia

Safe rewarming of a person who has developed hypothermia must be undertaken with care; patients may die several hours after arriving in the Emergency Department, even following an apparently successful rescue. This phenomenon, which has become known as 'after-drop', first came to prominence during the First World War during sea rescues of servicemen and women. After prolonged immersion in cold water, victims, alive when rescued and taken on board ship, died shortly afterwards despite receiving emergency rewarming treatment. These 'late' deaths after apparently successful rescue were a real tragedy and for many years were unexplained. It is now known, however, that 'after-drop' is a consequence of inappropriate rewarming. As the patient is warmed, blood vessels at the extremities dilate and a large volume of very cold blood flows from the extremities to the heart. This results in severe cardiac complications, e.g. ventricular fibrillation, and death follows.

The most appropriate way to rewarm a hypothermic patient after immersion in cold water also applies to the person subjected to cold exposure. The first step is to stop any further heat loss from the body, either by removing wet clothing or if this is not possible (due to the suspicion of a neck fracture for example) by wrapping the body in a blanket (e.g. a 'space' blanket), which prevents convective or evaporative heat transfer. This is called 'passive' rewarming and it allows core temperature to rise slowly by the gradual build-up of body heat resulting from natural heat production. Providing that all endogenously produced body heat is retained within the body, organ temperature will gradually rise. If core temperature is above 32°C, passive rewarming is the method of choice, for example with hypothermia following surgery. If core temperature is below 32°C and the patient is a young adult who has become hypothermic as a result of immersion in cold water or from exposure, 'active' rewarming of core tissues is required. There are a number of methods available, including:

- gastric lavage with warmed saline
- the introduction of warmed humidified oxygen in air via a ventilator
- the administration of warmed intravenous fluids
- warm peritoneal lavage.

It remains to be determined whether active or passive rewarming procedures are better in the treatment of accidental hypothermia in patients receiving intensive care (Vassal et al 2001).

In older patients, careful active rewarming is required (Ranhoff 2000). In all patients it is important to remember that if the skin surface is warmed first, blood flow to the extremities will be increased. For older people with pre-existing cardiovascular disease, this could precipitate a fall in blood pressure. With active rewarming, core temperature can rise from 0.6 to 1.9°C/h (Stoner & Randall 1990). Slow rewarming methods include intravenous solutions heated to 45°C (17 kcal/h), heated, humidified oxygen by mask (30 kcal/h or 0.7°C/h), warmed blankets (0.9°C/h), and heated, humidified oxygen via endotracheal tube (1.2°C/h). As core temperature rises, shivering may start and will become maximal at about 35°C.

Local cold injuries

Frostbite

When tissue freezes, ice crystals form and the substances in tissue fluid become concentrated. The ice crystals can be many times the size of the cell itself. The degree of cell death after freezing depends on the concentration of the solute. Tissue damage resulting from freezing very much resembles a burn injury. See website Box 22.7 for an account of the effects of exposure to extreme cold.

See website Box 22.7

The milder form of freezing injury is called 'frost nip'. The extremities, i.e. nose, ear lobes, cheeks, fingertips, hands and feet, can be affected, but treatment is by simple rewarming of the affected area. A more serious form of cold injury is frostbite. In this condition, blood vessels are damaged and blood circulation to the affected part stops. The congested blood causes agglutination of cells, resulting in thrombus formation. The severe conditions that result in frostbite can mean that the person is so cold that they neglect to care for the frostbitten tissues and that, if rewarming does occur because of improvements in weather conditions, the frostbitten areas become macerated.

Treatment for frostbitten limbs should aim to warm the core tissues first before treating the local damage. The affected limb can then be immersed in water at 10–15°C. The water temperature should then be raised every 5 min by 5°C to a maximum of 40°C. Antibiotics may be necessary if there is any evidence of infection, particularly if a risk of frostbite-associated tetanus is suspected. Booster injection in previously immunised individuals is recommended to prevent this potentially lethal syndrome. These should be supplemented with tetanus Ig, 250 U intramuscularly, if the patient is not fully immunised. Local treatment will require care of the wound together with early physiotherapy.

Raynaud's phenomenon

Raynaud's phenomenon develops most often in young women and is due to abnormal stimulation of vasoconstrictor nerves (see Ch. 2). The cause of this abnormal vasoconstriction is thought to be more complex than simply increased vasoconstriction on exposure to a change in air temperature and may involve microvascular changes in the endothelium (Gardner-Medwin et al 2001). The fingers are mainly affected; spasm of the digital arteries causes sluggish circulation in the fingers, which then become cyanosed. The intense vasoconstriction causes the arteries to empty of blood and this leads to the typical 'dead' white appearance of the fingers. When the vasoconstrictor spasm has passed, the circulation starts to flow again. At this stage the individual experiences tingling and throbbing followed by intense pain. In some people, vasoconstriction can be so severe and prolonged that the skin of the fingertips becomes ulcerated and necrosed, a condition known as 'Raynaud's disease'. Raynaud's phenomenon generally worsens in winter.

Nursing care of individuals with Raynaud's phenomenon should be directed towards helping them to avoid the stimuli which they know cause their fingers, and toes, to go 'dead'. For some people, simply wearing gloves may be sufficient precaution. Pocket hand warmers, often used by people involved in outdoor sports and pursuits, e.g. golfers and hill walkers, are very useful in preventing attacks but they should be used before the person goes out into the cold, as once the hands have become cold a pocket hand warmer is unlikely to be sufficient to reverse vasoconstriction. In severe cases, vasodilator drugs or sympathectomy may be necessary.

SUMMARY: KEY NURSING ISSUES

- The maintenance of a stable homeostatic environment is one of the most fundamental components of nursing observation.
- Measurement of temperature is a good example of how the nurses use their professional skills to appraise physiological stability.
- Due to circadian rhythms body temperature fluctuates in a characteristic pattern over a 24-h period. By the evening, body temperature may be as much as 1.0°C above the early morning temperature.

- The ability to make decisions to act on temperature deviation requires an understanding of the pathophysiology of human thermoregulation. However, as the interventions available to raise or lower body core temperature are numerous, the nurse is often confronted with making a decision about when/when not to intervene.
- The high body temperature associated with fever is due to an upward re-set in the central hypothalamic set-point temperature.
- The boundaries are beginning to blur with regard to the available therapies designed to protect the body in some patients, whilst in others the same therapies would be considered injurious. Distinctions should be made between the untoward effects of accidental hypothermia in the patient with systemic trauma and the potential benefit of therapeutic hypothermia in patients with brain damage.
- In brain-injured patients, a rise in temperature of 1–2°C above normal is linked to a poor neurological outcome. However, the evidence for an adverse neurological outcome due to raised temperature remains unproven.
- The young and the old are the most vulnerable to the effects of cold, particularly during the winter months. Older people do not have the same ability as young adults to generate heat within the body because the metabolic rate for heat production is reduced with age.
- Safe rewarming of a person who has developed hypothermia must be undertaken with care to prevent 'after-drop', which occurs when blood vessels at the extremities dilate and a large volume of very cold blood flows from the extremities to the heart. This results in ventricular fibrillation, and death follows.

⟳ REFLECTION AND LEARNING – WHAT NEXT?

- **Test** your knowledge by visiting the website 🖱 and answering the multiple choice questions and critical thinking questions.
- **Consolidate** your learning by looking at some of the further reading suggestions, references and specialist websites.
- **Revisit** some of the additional material on the website.
- **Consider** what you have learnt and how this will help your professional development.
- **Reflect** on how you can apply this knowledge to the care of your patients.
- **Discuss** your learning with your mentor/supervisor, lecturer and colleagues.

REFERENCES

Aschoff J, Wever R: cited in Stainer MW, Mount LE, Bligh J, 1984. *Energy balance and temperature regulation*, Cambridge, 1958, Cambridge University Press.

Bayley N, Stolz HR: Maturational changes in rectal temperature of 61 infants from 1–36 months, *Child Dev* 8(3):195–206, 1937.

BBC News Online: *Plan to cut deaths in cold homes*, 2001. Available online http://www.news.bbc.co.uk.

Brogan P, Childs C, Phillips BM, et al: Evaluation of a tympanic thermometer in children, *Lancet* 342:1364–1365, 1993.

Cannon B, Nedergaard J: Brown adipose tissue: function and physiological significance, *Physiol Rev* 84(1):277–359, 2004.

Childs C: Studies in children provide a model to re-examine the metabolic response to burn injury in children treated by contemporary burn protocols, *Burns* 20:291–300, 1994.

Childs C: Human brain temperature regulation, measurement and relationship to cerebral trauma. Part 1, *Br J Neurosurg* 22(4):486–496, 2008.

Childs C, Little RA: Acute changes in oxygen consumption and body temperature after burn injury, *Arch Dis Child* 71:31–34, 1994.

Childs C, Harrison R, Hodkinson C, et al: Tympanic membrane temperature as a measure of core temperature, *Arch Dis Child* 80(3):262–266, 1999.

Childs C, Vail A, Protheroe R, et al: Differences between brain and rectal temperatures during routine critical care of patients with severe traumatic brain injury, *Anaesthesia* 60:1–7, 2005.

Cole RP, Shakespeare PG, Chissell HG, et al: Thermographic assessment of burns using a non permeable wound covering, *Burns* 17:117–122, 1991.

Craig JV, Lancaster GA, Taylor S, et al: Infrared ear thermometry compared with rectal thermometry in children: a systematic review, *Lancet* 360:603–609, 2002.

Donaldson GC, Ermakov SP, Komarov YM, et al: Cold related mortalities and protection against cold in Yukutsk, Eastern Siberia: observation and interview study, *Br Med J* 317:978, 1998.

Edwards SL: High temperature, *Prof Nurs* 13(8):521–526, 1998.

Francis J, Zhang ZH, Weiss RM, et al: Neural regulation of the pro-inflammatory cytokine response to acute myocardial infarction, *Am J Physiol Heart Circ Physiol* 287(2):H791–H797, 2004.

Frayn KN: *Metabolic regulation – a human perspective*, Oxford, 1997, Portland Press.

Gardner-Medwin JM, Macdonald IA, Taylor JY, et al: Seasonal differences in finger skin temperature and microvascular blood flow in healthy men and women are exaggerated in women with Raynaud's phenomenon, *Br J Clin Pharmacol* 52(1):17–23, 2001.

Greer DM, Funk SE, Reaven NL, et al: Impact of fever on outcome in patients with stroke and neurologic injury: a comprehensive meta-analysis, *Stroke* 39(11):3029–3035, 2008.

Hoffman C, Boyd M, Briere B, et al: Evaluation of three brands of tympanic thermometer, *Can J Nurs Res* 31(1):117–130, 1999.

Houdas Y, Ring EFJ: *Human body temperature*, New York, 1982, Plenum Press.

Hull D: Temperature regulation and disturbance in the newborn infant, *Clin Endocrinol Metab* 5:39–54, 1976.

Jenney MEM, Childs C, Mahin D, et al: Oxygen consumption during sleep in atopic dermatitis, *Arch Dis Child* 72:144–146, 1995.

Kimberger O, Cohen D, Illievich U, et al: Temporal artery versus bladder thermometry during perioperative and intensive care unit monitoring, *Anesth Analg* 105(4):1042–1047, 2007.

Kirk D, Rainey R, Vail A, et al: Infra-red thermometry in neurocritical care: How reliable are tympanum and temporal artery measurements for predicting brain temperature? *Critical Care* 13(3):R81, 2009.

Klaus S: Adipose tissue as a regulator of energy balance, *Curr Drug Targets* 5(3):241–250, 2004.

Kluger MJ: *Fever: its biology, evolution and function*, Princeton, 1979, Princeton University Press.

Larsen SU: Reye's syndrome, *Med Sci Law* 37:235–241, 1997.

LeFrant J-Y, Muller L, Emmanuel Coussaye J, et al: Temperature measurement in intensive care patients: comparison of urinary bladder, oesophageal, rectal, axillary and inguinal methods versus pulmonary artery core method, *Intensive Care Med* 29:414–418, 2003.

Lim CL, Mackinnon LT: The roles of exercise-induced immune system disturbances in the pathology of heat stroke: the dual pathway model of heat stroke, *Sports Med* 36(1):39–64, 2006.

Lucas SM, Rothwell NJ, Gibson RM, et al: The role of inflammation in CNS injury and disease, *Br J Pharmacol* 147(Suppl 1):S232–S240, 2006.

Macqueen S: Clinical benefits of 3M Tempa-Dot thermometer in the paediatric setting, *Br J Nurs* 10(1):55–58, 2001.

Moran JL, Peter JV, Solomon PJ, et al: Tympanic temperature measurements: Are they reliable in the critically ill? A clinical study of measures of agreement, *Crit Care Med* 35(1), 2007.

Morley C, Murray M, Whybrew K, et al: The relative accuracy of mercury, Tempa-Dot and Fever Scan thermometers, *Early Hum Dev* 53:171–178, 1998.

Natale J, Joseph JG, Helfaer M, et al: Early hyperthermia after traumatic brain injury in children: risk factors, influence on length of stay and effect on short-term neurological status, *Crit Care Med* 28:2608–2615, 2000.

Ng PC, Lam CW, Li AM, et al: Inflammatory cytokine profile in children with severe acute respiratory distress syndrome, *Pediatrics* 113(1):e7–e14, 2004.

Passias TC, Meneilly GS, Mekjavic IB, et al: Effect of hypoglycaemia on thermoregulatory responses, *J Appl Physiol* 80(3):1021–1032, 1996.

Ranels HJ, Griffin JD: The effects of prostaglandin E2 on the firing rate activity of thermosensitive and temperature insensitive neurons in the ventromedial preoptic area of the rat hypothalamus, *Brain Res* 964(1):42–50, 2003.

Ranhoff AH: Accidental hypothermia in the elderly, *Int J Circumpolar Health* 59:255–259, 2000.

Sacho RH, Childs C: The significance of altered temperature after traumatic brain injury: an analysis of investigations in experimental and human studies: Part 2, *Br J Neurosurg* 22(4):497–507, 2008.

Soop M, Duxbury H, Agwunobe AO, et al: Euglycaemic hyperinsulinaemia augments the cytokine and endocrine responses to endotoxin in humans, *Am J Physiol Endocrinol Metab* 282:E1276–E1285, 2002.

Stainer MW, Mount LE, Bligh J, et al: *Energy balance and temperature regulation*, Cambridge, 1984, Cambridge University Press.

Stoner HB, Randall PE: The metabolic aspects of hypothermia. In Cohen RD, Lewis B, Alberti KGMM, Denman AM, editors: *The metabolic and molecular basis of acquired disease*, London, 1990, Baillière Tindall.

Talo H, Macknin ML, Medendorp SV, et al: Tympanic membrane temperatures compared to rectal and oral temperatures, *Clin Pediatr (Phila)* (Suppl):30–35, 1991.

Tortora GJ, Derrickson B: *Principles of anatomy and physiology*, ed 11, New York, 2006, John Wiley & Sons Inc.

Vassal T, Benoit-Gonin B, Carrat F, et al: Severe accidental hypothermia treated in an ICU: prognosis and outcome, *Chest* 120(6):1998–2003, 2001.

Ward MR: Reye's syndrome: an update, *Nurse Pract* 12:45–53, 1997.

Waterhouse J, Weinert D, Nevill A, et al: Some factors influencing the sensitivity of body temperature activity in neonates, *Chronobiol Int* 17(5):679–692, 2000.

Wilmore DW: *The metabolic management of the critically ill*, London, 1977, Plenum.

Wyllie FJ, Sutherland AB: Measurement of surface temperature as an aid to the diagnosis of burn depth, *Burns* 17:123–128, 1991.

FURTHER READING

Bernard SA, Gray TW, Buist MD, et al: Treatment of comatose survivors of out-of-hospital cardiac arrest with induced hypothermia, *N Engl J Med* 346:557–563, 2002.

Bland JM, Altman DG. Statistical methods for assessing agreement between two methods of clinical measurement, *Lancet* 327:307–310, 1986.

Bligh J: *Temperature regulation in mammals and other vertebrates*, Amsterdam, 1973, North Holland Publishing Company.

Childs C: Fever in burned children, *Burns* 14(1):1–6, 1988.

Clifton GL, Miller ER, Choi SC, et al: Lack of effect of induction of hypothermia after acute brain injury, *N Engl J Med* 344:556–562, 2001.

Crossmann AR, Neary D: *Neuroanatomy*, Edinburgh, 2005, Churchill Livingstone.

Fay T, Smith GW: Observations on reflex responses during prolonged periods of human refrigeration, *Arch Neurol Psychiatry* 45:215–222, 1941.

Guthrie JR, Dennerstein L, Hopper JL, et al: Hot flushes, menstrual status, and hormone levels in a population-based sample of midlife women, *Obstet Gynecol* 88:437–442, 1996.

Hutchison JS, Ward RE, Lacroix J, et al: Hypothermia therapy after traumatic brain injury in children, *N Engl J Med* 358:2447–2456, 2008.

MacLennan A, Lester S, Moore V, et al: Oral oestrogen replacement therapy versus placebo for hot flushes, *Cochrane Database Syst Rev* (1) CD002978, 2001.

Reith J, Jorgensen HS, Pederson PM, et al: Body temperature in acute stroke: relation to stroke severity, infarct size, mortality and outcome, *Lancet* 347:422–425, 1996.

Sharma HS, Syed F: Acute administration of 3,4-methylene-dioxymethamphetamine induces profound hyperthermia, blood–brain barrier disruption, brain edema formation, and cell injury. An experimental study in rats and mice usingbiochemical and morphologic approaches, *Ann N Y Acad Sci* 1139:242–258, 2008.

Stroud MA: Thermoregulation, exercise and nutrition in the cold: investigations on a polar expedition. In Kinney JM, Tucker HN, editors: *Physiology, stress and malnutrition: functional correlates, nutritional intervention*, Philadelphia, 1997, Lippincott-Raven, pp 531–548.

Stroud MA: *Survival of the fittest?* London, 1998, Jonathan Cape.

Tissue viability and managing chronic wounds

Jacqui Fletcher, Irene Anderson

Introduction

For most people, the word 'wound' conjures up thoughts of a cut, a graze or a surgical incision that heals without difficulty. For nurses, however, wound management is a complex aspect of patient care, requiring knowledge and expertise. Nurses care for patients with wounds in many settings, including patients with surgical incisions nursed in hospital or at home, those with chronic leg ulcers nursed at home, and patients with industrial injury or trauma treated at their workplace.

The impact of a wound on an individual can be considerable. Pain, fear and scarring are the most obvious, but individuals vary in their response to having a wound. For some, restriction in social activity, or the loss of earnings, should also be considered alongside the psychological effects of altered body image (Wilson 2000).

The presence of a wound will inevitably have some effect on well-being. There may be no difficulty when a wound is small and heals rapidly, but many patients experience anxiety relating to the wound (Atkinson 2002). This can disrupt sleep, increase pain perception and impair immune function. In more serious wounds, a disturbance of body image may also cause lasting distress, particularly if the patient is unprepared for this (Wilson 2000).

The healing process comprises a complex series of events that depend on a number of factors, and in order for it to proceed at its optimal rate the individual concerned should be in good health. In caring for patients with wounds, nurses have an important role in promoting health.

Clinical effectiveness and the delivery of evidence-based care are key to wound management.

Wound definition, types and classification

A wound is a defect or breach in the continuity of the skin. This is an injury to the skin or underlying tissues/organs caused by surgery, a blow, a cut, chemicals, heat/cold, friction/shear force, pressure or as a result of disease, such as leg ulcers and cancers.

There is no clear-cut method of classifying wounds. Some practitioners refer to wounds by anatomical site, e.g. abdominal wall wounds. Others classify wounds by their depth, e.g. epidermal loss, subcutaneous wounds. Another possible classification is by degree of tissue loss (Dealey 1999). In the first group, there are wounds with little or no tissue loss where the skin edges can be brought together and sutured. In the second, there is substantial tissue loss and the skin edges cannot be brought together. A further description may be to group wounds by their potential to heal, with wounds being described as acute or chronic (Fletcher 2008a).

Epidemiology

The epidemiology of wounds is not clearly documented. Because people with wounds can be found in almost every specialty, information relating specifically to wounds is not consistently collected. Posnett & Franks (2007) identify that there are over 200 000 individuals at any one time with a chronic wound in the UK, with costs estimated to be as high as £2.3–3.1 bn per year (at 2005/2006 prices), around 3% of total estimated expenditure on health (£89.4 bn). These figures do not address acute wounds which would add a considerable additional burden.

Physiology of wound healing

A number of cell types are involved in the healing process (Table 23.1).

Tissue repair

The wound healing process comprises a complex series of events whereby the continuity and strength of damaged tissues are restored by the formation of connective tissue and regrowth of epithelium. The process can be divided into four phases (Figure 23.1) but, since wound healing is a continuous biological process, there is some overlap between them.

Phase I – haemostasis

As soon as a wound occurs, it bleeds and blood initially fills the wound defect. Platelets aggregate and degranulate, resulting in clot formation and haemostasis. A fibrin clot forms as the blood coagulates and acts as a preliminary matrix or scaffold within the wound into which cells can migrate.

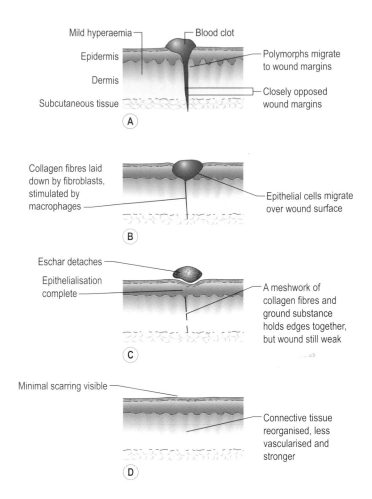

Figure 23.1 Wound healing by primary intention. A. Haemostasis. B. Inflammation. C. Proliferation/reconstruction phase. D. Maturation phase.

Phase II – inflammation

The fibrin clot begins to degrade and the surrounding capillaries dilate and become permeable, allowing fluid into the wound site. This activates the complement system, several interacting soluble proteins found in serum and extracellular fluid that induce lysis and destruction of target cells, such as bacteria. Cytokines and proteolytic fragments are also found in the wound space (Steed 1997), which initiate a massive influx of other cells. The two main inflammatory cells are neutrophils and macrophages:

- Neutrophils flood into the wound shortly after injury and reach peak numbers within 24–48 h. They destroy bacteria through the process of phagocytosis. Neutrophils have a very short lifespan and their numbers reduce rapidly 3 days post injury, provided there is no infection.
- Tissue macrophages, like neutrophils, destroy bacteria and debris through phagocytosis. However, the macrophage is also a rich source of biological regulators, including cytokines and growth factors, bioactive lipid products, and proteolytic enzymes, elements essential for the normal healing process (Slavin 1999).

This phase is one of biological 'cleansing'. It does, however, make considerable metabolic demands on the body. Much heat and fluid can also be lost. The shorter the

Table 23.1 Important cells in wound healing	
CELL	**FUNCTION**
Endothelial cells	Help to achieve haemostasis
Polymorphonuclear leucocytes ('polymorphs')	Take part in the initial inflammatory response
Macrophages	Digest debris and stimulate other cells to function; orchestrate wound healing processes
Fibroblasts	Produce collagen
Myofibroblasts	Aid wound contraction by producing mature collagen

duration of this phase, the better, because as it nears completion, proliferation or formation of new tissue can begin. Following the inflammatory phase, the wound site is prepared for the repair process to begin.

Phase III – proliferation/reconstruction

Tissue repair takes place during this phase. It usually begins at around day three and lasts for some weeks. Proliferation is characterised by the formation of granulation tissue in the wound space. This new tissue consists of a matrix of fibrin, fibronectin, collagens, proteoglycans and glycosaminoglycans, and other glycoproteins (Hart 2002). Fibroblasts move into the wound space and proliferate. Their function is to synthesise and deposit extracellular proteins, producing growth factors and angiogenic factors that regulate cell proliferation and angiogenesis (Stephens & Thomas 2002). Fibroblasts will multiply rapidly in the well-nourished individual and, to be most effective, need adequate amounts of vitamin C, iron, oxygen and nutrients. Granulation tissue also contains elastin, providing the wound with elasticity and resilience (Wysocki 2007).

Angiogenesis is the formation of new blood vessels in the wound space which are essential for the delivery of oxygen and other nutrients. The key cells involved in angiogenesis are the vascular endothelial cells, which arise from the damaged end of vessels and capillaries (Neal 2001). New vessels sprout from existing small vessels at the wound edge, endothelial cells detaching from these small vessels and penetrating the wound space. These sprouts are then extended in length until they meet other capillaries, connecting together to form new vascular loops and networks.

Re-epithelialisation begins a few hours after injury and continues as the wound begins to fill with granulation tissue. At the wound edges, epithelial cells divide and, gradually, epithelium migrates from the edges towards the middle of the wound. Epithelialisation of larger areas is achieved not only by migration, but also by rapid division of epithelial cells near hair follicles, which might be present deep in the dermis. Islands of epithelium appear wherever a follicle is present. Cells migrate from these islands to meet each other, while cells from the edges of the wound grow inwards to cover the raw surface.

The final feature of proliferation is wound contraction, beginning around day five. Wound contraction is a dynamic process where cells reorganise the surrounding connective tissue, reducing the amount of granulation tissue. This effect is mostly due to the activity of fibroblasts and myofibroblasts which, under the influence of cytokines, contract to pull the wound edges together.

Phase IV – maturation

Maturation usually begins around 7 days post injury and continues for many months or years, long after the wound looks to be closed or healed. The immature collagen laid down earlier is gradually replaced by a mature collagen. The formation of new collagen and the lysis of immature collagen are balanced so that the amount of collagen present remains constant. The immature collagen is laid down in a random, haphazard fashion, its function being to fill the wound defect as quickly as possible. The remodelling process involves the balance between synthesis and degradation of collagen, where the cells producing the different types of collagen are subjected to apoptosis (programmed cell death) (Tjero-Trujeque 2001). Mature collagen is laid down following lines of tension within the wound, and is cross-linked to give strength. Tensile strength at 14 days in sutured wounds is approximately 10% of the original strength of the skin. Within 3 weeks this increases to 20%, gradually reaching a maximum of 70–80% about 1 year later.

Healing by primary/first intention

Following wounding, treatment aims to effect complete healing as quickly as possible with minimal scarring. To achieve this, the method of choice is healing by primary intention, which occurs when wound edges are in apposition. There is minimal formation of granulation tissue and, once the wound has healed, only a thin scar remains. Healing by primary intention is only possible where there is adequate, mobile tissue and no complicating bacterial contamination. In situations where contamination is suspected, wound closure is accompanied by the use of prophylactic systemic antibiotics. For healing to take place by primary intention, the wound edges need to be closely approximated and held together until the wound has healed sufficiently. The skin may be closed by using tapes, clips, continuous or interrupted sutures, or glue (Figure 23.2).

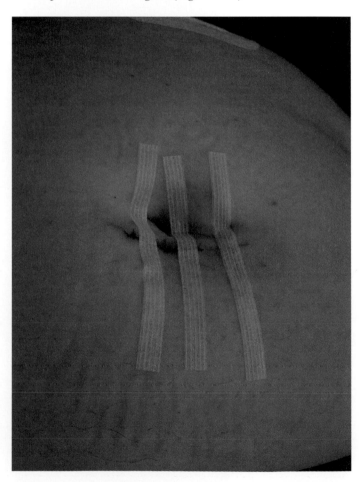

Figure 23.2 Wound healing by primary intention – wound edges in apposition, held by Steristrips®.

Healing by secondary intention

Where there is significant tissue loss and/or bacterial contamination, wounds are usually left open to heal by secondary intention through the formation of granulation tissue and, later, wound contraction (Figure 23.3). Due to the amount of tissue excised or lost during injury, wound healing by secondary intention is a longer process, taking weeks or even months to complete. The healing process proceeds in much the same way as for healing by primary intention. The proliferative phase is much extended, as this is when granulation tissue forms and fills the wound defect. It was established many years ago (Marks et al 1983) that, for some wounds, the length of time taken to heal depends on the original size, i.e. small wounds heal more quickly than larger ones, and it is therefore possible in some wound types (pilonidal sinus, abdominal and axillary wounds) to predict when wounds of a given size that are free from infection will heal.

Scar tissue

A scar is the mark that may remain after healing. It consists of relatively avascular collagen fibres covered by a thin layer of epithelium.

Most scars fade with time and the resultant cosmetic effect is generally acceptable, but abnormal scarring can lead to problems, as follows:

See website Figure 23.1

- *Stretching of scar tissue* – can occur where sutures have been removed prematurely, especially over areas that are under tension, e.g. the skin over the scapula and back.

- *Hypertrophic scar tissue* – collagen lysis and collagen production are out of synchrony and excessive tissue lies within the boundaries of the scar.
- *Keloid* – a protuberant, prominent scar resulting from excessive dermal collagen formation during connective tissue repair.

Hypertrophic and keloidal scarring are examples of excessive scar formation. Such scarring is more common in young people, especially during puberty and pregnancy, and also in dark skins, the peristernal area being particularly susceptible.

Box 23.1 outlines factors influencing scarring.

Factors that adversely affect healing

Many factors can adversely affect the normal rate of healing, slowing it down and, in severe cases, impairing it altogether. These factors can be described as pathophysiological (see below), psychological or practical (Harding 2007).

Pathophysiological factors

This section outlines intrinsic and extrinsic pathophysiological factors. These can be systemic factors such as malnutrition, or local wound factors including the presence of clot, devitalised tissue, foreign bodies, local hypoxia or infection.

Intrinsic factors

Advanced age

With advanced age the dermis gradually thins and the underlying structural support, collagen, reduces (see Ch. 34). Reduced collagen production results in loss of skin elasticity

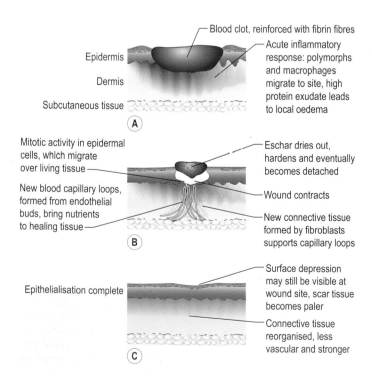

Figure 23.3 Wound healing by secondary intention. A. Haemostasis/inflammation. B. Proliferation phase. C. Maturation phase.

Labels for A:
- Epidermis
- Dermis
- Subcutaneous tissue
- Blood clot, reinforced with fibrin fibres
- Acute inflammatory response: polymorphs and macrophages migrate to site, high protein exudate leads to local oedema

Labels for B:
- Mitotic activity in epidermal cells, which migrate over living tissue
- New blood capillary loops, formed from endothelial buds, bring nutrients to healing tissue
- Eschar dries out, hardens and eventually becomes detached
- Wound contracts
- New connective tissue formed by fibroblasts supports capillary loops

Labels for C:
- Epithelialisation complete
- Surface depression may still be visible at wound site, scar tissue becomes paler
- Connective tissue reorganised, less vascular and stronger

Box 23.1 Information

Factors influencing scarring

Cause of injury
- Burn/trauma
  - The site – contractures can occur over joints.
  - Dirty injuries caused by gravel can cause pigmentation.
- Surgery
  - The skill of the surgeon.
  - The type of suture material used, i.e. non-absorbable sutures, alongside the wound.

Race
- Extreme hypertrophic scarring is common in dark-skinned people and rare in Caucasians.

Age
- In infancy and childhood, scars resolve quickly.
- During pregnancy, hypertrophic scarring is more common.

Wound site
- Scars that follow the body's natural lines of skin tension do best.
- Scars that cross skin folds do less well.
- Scars on the shoulders, sternal area and back produce unsightly scarring.

and its ability for elastic recoil, leading to creases and wrinkles. The amount of subcutaneous fat reduces, and there is less of a cushion for underlying bone. The natural moisture from sebum secretions lessens, leading to increasing dryness of the skin. The consequence of ageing is dry, thin, inelastic skin that is susceptible to damage, with a reduced metabolic rate and prolonged healing.

✋ See website Figure 23.2

These factors, together with poor circulation associated with older age, affect the tensile wound strength.

Malnutrition

Malnutrition may result in delayed wound healing and the production of weak, poor quality scars (Pinchcofsky-Devin 1994).

Protein–energy malnutrition (PEM) is caused by an absolute or relative deficiency of energy and protein that affects between 19 and 50% of hospitalised patients (McLaren 1997). Several factors contribute to PEM including a reduced intake of nutrients, reduced digestion and absorption of nutrients, and increased metabolic use. McWhirter & Pennington (1994) reported that 200 out of 500 patients admitted to hospital were undernourished, and just over 100 lost weight during their admission. Other research supports these findings. McLaren (1997) estimates that although 70% of patients admitted to hospital are malnourished prior to admission, the remaining 30% develop PEM during their hospital stay.

   Malnutrition can impede healing by reducing tensile strength, increasing wound dehiscence and the likelihood of infection.

Nutrient deficiency The European Pressure Ulcer Advisory Panel (EPUAP) (2003) recommends a minimum daily intake of 30–35 g/kg body weight, with 1–1.5 g/kg/day of protein and 1 mL/kcal/day of fluid intake. These guidelines also recommend that nurses consider the quality of the food that patients are offered, along with removing the physical or social barriers to its consumption. The latest guideline states 'Offer high-protein mixed oral nutritional supplements and/or tube feeding, in addition to the usual diet, to individuals with nutritional risk and pressure ulcer risk because of acute or chronic diseases, or following a surgical intervention' (European Pressure Ulcer Advisory Panel and National Pressure Ulcer Advisory Panel [NPUAP] 2009, p. 14).

   Some people may have difficulty in maintaining adequate nutrition, e.g. an older person living alone may lose interest in cooking or a patient having chemotherapy may be unable to eat due to nausea. The importance of diet cannot be overemphasised, and wherever possible the nurse should ensure that the patient receives all the nutrients required for healing. The advice of a dietitian may be sought in an attempt to improve or supplement the nutritional status of vulnerable individuals (see Ch. 21).

Dehydration

The normal metabolic processes of an individual require approximately 2500 mL of water every 24 h. Dehydration disrupts cell metabolism and this will adversely affect wound healing.

Disease

Many disease processes can delay healing, e.g. anaemia, cardiovascular disorders, diabetes mellitus, cancer, inflammatory disease, immune disease and organ failure, as in any other disease that impairs immune function. Importantly some patients, particularly older people, have co-morbidities.

Impaired blood supply to the area (ischaemia)

Where the blood supply to the wounded area is impaired, insufficient nutrients and oxygen are supplied and the healing is prolonged, for example in patients with peripheral arterial disease and lower limb ulcers. Slower healing is to be expected anywhere where gross oedema is present.

Smoking

Smoking adversely affects the healing process in a number of ways. Smoking and the absorption of nicotine has a vasoconstricting effect. The main influences of nicotine and carbon dioxide relate to the effects on peripheral tissues, with a reduction in tissue oxygen tension and the formation of thrombi. Nicotine has been demonstrated to inhibit epithelialisation (Waldrop & Doughty 2000) and the healing of abdominal wounds, the overall cosmetic effect of a scar being poorer in patients who were smokers (Siana et al 1992).

Extrinsic factors

Poor surgical technique Excessive handling of tissues during surgery can cause damage, resulting in haematoma formation. This can lead to an infection as the haematoma is broken down. A void (dead space) may also occur if tissues are not correctly approximated during surgery, again encouraging the development of infection. In addition, where sutures are inserted too tightly, the tissue becomes damaged and necrosis can occur.

Medication Several medications affect healing. Cytotoxic chemotherapy can destroy healthy as well as cancer cells. Ideally, its use is withheld until any wound healing is complete, usually a period of 4 weeks. Glucocorticosteroids also delay, or prevent, healing taking place and their use is closely monitored in individuals with wounds.

Inappropriate wound management The healing process may be adversely affected by the use of poor dressing technique, the wrong dressing material or unnecessary antiseptics. It is essential that the nurse is aware of what is required from a dressing material in order to ensure that each product is used cost-effectively.

Infection Of all the factors that can delay or prevent healing, infection is the most important (see below and Ch. 16).

Psychosocial factors

There is a close association between psychological and physical well-being. Stress and anxiety can impair immune function through elevation of stress hormones glucocorticoids and catecholamines (e.g. adrenaline, noradrenaline) (Webster Marketon & Glaser 2008). The same authors describe the effects of increased levels of stress hormones including reduced lymphocyte proliferation, reduced antibody production and decreased activity of natural killer (NK) cells. One of the many adverse effects of the changes to immune function is delay in wound healing (Webster Marketon & Glaser 2008). Sleep disturbances are linked to stress, and sleep is thought to be essential for healing and tissue repair (Dealey 1999).

Wound infection

It is inevitable that most wounds contain microorganisms, but it is only pathogenic organisms, usually bacteria, which delay healing and cause systemic illness (Carville et al 2008). Established infection in a healing wound often delays healing and may even cause wound breakdown, herniation of the wound or complete wound dehiscence. The clinical signs and symptoms of a wound infection are summarised in Box 23.2. Despite all the technological advances that have been made in surgery and wound management, the problem of wound infection persists with surgical site infections accounting for 13.8% of health care-associated infections (HCAIs) in acute settings (Hospital Infection Society 2007). It is suggested that at least 5% of patients undergoing surgery develop a surgical site infection. This relates to advances in surgical and anaesthetic techniques which have allowed patients with many co-morbidities and therefore greater risk levels to be considered for surgery (National Institute for Health and Clinical Excellence [NICE] 2008).

The wound environment itself can encourage bacterial growth. Anaerobic microorganisms, for example, thrive in wounds with a poor oxygen supply. A wound bed or area that is free from haematoma and dead tissue and is clean reduces the risk of infection.

The way in which the wound is managed can also affect infection. Bacterial contamination, through poor technique by the nurse, poor hygiene or loss of continence, can all increase the risk of wound infection. The consequences of wound infection vary depending upon the patient's condition and the environment in which they are being nursed: in hospital, a patient with a surgical wound infection poses a considerable risk to other patients with wounds on that ward; at home, that patient is less of a risk to the family and community, who are unlikely to be vulnerable.

Factors that predispose to wound infection

Factors may be associated with the patient or the hospital environment.

Factors associated with the patient

Several factors, in addition to delayed healing (see above), can predispose a patient to wound infection. These can be identified on first assessment:

- poor nutritional status – PEM has been linked to hospitalisation and impacts on all aspects of patient care, including developing pressure ulcers and influencing surgical site infection
- immunosuppression – with cancer treatments, diabetes mellitus, glucocorticosteroid therapy, etc., can lead to increased risk of infection
- excessive body weight
- advanced age.

Box 23.2 Information

Signs of wound infection (reproduced with permission from Principles of Best Practice: Wound Infection in clinical practice. An international consensus. London: MEP Ltd, 2008)

Acute Wounds, e.g. surgical or traumatic wounds, or burns

LOCALISED INFECTION	SPREADING INFECTION
Classic signs and symptoms: • new or increasing pain • erythema • local warmth • swelling • purulent discharge Pyrexia – in surgical wounds, typically 5–7 days post surgery Delayed (or stalled) healing Abscess Malodour	As for localised infection *plus* Further extension of erythema Lymphangitis Crepitus in soft tissue Wound breakdown/dehiscence

Notes:

Burns – also skin graft rejection, pain is not always a feature of infection in full-thickness burns.

Deep wounds – induration, extension of the wound, unexplained increased white cell count or signs of sepsis may be signs of a deep wound infection.

Immunocompromised patients – signs and symptoms may be modified and less obvious.

Chronic Wounds, e.g. diabetic foot ulcers, venous leg ulcers, arterial leg/foot ulcers, pressure ulcers

LOCALISED INFECTION	SPREADING INFECTION
New, increased or altered pain* Delayed or stalled healing* Periwound oedema Bleeding or friable (easily damaged) granulation tissue Distinctive malodour or change in odour Wound bed discolouration Increased or altered/purulent exudate Induration Pocketing Bridging	As for localised infection *plus* Wound breakdown* Erythema extending from the wound edge Crepitus, warmth, induration or discolouration spreading into periwound area Lymphangitis Malaise or other non-specific deterioration in patient's general condition

Notes:

In patients who are immunocompromised and/or who have motor or sensory neuropathies, symptoms may be modified and less obvious. For example, in a diabetic patient with an infected foot ulcer and peripheral sensory neuropathy, pain may not be a prominent feature.

Arterial ulcers – previously dry ulcers may become wet when infected.

Clinicians should also be aware that in the diabetic foot inflammation is not always indicative of infection. For example inflammation may be associated with Charcot's arthropathy.

*Individually highly indicative of infection. Infection is also highly likely if the patient has two or more of the other signs listed.

Factors specifically related to the hospital environment

- Adverse spatial arrangements – when too many patients are nursed in close proximity to each other, especially in an open ward, the wound infection rate increases. An increase occurs when more than 25 patients are being nursed in an open ward (NHS Estates 2002).
- Length of pre-operative hospital stay – the wound infection rate is linked to the length of time a patient spends in hospital prior to operation. The longer this period, the more likelihood there is of the individual being colonised by the pathogenic bacteria found in hospitals.
- Inappropriate pre-operative care – it is not usually necessary to shave the site pre-operatively (Williams & Leaper 1998). Where shaving is required, it should occur immediately prior to surgery to reduce the risk of bacterial growth on newly shaved skin (see Ch. 26). These precautions should result in a wound infection rate of less than 1%.
- Prolonged operative procedure – since 1980, research has suggested that the longer the operation, the greater is the risk of infection in clean wounds (Cruse & Foord 1980, Williams & Leaper 1998).
- Surgical contamination – in elective surgery, e.g. excision of breast lump, the rate of infection should be less than 5%, and with effective surveillance and control this can be reduced to less than 2% (Leaper & Harding 2000). In emergency surgery where the area is contaminated, e.g. bowel perforation, the rate soars to between 20 and 40% (Leaper & Harding 2000).
- Use of drains – used to close or minimise dead space in a wound or to evacuate haematomas or body fluids, in order to reduce infection risk (Bale & Leaper 2000). They should be used with caution, as all drains are foreign bodies and may cause tissue reactions.

As a wound infection develops, localisation of the infection leads to the formation of a wound abscess. This may drain through the suture line or into the wound in the case of cavities. Occasionally, if deep-seated, the abscess will need surgical incision to drain it properly. Where partial wound breakdown occurs, some wounds will be assessed as suitable for healing by secondary intention.

Sources of wound infection

Endogenous Organisms found on the patient's own skin are endogenous sources of wound infection. These organisms, usually *Staphylococcus aureus* or gut commensals, are either present under normal circumstances or are hospital pathogens that colonise the body after admission to hospital. Shortening the time between admission and surgery reduces the possibility of skin contamination by hospital-acquired bacteria (Dealey 1999).

S. aureus is found on the skin and sometimes in the upper respiratory tract. This organism does not normally affect the patient adversely, but when a wound has been created, *S. aureus* can invade the wound from adjacent skin or from the nose during exhalation.

Exogenous Exogenous infections occur following contamination of the wound from a source external to the patient. This may happen in theatre or later in the ward when pathogens are allowed to fall onto the wound and penetrate it. Bacteria such as *Pseudomonas aeruginosa* can be found in wet areas or where moisture is present, e.g. in water, other fluids or ventilators. *P. aeruginosa* is also found in flower vases, sinks and drains.

Accidental injuries are highly likely to have been contaminated by bacteria. *Clostridium tetani* and *Clostridium perfringens* present in the soil can be hazardous. People who receive minor injuries whilst gardening are at risk and the status of their tetanus immunity should be checked in case further treatment is required. Insect bites and stings can lead to cellulitis (diffuse, acute inflammation affecting the skin and subcutaneous tissue).

🖰 **See website Critical thinking question 23.1**

▷ Nursing management and health promotion: holistic wound care

All patients should have access to a minimum standard of care, regardless of where that care is provided or by whom, in order to optimise the chance of achieving a straightforward, uncomplicated and timely healing process (Fletcher 2008b). This should be a systematic process which is adapted to best suit the local circumstances, for example the care pathway proposed by Chadwick et al (2008, p. 7).

Although functioning best as a multidisciplinary specialty, wound care is frequently seen as the responsibility of nurses, with community nurses spending on average 50% of their time on wound care.

Research has been undertaken using different study designs to answer a diverse range of clinical questions, and to explore patients' views. Best available evidence is used not only to inform practice but also to develop clinical guidelines (NICE 2001, EPUAP 2003, EPUAP & NPUAP 2009).

Patient assessment

This should be patient-centred and comprehensive and should consider the physical and social environment.

Whether the patient is being cared for at home, other community setting or hospital, or is young or old, assessment of the patient's general condition should be undertaken. This is done to identify any of the factors that might impair the wound-healing process (pp. 636–638): for those factors seen as reversible, treatment should be sought; for those factors where no treatment is possible, some degree of delay in healing should be anticipated and allowed for in the care plan.

The patient's social environment can affect the treatment options. For example, when caring for a frail older person living alone, the nurse may need to select a dressing that is waterproof, in order that carers who come in to bathe the person need not disturb the wound unnecessarily.

Wound assessment

In assessment of the wound and surrounding skin, a range of wound criteria are considered which can help ensure that the patient receives the most appropriate care for their needs. A range of theoretical frameworks exist to guide this assessment for example: TIME – focuses on **T**issue type, **I**nfection/Inflammation, **M**oisture Balance and **E**dge/ Epithelialisation, Applied Wound Management which utilises the Wound Healing Continuum, the wound infection continuum and the wound exudate continuum. In practice these are translated into wound assessment charts which may vary from area to area but usually collect information around key parameters which suggest if the wound is healing/deteriorating or static. Key parameters to consider include:

- cause of the wound
- wound location
- measurements (e.g. length × width or surface area)
- description of the tissue type and percentage present, e.g. necrotic tissue, slough, granulation, epithelialisation
- volume of exudate
- odour
- pain
- condition of surrounding skin.

Where wound specific assessment tools are used, for example a leg ulcer assessment chart, other data such as the ankle brachial pressure index (see p. 650) would also be included. Once a thorough assessment has been completed objectives of care can be set in conjunction with the patient's needs and wishes.

Cause of the wound For many wound types identifying and addressing the cause of the wound will be the major factor in progressing a wound to healing, e.g. removing the cause of pressure damage is the most important factor in healing a pressure ulcer.

Wound location This is important to record not only because it makes it easier for successive practitioners to find but also because it may impact on treatment choices, for example sacral wounds are at high risk of contamination from urine and faeces, and wounds on the foot are difficult to dress because of high shear forces and limited space within footwear if the patient needs to remain mobile.

Wound measurement There are a variety of ways of measuring wounds; most commonly a simple length × width is recorded using a ruler. It is possible to convert this into a surface area; however, unless the wound is square or rectangular this is a very inaccurate measurement (Langemo et al 2008). A simple and more accurate practice is to trace the wound outline onto an acetate sheet with grid squares; these can then be counted and the area calculated.

🖱 **See website Figure 23.3**

In some areas this may be calculated digitally using a hand-held digital tablet or converted via a computer programme. Weekly measurement is often sufficient and steady progress should be evident.

Description of the tissue type Tissue types in a wound may be described in relation to colour (e.g. red, black, yellow) or terms such as granulating, necrotic, sloughy, or epithelialising. It is important to recognise that in most wounds there may be a combination of tissue types and for this reason the descriptor is usually accompanied by an approximate percentage.

🖱 **See website Figure 23.4**

Necrotic (black) tissue is dead (devitalised). It indicates the presence of hypoxia in the area and should be removed (unless there are other more pressing objectives) as its presence can encourage the development of infection.

Sloughy tissue, which may present from cream through to yellow, is a fibrinous covering which occurs as the dead cells from the wound healing process rise to the surface of the wound. Although it is generally removed its presence does not particularly indicate a problem in the healing process.

Granulation tissue is usually red and moist with an uneven granular appearance. It is formed by the creation of new capillary loops, which give the uneven, bumpy texture, and the laying down of ground substance and extracellular matrix. If the granulation tissue is a deep unhealthy red, friable (bleeds easily) or appears dehydrated this may be a sign of infection in the wound.

Epithelial tissue (pale pink) is the formation of new skin over the surface of the wound. Epithelial tissue can only be generated from epidermal cells which occur at the wound margin and from around any surviving hair follicles. This type of tissue is particularly fragile and requires protection and appropriate moisture balance.

Occasionally the wound may appear green in colour. This is a clear sign of clinical infection and wound swabs should be taken (Box 23.3).

Volume of exudate Recording the volume of exudate is difficult as it cannot be accurately captured in routine practice. Typically wound assessment charts record the volume as +, ++, +++ or use a range of subjective descriptors such as minimal, moderate, heavy. Being very subjective they do not assist in planning care. A more objective description is to record the frequency of dressing change, so if a dressing had previously needed changing twice daily and was now only requiring changing every other day it can be seen that the volume of exudate has reduced. Exudate can also be combined with other fluid; for example, in a patient with

---

Box 23.3 Information

Taking a wound swab

Points to remember:

- Use an aseptic technique.
- Use a sterile, microbiological cotton wool swab.
- This swab should be moistened in a transport medium before use.
- If the wound is flat or shallow, gently rotate the swab across the middle of the wound bed. Care needs to be taken not to contaminate the swab with skin flora from the edges of the wound.
- If the wound is deep, or has a recess, insert the swab into the depths of the wound. Bacteria present in the depths of a wound are different from and more likely to be pathogenic than bacteria on the surface of a wound.
- Carefully replace the swab directly into its storage tube containing culture medium.
- Deliver to the laboratory as soon as possible, but at the latest within 24 hours.
- Record antibiotic drugs being given and the site of the wound, together with any other information likely to be of help to the laboratory.

gross oedema of the lower leg and a leg ulcer it is not possible to determine what is truly exudate and what is leakage of the protein-rich fluid from the leg. Where water-based dressings such as hydrogels are used a similar situation occurs. In wounds that are progressing normally such as uncomplicated surgical wounds exudate levels decrease normally with time. In chronic wounds exudate levels may remain high due to a prolonged inflammatory phase. A sudden increase in exudate level in any wound, especially if accompanied by a change or increase in pain, is a strong indicator of the presence of infection.

Odour As with exudate, odour is difficult to assess/measure and is frequently recorded with +s or simply as 'malodour present'. Patients and inexperienced clinicians may consider the presence of malodour as a sign of infection; however, most wounds have a distinctive odour, as do some dressings, so care should be taken to distinguish what is normal but unpleasant from an indicator of infection. Several systems suggest evaluating the odour level by identifying when it can be detected, e.g. on entering the room, when close to the patient or only on dressing removal; this allows for a degree of objectivity. Consideration should also be given to the impact of the odour – for many patients a strong odour is the reason that they become increasingly isolated as visitors stop coming or the patient themselves chooses to withdraw from embarrassment.

Pain Pain should be assessed both to address patient comfort and also as an indicator of what may be happening in the wound. Several assessment tools exist to allow the patient to rate the severity of the pain. These may be numerical, e.g. how bad is the pain, when 0 is no pain and 10 is the worst pain imaginable, or be based on images of smiling/grimacing faces (see Ch. 19). Consideration should also be given to:

- pain location
- duration
- what it feels like
- what initiates or worsens pain
- what relieves pain (Vuolo 2009).

Changes in pain type and intensity may be related to a developing infection. Pain relating to dressing changes should trigger a review/evaluation of the management.

Condition of surrounding skin This is an indicator of general health, e.g. dry skin in a dehydrated patient, but may also reflect the efficiency of the wound management, for example the appearance of macerated skin when a dressing does not adequately control exudate levels.

Creating an environment for healing

Principles of moist wound healing

Healing proceeds at its optimal rate when the wound is enclosed in a warm, moist environment (Figure 23.4). Under these conditions, cellular activity is maximised; the benefits of such an environment have been recognised since the early 1960s (Winter 1962). This is true for the whole spectrum of wounds encountered, from superficial cuts and grazes to large, extensive granulating wounds. Exposure of a wound to the air precipitates drying out of the wound surface and scab formation. Nurses should consider the importance of providing a suitable environment for wound healing when choosing a wound management material. There are over 400 dressings available, but the availability of these changes constantly (Table 23.2). See also Further reading, e.g. JWC 2009, or Useful websites, e.g. World Wide Wounds.

Principles of cleansing

Sutured wounds rarely need cleansing unless leakage has occurred. In this situation the suture line can be gently, aseptically cleansed with sterile 0.9% sodium chloride solution. With open wounds, strict asepsis is not always required. Patients can bathe or preferably shower to irrigate the wound with warm water after 48 hours (NICE 2008). For patient comfort, wound cleansing fluids should be warmed to body temperature. The main reason for cleansing open cavity wounds is to remove any loose debris and excess wound secretions (see below). A shower is particularly useful as gentle flushing with the spray will remove any particles that are loose, and flushing for 10–15 s is usually sufficient. If bathing, the wound should be flushed by splashing water into it. Lower limb wounds can be bathed in a bucket (lined with a commercial bin liner) or bowl, gently splashing the wound to remove loose debris. A lining protects the bucket from contamination and makes cleaning of the bucket much easier, thus reducing the potential risk of cross-infection.

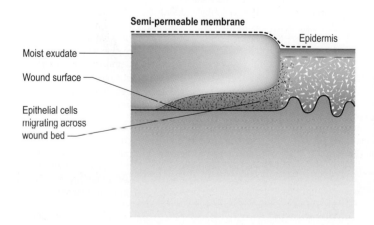
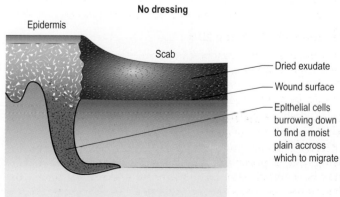

Figure 23.4 Healing of skin wounds with and without a semipereable membrane dressing. (Adapted from Winter 1962.)

Table 23.2 Dressings and topical wound products

MATERIAL	PRESENTATION	ACTION	INDICATIONS FOR USE	SPECIAL CONSIDERATIONS
Alginates (fibres of calcium or sodium alginate derived from seaweed)	Flat sheets, ropes and packing	Absorbent; gels in contact with exudate Non-adhesive, non-occlusive	Partial and full thickness wounds Moderate to heavily exuding wounds	Can be packed into cavities and sinuses Can be rinsed from wound bed, cavity or sinus Usually require a secondary dressing
Antimicrobial dressings (impregnated with iodine, silver, honey or other antimicrobials)	Flat sheets and packing	Have an antimicrobial effect on the wound bed	Heavily contaminated or infected partial and full thickness wounds Moderate to heavily exuding wounds as these products usually need exudate to activate the antimicrobial effect	Usually require a secondary dressing Silver products can cause staining of surrounding skin and clothing if not contained
Foams (hydrophilic polyurethane/polymer)	Flat sheets and cavity dressings Some are adhesive, some are semi-occlusive	Absorbent; some can retain exudate in foam	Partial and full thickness wounds Moderate to heavily exuding wounds	Removed in one piece Some can be cut to shape if necessary
Films (polyurethane or co-polymers)	Adhesive sheets	Transparent dressing Maintain a moist environment Impermeable to fluids and microorganisms	Superficial, dry or lightly exuding wounds as a primary dressing	Removed in one piece Can be used as a primary wound contact dressing or to hold other dressings in place (e.g. hydrogels or absorbent pads)
Hydrocolloids (hydrophilic colloid particles derived from cellulose, gelatins and pectins (constituents vary according to manufacturer) bound to a polyurethane foam backing)	Adhesive flat sheets in different thicknesses and shapes Also in gel or paste forms	Maintain a moist environment Provide an environment for autolysis Adhesive sheets are impermeable to fluids and microorganisms	Partial and full thickness wounds Dry to moderately exuding wounds	Sometimes leave a residue that can be malodorous Can be cut to shape
Hydrofibres (fibres of carboxymethyl-cellulose)	Flat sheets and packing	Absorbent product that gels on contact with exudate	Partial and full thickness wounds Moderately to heavily exuding wounds	Require a secondary dressing
Hydrogels (water- and glycerin-based crossed-linked hydrophilic polymers)	Sachets of gel Sheet forms and packing available	Maintain a moist environment Provide an environment for autolysis	Partial and full thickness wounds Dry to lightly exuding wounds Provide an environment for autolysis	Usually require a secondary dressing to hold gel in contact with wound bed May cause maceration of skin surrounding wound and so often not recommended for heavily exuding wounds
Low adherent dressings (woven mesh or net of polyamide)	Sheets often silicone coated to help reduce risk of adherence to the wound	Wound contact layers that wick exudate onto a retention dressing	Partial and full thickness wounds Moderately to heavily exuding wounds	Used under compression bandaging systems and in situations where a secondary dressing absorbs exudate

Continued

Table 23.2 Dressings and topical wound products – cont'd

MATERIAL	PRESENTATION	ACTION	INDICATIONS FOR USE	SPECIAL CONSIDERATIONS
Skin substitutes or equivalents (bioabsorbable matrix containing fibroblasts and/or keratinocytes)	Single or multilayers of living cells, transported on a mesh or medium	Replaces skin and provides wound coverage with cellular activity	Partial and full thickness wounds Usually indicated for chronic and slow or non-healing wounds such as diabetic foot ulcers and venous leg ulcers Have been used extensively in burns patients	Usually require specialist skills and facilities Require special transportation and storage as some products are provided frozen and others are incubated Some wound bed preparation is needed prior to application
Negative pressure therapy	Gauze or foam material placed in wound bed and attached to a sealed unit that exerts a negative pressure continuously or intermittently	Removes excess exudate, removes wound debris and microorganisms Stimulates granulation tissue	Full or partial thickness wounds, acute or chronic	Special techniques and precautions for some complex wound situations Appropriate training is necessary before using the device
Larvae (biosurgery, maggot therapy)	Free-range maggots applied to the wound surface or confined in a small bag and applied to the wound	Excretion of proteolytic enzymes that breaks down necrotic tissue Free-range maggots also have a physical action of breaking down tissue as they move around on the wound surface (Thomas et al 2002)	Used to debride necrotic and sloughy wounds	Patients and staff need to be carefully prepared for this procedure Larvae are applied for up to 3 days at a time and one or two applications only may be sufficient Not to be used if the wound is very wet, or very dry

NB: This table provides examples of the main groups of dressings and topical wound products. However, it is not an exhaustive list and other products are available as combinations or variations of these main groups.

The role of antiseptics and topical agents Antiseptics are rarely used for cleaning wounds unless they are heavily contaminated, for example a dirty traumatic wound, or at very high risk of infection, e.g. a sacral pressure ulcer when the patient has uncontrollable diarrhoea. For an overview of the role of antimicrobials in wound care see Useful websites, e.g. International Wound Infection Institute.

Wound cleansing The purpose of wound cleansing is to gently remove loose debris and other surface contaminants, so providing an optimal healing environment prior to applying a dressing. However, wound exudate bathes the surface of wounds and provides nutrients and cytokines essential for healing. Cleansing the surface of a wound removes exudate and in some cases this inhibits the healing process (Barone et al 1998). Nurses need to consider carefully why they are cleansing a wound and to balance the need to remove exudate because of harmful effects, against leaving it in place to enhance healing. Exudate needs to be removed if:

- it is causing maceration to the wound bed and/or surrounding tissues
- there are signs of infection
- foreign bodies are present
- devitalised tissue is present
- it has an unpleasant odour, which is embarrassing and making the patient feel nauseous

- it is excessive and is oozing through dressings and onto clothing/bedding/furniture.

Where the wound is healthy with minimal amounts of exudate, routine wound cleansing is of little benefit (Davies 1999).

Removal of devitalised tissue – debridement

Debridement, the removal of devitalised (dead) tissue, is most commonly achieved clinically by autolytic debridement, surgical and sharp debridement, and biosurgical debridement which is outlined in Table 23.2.

Autolytic debridement is the most commonly used method. Dressings are used which facilitate autolysis (the body's natural ability to remove devitalised tissues by leucocytes and lytic enzymes). These work best under moist conditions. Several types of wound dressing provide this moist environment that facilitates removal of devitalised tissue from the wound bed. These dressings can effectively remove devitalised and necrotic tissue without damaging either the skin surrounding the wound or healthy tissue within the wound. Included in these are the hydrogels and hydrocolloids (Table 23.2).

Surgical debridement is usually carried out in theatre where the surgeon removes devitalised tissue back to healthy bleeding tissue.

Sharp debridement is the removal of devitalised tissue using a scalpel and scissors. It is sometimes possible to excise devitalised tissue with or without local anaesthesia depending on the site and depth of the problem. If general anaesthesia is not indicated then careful consideration is needed to ensure that the patient has no pain or discomfort, and that the area is not painful. The advantages of this method are that debridement is instant and a healthy cavity results. Where patients are being cared for in the community, access to a surgeon or specialist nurse may be limited and this is not always a practical alternative for many patients. This procedure should not be carried out without specialised training and achievement of clinical competency.

Excessive granulation

From time to time, epithelialisation fails to take place due to the presence of excessive granulation tissue or 'proud flesh'. Treatment is needed to flatten the granulation tissue to a level with the epithelial edge, as new epithelium cannot migrate up over proud flesh. Silver nitrate (75%) stick should not be used to cauterise the tissue. A less traumatic method is the use of a cream containing a corticosteroid, although this should be used under medical supervision. Careful assessment is paramount in the successful treatment of cavity wounds. When planning a wound care programme, consideration of these factors should provide the nurse with an accurate picture of the needs of each patient and also provide some assistance with the dressing selection process.

Dressing techniques

Throughout the UK there are many different policies, procedures and protocols for dressing changes (Table 23.2, pp. 642–643). Standard infection control procedures must be adhered to when changing dressings (Parker 2000). This involves either clean or aseptic technique depending on the wound type, clinical setting and clinical considerations (Hampton 2002). Wound dressing packs no longer contain cotton wool to avoid fibres from the material becoming incorporated into wound tissue and perhaps causing an inflammatory reaction. Nor do the packs contain forceps, which were sometimes difficult to manoeuvre and risked causing trauma to the delicate wound bed. The sterile packs contain gauze to cleanse periwound skin and to dry around the wound after cleansing. The pack may contain a receptacle for cleansing fluid and a disposal bag for contaminated dressings and procedure debris. After handwashing the pack is opened and laid out using a non-touch technique. The disposal bag can act as a glove for the removal of the soiled dressing. Once the dressing has been removed the person carrying out the procedure washes and dries their hands and applies gloves prior to the dressing procedure.

A dressing needs to be changed when:

- there is a specific purpose, e.g. to remove sutures or when the maximum wear time for the dressing has been reached (see pack insert for individual dressings)
- clinical signs of infection are present
- wound discharge has leaked, or is about to leak, through the dressing (ideally a dressing should be changed before leakage occurs to reduce the risk of infection)
- special treatments are needed, e.g. burns dressings.

Clinical setting

Any differences in technique depend on the clinical setting. In hospitals, clinics or nursing homes for instance there may be an element of control over the environment in terms of cleanliness, equipment such as trolleys and clean surfaces and space. In this kind of environment there are many patients in close proximity to each other and often several members of staff moving around. This increases the risk of cross-contamination (cross-infection) and procedures need to take this risk into account. In a patient's home there are fewer people moving around but the nurse has to be mindful of cross-infection when moving from house to house, and equipment, space and cleanliness may be more of a challenge. However, many patients and their families go to great lengths to create a clean and safe working environment for wound care.

The two main methods of dressing change are aseptic or clean procedure techniques. Both require a sound knowledge of infection control principles including the use of aprons and gloves, cleansing of working surfaces, the careful washing and drying of hands and disposal of contaminated material. The practitioner must ensure that clinical protocols in relation to procedure clothing, hair and jewellery are strictly adhered to.

Aseptic technique

In some acute wounds or for particularly vulnerable patients an aseptic technique may be indicated (Box 23.4). The aseptic technique adopts a non-touch technique, the practitioner wears sterile gloves for the procedure and sterile fluids are used if the wound requires cleansing.

Box 23.4 Information

Principles of aseptic technique

- Perform the procedure in an area which is closed, clean and well ventilated at least 1 h after periods of activity where possible. Bed making and cleaning, for example, increase the circulation of dust particles and airborne microorganisms.
- Use a clean trolley – this should be thoroughly cleaned daily and wiped with an alcoholic solution before and after use.
- Wash hands (see Ch.16) before, after and at any point during the procedure should they become contaminated. The use of an alcoholic hand-rub can sometimes be substituted.
- Wear a clean plastic apron to protect the patient from bacteria on the nurse's clothing and to protect your clothing from wound debris and fluids.
- Use sterile equipment for the procedure – be aware of how your health trust/authority/board identifies equipment which is sterile and therefore safe to use.
- Discard equipment which has broken or damaged packaging.
- Use sterile fluids and dressing materials.
- Prepare equipment before dressings are removed.
- Use gloves to remove any dressings and dispose of both immediately. Alternatively insert your hand into the disposal bag using it like a glove. When turned the right way out it becomes a disposal bag for the rest of the procedure.
- Carry out the procedure using clean or sterile gloves depending on the procedure, discarding equipment as it becomes contaminated.
- Dispose of used equipment in the appropriate bin.

Clean procedure

This technique involves cleansing with tap water and the use of clean gloves. It is most commonly used for chronic wounds such as leg or pressure ulcers. People with leg ulceration may wash the wound in a container (see p. 641) or use a shower. The leg and the skin surrounding the wound is dried carefully using paper roll or a clean towel. This ensures the patient is socially clean and helps to ensure their skin is cared for. This type of cleansing is also beneficial from a psychological perspective, especially for people with long-term conditions (Moffatt et al 2007a). There is no evidence to suggest that the use of tap water from a clean source puts the patient at any higher risk of infection (Box 23.5, Fernandez & Griffiths 2008).

Involving patients in wound care

Wherever patients are cared for (home, community settings or hospital), there are many opportunities for the nurse to involve patients in wound management. This is important in empowering patients with a sense of independence and will help promote a return to normality. Patients with sutured wounds can be taught to monitor themselves for clinical signs of infection and in self-care areas such as nutrition, fluid intake, rest and avoidance of excessive movement of the affected area. In addition, they can be taught about the appearance of the wound surface and what to expect during the healing phase. In the community, patients and families can be taught the basic dressing-change technique where asepsis is not necessary, and the community nurse can assume a supervisory role. This obviously depends on individual circumstances and the patient's level of understanding, but certainly many patients with open wounds are able to play a major role in wound management. This is important as the patient begins to resume a more normal

---

Box 23.5 Evidence-based practice

Wound cleansing

Fernandez & Griffiths (2008) in a Cochrane Review on using water for cleansing suggest that there is little benefit in cleaning wounds with sterile solutions such as 0.9% sodium chloride solution (normal saline), particularly in the community setting.

Activity

- Access the review by Fernandez & Griffiths (2008) and consider the evidence.
- With your colleagues discuss why you think sterile saline continues to be the cleansing solution of choice for many nurses. You may want to consider the views of both the health care professional and the patient.
- Identify occasions when you would feel that tap water would be a better option and also times when you would only use sterile saline.

Resources

Fernandez R, Griffiths R. Water for wound cleansing. Cochrane Database of Systematic Reviews 2008, Issue 1. Art. No.: CD003861. http://www.cochrane.org/reviews/en/ab003861.html

---

Box 23.6 Reflection

Involving patients in wound care

Whilst you are caring for a patient with a wound, and if it is appropriate to do so, talk to them about their wound and how it impacts on their activities of daily living.

Activities

- Find out what they know about the cause and progress of their wound.
- What information have they been given about their treatment plan?
- Ask how easy is it for them to follow the plan and what they find challenging.
- Reflect on the areas of their treatment plan that they find challenging and discuss with your mentor how this could be addressed.
- Find out what wound care related information is available in your clinical area (e.g. information leaflets, DVDs, etc.).

---

lifestyle and it also avoids the need for routine frequent visits by the community nurse (Box 23.6).

Patients with chronic wounds, such as leg ulcers and pressure ulcers, need specific help and support, but it is very important to gain their cooperation. Patients with venous leg ulcers (see p. 651) require advice on leg elevation techniques and calf pump muscle exercises, which stimulate the circulation and aid drainage of the lower limb. Carers of patients with pressure ulcers (see pp. 647–649) need advice and training on manual handling, i.e. turning and repositioning the patient. Carers also need to know how the pressure-reducing aids work, so that these are used correctly at all times. Concordance is where patients and practitioners reach agreement on management regimens through open discussion and negotiation about what is desirable and what is manageable. Patient compliance is commonly referred to in the literature but often leads to conflict and is not easily sustainable in long-term conditions (Moffatt 2004). The patient, and where possible their carers, need to be involved in decisions and helped to feel that they have some control about what happens.

Nurse prescribing

Non-medical prescribing is now well established in the UK (Department of Health [DH] 2006) for community and hospital-based nurses who complete an approved education programme and period of supervised practice (Goswell & Siefers 2009). This has made a significant difference to patients with wounds who have more timely access to dressings and other therapies required for their care.

Wound management policies and guidelines

Most health care providers in the UK have developed wound treatment and prevention policies as well as wound selection formularies to help guide their staff towards safe and standardised care. Ideally, these are based on the best available evidence sourced from systematic reviews of the literature covering randomised, controlled trials, but other sources of evidence need to be included to ensure that patients' perspectives and experiences form part of the evidence base (Timmons 2008).

National and international guidance for wound care is produced by organisations including:

- Royal College of Nursing (RCN)
- Scottish Intercollegiate Guidelines Network (SIGN)
- National Institute for Health and Clinical Excellence (NICE)
- Department of Health (DH)
- Cochrane Collaboration
- European Pressure Ulcer Advisory Panel (EPUAP)
- European Wound Management Association (EWMA)
- Guidelines and Audit Implementation Network (GAIN), previously Clinical Resource Efficiency Support Team (CREST).

See Useful websites.

Expectations of outcome and effectiveness of treatment

Following individual patient and wound assessment, the nurse should have reasonable expectations regarding the prospects of achieving complete healing. In some wounds, complete healing is expected rapidly, as in primary wound closure following appendicectomy in a healthy young person. For others, the prognosis for healing is less good, e.g. an older woman with arthritis and a venous leg ulcer. The expected outcome affects the choice of treatment for individual patients. For patients with a poor prognosis for healing, treatment is often directed towards minimising symptoms and preventing further wound breakdown, such as in terminally ill patients with superficial pressure ulcers where the aim is to prevent the ulcer penetrating into deeper tissues. Patient comfort and convenience become the priorities and provide some measure of the effectiveness of the treatment. Where healing is expected, effectiveness means complete healing occurring in the minimum number of days with the fewest complications.

Cost-effectiveness

Efficacy is also measured by the cost of treatments. Hospital doctors, GPs, practice nurses or district nurses and the pharmacists who supply materials for wound management can be misled into believing that, because the initial cost of a material is high, then it follows that the total treatment costs will also be high. Modern wound dressing materials can be relatively expensive to buy per unit. However, these dressings can often be left on the wound for several days and, in some cases, for a full week.

It is important, when comparing the costs of dressing materials, to consider:

- how long the product can be left on the wound
- nursing time needed to change and apply dressings
- the benefits of using interactive products that stimulate tissue growth to achieve rapid healing or stimulate healing in chronic wounds
- how the dressing prevents damage to skin surrounding the wound, helping to reduce pain and discomfort, reducing ancillary product and analgesia costs
- the reduction of unnecessary pain, suffering and disruption for patients.

Specific wound types

This section covers pressure ulcers, leg ulcers, sutured wounds, traumatic wounds and malignant wounds (burn injuries are covered in Ch. 30).

▷ Nursing management and health promotion: pressure ulcers

A pressure ulcer is 'an area of localised skin damage caused by disruption of the blood supply to the area, usually caused by pressure, shear or friction, or a combination of any of these' (Dealey 1999). Pressure ulcers develop most commonly on the sacral area. Tissue damage ranges from superficial epidermal loss to damage to underlying structures, including muscle and bone (see below).

The prevention and management of pressure ulcers present major challenges for nurses. The pressure ulcer problem is widespread and persistent, affecting patients of all ages and with a range of illnesses. It reduces quality of life and causes distress to patients and carers and makes major financial demands on health services. As a result, in many community and hospital trusts, nurses are now supported by a tissue viability service (Dealey 1997). Particular difficulties arise in trying to identify patients who might develop a pressure ulcer, and when they are at risk of doing so.

Nurses have a basic responsibility to:

- Use a structured approach to risk assessment to identify people at risk of pressure ulcer development.
- Conduct a structured risk assessment on admission, and repeat as regularly and as frequently as required by patient acuity. Reassessment should also be undertaken if there is any change in patient condition.
- Document all risk assessments.
- Develop and implement a prevention plan when individuals have been identified as being at risk of pressure ulcer development (EPUAP & NPUAP 2009).

Aetiology

Pressure ulcers result from areas of previously healthy tissue becoming devitalised, resulting in localised tissue death. Pressure ulcers develop in a number of ways:

- from direct, unrelieved pressure of soft tissues against bone or another hard surface such as a catheter
- from friction occurring between the patient and the surface of a bed or chair; such as when the patient is moved and the skin is dragged over a sheet
- from shear forces that frequently accompany both direct pressure and friction; shear forces develop in tissues that are distorted and pulled, thus disrupting blood supply.

Classification

In order to assess the extent or degree of damage, a range of grading systems have been developed. Most recently EPUAP & NPUAP (2009) have classified four categories of damage:

Category I: Non-blanchable erythema

Intact skin with non-blanchable redness of a localized area usually over a bony prominence. Darkly pigmented skin may not have visible blanching; its colour may differ from the surrounding area. The area may be painful, firm, soft, warmer or cooler as compared to adjacent tissue. Category I may be difficult to detect in individuals with dark skin tones. May indicate "at risk" persons.

Category II: Partial thickness

Partial thickness loss of dermis presenting as a shallow open ulcer with a red pink wound bed, without slough. May also present as an intact or open/ruptured serum-filled or sero-sanguinous filled blister. Presents as a shiny or dry shallow ulcer without slough or bruising*. This category should not be used to describe skin tears, tape burns, incontinence associated dermatitis, maceration or excoriation.

*Bruising indicates deep tissue injury.

Category III: Full thickness skin loss

Full thickness tissue loss. Subcutaneous fat may be visible but bone, tendon or muscle are not exposed. Slough may be present but does not obscure the depth of tissue loss. May include undermining and tunneling. The depth of a Category/Stage III pressure ulcer varies by anatomical location. The bridge of the nose, ear, occiput and malleolus do not have (adipose) subcutaneous tissue and Category/Stage III ulcers can be shallow. In contrast, areas of significant adiposity can develop extremely deep Category/Stage III pressure ulcers. Bone/tendon is not visible or directly palpable.

Category IV: Full thickness tissue loss

Full thickness tissue loss with exposed bone, tendon or muscle. Slough or eschar may be present. Often includes undermining and tunneling. The depth of a Category/Stage IV pressure ulcer varies by anatomical location. The bridge of the nose, ear, occiput and malleolus do not have (adipose) subcutaneous tissue and these ulcers can be shallow. Category/Stage IV ulcers can extend into muscle and/or supporting structures (e.g., fascia, tendon or joint capsule) making osteomyelitis or osteitis likely to occur. Exposed bone/muscle is visible or directly palpable.

(EPUAP & NPUAP 2009, pp. 7–8)

In addition, in the US, two further categories – deep tissue injury and unstageable/unclassified – are used. These relate to the reimbursement system within the US health care system and the use of these categories is not currently recommended in Europe.

Assessment of risk

In an acute illness, even the most unlikely individual may become 'at risk' of developing a pressure ulcer; therefore, all patients should be assessed on admission to hospital, care/nursing home or a community nurse's caseload. A combination of disease and/or drug therapies or surgery, for example, can quite suddenly put an individual into an 'at risk' category.

The following are at risk of developing pressure ulcers:

- the very old or very young
- the immobile, e.g. paraplegic or after some orthopaedic surgery

- those with sensory loss, e.g. altered consciousness or diabetic sensory neuropathy
- those with systemic diseases, e.g. anaemia, peripheral vascular disease, cancer
- those having medication including anti-inflammatories, cytotoxics or corticosteroids
- those with loss of continence
- poorly nourished individuals
- those with BMI <20, or BMI >30.

Several scales and scoring systems have been devised for assessing risk; the most widely used in the UK is probably the Waterlow score (Waterlow 2005) (Figure 23.5).

There are other risk assessment scores available, though only some – the Norton Scale, the Braden Scale and the Central Begeleidings Orgaan (CBO) – have undergone validity testing (Braden 1997, Schoonhoven et al 2002). National (NICE 2001) and international (EPUAP & NPUAP 2009) guidelines have been produced to guide nurses towards an evidence-based approach to caring for patients (Box 23.7). Many health care providers have adapted guidelines for local use to suit their own patients' needs and as part of a pressure ulcer prevention policy. Guidelines are designed to rationalise and standardise patient care so that all patients receive a reasonable level of care. Guidelines also help to ensure that the available pressure-relieving equipment is used most efficiently. However, all health care professionals have a responsibility for taking action once risk is identified (Dealey 1997).

As part of guideline recommendations, risk assessment tools are designed to support nurses' clinical judgement and not to replace it (Braden 1997, NICE 2001). They are useful only if used regularly – on admission and again each time the patient's condition changes. The scores need to be accurately documented and then used to determine the most appropriate pressure-relieving devices to use.

Prevention of pressure ulcers

Once patients have been identified as being 'at risk', they should be nursed on the most appropriate surface. This includes not only the mattress on the bed but also any chairs they may use (Dealey 1999). Other areas worth considering are theatre tables and trolleys on which patients are transported around the hospital. Liaison with other professionals may be indicated, for example with the physiotherapist to assess the degree of mobility an individual has and where help and treatment can be given: '...repositioning should be considered in all at-risk individuals... to reduce the duration and magnitude of pressure over vulnerable areas of the body' (EPUAP & NPUAP 2009, p. 15).

Managing patients with established pressure ulcers

In addition to providing a suitable surface on which to nurse the patient, and ensuring adequate nutrition and using good handling techniques when moving a patient, local care of the pressure ulcer needs to be considered. The wound should be fully assessed and an appropriate dressing applied to manage the presenting symptoms. Removal of the cause of the damage is the most critical factor.

The management of patients with established pressure ulcers is costly in both economic and personal terms.

WATERLOW PRESSURE ULCER PREVENTION/TREATMENT POLICY
RING SCORES IN TABLE, ADD TOTAL. MORE THAN 1 SCORE/CATEGORY CAN BE USED

BUILD/WEIGHT FOR HEIGHT	♦	SKIN TYPE VISUAL RISK AREAS	♦	SEX AGE	♦	MALNUTRITION SCREENING TOOL (MST) (Nutrition Vol.15, No.6 1999 - Australia		
AVERAGE BMI = 20-24.9	0	HEALTHY	0	MALE	1	A - HAS PATIENT LOST WEIGHT RECENTLY	B - WEIGHT LOSS SCORE	
ABOVE AVERAGE BMI = 25-29.9	1	TISSUE PAPER	1	FEMALE	2	YES - GO TO B	0.5 - 5kg = 1	
OBESE BMI > 30	2	DRY OEDEMATOUS	1 1	14 - 49 50 - 64	1 2	NO - GO TO C UNSURE - GO TO C AND	5 - 10kg = 2 10 - 15kg = 3	
BELOW AVERAGE BMI < 20	3	CLAMMY, PYREXIA DISCOLOURED GRADE 1	1 2	65 - 74 75 - 80	3 4	SCORE 2	> 15kg = 4 unsure = 2	
BMI=Wt(Kg)/Ht (m)².		BROKEN/SPOTS GRADE 2-4	3	81 +	5	C - PATIENT EATING POORLY OR LACK OF APPETITE 'NO' = 0; 'YES' SCORE = 1	NUTRITION SCORE If > 2 refer for nutrition assessment / intervention	

CONTINENCE	♦	MOBILITY	♦	SPECIAL RISKS				
COMPLETE/ CATHETERISED	0	FULLY RESTLESS/FIDGETY	0 1	**TISSUE MALNUTRITION**	♦	**NEUROLOGICAL DEFICIT**		♦
URINE INCONT.	1	APATHETIC	2	TERMINAL CACHEXIA	8	DIABETES, MS, CVA		4-6
FAECAL INCONT.	2	RESTRICTED	3	MULTIPLE ORGAN FAILURE	8	MOTOR/SENSORY		4-6
URINARY + FAECAL INCONTINENCE	3	BEDBOUND e.g. TRACTION	4	SINGLE ORGAN FAILURE (RESP, RENAL, CARDIAC,)	5	PARAPLEGIA (MAX OF 6)		4-6
		CHAIRBOUND e.g. WHEELCHAIR	5	PERIPHERAL VASCULAR DISEASE	5	**MAJOR SURGERY or TRAUMA**		
SCORE						ORTHOPAEDIC/SPINAL		5
10+ AT RISK				ANAEMIA (Hb < 8)	2	ON TABLE > 2 HR#		5
15+ HIGH RISK				SMOKING	1	ON TABLE > 6 HR#		8
20+ VERY HIGH RISK				MEDICATION - CYTOTOXICS, LONG TERM/HIGH DOSE STEROIDS, ANTI-INFLAMMATORY MAX OF 4				

Scores can be discounted after 48 hours provided patient is recovering normally

© J Waterlow 1985 Revised 2005*
Obtainable from the Nook, Stoke Road, Henlade TAUNTON TA3 5LX
* The 2005 revision incorporates the research undertaken by Queensland Health.

www.judy-waterlow.co.uk

**REMEMBER TISSUE DAMAGE MAY START PRIOR TO ADMISSION, IN CASUALTY. A SEATED PATIENT IS AT RISK ASSESSMENT (See Over) IF THE PATIENT FALLS INTO ANY OF THE RISK CATEGORIES, THEN PREVENTATIVE NURSING IS REQUIRED A COMBINATION OF GOOD NURSING TECHNIQUES AND PREVENTATIVE AIDS WILL BE NECESSARY
ALL ACTIONS MUST BE DOCUMENTED**

PREVENTION
PRESSURE REDUCING AIDS
Special Mattress/beds:
10+ Overlays or specialist foam mattresses.
15+ Alternating pressure overlays, mattresses and bed systems
20+ Bed systems: Fluidised bead, low air loss and alternating pressure mattresses
Note: Preventative aids cover a wide spectrum of specialist features. Efficacy should be judged, if possible, on the basis of independent evidence.

Cushions:
No person should sit in a wheelchair without some form of cushioning. If nothing else is available - use the person's own pillow. (Consider infection risk)
10+ 100mm foam cushion
15+ Specialist Gell and/or foam cushion
20+ Specialised cushion, adjustable to individual person.

Bed clothing:
Avoid plastic draw sheets, inco pads and tightly tucked in sheet/sheet covers, especially when using specialist bed and mattress overlay systems
Use duvet - plus vapour permeable membrane.

NURSING CARE
General HAND WASHING, frequent changes of position, lying, sitting. Use of pillows
Pain Appropriate pain control
Nutrition High protein, vitamins and minerals
Patient Handling Correct lifting technique - hoists - monkey poles Transfer devices
Patient Comfort Aids Real Sheepskin - bed cradle
Operating Table
Theatre/A&E Trolley 100mm(4ins) cover plus adequate protection

Skin Care General hygene, NO rubbing, cover with an appropriate dressing

WOUND GUIDELINES
Assessment odour, exudate, measure/photograph position

WOUND CLASSIFICATION - EPUAP
GRADE 1 Discolouration of intact skin not affected by light finger pressure (non-blanching erythema)
This may be difficult to identify in darkly pigmented skin
GRADE 2 Partial thickness skin loss or damage involving epidermis and/or dermis
The pressure ulcer is superficial and presents clinically as an abrasion, blister or shallow crater
GRADE 3 Full thickness skin loss involving damage of subcutaneous tissue but not extending to the underlying fascia
The pressure ulcer presents clinically as a deep crater with or without undermining of adjacent tissue
GRADE 4 Full thickness skin loss with extensive destruction and necrosis extending to underlying tissue.

Dressing Guide Use Local dressings formulary and/or www.worldwidewounds

IF TREATMENT IS REQUIRED, FIRST REMOVE PRESSURE

Figure 23.5 The Waterlow pressure ulcer prevention/treatment policy. (Reproduced by permission of Judy Waterlow MBE SRN RCNT, http://www.judy-waterlow.co.uk/.)

Box 23.7 Evidence-based practice

Waterlow risk assessment

The EPUAP & NPUAP (2009) produced new guidelines on pressure ulcer prevention and treatment. Following a systematic review of the literature and consideration of the methodological adequacy of the studies they presented a list of factors which they felt were important in increasing patients' risk of developing pressure ulcers.

The unvalidated Waterlow risk assessment is one of several risk assessment tools available for use in clinical practice. It is a commonly used tool in the UK.

Activities

- Access the guideline from EPUAP & NPUAP (2009) and compare the evidence they present for inclusion of the individual risk factors to those used within the Waterlow Pressure Ulcer Prevention/Treatment Policy chart (Figure 23.5).
- Discuss with the trained staff how accurate they feel the Waterlow score is and what factors they feel are important in clinical practice.

Resources

European Pressure Ulcer Advisory Panel and National Pressure Ulcer Advisory Panel 2009 Prevention and treatment of pressure ulcers: quick reference guide. Washington DC: National Pressure Ulcer Advisory Panel. Available online http://www.epuap.org/guidelines/Final_Quick_Prevention.pdf

---

 Box 23.8 Information

Extract from an education leaflet: preventing pressure ulcers

As most pressure ulcers are the result of staying in one position for too long, the answer is to:

Relieve the pressure by changing position

Ideally, you should get up out of bed or your chair at least once every 2 hours during the day and take a short walk. This activity also helps your blood circulation and stops your muscles getting lax.

If you are confined to a chair, you should lift your bottom off the seat for a few moments every half an hour by pushing up on the arms of the chair.

If you have to stay in bed, then your bed may be fitted with a 'monkey pole' or rope ladder – the nurse will show you how to use this to lift yourself off the bed.

If your pressure ulcer is extensive or deep, or your movement is very restricted, a special movement chart will be devised for you by the nursing staff to keep you off the ulcer as much as possible, and you may be given a special bed or mattress.

(Reproduced with permission from Morison M, Moffatt C, Bridel-Nixon J, Bale S (eds) 1997 A colour guide to the nursing management of chronic wounds, 2nd edn. Mosby, London.)

Prevention of pressure ulcers is often far cheaper than management (Dealey 1997). Health service managers are able to cost the treatment of pressure ulcers more accurately, and as NICE (2005) requires that pressure ulcers of category 2 (II) or above are recorded as a critical incident more emphasis is being put on prevention with quality assurance systems such as root cause analysis being instigated when these reports are received. Pressure ulceration is also an important trigger for protection of vulnerable adults (POVA) activity.

Patient education

In the prevention and management of pressure ulcers, patients have an important role to play. All patients, including young people with chronic disabilities, can be taught methods of regularly relieving pressure by changing position (Colburn 1997). Patients who are not able to take such an active part in their own management can be taught the value of and need for the changes of position that nurses and other carers carry out for them. Concordance increases when patients understand why intervention is necessary.

Education leaflets, websites, etc., can also be useful. An extract from a typical patient information leaflet demonstrates how the nurse and the patient share in the prevention of pressure ulcers (Box 23.8).

Throughout the UK and mainland Europe guidelines for the prevention and treatment of pressure ulcers are produced in different languages for professionals, carers and patients (see Useful websites, e.g. EPUAP).

▷ Nursing management and health promotion: leg ulcers

Leg ulceration is a common problem, affecting between 1 and 2% of the population (Doughty & Holbrook 2007). Essentially a community-based problem, the day-to-day care of patients with these wounds is usually undertaken by district and practice nurses, supported by GPs, although there are an increasing number of specialist leg ulcer clinics in the community. The major cause of leg ulceration in the UK is chronic venous insufficiency associated with venous hypertension (70–75%). Between 20 and 30% of patients with a leg ulcer have some degree of ischaemia, with diabetes, vasculitis and trauma accounting for other causes of leg ulceration (Moffatt et al 2007b).

One of the most important stages in the assessment of patients is to diagnose the aetiology of the ulcer, as this dictates the most appropriate method of management. Such diagnosis is achieved by conducting a full patient assessment and a lower limb assessment in conjunction with the use of hand-held Doppler to ascertain the arterial flow to the lower limb (Royal College of Nursing [RCN] 2006).

Venous ulcers

This is the most common leg ulcer aetiology. Damage to the valves within the deep veins of the lower leg allows venous blood to flow the wrong way towards the foot. Because of this backflow the veins become congested with increased blood volume. This means that venous blood flows backwards through the perforator veins, between the deep and superficial system (Figure 23.6). Extra blood volume results in the superficial veins having to expand to deal with this

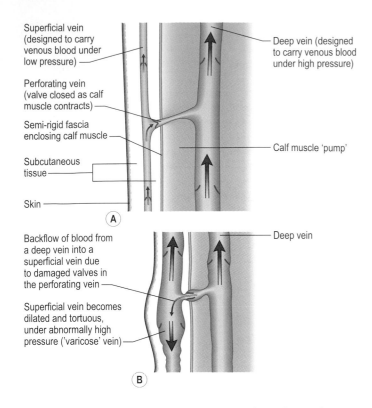

Superficial vein (designed to carry venous blood under low pressure)

Perforating vein (valve closed as calf muscle contracts)

Semi-rigid fascia enclosing calf muscle

Subcutaneous tissue

Skin

(A)

Deep vein (designed to carry venous blood under high pressure)

Calf muscle 'pump'

Backflow of blood from a deep vein into a superficial vein due to damaged valves in the perforating vein

Superficial vein becomes dilated and tortuous, under abnormally high pressure ('varicose' vein)

(B)

Deep vein

Figure 23.6 A. Healthy, intact valves prevent backflow of blood from the deep to the superficial veins. B. An incompetent valve in a perforating vein allows backflow of blood from the deep to the superficial venous system.

extra capacity. As the vein walls are stretched they leak plasma and red cells into the tissue of the lower leg which is visible as oedema and red/brown staining from blood pigments that are broken down in the tissue (Anderson 2009). Poor venous return affects the integrity of the skin and skin changes occur. As well as staining, the skin becomes dry and may become very sensitive to anything applied to it such as moisturisers, cleansing products and dressings, so extra care must be taken (Beldon 2009). Any knock or minor injury to the lower leg leads rapidly to breakdown of the skin and ulceration. Most commonly, ulceration occurs around the medial malleolus.

 See website Figure 23.5

The ulcers are shallow and can be painful, especially if there is ankle oedema and damage to the surrounding skin from exudate leakage. A typical past history reveals phlebitis, deep vein thrombosis (DVT), leg fracture or severe leg injury, or varicose veins (RCN 2006). It can take weeks or many months for venous ulcers to heal. Due to the poor condition of the tissues, ulceration can recur and patients need to wear compression hosiery, even after healing, to help maintain drainage of the affected limb.

Assessment

One of the primary aims of assessing a patient with a leg ulcer is to determine the cause. Nurses are the main health care professionals who carry out this assessment but input from other members of the health care team is important to ensure a full assessment with appropriate clinical investigations. Assessment includes:

- A comprehensive medical history which might indicate the presence of venous disease, e.g. previous DVT, vein surgery or pelvic trauma.
- A thorough clinical examination to support the medical history.
- Appropriate investigations, e.g. a Doppler assessment to ascertain the ankle pressure index which is used to detect the presence of significant arterial disease (Worboys 2006) (Box 23.9). Other investigations may include full blood count to exclude anaemia, erythrocyte sedimentation rate (ESR) to indicate inflammation, blood glucose to exclude diabetes mellitus, and wound swab where infection is suspected.

Sometimes further vascular investigations are indicated such as a Duplex scan to investigate arterial blockages, to identify venous disease if surgery is an option, or when the aetiology may be in doubt. A biopsy may be performed, particularly where malignancy is suspected.

Management

Bandaging The most important component in the treatment of venous ulcers is the use of compression therapy. This is normally in the form of compression bandages, sometimes with compression hosiery although hosiery is most often used to help prevent ulcer recurrence after healing. Compression bandages are designed to give graduated compression providing more support at the ankle and less at the knee to squeeze the veins and help the valves to close, thus

---

> ### Box 23.9 Information
>
> #### How to take the ankle:brachial pressure index (ABPI)
>
> - Lay the patient flat and allow the patient to rest quietly for 20 min. This is necessary to reduce the effects of gravity on the legs.
> - Place the sphygmomanometer cuff on the upper arm, and apply gel over the brachial artery. Hold the Doppler probe at a 45–60 degree angle and measure the systolic pressure. Repeat for the other arm and write down the highest of the two arm pressure readings.
> - Place the sphygmomanometer cuff around the malleolus (should the ulcer be sited here, cover the ulcer with protective material such as plastic film). Apply gel on at least two of the pulse points on the foot and take a systolic pressure reading from at least two of these points. Write down the highest reading.
> - The ankle:brachial pressure index is calculated by dividing the highest ankle pressure reading by the highest brachial pressure reading.
> - Do the same for the other leg, again using the highest brachial reading for the calculation.
>   *Normal ABPI ≥1 (1.3 is the upper limit of normal)* – full compression therapy may be applied.
>   *Abnormal ABPI ≤1 (this indicates a degree of arterial disease is present)* – if the patient assessment is satisfactory then full compression therapy may be applied.
>   *ABPI ≤0.8 and equal to or above 0.6 (arterial impairment is likely to be significant)* – reduced compression therapy may be used under specialist supervision.
>   *ABPI 0.5 or less (the patient has critical ischaemia)* – no compression is to be used.

preventing backflow. The bandages ease venous congestion, reduce oedema and allow improved blood flow to tissues. As the ulcer heals and the venous disease is controlled the skin condition should improve (Beldon 2009). The venous disease remains so it is important that the patient continues compression therapy even after healing. Bandages are most often multilayer systems using elastic materials or inelastic material (short stretch) (Figure 23.7). In the elastic system bandages are applied in a spiral with a 50% stretch and 50% overlap. Layer 3 (of 4) is applied as a figure of 8. In the inelastic system the bandage is unrolled onto the skin at a 100% stretch with a 50% overlap and application techniques can vary according to the size and shape of the leg. The principles of compression bandaging application are:

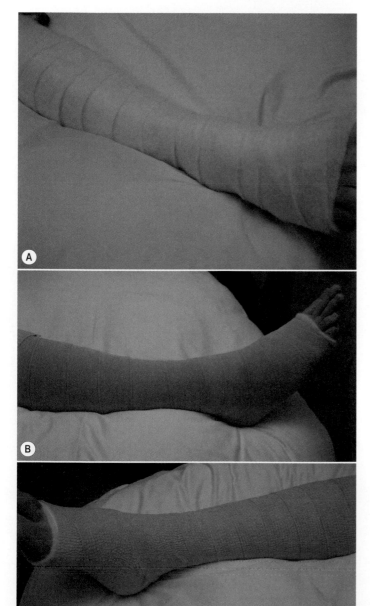

Figure 23.7 Compression bandaging. A. Padding. B. Short stretch bandage. C. Multilayer bandage.

- Ensure the lower leg is graduated in shape, i.e. a smaller circumference at the ankle than the calf (if this is not the case padding material is used to form the correct shape).
- The bandage is applied from toes to just below the knee (otherwise oedema will be pushed into the foot).
- Keep the tension of the bandage the same while the bandage is applied. The graduated shape of the leg will mean that more pressure is applied to the ankle and less as the circumference of the leg increases to the knee – 30–40 mmHg of pressure may be required at the ankle, graduating to 15–20 mmHg below the knee (Moffatt et al 2007c).
- Ensure that the bandage/hosiery does not slip, causing constriction of the limb.

Exercise and leg elevation Exercise and leg elevation are very important in managing venous disease. The most effective exercise to aid lower leg venous return is walking. If this is difficult then the patient must be taught and encouraged to rotate and flex the ankle joint as much as possible to create movement in the calf muscle. When the patient is sitting or lying they should be encouraged to have their feet higher than their hips to aid drainage of fluid from the lower leg. This can be uncomfortable when sitting and may be easier lying on a bed or couch.

Dressings Dressing management should be carefully considered once the factors outlined above have been successfully tackled. The ulcer should be assessed as for wounds (pp. 639–641) and the appropriate material then selected (pp. 641–643). Caution should be exercised with dressings and lotions as these patients quickly develop sensitivities to many of the commonly used products (Cameron 2007). The simplest treatments should be used first, e.g. non- or low-adherent textile dressings, as the most important part of management is compression. However, more interactive dressings may be selected depending on patient preference and clinical indications. For instance an antimicrobial, absorbent or pain-reducing dressing may be particularly indicated. A comprehensive patient assessment should aim to result in a complete treatment package. A suitable wound contact dressing and skin care combined with adequate compression therapy, exercise and leg elevation combined with patient education are most likely to produce the best patient outcomes.

See website Critical thinking question 23.2

Arterial ulcers

These are often the result of atherosclerosis (Doughty & Sparks-DeFriese 2007) affecting the arterial supply to the lower leg. The underlying disease processes are different from venous disease (Table 23.3). Damage to the arteries supplying the leg can occur and they gradually become occluded. Additionally, infarction of smaller arteries is caused by embolus formation, which causes ischaemia in the area of skin normally supplied by that artery. What follows is a very rapid breakdown of the skin.

The characteristics of these ulcers are a history of intermittent claudication and rapid onset of a deep ulcer that is often extremely painful. Relief may be gained by lowering the affected limb and hanging it over the edge of the bed or

Table 23.3 Characteristics of venous and arterial disease of the lower limb

CHARACTERISTIC	VENOUS DISEASE	ARTERIAL DISEASE
Site of ulcer	Around the 'gaiter' area, commonly above the medial malleolus	Anywhere on the lower limb including the foot, but commonly affecting the toes
Depth of ulcer	Shallow and spreading	Deep, with a punched-out appearance
Presence of oedema	Common, due to poor venous return	Often not detected
Onset	Gradual, unless precipitated by trauma	Rapid
Pain	Often uncomfortable, nagging in character, often worse if oedema increases. Related skin conditions can cause pain, discomfort and itching	Pain, sometimes made worse by elevation of limb relieved by lowering it (the blood flow is increased when the limb is in the dependent position). The pain of ischaemia can be unremitting
Temperature of foot	Warm and well perfused	Cool or cold and poorly perfused
Condition of the skin surrounding the ulcer	Varicose eczema, lipodermatosclerosis	Often shiny and hairless
ABPI	>0.8 (ABPI does not indicate venous disease)	<0.8 (indicates progressive arterial disease as index decreases)

NB: It is possible that a combination of both disease processes is present. It is important that a full assessment is conducted.

chair. These patients rarely go to bed to sleep, or if they do, they have to get up in the night because of the pain. They tend to sleep in a chair, which allows the affected limb to hang down optimising the arterial blood supply.

Arterial ulcers can occur anywhere on the lower leg, but usually present on the foot and lateral aspect of the lower leg. Foot pulses are often absent or very difficult to palpate. Doppler assessment reveals that the ABPI is significantly <0.8. There may also be a history of cardiovascular disease, typically hypertension, myocardial infarction, transient ischaemic attacks or stroke (RCN 2006).

Management

Surgical intervention may be necessary to improve the circulation or debridement of the ulcer, and skin grafting may be considered. Compression must be avoided as this would further impede an already poor blood supply to the area. Healing of these wounds is slow and the prognosis for eventual healing often poor. Treatment aims to keep the patient as comfortable as possible, to relieve pain and to achieve debridement and cleansing where necessary. Useful dressings include alginate or hydrofibre sheets if the wound is wet, hydrogel sheets for pain reduction if necessary (where the exudate level is not significant) and topical antimicrobial dressings if necessary.

Mixed aetiology ulcers

Around 20% of venous ulcers also have a poor arterial blood supply (Anderson & King 2006). This further complicates management, as oedema control is needed but without restricting the already compromised blood supply. Reduced levels of compression may be indicated to control oedema but if the arterial disease is progressing then optimising arterial flow must take precedence over managing venous

disease. In some cases a support bandage with sufficient underpadding can be used to control oedema but this must be under the direction of local protocols and a specialist nurse or doctor to ensure the patient is not harmed. Other types of leg ulcers are outlined in Box 23.10.

Patient education

Individual education regarding wound management can have a dramatic effect on progress. This aspect of care is particularly appropriate in patients with leg ulcers, especially venous leg ulcers. Patients who understand the cause of their ulcer and the rationale for the treatment and activities

Box 23.10 Information

Other types of leg ulcer

The following types of leg ulcer account for between 2 and 5% of lower limb ulcers:

- Vasculitic ulcers – these are due to connective tissue disease, e.g. rheumatoid arthritis, scleroderma, and also occur on the lower leg. They are unusual and extremely difficult to manage due to the underlying disease process and the medication that these patients require.
- Diabetic ulcers – these occur most commonly on the foot (see Ch. 5, Part 2). Again, due to the general condition of the patient, they heal slowly. It is worth noting that people with diabetes mellitus may give a falsely high reading on Doppler assessment due to peripheral hypertension.

The management of rheumatoid and diabetic ulcers is generally under specialist care and treatment is prescribed by the individual consultant.

- Miscellaneous causes – neoplastic and tropical ulcers are examples in this category.

(Based on data from Moffatt et al 2007a.)

they are asked to engage with are much more likely to have a concordant relationship with their practitioner. However, leg ulcers are long-term conditions and patients will need much support and encouragement to continue with treatment. Education can be helped by providing patients with appropriate information to be read at home (Box 23.11).

Sutured wounds

Common methods of wound closure are sutures, staples or adhesive glue. The decision which to use is often based on the extent, depth and site of the wound as well as patient circumstances. For instance there may be a risk of sensitivity to the material used, or the area may be subject to movement and flexion which may make adhesives less useful. Two Cochrane reviews which consider the merits of different closure methods conclude that each method has benefits in different circumstances and a holistic patient assessment must guide choice (Coulthard et al 2004, Farion et al 2002). Although the vast majority of sutured wounds heal without complication, there is a need for observation of both the patient and their wound for signs of infection by:

- Monitoring changes in vital signs, pulse, temperature, or malaise.
- Observing the wound for signs of infection after the initial inflammatory response has passed, i.e. redness, swelling, pain, discharge, heat.

The best time for removal of sutures depends upon:

- Wound site – wounds on the head and neck usually heal within 2 days due to the rich blood supply to the area, whereas wounds on the back may take 10–14 days to heal. The skin here is thicker and less vascular.
- Patient variation – if, during suture removal, the wound begins to gape then the nurse should stop and refer to the surgeon or a nurse specialist for advice. The skin edges can be pulled back together and held for a few more days with paper sutures.
- Cosmetic considerations – leaving sutures in for too long can cause excessive scarring.

In general, the principles for managing sutured wounds are to leave the wound undisturbed and the theatre dressing intact unless either the patient or the wound area shows signs which indicate the presence of infection (Bale & Jones 2006). Disturbing dressings unnecessarily can lead to the entry of bacteria into the wound or disturb newly forming epithelium. Local wound infection can slow down the rate of healing and also increase the amount of scar tissue produced. Careful postoperative observation is important. Ultimately a severe wound infection can spread into the tissues and also the bloodstream, causing life-threatening septicaemia (Williams & Leaper 1998).

Traumatic wounds

Patients presenting to the emergency department with traumatic wounds need special consideration. These patients may be shocked or have other injuries and their wounds are often contaminated due to the nature of the trauma (see Chs 18, 27).

These wounds are frequently irregular, with varying degrees of tissue loss (Whiteside & Moorehead 1999). Due to contamination, wound closure is often not attempted (Bale & Leaper 2000). Mechanical cleansing of the wound is undertaken to remove debris such as glass, wood or tarmac. Where wound closure is attempted, antibiotic cover is given to prevent infection, and the patient also needs to have prophylactic tetanus protection if they are not already covered (Bale & Jones 2006). Patients with extensive injuries are admitted for inpatient treatment. However, the majority of patients with wounds are discharged into the community. They may be instructed to care for the wound themselves or asked to return to the emergency department for any dressing changes, or the community nurse may be asked to manage wound care.

Malignant wounds

This is one group of wounds where healing is not always the expected outcome of wound management. Carcinomas and sarcomas are most likely to result in ulceration and fungation in the latter stages of the disease (Bale & Harding 2000). Such lesions may be associated with advanced breast cancer or malignant melanoma where the cancer ulcerates through the epithelium. The growth of tumours is a complex process that controls blood flow and tissue oxygenation (Grocott 1995). Tissue hypoxia causes tissue breakdown and encourages anaerobic and aerobic bacterial growth, producing malodour (Young 2005).

Problems encountered with malignant wounds (see Ch. 7) include:

- Wound site – often present in areas which are extremely difficult to dress in terms of keeping the dressing in place, e.g. the chest wall, groin and lower limb.
- Wound size and bulk – it may be difficult to find a dressing sufficiently large to cover the wound. The wound dimensions, shape and high exudate levels mean that dressings have to be bulky which adds to the difficulties patients have in managing both practically and psychologically (Young 2005).
- Exudate production – the exudate tends to be thick and sticky. Many dressings that do not adhere to other wound types will do so in the presence of this particularly viscous exudate. Hydrogel sheets and gel are very useful dressings for these wounds.
- Malodour – see Further reading, e.g. Draper 2005.
- Pain – where nerve endings are exposed, changing dressings and rubbing from dressings can be painful. Keeping the wound covered reduces the irritation to the nerve endings, and using gel dressings may help to reduce pain at dressing changes.

Where healing is not the ultimate aim, wound management should maximise convenience and minimise distress.

Box 23.11 Information

Leg Ulcer Forum: Patient information (Leaflet number 9) (reproduced with permission from the Leg Ulcer Forum)

How can I help my venous leg ulcer to heal?

I have a venous leg ulcer, how can I help it to heal?

You will be given a lot of information about wearing bandages and doing exercises. Your nurse will have discussed options with you so that you are involved in decisions which affect you. There are lots of things you can do to help your ulcer heal and make you feel better while this is happening.

Wear your bandages or compression hosiery

You have a problem with the circulation of blood in your veins. When the blood flow slows down it can cause your ankles to swell. Wearing bandages or hosiery keeps the blood moving efficiently and helps to reduce the swelling in your ankles. This is why you are asked to wear them all the time.

Do your exercises

Put your hand on the back of your calf and move your foot up and down. You will feel the muscle move and it is this movement which helps to keep the blood flowing in your legs. This happens when you walk but some people are not able to do this and everyone needs to do a little more exercise. The exercises are simple, you move your feet up and down and rotate your ankle. It is good to do this a few times every hour especially if you have been sitting down for a while. You may have been given a leaflet explaining exercise in more detail. If not ask your nurse or the person prescribing your care for a copy.

Put your feet up

Your ankles swell because of the slow blood flow. You will find that your ankles are less swollen when you have been in bed and it gets worse when you are sitting or standing. If you put your feet up so that they are higher than your hips, the swelling should be reduced.

Some people put their feet on the arm of the settee when they are sitting down, or put a cushion on a coffee table or footstool to rest their feet on. It does not matter as long as your feet are higher than your hips.

If you have stiffness in your hips it may be uncomfortable to sit with your feet up. It may be better to lie on the bed with a couple of pillows or cushions under your ankles. It is helpful to get into a routine for your rest time, perhaps when there is something you enjoy on the radio or television. It is best to have your feet up at least three times a day. When you do not have your feet up remember to do your exercises. It is important to do both.

Eat a healthy diet

As your ulcer heals it uses a lot of goodness from the food you eat. It is important that your diet contains protein, vitamins and minerals. These are found in a varied diet of meat, fish, eggs and cheese, as well as fruit and vegetables. Please ask your nurse for information on healthy eating.

It is important to watch your weight. If you are overweight you are putting an extra load on the veins in your legs.

Drink plenty of fluids

It is important to drink plenty of fluid during the day (unless you have been told not to by the doctor). This helps your ulcer to heal and helps to keep your skin healthy. Don't worry that this will add to the swelling in your ankles, the fluid here is different. Water is the best drink but you can have other drinks, but be careful not to have too many caffeine drinks or those high in sugar.

Take your medication

You may have been given medicine to help reduce the swelling in your ankles. It is important to take this and to wear your bandages or hosiery as well. If you have any questions about medicine you have been given, please discuss this with your doctor, nurse or pharmacist.

Skin care

The skin on your leg is very delicate. You may already apply cream to your face and you need to look after your legs just as carefully. While you are wearing your bandages the nurse will help you to wash your legs and apply a moisturiser. Only very gentle products should be used on your skin. Avoid using anything with lanolin (wool fat) or perfume. Some baby products contain these.

Keep in touch

When you have an ulcer you will see your nurse often. When the ulcer has healed you will still be advised to see the nurse from time to time. If you are worried about your legs it is important to tell the nurse as soon as possible. Problems might be a sore spot, itching or swelling. It is easier to sort problems out if they are found early.

Do other things

You might feel uncomfortable and that your ulcer is taking over your life. Try to do other things that you enjoy and discuss your worries with your nurse. It is important to get the ulcer healed as quickly as possible but any pain, discomfort or practical difficulties can also be dealt with along the way. This is much easier to do if you and your nurse work together.

Leaflets in the range

1. Venous disorders of the lower leg explained.
2. What is a venous leg ulcer?
3. Arterial disorders of the lower leg explained.
4. What is a Doppler ultrasound scan?
5. I am going for a Duplex scan.
6. Understanding compression bandaging.
7. Understanding compression hosiery.
8. Exercises to improve ulcer healing and help prevent recurrence.
9. How can I help my venous leg ulcer to heal?
10. Care of your skin.

Contact details of the person prescribing/providing your care

---

This leaflet is provided to offer advice but does not intend or claim to cover all eventualities.

If you are concerned you must seek professional help from your nurse or doctor or the person providing your care.

Leaflet sponsored by an educational grant from Smith & Nephew MARCH 2006

- Chronic and acute wounds have costs in terms of disruption to patients' lives, reduced quality of life and a huge financial cost in providing care.

- Nurses are key to the effective support and management of people with wounds; however, holistic wound care depends on the skills of many health professionals through interdisciplinary working.

- Evidence-based wound care requires an understanding of wound types and causes.

- Nurses must understand the physiology of wound healing in order to assess wounds.

- The prevention of problems by dealing with underlying factors such as nutritional assessment and optimal nutrition, maintaining continence, pressure relief, compression therapy, etc., are vital aspects of wound management.

- Developments in tissue viability and the management of chronic wounds proceed at a rapid pace and nurses have a professional responsibility to update their knowledge.

REFLECTION AND LEARNING – WHAT NEXT?

- **Test** your knowledge by visiting the website and answering the multiple choice questions and critical thinking questions.

- **Consolidate** your learning by looking at some of the further reading suggestions, references and specialist websites.

- **Revisit** some of the additional material on the website.

- **Consider** what you have learnt and how this will help your professional development.

- **Reflect** on how you can apply this knowledge to the care of your patients.

- **Discuss** your learning with your mentor/supervisor, lecturer and colleagues.

REFERENCES

Anderson I: What is a venous leg ulcer? *Wound Essentials* 4:36–44, 2009.

Anderson I, King B: Mixed aetiology leg ulcers, *Nurs Times* 102(16):45–50, 2006.

Atkinson A: Body image considerations in patients with wounds, *Journal of Community Nursing* 16(10):32–38, 2002.

Bale S, Harding K: Chronic wounds 2: diabetic foot ulcers and malignant wounds. In Bale S, Harding K, Leaper D, editors: *An introduction to wounds*, London, 2000, Emap Healthcare.

Bale S, Jones V: *Wound care nursing. A patient-centred approach*, ed 2, Edinburgh, 2006, Mosby.

Bale S, Leaper D: Acute wounds. In Bale S, Harding K, Leaper D, editors: *An introduction to wounds*, London, 2000, Emap Healthcare.

Barone EJ, Yager DR, Pozez AL: Interleukin-1 alpha and collagenase activity are elevated in chronic wounds, *Plast Reconstr Surg* 102:1023–1027, 1998.

Beldon P: Avoiding allergic reactions in skin, *Wound Essentials* 4:46–51, 2009.

Braden BJ: Risk assessment in pressure ulcer prevention. In Krasner D, Kane D, editors: *Chronic wound care*, Wayne, PA, 1997, Health Management Publications.

Cameron J: Dermatological changes associated with venous ulcers, *Wound Essentials* 2:60–66, 2007.

Carville K, Cuddigan J, Fletcher J, et al: *Principles of best practice. Wound infection in clinical practice. An International consensus*, London, 2008,

MEP Ltd. Available online http://www.mepltd.co.uk/pdf/Wound%20Inf%20S&N_English_WEB.pdf.

Chadwick P, Dowsett C, Findlay S, et al: *Best Practice Statement: Optimising Wound care*, Aberdeen, 2008, Wounds UK. Available online http://www.wounds-uk.com/best_practice.shtml.

Colburn L: Prevention of chronic wounds. In Krasner D, Kane D, editors: *Chronic wound care*, Wayne, PA, 1997, Health Management Publications.

Coulthard P, Esposito M, Worthington HV, et al: Tissue adhesives for closure of surgical incisions. *Cochrane Database Syst Rev* (2), 2004, CD004287. Available online http://www.cochrane.org/reviews/en/ab004287.html.

Cruse PJE, Foord R: The epidemiology of wound infection: a 10 year prospective study of 62,939 wounds, *Surg Clin North Am* 60(1):27–40, 1980.

Davies C: Cleansing rites and wrongs, *Nurs Times* 95:43, 1999.

Dealey C: The politicisation of pressure sores. In *Managing pressure sore prevention*, Guildford, 1997, Mark Allen.

Dealey C: The management of patients with chronic wounds. In *The care of wounds*, Oxford, 1999, Blackwell Science.

Department of Health (DH): *Improving patients' access to medicines: A guide to implementing nurse and pharmacist independent prescribing within the NHS in England*, 2006. Available online http://www.dh.gov.uk/en/Publicationsandstatistics/Publications/PublicationsPolicyAndGuidance/DH_4133743.

Doughty DB, Holbrook R: Lower-extremity ulcers of vascular etiology. In Bryant RA, Nix DP, editors: *Acute and chronic wounds: current management concepts*, ed 3, St Louis, 2007, Mosby, pp 258–306.

Doughty DB, Sparks-DeFriese B: Wound healing physiology. In Bryant RA, Nix DP, editors: *Acute and chronic wounds: current management concepts*, ed 3, St Louis, 2007, Mosby, pp 56–81.

European Pressure Ulcer Advisory Panel (EPUAP): EPUAP guidelines on the role of nutrition in pressure ulcer prevention and management, *EPUAP Review* 5(2):50–53, 2003.

European Pressure Ulcer Advisory Panel and National Pressure Ulcer Advisory Panel: *Prevention and treatment of pressure ulcers: quick reference guide*, Washington DC, 2009, National Pressure Ulcer Advisory Panel. Available online http://www.epuap.org/guidelines/Final_Quick_Prevention.pdf.

Farion KJ, Russell KF, Osmond MH, et al: Tissue adhesives for traumatic lacerations in children and adults, *Cochrane Database Syst Rev* (4), 2002, CD003326. Available online http://www.cochrane.org/reviews/en/ab003326.html.

Fernandez R, Griffiths R: Water for wound cleansing. *Cochrane Database Syst Rev* (4), 2008, CD003861.

Fletcher J: Differences between acute and chronic wounds and the role of wound bed preparation, *Nurs Stand* 20(22):62–68, 2008a.

Fletcher J: Optimising wound care in the UK and Ireland: a best practice statement, *Wounds UK* (4):73–81, 2008b.

Goswell N, Siefers R: Experiences of ward based nurse prescribers in an acute ward setting, *Br J Nurs* 18(1):34–37, 2009.

Grocott P: The palliative management of fungating malignant wounds, *J Wound Care* 4(5):240–242, 1995.

Hampton S: The appropriate use of gloves to reduce allergies and infection, *Br J Nurs* 11(17):1120–1124, 2002.

Harding KG: Understanding healing after skin breakdown. In Smith and Nephew Foundation, editor: *Skin Breakdown: the Silent Epidemic*, Hull, 2007, Smith and Nephew Foundation, pp 13–16.

Hart J: Inflammation 2: Its role in the healing of chronic wounds, *J Wound Care* 11:245–249, 2002.

Hospital Infection Society: *Third prevalence survey of healthcare associated infections in acute hospitals in England 2006*, 2007. Available online http://www.dh.gov.uk/en/Publicationsandstatistics/Publications/PublicationsPolicyAndGuidance/DH_078388.

Langemo D, Anderson J, Hanson D, et al: Measuring wound length, width and area: which technique? *Adv Skin Wound Care* 19(3):42–45, 2008.

Leaper D, Harding K: The problems of wound infection. In Bale S, Harding K, Leaper D, editors: *An introduction to wounds*, London, 2000, Emap Healthcare.

Marks J, Hughes LE, Harding KG, et al: Prediction of healing time as an aid to the management of open granulating wounds, *World J Surg* 7:641–645, 1983.

McLaren S: Nutritional factors in wound healing. In Morison M, Moffatt C, Bridel-Nixon J, et al, editors: *A colour guide to the nursing management of chronic wounds*, ed 2, London, 1997, Mosby, pp 27–52.

McWhirter JP, Pennington C: Incidence and recognition of malnutrition in hospital, *Br Med J* 308:945–948, 1994.

Moffatt CJ: Perspectives on concordance in leg ulcer management, *J Wound Care* 13(6):243–248, 2004.

Moffatt CJ, Martin R, Smithdale R: *Leg Ulcer Management*, Oxford, 2007a, Wiley-Blackwell.

Moffatt CJ, Franks PJ, Morison MJ: Models of service provision. In Morison MJ, Moffatt CJ, Franks PJ, editors: *Leg Ulcers: A problem based learning approach*, Edinburgh, 2007b, Mosby, pp 99–118.

Moffatt CJ, Partsch H, Clark M: Compression therapy in leg ulcer management, pp 169–198. In Morison MJ, Moffatt CJ, Franks PJ, editors: *Leg Ulcers: A problem based learning approach*, Edinburgh, 2007c, Mosby.

National Institute for Health and Clinical Excellence (NICE): *Inherited clinical guideline B: pressure ulcer risk assessment and prevention*, London, 2001, NICE.

National Institute for Health and Clinical Excellence (NICE): *The management of pressure ulcers in primary and secondary care. Clinical Guideline CG29, 2005*, Developed by the Royal College of Nursing. Available online http://www.nice.org.uk/nicemedia/pdf/CG029fullguideline.pdf.

National Institute for Health and Clinical Excellence (NICE): *Surgical Site Infection. Clinical Guideline CG74*, 2008. Available online http://www.nice.org.uk/nicemedia/pdf/CG74NICEGuideline.pdf.

Neal M: Angiogenesis: is it the key to controlling the healing process? *J Wound Care* 10:281–287, 2001.

NHS Estates: *Infection control in the built environment*, Norwich, 2002, TSO.

Parker L: Applying the principles of infection control to wound care, *Br J Nurs* 9(7):94–404, 2000.

Pinchcofsky-Devin G: Nutritional wound healing, *J Wound Care* 3(5):231–234, 1994.

Posnett J, Franks PJ: The costs of skin breakdown and ulceration in the UK. In Smith and Nephew Foundation, editor: *Skin Breakdown: the Silent Epidemic*, Hull, 2007, Smith and Nephew Foundation, pp 6–12.

Royal College of Nursing: *The nursing management of patients with venous leg ulcers*, 2006. Available online http://www.rcn.org.uk/__data/assets/pdf_file/0003/107940/003020.pdf.

Schoonhoven L, Haalboom JR, Buskens E, et al: Prognostic ability of risk assessment scales, *EPUAP Review* 4(1):17–18, 2002.

Siana JE, Frankild S, Gottrup F: The effect of smoking on tissue function, *J Wound Care* 1(2):37–41, 1992.

Slavin J: Wound healing: pathophysiology, *Surgery* 17(4):I–V, 1999.

Steed D: The role of growth factors in wound healing, *Surg Clin North Am* 77:575, 1997.

Stephens P, Thomas DW: The cellular proliferative phase of the wound repair process, *J Wound Care* 11:253–261, 2002.

Thomas S, Wynn K, Fowler T, Jones M: The effect of containment on the properties of sterile maggots, *Br J Nurs* 11(Suppl 12):S21–S28, 2002.

Timmons J: The RCT gold standard may be blinding us to the value of other research methods, *Wounds UK* 4(3):6, 2008.

Tjero-Trujeque R: Understanding the final stages of wound contraction, *J Wound Care* 10:259–263, 2001.

Vuolo J: Wound assessment and monitoring. In Vuolo J, editor: *Wound Care Made Incredibly Easy*, London, 2009, Lippincott Williams and Wilkins, pp 31–60.

Waldrop J, Doughty D: Wound-healing physiology. In Bryant RA, editor: *Acute and chronic wounds: nursing management*, ed 2, St Louis, 2000, Mosby.

Waterlow J: *The Waterlow Pressure Ulcer Prevention Manual*, 2005. Available online http://www.judy-waterlow.co.uk/the-waterlow-manual.htm.

Webster Marketon JI, Glaser R: Stress hormones and immune function, *Cell Immunology* 252(1–2):16–26, 2008.

Whiteside MCR, Moorehead JR: Traumatic wounds: principles of management. In Miller M, Glover D, editors: *Wound management*, London, 1999, NT Books.

Williams NA, Leaper DJ: Infection. In Leaper DJ, Harding KG, editors: *Wounds: biology and management*, Oxford, 1998, Oxford Medical Publications.

Wilson R: Massive tissue loss: burns. In Bryant RA, editor: *Acute and chronic wounds: nursing management*, ed 2, St Louis, 2000, Mosby.

Winter GD: Formation of the scab and rate of epithelialization of superficial wounds in the skin of the young domestic pig, *Nature* 193:293–294, 1962.

Worboys F: How to obtain the resting ABPI in leg ulcer management, *Wound Essentials* 1:55–60, 2006.

Wysocki AB: Anatomy and physiology of skin and soft tissue. In Bryant RA, Nix DP, editors: *Acute and chronic wounds: current management concepts*, ed 3, St Louis, 2007, Mosby.

Young CV: The effects of malodorous fungating malignant wounds on body image and quality of life, *J Wound Care* 14(8):359–362, 2005.

FURTHER READING

Bryant RA, Nix DP, editors: *Acute and Chronic Wounds: Current management concepts*, ed 3, St Louis, 2007, Mosby.

Dealey C: *The Care of Wounds: A Guide for Nurses*, ed 3, Oxford, 2005, Blackwell Publishing.

Draper C: The management of malodour and exudate in fungating wounds, *Br J Nurs* 14(11):S4–12, 2005.

JWC: *Wound Care Handbook 2009–2010*, London, 2009, Mark Allen Healthcare.

Morison MJ, Ovington LG, Wilkie K: *Chronic Wound Care*, Edinburgh, 2004, Mosby.

Morison MJ, Moffatt CJ, Franks PJ: *Leg Ulcers: A problem-based learning approach*, Edinburgh, 2007, Mosby.

Vuolo J, editor: *Wound Care Made Incredibly Easy*, Philadelphia, 2009, Lippincott Williams and Wilkins.

Wounds UK: Wound Essentials Journal series. Available online at http://www.wounds-uk.com/wound_essentials.shtml.

USEFUL WEBSITES

Cochrane Reviews (Systematic reviews of evidence related to wound care and infection control): www.cochrane.org/reviews/en/topics/96_reviews.html

Cochrane Wounds Group: http://wounds.cochrane.org/

Diabetic Foot Study Group: www.dfsg.org

European Pressure Ulcer Advisory Panel (EPUAP) (E.g. Resources/guidelines related to the prevention and management of pressure ulcers): www.epuap.org/glprevention.html

European Wound Management Association (EWMA) (Resources and position documents related to wound care including leg ulcer management): www.ewma.org/english/publications.html

Guidelines and Audit Implementation Network (GAIN), previously Clinical Resource Efficiency Support Team (CREST): www.gain-ni.org

Leg Ulcer Forum: www.legulcerforum.org

International Wound Infection Institute: www.woundinfection-institute.com

NHS Diabetes (E.g. Foot care guidance): www.diabetes.nhs.uk

Scottish Intercollegiate Guidelines Network (SIGN) (E.g. The Diagnosis and Management of Peripheral Arterial Disease, 2006): www.sign.ac.uk/pdf/sign89.pdf

Tissue Viability Society: www.tvs.org.uk

World Wide Wounds (Links to other wound care societies): www.worldwidewounds.com/Common/Links.html#Wound

Maintaining continence

Susan Walker

Introduction

Having control over urinary and faecal elimination is an expected norm within every society. In all but the very young, loss of continence is generally not viewed with sympathy and the real suffering it causes to individuals and their carers has not received the attention it deserves. Epidemiological research has shown that the number of people suffering from loss of continence in some form or other far exceeds the number of cases reported to health professionals. An underlying theme of this chapter is the need to acknowledge the extent of the problem and to promote continence by improving screening practices and raising public and professional awareness of preventive measures against incontinence and of the range of treatments available.

Loss of continence is a symptom that is often wrongly labelled as a disease. This chapter describes the underlying conditions that can prevent the acquisition of continence or provoke its loss. It is argued that a sound understanding of the causes and types of loss of continence is essential for its proper investigation, nursing management and treatment and that diagnostic assessment must recognise the individuality of each person. Similarly, where incontinence is intractable, assessment for aids and equipment must be sensitive to the values, needs and priorities of each person in order to ensure that an optimal quality of life (QoL) is achieved.

Throughout the chapter the emphasis is on a positive, problem-solving approach towards this often hidden problem, to reflect upon personal attitudes towards the subject of loss of continence, and to provide evidence-based care based on up-to-date research. Nursing management and health promoting activities aim to prevent the loss of continence, to help people to regain continence whenever possible and, when incontinence is intractable, to find solutions to problems that enhance the person's QoL. Nurses, working within the multidisciplinary team (MDT), fulfil a central role in the prevention of loss of continence.

CONTINENCE

The acquisition of continence in early childhood is a much valued developmental milestone. In the adult, the ability to control urinary and faecal elimination is largely taken for granted, and a loss of continence will have profound implications for the individual's ability to participate fully within society. While it may be deemed acceptable for a child to have an occasional 'accident', this is not generally the case for adults. The issue of loss of continence is one that many people find difficult to discuss openly, and one that is poorly understood.

The onus is on health professionals to foster a change in social attitudes by acquiring a clear understanding of how continence is attained and how loss of continence can develop. Nurses can make an important contribution to the promotion of continence among particularly vulnerable groups.

Defining continence

Continence may be defined in terms of the actions and abilities necessary for the appropriate management of urinary and faecal elimination. These include:

- recognising the need to pass urine or faeces
- identifying the correct place to pass urine or faeces
- delaying elimination until the appropriate place is reached
- reaching the correct place
- passing urine or faeces appropriately once a suitable place is reached.

Acquiring urinary continence

Urinary continence cannot be acquired until the nerve pathways necessary for micturition have matured. Once this has taken place, becoming continent is a matter of imitation, skill attainment and social conditioning.

The bladder acts as a reservoir for urine and it contracts to expel urine at the volition of the individual. Urine remains in the bladder as long as the intravesical (within the bladder) pressure does not exceed the urethral resistance.

In normal micturition, the contraction of the detrusor (expelling) muscle of the bladder induces the bladder neck to open while the pelvic floor muscles and the external urinary sphincter relax. For a child to obtain continence they must acquire control of the mechanisms that prevent the bladder from automatically emptying when it is full; this is usually achieved by the age of 3 years.

The neurological control of the bladder at birth involves a simple sacral reflex arc whereby automatic filling and emptying of the bladder are under the control of some sacral segments of the spinal cord. Nerve endings in the bladder wall are activated by stretch as urine accumulates. These relay impulses with increasing frequency through the parasympathetic nerves to the spinal cord until the motor parasympathetic nerve impulses cause the bladder muscle to contract and the urethral sphincters to open, whereupon reflex emptying occurs (Figure 24.1).

In order to achieve continence, a child needs to become aware of the sensation of bladder filling and through trial and error attempt to overcome the reflex emptying mechanism by using the pelvic floor muscles to keep the urethral sphincter

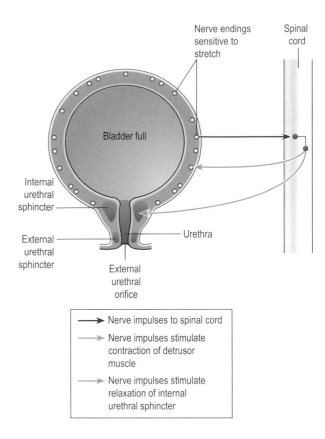

Figure 24.1 Reflex control of micturition when conscious effort cannot override the reflex action. (Reproduced from Waugh & Grant 2006 with permission.)

closed. Sensory impulses from the bladder travel in the spinal cord to the cerebral cortex, whereupon motor impulses from the cerebral cortex travel to the bladder to inhibit the bladder contractions; this requires practice as well as maturation of the central nervous system. Continence thus involves the active inhibition of nerve impulses. When micturition is initiated, the brain ceases to initiate inhibitory impulses, allowing the spinal reflex arc to be completed. Figure 24.2 illustrates the control of micturition once bladder control is established.

Normal patterns of micturition can vary markedly from one individual to another. Normally the adult bladder contains around 200–400 mL of urine before the urge to pass urine becomes too great. Most adults empty their bladder four to six times a day and have a bladder capacity of up to 600 mL (or more); this is influenced by age, fluid intake, medication, perspiration, body temperature, activity and stress. People who are anxious generally feel the need to empty their bladders more often; in the event of acute emotional distress or sudden shock, it is possible for involuntary bladder emptying to occur.

Acquiring faecal continence

Defecation is the expulsion of faecal matter from the rectum with the aid of peristaltic movements of the muscular walls of the intestine. As with urination, involuntary or autonomic reflex defecation occurs in the infant and young child, until voluntary control of the external sphincter is gained. Children usually gain this control in the second or third year of life.

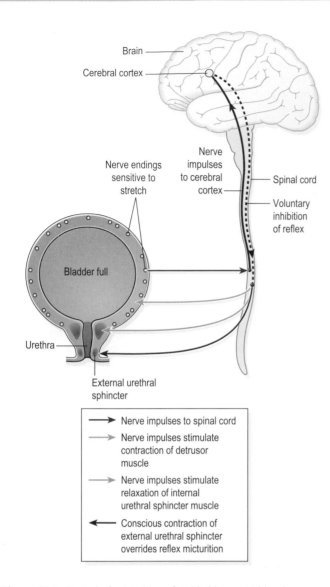

Figure 24.2 Control of micturition after bladder control has been established. (Reproduced from Waugh & Grant 2006 with permission.)

The rectum is stimulated to empty by strong peristaltic waves (mass movements) in the colon; these are initiated by the gastrocolic reflex (a sensory stimulus that happens when food enters the stomach). The need for defecation is felt as a response to distension of the sigmoid colon and the stimulation of the receptors.

Anxiety can produce an urge to defecate more often, and in situations of extreme crisis faecal control can be temporarily lost.

Attitudes towards loss of continence

In the UK, attitudes towards loss of continence are slowly changing. Loss of continence is becoming an acceptable subject for open discussion and began to be addressed openly in the media from 1985 onwards. Today, advertisements for absorbent products fill many magazine pages and television commercials. Nevertheless, certain myths still persist, such as the notion that incontinence is an inevitable consequence of old age, or that wearing pads is the only solution. Such myths must be dispelled in favour of seeking the underlying cause of incontinence in each individual case.

The psychosocial implications of incontinence are far-reaching. Social exclusion is common, as individuals with incontinence are often afraid to leave home, afraid they may be unable to access a lavatory in time, or experience an episode of incontinence in the presence of others. This can lead to depression. In older people this may contribute to a loss of mobility and can be a cause of falls (Teo et al 2006).

It is important for nurses to examine their own attitude towards bladder, bowel and continence care. It has been found that some nurses consider routine or service requirements to be more important than assisting people to use the lavatory (Morrow 2002, Nazarko 2003).

INCONTINENCE

This section of the chapter outlines the prevalence, types and causes of urinary and faecal incontinence and medical management.

Urinary incontinence

The International Continence Society (ICS) (2002) has coordinated the publication of a consensus document defining the terminology associated with the lower urinary tract, in which it defines urinary incontinence as 'a condition in which involuntary loss of urine is a social or hygienic problem'. However, it is only when the specific type and cause of the person's incontinence are known that appropriate treatment can be offered.

The prevalence of urinary incontinence in the UK is difficult to ascertain. Some estimates suggest that between 3 and 6 million people have some degree of urinary incontinence. Interestingly, the Bladder and Bowel Foundation (2008a) estimates that around one third of women are affected by stress urinary incontinence.

It is recognised that although urinary incontinence affects all age groups, male and female, its prevalence is greatest amongst women, particularly older women. In response to this fact the National Institute for Health and Clinical Excellence (NICE) (2006) developed guidelines on the management of urinary incontinence in women.

Types and causes of urinary incontinence

Stress urinary incontinence (SUI) results from a failure of the urethral sphincter to remain closed when a sudden increase in abdominal pressure on the bladder occurs, e.g. on effort or exertion, during coughing, sneezing or laughing. The weak pelvic floor allows the urethra to descend and the sphincter to open, releasing urine.

Urge incontinence results from the contraction of the detrusor muscle of the bladder as if to void, although the bladder may not be full. This may be caused by overactive detrusor function (motor urgency) or by hypersensitivity (sensory urgency).

Mixed incontinence is the involuntary leakage of urine associated with both urgency and exertion, effort, sneezing or coughing.

Overflow incontinence occurs as a consequence of urinary retention, which may in turn result from:

- obstruction, e.g. tumour, faecal impaction or prostatic enlargement
- underactive detrusor muscle, resulting in a flaccid bladder and thus failure to generate enough pressure to open the urethra
- failure of the urethra to open.

Reflex incontinence may occur as a result of damage to the spinal cord and loss of sensation associated with the desire to micturate, leading to failure to inhibit the simple reflex arc.

Enuresis refers to any involuntary loss of urine. Nocturnal enuresis is the term for urinary incontinence that occurs during sleep, in the absence of organic disease or infection (not to be confused with nocturia, which is being woken at night by the urge to pass urine). Enuresis may be primary or secondary. The number of adults afflicted with nocturnal enuresis is uncertain, due to the hidden nature of the problem, although Hjalmas et al (2004) quote the prevalence of enuresis as 0.5% in otherwise healthy adults aged 18–64. There are three conditions that may contribute to enuresis, often in combination:

- a reduced bladder capacity
- an inability to concentrate urine at night
- difficulty in waking when the bladder is full.

Functional incontinence An individual with this type of incontinence would, in favourable circumstances, be able to remain continent but is prevented by pre-existing disease or disability from gaining access to an appropriate place at an appropriate time to pass urine. Conditions that may affect mobility and dexterity, and therefore continence, include multiple sclerosis, spina bifida, arthritis and spinal cord injury. In addition, conditions associated with ageing, such as slowness of movement, pain, joint stiffness, inability to climb stairs or difficulty in manipulating fastenings, may all contribute to incontinence.

Faecal incontinence

According to NICE (2007), faecal incontinence is a not a diagnosis but is a symptom or sign. Reaching a consensus on a definition of faecal incontinence is difficult, but it can be classified by the symptom, such as faecal leakage. The prevalence of faecal incontinence in the UK is difficult to ascertain as it remains a taboo subject and people are reluctant to discuss their problems or seek help, due to embarrassment, anxiety and fear. It is estimated that faecal incontinence is experienced by 1–10% of the adult population living at home (NICE 2007). However, prevalence rates vary, from up to 13% for minor incontinence in the community, to up to 95% in nursing homes (Black 2007). It is known that faecal incontinence is more common in older people, particularly frail older women.

While urinary incontinence is more prevalent in the population than faecal incontinence, the latter is the more distressing problem. Faecal incontinence is socially even less acceptable than urinary incontinence and raises strong emotions among carers who have to deal with it. It is a source of discomfort and acute embarrassment for the sufferer, and contributes to feelings of helplessness, loss of self-esteem and social isolation.

Faecal incontinence, like urinary incontinence, is a symptom of an underlying pathology and with appropriate assessment and treatment many people will regain continence (Kenefick 2004).

Types and causes of faecal incontinence

The causes of faecal incontinence must be determined before treatment is instigated. Other than simple constipation, faecal impaction with overflow diarrhoea (spurious diarrhoea), the main cause of faecal incontinence is usually damage to the pelvic floor and anal sphincters (such as during childbirth, rectal prolapse or surgery), resulting in an inability to recognise that the rectum is full or to distinguish between flatus and faeces.

Causes of faecal incontinence in adults include:

- faecal impaction with overflow diarrhoea in very frail older people and often those with dementia and physical disability
- diarrhoea/intestinal hurry caused by gastroenteritis, inflammatory bowel disease (IBD) (see Ch. 4), and medications such as antibiotics, excessive use of laxatives and some foods
- neurological disease which may include spinal nerve injury, spina bifida, stroke and diseases such as Parkinson's and multiple sclerosis
- anal sphincter damage due to direct trauma caused during childbirth or surgery.

Rao (2004) states that many people who experience faecal incontinence refer to themselves as having diarrhoea or urgency as this seems more tolerable. Rao refers to faecal incontinence being graded in relation to its severity:

- Passive – involuntary discharge of faecal matter or flatus without awareness. The person may have impaired perception or impaired reflexes. There may also be sphincter dysfunction.
- Urge – involuntary discharge of faecal matter or flatus, in spite of active attempts to retain the bowel contents. This is usually related to sphincter disruption.
- Seepage – undesired leakage after a normal bowel movement. Mostly this is due to incomplete evacuation of the bowel contents and/or impaired rectal sensation. The sphincter function and the pudendal nerve are mostly intact.

Faecal incontinence or soiling in children is termed 'encopresis' and is defined as the passage of a normal consistency stool in a socially unacceptable place. The prevalence of children with faecal incontinence decreases from 1 in 30 children at age 5 years to 1 in 100 by the age of 12 years (Department of Health [DH] 2000).

Epidemiology of incontinence – prevalence studies

Seminal research into the prevalence of incontinence by Thomas et al (1980) found that whilst incontinence was most prevalent among older women, its occurrence was significant across all age groups. Stress incontinence was reported less often by nulliparous than by parous women of all ages, and was especially prevalent among those who had borne four or more children. Urge incontinence also occurred more commonly among parous than nulliparous women. No significant class differences were found among men or women, but individuals of African Caribbean or part African Caribbean descent were more likely to have some form of incontinence than those of Asian descent.

The most important finding of the study, however, was the 1:10 ratio of known to unknown cases of incontinence. This suggests that for every incontinent person who is known to health or social services professionals, there are 10 others who are unidentified. As further in-depth interviews revealed, many people try to 'cope' with moderate to severe problems of incontinence without professional support. These findings identify the need for health care workers to take advantage of all appropriate opportunities in all care settings to identify those who require assessment and treatment for incontinence.

The *Essence of Care Benchmark for Bladder, Bowel and Continence Care* recommends that nurses use a 'trigger' question to initiate conversation that may lead to further assessment of a person's continence, bladder and bowel status (DH 2010). It is recognised that the nurse asking a question provides an opportunity for the person to talk about this sensitive subject. An open question offers the opportunity for an in-depth answer, for example 'Tell me about any difficulties you have maintaining continence or with your bladder or bowel function'.

An audit of first assessments by community nurses found that district nurses were primarily assessing people with incontinence for absorbent products rather than assessing their incontinence with a view to improved management or regaining continence (Audit Commission 1999). There is a need not only to identify people who are incontinent, but also to improve public and professional understanding of incontinence, to evaluate services available for those requiring assessment and to improve methods of treatment and management (Scottish Intercollegiate Guidelines Network [SIGN] 2004). However, continence care seems to remain low on the list of nursing priorities, with a focus on containment rather than interventions to improve continence and QoL (Box 24.1).

Sociological factors in underreporting of incontinence

That incontinence remains to such a large extent a hidden problem among the general population can be attributed in part to the embarrassment felt by many people, leading to reluctance to admit to incontinence and seek treatment (Mason et al 2001). Several authors agree that the more severe the incontinence, the more likely a person is to seek medical help (Roe et al 1999, Shaw 2001). However, the severity of the symptoms is only one factor that influences the person in their choice to seek professional help or not. Shaw (2001) identifies other factors that influence this decision:

- lack of knowledge of causes, not considering incontinence to be a medical problem
- lack of knowledge of treatment options, not aware that incontinence is treatable

Box 24.1 Evidence-based practice

Do nurses promote continence in hospitalised older people? An exploratory study

Dingwall & McLafferty (2006) explored whether nurses working in older peoples' medicine and in acute medical settings promote urinary continence in older people or in reality use containment strategies.

The study demonstrated that untreated urinary incontinence in older adults can result in prolonged hospital admission and increased risk of admission to long-term care. It was recognised that little qualitative investigation into how nurses promoted urinary continence in older people was available.

Data were collected using focus groups and one-to-one semistructured interviews in two NHS regions in Scotland. Registered and non-registered nurses were invited to participate. Data were analysed thematically.

Their findings indicated that some nurses believe older people accept urinary incontinence as a result of ageing. Lack of assessment resulted in older people being labelled as incontinent of urine. Assessment strategies for older people tend to focus on product identification and management of incontinence, rather than identifying the cause. The study identified that although all nurses know the importance of promoting continence, the problem continues to be contained rather than treated.

Competing clinical priorities, varying staff approaches and deficits in education were cited as barriers to promoting continence.

Activities

- Access Dingwall & Lafferty's full paper. Discuss the main findings of their study with your mentor or a colleague.
- Which continence assessment tools have you seen used?
- Consider how you explore the views of older patients in your care with regard to their continence status.
- Have you been in a clinical area when the continence nurse specialist/advisor was consulted?

Resource

Dingwall L, McLafferty E: Do nurses promote continence in hospitalized older people? An exploratory study, *J Clin Nurs* 15(10):1276–1286, 2006.

- belief that incontinence is a long-term condition related to age and parity
- previous experience or experience of friends/family
- cultural background and attitudes to discussing such intimate problems
- personality of the person and their relationship with members of the health care team.

Many people prefer not to mention their incontinence to others (Roe et al 1999).

Incontinence may restrict employment, and educational and social activities, which in turn may compromise both physical and mental well-being.

It may also be true that, in women, the private nature of and, to some degree, secretiveness surrounding menstruation gives an easily transferable model of management to follow should incontinence develop. Many women conceal the leakage of urine as they have concealed menstruation previously.

For many people, incontinence is a source of embarrassment or shame rather than a signal to seek medical help. The dysfunction is seen mainly in terms of its social consequences rather than as a symptom of a possible underlying illness or disease process.

Personal and social attitudes towards incontinence are not, however, the only factors that account for the underreporting of this widespread health problem. The way that particular health services are marketed or presented can also influence an individual's decision whether to seek help or cope on their own. In the words of one person, 'I would find it too embarrassing to go to a special clinic…perhaps a home visitor would be more helpful' (Association for Continence Advice 2000).

It is therefore important that continence services reflect positive attitudes and approaches to promoting continence, and progress on this is demonstrated in the setting of standards by nurses and monitoring of services and treatment. It is vital that people and carers affected by incontinence are given every opportunity to regain their continence, to be empowered and to be involved in the development of targeted services. To this end, a *Charter for Continence* was developed by several professional organisations in 1995 (Box 24.2). Various government initiatives and other publications have assisted in the process.

In England and Wales, the DH (2000) issued guidance on continence services to the NHS. This provided targets for both inpatient and community care. The guidance also influenced the content of the 10-year programme of the National Service Framework (NSF) for older people

---

Box 24.2 Information

Charter for Continence

The Charter for Continence presents the specific needs and rights of people with bladder or bowel problems. It outlines the resources available and the standards of care that can be expected.

As a person with bladder or bowel problems you have the right to:

- Be treated with sensitivity and understanding
- Become continent if achievable
- Receive a thorough individual assessment of your condition by a doctor or nurse knowledgeable in this aspect of care
- Request specialist advice about continence care
- Be provided with a clear explanation of your diagnosis
- Participate in a full discussion of treatment options, their advantages and disadvantages
- Be provided with full, impartial information on the range of products which are available and how to obtain them
- Expect products to have clear instructions for use
- Receive regular reviews of treatment and be given the opportunity to change treatments if your condition has changed
- Be made aware of any treatments or products as they become available
- Be provided with a personal contact point able to give you ongoing advice and support.

Developed by The Continence Foundation, InconTact, Association for Continence Advice (ACA), the RCN Continence Care Forum, Education and Resources for Improving Childhood Continence (ERIC), the Spinal Injuries Association and the Multiple Sclerosis Society. (Produced by an educational grant from Bard Ltd, March 1995.)

(DH 2001). A supporting system redesign for older people is now underway to build on the progress of the NSF (DH 2009). The Essence of Care (DH 2010) benchmark statements ensured that specific areas of care, such as continence, could be audited and improved.

In Scotland, various guidance was published, for example, NHS Quality Improvement Scotland (NHSQIS) (2004), Nursing and Midwifery Practice Development Unit (NMPDU) (2002) and SIGN (2004).

In the last few years NICE has produced guidelines for both urinary and faecal incontinence and related treatments (NICE 2006, 2007).

The participation of those most affected by incontinence has been further strengthened by the inclusion of patients/carers on all the working parties for national continence publications, and including sections on patient information in those publications.

Factors contributing to incontinence

Incontinence is basically due either to a delay in achieving continence, or loss of established continence.

Delay in achieving continence

In childhood, the acquisition of the skills necessary to achieve continence may be delayed. Nocturnal enuresis may present as a primary or secondary feature; its cause is not known. Although it often spontaneously resolves, it is sometimes not resolved during childhood. In such cases, if it remains untreated, it may be a problem throughout life (Hjalmas et al 2004). Its impact on both individual and family has been researched by Morrison et al (2000).

Learning disability may also prevent a person from attaining continence. Professionals working with people who have learning disabilities should base their interventions on the assumption that, although the process of toilet training may be slow, continence will eventually be achieved provided interventions are tailored to the individual and their family's requirements (Rogers 1998). Physical difficulties can hinder the acquisition of continence. Some children cannot become continent without medical intervention, such as in some types of spina bifida. An infant or child who is continuously wet should always be investigated for either congenital fistula or failure to empty the bladder. Such symptoms should be taken seriously as failure of bladder emptying (with stasis of urine) can lead to vesicoureteric reflux (VUR). There is reflux of urine up the ureters following a rise of pressure within the bladder during voiding. The urine later runs back to the bladder and is not immediately voided, which in turn increases the risk of urinary tract infection (UTI). The constant reflux of infected urine into the ureters can lead to chronic pyelonephritis (reflux nephropathy) (see Ch. 8).

Factors affecting existing continence

A number of factors can affect continence. These include:

Physical factors
Age While incontinence is more prevalent among older people (especially women), it is not an inevitable consequence of growing older. However, with normal ageing

comes a decline in renal function; it is reduced by up to 50% by the age of 80 years, thus impairing the ability of the kidney to concentrate urine. This consequence of ageing occurs alongside a decrease in the bladder's urine-storing capacity (Hald & Horn 1998).

Ageing may also have some effect on the cerebral control of micturition; changes in cortical neurones can reduce their effectiveness in inhibiting the sacral reflex arc, so that involuntary emptying of the bladder occurs.

Ignoring the urge to urinate or defecate Ignoring the need to empty the bladder may lead to an episode of incontinence of urine, whilst ignoring the need to defecate may lead to constipation. Constipation is a common contributing factor to urinary incontinence and also retention of urine (see p. 670). Because of the anatomical proximity of the rectum and the urethra, it is possible for the urethra to be closed off by a faecal mass. This can result in incomplete voiding and stasis of urine, which in turn can encourage growth of bacteria and UTI.

Immobility Reduced mobility or a lack of mobility may mean that an individual is unable to get to the lavatory, or is dependent upon assistance. Should assistance not be available, or an individual be unable to manoeuvre themselves, they may be incontinent. Undoing zips or pulling down underwear may be difficult if manual dexterity is impaired. People may misguidedly attempt to reduce the need to micturate or defecate by reducing fluid and food intake, leading to dehydration and constipation.

Fluid/diet Eating and drinking play a significant part in the process of elimination. A lack of non-starch polysaccharides (NSPs or fibre) can cause constipation; fruit eaten in excess can result in diarrhoea. Increased fluid intake may increase the need to urinate, whilst reduced fluid intake leads to dehydration and constipation.

Hormones Constipation can occur during pregnancy.

Medications and other substances Diuretics, sedatives, laxatives, opioids, antibiotics, alcohol, etc., may influence elimination. For example, antibiotic-induced diarrhoea may lead to faecal incontinence.

Environmental/social/economic

- *Lack of facilities* – no toilet tissue or handwashing facilities.
- *Poor facilities* – cold, dirty, dark, too far away.
- *Lack of privacy/change in environment* – admission to hospital and having to use a bedpan/commode. Having to use communal facilities.
- *Costs* – need for adaptations to the home environment or aids to facilitate and promote independence with maintaining continence.

Psychological

- *Anxiety and stress* – can lead to diarrhoea.
- *Low mood, depression and dementia* – can be associated with constipation.
- *Life events* – bereavement and loss, a new sibling, change in a relationship, etc., can affect bowel habit.

Pre-existing conditions

- *Bladder or bowel disease* – UTIs (see Ch. 8) may cause frequency and urgency resulting in an episode of incontinence. Inflammatory bowel disease (see Ch. 4) may cause diarrhoea with incontinence. Functional bowel disorders may cause a number of problems including faecal incontinence and constipation.

See website for further content

- *Painful anorectal conditions* – e.g. haemorrhoids, fissure (see Ch. 4), cause people to 'put off' defecation leading to constipation which compounds the problem as it will cause even more pain on defecation.
- *Neurological conditions* – multiple sclerosis, paraplegia, stroke (see Ch. 9). For example, urinary and faecal incontinence is common following a stroke (Box 24.3). It is possible for continence to be regained with good nursing and rehabilitation (Nakayama et al 1997).
- *Systemic conditions* – thyroid disease can change bowel habit (see Ch. 5). Serious infection can lead to incontinence. Hyperglycaemia or hypercalcaemia can also lead to urinary incontinence.
- *Acute confusional state* – can precipitate urinary incontinence.

Medical management

Incontinence is best managed by an MDT comprising a specialist continence nurse, physiotherapist, pharmacist, general practitioner, specialist doctor and the person/carers. Many interventions that were previously the domain of the medical staff are now initiated or undertaken by specialist continence nurses. However, for clarity, medical history, examination, investigations, non-surgical and surgical interventions are outlined here.

History and examination

A full medical history is taken and the person is asked to describe the problem and how it affects their QoL. Listening to the person's lived experience is vital to reaching the correct diagnosis and ensuring acceptable outcomes. The person is examined by a health professional who has developed the appropriate knowledge and expertise (SIGN 2004). Explicit consent is required. In women, a vaginal examination can determine whether atrophic vaginal changes, vaginitis or painful excoriation are a problem, and whether cervicovaginal or uterovaginal prolapse is present (see Ch. 7). Examination in both men and women will determine whether rectal prolapse, painful anorectal conditions or constipation are present. An assessment of pelvic floor contraction strength should be undertaken before initiating a pelvic floor muscle re-education programme. Men should be examined for prostatic enlargement and to determine whether the bladder is palpable. If the bladder is palpable or the history suggests inability to empty the bladder completely, it may be necessary to ask the person to pass urine, after which a catheter can be introduced, or a portable bladder scanner used to assess the residual volume of urine.

If digital rectal examination is undertaken it also requires explicit consent and must be documented in the person's

Treatment of constipation and faecal incontinence in stroke patients

Despite the high prevalence of bowel dysfunction in stroke survivors, there is little clinical research conducted. This randomised trial by Harari et al (2004) evaluated the treatment of constipation and faecal incontinence in stroke survivors.

Stroke patients with constipation or faecal incontinence were identified by screening questionnaire (122 community, 24 stroke rehabilitation inpatients) and randomised to intervention or routine care (73 per group). The intervention was a single structured nurse assessment which included history taking and rectal examination, leading to targeted patient/carer education in the form of a booklet and provision of a diagnostic summary and treatment recommendations to the patient's GP/ward physician.

Results – The percentage of bowel movements per week graded as normal by participants in a prospective 1-week stool diary was significantly higher in intervention versus control patients at 6 months, as was the mean number of bowel movements per week. There was no significant reduction in faecal incontinence. At 12 months, intervention patients were more likely to be modifying their diets and fluid intake to control their bowels and to have visited their GP for their bowel problem. GP prescribing of laxatives and suppositories was significantly influenced at 12 months.

Conclusions – A single nursing educational consultation with recovering stroke patients effectively improved symptoms of bowel dysfunction up to 6 months later, changed bowel-modifying lifestyle behaviours up to 12 months later, and significantly influenced GP and physician prescribing patterns for laxatives and suppositories to this group of patients.

Activity

- Access the full paper by Harari et al and consider how their conclusions could be used to enhance your practice.
- Consider the discharge information given to patients regarding bladder and bowel continence in your clinical area.
- Are leaflets with health-promoting advice, useful websites and contact telephone numbers available to give to patients and carers on discharge?
- Discuss with your mentor or a colleague how the discharge information could be improved. If information leaflets are not available, consider what you think should be included in a bladder and bowel continence health promotion leaflet.
- Using Useful websites in the chapter, or by contacting your health promotion unit, find out what information on bladder and bowel care is available for members of the public.

Resource

Harari D, Norton C, Lockwood L, Swift C: Treatment of constipation and faecal incontinence in stroke patients: randomized controlled trial, *Stroke* 35:2549, 2004.

medical and nursing records. The Royal College of Nursing provides guidance on all aspects of digital rectal examination (RCN 2003, 2007).

Assessment of a person with faecal incontinence should include a history of the complaint and the person's normal bowel habit prior to the incontinence in order to establish the specific type of incontinence. Bleeding, loss of sensation,

feeling that defecation is incomplete, pain with defecation and the presence of mucus should all be investigated. A full description of the incontinence and its frequency are also important to the diagnosis. Liquid faecal leakage is quite different from true diarrhoea. Following a rectal examination by an appropriately trained and competent health professional other investigations may be necessary (see below).

Investigations

Investigations ordered will depend on the person's particular type of incontinence and situation. Those for urinary incontinence may include:

- *Urine testing* – observation for dark, cloudy or malodorous urine, and dipstick urine testing for protein, blood, glucose, etc., to exclude UTI and detect the possibility of other urinary pathology such as cancer or diabetes (see Chs 5, 8). NICE (2006) recommends that a urine dipstick test should be used for those presenting with urinary incontinence and/or symptoms that indicate infection. In people with symptoms of UTI and a positive urine dipstick test for leucocytes and nitrites, infection is likely.
- *Midstream urine (MSU)* sent for microscopy, culture and sensitivity.
- *Frequency volume charts.*
- *Urodynamic investigations* measure the pressure and flow relationships in the bladder and urethra (Table 24.1). They can aid diagnosis of the type of incontinence by showing sphincter incompetence, detrusor instability, urethral instability and problems with voiding due to obstruction or an underactive detrusor. The procedures are invasive, unpleasant and potentially very embarrassing, but generally not painful (see Further reading, e.g. Anders 2001).
- *Cystoscopy* allows inspection of the bladder and urethra, observing for tumours, stones, strictures and the condition of the mucosa.
- *Imaging:*
  - intravenous urogram (IVU), ultrasound scanning (USS) or magnetic resonance imaging (MRI). Used to detect structural abnormalities of the urinary tract, stones or cancer, and the extent of faecal impaction in the colon and to show any bowel narrowing or obstruction
  - cystography and cystourography. A urinary catheter is introduced and the bladder is filled to capacity with contrast medium and X-rayed, revealing any bladder abnormalities. The catheter is then removed to observe the function of the bladder and upper urethra during micturition – a micturating cystourogram.

Those for faecal incontinence may include:

- abdominal X-ray
- faecal occult blood (FOB)
- stool culture
- endoscopic examination – proctoscopy, sigmoidoscopy or colonoscopy to rule out serious pathology
- barium enema (used less often)
- specialist ultrasound investigations.

Table 24.1 Urodynamic investigations

TEST	TO ESTABLISH:	INDICATIONS
Post void residual urine (PVR)	the volume of urine remaining in the bladder after voiding	Should be done in all patients to exclude incomplete emptying and consequent recurrent infections, or damage to the upper urinary tract
Uroflowmetry	the rate of urine flow via the urethra	Advised for all patients to exclude voiding difficulties
Pressure/flow studies	voiding pressures (related to voiding, not incontinence)	Follow-up from abnormal PVR or uroflowmetry, to distinguish between possible causes, e.g. poor bladder contraction or urethral obstruction
Cystometry	the pressure/volume relationship within the bladder, detrusor activity, bladder capacity and bladder compliance	Basic urodynamic evaluation for patients experiencing incontinence to assess bladder function, especially prior to considering surgery
Urethral pressure profile	the closure pressure within the urethra available to counteract increase in bladder pressure	Suggested, though not proven, for individuals in whom urethral dysfunction is suspected
Leak point pressure	the bladder pressure at which involuntary leakage of urine from the urethra is observed (the rise in bladder pressure may be from detrusor contraction or increased abdominal pressure)	Detrusor leak point pressure estimations allow assessment of risk to the upper urinary tract. Abdominal leak point pressure assesses the increase in abdominal pressure that causes stress incontinence, and thus assesses the urethral contribution to continence
Surface electromyography	the efficiency of the pelvic floor muscles during the filling and voiding phases	Limited value in routine urodynamics
Videourodynamics	the simultaneous measurement of pressure and visualisation of anatomy	Useful in patients with a complex history, for example individuals with neurological disease
Ambulatory urodynamic monitoring	leakage, flow rates and bladder and abdominal pressure while the individual is ambulant	Useful to assess therapeutic effects of medication or to establish patterns that can not be exhibited in a clinic

Non-surgical intervention

An outline of non-surgical interventions is provided here, some of which are discussed in more detail in the nursing section below.

Urinary incontinence

- Prevention of constipation (see p. 670).
- Sufficient fluid intake.
- Drugs including:
  - antimuscarinics, e.g. oxybutynin hydrochloride, propiverine, fesoterodine; for urge incontinence
  - desmopressin, an antidiuretic analogue of vasopressin; for noctural enuresis
  - tricyclic antidepressants, e.g. amitriptyline; for nocturnal enuresis
  - duloxetine, an antidepressant that inhibits serotonin and noradrenaline re-uptake; licensed for moderate/severe stress incontinence in females
  - oestrogen pessaries/creams vaginally, or hormone replacement therapy if appropriate for atrophic vaginal changes.
- Pelvic floor training.
- Biofeedback.
- Electrical stimulation.
- Bladder retraining.
- Clean intermittent self-catheterisation (ISC).

Faecal incontinence

- Prevention of constipation.
- Pelvic floor training.
- Electrical stimulation.
- Biofeedback.
- Bowel retraining.
- Retrograde rectal irrigation (self-care).

McWilliams (2010) suggests that if biofeedback used alone has not improved the passage of faeces in people with functional bowel disorders, then rectal irrigation may be an option.

Surgical intervention

There are several surgical interventions that may be used when other modalities fail to alleviate the problem.

Urinary incontinence

Depending on the type of incontinence and the underlying cause, surgical interventions include:

- Procedures used for stress incontinence in women that prevent descent of the urethra:
  - retropubic mid-urethral tape procedures
  - colposuspension.
- Sacral nerve stimulation.
- Increasing bladder capacity – augmentation cystoplasty.
- Urinary sphincter surgery.

- Urinary diversion (see Ch. 8).
- Men with prostatic enlargement may experience overflow incontinence and other urinary problems. Transurethral resection of the prostate (TURP) may be required (see Ch. 8).

See NICE (2006) for further information.

Faecal incontinence

Depending on the type of incontinence and the underlying cause, surgical interventions include:

- Sacral nerve stimulation
- Repair of anal sphincter
- Artificial sphincter
- Appendicostomy (used for anterograde rectal irrigation), or continent colonic conduit
- Stoma formation (last resort).

See NICE (2007) for further information.

Nursing management and health promotion: promoting continence

Nurses working in many different settings will meet people who have continence problems. The aim is always to promote continence and to look for ways to improve the problems experienced.

It is important that nurses work with the person with a continence problem and carers, using their experiences and input from members of the MDT to inform the problem-solving approach – assessment, planning care and setting goals, implementation of care and evaluation of outcomes – to ascertain that the goals have been achieved.

Involving the person is empowering and increases their understanding, motivation and self-esteem. This encourages independence, control and effective coping skills.

This part of the chapter concentrates on urinary incontinence and outlines some issues concerning faecal incontinence.

Assessment

Assessment should be carried out in a manner that respects the person's privacy and dignity (*Essence of Care Respect and dignity*, DH 2010). It is vital that this assessment is conducted with a view to ascertaining the cause of any incontinence, for only then can the correct type of treatment be instigated (DH 2010). In collecting information from individuals, the nurse must have a clear understanding of the rationale behind the questions asked and of the implications for diagnosis and treatment of the person's responses (Table 24.2).

A full assessment should include:

- the person's/carer's account of the problem
- a detailed history
- recording of micturition and bowel movements, and incontinence over a few days.

See above for medical history, examination, investigations.

Assessment should take place in a private setting and allow adequate time for the person to air concerns and ask questions. In order to establish a good rapport with the person, it is important to meet their own agenda when discussing the potentially embarrassing topic of incontinence. Open questions such as 'Tell me about the problems with wetting that you have been having' will provide the person with a greater opportunity to relate the problem in detail than will closed questions requiring a 'yes/no' response. Sometimes, however, yes/no questions are useful with people who are embarrassed and cannot find a comfortable vocabulary to describe their problems.

The nurse's choice of language and sensitivity to the person's preferred terminology will be important to help to relax the person. People generally use terms such as 'passing water', 'peeing' rather than 'micturition' or 'voiding' and many find words such as 'accidents', 'wetting' or 'leaking' more acceptable than 'incontinence'. Where the person uses a euphemism or is vague, the nurse should seek clarification if there is any danger of misunderstanding, e.g. 'What do you mean by *'a little'*?'.

More specific questions may be indicated when the person has a pre-existing illness, or where bleeding, pain or discharge has occurred. Obviously, some questions, such as those concerning childbirth or prostate problems, will be gender specific. Supplementary questions can be asked by means of a written assessment form.

It is important that the nurse listens to the person's own account of their symptoms before asking specific questions.

Charting information

The person's history may yield enough information to determine the probable type and cause of the incontinence. A baseline chart, recorded over a few days, can confirm the accuracy of the history by supplying information indicating frequency of micturition and incontinence and, where required, the volume of urine passed. Charting such information again at intervals of a few weeks or at the end of treatment can be used to evaluate the intervention. Any chart provided should be straightforward and easily understood so that the person is encouraged to use it, as the success of any future treatment will depend upon their motivation. The times of voiding and times of wetting is the most important information. The before and after weighing of pads may also be considered for some patients (Groutz et al 2000).

Charts and diaries are also useful for those with bowel problems, to establish patterns. The *Bristol Stool Form Scale* (Figure 24.3) is the 'gold standard' resource for assessing and recording types of bowel movements, and is particularly useful as part of a bowel retraining programme.

For most people it is possible for the health care professional to diagnose the type of incontinence without the need for complex and invasive investigations (SIGN 2004). A thorough assessment will indicate the likely type, or cause, of the incontinence and a care/treatment plan can be devised.

Planning care strategies for promoting continence: an overview

Effective treatment can be implemented only when the type of incontinence has been correctly diagnosed. This may seem obvious, but people report instances where their continence problem has been dismissed as trivial, something they have 'to live with' rather than a symptom to be thoroughly investigated (Association for Continence Advice 2000).

Table 24.2 Urinary incontinence assessment questions

QUESTION	RATIONALE
How long have these symptoms been present?	The symptoms may have begun at a life crisis or on taking a new medication, or they may have had a long-standing problem, but some new development has prompted the person to ask for help
Are you wet every time?	It is important to establish the degree and frequency of wetting
How many times do you pass urine each day?	A baseline needs to be established in order for progress to be charted
Are you wet at night as well as by day?	This gives an indication of the degree of the problem as well as the type of incontinence
Are you aware of the need to go to the lavatory before you are wet?	This will determine whether signals are normal or absent
Do you have feelings of urgency to go to the lavatory?	This indicates whether signals are present and their degree of urgency
Do you lose urine if you laugh, cough, jump or run?	A positive response often indicates genuine stress incontinence
Do you pass small amounts of urine?	Passing small amounts of urine may be due to urge, stress or overflow incontinence. It may also be indicative of reduced fluid intake
Does the stream of urine seem normal or has it changed?	Passing a full stream suggests the bladder capacity is normal
Is the stream of urine poor?	The flow rate may indicate a degree of obstruction or the bladder's inability to contract
Does passing urine sting?	Stinging urine usually indicates infection or a sore or broken area
Is your urine dark and has it a strong smell?	Concentrated urine is often dark with a strong smell
Is your urine cloudy, does it contain blood or have an unpleasant smell?	Cloudy urine with blood and an unpleasant smell may indicate UTI
Does it hurt/burn when you pass urine?	Pain on micturition (dysuria) may indicate UTI
Do you have difficulty in starting to pass urine?	Hesitancy may be caused by an obstruction, e.g. prostatic enlargement
Do you dribble urine before or after going to the lavatory?	Dribbling before suggests overflow; dribbling after suggests a failure to completely empty the bladder or an incompetent sphincter
Do you need to use pads or other aids, and if so how many and how often?	The answer may indicate the degree of urine loss
How often do you pass faeces? Are you constipated?	Constipation is a common cause of urinary incontinence
Have you had any abdominal, gynaecological or urinary surgery?	Surgical trauma may be significant
Have you difficulty in getting to the lavatory, problems with undoing clothes or any sight problems?	If the person has problems with mobility or dexterity, clothes may need to be adapted and toilet seats raised. Supports to steady patients and aids to help them locate the toilet may be required
Are you taking any medication?	Many medications can affect the functioning of the urinary tract
Is the person mentally aware?	Dementia may be the cause of incontinence due to a failure to remember the routines of the day
Gender-specific questions	
Women should be asked about the number of children they have had and the type of labour and delivery	Stress incontinence is associated with childbirth
Men should be asked further specific questions to ascertain if they have prostatic enlargement, such as 'do you find it difficult to start passing water?' (see Ch. 8) *NB some of the routine questions will also be helpful*	An enlarged prostate gland is associated with several urinary problems, e.g. overflow incontinence

Strategies include advice on diet, fluid and caffeine intake, pelvic floor muscle training, biofeedback and other techniques, bladder retraining, medication, clean ISC and relieving underlying medical conditions, and surgical interventions (see pp. 665, 666, 668, 669). See Further reading, e.g. Getliffe & Dolman 2008.

Advice on diet, fluid and caffeine intake

Diet should be reviewed in relation to establishing and maintaining a regular bowel habit. The avoidance of constipation (see p. 670) is critical in preventing faecal incontinence and also will benefit urinary continence as an overfull rectum can

THE BRISTOL STOOL FORM SCALE

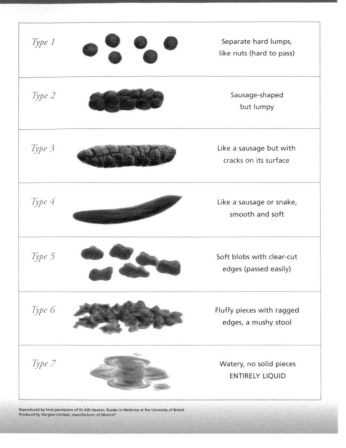

Type 1		Separate hard lumps, like nuts (hard to pass)
Type 2		Sausage-shaped but lumpy
Type 3		Like a sausage but with cracks on its surface
Type 4		Like a sausage or snake, smooth and soft
Type 5		Soft blobs with clear-cut edges (passed easily)
Type 6		Fluffy pieces with ragged edges, a mushy stool
Type 7		Watery, no solid pieces ENTIRELY LIQUID

Reproduced by kind permission of Dr KW Heaton, Reader in Medicine at the University of Bristol.
Produced by Norgine Limited, manufacturer of Movicol®

Figure 24.3 Bristol Stool Form Scale. (Reproduced by kind permission of Dr K W Heaton, Reader in Medicine at the University of Bristol. © 2000 Norgine Pharmaceuticals Ltd.)

distort the anatomical position of both the bladder and the pelvic floor. Many people are unclear about what constitutes appropriate fluid intake. Some will mistakenly restrict fluids in the hope of minimising incontinent episodes, others continually top up their cup or glass, generating such large volumes of urine that the bladder is unable to cope. Six to eight cups or glasses of fluid in 24 h is appropriate for most adults (Food Standards Agency 2010). There is evidence that caffeine increases the number of episodes of incontinence in those with a diagnosis of urge incontinence (Bryant et al 2002).

 See website Critical thinking question 24.1

Pelvic floor muscle training

Stress incontinence in men or women is the main problem for which pelvic floor muscle training may be used. Stress incontinence occurs when the pelvic floor muscles (Figure 24.4) are unable to counteract a sudden rise in abdominal pressure and allow the urethral sphincter to open, i.e. the intravesical pressure overcomes the intraurethral pressure.

Pelvic floor muscle training can also be useful for people with frequency and urge incontinence. Sitting down when strong 'signals' occur and carrying out pelvic floor muscle

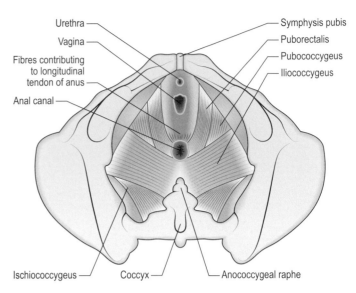

Figure 24.4 Pelvic floor muscles – levator ani, perineal aspect.

contraction can help to overcome the feeling of urgency and encourage the bladder to fill a little more before being emptied in a controlled way.

NICE (2006) recommends that pelvic floor muscle training should be offered to women during their first pregnancy as a strategy to prevent urinary incontinence. It is also useful following prostate surgery or other pelvic surgery in which the pelvic floor muscles may be weakened (Chartered Society of Physiotherapy [CSP] 2009) (Box 24.4).

Nurses work closely with specialist continence physiotherapists who provide pelvic floor muscle training. The first step is to ensure that the person can identify the pelvic floor muscles – levator ani (keeps the anal sphincter closed) and its anterior part the pubococcygeus (which stops the flow of urine). The CSP (2009) suggests that people imagine that they need to stop themselves passing 'wind' and at the same time to stop passing

---

Box 24.4 Reflection

Pelvic floor muscle training

The inability of the pelvic floor to maintain urinary continence can affect a wide spectrum of people, ranging from a 'new mum' to a person with a persistent cough associated with chronic obstructive pulmonary disease (COPD) (see Ch. 3) or someone who does heavy lifting at work.

Activities

- Access the publication *Personal training for your pelvic floor muscles* produced by the Chartered Society of Physiotherapy.
- Find out the causes of weak pelvic floor muscles.
- Reflect on the problems experienced by people with weak pelvic floor muscles.
- Discuss with your mentor or lecturer how you could use the information in your own practice.

Resource

Chartered Society of Physiotherapy (CSP): Personal training for your pelvic floor muscles. 2009. Available online http://www.csp.org.uk/uploads/documents/pelvic_floor_v5.pdf.

urine; they describe it as a feeling of 'squeeze and lift', and that men should notice a slight rise of the scrotum.

Once the physiotherapist has provided advice about pelvic floor muscle training, the nurse should ensure that the person has understood the programme. Importantly, the nurse offers support and encouragement for the person to continue with the training. They should understand that, like all training, it will be some months before any benefit is evident so sustained motivation is needed. An individual exercise regimen should be developed related to the person's current muscle strength and situation. An unrealistic regimen will be demotivating. The person should aim to do their training three times a day and should be reminded that they will need to continue with the exercises to prevent loss of muscle strength (CSP 2009).

Other techniques

Physiotherapists employ a range of equipment and techniques to help people to overcome stress incontinence. These include biofeedback, use of vaginal cones and neuromuscular electrical stimulation; those used for women are outlined in a *Quick Reference Guide* (Chartered Society of Physiotherapy 2003).

The person can be provided with biofeedback by a variety of methods, e.g. digital palpation, manometry or electromyography, which will demonstrate evidence of muscle strength and illustrate any improvement, providing positive reinforcement of the benefit of the training programme.

The use of cones of various weights, which are carried in the vagina, can support women in performing pelvic floor muscle training. However, there is no evidence that the use of vaginal cones is more beneficial than pelvic floor muscle training alone (SIGN 2004).

Neuromuscular electrical stimulation can be used to initiate muscle contractions, in the absence of a nerve impulse, by stimulating the muscle with a mild electric current. This is beneficial where a person is unable to perform a voluntary muscle contraction.

Nurse-led clinics providing treatment for faecal incontinence using electrical stimulation have been very successful (Norton & Chelvanayagam 2004).

Positive outcomes may be measured objectively by reviewing diary and chart recordings, and subjectively by the person's perceived improvement in continence or the number of visits to the lavatory for successful micturition or a bowel movement, or the number of pad changes required per day.

Bladder retraining

For urge incontinence, bladder retraining, in conjunction with antimuscarinic medication, is the main treatment. The aim of this treatment is for the bladder to 'learn' to increase its capacity and for the urethral sphincter to remain closed as the bladder fills, thereby lengthening the intervals between voiding.

Initially a baseline measurement is obtained of working bladder capacity, i.e. the amount of urine passed, and frequency of voiding at the time of assessment. In stages, the person learns to hold on for a few minutes more between the bladder signal and going to the lavatory. As each lengthened interval is achieved and maintained, new objectives are set for the next few days.

Antimuscarinic medication such as oxybutynin hydrochloride is a useful adjunct to bladder retraining, as it reduces the initial urge to void and thereby helps to increase bladder capacity. However, there are side-effects such as dry mouth, constipation (which may exacerbate incontinence) and sometimes difficulty in micturition. Modified-release oxybutynin has fewer side-effects. Newer antimuscarinics are available such as propiverine and fesoterodine.

When an acceptable social interval between visits to the lavatory and an adequate bladder capacity are reached the medication is reduced and eventually discontinued. The person then aims to maintain the same regimen as when taking the medication. Success is judged to be maintaining the same interval between voiding.

Timed and prompted voiding is referred to as habit training, and is a behavioural technique to improve continence status.

Whatever the degree of success of the treatment, toileting regimens will remain individual to each person. In order to evaluate progress, a further continence chart should be completed after a few weeks' treatment and again towards the end of treatment. Comparison of the charts, showing both voiding intervals and quantities, will allow an objective evaluation to be made as to the success of the treatment.

Specific strategies for nocturnal enuresis

It is important to chart the pattern of enuresis before treatment is commenced. Often a form of bladder training is tried initially, whereby the person learns to hold onto urine longer during the day, thus leading to an increased bladder capacity and increased ability to hold urine at night.

The main treatment for nocturnal enuresis for teenagers and adults is the use of an alarm system to assist with learning to wake in time to void. A small electrode attached to a battery alarm system about the size of a matchbox is attached to a region of the person's nightwear likely to become wet if enuresis occurs. When the first drop of urine touches the electrode, a signal is activated and wakes the person. The alarm system may be combined with short-term use of desmopressin (an antidiuretic analogue of vasopressin) given sublingually or orally. The antidepressant amitriptyline may be prescribed short-term.

Some people may benefit from a combination of an alarm and medication to begin the treatment programme and then gradually withdraw both as control is established (see Useful websites, e.g. Education and Resources for Improving Childhood Continence [ERIC]).

Clean intermittent self-catheterisation

Clean ISC can be used by people with voiding difficulties caused by conditions such as an atonic bladder or detrusor–sphincter dyssynergia, in which bladder contraction does not synchronise with opening of the urethral sphincter. It has also been of particular benefit to individuals with conditions that include multiple sclerosis, spina bifida and paraplegia (Bardsley 2000).

Clean ISC is a relatively simple strategy for incomplete bladder emptying, or for urinary incontinence that has not responded to other techniques. Assessment for ISC must include identification of the specific type of incontinence and an evaluation of the person's manual dexterity, mental ability and their motivation; there is a requirement that the person is able to identify the urethral opening. Children as well as adults have been successful in learning the technique. A small gauge catheter without a balloon is introduced into the bladder several times a day, dependent on individual requirements for assisted bladder emptying.

The procedure of self-catheterisation simulates normal voiding: the bladder is allowed to fill, the clean catheter is introduced and the bladder is then completely emptied. This prevents the build-up of residual urine in the bladder, which otherwise may cause:

- proliferation of bacteria in the bladder and UTI
- nerve damage
- overflow incontinence
- vesicoureteric reflux (VUR) of infected urine into the ureters and kidneys with the potential to cause chronic pyelonephritis (reflux nephropathy) (see p. 662).

Unlike long-term catheterisation, in which aseptic technique is of paramount importance, ISC may seem unhygienic. However, the clean technique is not associated with bladder infection, as the bladder is completely emptied each time a catheter is passed (NHSQIS 2004).

Catheters are available as pre-lubricated and non-lubricated. Pre-lubricated catheters are for single use only. Non-lubricated catheters can be used with or without separate lubrication depending on the person's preference. Non-lubricated catheters can be rinsed and reused, for a single person, for up to a week.

Most people find that inserting the catheter becomes easier with each attempt. Success can be measured in terms of the improved QoL it offers to people who previously were continually wet or who had to visit hospital emergency departments to seek relief from pain caused by failure to empty their bladder.

Managing symptoms related to conditions that exacerbate incontinence

The impact of some types of incontinence can be reduced by managing or preventing underlying conditions such as constipation and confusional states (UTI is discussed in Ch. 8).

Constipation

Constipation can be defined as 'the infrequent and difficult passing of hard stools'. It is a causative factor in urinary retention and subsequent incontinence. An investigation of the cause of the constipation must be undertaken to exclude serious pathology such as colorectal cancer, including a review of medication and concurrent conditions. Diet, fluid intake and exercise/mobility should also be assessed.

Constipation may be associated with headache, general malaise and lack of appetite, abdominal discomfort, rectal fullness and cramps. During physical examination, the abdomen can be measured for signs of increasing distension (Harari 2004).

In people with a normal bowel, constipation may be caused by any of the following:

- insufficient NSP intake
- insufficient fluid intake
- inactivity
- ignoring the urge to defecate

- anorectal pain, e.g. from haemorrhoids, etc., which may lead the person to avoid defecation
- immobility/inability to position oneself comfortably on the lavatory, leading to avoidance of defecation
- orodental problems, leading to intake of soft foods only
- the use of pads for urinary incontinence, leading to neglect of faecal elimination by person or staff where assistance is required
- opioid drugs (prescribed and illegal, see Ch. 33), sedatives or hypnotic medication
- unacceptable facilities – upstairs, outside, dirty, cold, used by others, lack of privacy, dependent on others such as asking for the commode
- unfamiliar surroundings or circumstances, leading to loss of habit
- inability to recognise social expectations, as in some cases of learning disability, dementia or substance misuse including alcohol.

Where no obvious cause is found for the constipation, the problem may be due to damage to the pelvic floor and anal sphincter or to some other pathology, such as loss of rectal sensation resulting from surgery, injury or tumour. Other contributing conditions include dehydration resulting from endocrine or metabolic disorders, and neurological damage.

Preventing constipation

People who are prone to constipation should be encouraged to be as active as possible. Requests by people to go to the lavatory should always be responded to as quickly as possible, in order to ensure that the gastrocolic reflex is never ignored. Once on the lavatory the person should be encouraged to sit for as long as is required. Structural adaptations may be necessary to make the lavatory more accessible, such as a raised seat.

A lack of privacy, time or comfort in a care setting can easily interfere with the maintenance of good bowel habits. Where people share facilities, nurses and carers must apply standards that maintain dignity and privacy (NHS Modernisation Agency 2003). Constipation can be prevented by the introduction of adequate NSP into the diet, in conjunction with a fluid intake of 8 cups/glasses a day. A dental check-up may be necessary to ensure that patients will be able to manage the raw or chewy food typical of a high-NSP diet. Individuals who are forced by dental problems to eat only soft foods will be susceptible to constipation, and therefore particular attention should be paid to their NSP intake, with addition to the diet as required.

A suitable laxative (oral or rectal) may be required to deal with the initial constipation and to prevent its recurrence.

Nurses must be alert to the possibility of spurious diarrhoea that can occur in severe constipation when liquid faeces leak around a hard mass of faeces causing faecal soiling/incontinence. It is essential that the exact cause is identified as it would be disastrous to treat faecal soiling with antidiarrhoeal medication, thus exacerbating the constipation.

Confusional states

For people with dementia or other confusional states, adherence to a regular routine will help to reinforce the need to go to the lavatory at particular times during the day. If an adequate intake of NSP and sufficient fluids is encouraged and usual patterns of defecation maintained, usually 30 minutes after breakfast, a hot drink or other meal, it should be possible to prevent constipation. It is preferable for people with dementia to be assisted to the lavatory at normal intervals rather than to be asked to adapt to new regimens such as using a commode.

Referring patients

The nurse is responsible for investigating the cause of a person's incontinence through assessment and knowledge application. Nurses in all areas of practice should take responsibility for their patients' continence assessments as part of a holistic care plan (NHS Modernisation Agency 2003). The findings from history taking can be supplemented with a baseline chart that records the times of elimination of urine and/or faeces. Having fully assessed the person's continence problem, the nurse should be in a position to initiate a plan of care aimed at restoration of continence. People with continence problems are best managed by the MDT, and the nurse who lacks specialist experience should liaise with a specialist continence nurse, continence advisor or specialist continence physiotherapist who can assist in interpreting the data obtained from the person's history and baseline elimination chart.

Should the person present with a complex history or be unresponsive to the treatment plan, the nurse should arrange referral to the appropriate professional. This may be a specialist continence nurse, specialist continence physiotherapist, occupational therapist (such as for home adaptations, ways of achieving specific tasks, etc.) gynaecologist, urologist, consultant in medicine for older people, neurologist or the mental health team.

In a busy setting, the significance of the person's incontinence may not be fully appreciated. The nurse, as their advocate, should make a case for further investigation, as the individual often feels embarrassed by the problem and may be unable to convince the doctor of its impact on their QoL.

Continence advisory services

More than a decade ago, *Good Practice in Continence Services* (DH 2000) recommended models of good continence services. People with continence problems and their carers are entitled to access professional organisations and specialist charities to ensure their needs and rights are met, in relation to accessing education, continence aids, services and support, both financial and practical.

As many people with continence problems are cared for in the community, the education of staff within residential care homes and nursing homes is essential so that continence care can be delivered within agreed protocols (NSF for Older People – DH 2001).

Most hospitals and primary care trusts provide the support of a specialist team including a specialist continence nurse and continence physiotherapists who work between the hospital and community to offer seamless care.

 ## Nursing management and health promotion: intractable incontinence

For some, the loss of continence will unfortunately be intractable. The key to successful management of their requirements for toileting programmes, aids and equipment is, as always, to determine individual needs and priorities with a view to improving QoL. The problem-solving approach should again be applied, taking into account:

- personal preference
- lifestyle
- home conditions
- family support
- the degree and frequency of micturition or defecation
- financial considerations.

Aids and equipment

The type of aid that should be recommended for an individual will depend upon the specific type of incontinence experienced. The assessment of a person's requirements for aids or equipment must be informed by an understanding of the cause of the incontinence.

Aids to enhance mobility and stability, raised lavatory seats, portable bidets or commodes and clothes that have been chosen or adapted for ease of access may be helpful to many individuals. Aids to personal cleansing can also be made available to help the person maintain independence and dignity.

Urinals can be used by both men and women. These are particularly useful for women who are, for example, confined to a wheelchair, have arthritis or are taking diuretics, for whom incontinence may result from an inability to get to the lavatory in time.

Additional equipment designed to enable men to contain urinary incontinence is available on prescription. Sheaths (urodomes) with varying types of adhesive fixings and drainage systems are continually being modified and the range available increased, to allow a more individual approach (Fader et al 2001). Urethral occlusive devices are available but should be used with caution. Y-front pants with a padded, waterproof-backed gusset are particularly useful for men with a retracted penis and dribbling problems.

A wide range of pads, pants and appliances is available for people who cannot achieve urinary control. The Bladder and Bowel Foundation (2008b) provides up-to-date, independent and unbiased information on continence products and appliances available in the UK. The person's local NHS continence service will be able to provide information on the availability of containment products in their locality. A range of absorbent products is provided through local health services. The availability of aids and collection or delivery service varies for each area (Morrow 2003). Whatever the local arrangements, the person and carers must be assured about continuity of supply and be provided with contact numbers in case of problems.

The choice of absorbent product for an individual will be influenced by factors such as the laundry facilities available, the role of any carer and the time available to that carer.

During assessment for such aids, the nurse should balance the person's wishes and the availability of laundry facilities, such as a washing machine, home help or laundry service, with the problems of soiled waste disposal, for example a limited weekly volume of waste collected by the local authority. A lack of supplies or aids will add to a person's anxiety, and may impact upon their ability to maintain continence. It is recognised that in the community incontinence is a prime reason for many people moving into nursing homes as relatives and carers feel unable to cope. During assessment for aids and equipment, it is advisable to consult an occupational therapist, physiotherapist or continence advisor on the range of supplies available in a particular health area. The person may also wish to investigate aids to daily living on view in regional centres or in specialist outlets. Accurate advice and support regarding continence products and services is essential for anyone living with loss of continence.

Long-term catheterisation

Long-term indwelling catheterisation is used in the management of incontinence only after all other treatment possibilities have been eliminated. It is associated with several complications, not least UTI.

🖰 **See website Table 24.1**

It should not be undertaken without due consideration of the person's lifestyle, preferences and likely level of concordance. The possible effects of long-term catheterisation on sexual relationships must be considered and discussed. Insertion of a suprapubic catheter may be preferable for some people. The person/carer should be made aware of what catheter management will entail before the procedure is carried out.

Catheter care is an important part of the nurse's role in all care settings; an understanding of the principles of catheter selection and closed drainage system management, together with skill in educating people/carers, are prerequisites for this. Leg drainage bags are provided for people with a catheter or a sheath who are up and about during the day. A care plan for teaching catheter management is provided on the website.

🖰 **See website Nursing care plan 24.1**

Emergency help and contact numbers All catheterised patients in the community should be given a 24-hour contact number through which to gain help in an emergency. Practical advice on what constitutes a real problem and what to do in certain emergencies should be given in writing to patients and carers (Getliffe 2003).

Chapter 8 provides detailed information about the management of an indwelling urinary catheter.

Preventing urinary tract infection

UTI accounts for nearly 20% of all health care acquired infections (HCAIs) in acute settings (Hospital Infection Society 2006). However, infection following urinary catheterisation is not inevitable and can be prevented when the potential entry points of microorganisms are properly managed (see Chs 8, 16 and Further reading, e.g. Gould & Brooker 2008). Bladder washouts should not be part of prophylaxis for UTIs. Getliffe & Dolman (2003) state that bladder washouts should only be used when absolutely necessary, for example if the washout is prescribed as a treatment or needed to remove a blockage in the catheter.

Supplying catheter equipment

Community nurses who have undertaken the required training may prescribe items, including catheters, drainage bags and sheaths, from the *Nurse Prescribers' Formulary for Community Practitioners* (British National Formulary 2010) for people in the community with an indwelling catheter. The person and carers should be given a list of all of their equipment, including sizes, types and capacity, as well as the name of a reliable pharmacist, retailer or mail order supplier.

Relationships – expressing sexuality

The impact of incontinence on self-esteem and the fear of wetting or soiling during intercourse can understandably have a negative effect on an individual's sex life (White & Getliffe 2003). MacKay & Hemmet (2001), in researching patient perceptions of incontinence, found that 16% of the respondents who considered their incontinence to be a significant problem had told no-one about their symptoms. This reluctance to discuss continence problems coupled with an avoidance of intimacy for fear of urinary leakage or faecal leakage will inevitably lead to relationship difficulties.

Although many professionals may not see this aspect of the person's well-being as a priority, people who have been sexually active and are suddenly faced with incontinence caused by injury, childbirth or disease, or those who are facing progressive incontinence as a result of chronic disease, will have to make difficult adjustments to changes in their sexual life. Problems of sexuality and incontinence affect both genders regardless of age (Cassels et al 2003).

Counselling with regard to the implications of incontinence for the individual's sexuality should be initiated only when the person signals that they are ready to address the issue. However, the nurse may need to introduce the subject and thereby give the person 'permission' to voice any concerns. Reluctance to discuss questions of sexuality may be due to the nurse's own inexperience or lack of self-awareness. Gregory (2000) warns that there is no justification in encouraging a person to divulge such personal and sensitive information if the nurse is not able to offer help or referral to the appropriate specialist.

Certain issues concerning sexuality and incontinence may be dealt with in a practical manner. For many women who are incontinent, orgasm produces further episodes of urine loss. Passing urine before sexual intercourse may help. Protecting the bed and discussing the problem with one's partner can help to make the wetting less of an issue. However, for people in a new relationship such a discussion is likely to be difficult.

People with a urinary catheter need not avoid intercourse. For men, the catheter may be strapped to the underside of the penis and, in some individuals with a degree of erectile dysfunction, may also help with rigidity (see Ch. 7).

In women, the catheter may be strapped to the inner thigh or up onto the abdomen. If clinically appropriate, sexually active people may opt for a urinary catheter which is inserted suprapubically.

The nurse should be able to provide the person with contact details for specialist sexual counselling should it be required.

SUMMARY: KEY NURSING ISSUES

- The number of people suffering from incontinence far exceeds the number of cases reported to health professionals.
- Loss of continence is embarrassing and affects every aspect of the person's life.
- Many factors affect a person's ability to gain continence and remain continent throughout life.
- The nurse's role in promoting urinary and faecal continence is critical.
- Incontinence is best managed by an MDT comprising a specialist continence nurse, physiotherapist, pharmacist, GP, specialist doctor and the person/carers.
- Over recent years, many interventions that were previously the domain of medical staff are now initiated or undertaken by specialist continence nurses.
- Positive communication and interpersonal skills are vitally important when assessing and assisting a person with continence, bladder or bowel problems.
- In all settings the nurse delivers care that is individual and considerate of a person's lifestyle, attitudes, beliefs and culture.
- Privacy and dignity should be promoted at all times during nursing interventions for continence, bladder and bowel care.

See website Critical thinking question 24.2

- Continence service provision is available to offer advice to those with continence, bladder and bowel problems. This service exists to ensure equity and quality in the service offered. The nurse has a responsibility to ensure that those who need it are aware of continence service provision and how it can be accessed.

REFLECTION AND LEARNING – WHAT NEXT?

- **Test** your knowledge by visiting the website and answering the multiple choice questions and critical thinking questions.
- **Consolidate** your learning by looking at some of the further reading suggestions, references and specialist websites.
- **Revisit** some of the additional material on the website.
- **Consider** what you have learnt and how this will help your professional development.
- **Reflect** on how you can apply this knowledge to the care of your patients.
- **Discuss** your learning with your mentor/supervisor, lecturer and colleagues.

REFERENCES

Association for Continence Advice (ACA): *Survey of patients. National Care Audit 1998/9*, London, 2000, ACA.

Audit Commission: *First assessment: a review of district nursing services in England and Wales*, London, 1999, Audit Commission.

Bardsley A: The neurogenic bladder, *Nurs Stand* 14(22):39–41, 2000.

Black D: Faecal incontinence, *Age Ageing* 36(3):239–240, 2007.

Bladder and Bowel Foundation (B&BF): *Stress urinary incontinence*, 2008a. Available online http://www.bladderandbowelfoundation.org/ bladder/bladder-problems/stress-urinary-incontinence.

Bladder and Bowel Foundation (B&BF): *Continence Products*, 2008b. Available online http://www.bladderandbowelfoundation.org/ bladder/methods-of-management/continence-products/.

British National Formulary (BNF): 2010. Available online http://www.bnf.org.

Bryant CM, Dowell CJ, Fairbrother G: Caffeine reduction education to improve urinary symptoms, *Br J Nurs* 11:560–565, 2002.

Cassels C, Geront M, Watt E: The impact of incontinence on older spousal caregivers, *J Adv Nurs* 42(6):606–616, 2003.

Chartered Society of Physiotherapy (CSP): *Clinical guidelines for the physiotherapy management of females aged 16–65 with stress urinary incontinence*, 2003. Available online http://www.csp.org.uk/uploads/ documents/csp_continence_QRG.pdf.

Chartered Society of Physiotherapy (CSP): *Personal training for your pelvic floor muscles*, 2009. Available online http://www.csp.org.uk/uploads/ documents/pelvic_floor_v5.pdf.

Department of Health (DH): *Good practice in continence services*, 2000. Available online http://www.dh.gov.uk/en/Publicationsandstatistics/ Publications/PublicationsPolicyAndGuidance/DH_4005851.

Department of Health (DH): *National Service Framework for older people*, 2001. Available online http://www.dh.gov.uk/en/Publicationsandstatistics/ Lettersandcirculars/Healthservicecirculars/DH_4004832.

Department of Health (DH): *National Service Framework for older people and system reform*, 2009. Available online http://www.dh.gov.uk/en/ SocialCare/Deliveringadultsocialcare/Olderpeople/ NSFforOlderPeopleandsystemreform/index.htm.

Department of Health (DH): *Essence of Care: Benchmarks for the Fundamental Aspects of Care*, 2010. Available online http://www.dh.gov. uk/

Fader M, Pettersson L, Dean G, et al: Sheaths for urinary incontinence: a randomized crossover trial, *BJU Int* 88:226–236, 2001.

Food Standards Agency: *Eat well, Be well*, 2010. Available online http:// www.eatwell.gov.uk/healthydiet/nutritionessentials/drinks/ drinkingenough.

Getliffe K: Catheters and catheterization. In Getliffe K, Dolman M, editors: *Promoting continence*, ed 2, London, 2003, Baillière Tindall.

Getliffe K, Dolman M, editors: *Promoting continence*, ed 2, London, 2003, Baillière Tindall.

Gregory P: Patient assessment and care planning: sexuality, *Nurs Stand* 15(9):38–41, 2000.

Groutz A, Blaivas J, Chaikin D, et al: Non-invasive outcome measures of urinary incontinence and lower urinary tract symptoms: a multicentre study of micturition diary and pad tests, *J Urol*, 164(3):698–701, 2000.

Hald T, Horn T: The human urinary bladder in ageing, *BJU Int* 82(S1):59–69, 1998.

Harari D: Bowel care in old age. In Norton C, Chelvanayagam S, editors: *Bowel continence nursing*, Beaconsfield, 2004, Beaconsfield Publishers.

Hjalmas K, Arnold T, Bower W, et al: Nocturnal enuresis: an international evidence-based management strategy, *J Urol* 171(6):2545–2561, 2004.

Hospital Infection Society: 2006, *The Third Prevalence Survey of Healthcare Associated Infections in Acute Hospitals*. Available online http://www. his.org.uk/.

International Continence Society (ICS): *Second international consultation on incontinence*, London, 2002, ICS.

Kenefick N: The epidemiology of faecal incontinence. In Norton C, Chelvanayagam S, editors: *Bowel continence nursing*, Beaconsfield, 2004, Beaconsfield Publishers.

MacKay K, Hemmet L: Needs assessment of women with urinary incontinence in a district health authority, *Br J Gen Pract* 51(471):801–804, 2001.

Mason L, Glenn S, Walton I, Hughes C: Women's reluctance to seek help for stress incontinence during pregnancy and following childbirth, *Midwifery* 17:212–221, 2001.

McWilliams D: Rectal irrigation for patients with functional bowel disorders, *Nurs Stand* 24(26):42–47, 2010.

Morrison M, Tappin D, Staines H: 'You feel helpless, that's exactly it': parents' and young people's beliefs about bedwetting and the implications for practice, *J Adv Nurs* 31(5):1216–1227, 2000.

Morrow L: Best Practice Statement: Adults with urinary dysfunction, *Nurs Times* 98(29):38–40, 2002.

Morrow L: The provision of absorbent garments, *Nurs Times* 99(1):63, 2003.

Nakayama H, Jorgenson HS, Pederson PM, et al: Prevalence and risk factors of incontinence after stroke; the Copenhagen Study, *Stroke* 28:58–62, 1997.

National Institute for Health and Clinical Excellence (NICE): Urinary incontinence: the management of urinary incontinence in women. Clinical guidelines 40 Quick reference guide, 2006. Available online http://www.nice.org.uk/nicemedia/pdf/word/CG40quickrefguide1006.pdf.

National Institute for Health and Clinical Excellence (NICE): Faecal incontinence: the management of faecal incontinence in adults. Clinical guidelines 49 Quick reference guide, 2007. Available online http://www.nice.org.uk/nicemedia/pdf/CG49QuickRefGuide.pdf.

Nazarko L: Auditing continence services, *Nurs Times* 99(19):15, 2003.

NHS Quality Improvement Scotland (NHSQIS): *Urinary catheterization and catheter care*, Edinburgh, 2004, NHSQIS.

Norton C, Chelvanayagam S: Conservative management of faecal incontinence in adults. In Norton C, Chelvanayagam S, editors: *Bowel continence nursing*, Beaconsfield, 2004, Beaconsfield Publishers.

Nursing and Midwifery Practice Development Unit (NMPDU): *Continence: adults with urinary dysfunction*, Edinburgh, 2002, NMPDU.

Rao SS: Practice guideline. Diagnosis and management of fecal incontinence, *Am J Gastroenterol* 99(8):1585–1604, 2004.

Roe B, Doll H, Wilson K: Help-seeking behaviour and social services utilization by people suffering from urinary incontinence, *Int J Nurs Stud* 36(3):245–253, 1999.

Rogers J: Promoting continence: the child with special needs, *Nurs Stand* 12(34):47–55, 1998.

Royal College of Nursing (RCN): *Digital rectal examination and the manual removal of faeces – the role of the nurse*, ed 3, Publication code: 000 934, London, 2003, Royal College of Nursing.

Royal College of Nursing (RCN): *Digital rectal examination. Guidance for nurses working with children and young people*, 2007. Available online http://www.rcn.org.uk/__data/assets/pdf_file/0009/78588/002062.pdf.

Royal College of Physicians (Clinical Standards Department): *National Audit of Continence Care. Combined Organisational and Clinical Report*, London, 2010.

Scottish Intercollegiate Guidelines Network (SIGN): *Management of urinary incontinence in primary care*, 2004 (updated 2005). Available online http://www.sign.ac.uk.

Shaw C: A review of the psychosocial predictors of help seeking behaviour and impact on quality of life in people with urinary incontinence, *J Clin Nurs* 10(1):15–24, 2001.

Teo J, Briffa NK, Devine A, et al: Do sleep problems or urinary incontinence predict falls in elderly women? *Aust J Physiother* 52:19–24, 2006.

Thomas TM, Plymet KR, Blannin J, et al: Prevalence of urinary incontinence, *Br Med J* 281:1243–1245, 1980.

Waugh A, Grant A: *Ross and Wilson Anatomy and Physiology*, ed 10, Edinburgh, 2006, Churchill Livingstone.

White H, Getliffe K: Incontinence in perspective. In Getliffe KA, Dolman M, editors: *Promoting continence*, ed 2, London, 2003, Baillière Tindall.

FURTHER READING

Anders K: Disorders of micturition. In Gangar EA, editor: *Gynaecological Nursing*, Edinburgh, 2001, Churchill Livingstone, pp 291–297.

Getliffe K, Dolman M: *Promoting continence*, ed 3, Edinburgh, 2008, Baillière Tindall.

Gould D, Brooker C: *Infection prevention and control. Applied microbiology for healthcare*, ed 2, Basingstoke, 2008, Palgrave Macmillan, pp 151–164, Ch. 7.

Royal College of Nursing: *Catheter Care RCN Guidelines for Nurses*, London, 2008.

Royal College of Physicians (Clinical Standards Department): *National Audit of Continence Care. Combined Organisation and Clinical Report*, London, 2010.

Soloman J: Eliminating. In Holland K, Jenkins J, Soloman J, editors: *Applying the Roper, Logan and Tierney Model in Practice*, Edinburgh, 2008, Churchill Livingstone, pp 229–264.

Walker S: Continence, bowel and bladder care. In Iggulden H, Macdonald C, Staniland K, editors: *Clinical skills: the essence of caring*, Maidenhead, 2009, Open University Press/McGraw-Hill Education, pp 167–187, Ch. 10.

USEFUL WEBSITES

Association for Continence Advice (ACA): www.aca.uk.com

Bladder and Bowel Foundation (B&BF) (previously The Continence Foundation): www.bladderandbowelfoundation.org

Chartered Society of Physiotherapy (CSP): www.csp.org.uk

Education and Resources for Improving Childhood Continence (ERIC): www.eric.org.uk

Health Information Resources (formerly National Library for Health): www.library.nhs.uk

International Continence Society: www.continet.org

NHS Quality Improvement Scotland: www.nhshealthquality.org

Outsiders (an organisation that supports social inclusion): www.outsiders.org.uk

Relate: www.relate.org.uk

The results of the National Audit of Continence Care published in September 2010 highlight that 'Overall, adherence to national guidance (NICE) for urinary and faecal incontinence is very variable . . .' and that 'Quality of care (assessment, diagnosis and treatment) is worse in older people (patients aged 65 years and over as compared with those aged <65) . . .' (Royal College of Physicians 2010, p. 6).

Promoting sleep

Andrée le May

Introduction

Sleep is a fundamental element of life. We know that everybody needs sleep and yet people find it difficult to describe exactly what sleep is. We are all intrigued, for instance, by what happens when we fall asleep, why we dream and why our sleep patterns alter. However, despite centuries of observing sleep, extensive and systematic research, and the creation of both physiological and behavioural theories to explain sleep, the mechanisms and functions of sleep still elude us. The aim of this chapter is to enable nurses to understand more about sleep by considering what is meant by sleep, to identify factors that impact on the ability to sleep and to think about the ways in which they can assess a patient's sleeping patterns. Reading this chapter should help nurses feel more confident in providing nursing care that helps patients to overcome some of the problems associated with sleeplessness.

Before reading on, reflect on the two scenarios detailed in Box 25.1. In the first, you are lying awake at home at 3 a.m. and in the second, you are awake in hospital. These two scenarios emphasise the importance that we attach to sleep. They also show how, in different situations, sleep means different things to different individuals, is affected by different environmental circumstances and the way we feel, and our ability to control how we help ourselves to sleep (Box 25.1).

What is sleep?

We spend so much of our lives asleep that one would expect it should be easy to define sleep but, paradoxically, once we are asleep, we remember little about it. One online dictionary definition (www.answers.com/topic/sleep) suggests that sleep can be defined as:

> *A natural periodic state of rest for the mind and body, in which the eyes usually close and consciousness is completely or partially lost, so that there is a decrease in bodily movement and responsiveness to external stimuli. During sleep the brain in humans and other mammals undergoes a characteristic cycle of brain-wave activity that includes intervals of dreaming.*

This definition seems to reflect what many of us remember from our own experiences of going to or waking from sleep and also our observations of others as they sleep. For the most part, modern scientific researchers have tended to use objective criteria to describe sleep, usually in terms of physiological events occurring during specific stages of sleep. These include changes in the electrical activity of the brain and fluctuations in the secretion of various hormones.

However, it is important to bear in mind that it is the individual's subjective experience of sleep that is of greatest importance in an assessment of the quality of sleep. Even when an electroencephalograph (EEG) indicates that sleep has been

Thinking about sleep

Scenario one

Imagine you are at home. You went to bed as usual at 11 p.m. but it is now 3 a.m. and you are still awake. There is nothing stopping you sleeping except the gentle workings of your mind: you are warm and comfortable, there is no noise to disturb you and you don't have anything to worry about...yet you still can't sleep. You know you need to, because you have to get up in the morning and go to work, be level headed and awake...you toss and turn with frustration then decide to get up and make a drink. You return to bed to sip it and slowly, very slowly, feel the drowsy sleepiness that you've been hoping for wash over you.

Scenario two

Imagine that you are awake during the night in hospital. You are too warm and your bed is unfamiliar. You can hear the constant breathing of other patients, the nurses as they walk past the bay and the intermittent ring of the telephone at the nurses' station, all of which keep interrupting the attempts to sleep. You are anxious about the results of the tests that have been taken and are due tomorrow. It seems as if everything is stacked against your sleeping: there is nothing that will help you to sleep without disturbing someone else or ringing for a sleeping pill and it is almost too late in the night to do that. You stare into the darkness willing sleep to overtake you, but it does not.

Activities

- Reflect on how the two scenarios are different.
- Consider whether being at home and able to make decisions such as putting on the light to read or making a drink would alter how you would feel about not sleeping. Consider how the hospital environment, your dependence on the nurses (for example for a hot drink), different anxieties and not wishing to disturb others would influence how you feel about not sleeping.
- If you have had sleepless nights, or had difficulty getting off to sleep, in what ways have you tried to deal with your sleeplessness? Try listing these, and then think how successful or otherwise your strategies were.
- Consider how patients you have nursed might deal with sleeplessness, and the various factors that might influence their ability to sleep – even the simple options you listed for yourself might be difficult for them to achieve.
- Access the paper by Cmiel et al (2004). Reflect on their innovative approach to sleep promotion in hospital and discuss it with your mentor or lecturer.

long and continuous, if the individual complains of sleeping badly, this cannot be contradicted. Conversely, if an individual habitually sleeps for only 2 hours during the night, but feels that this amount is adequate, leaving them rested and refreshed, then there is nothing wrong with their sleep. The most important element of any nursing assessment of sleep is therefore to find out and to respect the patient's experiences and interpretations of their own sleep/waking patterns.

In order to help us to understand patients' sleep difficulties and the implications of these in planning care, some basic knowledge about the structure and function of sleep is useful. A summary of the two distinct types of sleep – non-rapid eye movement (NREM) sleep and rapid eye movement (REM) sleep – and their function is briefly given below.

Non-rapid eye movement (NREM) sleep

NREM sleep comprises four stages associated with differing electrical activity of the brain.

- *Stage 0 or wakefulness* – a person is awake with their eyes closed.
- *Stage 1 or drowsing* – this is the lightest stage of sleep during which the pupils constrict and dilate at intervals of approximately 1–3 seconds. If asked, people may report feeling drowsy, but be awake. Even though the subject may feel fully alert, it is likely that observers will note reduced attentiveness.
- *Stage 2 or light sleep* – this phase of altered consciousness is such that, if awakened, most people recognise that they have been asleep. Body movements begin to diminish and dreams involving a storyline first appear. Dream recall on waking is far less vivid than for the second type of sleep, REM sleep.
- *Stage 3 or slow wave sleep* – body movements continue to diminish.
- *Stage 4 or slow wave sleep* – is associated with a high degree of immobility, and intense external stimuli are required to rouse a person in this stage of sleep.

Note: Stages 3 and 4 are often considered together and termed slow wave sleep (SWS).

Rapid eye movement (REM) sleep

REM sleep is characterised by dreaming, muscular relaxation and high levels of physiological arousal. During REM sleep, muscle tone is lower than in any other sleep stage. Blood pressure fluctuates, pulse and respiration rates increase and may become irregular, oxygen consumption increases, premature ventricular contractions may occur and there is penile tumescence in men and increased vaginal secretion in women.

The eye movement which occurs in REM sleep usually consists of rapid darting movements of the eyes under closed lids, occurring in bursts of 3–10 seconds at intervals of about 30–40 seconds. If people are woken up, they often say that they have been dreaming; consequently, REM sleep is frequently referred to as dreaming sleep.

During a night's sleep both REM sleep and all four NREM stages may occur many times, usually in a cyclical fashion (Figure 25.1). The first part of the night tends to contain more SWS, while the latter part of the night contains a higher proportion of REM. Interestingly, even during the day people have cycles of alertness and drowsiness although they are usually unaware of these.

Precisely how and why people sleep remains the subject of much research (see Further reading, e.g. Pocock & Richards 2006 and Widmaier et al 2007).

Functions of sleep

Despite enormous research efforts, the only universally agreed reason for sleeping is to avoid being sleepy! Interpretations of research findings vary, but it is generally considered that sleep appears to have a major role in the maintenance and/or restoration of physical and cerebral functioning (Moorcroft 1995). This may include:

Brain activity

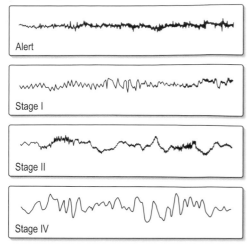

Stages of sleep

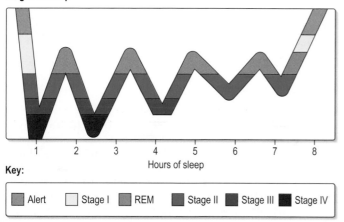

Figure 25.1 Sleep pattern. The electrical activity of the brain during various stages of sleep can be shown on electroencephalograms. During the night, people go through 3–5 90-minute sleep cycles. Each cycle includes a sequence of sleep stages. REM, rapid eye movement. (From Solomon EP, Schmidt RR, Adranga RJ 1990 Human anatomy and physiology, 2nd edn. Philadelphia: Saunders College, with permission.)

- the resetting of physiological systems
- growth
- energy conservation
- modulation of immune functions
- homeostatic restoration of brain function
- maintenance of inherited behaviours and creativity.

It has also been suggested, however, that sleep may be simply an instinctual behaviour, a genetic remnant of earlier days when immobility at night increased our chances of survival (see Further reading, Lee et al 2004).

Normal sleep

No matter what objective recordings of sleep might indicate about its duration, continuity or 'architecture', if the sleeper is satisfied with their sleep, then it may be considered to be normal. A good, restful night's sleep and a good day's refreshed and efficient wakefulness are, of course, inter-

related. Even though their relationship is not one of simple cause and effect, each depends on the quality of the other.

Individual requirements for sleep vary enormously. Russo (2005) highlights the differences in sleep required through the life course. For example, adults tend to need an average of 8 hours sleep each night, whereas older people generally seem to need less than this, with children and young infants needing more. Some people habitually take a nap during the day. Some are early risers, while others are more active in the evening and tend to go to bed late. Hospital routines, for instance early or late medication rounds and/or the taking of regular observations, tend to override these individual variations in behaviour, with a possible outcome of disturbed sleep patterns for some (Jarman et al 2002, Cmiel et al 2004).

Factors affecting normal sleep

There are many factors that may naturally affect and may disturb normal sleep, several of which are described below. These include, for example, age and gender, diet, noise, ambient temperature and pain. Each of these influences should be taken into account in nursing assessments of each patient's sleep, since the normal habits and needs of one person may vary from those of another.

Age

Changes in sleep patterns associated with age have been well documented, with neonates usually spending around 18 hours asleep in every 24, young adults sleeping for an average of 8 hours each night, and older people sleeping for 6 hours (see Further reading, Johnson 2006).

Problems such as getting to sleep or staying asleep also tend to be more common in older people (Rush & Schofield 1999); however, research reported by Klerman et al (2003) showed that although older people wake up more frequently than younger people, they do fall back to sleep at the same rate as their younger counterparts. These changes have been attributed to age-related loss of neurones and progressive fragmentation of circadian rhythmicity (Hood et al 2004). Older people also have increased amounts of wakefulness after sleep onset. Ersser et al (1999) attributed a high proportion of night-time awakenings among older people to pain and physical discomforts such as bladder distension and urinary urgency. Awareness of such problems should prompt nurses to alleviate discomfort as far as possible, to encourage regular bowel and bladder habits and ensure that optimal fluid intake is achieved by approximately 18.00 h. For those who enjoy tea or coffee, decaffeinated options should be encouraged for later in the day and evening.

Maher (2001) and Close (2006) discuss ways of assessing and improving disrupted sleep in older people.

For older people and their carers, the knowledge that changes in sleep patterns are commonly experienced and are therefore not necessarily pathological will be reassuring. Although some caution should be exercised, lest treatable problems relating to sleep are overlooked, nurses have an important role to play in educating patients and their carers about the predictable changes that occur in sleep habits with advancing age (Box 25.2). See Further reading, Maher (2004) and Close (2006).

> **Box 25.2 Reflection**
>
> **Older people and changes in sleep pattern**
>
> Think about the sleep patterns of older people you have cared for, or members of your own family.
>
> **Activity**
> - Discuss with your mentor any changes in sleep patterns that have been experienced by older patients in your care. Consider which may be due to inevitable age-related physiological changes and whether any adverse consequences are likely.

Gender

Research has shown that there are some interesting differences between men and women in terms of their satisfaction with sleep. Studies report that men have more disturbances in sleep than women from early adulthood onwards (Webb 1982), frequently due to nocturnal penile tumescence occurring during REM sleep, whilst others have highlighted that women, despite sleeping significantly longer than men, also report disturbances due to menstruation, pregnancy and climacteric (Krishnan & Collop 2006). Phillips et al (2007) remind us that women and men are differently affected by sleep disorders and also have their sleep disrupted differently by pain, depression and hormonal or psychological changes associated with major life events. These gender-based differences should be considered when assessing patients' sleeping patterns and views.

Heredity

Sleep quality and length appear to be influenced by genetic factors. De Castro (2002), in a study of self-reported sleep patterns in identical and fraternal twins, demonstrated significant genetic influences on the time individuals went to sleep and woke up, how often they woke up during the night, the duration of their sleep and wakefulness and their feelings of alertness both upon waking up and during the day. Familial clustering of narcolepsy (when sleep frequently intrudes into wakefulness) and idiopathic insomnia has also been observed. It is therefore worth noting in a nursing assessment whether there is a family history of sleep difficulties. It may not, however, always be possible to remedy inherited sleep problems by means of nursing interventions.

Body weight

Weight gain is associated with an increased duration of sleep, while weight loss is often associated with shorter sleep. This has been confirmed by several studies of people with anorexia, including one suggesting that anorexia and bulimia were both linked to sleep disorders (Della Marca et al 2004). As body weight falls, so does total sleep, which also becomes more broken and is interrupted by earlier waking.

Exercise

The effect of exercise on normal sleep is not straightforward and research studies have produced conflicting evidence: some have shown that exercise increases the duration of SWS, whereas some have found no effect and others a negative effect on sleep. Youngstedt et al's (1997) meta-analysis of 38 studies showed that exercise had different effects on different stages of sleep. The changes were somewhat modest, the greatest being an increase of 10 min on SWS. However, most of this research has focused on good sleepers. A randomised controlled trial of depressed older people showed that exercise had a more profound effect on poor than on good sleepers (Singh et al 1997).

Li et al (2004), also in a randomised controlled trial, studied the effectiveness of tai chi in improving sleep quality in older people who had disturbed sleep. Results demonstrated that older people who took part in the 6 month low to moderate intensity tai chi programme reported significantly improved sleep quality including shorter time to sleep onset and longer sleep duration.

A Cochrane Review of interventions for sleep problems in older age cites one study (Montgomery & Dennis 2005) which found that sleep quality improved after a short (16 week) exercise programme consisting of 30–40 min of walking or low impact aerobics four times a week when compared with no treatment.

It appears that, overall, exercise has a small sleep-promoting effect for many people, provided that it is not taken late in the evening.

Anxiety and depression

Anxiety and depression frequently interfere with sleep. Most people experience these at some time in their lives, associated with, for example, occupational stress, family tension, bereavement, illness or other traumatic events (Lavie 2001). Admission to hospital may be a major cause of anxiety, with all the accompanying worries with regard to illness, investigations or surgery. See Further reading, Carter (2003), Clark et al (2004) and Vena et al (2004).

Depressed patients tend to experience difficulty falling asleep, an increased number of awakenings during the night and early morning waking. Nursing staff should encourage depressed and anxious patients to discuss their feelings and, if possible, assist them to deal with underlying difficulties. Alerting medical staff to the apparent existence of anxiety and depression should ensure that the patient receives appropriate medical or psychological treatment.

See website Critical thinking question 25.1

Physical illness

Cardiac and pulmonary diseases often worsen during the night (Redeker & Hedges 2002, Sutherland et al 2003, Redeker et al 2004). For example, the incidence of asthma attacks increases during the latter half of the night, while angina, cardiac dysrhythmias and nocturnal dyspnoea are all likely to worsen during sleep (see Chs 2 and 3). Metabolic disorders such as Cushing's disease, Addison's disease, hyper/hypothyroidism and diabetes mellitus may disrupt normal sleep patterns (see Ch. 5). Diseases that mobilise the immune system, whether viral, bacterial or fungal, may be associated with increased sleepiness (see Ch. 16).

Since many areas of the brain are implicated in sleep regulation, any pathology impinging on these sites can cause problems (see Chs 9, 28 and 29). A rise in intracranial pressure, regardless of cause, increases sleepiness, sometimes leading to altered consciousness and death. Interference with the brain stem or hypothalamus may affect the onset and maintenance of sleep.

Pain

People who live with chronic pain commonly experience sleep problems (see Ch. 19). Some types of chronic pain, such as that from peptic ulceration or gastro-oesophageal reflux disease (GORD), have a circadian rhythm of increasing intensity at night. General practitioners tend to manage such pain by using medication, sometimes by aiming to relieve the cause, but more often providing symptomatic relief by means of analgesics or antacids. Sometimes the use of antidepressants, as adjuvant therapies, is successful in promoting sleep, since some chronic pain syndromes can be associated with depression.

Nurses are closely involved in giving pain-relieving agents in hospital because of their continuous contact with patients. There has long been an association between pain and sleep loss. Pain has been shown to be a major cause of sleep loss in intensive care units (Jones et al 1979) and the postoperative period (Box 25.3) (Closs 1992, Closs & Briggs 1997). Postoperative patients have strong views about sleep and pain (Closs 1991; Box 25.4).

If nurses are to be able to help patients cope with pain, they must perform an accurate nursing assessment of quality of sleep and be able to provide suitable interventions (see pp. 682–683 and Ch. 19). See Further reading, Tranmer et al (2003).

Diet

There has been a long history of research into the effects of diet on sleep. Brezinova & Oswald (1972) investigated the reasons why Horlicks® malted beverage seems to enhance sleep. A link was noted between habitual bedtime practices

Box 25.4 Information

What patients say about postoperative sleep and pain
Effects of tiredness on postoperative pain
- 'The pain is more nagging and it's harder to put up with if you're tired.'
- 'If you're tired, the pain's more draining, more severe, a down-puller. It can actually make you feel depressed.'
- 'If you're tired and in pain, you want to give up quicker. You could have shot me yesterday for all I cared.'

Effects of sleep on pain intensity
- 'If you've slept well, the pain isn't as bad a blow when you waken. If you don't sleep, you wonder when it'll ever end. It's a vicious circle.'
- 'If you're tired you're narky, if you're narky it hurts worse.'
- 'Sleep makes you relax and takes away some of the pain.'

Effects of sleep on coping with pain
- 'It's essential – you can't cope with anything unless you've slept, especially pain.'
- 'You're not so well able to cope if you're tired, you have a good attitude if you're rested.'
- 'It's impossible to cope properly if you haven't slept well.'

Effects of sleep on recovery
- 'Sleep is the best healer in the world. You know it's going to take longer to get better if you can't get your sleep.'
- 'You've got to get a good sleep before you get anything else. You feel fresh and don't get crabby, you can deal with the pain and everything else and it speeds up your recovery.'
- 'Sleep is a great healer – that's why I don't understand why they wake you up early in the morning. I think, why, what is it for? Certainly not for the patient. It makes you agitated. It's all done to their rules.'

From Closs (1991).

Box 25.3 Evidence-based practice

A study of patients' and nurses' assessments of sleep in hospital

In a study by Southwell & Wistow (1995), 454 hospital patients completed questionnaires about their sleep. This included patients on medical, surgical, care of older people and acute psychiatric wards. Questionnaires were also distributed to 129 nurses working on those wards. Patients and nurses then answered questions concerning the same nights in hospital.

Half of the patients reported that they could not sleep through the night and were consequently sleep deprived. The main factors which patients reported as disturbing their sleep were discomfort (including beds and pillows and particularly the use of plastic covers on these), pain, noise, being too warm and worries. Half were dissatisfied with both settling and waking times.

There were differences in emphasis between patients' and nurses' views of environmental factors disruptive to sleep. More patients than nurses reported noise outwith the ward, emergencies, patients making a noise, nurses' shoes and nurses talking to one another. More nurses than patients reported treatments, commodes/bedpans, toilets flushing and nurses talking with patients. Nurses were more aware of noise generated by their own

work and were largely unaware of the noise they caused by chatting to each other and from their shoes.

In view of the mismatch between nurses' and patients' perceptions, the authors emphasised the need to elicit patients' perspectives on care. However, the two groups were in agreement that patients did not get as much sleep as they needed. It was recommended that nurses, managers and others should take action to ensure that patients' sleep should be disrupted as little as possible. Nurses need to be aware when patients are awake, and take steps to ease pain, discomfort and worries. It is also important to minimise the wide range of possible disturbances during the night.

Activity

This piece of research was conducted over 15 years ago. Check whether it is still relevant by asking a small number of patients in your care and members of the nursing team on the ward what they think disrupts sleep in hospitals. Compare your findings to the ones found in this study.

Southwell MT, Wistow G: Sleep in hospitals at night: are patients' needs being met? *J Adv Nurs* 21(6):1101–1109, 1995.

and sleep rather than the content of the Horlicks®: those who normally ate little or nothing before bedtime had no improvement in sleep after having Horlicks®, while those who usually did have a bedtime drink slept better after Horlicks®. Hot milky drinks are provided in some hospitals in the late evening, but these may not suit everyone.

It should be remembered that many people prefer to take an alcoholic 'nightcap' at home, and if they are normally heavy drinkers they will suffer from withdrawal symptoms in hospital if they are not permitted to drink alcohol. Withdrawal from alcohol will result in disturbed sleep, as will withdrawal of hypnotic medication. It should be noted that alcohol is not a good hypnotic, since, although it accelerates sleep onset, it disturbs sleep patterns later on in the night and can cause early waking due to a full bladder. Tea, coffee, cola type drinks and chocolate contain caffeine and therefore act as stimulants, disturbing normal sleep patterns. As early as 1976, Karacan et al showed that coffee disturbed sleep, even in those who felt unaffected by it.

Whilst the biochemical effects of diet on sleep are unclear, avoiding stimulants and adhering to dietary routines appear to enhance sleep. Although research in this area has so far been inconclusive, community nurses might be able to help poor sleepers simply by giving them dietary advice, while hospital nurses should allow patients to eat or drink as they would at home prior to bedtime, as far as that is feasible.

🖰 **See website Critical thinking question 25.2**

Medications

There are many medications that affect sleep, hypnotics being perhaps the best known. In addition, there are many others that have side-effects on sleep, including antidepressants, antihistamines and anticonvulsants. L-dopa and beta-blockers may produce vivid dreams and nightmares, whilst diuretics increase urine production, leading to bladder distension and nocturia. Other medications, e.g. amfetamines, stimulate the central nervous system (CNS), delaying sleep onset and reducing total sleep time.

Sleep position and snoring

Sleep positions have been associated with objective and subjective sleep quality. Poor sleepers appear to spend a greater proportion of their time on their backs with their heads straight and to change position more frequently than better sleepers (Koninck et al 1983). Snoring has been associated with subjects who sleep flat on their backs. Since these symptoms are undesirable for the sleeper, and snoring may disturb others sleeping within earshot, nurses could perhaps encourage and assist poor sleepers to adopt alternative positions for sleeping. Many snorers may have problems such as sleep apnoea which are amenable to some types of treatment.

Breathing

Hypoventilation and breathing irregularities are common during normal sleep but may sometimes be clinically important. Normal changes include hypoxaemia (reduced oxygen in arterial blood) and hypercapnia (raised carbon dioxide tension in arterial blood) due to the slight reduction in metabolic rate that occurs during NREM sleep; in REM sleep irregular breathing is the norm.

Patients at home who have respiratory difficulties might benefit from advice regarding sleep position and the use of pillows to prop themselves up in order to maximise lung expansion and their carers should be advised of this. In hospital, nurses should ensure that anyone with respiratory difficulties, such as postoperative patients or those with chronic obstructive pulmonary disease (COPD) or respiratory tract infections, receives adequate support and assistance, particularly regarding oxygen administration, posture, deep breathing and coughing.

See Further reading, Carlsson & Mascarella (2003) and Gay (2004).

Temperature

Sleep patterns are affected by changes in temperature, either in ambient (room) temperature or in body temperature. Kendel & Schmidt-Kessen (1973) pointed out that unclothed and uncovered subjects awoke from cold at an ambient temperature of 26°C and below. Total sleep deprivation has also been shown to alter body temperature, resulting in a decrease in mean daily body temperature and an increase in subjective feelings of cold (Horne 1985).

Fever is associated with a greater number of awakenings, increased total waking time and reduced amounts of SWS and REM sleep. Elevated ambient temperature produces similar results. The duration of the REM phase is shortened in artificially induced fever as well as at high ambient temperature. These findings suggest that active management of pyrexial patients, perhaps by giving antipyretic medication, such as paracetamol for children, might improve their sleep.

Room temperature should be carefully monitored on general wards so that it may be maintained at a comfortable level, and patients should be encouraged to request more or fewer bedclothes as required. Older people are particularly vulnerable to fluctuations in room temperature, especially at home, since their ability to perceive temperature changes may be diminished. Community nurses are well placed to identify at least some of those individuals susceptible to hypothermia, and have a useful role in advising them about adequate clothing, bedding and heating in the home (see Ch. 22).

Noise

Noise can disturb sleep under all sorts of circumstances. In the home, mothers may wake at the slightest noise from their children, whilst in other circumstances they may sleep deeply through traffic or aeroplane noise. Conversely, those who live near a busy main road may have great difficulty sleeping in a quiet environment. Similarly, town dwellers might have problems sleeping for the first few nights of a quiet country holiday, or a patient who has had a long stay in a noisy hospital ward might have some difficulty readjusting to the quietness of their home environment. Individuals become habituated to the normal circumstances surrounding their sleep.

In hospital, noise poses a considerable problem, particularly in acute areas (Soutar & Wilson 1986, Aaron et al 1996). Patients' sleep may be disturbed by a wide variety of sounds, including noise made by other patients, nurses talking, footsteps, telephones, traffic, equipment alarms, squeaky doors, trolleys, rattling windows and many others

(Closs 1988, Southwell & Wistow 1995, Simpson et al 1996). While some noise is unavoidable at night, careful maintenance of equipment and precautions such as wearing soft-soled shoes can considerably improve the night-time hospital environment (Box 25.5). Where possible, nurses should acquaint the more long-term patients with the unfamiliar sounds on the ward, so that they become accustomed to these noises and develop the ability to sleep through them.

Having observed the detrimental effects of sleep deprivation in their patients, and become more aware of the amount of noise generated by ward activities at night, nurses in a surgical thoracic unit decided to set up a sleep promotion team within their unit in order to investigate these two related issues (Cmiel et al 2004). The team initiated a quality improvement project, the aims of which were, first, to make an objective pre-intervention measurement of noise levels on the ward, using a noise dosimeter. This instrument gave continuous recordings of decibel levels between 10 p.m. and 7 a.m. Secondly, subjective assessments of noise levels were obtained. In an innovative approach, two registered nurses each spent one night in an acute hospital setting, their bed areas containing the standard equipment and monitoring devices, to which they were connected, in a simulation of a normal patient's situation. Their report contained graphic descriptions of the noise levels and interruptions which disrupted their sleep. Patients were also surveyed about their sleep while in hospital. The sleep promotion team then carefully analysed the data obtained, following which various changes were implemented to improve the night-time environment for patients.

Common sleep disorders

Although the existence of sleep disorders has long been recognised, it is only in the past few decades that the seriousness of these has been acknowledged and a greater understanding developed. Insomnia is the most common complaint and has been defined by the US National Institutes of Health (2004) as 'experience of poor quality sleep, with difficulty in initiating or maintaining sleep, waking too early in the morning, or failing to feel refreshed'. Chronic insomnia is defined as insomnia occurring for at least three nights a week for 1 month or more. General practitioners have reported that around one third of the subjective complaints made by their patients are of difficulties in sleeping although it is worth noting that insomnia is often associated with other aspects of poor health and well-being (Walsh 2004). See Further reading, American Academy of Sleep Medicine The International Classification of Sleep Disorders: Diagnostic and Coding Manual (2005).

Sleep apnoea syndrome

This problem was first recognised over 25 years ago. The literal meaning of sleep apnoea is cessation of breathing during sleep. Often these episodes are repetitive and each may last up to a minute or even longer. Such apnoeas frequently cause the sleeper to wake, in some cases many times during the night. The main symptom resulting from this disorder is usually daytime sleepiness, although some sufferers complain of insomnia.

There are two main types of sleep apnoea: central sleep apnoea is caused by impaired neurological control of breathing, so that the intercostal muscles fail to contract; obstructive apnoea is the result of an obstruction of the airway, e.g. by large tonsils, a large or oedematous soft palate, fat deposits around the airway, retrognathia (backward displacement of the lower jaw) or micrognathia (a small lower jaw). The cause may be treated if the problem becomes severe. Obesity is common among these patients, in which case weight loss is usually the first approach to relieving the problem. For the more severe cases, continuous positive airway pressure (CPAP; see Ch. 29) during the night may help, while corrective surgery may be required for others. See Further reading, Barthlen (2002) and Centre for Reviews and Dissemination (2005).

Sleep-induced nocturnal myoclonus

This condition is characterised by repetitive twitching of the legs occurring at regular intervals of 20–60 s. These episodes may last from a few minutes to several hours, and one or both legs may twitch (Barthlen 2002). This does not always disturb the individual, unless they are a light sleeper or the twitching is severe enough to arouse them from 'deep' sleep. Associated with this condition is restless legs syndrome, where an unpleasant, crawling sensation is experienced in the calves or thighs. Nocturnal myoclonus has been

---

Box 25.5 Evidence-based practice

Nursing care at night

There is very little research about nursing at night and the impact that good care during this part of the 24 hours can have on people. This Swedish study, designed to evaluate nursing care provided at night in one hospital, focused on the perspectives of both patients ($n = 356$) and nurses ($n = 178$).

The study used a newly developed questionnaire known as the Night Nursing Care Instrument to gain the views of staff and patients, in order to make comparison between the nurses' assessments and the patients' perceptions of the nursing care provided at night. The researchers found that there were no significant differences between the two groups for areas of medical intervention and evaluation, but the two did differ around areas linked to nursing intervention, including the assessment of the patients' needs for nursing care at night.

The authors concluded by suggesting that night nurses need to improve their ability to assess patients' needs for nursing care at night, particularly in relation to their knowledge of which nursing actions promote patients' rest at night.

Oleni, M, Johansson P, Fridlund B: Nursing care at night: an evaluation using the Night Nursing Care Instrument. *J Adv Nurs* 47(2):25–32, 2004.

Activity

- Access the paper by Oleni et al, then think about how nurses in a clinical placement that you have just completed assess patients' needs for nursing care at night and what they do with these assessments in relation to providing care and communicating that care within the multidisciplinary team. This is relevant in the community as well as in hospitals or other residential care settings.

associated with the use of tricyclic antidepressant medication and chronic uraemia. Several remedies have been recommended, ranging from reduced caffeine and vitamin E supplementation to medication with ropinirole (Allen et al 2003).

Narcolepsy

This disorder occurs in approximately 4 in 10 000 people and can be described as an imbalance between wakefulness, REM sleep and NREM sleep. Sleep frequently intrudes into wakefulness and this change in conscious state is often triggered by strong emotions such as anger or laughter. It is REM sleep that intrudes, either partially or totally, producing the possibility of four different symptoms, as follows:

- excessive daytime sleepiness
- cataplexy, when only the muscular paralysis of REM occurs: the sufferer may be awake but is paralysed
- sleep paralysis, a type of cataplexy which occurs at sleep onset; paralysis which occurs on waking from REM is benign
- REM dreaming during wakefulness: hypnagogic hallucinations.

Parasomnias/partial arousals

Sleepwalking

This behaviour, when it occurs, commences during SWS, although the sleepwalker appears to be in a part-sleeping, part-waking state. Sleepwalking can be very dangerous: sufferers have been known to walk out of windows and to attack family members. During an episode of sleepwalking, the individual is usually uncommunicative and returns to bed spontaneously, rarely remembering the event the next morning. Sleepwalking is difficult to treat, so it is advisable, if a person does sleepwalk, to take precautions such as locking windows at night.

Night terrors and nightmares

Night terrors also arise during SWS and occur mostly in children. The sufferer often screams and shows signs of panic, such as a dramatic rise in heart rate, respiratory distress and sweating. They may be very difficult to arouse, but usually calm down within a few minutes, usually without waking up. Most people remember nothing about the incident. Nightmares occur during REM sleep and are often remembered very vividly on waking.

The effects of sleep deprivation

Total sleep deprivation, for as little as 48 hours, has been shown to result in changes in central nervous system function, such as behavioural irritability, suspiciousness, speech slurring and minor visual misperceptions. Increased suggestibility and/or a reduction in motivation and willingness to perform tasks may also accompany these. In hospital, this could impede a patient's willingness to mobilise and undertake aspects of self-care as well as to communicate. Detrimental psychological effects of sleep deprivation

sometimes observed in hospital patients include lethargy, irritability, confusion and, in more extreme cases, delusions and paranoia. Sleep deprivation for individuals in the community could reduce efficiency at work and affect social and family relationships.

 ## Nursing management and health promotion: sleep

Nursing assessment of sleep

The assessment of sleep is an important and integral part of the general nursing assessment of each patient and is particularly important to high-quality care during the night (see Box 25.5, p. 681). In order to make these assessments nurses rely mainly on a combination of their observations of sleep and their communication skills, both questioning patients carefully and listening to what they tell them. Assessment should take into account the patient's age, gender, diet, medical diagnosis and medical/surgical treatments, as well as paying specific attention to issues related to sleep (Fordham 1996) and the patient's immediate environment and how that might impact on their dignity and privacy (DH 2010). Possible questions in the nursing assessment of sleep include:

- Do you have a problem with sleeping? How long have you had a sleep problem?
- What is your usual going to bed and waking routine?
- What treatments, if any, have you used for your insomnia? How successful or otherwise did you find these?
- Do you take a little alcohol to help you sleep, and if so, how helpful or otherwise do you think this is?
- What things do you do to help you get to sleep?
- Do you have difficulty falling asleep and/or do you keep waking in the night? If you keep waking, what do you do to help you get back to sleep?
- What regular exercise do you manage to get?
- How much caffeine do you drink, and at what times during each 24 hours?

Adapted from Maher (2004).

Finding out about sleep

Although people are unable to give accurate reports of the actual time it takes for them to fall asleep, or how long they lie awake during the night, they can give reliable accounts of changes in their sleep patterns. Information can be gained from direct questioning, from non-verbal cues, the descriptions provided by relatives and carers, and from the nursing and/or medical records. Where patients are unable to answer direct questions due to age or incapacity, it may be possible to use a relatively new technique which employs a pictorial sleepiness scale on cartoon faces (Maldonado et al 2003).

Encouraging patients, where possible, to talk about themselves, their feelings and their needs is vital to the assessment of sleep. The use of open-ended questions and prompts can facilitate disclosure (Ersser et al 1999, Maher 2001, 2004) (see above). Nurses should ask both general questions about sleep, as well as more specific questions that could include details about time of settling down to sleep, time of morning waking, duration of sleep, night-time routines, diet, medication, pain and anxieties. The patient's disclosures should be recorded in the notes so that each nurse participating in their care is aware of their needs.

Body language is also important: patients are less likely to be forthcoming if the nurse speaks from an uncomfortable distance, looking as if they are about to leave for some more important task. Planned nurse–patient interactions can provide ample opportunities for discussion and nursing assessment.

Helping patients to sleep

Once an assessment of the patient's sleep has been made, nursing care and health promotion relevant to these sleeping habits/patterns can be planned. Fordham (1996) highlights several nursing interventions for sleep problems, including for:

- *psychological causes* – teaching, counselling and relaxation techniques
- *physical causes* – control or elimination of symptoms, e.g. nocturia, breathlessness or pain
- *medication-related causes* – assessment of the medication effects and of review with doctors or other prescribers
- *environmental causes* – controlling noise, temperature or light; maintaining dietary rituals as far as possible, e.g. where the person normally eats or what they do during meals, such as watch TV; considering exercise, activity or regularity in terms of sleep/waking patterns
- *scheduling difficulties* – postponement of sleep and discussion of regularity of sleep/wake patterns.

Nurses can also help by providing general information about sleep that enables patients and their carers/partners to have realistic expectations. The importance of including partners in the assessment and planning of care related to sleep disorders cannot be overemphasised since, as Strawbridge et al (2003) point out, a patient's sleep disturbances may impact on their partner's health and well-being.

Cultivating healthy sleep patterns

In addition, nurses can give advice for improving sleep through attention to behaviours and attitudes conducive to healthy sleep patterns. These might include:

- attitudes towards sleep
- the sleep environment
- attention to diet
- sleep scheduling
- pre-sleep activities and routines
- daytime sleep behaviours, e.g. napping.

More specifically, there are several points that should be borne in mind by nurses, on an everyday basis, as they assist patients to cultivate healthy sleep patterns. The information and advice to assist patients to cultivate healthy sleep patterns is available on the website.

See website for further content

Some people will have such serious sleep problems that they will require specialist treatments. If this is the case,

the nurse should alert the appropriate professionals. In the community, this may be the GP or clinical psychologist; in hospital, specialist support may be available.

Treatments for insomnia

The major treatments available for insomnia are pharmacological, although alternative approaches, e.g. developing good sleep habits, sometimes referred to as 'sleep hygiene', complementary and alternative medicine therapies (CAM) and cognitive behavioural therapies, may be the preferred first line of treatment for many people.

Pharmacological treatments

Pharmacological treatments include both hypnotic drugs and herbal remedies.

Hypnotic medications

Many hypnotics belong to the benzodiazepine group and include nitrazepam, temazepam and diazepam. Their use is dependent on the type of insomnia and associated symptoms, e.g. anxiety. Hypnotics provide temporary symptomatic relief but are not a cure. The sleep produced by these medicines does not resemble natural sleep: the duration of stage 2 sleep is increased at the expense of REM sleep and SWS. However, even though these medicines change the structure of sleep, most physiological processes associated with SWS continue as usual. It is difficult, therefore, to comment on the difference between the overall quality of sleep induced by hypnotics and that of normal sleep.

The effects of benzodiazepines vary, particularly with regard to their duration of action:

- Nitrazepam has quite long-lasting effects and is used less commonly than other forms, particularly for older people, in whom the medication's 'hangover effect' may cause loss of balance and result in falls.
- Temazepam acts for a shorter duration and has little or no 'hangover' effect.
- Diazepam is used for insomnia which is linked to daytime anxiety and is a long-acting drug which, in a single dose, may treat both insomnia and anxiety.

Other non-benzodiazepine hypnotics, such as zaleplon, zolpidem and zopiclone, act in a similar fashion to the benzodiazepines. Zaleplon is very short acting, with zolpidem and zopiclone having a longer duration of action. These three medications should not be used for long-term treatment since dependence has been reported in a small number of patients.

Generally, short-acting hypnotics are favoured, since they are less likely to produce hangover effects during the day. While hypnotics are initially effective in inducing sleep, their regular use produces some degree of 'tolerance'. As time goes on, the body requires increasing doses of the medication to achieve the same effect. The effectiveness of most hypnotics is diminished after 3–14 days of use.

Although hypnotics can provide short-term improvement in sleep, long-term use can result in more problems with sleep. After an initial improvement, hypnotics may actually cause tiredness because of the reduction in SWS and REM sleep. When hypnotics are withdrawn, the patient may suffer from rebound insomnia. This involves extreme feelings of edginess, greater difficulty in falling asleep and more intense dreams and nightmares. These symptoms gradually diminish over time. In spite of these drawbacks, the short-term use of hypnotics can be highly beneficial. For example, an anxious patient due to have surgery may benefit greatly from the limited use of hypnotics over, perhaps, 3 or 4 perioperative nights. See Further reading, the latest edition of the *British National Formulary* (www.bnf.org).

Herbal remedies

Although several herbs are claimed to have sleep-inducing properties, either when used as aromatherapy or dropped in bath water, e.g. lavender, geranium or rose oils, or taken as infusions or oral preparations, e.g. chamomile tea or St John's wort, valerian is the only one which has been scientifically evaluated (Centre for Reviews and Dissemination 2005a). It is believed that small doses of valerian act in several ways to affect sleep positively through reducing anxiety, exerting a calming influence, relieving stress and relaxing muscles. One of the stated benefits of using valerian is the lack of morning hangover that is commonly associated with other pharmacological preparations. However, noted side-effects include stomach upsets with small doses, and headaches and nausea with larger doses. See Further reading, Taibi et al (2007).

Despite the emphasis in the literature on valerian, other unproven herbal remedies may also be effective, not least by virtue of a placebo effect.

Psychological and behavioural treatments

While pharmacological treatments of insomnia are palliative, psychological treatments aim to deal with the cause of the sleeplessness. In some cases, insomnia may be attributed to physiological or psychological overactivity. Stress is a common cause of sleep disturbance and can be dealt with by a variety of techniques (see Ch. 17). However, some individuals who suffer from insomnia are constitutionally poor sleepers who are unlikely to respond to any treatment. They usually have difficulties sleeping throughout their lives, and the process of ageing is likely to reduce further the quality of their sleep. For those whose sleeplessness is associated with physiological or psychological hyperactivity, many non-pharmacological methods of treating insomnia have been attempted, with varying degrees of success. Four of the most widely known – relaxation therapy, paradoxical intention, associative learning technique and cognitive therapy – are discussed below. These therapies are mainly provided by clinical psychologists, whose choice of strategy depends on the cause of the sleeplessness and on the individual's temperament and personal preference. See Further reading, Montgomery (2003), Jacobs et al (2004) and Morin (2004), and search the DARE database at the Centre for Reviews and Dissemination (www.crd.york.ac.uk).

Increasingly, nurses are learning to provide some of these therapies, for example relaxation (Richards et al 2003) and music therapy (Johnson 2003), thus enhancing their already significant contribution to helping patients to sleep. Health visitors have for some time been involved in successful schemes designed to help adults with insomnia (Eaton 1996). Since sleep is such a fundamental activity of life and is essential to good health, this extension of the nurse's role would seem perfectly legitimate.

Relaxation therapy

Emotional problems such as anxiety can be modified using various types of relaxation therapy, which aim to reduce physical and mental tension. Autogenic training (Centre for Reviews and Dissemination 2005b) teaches people to concentrate on sensations of warmth and heaviness in their limbs by repeated suggestion. Progressive muscular relaxation achieves a similar effect by the alternate tensing and relaxing of a series of muscles. These methods have been successful in helping people to fall asleep and in increasing their satisfaction with sleep (Richards et al 2003).

A variety of alternative forms of relaxation have been studied, for example the use of music. In a study of the use of music to promote onset of sleep and sleep maintenance in 52 women over the age of 70, Johnson (2003) found that its use decreased the time to sleep onset and also the number of night awakenings, thus increasing the women's satisfaction with the quality of their sleep.

Paradoxical intention

Paradoxical intention has been used with success in the treatment of patients who are particularly anxious about their difficulty in falling asleep. This anxiety produces the opposite of the desired effect, making patients too tense to fall asleep. When such individuals are instructed to stay awake all night, their anxiety about falling asleep is reduced, paradoxically allowing them to relax and fall asleep (Ascher 1980).

Associative learning technique

This is a useful technique where the bed and bedroom have become associated in the patient's mind with sleeplessness. For such people, going to bed is an aversive stimulus that produces an aroused state. The method involves avoiding all behaviours in the bedroom not associated with sleep, such as reading, eating, watching television or just lying awake. Individuals are instructed to go to bed only when they are sleepy and to get up if they lie awake for more than 10 min. Eventually this re-establishes the psychological association between bed and sleep.

Cognitive therapy

An individual who is plagued by intrusive and repetitive thoughts that keep them awake can be taught to use cognitive refocusing. Usually these are problems and worries which the individual can learn to control, first by recognising that they cannot solve their problems by turning them over and over in their mind at night, and second, by learning to suppress the troubling thoughts, often by concentrating on alternative, benign thoughts. Other techniques employed by cognitive therapists include meditation and guided imagery.

SUMMARY: KEY NURSING ISSUES

- Despite sleep being a complex and universal behaviour that is prone to disruption by many internal and external influences, it remains an important individual experience.

- Every nurse needs to know how patients may be helped routinely to achieve the best sleep possible and how, in specific circumstances, to deal with individual sleep-related problems.
- Nurses have an important role to play in regulating individual and communal environments, in the hospital, nursing home or the patient's own home, so that they are as conducive as possible to the promotion of good sleep (Fordham 1996).
- The assessment of individual sleeping needs and of the environment within which patients are nursed should be a routine component of skilled nursing practice – you might find it useful to reflect on some of the cases where you have made a difference and where appropriate record this in your portfolio of learning.
- Many difficulties can be overcome by simple changes in lifestyle and by adjustments to the individual's expectations of sleep.
- Where more serious problems occur, help from other health care professionals should be sought.

➲ REFLECTION AND LEARNING – WHAT NEXT?

- **Test** your knowledge by visiting the website 🖰 and answering the multiple choice questions and critical thinking questions.
- **Consolidate** your learning by looking at some of the further reading suggestions, references and specialist websites.
- **Revisit** some of the additional material on the website.
- **Consider** what you have learnt and how this will help your professional development.
- **Reflect** on how you can apply this knowledge to the care of your patients.
- **Discuss** your learning with your mentor/supervisor, lecturer and colleagues.

REFERENCES

Aaron JN, Carlisle CC, Carskadon MA, et al: Environmental noise as a cause of sleep disruption in an intermediate respiratory care unit, *Sleep* 19(9):707–710, 1996.

Allen R, Picchietti D, Hening W, et al: Restless legs syndrome; diagnostic criteria, special considerations, and epidemiology. A report from the restless legs syndrome diagnosis and epidemiology workshop at the National Institutes of Health, *Sleep Med* 4:101–119, 2003.

Ascher LM: Paradoxical intention. In Goldstein A, Foa EB, editors: *Handbook of behavioural interventions: a clinical guide*, New York, 1980, Wiley, pp 266–321.

Barthlen GM: The brain: sleep disorders. Obstructive sleep apnea syndrome, restless legs syndrome, and insomnia in geriatric patients, *Geriatrics* 57(11):34–39, 2002.

Brezinova V, Oswald I: Sleep after a night-time beverage, *Br Med J* 2(5811):431–433, 1972.

Centre for Reviews and Dissemination: *Valerian for insomnia: a systematic review of randomized clinical trials*, York, 2005a, NHS Centre for Reviews and Dissemination, University of York.

Centre for Reviews and Dissemination: *Autogenic training: a meta-analysis of clinical outcome studies*, York, 2005b, NHS Centre for Reviews and Dissemination, University of York.

Closs J: Sleep and rest. In Redfern S, Ross F, editors: *Nursing Older People*, Edinburgh, 2006, Churchill Livingstone, pp 413–436.

Closs SJ: *A nursing study of sleep on surgical wards*, Nursing Research Unit report, Edinburgh, 1988, Department of Nursing Studies, University of Edinburgh.

Closs SJ: *A nursing study of patients' night-time sleep, pain and analgesic provision following abdominal surgery*, Nursing Research Unit report,

Edinburgh, 1991, Department of Nursing Studies, University of Edinburgh.

Closs SJ: Patients' night-time pain, analgesic provision and sleep after surgery, *Int J Nurs Stud* 29(4):381–392, 1992.

Closs SJ, Briggs M: *Evaluation of an intervention to improve post-operative sleep and pain control in orthopaedic patients at night*, Report for the NHS Executive Northern and Yorkshire, Hull, 1997, University of Hull.

Cmiel CA, Karr DM, Gasser DM, et al: Noise control: a nursing team's approach to sleep promotion, *Am J Nurs* 104(2):40–47, 2004.

de Castro JM: The influence of heredity on self-reported sleep patterns in free-living humans, *Physiol Behav* 76(4–5):479–486, 2002.

Della Marca G, Farina B, Mennuni GF, et al: Microstructure of sleep in eating disorders: preliminary results, *Eat Weight Disord* 9(1):77–80, 2004.

Department of Health (DH): *Essence of Care: Benchmarks for the Fundamental Aspects of Care*, 2010. Available online http://www.dh.gov.uk/

Eaton L: Health visitors tackle adult insomnia, *Health Visit* 69(8):312, 1996.

Ersser S, Wiles A, Taylor H, et al: The sleep of older people in hospital and nursing homes, *J Clin Nurs* 8(4):360–368, 1999.

Fordham M: *Patient problems: a research base for nursing*, Edinburgh, 1996, Churchill Livingstone.

Hood B, Bruck D, Kennedy G: Determinants of sleep quality in the healthy aged: the role of physical, psychological, circadian and naturalistic light variables, *Age Ageing* 33(2):159–165, 2004.

Horne JA: Sleep function with particular reference to sleep deprivation, *Ann Clin Res* 17(5):199–208, 1985.

Jarman H, Jacobs E, Walter R, et al: Allowing the patients to sleep: flexible medication times in an acute hospital, *Int J Nurs Pract* 8(2):75–80, 2002.

Johnson JE: The use of music to promote sleep in older women, *J Community Health Nurs* 20(1):27–35, 2003.

Jones J, Hoggart B, Withey J, et al: What the patients say: a study of reactions to an intensive care unit, *Intensive Care Med* 5:89–92, 1979.

Karacan I, Thornby JI, Anch M, et al: Dose-related sleep disturbances induced by coffee and caffeine, *Clin Pharmacol Ther* 20:682–689, 1976.

Kendel J, Schmidt-Kessen W: The influence of room temperature on night time sleep in man (polygraphic night-sleep recordings in the climate chamber). In Koella WP, Levin P, editors: *Sleep*, Basel, 1973, Karger, pp 423–425.

Klerman E, Davis J, Duffy J, et al: Older people awaken more frequently but fall back asleep at the same rate as younger people, *Sleep* 27(4):793–798, 2003.

Koninck J, De Gagnon P, Lallier S: Sleep positions in the young adult and their relationship with the subjective quality of sleep, *Sleep* 6(1):52–59, 1983.

Krishnan V, Collop N: Gender differences in sleep disorders, *Curr Opin Pulm Med* 12(6):383–389, 2006.

Lavie P: Sleep disturbances in the wake of traumatic events, *N Engl J Med* 345(25):1825–1832, 2001.

Li F, Fisher KJ, Harmer P, et al: Tai chi and self-rated quality of sleep and daytime sleepiness in older adults: a randomized controlled trial, *J Am Geriatr Soc* 52(6):892–900, 2004.

Maher S: Assessing age-related sleep disorders, *Nurs Older People* 13(3):27–28, 2001.

Maher S: Sleep in the older adult, *Nurs Older People* 16(9):30–35, 2004.

Maldonado C, Bentley A, Mitchell D: A pictorial sleepiness scale based on cartoon faces, *Sleep* 27(3):541–548, 2003.

Montgomery P, Dennis J: Physical exercise for sleep problems in adults aged 60+ (Cochrane Review). In *The Cochrane Library*, Issue 2, Chichester, 2005, Wiley.

Moorcroft WH: The function of sleep. Comments on the symposium and an attempt at synthesis, *Behav Brain Res* 69(1–2):207–210, 1995.

Oleni M, Johansson P, Fridlund B: Nursing care at night: an evaluation using the Night Nursing Care Instrument, *J Adv Nurs* 47(2):25–32, 2004.

Phillips B, Collop N, Drake C, et al: Sleep disorder and medical conditions in women. In *Proceedings of the Women and Sleep Workshop*, Washington, DC, March 2007, National Sleep Foundation.

Redeker NS, Hedges C: Sleep during hospitalization and recovery after cardiac surgery, *J Cardiovasc Nurs* 17(1):56–68, 82–83, 2002.

Redeker NS, Rugiero JS, Hedges C: Sleep is related to physical function and emotional well-being after cardiac surgery, *Nurs Res* 53(3):154–162, 2004.

Richards K, Nagel C, Markie M, et al: Use of complementary and alternative therapies to promote sleep in critically ill patients, *Crit Care Nurs Clin North Am* 15(3):329–340, 2003.

Rush S, Schofield I: Biological support needs. In Heath H, Schofield I, editors: *Healthy ageing: nursing older people*, London, 1999, Mosby, pp 119–158.

Russo M: *Normal sleep, sleep physiology and sleep deprivation: general principles*, 2005. Available online http://www.emedicine.com/neuro/topic444.htm.

Simpson T, Lee ER, Cameron C: Relationships among sleep dimensions and factors that impair sleep after cardiac surgery, *Res Nurs Health* 19(3):213–223, 1996.

Singh NA, Clements KM, Fiatarone MA: A randomized controlled trial of the effect of exercise on sleep, *Sleep* 20(2):95–101, 1997.

Soutar RL, Wilson JA: Does hospital noise disturb patients? *Br Med J* 292:305, 1986.

Southwell MT, Wistow G: Sleep in hospitals at night: are patients' needs being met? *J Adv Nurs* 21(6):1101–1109, 1995.

Strawbridge W, Shema SJ, Roberts RE: Impact of spouses' sleep problems on partners, *Sleep* 273:541–548, 2003.

Sutherland ER, Kraft M, Rex MD, et al: Hypothalamic-pituitary-adrenal axis dysfunction during sleep in nocturnal asthma, *Chest* 123(3 Suppl):405S, 2003.

US National Institutes of Health, cited by Clinical Evidence: *Bazian Ltd*, London, 2004, BMJ Publishing Group.

Walsh J: Clinical and socioeconomic correlates of insomnia, *J Clin Psychiatry* 65(Suppl 8):13–19, 2004.

Webb WB: Sleep in older persons: sleep structures of 50 to 60 year old men and women, *J Gerontol* 37:581–586, 1982.

Youngstedt SD, O'Connor PJ, Dishman RK: The effects of acute exercise on sleep: a quantitative synthesis, *Sleep* 20(3):203–214, 1997.

FURTHER READING

American Academy of Sleep Medicine: The International Classification of Sleep Disorders, Revised. Diagnostic and Coding Manual, 2005. Available online http://www.esst.org/adds/ICSD.pdf.

Barthlen GM: The brain: sleep disorders. Obstructive sleep apnea syndrome, restless legs syndrome, and insomnia in geriatric patients, *Geriatrics* 57(11):34–39, 2002.

British National Formulary: Available online http://www.bnf.org.

Carlsson BB, Mascarella JJ: Changes in sleep patterns in COPD – a new vital sign in the management of people with chronic obstructive pulmonary disease, *American Journal of Nursing* 103(12):71–72, 74, 2003.

Carter PA: Family caregivers' sleep loss and depression over time, *Cancer Nurs* 26(4):253–259, 2003.

Centre for Reviews and Dissemination: *Systematic review on obstructive sleep apnoea; its effect on health and benefit of treatment*, York, 2005, NHS Centre for Reviews and Dissemination, University of York.

Clark J, Cunningham M, McMillan S, et al: Sleep-wake disturbances in people with cancer. Part II: evaluating the evidence for clinical decision making, *Oncol Nurs Forum* 31(4):747–771, 2004.

Closs J: Sleep and rest. In Redfern S, Ross F, editors: *Nursing Older People*, Edinburgh, 2006, Churchill Livingstone, pp 413–436.

Gay PC: Chronic obstructive pulmonary disease, *Respir Care* 49(1):39–52, 2004.

Jacobs GD, Pace-Schott EF, Stickgold R, Otto MW: Cognitive behavior therapy and pharmacotherapy for insomnia: a randomized controlled trial and direct comparison, *Arch Intern Med* 164(17):1888–1896, 2004.

Johnson E: Epidemiology of insomnia: from adolescence to old age, *Sleep Medicine Clinics* 1(3):305–317, 2006.

Kalavapalli R, Singareddy R: Role of acupuncture in the treatment of insomnia: a comprehensive review, *Complement Ther Clin Pract* 13(3):184–193, 2007.

Lee KA, Landis C, Chasens ER, et al: Sleep and chronobiology: recommendations for nursing education, *Nurs Outlook* 52(3):126–133, 2004.

Maher S: Sleep in the older adult, *Nurs Older People* 16(9):30–35, 2004.

Montgomery P: A systematic review of non-pharmacological therapies for sleep problems in later life, *Sleep Med Rev* 8(1):47–62, 2003.

Morin CM: Cognitive-behavioral approaches to the treatment of insomnia, *J Clin Psychiatry* 65(Suppl 16):33–40, 2004.

Pocock G, Richards C: *Human Physiology: The Basis of Medicine (Oxford Core Texts)*, Oxford, 2006, Oxford University.

Taibi DM, Landis CA, Petry H, Vitiello MV: A systematic review of valerian as a sleep aid: safe but not effective, *Sleep Med Rev* 11(3):209–230, 2007.

Tranmer JE, Minard J, Fox LA, Rebelo L: The sleep experience of medical and surgical patients, *Clin Nurs Res* 12(2):159–173, 2003.

Vena C, Parker K, Cunningham M, et al: Sleep-wake disturbances in people with cancer. Part I: an overview of sleep, sleep regulation, and effects of disease and treatment, *Oncol Nurs Forum* 31(4):735–746, 2004.

Widmaier E, Raff H, Strang K: *Vander's Human Physiology*, Maidenhead, 2007, McGraw Hill.

USEFUL WEBSITES

National Sleep Foundation: www.sleepfoundation.org

Sleep (journal): www.journalsleep.org

Sleep Medicine (The Computerized Textbook of Sleep Medicine) Lists resources regarding all aspects of sleep including the physiology of sleep, clinical sleep medicine, sleep research and patient information. www.users.cloud9.net/~thorpy/

Nursing specific patient groups

SECTION

3

Nursing the patient undergoing surgery

Caroline E. Gibson, Ruth Magowan

Introduction

Surgery is one of the most frequently undertaken and important treatments offered in modern health care. The result of ongoing surgical and anaesthetic innovations means that an increasing number of medical conditions can now be alleviated or managed by surgical treatment. The aim of this chapter is to provide an overview of the nursing care of patients facing surgery. Nurses need to be able to help and support patients throughout their care pathway. Discussion will include not only those interventions immediately before, during and after the surgical procedure, but also the support needed by patients during the diagnostic period and their eventual rehabilitation at home. Patients undergo many types of surgery for a wide variety of reasons but the key principles of care can be generalised with reference to particular types of procedure.

Patterns of surgical care

National figures demonstrate that around 8 million surgical operations are carried out in the UK every year (National Patient Safety Agency 2008). In the past it was common to admit patients on the day prior to surgery and keep them in hospital beyond the acute phase of recovery. However, the length of time patients now spend in hospital preparing for, and recovering from, elective surgery has greatly decreased (Mitchell 2007a). Advances in surgical technology and anaesthesiology have allowed previously lengthy operations to be completed more quickly and recovery times have become shorter. Many procedures are now undertaken using laparoscopic, robotic and keyhole surgery. The use of lasers, angiographic stenting and ultrasound techniques has increased; for example, carotid artery stenting offers an alternative to carotid endarterectomy in patients at high risk of intra-operative complications (Zeebregts et al 2009). These techniques also allow interventions to be carried out at the same time as diagnosis, reducing the need for repeated anaesthesia. Improvements in anaesthesia techniques, such as regional anaesthesia and short-acting drugs with minimal side-effects (e.g. remifentanyl), allow larger numbers of patients to be ready for discharge in a matter of hours following surgery (Shnaider & Chung 2006).

Currently around 60% of surgical procedures are undertaken as outpatient or day cases (NHS Scotland 2010), and it is likely that in the future there will be further increases in the number and range of minimally invasive procedures available. Nurses must refine their skills and knowledge to be able to provide appropriate physical and psychological support to enable these patients to care for themselves following discharge (Mitchell 2007a).

An increase in the number of referrals for minor surgical procedures has also provided the opportunity to extend nursing roles to meet present and future demands. Martin (2002) describes the role of a nurse practitioner (NP) who provides a one-stop minor surgery clinic for the removal of moles, cysts, lipomas and papillomas using local anaesthetic. A patient satisfaction survey of this service reported that although 20% of patients had not expected a nurse to undertake their surgery, all patients found it acceptable to be operated upon by an NP. Developments in nurse-led initiatives such as pre-operative assessment units (Walsgrove 2006) and nurses carrying out endoscopies (Smith & Watson 2005) further expand the role of nurses in peri-operative care.

The demographic profile of the population in the UK is changing. With greater average life expectancy and improvements in treatments for chronic illness, there are now increasing numbers of older people in our society. This results in an increase of older adults presenting for surgery (Leung & Dzankic 2001, Sear 2003, McArthur-Rouse & Prosser 2007). Ageing affects all of the body systems and the most affected are the cardiovascular, renal and respiratory systems. This means that older patients may have reduced physiological reserves to maintain homeostasis during a period of acute illness such as surgery. Frail older adults are susceptible to hospital acquired, or nosocomial infections such as pneumonia, *Clostridium difficile* and complications of meticillin-resistant *Staphylococcus aureus* (MRSA). Leung & Dzankic (2001) found that approximately 21% of patients over the age of 65 develop one or more in-hospital postoperative complications involving the cardiovascular, neurological or respiratory systems. Older adults are also more likely to suffer from one or more co-existing diseases (known as co-morbidities) which also increases the risk of developing postoperative complications (Williams et al 2007). For example, patients with cardiovascular disease are more at risk of developing myocardial infarction (MI) or arrhythmias following surgery (Sear 2003).

Therefore patients nursed on acute surgical wards have increasingly complex health care needs. Structured care approaches such as protocols, clinical pathways and algorithms are frequently used to organise knowledge and guide patient care, but nurses must still be able to undertake accurate assessments and make decisions about patient management in order that complications are recognised early and expert assistance is sought rapidly (McArthur-Rouse & Prosser 2007). Pirret (2003) describes a pre-operative scoring system used by nurses to identify patients at risk of postoperative complications. Once identified, at-risk patients can be admitted electively to high-dependency (HDU) or intensive care units (ICU) to undergo close postoperative monitoring.

Nurses must also consider the additional burden of co-existing disease on the patient. In a study of 20 patients requiring total hip or knee joint replacement it was found that co-morbidity management was not consistently included in care plans during the acute phase of hospitalisation (Williams et al 2007). Patients with co-morbidities such as heart failure, diabetes or Parkinson's disease were expected to progress at the rate specified in standard clinical pathways, despite reporting higher rates of pain and fatigue postoperatively. Also, advice given on the day of discharge mainly focused on the joint surgery unless complications from the pre-existing conditions had arisen during the hospital stay. Peri-operative care of older surgical patients and those with co-morbidities is thus becoming an increasingly important part of nursing practice.

Patients are increasingly involved in their own care (Scottish Executive 2003). The patient facing surgery should be seen as a partner in the care process and participate in the planning and evaluation of health care (Edwards 2002). This may involve choosing where they receive surgery. In 2003 the Department of Health introduced a scheme to ensure that patients who are waiting for heart surgery or angioplasty receive their surgery more quickly and choose where they have this treatment (DH 2005). Patient participation is essential to the success of the enhanced recovery after surgery (ERAS) pathway for colorectal surgery (Wright et al 2009). Nursing staff spend considerable time with patients in the pre-operative period to ensure that they understand the goals of the programme which include early mobilisation and nutrition in the postoperative period. This laparoscopic-assisted colonic surgery has reduced most patients' stay from 7–10 days to 3–5 days (Kehlett & Wilmore 2002).

Integral to the care of patients facing surgery is the role of teamwork (Hughes & Mardell 2009). Nurses in surgical wards and departments must work collaboratively with many members of the interprofessional team so that continuous and high-quality care can be provided. Typically this will include surgeons, anaesthetists and theatre staff, but also allied health professionals such as physiotherapists and radiographers are often integral to the diagnostic and rehabilitation processes.

Pre-surgical care

Classification of surgery

Some patients experience periods of ill health or disability before undergoing an operation; others experience sudden illness or injury that necessitates immediate surgery. Around 15% of patients diagnosed with colorectal cancer are operated on following an emergency presentation (Taylor 2008), as in the case of Mr Shah.

🖱 See website Case study – Mr Shah

The degree of urgency of a surgical intervention is a useful criterion for its classification and prioritisation. A patient such as Sylvia who has uncomplicated gallstone disease would normally not be classified as 'urgent' but would be put on a waiting list and admitted 'electively'.

🖱 See website Case study – Sylvia

A given operation may be performed for different classifications of surgery. For example, surgery for a strangulated hernia will be handled as an emergency, whereas surgery for an irreducible hernia will be considered as essential, and surgery for a reducible hernia as elective. Patients requiring essential surgery will be admitted to hospital within a week or two of presentation at their outpatient appointment, but elective patients may have to wait for some considerable time.

Presenting for surgery

Personal definitions of health and ill health and the decision to seek treatment are influenced by factors such as previous experience, social context, perceived severity of illness and judgements as to whether treatment would be beneficial (Box 26.1).

In Box 26.2 Mr A had made a voluntary decision to seek treatment based on information obtained through the internet, and from talking with his partner. The accessibility of the internet has meant that more and more of the public use it as a source of information. Patients may present with an increasingly sophisticated level of knowledge about procedures. However, there are no standards guaranteeing the quality of information from the internet, and some of the information Mr A found may not be from a medical source or be research based.

Pathways and progress

Patients may be referred for surgery by different paths. Mr Shah, for example, was taken straight to the emergency department (ED) by ambulance without seeing his GP.

 See website Case study – Mr Shah

Patients may also be transferred from other wards. For example, a patient on a medical ward may undergo investigations

---

Box 26.1 Reflection

Presenting for surgery: stop and think

Ask a patient who has recently experienced surgery what signs and symptoms first brought the illness to their attention.

What was it that made them seek treatment?

Box 26.2 Information

Information on the internet

Mr A is a 41-year-old teacher who lives with his partner and four children. The youngest child is 18 months old. Mr A and his partner did not plan to have any more children. The last pregnancy had been a rather unplanned but welcome event! Mr A looked up some information on sterilisation on the internet on his home computer and was surprised at the amount of information that was available about vasectomy. He had not realised that it could be done as a short outpatient procedure and that it did not necessarily require a general anaesthetic. He discussed it with his partner and they decided that this was the most appropriate course of action.

His GP told them that, in their area, vasectomy could be undertaken at the local family planning clinic and that there was an opportunity to discuss the procedure and decision making in an appointment beforehand. Within a few weeks of the GP's referral to the clinic, a pack of information was sent out to Mr A's home along with a date for a vasectomy counselling appointment.

---

which lead to a diagnosis necessitating surgical treatment and therefore transfer to a surgical ward. A few patients admitted as emergencies may go straight to theatre from the ED and from there to the surgical ward following the operation. Some patients may need to go back to theatre or the intensive therapy unit (ITU) if their condition deteriorates or requires further intervention. Many hospitals now have specialist surgical high-dependency unit facilities where patients can be closely monitored for the first 24–48 h following their operation. These units usually have a higher ratio of nurses to patients than general ward areas. HDUs are thus often used for patients following major surgery or where pre-existing medical conditions predispose them to complications (DH 2000, Sheppard & Wright 2006). Occasionally, convalescence or rehabilitation may be required in another ward or hospital, e.g. following amputation or neurosurgery. However, increasingly these services can be provided by community health care teams.

A substantial morbidity exists among patients on waiting lists for surgery. Patients with gallstone disease requiring elective laparoscopic cholecystectomy make up a significant percentage of those awaiting surgery in the UK. Whilst on the waiting list, some patients may suffer recurrent bouts of severe abdominal pain and require emergency hospitalisation (Somasekar et al 2002, Lawrentschuk et al 2003). Waiting for treatment not only causes patients pain, distress and anxiety but can also have expensive consequences, e.g. absence from work and emergency hospital admissions (DH 2001a). In the case of Mr Rutherford he has experienced some episodes of temporary weakness and loss of vision that prompted him to see his GP.

 See website Case study – Mr Rutherford

He is likely to be extremely anxious because of this and concerned that his symptoms may worsen while awaiting surgery. His surgeon has started him on prophylactic antiplatelet medication to reduce the risk of thrombosis leading to occlusion of his carotid artery and stroke.

Informed decision making

The aim of this section is to introduce the issue of informed consent for surgery by discussing nursing responsibilities and highlighting areas for ethical debate.

The decision to operate

Once the outcome of investigations is known and the risks to the patient of surgery assessed, the surgeon can make a definite or provisional diagnosis and recommend a course of action. This may involve diagnostic, curative or palliative surgery, a combination of these, or no surgical intervention at all. If the patient can be treated as successfully without surgical intervention, then the relevant alternatives will be pursued. It may appear that it is the medical staff who make decisions about the course of treatment to be given. However, whereas the doctor decides what treatment appears to be the most appropriate, it is the informed patient who must make the final decision as to what treatment is accepted (Nursing and Midwifery Council [NMC] 2008).

Patients may feel pressure from family or health care professionals to undergo surgery if it offers the only chance of cure, and it is important to establish the true wishes of the individual (Myatt 2006).

Informed consent

Consent is a patient's agreement for a health professional to provide care (DH 2001b). The Nursing and Midwifery Council (NMC 2008) states that every adult has the right to consent or refuse treatment unless they are:

- unable to take in or retain information provided about their treatment or care
- unable to understand the information provided
- unable to weigh up the information as part of the decision making process.

When patients undergo any intervention or procedure, they must give consent. Touching someone without their consent and without lawful justification could be construed as trespass, civil assault or battery (Baxter et al 2002). In practice, it is preferable to obtain verbal rather than written consent from the patient for low-risk procedures, such as a chest X-ray or the administration of suppositories. However, when a patient is to undergo surgery or any invasive procedure, and when a general or local anaesthetic is required, it is advisable and standard practice to obtain written consent. As the medical team are in charge of these procedures, they are ultimately responsible for obtaining the written consent from the patient. Consent forms are traditionally used within hospitals and clinics to document that the patient and the medical staff have discussed and agreed the proposed treatment (Griffith & Tengnah 2008). However, a signed consent form does not give any indication of what the patient was told, what was consented to or whether there was a meaningful understanding as to what they were agreeing to (DH 2001b). The doctor signing the consent form with the patient has therefore to ensure that:

- the patient understands the information, and not just that it has been given and received
- the extent of the information is sufficient for that patient to make the decision.

It is suggested that a record of the discussion and an explanation of the treatment are recorded in the patient's notes to corroborate that consent has been obtained (Griffith & Tengnah 2008).

The role of the nurse

The nurse has an important role to play in obtaining consent prior to surgery. For a patient to give valid consent, they must comprehend fully what they are consenting to, i.e. their consent must be informed. The nurse can provide the team with knowledge of the individual's need for information and comprehension of the information given. The nurse will also provide the patient with information about the procedure and the recovery period, and may be able to clarify points previously discussed between patient and doctor. Where nurses do take consent, they should receive thorough training (NMC 2008). In Mr A's case (see Box 26.2), specialist family planning nurses provided pre-operative information and

obtained his consent for his vasectomy. There may also be occasions when the nurse is in charge of a particular procedure and must therefore obtain written consent from the patient, for example, where nurses undertake endoscopy (Smith & Watson 2005).

The need for informed consent raises legal and ethical issues for both nurses and patients. The current social climate emphasises consumerism and patients' rights. Patients have an increased desire to be 'partners in care', i.e. to be well informed and to take responsibility for their own health (Scottish Executive 2003). Patients have the right to be given an adequate explanation of proposed treatment, including any risks and alternative treatments. Nurses have a vital role to play in ensuring a patient's need for information is met and that full discussion takes place (Griffith & Tengnah 2008, NMC 2008).

However, there may be occasions when the patient is less than fully informed. The depth and complexity of information held by medical staff may be overwhelming for a lay person to absorb and understand. There is now heightened awareness of the need to explain the potential effects of treatments – adverse as well as beneficial. The risks of some procedures are now clearly stated on the consent form itself. When responding to specific questions about risks a health professional is required to answer fully and truthfully regardless of the likelihood of the risk materialising (Griffith & Tengnah 2008). Both the chance of occurrence and the severity of potential adverse effects of the procedure must be addressed.

Nurses who think that patients are insufficiently informed should discuss their concerns with the surgeon, but not in the presence of the patient. Booth (2002) suggests that nurses are in a good position to mediate between doctors and patients, to facilitate two-way communication, and to prevent patients becoming passive recipients of the doctor's expertise. However, it is more usual for nursing and medical staff to be sensitive to the individual needs of the patient and to work collaboratively with the patient and family.

In some cases, the patient may be too ill to comprehend what is proposed and thus to give informed consent. Also, within society there are groups of individuals who are unable to make decisions for themselves or who cannot communicate these decisions (Box 26.3). This inability is known as 'mental incapacity'. In Scotland, any issue relating to the

Box 26.3 Reflection

Decision making

How can nursing staff clarify where decision making responsibility lies in the following cases?

- A 25-year-old man with Down's syndrome is admitted to the ENT ward for elective tonsillectomy.
- An 81-year-old woman is admitted from a nursing home to the vascular ward with an ischaemic left foot. She has a 5-year history of dementia and is very confused. An embolectomy under local anaesthetic and sedation is proposed.
- A young motorcyclist is admitted to the Emergency Department following a motorcycle accident. He is unconscious and the CT scan reveals a subdural haematoma which requires emergency surgical evacuation.

welfare of an 'incapable adult' is governed by The Adult with Incapacity Act (Scotland) 2000 (HMSO 2000). Similar legislation has been introduced in England and Wales in the form of the Mental Capacity Act (2005) (Department for Constitutional Affairs 2007).

When an adult patient is unconscious or mentally incapacitated, it is necessary to find out whether a family member or friend has been given Power of Attorney, i.e. allowed to make decisions on the patient's behalf, or if the patient has previously indicated their wishes in an advance statement. An 'advance statement' is an expression of the patient's preference for treatment or care, given when they are legally competent. This may include the refusal of certain treatments such as surgical intervention or cardiopulmonary resuscitation. If there is no power of attorney, the court of protection may appoint a person, called a 'deputy', to make decisions on behalf of the patient.

Any refusal of treatment must be respected, provided the decision is appropriate in the circumstances. The patient's relatives have no legal right to give or, more importantly, to refuse consent. Lifesaving procedures can be performed without consent using the doctor's clinical privilege. A doctor has the power to take such action as is necessary, but only the minimal amount of treatment should be undertaken to alleviate the particular emergency, and should follow established practice (Griffith & Tengnah 2008). Good practice would suggest that the relatives are consulted and a decision is made in the patient's best interests.

Similarly, relatives have no legal rights in determining whether information should be given to or withheld from the patient. In fact, the doctor or nurse would be in breach of confidentiality if they were to tell the relatives first, or to tell them at all, without the patient's expressed consent. Where information is withheld from the patient, the patient cannot consent to its being divulged (NMC 2008). There is an NHS code of practice on protecting patient confidentiality (NHS Scotland 2003).

When a patient is too ill to be told, or cannot give informed consent, medical and nursing staff must carry out their professional duty to act in the patient's best interests, whilst considering the wishes of the relatives. *The Code: Standards of conduct, performance and ethics for nurses* (NMC 2008) provides guidelines on professional practice. Nurses are required to follow the Code in terms of acting to safeguard the patient's interests and to work in a collaborative and cooperative manner with other health care professionals. It is essential that nurses are familiar with the Code and apply it in practice. Guidelines on informed consent have also been produced for doctors and nurses (DH 2001b, General Medical Council 2008). A discussion of the implications of the Mental Capacity Act in relation to anaesthesia and critical care can be found in White & Baldwin (2006).

Pre-operative preparation

Pre-operative preparation might begin some time before the patient is admitted to a hospital ward or clinic. Patients arrive for surgery having experienced very different types of preparation. Mr Shah had little opportunity for psychological or physical preparation as he was taken to the ED

as an emergency. Mr A had already attended the family planning clinic where the vasectomy would be carried out and had discussed the procedure and after-care at length with one of the nurses. Meeting the needs of people with learning disabilities for elective surgery may require careful pre-operative planning.

♪ **See website Critical thinking question 26.1**

Pre-operative assessment begins when the decision to perform surgery is made (Scott et al 2007). Pre-preparation involves assessment and providing information. For more about the aims of pre-operative assessment and the role of pre-operative assessment clinics see Walsgrove (2006).

Assessment

Assessment of the patient is required to identify any special needs, to highlight potential problems and to provide a baseline against which to measure postoperative progress. The nurse will usually take a 'history', involving an interview where information is collected about the patient's demographic details and current health status. Nurses may also use sources of information, such as medical or nursing records, the patient's relatives and other health care professionals, to form a complete picture. Some pre-operative tests and investigations may be indicated prior to an operation, for example, a CT or PET scan to assess for tumour spread and pulmonary function tests in advance of a lung resection.

Blood samples are required prior to many surgical procedures; tests may include haemoglobin levels, clotting studies, urea and electrolytes. If a blood transfusion is anticipated, cross matching will be carried out. An audit of 100 patients at a pre-assessment clinic in England showed that many were unclear about the investigations they would undergo (Jolley 2007). Approximately half the patients (53%) realised that tests may be necessary but were not sure what was being checked. Only 11% of the sample understood why they needed investigations despite written information having been sent out in advance. Nursing staff should be able to give simple and specific information about pre-operative investigations.

The risk of surgery to the patient is determined by:

- the nature of the procedure (major or minor)
- patients' pre-existing health status.

The surgeon and anaesthetist will undertake an assessment of the patient and establish whether the risks are negligible, low, intermediate or high risk. A simple classification scale is produced by the American Society of Anesthesiologists (Box 26.4; ASA 2005).

As Sylvia is young and physically healthy she satisfies the recognised criteria for day surgery (Royal College of Surgeons of England 1992) and has been considered for a laparoscopic cholecystectomy in the day surgery unit.

♪ **See website Case study – Sylvia**

However, patients with a history of jaundice, abnormal liver function tests or a dilated common bile duct may be considered as 'high risk' and require an open cholecystectomy (Mitchell 2007b). Sylvia had attended a pre-assessment clinic at her local hospital prior to surgery where the nurse identified that Sylvia had difficulty in arranging childcare on the

Box 26.4 Information

Patient physical status (ASA classification 2005; adapted from Hughes & Mardell 2009)

P1 A normal healthy patient

P2 A patient with mild systemic disease

P3 A patient with severe systemic disease that restricts activity but is not incapacitating

P4 A patient with incapacitating systemic disease that is a constant threat to life

P5 A moribund patient who is not expected to survive without the operation

P6A Declared brain dead patient whose organs are being removed for donor purposes

---

scheduled date of surgery. The nurse was able to provide Sylvia with appropriate information about postoperative recovery, including the potential risks of driving on the day of surgery and advising her that another adult should stay with her overnight once she was discharged home. The nurse also explained that conversion to an open procedure was necessary for a few patients. This can be due to adhesions or if the surgeon has difficulty in visualising the anatomy of the gall bladder, or it was acutely inflamed (Graham 2008). If this was the case Sylvia would not be able to go home as planned on the same day. It is important that nurses undertake assessment of the patient's home circumstances to gain a full picture of their needs.

Giving information

The majority of patients are anxious on the day of surgery (Mitchell 2007a, Pritchard 2009). Hollaus et al (2003) suggest that pre-operative anxiety is prevalent regardless of the patient's diagnosis. Anxiety may result from fear of the unknown, separation from friends or family, fear of a diagnosis such as cancer or even fear of dying. Also patients may feel that they lack control in the unfamiliar clinical environment (Stirling 2006). Some patients reported that they feared a mask would be placed over their face to administer the anaesthetic (Mitchell 2007a). Nurses can reassure patients that induction of anaesthesia is usually administered intravenously. Anxiety may affect patients' vital signs, elevating the pulse, respiratory rate and blood pressure, providing baseline recordings that are not representative of usual values. If a patient appears anxious, particularly on admission, or immediately prior to theatre, it is wise to repeat any observations that are not within normal parameters. Patients who are very anxious may seek constant assurance and attention from the nursing staff. Pritchard (2009) warns that there may be a tendency for staff to label such patients as 'difficult' or 'demanding', when in fact they are frightened. Nurses should offer anxious patients support and attempt to relieve their concerns.

Reducing pre-operative anxiety and stress is not only desirable on humanitarian grounds, but it also promotes recovery. Giving the patient information and emotional support pre-operatively was shown to reduce pre- and postoperative anxiety substantially and reduce postoperative pain,

stress, anxiety and infection (Hayward 1975, Boore 1978). More recently it has been found that attending a standardised information session prior to hip surgery significantly reduces anxiety and is associated with less postoperative pain (Giraudet-Le Quintrec et al 2003). Garretson (2004) suggests that more pre-operative information programmes should be developed to enhance the patient experience but found that many centres still did not have formal policies on pre-operative information giving and patients were still arriving for surgery uninformed and anxious.

Lack of information has been found to be a major source of dissatisfaction among day-case patients. Costa (2001) investigated the lived experience of ambulatory surgery patients and suggested that many did not have a clear picture about what to expect pre-operatively, postoperatively and throughout their convalescence at home. Mitchell (2007a) found that 42% of day surgery patients in the UK were not offered a pre-assessment visit. Pre-admission information allows for emotional adjustment over a longer period and enables patients to share information with, and seek support from, their families.

Nurses are ideally placed to play a major role in reducing pre-operative anxiety and need to devise approaches to delivering effective pre-operative teaching in a reduced time frame (Pritchard 2009). Garretson (2004) suggests that a pre-operative information session should include the following elements:

- type of surgery
- length of surgery
- length of stay in hospital
- activities on morning of surgery (premed, preparation)
- meeting anaesthetic and theatre nurses
- what to expect in recovery.

However, it is also important that patients and family members receive information most useful to them for postoperative care activities at home after discharge. A literature review by Pieper et al (2006) identified that three main areas for which patients sought information were postoperative pain management, wound/incision care and activity guidelines. Patients may also be concerned about where they should report on the morning of surgery or whether they should arrive having fasted or bring their medications with them. Mitchell (2007a) outlines a useful framework for patient admission and discharge for day surgery.

Patients should receive information at an appropriate level and on matters that concern them – not simply on what the nurse assumes they will be anxious about. Giving patients large volumes of information will not necessarily lead to a reduction in anxiety for all patients. For some patients too much information may become confusing and lead to heightened anxiety (Mitchell 2007a). Information given should be dependent on the individual patient's preference and need, and be of high quality. Way et al (2003) describe the implementation of a group approach to pre-admission preparation of patients awaiting elective cardiac surgery. Patients reported that meeting and talking with other patients in advance of the operation helped them to cope with the surgery, and postoperative recovery was similar to patients who had received individual sessions. However, this approach may not be appropriate in other circumstances, such as emergency surgery, or when anxiety and pain interfere with the patient's ability to participate.

A small but increasing number of patients are undergoing surgical procedures whilst awake. A phenomenological study of patients undergoing awake craniotomy for intra-operative mapping of brain tumours by Palese et al (2008) highlighted that patients needed to feel in control of the situation and understand what is happening intra-operatively. Further research is required to explore the most appropriate information and planning for such patients.

Skilled, systematic and sensitive assessment is essential in determining what is important for the individual. Open questioning can determine what the patient already understands and what they would like to know more about. Simply giving a factual account of what will occur is insufficient. Patients want to know what to expect and how it will feel. They also need the opportunity to discuss their fears and worries. Nurses can use this opportunity to provide patient teaching on postoperative care issues such as the use of patient controlled analgesia (PCA) or deep breathing and leg exercises. When and how information is given will influence its effectiveness. Many patients have difficulty in remembering verbal information. While a personal, verbal explanation is invaluable in that it allows for feedback from the patient, it is difficult to recall over time (Mitchell 2007a).

Pre-admission booklets for surgical patients can be beneficial in reducing patient anxiety and improving outcomes. Information can also be presented using other media such as video (Garretson 2004). However, there may always be patients who do not wish to watch information videos about their proposed procedure immediately prior to surgery (Hyde et al 1998). Information leaflets or videos are not, therefore, a substitute for personalised explanation but do provide a constant reference source and can prepare patients to use their contact time with nurses more effectively. This allows the nurse to focus on areas of concern and to devote more time to counselling than to information giving, as in reality it is often difficult to complete both tasks well in the busy pre-operative period. Pre-operative information booklets should be easy to read without being patronising in tone (Markham & Smith 2003). Print size, reading ease and vocabulary should all be considered and the use of jargon avoided. Some departments produce their own booklets giving general information about wards and surgery and have leaflets about specific operations which can be given to the patient prior to admission.

Pre-operative education aims to produce a well-informed consumer, to promote healthy choices and to reduce anxiety. The informed patient is better equipped to make good decisions about their care and to discuss treatment fully and openly with staff. Information also serves to produce a more autonomous patient. One must then respect the view that the well-informed patient has the right to reject advice or treatment against professional judgement for personal reasons (Griffith & Tengnah 2008). What the professional advocates may conflict with what the patient wants. Simply informing someone of an objective fact that appears rational (e.g. smoking causes lung cancer) will be insufficient in some cases to promote healthy behaviour or coping mechanisms (Donovan & Ward 2001). It is also important to address the information needs of family members because they may have a role in providing support and care at home (Paavilainen et al 2001).

Safe preparation for anaesthesia and surgery

In the pre-operative assessment the patient's specific needs and potential problems may be identified. The general risks associated with anaesthesia and surgical intervention will also be taken into account in any related medical or nursing procedure. Patients undergoing surgery require medical assessment, the nature of which will depend on the extent of surgery, the age of the patient and on any pre-existing medical conditions. In some centres, an initial assessment is carried out by nursing staff so that patients most in need of anaesthetic review, such as those with poor exercise tolerance, asthma or previous problems during anaesthesia, are seen promptly (Hilditch et al 2003).

Minimising the risk of infection

There is a strong association between infection and surgery (SIGN 2008). Patients may develop infection at the site of their surgery (surgical site infection – SSI) which may include wound infections, infection of body cavities (e.g. peritonitis), bones, joints, meninges or any of the soft tissues involved in the operation. Infection can also occur at sites away from the operation, e.g. chest infection associated with hypoventilation at general anaesthesia, urinary tract infection from bladder catheterisation, or systemic sepsis following the bacteraemia of any invasive procedure. Attention to hygiene, asepsis, physiotherapy, antibiotics and bowel preparation (if appropriate) can help to minimise this risk. Advice about appropriate pre-operative antibiotic prophylaxis is available (SIGN 2008). Specific issues are considered below.

Minimising the risk of chest infection

The risk of chest infection is increased in patients who receive a general anaesthetic or who have prolonged periods of immobility. Smokers, and patients with pre-existing respiratory disease, are also more likely to develop perioperative respiratory problems such as pneumonia or bronchospasm (Warner 2006). Drugs and gases used in anaesthesia dry the respiratory tract and inhibit the action of the cilia. Secretions of mucus become thick and tenacious, causing partial obstruction of the lower airways. Cigarette smoking also damages and paralyses the cilia and leads to excess mucus production. The secretions eventually pool in the base of the lungs and plug the bronchioles. The retained secretions obstruct the lower airways, inhibiting gaseous exchange and providing a culture medium for bacteria.

General anaesthesia depresses respiration and, in the deep stage, breathing will actually cease. Artificial ventilation during the operation is at tidal volume and does not fully inflate the lungs (see Ch. 3). Normally, a person will sigh intermittently or increase demands for oxygen by activity, fully inflating the lungs and preventing stagnation and atelectasis. Changes of position, movement and coughing all serve to dislodge excess mucus or fluid, which is then expelled from the lungs as sputum. When under a general anaesthetic the patient will be lying still and unable to cough or sigh throughout the operation. There will also be a period of inactivity postoperatively and perhaps a reluctance to breathe deeply or cough if there is abdominal or thoracic pain. Opiates given for pain relief can also depress respiration (Baxter & Chinn 2006).

Current evidence suggests that patients should be advised to stop smoking prior to surgery (Warner 2006). Ideally patients should be encouraged to stop as soon as the surgery is scheduled because a longer period of pre-operative abstinence from smoking is associated with fewer respiratory complications (Warner 2006). This can also reduce other smoking-related problems such as peri-operative cardiovascular and wound-related complications. However, a study of 493 North American nurses (Houghton et al 2008) found that few regularly advised patients to quit or provided advice on doing so in the pre-operative assessment. While specialist smoking cessation services are available in the UK, all nurses should be able to offer support and advice to patients about stopping smoking. In fact, Houghton et al (2008) highlight that patients scheduled for a surgical procedure are more likely to stop smoking spontaneously than any other group in the general population. Advice about smoking cessation is available from the National Institute for Health and Clinical Excellence (NICE 2005).

All patients, regardless of whether they are smokers or not, should be taught deep breathing exercises and coughing. It can be difficult to teach a patient to contract the diaphragm in order to breathe deeply pre-operatively, let alone postoperatively. The tendency is to use intercostal and accessory muscles to lift the rib cage and draw the abdomen in. Although instruction may be the responsibility of the physiotherapist, it will still require reinforcement from the nursing staff. The need for early mobilisation can also be described to the patient.

Patients should also be informed that they may require oxygen therapy via a mask or nasal cannulae postoperatively to help maintain the level of oxygen in their bloodstream while recovering from the anaesthetic. They may also have an oxygen saturation probe clipped to their finger or ear lobe to continuously record the concentration of oxygen in their bloodstream. Oxygen therapy may have a drying effect on the mouth and the mucous membranes of the nose. Patients can be assured that ice chips or a mouthwash will be available to help relieve this until they are able to take fluids orally.

Reducing bacterial skin colonisation

The most significant cause of postoperative wound infection is the exposure to nosocomial pathogens, particularly *Staphylococcus aureus* (see Ch. 23). The risk can be reduced by shortening the length of hospital stay and the judicious use of standard infection control precautions by the nursing and medical team (Ch. 16).

Hair removal is considered by some clinicians, but shaving leaves small cuts and abrasions that harbour bacteria and may increase the risk of infection (Bockman & Putney 2008). Hair removal will only be necessary where sticking plaster is to be used, if the hair occludes the surgeon's view of the operation site, or if adhesive ECG leads, requiring a good skin contact, are to be applied. Day surgery patients should be asked not to shave the operative site (Bockman & Putney 2008). If hair removal is necessary, then the use of electric hair clippers is associated with fewer breaches of the skin than shaving (Bockman & Putney 2008). Clippers should be sterilised (Hughes & Mardell 2009) and hair removal should be undertaken as close to the time of incision as possible. However, loose hair clippings could fall into the surgical field and increase the risk of infection, therefore this procedure should not be performed in the room where the operation is to be carried out (Bockman & Putney 2008).

Pre-operative showering may be helpful. Day surgery patients are usually recommended to shower and wash their hair at home prior to admission. This removes surface dirt and microbes (Scott et al 2007). Inpatients will be required to wash using hospital facilities. A single pre-operative shower is unlikely to reduce the risk of infection and Murkin (2009) suggests that patients undergoing open surgical procedures below the chin should be asked to have two showers with chlorhexidine gluconate solution in the pre-operative period, as this reduces the level of resident skin flora. Patients will usually change from their own clothing into a clean theatre gown. It is unnecessary to change clean bed linen.

The maintenance of peri-operative body temperature in the range 36–38°C has been associated with a reduction in postoperative wound infection (Bockman & Putney 2008). The use of warmed blankets or a forced air warming system can help maintain patients' normal temperature (Bockman & Putney 2008). Moreover, a small study by Wagner et al (2006) found that patients reported feeling more comfortable and less anxious pre-operatively if they used a warming gown that allowed them to control their own temperature (Wagner et al 2006).

Bowel preparation

Prior to a procedure such as a colonoscopy or sigmoidoscopy effective bowel cleansing (bowel preparation) is important as it allows the endoscopist to accurately visualise the patient's anatomy and identify abnormalities. Current techniques used to clean the bowel include administration of oral preparations such as sodium picosulfate (Picolax), a phosphate enema or glycerine suppositories. Since many of these procedures are undertaken as outpatient or day cases, the bowel preparation is sometimes carried out by the patient at home. Therefore, patients must find the techniques easy and acceptable to use. A randomised controlled trial by Darroch et al (2008) found that phosphate enemas were well tolerated and provided the best overall bowel preparation; however, glycerine suppositories were found to be difficult to self administer. Until recently it was thought that vigorous pre-operative cleansing of the bowel, together with the use of oral antibiotics, reduced the risk of septic complications after colorectal operations. Pre-operative bowel preparation is time-consuming and expensive, unpleasant for patients, and even dangerous on occasion because of the increased risk of perforation and inflammation. Analysis of the evidence, however, shows no benefit in terms of bowel leakage, mortality rates, peritonitis, need for re-operation, wound infection, or other non-abdominal complications (Guenaga et al 2009). Consequently, there is no evidence that mechanical bowel preparation improves the outcome for patients.

Minimising the risk of aspiration pneumonitis

Patients who are undergoing a general anaesthetic, heavy sedation or a local anaesthetic with the possibility of proceeding to a general anaesthetic, are all at risk of aspiration pneumonitis. When a patient is anaesthetised or unconscious, the swallowing reflex is absent. From the point of induction of the anaesthetic, there is a risk that stomach contents may reflux and be inhaled through the open larynx into the lungs. This leads to the development of pneumonitis (lung inflammation) induced by stomach acid, which may become secondarily infected to become a pneumonia. Risks can be minimised, partly through the administration of certain drugs, but also by fasting the patient of both diet and fluids.

In young and healthy individuals pulmonary aspiration is a rare complication of anaesthesia (Crenshaw & Winslow 2002). However, elderly patients, those who receive opioids and those with diabetes may have reduced gastric motility (Woodhouse 2006). Patients with gastro-oesophageal reflux disease are also more at risk of aspiration, particularly when in a prone position. Gastric emptying is usually complete for most meals in 4–5 h but even fasting patients may still have residual fluid in the stomach (Woodhouse 2006). Taking this into account, the recommended minimum pre-operative fasting period is 2 h for water and 6 h for food. This is the '2 and 6' rule, and is summarised in Box 26.5 (RCN 2005).

While there is now a strong body of evidence and clear guidelines indicating acceptable minimum fasting times, research studies since the 1970s have consistently reported that pre-operative patients are often fasted for longer than necessary, with those on a morning list on average fasted for longer than those on the afternoon list (Jester & Williams 1999, Crenshaw & Winslow 2002). Prolonged fasting is associated with adverse effects (Crenshaw & Winslow 2002), mainly dehydration and electrolyte imbalance. The liver's glycogen stores are sufficient to maintain blood sugar levels for approximately 18 h but even a fast of 6–8 h can reduce the body's ability to cope with stressors such as blood loss or infection (Dean & Fawcett 2002). Older patients are particularly vulnerable to fasting. Depending on their pre-existing health status, older people are at risk of dehydration and confusion, potentially rendering them unfit for anaesthesia and surgery (Jester & Williams 1999). Fasting for patients with diabetes has additional risks, and maintenance of normal glucose levels may require a continuous dextrose/insulin infusion and regular checks of capillary blood glucose levels.

Box 26.5 Information

Pre-operative fasting in adults undergoing elective surgery – 'the 2 and 6 rule' (RCN 2005)

- '2' – Intake of water up to 2 h before induction of anaesthesia.
- '6' – A minimum pre-operative fasting time of 6 h for food (solids, milk and milk-containing drinks).
- The anaesthetic team should consider further interventions for patients at higher risk of regurgitation and aspiration.

It is suggested that in order to cope with workload in a busy surgical unit, where theatre times are always approximate, nursing staff may not always adopt an individualised approach to fasting (Dean & Fawcett 2002, Woodhouse 2006). For example, all patients who are on the morning list may be instructed to fast from midnight regardless of their place on the list. This sets a wide margin of safety, with all patients fasting for at least 6 h. However, a patient on the morning list may be fasted from midnight but may not go to theatre until 11.00 h. Thus they may have fasted for at least 11 h. Nurse-led pre-admission and care pathways offer opportunities for this to be tailored more closely to the patient's needs.

Minimising the risk of venous thromboembolic (VTE) events

Venous thromboembolic (VTE) events consist of deep vein thrombosis (DVT) and pulmonary embolism (PE).

DVT is the formation of a clot in the deep leg veins (femoral or popliteal veins), or in the deep veins above the leg (iliac veins or the inferior vena cava). The risk of this is that the clot can dislodge (or embolise) to the pulmonary artery or one of its branches, compromising lung function and sometimes causing death.

DVT is usually diagnosed 3–14 days postoperatively (Dougherty & Lister 2008). The signs are swelling in the calf or thigh, and redness of the skin which typically becomes tight and shiny (Ingram 2003). Patients may complain of pain in the calf, particularly on dorsiflexion of the foot. However, up to 80% of DVT cases are asymptomatic (Ingram 2003). DVT is important because it can lead to pulmonary embolism (PE) and this carries a high mortality rate (Walker & Lamont 2007). Prevention of the development of DVT is an important nursing consideration and should begin in the pre-operative period.

An intravascular clot or thrombus is most likely to occur when the following conditions, known as Virchow's triad, exist:

- trauma – damaged endothelium
- stasis – slow blood flow
- hypercoagulable blood.

Thrombus formation is initiated by the activation of factor XII in reaction to exposure to collagen filaments in the damaged endothelium. This results in platelet aggregation, formation of thrombin from circulating prothrombin, and stimulation of the production of insoluble fibrin from fibrinogen (see Ch. 11). It has been found that during surgery the veins of the lower leg distend. This distension leads to subluminal endothelial damage, which can provide a site for clot formation (Benkö et al 2001). In the soleal and gastrocnemius veins of the leg, the blood flow is highly dependent on exercise, and so these are often the sites of initial thrombus formation following prolonged periods of inactivity and lack of calf muscle pressure to assist venous return.

Fibrin clots may be broken down gradually by the enzyme plasmin in a process called fibrinolysis. However, the thrombus may persist, causing some degree of venous obstruction. In a small proportion of cases, a fragment of the clot breaks away, forming an embolus. The embolus may travel through the venous system, through the right side of the heart and into the pulmonary arteries. Here it becomes lodged at a point where the arteries become too small to allow the embolus to pass through. The extent of the resultant pulmonary infarct depends on the size of the vessel occluded.

All surgical patients are exposed to a number of risk factors for DVT. However, this risk may be increased depending on the individual patient history and the procedure performed. During the pre-operative assessment, the nurse should assess the patient for the presence of known risk factors (Box 26.6).

It is now generally accepted that all patients should use graduated elastic compression stockings (GECS) as these reduce the risk of developing DVT (Barker & Hollingsworth 2004). Although it is not fully understood how GECS work, these stockings create a decreasing pressure gradient in the leg from approximately 18 mmHg at the ankle to 8 mmHg at the thigh (full length) or to 14 mmHg at the calf (below-knee length). The gradient increases blood flow in the femoral vein, inhibits stasis of the venous circulation, stops build-up of any nidus of thrombosis formation and prevents the venous distension that causes endothelial damage (Parnaby 2004, Walker & Lamont 2007). GECS are inexpensive (Ingram 2003) and reduce the incidence of postoperative DVT by 50% (NICE 2007).

The role of the nurse is to ensure that a well-designed and well-fitting stocking is applied (Walker & Lamont 2007). Nurses should ensure that patients understand the importance of wearing GECS appropriately (Parnaby 2004). Stockings are fitted according to calf size and leg length and are available in a wide variety of sizes. If stockings roll down, a constricting band is created which may cause higher pressures, leading to an inverse gradient and delayed venous emptying. There are two lengths of stocking commonly available: thigh and knee length (Dougherty & Lister 2008). Thigh-length stockings are suggested to be more effective (SIGN 2002, NICE 2007) but below-knee stockings have been found to be more comfortable and compliance with therapy may therefore be better. They are also less costly than full-length stockings (Ingram 2003).

Inaccurately fitted stockings may offer no protection, or worse, lead to the development of ischaemic problems in the lower limb (Walker & Lamont 2007). Approximately 15–20% of patients are unable to wear GECS because of limb characteristics (Greerts et al 2001), marked leg oedema, severe peripheral arterial disease, dermatitis, severe peripheral neuropathy or other major leg deformity (SIGN 2002). The use of GECS is also contraindicated in patients with severe peripheral vascular disease or profound limb ulceration (Parnaby 2004, Walker & Lamont 2007). This emphasises the importance of accurate leg measurements and selection of the stockings. Nursing staff should also check the skin and circulation in the toes of any patient wearing GECS to detect complications, at least daily. If there are any concerns about correct fitting, the legs should be re-measured and new stockings applied. Patients should wear the stockings prior to surgery and up until discharge.

Other measures that should be encouraged where possible are early activity and hourly leg exercises. The patient should be taught to dorsiflex the foot pre-operatively. This will assist venous return by the action of the calf muscle compressing blood in the deep veins. Deep breathing exercises will also aid the respiratory pump, as deep inspiration reduces intrathoracic pressure and hence increases venous return. In addition, ensuring adequate hydration will reduce hypercoagulability.

Intermittent pneumatic compression stockings (IPCS) are mechanical devices that fill with air, periodically compressing the calf and/or thigh muscles of the leg and stimulating fibrinolysis. For patients at high risk of developing DVT, such as those undergoing orthopaedic and cardiac surgery, intermittent pneumatic compression of the legs has been shown to be particularly effective (SIGN 2002), although Arnold (2002) suggests that patients are often reluctant to participate in this treatment postoperatively. Patients may remove stocking sleeves or disconnect the pump because they find the stockings hot or uncomfortable (Murakami et al 2003).

Teaching leg exercises and applying GECS and/or IPCS devices reduce the risk of DVT by their action on two aspects of Virchow's triad: stasis and endothelial damage. Hypercoagulability can be avoided to some extent by adequate hydration but will be stimulated by the general adaptation to stress response and by the effects of surgery initiating clotting mechanisms. Medical staff will prescribe anticoagulants in the form of prophylactic low-dose heparin, often low molecular weight heparin, to minimise hypercoagulability. These anticoagulants are given daily or twice daily subcutaneously (NICE 2007). As full anticoagulation does not occur, the risk of increased intra-operative bleeding complications is minimal.

Premedication

The term 'premedication' (often abbreviated to 'premed') is used to describe drugs given to pre-operative patients before they leave the ward. These drugs constitute part of the

---

Box 26.6 Information

Patient-related risk factors for venous thromboembolism (adapted from SIGN 2002, NICE 2007)

- Spinal or epidural anaesthesia
- Surgery, especially major abdominal or orthopaedic surgery
- Active cancer or cancer treatment
- Active heart or respiratory failure
- Acute medical illness
- Age over 60 years
- Central venous catheter in situ
- Continuous travel of more than 3 h approximately 4 weeks before or after surgery
- Immobility (for example, paralysis or limb in plaster)
- Inflammatory bowel disease (for example Crohn's disease or ulcerative colitis)
- Nephrotic syndrome
- Obesity (body mass index >30 kg/m^2)
- Personal or family history of VTE
- Pregnancy or puerperium
- Recent myocardial infarction or stroke
- Severe infection
- Use of oral contraceptives or hormonal replacement therapy
- Varicose veins with associated phlebitis

Table 26.1 Common premedications

DRUG	USUAL ADULT DOSE	ROUTE	EFFECTS
Temazepam (most common)	10–20 mg	Oral	Sedative: reduces tension and anxiety. Induces drowsiness
Lorazepam	1 3 mg	Oral	Sedative: reduces tension and anxiety. Decreases muscle tone and potentiates non-depolarising muscle relaxants. Induces mental detachment and amnesia

For pre-emptive analgesia oral preparations are commonly used instead of i.m./s.c., e.g. paracetamol and ibuprofen, or oxycodone hydrochloride (long-acting opiate) 10 mg every 12 h.

anaesthetic and analgesia and are used to prepare the patient to receive a general or local anaesthetic (Table 26.1). They are often also used to relax the patient and relieve anxiety. However, research by Hyde et al (1998) found that, although often anxious about their surgery, many patients did not wish to be sedated in the immediate pre-operative period. Instead they would rather listen to music, read and be able to move about freely. The premed is prescribed by the anaesthetist after assessing the patient for the administration of the anaesthetic. The premed may be prescribed for a set time or 'on call', which means that the anaesthetist will telephone the ward to ask the nurse to administer the premed once it is clear how long it will take for the patient to be called to theatre. The nurse must ensure that the consent form has been signed, the patient has emptied their bladder and that all other pre-operative checks are complete before giving the premed. The patient should then be advised to rest and not get out of bed unsupervised if the premed contains a strong sedative or opioid. In day surgery premedication is not usually

prescribed because it can make the patient too drowsy to be discharged home (Mitchell 2007a).

Theatre safety

The nurse must carry out pre-operative checks before the administration of the premed, as the results of the checks may necessitate a delay in going to theatre. Moreover, the patient should not have received sedative or opioid agents before signing the consent form. Many hospitals have created their own checklists. Examples of criteria for checklists are given in Table 26.2.

For patients who rely on their hearing aids and/or glasses for communication, these can be labelled with adhesive tape and worn by the patient until anaesthetised. Equally they may wish to retain their false teeth until anaesthetised. A note should be made to this effect on the checklist or anaesthetic form.

During the immediate pre-operative period, the patient may feel extremely vulnerable and anxious (Pearson et al

Table 26.2 Pre-operative checklist

CRITERIA	ACTION	RATIONALE
Identification	Prepare two name bands with patient's full name, hospital unit number, date of birth, home address (as a minimum), plus ward and consultant	Correct identification of patient
	Clearly note allergies on the anaesthetic sheet and on wrist bands as well as the prescription chart	Avoidance of all allergens
	Ensure site is correctly marked with indelible ink	Correct identification of site
Documentation	Ensure that medical notes, nursing notes, signed consent form, X-rays and anaesthetic sheet accompany patient to theatre	Ready availability of all necessary information
Fasting	Document when patient last had anything to eat or drink	Prevention of aspiration pneumonia
Empty bladder	Ask patient to pass urine prior to administering premedication	To prevent damage to full bladder during surgery To enable complete bed rest after premed To prevent postoperative discomfort due to a full bladder
Risk of diathermy burns	Ask patient to remove all jewellery, hair pins and other items containing metal (wedding rings may be covered with tape)	To remove all metal that may concentrate the diathermy current
Prostheses	Ask patient to remove all prostheses, e.g. dentures, hearing aids, contact lenses, false eyes, glasses, etc.	To prevent harm caused by prostheses To prevent loss
Care of valuables	Offer to receive valuables into safekeeping for the patient	Patient will be away from the ward and unfit to be responsible for these valuables
Circulatory assessment	Ask patient to remove all makeup, lipstick and nail varnish	To facilitate observation of colour of skin, lips and nail beds

2004). They will be wearing only a flimsy gown, their dentures may have been removed, they may be unable to see well without glasses, and they may feel drowsy from the premed. Anxiety about the impending operation can be high, especially among patients placed in the later part of the operating list (Panda et al 1996). Reassurance by the nurse at this time and, for some patients, distraction, can be helpful. A family member or designated staff member offering support to the patient at this time may have a calming effect (Mayne & Bagaoisan 2009). Suggestions for managing this period in the day surgery setting are made by Mitchell (2007a).

Peri-operative safety

Caring for patients in the operating theatre

Patients may be brought to the theatre on a trolley but increasingly they are transferred on their bed accompanied by a nurse from the ward and a porter or operating department assistant (ODA). Once the patient transfers to the theatre table, the bed is taken to a holding area. The patient is then transferred back onto the bed at the end of the operation. This reduces the discomfort of transferring from trolley to bed in the ward, and reduces the amount of patient lifting by staff.

The anaesthetic or theatre nurse or ODA receiving the patient goes through the pre-operative check again (see Table 26.2) and, if possible, asks the patient to confirm details. The ward nurse will then usually return to the ward but if the patient is especially nervous or confused it can be comforting if a nurse or family member who knows them well can stay until the induction of anaesthesia (Mayne & Bagaoisan 2009). All patients must be supervised by a nurse in this pre-induction time, as the patient may have received premedication and is in an extremely stressful and unfamiliar environment. Many theatre nurses visit their patients pre-operatively to introduce themselves and also to give any information about patient care in theatre (Hughes 2002). In emergency cases, the theatre nurse may continue the pre-operative preparation.

The roles of theatre nursing staff are summarised in Box 26.7. Traditionally a surgeon is responsible for performing the surgery although Martin (2002) describes a nurse-led service in London where nurse practitioners perform minor surgical procedures using local anaesthetic. The anaesthetist will visit the patient pre-operatively in the ward to assess the patient's ability to tolerate the anaesthetic, give information and reassurance, and prescribe a premedication if required.

Operating department practitioners (ODPs) also work in operating theatres with anaesthetists, surgeons and nurses, providing care to patients (NHS Executive 2001). The role of the ODP may vary between hospitals, but many ODPs work in the anaesthetic room, assisting the anaesthetist, setting up and maintaining equipment. In recent years an increasing number of ODPs have been employed in the operating theatre itself and carry out similar roles to those performed by theatre nurses (Timmons & Tanner 2004). For further information about the role of the theatre nurse see Pidduck (2003).

Box 26.7 Information

The roles of the theatre nursing staff

The anaesthetic nurse
- Receives the patient in the reception area of the anaesthetic room
- Checks patient in, deals with any irregularities
- Helps to relieve patient anxiety
- Initiates routine monitoring of patient and assists with insertion of invasive monitoring devices if required
- Assists in the induction (and maintenance) of anaesthesia
- Performs emergency preparation of patients for theatre
- Uses and checks anaesthetic equipment
- Maintains patient safety and comfort

The circulating nurse
- Assists with the provision of equipment
- Maintains nursing records
- Positions the patient
- Ensures safety with regard to instruments and swabs
- Cleans and sterilises equipment
- Observes, measures and records vital signs

The scrub nurse
- Positions the patient
- Provides appropriate sterile equipment
- Assists the surgeon
- Protects the patient's dignity and changes drapes to avoid pooling of cleansing agents (e.g. povidone-iodine)
- Prevents diathermy and pressure injuries, and ensures no equipment is rubbing
- Ensures safety with regard to instruments and swabs
- Manages the high-risk patient

The recovery room nurse
- Maintains patency of the airway
- Observes patient for level of consciousness and safety
- Monitors vital signs: colour, respiration, temperature (core and peripheral), pulse, blood pressure, fluid intake and output, wounds and drainage
- Assesses pain and nausea and administers analgesics and antiemetics
- Reassures the patient and provides a quiet environment
- Provides total patient care
- Provides documentation and facilitates communication
- Ensures patient meets discharge criteria prior to transfer from recovery room

The emphasis of all roles in theatre is on patient safety and teamwork, and each professional has an important part to play in the patient's passage through theatre. Communication problems leading to information loss could compromise patient safety in the operating room (Christian et al 2006). Allard et al (2007) suggest that team briefings, involving all theatre staff, can promote effective teamwork and ensure there is a shared understanding of planned patient care priorities. The World Health Organization has published a 'surgical safety checklist' which allows surgical teams to document the completion of specific tasks before they proceed with an operation (National Patient Safety Agency 2008).

It may be difficult for a student nurse to appreciate the communication links in place, especially when some staff have half their faces covered with a mask. See Box 26.8 for suggestions for getting the best out of a theatre placement.

Environmental safety

The environment in the operating theatre is designed to minimise the risk of exogenous infection to the patient.

- Clean, filtered air is pumped into clean areas. Air pressure is higher inside the theatre than outside, in order to maintain an air flow from the theatre to the outside. This prevents potentially contaminated air from the rest of the hospital moving into the theatres. Waste anaesthetic gases are also removed via a scavenging system.
- Temperature is controlled through the ventilation system. This is to provide a comfortable working environment for staff and to prevent patients from developing intra-operative hypothermia.

Box 26.8 Information

Top tips for theatre placement (Veitch 2009)

- Be aware of the specialist area you are going to be working in. Having a good general knowledge of the physiology relating to the specialised area, for example orthopaedics or cardiothoracic, is an advantage as it means you have increased understanding of the surgical procedures taking place.
- Get to know the daily routine and layout of the theatres. Each theatre will differ slightly, but being aware of the patient pathway is helpful in learning when to get equipment ready for a procedure, whether as circulating nurse or scrub nurse.
- Know the dress code, even when socialising in the staff room. Scrubs, hat and clean shoes (which are only for theatre purpose) are essential. This is to prevent infection. When entering theatre, a mask is also needed and a lead overcoat may be necessary if X-rays are being taken. When scrubbed up, sterile overcoat, gloves, mask and glasses are essential.
- Work with different people – everyone will have differing experiences of working in theatres in terms of specialised areas, length of work time and trauma or elective theatre work.
- Be aware of the different stages of each procedure so that you can predict what implements may be needed, for example sutures or dressings.
- Participate in maintaining the theatre environment – cleaning after each patient, changing suction, wiping the whiteboard which contains information in relation to swab/suture counts, making sure correct equipment is available.
- If you are given the opportunity to scrub up, familiarise yourself with the basic trays and common sutures, alcoholic washes and dressings, so you are more likely to be aware of each instrument and their uses. Knowing the stages of the differing procedures is helpful here as you can predict which supplementary implements may be needed and what instruments the surgeon is likely to require. Knowing the basics can also help reduce anxiety when participating in the role of the scrub nurse, allowing for increased learning and enjoyment.

- Humidity is maintained at 50–55% (Ewart & Huntington 2007). This is to prevent a build-up of static electricity and the risk of sparks, if flammable anaesthetic gases are used. It also suppresses bacterial growth.
- Clean and dirty areas are delineated by doors or a line on the floor. All personnel moving into clean areas must be clean and appropriately dressed (see below). All items brought into clean areas must be clean. All dirty items leaving theatre should do so via dirty areas. It is essential that staff are aware which are the dirty and the clean areas and corridors.
- The numbers and movements of staff inside theatres are kept to an absolute minimum to reduce the number of skin scales shed and mixing of air (Mangram et al 1999).
- All staff entering clean areas are appropriately dressed. Clean theatre dresses or trouser suits are worn. Hair is completely covered by a bonnet-style cap and all jewellery, especially on the hands, is removed. Practice varies as to whether staff are able to leave the theatre area wearing theatre clothing. Some hospitals restrict staff to the theatre area when dressed in theatre clothing, while others allow for the wearing of gowns over scrub suits when personnel leave the theatre suite (Mangram et al 1999, Kaplan et al 2003).
- Masks are usually worn inside the theatre where sterile supplies are open and scrubbed personnel are located, to reduce airborne organisms (AORN 1998). However, there is evidence that face mask use varies (Lipp & Edwards 2010). A study by Webster et al (2010) advocates the use of masks by scrubbed personnel only. Masks, once applied, should be handled only by the tapes as the main fabric of the mask becomes contaminated with moisture and microorganisms which can then be transmitted to and by the hands.
- Appropriate theatre footwear should offer good protection from mechanical injury and body fluids and so should cover the toes fully. Staff must not wear theatre shoes outside the operating department, to prevent cross contamination (Ewart & Huntington 2007). Shoe covers may protect members of the surgical team from exposure to blood and body fluids (Mangram et al 1999).
- A sterile field is created around the patient. The patient and trolleys in this area are all covered with sterile drapes. The surgeon and scrub nurse wear sterile gloves and gowns to work within the sterile field.

Safety of the patient

The patient's safety in theatre is further ensured by the following precautions:

- Transfer to and positioning on the operating table are carried out with extreme care. The pre-operative visit by the theatre nurse enables the assessment of any potential problems, especially in relation to joint mobility and the risk of developing pressure ulcers. Surgical patients are at risk of developing pressure ulcers during the peri-operative phases of their care because of the combination of immobility while surgery is carried out and circulatory and metabolic changes resulting from anaesthesia and surgical trauma (Malan & McIndoe 2003). Patients who have epidural anaesthesia have reduced sensation in the lower extremities and impaired leg movement because of the effects of the anaesthetic mixture on the motor nerve pathways in the spinal cord. These patients are especially at risk of heel pressure ulcers because they may fail to change the position of their legs in bed, or feel the sensation of discomfort. Pressure-relieving padding, mattresses or overlays can be used can be used in high-risk patients to protect vulnerable areas such as elbows, heels and sacrum. Heel protectors may also be applied (Edwards et al 2006). Once patients are anaesthetised, they may lose muscle tone. Care should be taken with all limbs, as nerve damage can occur from compression or traction of a limb whilst the patient is anaesthetised. The nurse must also be aware when positioning patients on the operating table of limitations in movement that may result from previous joint replacement surgery; for example, hip flexion may be restricted in patients with a total hip replacement prosthesis. Patient position will depend on the requirements of the surgical procedure. Common surgical positions are supine, prone and lithotomy. A description of these positions and the physiological considerations required when caring for patients in different positions is found in Ewart & Huntington (2007, pp. 29–32) or Hughes & Mardell (2009, pp. 328–333).

- The diathermy pad is carefully positioned. A self-adhesive pad may be used and the pad is usually placed on the thigh to ensure good contact over the entire surface. Poor contact by only part of the surface may concentrate the current, causing it to leave a burn.
- Swabs, needles and instruments used during the operation are counted and checked throughout and at the end of the operation by the scrub nurse and circulating nurse. This ensures that all items used are accounted for and none left inside the patient.
- Allergies to drugs, skin antiseptics and dressings are assessed pre-operatively by the theatre nurse and anaesthetist, so the use of any allergens such as iodine or latex can be avoided (Murkin 2009).
- The patient's skin is cleaned at the start of the procedure with an antiseptic skin preparation (Murkin 2009). The most commonly used antiseptics are chlorhexidine gluconate, alcohol-based solutions and iodophors such as povidone-iodine. Current evidence suggests that 2% chlorhexidine gluconate in 70% isopropyl alcohol should be used for skin preparation as it is quick acting and produces a rapid reduction in bacterial counts on skin (Murkin 2009). Also, in comparison to iodine, its action is longer lasting (Murkin 2009). Once applied, alcohol-based solutions must be allowed to dry completely lest they ignite on contact with diathermy. Some surgeons also use a sterile plastic adhesive drape over the skin through which to make the incision. This prevents the surgeons' and nurses' sterile gloves being contaminated with the patient's skin flora. For a more detailed explanation of good practice in application of skin preparation solution see Murkin (2009, p. 668).
- Prophylactic antibiotics may be administered (usually intravenously) during the operation, or the site of the surgery may be irrigated with an antibiotic solution. These measures are usually taken only if there is a

specific risk of contamination, or if contamination from an abscess or the gastrointestinal tract is already present.

- During surgery the patient is at risk of primary haemorrhage. Bleeding during surgery is minimised by the use of clamps and ligatures, local pressure and diathermy to seal small vessels. To facilitate the surgeon's vision, the site of operation is kept free of blood by swabbing or suctioning. The circulating nurse may weigh the swabs and note the volume of blood in the suction bottle to estimate 'total blood loss'.
- Some additional precautions should be followed for the care of patients identified as carriers of blood-borne infectious diseases, such as HIV and hepatitis B (Mullerat & Winslet 2005). During the procedure the surgeon and scrub nurse may use two pairs of gloves and wear eye goggles or a visor. Their gowns or aprons may be impermeable to moisture to prevent soakage from body fluids, and water-resistant footwear/overshoes may be selected. Particular care must be taken in the use of sharps, in particular in the transfer between the surgeon and the scrub nurse in case of needlestick injury (Mullerat & Winslet 2005). To prevent cross infection and to reduce risks involved with cleaning and spillages, disposable equipment is used where possible. The patient should be operated on at the end of a theatre list to enable recovery in theatre and to allow thorough cleaning and disinfection of the theatre before it is used again. For further information on patient safety in theatre see *Standards and Recommendations for Safe Perioperative Practice* published by the Association for Perioperative Practice (2007).

Anaesthesia

An anaesthetic is used to block any sensations of pain during surgery. It may be applied locally or regionally to the area of surgery or generally throughout the body. A brief introduction to the use of anaesthetics is given here. For more information on medications used in anaesthesia, see Waller (2010) or Karch (2009).

Local anaesthesia

Local anaesthesia blocks transmission of pain from the region operated upon. In some cases, only the sensory receptors may be blocked; this is more correctly termed 'local analgesia'. Types and common uses of local anaesthetics are summarised in Table 26.3. Epidural or spinal anaesthetics may be used

Table 26.3 Types and common uses of local anaesthetics		
METHOD OF ADMINISTRATION	**EFFECT**	**EXAMPLE OF DRUGS AND THEIR USES**
Topical: solution or cream applied to skin or mucous membranes	Blocks local sensory nerve receptors	Lidocaine Amitop cream (topical) Minor ENT procedures Insertion of cannulae
Infiltration: injection into surgical site	Blocks local sensory nerve receptors	Lidocaine, bupivacaine E.g. removal of skin moles, insertion of Hickman line

when a general anaesthetic could be harmful or is undesirable, e.g. older patients with arteriosclerosis or diabetes, patients with respiratory disorders and those with hypertension. An infusion of epidural anaesthetic agents can also be continued after surgery to provide effective postoperative analgesia (see p. 710). The procedure causes hypotension and so should be avoided in patients with this condition.

Care must be taken to prepare the patient psychologically in order to reduce anxiety and ensure cooperation. Psychological support should continue throughout the operation and the nurse should ensure that the patient's vision of the procedure is adequately screened.

General anaesthesia

General anaesthesia is characterised by loss of consciousness, analgesia and muscle relaxation. These effects occur according to the stage of anaesthesia, as follows:

Stage 1 The pain is reduced or relieved, but the patient is still conscious. Heavy sedation can produce 'dissociative anaesthesia' and some muscle relaxation, while local analgesics supplement pain control as necessary. The patient may remain drowsy but conscious throughout the procedure. Entonox® (50% oxygen with 50% nitrous oxide) may be self-administered during childbirth or painful procedures such as large wound dressings to achieve stage 1 anaesthesia for pain control. This application is discussed with other methods of pain relief in Chapter 19.

Stage 2 Consciousness is lost, but the patient may exhibit wild movements and irrational behaviour. With intravenous induction of anaesthesia, this stage is passed through very quickly; it may be more in evidence when the patient is recovering from anaesthesia.

Stage 3 Breathing becomes regular and there is relaxation of the muscles along with loss of reflexes. This is the level of surgical anaesthesia. The degree of muscle relaxation required to facilitate surgery can be achieved by deepening this stage but this has undesirable side-effects such as fall in cardiac output, respiratory depression and liver damage. To overcome this problem, muscle relaxants can be administered to enable a relatively light anaesthetic to be used and so reduce the risks in older people and those with cardiovascular and respiratory complications.

Premedication can be used to relieve anxiety, induce a state of analgesia, reduce bronchial and salivary secretions, prevent vasovagal stimulation (mainly bradycardia) and make the patient less aware and somewhat drowsy. Usually, a sedative or anxiolytic is given orally (see Table 26.1).

The induction of anaesthesia is usually achieved with a short-acting intravenous agent administered with a short-acting muscle relaxant (see the website for examples of anaesthetic agents and muscle relaxants).

♫ **See website for further content**

This rapidly produces surgical anaesthesia, in which the patient is unable to maintain their own airway (due to lack of reflexes) and the muscles of breathing are paralysed. An endotracheal tube is passed through the relaxed larynx and artificial ventilation is maintained throughout the operation. For emergency patients who have not fasted, the anaesthetist may decide to use rapid sequence induction

with cricoid pressure (Graham et al 2003). As the patient becomes unconscious pressure is applied to the cricoid cartilage in the throat, which mechanically occludes the oesophagus and is thought to reduce the likelihood of aspiration of any regurgitated gastric contents. However, a review by Butler & Sen (2005) found that there was little evidence to suggest that cricoid pressure actually reduced incidence of aspiration, and may in fact interfere with airway management.

Anaesthesia can be maintained during surgery, usually by means of inhaled anaesthetics and a longer-acting muscle relaxant. At the end of the operation, the anaesthetic gas is discontinued and the effects of the muscle relaxant are reversed with the appropriate drug. The patient gradually regains consciousness, passing through stages 2 and 1 of anaesthesia (see p. 702) and regaining muscle tone, which enables independent breathing. During this time, the patient is transferred to the recovery room. The anaesthetist will hand over care of the patient to the recovery room nurse who will monitor the patient closely.

Recovery from anaesthesia

The patient will normally be nursed in the recovery room until the immediate effects of the anaesthetic have worn off. Regular and careful assessment of the patient is important at this time for early detection of any problems and to instigate immediate treatment. Recovery room nurses may follow principles of ABCD (Airway, Breathing, Circulation, Disability) assessment to structure their assessment (Resuscitation Council 2006).

Airway In the post-anaesthetic phase of care the nurse must ensure that the airway is kept open. This can be achieved by placing the patient in a lateral or semi-prone position, tilting the head backwards and pulling the mandible forwards, or inserting a Guedel (oropharyngeal) airway. If a Guedel airway is used it can be left in position until, as reflexes return, the patient expels it spontaneously. Anaesthetics, muscle relaxants, narcotics and severe pain itself can cause nausea and vomiting and so there is a risk of upper airway obstruction and aspiration pneumonia should the patient vomit while regaining consciousness. Therefore, suction equipment must be available.

Breathing Patients are usually prescribed supplementary oxygen until fully awake, in order to maintain PO_2 while there is still some respiratory depression due to anaesthesia. The recovery room nurse should observe the patient's respiratory rate, rhythm and depth closely for signs of hypoventilation due to secretions or uncontrolled pain, or respiratory depression due to opiates. Pulse oximetry (see Ch. 3) allows assessment of the saturation of haemoglobin in the blood (Francis 2006). Patients should be encouraged to commence deep breathing exercises as soon as consciousness is regained.

Circulation Close and frequent observation of pulse and blood pressure is required for the early detection of changes in the patient's condition. During surgery and anaesthesia the patient's blood pressure may have been reduced due to the effects of anaesthesia and blood loss. Hypotension is often induced during surgery due to anaesthetic agents and during the recovery period patients are especially at risk of reactionary haemorrhage as their blood pressure rises. A ligature or clot may become dislodged, leading to signs of haemorrhage and hypovolaemic shock (see p. 705). Observation of wound dressings and wound drainage will also aid assessment of any continued blood loss in the recovery period.

During surgery, the patient may have had a large surface area exposed, leading to loss of body heat. A high risk of hypothermia (a core temperature of less than 35°C) exists in older patients, in surgery where the peritoneal cavity is opened or when large amounts of unwarmed irrigation fluids are used (Scott et al 1999). Shivering will have been suppressed, due to the use of skeletal muscle relaxants. As well as feeling uncomfortable, the patient may also suffer adverse effects on postoperative recovery. A drop of 2°C during colorectal surgery has been shown to triple wound infection rates and to lead to an increased length of stay (Kurz et al 1996). Shivering in the recovery period increases oxygen demand and is distressing and painful for the patient (Scott et al 1999). Extra blankets, forced air system and warming of intravenous fluids can be used, but the nurse must be wary of warming the patient too quickly, as this can lead to peripheral vasodilatation and a consequent fall in blood pressure (see Ch. 22).

Disability The nurse should observe the patient's level of consciousness and be aware that a stage of excitement (stage 2 anaesthesia, see p. 702) may occur. Close observation and the use of side rails will be required. Pain management begins before, or as, the patient regains consciousness. The operation site may have been infiltrated with more local anaesthetic at the end of surgery. The anaesthetist may also prescribe some opioid analgesics and a simple oral analgesic for the patient's return to the ward. The patient's pain should be controlled before leaving the recovery room and many patients will receive their first dose of analgesic in the recovery room. This may be via the rectal, intramuscular, subcutaneous or intravenous route. In a partially conscious patient, a sudden rise in blood pressure and restlessness may indicate the presence of pain. The nurse must be aware that opioid analgesics may cause a fall in blood pressure and respiratory depression, and that severe pain in itself can lead to shock and shallow breathing.

The patient may spend several hours in the recovery room and will, in many respects, require the same care as an unconscious patient (see Ch. 28). As the patient regains consciousness, the nurse should bear in mind that hearing is usually one of the first senses to return. Verbal reassurance that the operation is over should be given. It may be appropriate to return hearing aids and spectacles at this point. The patient should be allowed to rest as quietly as possible during this period and will usually fall asleep after regaining consciousness. Most patients will require attention to their mouth, as mucous membranes will be dry due to oxygen therapy, fasting and perhaps dehydration, as well as to pressure areas.

The patient should be fully conscious, able to maintain a clear airway and be considered haemodynamically stable before transfer back to the ward (SIGN 2004). Pain should also be controlled and appropriate medication regimens prescribed. In some cases the patient will be transferred directly to the intensive therapy unit (ITU) while continuing to be intubated and their respiration is maintained by artificial ventilation. Alternatively, the patient may be ventilated in the recovery room overnight, hereby avoiding unnecessary admission to ITU.

The recovery room nurse will document the care given and provide a summary to the ward nurse who collects the patient so that continuity of care can be achieved. The role of the recovery room nurse is summarised in Box 26.7. Anaesthetic and surgical staff should document clear instructions for postoperative treatment and highlight possible complications.

Postoperative care

The postoperative phase of care is from when patients have regained stable vital functions in recovery until they are ready for discharge home (Allvin et al 2007). All patients require close observation during the immediate postoperative period in order to detect any complications. Close observation may be continued for hours or days for the patient requiring intensive nursing care, or, in day surgery, for a matter of a few hours.

Rehabilitation will be achieved at a different pace and to differing levels by each patient. The patient with a hip replacement may find that their joint pain is almost immediately reduced postoperatively and that their functional ability is far better than before the operation. Some patients may not be able to achieve the desired level of recovery and others may be seeking palliation rather than cure. For an analysis of the dimensions of postoperative recovery see Allvin et al (2007).

For purposes of clarity, this section will focus on the postoperative recovery, repair and rehabilitation most commonly experienced during the hospital stay, while the section on 'Rehabilitation' focuses on continued care after discharge from hospital. It is recognised, however, that many patients will still be recovering from the effects of the anaesthetic after discharge following day surgery. This can take up to 24 h to be eliminated from the body.

Postoperative assessment

Ward nurses should undertake a comprehensive assessment of the patient on their return from theatre. This provides a baseline against which subsequent recordings can be assessed. The collection of this data allows trends in the patient's condition to be identified. Action can be taken to identify and manage any problems before severe deterioration occurs. For an example of immediate postoperative care following a left hemicolectomy see Box 26.9.

The frequency of the recordings is determined by the patient's condition not merely as a routine procedure. Many surgical units have standard postoperative protocols in place which prescribe the frequency of routine recordings in the immediate postoperative period, for example every 15 minutes for the first hour, decreasing to 30 minutes over the next hour and hourly thereafter. It is important that nurses consider each patient's observations carefully, as the frequency of recordings may need to be escalated in response to changes in the patient's condition, for example if the patient has uncontrolled pain or becomes increasingly confused.

Box 26.9 Information

Immediate postoperative considerations – Mr Shah

Mr Shah was discharged to the postoperative ward from theatre recovery at 21.00 following a left hemicolectomy. On admission to the ward his observations were:

Pulse 100 bpm

BP 110/70 mmHg

Respiratory rate 23 bpm

SaO_2 level 95%

CVP + 4–5 mmHg

The dressings are dry and have no soakage.

He has one vacuum drain in situ.

There is 50 mL of bloodstained fluid in the vacuum drain.

Mr Shah had epidural analgesia in progress for postoperative pain and his pain score in recovery had been 2/10 on rest and 4/10 on movement. However, after 60 minutes on the ward his breathing became shallow and rapid (respiratory rate 28–30). His SaO_2 recordings were 92–93%. His pulse rate was tachycardic at 125 bpm but his blood pressure was unchanged. On questioning Mr Shah said he had pain that was decreasing his ability to take deep breaths, and although he was able to tolerate his pain when he lay still he was afraid to cough or expand his chest. He could feel he had something to cough up but did not want to bother the nurses. His pain appeared to be on his left side only. When the nurse checked his block level the epidural did not appear to be providing pain relief on his left side at all. The anaesthetist was called and Mr Shah received a 'top up' (bolus dose) of his epidural. Mr Shah's vital signs and pain score were observed at 5-minute intervals over the following 30 minutes in case he developed hypotension. Rapidly Mr Shah became more comfortable with a pain score of 0/10 on rest and 1–2/10 on movement. He was able to take deep breaths and cough. The nurse showed him how to support his wound with a pillow while coughing.

Interestingly, a study by Zeitz (2005) found that nurses in two hospitals with different postoperative recording protocols tended to collect vital signs from patients at similar frequencies, suggesting that these practices were based on routine rather than on the individual needs of the patient. Nursing and medical staff should agree acceptable parameters for the monitoring of postoperative patients and actions to be taken if the parameters being monitored change (SIGN 2004). A table of the key postoperative nursing considerations in the immediate postoperative period for Mr Shah is provided on the website (Box 26.10).

 See website Postoperative care plan – Mr Shah

Box 26.10 Reflection

Postoperative monitoring: deviation of vital signs

Mr Shah's change in pulse rate and respiratory rate were due to pain. What other causes of tachycardia would you would need to consider in a postoperative patient?

Shock and haemostasis

Nurses need to be vigilant for the signs and symptoms of shock; the key to successful management of shock is early identification and treatment to restore adequate tissue perfusion (Hughes 2004). The consequences of poor tissue perfusion include breakdown of surgical anastomoses, cerebral damage, renal failure, multiple organ failure and death (SIGN 2004).

Distinction should be made between hypovolaemic and other forms of shock, i.e. cardiogenic, septic, anaphylactic and neurogenic.

Cardiogenic shock is caused by failure of the heart to pump and maintain adequate cardiac output. Possible causes following surgery may be pulmonary embolus, causing massive resistance to the output from the right side of the heart, fluid overload and concomitant heart failure, anaesthetic depression of cardiac output or myocardial infarction. Careful patient assessment may reveal dilation of neck veins and a 12-lead ECG will detect arrhythmias and myocardial ischaemia associated with cardiogenic shock.

The patient may also be at risk of:

- neurogenic shock, usually due to severe pain
- anaphylactic shock, usually due to drug reactions
- septic shock, from infections following surgery; for a detailed discussion of the management of sepsis in the postoperative period see SIGN (2004).

Shock is discussed here with specific application to the care of surgical patients. For a wider discussion of the types and mechanisms of shock and their signs and symptoms, see Chapter 18.

Hypovolaemic shock

In the postoperative period there is a continued risk of reactionary haemorrhage for the first 24 h as the patient's blood pressure returns to normal. Hypovolaemic shock may also occur due to a slow, continuous loss of fluid; this might be a slowly bleeding vessel or the pooling of fluid in the gastrointestinal tract during the paralytic ileus (see p. 708) that occurs as a consequence of surgery. The loss of fluid may be detected as soakage on the dressing or blood in the wound drains, but if the patient is bleeding into a body cavity or losing fluid into the gut it may be less obvious.

Secondary haemorrhage can occur 1–7 days postoperatively due to vessel erosion by infection or from a long, slow bleed. The patient may collapse suddenly and will usually need to return to theatre.

The aim of nursing observations in the first 24 h following surgery is to detect changes that might indicate the initial stages of compensation to hypovolaemic shock. As the circulating volume falls, the nurse may see increased loss of blood on dressings or in wound drainage bags or bottles. There will be a slight rise in heart rate to maintain cardiac output but systolic blood pressure may remain unchanged, or even rise slightly. Peripheral vasoconstriction to conserve blood supply to vital organs (brain, heart and lungs) and secretion of sweat from the eccrine glands on the palms and forehead may lead to a pale, clammy appearance. The brain is extremely sensitive to hypoxia, the respiratory rate may be increased and the patient may also appear restless. In an average adult weighing 70 kg the body has ability to compensate for blood losses up to 750 mL and physiological signs can be difficult to detect at this early stage (Garretson & Malberti 2007). Blood pressure may be maintained because of the combination of vasoconstriction and increased cardiac contractility brought about by the sympathetic nervous system response. Vasoconstriction of the veins maintains diastolic (end) volume and therefore preserves stroke volume. This, along with increased cardiac contractility, can maintain blood pressure to at least pre-shock levels. It is not until fluid losses exceed 750 mL that changes in vital signs will occur as the body's compensation mechanisms deteriorate. Action should be taken immediately hypovolaemic shock is suspected. If nurses wait until the patient displays classic signs of tachycardia and profound hypotension, then blood loss is already significant.

If the blood or fluid loss continues, then these mechanisms will eventually fail to compensate effectively, leading to further vasoconstriction of the arterioles to increase peripheral resistance. There is also reduced parasympathetic activity to increase heart rate and stroke volume, resulting in increased cardiac output. At this point the heart rate increases further and blood pressure begins to fall. Urine output decreases rapidly, due to decreased renal perfusion over and above the effects of increased antidiuretic hormone (ADH) and aldosterone (see Ch. 8), as blood flow is conserved to maintain the brain, heart and lungs as a priority.

The patient appears breathless and centrally cyanosed and may be quite confused due to hypoxia. The signs and symptoms of the initial compensation and failing compensation are summarised in Box 26.11.

Oxygen therapy

Oxygen therapy is essential to reduce hypoxia. In hypovolaemic shock the lost fluid must be replaced or returned to the circulation. Some patients may have large amounts of

---

Box 26.11 Information

Signs and symptoms of the initial compensation and failing compensation

Initial compensation

- Appears clammy, pale
- Peripheral cyanosis
- Appears restless; may complain of feeling generally unwell
- Falling urine output but may remain above 0.5 mL/kg/h
- Increase in pulse rate
- Slight rise in systolic blood pressure
- Increased soakage of blood on wound dressings and in wound drains

Failing compensation

- Appears cold, clammy
- Central cyanosis
- Appears confused, often agitated, and then increasingly drowsy
- Urine output falls below 0.5 mL/kg/h
- Tachycardia
- Fall in blood pressure
- Capillary refill >2 seconds
- Large volumes of blood may be lost

---

fluid available in the body, as in paralytic ileus or peripheral oedema, but in the wrong body compartment. This fluid can be drawn back into the circulation by treating the cause and by raising the osmotic pressure of the circulation.

Fluid replacement

Crystalline fluids can be given intravenously but are soon lost from the circulation. Colloids such as dextran or fresh frozen plasma are given as plasma expanders. These raise the osmotic pressure and draw extracellular fluid into the circulation (Finlay 2004). Interstitial fluid also moves into the capillaries as hydrostatic pressure falls in response to lowered blood pressure and arteriolar constriction. However, some evidence suggests that colloids and crystalloids are of equal efficacy in the reduction of mortality and debate is ongoing as to which is the most appropriate to increase intravascular volume in hypovolaemic shock (Cotton et al 2006). In haemodynamic shock, rapid transfusion of blood may be required and should be given through a blood warmer (see p. 704). Central venous pressure measurements are of great value in assessing the volume of blood returning to the heart and the heart's ability to pump (see Ch. 18). A central venous catheter may be inserted as an emergency in a patient whose shock proves difficult to manage. Measurement of hourly urine volumes will also allow the nurse to monitor renal perfusion. See the website for a nursing care plan for Mr Shah, which illustrates the type of nursing care required to detect the early signs of shock.

 See website Postoperative care plan – Mr Shah

Fluid and electrolyte balance

Most patients experience some loss of fluid during surgery which may be compounded by electrolyte disturbances resulting from the illness itself or trauma during surgery. Nurses should also take account of other potential fluid loses such as gastrointestinal fluid loss through vomit, nasogastric tube or fistula. Pre-operative dehydration due to excessive fasting should be avoided (see p. 697). Patients having a general anaesthetic will be fasted postoperatively until they are fully conscious and cough and swallowing reflexes have returned. Some may be required to fast for longer than this if there is paralytic ileus (see p. 708) or after facial or laryngeal surgery. These patients require fluid and electrolyte replacement via the intravenous route to meet normal demands and some require over and above this volume to replace fluid lost during surgery. For patients undergoing bowel surgery see page 696.

Fluid and electrolyte balance can be significantly affected by the physiological response of the body to the stress of surgery. Glucocorticoid secretion increases reabsorption of sodium and water in the renal nephrons with a reciprocal loss of potassium and hydrogen ions. Elevated levels of ADH also increase water reabsorption and high aldosterone levels increase sodium reabsorption further. The net effect is to increase the extracellular fluid volume and reduce urine output. It would not be unusual for a well-hydrated patient to retain fluid and have a high positive fluid balance for the immediate postoperative period, although any patient with oliguria (low urine output) should be carefully monitored. The careful monitoring of urinary function is thus a key element of nursing observations in the postoperative period. Nurses must ensure that patients have passed urine in the hours following surgery

Many surgical patients complain of thirst and a dry mouth postoperatively. This is due partly to dehydration, to the drying effects of oxygen therapy and to the anticholinergic effects of drugs given during anaesthesia. As a result, thirst is an unreliable measure of hydration.

As a result of trauma to the tissues during surgery the intracellular electrolyte potassium is released; this is excreted in part-exchange for retained sodium. Therefore potassium levels should be closely monitored in patients who have undergone major surgery and appropriate replacement with intravenous fluids given.

Metabolic and stress responses

Surgery and general anaesthesia are major stressors which result in the 'general adaptation syndrome' (Selye 1976). The importance of adequate pre-operative education and counselling in minimising stress is discussed on page 692.

The physiological effects of stress can be reduced by minimising anxiety both pre- and postoperatively. In the immediate postoperative period, and up to 4 days after a major operation, the patient utilises protein (normally spared) as a source of energy along with fats and carbohydrates. The amino acids act as a source of glucose for the brain. Blood glucose levels can be elevated, resulting in glycosuria. Patients with diabetes may have difficulty in controlling their blood glucose levels postoperatively (Robertshaw & Hall 2006, Smiley & Guillermo 2006). Careful monitoring is required in patients with diabetes and those receiving parenteral nutrition. It is important that patients are in a nutritional state sufficient to withstand this period of catabolism and negative nitrogen balance.

If the patient has a poor nutritional status, and/or is undergoing major surgery with or without prolonged fasting, nutritional support such as total parenteral nutrition (TPN) is usually required. Chapter 21 describes nursing interventions to improve the nutritional status of the patient and provides a complete discussion of parenteral nutrition. Many patients become anabolic after 24–48 h and begin to rebuild proteins, while hormones released in stress decrease. A large diuresis and negative fluid balance may be seen at this point.

Patients should be given clear instructions about when they can restart normal eating and drinking, and largely this will depend on the type of surgery they have had. The link between nutrition and tissue repair is well established (Williams & Barbul 2003) and therefore resumption of a balanced diet is important for optimal wound healing.

Traditionally a period of fasting was commonplace following gastrointestinal surgery involving an intestinal anastomosis. Oral intake was restricted during this time to reduce the demands on the anastomosis, allowing it to heal, and to prevent postoperative nausea and vomiting, and possible aspiration pneumonia (Lewis et al 2001). Neither eating nor drinking was allowed until bowel sounds had returned or other signs of gastric motility were apparent, such as passing of flatus or stool. There is growing interest in the impact of early nutrition after surgery on wound healing and reduction in septic complications (Lewis et al 2001) (Box 26.12).

Most patients who have abdominal surgery may commence oral fluids on the first postoperative day (SIGN 2004) and progress to normal diet over the first 2–3 days. Field (2002) recommends a proactive approach, starting by giving patients milky drinks rather than water, which has no nutritional value. Also it should be emphasised that a key function of the nurse is to ensure that patients are provided with appetising food and assisted to eat if they have difficulty in feeding

---

 Box 26.12 Evidence-based practice

Postoperative nutrition following abdominal surgery

For the majority of patients recovering from major abdominal surgery early feeding is safe and well tolerated. A literature review of 15 studies between 1995 and 2004 by Quin & Neil (2006) was undertaken as a result of the observations in practice by one of the authors, that patients were still routinely fasted until they had passed flatus or stool following open colorectal surgery. This review concluded that early feeding after elective open colorectal surgery did not increase rates of postoperative ileus, vomiting or wound complications. There was also some evidence to suggest that when used as part of a multimodal approach early feeding is associated with a reduction in the length of hospital stay. However, the definition of early feeding varied across the studies examined. Some studies considered early feeding to be the commencement of fluids on the day of surgery while others did not start fluids until the first or second postoperative day. In addition, the nature of the oral intake varied among studies. The majority of studies administered clear fluids; however, three studies included protein drinks. The progression to solid foods appears to have been most common on the second postoperative day. However, the content of the diets was not consistent among studies. As this review only focused on patients undergoing elective surgery these findings cannot be directly applied to patients following an emergency procedure.

A Cochrane Database Systematic Review conducted by Charoenkwan et al (2007) advocated early feeding after major gynaecological surgery, concluding that early feeding is associated with reduced hospital stay. This review defined early feeding as having oral fluid or food within the first 24 h after surgery. In keeping with the conclusions of Quin & Neil (2006) this review found no differences in the rates of postoperative ileus, vomiting or wound complications between patients who had early or delayed feeing. However, this review found that early feeding was associated with increased nausea and suggested that further research opportunities should be sought to explore patient satisfaction and early feeding.

Activities

- Access the literature review by Quin & Neil (2006).
- Reflect on the practices you have observed in placement regarding the postoperative nutrition of patients following abdominal surgery.
- Consider the ways in which you can discuss recent evidence about safety and tolerability of early feeding with members of multidisciplinary surgical teams to improve nutritional care.

themselves (SIGN 2004). This will help patients to resume a normal food intake postoperatively.

Paralytic ileus

Surgical trauma to the gastrointestinal tract causes temporary paralysis of the smooth muscle, known as postoperative or temporary paralytic ileus (Bisanz et al 2008). This is manifest by the absence of bowel sounds and cessation of peristalsis. Bowel sounds are high-pitched gurgling noises caused by liquid and air moving through the gastrointestinal tract (Field 2002). Nurses should be vigilant for any symptoms, such as abdominal distension, nausea and vomiting, which suggest that the postoperative ileus has not resolved. Such patients may need a nasogastric (NG) tube to be inserted in order to drain the stomach contents and decrease tension on the anastomosis. Further oral intake should be withheld and intravenous fluids will be required to ensure the patient remains hydrated. Accurate fluid balance charting is important to document the drainage from the NG tube as losses can be substantial. Referral to the nutrition team may be indicated if it becomes apparent that feeding will be delayed for more than 7 days (Field 2002).

Pain

Postoperative pain deserves close attention in nursing practice, research and education because patients will experience significant physical and psychological effects if pain is not adequately treated (Layzell 2008). Issues relating to pain specifically in the postoperative period are discussed here. The reader is also referred to Chapter 19, where broader but equally pertinent issues are addressed.

Being in pain has been and remains the major pre-operative concern of many patients (Macintyre & Schug 2007). Patients may have very little knowledge of the nature of postoperative pain or the methods available to treat it (Iverson & Lynch 2006). While major thoracic and abdominal operations tend to cause most pain, Mitchell (2003) suggests that pain management is also a considerable issue for day surgery patients in the first 24 h postoperatively.

In 1990 The Royal College of Surgeons and College of Anaesthetists Working Party reported that health professionals working in acute care environments were not effectively managing and relieving pain. They also suggested that nurses lacked the knowledge and commitment to achieve satisfying postoperative pain control. Despite advances in pain management, recent studies suggest that under-treatment of postoperative pain is still a big problem (Dolan et al 2002, Brown 2008). Conclusions from a review by Dolan et al (2002) found that the overall incidence of severe pain after major surgery in the UK was 11%. Between 75 and 80% of patients still report moderate to severe pain postoperatively (Manias 2003). Dihle (2006) suggests that even if nurses possess theoretical knowledge about postoperative pain management they do not always implement appropriate pain-relieving measures. Macintyre & Schug (2007) identify a number of barriers to effective nursing management of pain including:

- perception that it is normal and acceptable for patients to have pain after surgery
- misconception that patients will become addicted to opioid analgesics

- underestimation of the severity when patients report pain and therefore failure to administer adequate analgesics to control pain
- failure to undertake regular assessment of pain and reassessment following administration of analgesics
- reluctance of some patients to ask for analgesics.

Iverson & Lynch (2006) found that patients often expect to experience pain, and may express satisfaction with pain management even if they are in pain, postoperatively. However, pain is not a 'natural, inevitable, acceptable or harmless consequence of surgery' (Macintyre & Schug 2007). Pain control after surgery is a prime concern on humanitarian grounds and it also has significant effects on other aspects of the patient's recovery. Good pain control allows for early activity, so minimising problems of immobility such as chest infection, urinary tract infection, deep vein thrombosis, pressure ulcers and muscle wasting. Pain after surgery has been cited as one of the main reasons for poor sleep (Mann 2003, Njawe 2003). Older patients are at an increased risk of the postoperative complications described above, and their subsequent recovery will be influenced by pain management.

Ineffective pain relief in the postoperative period can have serious psychological consequences for patients facing subsequent surgery and is also associated with the development of chronic pain (Kehlet & Holte 2002). The development of chronic post-surgical pain results in distress and disability for many patients. A variety of surgical procedures are associated with the development of chronic pain, including thoracic, breast and gall bladder surgery and amputations (Perkins & Kehlet 2000). Chronic pain is reported in 5–13% of patients undergoing dental surgery and in 5–33% of men following vasectomy (Macrae 2001). Chronic post-surgical pain occurs as a result of surgical injury to peripheral nerves and ongoing inflammation (Kehlet et al 2006). Nurses should be aware that uncontrolled postoperative pain can develop into a chronic condition and must ensure that pain is managed optimally.

Pain assessment and management

Nurses have two specific roles in the management of postoperative pain: pain assessment and provision of the means to alleviate the pain. Assessment is the cornerstone of care and accurate and systematic assessment of pain is essential. A small Swedish study by Ene et al (2008) found that nurses generally overestimated mild pain and underestimated severe pain, and 40% of the nurses in the study did not use a pain assessment tool. Visual analogue scales, verbal numerical rating scales and other assessment techniques are valuable and widely used but have limitations (Baxter & Chinn 2006) (see Ch. 19). Findings by Manias (2003) suggest that linear scales can be problematic where patients' first language is not English. For further discussion about pain assessment in the postoperative period see Brown (2008).

Postoperative pain can vary according to the site of the incision, being greater with midline, subcostal and intercostal incisions (Figure 26.1). The small incisions required for laparoscopic technique usually cause the least discomfort. However, patients can suffer extreme 'wind pain' following laparoscopic surgery which is disproportionate to the size of the incision, and 35–63% of patients complain of shoulder

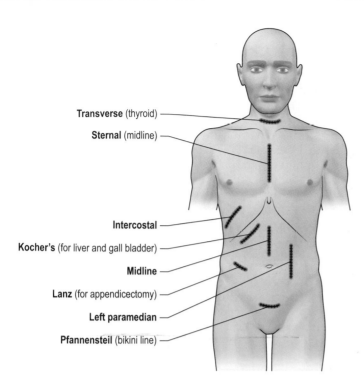

Transverse (thyroid)

Sternal (midline)

Intercostal

Kocher's (for liver and gall bladder)

Midline

Lanz (for appendicectomy)

Left paramedian

Pfannensteil (bikini line)

Figure 26.1 Some incision sites used in surgery.

number of days postoperatively and patients undergoing laparoscopy will require information and advice on how to control any pain following discharge.

Drain sites can also cause pain, at both change of dressing and during removal of the drains, which may require short-term pain relief (Baxter & Chinn 2006). Inhalation of Entonox® (50% nitrous oxide and 50% oxygen) works rapidly and allows patients to have a degree of control over their pain relief during short procedures (Baxter & Chinn 2006). Controlling pain in the immediate postoperative period is the responsibility of the anaesthetist and, increasingly, of the acute pain team. For a review of the role of the acute pain team in the UK see Nagi (2004).

The anaesthetist visits the patient pre-operatively to discuss the prevention and relief of pain and to make a full assessment of the individual's needs. Opioid analgesics are the mainstay of postoperative pain control. Some commonly used analgesics are given in Table 26.4. Opioid analgesics can be given via intramuscular, subcutaneous, intravenous or epidural routes.

Subcutaneous injection of the analgesic via a small cannula or 'butterfly' avoids the need for repeated skin punctures and the rate of absorption of morphine into the circulation is similar to that following an intramuscular injection. Best Practice Guidelines now recommend that this method of administration replace intramuscular injection (NHS Quality Improvement Scotland 2004a). Subcutaneous morphine can be administered hourly if required. The nurse should explain to the patient that the opioid is not absorbed to therapeutic levels immediately, so they should ask for an analgesic at the first indication of discomfort. The patient should be advised not to wait until the pain is unbearable (suffering the ill-effects of this pain) as they may continue to suffer for a further 15–20 minutes until the injection takes effect.

tip pain (Hong & Lee 2003). Pain following laparoscopic surgery occurs as a result of stretching of the peritoneum and irritation of the diaphragm by the CO_2 used to inflate the abdomen to allow visualisation of the internal organs (Wills & Hunt 2000). This pneumoperitoneum can persist for a

Table 26.4 Analgesics commonly used in postoperative pain control		
METHOD OF ADMINISTRATION	**EXAMPLE OF DRUG USED**	**EXAMPLE OF TYPES OF SURGERY**
Epidural infusion	Bupivacaine and lidocaine, fentanyl and bupivacaine mixture, diamorphine	Major pelvic or lower abdominal, e.g. colectomy
Intravenous infusion, for example PCA	Diamorphine, morphine sulphate, fentanyl, tramadol	Major surgery where moderate to severe pain expected
Intravenous or subcutaneous injection	Diamorphine, morphine sulphate, fentanyl, oxycodone	Major pelvic or abdominal, e.g. gastrectomy
Subcutaneous injection	Morphine, oxycodone	Many types of surgery, as for i.m. injection
Intramuscular injection	Morphine sulphate, tramadol Codeine	Many types, e.g. total hip replacement Specifically used in neurosurgery
Nerve blocks and local anaesthetic	Lidocaine with adrenaline Ropivacaine	Thoracic surgery, wound areas can be infiltrated after surgery Total knee arthroplasty
Oral	Diclofenac sodium (Voltarol) tramadol, co-codamol, paracetamol	Many products are available Used in continued recovery and rehabilitation or alone after minor surgery
Per rectum	Diclofenac sodium (Voltarol) paracetamol	Commonly used following minor surgery or as part of multimodal approach to pain relief following major surgery

For Further reading see Macintyre & Schug (2007).

Intravenous infusion can be advantageous as it enables the rate of infusion to be altered immediately, according to the patient's respiratory rate, as opioid drugs may depress respirations if too large a dose is given. Patients vary widely in their response to opioids. In adults, age is generally a more appropriate predictor of opioid requirements than weight. Intravenous opioids should be given carefully to older patients as their clearance and metabolism of analgesics are slower (Gagliese & Melzack 2006). In addition, reduction in cardiac output in the older patient means that intravenous doses of analgesic medications should also be given more slowly as peak blood concentrations after a single intravenous medication will be higher.

Nurses may encounter patients who have developed tolerance to opioids. This may be because they have a long history of opioid use for chronic pain relief (dependency) or they have a history of substance abuse (addiction). Such patients require special adjustments to their opioid administration and care in order that their postoperative pain is controlled effectively (D'arcy 2007, Bourne 2008).

Patient-controlled analgesia (PCA)

PCA allows the patient to control the administration of small boluses of intravenous analgesic (see Ch. 19). A special infusion pump is set to give a specific volume of solution (and therefore a set dosage according to the dilution of the drug) when the patient presses a hand-held button. The machine is programmed to provide a bolus only after a certain length of time has elapsed (lockout) and a maximum total number of boluses over a specified time period.

PCA can be very effective and many studies comparing PCA with conventional intramuscular or subcutaneous administration highlight better analgesic effects from PCA and enhanced patient satisfaction (Hudcova et al 2006). However, patients given PCA without sufficient explanation beforehand, or inadequately educated staff to support them while using the device, still may not achieve optimal pain relief (Macintyre 2001). Some patients are unable to understand the function of the system and press the button inappropriately. Therapeutic levels of opioid can fall while the patient is sleeping, leading to awakening in pain. Some patients experience unpleasant side-effects such as nausea and itching (Chumbley et al 2004), and antiemetic medication should be prescribed and administered appropriately. Patients need to be taught how to use the device prior to theatre if possible.

🖱 **See website Critical thinking question 26.2**

Epidural analgesia (EA)

EA is becoming increasingly common following major surgery, e.g. following radical prostatectomy or colonic surgery (Burch et al 2009). Major surgery places patients at significant risk of postoperative complications because of the effects on the lungs of prolonged anaesthesia and the creation of large incision sites. Patients may be unable to cough or breathe deeply postoperatively because of severe wound pain. EA is an effective form of postoperative pain relief for this group of patients because a solution of local anaesthetic and/or opiate is infused into the epidural space in the spine. This blocks the dermatomal nerves supplying the area of the wound (Weetman & Allison 2006). Such patients may have little or no sensation of pain at all in the immediate postoperative period and are able to carry out breathing exercises and get out of bed shortly after surgery, thus minimising the risk of complications (Burch et al 2009). EA is also associated with decreased levels of postoperative anxiety. There are, however, a number of complications associated with EA. These include side-effects from the analgesics used, such as hypotension and urinary retention, pressure ulcers and DVT from reduced mobility in the lower limbs, and infection such as dural abscess formation. For this reason patients should be nursed in areas where staff have special skills and knowledge in this form of pain relief, such as a high-dependency unit.

There is increasing interest in the use of patient controlled epidural analgesia (PCEA). A randomised controlled trial by Ferguson et al (2009) found that pain control with bupivacaine and morphine PCEA was superior to morphine intravenous PCA in women undergoing laparotomy for gynaecological cancer. Patients receiving PCEA reported less pain on the first day postoperatively and were able to cough more effectively. For further discussion about the use of epidural analgesia see Weetman & Allison (2006).

Nursing considerations in pain management

All opioid agents have similar side-effects, e.g. central nervous system and cardiovascular depression, the possibility of nausea and vomiting and the risk of addiction. Fear of respiratory depression can lead to doctors under-prescribing and under-administration by nurses (Macintyre & Schug 2007). Opioid agents can be reversed with naloxone should respiratory depression occur. It should also be remembered that respiration will, in fact, be hindered by inadequate pain control (see p. 708). The fear of addiction from the administration of opioids is largely unfounded. When opioids are administered only in the postoperative period less than 1% of patients will develop problems of addiction (D'arcy 2007).

The amount of opioid a patient requires can be reduced by the use of other medications and local anaesthetic agents. This is known as the multimodal approach. The use of non-steroidal anti-inflammatory drugs (NSAIDs) such as diclofenac sodium and ibuprofen, used in conjunction with opioids in the peri-operative stage, can result in a 20% reduction in opioid analgesic requirements (Lovett et al 1994) but is associated with undesirable side-effects including bleeding, renal failure and gastric ulceration. The role of one of the most common analgesics, paracetamol, should not be overlooked. Paracetamol can be used alone to treat mild pain, or in combination with opioids, because of its morphine-sparing properties. It can be given orally, via the rectal route and intravenously. A study by Hynes et al (2006) found that two doses of 2 g of intravenous paracetamol (pro-paracetamol, equivalent to 1 g oral paracetamol) was as effective as 75 mg intramuscular diclofenac following total hip arthroplasty.

Medications used in association with an opiate are most effective if given regularly or according to an algorithm rather than 'as required' or 'PRN' doses (NHS Quality Improvement Scotland 2004a). Other drugs may also be utilised; for example, hyoscine butylbromide (Buscopan), which has an anti-cholinergic effect causing smooth muscle relaxation, can be useful in the treatment of intestinal colic (Baxter & Chinn 2006). In day surgery, where side-effects such as respiratory depression, sedation and nausea can delay discharge, opioid-sparing strategies are particularly important (Segerdahl et al 2008). Patients should have their medication explained prior to going home and be given instructions about who to call in case the medication does not work (D'arcy 2007).

The variety of causes of postoperative pain and discomfort and the wide range of nursing interventions available clearly demonstrate that the nurse has a key role to play in alleviating postoperative pain (see the website for postoperative case studies for Mr Shah and Sylvia).

🖱 **See website Postoperative Case studies – Mr Shah and Sylvia**

A sensitive individualised approach to patient care will also improve the management of postoperative pain, as one experienced nurse can get to know the patient well. Detailed knowledge of the patient and their reaction to pain assists in planning and evaluating care, while the close relationship between nurse and patient instils trust and confidence. The therapeutic contribution of the nurse in relation to pain control is addressed in detail in Chapter 19. Comfort measures such as heat pads as well as complementary therapies such as foot massage and guided relaxation (Hattan et al 2002) can also be beneficial.

Postoperative nausea and vomiting (PONV)

PONV continues to be a common postoperative complication despite advances in anaesthetics and is experienced by 2–30% of patients (Jolley 2001). Zeitz (2005) reported that PONV is the most frequent complication in the first 24 h following surgery. PONV is unpleasant and distressing for patients (NHS Quality Improvement Scotland 2004a). The causes of PONV are multifactorial and complex, but include patient-related factors, the length and nature of surgery undergone and the anaesthetic agent used (Table 26.5).

PONV is exacerbated when patients have pain and inadequate pain relief (Thompson 1999). Quinlan (2002) reported that relief of postoperative pain is usually associated with relief of nausea. Unfortunately PONV is also a common side-effect of opioid analgesics. A period of prolonged starvation can cause PONV but so also can inadequate pre-operative fasting and the collection of secretions in the stomach. Paralytic ileus can lead to the accumulation of a large quantity of gastrointestinal secretions. Following some surgery, e.g. partial gastrectomy, patients may have some bleeding into the stomach postoperatively which can induce nausea. Postoperative hypotension is another common cause of PONV which can be avoided by helping patients to move in bed or sit up slowly.

Jolley (2000) advocates the use of a risk assessment tool by nurses and anaesthetists. Thomas et al (2002) compared two PONV risk assessment tools and found nurses greatly underestimated the actual incidence of PONV. The effect of unresolved PONV is significant. Patients are at risk of complications such as aspiration, dehydration, electrolyte imbalance and pain and may also suffer psychological effects such as distress, shame and embarrassment (Jolley 2001). Fear of PONV has been shown to heighten anxiety prior to subsequent surgery.

Treatment of established PONV is less effective than prevention. The cause of PONV should be identified and an appropriate antiemetic administered prophylactically and

Table 26.5 Risk factors for postoperative nausea and vomiting (PONV)

RISK FACTOR	EXPLANATION
Increased age	Older adults experience less PONV than younger adults
Female gender	Women are three times more likely to experience PONV than men (Jolley 2001)
Prior history of travel sickness	A history of motion sickness is associated with an increased incidence of PONV (Jolley 2001)
High pre-operative anxiety	Anxiety related to previous experience of PONV or general fears about a hospital admission can increase the likelihood of PONV occurring (Jolley 2001)
Type of surgery	Abdominal gynaecological procedures have an increased risk because of disturbance to the gut during surgery (Jolley 2000) In orthopaedic procedures the use of extradural infusions has been linked to the high incidence of PONV (Alexander & Fennelly 1997) Any surgical procedure of longer than 30 min places the patient at increased risk of PONV
Anaesthetic agent used	Patients receiving thiopental as an induction agent are more likely to experience PONV than those who receive propofol (Jolley 2001). Spinal and regional blocks are less likely to cause PONV than general anaesthetics
Smoking	Smokers are less at risk than non-smokers, although the exact mechanism for this is not understood (Hough & Sweeney 1998, Whalen et al 2006)
Obesity	Obesity may be a risk factor for PONV but the causes are not clearly understood. Jolley (2001) suggests that fat-soluble anaesthetic agents accumulate in adipose tissue and the anaesthetics are slowly released. Therefore, individuals with more adipose tissue will experience side-effects for longer

regularly (NHS Quality Improvement Scotland 2004a). Recent evidence suggests that PONV in the first 24 h following surgery may be reduced to 20% if combinations of prophylactic antiemetics are used (Jensen et al 2009). White et al (2007) reported that some gynaecology day surgery patients do not exhibit symptoms until after discharge and long-acting antiemetics may need to be considered. Caution must be taken with the administration of metoclopramide as this promotes gut motility and should be avoided in patients with bowel obstruction. Ming et al (2002) found that PONV can be reduced by the use of acupressure bands on the wrist. It is important, however, that patients are aware pre-operatively that PONV is not an inevitable outcome of anaesthesia, and that medication can and will be provided.

Sleep

Surgical inpatients often have very disrupted sleep patterns (Njawe 2003, Williams et al 2007). In addition to factors affecting the sleep of all hospital patients, surgical patients are exposed to pain, general discomfort and restricted positioning. Postoperative patients may experience hypoxia and hypercapnia due to anaesthetic sedation or shock, severely compromising CNS control of sleep patterns (see Ch. 25). Opioids can alter normal sleep patterns (Dawson et al 1999). Typically, patients report dropping off to sleep and feeling they have slept for hours, only to find that just a few minutes have passed. Some patients will be distressed by this and nursing staff can support and reassure them, explaining that this is a common but temporary side-effect of the analgesic. It is important to ensure that the patient does not stop using their PCA or asking for analgesics in an effort to relieve this symptom, because this will cause an exacerbation of pain. For many patients, the presence of a nurse during this wakeful period may be all that is required. For most patients, frequent observations and recordings are necessary, often into the first postoperative night. These disturbances, along with the general noise generated by procedures, new admissions and emergency action that may occur, all add to the disruption of patients' sleep.

Sleep is especially important for the postoperative patient as protein synthesis for optimal recovery takes place predominantly during sleep and rest. Growth hormone is secreted during periods of rapid eye movement (REM) sleep. Sleep and rest are therefore essential, not only for a feeling of well-being, but also for anabolism and tissue repair. Older patients are especially vulnerable as they have fewer physiological reserves and may have concurrent and chronic illness. Equilibrium is disturbed by lack of sleep and this may be related to development of delirium in some postoperative older patients (Bowman 1997).

In the longer term, fatigue may interfere with patients' ability to participate in exercises or activities required for postoperative rehabilitation, for example following cardiac surgery (Njawe 2003). Hunt et al (2000) reported that 17% of patients who responded to their survey complained of poor sleep quality one year after cardiac surgery. Williams et al (2007) investigated the experiences of patients with co-morbidities undergoing orthopaedic procedures. Pain associated with joint replacement surgery continued to impact on the sleep patterns of participants at 4 weeks following discharge and the subsequent fatigue interfered with general recovery and well-being.

Pain management and general comfort measures are paramount in promoting a good night's sleep. Bowman (1997) noted the impact made when nurses modified the environment to promote sleep, and suggests that warmth and effective pain control facilitate natural sleep in older patients. The measurement of O_2 saturation via pulse oximetry can be useful to indicate night hypoxia in vulnerable patients, e.g. those who have had thoracic or abdominal surgery. Nursing observations should be minimised to safe levels and noise reduced where possible.

Elimination

Postoperative constipation is a common problem which arises as a consequence of immobility, the use of opioid analgesics and dehydration. Conversely, diarrhoea can occur as postoperative temporary ileus resolves, but normal bowel function should resume spontaneously in a few days.

Patients may experience colicky pain due to flatus and muscle spasm; this can be reduced by increasing mobility and offering peppermint water or warm water. Ensuring adequate hydration and early activity helps prevent constipation before it becomes necessary to use oral laxatives.

All patients should be monitored to ensure that they pass urine in the hours following surgery to ensure return of normal bladder function and urine production. Urinary retention may occur due to immobility, the relaxation of bladder muscle tone caused by anaesthesia, or as the result of temporary ileus following abdominal or pelvic surgery. When urinary retention is anticipated, the patient should be catheterised in theatre to minimise discomfort. Otherwise, patients should be given the opportunity for privacy and assistance to assume a normal position to pass urine where possible. If retention leads to distension of the bladder and discomfort, or is a cause for concern, urinary catheterisation may be required.

Once the temporary ileus resolves, as detected by return of bowel sounds or passage of flatus or faeces, the urinary catheter is usually removed. If the catheter is required for monitoring urine output in haemodynamic shock, or retention due to immobility, it can be removed when monitoring is no longer required or the patient is sufficiently active to pass urine independently.

Use of urinary catheters should be avoided where possible due to the associated risk of infection (NHS Quality Improvement Scotland 2004b). The postoperative patient may also be at risk of urinary infection without catheterisation, as a result of immobility when a small volume of concentrated urine may remain in the bladder for prolonged periods, providing a medium for the growth of bacteria.

Following some surgical procedures on the bladder, for example transurethral resection of the prostate (TURP), continued blood loss and clot formation may obstruct the urethra. To prevent this, patients are catheterised with a three-way/triple lumen catheter and continuous bladder irrigation is given to wash out potentially obstructing clots or debris (see Ch. 8).

Wound care

The aim of wound care is to promote healing and minimise the risk of infection. Buggy (2000) argues that 9–27% of patients undergoing colorectal surgery acquire a wound infection. Methods of promoting healing depend on the individual patient's circumstances. Specific factors that should be considered in the surgical patient are glycaemic control, prolonged hypoxia due to shock, dehydration or local pressure, protein-calorie malnutrition, temperature and the local wound dressing. Factors to be considered in all patients with regard to wound healing are discussed in Chapter 23.

The mainstay of preventing hospital acquired infection is handwashing (SIGN 2004). Nursing staff must wash their hands before any patient contact. In addition to this, prevention of infection begins in the pre-operative period with skin cleansing and reduction of anxiety (see p. 696).

Asepsis in theatre reduces the threat of exogenous infection (see p. 701). Good tissue perfusion ensures that oxygen, neutrophils, nutrients for cellular regrowth and systemically administered antibiotics are carried to the incision site. However, tissue perfusion during surgery may be diminished because blood loss and manipulation of body structures aggravate the stress response, causing vasoconstriction of the skin, gut and renal vessels. The anaesthetist aims to reduce the impact of the stress response by maintaining the patient's tissue perfusion during the operation. This is done by increasing oxygen delivery during and after surgery, administering optimal fluid replacement therapy and avoiding hypothermia (Buggy 2000). Diabetic patients require careful management of blood glucose levels in the perioperative period to prevent hyperglycaemia as this is a risk factor for the development of infection (Smiley & Guillermo 2006).

The use of wound drains and aseptic technique, along with precautions against haematoma formation, will help to reduce wound infections postoperatively. However, some patients will be more at risk of infection than others, depending on the type of surgery and previous health status (Box 26.13). The patient's nutritional status and wound healing are closely linked. Patients who are malnourished preoperatively are at risk of delayed healing and have increased susceptibility to wound or systemic infection.

In the immediate postoperative period, the wound and any drains in the operation site must be checked frequently for signs of bleeding. Volume markings on drainage bottles and bags can give some indication of the amount of blood or fluid lost, although drains can become blocked with clots (Anderson 2003). Large volumes of bloodstained fluid may be due to the fluid used to wash out a cavity but this should still be reported. Wound dressings should not be changed if they become soaked with blood; instead, fresh pads should be added on top to promote clot formation beneath both dressings. To disturb dressings on the first postoperative day increases the risk of infection. Dressings on closed wounds should be left for 24–48 h if the dressing is clean and dry. Closed wounds usually heal by primary intention and are sealed by fibrin by this time (Prosser & McArthur-Rouse 2007).

Wound drains

The aim of wound drains is to drain blood and inflammatory exudates, to prevent haematoma formation and infection, and to give an indication of blood loss. Some drains may have suction applied to collapse the space left in the tissues after an operation. Drains can also indicate when an anastomosis has broken down by discharging blood, digestive or faeculent fluid and, when an abscess has resolved, the cessation of discharge of pus. Some examples

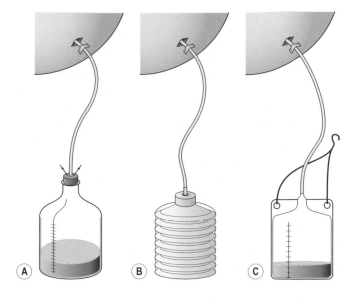

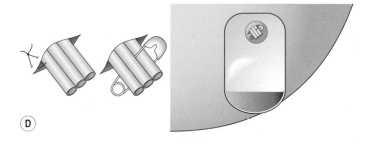

Figure 26.2 Common types of wound drains. A. Vacuum drain (prongs come together as vacuum is lost). B. Concertina-type drain. C. Simple tube/Penrose drain. D. Corrugated drain: secured by a suture and then a safety pin as the drain is shortened to prevent it from falling back into the patient. Fluid drains down the channels and into a bag.

of the more common types of wound drain are given in Figure 26.2.

To prevent infection, the entry site should be dressed aseptically and a closed drainage system maintained. If bags or bottles need to be changed, e.g. when the vacuum is lost or the receptacle is full or heavy, then asepsis must be maintained and sterile equipment used.

The decision to remove the drain is made by the doctor when there is minimal or no further drainage. Non-vacuum drains may be shortened before removal to encourage the space left behind to collapse and granulate, otherwise a cavity might be left that could fill with fluid and give rise to an abscess. Before a drain is removed, the procedure should be explained to the patient and careful assessment performed as analgesics may be required. Relaxation exercises can help to reduce the patient's anxiety and muscle tension. Vacuum drains should have their suction released and the securing sutures removed prior to removal. If the drain will not move smoothly this may be eased by rotating the tube slightly. Traction should not be applied if the drain has become fixed or tethered. Such cases must be referred to the medical staff.

After the first 24 h, the wound and drains should be checked to ensure optimal healing is occurring. The patient's

Box 26.13 Information

Patient factors that increase risks of postoperative infection

- Immune compromise (e.g. steroid use, cancer)
- Contamination of peritoneum (e.g. perforated bowel)
- Malnutrition
- Low cardiac output prior to surgery
- Increased age
- Diabetes

nutritional status and wound healing are closely linked (see p. 707). Patients who are malnourished pre-operatively are at risk of delayed healing and have increased susceptibility to wound or systemic infection. However, most wound infections typically do not appear until at least 3 days post-operatively. If infection is suspected (redness, swelling or production of pus) a wound swab should be obtained immediately and sent for culture and sensitivity. Signs of systemic infection such as elevated temperature and tachycardia should be identified early and antibiotic treatment instigated, as the development of sepsis can result in mortality rates between 20 and 40% (SIGN 2004).

Patients discharged within the first 2 days after an operation should be taught how to recognise a wound infection and advised to inform their GP if symptoms occur. Community and practice nurses may continue checks on patients with wounds who have been discharged home early.

After 48 h, wounds healing by 'primary intention' have laid down a layer of epithelium across the wound (see Ch. 23). The wound is effectively sealed from exogenous infection and may be left exposed, which allows for easy observation. Dressings are not necessary unless the wound has been closed with clips or staples that may catch on clothing or there is continued discharge from the wound. Some wounds may be left to heal by 'secondary intention' due to lack of tissue to close the wound or to the presence of infection in the tissues, where closure may well lead to abscess formation. Care of such of wounds is discussed in Chapter 23.

Wounds heal at different rates according to growth rate and blood supply of the local tissues and the patient's general physical condition. For example, subcuticular sutures in a carotid endarterectomy incision line would be removed at 3–5 days postoperatively, whereas abdominal sutures would not be removed until 10 days postoperatively. There is an increasing trend towards the use of absorbable continuous sutures where good healing is expected. This is especially useful when the patient is to be discharged home in the first few days. Most patients are also relieved to hear that their sutures do not have to be removed. Patients discharged home with non-absorbable sutures in situ may be referred to the community or practice nurse for their removal. Adhesive preparations are increasingly used in paediatric and trauma settings because of their impressive cosmetic results (Singer et al 2002). Chibbaro & Tacconi (2009) used this method for wound closure in open brain surgery, where tissue is thicker and the underlying bone structure is altered. The authors reported that wound complication rates for adhesive closures were similar to that for clips or sutures. The cosmetic outcome, and thus patient satisfaction, was higher in those with adhesive preparation. For further information about the removal of sutures see Lees (2007).

Potential complications

Virtually all surgical patients will be at some risk of developing deep vein thrombosis (DVT), pulmonary embolism (PE), chest infection and atelectasis. Prevention is the mainstay of care and is described on page 697. Preventive measures such as leg and breathing exercises, thromboembolic deterrent (TED) stockings and subcutaneous heparin are all continued throughout the postoperative recovery. Early mobilisation contributes significantly to the prevention of

these complications. Mr Shah's care exemplifies the type of proactive preventive measures required.

🖱 **See website Postoperative care plan – Mr Shah**

As with pain, pressure ulcers may deter patients from optimal return to normal activity.

Obese, immunocompromised and older patients are at risk of wound dehiscence, the separation and opening of the wound. Nursing management following abdominal wound dehiscence is to apply sterile pads that have been saturated with normal saline to prevent the abdominal organs from drying and becoming damaged. Assistance from the surgical team is required rapidly. Reassurance and support of the patient is vital as this can be both distressing and frightening and further surgical intervention is likely. Surgical dehiscence is a major complication of abdominal surgery, carrying with it considerable mortality and morbidity (Candido 2002). Moz (2004) presents a case study on the management of wound dehiscence.

Communication

When a patient recovers from a general anaesthetic, the first sense to return is that of hearing. Care of the patient in the recovery room can be enhanced by having aids to communication, such as their hearing aid and glasses, available. A number of patients, especially older people or the very ill, may become and remain confused postoperatively (Noimark 2009). This may be due to the effects of the anaesthetic or to a history of alcohol use and presence of co-morbidities. Efforts must be made to identify and treat the cause, and nursing measures to re-orientate and minimise confusion should be taken.

The use of anticholinergic drugs that cross the blood–brain barrier, such as atropine and hyoscine, should be avoided in older patients as they may cause confusion. Benzodiazepines are also associated with increased levels of delirium in older adults (Arora et al 2007). Opioid analgesics are undoubtedly the cause of delirium in some patients, and non-opioid analgesics might be employed.

Patients with provisional diagnoses are often anxious to speak to the doctor about findings in theatre and their prognosis. Patients are often reluctant to raise all their concerns with the consultant or registrar, possibly surrounded by an entourage of junior doctors and medical students on ward rounds. The nurse has an important role to play in clarifying the patient's understanding and answering questions where possible or referring the patient's queries to others. The nurse will need to support both patient and family at this anxious time, particularly if samples have been sent to pathology for diagnosis.

Good communication among professionals in the postoperative period is essential. Medical and nursing staff must rely on one another for information and advice in order to provide a coordinated plan of care. Other health professionals, such as physiotherapists and dietitians, also have an important role to play in a patient's postoperative recovery.

Body image

Body image is the mental picture we hold of our body and its functions. This is influenced not only by physical appearance but also by our attitude towards ourselves (Bredin 1999).

Price (1990) suggests that body image consists of three essential components:

- body reality – an individual's actual physical appearance
- body ideal – how an individual wishes their body to be
- body presentation – an individual's efforts to find a compromise between body reality and ideal; this may include the use of makeup and clothing to achieve a desired appearance.

Body image forms part of our total self-concept and, as such, can have enormous impact on psychological, sociocultural and physical concepts of self. Body image can be altered by a change in physical appearance, such as when a patient undergoes ileostomy formation (Sinclair 2009), or when something causes an individual to change their attitude towards their body, for example following a diagnosis of cancer (Bredin 1999), or a combination of both these factors. If this alteration leads to a negative self-concept, educational and psychological support will be necessary to help the patient regain a positive self-concept. Individuals may respond very differently to the same procedure. Sinclair (2009) explored the responses of young adults to ileostomy. Some reported the ileostomy as having a negative impact on their body image – one patient stated 'it was disgusting and the ileostomy was gross' (Sinclair 2009, p. 311); however, for another the ileostomy offered freedom from debilitating faecal incontinence and she felt able to wear light summer clothing for the first time in 10 years.

Sexuality and body image are linked issues (Borwell 2009). Some patients experience sexual dysfunction following surgery. This can be for a variety of reasons:

- Changes in body image can impact on sexual well-being. For example, a mastectomy for breast cancer may impact on a woman's sense of femininity or sexual identity and can lead to sexual difficulties (Keeton & McAloon 2002).
- A diagnosis of cancer, whether or not the tumour directly affects sexual organs, can adversely affect sexuality (Price 2009). Price (2009, p. 33) provides a patient account describing the impact of renal cancer on his sexuality and associated feelings of powerlessness.
- Sexual dysfunction may occur as a result of the physical changes brought about by the surgical procedure, for example, due to scarring or nerve damage (Borwell 2009).
- Psychological stress following surgery.

Patients need to be informed of potential effects of treatment on sexuality and sexual function in advance of the surgery. Borwell (2009) suggests that the needs of a wide range of individuals, such as single adults, people with mental health or learning disabilities and older adults, are often overlooked because nurses make incorrect assumptions about the nature of their sexual activity and orientation. Suggestions for enhancing nursing practice in this area are offered by Borwell (2009) and Holmes et al (2005).

Discharge planning

Discharge planning aims to provide a smooth transition from hospital to home for continued patient care, and should be considered from the time of admission. However, the growth of day surgery and decreasing lengths of hospital stay for major surgery have reduced the time available for nurses to meet patients' post-discharge needs (Pieper et al 2006).

Inadequate discharge planning can lead to patients being readmitted because they are unprepared for self-care or developing postoperative complications such as wound infections (Pieper et al 2006). Readmission and complications create inconvenience for patients and incur additional expense for the NHS. In a busy surgical ward there is often an urgent need for beds, which can lead to hasty and poorly planned discharge. All patients are referred to their GP on discharge from hospital by the surgeon. The nurse will decide whether the patient also needs to be referred to the community nurse. Referrals can be made for nursing interventions ranging from wound care to providing psychological support for the patient and family where there is a poor prognosis. If patients are able to attend the health centre or clinic for wound dressing procedures, then arrangements for an appointment can be made before discharge.

Communication is fundamental to the process of collaborative discharge planning. A personal telephone call to the relevant community nurses and a discharge summary outlining the patient's care can be useful in enhancing continuity. However, McKenna et al (2000) found that communication passed to the community carers on discharge was poor and documentation lacked detail. Interestingly, 56% of district nurses in this study were dissatisfied with the discharge documentation, whereas 41.4% of hospital nurses considered it to be very good. The role of a discharge coordinator who implements a discharge protocol can facilitate this process by providing consistent advice and initiating referrals (Maramba et al 2004).

Discharge education

Patient teaching for discharge should begin on or before the day of admission to hospital. Patients require specific information to continue their recovery from surgery, such as pain management, incision/wound care and guidelines on resuming activity (Pieper et al 2006). The opportunity for more general health education should also be taken.

Information may also be given to lay carers and relatives, with consent from the patient, to enable them to continue support at home (Mitchell 2003); also, the involvement of family members when giving discharge information appears to positively influence patient behavioural changes (Pieper et al 2006). Mitchell (2007a) advocates a telephone follow-up service for patients following laparoscopic cholecystectomy. This can allow nurses to address patients' questions about pain relief and to clarify any points in their postoperative recovery.

Some patients may be unsure, or have misconceptions, about how they should progress during their recovery at home. In day-case surgery it is essential that patients understand that the anaesthetic may take a full 24 h to be eliminated from the body. Therefore they must not drive home from hospital, should be accompanied for the first 24 h after surgery and should not drive to work the following morning in case they have a car accident (Chung & Assmann 2008). Some individuals expect to feel fully fit and to be able to care for themselves immediately on discharge. According to

Correa et al (2001), following day surgery, patients may be 'home ready' but not 'street ready'. Advice should include:

- Do not drink alcohol.
- Do not drive a motor vehicle.
- Have a responsible adult stay overnight with you.
- Do not make important decisions for 24 h following a general anaesthetic, regional anaesthetic and/or intravenous sedation.

Many patients will feel insecure without the presence of the nurse and feel anxious about their health (Mitchell 2002). Leahy et al (2005) suggest that taking home tape recordings made of their consultation for ready reference may be helpful for some patients facing heart surgery. All patients should be clear about seeking advice or treatment from the most appropriate source on discharge.

🖱 See website Postoperative Case studies – Mr A, Tom

In general the following principles are important when planning patient discharge:

- Discharge planning should begin at, or even prior to, admission and should be individualised to the patient, their condition and their specific home circumstances.
- Information is essential. This should be both written and verbal, and should include advice about pain, wound care and resumption of activities – particularly exercise and driving. It should also inform the patient about symptoms that might suggest that complications are developing.
- Multidisciplinary liaison, for example between hospital and community nurses, is of fundamental importance to safe continuity of care.

Rehabilitation

Rehabilitation can be a lengthy process, requiring continued support by community nurses, or a short event with minimal professional intervention. Successful rehabilitation centres on minimising impairment and disability and maximising well-being, social participation and recovery (Borwell 2009). Postoperative recovery requires energy, as the patient returns to pre-operative levels of dependence or independence and regains control over physical, psychological, social and habitual functions (Allvin et al 2007). Trends towards increased day surgery mean that an increasing number of patients are recovering from surgery at home. However, older and frailer patients may require additional time in hospital for specific tailored programmes of rehabilitation, for example following major surgery such as amputation, orthopaedic surgery and cardiac surgery.

Also, patients with co-morbidities may have delayed recovery as the acute care episode complicates pre-existing conditions (Williams et al 2007). A phenomenological study by Edwards (2002) provides an insightful glimpse into the difficulties experienced by a group of older patients following elective orthopaedic surgery. One patient felt the ward nurses had 'washed their hands' of after-care. Patients should not leave hospital feeling vulnerable and unsupported.

SUMMARY: KEY NURSING ISSUES

- Patients undergoing surgery require a range of care from nurses in the hospital and community settings, in both the pre- and postoperative periods.
- Whilst care may appear to be focused on performing tasks in a standardised manner, nurses are ideally placed not only to coordinate and humanise the surgical experience, but also to facilitate a safe and speedy recovery in an individualised manner.
- There is a trend towards minimally invasive procedures for many surgical conditions, and towards shorter hospital stay for most surgical operations.
- The increasing average age of surgical patients means that they often have more complex underlying medical problems including diabetes, obesity and cardiorespiratory disease.
- Careful pre-assessment and planning is very important in order to select the most appropriate surgical pathway and ensure patients are physically and psychologically prepared.
- In the pre-operative period nurses have a vital role in helping to anticipate problems and minimise complications, through effective physical and psychological preparation of patients.
- In the operating theatre, patient safety is essential. This includes meticulous pre-operative checks and coordinated intra-operative teamwork.
- Patient care in the recovery room includes careful assessment and management of airway, breathing and circulation.
- In the postoperative period the early identification of complications such as hypoxia, haemorrhage, ileus, sepsis and shock can be lifesaving.
- The patient's overall experience is likely to be very much better if the symptoms of pain and nausea are proactively managed.
- Discharge planning should begin at, or even prior to, admission and should be individualised to the patient, their condition and their specific home circumstances.

➡ REFLECTION AND LEARNING – WHAT NEXT?

- **Test** your knowledge by visiting the website 🖱 and answering the multiple choice questions and critical thinking questions.
- **Consolidate** your learning by looking at some of the further reading suggestions, references and specialist websites.
- **Revisit** some of the additional material on the website.
- **Consider** what you have learnt and how this will help your professional development.
- **Reflect** on how you can apply this knowledge to the care of your patients.
- **Discuss** your learning with your mentor/supervisor, lecturer and colleagues.

REFERENCES

Alexander R, Fenelly M: Comparison of ondansetron, metoclopramide and placebo as premedicants to reduce nausea and vomiting after major surgery, *Anaesthesia* 52(7):695–698, 1997.

Allard J, Bleakley A, Hobbs A, et al: Who's on the team today?' The status of briefing amongst operating theatre practitioners in one UK hospital, *J Interprof Care* 21(2):189–206, 2007.

Allvin R, Berg K, Idvall E, et al: Postoperative recovery: a concept analysis, *J Adv Nurs* 57(5):552–558, 2007.

American Society of Anesthesiologists (ASA): *Manual for anesthesia department organization and management*, Park Ridge, IL, 2005, ASA. Available online http://www.asahq.org/clinical/physicalstatus.htm.

Anderson ID: *Care of the critically ill surgical patient*, London, 2003, Hodder Arnold.

AORN: *American Operating Room Nurses. Standards, Recommendations, Practice and Guidelines*, Colorado, 1998, American Operating Room Nurses.

Arnold A: DVT prophylaxis in the perioperative setting, *Br J Perioper Nurs* 12(9):326–332, 2002.

Arora VM, McGory ML, Fung CH, et al: Quality indicators for hospitalization and surgery in vulnerable elders, *Journal of American Geriatric Society* 55(S2):S347–S358, 2007.

Association for Perioperative Practice: *Standards and Recommendations for Safe Perioperative Practice*, Harrogate, 2007, AfPP.

Barker SGE, Hollingsworth SJ: Wearing graduated compression stockings: The reality of everyday deep vein thrombosis prophylaxis, *Phlebology* 19(1):52–53, 2004.

Baxter CM, Brennan MG, Coldicott YGM, et al: *The practical guide to medical ethics and law*, Bodmin, 2002, MPG Books.

Baxter H, Chinn P: Pain management. In Sheppard M, Wright M, editors: *2006 Principles and Practice of High Dependency Nursing*, ed 2, Edinburgh, 2006, Baillière Tindall, pp 321–360.

Benkö T, Cooke EA, McNally MA, Mollan RA: Graduated compression stockings – knee length or thigh length, *Clin Orthop Relat Res* 383:197–203, 2001.

Bisanz A, Palmer JL, Reddy S, Cloutier L, et al: Characterizing postoperative paralytic ileus as evidence for future research and clinical practice, *Gastroenterol Nurs* 31(5):336–344, 2008.

Bockman T, Putney JL: Best practices to reduce infections, *OR Nurse* 2(4):14–15, 2008.

Boore JRP: *Prescription for recovery*, London, 1978, Royal College of Nursing.

Booth S: A philosophical analysis of informed consent, *Nurs Stand* 16(39):43–46, 2002.

Borwell B: Rehabilitation and stoma care: addressing the psychological needs, *British Journal of Nursing Stoma Care supplement* 18(4):S20–S25, 2009.

Bourne N: Managing acute pain in opioid tolerant patients, *Br J Perioper Nurs* 18(11):498–503, 2008.

Bowman AM: Sleep satisfaction, perceived pain and acute confusion in elderly clients undergoing orthopaedic procedures, *J Adv Nurs* 26(3):550–564, 1997.

Bredin M: Mastectomy, body image and therapeutic massage: a qualitative study of women's experience, *J Adv Nurs* 29(5):1113–1120, 1999.

Brown D: Pain assessment in the recovery room, *Br J Perioper Nurs* 18(11):480–487, 2008.

Buggy D: Can anaesthetic management influence surgical wound healing? *Lancet* 356(9227):355–357, 2000.

Burch J, Wright S, Kennedy R, et al: Enhanced recovery pathway in colorectal surgery 1: background and principles, *Nurs Times* 105(28):23–25, 2009.

Butler J, Sen A: Cricoid pressure in emergency rapid sequence induction, *Emerg Med J* 22:815–816, 2005.

Candido LC: Treatment of surgical wound dehiscence, *Dermatol Nurs* 14(3):177–178, 181, 2002.

Charoenkwan K, Phillipson G, Vutyavanich T, et al: Early versus delayed oral fluids and food for reducing complications after major abdominal gynaecological surgery, *Cochrane Database Syst Rev* (4), 2007.

Chibbaro S, Tacconi L: Use of glue versus traditional wound closure methods in brain surgery: A prospective, randomized controlled study, *J Clin Neurosci* 16(4):535–539, 2009.

Christian CK, Gustafson ML, Roth EM, et al: A prospective study of patient safety in the operating room, *Surgery* 139(2):159–173, 2006.

Chumbley GM, Ward L, Hall GM, et al: Pre-operative information and patient controlled analgesia: much ado about nothing, *Anaesthesia* 59(4):358–368, 2004.

Chung F, Assmann N: Car accidents after ambulatory surgery in patients without an escort, *Anesth Analg* 106(3):817–820, 2008.

Correa R, Menezes RB, Wong J, et al: Compliance with post operative instructions. A telephone survey of 750 day surgery patients, *Anaesthesia* 56(5):481–484, 2001.

Costa MJ: The lived peri-operative experience of ambulatory surgery patients, *Association of Peri-operative Registered Nurses' Journal* 74(6):874–881, 2001.

Cotton BA, Guy JS, Morris JA, et al: The cellular, metabolic and systemic consequences of aggressive fluid resuscitation strategies, *Shock* 26(2):115–121, 2006.

Crenshaw J, Winslow E: Preoperative fasting. Old habits die hard: research and published guidelines no longer support the routine use of 'NPO' after midnight but the practice persists, *Am J Nurs* 102(5):36–44, 2002.

D'arcy Y: Managing pain in a patient who's drug dependent, *Nursing* 37(3):37–40, 2007.

Darroch FJ, Page BP, Wakelin SJ, et al: A randomised controlled trial to determine the efficacy of bowel preparation with reference to the quality of endoscopic assessment and patient satisfaction at a one-stop colorectal clinic, *Br J Surg* 95(Suppl 3):39–40, 2008.

Dawson L, Brockbank K, Carr E, et al: Improving patients' postoperative sleep: a randomized control study comparing subcutaneous with intravenous patient controlled analgesia, *J Adv Nurs* 30(4):875–881, 1999.

Dean A, Fawcett T: Nurses' use of evidence in preoperative fasting, *Nurs Stand* 17(2):33–37, 2002.

Department for Constitutional Affairs: *Mental Capacity Act (2005) Code of Practice*, London, 2007, TSO Available online http://www.publicguardian.gov.uk/docs/mca-code-practice-0509.pdf.

Department of Health (DH): *Comprehensive critical care planning and managing critical care capacities. Detailed models can provide information for making good decisions*, London, 2000, TSO. Available online http://www.dh.gov.uk/en/Publicationsandstatistics/Publications/PublicationsPolicyAndGuidance/DH_4006585.

Department of Health (DH): *Inpatient and outpatient waiting in the NHS. Report by the Comptroller and Auditor General*, HE 221 Session 2001–2002. London, 2001a, National Audit Office.

Department of Health (DH): *Good practice in consent implementation guide: consent to examination or treatment*, London, 2001b, TSO Available online http://www.dh.gov.uk/en/Publicationsandstatistics/Publications/PublicationsPolicyAndGuidance/DH_4005762.

Department of Health (DH): Extending choice for patients, *Heart surgery* 2005. Available online http://www.dh.gov.uk/en/Publicationsandstatistics/Publications/PublicationsPolicyAndGuidance/DH_4106275.

Dihle A, Bjolseth G, Helseth S, et al: The gap between saying and doing in postoperative pain management, *J Clin Nurs* 15(4):469–479, 2006.

Dolan SJ, Cashman JN, Bland JM, et al: Effectiveness of acute postoperative pain management: 1 evidence from published data, *Br J Anaesth* 89(3):409–423, 2002.

Donovan HS, Ward S: A representational approach to patient education, *J Nurs Scholarsh* 33(3):211–216, 2001.

Dougherty L, Lister S: *The Royal Hospital Manual of Clinical Nursing Procedures*, ed 7, Oxford, 2008, Wiley-Blackwell.

Edwards C: A proposal that patients be considered honorary members of the health care team, *J Clin Nurs* 11(3):340–348, 2002.

Edwards JL, Pandit H, Popat MT, et al: Perioperative analgesia: a factor in the development of heel pressure ulcers, *British Journal of Nursing (Tissue Viability Supplement)* 15(6s):20–25, 2006.

Ene KW, Nordberg G, Bergh I, et al: Postoperative pain management – the influence of surgical ward nurses, *J Clin Nurs* 17:2042–2050, 2008.

Ewart L, Huntington S: The peri-operative phase. In McArthur-Rouse F, Prosser S, editors: *Assessing and Managing the Acutely Ill adult surgical patient*, Oxford, 2007, Blackwell, pp 17–37.

Ferguson SE, Malhotra T, Seshan VE, et al: A prospective randomised trial comparing patient-controlled epidural analgesia to patient controlled intravenous analgesia on post operative pain control and recovery after major open gynaecological cancer surgery, *Gynecol Oncol* 114:111–116, 2009.

Field J: Feeding patients after abdominal surgery, *Nurs Stand* 16(48):41–44, 2002.

Finlay T: *Intravenous therapy*, Oxford, 2004, Blackwell.

Francis C: *Respiratory care*, Oxford, 2006, Blackwell.

Gagliese L., Melzack R.: Pain in the elderly. In McMahon SB., Koltzenburg M, editors: *Melzack and Wall's Textbook of Pain*, 2006. Edinburgh, Elsevier, pp 1169–1179.

Garretson S: Benefits of pre operative information programmes, *Nurs Stand* 18(47):33–37, 2004.

Garretson S, Malberti S: Understanding hypovolaemic, cardiogenic and septic shock, *Nurs Stand* 50(21):46–55, 2007.

General Medical Council: *Consent: patients and doctors making decisions together*, 2008. Available online http://www.gmc-uk.org/static/documents/content/Consent_2008.pdf.

Giraudet-Le Quintrec JS, Coste J, Vastel L, et al: Positive effect of patient education for hip surgery: a randomized trial, *Clin Orthop Relat Res* 414:112–120, 2003.

Graham CA, Beard D, Oglesby AJ, et al: Rapid sequence intubation in Scottish urban emergency departments, *Emerg Med J* 20:3–5, 2003.

Graham L: Care of patients undergoing laparoscopic cholecystectomy, *Nurs Stand* 23(7):41–48, 2008.

Greerts WH, Heit JA, Claget CP, et al: Prevention of venous thromboembolism, *Chest (Suppl)* 119(1):132–175, 2001.

Griffith R, Tengnah C: *Law and professional Issues in Nursing*, Padstow, 2008, Learning Matters.

Guenaga KKFG, Matos D, Wille-Jørgensen P, et al: Mechanical bowel preparation for elective colorectal surgery, *Cochrane Database Syst Rev* (1), 2009.

Hattan J, King L, Griffiths P, et al: The impact of foot massage and guided relaxation following cardiac surgery: a randomized controlled trial, *J Adv Nurs* 37(2):199–207, 2002.

Hayward J: *Information: a prescription against pain*, London, 1975, Royal College of Nursing.

Hilditch WG, Asbury AJ, Crawford JM, et al: Preoperative screening: criteria for referring to anaesthetists, *Anaesthesia* 58(2):117–124, 2003.

HMSO: *The adult with incapacity Act (Scotland)*, 2000. Available online http://www.hmso.gov.uk/legislation/scotland/acts2000/20000004.htm.

Hollaus P, Pucher I, Wilfing G, et al: Preoperative attitudes, fears and expectations of non-small cell lung cancer patients, *Interact Cardiovasc Thorac Surg* 2:206–209, 2003.

Holmes L, Sharples J, Cooper S, Wright N, et al: Sexuality in gynaecological cancer patients, *Cancer Nursing Practice* 4(6):35–39, 2005.

Hong JY, Lee IH: Suprascapular nerve block or a piroxicam patch for shoulder tip pain after day case laparoscopic surgery, *Eur J Anaesthesiol* 20(3):234–238, 2003.

Hough M, Sweeney B: The influence of smoking on postoperative nausea and vomiting, *Anaesthesia* 53:932–933, 1998.

Houghton CS, Marcukaitis AW, Shirk ME, et al: Tobacco intervention attitudes and practices among certified registered nurse anesthetists, *Nurs Res* 57(2):123–129, 2008.

Hudcova J, McNicol E, Quah C, et al: Patient controlled opioid analgesia versus conventional opioid analgesia for postoperative pain, *Evid Based Nurs* 10(3):83, 2006.

Hughes E: Principles of post-operative patient care, *Nurs Stand* 19(5):43–51, 2004.

Hughes S: The effect of giving patients pre operative information, *Nurs Stand* 16(28):33–37, 2002.

Hughes SJ, Mardell A: *Oxford Handbook of Perioperative practice*, Oxford, 2009, Oxford University Press.

Hunt JO, Hendrata MV, Myles PS, et al: Quality of life 12 months after CABG surgery, *Heart Lung* 29(6):401–411, 2000.

Hyde R, Bryden F, Asbury AJ, et al: How would patients prefer to spend the waiting time before their operations? *Anaesthesia* 53(2):192–195, 1998.

Hynes D, McCarroll M, Hiesse-provost O, et al: Analgesic efficacy of parenteral paracetamol (propacetamol) and diclofenac in post-operative orthopaedic pain, *Acta Anaesthesiol Scand* 50:374–381, 2006.

Ingram JE: A review of thigh length versus knee length anti-embolism stockings, *Br J Nurs* 12(14):845–851, 2003.

Iverson RE, Lynch DJ: Practice advisory on pain management and prevention of postoperative nausea and vomiting, *Plast Reconstr Surg* 118(4):1060–1069, 2006.

Jensen K, Kehlet H, Lund C, et al: Postoperative recovery profile after elective abdominal hysterectomy: a prospective observational study of a multimodal anaesthetic regime, *Eur J Anaesthesiol* 26:382–388, 2009.

Jester R, Williams S: Pre-operative fasting: putting research into practice, *Nurs Stand* 13(39):33–35, 1999.

Jolley S: Post-operative nausea and vomiting: a survey of nurses' knowledge, *Nurs Stand* 14(23):32–34, 2000.

Jolley S: Managing post operative nausea and vomiting, *Nurs Stand* 15(40):47–53, 2001.

Jolley S: An audit of patients' understanding of routine preoperative investigations, *Nurs Stand* 21(22):35–39, 2007.

Kaplan C, Mendiola R, Ndjatou V, et al: The role of covering gowns in reducing rates of bacterial contamination of scrub suits, *Obstetrical and Gynaecological Survey* 58(9):582–583, 2003.

Karch AM: *Focus on Nursing Pharmacology*, ed 5, Philadelphia, 2009, Lippincott Williams and Wilkins.

Keeton S, McAloon L: The supply and fitting of a temporary breast prosthesis, *Nurs Stand* 16(41):43–46, 2002.

Kehlet H, Holte K: Effect of postoperative analgesia on surgical outcome, *Br J Anaesth* 87(1):62–72, 2001.

Kehlet H, Jensen TS, Woolf CJ, et al: Persistent post surgical pain: risk factors and prevention, *Lancet* 367(9399):1618–1625, 2006.

Kehlet H, Wilmore DW: Multimodal strategies to improve surgical outcome, *Am J Surg* 183:630–641, 2002.

Kurz A, Sessler D, Lenhardt R, et al: Perioperative normothermia to reduce the incidence of surgical-wound infection and shorten hospitalization, *N Engl J Med* 334(19):1209–1215, 1996.

Lawrentschuk N, Hewitt PM, Fracs PM, et al: Elective laparoscopic cholecystectomy: implications of prolonged waiting times for surgery, *Aust N Z J Surg* 73(11):890–893, 2003.

Layzell M: Current interventions and approaches to post operative pain management, *Br J Nurs* 17(7):414–419, 2008.

Leahy M, Douglass J, Barley V, et al: Audiotaping the heart surgery consultation: qualitative study of patients' experiences, *Heart* 91(11):1469–1470, 2005.

Lees S: The removal of sutures, *Nurs Times* 103(7):26–27, 2007.

Leung JM, Dzankic S: Relative importance of pre-operative health status versus intraoperative factors in predicting post-operative adverse outcomes in geriatric surgical patients, *J Am Geriatr Soc* 49(8):1080–1085, 2001.

Lewis SJ, Egger M, Sylvester PA, et al: Early enteral feeding versus 'nil by mouth' after gastrointestinal surgery: systematic review and meta analysis of controlled trials, *Br Med J* 323(7316):773–776, 2001.

Lipp A, Edwards P: Disposable surgical face masks for preventing surgical wound infection in clean surgery, *Cochrane Database Syst Rev* (3), 2010.

Lovett PE, Stanlon SL, Hennessy D, et al: Pain relief after major gynaecological surgery, *Br J Nurs* 3(4):159–162, 1994.

Macintyre PE: Safety and efficacy of patient-controlled analgesia, *Br J Anaesth* 87(1):36–46, 2001.

Macintyre PE, Schug SA: *Acute pain management: A practical guide*, ed 3, China, 2007, Saunders.

Macrae WA: Chronic pain after surgery, *Br J Anaesth* 87(1):88–98, 2001.

Malan T, McIndoe AK: Positioning the surgical patient, *Anaesthesia and Intensive Care Medicine* 4(11):360–363, 2003.

Mangram AJ, Horan TC, Pearson ML, et al: Guideline for prevention of surgical site infection, *Am J Infect Control* 27(2):97–134, 1999.

Manias E: Pain and anxiety management in the postoperative gastro-surgical setting, *J Adv Nurs* 41(6):585–594, 2003.

Mann E: Dealing with pain, managing pain, *Br Med J* 326:1320–1321, 2003.

Maramba PJ, Richards S, Larrabee JH, et al: Discharge planning process: applying a model for evidence-based practice, *J Nurs Care Qual* 19(2):123–129, 2004.

Markham R, Smith A: Limits to patient choice: examples from anaesthesia, *Br Med J* 326(7394):863–864, 2003.

Martin S: Developing the nurse practitioner's role in minor surgery, *Nurs Times* 98(33):39–40, 2002.

Mayne IP, Bagaoisan C: Social support during anesthesia induction in an adult surgical population, *AORN J* 89(2):307–320, 2009.

McArthur-Rouse F, Prosser S, editors: *Assessing and Managing the Acutely Ill adult surgical patient*, Oxford, 2007, Blackwell.

McKenna H, Keeney S, Glenn A, et al: Discharge planning: an exploratory study, *J Clin Nurs* 9(4):594–601, 2000.

Ming JC, Kno BIT, Lin JG, et al: The efficacy of acupressure to prevent nausea and vomiting in post-operative patients, *J Adv Nurs* 39(4):343–351, 2002.

Mitchell M: Guidance for the psychological care of day case surgery patients, *Nurs Stand* 16(40):41–43, 2002.

Mitchell M: Impact of discharge from day surgery on patients and carers, *Br J Nurs* 12(7):402–407, 2003.

Mitchell M: Psychological care of patients undergoing elective surgery, *Nurs Stand* 21(30):48–55, 2007a.

Mitchell M: Nursing intervention for day-case laparoscopic cholecystectomy, *Nurs Stand* 22(6):35–41, 2007b.

Moz T: Wound dehiscence and evisceration, *Nursing* 34(5):88, 2004.

Mullerat P, Winslet M: Surgery in carriers of HIV and hepatitis, *Surgery* 23(8):302–304, 2005.

Murakami M, Tandace L, Cindrick-Pounds L, et al: Deep venous thrombosis prophylaxis in trauma, improved compliance with a novel miniaturised pneumatic compression device, *J Vasc Surg* 38(5):923–927, 2003.

Murkin CE: Pre-operative antiseptic skin preparation, *Br J Nurs* 18(11):665–669, 2009.

Myatt RM: An introduction to thoracic surgery: assessment, diagnosis, treatment, *Br J Nurs* 13(17):944–947, 2006.

Nagi H: Acute pain services in the United Kingdom, *Acute Pain* 5:89–107, 2004.

National Institute for Health and Clinical Excellence (NICE): *Brief interventions and referral for smoking cessation in primary care and other settings*, 2005. Available online http://www.nice.org.uk/nicemedia/live/11375/31864/31864.pdf.

National Institute for Health and Clinical Excellence (NICE): *Reducing the risk of venous thrombo-embolism (deep vein thrombosis and pulmonary embolism) in patients undergoing surgery*, 2007. Available online http://www.nice.org.uk/nicemedia/pdf/VTEFullGuide.pdf.

National Patient Safety Agency: *UK surgical organisations sign up to World Health Organization challenge: Safe Surgery Saves Lives*, 2008. Available online http://www.npsa.nhs.uk/corporate/news/safe-surgery-saves-lives/.

NHS Executive: *The employment of operating department practitioners (OPDs) in the NHS*, Leeds, 2001, NHS Executive.

NHS Quality Improvement Scotland: *Best Practice Statement: Postoperative pain management*, 2004a. Available online http://www.nhshealthquality.org.

NHS Quality Improvement Scotland: *Best Practice Statement: Urinary catheterisation and catheter care*, 2004b. Available online http://www.nhshealthquality.org.

NHS Scotland: *NHS Code of Practice on Protecting Patient Confidentiality*, 2003. Available online http://www.nhshighland.scot.nhs.uk/Documents/Your%20Rights/Confidentiality/NHS%20Code%20of%20Practice%20on%20Protecting%20Patient%20Confidentiality.pdf.

NHS Scotland: *Inpatient, day case and outpatient activity*, Edinburgh, 2010, NHS Scotland. Available online http://www.isdscotland.org/isd/4158.html.

Njawe P: Sleep and rest in patients undergoing cardiac surgery, *Nurs Stand* 18(12):33–37, 2003.

Noimark D: Predicting the onset of delirium in the post-operative period, *Age Ageing* 38(4):368–373, 2009.

Nursing and Midwifery Council (NMC): *The Code: Standards of conduct, performance and ethics for nurses and midwives*, London, 2008, NMC.

Paavilainen E, Seppanen S, Asted-Kurki P, et al: Family involvement in perioperative nursing of adult patients undergoing emergency surgery, *J Clin Nurs* 10(2):230–237, 2001.

Palese A, Skrap M, Fachin M, et al: The experiences of patients undergoing awake craniotomy. In the patients' own words: A qualitative study, *Cancer Nurs* 31(2):166–172, 2008.

Panda N, Bajaj A, Pershad D, et al: Pre-operative anxiety, effect of early or late position on the operating list, *Anaesthesia* 51(4):344–346, 1996.

Parnaby C: A new anti-embolism stocking: use of below-knee products and compliance, *Br J Perioper Nurs* 14(7):302–307, 2004.

Pearson A, Richardson M, Peels S, et al: The care of patients whilst in the day surgery unit: a systematic review, *Health Care Reports* 2(2):22–54, 2004.

Perkins F, Kehlet H: Chronic pain as an outcome of surgery: a review of predictive factors, *Anesthesiology* 93(4):1123–1133, 2000.

Pidduck D: The theatre nurse role: a review of the literature, *Journal of Perioperative Nursing* 13(9):374–379, 2003.

Pieper B, Sieggreen M, Freeland B, et al: Discharge needs of patients after surgery, *J Wound Ostomy Continence Nurs* 33:281–291, 2006.

Pirret AM: A pre-operative scoring system to identify patients requiring postoperative high dependency care, *Intensive and Critical Care* 19:267–275, 2003.

Price B: *Body Image: Nursing concepts and care*, Hemmel Hempstead, 1990, Prentice Hall.

Price B: Understanding patient accounts of body image change, *Cancer Nursing Practice* 8(6):29–34, 2009.

Pritchard MJ: Managing anxiety I: the elective surgery patient, *Br J Nurs* 18(7):416–419, 2009.

Prosser S, McArthur-Rouse FJ: Post-operative recovery. In McArthur-Rouse F, Prosser S, editors: *Assessing and Managing the Acutely Ill Adult Surgical Patient*, Oxford, 2007, Blackwell, pp 39–59.

Quin W, Neil J: Evidence for early oral feeding of patients after elective open colorectal surgery: a literature review, *J Clin Nurs* 15:696–709, 2006.

Quinlan S: Sick and tired, *Nurs Stand* 17(13):24, 2002.

Resuscitation Council: *Advanced life support*, ed 5, London, 2006, Resuscitation Council (UK).

Robertshaw HJ, Hall GM: Diabetes mellitus: anaesthetic management, *Anaesthesia* 61:1187–1190, 2006.

Royal College of Nursing: *Perioperative fasting in adults and children. An RCN guideline for the multidisciplinary team*, 2005. Available online http://www.rcn.org.uk/__data/assets/pdf_file/0009/78669/002779.pdf.

Royal College of Surgeons and College of Anaesthetists: *Report of the working party on pain after surgery*, London, 1990, Royal College of Surgeons.

Royal College of Surgeons of England: *Guidelines for day case surgery*, HMSO, 1992, London. Available online http://www.rcseng.ac.uk/publications/docs/publication.2005-09-01.3078389478/.

Scott C, McArthur-Rouse FJ, McLean J, et al: Pre-operative assessment and preparation. In McArthur-Rouse F, Prosser S, editors: *Assessing and Managing the Acutely Ill adult surgical patient*, Oxford, 2007, Blackwell, pp 3–15.

Scott E, Earl C, Leaper D, et al: Understanding perioperative nursing, *Nurs Stand* 13(49):49–54, 1999.

Scottish Executive: *Partnership for care: Scotland's health, White Paper*, Edinburgh, 2003, TSO. Available online http://www.scotland.gov.uk/Publications/2003/02/16476/18730.

Scottish Intercollegiate Guidelines Network (SIGN): *Prophylaxis of venous thromboembolism*, Edinburgh, 2002, SIGN. Available online http://www.sign.ac.uk/pdf/sign62.pdf.

Scottish intercollegiate Guidelines Network (SIGN): *Postoperative management in adults*, Edinburgh, 2004, SIGN. Available online http://www.sign.ac.uk/pdf/sign77.pdf.

Scottish Intercollegiate Guidelines Network (SIGN): *Antibiotic prophylaxis in surgery*, 2008. Available online http://www.sign.ac.uk/pdf/sign104.pdf.

Sear J: Implications of aging on anesthetic drugs, *Current Opinion in Anesthesiology* 16(4):373–378, 2003.

Segerdahl M, Warren-Shomberg M, Rawal N, et al: Clinical practice and routines for day surgery in Sweden: results from a nationwide survey, *Acta Anaesthesiologica Scandinavia* 52:117–124, 2008.

Selye H: *The stress of life*, ed 2, New York, 1976, McGraw-Hill.

Sheppard M, Wright M: *Principles and Practice of High Dependency Nursing*, ed 2, Edinburgh, 2006, Baillière Tindall.

Shnaider I, Chung F: Outcomes in day surgery, *Current opinions in Anaesthesiology* 19:622–629, 2006.

Sinclair LG: Young adults with permanent ileostomies. Experiences during the first 4 years after surgery, *J Wound Ostomy Continence Nurs* 36(3):306–314, 2009.

Singer AJ, Quinn JV, Clark RE, et al: Closure of lacerations and incisions with octylcyanoacrylate: A multicentre randomised controlled trial, *Surgery* 131(3):270–276, 2002.

Smiley DD, Guillermo EU: Perioperative glucose control in the diabetic or non diabetic patient, *South Med J* 99(6):580–589, 2006.

Smith G, Watson R: *Gastrointestinal Nursing*, London, 2005, Blackwell.

Somasekar K, Shankar PJ, Foster ME, et al: Costs of waiting for gall bladder surgery, *Postgrad Med J* 78(155):668–671, 2002.

Stirling L: Reduction and management of perioperative anxiety, *Br J Nurs* 15(7):359–361, 2006.

Taylor C: Discharge after colorectal cancer surgery 1: an overview, *Nurs Times* 104(28):28–29, 2008.

Thomas R, Jones NS, Strike P, et al: The validity of risk scores for predicting postoperative nausea and vomiting when used to compare patient groups in a randomised control trial, *Anaesthesia* 57(11):1119–1128, 2002.

Thompson HJ: The management of postoperative nausea and vomiting, *J Adv Nurs* 29(5):1130–1136, 1999.

Timmons S, Tanner J: A disputed occupational boundary: operating theatre nurses and operating department practitioners, *Sociol Health Illn* 26(5):645–666, 2004.

Veitch H: *Top tips for Theatre Placement (Personal Communication)*, Edinburgh, 2009, Year 3 student nurse, Queen Margaret University.

Wagner D, Byrne M, Kolcaba K, et al: Effects of comfort warming on preoperative patients, *AORN J* 84(3):427–448, 2006.

Walker L, Lamont S: The use of antiembolic stockings. Part 1 A literature review, *Br J Nurs* 16(22):1408–1412, 2007.

Waller D: *Medical pharmacology and therapeutics*, Edinburgh, 2010, Elsevier Saunders.

Walsgrove H: Putting education into practice for pre-operative patient assessment, *Nurs Stand* 20(47):35–39, 2006.

Warner DO: Perioperative abstinence from cigarettes, *Anesthesiology* 104(2):356–366, 2006.

Way P, Fairbrother G, Grguric S, et al: The relative benefits of pre-operative clinic vs on admission approaches to preparing patients for elective cardiac surgery, *Aust Crit Care* 16(2):71–75, 2003.

Webster J, Croger S, Lister C, et al: Use of face masks by non-scrubbed operating room staff; a randomized controlled trial, *ANZ J Surg* 80(3):169–173, 2010.

Weetman C, Allison W: Use of epidural analgesia in post-operative pain management, *Nurs Stand* 20(44):54–64, 2006.

Whalen R, Sprung J, Burkle CM, Schroeder DR, et al: Recent smoking behavior and post operative nausea and vomiting, *Ambulatory Anaesthesia* 103(1):70–75, 2006.

White H, Black RR, Jones M, et al: Randomized comparison of two anti-emetic strategies in high-risk patients undergoing day case gynaecological surgery, *Br J Anaesth* 98(4):470–476, 2007.

White SM, Baldwin TJ: The Mental Capacity Act 2005, implications for anaesthesia and critical care, *Anaesthesia* 61:381–389, 2006.

Williams A, Dunning T, Manias E, et al: Continuity of care and general wellbeing of patients with comorbidities requiring joint replacement, *J Adv Nurs* 57(3):244–256, 2007.

Williams J, Barbul A: Nutrition and wound healing, *Surg Clin North Am* 83(3):571–596, 2003.

Wills VL, Hunt DR: Pain after laparoscopic cholecystectomy, *Br J Surg* 87(3):273–284, 2000.

Woodhouse A: Pre-operative fasting for elective surgical patients, *Nurs Stand* 20(21):41–48, 2006.

Wright S, Burch J, Jenkins JT, et al: Enhanced recovery pathway in colorectal surgery 2: post- operative complications, *Nurs Times* 105:29, 2009.

Zeebregts CJ, Meerwaldt R, Geelkerken RH, et al: Carotid artery stenting a 2009 update, *Curr Opin Cardiol* 24:1–4, 2009.

Zeitz K: Nursing observations during the first 24 hours after a surgical procedure: what do we do? *J Clin Nurs* 14:334–343, 2005.

FURTHER READING

Ayres U: Older people and hypothermia: the role of the anaesthetic nurse, *Br J Nurs* 13(7):3–6, 403, 2004.

Barthelsson C, Lutzen K, Anderberg B, et al: Patients' experiences of laparoscopic cholecystectomy in day surgery, *J Clin Nurs* 12:253–259, 2003.

Coll AM, Ameen JRM, Mead D, et al: Postoperative pain assessment tools in day surgery: literature review, *J Adv Nurs* 46(2):124–133, 2004.

Critical Care: Trouble down below: Understanding small bowel obstruction, *Nursing* 35(7):33–37, 2005.

DeLeskey K: The implementation of evidence based practice for the prevention of post-operative nausea and vomiting, *International Journal of Evidence based Healthcare* 7(2):140–144, 2009.

Farrar J, Kearney K: Acute cholecystitis, *Am J Nurs* 101(1):35–36, 2001.

Haynes AB, Weiser TG, Berry WR, et al: A surgical safety checklist to reduce morbidity and mortality in a global population, *N Engl J Med* 360:491–499, 2009.

Lowenstein L, Gamble T, Deniseko ST, et al: Sexual function is related to body image perception in women with pelvic organ prolapse, *Journal of Sexual Health Medicine* 6(8):2286–2291, 2009.

Mackintosh C: Assessment and management of patients with post-operative pain, *Nurs Stand* 22(5):49–55, 2007.

Makary MA, Sexton JB, Freishchlag JA, et al: Operating room teamwork among physicians and nurses: teamwork in the eye of the beholder, *Journal of American College of Surgeons* 202(5):746–752, 2006.

McMurray A, Johnson P, Patterson E, et al: General surgical patients' perspectives of the adequacy and appropriateness of discharge planning to facilitate health decision making at home, *J Clin Nurs* 16:1602–1609, 2007.

Mitchell L: The non-technical skills of theatre nurses, *Br J Perioper Nurs* 18(9):378–388, 2008.

Moos DD: Ineffective cricoid pressure: The critical role of formalised training, *British Journal of Anaesthetic and Recovery Nursing* 8(3):43–49, 2007.

Red Flag: Gallbladder woes: The passing stone, *Nursing Made Incredibly Easy* 3(5):51–55, 2005.

Rhodes L, Miles G, Pearson, et al: Patient subjective experience and satisfaction during the perioperative period in the day surgery setting: A systematic review, *Int J Nurs Pract* 12:178–192, 2006.

Taylor C: Discharge after colorectal cancer surgery 2: Planning, *Nurs Times* 104(29):30–31, 2008.

Wills V, Gibson K, Karihaloo C, et al: Complications of biliary T tubes after choledochotomy, *ANZ J Surg* 72(3):177–180, 2002.

USEFUL WEBSITES

Association for Perioperative Practice: www.afpp.org.uk

NHS Direct: www.nhsdirect.nhs.uk

NHS 24: www.nhs24.com

NICE: www.nice.org.uk

RCN Perioperative forum: www.rcn.org.uk/development/communities/rcn_forum_communities/perioperative

Royal College of Anaesthetists: www.rcoa.ac.uk

Royal College of Surgeons of England, information for patients: www.rcseng.ac.uk/patient_information

SIGN: www.sign.ac.uk

Nursing the patient who experiences trauma

Elaine Cole

Introduction

Trauma may be defined as 'blunt or penetrating external force exerted on the body resulting in injury' (Eckes-Roper 2003: 1). Trauma is not a new disease; however, it continues to be a leading cause of death and disability in all age groups, especially in the first four decades of life (Cole 2008).

Historically people have suffered traumatic injuries caused by modes of transport (the horse and cart for example), assaults, falls and work-related incidents. Conflict also causes death and disability due to traumatic injury. Contemporary trauma care was born out of wartime experience, and lessons learned from the two world wars and the Vietnam War have helped to shape current trauma practice, especially in relation to intravenous fluid therapy and surgical interventions (Cole & McGinley 2005).

Trauma patients are cared for by a variety of practitioners in many clinical settings – from the paramedic at the roadside, to the nurse in a rehabilitation unit; however, trauma is a relatively new specialty in its own right. In the late 1980s The Royal College of Surgeons of England carried out a retrospective review of 1000 trauma deaths in England and Wales (Anderson et al 1988). The report that followed identified that approximately one third of the deaths were preventable and were often due to treatable causes such as hypoxia and

haemorrhage, and organisational issues. Following this, the Advanced Trauma Life Support (ATLS) protocols (American College of Surgeons [ACS] 2004) were adopted by many Emergency Departments to guide trauma care and standardise patient management. However, in November 2007 the National Confidential Enquiry into Patient Outcome and Death (NCEPOD) launched *Trauma: Who Cares?* (Findlay et al 2007). This study has reported that nearly 50% of severely injured patients in the UK did not receive good-quality care. Deficiencies in organisational and clinical aspects of trauma care were identified and NCEPOD has called for significant improvements in pre-hospital and in-hospital trauma care.

Much of the trauma literature focuses on the care that the patient receives in the Emergency Department (ED). This is the area of the hospital where patients with unscheduled or unplanned injuries or illnesses are assessed and treated and was formerly known as the Accident and Emergency department (A&E). However, this is only one part of the patient's journey and does not really reflect the reality of contemporary trauma nursing. This chapter will outline the principles of care needed for the trauma patient, from pre-hospital care through to definitive care. Reflection boxes will help you to consider a trauma case history and reflect on the care needed. Contemporary evidence-based practice will be discussed, with links to web-based critical thinking exercises and further reading material.

Trauma: epidemiology and the need for injury prevention

Traumatic injury can be unintentional or intentional and continues to be a significant health problem. Trauma does not capture the public attention in the same way as other diseases such as cancer, cardiac disease or meningitis; however, traumatic injury *is* a disease. It has a host (the patient) and a mode of transmission (a vehicle, fire, knife) (ACS 2004) and the statistics are shocking. Trauma affects all age groups and it is the main cause of death in young people, under the age of 40. Annually in the UK, 14 500–18 000 deaths occur as a result of trauma, with 60 000 patients being admitted to hospital each year as a result of a road traffic collision (RTC) (Bonnett et al 2003). In the UK the incidence of severe traumatic injury is estimated at 4 people in every million per week. With approximately 60 million people in the UK, this means 240 severely injured patients per week (Findlay et al 2007).

The irony is that trauma in civilian settings is preventable. There is often a fatalistic 'accidents will always happen' attitude towards the cause of injuries; a death following a traumatic event, such as a car accident or a fall at work, is often publicly perceived as an unavoidable fatality (Chiara et al 2006). However, this is incorrect. Traumatic injury should not be thought of as an accident – this word implies a random circumstance, whereas injuries occur in specific, usually preventable patterns. Individuals in high-risk situations or environments, such as children playing near a busy road, adults driving a car at speed or following alcohol consumption, working without protective equipment or carrying a knife provide a chain of events that results in traumatic injury. Legislation such as seat belt laws, environment modifications such as road-calming measures and health promotion campaigns by organisations such as the Royal Society for the Protection of Accidents (RoSPA) have all helped to reduce death and disability, however more needs to be done. Trauma nurses who care for the injured are ideally placed to practise health promotion and injury prevention strategies, either during interactions with patients or by supporting injury prevention strategies such as the Safety and Risk Education Programme (RoSPA 2008).

Mechanism of injury

Following a traumatic event, information about the mechanism of injury may help identify up to 90% of a patient's injuries (ACS 2004). Mechanism of injury can be classified into four main groups (Greaves et al 2001a):

- blunt – such as a road traffic collision, assault, fall or sporting injury
- penetrating – such as a stab wound or impalement
- blast – caused by an explosive element, which may be intentional (a bomb) or accidental (an industrial incident)
- thermal – caused by extreme heat, such as a fire, or extreme cold, such as frost bite.

In general, 98% of the trauma in the UK is blunt, caused by injury, and other mechanisms make up the rest. However

this picture is changing in urban settings with penetrating injury becoming more prevalent.

Blunt trauma causes injury as a result of energy transfer leading to tissue compression and disruption (Eaton 2005). Common injuries include crushing, rupturing or shearing of organs or tissues, fractures (open and closed) and traumatic amputations (Middlehurst 2008). Blast injuries can cause a combination of blunt and penetrating injuries, due to the patient being thrown by the force of the blast, and surrounding objects or people being thrown at the patient.

Penetrating trauma causes injury when an object or missile with a small frontal area and high kinetic energy penetrates the skin and underlying tissues of the body (Eaton 2005). In general, penetrating forces are considered high and medium energy – firearms and fragments from blasts – and low energy such as knives, broken glass and other sharp objects (Middlehurst 2008).

The nurse assessing a trauma patient should consider the mechanism of injury, especially when it is suggestive of a serious, high-energy force. Patients may not appear to have sustained obvious injuries following a traumatic event, especially if the injury is internal. However, a high index of suspicion and careful assessment and reassessment of the patient is essential in every clinical setting to detect deterioration or the onset of complications (Middlehurst 2008).

Death following trauma

Death due to traumatic injury occurs in one of three time periods, described as the trimodal death distribution (ACS 2004) (Figure 27.1). This has significance for trauma nurses working throughout all the areas of trauma care.

The first period is where death occurs within seconds to minutes of sustaining the injury. Deaths are caused by very severe injuries such as major vessel (aorta, vena cava) disruption, severe traumatic brain injury, high spinal cord injury or apnoea. This period can only be significantly reduced by preventing the incident occurring in the first place.

The second period is where death occurs minutes to hours following the injury. Deaths are caused by injuries resulting in overwhelming hypoxia and hypovolaemia or a rapidly accumulating intracranial haematoma pressing on the brain. Nurses and practitioners working in pre-hospital and emergency care settings must carry out prompt assessment and resuscitation to recognise problems, seek expert help early and minimise death in this period.

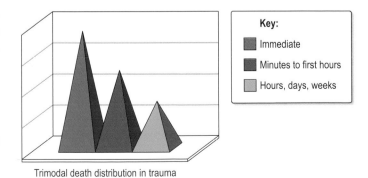

Trimodal death distribution in trauma

Figure 27.1 Trimodal death distribution in trauma.

The third period is where death occurs days or weeks after the initial injury. This is usually due to complex complications that have arisen such as multi-organ failure, coagulopathy (failure of normal clotting mechanisms), acute respiratory distress syndrome or overwhelming sepsis. Nurses working in definitive trauma care settings are responsible for assessment, monitoring and support of patients, in order to detect potential complications and maximise recovery.

Disability

It must be remembered that death is not the only outcome following traumatic injury. Worldwide, large numbers of people are left permanently disabled following intentional or unintentional injury, causing a huge financial and social burden on society (WHO 2008). Disabilities following injury include:

- physical and/or cognitive limitations due to neurotrauma
- paralysis due to spinal cord trauma
- partial or complete amputation of limbs
- physical limb deformation resulting in mobility impairments
- psychological trauma
- sensory disability such as blindness and deafness.

A combination of increased injury prevention awareness and better patient care can help to reduce the number of disabilities and provide better outcomes for society.

Pre-hospital care

Pre-hospital care is defined as the provision of skilled medical help at the scene of an accident, medical or other clinical emergency, and during transport of the patient to hospital (Noble-Mathews 2005). In most UK settings this will involve staff from an ambulance service, using road vehicles or possibly helicopters to assess, resuscitate and then transport trauma patients to hospital. Currently in the UK there are only a few pre-hospital care nurses working in the field of trauma, in comparison to the USA and other European countries.

As well as good clinical knowledge, pre-hospital care paramedics and nurses need specialist skills, such as ensuring scene safety or extrication of patients trapped in vehicles. This is achieved through education and training and also collaboration with other emergency services such as the police and fire and rescue teams.

Advanced notification

Pre-hospital care staff can provide essential information from the scene to the hospital teams waiting to receive the patient in the emergency department (ED). This advanced notification allows the receiving hospital to prepare the necessary equipment and personnel to ensure the best clinical care and outcome (Cole & McGinley 2005). Advanced notification may differ between ambulance services; however, it will generally include the following:

- age
- gender
- mechanism of injury (see p. 722)

- cardiovascular observations
- respiratory rate and oxygen saturations
- Glasgow Coma Scale (or level of consciousness)
- obvious and predicted injuries
- treatment given at scene or en route
- numbers of patients if more than one person is involved.

Hand over

Once in the ED the pre-hospital care staff will 'hand over' the patient to the hospital staff. This will involve the clinical aspects of the patient's injuries and care. If possible it should also involve information about the patient's relatives or next of kin (if known) and any police liaison that may be involved. Hand over will be given verbally but the pre-hospital care staff will also provide a written summary of their care that should form part of the patient's notes.

Emergency Department

Many Emergency Departments use a system of assessing (or triaging) the patients on arrival to determine the severity of their injury, and then streaming (or directing) them to the appropriate clinical area (Bickerton et al 2005). The ED is usually divided into sections where patients with minor injuries can be seen and treated in a designated area away from those who are more seriously ill or injured. The minor injuries section is where single system traumatic injuries such as ankle or wrist fractures, soft tissue injuries or uncomplicated wounds can be seen and treated.

Once the major trauma patient has arrived at the hospital they should be cared for in a resuscitation area. This is a clinical area which is designed to have the necessary equipment and space readily available to enable a trauma team to care for the patient efficiently and effectively. In the ED it is vital that there is a predetermined system, such as the Advanced Trauma Life Support (ATLS) protocols (ACS 2004), to guide personnel through the initial assessment of the patient. Using a systematic approach (A, B, C, D, E) helps the trauma team to identify life-threatening conditions quickly and to treat them appropriately (Box 27.1).

The trauma team

The trauma team is made up of clinicians (nurses, doctors, radiographers) who carry out pre-assigned roles so that several interventions can occur simultaneously (Cole & Crichton 2006). The aim of the trauma team is to promptly stabilise the patient, identify injuries and initiate a definitive

---

 Box 27.1 Information

Advanced Trauma Life Support (ATLS) Primary Survey Assessment

- Airway with cervical spine control
- Breathing and ventilation
- Circulation and haemorrhage control
- Disability and dysfunction
- Exposure and environment control

management plan. It has been shown that the most efficient resuscitation will occur if a 'horizontal organisation' approach is adopted (Bonnett et al 2003). This is when each member of the team carries out individual tasks simultaneously rather than sequentially (vertical organisation). This reduces the time taken to resuscitate a patient and initiate life-saving procedures, which will improve the patient's chances of survival. All members of the team should have received training in trauma care to ensure that they have the appropriate level of clinical knowledge and skills.

Trauma teams are usually alerted following the advanced notification information from the pre-hospital care staff. If the mechanism of injury and the status of the patient are suggestive of serious traumatic injury the Royal College of Surgeons/British Orthopaedic Association (2000) suggest that a trauma team should be called for:

- trauma victims with any of the following:
  - actual or potential airway compromise
  - signs of a pneumothorax (respiratory distress)
  - SpO_2 <90%
  - heart rate >100/minute (adults)
  - GCS <14 associated with a head injury
  - penetrating wound anywhere from the neck to the thighs
  - any gunshot wound
  - fall from >25 feet/8 metres
  - ejection from a vehicle
- children involved in a traumatic incident:
  - with an altered level of consciousness
  - with a capillary refill time of >3 seconds
  - with tachycardia
  - a pedestrian or cyclist hit by a vehicle.

Initial assessment and management of the patient: the primary and secondary surveys

Initial assessment and management of the trauma patient is usually performed in two stages: the primary survey and later the secondary survey (ACS 2004, Cole 2008).

The primary survey

The initial assessment (primary survey) has five components – 'A, B, C, D, E':

- Airway with cervical spine control
- Breathing and ventilation
- Circulation and haemorrhage control
- Disability and dysfunction
- Exposure and environmental control.

If any life-threatening condition is identified during the process, it is treated before moving on to the next stage. For example, if the patient is found to have a compromised airway, this is stabilised before the patient's breathing and ventilation are assessed. Each component is now discussed in detail.

Airway with cervical spine control

The first step of assessment is to find out if the patient has a patent airway (Box 27.2). Following a traumatic event the airway can become obstructed by bleeding in the mouth, swelling of the face, mouth or oropharynx, a reduced level of consciousness or vomiting and aspiration. Expert anaesthetic help

Box 27.2 Reflection

Emergency airway management

A 35-year-old man has been knocked off his bicycle by a motor vehicle. He appears to have sustained injuries to both legs and is very pale. On arrival to the ED he is drowsy but has a gag reflex. He does not appear to have had a head or face injury.

Activity

- Why is airway assessment and management so important and which airway adjunct should be used to maintain his airway?

should be sought immediately if there is any doubt about the patient's ability to maintain their own airway.

All nurses working with trauma patients should be able to perform a systematic approach to airway management. This is essential, as simple manoeuvres may be all that is required to keep the airway patent until anaesthetic help arrives. The sequential approach to airway assessment involves:

1. *Talking to the patient* – this helps to provide psychological support but also assesses the airway. If the patient is talking freely in a normal voice (i.e. no grunting or hoarseness) then it can be assumed that the airway is patent (Greaves et al 2001b). If there is no response or the patient is making noises from the airway then the next step should be followed.

2. *Look in the mouth* for signs of obstruction, such as vomit or blood. Suction with a rigid suction catheter attached will help to remove any foreign bodies, which once carefully removed may allow the patient to maintain their own airway.

3. *Open the airway* using a jaw thrust technique to pull the tongue and soft palate forward. This is used instead of the head tilt/chin lift because the neck must be kept still whilst the airway is opened as trauma patients are always at risk of a cervical spine injury.

4. *Insert an airway adjunct.* Airway adjuncts should be used in conjunction with an airway opening manoeuvre (jaw thrust) as they will not keep the airway open on their own in the unconscious patient lying supine (Cole 2008). The choice of airway is either an oropharyngeal airway (Guedel) in the unconscious patient without a gag reflex or a nasopharyngeal airway if a gag reflex is present (Greaves et al 2001b).
   a. Oropharyngeal airway. To ensure the correct size, an oropharyngeal airway is measured from the tragus of the ear to the corner of the mouth ('soft to soft') (see Figure 27.2). It is inserted upside down, rotated 180 degrees and then pushed into position. The flange should sit flush with the lips. If the patient gags or coughs during insertion the airway should be removed and a nasopharyngeal airway used instead.
   b. Nasopharyngeal airway. The size of a nasopharyngeal airway is chosen by ensuring that the diameter of the tube is smaller than the diameter of the nostril. The airway should be lubricated prior to introduction and inserted into the nose with a slight twisting motion. Nasopharyngeal airways extend from the nostril to the nasopharynx, with the wider end sitting at the nostril (Cole 2008).

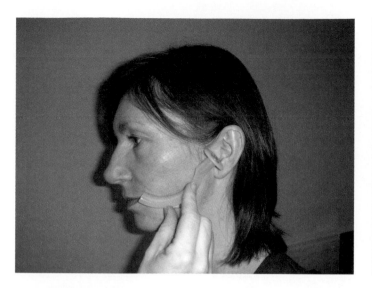

Figure 27.2 How to size an oropharyngeal airway.

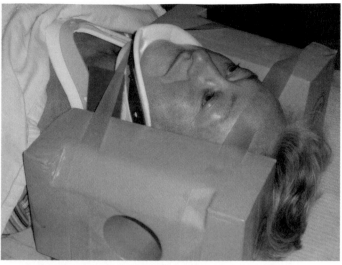

Figure 27.3 Cervical spine immobilisation.

5 *Definitive airway.* For patients who have more serious injuries or are unable to maintain their own airway, it may be necessary to protect the airway definitively. This means a secure airway that can remain in place until the patient is able to maintain their own airway, usually endotracheal intubation. This is done by an anaesthetist who will intubate the patient using a laryngoscope and endotracheal (ET) tube. Usually it will be necessary to sedate and paralyse the patient to facilitate this process. The anaesthetist will require a range of drugs and the nurse assisting with the procedure should be familiar with these and have them ready for immediate use. Once the ET tube is in place, a mechanism for ventilation will be required which must be attached to a high percentage of oxygen via a piped oxygen supply. Ideally, all this equipment should be pre-prepared for rapid use. For patients who have sustained massive facial injuries a surgical airway may be the only way to oxygenate them adequately. This requires specialist equipment (e.g. a scalpel, tracheal dilators, a small tracheostomy tube or ET tube that can be attached to a catheter mount), which should be readily available for immediate use in the ED.

For any trauma patient it is vital that the cervical spine is protected with in-line immobilisation until a senior clinician can rule out a cervical spine injury. This requires a correctly sized semi-rigid collar to be applied to the neck and manual immobilisation. Alternatively head blocks and tape (attached to an immovable part of the trolley) can be applied to immobilise the head and neck (Figure 27.3).

The nurse assisting with maintenance of the patient's airway must be vigilant in observing the patient for any signs of nausea or vomiting. With the cervical spine immobilised, the patient is unable to move. If vomiting is likely, the team will have to log roll the patient to protect the spine (Figure 27.4) and assist the patient with suction apparatus. In this case, an antiemetic should be prescribed and administered urgently.

Breathing and ventilation

The patient's respiratory rate must be measured and recorded to observe for the efficacy of ventilation, i.e. effective gaseous exchange taking place at the alveolar capillary membrane. Assessment should include the rate, depth and use of any accessory muscles (see Ch. 3). All patients who have a faster than expected respiratory rate (tachypnoea) should be considered to have had chest injury until proven otherwise.

Figure 27.4 The log roll technique. (Reproduced with permission from Lisa Hadfield-Law, Oxfordshire, UK.)

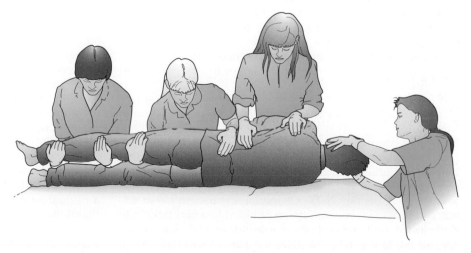

Table 27.1 Classification of major thoracic injury

THE LETHAL SIX	THE HIDDEN SIX
Airway obstruction	Traumatic aortic disruption
Massive haemothorax	Tracheobronchial tree injury
Tension pneumothorax	Oesophageal perforation
Open pneumothorax	Cardiac contusion
Cardiac tamponade	Pulmonary contusion
Flail chest	Diaphragmatic tear or rupture

Table 27.2 Changes in observations in response to haemorrhage

Pulse rate	Tachycardia due to adrenaline and noradrenaline release (tachycardia is an early sign) NB: Patients who are on beta blockers or patients who are very athletic will not appear to be tachycardic, although they may be hypovolaemic
Respiratory rate	Tachypnoea (increased respiratory rate) due to increased oxygen demand and compensatory mechanisms
Level of consciousness	Anxiety or confusion due to the reduction in oxygen delivery to the brain
Capillary refill time	Delayed >2 seconds due to systemic vasoconstriction
Blood pressure	Normal or raised due to compensation: systemic vasoconstriction (hypotension may be a late sign!)
Skin colour	Pale, cool peripheries due to systemic vasoconstriction
Urine output	Reduced urine output and increased urine concentration due to antidiuretic hormone and aldosterone production (part of the compensation process)

All patients who have sustained traumatic injuries are at risk of hypoxia and should receive a high flow of oxygen. This can be delivered via a mask with a reservoir bag (non-rebreathe mask) with a flow rate of 15 L/min (ACS 2004). By the addition of a reservoir bag the patient will receive up to 90% oxygen concentration compared to only 50% oxygen concentration with an ordinary oxygen mask (Resuscitation Council [UK] 2004). Pulse oximetry assists with monitoring of the patient's oxygenation saturation of arterial blood. An arterial blood gas sample may be taken if the patient is hypoxic or hypoventilating so that the clinician can gain an accurate picture of the patient's ventilatory status (Cole 2008).

Trauma patients must have their respiratory observations monitored regularly to detect any deterioration.

Major chest injuries can be divided into those that are immediately life threatening and those that are life threatening but are less obvious and often difficult to diagnose. The two groups of injuries have been described as the Lethal six and the Hidden six (Cole 2008) (see Table 27.1). In most cases the life-threatening chest injuries will need a chest drain inserted as part of the initial treatment. The nurse should be familiar with the equipment and assistance needed for chest drain insertion (see Ch. 3).

Circulation and haemorrhage control

Haemorrhage is the main cause of early trauma deaths (ACS 2004) and can contribute to problems such as clotting disorders or organ failure once the patient has reached definitive care. In severely injured patients hypovolaemia is common and it is the nurse's role to closely assess and monitor for signs of hypovolaemic shock (see Ch. 18). This includes regular measurement and recording of the patient's heart rate, blood pressure, capillary refill time and, where possible, urine output (catheterisation may be necessary to monitor this). Table 27.2 summarises the changes to observations in response to haemorrhage.

It is important to remember that *tachycardia is an early sign of haemorrhage*, whereas alteration of blood pressure is sometimes a later sign. This is because healthy adults and children may compensate during the initial stages of bleeding, and natural production of adrenaline and noradrenaline help to maintain the blood pressure within normal limits until approximately 30% of blood volume has been lost (Matthews & Bentley 2005). Observing the patient's skin colour can provide some indication of blood loss and talking to the patient will indicate their current mental status. The greater the blood loss, the paler the patient will look (in all

skin colours, however pallor may be easier to detect in the oral mucosa of patients with very dark skin) and as oxygen availability decreases in the blood supply, the patient will become increasingly confused, agitated and eventually unconscious (Bonnett et al 2003).

Common sites of haemorrhage following traumatic injury include the chest, the abdominal contents, the pelvis, the shaft of femurs and external haemorrhage from deep wounds. Internal haemorrhage can be difficult to detect by clinical examination and plain X-ray alone. Increasingly, diagnostic imaging such as ultrasound scans (known as FAST: Focussed Assessment with Sonography in Trauma) and computerised tomography (CT) scans are performed in the ED (or as close as possible) so that the source of bleeding can be found quickly. Trauma patients who are bleeding will need to be seen urgently by a senior surgeon to decide whether surgical or conservative treatment is necessary (Cole 2008).

Fluid resuscitation in early trauma The injured patient needs two wide-bore cannula inserted into large veins, such as those found in the crease of the elbow joint (antecubital fossa). At this point blood is taken for full blood count, clotting, urea and electrolytes and blood grouping (and if necessary cross matching for a transfusion). Intravenous fluid therapy may be necessary if the patient is hypovolaemic. Isotonic crystalloid fluids are recommended such as 0.9% saline or Hartmann's solution (ACS 2004). Colloids are not used in the early stages of trauma resuscitation as they have been shown to have a detrimental effect on blood clotting (Brohi et al 2003).

The volume of intravenous fluids required will depend on the cardiovascular status of the patient and the injuries that they have sustained. Traditionally, if a patient is bleeding, intravenous fluids are given to keep their blood pressure at a normal level. However, modern trauma practice suggests that if the patient is given a lot of fluids to maintain the blood pressure then there is a risk of causing clotting problems, hypothermia and further bleeding (Cole 2008). Therefore fluids need to be prescribed and administered following careful consideration of the patient's haemodynamic status and potential injuries. Once intravenous fluids have been commenced it is vital that cardiovascular observations are recorded every 5 minutes to determine whether the patient is responding. A patient who improves following intravenous fluids may not need urgent surgery, whereas a patient who only improves transiently or not at all is unstable and is likely to require an urgent blood transfusion. If the patient's own blood group and rhesus match is not available, O Rh-negative blood (the universal donor) will be used.

Disability and dysfunction: neurological assessment

If the patient has sustained a head injury or has a reduced level of consciousness a neurological assessment should be carried out. This can be done using two methods: AVPU and the Glasgow Coma Scale (GCS).

AVPU This is a simple acronym used to categorise the patient's response and level of consciousness:

* Is the patient Alert?
* Is the patient responding to your Voice?
* Is the patient only responding to Pain?
* Is the patient Unresponsive?

If the patient is anything less than Alert, further investigation should be carried out using the GCS.

Glasgow Coma Scale The Glasgow Coma Scale is an international scale used to assess and score level of consciousness. The patient's eye opening, verbal response and motor function are assessed and given a numerical rating between 3 (the worst score) and 15 (the best score). The nurse should also use a torch to assess the patient's pupils to see if they are equal in size and react to light. This should be documented as a baseline for future comparison. For more information about the Glasgow Coma Scale see Chapter 9.

Blood glucose level At this point, if not already done, a blood glucose measurement should be taken in order to rule out hypoglycaemia or hyperglycaemia as a cause of reduced level of consciousness.

Exposure and environmental control

Whilst the patient's dignity must be preserved as much as is possible, it is essential that all clothing is removed so that the entire body can be examined, front and back, to ensure that no injuries are missed. It is important to remember that exposure can cause rapid body heat loss, so the resuscitation room temperature should be warm enough to preserve the patient's body temperature. Blankets should be replaced between any procedure or examination, to help prevent further temperature drop. The log roll technique (see Figure 27.4) should be used to enable full examination of the patient's spine, and a rectal examination will be performed to assess sphincter tone (which may be altered with a spinal injury) and for signs of pelvic injury.

The secondary survey

The secondary survey is only started when the primary survey is complete and the patient's condition is stabilised. If the patient is critically injured, this secondary survey may not take place in the ED, as the patient is likely to require surgical intervention to stabilise their condition. However, if the patient's condition does permit, then the secondary survey involves a full head-to-toe examination and gives the nurse the opportunity to complete a thorough assessment, documenting wounds (location, surface area and depth), skin integrity, tetanus status, allergies, etc. Any wounds should be thoroughly irrigated. This may be with 0.9% saline or povidone iodine; however, current evidence suggests that potable (drinking) water is just as effective in cleaning traumatic wounds and removing contaminants (Svoboda 2008). Once clean, the wound should be covered with a sterile dressing until closure or exploration can be completed (Cole 2008). Fractured limbs may need to be splinted or immobilised until treatment of more urgent injuries has been carried out.

Pain management

Patients who have suffered traumatic injury will usually experience a great deal of pain. This can occur post injury, during the initial assessment, post operation or whilst recovering in definitive care. Pain is a physiological response to the injury and the stress response to this can have negative effects on the physical well-being of the patient, resulting in tachycardia, hypertension, immobility, etc. (Rayner-Klein & Rowe 2005). Additionally the emotional response to pain can cause altered behaviour which may be affected by previous experiences of pain, culture, fear, etc. It is essential that the nurse asks the patient if they are in pain, and observes for signs of pain such as groaning, facial expressions or a reluctance to move. Analgesics should be prescribed and administered to relieve or reduce the pain and should never be withheld on the grounds that the patient has a head injury or they may affect breathing (Jacobi et al 2002).

In the acute stages of trauma care an intravenous analgesic such as morphine is effective and may be given as a bolus, as an infusion or as patient-controlled analgesia. Once able to tolerate oral medication the patient may be prescribed a weak opioid such as co-codamol and/or a non-steroidal anti-inflammatory such as diclofenac or paracetamol. As well as observing for pain and monitoring the effect of the analgesic, nurses caring for the trauma patient should be aware of the side-effects of opiates such as respiratory depression, nausea and constipation, and ensure that these are prevented or relieved (Box 27.3).

Diagnostic imaging: the nurse's role

Most trauma patients need diagnostic imaging in the early stages of their care and consequently radiographers and radiologists are key members of the trauma service. Diagnostic imaging usually involves X-rays of the cervical spine, chest and pelvis; however, CT scans are increasingly being used to obtain more in-depth images.

At any stage of trauma care, accompanying an unstable or unwell trauma patient to the CT scan needs careful planning and preparation. Moving a patient to, from and within the CT scan is a high-risk procedure, especially if the patient's condition is unstable due to hypovolaemia, a head injury or overwhelming infection. Resuscitation equipment must be taken to and from imaging with the patient, and should include:

- oropharyngeal airways (unless the patient is intubated)
- oxygen – cylinder and masks
- bag-valve – mask device
- cardiac and blood pressure monitoring equipment
- fluids/blood products or medications as prescribed
- patient documentation (notes, charts, etc.) to enable observation recording throughout the procedure.

The nurse should explain to the patient about the need for movement from one area to another and what the CT scan will involve. Privacy, dignity and warmth must be maintained by ensuring that the patient is properly covered. It is also important to ensure that the correct number of staff are available to assist with a log roll (Figure 27.4) or sliding manoeuvre to move the patient to and from the imaging table.

Definitive care

Definitive care refers to the inpatient areas that the patient will be admitted to from the ED or theatres. Definitive care includes intensive care, the high dependency unit or a ward. Transfer between departments can be challenging and resuscitation equipment must accompany the patient (see above). Furthermore, clear communication is essential between the nurses working in each area that the patient may pass through. This will help to ensure that the receiving area has time to prepare for the patient's admission.

Theatres and operative care

Definitive treatment of traumatic injuries often involves surgical intervention (Cole & McGinley 2005). As trauma patients can present to the hospital at any time it is essential that there is an operating theatre available 24 hours a day for trauma emergencies. Trauma surgery, such as an emergency laparotomy to investigate internal bleeding, can be extremely challenging and requires consultant presence

within the operating theatre (Findlay et al 2007). Therefore the trauma theatre nurse or operating department practitioner (ODP) requires an in-depth knowledge of traumatic injuries and the surgery needed in order to assist the surgeon. Skilled theatre nurses are essential to care for the patient before, during and after operative procedures, from checking the patient as they arrive until discharge to the care of a unit or ward nurse. A trauma patient may need to return to theatre on more than one occasion if revision of surgery is needed. The theatre nurse can do much to relieve the anxiety of these patients by providing a reassuring presence and clear communication.

When collecting the patient following trauma surgery it is once again essential that the accompanying nurse has the necessary resuscitation equipment available (see above) to ensure a safe transfer.

Critical care

Many seriously injured patients will need to spend the first part of their definitive care in a critical care setting. This may be in an intensive care unit (ICU) or a high-dependency unit (HDU), depending on the patient's needs and the resources available. Critical care nurses need to be skilled and knowledgeable about caring for trauma patients in a high-technology environment. The remit of critical care in trauma is to provide (Cole & McGinley 2005):

- airway and ventilatory support (including physiotherapy)
- invasive monitoring (e.g. respiratory, cardiovascular, neurological, fluid balance)
- support for organ function when the patient cannot manage independently (e.g. the heart, the kidneys)
- delivery of powerful medication through central intravenous routes, such as inotropic drugs or antiarrhythmics
- pain management
- nutritional management
- maintenance of skin integrity and wound care
- psychosocial support
- care of the dying patient.

In general, a patient requiring intubation and ventilation and having multisystem problems will go to ICU for a period of one-to-one care and support. Surgical HDUs will generally admit patients who are not intubated (usually problems with only one system), but who may require invasive monitoring and organ support with inotropic drugs such as noradrenaline. These drugs help to maintain the blood pressure and preserve renal function in critically ill patients. Patients may also be admitted to HDU after being 'stepped down' from the ICU as their condition improves. For more on critical care see Chapter 29.

Trauma ward

It may be assumed that trauma patients are only cared for in the ED and ICU; however, the trauma patient will often spend the largest amount of their hospital admission on a ward. Trauma ward nurses care for patients with a range of problems including:

- orthopaedic injuries (such as fractures and postoperative care)

- plastics injuries (such as deep wounds, postoperative care and burn management)
- head and face injuries (such as head injury observation following concussion or postoperative care)
- vascular injuries (such as postoperative care or following angiography)
- a combination of these injuries.

Detecting patient deterioration

Considering this, trauma ward nurses need to have excellent assessment and nursing skills to look after a large number of injured patients with differing needs. Patients may deteriorate at any time, days or even weeks following the initial injury, for example following an infection, secondary haemorrhage or clotting problem.

See website Critical thinking question 27.1

In a busy ward environment it can be difficult to identify the deteriorating patient because signs of serious problems developing are often very subtle in the early stages. Therefore early warning systems (sometimes known as Early Warning Scores) need to be in place to assist the nurse in detecting such problems (Box 27.4), and to gain access to senior or specialist help as needed (Department of Health [DH] 2000, Cooper 2004). Early detection of any deterioration is vital to enable timely treatment and prevention of further deterioration. Early identification has been shown to help nurses and medical staff intervene when patients are at high risk of deterioration or death (Goldhill & McNarry 2004).

Rehabilitation

An important part of trauma ward care is to help with the process of rehabilitation, which starts soon after the injury has occurred as the treatment is commenced. This usually involves a multidisciplinary approach with physiotherapists to assist with mobilisation, occupational therapists to assist with functional needs and possibly social workers for financial/social support. The trauma ward nurse's role in rehabilitation may include administering analgesics prior to mobilisation or exercise, ensuring nutrition, hydration and elimination needs are met or working with the other disciplines to help the patient regain independence and confidence prior to discharge. Early links with community support teams are essential to ensure that the patient receives nursing, social care and rehabilitation input on leaving hospital. For more on nursing and rehabilitation see Chapter 32.

Box 27.4 Reflection

Early warning scores

Early warning scores can help nurses to identify the deteriorating patient.

Activity

- Reflect on how you identify a deteriorating patient. Think about which observations you would include in an early warning scoring system and why they are significant. Check your response with: http://student.bmj.com/issues/04/01/education/12.php

Psychological care

Traumatic injury, by the very nature of its mechanism, is nearly always an unexpected event. This means that the patient has no time to prepare for the ill health, incapacity and hospitalisation that will usually ensue. Many trauma patients are in the first four decades of life, and often this is the patient's first experience of inpatient health care, surgery and many other investigations and examinations. Therefore trauma is a very stressful, frightening experience and patients need psychological support and care from the outset (Mohta et al 2003). In the early stages of trauma care the patient may be unconscious, or intubated and sedated. Despite this it is essential that nurses and other members of the health care team talk to the patient, explaining and reassuring as if the patient was conscious. Some patients report flashbacks or nightmares of the events surrounding the injury which can be psychologically debilitating (Cole & McGinley 2005).

Once properly conscious, patients may find it difficult to comprehend what has happened or why they are in hospital; this may be due to their injuries or medication such as opiates. Again, clear, supportive communication is necessary and, if appropriate, non-verbal reassurance such as holding the patient's hand or touching the patient's arm to provide extra reassurance when talking to them. Some trauma patients will need extensive rehabilitation to try to gain either full or partial return to their pre-injury state. Injuries may leave the patient unable to carry out 'normal functions' such as walking and eliminating unaided, participating in sports, etc., and this can be psychologically devastating. Here the contribution of occupational therapists and physiotherapists cannot be underestimated. Moreover, many patients (and possibly their relatives) will need counselling or support from the mental health team to help them cope and come to terms with what has happened and what the future holds for them.

Post-traumatic stress disorder

Post-traumatic stress disorder (PTSD) is a common outcome for patients who have suffered psychological or physical trauma. PTSD causes the patient to suffer from overwhelming anxiety and it is hard for the person to get the trauma out of their mind (ptsduk.co.uk). If left unrecognised and untreated PTSD can have devastating consequences for the patient and the family. Patients can suffer from flashbacks of the injury (or hospital stay), insomnia, nightmares, and terror of facing the cause of the injury (e.g. getting into a car again, or travelling on a train after a train crash). It is difficult to predict who will suffer from PTSD. A recent study looked at severity of injuries compared to development of PTSD (Box 27.5) and suggested that careful community follow-up helps to identify these patients.

Care of relatives of the trauma patient

It is important from the beginning of the trauma patient's care that relatives or next of kin are considered. In the ED and during an operation it may be necessary for the relatives to be separated from their loved one. This can add to an already distressing situation and it is important that trauma

Box 27.5 Evidence-based practice

Post-traumatic stress disorder

Post-traumatic stress disorder (PTSD) is a common outcome following major traumatic injury; however, it is difficult to predict who will suffer from this condition.

A study by Harris et al (2008) aimed to examine the role of physical and psychosocial factors in the development of PTSD following major trauma. During the study period, all adult patients presenting to one major trauma centre in New Zealand with major trauma were identified. Their injury characteristics and clinical data were recorded from the hospital records and the hospital trauma database.

A questionnaire was posted to the patients at intervals between the first and the sixth year following the injury, asking them to complete a PTSD checklist (see below) and supply other data – employment, income, etc. Multiple linear regression (looking at the relationship between variables) was then used to identify significant independent associations with PTSD.

Three hundred and fifty-five patients (61%) responded to the questionnaire. Of those, 129 (36.3%) were classed as having PTSD. Symptoms of PTSD were not significantly related to how severe the injury had been, the time since the injury, education level, household income or employment status at the time of injury. PTSD was significantly associated with younger age, the presence of chronic illnesses, unemployment at the time of follow-up, use of a lawyer to try to settle a claim, blaming others for the injury and having an unsettled compensation claim. The authors concluded that PTSD following major trauma was not related to measures of injury severity, but was related to other factors, such as blaming others for the accident and the processes involved in claiming compensation.

Harris IA, Young JM, Rae H, Jalaludin BB, Solomon MJ 2008 Predictors of post traumatic stress disorder following major trauma. ANZ Journal of Surgery 78(7): 583–587

Significance for practice

Any trauma patient may go on to develop PTSD. As a result, two factors play an important role in their care. First, all major trauma patients who are to be discharged from hospital need to be taught about recognising the signs and symptoms of PTSD, and where to seek help if this occurs. Follow-up clinics should be offered, not only for the review of physical injuries, but also for a review of patients' psychological health and well-being.

Secondly, this study suggests that there is a role for community health and social care teams to provide follow-up for all major trauma patients, with a specific remit of carefully monitoring those patients in the identified high-risk groups. Neither of these initiatives is currently offered as a routine to all trauma patients in the UK.

Organisations such as www.ptsduk.co.uk can offer support and guidance for patients who are at risk of or who have developed PTSD.

For other useful information see: www.nhs.uk/Conditions/Post-traumatic-stress-disorder/Pages/Introduction.aspx?url=Pages/what-is-it.aspx

PTSD Checklist – Civilian Version

Patient's name: _____

Instruction to patient: Below is a list of problems and complaints that people sometimes have in response to stressful life experiences. Please read each one carefully, and, using the scale below, put a figure in the box to indicate how much you have been bothered by that problem in the past week

Not at all (1)

A little bit (2)

Moderately (3)

Quite a bit (4)

Extremely (5)

1. Repeated, disturbing *memories, thoughts, or images* of a stressful experience from the past? ☐
2. Repeated, disturbing *dreams* of a stressful experience from the past? ☐
3. Suddenly *acting* or *feeling* as if a stressful experience *were happening* again (as if you were reliving it)? ☐
4. Feeling *very upset* when *something reminded* you of a stressful experience from the past? ☐
5. Having *physical reactions* (e.g., heart pounding, trouble breathing, or sweating) when *something reminded* you of a stressful experience from the past? ☐
6. Avoid *thinking about* or *talking about* a stressful experience from the past or avoid *having feelings* related to it? ☐
7. Avoid *activities* or *situations* because they *remind you* of a stressful experience from the past? ☐
8. Trouble *remembering important parts* of a stressful experience from the past? ☐
9. Loss of *interest in things that you used to enjoy?* ☐
10. Feeling *distant* or *cut off* from other people? ☐
11. Feeling *emotionally numb* or being unable to have loving feelings for those close to you? ☐
12. Feeling as if your *future* will somehow be *cut short*? ☐
13. Trouble *falling* or *staying asleep*? ☐
14. Feeling *irritable* or having *angry outbursts*? ☐
15. Having *difficulty concentrating*? ☐
16. Being *"super alert"* or watchful or on guard? ☐
17. Feeling *jumpy* or easily startled? ☐

---

nurses use calm, caring and sensitive communication skills when talking to and supporting relatives. Open, honest, clear information is essential, and if the nurse caring for the relatives does not have the answers to questions then a senior member of staff should be sought. If the patient is in the critical care setting or a trauma ward, the relatives may want to participate in their care, and this should be encouraged and supported by the nursing team. The patient's relatives and friends play an important part in recovery and rehabilitation.

Care of relatives of the deceased trauma patient

A difficult situation for the trauma nurse may arise when resuscitative or treatment measures are not going to succeed. If staff know that the resuscitation attempts are likely to be futile and the family is present, it is important that the relatives are gently made aware of the situation by the nurse caring for them, who can outline the gravity of the situation. This provides the family with time, even just a few minutes, to internalise the seriousness of the situation. The decision to stop resuscitation or treatment efforts is a difficult one, and one that should be made after considering individual team members' views with the consultant in charge of the patient's care making the ultimate decision. If the relatives are present, it may be possible to offer them the option of seeing their loved one to say goodbye before the resuscitation efforts are stopped. Many emergency departments and critical care units operate a policy of witnessed resuscitation, where the relatives are allowed to stay at the bedside during resuscitation attempts (Fulbrook et al 2005). Traumatic injuries can be visually distressing and therefore it is important that a nurse or other health care professional stays with the relatives to support them during the process.

Following the death, if relatives wish to see their loved one, nurses can do much to help. If possible, those parts of the body that are exposed should be washed. One or (if possible) both of the deceased's hands should be left outside the sheets. The head of the trolley should be slightly raised; otherwise the face may seem distorted or discoloured when the family first sees the body. False teeth should be replaced if possible and the hair combed or smoothed. Where there are external injuries, bandages or dressings should be left in place and perhaps covered with a clean outer layer. A nurse should initially accompany the relatives, and, if they seem hesitant, can indicate that it is all right for them to touch the body, perhaps by doing so personally or by asking the family members if they wish to hold the loved one's hand. The nurse should then offer to withdraw. Not everyone will want to be left alone, but some may have private words of parting to say and should be given the opportunity to do so. Where a whole family is present, this chance should be given to each person individually. One family member may not feel able to ask for this for themselves, but when it is suggested by the nurse, they may gratefully accept. Relatives should also feel free to hug or kiss the body; in the case of a dead child, the parents should be able to take the child in their arms. This seems to help people to cope with the denial stage of grieving, especially in cases of sudden or traumatic death (Kubler-Ross 1984).

Early traumatic death is always unexpected and differs from an expected death in that the families have not had time to prepare for the event (Meisner 2008). Death at any stage of the patient's care in hospital is a difficult and sad time for relatives. Bereaved people sometimes have difficulty in remembering information so the nurse should consider writing information down or providing pre-prepared information about what has happened and what will happen next (e.g. the potential need for a post-mortem or when the body can be released from hospital). Trauma-related deaths may need to be reported to the coroner to determine the exact cause of death (Meisner 2008).

It is also important that the nurse is aware of the individual's religious and cultural beliefs, following a trauma death. Each health care trust should have direct access to religious ministers from different faiths who can offer advice or, if the family members request it, be present to support them during this difficult period. For more information on trauma-related deaths see Meisner (2008).

Organ and tissue donation following trauma death

Following a trauma-related death in the ED or critical care a family member may indicate to the nurse that the patient carried a donor card or had registered as a donor. It would at that point be appropriate for the consultant in charge of care to be informed and contact made with the local transplant coordinator. The transplant coordinator can then give advice and guidance, and can liaise with UK Transplant regarding would-be recipients. Continuing shortages of organs and tissue for transplantation have resulted in the UK Department of Health issuing a 10-year plan to maximise organ donation which includes looking at ways to recover organs from those who have died suddenly following a cardiac event or trauma (DH 2003).

Organs are most usually taken from patients who have been diagnosed with brain stem death by two senior doctors in the Intensive Care Unit where the potential for donation is recognised and the transplant coordinator is informed while the patient is being ventilated. These are called beating heart donors. In some EDs, patients who die in the department can donate kidneys, tissue and cells. The kidneys are preserved by inserting a femoral cannula and perfusing the kidneys with a preservative fluid. This allows time for family to be contacted and the deceased's wishes to be established. These are called non-heart beating donors (Meisner 2008). Many nurses find the concept of talking to relatives about donation challenging, especially at a time of grief and distress. It is essential that trauma nurses who are involved in this process have been trained to use the appropriate language and have the correct information to give the family.

There are only two conditions where organ donation is completely ruled out. A person cannot become an organ or tissue donor if they have human immunodeficiency virus (HIV) or have, or are suspected of having, Creutzfeldt–Jakob disease (CJD) (Meisner 2008).

Staff stress and grief

It is very difficult for staff (including students) to have worked hard to save a patient's life but without success. Feelings of inadequacy and failure may arise, especially when the patient is young or when the circumstances of the traumatic incident seem senseless. Repeatedly caring for patients and relatives in these circumstances may take its toll, both emotionally and physically, which means that the caregivers themselves may become casualties. It is important, therefore, to consider the grief that will be felt by staff who have been involved with the patient and/or the relatives. There should be a forum for expressing feelings and anxieties within the department. One method is a 'defusing' session which can be described as a short type of crisis intervention for staff involved in such an incident (Wright 1996). It allows staff to talk with one another about the experience in a relaxed atmosphere and provides an opportunity to give all staff the key information relating to the whole episode of the incident. This ventilation of feelings and re-run of events can be of benefit in two ways: it can allow staff to express their emotions, and it can highlight defects in the system or ways of improving practice in the future.

For particularly distressing incidents, a more formal type of debriefing may be required. Critical incident stress debriefing (CISD) (Ireland et al 2008) is a session which may be facilitated by someone who has knowledge of counselling skills. It usually takes place 24–72 h after the event and follows a structured format that focuses on the emotional consequences for staff involved in these types of incidents. Knowledge about stress and coping mechanisms will help staff and students recognise their own limitations and know when they themselves need help. Staff counselling should be offered for those who feel it necessary.

Medico-legal aspects of trauma care

Due to the nature of traumatic injury (road traffic collisions, assault, etc.), nurses are often required to work in close collaboration with the local police force. In order to investigate a traumatic incident or a trauma-related death the police may require information about the patient or clothing/blood samples for forensic evidence. This sometimes creates a conflict in the nurse's professional practice. All patients are entitled to confidentiality in respect of information pertaining to them and it is the nurse's responsibility to ensure that this right is respected (Nursing and Midwifery Council 2008).

There are exceptions where patient confidentiality may be broken because disclosure of information is required by the law, and this affects the public, not just nurses (Meisner 2008). This includes:

- Following a road traffic collision the Road Traffic Act 1991 requires any person to provide the police, when requested, with information that may identify the vehicle driver involved in a collision. The nurse must be sure of the facts as it is not always clear once the patient has arrived in hospital who was the driver.
- Under the Prevention of Terrorism Act 2000 any person who believes a person may have been involved in a terrorist act and has information to support this belief should inform the police.
- A court may order disclosure of information.
- Whilst injury involving firearms does not mandate disclosure, information may be given to the police in the public interest.

The nurse may be required to make a statement about the patient's care or injuries which will form part of the police investigation. It should be noted, however, that it may be several years before a case, whether criminal or civil, comes before the courts and the nurse is asked to write the statement. For this reason it is important that careful attention is paid to accurate documentation within the patient's nursing and medical records.

In the ED it is not uncommon for police officers to ask for a pre-transfusion blood sample to be taken and then given to them. However, unless the hospital has predetermined protocols allowing this, *blood samples must not be handed to police officers without a court order from a judge* (Meisner 2008). In some areas of the UK a police doctor, a forensic medical examiner, may come to the hospital to take blood from the patient.

The police may also ask for patients' clothing or any weapons that may have been brought to hospital. Anything that is handed to the police must be clearly documented in the patient's notes, with the police officer's name and number recorded.

Aggressive situations

A minority of patients (and/or their relatives) who have been involved in a traumatic incident maybe appear to be aggressive or potentially violent. It is important that nurses remember that aggression is seldom directed towards them personally. Many factors can contribute to the feelings of aggression towards a situation or person. These include frustration about the injury and a lack of information either about the condition of a relative or about the excessive waiting times. Waiting rooms in all clinical areas that have poor facilities can contribute to an individual's level of frustration, e.g. shabby decor, uncomfortable seating and an unwelcoming decor. *The attitude of staff to patients, particularly if it appears judgemental and unsympathetic, may contribute to the development of a confrontation between patient or relative and nurse.*

Sometimes the aggression is a result of physiological processes which cause acute confusional or combative states, e.g. pain, hypoxia or a head injury. In these situations the patient has no control over their actions and the cause of the altered mental state should be recognised and, if appropriate, treated.

It is essential that nurses are able to recognise when a patient is becoming aggressive if they are to prevent the situation escalating. Strategies that help to defuse difficult situations include the use of good verbal and non-verbal communication and the adoption of a calm, non-threatening, non-patronising approach. Other strategies include:

- Adopt an open appropriate body posture, arms unfolded, standing or sitting at arm's length away from the patient.
- Listen carefully, demonstrating a genuine interest in what the individual has to say. It is difficult not to shout back when being shouted at, but it is more effective if the pitch, tone and volume of the nurse's voice remain within a normal conversational range.
- Be sympathetic, offer clear explanations and an apology where necessary.
- Try to agree a plan. It is unwise to give false information or agree on solutions that are unachievable, as this will result in trust being lost and may cause further aggression at a later stage.
- Avoid physical risk. Ensure that you are talking in a private yet open environment where escape can be made if necessary.

It is important that, following any incident of aggression or violence, whether verbal or physical, an incident form is completed and that this is reviewed by the Trust risk management team. This monitors the escalating problem and may reveal patterns of aggression in the workplace, thereby allowing preventive strategies to be formulated. These may include education opportunities for the staff on communication and defusing techniques. If it is apparent that there is an increase in violent and aggressive situations, statistical evidence is useful when making a bid to management staff for more security staff or better protection.

Mass casualty trauma care: major incidents

Some traumatic incidents, such as a transport crash or a bomb blast, will involve more than one or two people. When considering large numbers of traumatically injured people that need immediate medical care, the term 'major incident' is used. There is no one standard definition of a major incident; however, Mackway-Jones & Carley (2005) suggest the following:

A major incident is an event, that owing to the number, severity, type or location of live casualties requires special arrangements (above and beyond the normal) to be made by the emergency and health services.

Most definitions are deliberately non-specific because what constitutes a major incident for a small rural hospital may have minimal impact in a large urban hospital. Similarly a large-scale disaster may affect only one hospital or may require the services of several hospitals within a region. The purpose of *emergency preparedness* (also known as emergency planning) for such situations within the NHS is to ensure that all the emergency services are able to work collaboratively and provide an effective response to any type of incident.

The increased risk of global terrorism has resulted in the planning for dealing with and preparing for major incidents having not only had to be re-thought (Hayward 2003) but re-appraised with each new incident, such as the London bombings in July 2005. It is essential that every hospital has a major incident plan, including a chemical decontamination plan (DH 2005, London Emergency Services Liaison Panel [LESLP] 2007). The ED plays a major role in this, as it is required to provide the rapid initial response. However, most of the departments and services within a hospital also have a role to play in a major incident. Ward and critical care areas will need to discharge or transfer patients quickly to make bed space available for the major incident patients. All routine surgery and clinics should be immediately cancelled so that theatre space and personnel are available for emergency surgery. Extra intravenous fluids, blood products, medication and other equipment will be urgently needed, with porters or runners available to transport these vital supplies. Non-clinical staff will provide essential roles for registering and admitting patients, maintaining communication networks, and providing support for patients being discharged and their relatives.

Types of major incident include:

- transport (train, aeroplane, motor vehicle crashes)
- explosions (industrial or bomb blasts)
- industrial incidents (explosions, fire, chemical leaks)
- sporting/entertainment events where large numbers of people are gathered (e.g. Hillsborough stadium disaster)
- environmental – natural (e.g. tsunami or earthquake) or collapse of a building or infrastructure
- chemical/biological spillages or deliberate releases
- radiation or nuclear incidents.

In the event of an incident, the police, fire service, ambulance service or local emergency planning officers may declare a major incident. In a large-scale incident where many casualties are predicted, more than one hospital will be involved in the response. The ED will be notified by the police or the local ambulance service, and informed of the type of incident that they are dealing with and the predicted number of patients. Usually, the nurse who receives the call will declare a hospital major incident through an emergency switchboard number. In order to prepare to receive the casualties, the department will be cleared as quickly as possible, restocking principal areas with extra equipment, such as decontamination equipment if dealing with a chemical incident, whilst calling in extra staff. Simultaneously, other areas and departments need to prepare to receive patients according to their local major incident plans.

The ED may be asked to provide an on-site mobile medical team (MMT). The MMT provided will depend on the local plan, and resources available at the hospital. Usually there will be some ED nurses, an ED doctor, a surgeon and an anaesthetist. However, in some areas there are dedicated pre-hospital care teams allied to a hospital (such as the Helicopter Emergency Medical Service in London) who will provide the MMT. It is vital that these staff are adequately trained in their role (DH 2005) and equipped with correct personal protective equipment as they will be required to support the ambulance service in difficult and potentially dangerous environments, such as a chemical or radiation spillage (Hayward 2003). If the major incident has a chemical, biological, radiological or nuclear (CBRN) involvement then ideally no casualty should leave the scene of the incident until they have been thoroughly decontaminated by the ambulance and/or fire service. Inevitably, some casualties may 'slip through the net' and will require immediate decontamination on arrival to the hospital; therefore all ED personnel should be trained and practised in decontamination procedures (DH 2005).

Due to the volume of patients, it is important that careful attention is paid to adequate identification of all individuals. The police documentation team, which will be based in the hospital, should operate a 'casualty bureau', where all information regarding patients is collated. Members of the public can contact the bureau for further information regarding casualties. The hospital staff will have to keep this unit updated with details of patients. Many relatives will arrive at the hospital seeking information and the media will require regular press statements, as in all public interest events. It is important that this does not interrupt the care of the patients. The hospital will need to ensure that adequate facilities and support staff are in place to care for friends and relatives waiting to see the injured, whilst establishing separate communication networks for the media. Once all the casualties have been cared for and transferred to other areas for their definitive care, the ED must resume its customary work as soon as possible. However, the hospital will probably remain on major incident alert as the patients may require hours of surgery following injury and days in the critical care or ward areas. All of this will disrupt the normal flow of a hospital and the impact of this cannot be underestimated.

Major incidents are not just an ED problem. The whole hospital or health care trust will usually have a role to play. Trauma nurses *must* know their role in a major incident,

Box 27.6 Reflection

The nurse's role in a major incident

A major incident can happen at any time. As a student nurse you may be on duty as a major incident is declared in your hospital. Would you know what to do?

Activity

Where is the major incident and chemical decontamination plan held in your hospital? Ask your mentor or link lecturer if you may see the plan, read the relevant local section and have an opportunity to discuss its content.

- **Reflect** on how you can apply this knowledge to the care of your patients.
- **Discuss** your learning with your mentor/supervisor, lecturer and colleagues.

regardless of the clinical setting in which they work (Box 27.6). Because of the relative infrequency of major incidents and the pattern of staff changes, it is recommended that hospitals carry out regular major incident exercises such as table top exercises or simulated incidents, together with the ambulance and other emergency services, so as to ensure a rapid and effective response (DH 2005).

SUMMARY: KEY NURSING ISSUES

- The trauma assessment framework 'A, B, C, D, E' is known as the primary survey: this helps to detect injuries and problems in the early stages of trauma care.
- Hypoxia and haemorrhage are common life-threatening problems for trauma patients.
- It is essential that nurses can identify abnormal observations, detect potential problems and access appropriate help promptly to avoid the patient deteriorating.
- Transferring or transporting trauma patients is a high-risk procedure that needs careful planning, preparation and the correct equipment.
- Trauma is a true multidisciplinary specialty where nurses work closely with medical staff, therapists, radiographers, etc. to ensure optimal care for the patient.
- Traumatic death is usually sudden and unexpected. This means that the nurse liaising with the patient's family should have clear, supportive communication skills.
- Trauma often has medico-legal implications and there are times when, by law, the patient's confidentiality has to be breached without their permission. The nurse must be absolutely certain of the facts before doing this.
- Major incident events resulting in large numbers of trauma patients need to be carefully planned for and practised.

REFLECTION AND LEARNING – WHAT NEXT?

- **Test** your knowledge by visiting the website and answering the multiple choice questions and critical thinking questions.
- **Consolidate** your learning by looking at some of the further reading suggestions, references and specialist websites.
- **Revisit** some of the additional material on the website.
- **Consider** what you have learnt and how this will help your professional development.

REFERENCES

American College of Surgeons: *Advanced trauma life support program for physicians*, ed 7, Chicago, 2004, American College of Surgeons.

Anderson ID, Woodford M, De Dombal FT, et al: Retrospective study of 1000 trauma deaths in England and Wales, *Br Med J* 296:1305–1308, 1988.

Bickerton J, Dewan V, Allan T: Streaming A&E patients to walk in centre service, *Emerg Nurse* 13(3):20–23, 2005.

Bonnett R, Gwinnutt C, Driscoll P: *Trauma resuscitation. The team approach*, ed 2, London, 2003, Taylor and Francis.

Brohi K, Singh J, Heron M, Coats T: Acute traumatic coagulopathy, *Journal of Trauma, Injury, Infection and Critical Care* 54(6):1127–1130, 2003.

Chiara O, Cimbanassi S, Pitidis A, Vesconi S: Preventable trauma deaths: from panel review to population based-studies, *World Journal of Emergency Surgery* 2006. Available online http://www.wjes.org/content/1/1/12.

Cole E, editor: *Trauma Care: Initial assessment and management of the trauma patient in the ED*, Oxford, 2008, Wiley-Blackwell.

Cole E, Crichton N: The culture of a trauma team in relation to human factors, *J Clin Nurs* 15:1257–1266, 2006.

Cole E, McGinley A: A structured approach to caring for the trauma patient. In O'Shea R, editor: *Principles and practice of trauma nursing*, Edinburgh, 2005, Elsevier, pp 37–60.

Cooper N: *Acute care: recognising critical illness*, 2004. Available online http://student.bmj.com/issues/04/01/education/12.php.

Department of Health: *Comprehensive critical care – a review of adult critical care services*, London, 2000, HMSO.

Department of Health: *Saving lives, valuing donors – a transplant framework for England*, London, 2003, HMSO.

Department of Health: *Emergency preparedness division*, 2005. Available online http://www.dh.gov.uk/en/Publicationsandstatistics/Publications/PublicationsPolicyAndGuidance/DH_4121072.

Eaton J: Kinetics and mechanics of injury. In O'Shea R, editor: *Principles and practice of trauma nursing*, Edinburgh, 2005, Elsevier, pp 15–35.

Eckes-Roper J: *Trauma Nursing Secrets*, Philadelphia, 2003, Hanley & Belfus.

Findlay G, Martin IC, Carter S, Smith N, Weyman D, Mason M: *Trauma: who cares? A report on the National Confidential Enquiry into Patient Outcome and Death (NCEPOD)*, London, 2007, NCEPOD, pp 10–14.

Fulbrook P, Albarran JW, Latour JM: A European survey of critical care nurses attitudes and experiences of having family members present during cardiopulmonary resuscitation, *Int J Nurs Stud* 42(5):557–568, 2005.

Goldhill DR, McNarry AF: Physiological abnormalities in early warning scores are related to mortality in adult inpatients, *Br J Anaesth* 92(6):882–884, 2004.

Greaves I, Porter KM, Ryan JM, editors: Mechanism of injury *Trauma Care Manual*, London, 2001a, Arnold, pp 99–114.

Greaves I, Porter KM, Ryan JM, editors: Patient assessment. *Trauma Care Manual*, London, 2001b, Arnold, pp 18–32.

Harris IA, Young JM, Rae H, Jalaludin BB, Solomon MJ: Predictors of post traumatic stress disorder following major trauma, *ANZ J Surg* 78(7):583–587, 2008.

Hayward M: Pre-hospital response to major incidents, *Nurs Stand* 17(30):37, 2003.

Ireland S, Gilchrist J, Maconochie I: Debriefing after failed paediatric resuscitation: a survey of current UK practice, *Emerg Med J* 25:328–330, 2008.

Jacobi J, Fraser GL, Coursin DB: Clinical practice guidelines for the sustained use of sedatives and analgesics in the critically ill adult, *Crit Care Med* 30:119–141, 2002.

Kubler-Ross E: *On death and dying*, London, 1984, Tavistock.

London Emergency Services Liaison Panel: *Major incident procedure manual*, ed 7, 2007. Available online http://www.leslp.gov.uk/docs/major_incident_procedure_manual_7th_ed.pdf.

Mackway-Jones K, Carley S: *Major Incident Medical Management and Support. The practical approach in the hospital*, Oxford, 2005, Blackwell.

Matthews W, Bentley P: Applied biochemistry pertaining to the trauma patient. In O'Shea R, editor: *Principles and practice of trauma nursing*, Edinburgh, 2005, Elsevier, pp 119–128.

Meisner S: Trauma related deaths. In Cole E, editor: *Trauma Care: Initial assessment and management of the trauma patient in the ED*, Oxford, 2008, Wiley-Blackwell.

Middlehurst T: Mechanism of injury. In Cole E, editor: *Trauma Care: Initial assessment and management of the trauma patient in the ED*, Oxford, 2008, Wiley-Blackwell.

Mohta M, Sethi AK, Tyagi A, Mohta A: Psychological care in trauma patients, *Injury* 34(1):17–25, 2003.

Noble-Mathews PM: Pre-hospital care. In O'Shea R, editor: *Principles and practice of trauma nursing*, Edinburgh, 2005, Elsevier, pp 61–70.

Nursing and Midwifery Council (NMC): *NMC code of professional conduct: standards for conduct, performance and ethics*, London, 2008, NMC.

Rayner-Klein J, Rowe CA: Analgesia and anaesthesia. In O'Shea R, editor: *Principles and practice of trauma nursing*, Edinburgh, 2005, Elsevier, pp 119–128.

Resuscitation Council (UK): *Advanced life support course. Provider manual*, ed 4, London, 2004, Resuscitation Council (UK).

RoSPA: *RoSPA safety and risk education*, 2008. Available online http://www.rospa.co.uk/safetyeducation/index.htm.

Royal College of Surgeons of England and British Orthopaedic Association: *Joint Report Better care for the severely injured*, London, 2000, RCS.

Svoboda SJ, Owens BD, Gooden HA, Melvin ML, Baer DG, Wenke JC: Irrigation with potable water versus normal saline in a contaminated musculoskeletal wound model, *Journal of Trauma – Injury Infection and Critical Care* 64(5):1357–1359, 2008.

WHO: *Injury-related disability and rehabilitation*, 2008. Available online http://www.who.int/violence_injury_prevention/disability/en/.

Wright B: *Sudden death: a research base for practice*, ed 2, Edinburgh, 1996, Churchill Livingstone.

FURTHER READING

Cole E, editor: *Trauma Care: Initial assessment and management of the trauma patient in the ED*, Oxford, 2008, Wiley-Blackwell.

NCEPOD Trauma: who cares: http://www.ncepod.org.uk/2007report2/Downloads/SIP_summary.pdf.

USEFUL WEBSITES

The Brain Trauma Foundation: www.braintrauma.org

Trauma.org: www.trauma.org

Nursing the unconscious patient

Catheryne Waterhouse

Introduction

The unconscious patient presents a special challenge to the nurse. Medical management will vary according to the original cause of the patient's condition, but nursing care will be constant. The unconscious patient is completely dependent on the nurse to manage all their activities of daily living and to monitor their vital functions.

High-quality nursing care is crucial if the patient is to relearn to perceive self and others, to communicate, to control their body and environment and to become independent. The nurse must have a good understanding of the mechanisms that can contribute to unconsciousness, as well as a sound knowledge of the potential and actual physiological, psychological and social problems that these patients may face in the future.

Not all patients will make a complete recovery; some will die and others will be left with varying degrees of physical and cognitive disability. The nurse plays a pivotal role working with the multidisciplinary team to plan, implement and evaluate specific treatment regimens, whilst providing emotional support and reassurance to the patient and their relatives.

Defining consciousness

Normal conscious behaviour is dependent upon the functioning of the higher cerebral hemispheres and an intact reticular activating system (see below). Impaired, reduced or absent consciousness implies the presence of brain dysfunction and demands urgent medical attention. In order to appreciate the importance of altered states of consciousness, a basic understanding of the physiology of consciousness is required.

Hickey (2003) defines consciousness simply as 'a state of general awareness of oneself and the environment' and includes the ability to orientate towards new stimuli. The individual is awake, alert and aware of their personal identity and of the events occurring in their surroundings. Deep coma, the opposite of consciousness, is diagnosed when the patient is unrousable and unresponsive to external stimuli; there are varied states of altered consciousness in between the two extremes (Box 28.1). Even during normal sleep, an individual can be roused by external stimuli, in comparison to the person in a coma.

Anatomical and physiological basis for consciousness

The reticular formation (RF) and the reticular activating system (RAS) (Figure 28.1) are responsible for collating and transmitting motor and sensory activities and controlling sleep/waking cycles and consciousness.

The reticular formation (RF)

The RF is a network of neurones within the brain stem (Waugh & Grant 2001) that connect with the spinal cord, cerebellum, thalamus and hypothalamus. The RF is involved in the coordination of skeletal muscle activity, including voluntary movement, posture and balance, as well as automatic and reflex activities that link with the limbic system.

The reticular activating system (RAS)

The RAS is a physiological component of the RF and the neurones which radiate via the thalamus and hypothalamus to the cerebral cortex and ocular motor nuclei. It is concerned with the arousal of the brain in sleep and wakefulness (Marieb 2004). Two main parts have been identified (Guyton & Hall 2000): the mesencephalon and the thalamus.

The mesencephalic area is composed of grey matter and lies in the upper pons and midbrain of the brain stem. Stimulation produces a diffuse flow of nerve impulses which pass upwards through the thalamus and hypothalamus, radiating out across the cerebral cortex to provoke a general increase in cerebral activity and wakefulness (see Figure 28.1). Signals from different areas in the thalamus initiate selective activity in the cortex protecting the higher centres from sensory overload (Marieb 2004). The reticular nucleus, which receives impulses from the RF, surrounds the front and sides of the thalamus. It is this nucleus that sends inhibiting messages back to the thalamic nuclei using the neurotransmitter γ-aminobutyric acid (GABA).

In order to function, the RAS must be stimulated by input signals from a wide range of sources. These are transmitted via the spinal reticular tracts and various collateral tracts from all the modalities of sensation, e.g. the specialised auditory and visual tracts (see Ch. 9). The RAS is also affected by signals from the cerebral cortex, i.e. the RAS may first stimulate the cerebral cortex, and the cortical areas responding to reason and emotion may 'modify' the RAS, either positively or negatively, according to the 'decision' of the cerebral cortex.

Sleep is induced by a hormone called melatonin which is synthesised from serotonin in the pineal gland. When an individual is in a deep sleep, the RAS is in a dormant state. However, almost any type of sensory signal can immediately activate the RAS and waken the individual, for example when daylight is detected by the retina of the eye, impulses are sent to the suprachiasmatic nucleus of the hypothalamus, activating sympathetic nerve fibres that will inhibit the secretion of melatonin in the pineal gland. This is called the 'arousal reaction' and is the mechanism by which sensory stimuli wake us

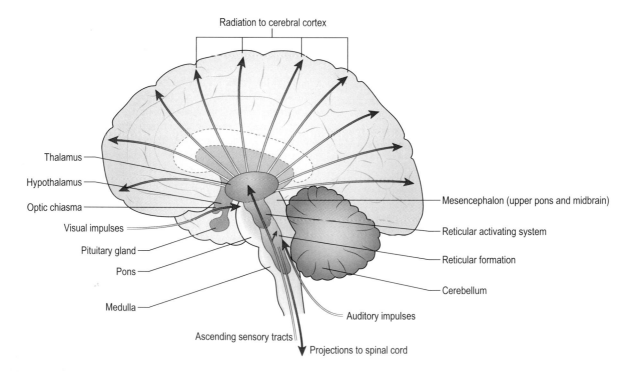

Figure 28.1 Mid-sagittal section of the brain, showing the reticular activating system and related structures.

from deep sleep (Guyton & Hall 2000). Lesions in this area can cause excessive sleepiness or even coma (Fitzgerald 1996).

There are numerous pathways to both mesencephalic and thalamic areas, arising from the sensory, motor and cortical regions of the cerebral cortex, that deal with a range of emotions. Whenever any of these areas becomes excited, impulses are transmitted into the RAS, thus increasing its activity. This is termed a 'positive feedback response'.

The feedback theory

The cerebrum regulates incoming information by a positive feedback mechanism (Guyton & Hall 2000). A second feedback cycle that stimulates proprioceptors in skeletal muscles is also shown in Figure 28.2.

After a prolonged period of wakefulness, the synapses in the feedback loops become increasingly fatigued, reducing the level of stimulation and activity directed to the reticular activating system and thereby inducing a state of lethargy, drowsiness and eventually sleep (Guyton & Hall 2000).

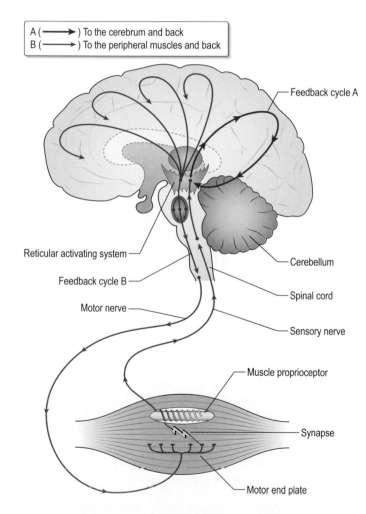

A (——→) To the cerebrum and back
B (——→) To the peripheral muscles and back

Feedback cycle A

Reticular activating system

Cerebellum

Feedback cycle B

Spinal cord

Motor nerve

Sensory nerve

Muscle proprioceptor

Synapse

Motor end plate

Figure 28.2 The feedback mechanism, showing two feedback cycles passing through the RAS. In cycle A, the RAS excites the cerebral cortex and the cortex in turn re-excites the RAS. This initiates a cycle that causes continued intense excitation of both regions. In cycle B, impulses are sent down the spinal cord to activate skeletal muscles. Activation of the muscle stimulates proprioceptors to transmit sensory impulses upward to re-excite the RAS. Consciousness results when the RAS, in turn, stimulates the cerebral cortex.

Box 28.2 Reflection

Causes of altered conscious level

The clinical condition of unconsciousness is one of complex physiology. Review the contributory causes of altered consciousness shown in Figure 28.3 and consider the underlying mechanism for each of them.

Figure 28.2 illustrates a number of activating pathways passing from the mesencephalon upwards.

The content of consciousness

The content of consciousness refers to the sum of cognitive and affective mental functions. It is dependent upon relatively intact functional areas within the cerebral hemispheres that interact with each other as well as with the RAS (Box 28.2).

Injury to, or disease of, the cerebral hemispheres may cause diffuse damage that can inhibit or block the signals from the RAS, depressing the level of consciousness. The damaged cortex is unable to interpret the incoming sensory impulses and therefore cannot transmit them to other areas for appropriate action.

Localised damage to the cerebral hemispheres can affect consciousness to a lesser degree. For example, a patient who has aphasia caused by a stroke may appear awake and alert; however, their inability to understand or to use language may decrease their full awareness of self and their environment. Such localised defects are not generally regarded as a true altered state of consciousness, but this example highlights the difficulties in defining true conscious behaviour.

States of impaired consciousness

There is no international definition of levels of consciousness but, for assessment purposes, differing states of consciousness can be considered on a continuum between full consciousness and deep coma (Hickey 2003) (see Box 28.1). Consciousness cannot be measured directly but can be estimated by observing behaviour in response to stimuli. The Glasgow Coma Scale (GCS) (Teasdale 1975) is widely used as an assessment tool and helps to reduce subjectivity during assessment of conscious level (see p. 741).

Impaired states of consciousness can be categorised as acute or chronic. Acute states, for example drug or alcohol intoxication, are potentially reversible whereas chronic states tend to be irreversible as they are caused by invasive or destructive brain lesions. Deterioration or improvement will depend on a number of factors such as the mechanism, extent and site of injury, age, previous medical history and length of coma. Common causes of altered level of consciousness are illustrated in Figure 28.3 (see www.headway. org.uk).

Signs of deterioration in a patient's level of consciousness are usually the first indications of further impending brain damage. The nurse must be able to assess and observe the patient accurately so that appropriate intervention can be instituted if the level of consciousness deteriorates. Signs and symptoms may include:

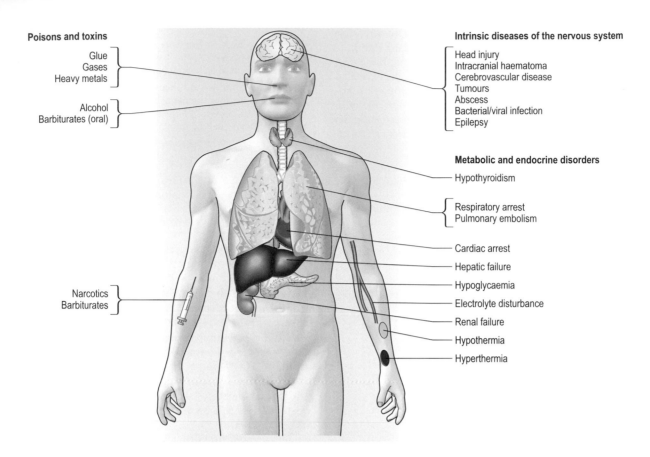

Figure 28.3 Common causes of unconsciousness.

- reduced awareness
- delirium
- illusions
- hallucinations
- delusions
- stupor
- coma.

Reduced awareness

Reduction in awareness reflects generalised brain dysfunction, as seen in systemic and metabolic disorders (see Figure 28.3). These disorders interfere with the integrity of the RAS, affecting the patient's arousal response.

In the early stage, subtle changes may occur in the patient's behaviour. They may exhibit signs of hyper-excitability and irritability, alternating with drowsiness, progressing to confusion and increased levels of disorientation. Minor disturbance such as irritability can easily go undetected and comments from a relative such as 'she does not seem to recognise me today' may denote a subtle change in behaviour that requires further investigation. Martin (1994) suggests that nurses who are expert in the care of head-injured patients can identify cues which indicate behavioural, cognitive, motor and sensory changes even in mild brain dysfunction.

Any new or acute change from the patient's normal baseline behaviour must be reported and documented. The patient's nursing care plan will also need to be re-evaluated and new goals for care set.

Cognitive disabilities, e.g. poor concentration or short-term memory problems, may only become apparent when a patient returns home. These can cause emotional distress for both the patient and family, particularly if they go unheeded and help is not provided. The primary care team plays a major role in supporting patients following acquired brain injury, facilitating referral to specialist agencies (see www.bann.org.uk).

Delirium

Delirium is a fluctuating mental state characterised by confusion, disorientation, fear and irritability. The patient may be talkative, loud, offensive, suspicious or extremely agitated. This behaviour reflects generalised brain dysfunction due to interference with the RAS, affecting the arousal mechanism (Siddiqi et al 2007). Patients will present with a range of symptoms including:

- *Illusions* – these are defined as misinterpretations of sensory material in the patient's environment. For example, a shadow on the wall may be perceived as an animal or a person; a noise can be misinterpreted as voices from strangers who have come to harm them.
- *Hallucinations* – these are defined as seeing or hearing something in the absence of the relevant sensory stimuli; for example, the patient will hear voices when no-one is present or see objects that do not exist in their environment. Other senses, such as touch, taste or smell, can also be affected.

- *Delusions* – these are defined as persistent misperceptions that are firmly held by a person, even though they are illogical or contrary to reality. Such illusions and hallucinatory experiences are common in patients with temporal lobe epilepsy (see Ch. 9). Perceptual disturbances and delusions can also occur in patients exposed to sensory deprivation or overload, e.g. in intensive care units or in sleep deprivation (Phipps et al 1999, Jones et al 2001, Hewitt 2002).

Delirium is very distressing for the patient and their relatives who may witness their altered behaviour. Early diagnosis and treatment with medication, and environmental changes such as reducing noise or sensory input may help to alleviate some of the symptoms.

Stupor

The term stupor describes a state whereby the patient is quiet and tends not to move, except in response to vigorous and repeated noxious stimuli (Hickey 2003).

Coma

Coma is an impaired state where the patient is totally unaware of themselves and their environment. It may vary in degree but in its worse stage, no reaction of any kind is obtainable from the patient. Always assume that an unconscious patient is able to hear and understand what you say, particularly if you need to discuss sensitive issues with their relatives. Hearing can often be the last sense to be lost and the first one to come back before they are able to respond.

Chronic states of impaired consciousness

The chronic states of impaired consciousness tend to be irreversible as they are caused by invasive or destructive brain lesions. They are:

- dementia
- vegetative state
- locked-in syndrome.

Dementia

This condition is caused by a generalised and progressive loss of cortical tissue in the brain. Mental functions progressively decline with global deterioration of memory, thought processes, motor performance, emotional responsiveness and social behaviour.

As the condition develops, speech and communication becomes difficult and behaviour becomes increasingly inappropriate until control of basic and vital processes is completely disorganised. Alzheimer's disease is the most prevalent type of progressive dementia but there are numerous other causes.

Although dementia is an irreversible condition, new drug therapies such as donepezil (Aricept®) are being used successfully to delay onset of the disease. Patients with normal pressure hydrocephalus may be helped by insertion of a ventricular shunt (Wilson & Islam 2004, Dalvi 2010; see also Life NPH in Useful websites, p. 756).

Vegetative state

Vegetative state (VS) is a term used to describe a condition that may occur following a severe brain injury, where there is extensive damage to the cerebral cortex. Although the patient has sleep/waking cycles, the higher centres of the brain are destroyed. Physiologically, the brain stem is functioning but the cerebral cortex is not, and patients can survive for several years requiring full-time nursing care. The British Medical Association (1996) recommends 'that the diagnosis of irreversible Permanent Vegetative State (PVS) should not be considered or confirmed (and therefore treatment not be withdrawn) until the patient has been insentient for 12 months'. Some neuro-rehabilitation units use a structured technique for assessing various sensory aspects of communication, movement awareness and wakefulness, known as SMART (sensory modality assessment and rehabilitation technique – www.smart-therapy.org.uk/), to enable clinicians to make a more accurate diagnosis of patients they suspect may be in PVS.

There is ongoing debate, both in the UK and other countries, about the moral, ethical and legal issues surrounding the care and treatment of these individuals and the dilemma posed by some patients to 'the right to die' and withdrawal of treatment has received considerable professional, public and political attention over recent years (Porter 2005) (see www.ethics-network.org.uk).

Locked-in syndrome

This occurs when there is damage to the pons in the brain stem, resulting from cerebral vascular disease or trauma, paralysing voluntary muscles without interfering with consciousness and cognitive functions. The patient is unable to speak and is sometimes unable to breathe spontaneously, the latter requiring mechanical ventilation and respiratory support. However, the patient is able to control vertical eye movements and blinking and may be able to use these movements to develop a simple communication system. It is important to remember that the patient is cognitively aware, even if they appear to be mentally and physically inert. For further information about PVS and locked-in syndrome, see Randall (1997), Smith (1997) and Royal College of Physicians (2003).

Assessment of the nervous system

The need to assess conscious level may arise at any time, in any ward, in any hospital. In 1974, Teasdale and Jennett developed the Glasgow Coma Scale (GCS), a process used throughout the UK and worldwide as part of the neurological assessment and ongoing observation of the patient (see Figure 28.4). It provides a standardised approach to observing and recording adverse changes in the patient's level of consciousness, so that appropriate action can be taken (National Institute for Health and Clinical Excellence [NICE] 2003) (Box 28.3).

The Neurological Observation Chart

The Glasgow Coma Scale

When monitoring the patient's conscious level, the functional state of the brain is assessed as a whole. The nurse observes and describes three aspects of the patient's behaviour:

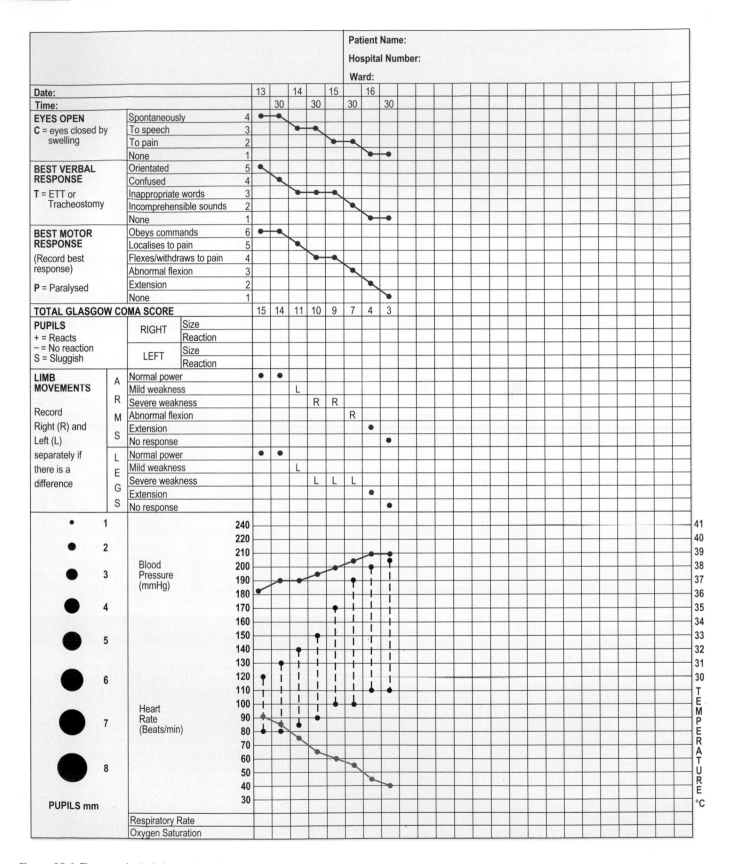

Figure 28.4 The neurological observation chart.

Box 28.3 Evidence-based practice

Head injury: triage, assessment, investigation and early management of head injury in infants, children and adults

The National Institute for Health and Clinical Excellence (NICE) developed clinical guidelines for 'Head injury: triage, assessment, investigation and early management of head injury in infants, children and adults' (2003), revised 2005. The documentation made recommendations for best practice including:

- pre-hospital management
- CT scanning based on presenting signs and symptoms
- frequent and consistent neurological assessment to identify early signs of neurological deterioration
- prompt referral and transfer to a specialist tertiary neurosurgical centre
- early identification and clearance of cervical spine fractures
- identification of non-accidental injuries
- discharge and advice about long-term problems and support services.

www.nice.org.uk/guidance/cg/published

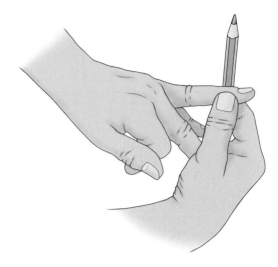

Figure 28.5 Applying a peripheral painful stimulus: fingertip stimulation.

- eye opening
- verbal response
- motor response.

Each of these is independently assessed and recorded on a chart (Figure 28.4). The patient's response is recorded with a dot joined with straight lines to form a graph, making it easier to assess whether the patient is improving or deteriorating. The frequency of recording will be based on the patient's clinical condition. The best response for each of the three aspects is recorded as a numerical score. In the case of eye opening, the best response would score a 4, the best verbal response would score a 5 and the best motor responses would score a 6. The lowest response for each of the three parameters is a score of 1. Thus the highest total score is 15 and the lowest is 3.

A score of 15 indicates that the patient is alert, orientated and able to obey commands; a score of 8 or less is generally considered to indicate that the patient is in a coma. However, it is important to consider each of the three responses (eye opening, verbal response and motor response) separately, taking into consideration any communication difficulties (e.g. deafness or paralysis) or if the patient is receiving muscle relaxants.

Eye opening

This assesses the integrity of the RAS in the brain stem and is observed and recorded using the following categories.

Spontaneously = scores 4. The patient opens their eyes when first approached, which implies that the arousal response is active.

To speech = scores 3. The nurse should speak to the patient by calling their name and asking them to open their eyes. It may be necessary to increase the level of the verbal stimulation to gain a reaction.

To pain = scores 2. A gentle shake of the patient's shoulder may be sufficient to elicit a response. If the patient still fails to open their eyes, a painful stimulus must be used. Pressure

is applied to the lateral inner aspect of the second or third finger using a pen or pencil, for a maximum of 15 seconds (Figure 28.5). Nail bed pressure is contraindicated as it will cause excessive bruising.

None = scores 1 . If the painful stimulus does not elicit any response from the patient this indicates a deep depression of the arousal system and the patient is recorded as having no eye opening.

Possible assessment problems The patient who is in a deep coma with flaccid eye muscles will show no response to stimulation. However, if the eyelids are drawn back, the eyes may remain open. This is very different from spontaneous eye opening and should be recorded as 'none'.

The nurse needs to be aware if the patient has any hearing deficits because if their eyes are closed, this will affect the initial response. Congenital deficits of the eye or previous enucleation (see Ch. 13) must also be taken into account. Inability to open the eyes due to bilateral orbital oedema, tarsorrhaphy (where upper and lower eyelids are sutured together), or ptosis (palsy of cranial nerve III) should be recorded as 'C' (closed) on the chart.

Opening of the eyes implies arousal, but it must be remembered that this does not necessarily mean that the patient is aware of their surroundings. This can be misleading and be a source of false optimism for relatives.

Verbal response

This assesses the area of the brain associated with receptive and expressive speech.

Orientated = scores 5. Patients are assessed as orientated in person, place and time if they can state their name, where they are and what the year and month are. Avoid asking them to state the day or the date as they are not easily remembered, especially after a period of time in hospital.

Confused = scores 4. The patient is able to produce phrases or sentences but the conversation is rambling and inappropriate to the questions being asked.

Inappropriate words = scores 3. The patient offers monosyllabic words, usually in response to physical stimulation. The words and phrases make little or no sense and may express obscenities.

Incomprehensible sounds = scores 2. The patient will moan or groan in response to painful stimulation. The verbal response may contain indistinct mumbling but no intelligible words.

None = scores 1. The patient is unable to produce any verbal response despite prolonged and repeated stimulation.

Possible assessment problems Patients may be unable to understand the nurse's questions or commands because they do not understand the language or may have a hearing deficit. The patient's verbal response may be impaired as a result of a speech deficit such as dysphasia. If appropriate, written instructions and replies can be used to assess the patient's language ability. The verbal response may also be compromised by the presence of an endotracheal or tracheostomy tube. This is indicated on the patient's chart as 'T'.

Motor response

This assesses the patient's best motor response. Only the best response from the arms is recorded as leg responses to pain are less consistent and may be confused with a simple spinal reflex. The responses described below are shown in Figure 28.6.

Obeys commands. Score = 6. The patient has the ability to follow instructions, for example, 'put out your tongue', 'lift up your arms', 'show me your thumb'.

Localises to pain. Score = 5. If the patient does not obey commands, an external stimulus must be applied. In the absence of any facial, orbital or skull fractures, pressure is applied with the flat of the nurse's thumb over the cranial nerve underlying the supraorbital ridge under the eyebrow (Figure 28.7a). Pressure is gradually increased for a maximum of 15 seconds. Providing the patient has not sustained a cervical fracture, the 'trapezius pinch' (Figure 28.7b) is a useful alternative; the trapezius muscle (the large triangular muscle of the neck and thorax) is squeezed between the nurse's fingers and thumb. The response is recorded as 'localising to pain' if the patient moves their arm across the midline, to the level of the chin, in an attempt to locate the source of the pain (Figure 28.6b). During the course of the day, the patient may display a localising response to other sources of irritation, e.g. suctioning, nasogastric tube or urinary catheter.

Flexion to pain. Score = 4. Following the application of a central painful stimulus, either the trapezius squeeze or supraorbital ridge pressure, the patient responds by flexing their arm normally by bending their elbow and weakly withdrawing their hand; no attempt to localise towards the source of the pain is made.

Abnormal flexion. Score = 3. In response to a painful stimulus, the patient bends their elbow with adduction of the upper arms and abnormal posturing of the wrist and fingers, otherwise known as decorticate posturing. This indicates more severe dysfunction of the brain and is a poor prognostic sign.

Extension to pain. Score = 2. Following painful stimulation, the patient responds by rigid extension, i.e. straightening the elbows and hyperpronation of the forearms, otherwise known as decerebrate posturing. The response usually includes spastic hand and wrist movements, with an inward rotation of the shoulders and forearms. The legs are generally straight, with the feet pointing outwards.

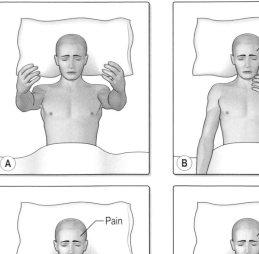
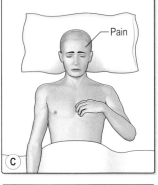
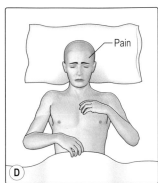
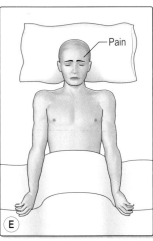

Figure 28.6 Motor responses. A. Obeys commands ('lift up your arms'). B. Localising to pain. C. Flexing to pain. D. Abnormal flexion. E. Extending to pain.

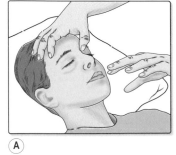
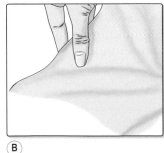

Figure 28.7 Applying a central painful stimulus. A. Supraorbital ridge pressure. B. Trapezius pinch.

None. Score = 1. This response is only recorded when sufficient painful stimulus has been applied to provoke a response and no detectable movement has been observed.

Possible assessment problems Variations in the motor response may occur during the assessment. Therefore, it is the best response that should be scored; for example, if the patient localises to pain on the left side but flexes to pain on the right, the localising response is recorded. Asymmetrical responses are significant, indicating that a focal neurological deficit is present, but overall brain function is more accurately reflected by the level of best response on the better side (see Limb movement, below).

When applying a painful stimulus, it is important to explain to the patient and their relatives what you are about to do and why you are doing it, otherwise they may feel that unnecessary trauma is being inflicted.

For further information about the use of the neurological observation chart and GCS in practice, see Woodward (1997a–d), NICE (2003), Waterhouse (2005) and Palmer & Knight (2006).

Recording other measurements

A neurological assessment includes the recording of additional measurements as follows:

- vital signs:
  - blood pressure
  - pulse rate
  - respirations
  - temperature
- pupil size and reaction
- limb movements.

Vital signs

Blood pressure and pulse A rising blood pressure (elevated systolic pressure), widening of the pulse pressures and a slowing pulse (see Ch. 9), known as 'Cushing's response', is a very late sign of raised intracranial pressure (ICP) and there may have been other signs such as subtle alterations in behaviour or fluctuating level of consciousness which could have indicated a deterioration in neurological status.

Respiration Factors that impair consciousness may also cause respiratory changes. The pattern and rate of respiration is directly affected by increasing brain injury that may produce an ataxic irregular or Cheyne–Stokes respiratory pattern characterised by periods of tachypnoea interspersed with periods of apnoea. It is important for the nurse to observe the ABCD approach to assessment, ensuring the patient has a clear airway, removing any obstructions (e.g. secretions or foreign bodies) and using airway adjuncts to maintain airway patency before assessing the rate, depth, rhythm and characteristics of breathing. Oxygen therapy should be commenced early and the patient's oxygen saturation levels monitored to reduce the risk of hypoxia.

Temperature A gradual elevation in temperature is likely to be an early sign of infection from the lungs, urinary tract or a wound. Rapid increases in body temperature are likely to be caused by damage to the hypothalamus (the body's temperature regulating centre). Each degree of rise in temperature increases the brain's metabolic rate, and must be treated urgently to prevent further neurological deterioration (see p. 753).

Pupil size and reaction

Abnormal pupillary size and reaction can indicate brain dysfunction and/or raised ICP. It is important to note any changes, particularly if they occur in conjunction with other changes in the neurological observations. The size of both pupils is measured in millimetres and recorded using the guide included in the neurological observation chart. Reaction to light is recorded by a plus (+); no reaction is recorded by a minus (−). Pupil reactions should be assessed in dim surroundings, using a small bright flashlight. To elicit the direct-light reflex, the nurse holds both of the patient's eyelids open, bringing the light in from the outer aspect of the eye and shining it directly into the eye. This should cause a brisk constriction of the pupil, and withdrawal of the light should produce brisk dilatation of the pupil. The size and reaction are observed and recorded on the chart. The shape of the pupils should also be assessed.

Limb movement

Disturbances of limb movement are an indication of localised (focal) brain damage and vary according to the site and extent of the damage; for example, the right arm and leg will be affected by a lesion in the left cerebral hemisphere due to the crossing over ('decussation') of most of the axons in the brain stem before they pass down the spinal cord. Diffuse brain damage will result in a greater disturbance of movement.

The nurse examines the arms and legs for movement and strength, and compares the right and left sides. When differences exist, right and left are recorded independently. Responses can be elicited by asking the patient to grip the nurse's hand, to lift up their arms or to bend their knees. To test strength in the legs, the nurse may ask the patient to push down against their hand. A painful stimulus is only applied if verbal requests fail to elicit a response.

Causes of unconsciousness

Unconsciousness occurs when the RAS is damaged or its function is depressed so that there is an interruption of the normal arousal mechanisms. This may be caused by a primary or secondary insult to the nervous system: primary insults are commonly caused by intrinsic diseases of the brain; secondary involvement is most often caused by metabolic, endocrine or toxic conditions, where the critical insult is manifested elsewhere in the body. Table 28.1 identifies some of the signs and symptoms of changes in level of consciousness and possible causes. The major causes of unconsciousness are shown in Figure 28.3 (see www.allaboutnph.org. www.npis.org).

Emergency care of the unconscious patient

Whatever the cause of unconsciousness and wherever the event occurs, the patient's life depends on the knowledge and skills of those who find and care for them. The first

Table 28.1 Clues to the cause of unconsciousness on general physical examination

SIGN OR SYMPTOM	POSSIBLE CAUSE
Elevated temperature	Infection Heat stroke
Subnormal temperature	Dehydration Excessive intake of alcohol Barbiturate intoxication Hypothyroidism Exposure to the cold
Bleeding from the mouth	Epileptic seizure Trauma
Pulse irregularities	Hypoxia from inadequate cardiac output
Slow, regular respirations	Hypothyroidism Morphine or barbiturate intoxication
Cheyne–Stokes respiration	Bilateral cerebral dysfunction Late stages of increased intracranial pressure Severe cardiopulmonary disease
Ataxic, irregular (cluster) respirations	Lesions of the brain stem – signifies impending apnoea
Breath odour	Excessive intake of alcohol Hepatic dysfunction Renal dysfunction Ingested poisons Diabetes mellitus – ketoacidosis
Skin	
Jaundice	Hepatic dysfunction
Cyanosis	Cardiopulmonary problems
Rash	Infection, drug reaction, meningitis
Needle puncture marks	Substance abuse
Hypertension	Raised intracranial pressure – tumours, abscess Intracranial haemorrhage – haematoma, stroke
Hypotension	Blood loss Septicaemia Myocardial infarction Pulmonary embolism

aid and care that the patient receives until consciousness is regained will help to determine the outcome.

A hospital emergency

An individual can be rendered unconscious by any of the causes shown in Figure 28.3. The measures a nurse should take on finding someone collapsed are as follows:

1 Press the emergency call button, shout or send someone for assistance.

2 Following the ABC principles (see Ch. 2), call the arrest team and initiate cardiopulmonary resuscitation (CPR) if the individual is not breathing and the carotid pulse is absent.

3 If the person is breathing and a pulse is present, place them in a semi-prone (recovery position, see Ch. 2) position. However, if spinal injury is suspected, maintain the patient's head, neck and spine in alignment until medical assistance arrives. Stay with the person until assistance arrives and they can be moved to an appropriate place for further treatment and investigation.

Planned admission

When an unconscious patient is to be admitted to hospital, prepare the bed area:

- Remove the top bedclothes and the head of the bed to facilitate easy transfer.
- Check that the oxygen supply and suction apparatus are functioning and that there is an adequate supply of relevant equipment.
- Ensure the following equipment is available for immediate use:
  - a resuscitation trolley containing the following:
    1 oropharyngeal (Guedel) airways (usually size 3 or 4 for an adult)
    2 Ambu bag with universal catheter mount
    3 laryngoscope and endotracheal (ET) tubes sizes 6.5–10.00 mm
    4 lubricating jelly; strapping or tape (to secure the ET tube); 5 mL syringe to inflate the ET tube cuff
    5 emergency drug box
  - intravenous infusion stand
  - nasogastric tube and associated equipment
  - neurological examination tray containing ophthalmoscope, reflex hammer, tuning fork, tongue depressor, sterile pin for assessment of sensation, cotton wool swabs to test corneal reflex
  - appropriate charts and admission forms.

Priorities of nursing management

The following checklist itemises the priorities of nursing management in an emergency situation.

1 Maintenance of a clear airway.
  a The patient's position – by positioning the patient correctly it is possible to minimise the risk of the tongue falling back and obstructing the pharynx. Avoid nursing the patient on their back (supine) as this increases the risk of developing a chest infection or pneumonia.
  b Artificial airways – these include airway adjuncts inserted into the mouth, through the nose or into the trachea to optimise breathing and facilitate clearance of bronchial secretions.
  c Suction – removes excess secretions and mucus from the trachea and lower airway when the patient's own cough is too weak to expectorate the secretions.
  d Oxygen – is used to prevent hypoxia (low blood oxygen) and hypercapnia (high levels of carbon dioxide).

e Nasogastric (NG) tube – inserted via the nose into the stomach to provide enteral feeding until the patient is able to commence oral feeding. The National Patient Safety Agency (NPSA 2007) has written guidance on the placement and safe management of the tube to reduce the risk of misplacement and aspiration.

2 Assessment of the central nervous system:
   a Glasgow Coma Scale
   b vital signs
   c pupillary reactions
   d limb movements.

3 Maintenance of fluid balance.
   a Intravenous infusion – maintains hydration until the patient is able to absorb enteral fluids or commence oral feeding. Crystalloid solutions of normal saline 0.9% are normally prescribed. Dextrose solutions are contraindicated in patients following a head injury as dextrose increases intracranial pressure and leads to cerebral ischaemia. Mannitol is an osmotic diuretic that reduces brain swelling associated with raised intracranial pressure, buying time for the underlying pathology to be treated or removed.
   b Catheterisation of the urinary bladder, if necessary, to allow accurate monitoring of hourly urine output.

Care of relatives A nurse who is not involved in the immediate care of the patient should be allocated to support the family/carers. It is a useful opportunity to gather the patient's biographical data and other information to help in planning the patient's care. A brief explanation of the management plan, supported with written information regarding hospital procedure or possible investigations, will help give some reassurance (Box 28.4) (see www.equip.nhs.uk/topic/neuro/injury.html).

Medical management

An unconscious patient is a medical emergency, unless the unconscious state represents the terminal stages of a progressive disease process. Although life support measures take priority such as provision of an adequate airway, control of haemorrhage, and fluid or blood replacement, the cause of the unconscious state must be determined before the most appropriate treatment can be delivered.

The medical history

The doctor or an experienced nurse will need to gain further information about the patient's medical history from the family or carers including the circumstances preceding and surrounding the onset of the unconscious state.

Box 28.4 Reflection

Support of families in critical care

Think about the relatives of critically ill or highly dependent patients.

What strategies might help to reduce their anxieties and enable them to be more involved with their relative's care?

The physical examination

The general physical examination of the unconscious patient should include:

- Airway – look for chest movement, listen for breath sounds or abnormal noise, feel at the mouth/nose for exhaled air.
- Breathing – rate, depth, pattern of respiration, odour.
- Circulation – vital signs, skin colour, temperature.
- Disability – neurological examination will include assessment of the cranial nerves, reflexes and motor and sensory function. A baseline assessment should be documented so that any future changes in the patient's condition can be observed.
- Exposure – other signs of trauma.

Laboratory tests

- Full blood count – measures haemoglobin levels, platelets and the number of red and white blood cells (neutrophils and lymphocytes).
- Blood glucose levels – to detect hypoglycaemia (low blood sugar levels) or hyperglycaemia (raised blood sugar levels).
- Urea and electrolyte levels – measures sodium, potassium and chloride levels in the blood that become deranged during periods of acute illness. If left untreated, abnormal levels can lead to confusion, cramps, irregular heart rhythm and ultimately death.
- Erythrocyte sedimentation rate (ESR) and C-reactive protein (CRP) are useful indicators for detecting acute and chronic inflammatory infection.
- Blood gas analysis – measures partial pressure of carbon dioxide ($PaCO_2$) and oxygen (PaO_2) to assess the effectiveness of gaseous exchange in the lungs.
- Toxicology – substance abuse or poisons.
- Urinalysis – for glucose, acetone, blood and infection.

Radiological studies and imaging

Once the patient has been resuscitated and their condition stabilised, radiological investigations are carried out:

- CT scan of head and cervical spine
- MRI scan to identify abnormalities in the soft tissue in the brain
- normal X-rays as appropriate if other injuries are apparent or suspected
- cerebral angiography (CT angiography or invasive radiology) to identify any aneurysms or congenital malformations.

Further investigations

Further investigations may be undertaken to aid diagnosis, e.g.:

- electroencephalogram (EEG) – records electrical activity within the brain, used in the diagnosis of epilepsy
- lumbar puncture (LP) – obtains cerebrospinal fluid and can be used diagnostically for signs of infection (meningitis, abscess) or therapeutically to relieve raised intracranial pressure
- electrocardiogram (ECG) – records the electrical activity of the heart and identifies a wide range of abnormalities
- positron emission tomography (PET scan) – uses a radioactive tracer to produce detailed images of the structure

and functioning of specific organs and tissues (often used in research)

- Doppler studies – ultrasound uses reflected sound waves to evaluate blood flow through a vessel, e.g. in deep venous thrombosis (DVT), stroke (see www.bbsf.org.uk).

Nursing management of the unconscious patient

Breathing

Alterations in the rate, rhythm and pattern of respirations can be caused by a number of factors including electrolyte imbalance, trauma to the cervical spine, drugs, e.g. narcotics or sedatives, pulmonary disease such as pneumonia or atelectasis (Ch. 3) or cardiac conditions (Ch. 2). To prevent cerebral ischaemia and infarction caused by hypoxia, the nurse must perform regular respiratory assessment including rate, depth, type, colour of the patient as well as oxygen saturation (PO_2). The priority must be to maintain a clear airway:

- Remove any obvious potential obstruction to the airway, such as dentures or dental plates. Take note of the presence of loose teeth, caps or crowns, as these could become detached and obstruct the airway.
- Bleeding into the oropharynx from head or facial injuries, vomit and aspirate should be removed with a Yankauer suction probe (insertion of a nasogastric tube will facilitate the emptying of the stomach reducing the risk of aspiration of gastric contents into the lungs).

Position of the patient

Unconscious patients and those with head injuries, unless their condition contraindicates, should be nursed in a semi-prone or lateral recumbent position with the head of the bed tilted slightly upwards (10–30 degrees). This prevents the tongue from obstructing the airway, reduces the risk of aspiration from secretions and saliva and aids cerebral venous drainage, helping to reduce intracranial pressure (Hickey 2003) (see Ch. 9). Patients with actual or suspected spinal injury will be maintained in a position of spinal alignment supported with pillows.

Artificial airways

The unconscious patient's cough reflex will be depressed or absent, affecting their ability to cough and clear their own airway. The use of artificial airways and suctioning may be required.

Oropharyngeal airway The Guedel airway is easy to insert and is available in varying sizes. It prevents the tongue from obstructing the throat and allows the patient to breathe through the device into the pharynx. It also allows easier access to facilitate suction of the oropharynx and trachea. An oropharyngeal airway can stimulate the gag and cough reflex, causing the patient to retch or cough, in which case it should be removed.

A nasopharyngeal airway may be better tolerated as this is passed through the nose and does not exert a stimulus on the rear part of the tongue.

Endotracheal tube An endotracheal tube is indicated if either the Guedel or nasopharyngeal airway proves inadequate or when mechanical ventilation is required. The tube is made of malleable plastic and has an inflatable cuff. The tube can be inserted orally or nasally into the trachea to the point just above the bifurcation of the bronchi. Breath sounds are determined immediately after insertion to make certain that the tube is properly positioned and is not obstructing one of the primary bronchi. An inflated cuff provides an airtight seal around the outside of the tube, preventing the aspiration of material from the mouth, nose and digestive tract into the lungs. The tube is usually left in place for no more than 5–7 days because of the increased risk of erosion of the tracheal wall.

Tracheostomy tube A tracheostomy, a surgical opening in the anterior wall of the trachea, is usually indicated if intubation needs to be prolonged, or if there are difficulties in inserting an endotracheal tube. The tracheostomy tube bypasses the nose, pharynx and larynx, enabling air to flow directly into the lungs, thus reducing dead space and the effort required by the patient to breathe, and facilitates suctioning of bronchial secretions (see Ch. 14).

A variety of different types and sizes of tracheostomy tube are available. The tubes may be cuffed or uncuffed, fenestrated or unfenestrated to facilitate weaning and communication. Cuffed tubes are made with high-volume, low-pressure, soft cuffs to reduce the risk of pressure trauma to the trachea. The amount of air in the cuff should be measured at least 8-hourly, using a pressure gauge. Pressures should be maintained between 15 and 25 cmH_2O unless otherwise directed by medical staff (Dikeman & Kazandijan 1995).

Most tracheostomy tubes consist of three parts: an obturator inside the tube to keep it rigid during insertion, an outer cannula and an inner cannula. The advantage of a tube with an inner cannula is that this can be removed every 2–4 hours for cleaning, reducing the risk of airway obstruction with excess secretions. The procedure can be carried out without disturbing the outer tube, reducing the frequency of outer tube changes, thus minimising the risk of trauma to the stoma and trachea.

The tracheal stoma must be cleaned using an aseptic technique, and a sterile, non-adherent dressing applied to minimise the incidence of infection caused by accumulation of secretions around the wound. For more on tracheostomy care see Chapter 14.

Suctioning

Tracheal or endotracheal suctioning is performed to remove excessive secretions from the oropharynx, trachea and bronchi. In a patient with raised ICP, the procedure can provoke transient raised ICP and should be performed with care. The nurse's assessment of the patient's colour, respiratory rate and pattern will indicate how often this is required. Suction must be applied if one or more of the following occurs:

- signs of cyanosis
- increased and irregular respirations
- noisy, gurgling respirations.

The following equipment is required:

- Suction device, collection jar with disposable liner, and disposable connecting tubing.

- Sterile suction catheters – catheter diameter should be less than half the internal diameter of the tube to allow airflow down the side of the catheter. Catheter size = (tube size − 2) × 2. For example, for a size 8 tracheostomy tube it will be 8 − 2 = 6 × 2 = size 12 FG catheter.
- Sterile plastic gloves. The use of a closed suction catheter system and disposable suction equipment is recognised as good practice.

Procedure Each hospital will have its own policy regarding suctioning, but the procedure described below is based on good practice and provides a general example (Buglass 1995, Laws-Chapman et al 2000).

1 Patients who are dependent on oxygen should continue with their therapy until immediately prior to insertion of the suction catheter and the supply must be replaced immediately afterwards.
2 Suction pressure is set below 16 kPa (120 mmHg) in adults.
3 Wash hands and pour the sterile normal saline into a sterile bowl, apply non-sterile examination gloves for your own protection.
4 Open the pack containing the sterile catheter and put a plastic sterile glove on the dominant hand.
5 Attach the catheter to the connecting tube, taking care not to contaminate the catheter.
6 Remove oxygen mask/nasal cannula from the patient.
7 Insert the catheter into the airway without applying suction and advance the catheter as far as it will easily pass, until resistance is met. This will usually cause the patient to cough.
8 Withdraw the catheter 1 cm and apply suction as the catheter is slowly withdrawn (Glass & Grap 1995, Laws-Chapman et al 2000).
9 Remove secretions within a time limit of 15 seconds.
10 Use the catheter once only and then wrap it around the gloved hand. Remove the glove with the catheter inside and discard both.
11 Rinse the suction tubing through with sterile water.
12 Give the patient at least 1 minute to recover before suctioning again. Give oxygen again, if prescribed.
13 If all the secretions have not been removed, repeat the procedure using a new sterile glove and sterile catheter.
14 If necessary use a new catheter to suction the patient's mouth and nose at the end of the procedure. Nasal suction is contraindicated if the patient has sustained a frontal skull fracture or has nasal leakage of cerebrospinal fluid (CSF rhinorrhoea).
15 The instillation of saline should not be routinely used (Ackerman 1996). A saline nebuliser which will deliver tiny droplets of moisture to the alveoli to optimise humidification is the preferred option.

Humidification

Normally the air drawn into the lungs is warmed, moistened and filtered through the nose and upper respiratory tract. To prevent irritation of the mucous membranes and production of dried tenacious secretions, patients with an endotracheal or tracheostomy tube must receive effective humidification, preferably through a heated system or nebuliser.

Oxygen

The amount of oxygen prescribed depends on the patient's clinical condition and the results from their arterial blood gases. A specimen of arterial blood is taken to ascertain the pH and partial pressures of oxygen (PaO_2) and carbon dioxide ($PaCO_2$). Severe deviations from normal are an indication for elective mechanical ventilation to ensure adequate oxygenation. Normal values are:

- pH, 7.36–7.44
- PaO_2, 11–15 kPa
- $PaCO_2$, 4.6–5.9 kPa.

There are various methods of administering oxygen and the doctor's prescription will include instructions about the rate of flow, duration of therapy and delivery system. The nurse must monitor the patients for complications (see Ch. 3).

Nursing and physiotherapy

The prevention of respiratory complications is a priority in the nursing management of the unconscious patient, but infection may occur despite every precaution being taken. Effective respiratory management is dependent on good communication, skill and cooperation between the nurse, physiotherapist and medical team. Antibiotics can be effective if organisms are cultivated from the patient's secretions.

Communicating

The patient

There is considerable anecdotal evidence of patients recalling, with startling accuracy, conversations they overheard whilst unconscious. It is important that conversations not intended for the patient should not be held in close proximity, as unguarded or misinterpreted information can cause distress.

It is imperative that the nurse explains clearly and simply to the patient every aspect of their care, whether it is related to procedures being carried out or to the patient's progress (Box 28.5). The explanations and reassurances should be repeated whenever a procedure is carried out. With the advent of ICP monitoring, several studies have been undertaken to determine the effects of verbal and physical interactions on ICP. Some interactions were shown to cause a rise in ICP, some a decrease and some no change (Treloar et al 1991, Chudley 1994).

Pain is common following traumatic brain injuries of all severities. Pain may arise from muscular skeletal injuries, spasticity or headache. The recognition and diagnosis of pain in the unconscious patient is difficult and further complicated by communication, cognitive and behavioural deficits. Most of

Box 28.5 Reflection

Possible barriers to effective communication

What do you understand by the term 'barriers to communication'?

List six potential barriers when caring for the unconscious patient and suggest strategies to enable you to cope with them.

the pain assessment scales, e.g. visual analogue or numerical rating scales, are inappropriate for the unconscious patient. It is important to be extra vigilant to the often subtle signs of pain. Analgesia must be administered cautiously as over-sedation can mask further signs of deterioration (pupil response, decreased respirations, decreased level of consciousness).

The family and others significant to the patient

Relatives and other visitors are likely to be distressed when they see the unconscious patient for the first time. A brief explanation of the immediate environment and the function of any equipment should be provided. Visitors should be encouraged to touch and speak softly to the patient. They should be given an opportunity to ask any questions and to speak with the doctor and nurse in charge of the patient's progress.

Rest and sleep

Providing adequate rest and sleep for a patient in the acute clinical environment is one of the most difficult challenges confronting the nurse, and given the associated hospital background noise, it is doubtful whether it is ever overcome (see Ch. 25). However, patients whose level of consciousness fluctuates may experience periods of sleep and periods of wakefulness even though they may not be responsive to external stimuli (Podurgiel 1990).

Treloar et al (1991), Chudley (1994) and Hickey (2003) mention the need to provide rest periods for patients between nursing and other activities. Nurses should consider this potential need when planning care. It can be detrimental to constantly stimulate the patient by undertaking frequent observations and procedures, and care should be planned with other members of staff who are attending to the patient.

Acutely ill patients in intensive care will receive enteral feeding 24 hours/day to preserve gut integrity, increase immune function and reduce the risk of sepsis. As the patient's clinical condition improves or stabilises, intermittent or bolus NG feeding allows the patient to rest overnight (Box 28.6).

Diet and hydration

The early commencement of fluid and nutritional support must be a high priority in the care of any unconscious patient. Failure to commence adequate fluid replacement and feeding can lead to dehydration and electrolyte imbalance, atrophy of skeletal muscle, increased risk of infection, immunosuppression and poor wound healing.

> **Box 28.6 Reflection**
>
> **Management of the clinical environment in critical care**
>
> What information do you have in your clinical area that addresses the physical and psychosocial needs of the highly dependent patients?
>
> Where will you find information to promote awareness of controlling the patient's environment in respect of noise, level of stimulation and avoidance of external noxious stimuli?
>
> Is there an opportunity to raise awareness by adding something to the notice board?

Fluids

In the acute stage, fluids are usually administered intravenously, either peripherally or via a central line, titrated against the patient's fluid balance and serum electrolyte levels. Intravenous fluids are also given to:

- maintain hydration
- administer medications
- maintain normal electrolytes and correct imbalances.

It is essential that the correct fluids are administered at the prescribed rate to maintain fluid balance and metabolic needs. An infusion device is usually used to ensure accuracy.

The patient may also have an arterial line to facilitate frequent blood sampling. The line must be clearly labelled to distinguish it from other multiple venous lines or ports (see Ch. 18).

Nutrition

Provision of adequate nutrition is particularly important in the unconscious patient. Even brief periods of malnourishment will weaken the immune system with loss of energy and muscle mass.

Daily nutritional requirements are calculated on the basis of body weight, gender, height and age. Unless the patient is nursed on a bed with an integral weighing scale, an estimated weight is often used.

Nasogastric feeding This is the most frequently used method of providing nutritional support, provided that the patient's alimentary tract is functional. The dietitian will assess the patient's nutritional requirements on a daily basis titrating against clinical need. If the patient has a suspected base of skull fracture, CSF rhinorrhoea or severe facial/nasal fractures, an orogastric tube is preferable.

The position of the tube must be checked according to local guidelines, which should reflect those of the NPSA (www.npsa.gov.uk).

Percutaneous endoscopic gastrostomy feeding Whenever possible, it is preferable to deliver food directly into the stomach to prevent the risk of translocation of bacteria from the unused gastrointestinal tract. Long-term feeding is better achieved by a percutaneous endoscopic gastrostomy (PEG) tube which has fewer associated complications than a venous line and is more comfortable for the patient. Relatives/carers can be taught how to administer feeds through the tube if the patient is later cared for at home.

As the patient regains consciousness, they should be assessed by the speech and language therapist (SALT) to ensure that the gag, cough and swallowing reflexes are present prior to giving any oral fluids or diet (see Ch. 21).

Parenteral nutrition Parenteral feeding is prescribed when the patient is unable to tolerate or fails to absorb enteral feeding. It is delivered either through a central venous line or a peripherally inserted central line (PICC line) (see Ch. 21). Patients who may benefit from parenteral nutrition include:

- patients with multiple trauma, particularly if there are gastrointestinal and/or facial injuries
- malnourished patients
- patients with sepsis or multisystem failure

- patients with inflammatory bowel disease which is extensive and life threatening
- patients in prolonged coma who are unable to tolerate enteral feeding.

For further information on enteral feeding and parenteral nutrition, see Chapter 21.

Elimination

The ability of the patient to control elimination is impaired due to their altered level of consciousness. Incontinence will lead to skin breakdown and loss of dignity. Initially, during the acute phase of admission, catheterisation will enable an accurate measurement of urinary output. Local protocols should be followed with regard to catheter care (see Ch. 8). Once the patient has stabilised, male patients may be able to manage with external penile collection devices such as a Uri-sheath.

The patient's bowel movements should be closely monitored. Stool softeners and aperients may be administered in order to produce a regular stool. It is important for the patient to avoid straining to defaecate as this will raise ICP. Diarrhoea should be quickly cleaned away and the skin inspected for signs of excoriation.

Personal cleansing and dressing

The unconscious patient is dependent upon the nurse to attend to all aspects of personal hygiene. A daily bed bath is necessary for most totally dependent patients, but care must be taken when turning the unconscious patient in bed as there is a danger that the airway may become compromised and the patient's chest movement may be impeded. To avoid this, turning should be planned and requires a minimum of two nurses to execute safely. If a mechanical hoist is available, the patient can be showered or bathed in a specifically designed bath. Many unconscious patients will require more than one bed bath a day to maintain their hygiene needs and personal comfort.

Hair washing may be difficult and, if the use of a wet shampoo is impossible, a dry shampoo may be used. Nails should be kept short and clean; referral to a chiropodist may be necessary for some patients. Male patients will require a daily facial shave. If the patient has a moustache or beard, this should be trimmed as necessary.

Eye care must be performed on a frequent basis because unconscious patients do not blink and the corneas become dry. Without adequate eye care this can quickly lead to corneal ulceration and permanent visual impairment. The eye and surrounding area should be cleaned with gauze and sterile normal saline, followed by the instillation of artificial tear drops at least four times a day. If the patient's eyelids do not close naturally, eye drops may need to be instilled more frequently. The eyes can be protected with a polyacrylamide hydrogel dressing or eye shield to prevent further damage to the cornea (Woodrow 2006). Electric fans directed towards the head and eyes can exacerbate corneal damage and must be avoided.

Oral hygiene should be maintained following thorough oral assessment to plan effective care (Eilers 1988, Huskinson 2009) (see also Ch. 15). The unconscious patient who has a Guedel airway or endotracheal tube in place may present with particular problems such as a dry mouth and difficult access to the oral cavity. A small toothbrush with a small amount of fluoride toothpaste and plain water should be used to clean the teeth, tongue and gums. Lubricants to prevent cracking of the lips and promote healing can also be useful (Dougherty & Lister 2008). Dentures must be stored dry in a covered container labelled with the patient's name and hospital number and should be cleaned again and rinsed in cold water before reinsertion.

Maintaining a safe environment

The unconscious patient is physically vulnerable to a range of complications, such as pressure ulcers and infection, and nursing staff must always be alert to the need to maintain a safe environment.

Infection

The unconscious patient is particularly at risk of respiratory and urinary infection. All wounds and drains are also potential sites for infection. Gram-negative bacillary pneumonia causes 40–60% of respiratory infections that are acquired in institutionalised settings. Most people are resistant to this organism, which is constantly present in the environment, but certain factors contribute to the breaking down of physiological and immunological defences. The unconscious patient is exposed to many of these, particularly the presence of invasive lines such as intravenous cannulae and urinary catheters. Antibiotic-resistant infections have become an increasing problem and patients are now all routinely screened on their admission for meticillin-resistant *Staphylococcus aureus* (MRSA), a potentially life-threatening organism. Routine screening of staff will be determined by local policy (Mackenzie 1997, Pellowe et al 2004) (see also Ch. 16).

The nurse needs to be aware of and conscientious about implementing trust policies in relation to standard infection control precautions (see Ch. 16). Handwashing has been comprehensively researched and is acknowledged to be the single most effective intervention to promote infection control in the clinical setting (DH 2001, Royal College of Nursing 2004a, Akyol et al 2006).

Medication

The types of medication most commonly used in the unconscious patient include analgesics, anticonvulsants (see Seizure, below), antibiotics and laxatives. The hazards of administering medications are well documented, but the risks are increased in the unconscious patient for two reasons:

- The routes that are used carry a greater risk for the patient. The simpler and safer oral route is contraindicated. Other methods of administration have to be utilised, including i.m. injections, i.v. infusions, via a nasal or orogastric tube and the rectal route.
- Patients cannot confirm their identity, so nurses must ensure that the right medication in the right dose is being given to the right patient via the right route at the right time.

Motor and sensory loss or impairment

The motor and sensory loss experienced by unconscious patients may be drug induced or part of an underlying disease process. Whatever the cause, the nursing intervention remains the same.

Motor loss See Mobility, below.

Sensory loss The sensory system is part of the body's defence system and the unconscious patient is unable to process sensory information. It is imperative that the patient is not exposed to extremes of temperature, particularly in localised area of the skin, e.g. when heating or cooling devices are used.

Care must be taken when moving and positioning the patient as they will not be aware of any adverse friction or pressure. The patient may have a reduced or absent sensation of pain or, if experiencing pain, may be unable to communicate that feeling.

Seizure

The main role of the nurse when the unconscious patient, or indeed anyone, has a seizure is to ensure that the patient does not harm themselves. Depending on the type of seizure the need for first aid may not be recognised, but always depends on the type and severity of the seizure (see www.epilepsy.org.uk).

- Do:
  - Stay calm.
  - Protect the patient from injury (especially the head).
  - Look for information/warning cards/jewellery.
  - Continually check the airway and remain with the patient until help arrives.
- Do not:
  - Restrain the patient in any way.
  - Try to move the patient (unless from immediate danger).
  - Give food or drink.
- Call an ambulance if:
  - This is the person's first seizure.
  - There is no sign of spontaneous recovery.
  - One seizure follows another.
  - A serious injury has occurred.

Status epilepticus (a prolonged seizure or a series of seizures without regaining consciousness) is always a medical emergency and demands urgent medical assistance. Further information about epilepsy can be found in Chapter 9.

Mobility

The nursing management of mobility and activity remains the same, whatever the cause of the unconsciousness. Lack of attention to mobility could lead to the development of:

- Contractures – permanent tightening of a muscle or tendon in response to increased muscle tone and involuntary movement preventing normal movement.
- Muscle atrophy/wasting – refers to a decrease in muscle mass following injury or disease to a nerve, e.g. polio, or occurs as a consequence of disuse due to immobility.
- Pressure ulcers – prevention is important for the comfort of the patient. Regular alteration of the patient's position and relief of pressure is paramount, particularly in the immobile, unconscious patient.
- Postural hypotension – a fall in blood pressure when the individual adopts an upright position after lying for long periods.

- Deep vein thrombosis (Ch. 2).
- Hypostatic pneumonia (Ch. 3).

Any one of these hazards will delay the patient's rehabilitation and cause additional pain and discomfort. Whilst the patient remains dependent, the nurse, working with the physiotherapists, is responsible for ensuring that the patient maintains a full range of movement. Correct positioning is important and the following should be considered:

- body alignment, especially if spinal injury is suspected
- use of aids such as pillows, foam pads or splints, to help to support weak or hemiplegic limbs
- avoidance of pressure, e.g. an arm trapped under the body, the pinna of the ear bent forward, bedclothes too tight
- changing the patient's position; this should be done frequently – at least every 2 hours is recommended
- avoidance of friction when moving the patient
- careful handling of joints and paralysed or weak limbs
- safety, e.g. if the patient is restless, padded bed rails may be required.

Safety/restraint

Many patients experience disorientation, confusion or aggressive behaviour as they recover consciousness. This may be due to their underlying illness and pathology, medication, sensory deprivation or the unfamiliar environment. Health care teams face difficult decisions about identifying strategies to prevent the patient inadvertently dislodging tracheostomy tubes, invasive lines or dressings (Box 28.7). Diversional therapy, involving the patient's family and friends, or providing one-to-one nursing supervision may be useful. Balancing the best interests of the patient to ensure safety and promote their well-being can be difficult and presents unique challenges. When all other alternative therapies have failed, and only as a last resort, short-term restraint may be necessary. A risk assessment must be completed and continuously re-evaluated to ensure the measures are discontinued at the earliest opportunity. No restraints should be applied without consultation with the patient, their family and the medical team involved with the patient's care (Department of Health [DH] and Welsh Office 1999, Royal College of Nursing 2004b, Nursing and Midwifery Council 2008). The Mental Health Act, article 5, relating to restraint, was amended in 2004.

 See website Critical thinking question 28.1

Recovery from coma

A multidisciplinary approach is essential to facilitate early mobilisation of the patient. Patients who have been nursed in bed for just a few days often experience dizziness and

> **Box 28.7 Reflection**
>
> **Managing challenging behaviour**
>
> Reflect on your experience and identify two issues about the ward environment or routine that may increase the risks to patients who are confused or disorientated or who may display challenging behaviour.
>
> Consider how these patients are managed and any interventions that might help to reduce these risks.

light-headedness due to postural hypotension when they sit up for the first time (see www.headway.org.uk).

The physiotherapist will normally carry out an initial assessment, taking into consideration the patient's sensory or motor deficits, balance and head and neck control. Initially, the patient may be unsure and apprehensive about the prospect of getting out of bed and will need constant reassurance. Once the patient is in a sitting position, the nurse should check the patient's vital signs and colour, and ask whether they are experiencing any untoward symptoms. If they are, an individualised mobility rehabilitation programme should be implemented at a slower rate. Specialist chairs are available that will provide additional support for highly dependent patients. It is more beneficial for patients to sit up for several short intervals rather than one long period (see Ch. 34).

Controlling body temperature

Body temperature is controlled by the heat-regulating centre in the hypothalamus, which acts like a thermostat (see Ch. 22), and must be maintained within a relatively constant range to sustain life, i.e. 36–37.5°C. Pyrexia (an abnormally high temperature) is more commonly seen in the unconscious patient than hypothermia (an abnormally low temperature) although hypothermia may be the primary cause of unconsciousness (see Ch. 22).

Pyrexia may be caused by damage to the hypothalamus, an infective process or a metabolic disorder. For each degree of temperature above the normal range, the cerebral metabolism significantly increases, adversely increasing the brain's oxygen demands, which can have serious implications for the patient's eventual recovery and prognosis. In the acute stages the nurse must monitor the patient's temperature continuously with an electronic probe, sited over the patient's skin, inserted rectally or integrated into the patient's urinary bladder catheter. Normothermia is achieved using cooling blankets, electric fans and anti-pyretic medication, e.g. paracetamol administered intravenously or as rectal suppositories.

Dying

Despite all intensive care measures, some patients will die. Active treatment may continue right up until the last moment or it may be decided that further active intervention would be futile. The emphasis would then move from curative to palliative care and the patient may be transferred to an 'End of Life' pathway (http://www.endoflifecareforadults.nhs.uk/eolc/). If the patient is on a mechanical ventilator they may fulfil the criteria required for assessing brain stem death.

Brain stem death

Some patients with severe and irreversible brain damage can continue to have their blood pressure, heart beat and respirations artificially maintained for a period of time by ventilation, drug therapy and other life support interventions. Some, however, will never recover and brain stem death testing has been developed to identify such patients, in order that therapy can cease.

Brain stem death may be clinically diagnosed by following a set of guidelines issued by the Working Group of the Conference of Medical Royal Colleges and their Faculties (1976, with revisions in 1979) and according to the concept of death endorsed by the Working Group of the Royal College of Physicians in 1995. The ventilated patient will already have been diagnosed as having irremediable structural brain damage; however, these tests can only be implemented after a series of preconditions have been fulfilled.

Preconditions All reversible causes of coma have been eliminated, including:

- drug intoxication, e.g. as the result of an overdose, neuromuscular blocking agents or sedation to facilitate intubation
- primary hypothermia
- metabolic or endocrine imbalances such as uncontrolled diabetes.

Testing brain stem function Two doctors perform the brain stem tests. Usually one is the consultant responsible for the patient and the other is of at least senior registrar status. If organ donation from the patient is being considered, neither doctor must be a member of the transplant team. There are six parts to the test:

1 The pupillary response to light is tested, using a bright torch; absence of response indicates loss of function. The examiner must be satisfied that a non-responsive pupil is not due to the instillation of paralytic eye drops or damage to cranial nerve III.

2 The integrity of the corneal reflex is tested by drawing a wisp of cotton wool across the exposed cornea. Absence of a blink response indicates loss of function, although the examiner should be satisfied that the presence of corneal oedema is not preventing the normal blink response.

3 Cranial nerve motor responses are tested by applying a painful stimulus at several sites (usually over the supraorbital ridge, compressing part of the trigeminal nerve). Again, no response indicates loss of function, although spinal reflexes can remain intact even in a brain-dead patient (Pallis & Harley 1996).

4 The cough and gag reflexes are tested by agitating the endotracheal tube back and forth or by applying a suction catheter to the oropharynx and observing the patient's response. No response would indicate loss of the pharyngeal and laryngeal reflexes.

5 Absence of the oculovestibular reflex rules out the existence of normally functioning anatomical pathways within the brain stem and is a very sensitive test of brain stem function. It is tested by syringing 20 mL of ice-cold water into the patient's ears in turn and noting any eye movement in response. This is called 'cold caloric testing'. Before testing, the examiner should use an auroscope to look directly at the tympanic membrane to ensure that it is intact and that there is no obstruction preventing the water from making contact with the membrane.

6 The final test is that for apnoea. Arterial blood gases are checked and $PaCO_2$ should be 5.33–6.00 kPa (40–45 mmHg). The patient is disconnected from the ventilator after providing a continuous flow of 100% intratracheal oxygen for 10 min. The patient's chest wall is observed closely for any respiratory movement and the $PaCO_2$ is allowed to rise above threshold level to stimulate breathing, usually to at least 6.65 kPa (50 mmHg).

The ventilator is then reconnected and the entire process is repeated (either immediately or after a few hours) before the patient is declared brain dead. If the patient has a donor card, and after consultation with the relatives, the patient is referred to the organ donor transplantation team who will assess the patient as a potential organ donor and discuss various options with the patient's family.

For further information on brain stem death, see Pallis & Harley (1996); on issues in organ donation and transplants, see www.uktransplant.org.uk; on organ shortage, see Meeting the Organ Shortage (1999); and on organ transplantation, see NHB Organ Transplantation (www.organdona-tion.nhs.uk).

Physical and psychological care

The patient The principles of care for the dying unconscious patient are the same as those for all patients requiring palliative care (see Ch. 33). The unconscious patient must be treated with dignity and sensitivity even though they are unable to respond.

The family A sensitive and coherent strategy for caring for the relatives is needed. The nurse should know what information has been given to the relatives by other members of staff, including doctors. This will enable the nurse to reaffirm what has been said and avoid confusing the family members at a time when their ability to process information is drastically reduced (Box 28.8). They need to see and feel that the patient, even if unconscious and unresponsive, is still being treated as a person, through the humane, caring attitude of the nurse (Sque et al 2003).

Some relatives may be helped by being encouraged to perform simple acts of care for the patient such as bathing them or combing their hair, reducing their feelings of passivity and helplessness.

Psychologically, this is a traumatic and emotionally distressing time for the patient's family, friends and/or those who have a significant relationship with the patient. They have perhaps spent the last few days (and in some cases, much longer than that) with the patient, in the unfamiliar technical surroundings. They may be relieved that an ending has been achieved or may find it difficult to accept the death, particularly if the patient has been artificially ventilated.

The support of a religious advisor may be appreciated, even if the patient or relatives have not previously held any particular religious beliefs. Bereavement counselling and support should be offered as well as practical information (preferably written) about registering the death and other formalities.

Inevitably, this chapter has focused on the care of unconscious people in hospital because, at the present time, only a small minority are cared for at home. Wherever the location of care, it is important for nurses to be sensitive to the fundamental needs of the unconscious patient and understand the emotional impact their condition has on their relatives, carers and friends. As noted at the outset of this chapter, caring for the unconscious person is a major challenge for the nurse and whatever the outcome, meticulous attention to nursing observations and care is vital.

🖱 **See website Critical thinking question 28.2**

SUMMARY: KEY NURSING ISSUES

- Loss of consciousness may occur gradually or suddenly and be a temporary or a permanent state. Patients will be totally reliant on the nurse to maintain their safety and bodily functions.
- An individualised care plan should be written ensuring all activities of living are supported and provided for.
- Ensure a patent airway is maintained and prevent hypoxia.
- Assess respiratory function – rate, depth, oxygen saturation – and use airway adjuncts and apply oral/tracheal suction to remove secretions.
- Maintain hydration and nutrition with intravenous fluids and monitor blood chemistry levels. Commence enteral feeding via a nasogastric feeding tube or PEG as soon as possible and assess swallow reflex before re-commencing oral feeding.
- Elimination – measure urine output with a urinary catheter if accurate urine output is needed. Apply sheaths and pads and other appliances to manage urinary incontinence. Monitor bowel function and avoid constipation.
- Monitoring and observations – record vital signs, pulse, blood pressure, respirations, temperature.
- Monitor level of consciousness using the Glasgow Coma scale and assess pupil reaction and limb movement.
- Maintain a safe environment by using bed rails and managing confused or challenging behaviour.
- Maintain personal hygiene with a bed bath at least daily and provide frequent eye and mouth care.
- Prevent pressure ulcers by risk assessment, use of pressure-relieving beds and equipment and adjusting the patient's position 2-hourly. Perform passive exercises and position limbs to reduce risk of contractures.
- Communicate with the patient as if he/she can hear and understand conversation and help the family to develop ways of communicating with the patient such as use of touch.
- Observe closely for signs of pain such as restlessness, vital signs, grimacing. Administer analgesia as prescribed.
- Maintain dignity and privacy by providing information for the patient and relatives in a confidential manner.
- Provide emotional support to the patient and family members.
- Promote sleep and rest and reduce stimulation, noise and external noxious stimuli where possible.

Box 28.8 Reflection

Brain stem death – breaking bad news

You have been asked to accompany the doctor when she informs the family that their relative is brain dead.

How will you feel? What strategies could you use to convey your compassion, empathy and concern for the relatives?

➡ REFLECTION AND LEARNING – WHAT NEXT?

- Test your knowledge by visiting the website 🖱 and answering the multiple choice questions and critical thinking questions.
- **Consolidate** your learning by looking at some of the further reading suggestions, references and specialist websites.

- **Revisit** some of the additional material on the website.
- **Consider** what you have learnt and how this will help your professional development.
- **Reflect** on how you can apply this knowledge to the care of your patients.
- **Discuss** your learning with your mentor/supervisor, lecturer and colleagues.

REFERENCES

Ackerman MH: A review of normal saline instillation: implications for practice, *Dimens Crit Care Nurs* 15(1):31–38, 1996.

Akyol A, Ulusoy H, Ozen I: Hand washing: A simple economical and effective method for preventing nosocomial infections in intensive care units, *J Hosp Infect* 62(4):395–405, 2006.

British Medical Association: *Treatment decisions for patients in persistent vegetative state*, London, 1996, British Medical Association. Available online http://ww.bma.org.uk.

Buglass EA: Oral hygiene, *Br J Nurs* 4(9):516–519, 1995.

Chudley S: The effect of nursing activities on intracranial pressure, *Br J Nurs* 3(9):454–458, 1994.

Conference of the Medical Royal Colleges: Diagnosis of brain death, *Br Med J* ii:1187–1188, 1976; also *Lancet* ii: 1069–1070.

Conference of the Medical Royal Colleges: Diagnosis of death, *Br Med J* i:332, 1979; also *Lancet* i: 261–262.

Dalvi A: *Normal pressure hydrocephalus*, 2010. Available online http://www.emedicine.com.

Department of Health: Standard principles for preventing hospital acquired infections, *J Hosp Infect* 47(Suppl):S21–S37, 2001.

Department of Health and Welsh Office: *Mental Health Act 1983 Code of Practice*, London, 1999, DH.

Dikeman KJ, Kazandjian MS: *Communication and swallowing management of tracheostomised and ventilator-dependent adults*, San Diego, 1995, Singular Publishing.

Dougherty L, Lister S, editors: *The Royal Marsden Hospital Manual of Clinical Nursing Procedures*, ed 7, Chichester, 2008, Wiley-Blackwell.

Eilers J, Berger AM, Peterson MC: Development, testing and application of the oral assessment guide, *Oncology Nurse Forum* 15(3):13–23, 1988.

Fitzgerald MJT: *Neuroanatomy – basic and clinical*, ed 3, London, 1996, W B Saunders.

Glass CA, Grap MJ: Ten tips for safer suctioning, *Am J Nurs* 95:51–53, 1995.

Guyton AC, Hall JE: *Textbook of medical physiology*, ed 10, London, 2000, W B Saunders.

Hewitt J: Psycho-affective disorder in intensive care units: a review, *J Clin Nurs* 11:575–584, 2002.

Hickey JV: *The clinical practice of neurological and neurosurgical nursing*, ed 5, New York, 2003, Lippincott Williams and Wilkins.

Huskinson W, Lloyd H: Oral health in hospitalised patients: assessment and hygiene, *Nurs Stand* 23(36):43–47, 2009.

Jones C, Griffiths RD, Humphries G: Memory, delusions and the development of acute post-traumatic stress disorder-related symptoms after intensive care, *Crit Care Med* 29(3):573–580, 2001.

Laws-Chapman C, Rushmer F, Miller R, et al: *Suction guidelines pack*, St George's Healthcare NHS Trust, Hythe, Kent, 2000, Portex Ltd.

Mackenzie D: MRSA: the psychological effects, *Nurs Stand* 12(11):49–53, 1997.

Marieb EN: *Human anatomy and physiology*, ed 6, San Francisco, 2004, Addison Wesley Longman.

Martin KM: When the nurse says 'He's just not right': patient cues used by expert nurses to identify mild head injury, *J Neurosci Nurs* 26(4):210–218, 1994.

Meeting the Organ Shortage: *Council of Europe. Meeting the organ shortage. Current status and strategies for improvement of organ donation*, Strasbourg, 1999, Council of Europe.

National Institute for Health and Clinical Excellence (NICE): *Head injury: triage, assessment, investigation and early management of head injury in infants, children and adults. Clinical Guideline 4*, London, 2003, NICE.

National Patient Safety Agency (NPSA): *Advice to the NHS on reducing harm caused by the misplacement of NG tubes*, London, 2007, NPSA. Available online www.npsa.nhs.uk/site/media/documents/856_Alert-FinalWeb.pdf.

Nursing and Midwifery Council (NMC): *The Code: Standards of Conduct, Performance and Ethics for Nurses and Midwives. Nursing and Midwifery Council*, London, 2008, NMC. Available online http://www.nmc-uk.org.

Pallis C, Harley DH: *ABC of brainstem death*, ed 2, London, 1996, BMJ Publishing Group.

Palmer R, Knight J: Assessment of altered conscious level in clinical practice, *Br J Nurs* 15:1255–1259, 2006.

Pellowe CM, Pratt RJ, Loveday HP, Harper P, Robinson N, Jones SRL: The epic project. Updating the evidence base for national evidence based guidelines for preventing healthcare associated infections in NHS hospital in England: a report with recommendations, *British Journal of Infection Prevention* 5:10–16, 2004.

Phipps WJ, Sand JK, Marek JF, editors: *Medical-surgical nursing: concepts and clinical practice*, ed 6, St Louis, 1999, Mosby.

Podurgiel M: The unconscious experience: a pilot study, *J Neurosci Nurs* 22(1):52–53, 1990.

Porter D: Advance Directives and the persistent vegetative state in Victoria: a human rights perspective, *J Law Med* 13(2):256–270, 2005.

Randall P: A stranger in the family, *Nurs Times* 93(39):32–33, 1997.

Royal College of Nursing: *Good practice in infection control. Guidance for nursing staff. Working Well Initiative*, London, 2004a, Royal College of Nursing. Available online http://www.rcn.org.uk/publications.

Royal College of Nursing: *Restraint revisited – rights, risk and responsibility. Guidance for nursing staff*, London, 2004b, Royal College of Nursing.

Royal College of Physicians: *The vegetative state – guidance on diagnosis and management*, London, 2003, Royal College of Physicians.

Siddiqi N, Holt R, Britton AM, Holmes J: Interventions for preventing delirium in hospitalised patients, *Cochrane Database Syst Rev* 2: CD005563, 2007.

Smith S: The outer edge of consciousness, *Nurs Times* 93(39):28–32, 1997.

Sque M, Long T, Payne S: Research notes on organ donation, *Nurs Stand* 17(34):21, 2003.

Teasdale G: Acute impairment of brain function: assessing conscious level, *Nurs Times* 71(24):914–917, 1975.

Treloar DM, Nalli BJ, Guin P, Gary R: The effect of familiar and unfamiliar voice treatments on intracranial pressure in head-injured patients, *J Neurosci Nurs* 23(5):295–299, 1991.

Waterhouse C: The Glasgow Coma Scale and other neurological observations, *Nurs Stand* 19(33):56–74, 2005.

Waugh A, Grant A: *Ross and Wilson's Anatomy and physiology in health and illness*, ed 9, Edinburgh, 2001, Elsevier.

Wilson J, Islam O: *Normal pressure hydrocephalus*, 2004. Available online http://www.emedicine.com.

Woodrow P: *Intensive Care Nursing*, ed 2, London, 2006, Routledge, Taylor & Francis Group.

Woodward S: Practical procedures for nurses. No 5.1. Neurological observations 1: Glasgow Coma Scale, *Nurs Times* 93(45), 1997a.

Woodward S: Practical procedures for nurses No 5.2. Neurological observations 2: pupil response, *Nurs Times* 93(46), 1997b.

Woodward S: Practical procedures for nurses No 5.3. Neurological observations 3: limb responses, *Nurs Times* 93(47), 1997c.

Woodward S: Practical procedures for nurses No 5.4. Neurological observations 4: case studies, *Nurs Times* 93(48), 1997d.

Working Group of Royal College of Physicians: Criteria for the diagnosis of brain stem death, *J R Coll Physicians Lond* 29:381–382, 1995.

USEFUL WEBSITES

British Association of Neuroscience Nurses: www.bann.org.uk

British Brain and Spine Foundation: www.bbsf.org.uk
    Freephone helpline: 0808 808 1000

Epilepsy Action: www.epilepsy.org.uk

Head and brain injuries: Equip (Electronic Quality Information for Patients): www.equip.nhs.uk/topics/neuro/injury.html

Headway – the brain injury association: www.headway.org.uk

Life NPH (Normal Pressure Hydrocephalus): www.allaboutnph.com

Mold-Help: www.mold-help.org/pulmonaryinfections

National Poisons Information Service: www.npis.org

Organ/tissue donation and transplants: www.uktransplant.org.uk

UK Clinical Ethics Network: www.ethics-network.org.uk

Nursing the critically ill patient

Helen Singh

Introduction

The term 'critically ill' is used to describe people who have acute, life-threatening conditions but who might recover if they are given prompt, appropriate, effective and often highly technical nursing and medical care. Critically ill patients, the conditions from which they suffer and the care and treatment they need are so varied that elements from every chapter in this book are relevant to their care. Patients who present in a critically ill state can be considered in three main categories:

- those who have never before had a significant illness and who have suffered a sudden, acute life-threatening event, e.g. extensive trauma, severe burns, near drowning, major childbirth complications or deliberate self-harm
- those who suffer from chronic illness, perhaps involving frequent previous hospital admissions, e.g. chronic pulmonary airways disease (COPD) or chronic pancreatitis, and who present as critically ill as a combination of their chronic illness with a life-threatening event
- those who have become critically ill as a result of surgery – in some cases, the life-threatening situation is not

expected, while in others, postoperative critical care is a recognised necessity.

Critical care is a constantly emerging and costly speciality that has grown as a response to developments in medicine and surgery (Department of Health [DH] 2000). The case mix is varied, and admission to critical care can result from trauma, disease adverse events or surgery. All patients will require some kind of organ support or intervention (DH 2005). Critical care is classified into three levels outlined in Box 29.1.

The term 'critical care' encompasses intensive care patients categorised as level 3, and high-dependency patients (level 1 and 2 in the Department of Health guidelines). Critical care in recent years has expanded to provide services throughout the hospital which are termed 'outreach services'. The service has been developed in many acute hospitals to meet the needs of critical care provision 'without walls'; this facilitates early identification of at risk patients and timely transfer to critical care services (Hancock & Durham 2007). The specialist teams made up of specialist nurses and medical staff are available to all wards and departments for advice and to review patients at risk of deterioration. Early warning scoring systems have been implemented in many hospitals to help identify patients at risk. These assessment tools use

Box 29.1 Information

Levels of critical care support (Department of Health 2000)

0. Patients whose need can be met through normal ward care in an acute hospital

1. Patients at risk of their condition deteriorating, or those recently relocated from a higher level of care, whose needs can be met on an acute ward with additional advice and support from the critical care team

2. Patients requiring more detailed observation or intervention including support for a single failing organ system or postoperative care and those 'stepping down' from a higher level of care

3. Patients requiring advanced respiratory support alone or basic respiratory support together with support of at least two organ systems. This level includes all complex patients requiring support for multi-organ failure

physiological parameters to assess the patient. An abnormal parameter such as a respiratory rate >30 would give a high score and identify to ward staff the need for support with the management of the patient. (See Further reading, ALERT Manual 2003. The text gives guidance of identifying at risk patients.)

Over recent years, critical care has expanded further to the community setting with the development of home ventilation services: patients with chronic diseases such as muscular dystrophy, motor neurone disease and high spinal injuries who require respiratory support are managed at home with input from specialised home ventilation nurse practitioners.

The nursing care of the critically ill patient is an extensive and specialised area of care that cannot be fully addressed in this chapter. The aim of this chapter is to provide an overview and, where appropriate, provide links to other chapters and more specialised texts and journals.

The primary responsibility of the nurse in the critical care setting is to provide physical and psychological care for patients and help prevent complications. There are a number of different models of nursing that have been adapted to deal with all aspects of care for these patients, and due to the nature of their condition, a *systems approach* is the most logical method of reviewing the care requirements for individual patients. Tools such as daily goals sheets, a multidisciplinary tool to ensure that all aspects of the patient's care are considered, are helpful.

 See website for an example of a daily review sheet

Patient safety

Patient safety is high on the agenda of Government and professional bodies. The acquisition of health care associated infections such as meticillin-resistant *Staphylococcus aureus* (MRSA) and *Clostridium difficile* receives a great deal of media attention, and developing strategies to avoid harm is crucial (NICE 2007). Critical care practitioners have developed evidence-based 'care bundles' in order to optimise care. Care bundles are a group of interventions related to a

disease process that, when executed together, result in a better outcome than when implemented separately (Fulbrook & Mooney 2003).

MEETING THE PHYSICAL NEEDS OF THE CRITICALLY ILL PATIENT

Respiratory needs and care

Many disease processes may lead to the need for ventilatory support (Box 29.2). Mechanical ventilation is the artificial support of, or assistance with, breathing when adequate gaseous exchange and tissue perfusion can no longer be maintained (see Ch. 3). Ventilatory support can be administered 'invasively' through an endotracheal tube or tracheostomy or non-invasively through a mask or hood. Both methods can maintain vital function; the type of support required depends on the patient's underlying condition. Patients with type I or type II respiratory failure or acute pulmonary oedema are likely to have a good response to non-invasive ventilation, which may avoid intubation (Tully 2002).

Ventilation modes

Practitioners must have specialist training in the equipment and processes involved in the care of patients requiring ventilation in order to deliver optimal care and recognise complications. The ventilation modes and care outlined below give a brief overview. The patient's underlying medical

Box 29.2 Information

Causes of respiratory failure (adapted from Weilitz 1993)

Acute respiratory failure without respiratory distress

• Central airway obstruction
• Decreased level of consciousness
  – head injury
  – sepsis
  – drug overdose
• Neuromuscular pathway impairment
  – Guillain–Barré syndrome
  – myasthenia gravis
  – postoperative diaphragmatic paralysis
  – trauma
• Cardiovascular impairment
  – acute myocardial infarction
  – cardiogenic shock

Lung parenchymal disease

• Asthma
• Pneumonia
• Acute lung injury (ALI)

Acute or chronic respiratory failure

• Exacerbation of chronic obstructive airways disease (COAD)
• Chronic neuromuscular disease

condition, age and weight, will determine the prescribed mode of ventilation.

Invasive modes

- **IPPV** (intermittent positive pressure ventilation). This delivers a preset tidal volume at a preset rate. It ignores the patient's own respiratory drive. Its use is restricted to heavily sedated or paralysed patients or those with central nervous system disturbance.
- **SIMV** (synchronised intermittent mandatory ventilation). The positive pressure breaths are synchronised with the patient's own breathing and the patient is able to breathe spontaneously.
- **BiPAP** (biphasic positive airway pressure). Used in invasive ventilation, this mode uses pressure control to deliver the tidal volume. It also allows spontaneous breathing and is often used in acute lung injury (ALI).
- **ASB/PS** (assisted spontaneous breathing/pressure support). This senses when a patient takes a breath and gives them additional preset support. It can be used with SIMV or alone.
- **PEEP** (positive end-expiratory pressure). PEEP increases functional residual capacity, i.e. the amount of air left in the lungs at the end of expiration. The pressure prevents small alveoli collapsing and allows a longer period of gas exchange. It is used as an adjunct to IPPV, SIMV and ASB/PS. High levels of PEEP can reduce venous return and reduce cardiac output.

The potential complications of mechanical ventilation are outlined in Box 29.3.

Non-invasive modes

- CPAP (continuous positive airway pressure). This is equivalent to PEEP but is delivered via mask or hood (see Figure 29.1) Airway pressure is maintained above

Box 29.3 Information

Potential complications of mechanical ventilation

- Damage to the airways/lung parenchyma
- Barotrauma, tension pneumothorax, disconnection/occlusion of the endotracheal tube
- Mechanical failure
- Subcutaneous emphysema
- Hypo/hyperventilation
- Pulmonary oedema/pleural effusions
- Nosocomial hospital acquired infection (HAI), consolidation
- Low cardiac output
- Cardiovascular depression
- Arrhythmias
- Water retention
- GI haemorrhage, aspiration of stomach contents, paralytic ileus
- Impairment of CNS, kidneys and liver function
- O_2 toxicity
- Altered body image
- Sleep deprivation
- Tracheal injury

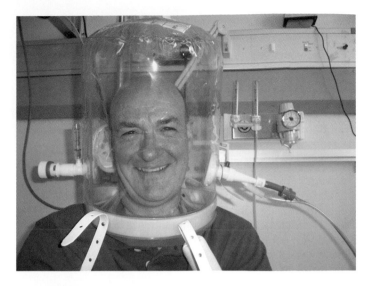

Figure 29.1 A CPAP hood.

atmospheric pressure throughout the ventilatory cycle by pressurisation in the ventilatory circuit. This makes breathing easier for the patient and facilitates gas exchange.
- NIV (non-invasive ventilation) supports the patient's breathing to a preset pressure level:
  - IPAP (inspired positive preset pressure). This is the pressure level the patient receives on inspiration. The patient initiates a breath, and this breath is then supported by the ventilator to the preset IPAP pressure.
  - EPAP (expired positive airway pressure). As the patient breathes out, the expired positive airway pressure prevents alveolar collapse.

This mode is frequently employed in type II respiratory failure or as a maximum treatment option if the patient is not suitable for invasive ventilation (British Thoracic Society 2002).

Non-invasive ventilation has become a popular choice for clinicians in recent years. It has the potential advantage over invasive methods of reducing the risk of infection and reducing length of stay (Tully 2002).

Close observations of the patient's face should be undertaken for pressure damage. Patients who are actively vomiting and those with gastrointestinal bleeds or facial trauma may not be suitable candidates for NIV. Clear explanations are required to ensure the patient understands the treatment. The patient is often anxious prior to treatment commencing due to feeling breathless, and the masks and hoods used can cause feelings of claustrophobia. The gradual implementation of treatment may be necessary to enable the patient to get used to the therapy.

 Nursing management and health promotion: respiratory care

Monitoring respiratory function and maintaining safe ventilation

Monitoring and maintaining safe ventilation is crucial and, once the patient is intubated (see Ch. 28) and receiving ventilation support, constant and thorough observations are required as there are many associated complications (see Box 29.3).

Chest auscultation This should be performed at the start of a shift, as a baseline, and thereafter at the discretion of the nurse. It can offer a wealth of information about the patient's air entry – from an expiratory wheeze requiring treatment with a bronchodilator, to areas of reduced air entry due to secretion retention, consolidation or pulmonary oedema. Using a systematic approach, this can detect trouble early and assure appropriate intervention.

Ventilator associated pneumonia A ventilator associated pneumonia (VAP) can be defined as a nosocomial airway infection that develops more than 48 hours after intubation (Westwell 2008). There is good evidence that implementing a ventilator care bundle can demonstrate a significant reduction of VAP (Arlene et al 2007).

Ventilator care bundle

The following components should be incorporated into the patient's daily care.

- Avoid the supine position; patients should be nursed at least 30 degrees head up to prevent oesophageal reflux and pulmonary aspiration (Drakulovic et al 1999).
- Sedation should be reviewed and if possible stopped each day in order to assess the patient's readiness to wean and prevent oversedation (Kress et al 2000).
- Patients should be assessed for readiness to wean each day. This daily screening reduces ventilator days and complications (Marelich et al 2000).
- Using chlorhexidine as part of daily mouthcare reduces oropharyngeal colonisation and VAP (Chlebicki & Safdar 2007).
- Use of subglottic secretion drainage in patients ventilated for more than 48 hours may prevent aspiration and lower airway colonisation (Lorente et al 2007). Potentially contaminated secretions collect in the patient's oropharynx above the cuff of the tracheal tube. Endotracheal and tracheostomy tubes are now available with an additional port so the subglottic secretions can now be cleared from the patient's oropharynx.

Each bundle element has its own set of exclusion criteria. Further information can be found on the Scottish Intensive Care Society website (www.sicsag.org.nhs.uk). An aide-memoire of the bundle is included on the website.

See website Figure 29.2

Humidification The oxygen used to ventilate the patient must be warmed, humidified and filtered artificially as the endotracheal tube bypasses the natural processes of the nasal passages. Exposing the lungs and airways to cold gas has a number of potentially harmful effects: it can increase mucus viscosity, depress ciliary activity and obstruct the airways due to the build-up of the tenacious secretions. Disposable heat moisture exchange filters (HMEF) are now widely used, primarily because they are cheap and disposable. Temperature-controlled water humidifiers may be used if patients have tenacious secretions.

Ventilator and endotracheal (ET) tubes The ventilator tubes must not be allowed to become kinked as this would reduce the desired respiratory effect. Patient comfort must be balanced with the safe and secure position of the ET tube in the patient's mouth. This is achieved by tying a crepe bandage around the patient's mouth to prevent movement of the ET tube. In the case of a patient with a head injury non-allergic adhesive tape should be used instead of a bandage to decrease the risk of raised intracranial pressure. Care should be given to pressure prevention and the position of the ET tube can be changed daily to facilitate this. Ventilator tubes must not be allowed to drag as this in turn pulls on the ET tube, thereby applying pressure to the lips. Ventilators usually have an 'arm' which will support the weight of the tubes. To prevent water from condensation in the tubing entering the ET tube and the lungs it is important that the tubes slope downwards from the patient towards the water traps. When turning the patient, care must always be taken to ensure that ET and ventilator tubes are guarded and supported.

Endotracheal cuff pressures These need to be checked regularly using an endotracheal cuff manometer. While cuff pressures of 30 mmHg are recommended, pressures of 17–23 mmHg have been shown to be adequate. Complications arising from prolonged excessive ET cuff pressures include tracheal oedema, loss of mucosal cilia, ulceration, ruptured tracheo-oesophageal fistula, stenosis, necrosis, sore throat and hoarseness (Wood 1998). Prevention of these complications is the reason why a tracheostomy is recommended after 12–14 days of oral intubation.

Ventilator observations

Continual observation of the patient should include:

- the patient's colour to check if well perfused or cyanosed
- oxygen saturation (SaO$_2$; see Ch. 3)
- level of consciousness, i.e. if sedated or whether drowsy due to CO$_2$ retention
- chest movements, i.e. are both lungs being ventilated?
- vital signs – changes in a patient's vital signs can indicate problems with ventilation; blood pressure, heart rate and rhythm, temperature, and respiratory rate and pattern should all be closely monitored.

Observations of the ventilator should include:

- fraction of inspired oxygen (FiO$_2$)
- the prescribed ventilatory setting
- the expired minute volume
- the patient's tidal volume
- airway pressures and respirations (spontaneous and ventilator breaths).

All observations should be recorded hourly allowing for continual respiratory assessment and the early detection and treatment of any problems.

Arterial blood gases (ABGs) Judicious analysis of ABGs (see Ch. 3) will most accurately reveal a patient's respiratory progress or deterioration and the adequacy of ventilatory support. Care must be taken not to oversample, to prevent iatrogenic anemia (Andrews & Waterman 2008).

Inhaled nitric oxide (NO) administration The administration of inhaled nitric oxide can improve oxygenation of patients with acute respiratory distress syndrome (ARDS). Whilst there is good evidence of improvement of oxygenation in the short term (Hsu et al 2008) the treatment shows no mortality benefit. Nitric oxide is a highly toxic environmental pollutant and so closed suction systems should always be used.

Positioning

The position of the patient will depend on where the pulmonary abnormality is, and the patient should be positioned to maximise the matching of ventilation and perfusion. In a case of a left lower lobe collapse, it may be helpful to nurse the patient on the right side, thereby optimising the treatment to the affected area. Regularly turning patients will not only assist in the prevention of pressure ulcers but also facilitate pulmonary postural drainage. Nursing the patient in a semi-recumbent position with a 30 degree head tilt reduces the risk of aspiration and ventilator associated pneumonia.

When a patient's oxygenation remains poor, despite high oxygen delivery and high PEEP levels (classically found in ALI), it may be decided to position the patient face down in the prone position. This manoeuvre increases lung compliance by recruiting underventilated areas of the posterior lung bases and improves oxygenation (Mancebo et al 2006).

Endotracheal suction

Together with hand ventilation (see below), ET suctioning is a procedure used to facilitate the clearance of secretions when a patient's normal cough mechanism is either inadequate or disrupted. This may occur where there is underlying respiratory or neurological disease or where the cough reflex is suppressed by sedation, muscle relaxants or anaesthetic agents during IPPV. Its purpose is the removal of pulmonary secretions, to avoid the problems associated with their retention, such as increased airway pressures, pneumothorax, cardiovascular instability, lobar consolidation, ventilation–perfusion mismatch, pneumonia, hypoxaemia and atelectasis. However, endotracheal suction can produce complications and carries with it hidden risks (see Box 29.4). Maintaining a patent airway involves endotracheal suctioning and, while it is essential to keep the airway clear of secretions, it is also important not to oversuction and thereby cause unnecessary trauma, irritation and hypoxia

Box 29.4 Information

Potential hazards of endotracheal suctioning
- Tracheal mucosal damage
- Hypoxaemia
- Atelectasis
- Arrhythmias
- Infections
- Excessive coughing
- Stress response
- Pain
- Aspiration of stomach contents

Box 29.5 Information

Some adverse effects of hand ventilation
Respiratory effects
- Pneumothorax
- Loss of the effect of PEEP
- Bronchospasm
- Decreased respiratory drive
- Rebreathing CO_2

Cardiovascular effects
- Decreased blood pressure due to decreased venous return caused by the IPPV of hand ventilation
- Increased blood pressure due to inadequate sedation or inadequate hand ventilation
- Vagal stimulation (causing bradycardia)

(Wood 1998). In order to minimise these risks certain principles should be adhered to; these are discussed in Chapter 28.

Hand ventilation (manual hyperinflation)

Manual hyperinflation is a manual form of positive pressure ventilation using a rebreathing bag. It is used primarily to stimulate a cough in patients with either a poor or absent cough reflex, or when there is atelectasis or excessive bronchial secretions. This intervention must be carefully assessed on an individual patient basis as it is not without severe adverse effects (see Box 29.5) and may have a negative effect on patients with raised intracranial pressure. Hand ventilation may be necessary when there is a ventilator fault, or during cardiopulmonary resuscitation.

Weaning

Weaning is the term used to describe the gradual transition from mechanical to spontaneous ventilation (self-ventilation). During the weaning phase, patients may alternate between these modes until they are able to cope continually on a reduced mode, ultimately achieving spontaneous breathing. It should be individually tailored and begun as soon as it is established that the patient is physically capable of maintaining respiration. The nurse has a key role to play in this. Patients who are likely to require ventilation over a longer period of time will be considered for a tracheostomy (see Chapter 14), which is more comfortable and the patient will require less sedation. It is good practice to allow the patient to rest overnight by giving them increased ventilatory support, which will also allow the patient's $PaCO_2$ to return to normal. Each patient should be assessed for readiness to wean each day, an example of an assessment tool can be found on the web.

 See website Figure 29.3

Extubation

When spontaneous respiration is successfully maintained, the next step is the removal of the ET tube, a procedure known as extubation. Prior to this procedure, ABGs, oxygen saturation, tidal volumes, respiratory rate and pattern, vital signs, any evidence of tiring, and the presence of a gag reflex together with a strong cough reflex must all be reviewed. Extubation should not be considered unless the patient can cough, swallow and protect the airway, and is sufficiently alert to co-operate. If possible, a planned extubation early in the day is ideal, with more staff on duty. Emergency equipment should be available in case rapid re-intubation is necessary.

Cardiovascular care

In critical care settings, monitoring systems are essential in order to evaluate any potentially fatal physiological derangements and to allow timely treatment to correct any abnormalities. The cardiovascular system can be monitored by the measurement of volume, flow, pressure and resistance in different areas. Chapter 2 covers haemodynamic aspects of care and should be referred to in relation to this section. Patients admitted to critical care units undergo monitoring to glean information about tissue perfusion, blood volume, tissue oxygenation and vascular tone. It is the nurse's responsibility to carefully monitor these parameters and identify changes.

Nursing management and health promotion: cardiovascular care

Monitoring heart rate and rhythm

The amount of information that can be gleaned from a three-lead ECG and, more importantly, a 12-lead ECG, must never be underestimated and a sound understanding of the heart's electrical activity facilitates this (see Ch. 2). Cardiac arrhythmias are commonplace in patients in critical care. Hypoxia, shock, electrolyte abnormalities, sepsis, vagal stimulation from ET suctioning, irritation from central venous or pulmonary artery catheters, and medication are responsible for the majority of cardiac arrhythmias; however, some will be the result of myocardial ischaemia in patients with underlying heart disease. Accordingly, where possible, the nurse needs to be aware of any cardiac impairment the patient may have. Monitoring should be continuous, to enable early detection and prompt treatment of underlying problems. For information about the conduction pathways of the heart, arrhythmias and their management, see Chapter 2.

Monitoring arterial blood pressure

Critically ill patients generally have an arterial line inserted for the accurate measurement of arterial blood pressure and the provision of easy access to arterial blood for blood gas analysis. Common sites for the insertion of arterial lines are (in order of preference): radial artery, brachial artery, femoral artery, dorsalis pedis artery (see Ch. 18 for care of patients with arterial lines). Together with the systolic and diastolic arterial pressure, the mean arterial pressure (MAP) is also recorded. This gives the measurement of perfusion pressure over the majority of the cardiac cycle. A MAP of 65–85 mmHg is generally the acceptable range. Below 50 mmHg is dangerous as it is inadequate to perfuse vital organs and tissues.

Box 29.6 Information

Complications associated with arterial lines

- Infection/potential sepsis. Infection can occur during insertion or at the site. Strict adherence to asepsis and the use of occlusive dressing and chlorhexidine to clean the site will reduce this risk
- Haemorrhage due to disconnection of the line. Check the Luer lock connections and ensure the line is not pulled when moving the patient
- Air embolism. If air gets into the system this could be 'flushed' into the patient. Care is required when setting up the transducer system
- Vascular occlusion/thrombosis (distal circulation should be assessed regularly)
- Ischaemia of the distal limb
- Poor reading. Lines should be re-zeroed each shift in order to calibrate the equipment to normal atmospheric pressure. The saline pressure bag should be maintained at 300 mmHg to maintain accuracy and the level of the transducer should be maintained at mid heart
- Spasm of the artery. This can be caused by forceful flushing of the line or aspirating samples of blood too vigorously
- Wrongful administration of medication. Arterial lines must be clearly identified to prevent them being confused with intravenous cannulae. Staff must be appropriately trained in their management to prevent this

Complications associated with arterial lines can and do arise (Box 29.6).

Monitoring central venous pressure (CVP)

Central venous access is generally preferred over peripheral access, because it enables assessment of the patient's circulating blood volume as well as allowing the administration of intravenous medication such as inotropes, specific antibiotics/antifungals and certain electrolyte supplements that can only be infused centrally. Monitoring the CVP also allows for the assessment of the tone of the vascular system and the ability of the right side of the heart to accept and expel blood, itself influenced by left ventricle function (see Ch. 18). The trend of readings, along with other clinical information, is more important than any one reading on its own. Insertion of invasive lines is not without its complications. A care bundle should be implemented to manage the care, and the elements are outlined in Box 29.7. The principles of this care bundle are applicable to all invasive lines.

Monitoring cardiac output

There are a number of tools that can give greater insight into the patient's cardiac performance.

Pulmonary artery catheter

A pulmonary catheter enables the assessment of the functioning of the left ventricle and very often becomes part of the monitoring profile in situations causing either circulatory failure or acute respiratory failure. Its use is considered when information is required about fluid status, cardiovascular function or oxygen delivery. It provides information

Box 29.7 Information

Central line bundle

Insertion bundle

- Hand hygiene and maximal barrier precautions
- Ensure the procedure is documented in the patient's notes
- Skin asepsis with 2% chlorhexidine
- Catheter site selection: the femoral site should be avoided where possible

Maintenance

- Assess patient daily to determine continued necessity for a central line
- Dressing should be intact, cleaning with chlorhexidine
- Needle-free access devices should be used

which guides the therapy of those patients on mechanical ventilation, circulatory assist devices or inotropic medication (see Ch. 18 for information on insertion of and care of pulmonary artery catheters).

The pulmonary artery wedge pressure (PAWP), or 'wedge', gives a more accurate indication of the fluid status of the patient. Elevated PAWP may be due to volume overload, left ventricular failure (LVF), mitral stenosis or regurgitation and cardiac tamponade. Abnormally low readings may be due to hypovolaemia (see Box 29.8).

Oesophageal Doppler monitoring

Oesophageal Doppler monitoring is now increasingly favoured in critical care, primarily because it is less invasive and offers a reduced risk of morbidity and mortality in comparison to the pulmonary artery catheter. An ultrasound probe is placed in the oesophagus running parallel with the descending aorta. The Doppler then measures the velocity of the blood flow in the descending aorta (Edwards 1998). This form of monitoring is not suitable for all types of patient; it is most useful as a guide in deciding when, what and how much fluid replacement to give in cases of hypovolaemia.

PICCO (pulse contour cardiac output index)

This method uses a standard central line with a temperature sensor on the distal lumen and a thermodilution sensor

Box 29.8 Information

Haemodynamic cardiac profile – normal readings

- Pulmonary artery pressure (PAP)
    - systolic: 15–25 mmHg
    - diastolic: 8–15 mmHg
- Pulmonary artery wedge pressure (PAWP): 6–12 mmHg
- Cardiac output (CO): 4–8 L/min
- Cardiac index (CI): 2.5–4.2 L/min per m^2
- Systemic vascular resistance (SVR): 900–1600 dyn/s per cm^5 (this measurement relates to the resistance to flow in the whole systemic circulation)
- Mixed venous oxygen saturations (SvO_2): 65–75%

Adapted from Coombs (1993).

arterial catheter in the femoral artery. Injection of cold fluid into the CVP line is sensed by the arterial line. The method allows calculations of cardiac output, cardiac index and stroke volume; it also gives an indication of extravascular lung water. It has the advantage of being less invasive than a pulmonary artery catheter.

Inotropic medication

Cardiac output monitoring is often used to determine inotropic therapy, as it clarifies whether there is a pressure problem (i.e. reduced blood pressure), a problem with the flow (i.e. decreased cardiac output), or a problem with oxygen delivery and consumption. Cardiac contractility can become impaired, either as a direct result of cardiogenic shock, or secondary to hypovolaemic and septic shock. In such cases, inotropic medication such as noradrenaline, dopamine and dobutamine, which improve cardiac contractility, is used to support the patient until such time as definitive treatment is administered or the patient recovers. Administration is always via a central vein and the effects of inotropic therapy are monitored closely. Different combinations of inotropic medication may be advocated in order to achieve the desired effect. It is common practice to titrate inotropic therapy against MAP, generally aiming for a MAP of between 65 and 85 mmHg; inotropic medication is always reduced slowly by 1 mL at a time before discontinuation.

Monitoring and regulating temperature

Despite a wide variety of heat-producing metabolic processes and the range of ambient temperatures to which the human body may be exposed, homeostatic mechanisms ensure that core body temperature is maintained with remarkable stability. However, critical illness can disturb temperature control, producing body temperatures at either end of the spectrum, i.e. hypothermia ($<35°C$) or hyperthermia/hyperpyrexia ($>38.5°C$). High temperatures can have an adverse effect on intracranial pressure of patients with unstable head injuries and these patients may be actively cooled (Price et al 2003). Patients who have suffered cardiac arrest may benefit from therapeutic cooling for brain protection (Collins & Samworth 2008). Chapter 22 explores temperature monitoring and regulation in depth.

Prevention of thromboembolism

Deep vein thrombosis (DVT) is a potentially fatal risk factor in any hospitalised patient and it is significantly increased in critical care patients where anticoagulation is often contraindicated. In addition to anticoagulation, compression stockings and pneumatic compression devices are effective in minimising risk (SIGN 2002). It is essential that the patient requirement for DVT prophylaxis is incorporated into the patient's daily assessment (Box 29.9).

Renal care and fluid balance

With the kidney normally requiring 25% of the cardiac output, physiologically compromised patients are at high risk of developing acute renal failure (ARF), a sudden and usually reversible failure of the kidneys to excrete the waste products of metabolism. This is a common problem in the Critical Care Unit. Sepsis is the most common cause of multi-organ dysfunction syndrome (Ronco 2006). ARF is characterised by a rapid decline in renal function over days or weeks, which results from the cessation of or decreased urine output and the accumulation of metabolites and electrolytes normally excreted by the kidney.

Other causes are divided into prerenal, renal and postrenal and are outlined in Chapters 8 and 20. Systemic manifestations may accompany the development of renal insufficiency and these can include lowered haemoglobin level, fluid overload, breathlessness, arrhythmias due to electrolyte imbalance, and confusion and itchy skin due to build-up of urea. The treatment of ARF is predominantly one of support until recovery occurs; the condition is nearly always recoverable.

Nursing management and health promotion: renal care

In susceptible patients, the primary goal must always be the prevention of renal impairment. This involves knowledge of the causes of ARF and meticulous monitoring of the following:

Urine output In addition to the monitoring of all fluid intake, hourly urine output volumes must be recorded, together with an accurate 24-h fluid balance of all fluid gains and losses. While a urine output of less than 0.5 mL/kg/h (oliguria) over a 24-h period is indicative of ensuing renal failure, it is also acknowledged that ARF can occur in the absence of oliguria (non-oliguric ARF).

Urea and electrolytes Daily assays of urea and electrolytes will indicate the degree of renal insufficiency present. Urea, creatinine and some electrolyte levels rise with developing ARF, leading to varying degrees of metabolic acidosis. It should be noted, however, that elevated urea on its own may indicate merely that the patient is dehydrated. The nurse must know the normal plasma values for urea, creatinine and the more common electrolytes and the significance of any deviations, as some electrolyte abnormalities can produce life-threatening arrhythmias.

Fluid therapy Intravenous fluid therapy should be considered carefully in the management of the critically ill patient. This is particularly so in conditions of sepsis, ALI or systemic inflammatory response syndrome (SIRS). In such situations,

the permeability of capillary endothelial cells increases and the vessels become 'leaky', allowing large protein particles to pass into the interstitial space, thus reducing the capillary osmotic pressure. This facilitates the movement of water together with further protein molecules into the interstitial space, depleting intravascular volume and impairing gaseous exchange. This results in peripheral oedema and, within the lungs, results in pulmonary oedema, causing hypoxaemia and consequently diminished oxygen delivery and consumption by peripheral tissues. Vascular volume must be restored. The three main groups of volume-expanding fluids are crystalloids, colloids and blood:

- Crystalloids are made up of non-ionic solutes such as sodium chloride added to water; they do not contain oncotic particles and will therefore eventually move out of the vascular compartment (see Ch. 20). These fluids, unlike colloids, are cheap to produce and are not associated with immunologically mediated reactions.
- Colloids, which contain oncotic particles, generating oncotic pressure, are mainly confined to the intravascular space, at least when first administered.
- Blood and blood products also exert an oncotic pressure due to the large protein particles they contain and so are less likely to contribute to interstitial oedema.

Cardiovascular status directly affects renal perfusion. It is recommended that the MAP is above 60 mmHg for renal perfusion to be ensured (Kishen 2002). Regular monitoring of the CVP, cardiac output and PAWP will indicate whether fluid input or inotropic support is required. The presence of peaked T waves on the ECG is suggestive of a rising plasma potassium level.

Nephrotoxic medication The use of nephrotoxics, e.g. gentamicin and non-steroidal anti-inflammatory drugs (NSAIDs), should be avoided in those with impending renal failure or in those whose renal function is precarious.

Immediate management of diminishing renal function

- Optimise fluid balance either by giving a fluid challenge if vital signs indicate hypovolaemia or by using diuretic therapy if there are clinical signs of fluid overload. Furosemide, a potent loop diuretic, is the drug of choice.
- Correct electrolyte imbalances as necessary.
- Maintain haemoglobin within the normal range.
- Ensure adequate nutritional input.
- Remove any known causative factors, e.g. nephrotoxic drugs.
- Exclude obstruction, e.g. make sure that the urinary catheter has not become blocked with sediment.
- Diuretic therapy. Diuretics will not alter the course of acute renal failure (Cleaver 2004), however they may help maintain fluid balance. Sumnall (2007) argues that diuretics should only be used when patients have had hydration status corrected and be limited in duration.

Renal replacement therapy

A small number of patients in critical care will require renal replacement therapy (RRT) to manage their ARF. While not providing a 'cure', it enables the critically ill patient to be supported pending recovery from the underlying disease process or injury. There are no set criteria for when RRT should be commenced, but it should be instituted before complications occur (Sumnall 2007). Hyperkalaemia, severe fluid overload, gross uraemia and metabolic acidosis are all indications for treatment. RRT administered with higher volume exchanges has shown some benefit for the treatment of sepsis syndrome (Ronco 2006).

Caring for patients with RRT is deemed part of the professional practice of experienced nurses working in the critical care. They require a thorough knowledge of the reasons for its use, the equipment involved, the problems that can arise and how to respond to them.

Haemofiltration

Technology has advanced significantly since the 1970s when the process of RRT was first introduced.

Continuous venovenous haemofiltration (CVVH) is generally the mode of choice in haemofiltration, as it allows the slow, steady removal of fluid volume. It also gives the venous system time to compensate for fluid lost from the interstitial spaces. Most importantly, it avoids the rapid shift of solutes and electrolytes, thereby preventing the risk of cardiovascular instability. A further advantage of CVVH is that it does not require arterial access. Access for CVVH is via a double-lumen catheter, often referred to as a Quinton line, which is inserted into a main vein. The blood is pumped through an artificial kidney where fluid, solutes and electrolytes are moved across a semi-permeable membrane by convection and ultrafiltration. A set amount of fluid is then added to the circuit to replace the removed fluid. Anticoagulation is necessary to prevent the blood clotting in the plastic circuit. The amount of fluid exchanged and replaced will be prescribed according to the urea and creatinine levels, fluid balance and stability of the patient.

Molecular adsorbent recycling system (MARS) MARS is a membrane-based blood purification system, also referred to as bioartificial liver support. It works directly with the CVVH in supporting liver function in severe liver failure, providing time for detoxification, hepatic regeneration or donor availability, and is used in patients with fulminant hepatic failure (FHF), e.g. after paracetamol and other drug overdose (Stange et al 2002).

Nursing responsibilities in haemofiltration

- **Fluid balance.** Accurate measurement of input and output of fluid is essential, and RRT is reviewed daily by the renal physicians. The nurse responsible for the patient should adjust filtration rates in accordance with the medical prescription.
- **Vital signs.** The recording of vital signs is imperative. At the start of CVVH, the patient's blood pressure may fall. The patient's temperature is also altered. It is generally believed that body temperature drops by 1°C with CVVH in progress. To prevent this, replacement fluid should be warmed to a suitable temperature. It should be noted that CVVH may mask developing sepsis, as a recorded temperature of 37°C may equate to a patient temperature of nearer 38°C.

- **Urea, electrolytes and arterial blood gases.** Regular assessment of urea, electrolytes and ABGs is necessary in order to assess acid–base balance. Electrolyte supplements are often required. Phosphate is normally elevated in ARF; however, it is removed very efficiently on CVVH and may require supplementation. Replacement fluids have different concentrations of potassium and are prescribed to meet patient need.
- **Monitoring the activated clotting time (ACT).** The time it takes for a small sample of blood to clot is of particular importance if the patient is receiving heparin as anticoagulation therapy while on the haemofilter. Heparin, the anticoagulant of choice, is administered to prevent clotting of the extracorporeal circuit (Urwin et al 2001). Some patients will not be able to tolerate the effects of heparin, as it is known to disrupt the intrinsic coagulation cascade and promote platelet aggregation. This is seen particularly in liver failure. In such cases, prostacyclin can be used as it preserves platelet function and number. It does, however, have strong side-effects, noticeably vasodilatation, causing facial flushing and significant hypotension. ACT is not required with prostacyclin.
- **Preventing infection and maintaining asepsis** are vital. Patients on haemofiltration are often immunocompromised and therefore are more susceptible to infection. Residual catheterisation is performed every 2–3 days, preventing stasis of urine in the bladder, a potential source for infection. If urine volume is 250 mL or more, the catheter is normally left in situ, as this can be indicative of the return of renal function.
- **Maintenance of patient safety** is the nurse's responsibility. If venous access is via the femoral vein, the limb must be carefully observed to ensure optimal perfusion is maintained. Furthermore, the prevention of air emboli, infection or haemorrhage, as a consequence of heparin use, should be borne in mind.

Neurological care

Altered states of consciousness of critically ill patients fall into two distinct types of causes:

- intracranial pathology, such as intracranial haemorrhage, cerebral hypoxia, tumours and abscesses
- systemic disease affecting the cerebral blood supply or oxygenation, such as sepsis, metabolic encephalopathy, hypoglycaemia, hepatic failure (hepatic encephalopathy), renal failure, pancreatitis, respiratory failure or hypo/hyperthermia, exogenous agents, such as drugs and toxins, and drug withdrawal.

 Nursing management and health promotion: neurological care

Neurological functioning is an important part of the overall clinical assessment and continuous care of those being nursed in critical care. The use of a standardised

Grades of encephalopathy (Gunning 2003)

I. Altered mood, impaired concentration and psychomotor function, rousable

II. Drowsy, inappropriate behaviour, able to talk

III. Very drowsy, may be agitated or aggressive

IV. Coma, may respond to painful stimuli

neurological assessment tool such as the Glasgow Coma Scale (GCS) is essential, enabling early detection of any deterioration and facilitating prompt treatment (see Ch. 28). In addition, patients with intracranial pathology may require invasive neurological monitoring of intracranial pressure (ICP) and cerebral perfusion pressure (CPP). This is often indicated in patients who demonstrate a GCS of 8 or less and/or a grade 3 or 4 encephalopathy (Box 29.10). As with the majority of clinical observations, it is the trend that is of greatest significance when monitoring ICP and CPP.

Monitoring neurological function

Glasgow Coma Scale (GCS) The GCS is the standard tool used in assessing neurological function. It is an objective way of measuring levels of consciousness (LOCs) and is discussed in Chapters 9 and 28.

Intracranial pressure monitoring (ICP) Intracranial pressure is the pressure exerted by the intracranial contents against the skull. Normally, brain tissue constitutes 80%, cerebrospinal fluid (CSF) 10% and blood volume 10% of the intracranial contents. Severe head injuries remain the most common cause of raised ICP, but it may also occur in patients presenting with problems such as hepatic encephalitis due to fulminant hepatic failure (Hawker 1996). This is increasingly seen nowadays as the consequence of paracetamol overdose. The level at which treatment of raised ICP will be necessary depends on the patient's condition, but is often set at around >20 mmHg. Medication of choice includes mannitol 20% given in conjunction with furosemide and albumin replacement; hypertonic saline (5%) is also effective in treating raised ICP. If ICP is unresponsive to these treatment modalities barbiturate therapy such as thiopentone may be necessary, which lowers ICP by reducing metabolism to a minimum and lowering blood pressure by reducing venous and arterial tone, thus reducing cerebral perfusion (Stanley & Hancox 2001).

Cerebral perfusion pressure (CPP) The value of monitoring the ICP is that it allows the CPP to be calculated. This is done by subtracting the ICP measurement from the mean arterial pressure of circulating blood within the cranial cavity (i.e. CPP = MAP − ICP). Generally the aim is to maintain CPP above 70 mmHg, thus preventing underperfusion of the cerebral tissue.

Computed tomography (CT) scan In relation to neurological functioning, CT scanning is usually performed in order to detect cerebral haematomas, oedema, infarctions, atrophy, hydrocephalus and tumours.

Jugular bulb oximetry (SJO$_2$) is an uncommon invasive monitoring system, but may be used to provide information about global cerebral oxygen consumption (Chatfield & Rees-Pedlar 2001).

Cerebral function analyser monitor (CFAM) This comprises a visual display unit and printer which allows the continual monitoring and display of cerebral activity. It is used continuously by the bedside to assess whether the patient is appropriately sedated and is commonly used with patients receiving paralysing agents in order to detect whether or not they are having seizures.

Nursing responsibilities and ICP

The maintenance of adequate ventilatory support is essential as hypercapnia and hypoxia will increase cerebral vasodilatation, causing raised ICP. Conversely a low $PaCO_2$ below 3.5 kPa can cause cerebral ischaemia and a target range of 4.0–4.5 kPa is standard for the majority of head-injured patients. Continual monitoring of the end-tidal CO_2 assists with this. To ensure adequate ventilatory support:

- Secure the ET tube with adhesive tape rather than a bandage around the neck to avoid restricting cerebral drainage.
- Ensure good head alignment, elevating the head of the bed to promote cerebral drainage.
- Keep all nursing procedures to a minimum. The nurse should give careful consideration to endotracheal suctioning. The procedure itself will cause a rise in ICP, however retained secretions will also have a negative impact on ICP.
- Check pupil size and reaction hourly and following all nursing and medical procedures.
- Maintain an accurate fluid balance chart. Monitor and be aware of electrolyte levels, e.g. both hypo- and hypernatraemia can contribute to raised ICP.
- Prevent cerebral ischaemia and maintain CPP above 60 mmHg. Inotropes are often administered to achieve this.
- Provide adequate nutritional support. Patients with ICP problems are often in a hypercatabolic state.
- Assess the need and extent to which pressure area care is appropriate.
- Maintain the patient's temperature at normothermia. Administration of antipyretics such as paracetamol and active cooling may be necessary to achieve this. In some cases of severe cerebral insult patients may require cooling to hypothermia.
- Seizures may occur after head injury due to direct brain irritation or secondary to hypoxia and hypotension (Price AM et al 2003). Close observation for seizure activity and administration of anticonvulsants is necessary.

A therapeutic flow chart on the management of acute head injury can be found on the website.

See website Figure 29.4 and Critical thinking question 29.1

Sedation and pain management

 ▷ **Nursing management and health promotion: sedation and pain management**

Pain has been identified as a major problem for patients in the ICU. Pain is a subjective experience and the control of pain will require regular assessment and clear documentation. The challenge is to provide the most appropriate form of pain relief. Pain control is covered extensively in Chapter 19 and therefore this section will focus primarily on the assessment of sedation required.

Assessing the need for sedation and analgesics

Most critically ill patients will, at some point during their stay, require sedation and/or analgesics. Sedation may be necessary to produce the respiratory depression required to facilitate adequate ventilation, to aid tolerance of the presence of the ET tube or to decrease anxiety in general. Views and practice have changed considerably over the years from the belief that patients should be heavily sedated and unaware of their surroundings to the current preferred state of lighter sedation while maintaining an optimal state of comfort (Shelley 1998). Sedation and analgesics can be administered continually or as a bolus, the prescribed regimen being tailored to the needs of each patient. The nurse must constantly assess the sedation level and a number of sedation scaling systems exist to assist with this (Box 29.11); this

requires a sound knowledge of the issues surrounding sedation in the ICU, i.e. sensory overload and sensory deprivation (see Meeting the psychosocial, cultural and spiritual needs of the critically ill patient). Optimal sedation should enable the patient to be rousable on stimulation but able to sleep/rest when undisturbed. Keeping the patient comfortable is a balance between under- and oversedation (Shelley 1998).

Daily sedation breaks

There has been a great deal of debate in the literature about nurse-led daily sedation breaks (Pinder & Christensen 2008). Patients are assessed each morning by the nurse, and if appropriate the sedation is stopped and the patient allowed to wake. If the patient is cooperative the sedation remains off, but if the patient is distressed or agitated it is recommenced at half the previous rate and titrated up until the optimal level is achieved. This intervention has been shown to reduce ventilator time and length of stay in critical care (SICSAG 2008). For an example of a combined sedation hold and weaning protocol see the website.

 See website Figure 29.5

Agitation and delirium

Agitation and delirium is common among critically ill patients and is multifactorial; the condition is also referred to as 'ICU psychosis'. Patients may experience anxiety, become paranoid and very disorientated to time and place, hallucinate and become agitated. It is physiological, treatment-related and associated with the physical environment; the causes are summarised in Box 29.12. Pharmacological intervention can assist with management of these challenging patients, however identification and correction of

---

 Box 29.11 Information

Richmond Agitation Sedation Scale (RASS) (Sessler et al 2002)

Score	Term	Description
+4	Combative	Overtly combative, violent, immediate danger to staff
+3	Very agitated	Pulls or removes tube(s) or catheter(s); aggressive
+2	Agitated	Frequent non-purposeful movement, fights ventilator
+1	Restless	Anxious but movements not aggressive vigorous
0		Alert and calm
−1	Drowsy	Not fully alert, but has sustained awakening (eye-opening/eye contact) to *voice* (**>10 seconds**)
−2	Light sedation	Briefly awakens with eye contact to *voice* (**<10 seconds**)
−3	Moderate sedation	Movement or eye opening to *voice* (**but no eye contact**)
−4	Deep sedation	No response to voice, but movement or eye opening to *physical* stimulation
−5	Unrousable	No response to *voice or physical* stimulation

Box 29.12 Information

Possible causes of agitation (reproduced with permission from Pinder & Christensen 2008)

Internal – associated with illness or physiology	External – associated with physical environment	Caused by treatment
• Infection • Sepsis • Fever • Encephalopathy • Hypoxaemia • Hypoglycaemia • Arterial hypotension • Inflammation • Brain injury • Acute renal failure and uraemia • Metabolic disturbance	• Sleep deprivation • Pain – surgical and less overt causes e.g. ET tube, urinary catheter position • Fear and disorientation	• Withdrawal from sedatives • Anxiety and disorientation • Alcohol and drug withdrawal • Medication and side-effects

underlying pathology is essential in management. The nurse has a key role to play in effectively communicating with and reorientating patients. Ensuring that communication aids such as glasses and hearing aids are worn and optimising the environment to ensure normal sleep patterns can be maintained are essential nursing interventions.

Pharmacological interventions

Four main groups of drugs can be used to enhance patient comfort:

Sedatives Propofol has anaesthetic properties and is commonly used to sedate patients who require short periods of mechanical ventilation. It is widely used as it provides a controllable level of sedation, which is easily maintained, and recovery is rapid, allowing weaning from the ventilator to progress. Midazolam has sedative, anxiolytic and amnesic properties and has a short half-life. However, it is largely hepatically metabolised and renally excreted and therefore could accumulate should these organs be impaired.

Analgesics Alfentanil is a valuable analgesic in the ICU, especially when short-term supplementation is required. It is short-acting with a short half-life. Morphine provides safe analgesia but should be used with caution in those with liver and renal impairment.

Neuromuscular blocking agents (paralysing agents, e.g. atracurium) are occasionally used in specific patient groups. They reduce O_2 consumption and stop respiratory drive in patients who have developed acute lung injury, and lower ICP in head injury.

Antidepressants (e.g. amitriptyline) Antidepressants are often prescribed in those showing depressive behaviour, often patients who have been critically ill for weeks, where weaning from the ventilator is slow, or in those with previous depressive illness. As well as improving mood, antidepressants can help to normalise the sleep pattern. Haloperidol is usually the medication of choice but should not be given before first assessing the patient's vital signs, clinical condition and the underlying cause of their behaviour.

Nutritional and gastrointestinal care

The nurse plays a key role in the nutritional management of the critically ill. Critical care patients are at risk of malnutrition, and the need for nutrition for critical care patients is well recognised. Where possible such nutritional support should be via the enteral route and started as soon as possible after admission. This will maintain the patient's gastrointestinal integrity, minimise translocation of organisms, decrease the incidence of infection and aid wound healing (Fulbrook et al 2007). The use of protocols is a useful tool in ensuring early establishment of enteral nutrition. Most patients in critical care can be fed enterally, the only absolute contraindication being true gut failure. Relative contraindications include bowel anastomosis distal to the feeding tube, pancreatitis or small bowel disease.

Nursing management and health promotion: nutritional and gastrointestinal care

Nasogastric (NG) feeding

The nurse has a responsibility to check the correct placement of the NG tube. The National Patient Safety Agency (2005) recommends this is done by regular checking of gastric pH using pH strips, or by radiography. Some patients may not absorb their feed due to factors such as opioids and immobility, which may be alleviated through the use of a wide variety of pharmacological agents such as metoclopramide, which stimulates gastric emptying, and erythromycin, which has been demonstrated to increase gastric motility (Bradley 2001a).

Naso-jejunal feeding

This involves the placement of a fine bore tube into the jejunum and may be an alternative for patients who are not tolerating NG feeding. However, an endoscopy is required to achieve this. Some companies have manufactured tubes that can be passed without the requirement of an endoscope, however the results are not fully consistent.

Parenteral nutrition

For patients who cannot be fed through the enteral route, parenteral nutrition (PN) is the alternative. It consists of a lipid-based substance that requires administration via a large central vein. Because of the high risk of sepsis PN should always be administered through a port on the central line that has not previously been used. Meticulous asepsis is required when changing the bags. Careful consideration of the patient's nutritional and electrolyte needs should be made; the dietician and pharmacist are helpful in assessing individual patient requirements. Critical care patients can undergo significant physiological stress and feeding can be a lifesaving intervention. Whilst the use of protocols shows positive results for ensuring early enteral nutrition, feeding regimens must be adapted to meet the patient's individual physiological needs.

Optimal glucose control

Critical care patients may have altered blood glucose levels due to acute disease processes, chronic diseases such as diabetes mellitus, and administration of inotropic medications, steroids and PN. Over the past few years research has indicated that keeping blood sugar within tight parameters reduces morbidity and mortality in the critically ill (Van den Berghe et al 2001). The role of hypoglycaemia in critical illness has been the subject of considerable debate in recent literature, and Parsons & Watkinson (2007) suggest the evidence is not as compelling as originally thought. The Institute for Healthcare Improvement (2008) recommend optimal control and recommend a more relaxed target of blood sugar maintenance between 3.5 and 8.5 mmol/L. The nurse has a key role in monitoring patients' blood sugar levels and administering insulin, usually according to a local protocol.

Maintaining GI integrity

Maintaining normal bowel function in critical care patients is a real challenge, with patients at risk of both diarrhoea and constipation. The nurse plays a key role in monitoring bowel function.

Constipation

Opioids, immobility, surgery and spinal injury can cause constipation, and pain and abdominal obstruction can be consequences. Many critical care units have bowel management protocols (Mckenna et al 2001) which can reduce the risk with early implementation of aperients and suppositories when required.

Diarrhoea

Enteral feeding, antibiotics and altered gut motility can cause patients to have diarrhoea, which is uncomfortable and embarrassing for patients as well as putting them at risk of dehydration and skin excoriation. Stool samples should be analysed to rule out any infective cause such as *Clostridium difficile*. Skin can be protected by the use of bowel management systems which use a soft tube inserted into the rectum. Close monitoring of the patient's fluid and electrolyte balance along with reassurance is a key nursing requirement for these patients.

Stress ulceration

This may develop due to damage to the mucosal layer of the gastrointestinal tract, often during a period of ischaemic anoxia as part of a shocked state (see Ch. 28). In addition, impaired production of gastric mucus, reduced epithelial renewal, disturbed acid–base balance, reflux of bile acids and the presence of uraemia all predispose the patient to gastric ulceration (Bradley 2001b). Enteral feeding acts as prophylaxis; however, in patients being supported by PN, prophylactic medication should be prescribed. Antacids and H_2-receptor blockers are thought to be equally effective as prophylactic agents for stress ulcers.

Hygiene, mobility and wound care

Critical care patients range from those who require assistance with all aspects of their care to the high-dependency patient who requires nursing input in the form of rehabilitation and mobilisation. Meticulous assessment skills and individualised nursing care are required in order to maintain optimal body tissue integrity and organ function.

▷ Nursing management and health promotion: hygiene, mobility and wound care

Personal hygiene

Assisting with the maintenance of personal hygiene not only promotes comfort and dignity, but also represents an opportunity for thorough assessment of the patient, including skin integrity, any potential sites of infection, e.g. cannula insertion site, and the peripheral circulation. The nurse should maintain the dignity of the critically ill patient at all times.

Oral hygiene

Most seriously ill patients will encounter oral problems, some specific to the disease and others associated with the medication. There is, for example, an increased risk of mouth ulcers, dry, cracked oral mucosa or yeast growth in those with diabetes mellitus, acute or chronic breathing difficulties and thyroid dysfunction. Furthermore, with the use of certain antibiotics, diuretics or morphine and procedures such as intermittent suction, the potential for oral hygiene problems is heightened. In accordance with the VAP prevention bundle (see p. 760), ventilated patients should have 2% chlorhexidine gel administered 4 times per day (Chlebicki & Safdar 2007) (see Ch. 15 for more on oral hygiene).

Eye care

Critical care patients have reduced ability to use their protective blink reflex and poor eyelid closure. Artificial ventilation causes reduced tear production and decreases venous return leading to conjunctival chemosis (Dawson 2005). Microbial keratitis and corneal exposure are also risks in the ventilated and sedated patient. To prevent such complications it is essential that the eyes are kept lubricated and eyelid closure is maintained. Polyacrylamide gel is a commonly used substance to achieve eyelid closure. The sterile clear substance is gently placed over the patient's eyes and changed 4 hourly. Patients must be adequately sedated if using this method, otherwise they will become very anxious as the gel prevents eye opening.

Maintaining skin integrity and promoting wound healing

A sound knowledge is necessary of the factors involved in successful wound healing and those that adversely affect its progress (see Ch. 23). The main types of wound encountered in the ICU are surgical wounds (see Chs 23 and 26), traumatic wounds and pressure ulcers (Chs 23 and 30).

Pressure ulcers

Prevention is always better than cure and this is certainly the case when it comes to pressure ulcers. However, with the critically ill patient, the main priority is ultimately to maintain haemodynamic stability and optimise ventilation, and in some cases this may be jeopardised by turning or rolling the patient. Therapeutic pressure relieving beds are regularly required for the maintenance of skin integrity. There is also a risk of tissue damage due to pressure from equipment, such as an ET tube pressing on the lip, a tightly taped three-way tap or tube pressing on the skin. Pressure ulcers may delay recovery, pose increased infection risks and entail much discomfort for the patient. Assessment of the patient's risk of developing pressure ulcers should be undertaken daily using a standardised tool such as the Waterlow pressure sore prevention/treatment policy (see Ch. 23).

Promoting and maintaining normal tone, power and movement of the musculoskeletal system

As well as regularly positioning the patient to optimise air entry and ventilation and maintain skin integrity, passive and active exercises should be carried out. In patients who have limited movement or who are unable to move at all, a regimen of passive movements can be implemented which will progress to active/assisted movements as the patient's condition improves. This can counteract effects of bed rest, e.g. deep venous thrombosis (DVT), contractures and foot drop. Physiotherapists play a vital role in assisting with mobilisation as the patient's condition gradually improves.

Prevention of health care associated infection (HAI)

HAI currently attracts a great deal of media attention and its prevention is rightly high on the Government's agenda. Critical care patients are at high risk of acquiring infection due to their immunocompromised state secondary to the disease process, and multiple tubes and invasive lines create access points for bacteria (Box 29.13). The nurse plays a key role

Box 29.13 Reflection

Mrs T is a 67-year-old lady who was admitted to critical care following a craniotomy and evacuation of subdural haematoma. On arrival from theatre she was ventilated and had intravenous access and an arterial line. A central line was inserted in order to support Mrs T's blood pressure with the administration of inotropic medication. She had an indwelling urinary catheter and was commenced on antibiotic treatment.

Mrs T had a past medical history of chronic atrial fibrillation which was treated with warfarin. She also had gastric ulcer disease and was on long-term omeprazole, a protein pump inhibitor. Mrs T also had a hiatus hernia and it was technically very difficult to put down a nasogastric tube to allow enteral feeding to commence.

Mrs T was ventilated for 5 days and discharged on day 6.

What factors put Mrs T at risk of getting an infection?

Answer

- Mrs T had 5 days on a ventilator. Any ventilated patient is at risk of VAP. Neurological patients are also twice as likely to get a VAP as general patients
- Presence of invasive lines – central lines, intravenous cannulae, arterial lines and urinary catheters
- Bacterial translocation. The passage of indigenous bacteria from the intestinal tract to other areas of the body which can cause sepsis and multi-organ failure in critical care patients. This risk can be reduced by early enteral feeding
- Recent major surgery. Neurological surgery carries a risk of meningitis or, as with any operation, surgical site infection
- Antimicrobial treatment. The widespread use of antibiotics also puts patients at risk of developing resistances. It also can alter the ecosystem in the patient's gut leading to overgrowth of some pathogens such as *C. difficile*. Mrs T is at increased risk of this infection due to being on a long-term PPI
- Immunological competence. The majority of critical care patients develop a degree of immunological compromise due to their underlying conditions
- Nutritional depletion. It is good practice in critical care to implement enteral nutrition early to reduce nutritional depletion, which is a significant factor in the body's ability to fight infection. In the case of Mrs T, this did not happen due to mechanical problems of siting a nasogastric tube
- Staff. Critical care has a large number of staff. The importance of handwashing cannot be stressed enough

in its prevention. Excellent nursing care and the use of central line and VAP prevention bundles help in the prevention strategy and isolation of patients with MRSA and *C. difficile*. However, the single most important prevention strategy is handwashing. Nurses not only play a key role with their own practice, but are also in a key position to remind other members of the multidisciplinary team to adhere to policy.

Meeting the psychosocial, cultural and spiritual needs of the critically ill patient

 ## Nursing management and health promotion: meeting the psychosocial, cultural and spiritual needs of the critically ill patient

It is important to support the patient psychologically and minimise the stress of the ICU environment. This can be achieved by:

- providing adequate information, reassurance and encouragement
- preventing sensory overload or sensory deprivation
- maintaining natural biorhythms/sleep patterns.

Providing adequate information, reassurance and encouragement

One of the most challenging aspects of critical care nursing is caring for the patient's psychological needs. The presence of ET tubes and underlying medical conditions makes communication more difficult but good communication may enable patients to see monitoring equipment as helpful rather than frightening, even if they do not always remember being told about it.

Preventing sensory overload or sensory deprivation

Critical care is a very foreign and strange environment to patients, and they are prone to experiencing sensory deprivation. Ensuring that patients have their spectacles and hearing aids available is an important nursing role. As patients are recovering, radios and televisions will help 'normalise' the environment.

Support for each patient is most likely to be optimised when nurses, visitors and the patient collaborate to achieve effective and sensitive communication. It is recognised that nurses who are known to the patient and those in whom they have confidence reduce levels of anxiety and panic (Price 2004).

Maintaining natural biorhythms/sleep

Human beings have biological or circadian rhythms that are normally related to the sleep/wake cycle, including fluctuations in body temperature, blood pressure, heart rate and plasma levels of various hormones (see Ch. 25). In critical care there is always a concern that activity and lighting may be more or less constant because of the need for constant observation and frequent treatment, leading to lack of sleep for patients and disturbance of their biological rhythms, and also contributing to the sensory–perceptual alterations and delirium known to affect a considerable proportion of critically ill people. Diminishing the amount of light, noise and disturbance as far as possible at night can help to minimise such potential problems. It is clear that nursing requires the application of sound knowledge, judgement and skill. Practice must be sensitive, relevant and responsive to the needs of the individual, and nowhere more so than when preventing sleep deprivation.

Cultural needs and spiritual care

Spiritual health relates to having a sense of meaning, hope and purpose in life, not simply to having a religious faith. Cultural and personal values are relevant to purpose in life and should be considered in assessment and care. Some critically ill patients lose hope and 'give up', ceasing to fight for life, particularly when ill for days or weeks. This can contribute not only to their current physical and emotional experience but also to the outcome of the illness. Anything a nurse can do, either directly or with the help of the patient's family or friends, to help the patient draw on their usual resources and sources of support must be helpful (Hupcey 2001). Many former patients have indicated that faith is an important part of a person's life and provides comfort in a crisis (Ashworth 1987).

The role of family and friends

Family and friends play an important role in relieving social isolation, depersonalisation and disorientation for patients. Yet family and friends are unable to be of maximum help to patients unless they themselves are assured of any necessary help from the nurses in the form of access, information and emotional support. Nurses have a great influence on the extent to which family and friends can support the sick patient during intensive care, after transfer to a ward and then home. Families themselves need significant support when their relative is in critical care, and their anxiety can be relieved by clear explanations. Many critical care units have an open visiting policy which is welcomed by families. Due to the nature of critical illness, death rates are high in critical care. The nurse has an integral role in guiding families through difficult processes of treatment withdrawal, brain stem death and organ donation.

SUMMARY: KEY NURSING ISSUES

- Care of the critically ill patient is a diverse and ever-expanding field with advances in medicine and technology.
- Patient care is designed to support patients both mentally and physically through this life-threatening time and prevent further complications of infections or secondary complications.
- To be effective, nurses must have a sound knowledge and understanding of physiology and other sciences and how the body works in health as well as in illness.
- The practitioner has a responsibility to ensure that evidence-based care is used to prevent secondary complications to achieve the best possible care for patients and their families. One of the most

effective ways of achieving this is by the implementation of care bundles where groups of interventions can be effective in improving patient outcome.

REFLECTION AND LEARNING – WHAT NEXT?

- **Test** your knowledge by visiting the website and answering the multiple choice questions and critical thinking questions.
- **Consolidate** your learning by looking at some of the further reading suggestions, references and specialist websites.
- **Revisit** some of the additional material on the website.
- **Consider** what you have learnt and how this will help your professional development.
- **Reflect** on how you can apply this knowledge to the care of your patients.
- **Discuss** your learning with your mentor/supervisor, lecturer and colleagues.

REFERENCES

Andrews T, Waterman H: What factors influence arterial blood gas sampling patterns? *Nurs Crit Care* 13(3):132–137, 2008.

Arlene F, Tolentino-DelosReyes AF, Rupert SD, Shiao SPK: Evidence based practice: Use of ventilator care bundle to prevent ventilator associated pneumonia, *Am J Crit Care* 16:20–27, 2007.

Ashworth P: The needs of the critically ill patient, *Intensive Crit Care Nurs* 3(4):182–190, 1987.

Bradley C: Drug therapy review: erythromycin as a gastrointestinal prokinetic agent, *Intensive Crit Care Nurs* 17(2):117–119, 2001a.

Bradley C: Drug therapy review: stress ulcer prevention – the controversy continues, *Intensive Crit Care Nurs* 17:58–59, 2001b.

British Thoracic Society: Non-invasive ventilation in acute respiratory failure, *Thorax* 57:192–211, 2002.

Chatfield D, Rees-Pedlar S: Jugular venous oxygen saturation: is it relevant to the nurse? *Nurs Crit Care* 6(4):187–191, 2001.

Chlebicki MP, Safdar N: Topical chlorhexidine for prevention of ventilator-associated pneumonia: A meta-analysis, *Crit Care Med* 35:595–602, 2007.

Cleaver N: Drugs used to promote diuresis a treatment for fluid balance chart? *Nurs Crit Care* 9:80–85, 2004.

Collins TJ, Samworth PJ: Therapeutic hypothermia after cardiac arrest: a review of the evidence, *Nurs Crit Care* 13(3):144–151, 2008.

Coombs M: Haemodynamic profile and the critical care nurse, *Intensive Crit Care Nurs* 9:11–16, 1993.

Dawson D: Development of new eye care guidelines for critically ill patients, *Intensive Crit Care Nurs* 21(2):119–122, 2005.

Department of Health (DH): *Comprehensive Critical Care: a review of adult critical care services*, London, 2000, DH.

Department of Health (DH): *Quality Critical Care – Beyond 'comprehensive critical care': A report by the critical care stakeholder forum*, London, 2005, DH.

Drakulovic MB, Torres A, Bauer TT: Supine body position as a risk factor for nosocomial pneumonia in mechanically ventilated patients: a randomised trial, *Lancet* 354:1851 1858, 1999.

Edwards S: Determining hypervolaemia using trans-oesophageal Doppler monitoring, *Nurs Crit Care* 3(4):176–181, 1998.

Fulbrook P, Mooney S: Care bundles in critical care: a practical approach to evidence based practice, *Nurs Crit Care* 8(6):249–255, 2003.

Fulbrook P, Bongers A, Albarran JW: A European survey of enteral nutrition practices and procedures in adult intensive care units, *J Clin Nurs* 16(11):2132–2141, 2007.

Gunning KEJ: Acute Liver Failure, *Anaesthesia and Intensive Care Medicine* (2):112–113, 2003.

Hancock HC, Durham L: Critical care outreach: The need for effective decision making in clinical practice (Part 1), *Intensive Crit Care Nurs* 23(1):15–22, 2007.

Hawker FH: Intensive care nursing management of fulminant hepatic failure. In Dellinger RP, Burchardi H, Dobbs GJ, Bion J, editors: *Current topics in intensive care*, London, 1996, WB Saunders, Ch. 9.

Hsu CW, Lee DL, Lin SL, Chang HW: The initial response to inhaled nitric oxide treatment for intensive care unit patients with acute respiratory distress syndrome, *Respiration* 75(3):188–295, 2008.

Hupcey J: The meaning of social support for the critically ill patient, *Intensive Crit Care Nurs* 17(4):206–212, 2001.

Institute for Healthcare Improvement: *Establish a glycemic control policy in your ICU*, 2008. Available online http://www.ihi.org/IHI/Topics/CriticalCare/IntensiveCare/Changes/IndividualChanges/EstablishaGlycemicControlPolicyinYourICU.htm.

Kishen R: Managing acute renal failure in the critically ill: where are we today? *Care of the Critically Ill* 18(6):170–171, 2002.

Kress JP, Pohlman AS, O'Connor MF, Hall JB: Daily interruption of sedative infusions in critically ill patients undergoing mechanical ventilation, *N Engl J Med* 342:1471–1477, 2000.

Lorente L, Lecuona M, Limenez A, Mora ML, Sierra A: Influence of an endotracheal tube with a polyurethane cuff and subglottic secretion drainage on pneumonia, *Am J Respir Crit Care Med* 176:1079–1083, 2007.

Mancebo J, Fenandez R, Blanch L, Rialp G: A multicenter trial of prolonged prone ventilation in severe acute respiratory distress syndrome, *Am J Respir Crit Care Med* 173(11):1233–1240, 2006.

Marelich GP, Murin S, Battistella F: Protocol weaning of mechanically ventilation in medical and surgical patients by respiratory care practitioners and nurses: effect on weaning time and incidence of ventilator associated pneumonia, *Chest* 118:459–467, 2000.

Mckenna S, Wallis M, Brannelly A, Cawood J: The nurse management of diarrhoea and constipation before and after the implementation of a bowel management protocol, *Aust Crit Care* 14(1):10–16, 2001.

National Institute for Health and Clinical Excellence (NICE): *Patient safety solutions pilot: pilot project summary*, 2007. Available online http://www.nice.org.uk/patient safety.

National Patient Safety Agency (NPSA): *Patient safety alert: Reducing the harm caused by misplacement of nasogastric feeding tubes*, 2005, National patient safety agency UK. Available online http://npsa.nhs.uk/site/media/documents/856-Alert-Finalweb.pdf.

Parsons P, Watkinson P: Blood glucose control on critical care patients – a review of the literature, *Nurs Crit Care* 12(4):202–210, 2007.

Pinder S, Christensen M: Sedation breaks: are they good for the critically ill patient? A review, *Nurs Crit Care* 13(2):64–70, 2008.

Price A: Intensive care nurses' experience of assessing and dealing with patients' psychological needs, *Nurs Crit Care* 9(3):134–142, 2004.

Price AM, Collins TJ, Gallagher A: Nursing care of the acute head injury: a review of the evidence, *Nurs Crit Care* 8(3):126–133, 2003.

Price T, McGloin S, Izzard J, Gilchrist M: Cooling strategies for patients with severe cerebral insult in ICU (Part 2), *Nurs Crit Care* 8(1):37–45, 2003.

Ronco C: Recent evolution of renal replacement therapy in the critically ill patient, *Crit Care* 10(1):123–127, 2006.

Sessler CN, Gosnell M, Grap MJ: The Richmond Agitation-Sedation Scale: validity and reliability in adult intensive care patients, *Am J Respir Crit Care Med* 166:1338–1344, 2002.

Shelley MP: Sedation in the ITU, *Intensive Crit Care Nurs* 14(3):85–88, 1998.

Scottish Intensive Care Society Audit Group (SICSAG): *VAP Prevention Bundle, Guidance for implementation*, 2008.

Scottish Intercollegiate Guidelines Network (SIGN): *Prophylaxis for thromboembolism (SIGN 62)*, 2002. Available online http://www.sign.ac.uk.

Stange J, Hassanein TI, Mehta R, Mitzner SR, Bartlett RH: Molecular adsorbents recycling system as a liver support system based on albumin dialysis: a summary of preclinical investigations, prospective, randomized, controlled clinical trials and clinical experience from 19 centers, *Artif Organs* 26(2):103–110, 2002.

Stanley IR, Hancox D: Initial management of severe head injuries: is cerebral perfusion pressure maintained? *Care of the Critically Ill* 17(5):166–167, 2001.

Sumnall R: Fluid management and diuretic therapy in acute renal failure, *Nurs Crit Care* 12(1):27–33, 2007.

Tully V: Non-invasive ventilation: a guide for nursing staff, *Nurs Crit Care* 7(6):296–299, 2002.

Urwin S, Leary TS, Fletcher S: Haemofiltration II, *Care of the Critically Ill* 17(3):99–104, 2001.

Van den Berghe G, Wouters P, Weekers F, et al: Intensive insulin therapy in critically ill patients, *N Engl J Med* 345(19):1359–1367, 2001.

Weilitz PB: Weaning a patient from mechanical ventilation, *Crit Care Nurse* 13(4):33–40, 1993.

Westwell S: Implementing a ventilator care bundle in an adult intensive care unit, *Nurs Crit Care* 13(4):203–206, 2008.

Wood C: Endotracheal suctioning: a literature review, *Intensive Crit Care Nurs* 14(1):124–136, 1998.

FURTHER READING

ALERT Acute Life-Threatening Events Recognition and Treatment: *Learning media development*, 2003, University of Portsmouth.

Scottish Intercollegiate Guidelines Network: *Prophylaxis for thromboembolism (SIGN 62)*, 2002. Available online http://www.sign.ac.uk.

USEFUL WEBSITES

Scottish Intensive Care Society: www.sicsag.org.nhs.uk

CHAPTER 30

Nursing the patient with burn injury

Breeda McCahill

Introduction

Imagine for a moment having lost everything: your loved ones; your home and possessions, including mementoes from the past; your health and ability to function normally; your appearance – in other words, yourself. This not infrequently occurs when people are victims of a house fire.

Most people experience minor burns more than once in their lifetime but few have any conception of the horror associated with severe burns injury. Extensive burns injury is catastrophic, both physically and psychologically, for the patient and their family. It is also one of the most challenging and arduous types of injury to treat. In order to help the patient and their family to achieve optimal function, the responsibility of care must be distributed throughout the multidisciplinary team. However, the nurse, being the only professional in 24-h attendance, will play an especially important role. Nurses also attend to many patients whose burns are not extensive, providing care in the community, in emergency departments (ED) and in general surgical wards. This chapter provides information which will help nurses care for patients with burn injuries in all settings.

Prevention of burn injuries

Burns are frequently described as being among the most serious of injuries because of the long-term problems which are often associated with them. Advances in treatment and improved facilities have led to a reduction in mortality rates (Pereira et al 2004), but the resultant morbidity is such that prevention is the responsibility of all health care personnel.

Studies emphasise that, in order to be effective, burn prevention programmes should involve assessment of the incidence of burn injuries, followed by planning, implementation and evaluation of appropriate interventions (Liao & Rossignol 2000).

Assessment

This includes identifying the extent of the problem, its causative agents and any predisposing factors.

The extent of the problem

It is estimated that, in the UK, 112 000 people attend emergency departments annually suffering from the effects of burn injuries, with a further 250 000 presenting at GP services; approximately 7765 people require hospital admission and 211 people die each year as a result of burn injury (Benson et al 2006). Although statistical data on burn mortality are generally available, the incidence of burn morbidity is difficult to estimate.

Causative agents

Scalds or flame burns are the most common type of burn injury. Contact burns (touching hot objects) also have a high incidence. Chemical and electrical burns occur less frequently.

The Office of the Deputy Prime Minister (2003), previously responsible for collating fire statistics, identified the most common cause of death in domestic fires as careless handling of fire and hot substances, mainly smokers' materials. Non-fatal burn casualties result from the misuse of equipment or appliances, most commonly cooking appliances. Hot water in plumbing systems is also a considerable cause for concern in countries where there is no legislation governing the upper limit of plumbed water temperature. Although many authorities advocate a temperature of 50°C (which would take 2–3 min to cause a burn), because of altered sensation and reduced mobility in older people, this figure has been reduced to 43°C in residential accommodation for older people (Stone et al 2000).

Predisposing factors

Epidemiological studies identify toddlers as being at greatest risk of burn injuries, with scalds accounting for most of these (Tse et al 2006). Adult high-risk groups include those with epilepsy (Unglaub et al 2005) and those who smoke tobacco, drink alcohol in excess and take prescribed psychotropic medications (Anwar et al 2005). Older people have also been identified as being more susceptible to burn injury and as having a higher mortality rate following injury (DeSanti 2005). Studies agree that males of all ages are at higher risk than females.

The common denominator of predisposition to burn injury appears to be a combination of reduced awareness of danger and decreased mobility.

Planning and implementation

Planning for a burns prevention programme must be realistic. While it is impossible to modify certain risk factors, e.g. gender and age, having identified the groups most at risk, it should be possible to alter some of the related predisposing factors.

There are already numerous health education/promotion campaigns aimed at persuading the public not to smoke and to only drink alcohol in moderation. It seems unlikely that those who do not comply would be influenced by the knowledge that smoking and drinking alcohol increase their risk of burn injuries. Tones and Tilford (2001) state that, unlike the promotion of commercial products, which is based on enhancing pleasure and promising immediate gratification, health promotion usually urges people to stop doing something which they find pleasurable in the hope of long-term benefit. They also state that people have a right not to be unreasonably frightened. Blatant shock tactics are therefore considered unacceptable and are likely to make people 'switch off'. More subtle, but potentially potent, messages may be conveyed, e.g. by incidental reference in popular television series.

Identification of the burn agent or energy source results from epidemiology studies. The agent may be a result of poor design of equipment, e.g. the hot water jug with a higher centre of gravity than a kettle, or a radiator which produces a high surface temperature. Once the problem has been recognised, design modification may be sufficient to eradicate the danger.

Product modification may be carried out voluntarily by manufacturers; however, legislation is often required. Since 1990, it has been against the law to sell new or re-upholstered soft furnishings which are padded with foam that is not combustion modified or which are covered with fabric that does not resist ignition tests for both smouldering cigarettes and match-like flames.

Previous legislation and regulations include the prohibition of the sale of highly flammable children's nightwear and the requirement that all new gas or electric fires and radiant oil-burning stoves are fitted with a fireguard which passes British Standards specifications.

With regard to the environment, probably the greatest single factor in reducing death and injury by fires in the home has been the introduction of smoke detectors/alarms. In North America, their installation into both new and established domestic properties is legally required. In the UK, legislation is more arbitrary and installation into established properties is voluntary. It must be recognised that the groups at highest risk of burns, i.e. older or disabled people, may be less able than others to buy safer soft furnishings and heating appliances. Smoke detectors may be bought for as little as £5, but their fitting, although simple for the able-bodied, may be impossible for older or disabled individuals.

Health care workers, therefore, not only have a responsibility to disseminate information on the prevention of burn injuries, but also must work closely with other interested groups such as the Fire Service, The Royal Society for the Prevention of Accidents (Useful websites) and both local and national government in order to lobby for more effective legislation and regulations (Box 30.1). Nurses working in the community have the opportunity to observe the environment and to give specific advice relating to burns prevention.

First aid treatment of burns

Burn injuries result from the transfer of energy from a heat source to vulnerable tissues. The higher the temperature of the heat source and the longer it is in contact with the tissues, the greater will be the destruction.

The first priority of first aid treatment is to remove the individual from the source of heat. If the causative agent is electricity, it is important to switch off the supply, if possible, or to use non-conducting material to rescue the person.

Frequently, there is a continuing source of heat if the individual's clothing is on fire or saturated by a hot liquid. The most effective way to remove this continuing heat source is to throw cool liquid, which is neither flammable nor corrosive, over the affected material, thus dousing the flames or reducing the temperature of the scalding liquid. If no such cool liquid is immediately to hand, rapid removal of hot

Box 30.1 Reflection

Reducing burn injuries

Will and some friends returned home after a night out and, feeling hungry, decided to have some chips. Will put the chip pan on the stove, leaving the fat to heat whilst he checked his e-mail and put on some music. Sometime later, smelling smoke, Will rushed back to the kitchen to find the saucepan in flames. In his panic he tried to douse the flames by smothering them with a towel, which promptly caught fire. He then remembered to put the lid on the saucepan and turn off the stove. The noise alerted his friends, who phoned 999 for an ambulance and the fire service. Will was rushed to the nearest emergency department, where, on examination, he was found to have a total of 8%, mainly superficial, burns to his hands, forearms, chest and face.

Activity

- Reflect on the potential reasons why this burn injury occurred and why the chip pan was well alight before Will and his friends were aware of the fire.
- Visit the Fire Service website (www.fireservice.co.uk/safety/chippans.php) and discuss with your mentor how you could use the Fire Service information to reduce burn injury caused by chip pan fires.

saturated clothing will arrest the heat transfer. Where clothing is on fire, it is important to stop the person running around as this will fan the flames. The person assisting should lie the victim on the ground and use heavy material such as a coat or blanket to smother the flames. If chemicals are the causative agent, prompt sluicing with copious amounts of water will dilute the strength of the agent and limit the penetration of the chemical into the skin, where it will continue to cause damage for many hours. Hojer et al (2002) demonstrate the advantage of taking this universal first aid measure rather than taking time searching for specific neutralising agents. In the clinical situation, a useful means of identifying whether a chemical is acid or alkaline is to apply a urine testing strip, as this will give a pH reading.

After removal of the heat source from the skin, the next measure is to cool the superheated tissues. The easiest means of doing this is to place the affected part in cold water. For the face, however, cold soaks should be applied. The application of ice or chilled water below 8°C is contraindicated, as Venter et al (2007) found that this was associated with increased likelihood of tissue damage. There is no doubt that continued cooling reduces pain from the burn wound, but if a large area of the body surface is involved there is a risk of hypothermia.

Since patients with extensive burns have problems retaining body heat, the use of space blankets or other heat-retaining coverings is advised during transfer to hospital.

Many burns units in the UK are now advising that the temporary wound dressing of choice is polyvinyl chloride film, e.g. cling film (Hudspith & Rayatt 2004). The reasons for this are:

- The film is sterile on the inner rolled surface.
- It does not adhere to the wound surface and cause pain on removal.
- It conforms closely to the body contours and excludes air, thus reducing pain.

- The wound can be viewed without removal of the transparent film.

This kind of material is often available in the home but, if not, a clean cloth should be used as a temporary cover. The use of ointments, lotions and powders should be avoided as they may change the appearance of the wound and thus impair the assessment of the burn.

To summarise, first aid treatment of burn injuries consists of:

- separating the individual from the source of injury
- immersion of the affected part in cold water for 10 min or application of cold soaks to the face
- application of cling film or a clean cloth to the wound; cold soaks may be used for wounds which are not extensive.

Assessing the severity of burn injuries

The majority of patients with burn injuries do not require hospitalisation. The UK National Burn Injury Referral Guidelines (2001) recommend that when deciding whether to refer patients to a burn unit, consideration should be given to the complexity of the burn injury rather than simply to the size of the burn wound. The categories of patients for whom admission or referral to a regional burns unit is advisable include those:

- under 5 years or over 60 years of age
- whose burns exceed 5% of the body surface area
- with burns on functionally important areas such as face, hands, feet, perineum, joints or flexor surfaces
- with electrical or chemical burns
- with infected wounds or evidence of infection
- with small, full-thickness burns which would benefit from early excision and grafting
- whose injury limits their capacity to care for themselves at home
- with associated injuries, e.g. smoke inhalation, crush injuries, fractures
- with other medical conditions, e.g. epilepsy, diabetes mellitus
- where there is doubt, either suspected non-accidental injury or uncertainty about the depth of the burn.

For patients who do not fall into any of these categories, relief of pain and local treatment of the burn wound are generally all that is required. Both interventions will be described later (p. 782).

The UK guidelines also suggest that in the post-acute phase of burn injury, practice nurses and district nurses should refer patients whose burn has not healed within 14 days, as any resulting scarring may have significant impact on the subsequent physical and psychological rehabilitation of the patient.

Assessment of the severity of the burn injury involves estimation of the:

- extent of body surface area involved
- depth of tissue damage
- probability of associated respiratory tract injury.

Knowledge of the circumstances of the accident, e.g. whether electricity was involved, and information about the individual's general health and domestic situation will help in deciding whether the patient may, or may not, be managed by the primary health care team.

Extent of burn

Whenever tissues are traumatised, the inflammatory response occurs, resulting in increased circulation to the area (hyperaemia) and increased movement of fluids from intravascular to interstitial compartments. If this occurs in a small area, i.e. over less than 5% of the body surface, the effects are localised. However, when a larger percentage of the body surface is injured, there is a massive shift of fluids into the tissues with a corresponding reduction in circulating volume. It is generally accepted that children with burns involving more than 10%, and adults with burns of more than 15%, of body surface area will suffer from hypovolaemic shock unless there is prompt intravenous replacement of fluid (see Ch. 18).

In order to estimate the percentage of body surface affected, the simplest and most easily remembered method is the long established 'rule of nines' introduced by Wallace in 1951 (Figure 30.1). In this method, the head and upper limbs each equal 9%, while the anterior trunk, the posterior trunk and the lower limbs each equal 18%. The remaining 1% is usually applied to the perineum. Another rapid approximation of the percentage can be made by using the palmar aspect of the patient's hand (with fingers together) as 1% of the body surface area.

The rule of nines should never be used for estimating burn percentage in young children as it does not allow for the different proportions of head and lower limbs in infants and toddlers. Under the age of 1 year the child's head equals 19% of the body surface area and the lower limbs are correspondingly smaller. A more accurate chart which allows for the changing proportions of different age groups and which shows percentages applicable to smaller, more specific areas

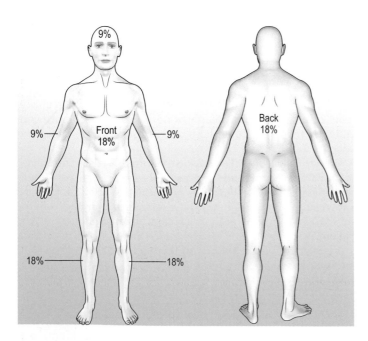

Figure 30.1 Wallace's rule of nines.

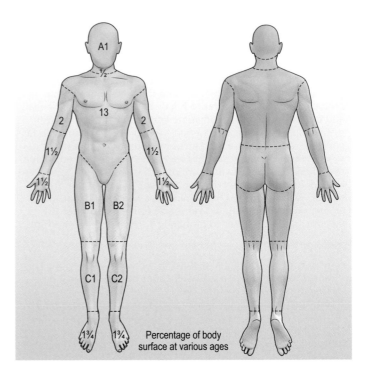

Percent of areas affected by growth

	0	1	5	10	15	Adult age
A = ½ head	9½	8½	6½	5½	4½	3½
B = ½ one thigh	2¾	3¼	4	4¼	4½	4¾
C = ½ one leg	2½	2½	2¾	3	3¼	3½

To estimate the total of the body surface area burned, the percentages assigned to the burned sections are added. The total is then an estimate of the burn size.

Figure 30.2 The Lund and Browder burn chart.

of the body surface is the Lund and Browder (1944) burn chart (Figure 30.2). This is generally in use in specialist units and is available in EDs throughout the UK.

Burn depth

The depth of a burn influences the rate at which the wound will heal spontaneously. The longer the wound takes to heal, the greater the probability of infection and the worse the scarring and loss of function. There are a number of methods of classifying burn depth. In the UK, the most popular is to differentiate between partial-thickness and full-thickness skin destruction. Partial-thickness burns involve the epidermis and part of the dermis. Full-thickness burns destroy the epidermis and all of the dermis.

See website Figures 30.1 and 30.2

Full-thickness burns may also involve deeper structures such as fat, muscle and bone. Partial-thickness burns are classified as 'superficial' or 'deep', depending on the amount of dermis involved. As a general rule, deep partial thickness and full-thickness burns require skin grafting.

As may be seen from Figure 30.3, the more superficial the injury, the greater the number of surviving epithelial sources from which cells migrate across the wound surface; thus a more superficial burn heals more rapidly and causes less

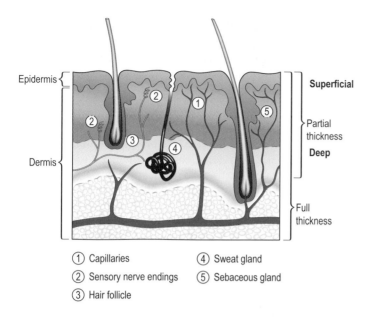

Epidermis

Dermis

Superficial

Partial
thickness

Deep

Full
thickness

① Capillaries
② Sensory nerve endings
③ Hair follicle
④ Sweat gland
⑤ Sebaceous gland

Figure 30.3 Classification of burn depth.

wound contraction. The effects of superficial partial-thickness burns and full-thickness burns are described below and in Table 30.1.

Superficial partial-thickness burns

These burns are very painful as the sensory nerve endings are stimulated by the injury or exposed to air. They are characterised by oedema, blister formation and serous exudate where the blisters burst. The blistering results from the increased permeability of the capillary walls, with fluid leaking into the interstitial spaces and from the wound surface. This fluid collects into blisters beneath the non-germinating layers of the epidermis. Heat radiates from the wound surface due to arteriolar dilatation and increased blood flow and as part of the inflammatory response. This also causes the typical bright pink appearance of the wound, which will blanch on pressure. On removal of the pressure the hyperaemia is restored.

Full-thickness burns

These burns are insensate (without sensation), as the sensory nerve endings have been destroyed. There is normally no blister formation and the wound surface is dry. There is no overt oedema, the wound surface is cool to the touch and the colour may be white, brown or bright red with no blanching on pressure.

⌐ **See website Figures 30.1 and 30.2**

These characteristics are all due to the fact that there is no surviving circulation within the dermis. The brown or red colour is due to the release of haem pigments from destroyed erythrocytes. The area may appear translucent with thrombosed vessels being apparent. It is important to recognise that there is an inflammatory response in deeper tissues affected, but this is masked by overlying necrotic tissue. High temperatures (>60°C) cause coagulation of the tissue proteins and water is lost from the cells, interstitial spaces and blood vessels, resulting in a degree of contraction of the affected tissues. Destruction of the dermis renders the skin inelastic and the texture becomes firm and leathery. This is known as eschar.

Table 30.1 Indications of burn depth		
DEPTH	**SIGNS AND SYMPTOMS**	**RELATED ANATOMY/PHYSIOLOGY**
Superficial partial-thickness burns	Very painful	Sensory nerve endings in the dermis are stimulated by the injury and/or exposed to air
	Oedema, blister formation, serous exudate where blisters have burst	As a result of the inflammatory response, the capillary walls are more permeable and fluid leaks into the interstitial spaces of the dermis, collecting below the non-germinating layers of the epidermis or exuding from the wound surface
	Wound surface warmer than unburned skin	Also due to the inflammatory response; arteriolar dilatation causes increased blood flow
	Wound appears bright pink and blanches with pressure	Due to increased blood flow Pressure greater than capillary blood pressure occludes the flow of blood
Full-thickness burns	Painless, no sensation	Sensory nerve endings in the dermis are destroyed
	Wound surface dry. No blistering	Cessation of blood flow through dermal capillaries
	No overt oedema	Necrosis of dermis renders it inelastic
	Wound surface cooler than unburned skin	Cessation of blood flow through dermal capillaries
	Wound colour may be white, brown, translucent showing thrombosed vessels, or bright red (does not blanch on pressure)	Cessation of blood flow through dermal capillaries. Brown or red appearance is caused by release of haem pigments from the destroyed erythrocytes (red blood cells)

Deep partial-thickness burns

As the depth of destruction in this type of burn is between those of superficial partial-thickness and full-thickness burns, the presenting signs and symptoms are between the extremes in sensation, blistering, temperature and colour.

Problems in assessment

The assessment of burn depth is an inexact science, although much work has been carried out to make it more exact in recent years. The use of a hypodermic needle to test for pin-prick sensation was first described by Bull and Lennard-Jones (1949). More recently, McGill et al (2007) found that both laser Doppler imaging and video microscopy may be used successfully in aiding assessment of burn depth; however, these options are not readily available outwith specialist burn units. Frequently, assessment of burn depth is dependent on the visual characteristics of the wound, the information regarding the circumstances of the accident, the agent involved and the first aid measures carried out.

Burn-associated respiratory tract injury

Inhibition of respiratory function may result from thermal injury to the skin of the trunk and neck. Hidden oedema formation below the leathery, inelastic eschar of circumferential full-thickness burns causes pressure on the deeper structures. In deep burns of the neck, this may cause compression of the trachea and, if there is involvement of the chest and upper abdomen, will inhibit expansion of the thoracic cavity. Decompression by escharotomy will be required (Box 30.2).

Inhalation of smoke and hot toxic gases is frequently associated with burn trauma. The main types of inhalation injury are:

- intoxication and hypoxaemia (reduced oxygen in arterial blood)
- thermal damage to the airways
- respiratory tract injury due to irritants.

Box 30.2 Reflection

Escharotomy

Where full-thickness burn injury occurs circumferentially around a limb, the combination of a firm inelastic eschar and the inflammatory response in the subcutaneous tissues will cause compression of the deeper structures, especially the blood vessels. Incisions through the eschar to allow decompression are carried out by the surgeon and are termed escharotomy.

Escharotomy may also be carried out when full-thickness burn injury of the chest and upper part of the abdomen inhibits rib or diaphragmatic movement, causing respiratory difficulty.

Monitoring of circulation to distal parts of limbs involved or of respiratory ease is required when full-thickness burns are suspected in either site.

Activity

- Think about how a patient and their family might feel if the surgeon tells them that escharotomy is needed.
- Consider which observations would be appropriate to monitor the circulation of the distal part of a limb affected by circumferential burn injury. Discuss the observations with your mentor and decide how often they should be performed.

Intoxication and hypoxaemia

Intoxication and hypoxaemia most commonly result from inhalation of carbon monoxide and/or hydrogen cyanide produced by burning plastics.

Carbon monoxide (CO), produced by the combustion of carbon and organic materials in a limited oxygen supply, has an affinity for haemoglobin many times that of oxygen. Therefore, following inhalation of CO there is displacement of oxygen from haemoglobin and the production of carboxy-haemoglobin (COHb) with resulting generalised hypoxia (reduced oxygen in the tissues). The symptoms of CO poisoning are related to the concentration of the inspired gas and to COHb levels and are recognised as mild headache, dizziness, confusion, irritability, nausea, vomiting and fainting. At higher levels there will be convulsions, altered consciousness, respiratory failure and death. Diagnosis is suggested by the typical cherry pink appearance of the patient and confirmed by checking COHb levels. The formation of carboxyhaemo-globin can be reversed by the administration of high concentrations of oxygen.

Hydrogen cyanide is rapidly absorbed through the lungs and inhibits cell function that results in metabolic acidosis. It causes loss of consciousness, neurotoxicity and convulsions.

Thermal damage

The upper airway may be damaged by the inhalation of hot gases, hot vapours or combustible gas mixtures. Mucosal oedema will narrow the lumen of the airway. The diagnosis is suspected where there is a history of explosion, burns of the face, singed nasal hairs, erythema and ulceration of the oropharynx. Hoarseness and inspiratory stridor (harsh breathing sound due to turbulent airflow through narrowed airways) may present later. As signs of upper airway obstruction may take several hours to become apparent, constant supervision is required.

Hot, dry air seldom causes burns of the airway below the level of the epiglottis as the respiratory tract has an excellent heat exchange capability. Injury to the lower airway is most commonly caused by inhalation of toxic chemicals.

Inhalation of irritant chemicals

The combustion of various materials produces a wide spectrum of irritant chemicals, including chlorine, formaldehyde and phosgene. The extent of the resultant damage to the respiratory system is determined by the density of the smoke and the duration of exposure. Patients who are asleep or under the influence of drugs or alcohol at the time of the fire will tend to have a longer exposure time, as will those who have restricted mobility, e.g. older or people with a disability.

When irritant chemicals bound to carbon particles settle on the respiratory endothelium, the following events occur:

- inflammatory response
- inflammation of the alveolar capillary membrane
- bronchospasm
- chemical denaturation (change in basic structure or nature) of proteins
- loss of surfactant production by type II alveolar cells.

Surfactant normally lowers the surface tension of the alveolar walls, thus preventing collapse, and also prevents the transudation of fluid from capillaries into the alveoli. Loss of surfactant production will therefore lead to atelectasis (see Ch. 3).

In summary, the pathophysiological results of the inhalation of irritant chemicals may include tracheobronchitis (inflammation of the trachea and bronchi), pulmonary oedema, atelectasis and airway obstruction. These are frequently compounded by infection.

In cases where the patient survives long enough for admission to hospital, the respiratory damage related to inhalation of smoke may take several hours or even days to become manifest. Suspicion should be aroused where:

- The fire occurred within an enclosed space, especially at night.
- The history suggests exposure to smoke, especially if the patient required bodily rescue.
- The patient's breath and clothing smell of smoke.
- The conjunctivae are inflamed.
- Carbon particles are present in clothing, wounds, nose, mouth and sputum.

Other injuries

The appearance of a patient with extensive burns may be so visually dramatic as to distract the assessor from checking for other, less obvious, injuries. Fractures, internal injuries and spinal cord damage may have been sustained, especially if the burn was a result of a road traffic accident, an explosion or high tension electricity, or if the patient jumped from a burning building.

The patient with extensive burns

Early problems and nursing care

The patient with extensive burns has multiple problems, the relative urgency of which will vary during the perhaps very prolonged period following injury. There is increasing awareness that extensive burn injury causes a systemic inflammatory response syndrome (SIRS) in which there is widespread disorganisation of the immune system, eventually resulting in multiple organ dysfunction syndrome (MODS) (Chs 18, 29) (Bhatia & Moochhala 2004).

During the first 36–48 h, however, the most life-threatening problem, except where inhalation injury is present, will be burn shock. Shock is covered in Chapter 18, but a summary of events which have particular relevance to burns injury is given here (Table 30.2).

The initial physiological response to a burn injury results in plasma loss from the circulation (pp. 781, 782). This is accompanied by:

- Gross oedema of the affected tissues.
- Hypovolaemia – as in all types of shock, this results in decreased circulation to the skin, muscle and internal organs. Cerebral and coronary perfusion, being of greatest priority, are temporarily maintained.
- Haemoconcentration – unlike the hypovolaemia which results from haemorrhage, the loss of plasma alone from the

Table 30.2 Pathology and related signs and symptoms of burn shock

PATHOLOGICAL CONDITION	CLINICAL SIGNS AND SYMPTOMS
Hypovolaemia	Thirst Rapid, weak pulse Hypotension Peripheral and splanchnic (relating to the viscera) vasoconstriction
Peripheral vasoconstriction	Pale skin and mucosa Extremities feel cold Patient complains of feeling cold
Reduced perfusion of kidneys	Oliguria, anuria Impairment of renal function Metabolic acidosis Renal failure may occur
Red cell haemolysis	Haemoglobinuria (haemoglobin in the urine) Renal failure may occur
Reduced perfusion of lungs	Rapid, shallow breathing Air hunger – gasping
Reduced perfusion of gastrointestinal tract	Reduced absorption and intestinal stasis Vomiting, loss of electrolytes and fluid Paralytic ileus, lack of bowel sounds Bacterial translocation through mucosa
Hypoxaemia/electrolyte imbalance	Restlessness, disorientation, confusion May lead to altered consciousness and death

intravascular compartment causes an increase in the ratio of blood cells to plasma in the circulation, a raised packed cell volume (haematocrit). This increases the viscosity of the blood, further reducing the flow through the capillaries.

In addition to suffering from burn shock, the patient may be emotionally shocked, in great pain and have extensive destruction of the skin and, possibly, deeper structures. There may be associated injuries, especially inhalation of smoke, and a pre-burn illness may be present.

Haemoglobinuria (haemoglobin in the urine) may develop in patients who have been badly burned, as thermal injury destroys red cells (intravascular haemolysis). The resultant free haemoglobin in the blood will damage the kidneys and can cause renal failure, especially if renal perfusion is poor due to hypovolaemia.

The emergency department (ED)

To those unfamiliar with burns, the patient with extensive burns may not appear to be critically ill. The loss of plasma from the circulation is less rapid than haemorrhage from ruptured vessels and the patient may appear quite well. Inexperienced staff should consult with the regional burns unit to ensure that treatment is appropriate to the severity of the injury.

The Australia and New Zealand Burn Association Ltd (UK) (1996) identifies the following principles of primary assessment and management by medical personnel:

A   Airway maintenance and cervical spine control
B   Breathing and ventilation
C   Circulation; cardiac status, with control of haemorrhage if present
D   Disability, neurological status
E   Exposure with environmental control; evaluation of extent and depth of injury, including removal of jewellery and keeping the patient warm
F   Fluid resuscitation; intravenous (i.v.) fluid replacement, including introduction of a urinary catheter for monitoring output, and insertion of a nasogastric tube.

These are followed by X-ray of the cervical spine, chest and pelvis to exclude associated injury.

After life-threatening conditions have been excluded or treated, the secondary survey should be commenced. This includes a patient history, description of the incident and complete examination.

Except in instances where nurses are specially educated, the role of nursing staff is to assist with the above procedures, to support the patient and their relatives and to keep meticulous records of fluid balance and of medications given.

 See website Critical thinking question 30.1

Transfer of the patient with extensive burns

The patient should be prepared for transfer with the application of a temporary wound dressing, preferably cling film, and covered with a space blanket or layers of ordinary blankets. As described earlier, there is a high risk of hypothermia, especially during transfer, and wet dressings should not be used. If there are airway problems the patient must be accompanied by an experienced nurse, as well as by a member of the medical staff. Monitoring of vital signs and maintenance of the intravenous fluids are usually carried out by the nurse. The speed of travel is frequently rapid, which will make the task of monitoring and recording fluid balance and vital signs very difficult; nonetheless these records are important and, along with the ED file, should be given to the staff of the burns unit on arrival.

Admission to a regional burns unit

Reception of the patient

When the patient arrives at the unit, they should be greeted sensitively and orientated as to place, as many regional burns units receive patients from a wide catchment area. Where possible, the patient should be reassured and given a simple explanation of what is being done at every stage of the admission procedure and thereafter, throughout their stay in the unit. The appearance and smell of the burn wounds may be very upsetting, not only for the patient but also for inexperienced staff. It is important for staff to appear calm and confident, thus helping to reassure the patient.

The receiving staff must use personal protective equipment (PPE), e.g. waterproof gowns, plastic aprons or tabards and gloves. This is to protect staff against contact with wound exudate and blood and the patient against wound contamination (Weber et al 2004).

The patient should be received into a single room warmed to a temperature of 28°C, as heat loss from the inflamed wounds, in addition to evaporative heat loss from the wound exudate, can be extensive.

Maintaining the airway

If the patient has inhalation injury, endotracheal intubation and assisted ventilation may have been instituted in the ED or may be required at the time of admission to the unit. In any case, all nursing care and observations relative to this treatment must be carried out (see Chs 3, 29).

Constant observation of respiratory rate and ease, and of the colour of unburned skin and mucosa, must be carried out and recorded. Humidified air or oxygen administered by face mask or nasal catheter may be required.

Weighing the patient

If possible, an accurate body weight in kilograms should be obtained as this is one of the baseline measurements on which the volume of fluid replacement is calculated. Estimation of weight is sometimes carried out but, unless the person doing so is experienced in this, gross over- or under-transfusion may result. In many units the patient is weighed on a special bed or sling, still covered in the blankets and temporary dressings used for the transfer; these are then gently removed and the patient laid on and covered with sterile sheeting, e.g. linen, foam or cling film. The original coverings are then weighed and their weight subtracted from the total in order to get a naked weight. It is important to record the weight immediately as the exact figure may easily be forgotten, especially if there is a great deal of activity in the room.

Wound assessment

Medical staff will estimate the depth of the burn wounds and chart their position and extent. Colour photographs will usually also be taken for recording purposes. In addition to being useful baseline records of wound appearance and distribution, the photographs may, with the patient's permission, be used in evidence in any subsequent criminal or civil proceedings relating to the circumstances of the burn injury. Whilst the wounds are exposed, the nurse can take swabs for bacteriological examination from each wound site, e.g. right hand, left hand, chest, neck. This reduces the possibility of wound contamination and the discomfort and possible loss of dignity suffered by the patient during repeated removal of the coverings. The initial wound swabs usually show no bacteriological contamination but provide a useful baseline for further monitoring. The wounds are then covered with a temporary dressing. Specific care will be carried out once the patient's condition has been stabilised.

Bacteriology swabs from nose and throat are also obtained in order to identify commensals which may act as wound pathogens (Ch. 16).

Analgesics

Intravenous analgesics, usually in the form of morphine, are administered by infusion pump, giving an initial dose and then at an hourly rate of 20–30 µg/kg. The intramuscular route is never used if the patient is in shock, as the medication will not be absorbed owing to the peripheral vasoconstriction.

Intravenous fluid replacement

Once an accurate body weight has been obtained and the percentage area of the burn estimated (Figures 30.1, 30.2), the medical staff will calculate the volume of intravenous therapy required. There are a number of different formulae in current use (e.g. Parkland, Muir & Barclay) but most depend on these two parameters for calculation of the volume to be infused. Regulation of the rate of flow and recording of the volume transfused, as well as care of the intravenous cannula site, is the responsibility of the nurse. A volumetric intravenous pump provides accuracy for the infusion of volumes required in each period which may be very large.

Monitoring urine output

If this has not been carried out in the ED, an indwelling urinary catheter is inserted, the bladder emptied and the urine volume measured. A specimen is tested for specific gravity and tested using a urine testing strip. The appearance is noted. A urimeter which allows hourly measuring and sampling whilst maintaining a closed system is attached to the catheter. Williams (2008) emphasises the importance of monitoring renal function through regular, frequent measurement of volume and composition of the urine. A volume of 0.5–1.0 mL/kg body weight hourly is generally accepted as indicating that intravenous fluid replacement is satisfactory, although urine concentration, measured by specific gravity or osmolality, must also be estimated in order to assess renal function.

The appearance of the urine is monitored for indications of haemoglobinuria, such as dark coloured urine and, if this is present, for indications that it is diminishing. It is important that the nurse inform the medical staff at the first indication of haemoglobinuria, as it is usual for a solution of sodium bicarbonate and an osmotic diuretic, e.g. mannitol, to be prescribed in order to clear the pigments.

Monitoring vital signs

Pulse If the patient is shocked, the pulse will be rapid and weak. This, combined with generalised oedema, can make manual counting very difficult and mechanical aids are normally used.

Blood pressure Where all four limbs have been burned, it is not usual practice to record blood pressure. Indeed, even if one limb is unaffected it has been considered more important to ensure effective intravenous access and fluid replacement than to repeatedly constrict the vessels with a blood pressure cuff.

The routine measurement of central venous pressure or arterial pressure is not recommended in most UK burns units because of the risk of systemic infection associated with such invasive techniques, especially if the site of entry of the catheter is close to the burn wound.

Temperature A good indicator of the state of peripheral perfusion is the difference between core and shell temperatures (see Ch. 22). In the normal person, under warm conditions, the temperature of a toe is 1–4°C lower than rectal temperature, but in the patient suffering hypovolaemic shock the vasoconstriction is such that the difference may be as much as 15°C. Temperature monitoring is usually facilitated by the use of thermistor probes in preference to the repeated insertion of a rectal thermometer. In some units, a specially designed probe is inserted into the external auditory meatus in preference to using the rectum. If thermistor probes are not available, it is possible to gauge the shell temperature by feeling the temperature of the peripheries, especially the toes or the tip of the nose.

In addition to monitoring the difference between a normal core temperature and changes in the shell temperature, measuring the core temperature will, of course, also indicate a trend towards hyperpyrexia or hypothermia (see Ch. 22).

Oral intake

Because of the reduction in gastrointestinal tract perfusion which results from hypovolaemia, it is necessary to restrict the volume of oral fluids initially, even if the patient is very thirsty, until it has been established that there is no nausea or vomiting. If there is persistent vomiting, a nasogastric tube is passed and is either allowed to drain freely or aspirated hourly before small amounts of water are given. In some units, a nasogastric tube is passed routinely in all patients with burns greater than 35% of the body surface.

Patient behaviour

In addition to recording clinical measurements as described above, it is useful for the nurse to keep a record of the patient's behaviour, noting for example, restlessness, confusion, distress or apathy, as these, along with the measured recordings, will give a more complete picture of the patient's condition. If there is cause for concern, monitoring of neurological status is facilitated by use of the Glasgow Coma Scale (see Ch. 28).

The post-shock phase

After the first 36–48 h following injury, the fluid in the interstitial spaces is reabsorbed into the circulation and, although there is continuous fluid loss through exudate and evaporation from the wound surface, there is normally no longer a need for intravenous replacement of fluids. Unless complications arise (Box 30.3), the intermediate stage of management will have been reached.

Nursing management during the intermediate stage of burn injury recovery follows the basic principles of burn care whatever the extent of body surface involved. Thus nursing priorities include:

- pain relief (p. 782)
- hydration and nutrition
- prevention of infection and local wound care
- psychosocial support for patients and relatives (pp. 785–786).

Box 30.3 Information

Complications of burn injuries

In some patients with extensive burns, recovery from the initial injury may be complicated by severe episodes of conditions that include (see Chs 18, 29):

- severe sepsis
- acute/adult respiratory distress syndrome (ARDS)
- disseminated intravascular coagulation (DIC)
- gastrointestinal ulceration and haemorrhage
- systemic infection of the respiratory system or urinary tract, wound infection
- wound contraction and scar formation

Hydration and nutrition

Until wound closure is complete, there will be continuous loss of the water, protein and electrolytes which comprise the wound exudate (see Ch. 20). In addition, nutritional requirements will be increased because of the elevation in the metabolic rate resulting from trauma, as well as the cellular requirements of wound healing. In patients whose burn area is less than 20% of the body surface, oral intake of a normal diet, perhaps supplemented with high-protein, high-calorie drinks, should be all that is required. However, dietary intake should be monitored to allow assessment by the dietitian and the patient should be weighed weekly. The patient should be encouraged to take fluids and the fluid balance should be monitored and charted.

In more extensive burns, metabolic requirements will be greatly increased, making enteral nutrition via a nasogastric tube necessary (Lee et al 2005). There are a number of proprietary preparations of enteral feeds available and the dietitian will prescribe the type, volume and rate of administration for each individual. If there is a problem with using the nasogastric route, percutaneous endoscopic gastrostomy (PEG) may be performed; Kreis et al (2002) found that the placement of PEG tubes through wound areas did not precipitate wound complications. Parenteral nutrition is reserved for patients who are unable to achieve adequate nutrition by the preferred enteral route (see Ch. 21) because of the danger of infection associated with the introduction of central lines; peripheral lines are usually impractical because of the limited availability of peripheral veins.

Prevention of infection

Both non-specific and specific mechanisms of the immune system are impaired in patients with extensive burns (see Chs 6, 16).

Because of the large areas of skin destruction and the presence of exudate and necrotic tissue, burn wounds rapidly become colonised with bacteria. It has been found that most of the bacteria are acquired from other contaminated patients or equipment in the ward or unit and therefore meticulous attention must be paid to the prevention of cross-infection (Tredget et al 2004) (see Ch. 16). When possible, the patient should be nursed in a single room and standard infection control precautions implemented. Once the patient's wound becomes colonised with an organism, it will soon be found on their bedclothes, personal clothing and on the surface of dressings. PPE must be worn whenever the patient is attended to; this normally consists of plastic tabards or water-resistant gowns. The wearing of masks and caps is usually not necessary, except when the wound is exposed. Gloves should be worn during any direct contact with the patient and the immediate surroundings; clean rather than sterile gloves may be used for most procedures, apart from those requiring an aseptic technique. Adherence to good handwashing practice requires frequent emphasis (Weber et al 2004).

The bacteriological status of the wounds should be monitored regularly by obtaining wound swabs during dressing changes.

The burn wound

As for any wound, the aim of management is to provide the optimal environment for the natural healing processes to take place (see Ch. 23). However, most burn wounds involve larger areas of the body surface than is common in other types of wound and this presents many problems in wound management.

See website Critical thinking question 30.2

Most burn wounds exude copious amounts of fluid. This is evident in superficial partial-thickness wounds from the outset. In deeper wounds, the surface is initially dry and, depending on the depth of tissue destruction, it may take days before the eschar becomes saturated with fluid leaking from the damaged capillaries in the deeper tissues. Unless the superficial partial-thickness burn wound becomes infected, or is subjected to further trauma, it should re-epithelialise in 7–10 days. As migration of the epithelial cells occurs, the exudate will gradually diminish. Greenhalgh (2007) describes the major aim in burn wound care to be obtaining wound closure as soon as possible with the least amount of scarring thus maximising functional and cosmetic outcome. In order to meet this goal, management must entail:

- meticulous cleansing and debridement of devitalised tissue in order to prevent infection
- facilitating re-epithelialisation or granulation in preparation for any necessary wound grafting
- promoting patient comfort.

Pain relief

It is generally agreed that patients with burns experience the greatest pain during therapeutic procedures (Patterson et al 2004). Pain-relieving strategies used in wound care include:

- the administration of morphine and other similar opioids timed to ensure optimal cover during the procedure
- patient-controlled analgesia by inhalation administration, e.g. Entonox® (nitrous oxide and oxygen)
- relief of anxiety through explanation, and if necessary complementary and alternative medicine therapies (CAM) (e.g. hypnosis) and other psychological coping strategies.

The degree of discomfort the patient experiences will be strongly related to the skill of the nurse to recognise and appreciate the individual's pain tolerance (see Ch. 19).

Wound cleansing and debridement

Burn wound cleansing can be very time consuming and, where wounds are extensive, will require a number of staff. In some units, patients with extensive burns will have dressings changed under general anaesthesia with the involvement of a full surgical team.

Depending on the size and site of the wound, other methods include irrigation via a syringe, showering or immersion in a special tub. What is important for both patient comfort and to limit heat loss, especially when the wounds are extensive or on the trunk, is to ensure that the solution used is warmed to body temperature.

Following cleansing, loose devitalised tissue is trimmed using sharp scissors. Specialists vary in their approach to the management of blisters: Flanagan & Graham (2001) advise that they be left intact, whereas DuKamp (2001) advocates this approach only if the blister does not restrict joint movement, recommending aspiration of the blister with a needle and syringe in this instance. However, as this method does not allow for accurate assessment of the wound surface, many authors agree that this subject warrants further research and investigation (Box 30.4).

Promotion of re-epithelialisation or granulation and the prevention of wound contamination are normally facilitated either by applying dressings or more infrequently by exposing the burn wound.

Exposing the burn wound

This method is currently most commonly used for burns of the face. The aim of the exposure method is to provide a dry, intact scab under which re-epithelialisation will take place. Relevant nursing management is described later in the section dealing with facial burns.

Dressing the burn wound

One of the main problems presented by the burn wound is the copious amount of exudate it produces. This strongly influences the choice of dressing material used. Many modern materials are designed to create the optimal environment for healing, i.e. warmth and moisture, whilst removing excess exudate. This may be accomplished by highly absorbent materials, such as alginates, hydrocolloids or hydrophilic foams, or by materials which allow rapid transmission of water vapour. These types of dressing can

be used successfully in burns affecting a relatively small area, but a substantial margin must be in contact with unburned skin to prevent leakage of exudate. Thus their use is often not feasible for large wounds.

For extensive burns in the initial stages of injury conventional dressings which comprise of an inner layer of mesh, usually impregnated with paraffin and thick layers of cotton gauze, are usually used (Bessey 2007). The materials may be retained with cotton conforming bandages, or on the trunk by stitching or stapling. The aim of conventional dressings is to allow exudate to filter through the layers and for water to evaporate from the surface of the dressing, thus preventing maceration of the wound. It is important, therefore, that the surface of the dressing is not occluded with a nonporous material, such as many of the adhesive tapes used to retain bandages. If the outer surface of the dressing does become moist, the outer layers only are changed under aseptic conditions. To change the whole dressing unnecessarily exposes the burn to contamination from the atmosphere and may disrupt healing. The frequency of scheduled dressing changes depends on the depth and state of the wound and on the properties of any medication incorporated in the innermost layer. Superficial partial-thickness burns may have their dressings left undisturbed for 7–10 days, the estimated time of healing, unless there are indications for investigating the wound, such as signs of infection. More frequent changes, daily, every second day or twice weekly are required in deeper burns as the presence of necrotic tissue increases the likelihood of bacterial growth. In such cases, antibacterial agents are normally used. For many years, silver sulfadiazine cream, in the UK Flamazine®, was a popular antibacterial application for burn wounds throughout the developed world. However, because of its tendency to change the appearance of the wound and to macerate non-viable tissue, making surgical excision difficult, other silver-containing wound products including Aquacel® Ag (Caruso et al 2006) and Acticoat® (Dunn & Edward-Jones 2004) are now regularly used in burn wound management. Silver sulfadiazine with cerium nitrate is also used in some UK burn units for treating extensive burns where the patient's medical condition does not allow for early excision and skin grafting to occur (Garner & Heppell 2005). The ideal wound cover is the patient's own skin in the form of an autograft which 'takes' to provide wound closure. Other types of skin graft, i.e. from other humans, an allograft, or from animals, a xenograft, provide only temporary cover except in the case of identical twins. Sheets of epidermal cells (keratinocytes) may be cultured from the patient's own skin but it may take some weeks before sufficient material is available (Atiyeh & Costagliola 2007). However, there are now also many bioengineered skin substitutes widely available for the treatment of extensive burn wounds (Pham et al 2007).

Care of burn wounds prior to skin grafting

The necrotic tissue has to separate from the wound bed before granulation tissue, suitable for skin grafting, is produced.

Surgical removal of necrotic tissue is carried out usually within the first 4 days following injury. The tissue is either excised with a scalpel or shaved down to a viable (bleeding) surface with a skin grafting knife. This procedure can result

---

 Box 30.4 Evidence-based practice

Blister management

Specialists vary in their approach to the management of blisters – the two examples below suggest very different management.

Activity

- Access and read the articles by Flanagan & Graham (2001) and DuKamp (2001).
- Search the literature to see if further research about blister management has been published since 2001 and discuss your findings with your mentor.

in extensive blood loss, and multiple blood transfusions may be required. The freshly prepared wound bed is usually skin grafted immediately.

A skin graft 'takes' by the ingrowth of capillaries from the wound into the graft, a process which takes only a few days. This will be disrupted if there is any blood, serum or pus preventing contact between graft and wound. Other factors which can cause disruption of the graft include any shearing of the graft/wound interface and the presence of β-haemolytic *Streptococcus*, group A (*S. pyogenes*) bacteria which produce streptokinase, an activator of plasmin which is fibrinolytic. Sometimes the surgeon will choose not to apply a dressing to a newly grafted area. Nursing staff will be responsible for ensuring that there is no collection of fluid under the graft. This is done by gently rolling a rolled-up swab from the centre to the margins of the graft, thus expressing any blood or serum. An aseptic technique is employed and great care is required to prevent the graft shearing on its bed.

The skin graft donor area is a superficial wound and, as a result, can be very painful. For the first 48 h or so it produces large amounts of bloodstained exudate and is usually dressed with calcium alginate followed by a conventional dressing, which is managed in the same way as that covering a superficial partial-thickness burn. The speed of re-epithelialisation depends on the depth of dermis removed along with the epidermis but is normally between 10 days and 2 weeks.

Ideally, the dressing is left intact until it falls off. Injudicious early investigation will cause further trauma, delay healing and lead to risk of infection.

The alginate dressing dries out as epithelialisation occurs but readily regains its gel consistency when soaked with normal saline.

Care of special areas

Face The most common method of managing facial burns is that of exposure.

The face becomes very oedematous and the head should be elevated as soon as the patient's condition allows. Drying out of the exudate is encouraged in order to produce a thin scab.

Once the scab has formed, it will be similar to a cosmetic face mask and greatly restrict facial movement. Because of this it is usual practice in some units to apply a thin layer of liquid paraffin to facial burns (Hudspith & Rayatt 2004), in particular to the areas around the eyes and mouth, as mobility of these areas is most important The resultant stickiness may allow adherence of debris and it is important to cleanse these areas gently with saline on a regular basis.

Oedema of the periorbital region can cause closure of the eyelids. As this can be very frightening for the patient, the nurse should warn the patient that eyelid closure may occur but reassure that the swelling will lessen in a few days. Eye drops or ointment will be prescribed in order to reduce the possibility of conjunctivitis. The use of artificial tears will make the patient more comfortable.

Oedema of the lips may cause eversion of the oral mucosa, which should not be allowed to dry out. The skin of the lips should be kept lubricated with yellow soft paraffin and care

must be taken when oral hygiene is performed. The use of a soft toothbrush, by patient or nurse, will help to maintain normal mouth care and, if the patient is unable to eat, regular mouthwashes should be given. If oral intake is allowed, the patient may experience difficulty in drinking from a normal cup; a feeding cup with a spout is preferable to using a straw as the patient may find it difficult to exert just the right pressure to allow suction without collapsing the straw.

Oedema of the ears may cause them to jut out at right angles to the head, making them more susceptible to further trauma. If the pinna produces exudate, this is liable to trickle into the external auditory meatus, where it will collect and dry out at the level of the ear drum, reducing the patient's ability to hear. This may not be detected until some time later, in which case it may prove very difficult to evacuate the plug. It is easy to avert this problem by inserting a small piece of gauze just at the opening of the meatus to absorb the exudate, changing it as necessary. The ears may be dressed lightly with a conventional dressing or have gauze spread with an antibacterial ointment, e.g. Flamazine®, gently applied.

Nostrils (anterior nares) should be kept free of exudate build-up by regular cleansing with a dampened cotton bud. If exudate dries on the nasal hairs, the crust will occlude the nostrils and its removal will be very painful indeed. This problem may be prevented by the application of a light smear of soft yellow paraffin just inside the nostrils.

Beard area In male patients hair becomes incorporated in the crust as it grows. This does not usually present problems until the scab is separating from the newly epithelialised facial skin; in the case of deep burns, the hair follicles will be destroyed and no hair growth will occur. Once the scab starts to lift it may be rehydrated using a moisturising lotion or hydrogel; this causes swelling of the scab, which no longer fit the contours of the face, and softens it to allow painless removal.

Scab removal As the scab lifts on the rest of the face, loose areas should be trimmed with care. There may be a strong temptation on the part of both nurse and patient to remove as much as possible, as the satisfaction of revealing nice pink skin can prove irresistible. However, it must be borne in mind that removing adherent crust causes trauma and may increase the possibility of scar formation. Newly epithelialised skin needs to be moisturised regularly with a bland cream to keep it from drying out.

Hands Burns involving the majority of the hand usually cause excessive swelling to the hand and are most commonly treated by the application of polythene bags or gloves, with or without the addition of an antibacterial cream, in order to facilitate movement and thus prevent joint stiffness and allow the patient a degree of independence. Because the polythene does not allow evaporation of water, the wound environment is very moist and the non-burned skin will become macerated. As large volumes of exudate will collect, it is usual, before applying the bag, to apply several layers of gauze around the wrist to absorb some of the exudate. The bags should be changed on a daily or more frequent basis, and the hand gently cleansed at each change. Minor burns to the hand are treated with lighter dressings, which should not restrict mobility.

Limbs In order to reduce oedema formation, burned limbs are elevated and exercised on a regular basis, unless freshly laid skin grafts preclude movement.

Joints Wound contraction is an integral part of the healing process, but excessive contraction leads to dysfunction and deformity. As flexor surfaces are more liable to contract, joints must be correctly positioned, with compensatory hyperextension especially of the wrists and neck. Physiotherapy should be carried out regularly, with adequate analgesic cover, to maintain a full range of movement of all joints. However, splinting may be necessary to arrest or correct contracture formation.

Scar formation

Scar formation is part of the maturation phase of the healing process. In wounds healing by secondary intention (see Ch. 23), the scar often appears red and is raised above the level of the surrounding skin (hypertrophic). Hypertrophic scarring is a well-known complication following burn injury and the resulting disfigurement causes great distress. The most common means of prevention is the application of external pressure, usually effected by the use of specially designed elasticated garments which can be made to fit any anatomical part. The garments should be worn, apart from bathing and skin care, for 24 h/day; treatment should continue for at least 9 months and a pressure of at least 24 mmHg is necessary for the treatment to be effective. Patients are provided with at least two sets of garments, which are alternately washed and worn.

Elastic garments are not very effective for applying pressure to concavities on the body surface, especially on the face around the nose and mouth. For treatment of these areas, a rigid, or semi-rigid, transparent face mask can be made. One technique which does not rely on pressure to reduce the hypertrophy and redness of scars is the use of silicone gel sheets (Mustoe et al 2002). These need to be retained in place with light bandages or adhesive tape and must be removed regularly for washing as they are reusable for a few applications.

Psychological effects of burn injuries

The disfigurement and impaired function which result from wound contraction and scar formation are generally accepted as the major sequelae of burn injuries, causing great distress and psychological problems for the patient and their loved ones. This, however, describes the long-term view and does not take into account that, for the patient and their family, the psychological effects start at the time of injury.

Many patients voice their relief at being alive in the immediate period following the accident, but as the implications of their injury sink in, their emotions and behaviour may begin to go through a series of changes.

Badger (2001) described three psychological phases experienced by patients hospitalised following burn injuries:

- acute
- subacute
- chronic.

The acute phase

During the early stages of treatment, the patient will be preoccupied by bodily feelings and by the care provided by nursing and medical staff. If the wounds are extensive and complications arise, the patient will be cared for in ICU, perhaps for long periods, which may result in various mental health problems (see Ch. 29). Nightmares associated with the accident are common at this stage, as are fears of dying. A constant presence, reassurance and reorientation may be necessary.

The subacute phase

When the patient reaches this stage, anxiety related to survival is replaced with fears for the future, both short and long term. In the short term, stress is related to anticipation of pain and many patients become depressed or are hostile towards the nursing staff. They may regress in their ability to cope with activities of living and demand care and attention. This is perhaps the most difficult phase for the unit staff to cope with. Pain control helps to reduce patient anxiety related to wound care, and physiotherapy and monitoring of pain should continue throughout the period of hospitalisation.

Longer-term anxieties include the fear of disfigurement (Box 30.5) and of losing function and former roles. Nursing staff can help the patient come to terms with their changed situation by being honest and supportive and allowing them to grieve. The first look in the mirror should not be accidental but a planned occasion with the patient making the choice whether to be alone or to be accompanied by nursing staff or loved ones. Although the patient may have some idea of their changed appearance from watching the reactions of visitors, the true extent of disfigurement may only be seen on first looking in a mirror. If the hands are not injured, the patient may gauge contour and textural changes through touch, but the reality of their changed appearance will still be a great shock.

Box 30.5 Reflection

Coping with disfigurement

The disfigurement caused by burns injury causes psychological problems for patients and their family and friends. Disfigurement affecting the face and hands is obvious all the time, but scarring present on other body areas causes problems, such as with relationships or undressing in a communal changing room.

Activity

- Think about, or discuss with colleagues, how you might feel about obvious disfigurement. How would it change your life? For instance would you want to continue with your nursing course/career?
- Investigate the information, advice and services offered by the British Association of Skin Camouflage (BASC) (www.skin-camouflage.net/) and Changing Faces (www.changingfaces.org.uk/), for example, physical means to reduce the impact of disfigurement, the problems of discrimination at work and the relevant legislation.

Regression in physical ability may also be managed by behavioural modification, with the patient being set easily achievable tasks, such as pouring a drink from their own water jug and being encouraged to feel a sense of achievement on doing so. Many patients regress when there is a sudden, unexplained reduction in the amount of nursing care they receive. Explanation about their improving condition, and patient involvement in identifying needs and planning the reduction of care can help to alleviate this problem.

The chronic phase

This phase is marked by the patient rediscovering former interests and pleasures. The patient may, for example, take more notice of the activity in the unit and of the other patients. When possible, mixing with the other patients should be encouraged; the patient's involvement in small tasks, such as distributing newspapers, will also aid independence and self-esteem. When disfigurement is highly visible, such as on the face and hands, the patient may not wish to mix with others and will require a great deal of support from staff as well as from family and friends.

Prior to discharge patients frequently experience ambivalence about leaving the safe confines of the unit where they are known and accepted. The actual discharge may be graduated by the introduction of visits home and by giving the patient the opportunity to discuss the pleasures and problems encountered. Liaison with the primary health care team will ensure continuity of care, and involvement of social workers and occupational therapists in the community will provide financial and practical help in the resumption of home life.

After discharge

It is possible that the patient will need to return to hospital for clinic appointments and, later on, for plastic surgery to improve appearance and function, a process which may involve many operations over a number of years. Many patients suffer long-term psychological problems including depression, anxiety and other post-traumatic stress symptoms.

No matter how high the standard of care provided, the patient who suffers extensive burns may never return fully to their former physical or emotional functioning – a fact which can only serve to emphasise the need for greater effort in the field of burn prevention.

SUMMARY: KEY NURSING ISSUES

- Burn prevention and health education is the most effective way of decreasing burn mortality and morbidity.
- Accurate assessment of depth and extent of burn wound is necessary to initiate the most appropriate evidence-based treatment thus giving the burn patient the best possible chance of survival as well as decreasing any long-term effects of scarring or contracture.
- Nursing patients with burn injury requires skill and can be challenging. A holistic approach is essential to achieve optimal outcomes. This includes assessment, fluid replacement, pain relief,

wound care (when many wound care products are not feasible for extensive burns), nutrition, prevention of complications, etc.
- Psychological effects of burn injury can often occur and can result in long-term psychological damage to the individual and the family. Nurses have a vital role in providing information and support.

➡ REFLECTION AND LEARNING – WHAT NEXT?

- **Test** your knowledge by visiting the website 🖱 and answering the multiple choice questions and critical thinking questions.
- **Consolidate** your learning by looking at some of the further reading suggestions, references and specialist websites.
- **Revisit** some of the additional material on the website.
- **Consider** what you have learnt and how this will help your professional development.
- **Reflect** on how you can apply this knowledge to the care of your patients.
- **Discuss** your learning with your mentor/supervisor, lecturer and colleagues.

REFERENCES

Anwar M, Majunder S, Austin O, et al: Smoking, substance abuse, psychiatric history, and burns: Trends in adult patients, *J Burn Care Rehabil* 26(6):493–501, 2005.

Atiyeh B, Costagliola M: Cultured epithelial autograft (CEA) in burn treatment: Three decades later, *Burns* 33(4):405–413, 2007.

Australia and New Zealand Burn Association Ltd (UK): *Emergency management of severe burns course manual*, 1996, UK version for The British Burn Association.

Badger J: Burns: The psychological effects, *Am J Nurs* 101(11):38–42, 2001.

Benson A, Dickson W, Boyce D: ABC of wound healing, *BMJ* 332:649–652, 2006.

Bessey PQ: Wound Care. In Herndon D, editor: *Total Burn Care*, ed 3, Philadelphia, 2007, Saunders, pp 127–134.

Bhatia M, Moochhala S: Role of inflammatory mediators in the pathophysiology of acute respiratory distress syndrome, *J Pathol* 202(2): 145–156, 2004.

Bull JP, Lennard-Jones JE: The impairment of sensation in burns and its clinical application as a test of the depth of loss, *Clin Sci* 8:155, 1949.

Caruso D, Foster K, Blome-Eberwein S, et al: Randomised clinical study of hydrofiber dressing with silver or silver sulfadiazine in the management of partial-thickness burns, *J Burn Care Res* 27(3): 298–309, 2006.

DeSanti L: Pathophsiology and current management of burn injury, *Adv Skin Wound Care* 18:333–334, 2005.

DuKamp A: Deroofing minor burn blisters – what is the evidence? *Accid Emerg Nurs* 9(4):217–221, 2001.

Dunn K, Edward-Jones V: The role of Acticoat® with nanocrystalline silver in the management of partial thickness burns, *Burns* 30(Suppl 1): S1–S9, 2004.

Flanagan M, Graham J: Should burn blisters be left intact or debrided? *J Wound Care* 10(2):41–45, 2001.

Garner J, Heppell P: The use of Flammacerium in British burn units, *Burns* 31(3):379–382, 2005.

Greenhalgh D: Wound healing. In Herndon D, editor: *Total Burn Care*, ed 3, Philadelphia, 2007, Saunders, pp 523–535.

Hojer J, Personne M, Hulten P, Ludwigs U: Topical treatments for hydrochloric acid burns: a blind controlled experimental study, *Journal of Toxicology* 40(7):861–866, 2002.

Hudspith J, Rayatt S: First aid and treatment of minor burns, *Br Med J* 328 (7454):1487–1489, 2004.

Kreis BE, Middelkoop E, Vloemans AF, Kreis RW: The use of a PEG tube in a burn center, *Burns* 28(2):191–197, 2002.

Lee JO, Benjamin D, Herndon DN: Nutrition support strategies for severely burned patients, *Nutr Clin Pract* 20(3):325–330, 2005.

Liao CC, Rossignol AM: Landmarks in burn prevention, *Burns* 26(5):422–434, 2000.

Lund CC, Browder NC: The estimation of areas of burns, *Surg Gynecol Obstet* 79:352–354, 1944.

McGill D, Sorensen K, MacKay I, et al: Assessment of burn depth: A prospective, blinded comparison of laser doppler imaging and videomicroscopy, *Burns* 33(7):833–842, 2007.

Mustoe TA, Cooter RD, Gold MH, et al: International clinical recommendations on scar management, *Plast Reconstr Surg* 110(2):560–571, 2002.

National Burn Injury Referral Guidelines: *National Burn Care Review Committee, Standards and Strategy for Burn Care*, , pp 68–69. Available online http://www.britishburnassociation.org/Downloads/2001-nbcr. pdf.

Office of the Deputy Prime Minister: *Fire statistics, United Kingdom – 2001*, London, 2003, ODPM.

Patterson DR, Hoflund H, Espey K, et al: Pain management, *Burns* 30(8):10–15, 2004.

Pereira C, Murphy K, Herndon D: Outcome measures in burn care. Is mortality dead? *Burns* 30(8):761–771, 2004.

Pham C, Greenwood J, Cleland H, et al: Bioengineered skin substitutes for the management of burns: A systemic review, *Burns* 33(8):946–957, 2007.

Stone M, Ahmed J, Evans J: The continuing risk of domestic hot water scalds to the elderly, *Burns* 26(4):347–350, 2000.

Tones K, Tilford S: *Health promotion: effectiveness, efficiency and equity*, Cheltenham, 2001, Nelson Thornes.

Tredget H, Shankowsky R, Rennie R, et al: Pseudomonas infections in the thermally injured patient, *Burns* 30(1):3–26, 2004.

Tse T, Poon HY, Tse KH, et al: Paediatric burn prevention: An epidemiological approach, *Burns* 32(2):229–234, 2006.

Unglaub F, Woodruff S, Deimer E: Patients with epilepsy; a high risk population prone to severe burns while showering, *J Burn Care Rehabil* 26:526–528, 2005.

Venter T, Karpelowsky J, Rode H: Cooling of the burn wound: The ideal temperature of the coolant, *Burns* 33(7):917–922, 2007.

Wallace AB: The exposure treatment of burns, *Lancet* i:501–504, 1951.

Weber J, McManus A: Nursing Committee of the International Society for Burn Injuries: Infection control in burn patients, *Burns* 30(8):16–24, 2004.

Williams C: Fluid Resuscitation in Burn Patients 2: Nursing Care, *Nurs Times* 104(15):24–25, 2008.

FURTHER READING

Herndon D, editor: *Total Burn Care*, ed 3, Philadelphia, 2007, Saunders.

Williams C: Fluid Resuscitation in Burn Patients 1: Using Formulas, *Nurs Times* 104(14):28–29, 2008.

USEFUL WEBSITES

British Association of Skin Camouflage (BASC): www.skin-camouflage.net

Changing Faces: www.changingfaces.org.uk

Fire Service: www.fireservice.co.uk

The Royal Society for the Prevention of Accidents (RoSPA): www.rospa. com

Nursing the patient with cancer

Susanne Cruickshank, Karen Campbell

Introduction

Cancer remains one of the top priorities in health care alongside heart disease, stroke and diabetes. It can profoundly affect every aspect of life, encompassing physical, psychological, social or spiritual aspects. Cancer care is changing rapidly with advances in technology and emerging treatments improving survival rates. Nurses are now at the forefront of care for cancer patients and their families.

Despite improvements in survival, the term 'cancer' impacts on the attitudes and beliefs of practitioners and patients, instilling thoughts about pain, uncertainty and death (Box 31.1). Government policy in prevention and predictions about the nature and cause of cancer can appear controversial and contradictory. This creates misinformation and inconsistency surrounding the disease.

✎ See website for further content

Cancer is a serious social problem, costing much in human and financial terms. One in three people in the UK risk developing cancer in their lifetime. One in four deaths are attributable to cancer (Cancer Research UK 2009). The incidence of different cancers and the death rate associated with them can vary both within the UK and globally. (See Useful websites Cancer Research UK, World Health Organization.)

Oncology as a specialty

The UK political and health care agenda has recognised cancer as a high priority area for over a decade. The first important documentation to drive organisational change in cancer services across the country was initiated by the publication of the Calman–Hine/Calman Report (Department of Health 1995). The Calman Report focused around the patient and their family, care being delivered in specific designated cancer centres and cancer units in partnership with each other. The report recommended a seamless service integrating primary, secondary and tertiary care, with real commitment to psychosocial as well as medical needs. It also provided the opportunity to think about cancer control, early screening and detection programmes.

Subsequent policy documents have influenced the progression of cancer services and, following devolution, England, Wales and Scotland have set out their own policy directions for health (Department of Health 2004, Scottish Government 2008). Comprehensive long-term strategies are continually being developed to shape cancer services, focusing on all aspects of the patient's cancer journey, ensure equity of care and invest in equipment and the cancer workforce. Nursing plays a key role in this development and both student nurses and newly qualified health care professionals need to understand the multidisciplinary nature of cancer management within and outside the hospital, appreciating the roles of all those providing patient care.

The fundamental process of cancer

The formation of cancer is a very complex process which involves the disruption of the regulation of growth of normal cells in the body. The process is called carcinogenesis. Any organ within the body has the potential to become cancerous, however some cancers are more common and potentially linked to a known carcinogen exposure.

In recent decades, molecular biology has made great progress in unravelling the steps involved in this process of cell transformation and is improving our ability to understand, classify, diagnose and treat cancer. A critical component in understanding the cancer process and rationale for treatment is a knowledge of the structure and function of cells, the role of deoxyribonucleic acid (DNA) and the cell cycle. (See Further reading, e.g. Martini & Nath 2009 and Useful websites, e.g. Cancerquest.)

To maintain functional cells through cell division the normal regulatory function of the cell will employ chemical signals to drive and halt growth; this is controlled by genetic components of the cell. The chemical signals are protein components of growth factors, receptors, and messenger and regulatory proteins. The chemical signals act within individual cells and are also utilised when communicating with neighbouring cells in regulating growth. Damage to the genetic components of the cells can result in loss of function and ability to regulate growth. As the scientific evidence for the chemical signals is complex this text will concentrate on the key genetic components involved.

During scientific research on viruses and how they propagate and reproduce within their host, scientists discovered extremely important genes involved in regulation of cell growth. These genes were called proto-oncogenes and had the ability to promote cell growth (switch on). When one of these genes becomes damaged and permanently switched on it is referred to as an oncogene. The ability of the cell to inhibit (switch off) growth is regulated by a tumour suppressor gene, the activity of which was revealed when investigating the childhood hereditary cancer retinoblastoma. When this gene is damaged the function is lost and the cell can no longer switch growth off. Another gene implicated in the replication repair process is called the mismatched repair gene. This gene repairs damaged DNA after replication. When this gene is damaged the cell accumulates lots of mismatched DNA which in turn promotes cell growth. The last essential gene controls the process of apoptosis (programmed cell death) – when the cell has divided a certain number of times it commits cell death. Therefore damage in this gene results in an inability to programme the cell to die. Such damage may occur from either error in DNA replication during mitosis or exposure to environmental agents. In the transformation to a cancerous growth, there is a progressive series of mutations of genes regulating cell division and differentiation.

Cancers develop when the cell can no longer regulate its own growth, resulting in the cells being able to divide rapidly. To survive within the host the forming tumour seeks out a new blood supply to maintain its growth which results in small fragments of tumour splitting off and travelling to distant sites to form secondary tumours (metastases); the cancer is said to have metastasised.

Tumours grow by repeated cell divisions; their rate of growth is often defined in terms of doubling time. Tumours vary greatly in their doubling time but, contrary to popular belief, their growth is not as rapid as that of normal tissues. For a tumour growth to exceed 1 or 2 mm, it requires a blood supply for survival; therefore the formation of a capillary network from the surrounding host tissue is initiated by proteins or angiogenic factors, e.g. fibroblast growth factor (FGF) and tumour necrosis factor (TNF).

Tumour pathology

A tumour may be benign or malignant. 'Cancer' is a general term used to describe all malignant neoplasms, i.e. a new growth of tissue, or tumour.

Usually benign tumours are:

- well differentiated – still closely resemble the host tissue
- slow growing
- enclosed in a capsule
- non-invasive – do not invade locally or metastasise.

Once removed, benign tumours rarely recur. However, a benign tumour can cause problems or even death in certain sites. For example, a benign brain tumour can cause pressure on the brain (see Ch. 9) and some benign tumours cause problems in other ways, such as bleeding or secreting excess hormones.

Malignant tumours grow at the expense of the host. They are characterised by:

- various degrees of cell differentiation – well differentiated to totally undifferentiated
- variable growth rate – may be uncoordinated; some are slow growing
- having no enclosing capsule
- their invasive nature – locally by infiltration and by metastatic spread to other sites.

Malignant tumours destroy vital structures, cause severe weight loss and debility (cancer cachexia syndrome) and result in death without effective treatment. It is, however, important to remember that as survival times continue to improve many more people will be 'living with cancer'.

Understanding the molecular biology of cancer is very important to identify and obtain a definitive cancer diagnosis and thus predict prognosis. Increasing knowledge about newer biological factors such as HER2/neu receptors and proliferative index (rate of cell division in the tumour) has altered the way adjuvant treatments (see p. 812) are prescribed and these indicators are increasingly used to predict prognosis. The HER-2/neu receptor belongs to the epidermal growth factor receptor family which is one of the receptors critical in controlling the pathway for epithelial cell growth and differentiation, and possibly angiogenesis (Karunagaran et al 1996). Overexpression of the HER-2/neu protein is observed in 15–20% of breast cancers (Slamon et al 1989), and it is now accepted that high levels of expression of HER-2/neu identify those patients most likely to respond

Table 31.1 Examples of molecular genetic markers used in cancer diagnosis and prognosis

CANCER	GENETIC MARKER	PRINCIPAL APPLICATION
Chronic myeloid leukaemia	Philadelphia chromosome t(9;22)(q34;q11) [BCR/ABL]	Primary diagnosis, detection of residual disease after treatment
Non-Hodgkin's lymphoma 　Follicular 　Burkitt's	l(14;18)(q32;q21) [BCL2/IGH] t(8;14)(q24;q32)	Primary diagnosis, detection of residual disease after treatment As above
Neuroblastoma	MYCN amplification	Prognosis
Breast cancer	HER2-neu/ERB2 amplification	Prognosis
Familial cancers		
Breast	BRCA1, BRCA2	Diagnosis of hereditary predisposition
Colon	APC, MSH2, MLH1	As above
Wilms' tumour	TP53 mutation	As above
Retinoblastoma	RB mutation	As above

to trastuzumab in both the adjuvant and metastatic disease setting.

Identification of the steps involved in carcinogenesis has led directly to the discovery of molecular tumour markers (Table 31.1). Among the cancers for which molecular diagnostics has had an impact is chronic myeloid leukaemia (CML). The marker of this disease is the Philadelphia chromosome, which is detectable in 95% of cases. This additional information enhances the ability to accurately diagnose and determine prognosis.

Tumours may be classified not only by their biological behaviour but also traditionally by their tissue of origin. Most tumours retain sufficient characteristics of the normal differentiated cell to allow recognition of the type of tissue from which they were derived, which is the basis for the classification of tumours by tissue type (Table 31.2).

The physical effects of cancer

The manifestations of cancer depend directly or indirectly on the location, size and type of tumour involved and the site of any metastases present. The most common sites of metastatic deposits are the lungs, bones, brain and liver.

Direct tumour effects include the following:

* obstruction of duct and tracts, e.g. the oesophagus, causing dysphagia
* compression of major blood vessels such as the superior vena cava, causing ischaemia, oedema of the head, neck and right arm, and dyspnoea
* compression of neighbouring tissues and organs, e.g. brain metastases may cause pressure and local oedema, which can compromise brain function and level of consciousness
* pressure on regional nerves, causing pain and/or paralysis, e.g. metastases in the vertebrae may cause spinal cord compression (SCC) and result in pain or loss of sensation and paralysis – an oncological emergency

* invasion of small local blood vessels, causing chronic bleeding and anaemia; when major vessels such as the carotid artery erode, a haemorrhage may be sudden and fatal
* uncontrollable growth causing necrosis or ulceration which may be internal or external – often termed 'a fungating tumour'
* infiltration by the cancer cells into the bone marrow compromising haemopoiesis (blood cell production) and leading to increased susceptibility to infection
* metabolic alterations – there are many tumour-specific metabolic imbalances such as those affecting the kidneys, liver and pancreas. Hypercalcaemia is the most common oncological emergency and is associated with cancer of the breast, bone, lung and kidney. It is caused by local bone metastases directly stimulating osteoclast activity (causing breakdown of bone structure) and the release of humoral hypercalcaemia factors. (See Further reading e.g. Scott-Brown et al 2007.)

Indirect tumour effects A group of rare degenerative disorders broadly termed as 'paraneoplastic syndromes' may be the presenting features before diagnosis in 10–15% of patients (Armstrong 2005). Early detection is important as these symptoms can often be ameliorated.

📖 **See website for further content**

Cancer recurrence

The exact manner in which a cancer moves from being a carcinoma in situ to one which is capable of invasion and spread to other organs or tissues is not clear; however, it is thought to be partly due to physiological changes occurring in tumour cell membranes which reduce their adhesion to other cells. Tumours also produce proteolytic (protein-dissolving) enzymes, which may assist in the invasion of normal tissue. Malignant cells also seem to lose contact inhibition, failing to recognise their boundaries and to cease

Table 31.2 Classification by tissue type of malignant tumours

TISSUE OF ORIGIN	MALIGNANT TUMOUR
Epithelial	**'Carcinoma'**
Squamous: surface epithelium, cell lining covering body cavities, organs and tracts	Squamous cell carcinoma, e.g. lung, skin, stomach
Glandular: glands or ducts in the epithelium	Adenocarcinoma, e.g. breast, lung, colon
Transitional cells: bladder lining	Transitional cell carcinoma, e.g. bladder
Basal cells: skin layer	Basal cell carcinoma (BCC), 'rodent ulcer'
Liver	Hepatocellular carcinoma
Biliary tree	Cholangiocarcinoma
Placenta	Choriocarcinoma
Testicular epithelium	Seminoma, teratoma, embryonal carcinoma
Endothelial cells	Angiosarcoma
Mesothelial: covering the surface of serous membranes	Mesothelioma, e.g. pleura, peritoneum
Connective tissue	**'Sarcoma'**
Bone	Osteosarcoma
Cartilage	Chondrosarcoma
Fatty tissue	Liposarcoma
Fibrous tissue	Fibrosarcoma
Lymphoid tissue	Lymphomas
Bone marrow	Leukaemias, e.g. ALL, CML
Muscle	**'Myosarcoma'**
Smooth muscle	Leiomyosarcoma
Striated muscle	Rhabdomyosarcoma
Cardiac muscle	Cardiac sarcomas
Neural	
Meninges	Meningeal sarcoma
Glia	Glioblastoma multiforme
Neurones	Neuroblastoma, medulloblastoma
Germ cells	
Testes or ovary	Teratoma, germ cell

ALL, acute lymphoblastic leukaemia; CML, chronic myeloid leukaemia.

growth on meeting a different tissue type. For example, tumours of glandular lung tissue may continue invasion through the pleura to the chest wall. The risk of cancer recurrence is always present when a diagnosis has been given. Two thirds of patients develop metastases and most deaths from cancer are due to metastases that are resistant to conventional therapies (Fidler 1997). (See Useful websites, e.g. Cancerquest; tumour biology.)

Metastatic invasion (spread) may occur in one of four ways (see Figure 31.1):

- via the lymphatic system
- via the bloodstream (arteriovenous)
- via serous cavities
- via the cerebrospinal fluid (CSF).

Lymphatic spread Tumour cells may invade the lymphatic vessels and grow in clumps and cords, establishing themselves en route in local lymph nodes. This is termed 'regional spread'.

Arteriovenous spread Tumour cells enter blood vessels near the primary tumour or are shed into the blood via the thoracic lymph duct. They then become enmeshed in the next capillary network they encounter. For example a gastrointestinal tumour will typically spread via the hepatic portal vein, initially to the liver.

Serous cavity spread Serous membranes such as the pleura or the peritoneum may be invaded by tumours, either locally from the primary tumour or from nearby metastases. This can cause excess serous fluid to be produced and the formation of malignant pleural effusions or ascites. This process is commonly known as 'seeding'

CSF spread Tumour cells may spread directly in the CSF. Some brain tumours metastasise along the spinal cord in this fashion.

Survival is referred to in 5-, 10- and 15-year intervals and, while more cancer patients are surviving, the term 'cure' is used with caution. It is important for health care professionals to clarify their meaning for patients, as the uncertainty surrounding cancer and cancer recurrence creates distress for the patient and their family.

The psychosocial impact of cancer

There are psychosocial implications for patients and families from diagnosis, through treatment, the development of recurrence and end of life. It is now widely accepted that quality of life in cancer patients is an important consideration and may be improved by psychological interventions at specific stages (Cruickshank et al 2008). These important areas are explored further in this chapter.

Epidemiology of cancer

Epidemiological studies provide data about possible causes of different forms of cancer and inform the strategies for cancer prevention and screening. The most commonly diagnosed cancers in the UK are breast, lung, colorectal and prostate; together these four cancers make up over 50% of all new cancers each year (Cancer Research UK 2009). The 20 most commonly diagnosed cancers are shown in Figure 31.2.

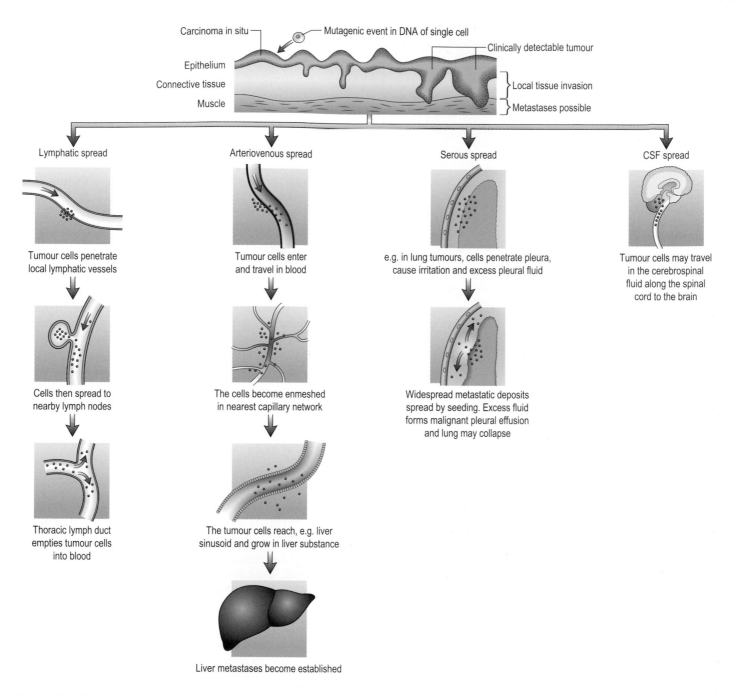

Carcinoma in situ — ⭕ ← Mutagenic event in DNA of single cell

Epithelium

Connective tissue

Muscle

Clinically detectable tumour

Local tissue invasion

Metastases possible

Lymphatic spread

Tumour cells penetrate local lymphatic vessels

Cells then spread to nearby lymph nodes

Thoracic lymph duct empties tumour cells into blood

Arteriovenous spread

Tumour cells enter and travel in blood

The cells become enmeshed in nearest capillary network

The tumour cells reach, e.g. liver sinusoid and grow in liver substance

Liver metastases become established

Serous spread

e.g. in lung tumours, cells penetrate pleura, cause irritation and excess pleural fluid

Widespread metastatic deposits spread by seeding. Excess fluid forms malignant pleural effusion and lung may collapse

CSF spread

Tumour cells may travel in the cerebrospinal fluid along the spinal cord to the brain

Figure 31.1 The cancer process.

Cancer is associated with increasing age. Around 75% of people diagnosed with cancer are aged 60 years and over (Cancer Research UK 2009). Cancer is very rare in children; approximately 1% of cancers are diagnosed in children, teenagers and young adults (Cancer Research UK 2009). (See Further reading, e.g. Baggott et al 2002.)

The incidence of cancer in the UK is one of the highest in the northern hemisphere. Predominantly, cancer is a disease of well-resourced countries but it is clear that patterns of cancer are set to increase in developing countries over the next decade (Ferlay et al 2007). The greater incidence in the northern hemisphere may be partly attributed to the availability of screening, diagnostic and reporting procedures,

improved overall life expectancy and diet. Geographical variations across the world in the incidence of cancer provide clues to the lifestyles of different populations.

In Mozambique a high incidence of liver cancer is thought to have been associated with aflatoxin from mould found on stored peanuts. Since the introduction of more appropriate storage practices, the incidence of liver cancer has been falling. The Japanese have a low incidence of breast cancer in comparison to the UK and USA but a high incidence of stomach cancer.

Epidemiological investigation of genetic predisposition to cancer is growing rapidly as developments in molecular biology make it possible to study genetic markers in large

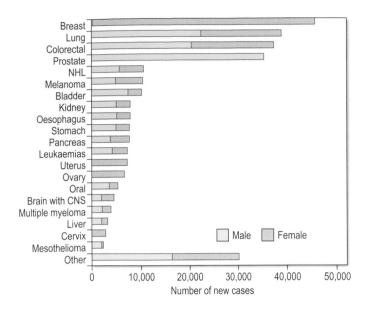

Figure 31.2 The 20 most commonly diagnosed cancers (ex NMSC), UK, 2006 (Cancer Research UK, http://info.cancerresearchuk.org/cancerstats/incidence/commoncancers/ June 2009). CNS, central nervous system; NHL, non-Hodgkin's lymphoma.

populations. The completion of the Human Genome Project is accelerating the discovery of such markers (see Useful websites).

Aetiology of cancer

The cause of cancer is the combined interaction of genetic and environmental factors and it is difficult to separate the two completely. Although all cancers have a genetic origin at the cellular level, this does not mean that all cancer is inherited. Genetic changes or mutations may be either *somatic* (acquired) or *germline* (inherited).

- *Germline mutations* are those present in the gamete (oocyte or spermatozoon) of a parent that can be passed to the offspring. The mutation is present in every cell of the body.
- *Somatic mutation* is when an individual body cell, post conception, acquires a gene alteration. If not repaired, the mutation is passed on to all future cells through mitosis. These clonal changes are unique to the cells in that particular tissue and are not inherited.

Many questions remain to be answered regarding the exact mechanisms involved in the cellular mutations that lead to cancer. However, epidemiological studies have identified certain causative factors, termed 'carcinogens'.

Carcinogens are factors that both initiate and promote changes in the cell which lead to cancer. Both are required to cause the cancer:

- *Initiation* – a mutagenic event occurs in the DNA of a single cell.
- *Promotion* – repeated exposure to carcinogenic agents may or may not cause this initiated cell to proliferate to form a tumour.

Carcinogenic factors and substances can be either intrinsic or extrinsic.

Intrinsic factors

Heredity Inherited cancers constitute 5–10% of all cancers. Several genes have now been identified that are responsible for predisposing individuals to develop certain cancers. Cancers that occur with increased frequency in families are components of various hereditary cancer syndromes, e.g. hereditary non-polyposis colon cancer (HNPCC).

Cancer susceptibility genes such as BRCA1 and BRCA2 have been identified in breast and ovarian cancer. Women who inherit a mutation in these genes may face a 50–85% lifetime risk of developing breast cancer including an increased risk for ovarian cancer (Calzone & Biesecker 2002). Testing for these particular genes and others is now available commercially.

Hormones Certain hormones are thought to promote some tumours. Early menarche, late menopause and nulliparity are associated with an increased lifetime risk of breast cancer. The Million Women Study (2003) found that the use of combined oestrogen plus progesterone hormone replacement therapy (HRT) also increases the risk of breast cancer. High testosterone levels have been related to increased risk of prostate cancer (Ross et al 2003).

Immunity Individuals with impaired immunity are more susceptible to cancer; for example, people with HIV disease have a higher incidence of Kaposi's sarcoma than the normal population (see Ch. 35). It is the prolonged immunosuppression that may predispose these patients to cancer rather than the infectious agent per se.

Pre-existing disease Any tissue subjected to constant irritation or to a disease process has an increased susceptibility to malignant change.

Age The increased incidence of cancer with age is thought to be attributable to:

- prolonged exposure to carcinogens
- decreased resistance to carcinogens
- hormonal changes that occur with age.

Extrinsic factors

At least 70% of cancers occur in epithelial cells which are constantly exposed to external, ingested or inhaled substances. Extrinsic factors related to lifestyle and the environment are important in the process of carcinogenesis. These factors include physical agents, chemical agents, viruses and diet.

Physical agents

Radiation is known to cause cellular mutations and cancer. Survivors of the atomic bomb explosions in Hiroshima and Nagasaki in Japan experienced a high incidence of leukaemia and skin cancer. Early research has shown an apparent increase in the incidence of leukaemia among the children of fathers working in the nuclear industry, possibly due to germ cell mutations (Gardner et al 1990). Repeated exposure to therapeutic doses of radiation is not thought to be harmful, although stringent precautionary regulations must be followed for the protection of all exposed workers. Therefore, it is not routine discharge of radioactivity by the nuclear industry that should be feared, but rather the catastrophic event, such as occurred at Chernobyl in 1986.

Ultraviolet light (UVL) There is overwhelming evidence that repeated exposure to solar UVL is the primary cause of basal and squamous cell carcinoma (see Ch. 12). Data establishing a direct causal relationship with sunlight are more complex, but suggest a promotional role of sunlight in the cause of melanoma. Light-skinned or freckled individuals who are unable to manufacture sufficient protective melanin are particularly at risk (see Ch. 12).

Chemical agents

Tobacco Ninety per cent of all lung cancers can be attributed to tobacco smoking. The temporal relationship between smoking and lung cancer was defined in the 1950s by studies undertaken by Doll & Hill (1954). Cigarette smoking has now clearly been identified as a major cause of cancers of the mouth, pharynx, larynx, bladder and pancreas, whilst contributing to many others. Risk is more dependent on duration of smoking than on consumption. Smoking 20 cigarettes a day for 40 years is eight times more hazardous than smoking 40 cigarettes a day for 20 years. People who stop smoking even well into middle age avoid most of their subsequent risk of lung cancer, and stopping before middle age avoids more than 90% of the risk attributable to tobacco (Peto et al 2000). It is also evident that non-smokers are at risk from exposure to other people's smoke: one-quarter of lung cancer cases in non-smokers are estimated to be due to passive smoking (International Agency for Research on Cancer [IARC] 2004).

Alcohol Excessive alcohol, ingested over long periods of time, contributes to cancers of the mouth, pharynx, oesophagus and liver. Those who drink spirits as opposed to wine and beer and those who smoke as well as drink are particularly at risk.

Other chemicals Carcinogenic chemicals present occupational hazards. Some of these, but by no means all, are now subject to control through regulation or ban. These controlled substances, and associated cancer sites, include:

- asbestos (lung, mesothelium and larynx)
- vinyl chloride (liver)
- certain chemical dyes (bladder)
- arsenic (lung and skin)
- some hardwood dusts (nasopharynx).

Viruses

Although cancer is not contagious, some cancers are associated with viral infections. For example, the Epstein–Barr virus (EBV) causes a systemic infection that may precede Burkitt's lymphoma, a malignant disease common in parts of Africa. Patients with chronic hepatitis B are more susceptible than others to liver cancer. The human papilloma virus (HPV), which may be sexually transmitted, is associated with cervical cancer, and the development of vaccines against some types of HPV has created opportunities to prevent some cases of cervical cancer (see p. 812).

Diet

Epidemiological studies that isolate diet as a causal factor in the development of cancer are extremely problematic to undertake. Nevertheless, dietary factors have been implicated as a major cause of the high incidence of cancer in the West. Countries where the average diet is high in fat and protein appear to have a high incidence of breast cancer, and low-fibre diets are thought to contribute to bowel cancer.

Cancer prevention and screening

Prevention of cancer is a major focus of research and education. The goal of primary prevention is to reduce the risk of the healthy population developing cancer. Secondary prevention aims to detect early-stage, curable cancer. Primary prevention is therefore the most effective and economic method of controlling cancer.

Nurses now have a responsibility to incorporate health promotion, health education and disease prevention in their role as well as the care of those who are ill. This wider role is reflected in their initial and post-registration education. Community health practitioners work in health centres offering a range of health promotion programmes, as well as screening for ill health. Antenatal care, well-woman or well-man clinics, sexual health and family planning centres and other health screening clinics all provide opportunities for the promotion of cancer prevention. Within hospitals, clinical nurse specialists incorporate cancer awareness and prevention in their roles, with many involved in local and national initiatives such as cancer site-specific awareness weeks and health promotion in schools.

Primary prevention

Primary cancer prevention includes activities such as:

- identifying risk factors in individuals or groups
- counselling high-risk individuals to promote behaviour modification
- genetic screening
- implementation of new cancer prevention programmes, e.g. smoking cessation, healthy eating.

Media reporting of cancer risk development requires cautious interpretation and should be put into perspective by reference to the original studies on which it is based. It is important to remember that substances that are carcinogenic in animals are by no means always so in humans. Moreover, everyday exposure to some substances implicated is so minimal as to make risk insignificant. Some media scares do little to promote health; fear of cancer, after all, is one of the most common reasons why people avoid screening or fail to present with symptoms.

Health promotion programmes

Health promotion/education programmes have some measure of success. Several government publications have taken on 'The Cancer Challenge', with measures to promote a 'pro-health' culture (Department of Health 2000, Scottish Executive Health Department [SEHD] 2004). Projects have been developed to assist smokers to quit, particularly in areas with high levels of deprivation, prisons, the army and working men's clubs. Political action has included a comprehensive ban on tobacco advertising, a smoking ban in public places and the workplace, the setting up of new stop-smoking clinics and a smokers' helpline, nicotine replacement patches and bupropion available on prescription, as well as a major health education campaign in schools aimed at preventing youngsters from starting to smoke (Department of Health 2000, SEHD 2004).

Box 31.2 Reflection

Lifestyle and cancer: reducing the risk

Access the European code against cancer and Cancer Research UK websites and consider their advice on reducing cancer risk.

Activities

- Reflect on how you could modify your own lifestyle to reduce cancer risk.
- Discuss with your mentor how you could use the European code against cancer when talking with patients about reducing cancer risk.

Resources

European code against cancer – http://www.cancercode.org/index.html

Cancer Research UK – http://info.cancerresearchuk.org/healthyliving/

Through working partnerships with the community and the food industry, strategies to promote healthy eating include a national 'Five a Day' programme, improving accessibility to affordable fresh fruit and vegetables, and advocating five portions of these daily (see Ch. 21) (Box 31.2).

Attitudes

Psychologists have developed a Health Belief Model (Strecher & Rosenstock 1997) to predict an individual's preventive health behaviour and account for some of the factors which determine attitudes to health and illness. The Health Belief Model states that an individual feels vulnerable to a disease if they believe they are susceptible to developing it and believe the disease to be serious. Preventive action will be taken only after the individual has balanced the benefits of that action against its physical, psychological and financial costs (Smith 2005).

Despite being taught about the risks of smoking, teenage smokers may consider themselves to be young and healthy and therefore not 'at risk'. Young people in general are motivated by short-term rather than long-term rewards. Smoking in some subcultures and families is associated with attributes such as maturity or rebelliousness, which the young person and their peer group may value. Later, the physical addiction to nicotine becomes a coping mechanism for life's stresses and social deprivation. For such people, possible avoidance of lung cancer is not worth the cost of surrendering the immediate gratification and social status offered by smoking.

Clearly, consideration of the wider causes of individual behaviour would lead those involved in health promotion to an awareness of the social and political action necessary. The causes of social deprivation need to be considered alongside individual behaviour. Preventive services must be readily accessible, based on the expressed needs of the community and client-centred.

The concepts of health and ill health are open to wide interpretation. An essential aspect of communication is that everyone understands and attaches the same meaning to language used. If adherence to health care programmes is to be achieved, nurses need to understand an individual's personal health beliefs and how information is interpreted.

Secondary prevention: screening

The prognosis and outcome of patients with cancer is improved considerably if the tumour is detected at an early stage. Complete cure can only be assured if pre-cancerous tissue can be identified and treated, as in the case of cervical intraepithelial neoplasia (CIN).

Cancer screening difficulties

The development of an accurate and cost-effective method of screening at-risk sections of the population is problematic for several reasons. The test must have both a high degree of sensitivity, reducing the risk of false-negative results, and specificity, reducing the psychological trauma and expense of treating false-positive results.

It must be possible to identify an at-risk group; otherwise the cost of screening becomes prohibitive. Finally, and most problematically, it must be determined whether detecting the cancer type at an early stage will prolong life (Segnan et al 2004).

The general cancer screening programmes currently offered (in the UK) are:

- breast cancer screening
- cervical cancer screening
- colorectal cancer screening.

Plus the Prostate Cancer Risk Management.
(See Useful websites NHS Cancer Screening Programmes.)

Breast cancer screening

Despite recent debates about the quality of over 40 years of trials, it is generally agreed that there is a clear benefit and reduction in mortality from breast cancer from screening women over the age of 50 years by mammography every 2 years (IARC 2002). In the UK mammography is routinely offered every 3 years to women aged between 50 and 70 years. However, the age range for routine invitation for screening is to be extended to include women aged 47 to 73. Accepted screening techniques include mammography and clinical breast examination, although Baxter (2001) has concluded that breast self-examination is of no benefit in routine screening. The value of screening women of 40 years or younger remains controversial, consequently professional clinical judgement and a woman's choice should guide decision-making. The denser breast tissue of premenopausal women makes mammograms difficult to interpret in this age group. In future, genetic screening and new technologies such as digital mammography may be of benefit.

Cervical cancer screening

Cervical cancer is one of the most common female cancers in under-resourced economies. Since the introduction of the Papanicolaou ('Pap') smear test in the mid 1960s, there has been a steady decline in mortality rates in the UK. Women in the UK are first offered screening at age 25 years. This continues every 3 years until they reach the age of 49 years. Thereafter the test is offered at 5-year intervals until women reach the age of 64. Women aged 65 or over are only offered a smear test if they have not had a smear since they reached 50 or have recently had an abnormal smear. However, some GPs may offer early screening as part of their consultation with women regarding sexual health.

Uptake of the service by groups at highest risk, i.e. women over the age of 40, of lower socioeconomic status and in minority ethnic groups, could be better. Barriers to cervical screening include lack of sensitivity and trust in health professionals, possible feelings of guilt and embarrassment, judgemental attitudes, and a lack of privacy and supportive care in clinics (Fitch et al 1998). It is important for staff working in screening services to have well-developed interpersonal and communication skills to alleviate any fears or anxieties. In addition, clinic schedules should allow time to provide support.

Intervention strategies based on individual respect, health care provider relationships and inclusion of significant others may increase adherence to cancer screening guidelines (Steven et al 2004).

Colorectal cancer screening

The natural history of colon cancer with the relatively long time from biological onset to the development of cancer makes it a good candidate for screening. A national bowel screening programme based on faecal occult blood (FOB), using a home screening kit, was rolled out in 2006 (England) and 2007 (Scotland). The service became available throughout the UK in 2009.

Screening is routinely offered every two years to people aged 60–69 years (in England) and 50–74 years (in Scotland). However, people aged over 70 years in England can request a screening kit (NHS Cancer Screening Programme 2009a). People with an unclear result will have the FOB test repeated. Where an abnormal result occurs the person is offered an appointment with a specialist nurse to discuss colonoscopy (see Ch. 4). Campaigns by Colon Cancer Concern have been initiated to promote a greater awareness of the early warning signs of colon cancer (see Ch. 4).

Screening options for other cancers

Screening programmes for the cancers below are being reviewed, including:

- prostate cancer
- ovarian cancer
- lung cancer.

Prostate cancer There is at present no consensus regarding the most appropriate screening method. There are three main screening modalities: digital rectal examination (DRE), serum prostate-specific antigen (PSA) and transrectal ultrasonography (TRUS). There are wide ranges in the estimates of sensitivity and specificity. Interest in PSA (a blood test) emerged in the late 1980s. However, PSA may be elevated in men with non-cancerous conditions. There is currently no evidence that prostatic screening improves clinical outcomes; in fact, there are issues of uncertainty surrounding the appropriateness and type of treatment for men with early-stage prostatic cancer, since it has a long asymptomatic latency period. It is therefore important to consider that there might be an adverse psychological impact as a result of prostate screening although, for those men at risk, it may provide some reassurance (Cantor et al 2002).

A *Prostate Cancer Risk Management* programme is available to improve men's understanding of the benefits and limitations of PSA testing (NHS Cancer Screening Programme 2009b).

Ovarian cancer This cancer is sometimes referred to as the 'silent killer' because it often presents late and has the highest mortality rate of all malignant gynaecological cancers. Transvaginal ultrasound and detection of a raised cancer antigen (CA125) in the blood provide two possible techniques for the screening of ovarian cancer. However, as with PSA, CA125 may be elevated in non-malignant conditions. A UK collaborative trial of ovarian cancer screening (UKCTOCS) is underway to answer the question of whether or not early detection will save lives. The effectiveness of different screening technologies is being examined. A report is expected in 2010 and will make recommendations about ovarian cancer screening for the whole population (Menon et al 2009).

Women known to have a high familial risk of developing ovarian cancer are offered annual screening as part of a national familial ovarian cancer screening study.

Lung cancer It has been shown that low-dose spiral computed tomography (CT) scanning can identify lung cancer in high-risk but asymptomatic individuals (Gohagan et al 2005). Whilst this may be a useful screening test, further evidence is required to see if early detection is linked with a decrease in mortality.

Medical intervention and the nurse's role

Diagnosis and staging

Patients present with cancer at different stages of the disease and may be asymptomatic or symptomatic.

The staging of a cancer is the process whereby the extent of the disease is established; this involves a variety of tests (see the appropriate chapter for the staging of a particular tumour site). The diagnosis and staging can be long, complex and tedious for the patient and their family, raising many issues of uncertainty. However, accurate staging of the extent of the disease is vital for the following reasons:

- Different forms of treatment are known to be effective for specific tumours and at specific disease stages. For example, thoracic surgery for a patient with disseminated small cell lung carcinoma (SCLC) and metastases in the ribs would be inappropriate given the metastatic spread of the disease. Staging avoids human and financial cost of using inappropriate treatment.
- It provides a better estimation of prognosis.
- It allows clinicians to determine a patient's eligibility to enter a clinical trial of a new treatment.

The tumour, node (lymph) and metastasis (TNM) system

The most common internationally used method of defining disease stage is the TNM system (Sobin & Wittekind 2002), in which:

- T denotes the size or extent of local invasion of the primary tumour.
- N refers to the spread to local lymph nodes
- M refers to the presence of metastases.

Agreed staging criteria exist for each cancer, such as those staging systems used for lung cancer (Box 31.3), gynaecological, testicular cancers, etc. (see Chs 3, 7). Box 31.4 illustrates the

Box 31.3 Information

Summary of the TNM staging system for lung cancer

T (primary tumour)

TX	Positive cytology only
Tis	Carcinoma in situ
T1	Tumour ≤3 cm in diameter. No proximal invasion
T2	Tumour >3 cm in diameter, within 2 cm from carina or invading the visceral pleura or partial atelectasis
T3	Tumour of any size extending into the chest wall, diaphragm, pericardium, mediastinal pleura or within 2 cm of carina, total atelectasis
T4	Tumour of any size with invasion of mediastinal organs or vertebral body, malignant pleural effusion

N (lymph nodes)

N0	Nodes negative
N1	Positive nodes in ipsilateral hilar nodes
N2	Positive ipsilateral, mediastinal and subcarinal nodes
N3	Positive contralateral mediastinal or hilar nodes, scalene or supraclavicular nodes

M (distant metastases)

M0	No metastases
M1	Metastases present

The disease is then staged using the above information, as follows:

Stage IA	T1	N0	M0
Stage IB	T2	N0	M0
Stage IIA	T1	N1	M0
Stage IIB	T2	N1	M0
	T3	N0	M0
Stage IIIA	T1–3	N2	M0
Stage IIIB	T4	Any N	M0
Stage IV	Any T	Any N	M1

Adapted from Sobin & Wittekind (2002).

staging system through the experience of a young man with testicular cancer.

Some types of cancer – usually those that are disseminated at presentation – cannot be effectively staged with the TNM system and have necessitated the development of other systems.

During the course of their illness, patients may be restaged in order for their response to treatment, or the extent of disease recurrence, to be assessed.

 See website Critical thinking question 31.1

Psychological impact of diagnosis and staging

Primary diagnosis

It is very common for patients to be aware that they have cancer before they are told formally of their diagnosis. This awareness derives from their experience of symptoms, tests and, in some cases, surgery and from the non-verbal communication of staff or relatives. How to inform patients *in full* of their diagnosis, and when this should be done are ongoing issues of ethical debate (Box 31.5).

Box 31.6 provides an opportunity for you to reflect on patient experiences of being given a diagnosis of cancer.

Even if they suspect their diagnosis, patients often cling to hope or use denial as a coping mechanism. These are the early emotional reactions experienced by people facing any actual or potential life crisis or loss, as described by Kübler-Ross in her seminal text (1973).

Disease recurrence

The discovery that the disease has recurred after a symptom-free period may provoke further psychological distress, as the patient realises there is no hope of cure. The period of waiting for test results, whether at initial diagnosis or at recurrence, can cause anxiety to both the patient and their family.

Psychological support

The nurse has an important role providing both practical information prior to and following each test, and emotional support. It is important to know why each test is being

Box 31.4 Reflection

Staging Dan's testicular cancer

Staging system generally used in the UK

Stage I	Tumour confined to testes
Stage II	Pelvic and abdominal lymph node involvement
Stage III	Mediastinal and/or supraclavicular lymph node involvement
Stage IV	Distant metastases, e.g. lung

Dan, a 22-year-old student, discovered a testicular swelling but chose to ignore it, initially because he misinterpreted it as a sports injury and he was busy with exams, and later because he felt embarrassed and frightened. Nine months later he presented to the student health centre because he was becoming breathless far more readily than usual and suffered a constant backache. These symptoms were due to lung metastases and referred pain caused by metastases in the para-aortic lymph nodes.

Dan was admitted to a surgical ward, where a biopsy under anaesthesia was performed. A frozen section taken for histology showed a testicular teratoma. A left orchidectomy was then performed.

Following postoperative recovery, Dan was transferred to an oncology ward for staging. Dan lived too far away to travel to the department each day; otherwise the necessary tests could have been performed while he was an outpatient. Dan wanted to know why staging was needed and the specialist nurse explained the purpose of staging and outlined the tests that would be necessary. The tests were carried out and their results were as follows:

- chest X-ray: showed multiple lung metastases
- thoracic computed tomography (CT) scan: confirmed lung metastases
- abdominal CT scan: showed a large para-aortic lymph node and no liver metastases

Continued

Box 31.4 Reflection – cont'd

- blood samples for full blood count, urea, creatinine and electrolytes, liver function and tumour markers (alpha-fetoprotein [AFP] and human chorionic gonadotrophin [hCG]).

These tests showed that Dan had stage IV testicular teratoma (see staging system above). Dan asked the specialist nurse to explain the results and treatment options to him and his parents who were extremely concerned.

Even extensive disease is curable with cisplatin-based chemotherapy. Accordingly, this was the treatment course chosen following further discussion with Dan.

Note. Creatinine clearance measures the rate at which the kidneys are able to clear creatinine (a byproduct of metabolism) from the blood. It is calculated from the serum creatinine using an equation

that includes age, gender, and lean body weight to establish baseline measurements for subsequent assessment of any nephrotoxicity (damage to kidney tissue or function) induced by platinum compounds.

Activities

- Consider how you would react if you discovered a lump in a testis or a breast. Would you seek medical advice quickly, assume it to be completely innocent and forget it, or would you think it could be cancer but wait and hope the lump goes away?
- Discuss the role of the specialist nurse in supporting patients during the staging phase of a cancer with your mentor.

Box 31.5 Information

Informing patients of their diagnosis: ethical considerations

Two ethical principles are central to the discussion of whether it is always right to tell a patient the whole truth about their diagnosis: these are the principles of autonomy and of beneficence (see further reading, e.g. Thompson et al 2006).

Autonomy

Patients have a right to autonomy, or self-determination. They cannot make decisions about their treatment or the future if they are not fully aware of their diagnosis. However, research has suggested that denial as a coping mechanism is sometimes necessary for the preservation of well-being during a crisis, allowing an individual time to mobilise the resources to cope with the seriousness of their disease (Moyer & Levine 1998). Unlike years ago, patients are now normally told their diagnosis, with a discussion of prognosis – often a medical uncertainty – and the level of information is tailored to the individual's needs. There is no evidence to suggest that acceptance correlates positively to survival in cancer (Spiegel 2001).

Beneficence

The principle of beneficence obligates health care professionals to prevent harm and 'do good' for their patients. It may seem obvious that to tell lies or withhold the truth is wrong. Patients may suffer severe psychological problems if they continue to feel unwell despite the optimistic messages they receive from others, and may even blame themselves for their symptoms. They may also lose trust if and when they discover the 'conspiracy'.

Discussion

The matter is seldom as simple as the choice between lying and truth-telling, and each case must be considered individually. Relatives may ask that their family member be protected from the *whole* truth. However, respect for the patient's autonomy should, whenever possible, override such a request, but the relatives and patient need to be supported when such information is given, and their issues and concerns addressed.

Tension can arise within the health care team when medical staff fail in their responsibility to disclose appropriate information to those patients who clearly wish to know more. Other staff – nurses in particular – who spend more time with patients become frustrated in their attempts to meet the psychological needs of individuals who lack awareness of the reality of their situation. There must be an open staff forum for the discussion of such problems.

In most cancer centres, the issue is not whether, but how and when, to inform patients of diagnosis and prognosis. A study by Schofield et al (2003) showed that clinical practices that are linked to lessening anxiety include preparing the patient for a possible cancer diagnosis, having significant others present at diagnosis, being given as much information as desired in understandable language, having questions answered, talking about feelings and being given reassurance. It would seem appropriate that a nurse is present at such discussions because they can follow up the conversation and help the patient to strike a balance between realistic hope and the acceptance of reality.

Box 31.6 Reflection

Supporting patients and families at diagnosis

Listen to some patients talking about their diagnosis at Health talk online (2008) lung cancer stories – http://www.healthtalkonline.org/Cancer/Lung_Cancer

Activities

- Write a few notes about how you felt listening to the patients talking about their diagnosis.
- How can you as a nurse support this period for patients and their families?

performed and what it will entail for the patient. Findings from research suggest that a substantial proportion of the lay public do not understand phrases used in cancer consultations. One study found that only 52% understood that the phrase 'the tumour is progressing' was not good news and less than a third understood what was meant by 'seedlings' (Chapman et al 2003). The nurse, acting as patient advocate, should ensure they are present when doctors explains test results so they are able to offer additional support and revisit this information again with the patient if necessary. The patient may have fears they wish to express and an opportunity to discuss these openly is important. The nurse is well placed do this.

Aims of treatment

Cancer treatments can be broadly described as:

- curative – given with the intention of eradicating the disease
- palliative – given with the intention of controlling the disease and distressing symptoms.

Adjuvant treatments, such as a drug, that assist or increase the action of other drugs or therapies are often used in cancer treatment, for example cytotoxic drugs used after removal of the tumour by radiotherapy or surgery. The aim is to enhance the chance of cure and prevent recurrence.

Treatments, such as radiotherapy, used to reduce tumour size before other treatment (e.g. surgery) are termed *neoadjuvant*. The aim is to improve the outcome of surgery and to reduce the risk of metastatic spread.

The transition from cure to palliative therapy may occur gradually over time but should always be discussed openly with the patient. Treatments for cancer vary considerably and can include surgery, radiotherapy, chemotherapy and hormonal agents or all of these treatments.

Response to treatment

Response to treatment can be described as:

- complete – the tumour has disappeared

- partial – the tumour has decreased by at least 50%
- minimal or stable – there is very little change in tumour volume
- progressive – 25% increase in tumour volume.

Unfortunately, cancer treatments can have side-effects which may seriously reduce quality of life. Figure 31.3 outlines the side-effects of both chemotherapy and radiotherapy, and further coverage is provided in the appropriate sections below. Thus, the decision to treat a patient must be carefully balanced between the costs and benefits of treatment for the patient and should ideally be taken jointly by the health care team and the patient.

Treatment modalities

The principal forms of cancer treatment are:

- surgery
- radiotherapy
- chemotherapy – both cytotoxic chemotherapy and biological response modifiers (BRMs).

Surgery

Surgery remains the most successful method of achieving long-term cure for patients with various types of localised tumour. Surgical removal of tumours of the skin (non-

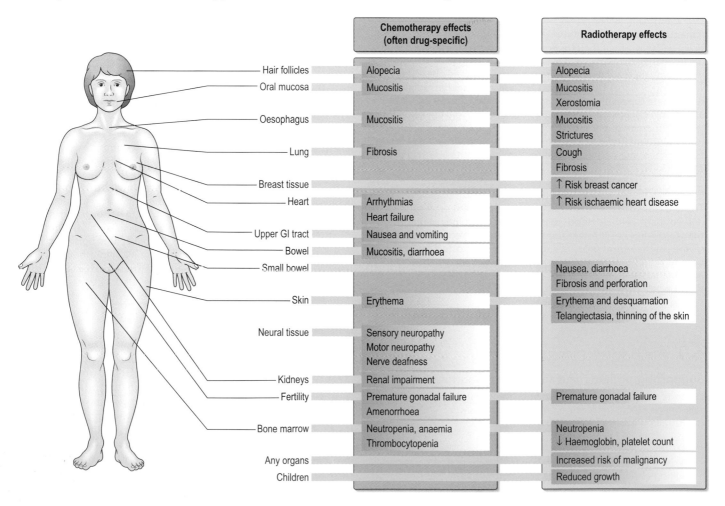

Figure 31.3 Side-effects of chemotherapy and radiotherapy – acute (in pink) and late (in blue). (Reproduced from Boon et al 2006 with permission.)

melanoma), thyroid gland, uterus, colon and rectum (early stage) are associated with an excellent chance of cure. Tumours which have disseminated at presentation are inoperable.

Surgery can also be used as an adjuvant treatment, e.g. in the resection of diseased bone after radical chemotherapy for osteosarcoma, or as palliative surgery, e.g. a stent insertion or bypass of the common bile duct can be performed to relieve jaundice in cancer of the head of the pancreas, leading to an improved quality of life.

Psychological support

Surgical techniques, pre- and postoperative nursing care, and the psychological problems associated with undergoing surgery are discussed in Chapter 26. Important issues for nurses to consider around surgery are the possibility of the patient receiving the diagnosis during the perioperative period, alterations to body image and slower recovery time if treated with chemotherapy or radiotherapy prior to surgery. Box 31.7 provides an opportunity for you to reflect upon a patient's experiences having breast surgery.

Radiotherapy

Radiotherapy is the use of ionising radiation to destroy cancer cell populations. Approximately 70% of all patients with cancer receive radiotherapy. Note that radioactive substances may also be used for some non-malignant conditions, such as hyperthyroidism (see Ch. 5, Part 1).

Radiation physics and biology are complex topics which are subject to intense research and development. (See Further reading, e.g. Faithful & Wells 2003.)

There are two kinds of radiation:

- particle radiation, e.g. alpha particles, beta particles, electrons, protons, neutrons which have a mass, limiting their depth of penetration
- ionising electromagnetic radiation, e.g. gamma (γ) rays and X-rays – these are similar to light, radio or microwaves, but have a very much higher energy level and are deeply penetrating.

Alpha particles are of low energy; they can be absorbed by a sheet of paper and are too weak to kill cancer cells. Electrons are of higher energy and can penetrate anything up to the density of wood. In radiotherapy, electrons are used to treat superficial areas located a few centimetres beneath the skin, e.g. a 'booster' treatment to the site where the tumour was in breast cancer is known to prevent local recurrence. Gamma rays are short, very powerful waves that require lead or concrete to absorb them. They are emitted from the nuclei of radioactive elements, e.g. caesium and cobalt, and are able to penetrate deeply into the body tissues.

The most common form of radiotherapy now is the X-ray. These rays are artificially generated when a stream of electrons bombard tungsten metal targets, releasing energy in the form of X-rays.

Radioactivity

Understanding ionising radiation requires a basic understanding of subatomic, atomic and molecular structure. All matter is made up of atoms, which consist of a central nucleus containing positively charged protons and uncharged neutrons, orbited by negatively charged electrons, equivalent in number to the protons. The negatively charged electrons (−) orbit the

---

Box 31.7 Reflection

A patient's view of care prior to and following breast cancer surgery

These extracts are taken from a paper written by Niven & Scott (2003) in which they consider the appropriate use of nurse resource and the importance of 'hearing the patient's voice'. What makes this account so powerful is that the patient is a nurse and co-author of the paper.

'Being "prepped" consisted of having my breast, axilla and back painted. The sensation was pleasant; the last pleasant sensation there would be for a breast that had, in its time, been appreciated by baby and lover alike. There was no avoiding the issue, this was what I was going to lose. The nurse and I didn't talk. She didn't fill the moment with idle chit chat or pseudo empathy, which I would have found offensive and would have demanded social responses from me that I would have struggled to make. The nurse treated the task and thus me and my soon to be no more breast, with respect. While sharing none of the horrors of pubic shaving, this pre-operative preparation was an activity that called for high calibre nursing skills. I was very grateful for the way it was managed; it preserved my dignity, did not exacerbate an intrinsically distressing situation and gave me a sense of, literally "being in good hands".

On return from theatre it was trained staff who washed me, made me comfortable, gave me iced water to drink while checking heart rate, blood pressure, oxygen saturation, drain and wound. The

sense of being completely cared for when I was in that post anaesthesia dependency state was wonderfully comforting and reassuring. For a short while I was completely in their hands and their competence was very obvious. Each task done well reinforced the sense of that competence. So it was as important that the water from the face cloth didn't run down my front as that the drain wasn't pulled or the wound exposed, forcing me to look at it rather than letting me choose my moment. These demonstrations of hands on competence created a climate of confidence in the nurses' expertise.' (Niven & Scott 2003, pp 202–203)

Activities

- Consider the extract above, especially the patient's response to the supportive and competent care provided by the trained staff.
- Access and read the full paper.
- Reflect on the patient's account of her first postoperative shower (Niven & Scott 2003, p. 203). A seemingly 'basic' activity delegated to a nursing assistant, which the patient regarded as a key nursing activity.
- Discuss with your mentor the patient's observations on the lost opportunities for a trained nurse to monitor the wound and assess the patient's psychological state such as her readiness to look at the wound, etc.

nucleus, being held in place by the attractive force of the positively charged protons (+); hence a stable state is maintained.

However, as the number of protons increases, an excess number of neutrons are required in order to hold the nucleus together. This imbalance causes the spontaneous disintegration of the nucleus with an associated emission of charged particles and radiation energy.

Some elements exist in a variety of states, depending on the number of neutrons in the nucleus. These are termed the isotopes of an element. Two isotopes of iodine (I), for example, are ^{127}I and ^{131}I. The latter is a radioisotope (also known as radionuclide), i.e. it is unstable, because the nuclei of its atoms have a disproportionate number of neutrons. Radioisotopes may be naturally occurring, such as radium-226 (^{226}Ra), which is now seldom used in radiotherapy, or artificially manufactured by bombarding elements with neutrons in a nuclear reactor, e.g. cobalt-60 (^{60}Co).

The effects of radiation

Radiation kills cancer cells by:

- a direct hit – when the radiation damages DNA directly; or
- an indirect hit – when the radiation produces free radicals in water adjacent to the DNA, which then damage the DNA.

Radiosensitivity of a given tumour is closely related to cell proliferation activity. As malignant cells are constantly dividing, they are all radiosensitive, although to varying degrees. Unfortunately, rapidly dividing healthy cells, such as those of the skin, the epithelium of the gastrointestinal and urinary tracts, the gonads and the bone marrow, are also vulnerable to radiation damage; this accounts for the unwanted side-effects of radiotherapy (see pp. 803–807). Figure 31.4 illustrates the

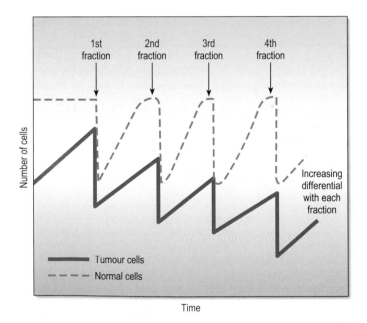

Figure 31.4 The difference between normal and tumour cell kill and recovery in radiotherapy. Normal cells have the capacity to recover to their previous population level more rapidly than malignant cells. Therefore, successive treatments given after normal cell population recovery but before malignant cell population recovery will result in minimal damage to normal tissue but successive reductions in tumour size.

difference between the radiation responses of tumour cells and normal cells.

In theory, all tumour cells could be eradicated by radiotherapy. However, the often narrow difference between the dose required to produce lethal damage to the tumour and that which causes irreversible damage to normal tissue (therapeutic ratio), makes it difficult to achieve optimal dosing without causing unacceptable side-effects.

Radiotherapy is prescribed as an 'absorbed dose'. The unit used is the gray (Gy), where 1 Gy = 1 joule as absorbed by 1 kg of body tissue. The dose prescribed will vary, depending on several factors such as the volume and site of the area to be treated, sensitivity of the surrounding normal tissue, radiosensitivity of the particular tumour and also treatment intent, i.e. curative or palliative.

Sources of radiation

Radiotherapy is given in a variety of ways, according to tumour type and stage and, occasionally, the patient's condition. Teletherapy (from the Greek téle – 'far'), sometimes called 'external beam therapy', is the most common method of treatment. Brachytherapy (from the Greek brachys – 'short') is administered via radioactive sources placed within a body cavity or tumour bed.

Teletherapy External beam radiotherapy is administered by machines which are categorised according to the level of energy of radiation produced and depth of penetration (kilovoltage, orthovoltage, megavoltage, cobalt machine). The linear accelerator or 'linac' is the predominant teletherapy equipment in use throughout the world. Machines delivering lower voltages are still used to treat superficial lesions, such as skin cancers. The total prescribed radiation dose, if administered in one session, may be far too toxic to normal tissue and possibly even fatal to the patient. Hence treatment is often administered in daily 'fractions' of the total dose, so as to take advantage of the four 'Rs' of radiobiology – repair, reproduction, redistribution and reoxygenation. Repair of sublethal cell injury generally occurs within 24 h, but possibly in as little as 30–90 min. Normal cells can therefore repair between daily doses of radiation. Tumour cells may do so initially but become less capable as treatment is protracted.

Two strategies have been developed involving multiple fractions per day: hyperfractionation and continuous hyperfractionation accelerated radiotherapy (CHART). Hyperfractionation is the use of several smaller than standard doses given two to three times daily. The accumulative daily and total doses are usually greater than for conventional treatment. Accelerated hyperfractionation refers to an overall shortened treatment time, achieved by increasing the number of fractions per day and treating continuously including weekends. In both approaches, 6 h between doses must be allowed for repair of sublethal damage from the first dose before the second is given. CHART has significantly better tumour control but implementation requires considerable changes in working practice (Adamson 2003).

The patient's initial visit to the department involves a planning session (simulation) which, if complex, may necessitate more than one visit. Extreme accuracy in devising the unique plan for each patient is vital, the aim being adequate dosage to the tumour and minimum exposure of healthy tissues and organs. Localisation of the tumour is made using an X-ray simulator, which mimics the treatment machine, and information from CT or magnetic resonance imaging (MRI) scans. This information is then used by the planning computer staff to determine a beam configuration that conforms precisely to the target organ or site. Patient immobilisation is important, particularly for patients with head and neck tumours. A close-fitting individualised Perspex shell is made in the mould room, which is worn throughout treatment. Some individuals may find this claustrophobic.

In most centres, the treatment field, or reference points, are marked out on the patient's skin using small permanent tattoos.

Brachytherapy This form of treatment is less common than teletherapy. It is the temporary or permanent placement of a radioactive source (radioisotope), either in close proximity to or within a tumour. It offers the advantage of delivering a continuous dose of radiation to a specific tumour volume. The most common methods used include interstitial implants, intracavitary treatment and systemic therapy. In an interstitial implant, the radioactive source is contained in the form of a needle, seed, wire or catheter that is implanted directly into the tumour (e.g. iridium – breast, prostate, head and neck cancer). In intracavitary treatment, the radioactive source is placed directly into the body cavity by remote control and held in place by a prepositioned applicator (e.g. caesium – cervical, endometrial, vaginal and lung cancer). In systemic therapy an unsealed radioactive source is given orally or intravenously (e.g. iodine – hyperthyroidism).

Stereotactic radiotherapy has been developed to deliver a precise dose of radiotherapy to a small area (millimetres). It is a complex and highly specialised treatment, initially used for the treatment of benign brain tumours of poor surgical risk.

Radiotherapy treatment intent

This may be:

* curative
* adjuvant
* palliative.

The goal of radiotherapy in early-stage cancer is curative. Certain tumours such as skin cancer, Hodgkin's lymphoma, cervical cancer, cancer of the larynx and seminoma (germ cell tumour, testicular in origin) are particularly radiosensitive. Treatment can take up to 30 days and is associated with side-effects but prognosis is very good long-term.

Adjuvant radiotherapy Radiotherapy is commonly used as an adjuvant treatment which forms part of the treatment plan. It is given either pre- or postoperatively, and increasingly alongside chemotherapy especially for cancer of the breast, prostate, colon and rectal cancer. Chemotherapeutic agents such as cisplatin, 5-fluorouracil (5-FU), doxorubicin or mitomycin C are given alongside radiotherapy in cancers of the cervix, anus, head, neck and lung to achieve a greater cell kill.

Palliative radiotherapy Cancers at a more advanced stage where cure or eradication is not possible constitute 50% of all radiotherapy treatments given (Blyth et al 2001). It involves a shorter course of treatment at much lower doses than either radical or adjuvant therapy. Its aim is to maximise symptom relief and quality of life and minimise side-effects. Examples include haemoptysis in lung cancer or rectal bleeding in rectal cancer and spinal cord compression (SCC) which presents as an emergency whereby the use of radiotherapy may alleviate symptoms and further distress for the patient.

Large field radiotherapy

Radiotherapy is given to much larger areas of the body for conditions such as leukaemia. Total body irradiation (TBI) is used to eradicate all tumour cells from chemotherapy-resistant tissues. This treatment must be followed by a haemopoietic stem cell transplantation (HSCT; bone marrow transplant [BMT]) to restore bone marrow function (see Ch. 11). Hemibody (half body) radiation provides effective palliation for patients with extensive bone metastases, as are common, for example, in prostatic cancer.

The decision making and planning surrounding any course of radiotherapy involve a team approach. Informed consent is essential as is patient and carer education. Incorporation of the principles of physics, radiobiology, dosimetry, treatment technique, anatomy, physiology, psychosocial and patient/family care requires a multidisciplinary approach.

Radiation protection

There is much fear and misconception amongst both professionals and lay people about the dangers of radiation exposure. Indeed, radiation is potentially extremely hazardous, and exposure to high doses can cause several side-effects, together with cell mutations that may lead to carcinogenesis, or to congenital abnormalities if pregnant women are exposed.

Every institution dealing with radiation is legally obliged to appoint a radiation protection officer, to follow stringent guidelines for radiation monitoring and to provide education for staff and patient protection. If these are adhered to, radiation damage risk is negligible. Staff most at risk are those working constantly with unsealed sources. Staff working in areas of potential radiation exposure should wear personal dosimeters or film badges to monitor their individual exposure (see Further reading, e.g. Royal College of Nursing 2006).

Side-effects of radiotherapy (see Figure 31.3, p. 800)

Side-effects occur when normal tissue is irradiated. Manifestation of side-effects varies greatly from patient to patient, depending on the location and amount of tissue being irradiated, the dose and its fractionation, and the patient's physical and psychological state. Treatment techniques are constantly being developed to improve accuracy of delivery and minimise side-effects. Patients may suffer from systemic side-effects such as fatigue, lethargy, nausea, anorexia and headaches but in general, radiotherapy affects only those tissues being irradiated. For example, a patient receiving treatment for bladder carcinoma will experience localised bladder irritation while radiotherapy to the brain will cause loss of hair on the head.

Side-effects may be 'early' (acute), occurring within days of commencing treatment, continuing for a period of weeks following treatment completion. Long-term or 'late' side-effects usually present 18 months to 2 years after treatment. Acute problems manifest in areas of rapid cell growth and division and are usually reversible. The nursing management of the most common side-effects forms a major part of the nursing role in the radiotherapy department (Table 31.3).

Table 31.3 Nursing management of the side-effects of radiotherapy

IRRADIATED BODY PART/ORGAN	RADIATION EFFECT	NURSE INTERVENTION	RATIONALE
General	Fatigue	Forewarn patients of fatigue during and after radiotherapy. Provide appropriate information about pattern of symptoms	To foster independence, encouraging energy-saving activities To prevent feelings of social isolation, low mood and to decrease anxiety
		Assess and promote self-care strategies. Refer to appropriate healthcare professional as necessary	
		Assess baseline fatigue levels prior to treatment starting	To monitor changes over time and need for further intervention
		Check for physical, biochemical and psychological causes of fatigue	Electrolyte imbalances/anaemia may be corrected. Appropriate psychological support can be given
		Encourage patients to maintain a daily record of fatigue levels and the relationship to activities	Enhances the ability to control activities or plan ahead, goal setting and prioritising
Skin (See Further reading NHS Quality Improvement Scotland 2004) Particularly areas where the skin is thin, moist, e.g. skin folds, axilla, groin, breast and perineum. Light skin is especially sensitive	Three-stage reaction: 1. Erythema: redness, heat, itchiness	No metal-containing skin preparations	Metal may intensify radiation reactions
		Gentle washing with warm water and gentle drying, no rubbing	Friction causes irritation. Ink marks must not be washed off
		Application of simple moisturiser	Soothing and minimises friction, keeps skin supple
		If itchy, an antihistamine cream may be prescribed. Apply 1% hydrocortisone	To alleviate discomfort and itch
		Avoid exposure to the sun and extremes of heat and cold	UV light may intensify any reaction
		Encourage non-constrictive clothing in lightweight, natural fabrics: no tight or elastic clothing	Reduces sweating and friction
	2. Dry desquamation: dryness, scaliness, tight feeling, pain on movement	1% hydrocortisone or lanolin cream (centres vary in their recommendations)	Soothing emollient and/or anti-inflammatory
		Expose skin to fresh air or cool fan	Cooling has a short-term analgesic effect
		For moderate to severe reaction, or if skin folds involved, consider application of a non-adhesive tape, ensuring it is removed with baby oil	Preventive measure and promotes wound healing as is permeable. Removing with oil ensures the skin is not damaged
	3. Moist desquamation: blisters, loss of surface epithelium, pain, susceptibility to infection Occasionally progresses to necrosis	A break in treatment may be required Analgesics	To prevent further skin breakdown and discomfort
		Observation for signs of infection	Infection exacerbates skin damage and may become systemic
		Use of hydrogel/hydrocolloid/alginate dressings	To promote wound healing
		Dressing plan: assessment, dressings, evaluation using wound care principles	To record any changes, evaluating the effectiveness of the intervention applied
Scalp	Alopecia (in treatment field only) Loss of any body hair occurs from weeks 2–3	Reassure the patient that hair will usually grow back in 2–3 months, although it may be of a different texture and colour	Hair loss poses a very stressful threat to body image, especially for women
		Organise provision of a wig Wearing of scarf/turban at night	Prevents distress of hair on pillow
Brain	Cerebral oedema (within week 1 of treatment) (see Ch. 9)	Administer prescribed corticosteroids	Anti-inflammatory
		Observe and report alterations in mental status	Enables prompt medical intervention
		Ensure patient safety	

Continued

Table 31.3 Nursing management of the side-effects of radiotherapy – cont'd

IRRADIATED BODY PART/ORGAN	RADIATION EFFECT	NURSE INTERVENTION	RATIONALE
Mouth (see Useful websites, e.g. Multinational association of supportive care in cancer)	1. Mucositis due to damaged, sloughed oral mucosa	Comprehensive dental review prior to treatment	To identify potential infection risks and carry out any necessary dental work, giving time for wound healing
	Opportunistic infection may ensue, e.g. candidiasis ('thrush')	Regular use of an oral assessment tool	To monitor any changes, evaluating interventions
		Teaching and encouraging frequent routine systematic oral hygiene, initiated prior to treatment if possible	To reduce the amount and severity of mucositis and encourage compliance. Also to minimise the risk of infection
		Use of a soft toothbrush, fluoride toothpaste and regular 0.9% sodium chloride mouthwashes	To minimise damage to the oral mucosa and prevent build-up of plaque
		Use of antibacterial/antifungal preparations, e.g. chlorhexidine, nystatin	To prevent or treat infection
		Regular analgesics: topical, e.g. benzydamine, and systemic including opiates	Oral pain is excruciating and always to the forefront of consciousness
		Use of cellulose film-forming agents to line the mucosa	Forms a thin protective film which relieves pain and discomfort
		Observe for signs of dehydration and inadequate nutrition, liaising with the dietitian (see Useful websites, e.g. National Cancer Institute)	Prompt parenteral hydration and dietary supplements or enteral feeding may be commenced
	2. Xerostomia (dry mouth) due to altered salivary gland function. May be permanent. Causes difficulty in chewing, swallowing and talking	Frequent mouth rinses with 0.9% sodium chloride and sodium bicarbonate	Comforting, aids swallowing, buffering of oral environment
		Frequent sips of water	
		Use of artificial saliva	Lubrication of mucosa
		Moist soft diet	
		Avoidance of spices, alcohol, smoking, extremes of temperature	Easier to tolerate. These are mucosal irritants
	3. Taste changes due to xerostomia and damaged tastebuds	Assist patients to experiment with other foods	To maintain nutritional intake
	4. Dental decay due to xerostomia and radiation gingivitis	Pre-treatment dental referral	Any caries will be exacerbated by radiation and form foci for infection
		Avoidance of high sugar content foods and fluids	Sugar alters natural slightly alkaline pH of oral environment and demineralises teeth
Neck area	1. Pharyngitis, laryngitis, causing pain, hoarseness, loss of voice, dry cough and occasionally respiratory stridor	Discourage smoking	Mucosal irritant
		Encourage patient to rest voice	
		Observe respiratory status and colour	Medical intervention: corticosteroids or even a tracheostomy may be necessary
		A cough suppressant	Prevents mucosal irritation caused by coughing
		Topical analgesics prior to food, e.g. aspirin gargles, anaesthetic throat spray; systemic analgesics	Promotes comfort and aids swallowing
	2. Oesophagitis (upper one third) causing dysphagia	Maintain nutrition. Soft diet, referring to the dietitian for supplements	These patients are often already malnourished
		Avoid irritant foods, strong alcohol and smoking	
Thorax	1. Oesophagitis (lower two-thirds) causing 'heartburn'	As above; also administer antacids prior to food. Some antacids also contain topical anaesthetics	Lines oesophagus and prevents pain and trauma of swallowing and from gastric acid reflux

Continued

Table 31.3 Nursing management of the side-effects of radiotherapy – cont'd

IRRADIATED BODY PART/ORGAN	RADIATION EFFECT	NURSE INTERVENTION	RATIONALE
	2. Pneumonitis due to inflammation. May cause dyspnoea, productive cough and haemoptysis	Discourage smoking Observe for signs of infection: pyrexia, cough, purulent sputum Oxygen as prescribed Assessment and management of breathlessness	Irritant Enables prompt commencement of antibiotics Patient comfort and integrated approach to managing this distressing symptom
	3. Dyspepsia, nausea and vomiting (less severe than with abdominal radiation)	(see below)	
Abdomen and pelvis	1. Nausea and vomiting due to inflammation of gastrointestinal epithelium; also a generalised radiation reaction	Encourage a small meal 3 h before treatment and light snacks after Regular and appropriate antiemetics Distraction/relaxation techniques Monitor fluid and food intake	Some patients are unable to eat after treatment due to nausea Regular administration required to prevent and relieve nausea There may be a contributing psychological factor in nausea To avoid fluid balance problems and malnutrition
	2. Diarrhoea, possibly accompanied by rectal bleeding	Maximise privacy Administer antimotility medication as prescribed Low-residue, bland diet, low fat Observe for dehydration (see Ch. 20) Maintain high fluid intake Observe perianal skin: gently apply barrier cream after washing if necessary	 Better tolerated by damaged mucosa Avoid dehydration To prevent skin excoriation
	3. Cystitis due to inflammation of bladder epithelium. Predisposition to urinary tract infection (UTI)	Encourage high fluid intake (3 L daily) Encourage and/or assist with personal hygiene Regular collection of urine specimens for microbiology	Prevents stasis of urine and sloughed epithelium Helps prevent ascending urinary tract infection Enables prompt antibiotic treatment of UTI
	4. Altered sexual function (depends on treatment site and dosage)	Psychological support and counselling Include partner in discussion if patient wishes Assess the need for psychosexual counselling	Loss of any degree of sexual function is very threatening to most people's self-image; opportunity to talk this through is vital To gain understanding and support and minimise body image problems To maintain a healthy relationship and sexuality
	Men: Erectile dysfunction (usually temporary)	Psychological support	To explore possible options to help with erectile difficulties
	Sterility (usually permanent) Decreased libido	Offer sperm banking if appropriate Monitor hormone levels Testosterone replacement therapy Patient/couple education and psychological support	To enable sperm to be used for artificial insemination To improve libido and promote healthy sexuality
	Women: Sterility (if ovaries are irradiated). May be temporary or permanent	Advise continued contraception during and for several months after treatment. Hormonal contraception is contraindicated with some cancers, e.g. breast	Fertility is not always immediately affected and any pregnancy may not be viable
	Dyspareunia due to vaginal fibrosis and dryness	Advise use of vaginal lubricant	To promote comfort and ease of penetration

Continued

Table 31.3 Nursing management of the side-effects of radiotherapy – cont'd

IRRADIATED BODY PART/ORGAN	RADIATION EFFECT	NURSE INTERVENTION	RATIONALE
		Use of barrier contraceptives, e.g. condom during intercourse	There may be a burning sensation associated with semen and this will help to decrease irritation.
		Education and use of vaginal dilators during (if tolerated) and for up to 2 years after treatment	To prevent vaginal stenosis and post-coital bleeding
	Loss of libido	Patient/couple education and psychological support, sensitively explaining that this is usually temporary	To maintain healthy sexual relationships
	Premature menopause (if ovaries irradiated)	Inform of possibility and potential menopausal symptoms	To help women manage menopausal symptoms
		Discuss possible strategies in managing the hot flushes, preventing osteoporosis, etc.	
		Hormone replacement therapy should be discussed if appropriate	

Skincare is particularly important during and after a course of radiotherapy (see Further reading, e.g. NHS Quality Improvement Scotland 2004).

Late side-effects occur as, due to DNA damage, slowly dividing cells fail to replicate. Problems are most often a consequence of damaged vasculature and are usually permanent. Examples include fibrosis of the lung, chronic bowel inflammation, and lymphoedema. Monitoring of late side-effects is undertaken during follow-up outpatient clinics.

Psychological and supportive care

Radiotherapy patients are often perceived as the self-caring 'walking wounded'. Their problems and needs are often hidden as treatment is mostly on an outpatient basis with the added stress of daily travel to and from the department. It is important to remember that radiotherapy treatment is not always an isolated event but usually precedes or follows other forms of cancer treatment. Although it brings its own problems and side-effects, its impact needs to be considered in the context of the patient's overall experience. That experience may be affected by existing psychosocial, physical and functional needs related to other existing disease or to financial or social constraints.

Myths and fears

Few therapeutic modalities in medicine induce more misunderstanding, confusion and misapprehension than radiotherapy. For many patients, the news that they are to receive radiotherapy comes soon after knowledge of their cancer diagnosis when they are already coping with multiple stressors and feelings of loss. Myths and fears compound these stresses. Hammick et al (1998) examined patients'

knowledge and perceptions of radiotherapy and radiation. Outside of medical usage, radiation was commonly perceived in terms of nuclear weapons. Media coverage often highlighted problems in terms of overdosages, burns and permanent damage. From observations in clinical practice it is apparent that media reports do influence patients' anxiety levels regarding treatment. This became evident at the time of publicity surrounding patients belonging to RAGE (Radiation Action Group Exposure), where women had developed long-term toxicity as a result of radiotherapy to the brachial plexus following treatment for breast cancer. To manage fears and increase the provision of information, most radiotherapy units have nurse-led or radiographer-led clinics to assess patients on a daily basis (see also Box 31.8).

 Box 31.8 Reflection

Starting treatment at the radiotherapy unit

Look at the Radiotherapy Treatment for Breast Cancer virtual tour on the website http://www.scan.scot.nhs.uk

This will allow you to see what radiotherapy machines look like.

Activities

- Find out where your nearest radiotherapy unit is and whether there is a virtual tour for staff and patients to view.
- Consider the benefits of this form of visual information for patients and their families.
- Reflect on how a patient might feel arriving at the department for their first treatment. Compare your impressions with those of another student.

Nursing management and health promotion: radiotherapy

Nurses can do much to alleviate the patient's fears and anxieties, helping to make the experience of radiotherapy more tolerable. Supportive care relies on the understanding of the impact of cancer and its treatment viewed from the perspective of the patient. A thorough needs assessment is fundamental to enable effective interventions to support the patient and their family throughout treatment. A study by Bonevski et al (2000) used a questionnaire to allow patients to identify needs they may have experienced in the last month as a result of having cancer. It considered needs associated with psychological, health system and information, physical and daily living, patient care and support, sexuality, and financial issues. The authors found real benefits for both patients and clinicians in using this tool to assess the magnitude of needs which occur in clinical oncology settings. Supportive care may also involve simple behavioural strategies such as simply being there: actively listening, talking, preserving the patient's individuality and providing information.

Information is seen as crucial for successful interactions between patients and health care professionals, relieving anxiety and promoting a sense of control (Association of the British Pharmaceutical Industry [ABPI] 2005, Van der Molen 1999). Nurses are responsible, therefore, for becoming accurately informed themselves – about radiotherapy in general, and about each patient's individual treatment plan and likely side-effects in particular.

Good practice advocates that written information should be accompanied by verbal explanation wherever possible. There are now a comprehensive range of patient information materials from a wide range of support agencies such as Macmillan Cancer Support and Tenovus (see Useful websites), alongside telephone information helplines. Managed clinical networks are also involved in the development of local information, ensuring patients receive accurate information at the appropriate time across all care settings. The internet has many sites providing high-quality information but caution must be taken that they are trusted sites otherwise they can cause more harm than good.

Studies have also shown that the vast majority of patients want as much information as possible to enable them to prepare for treatment, decrease their fears and anxieties, and increase their understanding of treatment. Information requested includes:

- how treatment works
- the effectiveness of treatment
- likely side-effects
- preventive and self-care strategies
- impact of treatment on their lives and their families (Skalla et al 2004).

Nurses have an increasingly important role in radiotherapy care, with both nurses and therapy radiographers developing advanced practitioner roles through which innovative approaches to care are more and more evident. The central components of these roles include assessment, education, knowledge, prevention of side-effects, psychosocial support, liaison with other health care professionals and rehabilitation. Employment of both nurse specialists and therapy radiographers to provide information and

counselling services, practitioner-led review and follow-up clinics, telephone follow-up and nursing interventions for side-effects can make a positive contribution to patient care (Koinberg et al 2004). (See Further reading, e.g. Faithful & Wells 2003.)

Systemic treatment: chemotherapy

Chemotherapy literally means 'treatment with chemicals' and therefore can refer to any form of medication therapy, but especially drugs used to treat cancer and antimicrobial drugs. However, in common usage the term refers to cytotoxic drugs. Cytotoxic (toxic to cells) chemotherapy involves the use of medication to disrupt the cell cycle and thus ultimately kill malignant cells.

Cytotoxic drugs, like radiation, are toxic to both healthy and malignant dividing cells and interfere with cell reproduction (see Figure 31.3, p. 800). There are many different cytotoxic agents, each with a different mode of action and function at different phases in the cell cycle (see Useful websites, e.g. British National Formulary, and Further reading, e.g. Brighton & Wood 2006, Tortora & Derrickson 2009).

Cytotoxic drugs are usually classified according to their chemical structure, cell cycle activity and primary mode of action. The classic categories include:

- alkylating agents
- antimetabolites
- antitumour antibiotics
- vinca alkaloids (plant alkaloids)
- taxanes
- miscellaneous compounds.

The action of some of these is described in Box 31.9. (See Further reading, e.g. Brighton & Wood 2006.)

Modes of cytotoxic chemotherapy treatment

Cytotoxic chemotherapy differs from radiotherapy in that it is a systemic rather than a localised treatment modality. It is useful for treating any cancer which has a risk of metastasising. Despite reports of newer drugs, many of the drugs used in current practice date back to the 40s, 50s and 60s. Complete responses are seen in up to 20% of adults with Hodgkin's lymphoma, and 70% of childhood leukaemias. Chemotherapy is used mainly as an adjuvant treatment in solid tumours to prevent future recurrence.

Adjuvant and palliative chemotherapy For the most part, chemotherapy is used:

- as the sole, or most important, treatment
- as a means of reducing the size of the tumour to aid the success of subsequent surgery or radiotherapy, i.e. 'debulking' of tumours, such as those of the head, neck and bladder
- following radiotherapy or surgery to eradicate remaining tumour cells or any micrometastases; this is common in breast, colorectal and ovarian cancer
- to treat a recurrence
- for palliation of symptoms – some tumours are partially chemoresponsive, so that treatment may relieve symptoms and improve the quality of, and possibly lengthen, life
- for investigation of the usefulness of a new medicine.

Classification of cytotoxic agents

Alkylating agents

Alkylating agents are highly reactive and are cell cycle phase non-specific (CCPNS). Their primary mode of action is to join together or cross-link the two strands of DNA, preventing them from separating and therefore replicating. Cyclophosphamide is an example of a cytotoxic which acts in this way. Another group of alkylating agents are platinum-based compounds, e.g. cisplatin and carboplatin, which cause interstrand and intrastrand linkages.

Antimetabolites

These are cell cycle phase specific (CCPS), exerting their effect in the S phase. They are structural analogues of normal intracellular metabolites essential for cell function and replication and so are used to disrupt cellular metabolism. Methotrexate, for example, inhibits the enzyme necessary for the conversion of folic acid to folinic acid. Folinic acid is necessary for the formation of purines and pyrimidines, components of DNA. Folinic acid rescue, in the form of folinic acid replacement, is necessary 12–24 h after the administration of methotrexate to prevent the death of too many healthy cells. Other antimetabolites include 5-fluorouracil (5-FU) and cytosine arabinoside.

Plant alkaloids

Many plants and plant extracts continue to be screened to identify new cytotoxic agents. To date these include the vinca alkaloids, taxanes and topoisomerase inhibitors. Mitotic inhibitors include vincristine, vindesine and vinblastine, which are CCPS acting in the mitosis phase. They bind to microtubule proteins, blocking spindle formation and preventing cell separation.

The taxanes (docetaxel and paclitaxel), on the other hand, promote assembly of the microtubule which results in a very stable microtubule that is non-functional.

Topoisomerase inhibitors (etoposide, teniposide, irinotecan and topotecan) interfere with DNA replication by binding to DNA and the topoisomerase enzymes.

Antitumour antibiotics

Some classes of antibiotic have been found to be cytotoxic. In general, they are CCPNS and interfere with DNA function, although several other mechanisms of action may occur, such as alteration of the cell membrane or inhibition of certain enzymes. The most widely used is doxorubicin because it has a broad spectrum of activity; others include mitoxantrone and bleomycin.

Cytotoxic agents are constantly being researched and developed. There are several which do not fit into the above categories and whose action may not be fully understood.

Combination chemotherapy This is the use of a variety of agents. The purpose is to use a combination of drugs with different modes of action to reduce the risk of drug resistance. This interaction is more effective than using the drugs separately. It also allows drugs with different toxicities to be given at a maximum dose without causing unacceptable or irreversible toxicity.

Administration of chemotherapy

Chemotherapy is scheduled at regular intervals, sometimes called 'pulses' or 'cycles'. The purpose is to prevent the cancer cells recovering and repairing. The specific regimen or protocol of drugs to be used is then calculated based on the patient's body surface area (BSA). The goal is to provide a concentration of the drugs that is sufficient to achieve a therapeutic cytotoxic effect without causing too much toxicity to normal cells. Numerous routes are used in the administration including:

- oral
- subcutaneous
- intramuscular
- intravenous
- directly into blood vessels supplying the cavity containing the tumour or into the tumour itself; such routes include intrahepatic, intra-arterial, intrapleural, intraperitoneal and intrathecal.

Intravenous administration may be delivered as a 'bolus', a short infusion or as a continuous infusion. Continuous infusions may be delivered using a medication delivery pump via a vascular access device (VAD) such as a skin-tunnelled catheter (STC), a totally implanted port (TIP) or a peripherally inserted central catheter (PICC). (See Further reading, e.g. Dougherty 2006.)

Side-effects of chemotherapy

Chemotherapy causes an array of side-effects affecting a patient both physically and psychologically. It is nurses who deliver the majority of chemotherapy in outpatient departments and the community, thus there is a consensus that this requires special chemotherapy education requirements to fulfil this role (Royal College of Nursing [RCN] 1998) (Box 31.10).

Each cytotoxic agent causes different side-effects, varying in intensity with dosage and method of administration (see Useful websites e.g. British National Formulary, and Further reading, e.g. Brighton & Wood 2006) (Box 31.11). Nursing management of the potential side-effects requires an in-depth knowledge of the common and uncommon toxicity profiles of each agent given in the regimen.

Physical and emotional responses to chemotherapy vary greatly between patients and it is important that nurses consider both of these when assessing the patient (Mitchell 2007). A toxicity assessment tool is widely used in outpatient chemotherapy units to provide a consistent approach to care and encourage patients to participate in this care. The following is a brief summary of some of the potential physical side-effects of chemotherapy. (See Useful websites, e.g. British National Formulary, Multinational association of supportive care [2006], National Cancer Institute.)

Myelosuppression is the most common dose-limiting toxicity of chemotherapy but also potentially the most lethal. To understand the potential damage that chemotherapy may cause to the bone marrow, it is helpful to review normal blood cell development (see Further reading, Tortora & Derrikson 2009). The suppression of the production of blood constituents by the bone marrow occurs to varying degrees after almost all types of cytotoxic chemotherapy.

Box 31.10 Information

Safe administration of chemotherapy

Cytotoxic agents can be dangerous if they are not handled appropriately. A joint proposal to develop national guidelines for the administration of chemotherapy was initially funded by the NHS Executive (1995). From this, the Royal College of Nursing (1998) and the Scottish Cancer Care Pharmacy Group (2000) have issued guidelines for the safe use of cytotoxic chemotherapy in the clinical environment. These guidelines are to assist practitioners in defining and demonstrating high standards of practice, reducing unacceptable variations.

Extravasation

Some cytotoxic agents, e.g. doxorubicin and vincristine, are termed 'vesicants' and can cause severe burns and tissue damage if they leak from the vein into the subcutaneous tissue (Figure 31.5).

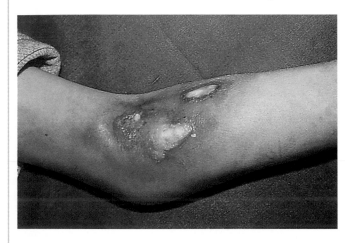

Figure 31.5 Extravasation. Skin necrosis due to extravasation of anthracycline chemotherapy (e.g. doxorubicin). (Reproduced from Boon et al 2006 with permission.)

If extravasation is suspected, the infusion should be stopped and an experienced clinician informed immediately. There are various antidotes available, but more scientific research is required (see Further reading, e.g. Brighton & Wood 2006, and Useful websites, e.g. National Extravasation Information Service [NEIS]).

Staff protection

There has been concern for many years regarding the potential exposure and subsequent effects in health care workers. The scientific evidence indicates that staff handling these medications do so with extreme caution. It is known that at therapeutic doses these substances can cause carcinogenesis, cell mutations and embryonic/fetal damage. Staff handling cytotoxic medicines should be educated about exposure risks, safe handling procedures and appropriate clothing, i.e. wearing aprons and latex gloves, as risk management strategies have been shown to minimise exposure (Ziegler et al 2002). More research is required to evaluate occupational surveillance. A register for those at risk should be kept and safe practice needs to be regularly audited. Chemotherapeutic agents should be prepared in a specially designed pharmacy unit (laminar air flow/isolator). Staff should always wear gloves when handling oral preparations and should mop up spillages immediately, using large amounts of water and wearing protective clothing. Spillage kits should be available in all the areas where chemotherapy is administered. On seeing the precautions necessary, patients may be alarmed that such dangerous substances are required to control their disease. They should be reassured that these measures are necessary to protect those who are constantly dealing with cytotoxic agents.

Handling body fluids

Many cytotoxic agents are excreted unchanged in urine and faeces, and both should be treated as hazardous for at least 48 h and up to 7 days. It is therefore important to wear gloves when handling the body fluids of patients receiving chemotherapy, and also to teach patients and their families to take appropriate precautions.

Box 31.11 Reflection

Anticipating the side-effects of chemotherapy

Listen to a patient who is receiving combination chemotherapy at Health talk online (2008) lung cancer stories http://www.healthtalkonline.org/Cancer/Lung_Cancer

Activities

- Write a few notes about how you felt listening to the patient's experience of side-effects such as nausea/vomiting, or hair loss.
- Next time you are helping to care for a patient who is having chemotherapy, find out the usual doses and the emetogenic (ability to cause nausea and vomiting) potential of each of their drugs. Are there other side-effects and how are they managed?

Resources

- Guidelines from the manufacturers' instructions
- Your hospital pharmacy cytotoxic manual
- British National Formulary (www.bnf.org.uk)
- Further reading, e.g. Brighton & Wood 2006

CCPS specific agents (e.g. antimetabolites, natural products) tend to cause a rapid decline to a low point (nadir) in the marrow cells, usually 7–10 days after drug administration, although with some drugs the nadir may be reached earlier. CCPNS drugs (doxorubicin, cisplatin) have nadirs around 10–14 days, while with others the nadir is 26–30+ days. Such factors need to be considered in the planning of treatment regimens. Since the prime function of neutrophils is phagocytosis, neutropenia eliminates one of the body's prime defences against bacterial infection (see Ch. 11). The longer the nadir period, the greater the opportunities to develop infections. Thrombocytopenia is usually delayed but, if active bleeding occurs, transfusions of platelets may be given. In view of the significant problems associated with bone marrow suppression, therapeutic use of haemopoietic growth factors such as granulocytic colony-stimulating factor (GCSF) is normal practice (Cappozzo 2004). Studies have shown that these factors can significantly reduce or prevent myelosuppression induced by chemotherapy (Gatzemeier et al 2000).

 See website Critical thinking question 31.2

Stomatitis/mucositis induced by chemotherapy is strongly associated with myelosuppression. It occurs in a two-stage process. First, some cytotoxic agents have a direct effect on the oral mucosa, causing thinning and ulceration within 4–7 days of administration. Patients may experience mild redness and swelling along the mucocutaneous junction of the lip, mouth dryness and a burning sensation in the lips. Nausea, vomiting and a reduced food and fluid intake compound this effect, making the mucosa an ineffective barrier to opportunistic infection. Within 10–16 days, myelosuppression causes the already compromised mucosa to be even more susceptible to infection and haemorrhage. Regular thorough assessment and care of the oral mucosa is a vital part of a supportive care strategy (Miller & Kearney 2001). A meaningful and validated assessment tool should be used at least daily and more often if mucositis is severe. It will contain questions about eating, swallowing, pain, etc.

Oral care interventions should aim to provide adequate pain relief, prevent or treat infection and promote healing. (See Ch. 15 and Further reading, e.g. Brown & Wingard 2004, Daniel et al 2004, Epstein & Schubert 2004, Peterson et al 2004, Sonis 2004.)

Nausea and vomiting Chemotherapy drugs can be characterised as having mild, moderate or severe emetogenic potential and therefore antiemetic medication should be prescribed accordingly. There are three types of nausea/vomiting that patients may experience:

- anticipatory
- acute
- delayed.

Antiemetics such as the 5-HT$_3$ antagonists (e.g. ondansetron, granisetron) have vastly improved the management of chemotherapy-related nausea and vomiting. However, studies continue to show that nurses are markedly underestimating this side-effect and patients report the negative impact such symptoms have on their quality of life (Miller & Kearney 2004). These medications have their own side-effect profile, including constipation (ondansetron) and headaches (granisetron). Corticosteroids such as dexamethasone potentiate the effect of these antiemetics and are most effective in delayed vomiting. Again they have their own toxicity profile, such as indigestion, hyperactivity and mood disturbance, and may mask signs of infection in myelosuppressed patients. Relaxation, meditation and sedatives such as lorazepam have also been found to be helpful for some patients, especially with anticipatory nausea/vomiting.

Alopecia is caused by particular chemotherapy agents such as doxorubicin, taxanes and topoisomerase inhibitors, and may range from slight thinning to complete hair loss. The severity of hair loss is directly related to the specific drug, dose and regimen. It usually occurs approximately 2 weeks after therapy has started and is temporary, with hair regrowth occurring about 6 weeks after the completion of treatment. Hair loss includes complete loss of eye brows, eye lashes, body and facial hair. Patients should be offered the choice of a wig prior to any hair loss to enable close matching to their own hair. Promoting a positive self-image by offering advice to minimise hair loss, the use of fashion accessories and offering the opportunity to speak with other patients is important, as the psychological impact of alopecia should not be underestimated (Batchelor 2001).

Scalp cooling techniques have been developed with varying degrees of success (Massey 2003). Earlier scalp cooling techniques involved wetting the scalp and applying ice packs, but more sophisticated refrigeration systems are now available which offer a more uniform cooling at a constant rate (Massey 2003). Observations from clinical practice suggest that scalp cooling can slow down the rate of hair loss when used with single-agent drugs with a short half-life at low dosages, e.g. doxorubicin, cyclophosphamide, docetaxel.

Sexual dysfunction may occur due to vascular changes and hormonal imbalance. Amenorrhoea and menopausal symptoms may be induced due to ovarian failure and follicle destruction. Women under 35 years of age have a greater chance of resumption of the menses on completion of treatment; however, this may not occur for 6–12 months.

Infertility may occur, depending on the agent, its dosage, the patient's age and gender, and other as yet unknown factors. Infertility may be temporary or permanent. Alkylating agents such as cyclophosphamide, chlorambucil and the nitrosourea compounds are certain to induce infertility. Patients should be informed about this side-effect. However, barrier methods of contraception are encouraged, as the exposure of a fetus to cytotoxic agents may result in congenital abnormalities or loss of the pregnancy.

In certain circumstances, some patients may receive counselling for sperm banking or oocyte harvesting. These options raise emotional and ethical dilemmas which may compound patients' existing stress concerning their diagnosis and treatment. This is an area of nursing that provides new challenges in terms of psychological support for patients and their partners.

Other side-effects It is not possible to address all the potential side-effects of chemotherapy in this chapter. (See Further reading, e.g. Brighton & Wood 2006 and Useful websites, e.g. British National Formulary.) However, apart from the more common ones mentioned above, it is important to remember the long-term effects which include cardiotoxicity, pulmonary fibrosis, myalgia, neuropathy and renal toxicity. In addition, much nursing research has focused attention on fatigue and the need to develop positive interventions such as energy conservation. (See Further reading Coackley et al 2002.)

Biological response modifiers

Biological response modifiers (BRMs), often referred to as the fourth treatment modality, involve the therapeutic use of substances known to occur naturally in the body. Most of these are involved in some way in the immune response (see Ch. 6), controlling cell-mediated and humoral responses; hence some of these developments are termed 'immunotherapies'. The theory behind these treatments is that it may be possible to manipulate the immune system such that it recognises tumour cells as antigens and causes the body to reject them.

Cytokines

Cytokines are substances released from an activated immune system. Interferon α_{2a}, for example, is an activator of natural killer cells and protects host cells against viruses. It has been found to maintain remission in hairy cell leukaemia and is being used with some success in certain patients with renal cancer and AIDS-related Kaposi's sarcoma. Side-effects include flu-like symptoms and mood disturbances, which may be very unpleasant. Other similar substances include tumour necrosis factor (TNF) and interleukin 2 (IL-2).

Monoclonal antibodies

During the 1980s, significant strides were made in the field of antibody therapy, which promotes specific targeting of cells through an antigen–antibody response. Tumour cells have antigens on their surface, and monoclonal antibodies to these antigens can now be manufactured commercially. Examples of monoclonal antibodies used in the clinical setting are rituximab and trastuzumab. Rituximab is directed against the CD20 antigen expressed in over 90% of B cell lymphomas and chronic lymphocytic leukaemia (CLL). Trastuzumab is directed against the human epidermal growth factor HER2-neu (c-erb2) proto-oncogene. In clinical studies, HER2 protein overexpression and gene amplification have been associated with a higher frequency of tumour recurrence and a reduction in overall survival time. Trastuzumab is presently used alongside other chemotherapy agents for the treatment of women with both primary and metastatic breast cancer whose tumours overexpress the HER2-neu protein (see Ch. 7, Part 2).

Cancer vaccines

Based on the antibody–antigen response mechanism, several vaccines have been developed for use in melanoma and trialled with encouraging responses. Vaccines against some types of the HPV, a risk factor for cervical cancer, have recently been developed and are recommended for widespread administration among 11–26-year-olds (Friedman et al 2006). Currently, one vaccine protects against HPV types 16 and 18, whereas a second vaccine protects against types 6, 11, 16 and 18. The HPV vaccine is included in the routine immunisation schedule in the UK.

Biological therapies have very different toxicity profiles from those of chemotherapy and include infusion syndrome, flu-like symptoms such as fever, chills, headache, malaise, arthralgia and fatigue. These symptoms require additional knowledge by the nurse as the timing of appropriate interventions such as premedications is important to safely administer these drugs. (See Further reading, e.g. Gale 2003, Liu 2003, Mautner & Huang 2003, Muehlbauer & Schwartzentruber 2003 and Schhmidt & Wood 2003.)

Psychological support during chemotherapy and BRM

There is increasing recognition, supported by research, that chemotherapy can lead to psychological distress and thus affect an individual's quality of life (Del Mastro et al 2002). In a study, nurses reported that patients were often anxious, distressed or frightened and emphasised that patients required individualised, clear information about their disease and treatment. Psychological, social and financial support for themselves and their families was also seen to be important. Nurses perceived that patients required more psychological support at the beginning and at the end of treatment, which may be difficult times for patients. The importance of talking and providing information was seen as an essential intervention for meeting patients' psychological needs (Arantzamendi & Kearney 2004).

Nurses in most oncology centres and some cancer units have their own patient caseload where care priorities include assessment of treatment toxicities, cannulation, administration of bolus and intravenous chemotherapy, and coordinating the chemotherapy/BRM regimens in collaboration with the oncologist. The continuity of care engendered by this approach allows a trusting supportive relationship to be built between nurse and patient.

Some areas in the UK offer home chemotherapy. Specialised nurses, who may be hospital or community based, deliver chemotherapy to patients in the comfort of their own homes. Some projects are nurse led, and others are collaborative schemes involving both statutory services and private sector companies (Pattison & Macrae 2002).

Hormonal agents

Hormonal agents are used to treat specific cancers. They are specifically used with tumours that are affected by hormones. The first stage may be surgical removal of the ovaries (oophorectomy) or testes (orchidectomy) to reduce the growth stimulus to tumours of the breast or prostate provided by oestrogen and testosterone, respectively, or this may be achieved by the use of medication such as tamoxifen. Tamoxifen blocks the action of oestrogen by binding to oestrogen receptor sites on the tumour cells. However, aromatase inhibitors such as anastrozole, letrozole and exemesterone are adding to the treatment options available for postmenopausal women. They act on the cancer cells differently from tamoxifen, by preventing rather than blocking the effect of oestrogen.

Corticosteroid hormones, such as prednisolone and dexamethasone, are also widely used, the former in conjunction with cytotoxic medication as primary treatment, usually for lymphomas, and the latter for its anti-inflammatory action in symptom control and the control of emesis.

Clinical trials

Despite an enormous amount of worldwide investment in research, cancer remains on the whole an incurable disease.

Most cancer centres are involved in multiple research trials, and through the clinical networks it has been possible to recruit patients from units. Nurses should be familiar with the clinical trials available in their area in order to understand the implications, support patients' decisions and provide nursing care.

New treatment methods for cancer are tested on fully informed and consenting patients by means of a series of trials termed phase I, II and III trials. During phase I, the maximum tolerable dose is established and information is obtained about the drug's toxicity profile; phase II trials discover which type of cancer is most responsive; and finally, phase III trials discover the extent to which the treatment improves survival. In phase III trials, patients from the target group are randomly selected to receive either the new treatment or the best established one. Phase IV trials continue once the drug has approval for clinical use in order to monitor, report and collate adverse and other reactions not reported in earlier phases. Survival rates are then compared.

New approaches to using radiotherapy, chemotherapy and biological agents are constantly being tested in this way.

Complementary and alternative medicine (CAM) therapy

The uncertainty that surrounds cancer and the impact it has on daily life has seen an increasing interest in CAM therapies. Based on the connection between body and mind, these therapies focus on a more 'holistic' approach to health in which the individual is encouraged to take control of their own life, both mentally and physically. Such therapies include homeopathy, acupuncture, therapeutic touch, massage, aromatherapy, relaxation techniques, yoga, hypnotherapy, nutrition, self-help groups and stress management.

Little research exists to support their use as alternatives to orthodox treatments (Fitch et al 1999). However, evidence is accumulating that some interventions may contribute positively to both psychological and physical health outcomes. Data from eight randomised controlled trials in a Cochrane Review of the use of massage and aromatherapy for symptom relief in patients with cancer found short-term benefits. The authors concluded that longer follow-up studies are required to determine whether these benefits persist (Fellowes et al 2004).

It is important that health professionals respect an individual's beliefs and choices, recognising the potential benefits of a combined approach to cancer treatment. In order to avoid potential harm, only certified practitioners with knowledge of interactions or contraindications should deliver complementary therapies. Recent surveys confirm that a substantial proportion of patients are using herbal medicines, which have the potential to cause adverse reactions (Werneke et al 2004).

Nursing management and health promotion: cancer care

The cancer nurse

Cancer and its treatment have a unique impact on an individual's life. Although the physical problems experienced by cancer patients may be similar to those of patients with many non-malignant conditions, the combination of these problems with the chronic nature of cancer, the highly toxic effects of treatment and the profound psychological impact of the disease mean that cancer nurses require specialised knowledge and skills. Cancer nursing as a specialty has been in existence for many years in the UK and is continually developing. Key skills in cancer nursing are those that help the cancer patient and their carers to adapt to the reality of living with cancer while maximising quality of life.

Hospital–community liaison

Cancer is a chronic illness characterised by remissions, exacerbations and progressive physical changes. More patients with cancer are living longer. Health professionals caring for cancer patients should view care as a continuous process, whether it takes place in the hospital or in the community setting. Supporting the patient through the cancer journey requires the skills of all members of the multiprofessional team in conjunction with the patient and family. Shared care protocols, a relatively new concept in cancer care, came about in response to the recognition of unfulfilled needs of patients receiving active treatments at home, e.g. immunotherapy or continuous chemotherapy infusions. Such protocols promote the philosophy of continuity of care between hospital and community. Effective communication and discharge planning are essential to optimal care. Without proper coordination and integration of services, the cancer patient's 'journey' through the health care system can be a bewildering and demoralising experience. Box 31.12 illustrates the need for good discharge planning and liaison between hospital and community nurses.

Cancer patients spend most of their lives at home, interrupted by short hospital admissions. As a result, much of the psychological and physical adjustment to cancer takes place at home. Community initiatives and services are set up to support patients, their families and other carers from diagnosis to terminal illness and end-of-life care, helping patients in decision making and achieving optimal independence and quality of life.

Cancer care in the community

Community nursing staff are involved in cancer care during five phases:

- prevention programmes
- diagnosis
- treatment-related support
- rehabilitation following initial cancer treatment
- palliative care and end-of-life care.

GPs, practice nurses, community nurses, liaison nurses and health visitors are generally involved in prevention schemes. District nurses coordinate and carry out a needs assessment for patients throughout their time in the community. In some areas, initiatives are being developed to support patients in the community at diagnosis and during treatment with the introduction of community cancer care nurses with specialist oncology knowledge and skills (Gorman et al 2000). Towards the later stages of the disease, symptoms may become more problematic and place more strain on carers; at this stage, Macmillan Cancer Support, Marie Curie or community palliative care nurses who have close links with the hospice and hospital-based palliative care teams may become involved. These nurses have specialist skills in managing complex symptoms, providing psychosocial support and planning care in conjunction with the district nurse and other members of the primary care team.

The role of the district nurse

The role of community staff is one of partnership with the patient and their family, who constitute the main 'unit of care' (Kennedy 2002). Providing information, support and advice is often as important as assistance with physical care.

Another major role of the district nurse involves coordination of the primary care team and integration of statutory and non-statutory services. Because of the nature of cancer, the need for these services is considerable. The statutory services available include all of those necessary for the care of long-term illness in the community (see Ch. 32).

Non-statutory services in the community

Non-statutory services for cancer patients are particularly comprehensive in their provision and include the following.

Box 31.12 Reflection

Joined up cancer care

Bob, a 58-year-old head teacher, is married to Margaret and has two grown-up children: a daughter in Australia and a married son with two small children who live nearby.

He presented to his GP with urinary hesitancy and frequency. Examination and subsequent referral to an urologist revealed a locally invasive tumour of the prostate with no metastases. A biopsy of the tumour and a bone scan were performed with Bob as an outpatient. Following a full discussion of the options with the urologist and specialist nurse, Bob opted for 4 weeks of radical radiotherapy rather than a prostatectomy. Because he lived in a small town 50 miles away from the nearest radiotherapy department, he became an inpatient, going home at weekends. During his recovery at home, a health visitor visited twice.

Two years later, 1 week after his retirement, rib pain necessitated a further bone scan. This showed metastatic deposits in the ribs and spine. At Bob's local hospital, a bilateral orchidectomy was performed to reduce hormonal stimulation of tumour growth. Bob was then readmitted to the radiotherapy department. One week of palliative radiotherapy and the commencement of opiate analgesics enabled discharge and 6 months of reasonably independent life.

However, a fall whilst Bob was gardening resulted in the collapse of the third thoracic vertebra, with resultant severe pain and paraplegia due to SCC. High-dose corticosteroids initially, emergency radiotherapy and intensive physiotherapy restored some function, but Bob was now confined to a wheelchair and had no bladder or bowel control.

Margaret was fit and very determined to cope at home with the help of her son and his wife. Prior to Bob's discharge, the community occupational therapy department oversaw the installation of a wheelchair ramp, bath aids and a hoist in Bob and Margaret's bungalow. District nurses visited regularly and referred Bob to social services to provide support with washing and dressing. The Macmillan nurse provided psychological support and complex symptom management, linking Bob in with the local hospice.

Within 6 weeks a further admission, this time to the local hospital, was necessary due to hypercalcaemia, which was treated with intravenous bisphosphonates. Gradually Bob's condition deteriorated and he was generally too weak to get out of bed. District nurses now visited him twice a day and the Macmillan nurse specialist visited regularly to provide additional advice for pain and symptom control. It was arranged for Marie Curie nurses to care for Bob at night, in order to allow the family to rest and sleep. Bob died peacefully at home with his wife and both children with him.

Activities

- Consider the roles of the many health professionals involved in the care of Bob and his family.
- Reflect on the skills needed to provide coordinated integrated services for cancer patients.
- Discuss with your mentor how hospital-based staff, community staff and the cancer charities work together in your locality to provide such services.

Support and self-help groups Such groups can reduce the isolation of the cancer experience. The sharing of feelings and experiences provides emotional support, fosters hope and encourages a sense of self-worth and purpose. Many local groups exist for patients and/or their carers.

Support and information centres Empowerment of individuals, thereby allowing them to help themselves, is the basis of psychoeducational intervention programmes advocated by Fawzy et al (2000). Information, emotional support, relaxation and stress management are provided in thoughtfully designed environments for those affected by cancer, including carers, partners, relatives and friends. Programmes have been developed to provide opportunities for people to live and cope with a cancer diagnosis. Maggie's Cancer Caring Centres and Macmillan Information Centres are just two examples. Many other UK cancer support centres provide similar assistance and access to CAM therapists.

Counselling services Counselling may be necessary to assist the patient and their family to adapt emotionally to cancer and can help to relieve anxiety and depression. The Cancer Counselling Trust provides this service by telephone and in person.

Financial aid The Macmillan Cancer Support fund can provide financial aid to meet the cost of aids, appliances, heating, bedding, holidays and other special needs.

Nursing services Marie Curie Cancer Care charity provides nursing staff, including a night nursing service, to allow carers some respite or sleep.

Nursing frameworks for cancer care

No one framework or model of nursing can be suitable for every cancer patient or care setting. Integrated care pathways (ICPs) are an example of a framework which aims to integrate evidence-based practice through a documented plan of anticipated care for a group of patients with a particular diagnosis or set of symptoms. Each professional involved in the patient's care has a clearly defined role and the plan of care leads the patient towards a required goal, for example, the Liverpool Care Pathway for the Dying (see Useful websites, e.g. www.mcpcil.org.uk/liverpool_care_pathway).

Family coping

A cancer diagnosis can have a drastic effect on the patient's family and loved ones in the following ways:

- Cancer can disrupt patterns of familial and other interpersonal interaction. Reactions vary from overprotection and excessive vigilance to distancing behaviour and even the complete breakdown of relationships. Many patients, especially in the early stages of the disease, may feel that they have to be the strong one emotionally, supporting and holding the family together. A study by Schmid-Buchi et al (2008) found partners want information concerning the patient's condition and how to support their loved one from different threats while both parties needed support about the prognosis.
- Cancer disrupts planning for the future. The uncertainty involved disrupts family plans and dreams for holidays,

retirement, parenthood and so forth. Roles within the family change, particularly if the patient is a breadwinner or parent. Such change is stressful and can undermine the patient's sense of self-worth and purpose. Loss of income and increased expenditure due to the illness can create financial hardship, isolation and feelings of low esteem.

Nursing interventions After assessment of family dynamics and needs, the following nursing interventions may help to alleviate some of the above problems:

- Providing regular information about the patient's status and plans for care, preferably facilitating open communication between the patient and their family, which is associated with lower anxiety levels (Edwards & Clarke 2004). Shared information helps to promote a positive attitude and improves adaptation and communication within the hospital setting and at home.
- Encouraging relatives to express their feelings of fear, loss, guilt and exhaustion.
- Encouraging realistic, mutual goal-setting, e.g. the timing and planning of holidays.
- Encouraging family members to adapt the patient's role within the family to maintain a sense of belonging and worth, e.g. by exchanging physical tasks for clerical ones.
- Referring families promptly to the social work department for financial assistance and, if necessary, rehousing.
- Recognising signs of exhaustion in carers, giving them 'permission' to take time off and arranging respite care or hospital/hospice admission for the patient if necessary.
- Encouraging continued social involvement, suggesting appropriate activities if necessary.
- Suggesting referral to a psychologist or Relate counsellor if family relationships appear to be breaking down.

Diet and exercise

Up to 85% of cancer patients, due to a variety of complex factors, are malnourished (Shaw 2002). These are usually patients with advanced disease as patients with primary disease, particularly breast cancer patients, can often gain weight during treatment.

Cancer patients lose weight because of metabolic changes caused by the tumour; this is referred to as cancer cachexia syndrome (Boon et al 2006). The associated weight loss can have a negative impact on a patient's body image and sexuality; it represents a major source of concern for both patient and family, often acting as a barometer of the patient's condition.

Causes of malnutrition and weight loss in cancer patients include the following:

- Reduced food intake due to:
  - anorexia: due to multiple causes, e.g. release of cytokines such as TNF and IL-1 is thought to delay gastric emptying, thus delaying digestion, suppressing the appetite and causing satiety (Shaw 2002)
  - taste changes: may occur in any cancer patient; they are most common following radiotherapy to the head or neck due to destruction of salivary tissue. These changes involve a lowered threshold for bitter tastes, and therefore aversion to meat; raised threshold for sweet tastes, and hence many foods taste bland and 'cardboard-like'; alteration of the taste of tea and coffee
  - early satiety: metabolic abnormalities directly related to tumour burden may result in early satiety, a premature feeling of fullness, usually progressing over the day
  - other symptoms: such as pain, nausea, vomiting and drowsiness
  - physical difficulties: due to oral prostheses or badly fitting dentures; also to the tumour and treatment, e.g. oesophageal obstruction, chemotherapy-induced mucositis
  - anxiety and depression.
- Malabsorption due to:
  - resection of tumours of the gastrointestinal tract, leading to decreased enzyme production and increased transit time
  - impairment of nutrient absorption resulting from chemotherapy and abdominal radiotherapy.
- Excess expenditure of nutrients, due to:
  - in many patients, raised basal metabolic rate (BMR), partly due to the demands of the tumour
  - loss of body protein due to vomiting, diarrhoea, haemorrhage, oedema, from stomas, fistulae and in exudates from ulcerations.

Nursing interventions Actions that the nurse can take to help the patient overcome or manage difficulties with eating and drinking include the following:

- Use a screening tool such as Malnutrition Universal Screening Tool (MUST) to assess the patient's current nutritional status and potential for further deterioration (British Association for Parenteral and Enteral Nutrition [BAPEN] 2003). Weekly weighing is adequate; more frequent weighing may cause the patient to become anxious and demoralised.
- Identifying the major factors that contribute to the nutritional deficit.
- Referring 'at-risk' patients to a dietitian.
- Referring to a speech and language therapist (SLT) those patients with an identified swallowing or aspiration problem.
- Referring to an occupational therapist (OT) to assist with functional or practical difficulties.
- Referring to a social worker for a care package to assist with shopping and meal preparation.
- Enlisting the help of relatives and friends to offer the patient's favourite foods whilst respecting autonomy. However, it is important to explain that there are very real reasons for the patient's reluctance to eat. Provision of dietary information, recipes and self-care measures may be helpful.
- Offering frequent, small, high-calorie attractive meals and snacks throughout the day; negotiating with the catering department for flexibility in portion size and for a supply of nutrient-rich foods to be kept at unit/ward level.
- Encouraging patients to take fluids in the form of high-energy drinks; discouraging drinking at mealtimes, to avoid early satiety.

- Decreasing satiety by the avoidance of high-fat foods which delay gastric emptying; the use of drugs, e.g. metoclopramide, may promote gastric emptying.
- Reassuring the patient that taste changes are to be expected and may disappear in time; offering taste-enhancing herbs, spices, marinades (unless mucositis is a problem) and alternatives to tea and coffee.
- Supporting the patient if there is further weight loss despite sufficient calorie intake, due to abnormal metabolism.
- Using gentle exercise, relaxation or modest amounts of alcohol to stimulate the appetite.
- Controlling other symptoms. Antiemetics and analgesics (topical and systemic) should be administered 30 min before meals.
- Encouraging regular oral care, such as mouthwashes, before and after meals.
- Eliminating nauseating environmental stimuli at mealtimes, such as bedpans, odours and disturbing procedures.
- If intake is consistently inadequate and/or weight loss continues, commencing other forms of feeding: enteral feeding by nasogastric tube if absorption is adequate; parenteral if not (see Ch. 21).

Expressing sexuality

Following treatment for cancer, up to 50% of patients who were sexually active before the illness report some reduction in sexual interest or activity. Health care professionals fail to take the initiative in addressing their patients' sexual problems within the context of treatment for chronic and life-threatening illness. The reticence of some nurses may be due to embarrassment, but a lack of relevant knowledge and counselling skills has also been reported (Guthrie 1999).

Sexuality involves more than sexual intercourse. It includes self-image in relation to gender, role behaviour within a partnership, and many forms of love and affection between partners. Partners are also affected by the experience of cancer and in some cases report higher levels of psychological distress and psychosexual concerns than patients (Carlson et al 2000). A cancer patient's sexuality may be altered for many reasons, including:

- the physical effects of the tumour, e.g. lesions of the spinal cord may interfere with the nerve pathways necessary for sexual sensation or motor function
- symptoms caused by the tumour, e.g. pain, immobility, nocturia, dysuria, vaginal or rectal bleeding and fatigue can all contribute to a decrease in desire for sexual intimacy
- the physical effects of treatment, e.g. hormone manipulation may alter sexual function; surgery may alter the anatomy, for example prostate surgery may cause pelvic nerve damage resulting in erectile dysfunction; pelvic irradiation may reduce vaginal lubrication causing painful intercourse (dyspareunia)
- body image problems, e.g. following mastectomy or stoma formation; less obvious changes may also contribute, e.g. varying degrees of weight loss or hair loss
- anxiety and depression related to the cancer diagnosis resulting in low self-esteem.

Nursing interventions The nurse can provide support for the cancer patient experiencing problems with the expression of sexuality in the following ways:

- Initiating discussion in order to give the patient 'permission' to voice their concerns. Once the discussion is initiated, the patient will indicate whether or not they wish to pursue the topic.
- Anticipating problems before treatment: explaining how long problems will last and that they are to be expected; describing measures that can be used to relieve them (see Table 31.3, pp. 804–807, for examples of interventions for patients receiving radiotherapy).
- Opening discussion with non-threatening subjects such as contraceptive advice or the alterations in partnership roles due to illness. This will aid progression to potentially more personal issues.
- Ensuring that anxiety and depression are treated and body image problems addressed. Severe body image problems may require psychological therapy.
- Involving partners in discussion and physical care as appropriate.
- Facilitating the privacy of couples in hospices and hospitals.

Communicating

From the cancer patient's perspective, patient-focused communication can be the most important aspect of treatment, in part because of its capacity to exacerbate or allay the fear that often accompanies cancer (Fallowfield & Jenkins 1999). Communication encompasses three areas of activity, which may be described as:

- cognitive – the giving and receiving of information
- emotional – the feeling and expression of psychological responses
- spiritual – the expression and feeling of thoughts relating to existential issues beyond the self.

Although this division can help in identifying specific nursing activities, the three areas are interrelated. Providing information in a sensitive, caring manner affords emotional support, and many people do not consciously make the distinction between the emotional and spiritual dimensions.

Cognitive activity

The patient's need for information in relation to diagnosis and treatment has been examined in earlier sections of this chapter. To this discussion the following observations may be added:

- Knowledge is power: power that enables independence, choice, autonomous decision making and realistic goal-setting for patients and their families. Information promotes the patient's sense of control over their life.
- Studies of patients' perceived needs rank information as a key component for coping with cancer (Van der Molen 1999).
- Lack of information can deepen a depressive reaction to a cancer diagnosis.
- Specific information about diagnosis and prognosis can encourage active participation by patients in their own

care, and in fact generates rather than negates hope (Skalla et al 2004).

- Patients have traditionally expected their needs for information to be met by doctors, and their needs for support to be met by nurses. However, in practice, particularly with the evolution of specialist nurses, this is changing. Patients will choose the person they wish to obtain information from depending on their needs.
- Nurses, by their behaviour and non-verbal communication, may indicate they are too busy to answer questions at that particular time. They may also feel they lack the information the patient is seeking, or fear that information-giving may lead to an emotional unburdening by the patient, for which they may lack the personal resources necessary to cope.
- Patients and their families need information on the cause of the cancer, the possible course of the disease, treatment options, the role of the health care team, available services and sources of further information.
- Patients vary greatly in their desire for, and receptivity to, information. For example, patients who actively deny their cancer are unlikely to listen to information about community nursing support on discharge, and patients with a fatalistic attitude may not be interested in information about self-help groups or complementary therapy.

Nursing interventions The following advice may assist the nurse to meet the patient's communication needs:

- Be equipped with the information that the patient needs. Be assertive in obtaining this information from other members of the health care team so that consistent information is given to the patient.
- Be present at as many interactions between the patient and the doctor as possible. Afterwards reinforce messages and ensure that the patient has understood.
- Find out what the patient already knows and has been told, and what they want to know. In general, follow the patient's agenda.
- Bear in mind that when receiving information most people remember only three specific points; the first three points made are those most likely to be remembered.
- Avoid jargon: *'your white cell count will fall'*, for example, may mean nothing to most patients. Information about how they will feel and what they will experience is most important to most patients.
- Be prepared for the patient to forget or deny receiving the information given.
- Reinforce verbal information with written information. CancerBACUP (now merged with Macmillan Cancer Support) and many oncology centres produce patient literature on a wide range of subjects.
- Be prepared for information-giving to lead to emotional issues. Allow time for this or promise to return at an arranged time – and do so.
- Give the patient and their relatives the same information. Give each the opportunity to receive this information both together and separately, so that personal anxieties can be expressed privately and within the family group.

Emotional activity

Enabling patients and their families to cope with the emotional impact of cancer demands effective listening skills and is an essential component of counselling (Box 31.13).

The following considerations should be borne in mind by the nurse in addressing the cancer patient's emotional needs:

- During any stage of the disease, the cancer patient is suffering the effects of various actual or potential losses. These may include loss of a body part or function, loss of self-image, loss of work or leisure activities, loss of family or social role, loss of control over life, loss of goals and dreams for the future and, ultimately, loss of life itself. Loss is the predominant factor in all sadness and depression.

Box 31.13 Reflection

Communication skills in the care of Lara

This is an example of how one nurse offered her support to a young woman with acute leukaemia and her family.

'While waiting for confirmation of the diagnosis, I did a lot of listening. I listened to the expression of shock, fear and guilt. I did not negate their concerns or try to offer false assurances.

It was clear that one of the most useful things I could do for this distraught family, who were in a strange and overwhelming place, was to assist them, little by little, in gaining control over their experiences. This involved helping them to anticipate and be prepared for what was to come, for how it might feel or look physically or emotionally. It also involved helping them to continue in their usual roles as much as possible, and engaging them in the decisions affecting Lara's care.

Although she knew that she had less than a 50% chance of survival, Lara concentrated on the here and now: the pain associated with frequent intravenous therapies, bone marrow and lumbar punctures; the embarrassment of hair loss; the isolation from her friends; and the nausea and vomiting associated with her chemotherapy. I followed her lead by responding to her immediate concerns.

I used a variety of approaches in working with her, depending on what kind of day she was having. Sometimes we would just joke around; other times we would talk about more serious issues – not just her illness but her personal life, as well as my own.

I was always open with her, accepted her feelings, and never made light of them. I did not assure her that "it would get better soon" or that "I knew how she must be feeling" because I truly did not know whether she would get better or how she actually felt.

Lara was just plain miserable. All I could do was to listen, acknowledge how awful it must be, and honestly say that she must feel like crying. Permission to cry was all she needed to let the tears flow. One day, she looked me directly in the eyes and said, "I'm so sick, am I going to die?". Although it was a matter of seconds before I answered, it seemed like hours as my mind groped for the right words. I did not avert my gaze and answered from my heart: "I'm afraid Lara, you are so sick that you could die".'

Activities

- Reflect on how the nurse followed the agenda set by Lara and responded to the situation as it developed, rather than imposing a preconceived structure for communication.
- Discuss with some fellow students how you would feel if a patient asked 'I'm so sick, am I going to die?'.

- There are many uncertainties involved in cancer; uncertainty leads to anxiety.
- While the majority of cancer patients adjust emotionally and cope reasonably well with loss and uncertainty, there is psychological distress and even psychiatric illness among this client group. A study by Zabora et al (2001), examining the prevalence of psychological distress in 14 cancer sites ($n = 4496$), found the overall prevalence rate of distress to be 35.1%.
- A great deal of this emotional turmoil, anxiety and depression passes undetected and unrelieved (Fallowfield et al 2001). Some research has focused on prediction and early detection of affective disorders, through screening and improving communication skills of health professionals as well as therapeutic interventions (Maguire 1995).
- Emotional support is not a luxury in nursing care. Emotional distress may result in somatic symptoms such as confusion, immobility, insomnia and pain. As previously suggested, long-term distress may exacerbate disease progression (Brown et al 2003).
- Patients' reactions to cancer vary greatly, depending on personality, past experience and learned coping strategies.

Nursing interventions The following strategies can be employed to give patients support as they adjust emotionally to their illness and treatment:

- Give the patient 'openings' to state what is on their mind, e.g. by concluding an information-giving session by asking them how they feel about the information, or by remarking upon a worried or sad expression.
- Do not be afraid of saying the wrong thing. A desire to understand and an attitude of concern are the important factors (Hinds & Moyer 1997).
- Learn and apply interviewing techniques used in counselling, e.g. reflecting a patient's question or statement. This gives the patient the chance to realise what has been said and to expand on it, and the nurse time to reflect on what is meant. Constant reflection of questions, however, will irritate patients. Once the patient's main concerns have been established, it may be time to give direct answers.
- Resist giving 'pat' answers and false reassurances. Many of the dilemmas faced by cancer patients have no ready solution. Do not be afraid to admit that answers cannot be given to all the patient's questions about the future. Try, however, to leave the patient with some hope: help the patient to identify something positive in their situation on which to focus.
- Assist the patient to identify realistic goals in order to foster hope. These goals should originate from the patient but often need an objective person to identify them. Examples may be the goal of fighting the disease, of living until a daughter's wedding or returning to work part-time.
- A certain degree of worry and sadness is to be expected. Be alert to signs of disabling anxiety (somatic stress symptoms, lack of concentration, feelings of panic) or depression (a 'flat' mood, an exaggerated feeling of guilt and self-blame, suicidal ideation) (see Ch. 17). If these are noted, refer the patient to a psychologist or psychiatrist. Anxiolytic and antidepressant medication and various forms of

psychological therapy may be required before other forms of counselling therapy can be effective (Strong et al 2004).

- Patients may react to their disease with denial, anger, bargaining, depression and acceptance (Kübler-Ross 1973). Counselling cannot force the patient to move from one stage to another, but it does allow them to express feelings and perhaps make progress. The nurse should give patients permission to express their feelings in any safe way they choose and should not feel a sense of failure when a patient becomes emotionally distraught. The expression of emotions is therapeutic and is an important part of psychological adaptation.
- Supporting patients and their families through the cancer experience is very demanding emotionally. It is important for nurses to recognise the resultant stress in themselves and their colleagues and to seek and offer active support (see below).

Spiritual activity

A full consideration of the cancer patient's quality of life must recognise the spiritual dimension of the experience, which might be described, in the most basic terms, as the search for meaning and purpose. Because spirituality involves the contemplation of things that affect us but lie beyond our control, cancer has the capacity to precipitate a spiritual crisis. (See Further reading, e.g. NHS Education Scotland 2009.)

Stress in cancer nursing

In 1988, Speck stated that the most important ethical choice made by cancer nurses is whether or not to engage in '*an intense, personalised involvement*' with their patients in response to human need. A degree of emotional involvement is inevitable, and even necessary, to achieve excellence in cancer care. But such involvement, particularly as it may be terminated by the patient's death, results in considerable occupational stress. This emotional involvement is simultaneously a great asset and a point of vulnerability for nurses (Haylock 2005).

The picture that emerges from the research and literature related to stress, burnout and the emotional labour of cancer nursing is mixed (Magnusson & Robinson 2000). A focus group found that patient care or contact was the greatest source of job satisfaction for cancer care workers. Oncology was felt to be a special environment because of the type of relationship established with patients and their families. However, over a third of participants demonstrated high levels of emotional exhaustion and low levels of personal accomplishment (Grunfeld et al 2005).

The constructive expression of emotions is as important as stress control. Establishing an environment of trust and mutual respect where it is safe to admit to colleagues feelings of inadequacy, grief and guilt, and even personal fears about cancer and death, is beneficial in relieving stress. Such support should also be provided on an organised basis in the form of support groups and counselling services, as formal support groups are often catalysts for social support, problem solving and task sharing (Tschudin 1996) (Box 31.14). Reflective practice, clinical supervision and mentorship are also important concepts that enable and empower individuals within their nursing practice. Nurses continue to describe emotionally charged areas of care as being the

Box 31.14 Reflection

Stress in cancer nursing

Caring for cancer patients and their families is intensely rewarding but the emotional involvement required can have negative consequences for the nurse.

Activities

- Think about a patient with cancer that you have cared for on placement. Reflect on the positive aspects of your professional relationship with the person – for the patient and for your professional development.
- How were you affected by caring for this person? Discuss your thoughts with a fellow student or your mentor.
- Find out what support services are available in your area for nurses and other health professionals who care for cancer patients.

most difficult and stressful; however, Wilkinson et al (2002) have shown that an integrated approach to communication skills improves nurses' expertise in this area.

An active life and supportive relationships outside of work are also vital in maintaining a realistic perspective on life. Without external interests, it may be easy for the nurse to imagine that cancer is far more prevalent than it is. Fields et al (1997) introduced stress reduction therapies such as a 10-minute massage, listening to music, visual imagery and social support group sessions and found that nurses experienced increased vigour and decreased anxiety and fatigue.

A commitment to continuing education by nursing management is essential in stress control. However, as Tschudin (1996) concludes: '*nurses themselves need to take on more direct responsibility for their own psychological care*', and in campaigning for support and education.

See also Chapter 17.

New directions for cancer care

Seminal work by Slevin et al (1990) pointed out that those who do not have cancer, whether they are lay people or professionals, have very little concept of the experience of cancer or of how the cancer patient perceives quality of life, their future and the decisions that must be made. Cancer is a chronic illness and more patients are surviving and living with their disease than previously. These patients have needs and expectations – physical, psychosocial and spiritual. While they may survive they may not necessarily thrive. In this situation, cancer rehabilitation is paramount to support patients in effectively managing their illness on a day-to-day basis.

This millennium will see an increase in strategies aimed at self-care management, with individuals, families and communities playing a larger role in determining and meeting their own health needs. The internet has empowered patients by providing access to information about their disease and treatment, and opening up communication links with fellow patients. Advances in molecular biology may lead to the identification of high-risk groups and better targeted prevention and screening as well as treatment. New challenges lie ahead for nurses in all fields for role development, research and education to support patients and their families through the cancer experience.

SUMMARY: KEY NURSING ISSUES

- Cancer is a major health care problem. One in three people in the UK risk developing cancer in their lifetime.
- The term 'cancer' evokes a variety of emotions for people and families including shock, disbelief and a fear of pain and death. Many people with cancer are surviving longer but this is not universal. Although cancer management and treatment involves a large team of health and social care professionals and the voluntary sector, nurses are at the forefront of prevention and early detection, delivery of cancer treatments and providing supportive care.
- Nurses need to understand the biology of cancer – how it develops and why it spreads – and recognise the features associated with common cancers.
- Patients need accurate information about their cancer and treatments. Nurses have an important role in providing general information but for more specialist information it is important to seek help from a cancer nurse or palliative care specialist.
- Cancer affects not only the patient but also their family, partners and friends.
- Cancer can be extremely debilitating. Nurses must listen to the patient and act on their symptoms. Distinguishing between cancer symptoms and those of treatment is very important.
- The psychological impact of a cancer diagnosis and subsequent treatment can be very difficult for patients. Nurses are often witness to this. Nurses are not the sole providers of care and support and they must be mindful that there are many other professionals, such as psychologists, social workers, GPs and voluntary cancer services, who can also support patients. Nurses are often in a position to help patients to access these services.

REFLECTION AND LEARNING – WHAT NEXT?

- **Test** your knowledge by visiting the website and answering the multiple choice questions and critical thinking questions.
- **Consolidate** your learning by looking at some of the further reading suggestions, references and specialist websites.
- **Revisit** some of the additional material on the website.
- **Consider** what you have learnt and how this will help your professional development.
- **Reflect** on how you can apply this knowledge to the care of your patients.
- **Discuss** your learning with your mentor/supervisor, lecturer and colleagues.

REFERENCES

Adamson D: The radiobiological basis of radiation side effects. In Faithful S, Wells M, editors: *Supportive care in radiotherapy*, Edinburgh, 2003, Churchill Livingstone, pp 71–95.

Arantzamendi M, Kearney N: The psychological needs of patients receiving chemotherapy: an exploration of nurse perceptions, *Eur J Cancer Care (Engl)* 13(1):23–31, 2004.

Armstrong TS: Paraneoplastic syndromes. In Yarbro CH, Frogge MH, Goodman M, Groenwald SL, editors: *Cancer nursing: principles and practice*, ed 5, Boston, 2005, Jones and Bartlett, pp 808–824.

Association of the British Pharmaceutical Industry (ABPI) in partnership with CancerBACUP: *The cancer information maze*, 2005. Available online http://www.abpi.org.uk/Details.asp?ProductID=300.

Batchelor D: Hair and cancer chemotherapy: consequences and nursing care – a literature study, *Eur J Cancer Care (Engl)* 10(3):147–163, 2001.

Baxter N: Preventive healthcare, 2001 update: should women be routinely taught breast self examination to screen for breast cancer? *Can Med Assoc J* 164(13):1837–1846, 2001.

Blyth CM, Anderson J, Hughson W, et al: An innovative approach to palliative care within a radiotherapy department, *Journal of Radiotherapy in Practice* 2:85–90, 2001.

Bonevski B, Sanson-Fisher R, Girgis A, et al: Evaluation of an instrument to assess the needs of patients with cancer. Supportive Care Review Group, *Cancer* 88(1):217–225, 2000.

Boon NA, Colledge NR, Walker BR: *Davidson's Principles and Practice of Medicine*, ed 20, Edinburgh, 2006, Churchill Livingstone.

British Association for Parenteral and Enteral Nutrition (BAPEN): *Malnutrition Advisory Group. The malnutrition universal screening tool (MUST)*, 2003. Available online http://www.bapen.org.uk/pdfs/must/must_full.pdf.

Brown K, Levy AR, Rosberger Z, Edgar L: Psychological distress and cancer survival: a follow up study 10 years after diagnosis, *Psychosom Med* 65(4):636–643, 2003.

Calzone KA, Biesecker BB: Genetic testing for cancer predisposition, *Cancer Nurs* 25(1):15–25, 2002.

Cancer Research UK: *Cancer incidence for common cancers – UK statistics*, London, 2009, CRUK. Available online http://info.cancerresearchuk.org/cancerstats/incidence/commoncancers/.

Cantor SB, Volk RJ, Cass AK, et al: Psychological benefits of prostate screening: the role of reassurance, *Health Expect* 5(2):104–113, 2002.

Cappozzo C: Optimal use of granulocyte-colony-stimulating factor in patients with cancer who are at risk for chemotherapy induced neutropenia, *Oncol Nurs Forum* 31(3):569–576, 2004.

Carlson LE, Bultz BD, Speca M, et al: Partners of cancer patients. Part I. Impact, adjustment and coping across the illness trajectory, *Journal of Social Oncology* 18(2):39–63, 2000.

Chapman K, Abraham C, Jenkins V, et al: Lay understanding of terms used in cancer consultations, *Psychooncology* 12(6):557–566, 2003.

Cruickshank S, Kennedy C, Lockhart K, et al: Specialist breast care nurses for supportive care of women with breast cancer, *Cochrane Database Syst Rev* (1):CD005634, 2008.

Del Mastro L, Costantini M, Morasso G, et al: Impact of two different dose-intensity chemotherapy regimens on psychological distress in early breast cancer patients, *Eur J Cancer* 38:359–366, 2002.

Department of Health: *A policy framework for commissioning cancer services: a report by the Expert Advisory Group on Cancer to the Chief Medical Officers of England and Wales*, London, 1995, HMSO.

Department of Health: *The nursing contribution to cancer care: a strategic programme of action in support of the national cancer programme*, London, 2000, DH.

Department of Health: *Manual for cancer services*, London, 2004, DH. Available online http://www.dh.gov.uk/en/Healthcare/Cancer/Treatment/DH_101998

Doll R, Hill AB: The mortality of doctors in relation to their smoking habits. A preliminary report, *Br Med J* 1:1451–1455, 1954.

Edwards B, Clarke V: Psychological impact of a cancer diagnosis on families: the influence of family functioning and patients' illness characteristics on depression and anxiety, *Psychooncology* 13(8):562–576, 2004.

Fallowfield L, Jenkins V: Effective communication skills are the key to good cancer care, *Br J Cancer* 35:1592–1597, 1999.

Fallowfield L, Ratcliffe D, Jenkins V, et al: Psychiatric morbidity and its recognition by doctors in patients with cancer, *Br J Cancer* 84(8):1011–1015, 2001.

Fawzy F, Fawzy N, Canada A: Psychoeducational intervention programs for patients with cancer, *Psychologische Beitrage* 42(1):95–118, 2000.

Fellowes D, Barnes K, Wilkinson S: Aromatherapy and massage for symptom relief in patients with cancer, *Cochrane Database Syst Rev* (3): CD002287, 2004.

Ferlay J, Autier P, Boniol M, et al: Estimates of the cancer incidence and mortality in Europe in 2006, *Ann Oncol* 1–12, 2007. doi: 10.1093/annonc/md1498.

Fidler IJ: Molecular biology of cancer: invasion and metastases. In DeVita VT, Hellman S, Rosenberg SA, editors: *Cancer: principles and practice of oncology*, Philadelphia, 1997, Lippincott-Raven.

Fields T, Quintino O, Henteleff T, et al: Job stress reduction therapies, *Alternative Therapies* 3:54–56, 1997.

Fitch MI, Greenberg M, Cava M, et al: Exploring the barriers to cervical screening in an urban Canadian setting, *Cancer Nurs* 21:441–449, 1998.

Fitch MI, Gray RE, Greenberg M, et al: Nurses' perspectives on unconventional therapies, *Cancer Nurs* 22(3):238–245, 1999.

Friedman LS, Kahn J, Middleman AB, et al: Human papillomavirus (HPV) vaccine: a position statement of the society for adolescent medicine, *J Adolesc Health* 39:620, 2006.

Gardner MJ, Snee MP, Hall AJ, et al: Results of case control study of leukaemia and lymphoma in young people near Sellafield nuclear plant in West Cumbria, *Br Med J* 300:423–429, 1990.

Gatzemeier U, Kleisbauer JF, Drings P, et al: Lenograstim as support for ACE chemotherapy for small cell lung cancer: a phase III, multicentre, randomized study, *Am J Clin Oncol* 23(4):393–400, 2000.

Gohagan JK, Marcus PM, Fagerstrom RM, et al: Final results of the lung screening study, a randomized feasibility study of spiral CT versus chest X-ray screening for lung cancer, *Lung Cancer* 47(1):9–15, 2005.

Gorman DR, Mackinnon H, Storrie M, et al: The general practice perspective on cancer services in Lothian, *Fam Pract* 17(4):323, 2000.

Grunfeld E, Zitzelsberger L, Ciristine M, et al: Job stress and job satisfaction of cancer care workers, *Psychooncology* 14(1):61–69, 2005.

Guthrie C: Nurses' perceptions of sexuality relating to patient care, *J Clin Nurs* 8(3):313–321, 1999.

Hammick M, Tutt A, Tait DM: Knowledge and perception regarding radiation in patients receiving radiotherapy: a qualitative study, *Eur J Cancer Care (Engl)* 7(2):103–112, 1998.

Haylock P: Oncology nursing and professional advocacy. In Yarbro CH, Frogge MH, Goodman M, Groenwald SL, editors: *Cancer nursing: principles and practice*, ed 5, Boston, 2005, Jones and Bartlett, pp 1814–1824.

Hinds C, Moyer A: Support as experienced by patients with cancer during radiotherapy treatments, *J Adv Nurs* 26:371–379, 1997.

International Agency for Research on Cancer (IARC): *IARC handbooks of cancer prevention: Breast Cancer Screening; 7*, Lyon, 2002, IARC Press, pp 100–101.

International Agency for Research on Cancer (IARC): *Tobacco smoking and involuntary smoking*, IARC monographs on the evaluation of carcinogenic risks to humans; 83, Lyon, 2004, IARC.

Karunagaran D, Tzahar E, Beerli RR, et al: ErbB-2 is a common auxiliary subunit of NDF and EGF receptors: implications for breast cancer, *European Molecular Biological Organization* 15(2):254–264, 1996.

Kennedy CM: The work of district nurses: first assessment visits, *J Adv Nurs* 40(6):710–720, 2002.

Koinberg IL, Fridlund B, Engholm GB, Holmberg L: Nurse-led follow-up on demand or by a physician after breast cancer surgery: a randomised study, *Eur J Oncol Nurs* 8(2):109–117, 2004. discussion 118–20.

Kübler-Ross E: *Death, the final stage of growth*, New York, 1973, Prentice Hall.

Magnusson K, Robinson L: The practice base of cancer nursing. In Kearney N, Richardson A, Di Guilio P, editors: *Cancer nursing practice: a textbook for the specialist nurse*, Edinburgh, 2000, Churchill Livingstone, pp 19–38.

Maguire P: Psychosocial interventions to reduce affective disorders in cancer patients: Research priorities, *Psychooncology* 4:113–119, 1995.

Massey CS: A multicentre study to determine the efficacy and patient acceptability of the Paxman scalp cooler to prevent hair loss in patients receiving chemotherapy, *Eur J Oncol Nurs* 8(2):121–130, 2003.

Menon U, Gentry-Maharaj A, Hallett R, et al: Sensitivity and specificity of multimodal and ultrasound screening for ovarian cancer, and stage distribution of detected cancers: results of the prevalence screen of the

UK Collaborative Trial of Ovarian Cancer Screening (UKCTOCS), *Lancet Oncol* 10(4):327–340, 2009.

Miller M, Kearney N: Oral care and patients with cancer: a literature review, *Cancer Nurs* 24(4):241–254, 2001.

Miller M, Kearney N: Chemotherapy-related nausea and vomiting – past reflections, present practice and future management, *Eur J Cancer Care (Engl)* 13:71–81, 2004.

Million Women Study Collaborators: Breast cancer and hormone replacement therapy in the million women study, *Lancet* 362 (9):419–427, 2003.

Mitchell T: The social and emotional toll of chemotherapy – patients' perspectives, *Eur J Cancer Care (Engl)* 16:39–47, 2007.

Moyer A, Levine EG: Clarification of the conceptualization and measurement of denial in psychosocial oncology research, *Ann Behav Med* 20:149–160, 1998.

NHS Cancer Screening Programme: *NHS Bowel Cancer Screening Programme*, Sheffield, 2009a, NHSCSP. Available online http://www.cancerscreening.nhs.uk/bowel/index.html.

NHS Cancer Screening Programme: *Prostate Cancer Risk Management*, Sheffield, 2009b, NHSCSP. Available online http://www.cancerscreening.nhs.uk/prostate/index.html.

NHS Executive: *A policy framework for commissioning cancer services*, London, 1995, DH.

Niven CA, Scott PA: The need for accurate perception and informed judgement in determining the appropriate use of nursing resource: hearing the patient's voice, *Nurs Philos* 4:201–210, 2003.

Pattison J, Macrae K: Home chemotherapy: NHS and independent sector collaboration, *Nurs Times* 98(35):34–35, 2002.

Peto R, Darby S, Deo H, et al: Smoking, smoking cessation and lung cancer in the UK since 1950: combination of national statistics with two case-control studies, *Br Med J* 321:323–329, 2000.

Ross RK, Makridakis NM, Reichard JK, et al: Prostate cancer: epidemiology and molecular endocrinology. In Henderson BE, Pender B, Ross RK, editors: *Hormones, genes and cancer*, Oxford, 2003, Oxford University Press, pp 273–287.

Royal College of Nursing (RCN): *The administration of cytotoxic chemotherapy – clinical practice guidelines. Recommendations*, London, 1998, RCN.

Schmid-Buchi S, Halfens RJG, Dassen T, et al: A review of the psychosocial needs of breast cancer patients and their relatives, *J Clin Nurs* 17(21):2895–2909, 2008.

Schofield P, Butow PN, Thompson JF, et al: Psychological responses of patients receiving a diagnosis of cancer, *Ann Oncol* 14:48–56, 2003.

Scottish Cancer Care Pharmacy Group: *Guidelines for the safe use of cytotoxic chemotherapy in the clinical environment*, Edinburgh, 2000, The Association of Scottish Trust Chief Pharmacists.

Scottish Executive Health Department (SEHD): *Cancer in Scotland: action for change – where we are now*, 2004. Available online http://www.scotland.gov.uk/Publications/2004/05/19344/36946.

Scottish Government: *Better Cancer Care*, 2008. Available online http://www.scotland.gov.uk/Publications/2008/10/24140351/0.

Segnan N, Armardi P, Sancho-Garnier H: Screening. *Evidence-based cancer prevention: strategies for NGOs – a UICC handbook for Europe*, Geneva, 2004, UICC. Available online http://www.uicc.org.

Shaw C: Therapeutic aspects of nutrition in cancer patients. In Souhami R, Tannock I, Hohenberger P, et al, editors: *Oxford textbook of oncology; 1*, Oxford, 2002, Oxford University Press, pp 1007–1016.

Skalla KA, Bakitas M, Furstenberg CT, et al: Patients' need for information about cancer therapy, *Oncol Nurs Forum* 31(2):313–319, 2004.

Slamon DJ, Godolphin W, Jones LA, et al: Studies of the HER-2/neu protooncogene in human breast and ovarian cancer, *Science* 244(4905):707–712, 1989.

Slevin ML, Stubbs L, Plant H, et al: Choices in cancer treatment: comparing the views of patients with cancer with those of doctors, nurses and the general public, *Br Med J* 300:1458–1460, 1990.

Smith JJ: Dynamics of cancer prevention. In Yarbro CH, Frogge MH, Goodman M, Groenwald SL, editors: *Cancer nursing: principles and practice*, ed 6, Boston, 2005, Jones and Bartlett, pp 95–107.

Sobin LH, Wittekind C, editors: *TNM classification of malignant tumours*, ed 6, New York, 2002, Wiley-Liss.

Speck PW: Ethical issues in cancer care. In Webb P, editor: *Oncology for nurses and health care professionals*, ed 2, London, 1988, Harper and Row, pp 36–48.

Spiegel D: Mind matters – group therapy and survival in breast cancer, *N Engl J Med* 345:1747–1768, 2001.

Steven D, Fitch M, Dhaliwal H, et al: Knowledge, attitudes, beliefs and practices regarding breast and cervical cancer screening in selected ethnocultural groups in Northwestern Ontario, *Oncology Nurses Forum* 31(2):305–311, 2004.

Strecher VJ, Rosenstock I: The health belief model. In Glanz K, Lewis F, Rimer B, editors: *Health behaviour and health education*, ed 2, San Francisco, 1997, Jossey-Bass, pp 41–59.

Strong V, Sharpe M, Cull A, et al: Can oncology nurses treat depression? A pilot project, *J Adv Nurs* 46(5):542–548, 2004.

Tschudin V, editor: *Nursing the patient with cancer*, ed 2, Hemel Hempstead, Herts, 1996, Prentice Hall.

Van der Molen B: Relating informational needs to the cancer experience: information as a key coping strategy, *Eur J Cancer Care (Engl)* 8:238–244, 1999.

Werneke U, Earl J, Seydel L, et al: Potential health risks of complementary alternative medicines in cancer patients, *Br J Cancer* 90:408–413, 2004.

Wilkinson S, Gambles M, Roberts A: The essence of cancer care: the impact of training on nurses' ability to communicate effectively, *J Adv Nurs* 40(6):731–738, 2002.

Zabora J, Brintzenhofeszoc K, Curbow B, et al: The prevalence of psychological distress by cancer site, *Psychooncology* 10:19–28, 2001.

Ziegler E, Mason HJ, Baxter P: Occupational exposure to cytotoxic drugs in two UK oncology wards, *Occup Environ Med* 59:608–612, 2002.

FURTHER READING

Baggott CR, Patterson-Kelly P, Fochtman D, et al, editors: *Nursing care of children and adolescents with cancer*, ed 3, London, 2002, Association of Paediatric Oncology Nurses/Saunders.

Brighton D, Wood M: *The Royal Marsden Handbook of Cancer Chemotherapy*, Edinburgh, 2006, Churchill Livingstone.

Brown CG, Wingard J: Clinical consequences of oral mucositis, *Semin Oncol Nurs* 20(1):16–21, 2004.

Calzone KA, Masny A: Genetics and oncology nursing, *Semin Oncol Nurs* 20(3):178–185, 2004.

Coackley A, Hutchinson T, Saltmarsh P, et al: Assessment and management of fatigue in patients with advanced cancer: developing guidelines, *Int J Palliat Nurs* 8(8):381–388, 2002.

Daniel BT, Damato KL, Johnson J: Educational issues in oral care, *Semin Oncol Nurs* 20(1):48–52, 2004.

Department of Health: *Improving Outcomes: A Strategy for Cancer*, London, 2011, DH. Available online http://www.dh.gov/publications/

Dougherty L: *Central venous access devices. Care and Management*, Oxford, 2006, Wiley-Blackwell.

Epstein JB, Schubert MM: Managing pain in mucositis, *Semin Oncol Nurs* 20(1):30–37, 2004.

Faithful S, Wells M: *Supportive care in radiotherapy*, Edinburgh, 2003, Churchill Livingstone.

Gale DM: Molecular targets in cancer therapy, *Semin Oncol Nurs* 19(3):193–205, 2003.

Greco KE, Mahon S: Common hereditary cancer syndromes, *Semin Oncol Nurs* 20(3):164–177, 2004.

Jenkins J: Genomics: offering hope for oncology care, *Semin Oncol Nurs* 20(3):209–212, 2004.

Kwitkowski VE, Daub JR: Clinical applications of genetics in sporadic cancers, *Semin Oncol Nurs* 20(3):155–163, 2004.

Liu K: Breakthroughs in cancer gene therapy, *Semin Oncol Nurs* 19(3):217–226, 2003.

Loud JT, Hutson PS: The art and science of cancer nursing in the genomic era, *Semin Oncol Nurs* 20(3):143–144, 2004.

Lowrey K: Legal and ethical issues in cancer genetics nursing, *Semin Oncol Nurs* 20(3):203–208, 2004.

Martini F, Nath J, editors: *Fundamentals of Anatomy and Physiology*, ed 8, San Francisco, 2009, Pearson Benjamin Cummings.

Mautner B, Huang D: Molecular biology and immunology, *Semin Oncol Nurs* 19(3):154–161, 2003.

Muehlbauer PM, Schwartzentruber DJ: Cancer vaccines, *Semin Oncol Nurs* 19(3):206–216, 2003.

NHS Education Scotland: Spiritual Care: 2009. Available online http://www.nes.scot.nhs.uk/spiritualcare/.

NHS Quality Improvement Scotland: *Best Practice statement; skin care of patients receiving radiotherapy*, 2004. Available online http://www.nhshealthquality.org/nhsqis/files/20373_NHSQISBestPractice.pdf.

Peterson DE, Beck SL, Keefe DMK: Novel therapies, *Semin Oncol Nurs* 20(1):53–58, 2004.

Rieger PT: The biology of cancer genetics, *Semin Oncol Nurs* 20(3):145–154, 2004.

Royal College of Nursing (RCN): *Best practice guidance on radiation protection and the use of radiation protective equipment*, London, 2006, RCN.

Schmidt KV, Wood BA: Trends in cancer therapy: role of monoclonal antibodies, *Semin Oncol Nurs* 19(3):169–179, 2003.

Scott-Brown M, Spence RAJ, Johnston P: *Emergencies in oncology*, Oxford, 2007, Oxford University Press.

Sonis S: Pathobiology of mucositis, *Semin Oncol Nurs* 20(1):11 15, 2004.

Thompson IE, Melia KM, Boyd KM, Horsburgh D: *Nursing ethics*, ed 5, Edinburgh, 2006, Churchill Livingstone.

Tortora GJ, Derrickson B: *Principles of Anatomy and Physiology*, ed 12, New York, 2009, John Wiley & Sons, Inc.

Vadaparampil ST, Permuth-Wey J, Yeomans-Kinney A: Psychosocial aspects of genetic counselling and testing, *Semin Oncol Nurs* 20(3):186–195, 2004.

USEFUL WEBSITES

About the Human Genome Project: www.ornl.gov/sci/techresources/Human_Genome/project/about.shtml

British National Formulary: www.bnf.org.uk

CancerBACUP (now merged with Macmillan Cancer Support): www.cancerbackup.org.uk

CancerHELP UK: www.cancerhelp.org.uk

Cancer Index: www.cancerindex.org

Cancerquest for further biology: www.cancerquest.org/index.cfm?page=3102

Charitable organisation that funds research, prevention/education, counselling and care for cancer patients and their families.

Clearly sets out information on different cancers, lifestyle issues, treatments and prevention.

Cancer research UK: info.cancerresearchuk.org/cancerstats/incidence/commoncancers/ and info.cancerresearchuk.org/healthyliving

European Code Against Cancer (for UK incidence and survival): www.cancercode.org/index.html

Guide to internet resources for cancer; provides over 100 pages and more than 1000 links to cancer-related information that is regularly updated.

Health talk online (2008) lung cancer stories: www.healthtalkonline.org/Cancer/Lung_Cancer

Liverpool Care Pathway for the Dying Patient (LCP): www.mcpcil.org.uk/liverpool_care_pathway

Up-to-date information on cancer symptoms such as anorexia, pain, depression, neutropenia including interventions in their management.

Macmillan Cancer Support: www.macmillan.org.uk

Maggie's Centres: www.maggiescentres.org

Marie Curie Cancer Care: www.mariecurie.org.uk

Multinational association of supportive care in cancer: www.mascc.org

National Cancer Institute (NIC): www.cancer.gov/cancertopics

A US government site with, for example, information about nausea and vomiting:

www.cancer.gov/cancertopics/pdq/supportivecare/nausea/healthprofessional

and oral complications of chemotherapy and head/neck radiation PDQ:

www.cancer.gov/cancertopics/pdq/supportivecare/oralcomplications

National Extravasation Information Service (NEIS): www.extravasation.org.uk/home.html

NHS Cancer Screening Programmes: www.cancerscreening.nhs.uk

Information about cancer screening programmes in England.

Oncology Nursing Society: www.cancersymptoms.org

Provides expert information, advice and publications.

South East Scotland cancer network: www.scan.scot.nhs.uk

Supports all those affected by cancer through provision of information, psychological support, relaxation and stress management in purpose built environments.

Tenovus: www.tenovus.org.uk

World Health Organization: www.who.int/topics/cancer/en

Care and rehabilitation of people with long-term conditions

Erica S. Alabaster

Introduction

Medicine's traditional cure orientation has long influenced health service development, resulting in long-term conditions assuming low priority. In these terms, working with people who had no prospect of full recovery carried little prestige and represented the antithesis of skilled practice. This, and the dominance of acute care provision, is changing. Contemporary drivers, including changes in demography and morbidity, shifting emphasis towards community services and evolving roles, mean that nurses in all settings need to be prepared to care for people who are living with long-term conditions. Those people will be experiencing differing stages of disease processes or injuries, levels of impairment and degrees of disability and a variety of life circumstances.

Developing a long-term condition is life changing, and meeting the challenges of promoting and restoring optimal health among a disparate client group requires a range of knowledge and skills, with those enabling self-management and rehabilitation having particular relevance. Nursing involvement is influenced by diagnostic labelling and the way services are organised but directed by what is meaningful to the individual and interdisciplinary input. The role is, therefore, collaborative and contextual in nature. This context also includes the nature and prevalence of long-term conditions, their impact on personal experience and functioning, and the relationship between individuals, their carers and care agencies. Perhaps the best place to begin is to consider how long-term conditions are defined.

What is a long-term condition?

Although capturing their complexity is difficult, a number of attempts have been made to describe both congenital and acquired conditions that are 'long term and have a profound influence on the lives of sufferers' (Locker 2008). Although the terms 'long-term condition', 'life-long condition', 'chronic disease and 'chronic illness' are often used interchangeably, the way these are applied reveals assumptions about enduring conditions and the individuals who experience them. For example, the seminal North American definition proposed by the Commission on Chronic Illness in the 1950s (cited by Daly 1993) focuses on pathology and identifies chronic illness as being a deviation from the norm. This raises questions as to what constitutes a 'normal' state, as well as suggesting that people with such conditions are 'less than normal'. More recently, Larsen (2009) offered Curtin & Lubkin's (1995) definition to contend that from a nursing perspective: 'Chronic illness is the irreversible presence, accumulation, or latency of disease states or impairments that involve the total human environment for supportive care and self-care, maintenance of function, and prevention of further disability'. This reflects growing interest in person-centredness and attending to the totality of individual circumstances.

Does it matter what we call it?

Terminology

Some definitions of long-term conditions are concerned with disease rather than illness. Distinction can be made between these terms, such that 'disease' is a biomedical conception of abnormality as indicated by its presenting features, whereas 'illness' is the individual's subjective response to feeling unwell. Although it is possible to feel ill without having a disease, and vice versa, 'illness' and 'disease' are not separate phenomena but, rather, operate at different levels of human experience. Their relationship is complex because this depends on the nature and severity of the condition and coexisting psychosocial variables. Long-term conditions are associated with the presence of protracted disease processes or consequences of trauma which are not amenable to treatment, are responsible for impairment or disability and thus have a sustained influence on the individual's functioning and lifestyle.

Biomedical classifications of disease do not necessarily account for the psychological and social consequences of living with a long-term condition. For example, depression experienced in rheumatoid disease might be related to an individual's response to diagnosis and social stress, rather than directly to the severity of their physical problems. The terms 'impairment', 'disability' and 'handicap' are commonly associated with long-term conditions and are used in a variety of ways, whether their definitions are stated explicitly or merely implied. Their use has sociocultural and historical dimensions, is influenced by how disability is viewed in itself and has significant implications which can be illustrated with reference to models of disability.

Models of disability

Models of disability are often represented as opposing medical and social models. The medical model regards disability as a problem which is intrinsic to the person and caused directly by disease, a health condition or trauma. Here, 'impairment' is not only used to describe disturbance in the body's structure and function. It is also seen as responsible for preventing the individual's participation in normal society and, therefore, disabling them. This means that management of disability is diagnosis-related and cure-oriented, led by professionals, and aims either to improve the individual's functional ability to engage in society according to its norms or to make separate (segregated) provision for them. Conversely, the social model is based on the assumption that disability exists where attitudinal or environmental barriers exclude people with impairments from full engagement in mainstream activities. This defines it as a socially created problem which is distinct from and superimposed on impairment. From this standpoint disability can be managed collectively by social action. This seeks to remove and change barriers, whether present though society's intent or omission, and to support individuals in dealing with them (WHO 2001).

There is a danger of seeing the above models as absolutes, for example in judging services simplistically as either focusing on medical intervention or not. The social model arose from the British disability movement and, in characterising disabled people as an oppressed group, has been central to its civil rights agenda. As Shakespeare & Watson (2002) comment, however: 'Most activists concede that behind closed doors they talk about aches and pains and urinary tract infections, even while they deny any relevance of the body while they are out campaigning'.

While the medical model might be criticised for defining people by their impairments and medicalising their lives, the social model arguably downplays the impact impairment has on daily personal experience and that most impairments have some medical implications.

The WHO's (2001) International Classification of Functioning, Disability and Health (ICF) was developed with the intent of synthesising the above models via a bio-psychosocial approach. Its aims included establishing a common language to improve communication between service stakeholders and a framework that would allow international comparison. In so doing, it provides a conceptual basis for defining, measuring and formulating policy for health and disability. Using this gives nurses the potential to understand disability's social, political and cultural dimensions and provides a platform for working collaboratively with disabled people and other health professionals (Kearney & Pryor 2004).

The ICF (WHO 2001) comprises two parts, each being made up of two components. Part One is concerned with functioning and disability, encompassing body structures and functions, activities and participation; Part Two addresses contextual environmental and personal factors. As shown (Figure 32.1), these elements have an interactive and dynamic relationship.

This work supersedes the International Classification of Impairments, Disability and Handicaps (ICIDH) (WHO 1980). The term 'handicap' was then used to describe comparative disadvantage and role loss but is now perceived

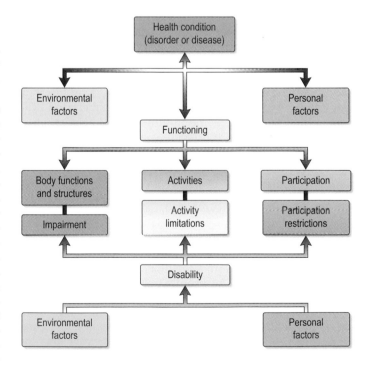

Figure 32.1 Interactions between the components of the international classification of functioning, disability and health. (Adapted from WHO 2001, with permission.)

Box 32.1 Reflection

The impact of language used to describe disability
(see also website)

If you are able-bodied or able-minded, how do you feel about being described as an 'abled' or 'normie'? Think about how this makes you feel about terms you have used to describe disabled people.

as pejorative and generally avoided. In North America, however, the term is used in the same way as 'disabled' is in Britain (e.g. designation of handicap parking spaces).

Disabled people are divided over the use of other collective descriptors of themselves. For example, some choose to use the term 'crip', reclaiming the term 'cripple' in their identity, whereas others feel it offensive. Importantly, being referred to in this way by non-disabled people and without permission is regarded as offensive. Similarly, some disabled people draw distinctions between themselves and those without disability by referring to them as 'AB/AM' (able-bodied/able-minded) or 'normie' (Box 32.1).

Social perceptions of long-term conditions and disability

Lifestyle and blame

Clear associations can be made between aspects of lifestyle and some long-term conditions; for example, smoking is linked with lung cancer, and a diet high in saturated fats with coronary heart disease. Awareness of such relationships might result in individuals being judged to have caused their own disease and suffering. There is also an implication that they have failed to respond to preventive health education campaigns. Attribution of blame has a strong moral influence where links can be alleged between diseases and sexual behaviour, such as that between HIV/AIDS and promiscuity. Beliefs concerning the origin of long-term conditions and disability appear, therefore, to reflect a combination of moral ideology and scientific principles (Box 32.2).

Disability and unemployment

Economic survival in pre-industrial society largely depends on the capacity to engage in physical labour. Individuals restricted by the effects of protracted disease or impairment would thus have a limited function in their social group. This, together with likely dependency on others, could result in the perception that disabled people are of less value than their able-bodied counterparts.

Box 32.2 Reflection

Health behaviours and individual responsibility

Given the association between cigarette advertising and tobacco consumption and that tobacco companies appear to be accepting the addictive nature of their products, can individuals be blamed for their behaviour? What other factors influence personal health choices?

In an industrialised society, however, technological developments and diversification of working practices should create opportunities for those with a wide range of disabilities to gain employment. Nonetheless, disabled people encounter discrimination. One in five people of working age can be defined as disabled, yet 52.6% of disabled people are unemployed and they are three times more likely to be economically inactive than other groups. UK legislation has not fully addressed this because the Disability Discrimination Act (DDA) 1995 and its subsequent amendment (2005) are subject to interpretation while the impact of the Equality Act (2010) remains to be seen. For example, this now prevents employers asking about an applicant's health before offering them work but does allow them to ask questions regarding assessment and need for reasonable adjustment. Also the onus is on individuals to demonstrate that they are disabled under the terms of the Act and assert their rights. Decline in employment rates for disabled people since introduction of the Act could be due to employers' lack of awareness and perceived added costs of recruiting or retaining disabled staff (Bambra & Pope 2007). Thus applicants for posts that match their skills and experience might still not be short-listed, with reasons other than disability used to explain why their profile is not considered appropriate. Some issues around employment will be explored later in this chapter.

Work and the state benefit system

Despite evidence that many economically inactive people with long-term conditions want to work (Disability Rights Commission 2006), some believe instead that they are malingerers who choose not to (Scambler 2008). When this view predominates, programmes for the alleviation of poverty concentrate on reforming attitudes, promoting simplistic models of condition management, implementing workfare-style schemes and subjecting individuals whose impairments are well established to repeated, rigorous testing to 'prove' incapacity (Ravetz 2006). Accessing state benefits is further complicated by their administration, range, difficulty in obtaining definitive information and varying criteria for eligibility. Media representations of the benefits culture and fraudulent claims can leave people with long-term conditions feeling that they are perceived as 'spongers', yet entitlement to some payments assumes an all-or-nothing approach to fitness for work and limits the hours and the time recipients can engage in 'permitted work' without losing their entitlement. This traps individuals into remaining on benefits because it prevents them from testing their capabilities, gaining confidence and accumulating experience to assist in obtaining paid employment.

Stigma

According to Goffman's (1963) seminal text, the word 'stigma' was originally used with reference to visible signs inflicted to brand individuals (including slaves or criminals) unfit for participation in normal social interaction. These signs had moral and judgemental implications, such that the disgrace and shame of the stigma assumed more importance than its physical presence. The stigma attached to a long-term condition relates to deviation from the perceived norm and depends on the body part involved, visibility, controllability and diagnostic labelling. Dependency can also be stigmatising. Reliance on services, state benefits or other people means that individuals with long-term conditions are in a position of receiving without being able to contribute in return. To be labelled with a long-term condition is to be deemed exceptional and, in many cases, marginalised. People in this situation engage in constant efforts to make themselves acceptable and their stigmatising condition often dominates their social identity and relations with others (Box 32.3).

People with less visible conditions such as epilepsy experience 'felt stigma' which increases the stress of managing their condition (Jacoby et al 2005). The problem of constantly concealing part of oneself in order to pass as normal and avoid being found out is added to by difficulties in gauging which details to share with whom, so that relationships can be maintained. Relatives also experience stigma by association and this affects their relationship with the individual and wider society. Cultural and ethnic dimensions also have relevance here, as illustrated by Chadha's (2003) experience of living with multiple sclerosis (MS). Because this is seen by the UK's Asian community as a disorder more likely to be found in the indigenous white population, it left him isolated, misunderstood and 'made to feel that my immediate family and I were responsible'.

Others' behaviour towards people with long-term illness reinforces stigma when they generalise or make assumptions about impairments. For example, they might treat a wheelchair user as if incapable of reasoning, speak loudly to someone with visual impairment or communicate with others accompanying a disabled person rather than to the individual directly. This 'does he take sugar?' approach leaves people feeling less than adult. For example, C, an office administrator

with cerebral palsy, described the public humiliation felt when waiting with a friend at a crowded supermarket checkout. The sales assistant confirmed the purchase with the friend before reluctantly taking C's money and then made a point of handing the friend the bagged items, change and receipt.

Health care workers share society's view of disability. Reflecting this in their interactions with disabled people can compromise effective care (Seccombe 2007). Perceiving disabled people to be dependent or to be pitied gives rise to an approach which gives them a sense of being patronised, demeaned and disempowered, adds to their feelings of inferiority and reduces confidence in the caregiver. Nurses working with people who have long-term conditions will naturally experience a range of emotions when confronted with very real manifestations of human vulnerability. Distancing might provide short-term protection in shielding these emotions but accentuates the space between nurses and stigmatised people.

Public awareness campaigns

Groups have been established to raise awareness of long-term conditions. The amount of popular support they receive depends on how society views the circumstances to which they are related, that is, whether people are likely to have direct experience of a disorder or, in the case of war veterans, if they are associated with controversial campaigns.

Some groups draw attention to specific conditions and their effects. Independent from formal agencies, these organisations function as a resource for people with long-term conditions, their families and professionals, lobby to influence policy, and raise funds for facilities and research. Groups operating without the active participation of affected individuals risk addressing assumed, as opposed to actual, need. In addition, disability activists assert that fundraising events reinforce the notion that an automatic relationship exists between disability and handouts. Members of these groups advocate the principle of 'nothing about us without us' and believe that disabled people should avoid passivity and the socialised dependency that results. Their practice of self-advocacy, use of direct action and insistence upon parity rather than charity contrasts sharply with the conventional image of 'the disabled' as recipients of care.

 See website Critical thinking question 32.1

See website Critical thinking question 32.1

How prevalent are long-term conditions and disability?

The prevalence of long-term conditions and disability is difficult to establish. This is due in part to their inherent interactive, dynamic, multidimensional and subjective natures. Estimates in the UK are also not definitive, given differences in definitions, sampling and data capture. Although separate registers are maintained by local authorities and the Department of Health (DH) for those who are 'sight impaired/partially sighted' or 'severely sight impaired/blind' (see Ch. 13), there is no single register of disabled people and individuals do not have to be registered with local authorities to be defined as disabled or to receive services. In addition,

---

Box 32.3 Reflection

Living with a visible long-term condition

D is 44 years old, is employed as a hotel receptionist and has had psoriasis for some years. He experiences periods of exacerbation and at present his scalp is covered in a thick, hardened layer of scales. When these areas are detached, his scalp surface weeps and becomes painful. Scales are also deposited on his clothing and in his immediate vicinity. D is conscious that people stare and look at his affected skin rather than making eye contact. When his children were small, one of them asked him not to attend a school play and eventually admitted it was due to being embarrassed by his appearance. D thinks that some people think his condition is contagious or caused by poor personal hygiene and believes this explains why bus passengers rarely occupy the space next to him until the vehicle becomes crowded.

D feels that he is managing his problems well. Since his job involves public contact, he has learned to project an outgoing and friendly image which he feels is stronger than the visual impression of the condition. Other people's behaviour still makes him uncomfortable and affects his confidence but he has learned to accept it as something he must live with.

Activity

Reflect on D's sense of stigmatisation. Consider the daily experience of someone with an obvious skin condition. Have you have ever felt embarrassed or uncomfortable when you encountered someone like this? How did you react?

sampling only private households excludes people living in communal establishments, a situation more likely for people severely impaired by long-term conditions. Not all disabled people claim benefits, so capturing data only from recipients of these also provides a limited picture.

Individuals are considered disabled if their situation comes under the Disability Discrimination Act (DDA). This defines the person with disability as having 'a physical or mental impairment which has a substantial and long-term adverse effect on his ability to carry out normal day-to-day activities'.

The DDA 2005 changed the definition of disability so that people with cancer, multiple sclerosis and HIV are covered by its provision automatically from the point of diagnosis, as opposed to when their conditions affect them adversely day to day. Conditions otherwise covered can include cardiac disorders, hearing or sight impairments, significant mobility difficulty, mental health conditions and learning difficulties (Equality and Human Rights Commission 2007). Despite reference to impairment, this definition is, therefore, allied to the medical model. It is possible that individuals with the conditions named might not identify themselves as disabled and be missed from data collection.

Some indication of prevalence can be derived from studies accounting for variables including demography and morbidity but the complexity of this issue is mirrored in a review commissioned by the UK Department of Work and Pensions (DWP). This provides a flow chart for choosing the most appropriate estimate of disability according to purpose, via age grouping and definitions. The latter include health status, capacity for paid work, and coverage under the DDA or the WHO classification mentioned above (Bajekal et al 2004).

Consequences of changing morbidity and mortality

Improvements in public health have almost eradicated some infectious diseases, while others have been largely controlled by vaccination programmes. In addition, infectious diseases are generally amenable to treatment and therefore long-term rather than infectious disease remains the major cause of death and disability (Health Protection Agency [HPA] 2005). However, it must neither be assumed that infection has been eliminated from Western societies nor that long-term conditions cannot be infectious; AIDS is the result of infectious disease, yet to contract it means living with a long-term condition.

Continuing decline in mortality from infectious disease is reflected in an increased expectation of life for all age groups, a trend liable to continue. This has implications for the number of people experiencing long-term conditions and disabilities because the prevalence of these rises with advancing age. Confirmation of this can be found in data from sources such as the UK Census, General Household Survey (GHS) (latterly known as the General LiFestyle Survey or GLF) and Labour Force Survey, all of which use variants of the most widely used method of assessing activity limitation – the self-reported limiting long-term illness (LLTI) or disability question (ONS 2004, 2006). This generally involves asking respondents whether they have any long-standing illness, health problem or disability and whether this limits their activities in any way.

The national picture

In the 2001 Census, an LLTI or disability was reported by 10.86 million people, representing 18.47% of the UK population. Of these, 10.3 million lived in private households and the remainder in communal settings. Rates of LLTI or disability increased steadily with age, though gender differences were relatively small until the age of 60. Just over 10% of males and females aged between 35 and 39 years reported an LLTI, while in the 60–74 age group, 41% of males and 38% of females fell into this category. Rates among those aged over 90 were 69% and 78% respectively. Geographical comparison across the UK shows that England has the lowest rates, with Wales and Northern Ireland having the highest (www.statistics.gov.uk/census).

Census data reveal other social inequalities. Of working people, those connected with routinised occupations were most likely to report LLTIs but prevalence was greatest among economically inactive respondents. Among ethnic groups, Asians have the highest rate of LLTIs at 20%. Rates in those identified as Mixed or Black are both higher than found in the White population, while people of Chinese and other backgrounds have the lowest rate overall.

Census questions have not concerned types of long-term conditions and disabilities experienced or how these limit activities. Although the GHS samples only private households, it asks about the nature of health problems, coding replies according to the International Classification of Disease. Data from the 2002 survey show the prevalence of long-standing illness in children and adults to have risen from 21% to 35% between 1972 and 2002, while LLTIs have increased from 15% to 21% (www.statistics.gov.uk/ghs).

Adults reporting a long-standing illness most frequently identified musculoskeletal, circulatory, respiratory, endocrine, digestive and nervous system disorders. With the exception of skin disorders, prevalence of all conditions rose with advancing age. For example, 7.6% of 16–44-year-olds had a musculoskeletal disorder, compared with 36.3% of those aged 75 and over. The number of conditions identified per person increased similarly, being 1.3 for those aged 16–44 years and 1.8 for those aged 75 years and above. Musculoskeletal, circulatory and respiratory disorders were also the most common limiting conditions, affecting respectively 34%, 19% and 10.5% of respondents with LLTIs.

There is striking similarity between the proportions of men and women experiencing various long-standing conditions, with the following two exceptions among those aged 75 years and over. First, 27% of men stated they had a long-standing musculoskeletal disorder, compared with 42% of their female counterparts. This could be partly due to women's longevity. Secondly, 11% of males identified themselves as suffering from respiratory disease, whereas only 7% of women characterised themselves in the same way. Differences in lifetime smoking behaviour are reflected here, although occupational factors could also be significant (Box 32.4).

Box 32.4 Reflection

Long-term conditions, disability and health

Reflect on what health means to people with long-term conditions or disabilities. Can they be 'healthy'?

The 2002–3 Family Resources Survey (www.statistics.gov.uk/surveys) asked respondents with LLTIs to identify their limitations or disability from eight categories offered. Mobility was most commonly named by over 60%, a similar percentage had difficulty with lifting, carrying or moving objects, and 25% experienced this with manual dexterity. Problems with memory, concentration and learning, continence and communication were less prevalent.

The findings of these surveys support the notion that, while long-term conditions are widespread, only a proportion of those affected might be significantly impaired or disabled. It is, however, important to recognise that the results need to be interpreted in the light of improved diagnostics and treatment leading to an increased number of people being diagnosed and living with long-term conditions than previously. Data are also based on respondents' own assessments; people might not define their illnesses as long-term and older people are liable to under-report limitations because they perceive these to be normal features of ageing.

Features of living with long-term conditions

While prevalence data are helpful in predicting the demand for resources, they give no indication of the impact of long-term conditions on daily life. Overemphasis on diagnosis and disease conceals both the psychosocial problems shared by people living with them and the uniqueness of individual experience. It is only when aware of these that nurses can begin to appreciate the profound effect such conditions have on individuals, relatives/friends and health workers. In their seminal work, Strauss et al (1984) identified seven features of chronic illness and developed a framework to enable its impact to be understood more clearly and empathically (Figure 32.2). This was furthered in the subsequent development of a trajectory model which aimed to give insight into experience over the course of an illness over time (Corbin & Strauss 1991; Figure 32.3). These models are drawn on in the next section of this chapter.

Endurance

The time span of acute illness contrasts markedly with that of long-term conditions. Once treatment is initiated, acute illness is generally resolved within a short period and life is resumed as before, whereas the duration of long-term conditions is indefinite. Their presentation is as varied as the conditions involved. For example, some might be evident at birth, while the onset of others results from injury or occurs over time. Regardless of this, individuals and their families are faced with adjusting life to accommodate the presence, unpredictable course and treatment of something which might be controlled but never cured. Building on Curtin & Lubkin's (1998) metaphor, this can be likened to a stranger arriving at someone's home unexpectedly and announcing that they are taking up permanent residence, regardless of whether there is a vacant spare room.

Although diagnostic labels often come as a relief because they explain symptoms and validate individuals' feelings that

Salient features of chronic illness

- Chronic illnesses are long-term by nature
- Chronic illnesses are uncertain
- Chronic illnesses require proportionately great efforts at palliation
- Chronic illnesses are multiple diseases
- Chronic illnesses are disproportionately intrusive
- Chronic illnesses require a wide variety of ancillary services
- Chronic illnesses are expensive

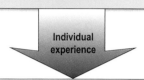

Individual experience

Key problems

Chronic illnesses cause multiple key problems for daily living, including;
- Prevention and management of medical crises
- Control of symptoms
- Carrying out prescribed regimens and management of related problems
- Prevention of, or living with, social isolation
- Adjustment to changes in the course of the disease
- Attempts at normalising interaction with others and style of life
- Funding – finding money to survive partial/complete loss of employment or pay for treatment
- Confronting psychological, marital and familial problems

Basic strategies

- Individuals and families need to develop basic strategies (standard methods or techniques) to manage key problems

Organisational and family arrangements

- Basic strategies require the assistance of others acting as *agents* (family, friends, acquaintances or strangers who act in a rescuing or protective capacity)
- Agents' arrangements must coordinate efforts, understandings and agreements, relying on trust, interactional skill and financial, medical and familial resources

Consequences

- The way organisational and family arrangements are carried out influences how problems are managed, with consequences for individuals and their families

Figure 32.2 Strauss et al's (1984) features of chronic illness and framework for understanding individual experience.

'something isn't right' (Locker 2008), labelling also represents a defining moment in the trajectory from person to patient. For example, after being told he had Addison's disease, one man told of a heightened sense that 'things would never be the same again', while a horse rider who sustained a spinal cord injury in a fall felt this when the trauma team started talking about her transfer to a spinal injuries unit.

Chronic illness trajectory: stages of chronic illness

- Pre-trajectory – before the onset of symptoms and formal diagnosis. Genetic or lifestyle factors for the development of a long-term condition are in place
- Onset – symptoms appear, the diagnosis is made and the individual starts to learn how to manage its implications
- Stable – the individual manages life activities within limitations and symptoms are controlled, with care taking place in the home
- Unstable – symptoms cannot be controlled or the condition reactivates, life is disrupted and the individual experiences difficulty managing activities. Care takes place at home
- Acute – severe, unrelieved symptoms or complications require acute intervention, hospitalisation and temporary reduction or suspension of life activities
- Crisis – a life-threatening episode requiring urgent intervention, with life activities suspended until resolution is achieved
- Comeback – the individual's efforts result in gradual return to relative stability and an acceptable way of life
- Downward – gradual or rapid deterioration, increasing disability and difficulty in managing symptoms
- Dying – the terminal stage where body processes begin to shut down, the individual relinquishes life activities and prepares for death

Figure 32.3 Stages of chronic illness, as featured in the trajectory model. (After Corbin & Strauss 1991 and Ballard 2007.)

Adulthood is a dynamic period usually associated with autonomy and control. It is a time of life in which people expect to nurture others, rather than to be nurtured. The limitations imposed by long-term conditions and need for ongoing care conflict with these expectations and can be damaging to the individual's self-esteem. Accepting help can be difficult enough; however, disabled people can be offered unnecessary assistance based on presumed need and their preferences overlooked. For example, a wheelchair user described wheeling manually through a town centre on her way to meet a friend and suddenly finding herself moving at speed towards a department store. A helpful member of the public had thought this was her destination, decided that it would be easier for her to be pushed, ignored her requests to stop and took her response as a personal rejection: 'I was disoriented and motion sick. But what really got me was they acted like I was ungrateful and being too independent! My chair is part of me – it's the same as pulling their legs out from under them and dragging them off without permission'. Unsurprisingly, some users prefer not to have grab handles on their chairs.

Living with a long-term condition impinges on domestic, work-related and social activities. Experience leads individuals to develop a repertoire of strategies for managing their conditions around these. For instance, when attending events where food and drink are available, some people with diabetes mellitus are guided by their condition, rather than purely by desire. If they do not wish to bring this to wider attention, they might avoid alcoholic drinks on the pretext of wanting to 'keep a clear head'. Conversely, others might learn to alter their insulin injections to allow for indulging in food and drink which they actually prefer. Creative non-adherence (Taylor 2008) to treatment or 'intelligent cheating' is common in long-term conditions. It can result in errors but careful adaptation actually reflects individuals' assertion of control, successful renegotiation of life situations in their own context. Strategies used can require the ongoing assistance of relatives, friends, acquaintances or strangers who might function in various ways to assist in maintaining treatment programmes or protect the individual from harmful effects of the disorder. For example, someone with epilepsy might need help from workmates such that harmful objects are moved should an unexpected seizure occur.

The enduring nature of long-term conditions also results in repeated interaction between individuals and service providers, perhaps over a period of months or years. This leads to individuals becoming familiar with organisations and staff with whom they come into contact, having implications for the development of complex relationships between them. Familiarity helps staff in monitoring self-management and detecting subtle changes in health but can make maintaining social boundaries difficult. Frequent attendance with problems that are vague or irresolvable can also mark patients as unpopular. Individuals might be encouraged to relinquish control to health workers, though this stance is opposed in patient-focused rehabilitative care and by policies emphasising the importance of self-management in long-term conditions (Jester 2007). Depending on the dominant approach in a particular setting, either asserting oneself or passivity can be regarded as resistance to adopting the patient role and result in individuals acquiring a reputation for being 'demanding' or 'difficult'.

Uncertainty

Living with a long-term condition means living with uncertainty. Obtaining a diagnosis is sometimes lengthy and complicated due to the ambiguity of symptoms experienced and insidiousness of onset. Repeated visits to GPs and outpatient clinics might be necessary and people sometimes feel it hard to convince health workers of the legitimacy of their condition. Difficulty in establishing a prognosis is also problematic, since only the progress of the condition itself suggests a likely timescale of events for a particular individual.

Adulthood is associated with the achievement of socially and culturally specified life goals such as leaving the parental home, beginning a career and finding a partner (Schaie & Willis 2001). The restriction, discomfort and possible dependence that accompany long-term conditions may force the individual to forgo these or adopt an alternative lifestyle. Biographical disruption (a term used to describe the way individuals with chronic illness are faced with losing life as lived previously, sense of self in relation to this and their vision of the future) leads to grieving for previously taken-for-granted opportunities and ambitions (Box 32.5).

Fear of dependence, which in itself causes uncertainty, is a fundamental human concern in cultures valuing self-reliance and physical and economic independence. Following diagnosis this problem is shared to an extent by health workers who must decide how much to share regarding the likely course of conditions and difficulties of treatment. Although it is seen as important to provide sufficient information to enable patients to exert maximum control over their situation, staff might question this in situations where only limited solutions can be offered. They might also withhold information to avoid destroying hope, for example when presenting the realistic survival gain of palliative chemotherapy (Audrey et al 2008).

The impact of fluctuation

Fluctuations in symptoms, and energy to manage them, make it impossible to forecast the occurrence of 'good days' and 'bad days' and this is compounded because a 'good day' can turn abruptly into a 'bad day' and vice versa. Uncertainty is also present because many long-term conditions are episodic, involving recurrent unpredictable exacerbations, followed by periods of remission or control. Since the onset and duration of exacerbations cannot be anticipated, individuals and their carers must be vigilant for them and ready to respond at any time. This means that

individuals and their families can find it difficult to maintain continuity or plan their activities ahead and, as a result, cannot participate fully in community life. Friends might, for instance, eventually hesitate to extend invitations when people have repeatedly refused or withdrawn from events. Regret, resentment and social isolation can follow as activities are curtailed (Biordi & Nicolson 2009).

Fluctuation in long-term conditions also influences the way in which individuals perceive themselves and are perceived by others. Crucially, the invisibility of some conditions can cause others to question the reality of their experience and even doubt that it exists. For example, when people comment 'but you look so good for someone who has MS...if they can't see it, there really isn't anything wrong with me' (National Multiple Sclerosis Society 2007), the subtext is 'You can't be sick, you're just faking it' (Anon 2007). This means that the consequences of living with a long-term condition are disregarded. Individuals are believed to be directly affected only when it becomes noticeable, so variation in ability, during a particular day or period of exacerbation, is misunderstood. Nurses lacking knowledge of long-term conditions can be quick to make judgements as to why people could perform activities yesterday but not today or cannot be certain of their capability for tomorrow. This can have harmful consequences. For instance, staff caused an immobile man with Parkinson's disease considerable distress when they implied he was lazy because they had seen him walking previously. He was actually unable to move due to the unpredictable 'on-off effect' associated with his response to long-term medication.

Beneficial effects of uncertainty

Paradoxically, uncertainty in long-term conditions can be perceived positively as an opportunity to reappraise life's possibilities (Bailey et al 2007). Whether of sudden life-changing onset or signalling that changes will occur, diagnosis can prompt individuals to reflect on the way life had been lived and to search for new meaning in exploring events, reprioritising and seeking new challenges. As one person explained: 'If anyone asks, I tell them I wouldn't do away with having had my stroke now. Yes, I'd do away with its problems but I've learned who my real friends are, that I don't want to spend all my waking hours in the office and discovered I can do things I'd never thought of as "me" before too – like disability sport and joining a service users' group'. Uncertainty can also motivate concordance with treatment, since this provides a tool for maintaining some stability.

Palliative emphasis

As the prospect of cure is remote in long-term conditions, measures to improve or maintain quality of life assume primary importance. More emphasis is placed on palliation, i.e. alleviating pain, discomfort and nausea, providing symptomatic relief and addressing problems created by restricted activity. Palliation is of greater significance than in acute illness because people with long-term conditions must live with both the conditions' features and the cumulative side-effects of the treatment. This has other implications: for example, someone taking long-term medication for HIV can experience side-effects including hypercholesterolaemia, cardiac disease and diabetes, all of which are compounded by ageing – something which the treatment itself has enabled the person to do.

Decisions as to which palliative measures are suggested depend on their availability, acceptance by individuals and the medical profession, evidence base, perceived benefit and financial constraints. Improvements in quality of life following palliation are difficult to measure objectively and this has implications for the allocation of resources, as discussed later.

Individuals have considerable personal resources and many use these to try to resolve problems before seeking official help or as an adjunct to it, particularly if these agencies cannot provide palliation or the side-effects of treatment are intolerable. Complementary therapies are used commonly by people who feel that orthodox medicine has nothing further to offer but, in long-term conditions, this also represents assumption of control where it otherwise seems to have been lost. Furthermore, in contrast with conventional care, there is a possibility of accessing person-centred treatments which are inherently pleasurable, providing individuals with the potential for taking responsibility for their well-being in its wider sense and developing skills to manage a range of stressors (Cartwright & Torr 2005). This is important because stress both results from the experience of living with long-term conditions and exacerbates symptoms, being associated with relapse. Mental distress can also lead to the development of anxiety-related and depressive disorders. Stress management is aided by therapies that pay explicit attention to the mind–body relationship, and approaches that mobilise individuals' inner resources, such as mindfulness-based interventions (Kabat-Zinn 2001), are also practised alongside conventional treatment. Management strategies can also be learned through experience and membership of self-help groups.

The UK Government's Expert Patients Programme (EPP) initiative is integral to policies aimed to modernise the NHS. It stems from recognition that traditional cure-oriented services have not dealt comprehensively with problems faced by people with long-term conditions and that partnership enhances self-efficacy (DH 2001a). Consistent with this, EPPs are led by lay people rather than health care professionals. Depending on local health service targets, they can be organised along generic lines or for condition-specific groups, although the latter limits participation and marginalises people with other diagnoses. EPPs aim to increase people's confidence, resourcefulness and control, thereby improving quality of life and reducing service use. Underlying principles are reflected in service development and governance, for example the English National Service Framework (NSF) for long-term (neurological) conditions (DH 2005) and other disorder-specific strategies. Examples of such frameworks for diabetes may be found across the UK (DH 2001b, Scottish Executive 2002, Clinical Resource Efficiency Team [CREST] 2003, Welsh Assembly Government 2003).

Co-morbidity

The systematic and degenerative effects of many long-term conditions mean that the failure of one organ or system leads eventually to the involvement of others. For example,

the complications associated with diabetes mellitus include vascular damage, which might result in renal and visual impairment, and an increased risk of myocardial infarction. Impaired circulation to the lower limbs also predisposes to the development of gangrene, the onset of which is, in turn, influenced by degeneration of the nervous system and greater susceptibility to infection (Crumbie 2002a). Amputation of an affected limb leads to further alteration of physical, psychological and social functioning. Clearly, the effects of long-term conditions are compounded by the consequences of treatment used. Efforts to adjust to reduced activity are also complicated by multiplication of symptoms and resulting impairment. For example, chronic pain both inhibits movement and correlates with atrophy in the brain's prefrontal cortex, which impairs decision making.

Since contemporary medical services are organised by area of specialisation, people in this situation require referral to physicians in diabetes and renal medicine, an ophthalmologist and a vascular surgeon. Defining specialists' boundaries and intra-service communication are not always straightforward, so individuals have difficulty in identifying from whom to seek advice for different aspects of their condition and whose recommendations should take precedence at any one time.

To be confronted with the inevitability of deterioration is a substantial psychological challenge to individuals and their carers. Those fearing the prospect of total disability might regard any development of their condition with anxiety and anger, directing these emotions towards others. Carers are faced with difficulties in dealing with this, at the same time as they face increased demands to compensate for the individual's failing abilities. These demands may include seeking information about services, learning new skills and accommodating more physical activity when managing care. This has considerable impact because care giving is carried out in the context of other competing domestic and work-related activities.

Health care professionals can be perceived as being incapable of resolving certain issues or, in the case of problems arising from treatment, as actually responsible for them. This has obvious implications for the quality of nurse–patient relationships, which to be genuinely therapeutic must be characterised by mutual trust and cooperation (Box 32.6).

Intrusiveness

A significant aspect of living with long-term conditions is the 'daily grind' of monitoring and managing their features (Locker 2008). Such work is unrewarding, unrelenting and inescapable. As someone with chronic fatigue syndrome (CFS) explained: 'For one wonderful moment when you wake up you forget. But there it is. Again. Any novelty around pills and things has gone and there's no time off'. Becoming accustomed to this is challenging because it involves a fundamental shift from the former self and life towards recognition and acceptance of a 'new normal' (Fennell 2003).

Loss, grief and adaptation

Grief experienced in long-term conditions resembles that in bereavement. It can be associated with loss of a body part, image, function, social status or role and can occur suddenly

Box 32.6 Reflection

Different approaches to managing a long-term condition

Until recently L, a 60-year-old who has COPD (chronic obstructive pulmonary disease), was making progress in managing his condition but he had recently been under pressure at work and become depressed. He was reluctant to disclose his feelings to his GP but was reassured to be received positively and told that commonly prescribed medication should help. L added this to his drug regimen; however, he was distressed to find he was gaining weight and now had sexual dysfunction. These developments deepened L's sense of hopelessness; he felt a failure and related stress exacerbated his dyspnoea.

L began to fear what might happen next and his trust in the health care team was badly shaken. This was underlined when, during his next GP visit, the issues seemed to be put down to his mental ill-health and the importance of its continued treatment was emphasised. The consultation was short and it seemed to L as though he was expected to comply with what was deemed to be in his best interests without any discussion or acknowledgement that, from his perspective, the side-effects of treatment were making his situation much worse.

Despite having lost motivation to attend, L decided to keep his forthcoming appointment with the practice nurse at the COPD clinic. This was because, while other health care team members seemed to be 'always on at him' about condition management, her previous approach to his smoking cessation had involved listening without judgement to difficulties he was having, identifying his personal barriers and considering pros and cons around genuinely realistic solutions. L reasoned that it would be easier to explain to her that this experience was more than he could tolerate and to ask about other treatment options.

Activities

Reflecting on L's circumstances:

- Why should people be aware of both the benefits and drawbacks of treatment?
- What could happen to an individual's long-term condition management if they are unable to share their views with the health care team?
- Identify why L perceived his relationship with the nurse positively. You could think about organisational issues such as availability and continuity, together with attributes such as knowledge of long-term conditions, being open to patients' insights, skilled interaction, developing rapport and demonstrating empathy.

when a long-term condition is acquired or over time as it progresses. People can also experience loss of identity because it reflects their previous, non-impaired self and they feel they have become less of a person than they were. Awareness of models of grief or response towards threat to self-integrity (e.g. Kubler-Ross 1969 and Morse 1997 respectively) guides nurses in supporting individuals to work towards adaptation to unwanted change. However, care must be taken not to apply these prescriptively because personal reactions differ. Falvo (2008) identifies a general path beginning with shock, numbness and disbelief, when the diagnosis or the severity of the condition is denied. This is followed by acknowledgement of the situation's reality, when grief intensifies. Continued exposure to the loss can

lead individuals to adjust and come to emotional acceptance but this is not guaranteed. The process is painful, unpredictable and fluctuates in their struggle to manage the powerful reactions created, as shown in Rushby-Smith's (2008, p. 210) thoughts on life after spinal cord injury. 'For most of the day I'm in pain. I get frustrated that I can't reach things, climb things, negotiate stairs, step over things, bounce my daughter on my knee [...] At the end of every day I am filled with a mixture of rage and utter debilitating terror, as I struggle to accept that this is me this is happening to, and that I will never get back my life as I knew it.'

For some, grief remains unresolved and can be more disabling than the condition itself. Here, it is essential for nurses to recognise the meaning of what has been lost and understand that addressing this is key to renewing self-identity (Telford et al 2006). Again, this means considering bio-psychosocial issues beyond diagnostic labels and accounting for other health problems present. For example, following traumatic injury, a researcher adjusted to physical impairment with relative ease but had difficulty in accepting the continuing impact of a stress-related anxiety disorder. He felt profoundly diminished by the realisation that his hard-worked-for career would not progress as planned, having to regard as a real achievement the completion of workplace activities he previously undertook without thinking and depending on his partner for reminders about household tasks. This was compounded by a nurse saying he was fortunate: 'but my ability to rely on my mental sharpness and function under pressure is important – it's who I am. I just can't get past that. I feel like a champion runner who battles daily to stumble round the block and is expected to be grateful for it'.

It can be seen from this that adaptation is complicated, particularly because 'good' adaptation is judged by others. The emotional burden involved can be increased by shame and guilt at failing to recover or adjust as quickly as expected. Health workers need to bear this in mind if attempting to encourage individuals by comparing them with others who have adapted successfully despite being 'worse off', for instance having shorter life expectancy or being socio-economically disadvantaged. Creating artificial hierarchies of suffering and invalidating someone's experience are unhelpful. Although it is not truly possible to walk in another's shoes, trying to understand the person's own perspective is paramount. Individuals can feel responsible for not doing better, in the light of images of disabled people as 'brave' with an innate capacity to tolerate adversity, or assumptions that they must simply adjust to the obvious. Pressure can be added where media portrayals of triumph over tragedy create models of behaviour which individuals feel they must live up to. As someone with lymphatic cancer recalled: 'Everything and everyone, everywhere, tells you to think positively. So, when a tumour came back I thought it was my fault. I hadn't thought positively enough'.

Others can also compound feelings of difference. Disabled people are commonly treated as if public property, being subjected to staring and unsolicited comments. This can be shocking when acquiring a long-term condition. For example, one person described her eagerly awaited first post-stroke holiday being ruined when passers-by overtook her moving slowly up a station stairway and observed loudly 'People like that shouldn't be allowed out'. Questions such as 'What's wrong with you?' and 'Why are you using that stick?' are invasions of privacy, yet strangers and acquaintances feel justified in posing them out of apparent interest. Their persistence can make individuals feel obliged to explain their situations, even though this involves revealing intimate details. Reacting assertively to nosiness or society's exclusion results in blame being handed back to the disabled person and labelling them pejoratively as a 'crip with a chip'.

In acute illness it is feasible and acceptable to gain temporary exemption from normal social obligations; however, this is not always possible for people with long-term conditions. Parson's (1951) conceptualisation of the sick role makes sense of illness as a social state, but its applicability is questionable in this context, since it implies a duty to recover. The sick role does, however, grant medically mediated access to services and explains why the concordance of people with long-term illness with treatment is expected in the same way as those who are acutely ill (Field & Kelly 2007).

Impact on home life and relationships

Long-term conditions often impose changes to normal domestic routines to allow for physical limitations and the sustained requirements of treatment programmes. Structural alteration of housing might also be required to install equipment and reassign room space for access to facilities. These adaptations, together with alterations in appearance and behaviour associated with the condition, will impact on other members of the household. Families' daily activities are often centred on supporting individuals and it might not possible for them to pursue interests they once enjoyed together. Providing ongoing care changes relationships and compels those who have assumed an unexpected caring role to make fundamental changes to their lifestyle. The strategies used to manage conditions can have implications for everyone taking part. For example, the paced schedule of activities that enables people with COPD to accommodate oxygen deprivation and recovery times between tasks may give little opportunity for flexibility. Previously taken for granted events, such as visits to the hairdresser, can disrupt well-established routines and individuals and carers are faced with developing a lifestyle structured by the demands of the presenting condition, within which spontaneity has no place.

Adopting the roles of carer and cared for also impacts on established relationships. For example, it can be difficult for a disabled person to blend the role of partner with that of someone now needing support to manage incontinence from the other in a relationship. Marriott's (2009) insight into the all-consuming consequences of caring for a partner with Huntington's disease and the 'emotional whirlpool' entered into, is helpful in illuminating the resulting stresses, for instance the conflict experienced when carers sense that their lives are no longer their own but think themselves selfish to resent this (Box 32.7).

Legislation emphasises the importance of recognising informal carers as partners in the care process, for example entitlement to a separate needs assessment. However, this has not yet been translated into practice due to failure to offer assessments, confusion as to who is responsible for conducting them, ineffective recording of needs, subjective interpretation of eligibility for support and insensitivity to the demands of their role and relationship with the cared

for (Seddon et al 2007). Carers experience considerable difficulty in navigating though convoluted support systems administered by local and central government, seeing the care reform agenda as presenting bureaucratic and financial hurdles rather than aiding them in their role. Dealing with this is stressful and demands resources which, by nature of their activities, carers simply do not have.

Financial and employment issues

Long-term conditions also have economic implications. Even if the person is not totally incapacitated, continued employment might be impossible because of the demands that disorders and their treatment make on time, strength and stamina. Difficulty in adhering to work schedules and non-attendance during exacerbations can give the impression that individuals are unreliable, while employers' inclusion of related absences in cumulative records of sick leave and offering incentives to reward low absenteeism disadvantages disabled people. Individuals might also be assigned less demanding roles and be overlooked for training or promotion because they are perceived to have limited potential, so are not deserving of the investment (Taylor 2008). Gaining employment is problematic in itself; employers may see the prospect of incapacity and variable function as risk and hidden costs, including lost production and redeployment of other workers.

It is understandable that, despite there being advantages in disclosing health status to an employer, people with long-term conditions are often reluctant to do so. Disclosure affects their workplace identity, as in the case of a woman who maintained silence for 8 years to avoid being 'stuck with the MS label, to become Sukie with MS as opposed to just Sukie' (Freeman 2002). It can also lead to an individual's competence being doubted, reduces self-esteem and gives rise to guilt and fear of letting others down. This can result in individuals working harder than others to prove their worth when the effort needed to manage their conditions means that their energy margins are already tight. Employers do not always recognise the implications of this or of the 'reasonable adjustments' required by the DDA. For example, someone who had explained their concentration and fatigue issues to their employer still found themselves expected to attend meetings held towards the end of the working day. These inevitably over-ran and left them exhausted. Having to remind their employer of this and focus repeatedly on what they could not do was difficult enough; however, the solution offered was not to begin meetings at differing times to meet everyone's needs but that the individual should leave on time. This meant drawing attention to themselves by departing during business and inviting those unaware of their condition to question their commitment to work.

Effect on social activities

Long-term conditions affect the ability to participate in social activities. The impact of this depends in part on the strategies people use to deal with the features of their disorder. For example, urgent, frequent episodes of diarrhoea, soiling clothes and odour are major social concerns for people with ulcerative colitis (National Association for Colitis and

Box 32.7 Evidence-based practice

Informal caring – the impact of supporting people with long-term conditions

The Office for National Statistics (ONS 2002) used data from the GHS (see p. 827) to explore trends in care-giving. For the purpose of the survey 'carers' were defined as individuals who looked after or provided a regular service for sick, disabled or older people living in their own or another household. The following are among the results:

- Twenty-one per cent of households contained a carer.
- Women were more likely to be carers than men – 18%, compared with 14%.
- Eight per cent of 16–29-year-olds have caring responsibilities, compared with 24% of those aged 45–64 and 16% of people of 65 and above.
- Carers included 13% of adults in full-time work, 17% in part-time work and 15% of unemployed people.
- Almost a third of married or cohabiting women aged 45–64 were carers.
- A third of carers were the only support for the main person cared for.
- Twenty-eight per cent of carers spent at least 20 hours a week on their caring responsibilities, while 1% spent 50 hours or more.
- Half of those spending 20 hours or more on caring weekly were looking after someone needing constant attention and who could not be left for a few hours.
- Thirty-five per cent of those devoting at least 20 hours per week to caring reported an LLTI, rising to 47% among older carers.
- Thirty-nine per cent reported that their physical and mental health had been affected as a result of caring.
- Twenty per cent of carers reported feeling tired, 20% experienced stress, 17% were short-tempered, 14% felt depressed and 14% had disturbed sleep.

A report by Carers UK and the University of Leeds (Buckner & Yeandle 2007) added to this by using an actuarial formula to demonstrate that the replacement cost of unpaid care would be £87.01 billion per year, representing £15 260 per carer. However, in the UK, the Carer's Allowance remains lower than other working age benefits and is less than the minimum wage, at £53.10 per week for people providing at least 35 hours of support (carers are eligible if aged 16 or over and the person cared for receives certain benefits but not if the carer is in full-time education with 21 hours or more a week of supervised study or earns more than £95 a week after certain deductions have been made; Carer's Allowance can also be reduced by the amount of some other benefits received). The report contains recommendations for policy measures to ensure that carers' value is recognised.

References

Buckner L, Yeandle S: *Valuing carers – calculating the value of unpaid care*. London, 2007, Carers UK.

Office for National Statistics: *Carers 2000*. London, 2002, TSO.

Activities

- Access the reports to discover more about the extent and nature of care-giving.
- Consider how data like these help you to appreciate the experience of long-term conditions from the carers' perspective and why some people might assume and continue the caring role, despite its impact.

Your answer could include issues such as:

- Research of this nature can provide a means of accessing information about the experience of an otherwise hidden group. By their very nature, caring activities are liable to take place behind closed doors.
- Collated data build a picture of carers' diversity, revealing shared characteristics and differences and reveal the pervasive implications caring has for the quality of their lives.
- Learning about the demands of caring can assist others to appreciate which forms of support might be helpful in a given situation.
- Assumption of the caring role can be associated with an extension of an existing relationship, love or emotional attachment, reciprocity (e.g. a child taking on the role of caring for their parent), moral or social obligation, desire to help, concern for the well-being of another individual, expectation or preferred option of the cared for, expectation of others (e.g. health workers may expect someone to care for a partner), being accustomed to caring and not having considered doing otherwise, aiming to prevent the cared for from being admitted to a long-term care facility.

Crohn's Disease 2008). Individuals may respond by withdrawing from interaction or planning outings carefully, using known venues with accessible toilets and using a 'Can't wait' flashcard to alert others to their needs. Some people might resort to avoiding intimate relationships because anxiety regarding possible faecal incontinence or emission of flatus during sexual activity makes relaxation difficult. Others learn to institute strategies such as keeping unobtrusive towels at the bedside, behaving spontaneously to lessen anticipatory fear or increasing their sense of control through tactical use of prescribed anti-diarrhoeals.

Complex service use

An abundance of statutory, voluntary and independent agencies are concerned with supporting people with long-term conditions in the UK. The NHS, the Department of Work and Pensions (DWP) and local authority social services are principal sources of statutory support. Provision can be fragmented due to the number of medical specialities and personnel involved, ineffective interagency coordination, differing access criteria and service targets. Transfers between care settings or the UK's administrative areas can add to this. For example, where an individual's relocation means that they cross regional boundaries and move into an area administered by another agency, it is likely that they will have to make a new application for services or equipment that they received previously. There is a risk of refusal if their needs are deemed inconsistent with priorities in the new locality and can have a detrimental effect on independence and quality of life.

Definitions used by formal agencies to categorise individuals and allocate resources lack compatibility with disabled people's experience. For example, assessment to determine eligibility for benefits and services might fail to acknowledge that long-term conditions fluctuate. If assessed during a period of relative wellness, the type and level of support required at other times might not be apparent. Some benefit claim forms acknowledge this but completing them can be dispiriting because their lengthy 'I need help with...' approach throws what individuals cannot do into sharp focus. This also discourages claims from those who are able to perform activities to some degree but with considerable difficulty, for example being able to prepare a simple main meal independently even though problems with manual dexterity, pain, fatigue and managing spillages mean this takes several hours. The situation is compounded by having to reapply for benefits when only time-limited awards are made, despite the well-established existence of a long-term condition.

People might avoid seeking support because they perceive the organisation of services to be complex and arbitrary or fear that this could trigger state interference in their lives, whereas appealing against the refusal of awards requires energy which individuals might not have. Ineffective communication presents an obstacle when those entitled to benefits lack information or have difficulty interpreting the information given. In addition, some people might be reluctant to seek or accept help because to do so would conflict with cultural values regarding responsibility and self-sufficiency.

Systems for care delivery are complex, with variation across the UK. Cross-party commitment to the concept of community care since the 1960s has been formalised in legislation and is a feature of central government's modernisation agenda. The latter also aims to improve interagency working, so that integrated health and social care is user focused (DH 1998a,b, 2001c). This reflects trends towards casting the service user as consumer. Key reforms implemented from the 1990s include splitting the commissioning and provision of care and dominance of the market by the independent and voluntary sectors. Related initiatives, including the introduction of shared health and social assessments, have enabled the development of creative and flexible care packages. In addition, social care proposals favour more personalised care via the provision of individual budgets which would pool resources from local authority and DWP funding steams, allowing people to purchase according to their needs (Glendinning & Means 2006).

The responses of many agencies remain ineffective, however, due to differences in priorities and practices, as exemplified in the provision of 'free' nursing, personal and continuing care in care home and domestic settings across the UK. Funding of health and social care are devolved functions but varying degrees of devolution have resulted in diversity (Community Care and Health [Scotland] Act 2002, Northern Ireland Assembly 2002, Welsh Assembly Government [WAG] 2007, DHI 2007).

Differing practices have significant implications for quality of life. For example, giving priority to individuals who have complex needs and are at risk of admission to institutional care means withdrawing low-level support from others who, in turn, become more dependent on their informal carers. An emphasis on personal or physical care also results in classifying social needs as lesser wants (Means et al 2003). Carers might accept this because they take caring as the natural order of things and it is expected that they have assumed the role willingly. People with long-term

conditions and their families may not, therefore, receive the support that they believe would be of greatest help to them. This is liable to result in involuntary social isolation affecting individuals and their close associates (Biordi & Nicolson 2009).

Strategies adopted to manage an individual's problems also require the coordinated effort of everyone involved. The establishment and maintenance of arrangements relies on trust, skilled interaction, sufficient resources and realistic negotiation of the roles, responsibilities and expectations of all concerned. This does not only apply to formal care. Someone whose mobility is severely limited, for instance due to long-standing arthritis, might have an array of relatives and friends to do shopping, pick up drug prescriptions, change light bulbs or batteries and walk their dog. The continued success of this depends on each person involved having a clear appreciation of what actually is required, as well as an understanding of their own contribution to the individual's chain of support.

Intensive use of resources

The direct and indirect costs of long-term conditions are high. While expensive technological intervention is not always required, monitoring the effectiveness of treatment and rehabilitation programmes involves regular encounters with members of health care teams and ongoing input intensifies as disorders progress or complications arise. Long-term medication to control or palliate symptoms has significant financial and ethical implications. Rationing of health care has become more explicit in the face of growing demand and the increased availability of treatment options, coupled with pressure to reduce expenditure (Terry 2007). Limited resources mean that decisions are concerned with identifying the potential benefit to individuals and justifying whether such expenditure on a single patient is warranted or making population-based cost:benefit calculations, for example per quality adjusted life year (QALY). The latter approach has, however, been criticised for discriminating against people with long-term conditions and older individuals whose life expectancy is by definition limited, and where quality of life measures 'perfect health' rather than what it means to individuals against the background of their specific life circumstances (Box 32.8).

Additional medications can be required as long-term conditions evolve and to compensate for side-effects of treatment or medication already prescribed. Changes in treatment can

Box 32.8 Reflection

Ethical issues and resource allocation

Where resources are limited, it could be argued that efforts should be directed towards patients for whom improvement can be assured, rather than those who have long-term conditions or are disabled.

Activities

• Using ethical principles to underpin your thinking, reflect on why patients with long-term conditions should be given equal or priority consideration.

also be initiated by relapse. Repeated hospital admissions and the increased use of support services during such times is a source of considerable expense. Interdisciplinary involvement is essential in view of the effect long-term conditions have on all aspects of individuals' lives. Cost containment in health care has reduced the length of acute hospital stays; however, the presence of acute illness superimposed on a long-term condition inevitably results in a longer stay or more intensive home care. As indicated above, the cost of long-term conditions in comparison with that of acute illness is very high in respect of lost employment, reliance on state benefits and social exclusion.

Treatment intended to inhibit the development of conditions, but which does not necessarily cure or save lives, can be costly. Expenditure can be difficult to justify where outlay is high, interventions are controversial and outcomes uncertain. Attempts have been made to address this. For example, individuals with either relapsing–remitting MS (a pattern of disease characterised by at least two attacks of neurological dysfunction over the preceding 2-year period followed by complete or incomplete recovery) or relapse-dominant secondary progressive MS (where function decreases progressively after an initial relapsing–remitting course) can be prescribed disease-modifying drugs. These might decrease the frequency of relapses and prevent the accumulation of neurological damage but are also expensive. The UK's health departments responded by implementing the first NHS risk-sharing scheme, the aims of which are to obtain treatment cost-effectively and appraise its long-term clinical impact.

This scheme involves prescribing the drugs to a cohort of patients who meet defined criteria and monitoring their disease progression over 10 years. Annual treatment costs are estimated at £50 million but prices paid to the pharmaceutical companies depend on whether the patients benefit, with adjustments being made at intervals. This means that, if benefit equates to or exceeds expectations, the NHS makes payments at fixed rates. However, should outcomes fall short of targets, payments are reduced using a sliding scale to achieve an agreed average cost per QALY of no more than £36 000 for the remainder of the scheme (DH 2002). Criticisms of the scheme include its lack of a robust scientific approach towards gathering and evaluating data, reliance on existing NHS funding, reducing resources available for use elsewhere, and the idea that associated activity can be absorbed by the existing service without compromising patient care (Sudlow & Counsell 2003).

Clinical governance

Clinical governance should aid people with long-term conditions by eradicating inequalities in care and raising standards, although frameworks and working practices differ among UK countries (Department of Health, Social Services and Public Safety Northern Ireland [DHSSPSNI] 2006, NHS Quality Improvement Scotland 2007, NHS Clinical Governance Support Team [CGST] 2008, WAG 2008). The Care Quality Commission, which replaced the Healthcare Commission in 2009, carries out clinical governance reviews in England and some related activities in Wales, alongside the Healthcare Inspectorate Wales (HIW), while NHS Quality Improvement Scotland and the Regulation and Quality

Improvement Authority (RQIA) review the quality of services in Scotland and Northern Ireland respectively. These bodies review implementation of NSFs and guidance from the National Institute for Health and Clinical Excellence (NICE), with contextual advice as appropriate from the Scottish Intercollegiate Guidelines Network (SIGN) and the DHSSPSNI (NICE 2007). NICE recommendations are intended to inform professionals' decisions without overriding patients' individual circumstances. The extended time taken to appraise some treatments has, however, been criticised. For example, delays in implementing a UK-wide risk-sharing scheme for beta-interferon use in MS (see above) resulted in prolonging the 'postcode lottery' and frustrated individuals who feared that progression of their symptoms in the meantime would disqualify them from prescription. Balancing the interests of stakeholders, including doctors, the pharmaceutical industry and self-help groups lobbying for access to treatment, is a complex process.

Nursing management and health promotion

Location and management of care

Government policy in the UK reflects the imperative that improving services in this area involves more than simply treating the clinical features of long-term conditions and is 'about delivering personalised, responsive, holistic care in the full context of how people live their lives [...] evidence compels us to do this' (Colin-Thomé 2008, p. 5). Nurses encounter adults with long-term conditions in a range of community and institutional settings including the person's own home, care homes and hospitals providing acute, rehabilitative, intermediate or continuing care. Statutory and other agencies have responded to the shift towards user-focussed community care by attempting to meet rising demand, while accounting for the shortcomings of long-term institutionalisation. Home-based care is viewed as resource effective, while also being preferable for and preferred by individuals. Community nursing is essential to this and visits can continue over many years. Carers' needs have not always been a focus of intervention in this setting; however, changes have resulted in nurses acting as co-experts with them. In addition, NHS reforms across the UK are diverting resources towards primary care and nurses' involvement with long-term conditions, providing a platform for promoting health and working with family units in this setting.

Intermediate care, reablement teams, telehealth and telecare initiatives support this home-based approach. For example, reablement teams provide intensive time-limited intervention to assist people in regaining skills and independence on return home from hospital or residential care. Telecare offers automated remote or enhanced service delivery via telephone or internet-based systems and has wide-ranging uses. These include safety monitoring, medication reminders, providing access to information, asking individuals questions to check and improve their knowledge of self-management and collecting physiological data (Brownsell 2008). The latter can involve sending data from devices such as pulse oximetry or blood glucose monitors to a central server, where they are compared against patient norms and clinicians alerted if needed. Importantly, ongoing data capture also enables the effects of treatment and lifestyle changes to be monitored over time.

People with long-term conditions have diverse needs which sometimes cross, or fall between, traditional service boundaries, resulting in inappropriate and uneven provision. This is being addressed in part by the introduction of Single (England and Northern Ireland), Unified (Wales) and Single Shared (Scotland) assessment processes. The introduction of nurse-led case management aims to use a whole systems approach in providing proactive, coordinated care for people with complex health and social needs. This involves identifying those most at risk of repeated unplanned hospital admission and using intensive home-based care preventively or to aid them to return home more quickly and improve quality of life. To achieve this, nurses working as community matrons or case managers need to work collaboratively with other primary, acute, mental health and social care providers (DH 2008).

Moving into a care home can be perceived negatively as a last resort but can come as a relief when, for instance, someone is unable to maintain their desired lifestyle, an inflexible care package is in place or services no longer meet their needs. As one man with motor neurone disease (MND) put it: 'things just got too much, my home wasn't really mine. I'd lost count of the number of care workers who'd been in my underwear drawer or gone upstairs without asking and didn't want to count any more'. Nurses have an important role in supporting individuals and their carers in considering options, adjusting to new environments, grieving for their past life and constructing a future (Jarrett 2003), such that they feel 'at home' in every sense and consider theirs a place for living. The quality of daily life in care homes depends on whether staff recognise residents' adult status, enable them to maintain a sense of identity, exercise choice and avoid socialised dependency, help them to preserve links with the wider social world, provide opportunities for meaningful activity and involve them in decision making about their community (Owen & NCHRDF 2006). This should be enhanced by the introduction of standards for care homes (e.g. DH 2003a,b, WAG 2004, Scottish Government 2007) which are, arguably, more stringent than those applied to statutory agencies. Issues around implementing these standards, securing fees for residents reliant on state funding and the low returns such arrangements offer to care homes have, however, resulted in the closure of some establishments. This has reduced choice for those seeking places and delayed admissions from home or hospital, presenting nurses with additional challenges in supporting individuals and their carers through what can be a difficult life transition.

Service contact with people who have long-term conditions can occur intermittently and recurrently in relation to establishing diagnoses, managing exacerbation or when conditions necessitate rehabilitation, stabilisation or palliation. It is also important to remember that it might result from the development of unrelated health problems: so, for example, nurses working in an ambulatory care unit will need to adapt their approach to care for someone with an acquired brain injury who has been admitted for laparoscopic surgery. Likewise, practice nurses will need to consider how cervical cytology screening can be made accessible for disabled women who are unable to adopt the customary position on the couch.

Care management in the form of integrated care pathways (ICPs) has particular relevance in long-term conditions because these present a structured means of planning and delivering coordinated, patient-oriented care as part of a sequential journey, instead of as a series of separate episodes. There is, however, a danger that rigid adherence to protocols may actually prevent individuals having a say in their treatment (Hunter 2000). In addition, evidence supporting the use of ICPs in rehabilitation is equivocal. Although they have value in the acute phase of long-term conditions, for example by ensuring that appropriate interventions are delivered in a timely manner, ICPs have less to offer where recovery is variable or unpredictable. ICPs may also have a limited role in dedicated rehabilitation units, since their well-established processes of interdisciplinary and team working are more adaptable, are supported by shared values and have greater capacity to address fully patients' and carers' diverse bio-psychosocial needs (Kalra & Langhorne 2007, Allen et al 2009).

What is rehabilitation?

Definitions of rehabilitation vary, in line with its perceived purpose, but it is best described as an ongoing process that begins as soon as individuals are clinically stable, is independent of the location of care, reflects a transferable underpinning philosophy and involves shifting degrees and forms of support. This means that rehabilitation takes place wherever the patient is (and not on the ward next door, the unit downstairs or in the hospital across town). As a 'person-centred, active and creative process that involves adaptation to changes in life circumstances' and 'a shared activity between the...person, people close to them, and multiprofessional teams who recognise the contribution of all concerned' (Royal College of Nursing [RCN] 2000), rehabilitation has clear significance for long-term conditions. It should be recognised, however, that individuals require rehabilitation in relation to:

- recovery from acute conditions, e.g. straightforward traumatic injury
- recovery from surgical intervention, e.g. hysterectomy for menorrhagia
- long-term conditions with acute onset, e.g. myocardial infarction, stroke, spinal cord injury, traumatic amputation and some cancers
- long-term conditions with gradual onset and a relapsing–remitting or progressive course, e.g. MS, osteoarthritis and some cancers.

Rehabilitation is frequently associated with 'restoration' but, as can be seen from the discussion above, this does not necessarily equate with returning someone to their former life. Rather, it implies enabling individuals to acquire the knowledge and skills needed for optimal bio-psychosocial functioning, so that they can manage their impairments and reconstruct their lives. This requires an approach that embraces autonomy, independence, empowerment, problem-solving and learning because taking a purely functional view can fail to address the qualitative aspects of living with impairment. For example, Oakley's (2007, pp. 91–92) account of the long-term neurological consequences of her injured arm demonstrates that the medical team were satisfied with the motor function but were indifferent to the impact of sensory loss – she could not feel her limb and was unaware of where it was: 'Restoration of function is what counts [...] They looked at my arm and my hand, and assessed the function of them both, according to their own "objective" tests, but they never inquired what they felt like to me or what it was like to live in a body with these disabilities'.

Similarly, some people find it hard to understand why care teams persist in promoting walking as a functional goal when they feel they no longer have the stamina required and that, far from being an indication of failure, wheelchair use would actually improve their mobility and provide a sense of liberation through increasing independence and reducing pain.

The rehabilitative process

The principles of rehabilitation apply to the care of people with long-term congenital or acquired conditions, though the emphasis given to it will depend on the individual's position relative to life-threatening or acute ill-health and differs between settings. A stroke, for example, is a medical emergency, so initial care would focus on optimising homeostasis and survival but would shift subsequently to minimising the stroke's impact and risk of complications (Warlow et al 2008) or to palliative care.

Davis & Madden's (2006) continuum of rehabilitation can be applied here (Figure 32.4), demonstrating that goals and interventions evolve according to the stroke survivor's needs and degree of impairment.

Thus, during the initial stage when individuals are unconscious, rehabilitative care might involve providing stimulation, coming to know about them as people and supporting relatives/friends. Once individuals are fully responsive, have regained physical function and enter the second stage, interventions could include continual assessment of functional and cognitive ability, managing challenging behaviour, re-establishing daily activities, offering choice and involving relatives/friends in care. A more active rehabilitative programme assumes prominence in the third stage, with care in specialist settings concentrating on the individual's level of participation and quality of life. Interventions entail empowerment though shared goal planning, facilitating movement towards maximum potential in daily living, providing a coordinated rehabilitation programme and psychologically supporting all concerned. Having achieved this, the fourth stage focuses on maintaining quality of life and enabling individuals to live with their impairments, perhaps through outpatient care, reassessment and problem-solving.

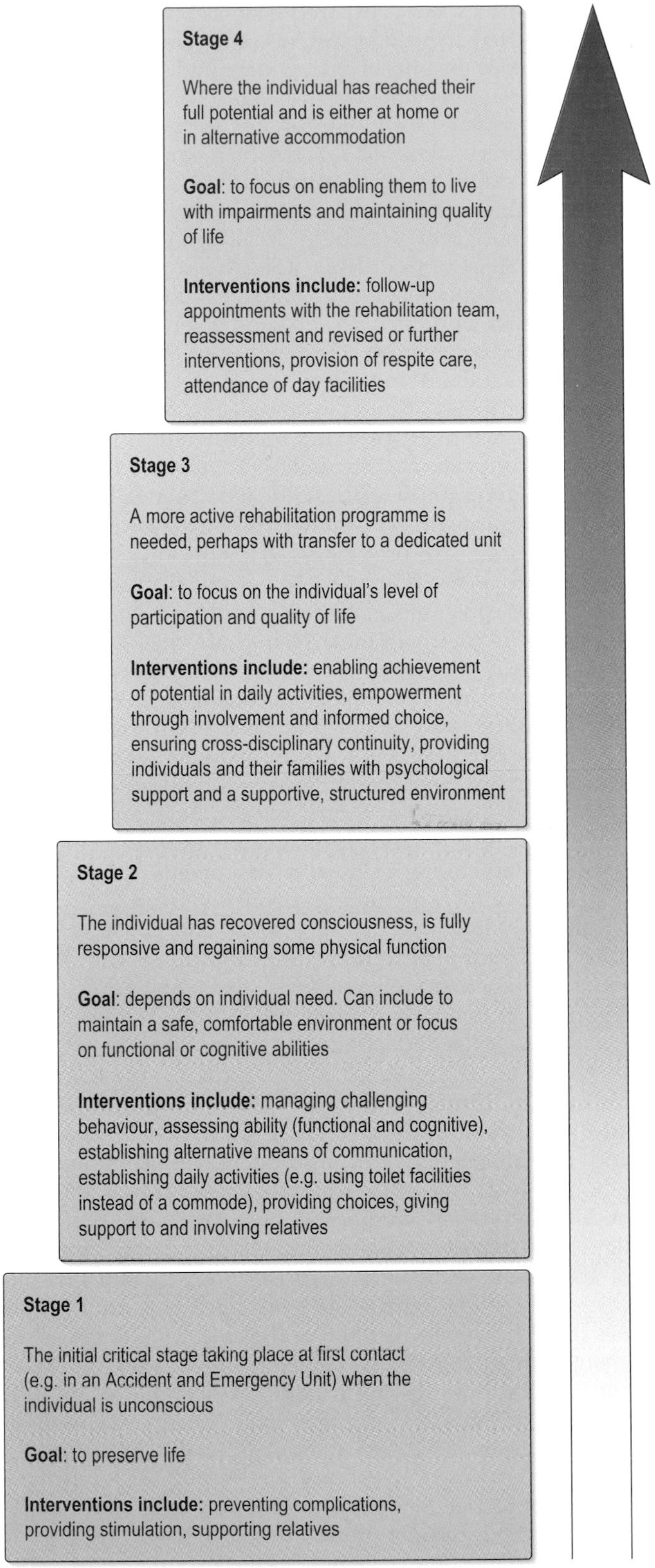

Team-working

Effective rehabilitation requires input from several disciplines, and team-working is generally accepted as central to this. Contributory characteristics include clear communication, acceptance of collective responsibility and purpose, understanding each other's roles and overlap, goal-directedness, flexibility, valuing the perspective of others and willingness to resolve conflicts (Long et al 2003). The terms used to describe teams reflect their ways of working, for example whether they are

Stage 4

Where the individual has reached their full potential and is either at home or in alternative accommodation

Goal: to focus on enabling them to live with impairments and maintaining quality of life

Interventions include: follow-up appointments with the rehabilitation team, reassessment and revised or further interventions, provision of respite care, attendance of day facilities

Stage 3

A more active rehabilitation programme is needed, perhaps with transfer to a dedicated unit

Goal: to focus on the individual's level of participation and quality of life

Interventions include: enabling achievement of potential in daily activities, empowerment through involvement and informed choice, ensuring cross-disciplinary continuity, providing individuals and their families with psychological support and a supportive, structured environment

Stage 2

The individual has recovered consciousness, is fully responsive and regaining some physical function

Goal: depends on individual need. Can include to maintain a safe, comfortable environment or focus on functional or cognitive abilities

Interventions include: managing challenging behaviour, assessing ability (functional and cognitive), establishing alternative means of communication, establishing daily activities (e.g. using toilet facilities instead of a commode), providing choices, giving support to and involving relatives

Stage 1

The initial critical stage taking place at first contact (e.g. in an Accident and Emergency Unit) when the individual is unconscious

Goal: to preserve life

Interventions include: preventing complications, providing stimulation, supporting relatives

Figure 32.4 Continuum of rehabilitation. (After Davis & Madden 2006.)

multi-, inter- or trans-disciplinary. Interdisciplinary working implies greater commitment to shared decision making, authority and responsibility. This approach is adopted more commonly in specialist rehabilitation settings and is achieved though collaborative setting of person-oriented goals, using integrated pathways and records, transcending professional or role boundaries and leadership based on skill, as opposed to professional grouping. Obstacles to this can be attitudinal, for example perceived loss of professional autonomy or status, and organisational, such as uniprofessional education, different working patterns and lines of accountability (Booth & Jester 2007). In Wade's (2002) view, the efficacy of rehabilitation rests on specialised teams taking a carefully structured and standardised approach to common problems, enabling them to anticipate and avoid complications. Associated with this are person-centred problem-solving processes, targeted evaluation of interventions and the ability to deliver evolving, multifocal care.

The foundation for nursing roles

While the contribution of health professionals is crucial during diagnosis, rehabilitation and exacerbation, individuals and their carers are responsible for managing conditions on a daily basis. The nursing role is, therefore, far from restricted to the delivery of direct care. For example, people's cognitive and physical ability to develop required practices must first be assessed. It is also vital to ensure that the information that they need to manage home care has been successfully communicated.

In aiming for optimal self-management, the nurse must also be prepared to adopt a flexible approach. During some phases of long-term illness it may be necessary to act for patients and carers, while, at other times, support will focus on facilitating the performance of self-care activities, imparting knowledge, teaching practical skills or giving emotional support to aid adaptive behaviour. This echoes issues raised above, in that nurses need to be committed to forming and maintaining collaborative, empowering relationships (Crumbie 2002b). In rehabilitative care, nurses also need to adopt an approach which is more 'hands off' than 'hands on' in caring *about* individuals and not *for* them (RCN 2007). Individuals can be disabled where nurses are accustomed to acting as 'doer' by, for instance, considering someone's request to go to a ward day room in isolation from their overall plan and as something to be accomplished quickly, so pushing them in a wheelchair instead of coaching their efforts to use a walking aid and reach it independently.

Empowerment

The notion of empowerment has particular value for people living with long-term conditions because they are likely to have lost control and confidence in their own abilities. Empowerment is an enabling process that enhances personal control and facilitates the process of recreating self. Although self-management groups and EPPs (see p. 831) provide a means of empowerment, they also reflect preparedness to assert the value of experiential knowledge and to question that of medicine. This opposes traditional roles and leads professionals to control information and dismiss patients' efforts to theorise about or explain their conditions (Fox et al 2005).

Conversely, patients can feel coerced into partnership, experiencing tension at being expected to both drive their care and 'do as they are told' in accepting this. Rehabilitation is a difficult process to enter into and requires individuals to

be receptive and committed to intensive, new learning at a time when they are dealing with the physical impact of disability and related psychosocial issues. As such, moving from 'I cannot do' to 'I am newly abled' involves relentless hard work (Papadimitriou 2008). In Shakespeare's (2008) experience, rehabilitation '...isn't glamorous. It's boring, and difficult, and frustrating. Progress, I have discovered, is glacially slow. One day, I manage to sit up without assistance: result!'.

Nurses need to recognise that not all individuals are motivated to participate actively in their rehabilitation and that support and patience are needed to enable them to work towards their potential at their own pace (Pellatt 2006) (Box 32.9).

The complexity of long-term conditions and their impact on lifestyle and functioning have already been emphasised. It is all too easy for nurses to make assumptions about the problems experienced by individuals on the basis of medical diagnosis alone. There are additional implications arising from classifying people as '*the* long-term ill' or '*the* disabled' Overuse of these labels can give the impression of homogeneous groups for whom care can be planned unilaterally. It also opposes the idea that individuals with long-term conditions should be regarded as team members in shaping the rehabilitation process.

Nursing roles in rehabilitation

Rehabilitation nursing is recognised as a speciality but roles are not clearly defined and nurses do not always feel their contribution is recognised by other team members. McPherson (2006) argues that skills claimed in areas such as teamworking, communication, assessment, facilitating independence in activities of living, health promotion, working with person-centred goals, empowerment and acting as advocate for individuals and their families, apply equally to roles of others working in the field. That they maintain a 24-hour presence is not reason enough to assert nurses' unique role but this does provide opportunities for them to 'close the circle in the rehabilitation process' by encouraging people to incorporate new skills and therapeutic activity into daily life (therapy 'carry-on'), leading, educating, coordinating and sharing their ongoing observations with team members whose decision making might otherwise be based on snapshot evaluation (Jester 2007, p. 15).

Box 32.9 Reflection

Partnership working – myth or reality?

People with diabetes in Paterson's (2001) study observed that members of the health care team talked of empowering patients but used a range of contradictory behaviours and practices that prevented this aim from being realised.

Activities

- Reflect on your experience of caring for people with long-term conditions. Why might nurses feel that sharing information and offering choice threatens their power in the caring situation or somehow undermines their professional role?

In addition, nurses integrate the management of pain, continence, nutrition, tissue viability and the need for balanced rest and stimulation into the individual's overall rehabilitation programme. The important thing here is not so much what nurses do but the way care is provided. Rehabilitation is not effective because it provides life-saving interventions but by focusing on enabling individuals to achieve their own goals by identifying how barriers can be overcome (Pellatt 2006). This also involves 'being with' the person and sharing their journey through the development of a supportive, empathic relationship. In underlining the role of patients as co-workers, rehabilitative care has particular resonance with initiatives to provide patient-focused benchmarks of practice, such as the Essence of Care (DH 2001d) and Fundamentals of Care (WAG 2006). Consultant nurse and rehabilitation specialist nurse posts enable expert practitioners to play an important part in service development, driving change and quality improvement initiatives (RCN 2007).

Using frameworks and models to guide practice

As discussed earlier, although a variety of characteristics are shared by people with long-term conditions, there is considerable diversity in their response. A nursing approach that recognises explicitly the uniqueness of individuals and enables the totality of their situation to be understood must therefore be adopted. The use of a formalised framework to guide practice is also valuable in providing a systematic prescription for action, encompassing a sound theoretical base and acting as a learning tool – for example, in developing problem-solving skills and applying evidence to practice.

Various conceptual models have been devised to articulate beliefs about nursing's essential components and underpinning theory. In representing the reality of practice, concepts of person, environment, health and nursing are central to them. These models offer a foundation for the development of nursing as a discipline (Fawcett 2003) and, if adopted by a nursing team, promote consistency and continuity of nursing action. The selection of a particular model for practice depends largely on the extent to which it reflects the nursing team's own values and perceived goals.

While a number of models have relevance for nursing people with long-term conditions, three identified below might have particular interest for those working in this area. Discussion of the models is necessarily brief in this chapter and readers are encouraged to refer to the referenced sources to gain a better understanding.

Orem's self-care model

The self-care deficit nursing theory (SCDNT; Orem 2001) is likely to appeal to nurses who consider its emphasis on client autonomy and motivation to be consistent with the aim of helping individuals to accept responsibility for themselves. This might seem appropriate, given the role people with long-term conditions play in managing their condition. Its concern with independent action is, however, more complex than face value suggests. The concept of self-care must be seen in the context of the model's other components, so that underlying theory can be understood and the whole operationalised.

Self-care is the contribution people make to their own continued existence and involves practising activities to maintain health and well-being. Nurses assist patients and their associates to achieve self-care, taking individual ability and need into account. Following negotiation with all concerned, care is organised in terms of one of three nursing systems. These are wholly compensatory, partly compensatory or supportive–educative, i.e. the nurse may perform activities for the individual, assist the individual in carrying out shared activities, or help them to develop the ability to act on their own behalf. The decision to use a nursing system or a combination of systems is not static but changes in response to patient need over time.

Orem's model can be used in a variety of settings. The importance of partnership with patient and carers is acknowledged and their involvement in planning nursing interventions considered essential. Attention is given to the notion that people are active in learning to live with the effects of long-term conditions and exploits their motivation to do so. The variation in nursing activity necessary to address the range of problems likely to be experienced during the course of such disorders is also accounted for.

Roy's adaptation model

Roy's adaptation model (Roy & Andrews 2008) might be thought suitable in long-term conditions because it views human behaviour as being influenced by an interrelated set of biological, psychological and social systems, each of which is directed towards achieving a state of relative balance. This will, as far as possible, promote regularity of function and aid the individual to adapt positively to environmental stimuli (or stressors).

Roy identifies three types of stimuli to which individuals are exposed: focal, contextual and residual. A focal stimulus is something that has an immediate effect on the person, a contextual stimulus is a contributory circumstance, and a residual stimulus arises from beliefs or attitudes relating to past experiences. Maladaption occurs where the effect of any stimulus exceeds someone's capacity to make a positive response. This results in a threat to continued health and well-being. Roy's model accepts that individuals possess a unique capacity to deal with stimuli, such that people react differently when faced with the same events. The ability to adapt thus varies from person to person.

Nursing intervention is needed when an individual's usual methods of coping with stressors prove ineffective. The nursing role centres on promoting adaptation in maintaining health and during periods of illness, and is concerned with manipulating stimuli, enabling people to respond positively.

This model also has value for care in long-term conditions in a variety of settings. Its focus is congruent with the belief that individuals manage and adapt to the same events differently, considers it desirable for them to develop the ability to live with the effects of their conditions and engages them collaboratively in their care. Nurses are encouraged to consider factors that influence the individual's context, not merely the immediate problems confronting them. In this way it is possible for nurses to appreciate the effects of a condition over time and how the individual feels about this. The model assists nurses in identifying successful past coping mechanisms and elements likely to impede future adaptation, so that intervention may be planned with realisable goals. Care can therefore be tailored in relation to individual resources.

The Roper–Logan–Tierney (RLT) model

A more detailed exploration will be made here of caring for people with long-term conditions using the Roper et al model for nursing (Roper et al 2000, Holland et al 2008). This model has been widely adopted in the UK and thus is one with which many nurses are familiar. In addition, it is based on ideas drawn directly from practice. Roper et al's portrayal of an uncomplicated view of nursing is a deliberate attempt to provide a flexible framework that can be applied across settings. In this model, the focus of nursing intervention is on assisting individuals in the prevention, resolution and management of problems. Problems are defined as actual or potential, as nurses are concerned not only with problems that actually exist but, also, with preventing the development of others.

The RLT model applies readily to long-term conditions because it is grounded on a model for living, demonstrating that health status and lifestyle are closely related. An awareness of this helps nurses to perceive their role in terms of health promotion and maintenance, as well as dealing with acute condition-oriented problems. The model's purpose of equipping practitioners with a means to plan and deliver individualised care in relation to both nurse-initiated and multiprofessional activity facilitates collaboration. Figure 32.5 outlines the model's five components. These will be considered in turn and applied to the care of people with long-term conditions.

Activities of living (ALs)

Living can be described as a fusion of the 12 ALs (Figure 32.5), which individuals experience and carry out differently. Although the ALs are the core of the RLT model and present a framework for assessment, there is a danger that some nurses use it simply as a 12-point checklist and the model's other dimensions may be overlooked as a result. For example, identifying an older woman who has osteoporosis and is admitted to hospital following a fall as simply 'having problems mobilising' would not necessarily take into account issues such as the systemic effects of her condition, the effectiveness of her existing long-term pain management strategies, the psychological impact of not being able to go out from her first-floor flat as before, having to accept help as someone who has been fiercely independent and a caregiver to her neighbour, inactivity making her feel colder, difficulty paying utility bills and avoidance of claiming benefits because she views this as 'something more deserving people do'.

The performance of any AL requires the coordination of a complex pattern of behaviour. The ability to communicate, for example, relies on skills including the reception and interpretation of information and the formulation and transmission of appropriate verbal and non-verbal responses. This is influenced by many variables, such as the efficiency of physiological and psychological functions. Thus there is considerable scope for error and it is likely that people with long-term conditions will experience a wide range of associated problems. For instance, some individuals may not understand or express ideas verbally following a stroke, while others find no difficulty in this area but are unable to articulate words clearly (see Ch. 9). In either case, individuals will be limited in their ability to make their thoughts and feelings known and this will cause frustration for all concerned.

Speech deterioration also takes place in, for example, Parkinson's disease where communication can be further inhibited by memory impairment and loss of facial expression. The latter provides the listener with poor feedback and results in the absence of important non-verbal cues. As mentioned above, alteration in the person's physical appearance can also present a barrier to communication, in that people might avoid casual social contact with them or make assumptions about their mental state.

It is common for people with long-term conditions to find that disruption in the performance of one AL leads to difficulty in the performance of others. For instance, someone who has COPD who experiences shortness of breath might also find their capacity to communicate, eat and drink, reach the toilet, attend to personal hygiene, walk, work, socialise and sleep compromised.

Lifespan

This component of the model represents the passage through life from conception to death. The progression along the lifespan is marked by continual change, as the individual moves through a series of developmental stages, each of which is associated with the expression of different levels of physical, cognitive and social function. As mentioned previously, adulthood is generally characterised by self-reliance centring on occupational and family interests but there is, of course, considerable diversity in individual lifestyle and behaviour during this life stage. Chronological age alone does not give the nurse sufficient information to appreciate the likely impact of long-term conditions. Rather, the nurse will need to gain an understanding of which developmental tasks someone has already achieved, those

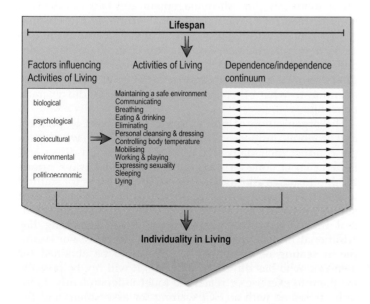

Figure 32.5 The Activity of Living (AL) model. (Holland et al 2008, with permission.)

they aspire to and the value placed on each by the individual and those close to them.

Obtaining this kind of information reveals the existence of actual or potential problems requiring nursing intervention. For example, a woman who has MS and wishes to become pregnant may have to confront issues such as sexual dysfunction, the impact of discontinuing disease-modifying or other medication and whether her functional impairment would present difficulties in meeting the needs of a newborn. Once the nurse recognises this as causing emotional distress, it can be accounted for in the care planning process; for example, the woman's need for accurate, evidence-based information may be met by referral to a specialist nurse and a suggestion that she obtain peer support from the MS Society.

The dependence/independence continuum

This component acts as a reminder that individuals are not always able to perform each AL unaided (Holland et al 2008). Some people have yet to acquire the necessary skills or do not have the means to develop them, whilst illness or trauma causes others to lose abilities they once had.

No single measure reflects the capacity for independent function in all ALs, since it can be argued that few people, if any, are truly self-sufficient. In addition, the concepts of dependence and independence have meaning only when considered in relation to each other. For these reasons, any form of assessment will have a subjective bias which is determined by the nurse's interpretation of an individual's abilities in comparison with clinical, developmental and social norms. This means, for example, that assumptions about the inevitability of universal deterioration in advancing age need to be questioned.

The interactive nature of the ALs and the fact that difficulty in carrying out one can affect adversely the performance of others have implications for the maintenance of independent action in long-term conditions. In recognition of this, it is essential that attention is paid to each of them when assessing a patient's dependence/independence status. For example, altered mobility associated with systemic lupus erythematosus (SLE or lupus) can also interfere with shopping for and preparing meals, while sports activity and keyboard skills might be made difficult by reduced physical dexterity.

Factors influencing the Activities of Living

Individual differences can be identified in the way that ALs are performed, regardless of the point reached in the lifespan or the level of dependence held. Knowledge of five influential factors assists nurses in taking a holistic view of an individual's situation:

- biological
- psychological – incorporating intellectual and emotional factors
- sociocultural – incorporating spiritual, religious and ethical factors
- environmental
- politicoeconomic – incorporating legal factors.

These factors, acting singly or in combination, influence each AL to some degree. It is not always easy to distinguish the influence of one from that of another, since they are interrelated and share several areas of concern. Consideration of these factors during assessment provides the basis

for a deeper understanding of the cause of an individual's difficulties, as well as indicating likely outcomes.

This has particular relevance for people with long-term conditions, given the timescales involved, the multiple effects of such disorders and the pattern of relapses associated with them. For example, knowledge of normal anatomical structure and physiological function enables the nurse to appreciate the effects of spinal cord injury (SCI). This is useful both in guiding immediate action to alleviate existing problems and in devising care to prevent the onset of anticipated complications, such as autonomic dysreflexia, constipation and pressure ulcers. An exploration of psychological status will reveal someone's capacity to acquire further information and motivation to develop the skills necessary for self-management.

Everyday behaviour related to health promotion and the management of long-term conditions has strong social and cultural determinants. The nurse should attempt to understand how the condition has affected the individual's accustomed roles and in what respect this has influenced relationships with others. A man who develops Guillain-Barré syndrome (GBS), for instance, may perceive that his role as provider and protector of the family group is threatened when he is no longer earning and requires help to perform basic living activities.

Environmental factors such as noise, climate and atmospheric pollution can affect the performance of ALs. For example, people with COPD experience worsening of their symptoms during periods of poor air quality and disturbed sleep if their home is located in a noisy neighbourhood. The structure and layout of buildings in which activities are performed are also of significance here. Someone in this situation who lives in a top-floor flat without a lift might not be able to negotiate the stairs easily. This would further limit their activities and worsen their health in broad terms. Access to GP surgeries can be difficult if they are sited at some distance from public transport or on uneven terrain and the interior of older facilities might not be optimally disabled-friendly. This may discourage users from attending and result in inadequate monitoring of self-management and lack of attention to some features of their conditions. Admission to hospital can present an additional source of anxiety because the distance between facilities, and the need to share bathroom and sleeping accommodation can interfere with an individual's routine performance of a number of ALs or draw attention to what others might consider to be idiosyncratic behaviour.

The organisation of public services is subject to political and economic influences, affecting the manner in which people conduct their daily lives. Despite their high direct and indirect costs, long-term conditions are not always prioritised in resource allocation. This has implications for staffing levels and the provision of equipment, and hence the level of support individuals are offered as they strive to attain optimal functioning and independence. Poor resourcing has additional implications for individual lifestyles. For example, if seating of a suitable height cannot be obtained for someone who has difficulty standing, it will not be possible for them to exercise or reach the toilet independently. Similarly, someone with an SCI waiting for assessment and the delivery of a suitable wheelchair can experience considerable difficulty using a temporary chair that does not meet their needs, forces the adoption of an uncomfortable posture and is heavy to manoeuvre.

Individualising nursing

As noted, the way each person carries out the ALs is unique. This arises from the complex interaction between the components described above and is apparent in the frequency, location and timing of activities, rationale for using particular practices, and the knowledge, beliefs and attitudes of the person concerned. An appreciation of this underpins individualised nursing. The process of nursing can be used as a vehicle to translate the RLT model into practice and to systematise the delivery of care (Holland et al 2008).

Applying the Roper–Logan–Tierney model using the nursing process

Assessment

This stage of the nursing process is a dynamic and ongoing activity, rather than a single event that takes place when first encountering an individual. Initial assessment is important in long-term conditions because it presents a structured method of data collection, which will create a total picture of the person and, thus, provide a baseline against which change can be measured. In some cases, for example in the immediate aftermath of trauma or a stroke, priority will necessarily be given to managing threat to life or pain and distress, with more comprehensive details of daily activities gathered over time. It must be emphasised, however, that circumstances are seldom static in long-term conditions, so continued assessment is essential and should be considered at any stage of the nurse–patient relationship.

Assessment in rehabilitative care prompts people to become involved in and drive the process by encouraging them to focus on their own needs and enabling staff to recognise these. In specialist units the format taken is based on a shared interdisciplinary, as opposed to nursing, model and could include aspects such as activities of daily living, current level of dependence and expectations for independence. Issues considered might be bowel and bladder management, mobility, nutrition, communication and psychological and social needs. The aim of this would be as above and, similarly, requires a systematised approach and comprehensive history taking (Booth & Jester 2007).

A number of issues require attention during the assessment of people with long-term conditions, regardless of the setting, some of which relate directly to traumatic or disease processes and include the type and duration of the presenting condition. For those with an established condition, information about strategies used for managing its features and ongoing treatment will be needed. This will help nurses understand how individuals and their carers incorporate these into daily life and the degree of efficacy achieved. The collation of objective and subjective data is crucial here. For example, spasticity (uncoordinated, involuntary muscle contractions associated with painful spasms, stiffness and changed movement) is an observable phenomenon in MS and this can prompt nurses to explore how it affects individuals, whereas invisible problems, such as fatigue, might

not be evident unless patients explain their impact. Its subjective, experiential nature means that fatigue is poorly recognised, so nurses need to be prepared to assess how this presents for individuals (e.g. 'so debilitated', 'completely wiped out') to enable exacerbating factors to be identified. These might include finding out that someone tires themselves by undertaking periods of intensive activity without rest periods in a misguided, but understandable, effort to complete tasks before energy is lost (Peniket & Grove 2007) (see Critical thinking question 32.2).

See website Critical thinking question 32.2

When using the RLT model, assessment involves collecting data pertaining to biography, health history and the ALs. It is likely that these elements will be closely related in long-term conditions; for example, an individual's lifestyle and their perception of health status will shape the performance of some activities. Review of biographical data provides an opportunity to explore the individual's pre-morbid lifestyle (that which existed prior to the condition's onset) and to appreciate the changes imposed by their long-term condition in this context. The consequences of these should be reviewed with reference to the ALs, while bearing the model's other components in mind. Each AL should be considered so that specific relevance and relationships between them can be identified. For example, some people can be concerned that their condition hastens the prospect of dying and how this might occur, while others express profound grief at social exclusion resulting from loss of roles.

The RLT model prompts nurses to consider the individual's abilities as well as impairments in carrying out the ALs, through reference to the dependence/independence continuum. Any equipment used to assist independence can be identified and carer involvement, resource use and support services can be explored. Independence needs to be judged in terms of whether activities can be completed safely and if individuals can direct them when unable to act unaided. In this way, for instance, someone with significant physical impairment due to SCI can be assessed as having task independence because they are in a position to instruct others in the correct management of their care (Kennedy et al 2003). This part of the assessment can also help to determine whether people have a realistic idea of their situation.

Although much of the assessment data can be obtained from patients, other sources of information must be included. The views of formal and informal carers should be used to build up a more detailed impression of behaviour and events. For example, when someone with MND is admitted for respite care, a community nurse might share an observation that during recent months there has been a marked deterioration in the relationship between the patient and their partner, although the couple strenuously denies that this has taken place. This could then be interpreted with reference to the features of MND, progression of the condition and demands on the carer, so that key problems are identified and accounted for in the plan for care (Box 32.10).

Planning

Care is planned to address the actual and potential problems identified in the course of assessment. The priority given to each depends on the individual's situation, though, again,

Box 32.10 Reflection

Recognising the importance of individual experience

Living with long-term conditions is influenced by a range of interacting physical, psychosocial, politicoeconomic and spiritual factors. It is also clear that people share some experiences of long-term conditions but have individual approaches to living with and managing them.

Activities

- Reflecting on your experience, think about two people with long-term conditions whom you know or have met in your practice. Identify examples of physical, psychosocial, politicoeconomic and spiritual factors affecting each of their lives.
- Which similarities and differences do you see?
- Consider how coming to know the individual could enhance their care.

life-threatening or distressing problems assume precedence over those with a less immediate impact. Aside from this, priority setting in long-term conditions should always be negotiated by the nurse, patient and main carer. An open discussion is useful in clarifying the meaning of each problem to the individual, determining how problems are related to each other, discussing options for addressing them and creating a shared awareness of difficulties. This helps to foster collaborative relationships and enhances the commitment of all concerned.

The aim of the care plan is to assist the patient in preventing, solving, alleviating or managing problems as far as is possible by using best practice. Goals are set for each problem and appropriate strategies devised to attain them. In long-term conditions it is particularly important that goal-setting reflects the individual's capacity for achievement, is meaningful and is consistent with personal values and priorities. Both short- and long-term goals can be specified. However, given the instability of long-term conditions, it might be inappropriate to select broad objectives for eventual achievement, such as acceptance of the condition and total self-management. It is preferable to simplify these by dividing them into a series of short-term goals, so that progress can be achieved and motivation maintained. This provides patients with a stimulus and sense of purpose (Holland et al 2008). Goals must also be expressed in understandable, measurable terms so that their attainment is obvious to patient and carer. This is furthered in specialist rehabilitative care, where regular goal planning meetings are held with individuals, their carers and other interdisciplinary team members to identify needs, set specific, measurable, achievable, realistic and time-framed goals and review progress.

The way in which ALs are addressed during assessment, whether related problems are identified and how care is planned depends on social and cultural issues and nurses' knowledge, skill and approach. For instance, although promoting sexual health is generally agreed to be part of their role, nurses do not necessarily address this proactively and prefer to wait for patients to voice related concerns (Higgins et al 2006). Given its intimate nature, however, patients might be reluctant to do this. This means that sexual expression risks

being neglected, whether this concerns the sexual act, relationships or how individuals dress and present themselves.

This is particularly important in long-term conditions because associated changes in appearance, body image or function have significant effects on sexual health. For example, impaired mobility can prevent attention to personal hygiene and preferred management of body hair, limit clothing choices, restrict body positioning, cause pain and dominate one's appearance as a disabled person. Incontinence causes embarrassment and sensory alteration affects stimulation and perceived pleasure from physical contact. Chronic pain is associated with depression which decreases libido, as does some antidepressant medication (see Box 32.6). Specific conditions also influence sexual expression directly. Gynaecological, breast and male reproductive cancers have an obvious relationship with this activity. Acquired brain injury can be followed by changes in libido, erectile dysfunction and inability to orgasm. Changes in male fertility might occur here and in SCI, where ejaculatory failure, retrograde ejaculation, raised testicular temperature and chronic infection are implicated (Pellatt 2006). Not all nurses are in a position to give advice on sexual health management but they should provide support by having an awareness of potential problems, being sensitive, being willing to present patients with an 'open door' to discuss them when ready and by planning for specialist referrals.

Care plans should describe prescribed interventions and patient participation in detail, communicating clearly what can be expected from everyone involved. This offers a means of ensuring continuity of care and can help to prevent confusion, such as when individuals are learning to develop a routine for renal dialysis in a domestic setting. It also articulates nursing's contribution to interdisciplinary planning, for instance with reference to care pathways. Where collaborative plans are used, it is important to identify which team member is best placed to support progression towards each goal and to ensure that everyone concerned is committed to the agreed process and outcome (Booth & Jester 2007).

 See website Critical thinking question 32.3

Implementation

The actions proposed in the care plan are realised in this phase of the nursing process. It is tempting to believe that the majority of nurses will experience little difficulty in this area because they are familiar with the idea of 'doing'. While there may be some truth in this assumption, there is a tendency for ease of performance to conceal the depth of knowledge and the complex array of skills needed to meet the needs of people with long-term conditions effectively.

The delivery of care in relation to the ALs should be consistent with the way in which individuals with long-term conditions usually behave, whether or not they normally require assistance. As in Orem's (2001) model, this may require the nurse to act for the patient, to supplement and develop the person's self-care capability or in promoting health to aid learning. Determining the emphasis to be placed on each of these approaches in a given situation requires nurses to be responsive to the individual's experience of their condition in the light of issues considered in the first part of this chapter, while being aware of the possibilities of nursing roles.

Rehabilitation has a conserving function in maintaining normal function, preventing trauma or complications and meeting fundamental needs (Pellatt 2006). Williams et al's (2007) exploration of the Northwick Park Dependency Scale and Care Needs Assessment illustrates the range of nursing knowledge and skill required to implement care in line with this, in relation to what are defined as 'Basic Nursing Needs' (mobility, transfers, toileting, hygiene and dressing, nutritional support including enteral feeding, drinking, positioning, safety awareness and communication) and 'Special Nursing Needs' (tracheostomy care, wound care, medication, assisting interdisciplinary team members, routine checks and observations, collecting specimens, applying splints and miscellaneous support functions). Effective fulfilment of these relies on nurses' understanding of normal and abnormal physiological functioning and evidence-based interventions, together with an ability to combine sensitively the performance of personal and technical care with empowering individuals for self-management, for example, in maintaining someone's dignity and sense of worth when working with them to manage continence using self-catheterisation, doing this in the context of their being a sales person who undertakes frequent long-distance travel and collaborating with specialist nurses to obtain advice or products most suited to their lifestyle.

Implementation also involves supporting patients to optimise their strengths in developing their own knowledge and applying skills learned during therapy sessions. Peer support and learning from others who have moved further in the rehabilitative process can be invaluable here, however, practices need to be adapted to fit individual impairments and preferences. For example, many people with long-term conditions have limited movement. Universal risk assessment will identify those most liable to develop pressure ulcers but tissue viability is of greater concern to people with paralysis and sensory deficit, such as following SCI. Here, instinctive movements to ensure circulation and prevention of pressure damage cease, while the lower body's skin quality and muscle bulk decline. This means that individuals need to learn the serious consequences of pressure ulcers and take responsibility for avoiding them by incorporating careful movement and transfers, turning and skin inspection into daily life. However, as Prince (2009, p. 9) commented: 'the difficult part is learning the routines [...] and sticking to them rigorously, however inconvenient it may be to do so. No two individuals are the same and you need to learn for yourself what your body can tolerate'.

Psychological factors will also influence patients' level of engagement and, thus, determine when intervention would be most appropriate. The development of a therapeutic relationship with individuals and their carers is a sound basis from which to work. Individuals can discern quickly whether nurses have a genuine interest in their well-being and are more likely to be responsive to them. For instance, a simple act of communication shaped McCrum's (2008) feelings of being cared for after a stroke, while a nurse's focus on her own religious beliefs alienated Rushby-Smith (2008) following his SCI.

It is important for nurses to gain patients' trust and to recognise that, under normal circumstances, they and their carers have – or will have – responsibility for managing their condition and daily life. In both hospital and community settings, nurses must enable people to retain control of their situation rather than expecting them to conform to alien norms and expectations.

In long-term conditions, nursing intervention is far from restricted to the delivery of physical care, although the value of this should not be underestimated. Assisting another person in carrying out any activity, such as washing and dressing, requires more than the ability to reproduce simple practical actions. The promotion of health and self-care capability requires an understanding of an individual's developmental level as well as of effective teaching techniques. This involves the use of refined communication skills, as does the role of counsellor and supporter to both patients and carers.

The ability of family members to participate in rehabilitative programmes and long-term care varies. Involving them actively in goal planning and care delivery can give an indication of this and provides them with opportunities to gain information and training for the role. Culture influences the way they view illness, disability, gender roles, religious adherence and the performance of daily activities. Their involvement also depends on existing family dynamics, structure, location and culture. An extended family might provide several carers whose availability makes role sharing feasible, while family members who are geographically distant could perhaps offer some direct assistance during times of hospitalisation, transition and relapse or remote support using phone and online contact.

Some carers might have unrealistically high expectations of an individual's independence or, conversely, hinder their progress by being overprotective and performing activities for them. Nurses need to be prepared to help patients to express their needs and, if necessary, advocate for them in liaising with carers. They should, however, acknowledge that personal characteristics and poor relationships can make caring inappropriate. Carers can feel pressured to participate or guilty at not being able to, even though they have the right to refuse engagement or to continue caring, and sharing this with nurses is difficult. It is important to try to understand people's decisions and avoid making judgements. Family members might care very much for an individual but just not as others expect.

When helping an individual to adapt to living with a long-term condition, nurses should present explanations honestly and positively, to foster realistic hope for the future. Non-verbal communication, especially touch, can be a helpful way to strengthen a caring relationship, providing this is culturally, age and gender appropriate.

Extending traditional nursing skills in relation to touch has significant benefits for people in this situation. The provision of massage, for example, can be of value in assisting individuals to deal with stress, enhance self-worth, contribute to palliation and facilitate sympathetic reconnection with a body that has 'let them down'. As with all complementary therapies, nurses should ensure that the care provided is safe, in patients' best interests, that they are trained and competent to practice, have involved interdisciplinary members in decision making and obtain informed consent (Nursing and Midwifery Council 2008).

Evaluation

The effectiveness of nursing interventions can be judged by evaluating whether or not goals have been achieved. This phase of the nursing process lends meaning to those that precede it. The extent to which goals have been achieved should be measured objectively where possible. For example, successful self-management of insulin-dependent diabetes can be demonstrated by HbA_{1c} measurement (Heisler et al 2005). It is also possible to identify movement on the dependence/independence continuum in response to teaching programmes or how patients manage symptoms.

The evaluation of some aspects of care is, however, largely dependent on subjective data. For instance, it is difficult to measure to what extent an individual has adapted to the idea of having a long-term condition. Evaluation in this area could be guided instead by interpreting behavioural cues, for instance by observing whether they are active in information-seeking and practising new skills, appear depressed or avoid discussion of the condition and its related problems. It is essential to combine observation with listening to what the person says about their experience. The use of tools such as symptom diaries and pain scales can be helpful in mapping patient experience and identifying trends. Measuring functional outcomes without acknowledging their context provides an inadequate indicator of progress. An individual might, for example, be able to get up, shower and dress but take until 10.30 a.m. to do so. This might be judged as successful in some respects but not in others. The person can perform the named activities independently but when 'bodily housekeeping' becomes a job in itself, paid employment is not possible and forces reliance on state benefits.

The achievement of any goal relies on wide-ranging situational variables. It is therefore sometimes difficult to identify whether strategies have been successful. The contribution of human, material and environmental factors can all influence outcomes. Not all nursing interventions will be effective, even if they proved so when caring previously for people with similar impairments. Non-achievement should not be viewed as 'failure', as this has negative connotations and is liable to demotivate, but should be considered a stimulus for reassessment and an opportunity to revise better targeted problem statements and to set new goals. Nurses have to think creatively when identifying why goals were not achieved and in searching for solutions (Box 32.11).

The importance of the nurse's own self-evaluation must not be forgotten. Caring for people with long-term conditions engenders considerable emotional labour for a number of reasons. As noted earlier, nurses sometimes find it difficult to work within the boundaries of their occupational role where relationships develop with individuals and their families over time. They can find it difficult to accept the inevitability of the patient's decline and to have a meaningful role where medicine deems that nothing more can be done. It is also possible that they will identify with the patient, particularly if they occupy the same stage of the lifespan. Some nurses will be unable to form close protracted relationships due to differences in personality, culture and attitude. Individual nurses must recognise that they cannot be all things to all people. Exposure to another's traumatic experience is a source of vicarious stress and the cumulative

Box 32.11 Reflection

Case history: the importance of understanding the individual's perspective of their rehabilitative experience

Team members working with 51-year-old B aimed to reduce her risk of falling post traumatic injury. Care included advising her to consider safety a priority by focusing consciously on balancing during activity, wearing orthoses (braces, splints or in-shoe devices used to support and correct limb function), using a stick and avoiding simultaneous movement and talking when practising stairs.

On evaluation, staff found it hard to understand why B felt that the goal of being able to manage this confidently had not been achieved; after all, she had fallen less frequently since the plan had been implemented and was observed to be moving more steadily.

In later discussion with a nurse, B agreed that this was true when walking in sports shoes on even surfaces in a hospital setting but it had raised awareness that she would not be able to wear high-heeled footwear and dress as before, so would feel out of place at business and social events. This had upset her but she had not mentioned it to the team because it felt comparatively petty.

The nurse reassuringly explained that what was meaningful to B was important for her rehabilitation. The team reviewed B's specific circumstances and the timescale for the goal was revised. It was also suggested that that she obtain a more stylish stick, as suitable for her height and weight, and consider suitable compromises for the future, such as searching for fashionable orthotic-friendly shoes with laces or other 'stay put' closures, taking high-heeled shoes for changing into once seated at events and checking with the orthotist whether it would be acceptable to wear less substantial flat evening shoes without orthoses for occasional short distances 'car to bar'. Practical issues, including wearing flat footwear when negotiating her way to the toilet, were explored in the interests of helping B to seek the best and safest solution for herself.

Activity

- Reflecting on assessment and planning processes, how might the problem noted at the evaluation stage of B's care have been avoided?

impact of working with long-term conditions adds dimensions to this. Nursing teams should be supportive of their members in enabling them to share feelings of vulnerability or emotional distress without fear of disapproval, to develop strategies for managing their own experience of sharing difficult journeys while working in restrictive service environments and offer genuine opportunities for clinical supervision and reflection.

SUMMARY: KEY NURSING ISSUES

- Long-term conditions are congenital or acquired, associated with a protracted disease processes or the consequence of trauma, might be controlled or palliated but not cured, and impact profoundly on all aspects of people's lives.
- Related impairments can result in disability, stigmatisation and, in turn, marginalisation. Society's perception of disabled people as dependent, incapable or objects of pity and curiosity are shared to some extent by health workers.

- Developments in screening, diagnostic methods, treatment and care delivery, together with an ageing population and policy drivers, mean that, regardless of the setting in which they work, most nurses will encounter people with long-term conditions.

- Living with a long-term condition is characterised by accommodating its lifelong presence in daily activities, identifying the need for and obtaining appropriate support and dealing with uncertainty.

- Managing impairments and controlling a condition's features and the side-effects of treatment are complicated by deterioration over time, unpredictable relapses and multiple pathology.

- Effective, evidence-based care requires not only a full understanding of specific conditions but, also, grounding in human and physical sciences, so that individual experiences and priorities can be understood.

- Nursing roles in long-term conditions are collaborative and enabling in nature, involving the expression of technological, rehabilitative, caring and interpersonal skills which are transferable across settings.

- Despite many conditions requiring complex and varied service use, individuals and their carers are responsible for their day-to-day management.

- Integrating principles of inclusivity and individuality into approaches to all patients as a matter of course means that differences will be anticipated and positive responses made naturally, instead of dealing with differences reactively and leaving disabled people's needs unmet.

- Self-management of long-term conditions differs from traditional approaches to care and requires nurses to be provided with knowledge and skills to deliver person-focused interventions, promote self-care of conditions and their psychosocial implications and enable patients to exercise control in decision making.

➡ REFLECTION AND LEARNING – WHAT NEXT?

- **Test** your knowledge by visiting the website 🖱 and answering the multiple choice questions and critical thinking questions.

- **Consolidate** your learning by looking at some of the further reading suggestions, references and specialist websites.

- **Revisit** some of the additional material on the website.

- **Consider** what you have learnt and how this will help your professional development.

- **Reflect** on how you can apply this knowledge to the care of your patients.

- **Discuss** your learning with your mentor/supervisor, lecturer and colleagues.

REFERENCES

Allen D, Gillen E, Rixson L: Systematic review of the effectiveness of integrated care pathways: what works, for whom, in which circumstances? *International Journal of Evidence-based Healthcare* 7:61–74, 2009.

Anon: *But you look so good,* 2007. Available online http://multiplesclerosissucks.com/aphorism.html.

Audrey S, Abel J, Blazeby JM, Falk S, Campbell R: What oncologists tell patients about survival benefits of palliative chemotherapy and implications for informed consent: qualitative study, *Br Med J* 337:492–496, 2008.

Bailey DE, Wallace M, Mishel MH: Watching, waiting and uncertainty in prostate cancer, *J Clin Nurs* 16:734–741, 2007.

Bajekal M, Harries T, Breman R, Woodfield K: *Department of Work and Pensions in-house report 128: review of disability estimates and definitions,* London, 2004, DWP.

Ballard KA: Clients with chronic mental illness. In O' Brien PG, Kennedy WZ, Ballard KA, editors: *Psychiatric Mental Health Nursing: An Introduction to Theory and Practice,* Sudbury, 2007, Jones & Bartlett, pp 537–547.

Bambra C, Pope D: What are the effects of anti-discriminatory legislation on socioeconomic inequalities in the employment consequences of ill health and disability? *J Epidemiol Community Health* 61:421–426, 2007.

Biordi DL, Nicolson NR: Social isolation. In Larsen PD, Lubkin IM, editors: *Chronic Illness: Impact and Interventions,* ed 7, Sudbury, 2009, Jones and Bartlett, pp 85–116.

Booth S, Jester R: The rehabilitation process. In Jester R, editor: *Advancing Practice in Rehabilitation Nursing,* Oxford, 2007, Blackwell, pp 1–13.

Brownsell S: *Supporting long-term conditions and disease management through telecare and telehealth: evidence and challenges,* London, 2008, Care Services Improvement Partnership.

Cartwright T, Torr R: Making sense of illness: The experiences of users of complementary medicine, *J Health Psychol* 10:559–572, 2005.

Chadha S: 2003, *Sanjay Chadha: My Multiple Sclerosis (MS) Journey So Far.* Available online http://www.redhotcurry.com/archive/health/news2004/asians_with_multiple_sclerosis.htm.

Clinical Resource Efficiency Support Team: *Executive summary of the report of the Northern Ireland task force on diabetes: a blueprint for diabetes care in Northern Ireland in the 21st century,* Belfast, 2003, CREST.

Colin-Thomé D: Foreword. In *Raising the profile of long term conditions care: A compendium of information,* London, 2008, DH.

Community Care and Health (Scotland) Act: London, 2002, HMSO.

Corbin JM, Strauss A: A nursing model for chronic illness management based upon the trajectory framework, *Sch Inq Nurs Pract* 5:155–174, 1991.

Crumbie A: Diabetes. In Crumbie A, Lawrence J, editors: *Living with a Chronic Condition: A Practitioner's Guide to Providing Care,* Oxford, 2002a, Butterworth-Heinemann, pp 59–81.

Crumbie A: Patient–professional relationships. In Crumbie A, Lawrence J, editors: *Living with a Chronic Condition: A Practitioner's Guide to Providing Care,* Oxford, 2002b, Butterworth-Heinemann, pp 3–15.

Curtin M, Lubkin IM: What is chronicity? In Lubkin IM, editor: *Chronic illness: Impact and Intervention,* Boston, MA, 1995 Jones and Bartlett, pp 3–25.

Curtin M, Lubkin IM: What is chronicity? In Lubkin IM, Larsen PD, editors: *Chronic Illness: Impact and Interventions,* ed 4, Sudbury, 1998, Jones and Bartlett, pp 3–25.

Daly BJ: Managing the hospitalized chronically ill. In Funk SG, Tornquist EM, Champagne MT, Wiese RA, editors: *Key aspects of caring for the chronically ill: hospital and home,* New York, 1993, Springer, Ch. 3.

Davis S, Madden S: Rehabilitation at a macro and micro level. In Davis S, editor: *Rehabilitation: The Use of Theories and Models in Practice,* Edinburgh, 2006, Churchill Livingstone, pp 3–22.

Department of Health: *Modernising social services: national priorities guidance 1999/00–2001/02,* London, 1998a, TSO.

Department of Health: *Modernising social services: promoting independence, improving protection, raising standards,* London, 1998b, TSO.

Department of Health: *The expert patient: a new approach to chronic disease management for the 21st century,* London, 2001a, DH.

Department of Health: *The National Service Framework for diabetes,* London, 2001b, DH.

Department of Health: *Health and Social Care Act 2001,* London, 2001c, DH.

Department of Health: *Essence of care,* London, 2001d, DH.

Department of Health: *Health Service circular: cost effective provision of disease modifying therapies for people with multiple sclerosis,* London, 2002, DH.

Department of Health: *Care homes for adults (18–65) and supplementary standards for care homes accommodating young people aged 16 and 17 national minimum standards care homes regulations*, London, 2003a, TSO.

Department of Health: *Care homes for older people: national minimum standards and the care homes regulations 2001*, London, 2003b, TSO.

Department of Health: *The National Service Framework for long-term conditions*, London, 2005, DH.

Department of Health: *The National Framework for NHS continuing healthcare and NHS funded nursing care*, London, 2007, DH.

Department of Health: *Case management*, London, 2008, DH.

Department of Health, Social Services and Public Safety Northern Ireland: *Governance in HPSS*, Belfast, 2006, DHSSPSNI.

Disability Discrimination Act: London, 1995, HMSO.

Disability Discrimination Act: London, 2005, HMSO.

Disability Rights Commission: *DRC disability briefing, March 2006*, London, 2006, DRC.

Equality Act: London, 2010, HMSO.

Equality and Human Rights Commission: *Disability*, London, 2007, EHRC.

Falvo DR: *Medical and Psychosocial Aspects of Chronic Illness and Disability*, ed 4, Sudbury, 2008, Jones & Bartlett.

Fawcett J: On bed baths and conceptual models of nursing, *J Adv Nurs* 44:229–230, 2003.

Fennell PA: *Managing Chronic Illness Using a Four-Phase Treatment Approach: A Mental Health Professional's Guide to Helping Chronically Ill People*, New York, 2003, Wiley.

Field D, Kelly MP: Chronic illness and physical disability. In Taylor S, Field D, editors: *Sociology of Health and Health Care*, ed 4, Oxford, 2007, Blackwell, pp 137–158.

Fox NJ, Ward KJ, O'Rourke AJ: The 'expert patient': empowerment or medical dominance? The case of weight loss, pharmaceutical drugs and the Internet, *Soc Sci Med* 60:1299–1309, 2005.

Freeman H: Should you reveal your health status? *The Guardian*, 2002. Available online http://www.guardian.co.uk/money/2002/apr/20/careers.students2.

Glendinning C, Means R: Personal social services: developments in adult social care. In Bauld L, Clarke K, Maltby T, editors: *Social Policy Review 18: Analysis and Debate in Social Policy, 2006*, Bristol, 2006, The Policy Press, pp 15–32.

Goffman E: *Stigma*, Harmondsworth, 1963, Penguin.

Health Protection Agency: *Health protection in the 21st century: understanding the burden of disease; preparing for the future*, London, 2005, HPA.

Heisler M, Piette JD, Spencer M, et al: The relationship between knowledge and recent HbA1c values and diabetes care understanding and self-management, *Diabetes Care* 28:816–822, 2005.

Higgins A, Barker P, Begley CM: Sexuality: the challenge to espoused holistic care, *Int J Nurs Stud* 12:345–351, 2006.

Holland K, Jenkins J, Solomon J, et al: *Applying the Roper–Logan–Tierney Model in Practice*, ed 2, Edinburgh, 2008, Churchill Livingstone.

Hunter DJ: Disease management: has it a future? *Br Med J* 320:530, 2000.

Jacoby A, Snape D, Baker GA: Epilepsy and social identity: the stigma of a chronic neurological disorder, *Lancet Neurol* 4:171–178, 2005.

Jarrett L: Attitudes to long-term care in multiple sclerosis, *Nurs Stand* 17:39–43, 2003.

Jester R: The role of the specialist nurse within rehabilitation. In Jester R, editor: *Advancing Practice in Rehabilitation Nursing*, Oxford, 2007, Blackwell, pp 14–28.

Kabat-Zinn J: *Full Catastrophe Living: Using the Wisdom of Your Body and Mind to Face Stress, Pain and Illness*, London, 2001, Piatkus.

Kalra L, Langhorne P: Facilitating recovery: evidence for organized stroke care, *J Rehabil Med* 39:97–102, 2007.

Kearney P, Pryor J: The International Classification of Functioning, Disability and Health (ICF) and nursing, *J Adv Nurs* 46:162–170, 2004.

Kennedy P, Evans MJ, Berry C, et al: Comparative analysis of goal achievement during rehabilitation for older and younger adults with spinal cord injury, *Spinal Cord* 41:44–52, 2003.

Kubler-Ross E: *On Death and Dying*, New York, 1969, Macmillan.

Larsen PD: Chronicity. In Larsen PD, Lubkin IM, editors: *Chronic Illness: Impact and Interventions*, ed 7, London, 2009, Jones & Bartlett, pp 3–24.

Locker D: Living with chronic illness. In Scambler G, editor: *Sociology as Applied to Medicine*, ed 6, Oxford, 2008, Saunders Elsevier, pp 83–96.

Long AF, Kneafsey R, Ryan J: Rehabilitation practice: challenges to effective team working, *Int J Nurs Stud* 40:663–673, 2003.

Marriott D: *The Selfish Pig's Guide to Caring*, London, 2009, Piatkus.

McCrum R: *My Year Off: Rediscovering Life After a Stroke*, London, 2008, Picador.

McPherson K: Rehabilitation nursing: final frontier? *Int J Nurs Stud* 43:787–789, 2006.

Means R, Richards S, Smith R: *Community Care: Policy and Practice*, ed 3, Basingstoke, 2003, Palgrave Macmillan.

Morse J: Responding to threats to integrity of self, *Adv Nurs Sci* 19:21–36, 1997.

National Association for Colitis and Crohn's Disease: *Information sheet: managing diarrhoea*, St Albans, 2008, NACC Available online http://www.nacc.org.uk/downloads/factsheets/FAQdiarrhoea.pdf.

National Institute for Health and Clinical Excellence (NICE): *NICE and the NHS*, 2007. Available online http://www.nice.org.uk/cat.asp?c=137.

National Multiple Sclerosis Society: *'But you look so good': managing specific issues*, Denver, 2007, NMSS.

NHS Clinical Governance Support Team: *About clinical governance*, Leicester, 2008, CGST.

NHS Quality Improvement Scotland: *Specialist units*, Edinburgh, 2007, NHSQIS.

Northern Ireland Assembly: *Report on the Health and Personal Social Services Bill (NIA Bill 06/01), Session 2001/2002 third report*, NIA, Belfast, 2002, Committee for Health, Social Services and Public Safety.

Nursing and Midwifery Council: *Complementary therapies and homeopathy*, London, 2008, NMC.

Oakley A: *Fracture: Adventures of a Broken Body*, Bristol, 2007, The Policy Press.

ONS: *Living in Britain 2002*, London, 2004, TSO.

ONS: *Focus on health 2006 edition*, Basingstoke, 2006, Palgrave Macmillan.

Orem DE: *Nursing: Concepts of Practice*, ed 6, St Louis, 2001, Mosby.

Owen T: National Care Forum and the National Care Homes Research and Development Forum: *My home life: quality of life in care homes*, London, 2006, Help the Aged in association with the NCHRDF.

Papadimitriou C: 'It was hard but you did it': the co-production of 'work' in a clinical setting among spinal cord injured adults and their physical therapists, *Disabil Rehabil* 30:365–374, 2008.

Parsons T: *The Social System*, London, 1951, Routledge and Kegan Paul.

Paterson B: Myth of empowerment in chronic illness, *J Adv Nurs* 34:574–581, 2001.

Pellatt G: The patient in need of rehabilitation. In Alexander MF, Fawcett JN, Runciman PJ, editors: *Nursing Practice: Hospital and Home: the Adult*, ed 3, Edinburgh, 2006, Churchill Livingstone, pp 1117–1130.

Peniket D, Grove R: Rehabilitation of patients with an acquired brain injury or a degenerative neuromuscular disorder. In Jester R, editor: *Advancing Practice in Rehabilitation Nursing*, Oxford, 2007, Blackwell, pp 123–157.

Prince K: quotation. In *Spinal Injuries Association Factsheet – pressure care management*, Milton Keynes, 2009, SIA, p 9.

Ravetz A: *A summary critique of the Government Green Paper 'Empowering People to Work'*, 2006. Available online http://www.leeds.ac.uk/disability-studies/archiveuk/ravetz/GP%20critique%20summary.pdf.

Roper N, Logan W, Tierney AJ: *The Roper, Logan and Tierney Model of Nursing*, Edinburgh, 2000, Churchill Livingstone.

Roy C, Andrews HA: *The Roy Adaptation Model*, ed 3, Englewood Cliffs, 2008, Prentice Hall.

Royal College of Nursing: *Rehabilitating older people: the role of the nurse*, London, 2000, RCN.

Royal College of Nursing: *Role of the rehabilitation nurse*, London, 2007, RCN.

Rushby-Smith T: *Looking Up*, London, 2008, Virgin Books.

Scambler G: Deviance, sick role and stigma. In Scambler G, editor: *Sociology as Applied to Medicine*, ed 6, Oxford, 2008, Saunders Elsevier, pp 205–220.

Schaie KW, Willis SL: *Adult Development and Aging*, ed 5, Englewood Cliffs, 2001, Prentice Hall.

Scottish Executive: *Scottish diabetes framework*, Edinburgh, 2002, Scottish Executive.

Scottish Government: *National care standards: care homes for older people revised 2007*, Edinburgh, 2007, Scottish Government.

Seccombe JA: Attitudes towards disability in an undergraduate nursing curriculum: a literature review, *Nurse Educ Today* 27:49–65, 2007.

Seddon D, Robinson C, Reeves C, et al: In their Own Right: Translating the Policy of Carer Assessment into Practice, *Br J Soc Work* 37:1335–1352, 2007.

Shakespeare T: *They tried to make me go to rehab, I said Yes! Yes! Yes! BBC Ouch*, London, 2008, BBC. Available online http://www.bbc.co.uk/ouch/columnists /tom/220908_index.shtml.

Shakespeare T, Watson N: The social model of disability: an outdated ideology? *Research in Social Science and Disability* 2:9–28, 2002.

Strauss AL, Corbin J, Fagerhaugh S, et al: *Chronic Illness and the Quality of Life*, St Louis, 1984, Mosby.

Sudlow CLM, Counsell CE: Problems with UK government's risk sharing scheme for assessing drugs for multiple sclerosis, *Br Med J* 326:388–392, 2003.

Taylor SE: *Health Psychology*, ed 7, New York, 2008, McGraw-Hill.

Telford K, Kralik D, Koch T: Acceptance and denial: implications for people adapting to chronic illness: literature review, *J Adv Nurs* 55:457–464, 2006.

Terry L: Ethics and contemporary challenges in health and social care. In Leathard A, McLaren S, editors: *Ethics: Contemporary Challenges in Health and Social Care*, Bristol, 2007, The Policy Press, pp 19–34.

Wade D: Rehabilitation is a way of thinking, not a way of doing, *Clin Rehabil* 16:579–581, 2002.

Warlow C, Sandercock P, Hankey G, et al: *Stroke: Practical Management*, ed 3, Oxford, 2008, Blackwell.

Welsh Assembly Government: *National Service Framework for diabetes in Wales: delivery strategy*, Cardiff, 2003, WAG.

Welsh Assembly Government: *National minimum standards for care homes for older people*, (revised March 2004), Cardiff, 2004, WAG.

Welsh Assembly Government: *Fundamentals of Care*, Cardiff, 2006, WAG.

Welsh Assembly Government: *National Framework for continuing NHS health care*, Cardiff, 2007, WAG.

Welsh Assembly Government: *Clinical governance support and development unit*, Cardiff, 2008, WAG.

Williams H, Harris R, Turner-Stokes L: Northwick Park Care Needs Assessment: adaptation for inpatient neurological rehabilitation settings, *J Adv Nurs* 59:612–622, 2007.

World Health Organization: *International classification of impairments, disabilities and handicaps (ICIDH)*, Geneva, 1980, WHO.

World Health Organization: *International Classification of Functioning, Disability and Health (ICF)*, Geneva, 2001, WHO.

FURTHER READING

Burton CR: Re-thinking stroke rehabilitation: the Corbin and Strauss chronic illness trajectory framework, *J Adv Nurs* 32:595–602, 2000.

Campling F, Sharpe M: *Living with a Long-term Condition*, Oxford, 2006, OUP.

Carrier J: *Managing Long-term Conditions and Chronic Illness in Primary Care*, Abingdon, 2009, Routledge.

Donaghue PJ, Siegel ME: *Sick and Tired of Feeling Sick and Tired: Living with Invisible Chronic Illness*, ed 2, New York, 2000, Norton.

Neal LJ, Guillett S: *Care of the Adult with a Chronic Illness or Disability: A Team Approach*, St Louis, 2004, Mosby.

Snyder M, Lindquist R: *Complementary/alternative therapies in nursing*, ed 5, New York, 2006, Springer.

USEFUL WEBSITES

Organisations for a variety of long-term conditions can be found easily by using an internet search engine and using the condition's name and preferred country/countries of location.

Carers UK: the voice of carers (information and advice on carers' rights): www.carersuk.org

Healthtalkonline (based on qualitative research, with personal stories enabling readers to share individuals' experiences): www.healthtalkonline.org

Skills for health (a resource intended to support service development in promoting self-care and management): www.skillsforhealth.org.uk/~/media/Resource-Library/PDF/CommonCorePrinciples.ashx

Nursing patients who need palliative care

Patricia Black, Karen Strickland

Introduction

Caring effectively for people with a progressive, life-limiting illness presents a number of challenges for the multiprofessional team. Nurses have an important role to play in assessing care needs and managing the impact of an incurable illness on the patient and their family. Nursing knowledge and skills are vital contributions to the delivery of high-quality palliative care that enables patients to experience a good quality of life and a peaceful, dignified death, and their family to cope with bereavement.

The first part of this chapter defines palliative care and explores the fundamental principles of this approach. Consideration is given to how palliative care is provided within different settings and the range of services and teams which may be involved. The middle section has two parts: first it focuses on how the principles of palliative care may be applied in clinical practice, including communication with patients and families, and secondly on the evidence-based strategies for the management of common, distressing symptoms. The chapter concludes by exploring issues specific to the final phase of the patient's illness and considering how these may be addressed by effective end-of-life care.

What is palliative care?

The most widely accepted definition of palliative care was first provided by the World Health Organization (WHO) (1990). The most recent version states:

Palliative care is an approach that improves the quality of life of patients and their families facing the problems associated with life-threatening illness, through the prevention and relief of suffering by means of early identification and impeccable assessment and treatment of pain and other problems, physical, psychosocial and spiritual.

This clearly portrays palliative care as an active approach to assessing and managing care needs, far from the perspective that 'nothing more can be done' for the patient when their illness cannot be cured. The aim is to support the patient in living as comfortable and fulfilling a life as possible as their illness progresses towards death. It is important for health care professionals to recognise that dying is more than a physical experience and that suffering has psychological, social and spiritual dimensions which can also envelop those closest to the patient. This requires consideration not just of the physical disease process, but also the effects on the patient as an individual and their family when planning

Box 33.1 Reflection

Principles of palliative care

The World Health Organization sets out what palliative care involves, for example relieving pain and other distressing symptoms, and a holistic approach through the integration of the physical, psychological and spiritual aspects of care (WHO 2009).

Effective palliative care is essential, especially so when you consider that in most countries the majority of people will first access medical services when their illness is already advanced (WHO 2009).

Activities

- Access the website below and consider the components of palliative care.
- Reflect on the palliative care provided for patients and their families that you have cared for or witnessed in practice.
- Did the care provided fulfil the principles as set out by the WHO?
- Discuss your thoughts with your mentor or another student.

Resource

World Health Organization (WHO) – WHO Definition of Palliative Care, 2009. Available online http://www.who.int/cancer/palliative/definition/en/.

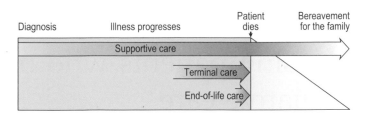

Figure 33.1 The scope of palliative care.

includes all stages of the disease trajectory including whilst the patient is receiving treatments which, although cure is not possible, may prolong their life or help control symptoms. Supportive care is integral to the palliative approach in helping the patient and family cope with the impact of the disease and the uncertainties and losses of the dying process. Terminal care refers to the last stage of the patient's illness, where there is increasing disability and dependence and death is anticipated in the near future. End-of-life care is delivered in the last days of the patient's life and will be considered in more depth later in this chapter.

The development of palliative care

In the United Kingdom, the palliative care approach was pioneered by Dame Cecily Saunders, attributed as founding the modern hospice movement with the opening of St. Christopher's Hospice, London, in 1967. This was a milestone in the history of palliative care, from which has evolved the person-centred, holistic approach underpinned by research and evidence-based practice that is now recognised worldwide.

In 1987, twenty years after the opening of St. Christopher's Hospice, palliative care was awarded the status of a medical specialty by the Royal College of Physicians in recognition of the growing body of knowledge and expertise in care of the dying generated within the hospice setting. Since then there have been further significant advances in clinical practice, research and education for health care professionals. As a result, there is now a substantial evidence base underpinning palliative care and greater expectations from both professionals and the public that suffering can be alleviated and a 'good death' achieved.

This is reflected in the wide range of guidelines, protocols and standards available to guide clinical practice and the delivery of care, including those from government advisory bodies and regulatory organisations such as the National Institute for Health and Clinical Excellence (NICE), NHS Quality Improvement Scotland (NHS QIS), the Care Quality Commission (CQC) (in England) and the Scottish Commission for Regulation of Care (SCRC).

The need to apply the principles of the palliative care approach developed within hospices to the care of patients dying in their own home, hospitals and nursing homes has received increasing attention. From reviewing place of death within England and Wales over the past 30 years, Gomes & Higginson (2008) highlight that most people with a life-limiting illness are cared for and die in these settings. The full breakdown of place of death is approximately:

- 5% within a hospice
- 17% within a care or nursing home, or other residential setting

and delivering care. The palliative care approach is therefore person-centred, holistic and multidimensional (Box 33.1).

Historically, a number of terms have been associated with palliative care. These include 'care of the dying', 'hospice care', 'supportive care', 'terminal care' and 'end-of-life care'. Birley & Morgan (2005) highlight that these terms are often used interchangeably and thus are open to misinterpretation.

A number of factors may have contributed to the varied terminology used to describe palliative care. Improved health and social care alongside advances in medical technologies have caused an epidemiological shift in the main causes of death within the developed world. From the late nineteenth century onwards, mortality rates from infectious diseases, childhood illnesses and maternal deaths have gradually declined. As a result, the average life expectancy has significantly increased and has now reached the highest level on record for both men and women (Office for National Statistics 2008). This has led to a steady rise in the incidence of life-limiting illnesses with more prolonged disease trajectories such as cancer, chronic respiratory and cardiovascular disease, for which more sophisticated diagnostic and treatment options have improved prognosis and length of survival. This means that an increasing number of people are living longer with progressive and ultimately fatal conditions. Kellehear (2007) provides a comprehensive and thought-provoking account of how in modern society the predominant conception of dying has shifted from an event characterised by a rapidly fatal or sudden demise, to that of a process of transition. This is now commonly referred to as 'living whilst dying' and 'the dying process', which can extend over weeks, months, even years.

Following the World Health Organization definition, the palliative approach is applicable from the time a life-limiting illness is diagnosed, throughout the patient's illness and into bereavement support for the family (Figure 33.1). This

- 18% at home
- 58% in hospital
- 2% other.

Furthermore, Gomes & Higginson (2008) project that, in line with an aging population, the demand for palliative care in general hospitals and the community setting will rise significantly by 2030.

As the majority of care for the dying is delivered within hospitals, the community and nursing homes, palliative care is a core responsibility of all health and social care professionals in these settings. Yet, increasing societal awareness and expectations of palliative care contrast sharply with reports of variation and deficiencies in care provision and the unmet needs of dying patients (Costello 2004, National Audit Office 2008). This has prompted development in two main areas:

- the expansion of hospice and specialist palliative care services
- introduction of frameworks to support professionals in delivering palliative care within mainstream services in both hospital and community settings.

The expansion of hospices and specialist palliative care services

Hospices were the first specialist palliative care services and there are currently over 200 inpatient units in the UK (Audit Scotland 2008, National Council for Palliative Care 2007). Patients may be admitted for a variety of reasons including assessment, rehabilitation and symptom management, respite stays to give families and carers a short break, and terminal care.

From the 1990s onwards, the specialty of palliative care expanded with the development of services within the hospital and community. These include specialist hospital palliative care teams, day hospices and community palliative care teams. Some of these specialist services are partly funded and hosted by independent and charitable organisations, such as Marie Curie Cancer Care, whilst others are fully funded and based within the NHS. Charities such as Macmillan Cancer Support have provided the financial backing to initiate a number of specialist posts and developments to support the delivery of palliative care within general, mainstream services. The contribution of these charities is recognised by the continued use of their name and this has led to a plethora of titles for similar posts, for example clinical nurse specialists in palliative care may also be known as Macmillan Nurses and Marie Curie Homecare Sisters.

The core dimensions of specialist palliative care services are:

- Multiprofessional teams of health and social care professionals with advanced knowledge and skills in palliative care, having completed post-qualification accredited education and substantial clinical experience. They include palliative medicine consultants and clinical nurse specialists, together with a range of expertise provided by physiotherapists, occupational therapists, dietitians, pharmacists and social workers.
- The provision of specialist interventions and direct care for patients and families with moderate–high complexity of palliative care needs.

- The provision of advice and support for other professionals within general hospital and community care settings in applying the principles of palliative care in clinical practice.
- Advancing the specialty of palliative care through research, audit, education and practice development initiatives (National Council for Hospice and Specialist Palliative Care Services 2002, NHS Quality Improvement Scotland [NHS QIS] 2004).

Specialist palliative care services are not involved in the care of all patients with a life-limiting illness but operate on an advisory and referral basis. Other health and social care professionals, such as GPs and district nurses in the community and ward teams in hospitals, can request advice regarding how to address the needs of patients and families under their care. They can also refer patients and families with more complex needs for specialist assessment and direct intervention, for example in managing difficult pain and other symptoms, and psychological and spiritual distress. In this way, the expertise of the specialist team is shared through joint-working to address palliative care needs, although the referring team retains overall clinical control and responsibility for the patient (Box 33.2).

Supporting general palliative care within community and hospital settings

Current health care strategy emphasises the need to ensure access to a high standard of palliative care for all patients with a life-limiting illness within all care settings (Department of Health [DH] 2008a, Scottish Government 2008). Traditionally, hospices have provided care predominantly for people with cancer. It would appear that this is generally still the case from reports that during 2006–2007, 93% of those referred to specialist palliative care services across the UK had a diagnosis of malignancy (National Council for Palliative Care 2007). Cancer remains a leading cause of death in the developed world (see Ch. 31). Studies have identified, however, that people dying from non-malignant life-limiting illnesses such as advanced cardiac and respiratory diseases, dementia and stroke have just as great a need for palliative care as those with cancer (Solano et al 2006).

Box 33.2 Reflection

Availability of specialist palliative care services

Specialist palliative care services vary from area to area. For example, the provision of services in a city may be quite different to those provided in a sparsely populated rural area.

Activities

- What specialist palliative care services are available in your area?
- What are the criteria for referring patients to these specialist palliative care services?
- Reflect on the range of services offered and the benefits to patients and their families.

Resource

Help the Hospices: Directory of Hospice and Palliative Care Services – www.helpthehospices.org.uk.

It has already been highlighted that the incidence of both malignant and non-malignant life-limiting illnesses is rising, with a corresponding increase in demand for palliative care. In addition, greater awareness of inequity of access to effective care across settings and for some patient groups has made strengthening the delivery of palliative care within mainstream hospital and community services a priority. Developments towards this include the introduction of The Gold Standards Framework (Thomas 2003) and the Liverpool Care Pathway for the Dying (Ellershaw & Wilkinson 2003) to support the delivery of a high standard of palliative care in all settings.

The palliative care approach in practice

This part of the chapter considers the palliative care approach in clinical practice. A model of palliative care is presented which can be used as a guide to applying the principles of palliative care when caring for patients and families.

The palliative care approach – a model for practice

The model for practice is presented as a guide for the clinical nurse in the twenty first century (Figure 33.2). In accordance with the Nursing and Midwifery Council (2008) *The Code: Standards of Conduct, Performance and Ethics for Professional Practice,* this nurse is a critical thinker. This means challenging assumptions and looking for creative and workable solutions to problems, critically reading literature and appraising research and, in partnership with the multiprofessional team, implementing reflective, evidence-based practice.

Each dimension of the model is presented and discussed. It is important to recognise that these dimensions are interrelated and interdependent.

Fundamental to person-centred palliative care is *therapeutic communication with the patient and family*, therefore this forms the core of the model. *Holistic assessment and care management* relates to the overarching aim of palliative care and

the patient experiencing a quality of life and a dignified death. This requires consideration of the wide range of physical, psychological, social and spiritual issues which may arise from a life-limiting illness and the individual responses of the patient and family to their situation. *Multiprofessional teamwork* emphasises that the knowledge and skills of different health and social care professionals are vital contributions to the provision of holistic palliative care. *Effective symptom control* maximises independence and comfort and thus allows both the patient and family to focus on goals and activities which are important to them. The dimension of advance care planning identifies palliative care as a proactive approach to care as well as responsive to the current needs of the patient. Planning ahead for anticipated changes in condition allows the patient's wishes to be considered regarding their future care and treatment, a quality of life to be maintained and the distress of unnecessary hospital admissions avoided.

Therapeutic communication

Effective communication with the patient and family is central to the delivery of palliative care. Knowing how the illness affects the person, what they think and how they feel about their situation provides the basis for care appropriate to their individual needs and goals. If a key aim of palliative care is that the patient experiences a quality of life, then professionals need to understand exactly what that means for them. Quality of life is a subjective experience and therefore we need to consider what is important to the patient and what gives their life meaning. How do they perceive the illness affects them, their family and their quality of life?

Eliciting this information requires effective and sensitive communication between professionals and patients. This can be termed therapeutic communication, which differs from the social communications integral to everyday life in relation to context, purpose and the communication skills used by the professional.

The purpose of therapeutic communication is primarily supportive to the patient and family in the context of care provision and provides the medium by which professionals can gain an accurate understanding of care needs. Therapeutic communication also allows information needs to be identified and addressed, at a level appropriate to the individual patient and family to ensure their understanding. From summarising research in this area, Duke & Bailey (2008) report that the effective provision of information has been shown to reduce distress and enhance compliance with treatment and the ability to cope with the practicalities of living with and dying from a life-limiting illness. Professionals have a responsibility to be aware of how well they communicate with patients and families, and this can be supported by critical reflection on practice. This responsibility extends to then developing the necessary knowledge, skills and confidence in the use of strategies which support effective interaction with the patients and families under their care.

A full discussion regarding skills and strategies for therapeutic communication is beyond the scope of this chapter, however some key points are considered below.

Therapeutic interaction with patients and/or families may take the form of an assessment interview, a one-to-one discussion or interaction with patient and family together.

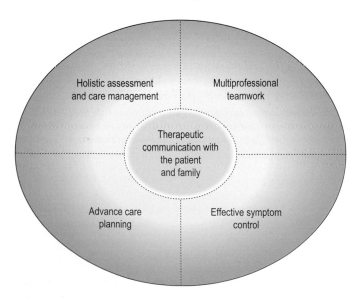

Figure 33.2 The palliative care approach – a model for practice.

Preparation is important in ensuring that the nurse has as much information as is available regarding the patient's condition, history and circumstances. Patients often feel they have to repeat information over and over again to different professionals and this can be frustrating and extremely tiring for those already fatigued because of their illness. The patient's case notes should be read, as they may contain a great deal of the required information regarding diagnosis, previous treatment, current issues and problems. Members of the multiprofessional team may be able to provide further details, including those in other care settings: for example the district nurse may be able to provide useful information for hospital staff regarding the care needs of the patient at home and any family issues. It is wise to remember, however, that the nature of a life-limiting illness means that issues and problems change over time and that how they are perceived by the team caring for the patient may be different from those causing the greatest concern for the patient. This means the nurse should work from an informed basis but check and expand their understanding of the patient's situation and importantly, related perceptions and concerns.

The ideal situation for therapeutic communication is one in which privacy is provided without interruption. The patient's physical comfort should be attended to. The purpose should be made explicit and the patient's consent obtained to proceed. Patients and families need to feel secure that confidentiality will be maintained. It is often believed that patients realise that they are being cared for by a multiprofessional team and that they therefore implicitly agree that information given to one professional may be openly shared with others. This should not be assumed. It is useful to remind patients and families that information which is relevant to their care is shared within the multiprofessional team and to emphasise that they do not have to talk about areas they prefer to keep private. The ethics of confidentiality are beyond the scope of this chapter (see Nursing and Midwifery Council 2008 and Further reading, e.g. Dimond 2008, Griffith & Tengah 2008).

Attention to non-verbal behaviours such as maintaining appropriate eye contact, sitting rather than standing beside the patient and adopting an open posture, slightly leaning forward rather than sitting back with crossed arms and legs, can display warmth and respect. The use of paralinguistic responses can encourage the patient to continue to talk and shows the nurse is paying attention. Active listening is a key skill and incorporates close attention to not just what the patient is saying verbally, but their facial expression, tone of voice and behaviour, which can convey the meaning and emotion behind their words.

The flow of discussion should be paced according to the patient, who is encouraged to talk about their main problems and concerns. Open questions such as 'Can you tell me how this affects your day-to-day life. . .?' give the patient the opportunity to provide rich and detailed information from their perspective. In contrast, closed or focussed questions such as 'How many times a day does this happen?' provide more specific information, particularly when clarification is needed or when the patient is too tired or breathless for a lengthy discussion.

From skilful use of questioning it should be possible to appraise the patient's understanding of their illness and expectations regarding care. Patients are individuals in how they cope with a life-limiting illness. This includes what they understand about their illness from the information provided by professionals, how they interpret changes in their condition and their social circumstances and their psychological coping style. This can also influence what they wish to discuss and when, and their choice to do so should be respected. Asking an open question such as 'Can you tell me what you understand about. . .?' allows the patient to exert some control over what is discussed and how they respond. If the patient becomes tired or upset at any time, the nurse must enquire if they wish to stop. The patient may wish to conclude the interview or, where the expression of the emotions is appropriate and needed by the patient, they may simply wish some time. In this situation, the importance of sensitivity and the nurse's presence should not be underestimated. An upset or distressed patient should not be abandoned. If, however, they require some private time alone or with their family, then reassurance should be given that the nurse will return at an agreed time in the very near future or sooner, should they request.

There may be occasions where the nurse does not have the information required to answer a question or address a concern. Honesty is the best policy, alongside acknowledgement that the question or concern is important to the person. Reassurance can be given that the nurse will direct their question or concern to an appropriate member of the multiprofessional team. Dying patients and their families do not expect every professional to have all the answers; however, dishonesty or failing to acknowledge their concerns can undermine their trust, confidence in and openness with the multiprofessional team (Costello 2004).

When speaking to families it is important to note that where the patient has capacity their permission and wishes should be ascertained regarding disclosure of information. Family members can offer useful information regarding care needs and may be the greatest source of support for the patient, including supporting their wish to be cared for at home. Family dynamics do vary, however, and therefore an understanding of roles and relationships ensures that the patient's wishes can be respected whilst addressing the concerns of the family, reinforcing the principle that family support is an integral part of palliative care (Payne 2007).

In concluding the interaction, summarising key points which have been discussed is a useful strategy. This lets the patient and/or family see that the nurse has listened and understood what they have said and provides the opportunity for them to add more detail or correct any misunderstandings. The summary should include agreeing any required actions or changes to plan of care and allows the nurse to ensure their understanding of any information given. Screening for any other issues gives patients and/or families the opportunity to raise any concerns which they have not yet mentioned. Following such interactions, the nurse will clearly and succinctly document relevant information and communicate any immediate issues to the appropriate multiprofessional team member. In this way, care is patient-centred and consistent whilst avoiding the need for patients to repeatedly provide the same information to different team members.

Holistic assessment and care management

Holistic assessment is a key activity in palliative care and directs the use of appropriate strategies for care needs associated with the physical, psychological, spiritual and social impact of the illness on the patient and family. A number of approaches may be used. These include quantitative measures such as rating scales to measure the severity of a symptom, for example pain assessment tools (see Ch. 19), and more qualitative approaches such as history taking. Whatever approach is used it is imperative that it is multidimensional so that the assessment captures a full and comprehensive picture of the palliative care needs of the patient and family. Some key assessment questions which can be adapted for a holistic assessment include:

- Can you describe what ...... is like?
- How bad is it – at worst/at best?
- How often does ...... happen?
- What makes ...... better/worse?
- What do you think is causing ......?
- How does ...... make you feel?
- What does ...... mean to you?
- How does ...... affect your day-to-day life?

A plan of care can then be devised which reflects the principles of palliative care. Attention to detail is important, as is continuous review because of the complex and progressive nature of the dying process.

Multiprofessional teamwork

From review of the principles of palliative care it can be identified that no one profession can meet all the care needs of the patient and family. A holistic approach requires the skills and expertise of different professionals. Nurses play a central role within the multiprofessional team which includes facilitating communication and coordinating the input of other team members in patient care. This may include a range of professionals including the physiotherapist, occupational therapist, chaplain, social worker and dietitian.

Effective multiprofessional teamwork is, however, more than just a group of professionals involved in the care of the same patient and family. Speck (2006) outlines a number of challenges for the multiprofessional team in palliative care. These include ensuring a shared understanding of goals and objectives and that a blurring of traditional role boundaries can occur when all professionals share a holistic perspective. Effective communication and coordination of activity across a wide team is essential to avoid the risk of fragmented care and key needs not being identified and properly addressed.

Advance care planning

A thorough understanding of the pathophysiology of the patient's illness offers direction for anticipating likely disease progression and associated issues. Effective palliative care requires consideration of what problems may arise and, where possible, the instigation of measures to prevent them or facilitate their timely management. This includes ensuring adequate medications are available, including on a prn 'as required' basis should the patient's symptoms worsen. Unnecessary hospital admissions can potentially be avoided by providing ready access to equipment and increased social support should the patient's condition deteriorate and ensuring that out-of-hours services have essential access to information.

Ascertaining the wishes of the patient regarding future care and treatment is an important part of care planning and nurses play a key role in acting as the patient's advocate

and supporting an informed choice. This may include decisions concerning resuscitation which can present a number of ethical and practice issues for nurses. The General Medical Council GMC (2010) and the Scottish Government (2008) have produced guidance regarding this sensitive area of care.

The patient's preferences regarding place of care during their illness and at the end of life should also be explored using therapeutic communication. Patient's wishes may change over time and therefore decisions should be sensitively revisited as appropriate when circumstances change. Recently, the use of the *Preferred Place of Care* document to communicate and support patient choice across care settings has been advocated in England and Wales (Department of Health 2008b).

Effective symptom control

The key components of symptom control in palliative care are well described (see Further reading, e.g. Hanks et al 2009). In summary, the multiprofessional team must work with the patient to:

- make a thorough assessment of each symptom
- discuss causes and treatment options
- plan symptom management in light of the patient's expectations and priorities
- evaluate regularly with changing condition and progressive disease.

When administering medications for symptom control the most appropriate route for the patient must be considered. If, for example, the patient is regularly nauseated or is vomiting, then they are unlikely to fully absorb oral medications and likewise, if drowsy at the end of life, may be unable to swallow. In such situations parenteral administration is appropriate, usually via continuous subcutaneous (s.c.) administration by syringe driver. This avoids the need for repeated injections and is less invasive than the intravenous route. Patient choice must also be considered: for example, some patients with stable pain may prefer an adhesive transdermal analgesic patch which is changed every 3 days to taking oral analgesics regularly by mouth.

The effective control of some common distressing symptoms is discussed below.

 ## Nursing management and health promotion: common distressing symptoms

This part of the chapter focuses on the management of four common distressing symptoms: pain, nausea and vomiting, constipation and breathlessness. See Further reading (e.g. NHS Lothian 2008, Fallon & Hanks 2007) for information about other symptoms, such as cough, hiccup, delirium, etc.

Pain

Pain is one of the most feared symptoms of a terminal illness and is estimated to occur in up to 70% of patients with cancer and 65% of patients dying from non-malignant diseases (Fallon & McConnell 2006). Despite the complexity of this symptom, a vast amount of knowledge is available regarding strategies for effective management. However, pain that is not identified will not be treated, and pain will not be treated vigorously enough if its severity is underestimated.

It has now been accepted that the patient's self-report is the most reliable indicator of pain. However there are challenges to this in practice. Self-report of pain may not be an option in the confused or non-verbal patient. Observation of behaviour and proxy reporting from carers then becomes the main method of assessing the pain of these individuals (Royal College of Physicians, British Pain Society and British Geriatrics Society 2007).

In addition, there are personality, attitudinal and cultural reasons why people do not reveal their pains. These range from being loath to admit to an increase in pain as they perceive this may signify progression of their disease, to being unwilling to admit that the best efforts of the multiprofessional team have been to no avail.

Patients who are dying commonly have more than one pain. The nurse committed to helping the patient must therefore systematically assess and document the following information about each pain the patient is experiencing:

- location
- severity
- radiation – does the pain move or travel from its original site?
- type – is the pain described as dull/gnawing/shooting/ burning/spasmodic?
- when started
- aggravating factors
- alleviating factors.

The severity of pain can be assessed using visual or numerical analogue scales, for example by asking the patient to score their pain on a scale of 1–10 where 0 equals no pain and 10 equals the most severe pain possible (see Ch. 19). Some patients may prefer rating their pain as none/mild/ moderate/severe or simply using their own terms. It is important to find a way of rating pain severity that is clearly understood by both the patient and the multiprofessional team. From this shared understanding of how bad the pain feels, management strategies can be targeted most effectively and patient distress minimised. Professionals must remember that in a palliative context, the patient may have been experiencing pain for some time. The physiological indicators common to those with acute pain, e.g. tachycardia and raised blood pressure, may therefore be absent.

It is also important to ask the patient about their pain *now* and when *at its worst*. This can detect the presence of 'incident pain' which is pain that only happens at certain times or is triggered by specific events, for example the patient may rate their hip pain as 0 out of 10 when sitting at rest but 9 out of 10 when trying to walk or bend. This has obvious implications for the patient's quality of life and maintaining their independence for as long as possible.

How the patient describes the character of their pain helps determine the type of pain they are experiencing. Pain which is described as shooting or burning may denote nerve or neuropathic pain whilst aching and gnawing pain over a joint may indicate bone pain from secondary cancer or severe arthritis. The type of pain is a key factor in selecting the most appropriate choice of analgesics and interventions.

The nurse should discuss the findings from the assessment with medical staff and other relevant members of the multiprofessional team, such as the physiotherapist. It is essential that this be done in an informed manner by giving a detailed description of the pain as outlined above. It is poor practice when requesting medical attendance or input from other professionals for the nurse just to give the blank statement that the patient is in pain.

An accurate diagnosis of new pains is usually derived from observation, discussion and physical examination by the doctor. A full assessment is essential, as new pains may require laboratory or radiological investigations and other treatments, as well as analgesics.

Analgesic medications, given regularly to prevent the recurrence of pain, are central to effective pain management in palliative care. It is essential that an adequate, regular dose is calculated and administered, enabling the patient to be as comfortable as possible without being drowsy.

Principles have been established by the WHO (1986, 1996) to guide health care professionals in the effective management of pain. In addition, guidelines such as the Scottish Intercollegiate Guidelines Network (SIGN) (2008) publication *Control of Pain in Adults with Cancer* are readily available online. Registered nurses must have a working knowledge of these principles and guidelines to promote good multiprofessional understanding and patient confidence.

WHO Key principles of pain control and the analgesic ladder

The key principles of the WHO approach are that analgesics be given by the mouth, by the clock and by the ladder.

By the mouth

This convenient and easy route of administration should be the method of choice for as long as possible. When the patient can no longer tolerate oral medicines, the s.c. route is most frequently used by setting up a syringe driver.

By the clock

Persistent pain must be prevented; it is inhumane to simply wait for pain to return before administering the next dose, and regular analgesia is necessary to achieve stable pain control. This requires that professionals are knowledgeable about the duration of action of different analgesic preparations. For example, normal release morphine solution is effective for 4 h, therefore it *must* be administered regularly every 4 h. Other controlled-release preparations, such as MST Continus®, last 12 h and so are administered every 12 h to provide stable levels of background analgesia. In an inpatient setting, care must be taken that the patient receives their analgesics at an appropriate time and does not have to wait for drug rounds for the analgesics they need to control their pain.

By the ladder

The analgesic ladder developed by the WHO (1996) details a three-step approach to using mild to strong analgesics to control pain (see Useful websites, e.g. WHO Pain ladder). This was developed for cancer pain but is now commonly applied to those with non-cancer life-limiting illness. The ladder combines primary analgesics and adjuvant therapies.

The WHO (1996) recommends that the strength of analgesia required should be matched with the severity of the pain and from this they developed the analgesic ladder. Commonly used analgesics are outlined in Box 33.3.

Box 33.3 Information

Analgesic medications commonly used for cancer pain

Step 3

Opioids for moderate to severe pain

Morphine normal release – as an oral solution, e.g. Oramorph® or tablets, e.g Sevredol®

Morphine controlled release, e.g. MST Continus® or MXL®

Morphine or diamorphine by s.c. injection

Oxycodone normal release as an oral solution or capsule e.g. Oxynorm®.

Oxycodone controlled release, e.g. Oxycontin®

Oxycodone by s.c. injection

Step 2

Opioids for mild to moderate pain

Codeine often combined with paracetamol, e.g. co-codamol 30/500

Step 1

Non-opioids for mild pain

Paracetamol or non-steroidal anti-inflammatory drugs (NSAIDs)

If the patient's management starts on *step 1* of the ladder (mild pain), paracetamol may be given until the ceiling of 4 g in 24 h has been reached, i.e. the upper dose limit of this drug. If it does not control the pain then a drug on *step 2* (mild to moderate pain) will be prescribed. Co-codamol 30/500, a combination of paracetamol and the step 2 opioid codeine, is commonly used. It is referred to as co-codamol 30/500 as each tablet contains codeine 30 mg and paracetamol 500 mg. It will be given up to the ceiling of two tablets 6-hourly. When that is ineffective in controlling the patient's pain, the step 2 opioid is stopped and a drug on *step 3* (moderate to severe pain) will be prescribed. It is essential to note that paracetamol may be continued simultaneously with a step 3 opioid as the analgesic action is different from opioids and the combination can therefore be synergistic in relieving pain. The decision to use a step 3 opioid should be based on patient need and the severity of pain and not their prognosis. The outdated practice of saving morphine for the last few weeks of life is misinformed.

A normal release oral preparation of morphine, such as Oramorph® liquid or Sevredol® tablets, will be prescribed with the intention of establishing a regimen that will relieve the pain without causing oversedation. This process is known as titration. A common starting dose of normal release morphine is 5–10 mg, except in older, frail or cachexic patients when 2.5 mg might be the starting dose. It will be prescribed to be taken 4-hourly round the clock, for example at 06.00, 10.00, 14.00, 18.00, 22.00 and, if awake, at 02.00 h.

Should the patient be in pain between doses, a breakthrough dose equivalent to the standard 4-hourly dose will be given. If a breakthrough dose is given, the timing of the next regular dose must not be altered. For example, if a patient has Oramorph® at 06.00 h and requires a breakthrough dose at 09.00 h, the dose due at 10.00 h will still be given on time. Once a stable dose of analgesic has been reached for 24–48 h the dose of normal release medication can be converted into a sustained release preparation. For example, the patient receives 10 mg of normal release morphine every 4 h, therefore over a 24-h period they receive 6 doses × 10 mg = 60 mg in total. This can be converted to an equivalent dose of MST Continus® = 30 mg MST Continus® every 12 h. Guidance for transferring patients from oral morphine to s.c. diamorphine and other step 3 opiates is available from Scottish Intercollegiate Guidelines Network (SIGN) (2008). It is essential that nurses are aware that patients may have more than one pain and that different analgesics may well be required for effective pain relief (Box 33.4).

Some common side-effects might be expected when a patient commences on step 3 opioids. Transitory effects may be slight

---

Box 33.4 Reflection

Michelle: assessment and management of pain

Michelle is a 39-year-old mother of two (Jack aged 9 and Sophie who is 7 years of age). Her mother (Kate) is caring for the children and visits Michelle every day. Michelle is a company director and is separated from her husband. She has advanced breast cancer with metastases to bone, liver and brain. Whilst you are helping Michelle to wash one morning, she complains of pain. On further questioning, she describes three pains.

- First, she rubs the upper right quadrant of her abdomen and states that a feeling of extreme pressure builds up from deep inside her body. It has been getting steadily worse over the last few weeks, especially if she tries to lie on her right side.
- Second, Michelle describes the tight band of headache that is frequently worse on waking in the morning.
- Third, Michelle grimaces as the skin over her right femur is washed. When encouraged, she points with her finger to a specific area of pain in the bone that is causing discomfort.

The first pain is visceral pain caused by the liver being enlarged with metastases and a stretched liver capsule. Michelle has been prescribed diamorphine by continuous s.c. infusion and the adjuvant medication dexamethasone for this pain. Before admission, Michelle was trying to take MST Continus® 60 mg 12-hourly for this pain; however, nausea and vomiting affected concordance. Cyclizine, an antiemetic, has been added to the diamorphine by s.c. infusion to alleviate the nausea/vomiting whilst assessment as to cause is undertaken.

The second pain around Michelle's head is likely to be caused by pressure from the oedema due to cerebral metastases. The dose of dexamethasone already prescribed for her liver pain has been increased to reduce the oedema. In addition, paracetamol 4 g in 24 h will now be prescribed to help relieve this headache. The doctor has discussed with Michelle the role of palliative radiotherapy in treating this problem. Pain from extensive bone metastases was a considerable problem almost 1 year previously although successfully managed with hemibody radiotherapy.

It is likely that the third pain in Michelle's femur is due to bone metastases. The paracetamol being commenced for her headaches may also help to relieve bone pain. In addition, NSAIDs, which can bring considerable relief, should be considered.

Continued

Box 33.4 Reflection – cont'd

Michelle reports that she feels less able to cope with her pain when she is tired and feels low in mood, particularly when she cannot do the things she previously enjoyed, including as part of caring for her children.

Activities

• Reflect on the complex nature of Michelle's different pains and discuss with your mentor the importance of a thorough pain assessment for patients who need palliative care.

• Consider how analgesics (primary and adjuvant), adjuvant drugs and non-pharmacological treatment all have a role in relieving Michelle's pain.

• Consider the guidance on transferring patients from oral to s.c. analgesia (Scottish Intercollegiate Guidelines Network (SIGN) 2008).

sleepiness and nausea; these usually pass in a few days. More troublesome are constipation (see also pp. 860–861) and a dry mouth. Constipation *must* be treated prophylactically; a laxative such as co-danthramer (dantron and poloxamer) or a macrogol (polyethylene glycols) such as Movicol® must be prescribed at the same time as the opioid (see also p. 861).

Occasionally unacceptable side-effects may occur. 'Opioid toxicity' is a term used to denote a range of side-effects which can be distressing and, if untreated, life-threatening. Early signs are subtle and include vivid dreams, seeing shadows moving at the periphery of their visual field and mild confusion. This can progress to worsening confusion, agitation, muscle twitches and hallucinations. Opiate toxicity may arise where the dose of opioid has been rapidly escalated or, alternatively, where dehydration or renal failure occurs and opioid metabolites normally excreted via the kidneys accumulate in the bloodstream. Such side-effects must be reported to the medical team as soon as detected. The dose of opioid will be reduced and intravenous fluids may be required to help excretion of metabolites. Opioid toxicity from morphine and other intolerable side-effects including intractable constipation might cause the physician to prescribe a second-line opioid such as oxycodone, fentanyl or alfentanyl. This is referred to as opioid switching or rotation and should be done under the guidance of specialist palliative care services (Colvin et al 2007).

Adjuvant medications are frequently given along with analgesics in the effective management of pain (see Ch. 19) and may be given in conjunction with a primary analgesic on any step of the ladder (Table 33.1). Some pains do not respond well to the primary analgesics codeine, morphine and the medications that are collectively known as opioids. Bone pain and neuropathic pain present particular challenges and commonly require adjuvant analgesics (Callin & Bennett 2008).

Approximately 80–90% of pain due to cancer can be relieved with oral analgesics and adjuvant medications following the WHO guidelines (Colvin et al 2007). The remaining percentage of pain can be challenging to manage and may require input from specialist palliative care or pain services. For detailed information on complex pain problems see Scottish Intercollegiate Guidelines Network 2008, Cherny 2009 and Gordon-Williams & Dickenson 2009.

Fear of addiction

One barrier to effective pain control in palliative care is the fear that patients, families and some health care professionals have of addiction to opioids. This fear is unfounded when the

Table 33.1 Adjuvant analgesics commonly used for cancer pain		
MEDICATION	**EXAMPLE**	**INDICATIONS**
Non-steroidal anti-inflammatory drugs (NSAIDs)	Diclofenac	Bone pain, inflammatory pain, soft tissue infiltration
Corticosteroids	Dexamethasone Prednisolone	Raised intracranial pressure (see Ch. 9) Neuropathic pain from nerve compression or destruction Soft tissue pressure or infiltration Hepatomegaly (enlarged liver)
Tricyclic antidepressants	Amitriptyline	Neuropathic pain from nerve compression or destruction Paraneoplastic neuropathies
Anticonvulsants	Gabapentin	Neuropathic pain from nerve compression or destruction Paraneoplastic neuropathies
Bisphosphonates	Pamidronate	Bone pain

patient has physical pain. The confusion frequently arises when the patient on opioids requires increasing doses to relieve the physical pain arising from progressive disease.

An understanding of the terms 'addiction', 'tolerance' and 'dependence' is useful to reassure the patient and family. Addiction, i.e. psychological dependence and craving, is usually seen in individuals who are taking morphine in the absence of physical pain. In contrast, tolerance is an involuntary physiological response when, having taken the opioids for some time, the patient requires larger doses to benefit from the same analgesic effect. Physical dependence is another physiological response which patients may experience when an opioid is stopped suddenly, such as flu-like symptoms which can be avoided by gradual dose reduction. Tolerance and physical dependence are not the same as addiction and it is important to note that the requirement for increasing doses is most commonly due to disease progression and not pharmacological tolerance (Fallon et al 2007).

Nausea and vomiting

Nausea and vomiting are common and distressing symptoms in palliative care. The pathophysiology of nausea and vomiting is complex and incompletely understood. There is no antiemetic ladder to guide the multiprofessional team, but efforts have been made to identify a logical approach to these symptoms (Kinley 2005, Mannix 2007).

An understanding of the pathophysiology of nausea and vomiting is important to allow the nurse to participate actively in planning care and to explain care to patients and their families.

In order for vomiting to occur, there must be detectors to identify the need to vomit, a coordinating centre and effectors which make the vomiting take place. The main receptors involved in controlling the experience of nausea and need to vomit are located in the:

- gastrointestinal tract
- chemoreceptor trigger zone (CTZ), a specialised area of the brain on the floor of the fourth ventricle
- inner/middle ear
- higher brain centres.

Figure 33.3 illustrates the location of these receptor sites. Messages from each of these receptor sites are transmitted to the vomiting centre in the medulla (part of the brain stem), which coordinates vomiting. Transmission from the gastrointestinal tract to the vomiting centre is via the vagus nerve. As this nerve innervates other tissues, vomiting may be stimulated by disease or trauma to other organs, e.g. the pharynx, liver or bladder. Direct stimulation of the vomiting centre by pressure, trauma or disease may also cause vomiting.

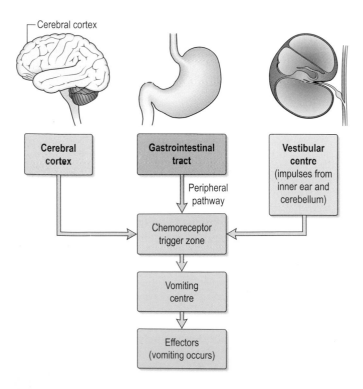

Figure 33.3 The vomiting reflex. (Adapted from Bruce & Finlay 1997 with permission.)

In advanced cancer the vomiting centre can be activated in a number of ways:

- vagal stimulation caused, for example, by gastric or bowel distension, liver capsule stretch, mediastinal disease or genitourinary problems
- stimulation from the CTZ caused by chemical abnormalities in the blood, e.g. uraemia, hypercalcaemia (excessive calcium level in the blood), drugs or bacterial toxins
- stimulation from the inner/middle ear due to infection, movement or local tumour
- stimulation from higher central nervous system centres by anxiety, fear or revulsion
- direct stimulation from raised intracranial pressure.

Many neurotransmitter receptors have been identified as playing a part in vomiting pathways (Mannix 2007) and understanding of this is developing. What is important in terms of patient care is to appreciate that particular antiemetics are thought to block messages about the need to vomit at specific points along the vomiting pathways. It is this action which produces improvement or control of nausea and vomiting. Some of the commonly used antiemetics in palliative care act centrally at the vomiting centre, vestibular centre and/or the CTZ. Some antiemetics act peripherally in the gastrointestinal tract and some act at both levels (NHS Lothian 2008). Specific antiemetics must therefore be selected for specific causes of nausea and vomiting. Further information regarding antiemetic medication and prescribing may be found in the *Lothian Palliative Care Guidelines* (NHS Lothian 2008) and the *British National Formulary (BNF)* (see Further reading, e.g. Mannix 2009, and Useful websites, e.g. Palliativedrugs.com). A table outlining the commonly used antiemetic drugs is also provided on the companion website.

See website for further content

Careful assessment is crucial. Working with the patient, the team puts together a detailed picture of these symptoms. The importance of the clinical picture in assessing and managing nausea and vomiting has been recognised (NHS Lothian 2008). The challenge for the multiprofessional team in caring for a patient who is vomiting is to tailor symptom management to the patient's problems, expectations, priorities and wishes. The doctor's comprehensive physical examination of the patient is another important source of information. Blood tests may be requested to measure serum urea, calcium and other electrolyte levels, which in some cases may be contributing to nausea/vomiting or be deranged as a result of this.

The multiprofessional team may also consider non-pharmacological measures. The potential benefits of non-pharmacological interventions such as transcutaneous electrical nerve stimulation (TENS), acupuncture and guided mental imagery are acknowledged in the literature (Mannix 2007), but more research is required. Nursing measures are important, such as encouraging fluid intake, avoiding exposure to strong smells, ensuring good oral hygiene and providing small portions of food.

See website Critical thinking question 33.1

Constipation

Constipation is a very common problem for patients in the palliative phase of illness and can cause abdominal pain, nausea and embarrassment. It may lead on to other serious problems such as faecal impaction, overflow diarrhoea, urinary dysfunction, vomiting and even confusion (Sykes et al 2007). Careful assessment, management and documentation of this symptom may make the difference between the patient staying at home and hospital admission. The nurse's role in this is crucial. Evidence-based guidelines for the assessment and management of constipation in palliative care are available in the *Lothian Palliative Care Guidelines* (NHS Lothian 2008).

Many factors may work together to cause constipation. Sometimes constipation is disease related. For example, for the patient with cancer, the site of the tumour or the presence of hypercalcaemia may be contributing causes. Eating very small helpings of food with little fibre, drinking considerably less than before and restricted mobility may all contribute to the development of constipation. If the patient is nauseated or experiencing vomiting then they may be reluctant to eat and drink. When opioids are added to this scenario, constipation becomes a certainty. Opioids have a number of effects on the bowel. They reduce peristalsis, inhibit fluid secretion (Regnard & Hockley 2004), increase sphincter tone and diminish sensitivity to rectal distension (Sykes et al 2007). In this way, the patient can quickly become constipated, struggling to expel small, dry, hard stools.

Anticipation and assessment of this symptom forms the basis for effective management. In other words, the nurse does not wait until the patient complains of constipation, but is constantly alert to this possibility, reviewing the situation each day. As part of the holistic assessment of the patient, the nurse needs to take a careful and sensitive history including:

- previous bowel habits
- the most recent stool (when it was passed, what it was like, any problems experienced)
- intake of diet and fluids
- compliance with laxative regimen
- other medications taken
- accessibility and acceptability of toilet arrangements.

Where constipation is suspected, abdominal and digital rectal examinations are indicated. Depending on local policy and practising within the *The Code: Standards of Conduct, Performance and Ethics for Professional Practice* (Nursing and Midwifery Council 2008), a competent registered nurse may perform a digital examination of the rectum. A plain X-ray of the abdomen may be useful in assessing the extent of constipation (Sykes et al 2007).

The management of constipation requires more than prescribing and administering laxatives. It involves attention to the relief of pain and other symptoms, to fluids and diet and to adapting toilet facilities to ensure accessibility, comfort and privacy.

An understanding of laxatives is vital, especially for nurse prescribers. Oral and rectal laxatives may be classified as:

- stimulant laxatives, e.g. bisacodyl (oral and suppositories), docusate sodium (oral or microenema; note, docusate sodium most likely has both stimulant and softener properties, BNF 2009), senna, glycerol suppositories, dantron (danthron)
- faecal softeners, e.g., docusate sodium, arachis oil (peanut oil, groundnut oil) retention enemas

- bulking agents, e.g. ispaghula husk, are rarely used in palliative care because they are unpalatable, require to be taken with a large volume of fluid and may complete an incipient intestinal obstruction
- osmotic laxatives, e.g. macrogols, lactulose, phosphate or sodium citrate enemas
- a peripheral opioid-receptor antagonist, such as methylnaltrexone bromide, can be used with other laxatives for the management of constipation associated with opioid analgesics in palliative care under guidance of specialist palliative care services.

A combination of a stimulant and faecal softener, e.g. co-danthrusate (dantron/docusate sodium) or co-danthramer (dantron/poloxamer) gives the most favourable results, at an acceptable dose and with a minimum of unwanted side-effects. The dose should be titrated against patient response. Recently, macrogols such as Movicol® have grown in popularity.

As the majority of patients prefer oral to rectal measures, the nurse should endeavour to keep the use of enemas and suppositories to a minimum. All rectal measures act to a greater or lesser extent by stimulating the anocolonic reflex. When rectal treatment is given, the prescriber should review the oral laxative prescription and increase the dose as appropriate. Many teams will have devised a multiprofessional protocol for the use of oral and rectal laxatives similar to the Lothian Palliative Care Guidelines (NHS Lothian 2008). A case history of a patient with constipation (Ziyad) is also provided on the companion website, which you might want to use for discussion with your mentor.

 See website for further content

Breathlessness

Breathlessness is a common and distressing symptom of many life-limiting illnesses, including advanced cancer, chronic obstructive pulmonary disease (COPD) and heart failure. Ascertaining the subjective experience for the patient is a vital part of the holistic assessment, as measurable signs such as increased respiratory rate and oxygen saturation are inadequate for fully understanding the total experience of breathlessness for the patient. Patients commonly report feeling such as having to 'fight for air' and that an acute episode can be like choking or suffocating as if 'they are not going to get another breath'. Anxiety and fatigue are therefore commonly associated with breathlessness.

It is always important to exclude reversible causes of breathlessness, such as infection or pulmonary embolus (Brown 2006). For many patients, their breathlessness is part of a progressive disease process and ongoing management includes both medication and non-pharmacological strategies including breathing control techniques, relaxation and anxiety management, which help to maintain steady breathing during exertion and avoid precipitating an acute attack. Pacing and prioritising activities helps patients to manage their energy and achieve daily tasks which are important to them with as little energy expenditure as possible. The occupational therapist and physiotherapist can play key roles in helping the patient to control their breathing and to remain as independent as possible using these strategies.

Nurse-led clinics are available in some areas and offer support to patients in coping with the meaning and the distress associated with breathlessness as well as practical advice regarding the strategies described above. This integrative approach has been shown to reduce distress, maximise the patient's functional ability and thus maintain their independence for a greater length of time (Zhao & Yates 2008). It is important not to forget that supportive measures such as ensuring a well-ventilated room, the use of a fan and not rushing the patient can reduce the labour of breathing whilst providing small, easily taken meals can help maintain energy levels.

Medication plays an increasing role in managing breathlessness as the illness progresses. Opioids such as morphine and diamorphine are commonly used via oral and parenteral routes and have been shown to be effective in relieving the sensation of breathlessness (Jennings et al 2001). A normal release preparation such as Oramorph® liquid may be given as a trial dose and according to response can be titrated. Patients usually require lower doses than when given for pain and the interval between doses may be longer. A starting dose may be 2.5 mg of Oramorph® taken on a prn or as required basis. This can be taken before exertion and situations where breathlessness can be anticipated. Where the patient is continually breathless at rest, a regular normal release preparation or a sustained preparation such as MST Continus® can be taken, or when the oral route is not viable this can be administered via continuous s.c. infusion by syringe driver. The patient must be monitored for opiate side-effects such as drowsiness, nausea and constipation and unfounded fears of addiction or hastening disease progression elicited and addressed.

Anxiolytics are another group of commonly used medications for breathlessness and work by relieving feelings of anxiety. There are short-acting preparations such as the benzodiazepines, for example lorazepam which is administered buccally or sublingually and so rapidly absorbed to relieve intermittent episodes of acute panic and anxiety. Midazolam is a short-acting parenteral benzodiazepine which can be given by injection or added to an infusion by syringe driver. Other preparations such as diazepam are longer acting and so useful for continuous or background anxiety, and diazepam can be administered rectally (p.r.).

The use of oxygen in clinical practice is contentious (Brown 2006). When the patient is breathless due to a lack of oxygen the administration of this drug can help. In advanced illness, patients may be breathless without lacking oxygen and therefore this is unlikely to help. Careful assessment of need is required as inappropriate use is unlikely to help, can cause dry uncomfortable oral or nasal mucosa and ties the patient to nasal cannulae or oxygen mask and tubing. In addition there can be health and safety issues which must be considered, including the inflammability of oxygen which may be a particular concern in the home setting, where relatives may smoke. Booth et al (2004) provide useful guidance regarding the appropriate use of oxygen to manage breathlessness in palliative care.

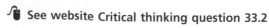 **See website Critical thinking question 33.2**

 ## Nursing management and health promotion: care of the dying patient and their family

This section of the chapter will focus on the terminal phase of the patient's illness including end-of-life care and the provision of bereavement support for families and carers.

Caring for a patient who is facing their own mortality and supporting their family and carers through this difficult time can be challenging for health and social care professionals (Copp 1998). This time requires careful consideration and skilled communication to enable the patient and family to come to terms with the reality of expected death. Making the adjustment from thinking of oneself as a relatively healthy person who will die someday in the future, to thinking of oneself as an ill person who is dying right now, is a very big step. Theorists have described the potential emotions and behaviours of people in this situation. Many variables influence the responses of the dying patient and the family, the most notable being personal characteristics, level of social support, past experience of illness and death, age, culture, religious belief and the characteristics specific to the illness. Several theories of the bereavement process have been proposed. Bayliss (2008) and Greenstreet (2004) review a number of seminal theories you may be familiar with and also some of the more contemporary perspectives.

Loss is an abiding feature in the life of a person who is dying – loss of future, loss of role, loss of independence. This period in the palliative care patient's life has been compared to bereavement. Many patients perceive that those who are dying are shunned by health professionals because they cannot be cured. The nurse caring for the dying person needs to be aware of this and must demonstrate the importance of the individual by displaying interest and respect, for example by consulting the patient about their wishes, needs and priorities and thereby helping to maintain self-esteem.

A useful starting point for understanding an individual's response to a life-threatening illness is to consider the question: 'What does this illness mean to this person?'.

Suffering

Pain and suffering are terms that are sometimes used as if they had the same meaning; this demonstrates a deep misunderstanding of the experience of human suffering. Physical pain can usually be controlled or reduced, whereas suffering is a much more complex phenomenon, encompassing emotions and psychosocial concerns that, in some instances, may elude control (Nyatanga 2005).

Patients and families may suffer because of unresolved issues from the past. There may be guilt, remorse, loss of hope and fear of the future. People who are dying have lost control over their future, may have suffered multiple losses in relation to their previous lifestyle and are often witnessing their decline into total dependence on others. In addition, they may be suffering through observing the effect their imminent demise is having on their family, and may be worried about how their survivors will cope. Family members may suffer by watching their loved one's decline and feeling unable to help. Previous experience of poor symptom control in a dying relative or friend may be the cause of considerable anxiety for both patient and family in anticipating the future.

Coping styles have attracted much interest in the literature. There is no doubt that some people cope much more effectively than others in stressful situations. Some, but not all, individuals are flexible in being able to change their lifestyle to their new circumstances, to seek information, to be involved in decision making, to maintain hope and to preserve their self-worth.

Many factors are involved. These are as diverse as personality, the manner in which the bad news of the diagnosis was broken, and the social support available. A previous coping style is not always useful in relation to facing a life-threatening illness. This can be very distressing for patients and families as they struggle with new and fearful situations. For example, a person who tends to cope with stressful life events by being very busy, active and organisational, who needs to feel 'in control' of what's going on around them, may struggle with the constraints imposed by their illness and treatment and lack of control over their day-to-day life. The physical effects of their illness including fatigue and reduced functional ability may preclude the busyness by which they usually avoid dwelling on more emotive issues whilst dependence on others may seem intolerable. How the person sees themselves may change markedly from employee, provider for the family, parent and this can reduce self-worth. Responses such as emotional withdrawal or strong emotions such as anger due to frustration can be difficult for both family and professionals to deal with and can result in the patient feeling very isolated. In this situation, helping the patient to remain as in control of their situation as possible is needed, including their involvement in decision making related to the planning and organisation of care. Through therapeutic communication, the nurse can gently acknowledge the person's distress and loss but also work with them to identify realistic and achievable goals that are personally important and meaningful. Fulfilling such goals may require the involvement of other team members. The occupational therapist may provide equipment which will allow the patient to retain a greater degree of independence or the social worker may be able to address financial issues due to inability to work which relieves the pressure of providing for the family. Identifying the essence of what is important to the patient and how this can be achieved in another way can have a profound effect on the patient's quality of life. For example, a father who highly values playing football with his son as important to their father–son relationship and who can no longer participate due to the physical effects of the illness, may find satisfaction and worth in this role by spending time with his son in another way, such as doing his homework with him – something he could never do before his illness because he was working.

Changing coping styles within the time limitations of a life-limiting illness is not generally an option. What is recommended is to adapt existing strategies and provide extra, positive coping strategies to enable individuals to achieve some relief from their suffering.

The assessment of psychological needs, coping styles and how the person is adapting to their situation is integral to holistic assessment. Therapeutic communication forms the basis of this, alongside observation of behaviour and social interactions with others, including family and friends. Whenever the patient is consistently anxious or distressed or when the usual approach to pain management does not appear to be having the desired effect, the nurse caring for the dying patient and their family must consider whether all avenues have been explored to alleviate suffering. Where measures by the multiprofessional team caring for the patient and family appear not to be fully addressing suffering and psychological distress, referral for more specialist input is required. This may be, for example, to specialist palliative care services (see pp. 864, 866), a psychologist, social worker or chaplain. Within the multiprofessional team, it is the nurse that usually spends more time with the patient and family than any other professional group and plays a key role in coordinating the input of other team members. The nurse should therefore be alert to the need for further referral for the patient and family and aware of what resources and services are available in their area should such a situation arise.

Realising the enormity of suffering that may be experienced by both patient and family can be daunting when providing palliative care; however, help and support can and should be offered. By building up a supportive relationship with the patient and the family and through therapeutic communication, the nurse may gain some insight into what would be useful for the individual.

Regular communication with the family is a good method of giving support. Family members should never feel they have to constantly search for someone to talk to about the patient or that the nurse or doctor is always too busy. A conscious effort must be made to show respect for family members which can include knowing and using their names and displaying warm body language towards them. Regularly approaching the family and listening to their concerns is important, and exploring who they have outwith the family circle to give support can help them identify practical solutions to easing the stresses of their caring role. Practical solutions within clinical areas may include providing privacy for the patient and family to talk and so maintain the interpersonal contact between patient and family essential for maintaining family bonds and ties.

Mind and body are inextricably linked. The stresses caused by suffering may evoke physiological effects on the body, such as muscle tension which can exacerbate pain, anxiety which interferes with sleep, and nausea which reduces appetite. Complementary and alternative medicine (CAM) therapies may be of benefit to patients in this respect. Relaxation, massage, music therapy and other distractions may help to relieve the stresses of dying and should be available alongside mainstream medicine (Deng & Cassileth 2009).

It is important to remember that a life-limiting illness can affect the very meaning individuals attach to their life and raise a number of spiritual concerns. Spirituality and religion are commonly considered to be the same. A person's religion may be integral to their spirituality, however 'spirituality' is a much wider term which includes the meaning patients attribute to their illness and the dying process. Thought-provoking accounts of this aspect of care are given in a number of texts (see Further reading, e.g. Byrne 2008, Puchalski 2006).

Whenever the patient is consistently anxious or distressed or when the usual approach to pain management does not appear to be having the desired effect, the nurse caring for the dying patient and their family must reconsider whether there is a requirement for specialised support from a chaplain, counsellor or clinical psychologist.

End-of-life care

When it is recognised that the patient has entered the last phase of their illness, there is a shift in the priorities and the organisation of care. The focus moves from achieving a quality of life and supporting the patient in 'living whilst dying' whilst their illness is progressing, to ensuring a peaceful death and supporting the family in coping with their impending loss.

Recognising that the patient has entered the terminal phase of their illness allows the multiprofessional team to plan end-of-life care. This includes consideration of the patient's expressed wishes regarding care and where they wish to die. It is important to recognise however that the patient's wishes can change over time as their circumstances change. Perspectives change between thinking of dying as something that will happen in the future and when later faced with the reality of this in the immediate future. Sensitive revisiting of such issues may therefore be required, as appropriate to the patient's condition and their ability to participate in such discussions.

Over recent years, defining criteria for diagnosing that the patient is in the terminal, dying phase has received considerable attention (Murray et al 2005, Dy & Lynn 2007). This follows recognition that the trajectories of different illnesses can vary markedly. The typical cancer trajectory, for example, is a steady decline where the patient becomes progressively weaker, usually over a period of months, with a period of rapid escalation in the last few weeks of life. This makes the terminal phase of the illness recognisable as the patient becomes progressively weaker and more dependent, is bed bound, eats and drinks less and sleeps for longer periods. In contrast, patients with organ failure including heart failure and chronic respiratory disease most commonly experience this deteriorating condition over two to three years; however, this is also punctuated with increasingly frequent acute exacerbations. The outcome of these exacerbations becomes more unpredictable as the illness progressively fails to respond to treatments, and death can occur suddenly during an acute exacerbation or may occur following a period of general decline.

A third trajectory, most commonly experienced by people with dementia and general ageing is the longest trajectory of palliative care and is that of progressive decline which may last over a few years. Patients can be very frail and dependent for some time and this can result in professionals failing to recognise that the illness has now reached the stage where the patient is in the terminal phase of their illness and imminently dying. Patients are at risk of pneumonia and other such conditions which may act as a terminal event which precipitates their death.

This emphasises that, to provide palliative care, nurses must therefore have a sound understanding of the pathophysiology of the patient's illness and the likely disease trajectory. The decision that the patient is in the terminal phase

and at the end of life should be made in a multiprofessional team context. Commonly used criteria include:

- The patient is bed bound and semi-comatose/comatose.
- The patient is unable to take oral tablets and fluids/only sips of fluids.
- Reversible causes of deterioration in the patient's condition have been excluded.

In recent years, an integrated care pathway known as the *Liverpool Care Pathway for the Dying* (LCP; Ellershaw & Wilkinson 2003) has been developed to provide an evidence-based structure to planning, delivering and evaluating care in the last days of the patient's life. This pathway aids professionals in decision making with regard to choosing appropriate interventions to ensure the comfort of the patient in the dying phase and that the needs of the family are considered. The pathway was developed by a multiprofessional group and is recommended for use in all care settings, with adaptation as appropriate to local needs.

Essential features of end-of-life care contained within the LCP include stopping inappropriate interventions such as blood tests and antibiotics. The patient's medications should be reviewed to ensure that any unnecessary medications are withdrawn and the patient only receives those that will help to make them more comfortable. Essential medications directed at controlling symptoms and ensuring comfort, such as analgesics and antiemetics which the patient was previously taking by mouth, may require to be given parenterally via continuous s.c. infusion by syringe driver. Anxiolytic medications such as the benzodiazepines, e.g. temazepam, lorazepam and midazolam, are frequently prescribed in palliative care to help the patient sleep at night and to relieve anxiety, terminal agitation or distress (Adam 2007).

It must be noted, however, that the patient's symptoms can change at the end of life and prn medications must always be available in case of any breakthrough symptoms. Appropriate anticipatory prescribing means that if medication is required there is no delay due to waiting for prescriptions to be written. This is also necessary to consider for patients who may never have experienced any symptoms before, as symptoms may occur during this phase. The following medications may be prescribed for intermittent s.c. injection:

- analgesia – usually morphine or diamorphine as first line
- a broad spectrum antiemetic, e.g. levomepromazine
- an anxiolytic in case of terminal anxiety and distress, e.g. midazolam
- an anti-secretory medication, e.g. hyoscine butylbromide or glycopyrronium, in case respiratory secretions become problematic.

A common symptom in the last days of life is increased or retained secretions that accumulate in the oropharynx or bronchial tree, which the patient close to death cannot clear by coughing or swallowing. This causes a gurgling noise when the patient breathes in and out which is commonly termed 'the death rattle'. This noise can be distressing for families to hear, therefore explanation and reassurance is essential. Unless secretions are purulent and copious, suctioning usually has limited effect and the administration of anti-secretory medications is required. Careful positioning can also help, with the patient's head to the side supported by pillows and avoiding semi-recumbent or supine positions.

In addition to supporting care for the patient, attention to the psychological and spiritual care of the patient and family is also a key feature of the LCP. The LCP contains prompts for discussions to take place with the family to ensure that they are informed of changes in the patient's condition and can prepare themselves that the patient will die very soon. Care at this time includes supporting the family in spending as much time with the patient as is wished and sensitively answering any questions they may have. This may include explaining what is happening and the physical changes they see as the patient is dying.

Attention to and respect for religious and cultural beliefs is an essential dimension of palliative care throughout the patient's illness. In relation to end-of-life care and following the patient's death there may be customs and traditions important to the patient and family which must be followed. A useful resource is the *A Multi-faith Resource for Healthcare Staff* which can be accessed from the NHS Education for Scotland spirituality page (see Useful websites).

The LCP is a part of the Gold Standards framework (Thomas 2003) which outlines good practice in relation to the provision of palliative care in community settings, including the patient's own home, nursing homes and community hospitals. The aim is to support local processes of care delivery by GPs and primary care teams. There are seven standards for the provision of palliative care, referred to as the seven Cs:

- communication
- coordination of care
- control of symptoms
- continuity including 'out of hours'
- continued learning for the multiprofessional team
- carer support
- care in the dying phase.

Implementation of the LCP and Gold Standards framework or equivalent have been identified as a requirement by both the Scottish Government and Department of Health in their respective strategies for palliative care: *Living and Dying Well: A National Action Plan for Palliative and End-of-Life Care* (Scottish Government 2008) and the *End-of-life Care Strategy* (Department of Health 2008a). Box 33.5 provides an opportunity to reflect on end-of-life care.

The needs of the professional

It is important to recognise one's limitations and feelings towards mortality when caring for people who are approaching death. A number of research studies including that of Ekedahl & Wengstrom (2007) have identified that nurses also experience existential concerns and other stressors in caring for people who are dying. Often it is useful to reflect with a colleague or clinical supervisor how one feels regarding this type of care giving. This is not a sign of weakness or inability. To the contrary, acknowledgement of one's own feelings may help develop an empathic understanding of what the patient and family are experiencing at this time and positive strategies for coping with the emotional cost of caring. Failure to do so can result in

Box 33.5 Reflection

End-of-life care

Access the information available on the Liverpool Care Pathway and Gold Standards framework websites. Reflect on the principles of palliative care (Box 33.1, p. 852) and consider the following.

Activities

- How do you think these tools could support nursing practice?
- What may be the benefits to (a) patients, (b) families, (c) the multiprofessional team in using these tools to support palliative care?

Resources

Liverpool Care Pathway – www.mcpcil.org.uk/liverpool_care_pathway.

Gold Standards framework – www.goldstandardsframework.nhs.uk/.

nurses distancing themselves as a protective mechanism which can interfere with therapeutic communication and leave patients and families feeling isolated. The multiprofessional team may also suffer (Davis 2005) and a culture of mutual support must be developed by those caring for the dying.

Bereavement support

Bereavement support for the family begins before the patient dies, in supporting family members in adjusting to the impending death of the patient. Care around the time of death plays a crucial role in facilitating adjustment to loss and a future without the patient. This includes allowing the family time to be with the patient, to say goodbye and to ventilate their grief where wished.

Many people go through the bereavement process with no professional support, finding that informal support from family and friends is sufficient. For a minority of individuals, professional help is however required. Recognised risk factors for a complicated bereavement include sudden, unexpected death, traumatic death, an ambivalent relationship with the deceased and previous mental health, drug or alcohol issues.

As the nurse working in the hospital setting who has cared for the patient until death your involvement with family members may end here; however, in other settings such as the community or hospice settings your involvement may also extend to bereavement care of the family. Relatives of those you have cared for in practice may also ask you where they can receive support. It is therefore helpful to be ready to answer these questions promptly and accurately. The nurse should also be able to identify those at risk of a complicated bereavement and ensure they know where to access support where required.

Sources of bereavement support

There are a number of agencies available to provide professional bereavement services, however they are individual to regions and countries (in the UK). Examples include hospital-based services, chaplaincy or psychologist/psychiatric services, local hospices, Cruse Bereavement Care, and Macmillan Cancer Support as well as GP surgeries and hospital palliative care teams. Some of these may also provide information for grieving children and adolescents.

Increasingly information is being provided online, making it easy for those with computer skills and Internet access to gain information and support. However, these are open to interpretation and some may include chat rooms. A selection of reliable sources is provided on the companion website.

🖱 See website for further content

The advantages of online help include its availability 24 hours a day, so the individual may access this source as and when is convenient to them. Each site offers practical advice as well as some offering discussion boards. Discussion boards may help the bereaved identify with others who are experiencing similar feelings regardless of whether they participate in posting messages or not.

However, there are disadvantages. People who prefer to talk to someone about their feelings may not find this method helpful but they may be able to access sources where they may talk over the phone or in a local group/individual setting. Not everyone has computer/internet access or the reasonable level of navigation skill required.

Health promotion in palliative care

For many, including the general public, applying the term 'health promotion' to care of dying patients may seem inappropriate. Yet it should be apparent from reading this chapter that health promotion is a key aspect of palliative nursing care. This includes providing information, equipment and support for patients and families to enable them to retain as much independence as possible and to focus on a quality of life throughout their illness. Specific examples include addressing patient concerns regarding addiction when taking morphine, ensuring they know that normal release morphine preparations should be taken every 4 hours and how to avoid opiate-induced constipation by concurrent use of laxatives, facilitating compliance, reducing anxiety and alleviating pain. Effective management of pain contributes to avoiding suffering and distress which can lead to depression and enhances the person's ability to be physically active, so reducing the risks of immobility such as pressure ulcers (see Ch. 23). Advance care planning and therapeutic communication can support the patient in accepting the reality of their situation and making decisions which are important to them with regard to treatment and place of care/death, avoiding later distress from unfinished business. Supporting the family in coping with loss and preparing for the patient's death, including identifying and utilising positive coping mechanisms, can facilitate successful adjustment to their bereavement and thus is also a key dimension of health promotion.

Recently the need to address public awareness and attitudes towards death and dying has been recognised. Changing societal perspectives are described by Kellehear (2007) and the requirement to consider these in service planning is outlined within national strategy (Department of Health 2008a, Scottish Government 2008).

SUMMARY: KEY NURSING ISSUES

● This chapter has introduced you to the philosophy of palliative care which includes the assessment and management of the symptoms of advanced illness as well as the provision of compassionate care for the patient and family ensuring their psychological and spiritual needs are met.

● A model of palliative care was introduced which outlines the need for *therapeutic communication* with the patient and their family, *holistic assessment and care management, effective symptom control, good multiprofessional team working* and *advance care planning.*

● Adoption of this model may help the nurse to apply the philosophy of palliative care within any care setting.

● Palliative care undeniably requires a multiprofessional approach; however, nurses fulfil key responsibilities as palliative care is an integral aspect of their role.

● When cure is not possible care takes precedence, and caring is considered to be the very essence of nursing.

➡ REFLECTION AND LEARNING – WHAT NEXT?

● **Test** your knowledge by visiting the website 🖱 and answering the multiple choice questions and critical thinking questions.

● **Consolidate** your learning by looking at some of the further reading suggestions, references and specialist websites.

● **Revisit** some of the additional material on the website.

● **Consider** what you have learnt and how this will help your professional development.

● **Reflect** on how you can apply this knowledge to the care of your patients.

● **Discuss** your learning with your mentor/supervisor, lecturer and colleagues.

REFERENCES

Adam J: The Last 48 Hours of Life. In Fallon M, Hanks G, editors: *2007 ABC of Palliative Care*, ed 2, London, 2007, BMJ Books, Blackwell Publishing, pp 44–47.

Audit Scotland: *Review of Palliative Care Services in Scotland*, Edinburgh, 2008, Auditor General for Scotland Office, Scottish Government. Available online http://www.audit-scotland.gov.uk.

Bayliss J: Rethinking Loss and Grief. In Nyatanga B, editor: *Why is it so difficult to die?* ed 2, London, 2008, Quay Books, pp 241–254.

Birley J, Morgan G: Written Words: Hidden Meanings. In Nyatanga B, Astely-Peper M, editors: *Hidden Aspects of Palliative Care*, London, 2005, Quay Books, pp 1–10.

Booth S, Anderson H, Swannick M, et al: The Use of Oxygen in the Palliation of Breathlessness: A report of the Expert working group of the scientific committee of the association of palliative medicine, *Respir Med* 98:66–77, 2004.

British National Formulary: 2009. Available online www.bnf.org/bnf/.

Brown D: Palliation of breathlessness, *Clin Med* 6(2):133–136, 2006.

Bruce L, Finlay T, editors: *Nursing in gastroenterology*, Edinburgh, 1997, Churchill Livingstone.

Callin S, Bennett M: Diagnosis and management of neuropathic pain in palliative care, *Int J Palliat Nurs* 14(1):16–21, 2008.

Cherny NI: Pain assessment and cancer pain syndromes. In Hanks G, Cherny NI, Christakis NA, et al, editors: *Oxford textbook of palliative medicine*, ed 4, Oxford, 2009, Oxford University Press, pp 599–625.

Colvin L, Forbes K, Fallon M: Difficult Pain. In Fallon M, Hanks G, editors: *ABC of Palliative Care*, London, 2007, Blackwell Publishing, pp 8–12.

Copp G: A Review of Current Theories of Death and Dying, *J Adv Nurs* 28(2):382–390, 1998.

Costello J: *Nursing the Dying Patient: Caring in Different Contexts*, Hampshire, 2004, Palgrave Macmillan.

Davis H: The emotional load of caring: care for those for whom there is no cure. In Nyatanga B, Astely-Peper M, editors: *Hidden aspects of Palliative care*, London, 2005, Quay Books, pp 143–158.

Deng G, Cassileth BR: Complementary therapies in palliative medicine. In Hanks G, Cherny NI, Christakis NA, et al, editors: *Oxford textbook of palliative medicine*, ed 4, Oxford, 2009, Oxford University Press, pp 1519–1526.

Department of Health (DH): *End-of-life Care Strategy–promoting high quality care for all adults at the end-of-life*, London, 2008a, DH. Available online http://www.dh.gov.uk/en/Healthcare/IntegratedCare/Endoflifecare/index.htm.

Department of Health (DH): *End-of-life care programme*, London, 2008b, DH. Available online http://www.endoflifecareforadults.nhs.uk/.

Duke S, Bailey C: Communication with the patient and family. In Payne S, Seymour J, Ingleton C, editors: *Palliative Care Nursing Principles and Evidence Base for Practice*, ed 2, Maidenhead, 2008, Open University Press, pp 145–161.

Dy S, Lynn J: Getting Services Right for Those Sick Enough to Die, *Br Med J* 334(7592):511–513, 2007.

Ekedahl M, Wengstrom Y: Nurses in Cancer Care – Stress when Encountering Existential Issues, *Eur J Oncol Nurs* 11(3):228–237, 2007.

Ellershaw J, Wilkinson S: *Care of the dying: a pathway to excellence*, Oxford, 2003, Oxford University Press.

Fallon M, McConnell S: The principles of cancer pain management, *Clin Med* 6(2):136–139, 2006.

Fallon M, Hanks G, Cherney N: The Principles of Control of Cancer Pain. In Fallon M, Hanks G, editors: *2007 ABC of Palliative Care*, London, 2007, Blackwell Publishing, pp 4–7.

General Medical Council (GMC): *Treatment and care towards the end of life: good practice in decision-making*, London, 2010, GMC. Available online http://www.gmc-uk.org/guidance/ethical_guidance/6858.asp.

Gomes B, Higginson I: Where people die (1974–2030) Past Trends, Future Projections and Implications for Care, *Palliat Med* 22(1):33–41, 2008.

Gordon-Williams RM, Dickenson AH: Pathophysiology of pain in cancer and other terminal illnesses. In Hanks G, Cherny NI, Christakis NA, et al, editors: Oxford textbook of palliative medicine, ed 4, Oxford, 2009, Oxford University Press, pp 587–598.

Greenstreet W: Palliative Care Nursing. Why Nurses Need to Understand the Principles of Bereavement Theory, *Br J Nurs* 13(10):590–593, 2004.

Jennings A, Davies A, Higgins J, et al: Opioids for the palliation of breathlessness in terminal illness, *Cochrane Database Syst Rev* (3) CD002066.

Kellehear A: *A Social History of Dying*, Cambridge, 2007, Cambridge University Press.

Kinley J: Controlling Nausea and Vomiting in Palliative Care, *Nurse Prescribing* 3(4):141–150, 2005.

Mannix K: Nausea and Vomiting. In Fallon M, Hanks G, editors: *ABC of Palliative Care*, London, 2007, Blackwell Publishing, pp 25–28.

Murray S, Kendall M, Boyd K, Sheikh A: Illness Trajectories and Palliative Care, *Br Med J* 330(7498):1007–1011, 2005.

National Audit Office: *End-of-Life Care: Report by the Comptroller and Auditor General*, London, 2008, The Stationary Office (TSO). Available online http://www.nao.org.uk/publications/0708/end_of_life_care.aspx.

National Council for Hospice and Specialist Palliative Care Services: *Definitions of Supportive and Palliative Care*, Briefing paper no 11, London, 2002, National Council for Hospice and Specialist Care Services.

National Council for Palliative Care: *National Survey of Specialist Palliative Care Services*, 2007. London Available online http://www.ncpc.org.uk.

NHS Lothian: *Palliative Care Guidelines–Symptom Control*, Edinburgh, 2008. Available online http://www.nhslothian.scot.nhs.uk/ourservices/palliative/palliative_care_guidelines/symptom_control/.

NHS Quality Improvement Scotland (NHS QIS): *Standards for Specialist Palliative Care: National Overview*, Edinburgh, 2004. Available online http://www.nhshealthquality.org.

Nursing and Midwifery Council (NMC): *The Code: Standards of conduct, performance and ethics for nurses and midwives*, London, 2008, NMC. Available online http://www.nmc-uk.org.

Nyatanga B: The Concept of Suffering: A Hidden Phenomenon. In Nyatanga B, Astely-Peper M, editors: *Hidden aspects of Palliative care*, London, 2005, Quay Books, pp 58–73.

Office for National Statistics: *Life Expectancy*, 2008. Available online http://www.statistics.gov.uk/cci/nugget.asp?id=168.

Payne S: Resilient Carers and Caregivers. In Monroe B, Oliviere D, editors: *Resilience in palliative care*, Oxford, 2007, Oxford University Press, pp 83–98.

Regnard C, Hockley J: *A guide to symptom relief in palliative care*, ed 5, Abingdon, 2004, Radcliffe Medical Press.

Royal College of Physicians, British Pain Society and British Geriatrics Society: *The Assessment of Pain in Older people: National guidelines*, London, 2007, RCP. Available online http://www.rcplondon.ac.uk/pubs/contents/ff4dbcd6-ffb7-41ad-b2b8-61315fd75c6f.pdf.

Scottish Government: *Living and Dying Well: A national action plan for palliative and end-of-life care in Scotland*, Edinburgh, 2008. Available online http://www.scotland.gov.uk/Publications/2008/10/01091608/0.

Scottish Intercollegiate Guidelines Network (SIGN): *Control of Pain in Adults with Cancer*, Edinburgh, 2008. Available online http://www.sign.ac.uk/pdf/SIGN106.pdf.

Solano JP, Gomes B, Higginson IJ: A Comparison of Symptom Prevalence in Advanced Cancer, AIDS, Heart Disease, Chronic Obstructive Pulmonary Disease and Renal Disease, *J Pain Symptom Manage* 31(1):58–69, 2006.

Speck P: *Teamwork in palliative care: Fulfilling or Frustrating?* Oxford, 2006, Oxford University Press.

Sykes N, Ripamonti C, Bruera E, et al: Constipation, diarrhoea and intestinal obstruction. In Fallon M, Hanks G, editors: *ABC of Palliative Care*, Oxford, 2007, Blackwell Publishing, pp 29–35.

Thomas K: Department of Health: *The Gold Standards framework*, 2003. Available online http://www.goldstandardsframework.nhs.uk/.

World Health Organization (WHO): *Cancer pain relief*, Geneva, 1986, WHO.

World Health Organization (WHO): *Cancer pain relief with a guide to opioid availability*, ed 2, Geneva, 1996, WHO.

World Health Organization (WHO): *Cancer pain relief and palliative care, Report of a WHO Expert Committee*. Technical Report Series No 804, Geneva, 1990, WHO.

World Health Organization (WHO): *Palliative Care*, Geneva, 2009, WHO. Available online http://www.who.int/cancer/palliative/en/.

Zhao I, Yates P: Non Pharmacological Interventions for Breathlessness Management in patients with lung Cancer A Systematic Review, *Palliat Med* 22:693–701, 2008.

FURTHER READING

Byrne M: Spirituality in palliative care What language do we need? *Int J Palliat Nurs* 14(6):274–285, 2008.

Costello J: *Nursing the Dying Patient: Caring in Different Contexts*, Hampshire, 2004, Palgrave Macmillan.

Dimond B: *Legal Aspects of Death*, London, 2008, Quay Books.

Ellershaw J, Wilkinson S: *Care of the dying: a pathway to excellence*, Oxford, 2003, Oxford University Press.

Fallon M, Hanks G: *ABC of Palliative Care*, London, 2007, Blackwell Publishing.

Griffith R, Tenga C: *Law and Professional Issues in Nursing*, Exeter, 2008, Learning Matters.

Hanks G, Cherny NI, Christakis NA, et al, editors: *Oxford Textbook of Palliative Medicine*, ed 4, Oxford, 2009, Oxford University Press.

Mannix KA: Palliation of nausea and vomiting. In Hanks G, Cherny NI, Christakis NA, et al, editors: *Oxford Textbook of Palliative Medicine*, ed 4, Oxford, 2009, Oxford University Press.

National Council for Hospice and Specialist Palliative Care Services: *Definitions of Supportive and Palliative Care*, London, 2002. Briefing paper no 11.

NHS Lothian: *Palliative Care Guidelines–Symptom Control*, Edinburgh, 2008. Available online http://www.nhslothian.scot.nhs.uk/ourservices/palliative/palliative_care_guidelines/symptom_control/.

NHS Quality Improvement Scotland (NHS QIS): *Standards for Specialist Palliative Care: National Overview*, Edinburgh, 2004. Available online http://www.nhshealthquality.org.

Nyatanga B: *Why Is It So Difficult to Die?* London, 2008, Quay Books.

Nyatanga B, Astely-Peper M, editors: *Hidden Aspects of Palliative Care*, London, 2005, Quay Books.

Payne S, Seymour J, Ingleton C, editors: *Palliative Care Nursing Principles and Evidence Base for Practice*, ed 2, Maidenhead, 2008, Open University Press.

Puchalski C: *A Time for Listening and Caring: Spirituality and the Care of the Chronically Ill and Dying*, Oxford, 2006, Oxford University Press.

Speck P: *Teamwork in palliative care: Fulfilling or Frustrating?* Oxford, 2006, Oxford University Press.

Thomas K: *Caring for the Dying Patient at Home Companions on the Journey*, Abingdon, 2003, Radcliffe Medical Press.

Worthington R, editor: *Ethics and Palliative Care: A Case Based Manual*, Oxon, 2005, Radcliffe Publishing Ltd.

USEFUL WEBSITES

British National Formulary: www.bnf.org/bnf

Cancernursing.org: www.cancernursing.org
Provides a range of interactive educational materials including an online tutorial on the use of the syringe driver for palliative care and lectures and videos on a wide range of palliative care topics. Free to access but requires registration.

Cruse Bereavement Care: www.crusebereavementcare.org.uk

Department of Health – Bereavement Website: www.dh.gov.uk/en/Healthcare/Secondarycare/Bereavement/index.htm

Department of Health – End-of-life Care Programme: www.endoflifecareforadults.nhs.uk/eolc

Gold Standards framework: www.goldstandardsframework.nhs.uk

Liverpool Care Pathway for the Dying Patient: www.mcpcil.org.uk/liverpool_care_pathway

Macmillan Cancer Support (incorporating CancerBACUP): www.macmillan.org.uk

Marie Curie Cancer Care: www.mariecurie.org.uk

National Institute for Health and Clinical Excellence: www.nice.org.uk

NHS Education for Scotland – A Multi-faith Resource for Healthcare Staff which can be accessed from the spirituality page: www.nes.scot.nhs.uk/spiritualcare/default.asp

Palliativedrugs.com: www.palliativedrugs.com
Provides a formulary of medications used for palliative care and a discussion forum used by experts in palliative care from around the world. Access is free although registration is required.

Scottish Intercollegiate Guidelines Network: www.sign.ac.uk

Scottish Partnership for Palliative Care: www.palliativecarescotland.org.uk

Sue Ryder Care: www.suerydercare.org

The National Council for Palliative Care: www.ncpc.org.uk

The International Association of Palliative and Hospice Care: www.hospicecare.com
Provides a wide range of resources which include a list of (and direct access to) pain and palliative care assessment tools.

World Health Organization – Pain ladder: wwwwho.int/cancer/palliative/painladder/en

World Health Organization – Palliative Care: www.who.int/cancer/palliative/en

CHAPTER 34

Nursing older adults

Cheryl Holman

Introduction

Old age has always been a possibility but it is now an increasing probability, at least in the developed world (McKevith 2009). The medical, social and economic advances of the last century have largely eradicated a range of 'killer' diseases that robbed people of life in their childhood (Vincent 2003). Infectious diseases, for example, and the widespread use of antibiotics have accounted for a dramatically decreased mortality from infections that would previously have proved fatal. At the same time, nutrition has improved, people generally live in better housing and health and safety has become more important in the workplace (Vincent 2003, McKevith 2009). Some of the more dangerous occupations such as coal mining have been made safer or have largely disappeared due to changing economic circumstances. The outcome of the above changes is that more people are living longer.

Consequences of an ageing population

The increase in longevity is an indicator of success in health and social circumstances but the complex issues of an older population have to be faced by governments and planners. Economic consequences are relevant as this sector of the population is not, generally, economically active (Vincent 2003) and the issues of retirement and pension payments are significant for individuals and the wider society.

Importantly for health care providers, there has been an increase in the prevalence of diseases that are, largely, associated with old age (Armour & Cairns 2002). These include cancer, heart disease and dementia. The likely impact on health and nursing services, and how this should be addressed, was recognised in the UK when the Royal Commission on Long Term Care (1999) reported to the UK government at the end of the last century. The increasing, but not inevitable, likelihood of developing particular diseases with age demands health service resources at the primary and secondary levels. It is the job of governments to introduce policies to address these facts and ensure older people have fair access to financial and health resources. It is the job, increasingly, of nurses and other members of the multidisciplinary team, to work with individual older people who have health needs. It is important that health care workers such as nurses, doctors, social workers and therapists work together to coordinate appropriate care of a high standard.

In one sense, older people are no different from other people nurses come into contact with in the course of their work, despite the negative images that are often used to portray older people in our society (Carrigan & Szmigin 2000). Like any patient, the older person requires sensitivity, tact and professionalism. In relation to the media and advertising, one could be mistaken for assuming that the best things in life are only available for younger people (Loretto et al 2000). Advertising of clothes, cars and cosmetics, albeit that many of these are designed to hide the signs of ageing, is conveyed as purely of interest to younger people. If the subject of an advertisement is not pensions and retirement issues, the target audience is almost exclusively younger people (Carrigan & Szmigin 2000). Nurses are part of society and it is understandable that they too may have negative images of older people. Such images will not be dispelled by propaganda on behalf of older people but by evidence and an understanding of the ageing process and the facts about ageing. Nurses should avoid, in particular, holding and conveying stereotypes. One popular stereotype, for instance, is that older people are either no longer interested in sex or are incapable of sexual relations. There is plenty of evidence to the contrary (Gott & Hinchliff 2003, Araujo et al 2004), but the stereotype persists (Box 34.1).

What happens when we age?

That ageing takes place is beyond dispute (British Society of Research on Ageing [BSRA] 2004), despite the efforts of people to deny this or to hide the effects of the ageing process. Most of what is considered ageing is quite superficial. Aspects of the ageing body, such as the loss of elasticity in the skin leading to wrinkling and the loss of hair colour and thinning of the hair, have little or no clinical significance (BSRA 2004). They are external indicators that ageing is taking place but people age very differently. Some people retain their hair into old age, whilst others become grey haired prematurely. Of course, external factors may play a part in the appearance of ageing. For example, sunbathing and smoking are almost guaranteed to lead to premature ageing of the skin (Ferrini & Ferrini 2008). The changes of ageing not only depend on an individual's makeup and external environment but also how they perceive and experience ageing changes. The complex interplay of these factors can result in deficits that lead to the older person becoming unstable and vulnerable. In this state the older person may be described as frail (Nicholson 2007). The next section describes possible physical and psychological changes that may take place in later life, but it should be remembered that these

are only a guide to what may occur, rather a blueprint of what will happen.

Changes in blood pressure control

In later life, the blood vessels are less adaptable because of structural alteration; this can lead to increased blood pressure. The heart and blood vessels become less responsive to adrenaline and noradrenaline, which means that the homeostatic mechanisms for maintaining blood pressure become less efficient (Herbert 2006). One tangible outcome of this is a tendency towards postural hypotension, whereby a sudden change in position from sitting to standing is less well tolerated and blood pressure remains low, leading to dizziness or even fainting due to cerebral insufficiency (Watson & Fawcett 2003). Another consequence of changes in the cardiovascular system, through a combination of arterial disease and raised blood pressure, is a greater tendency in older people to suffer from cerebrovascular accidents, more commonly known as stroke (Department of Health [DH] 2001a). Deterioration in the blood supply to the brain can also lead to more chronic cerebrovascular disease which may lead to ischaemic dementia (McKeith & Fairbairn 2001), transient ischaemic attacks, or a fully evolved stroke (see Ch. 9).

Changes in exercise tolerance

Along with changes in the cardiovascular system there are changes in the respiratory system such that it becomes less efficient at extracting oxygen from the blood (Herbert 2006). This is not usually a problem but it does lead to exercise intolerance. The older person may well be able to go about their normal level of activity as these systems have considerable reserve capacity but will, for instance, be less able to run to catch a bus than they were when they were younger.

Changes in muscles, bones and teeth

With age our muscles atrophy, tendons and ligaments become less flexible and the skeleton becomes weaker due to the fact that less bone material is laid down in the skeleton (Herbert 2006). This is particularly marked in postmenopausal women but some men may also suffer from osteoporosis (NIH Consensus Development Panel 2001). The combined effects of osteoporosis and thinning of the cartilaginous discs between the vertebrae lead to a more stooped posture and this, in conjunction with the atrophy of skeletal muscle and a loss of elasticity in the lungs, can contribute to the reduced efficiency of the respiratory system (Herbert 2006). Teeth also change in later life. They lose their enamel covering and become worn and more brittle (Clay 2000). Combined with receding gums and poor hygiene this can lead to decay and eventual tooth loss.

Changes in reaction to temperature

Older people take longer to acclimatise when they move between climates of extreme temperature (Schofield 2000). This is due to the fact that acclimatisation is achieved by changes in the levels of circulating thyroxine: levels of thyroxine increase in cold climates and decrease in warmer

Box 34.1 Reflection

Attitudes towards older people

Think of a man or woman in public life who you believe is older than 70; it might be a politician, faith leader, journalist or entertainer.

Activities

- Write down 10 words that describe him or her.
- Look at your list and see if any of your words are age stereotypes. For most older people their age is a less important aspect of their identity than their personality, achievements and aspirations.
- Look at your list again. Are there any words that are not age related but more about the person's personality, achievements or aspirations?

climates. With age, the pituitary–thyroid axis is less sensitive to these changes, leading to slower acclimatisation in older people (Schofield 2000).

Changes in resistance to infection

The changes in the immune system that occur with age are complex. The overall levels of immunoglobulins remain relatively stable with ageing but the composition of these immunoglobulins changes and more immature T cells are produced (Ferrini & Ferrini 2008). This may lead to decreased defences against infections and also to the phenomenon in some older people whereby they do not necessarily exhibit pyrexia when they have a bacterial or viral infection (Adams & Herbert 2006). Instead, the presence of an infection may only be noticed when it is quite advanced, when confusion and drowsiness may occur. In old age, the immune system may become less able to distinguish 'self' from 'non-self', leading to autoimmunity whereby the immune system begins to attack its own tissues. Type 2 diabetes is, for example, a disease with autoimmune components and is definitely associated with ageing. The immune system also plays a key role in keeping cancer cells under check via immune surveillance, which becomes less effective with age (Ferrini & Ferrini 2008).

Changes in sensory perception

Despite misconceptions, the nervous system remains relatively unchanged with ageing (Ferrini & Ferrini 2008) but there are changes that affect the way older people perceive and make sense of their surroundings. There is an inevitable decline in vision as we age and this is due to changes in the eye, rather than in the neural conduction system from the eye to the brain. With age it is common for the lens to become more opaque (Wolf 2004) and some older people suffer from cataracts which, if untreated, severely limit their vision (see Ch. 13). In the ear, the bones that transmit sound waves from the outer to the inner ear tend to become fused together, thereby reducing their ability to transmit sound, leading to reduced hearing – presbycusis (Herbert 2006). This does not mean that all older people are blind and deaf but this reduction in hearing and vision has to be taken into account when considering their care and support. Similarly, it is clear that older people can suffer from pain. Seers (2006) argues that older people may experience pain differently to younger people and it is important that they are encouraged to describe their pain so that it can be managed effectively.

Changes in thought processes

Older people are no less intelligent, no less able to remember and recall and no more stubborn than their younger counterparts. The facts are plain; other than in neurodegenerative conditions such as dementia, memory and intelligence remain relatively intact with age and the personality we are born with is usually the one we take into old age. There is some change in short-term memory with ageing (Ponto 2006) but this does not usually interfere with leading a normal life. Some older people do suffer from age-associated memory impairment (Ferrini & Ferrini 2008); however, it is unclear whether or not this is a precursor to dementia. Intelligence, measured using standard IQ tests, does not decline with age. There is some change in intelligence, with a decline in fluid intelligence (e.g. problem solving) and an increase in crystallised intelligence (the application of learning to new problems), but these changes do not have a significant impact on daily living (Ponto 2006).

Changes in emotional life

There are theories that relate to psychological and sociological changes in later life. Erikson et al's classic study (1986) identified stages of ageing during which the ageing person either manages or fails to come to terms with their life in order to develop as a person. The ultimate stage during later life leads to the older person being at peace with life and reconciled to what they have, or have not, done and experienced. The activity theory of ageing and the disengagement theory of ageing (Ponto 2006) acknowledge psychosocial changes with ageing: the former that as people age they give up certain activities and take up others, and the latter, that as people age they give up activities and gradually withdraw from life and from society. Broadly speaking, these types of theories try to explain how people sustain themselves and grow whilst negotiating losses that may be incurred through ageing. Sometimes this relates to social or culturally determined losses such as retirement or the family position of grandparents, whilst other losses are brought on by individual circumstances such as illness and physical dependence. It can be argued that much of ageing depends on the ability to negotiate and transcend loss and grief and ultimately to face the end of one's life (Box 34.2).

 See website Critical thinking question 34.1

Working with older people

As a nurse working with adults you will inevitably encounter older people in the course of your practice. You will have much to offer each older person you meet and they, in turn, will have much to offer you. Nurses increasingly work with older people whether or not they specialise in this area (Standing Nursing and Midwifery Advisory Committee [SNMAC] 2001). Some nurses choose to work exclusively with older people in hospitals and the community. However, with the increasing proportion of older people in our society, unless the choice is made to specialise in working with children or

---

 Box 34.2 Reflection

Changes in later life and nursing assessment

Read the section 'What happens when we age?' again (see p. 870).

Activities

- List the specific considerations for assessing an older person based on your knowledge of what happens when we age.
- For each subheading, write a nursing action that should be carried out when assessing an older person. State your reasons for identifying the nursing actions based on the changes that occur in later life.

in maternity care, nurses will meet older people in general medical and surgical wards, in the community and in many specialist areas. In hospitals, two thirds of beds are now occupied by people aged over 65 years and there has been an increase in emergency admissions of people aged over 75 years, over half of whom suffer from ill-defined conditions (SNMAC 2001). Care is provided for older people in many different settings by a range of health care professionals and those who provide personal and social care.

The organisation of care is complex and it is important that it is coordinated and tailored to meet the needs of the individual (SNMAC 2001). For example, if an older person living in a residential care home has a fall they might have support from their family and the staff who work there. They may have an assessment by a general practitioner or district nurse and be referred to a falls clinic provided by a local hospital or community services. In addition the person might access privately funded services such as chiropody or optometry as well as needing advice about making adjustments to their living conditions from social services. The role of the nurse working with older people is not only about the provision of care; it also involves liaison with other members of the multidisciplinary team, coordinating care packages and providing education for patients, families and carers about the caring skills needed to sustain a more independent lifestyle (Box 34.3).

Key policies and frameworks

In 1998, with specific reference to the care for older people in acute wards in general hospitals, the Health Advisory Service [HAS] 2000 produced a pivotal report entitled *Not Because They Are Old* (HAS 2000). The HAS report can be described as 'pivotal' because it gave rise to two further influential reports: *Caring for Older People: A Nursing Priority – Integrating Knowledge, Practice and Values* (SNMAC 2001) and the *National Service Framework for Older People* (DH 2001a), which outlines UK government policy with regard to the care of older people. *Not Because They Are Old* catalogued the lamentable level of care that many older people experience in hospital. Amongst other things, the HAS 2000 report recommended the following:

- Older people themselves and their relatives must be more involved in the care of older people in hospital.
- There must be more clarity about who is responsible for the nutrition of older people in hospital.

Box 34.3 Reflection

Networks of care for older people

Think about an older person for whom you have helped provide care.

Activities

- List all the health care professionals that were involved in their care. Now list all non-professionals who were involved in their care.
- Look at your lists and decide in each case whether the nurse's role was to liaise, coordinate or educate.

- Better education is needed for staff, including nurses, about the specific needs of older people in hospital.

As a response to the need for better education of nurses highlighted by the HAS (2000), in 2001 the Standing Nursing and Midwifery Advisory Committee (SNMAC) commissioned research into the care of older people, as it related to nurse education, and produced a report (SNMAC 2001). It was noted that older people comprise the majority of all patients in acute settings and that they and their carers were the least satisfied of all groups with the care they received. In particular the care for older people was deficient in the fundamental aspects of care, often failing to meet basic needs for food, fluid, rest, activity and elimination (SNMAC 2001). The *National Service Framework for Older People* produced by the UK Department of Health in 2001 (DH 2001a) provides a guide for care for older people and used the research findings to set standards in key areas:

- rooting out age discrimination – ensuring older people get fair treatment regardless of their age
- person-centred care – ensuring older people have their individual needs met
- intermediate care – ensuring services are flexible and can help older people maintain their independence
- general hospital care – ensuring hospital care for older people is dignified and of an appropriate standard
- stroke – ensuring older people can access specialist stroke teams
- falls – ensuring services are provided to prevent falls in the older population
- mental health in older people – ensuring older people can access a full range of mental health services
- the promotion of health and active life in old age – ensuring services are provided to maximise people's chances in fulfilling their potential in later life.

Long-term conditions

The effects of long-term conditions have been identified as having significant impact on an older person's life (DH 2001a). The common long-term conditions of old age include cancer, heart disease, diabetes, stroke and Alzheimer's disease. As a disease progresses or the individual develops other concurrent illness, nurses and carers can support and care for the person and help them develop coping skills in order to adapt. The reasons why older people need nursing care are complex: they are often unrelated to a single medical diagnosis and more related to the poorly defined concept of frailty (Markle-Reid & Browne 2003). Frailty occurs not only as the result of one or more medical condition but also as a result of the difficult losses sometimes experienced in later life.

Nursing management and health promotion: working with older people

In this section important aspects of nursing care are discussed. The issues have been identified by the National Service Framework for Older People (DH 2001a) or subsequent reports and explore the complexity of care provision. It is not possible to cover all relevant topics so there is a list of resources at the end of the chapter where further information can be found.

Equity, dignity and care for older people

It is important that care offered to older people is equitable to the care given to younger people. This means that decisions about access to treatment and care should not be based on age and that it is not appropriate to restrict specific services to certain populations based on age criteria (DH 2001a). Diverse needs in relation to culture, ethnicity, religion, gender, sexuality and disability should be considered and respected in an older client group as in any other (Nursing and Midwifery Council [NMC] 2009). It is important to address issues that affect particular groups, for example health promotion material needs to recognise that black and Asian elders are at higher risk of diabetes. Services also need to be sensitive to people whose needs may be overlooked such as lesbian and gay residents in care homes.

Equitable care also means that the care services predominantly offered to older people should be of a similar quality to other services. A particular area of concern for older people themselves is that care offered to older people should sustain or promote dignity (DH 2006). The notion of dignity is complex and involves many overlapping concepts (Cass et al 2009). Dignified care should promote a person's self-respect and usually involves giving respect. At the simplest level this can mean older people's care environments have proper toilet facilities and that curtains are clean and of sufficient quality to provide privacy. At the more complex level it means developing a culture of care that respects the personal needs of individuals. This is sometimes called 'person-centred care' (DH 2001a). Developing person-centred care can be challenging when there are competing demands on the nurses' and carers' practical and emotional resources. It is important that nurses and carers receive meaningful and regular supervision so they can understand the emotional component of their work and provide practical care that prioritises the person in their care (Davenhill 2009).

Person- and relationship-centred care

In person-centred care, nurses and carers get to know the patient, client or resident in a more intimate way. It is still important to plan care to meet the clinical needs of the older person, but this is in the context of the whole person, including their life history (Ashburner et al 2004). By taking this approach, communication and care interactions are more likely to prioritise the older person's needs rather than those of the care organisation. A criticism of person-centred care is that it ignores the fact that caring is a two-way process and that the needs of the carers play a significant role in how they can carry out their work. Nolan et al (2001) identified a relationship-centred care framework that acknowledges the needs of those delivering care (Table 34.1). This shifts the focus to the organisation of care rather than just the individuals providing it. Nolan et al (2001) suggest that where care delivery is of an optimal standard, the culture of an organisation provides a certain atmosphere or feeling. They suggest that the organisation should promote a sense of security, continuity, belonging, purpose, fulfilment and significance. Importantly, these senses should not only be felt by the older people being cared for, but also the staff working with them. Table 34.1 illustrates how the senses framework applies to older people and their carers.

Consent and older adults

In poor health, in a state of confusion or when dying, older people may become vulnerable. This does not mean that their rights can be overridden, even in the apparent pursuit of the older person's best interests; action taken must not cause an affront to dignity. Wherever possible, the consent of an older person to treatment or even a seemingly innocuous nursing intervention, is required; treatment, including life-saving treatment, cannot be forced on an older person without consent (DH 2001b). In particular, restraint should not be applied unnecessarily to an older person who is confused and who may be wandering or aggressive due to confusion. Clearly, patient and staff safety are paramount considerations but restraint has such harmful consequences (McCreadie & Penhale 2006) that it should only be applied under very controlled conditions for which the Royal College of Nursing (RCN) (2008) has produced relevant guidelines. Related to restraint is the issue of elder abuse. Nurses should be able to recognise signs of abuse and know what action to take (NMC 2009).

Communication and older people

Communication with older people, especially those who have sight and hearing impairment, can be made more effective by the following (Holman et al 2005a):

- Make time to listen to the older person's ideas, concerns and point of view.
- If you want the person to talk, especially about sensitive issues, ensure privacy and give them your full attention.
- If the person has a communication difficulty make sure your face can be seen and do not cover your mouth when speaking.
- If the older person wears a hearing aid and/or glasses make sure they are accessible and in working order.
- Remember, anxiety, pain or confusion is likely to interfere with the ability to communicate. You will need to adapt your communication to the individual's needs. You may need to administer analgesics to control the pain before giving information or have a family member present to help the person cope with their anxiety.
- Be aware of cultural differences, for example in some cultures it is a sign of respect to make eye contact, in others it is a sign of disrespect.
- If the older person does not understand you, choose different words and avoid jargon where possible.
- Visual cues may be helpful, especially if you are trying to explain a complex issue. Charts and pictures can be helpful and interpreters may be necessary for deaf people or people who do not speak English.
- Be mindful of the environment, for example consistent lighting can be helpful for the visually impaired and reduce background noise if the person has a hearing impairment.

Perhaps the most important form of communication between nurses and older people in their care is the indirect communication made via the relationships they form. Bridges et al (2009) suggest that older people prefer nurses to try and make a meaningful connection with them and to

Table 34.1 The senses framework	
A sense of security	
For old people	Attention to essential physiological and psychological needs, to feel safe and free from threat, harm, pain and discomfort. To receive competent and sensitive care
For staff	To feel free from physical threat, rebuke or censure. To give secure conditions of employment. To have the emotional demands of work recognised and to work within a supportive but challenging culture
For family carers	To feel confident in knowledge and ability to provide good care without detriment to personal well-being. To give adequate support networks and timely help when required. To be able to relinquish care when appropriate
A sense of continuity	
For older people	Recognition and value of personal biography. Skilful use of knowledge of the past to help contextualise the present and future. Seamless, consistent care delivered within an established relationship by known people
For staff	Positive experience of work with older people from an early stage of career, exposure to good role models and environments of care. Expectations and standards of care communicated clearly and consistently
For family carers	To maintain shared pleasures/pursuits with the care recipient. To be able to provide competent standards of care, whether delivered by self or others, to ensure that personal standards of care are maintained by others, to maintain involvement in care across care environments as desired/appropriate
A sense of belonging	
For older people	Opportunities to maintain and/or form meaningful reciprocal relationships, to feel part of a community or group as desired
For staff	To feel part of a team with a recognised and valued contribution, to belong to a peer group, a community of gerontological practitioners
For family carers	To be able to maintain/improve valued relationships, to be able to confide in trusted individuals, to feel that you're not 'in this alone'
A sense of purpose	
For older people	Opportunities to engage in purposeful activity facilitating the constructive passage of time, to be able to identify and pursue goals and challenges, to exercise discretionary choice
For staff	To have a sense of therapeutic direction, a clear set of goals to which to aspire
For family carers	To maintain the dignity and integrity, well-being and 'personhood' of the care recipient, to pursue constructive/ reciprocal care
A sense of achievement	
For older people	Opportunities to meet meaningful and valued goals, to feel satisfied with one's efforts, to make a recognised and valued contribution, to make progress towards therapeutic goals as appropriate
For staff	To be able to provide good care, to feel satisfied with one's efforts, to contribute towards therapeutic goals as appropriate, to use skills and ability to the full
For family carers	To feel that you have provided the best possible care, to know you've 'done your best', to meet challenges successfully, to develop new skills and abilities
A sense of significance	
For older people	To feel recognised and valued as a person of worth, that one's actions and existence are of importance, that you 'matter'
For staff	To feel that gerontological practice is valued and important, that your work and efforts 'matter'
For family carers	To feel that one's caring efforts are valued and appreciated, to experience an enhanced sense of self

First published in Nolan et al (2001). Reproduced with permission of the authors.

involve them in their care. In Box 34.4 the findings of the study are summarised and the key positive features of relationships with older people are identified.

Providing this sort of caring relationship can be very challenging when there are competing demands on the practical and emotional resources available in particular care environments (Holman & Crowhurst 2009). Making time to listen to older people and find out about their life history, their family lives and their hopes and concerns is skilled work and a very important role for the nurse working with older people. It is important that staff are supported so they can develop the skills and resources to be able to do this (Box 34.5).

Depression and older people

Depression is a common mental health problem in later life (Waugh 2006). It is difficult to get an accurate picture of how many older people suffer with depression due to under diagnosis but it is a significant problem that affects people's quality of life and in its severest form can lead to suicide (Minardi & Blanchard 2004, Waugh 2006). The incidence of depression increases considerably when older people enter a care home (Waugh 2006). Depression is said to occur when a person's mood is lowered, there is a decrease in their enjoyment of their usual activities and there is a reduction in their levels of energy and activity for a period of at least

Box 34.4 Evidence-based practice

Older people and their relatives' experiences of acute care

A hospital admission can have a significant impact on an older person and their relatives. There are many smaller-scale studies that examine in depth older people and their relatives' views and experiences of acute hospital admission. Bridges et al (2010) systematically reviewed 42 of these qualitative research studies in order to identify common themes in older people and their relatives' experiences of acute care. They concluded that older people and their relatives rated relationships and the atmosphere of the care environment as highly important. They identified key features that make a positive impact on older people's experience in hospital from the older person's perspective. These are:

- Connect with me: reciprocal and trust based relationships.
- See who I am: relationships based on a knowledge of the individual and their personal identity.
- Include me: relationships where decision making is shared.

Bridges J, Flatley M, Meyer J Older people's and relatives' experiences in acute care settings: Systematic review and synthesis of qualitative studies, *Int J Nurs Stud* 47:87–107, 2010.

Box 34.5 Reflection

The importance of relationships when caring for older people

Think about a time you were involved in the care of an older person.

Activities

- Do you feel you got to know them well?
- What questions could you have asked to find out more about their background or family circumstances?
- Are there any topic areas you would avoid asking about?

2 weeks (World Health Organization 2003). It is important that nurses and carers understand depression in old age, so that older people have proper assessment and access to appropriate care. A key issue is to recognise that whilst anxiety and confusion may be conditions that are experienced separately, they can be linked to depression and require thorough investigation.

There are significant risk factors to depression in old age. These include a history of previous episodes of depression, being isolated, moving to long-term care, poor access to support and resources, physical illness, feeling out of control and loneliness (Waugh 2006). There are also factors that protect older people from depression such as a high degree of self-esteem, the presence of a confidant and access to high-quality support (Minardi & Blanchard 2004). Older people are vulnerable to depression when the risk factors overwhelm their protective resources.

Psychologically based therapies such as psychodynamic, systemic, cognitive behavioural or interpersonal therapy may be helpful for depressed older people (Minardi &

Blanchard 2004). Less formal interventions such as activity-based programmes, for example drama therapy, may also be helpful (Porter 2000). A criticism of mental health care for older people is that there is an over reliance on medications as a treatment and lack of referral for psychologically based interventions (Minardi & Blanchard 2004). Worse still, there is sometimes a complete focus on the physical needs of older people at the expense of their emotional well-being (Waugh 2006). Waugh (2006) suggests that nurses should be aware of the risk factors of suicide. These include one or more of the following: helplessness, worthlessness, guilt, being male, lack of feelings of pleasure, being withdrawn and any gestures of self-harm or an apparent wish to die. Severe depression can lead to suicide and a referral to specialist services should be made if an older person appears to be at risk.

Confusion, delirium and dementia

Older people are at greater risk of being confused. Confusion is evident when a person seems disorientated about time and place and appears unable to identify people (RCN 2006). Nurses and carers need to know the difference between delirium (an acute confusional state) and dementia. Delirium is a disturbance of a person's awareness and thought processes. This usually results in a change in a person's behaviour, typically becoming disturbed or agitated, although people can sometimes become withdrawn and sleepy (Schofield 2008). Delirium usually develops over a short period of time, hours or days, and is generally caused by a medical condition such as infection or disorders of fluid or electrolyte balance that are often reversible (Farley & McLafferty 2007). In contrast dementia is caused by specific illness that results in progressive confusion, for example Alzheimer's disease. Dementia is unlikely to be significantly reversed and it is gradual in onset. The symptoms of memory loss causing an inability to perform usual activities of living take months and years to progress (RCN 2006).

Causes of delirium might be physical, emotional or social. In some cases the underlying cause may be a complex combination of factors (Farley & McLafferty 2007). Common causes include infection, constipation, dehydration, medication imbalance, malnutrition and depression (Farley & McLafferty 2007). Whilst a person is in a state of delirium they are likely to be anxious as they cannot understand their surroundings. The principles of care include finding out the cause of the delirium and treating it, reassuring the person whilst they are anxious and ensuring their safety (RCN 2006).

Dementia is caused by disease processes such as Alzheimer's or vascular degeneration in the brain. Dementia is a severe and devastating disorder. There are approximately 700 000 people with dementia and in the next 30 years this figure is expected to double (DH 2009). The government has developed a strategy to address this, set out in *Living Well with Dementia: A National Dementia Strategy* (DH 2009). Although dementia is a terminal disorder, many people can live for 7–12 years after diagnosis. Care services can make a significant impact on the quality of life for people with dementia and their families.

Initially, symptoms of dementia include impaired memory, disorientation, poor concentration, emotional changes and a loss of language skills (RCN 2006). It is important for people in confusional states to undergo psychiatric assessment. Early diagnosis of dementia allows people to access appropriate services as well as advice and help with memory loss and appropriate medication (DH 2009). This can preserve memory and function and enhance coping strategies. The Alzheimer's Society (2010) provides practical tips to help the memory and recommends providing verbal cues rather than asking questions. Ordinary questions may be distressing for the person with dementia as they might feel 'put on the spot'. For example, it is better to say: 'Look – here is David your nephew, who has come to see you', rather than 'Do you remember who this is?' (Alzheimer's Society 2010). It is important to listen to the person with dementia, to hear their feelings and help them come to terms with their illness.

Over time, dementia can result in severe disability and loss of function (Cunningham & Archibald 2006). Care practices should preserve the person's dignity and sense of self-worth by treating them as an individual and encouraging them to be independent. The Alzheimer's Society provides good information about issues such as helping the person with dementia to eat, drink, dress and wash. For example, laying out clothes on the bed for the person with dementia will remind them of dressing activities and provide the optimal opportunity for choice and independence (www.alzheimers.org.uk) (Box 34.6).

The progression of dementia takes a long time and it is important that nurses and carers are sensitive to the changes and losses involved. Care plans need frequent review and appropriate referral to relevant members of the multidisciplinary team as necessary. Underpinning this are the needs and wishes of the person with dementia and their family. It is a key role of the nurse to provide practical and emotional support to relatives and informal carers (Box 34.7), give information, coordinate resources and assess the needs of relatives and carers of older people, see Box 34.8.

Preventing falls in older people

An important concern for older people is the risk of having a fall. Falls in old age are common, costly, cause anxiety and impact on a person's ability to function independently (Wang & Wollin 2004). The National Institute for Health and Clinical Excellence (NICE) (2004) has published a clinical guideline for the assessment and prevention of falls in older people and makes recommendations for practice (Box 34.9).

Central to best practice is an assessment of multiple factors including the person's individual circumstances and environment. The purpose of the assessment is to identify risk factors

Box 34.6 Reflection

Providing good care for people with dementia

Think about other ways to promote and stimulate the person's memory so they have more choice and independence.

Activities

- List ways you can improve your care for people with dementia.
- Go to the Alzheimer's Society website and look at the examples they give. How did yours compare?

Box 34.7 Reflection

Advice and support for older people and their carers

Consider how confident you are in your role as information provider. Advice and support for older people with dementia and their carers is provided by the charity For Dementia (www.fordementia.org.uk) and for more generally for carers by the charity Carers UK (http://www.carersuk.org). Both charities have a helpline.

Activities

- Identify ways you can improve your role as information provider.
- What sort of questions do you think carers and relatives ask the helpline?
- How can you help carers and relatives find out information?

Box 34.8 Evidence-based practice

The craft of care

Family caregivers provide care for their loved ones in all sorts of circumstances. When an older person develops a long-term condition such as dementia it often means that a family member has to develop complex skills to overcome challenges. De la Cuesta (2005) interviewed 18 family caregivers to find out about their experiences. She adopted a grounded theory approach that involved detailed and systematic analysis of the interviewees' accounts in order to identify categories of their caring skills. She found that family carers developed sophisticated skills and strategies to overcome the difficulties of looking after a person with dementia. She called this 'the craft of care'. For example, she found that carers developed ways of getting round the person with dementia's memory loss and they adapted their communication style to overcome practical problems.

De la Cuesta C: 2005 The craft of care: family care of relatives with advanced dementia. *Qual Health Res* 15(7): 881–896.

Box 34.9 Information

Principles of practice in the prevention of falls (NICE 2004)

- There should be a person-centred approach.
- There should be a multidisciplinary approach to care.
- Organisational issues such as education, training and audit should be integral to falls prevention strategies.
- Individuals contacting health care professionals should be assessed for risk routinely.
- Assessment of older people's risk of falling should be multifactorial.
- Interventions should be multifactorial.
- Exercise and strength training is recommended.
- Home hazard and safety intervention should be in place on discharging older people at risk.
- Assessment of medications should be integral to falls prevention strategies.

with the view to developing a strategy to reduce the risk (Chang et al 2004, Gates et al 2008). It is not possible for risk to be completely eliminated but it is important to identify potential hazards and educate the person at risk. Often the anxiety about falling has emotional significance so sensitivity, good communication and careful listening are required (Davenhill 2007). Wang & Wollin (2004) identify the following common factors that suggest a risk of falling.

Intrinsic factors These include gait disorders, poor muscular strength, impaired balance and general weakness, confusion, poor visual acuity and poor hearing. In addition a history of falls, medication side-effects, increased age and concurrent illnesses should be considered in an assessment of risk.

Environmental factors that may suggest hazard are poor lighting, poor colour distinction in furniture, objects and surrounding environments, unsuitable footwear and the use of restraint, especially bed rails.

These risk factors rarely exist in isolation so assessment needs to acknowledge the complexity of people's lifestyles, personalities and the environments in which they live (Kelly & Dowling 2004).

Medications and falls

It is important to review older people's medications regularly. This is especially relevant as the combination of drugs and specific medications such as sedatives and those prescribed for mobility problems can increase the risk of falling if not properly monitored. It is good practice to keep the dose and the number of medications prescribed to a minimum where possible (McGavock 2003). It is also important that older people understand their medications to maximise their effectiveness. They should be given a full explanation of what the medication is for, the possible unwanted side-effects and how to get help if they do experience side-effects. For example, if a person is prescribed diuretics they may suffer dizziness and loss of balance when getting up (postural hypotension). If they are aware of the potential for this happening they might adjust their behaviour by getting up slowly and feel less anxious should it occur (Kelly & Dowling 2004). The older person will also need to know what to do when they require another prescription or how to dispose of their medications should they go out of date (DH 2001c). The Department of Health identifies issues to be considered in relation to older people's needs and their medications (Box 34.10).

Exercise and fall prevention

Exercise can reduce the fall rate in groups of older people. In particular, exercises that improve muscle strength, gait and balance enhance rehabilitation from falls and may improve confidence and stability (Kelly & Dowling 2004). Falls commonly occur in the bedroom and involve the process of transferring from bed to chair. Some exercise classes specifically target this activity whereas others are more general and include walking and low-impact weightbearing exercise. Sustained exercise in later life is helpful for general well-being and preventing falls.

Attention to environmental factors is also important (Kelly & Dowling 2004). Areas of high risk such as bathrooms and bedrooms can be adjusted to ensure there is enough space and

Box 34.10 Information

Medicines and older people: issues identified by the Department of Health (2001c)

- Many adverse reactions can be prevented.
- Some medicines that could benefit older people are underused.
- Medicines are not taken because older people and their carers have not been involved in making decisions about their treatment.
- Medicines are wasted due to some repeat prescription practices.
- GPs change medication after older patients are discharged from hospital.
- Primary and secondary care communication is poor.
- Labels on some medications are inadequate.
- Getting to the surgery or the pharmacy can be a problem for some older people.
- The contribution that carers could make in helping older people with their medication is often not addressed.
- Medication review could reduce costs.
- Some long-term medications could be withdrawn without adverse effects.

clutter is removed. Aids to provide physical support such as hand rails can be fitted. Preventative measures such as removal of loose-fitting carpets and effective cleaning after spillage can be effective. In organisations such as care homes and hospitals a record analysis can identify whether particular times or activities influence the rate of falls. For example, practices can be adjusted to improve supervision at busy times and identify moving and handling training needs.

Nutrition and older people

Older people generally suffer from more problems with nutrition than younger people, and older people in institutions are at even greater risk (Denny 2007). Mainly, although not exclusively, older people suffer from undernutrition, which leads to weight loss and vulnerability to secondary problems of infection, skin breakdown and poor recovery from illness and surgical procedures (Watson 2003). The reasons why older people suffer from poor nutrition are varied and encompass not only some of the biological problems that may be associated with age (e.g. lack of teeth and a reduced sense of smell and taste), but also factors such as being immobile or having reduced mobility due to a fall (Denny 2007). This may prevent the older person from being able to prepare food or from being able to shop for appropriate food. However, there are also social and economic reasons why older people may become poorly nourished. Older people in retirement may have reduced incomes compared to their working years and this may lead them to reduce their food intake or to eat foods that are less nutritious than they require (Denny 2007). Older people with cognitive impairment related, for example, to dementia are particularly at risk of undernutrition, especially in the terminal stages. In Alzheimer's disease weight changes can become apparent even in the very early stages (Hallpike 2008).

Nurses have a considerable responsibility in hospital and at home to assess the nutritional status of older people (Heath & Sturdy 2009). The nurse should to be able to screen for nutritional problems and pass this information to the doctor or the dietitian as appropriate. Principles of nutritional screening include gathering nutritional measurements such as height, weight, body mass index, and noting any unplanned weight loss and the effects of acute illness. Screening tools can ensure the assessment is systematic and evidence based (Heath & Sturdy 2009). A more thorough assessment should investigate whether the older person is dehydrated by asking them about their fluid intake and observing them for signs of dehydration such as dry or discoloured skin, concentrated urine and change in urine output. Nurses and carers should also be aware of medications such as diuretics that affect fluid and electrolyte balance (Holman et al 2005b) and have a basic knowledge of nutrition to be able to identify basic food groups in order to advise on adequate nutritional intake (Holman et al 2005c). Nurses also need to be aware of people with conditions such as dysphagia (difficulty swallowing), which require a more specialised assessment (Heath & Sturdy 2009).

It is important to ensure that mealtimes are a time when people can eat their meals without unnecessary interruptions and that people with special needs receive adequate support and practical help (Heath & Sturdy 2009). Careful planning around the support of people with problems that may impact on their ability to eat, such as confusion or difficulties with fine movements of the hand, need to be incorporated into the organisation of care.

Staff need to understand the importance of good nutrition and be able to use relevant equipment, aids and any dietary supplements prescribed by the doctor or dietician. They should consult with relatives and involve the older person in order to find out their individual preferences. The Alzheimer's Society offers further guidance about practical care at mealtimes.

Continence and older people

First of all, the myth must be dispelled that older people commonly suffer from incontinence. People can suffer from incontinence at any age but, as with many physical problems, there is an association between incontinence and ageing (Norton 2006). When referring to incontinence, it is usually urinary incontinence that is being implied; faecal incontinence is relatively rare. Urinary incontinence is more prevalent in women than in men but the frequency of incontinence rises in both men and women with age (Heath & Watson 2003). Urinary incontinence can lead to multiple problems that span the psychological, the social and the physical. People find urinary incontinence profoundly embarrassing and can become socially isolated as a result, with the condition completely dominating their lives (White & Getliffe 2003). Urinary incontinence can arise for several reasons and can usually be classified as follows (Norton 2006):

- Detrusor dysfunction arises from an inability to suppress spontaneous contractions of the bladder leading to voiding of urine (urge incontinence).
- Stress incontinence arises through incompetence of the pelvic floor muscles and, while this is common in women

following childbirth, it can arise in men following pelvic surgery.
- Outflow obstruction arises when there is something blocking outflow of urine from the bladder; for example, it may arise in constipation, prostatic hyperplasia or as a result of a tumour. This leads to urine overflowing periodically under the pressure in the bladder.
- Neurogenic bladder arises when the peripheral nervous supply to the bladder has been damaged; a common cause of this is dementia.

Urinary incontinence in older people is difficult to resolve unless the cause is obvious and easily obviated, such as an obstruction to outflow which can be removed or a urinary tract infection causing urgency and frequency, which can be treated. When a person is incontinent it is important to collect data about when and how often the incontinence occurs as well as any associated symptom. This requires sensitivity but should include specific questions to obtain the relevant information. Wagg (2009) suggests that specific questions will identify certain types of incontinence. For example, answering 'Yes' to the question 'Do you get so desperate to pass water that you find it hard to hold on?' may indicate that the person has urge incontinence. Answering 'Yes' to the question 'Do you leak urine if you cough, laugh or exert yourself?' is likely to indicate stress incontinence. A thorough assessment is important to establish the right approach to care and treatment. The person with the continence problem can be asked to keep a diary to establish patterns of incontinence, and investigations into other underlying problems such as confusion or diabetes may be necessary.

In the absence of effective treatments, nurses should approach older people suffering from urinary incontinence with sensitivity, tact and the hope, in the absence of a cure, that life with urinary incontinence can be made more bearable. It is beyond the scope of this chapter to provide detailed guidance regarding the management of urinary incontinence but it should be noted that a variety of appliances, some specific to men and some to women, is available and that technology in this area has vastly improved in recent years with the introduction of highly absorbent gels that help to keep the person with incontinence dry and free from odour (see Ch. 24).

End of life care

End of life care usually refers to the support and care given to a person during the time when they are living with the practical and emotional concerns about dying although their death is not obviously imminent. Terminal care usually means the care provided immediately preceding a person's death – perhaps in the last few hours or days of life (Nicholson 2007). End of life care is significant for older people because it can be supportive and validate a person's life. The physical and emotional aspects of the end of a person's life vary and are difficult to predict (Field & Froggatt 2003).

Honest and sensitive communication is a key skill in providing end of life care. For instance, it is important to establish what the older person would prefer to happen should their condition deteriorate or should they suffer a cardiac arrest (NMC 2009). When a nurse or carer talks about these issues with the older person, they should try to explain the possible limits of the medical intervention and clarify the older person's expectations (Holman & Crowhurst 2009). If the nurse does not feel able to talk about dying in this way it is essential to refer to a more experienced nurse or another member of the multidisciplinary team so that the older person is helped to express their hopes and fears.

Older people often experience a complex array of losses towards the end of their lives. There are many frameworks that explain the experience of grief following a loss. One that is familiar to nurses is described by Kubler-Ross & Kessler (2005). They suggest that when a person is faced by significant loss such as death or losses related to increased dependence, they have to grieve. They describe five stages of grief: denial, anger, bargaining, depression and acceptance. Nurses and carers have a role in supporting older people to work through the feelings that can be stirred up as part of the grieving process. For example, when circumstances necessitate moving to continuing care it is important for nurses and carers to help the older person identify, express and acknowledge their feelings in order to make the appropriate transition.

Nurses and carers can be supportive by developing a therapeutic relationship with the person and using the communication skills outlined earlier in the chapter (p. 873). They should also be alert to recognise when symptoms persist and intensify as this can indicate that the person may be experiencing depression. In this case an appropriate referral should be made for specialist help from mental health services (Minardi & Blanchard 2004).

A palliative care approach is helpful in making sure the person can maintain optimal levels of independence whilst being comfortable and free of other distressing symptoms (Hockley 2002). Practical support for older people at the end of their lives should prioritise pain relief, aid coping with chronic fatigue and assist with any problems related to eating and drinking. In older people's care, palliative approaches are often appropriate over long periods of time and should be integral to the organisation of care. Community and care home staff should have the relevant training and support to ensure that high levels of communication and clinical care are delivered appropriately.

SUMMARY: KEY NURSING ISSUES

- Old age is a varied and interesting aspect of life, and nursing older people is important and rewarding. Making time to listen to older people and find out about their life history, their family lives and their hopes and concerns is the most skilled and most important role of the nurse working with older people.

- Older people are no different from other people nurses come into contact with in the course of their work; like any patient, the older person requires sensitivity, tact and professionalism.

- Dignified care should promote a person's self-respect and usually involves giving respect. At the simplest level this can mean proper toilet facilities and curtains to provide privacy. At the more complex level it means developing a culture of care that respects the personal needs of individuals.

- The physical and psychological changes of ageing not only depend on an individual's makeup and external environment but also how they perceive and experience ageing. Most people experience some physical, psychological and social changes in later life.

- Changes in blood pressure control, exercise tolerance, muscles, bones and teeth, reaction to temperature, sensory perception and resistance to infection are common but by no means inevitable.

- The effects of long-term conditions have a significant impact on an older person's life. The common long-term conditions of old age include cancer, heart disease, diabetes, stroke and Alzheimer's disease.

- Older people generally suffer from more problems with nutrition than younger people, and older people in hospital suffer greatly from nutritional problems. Undernutrition leads to weight loss and vulnerability to secondary problems of infection, skin breakdown and poor recovery from illness and from surgical procedures.

- Relationship-centred care is central to quality care for older people. It acknowledges the needs of those delivering care and shifts the focus to the organisation of care rather than just the individuals providing it. The organisation should promote a sense of security, continuity, belonging, purpose, fulfilment and significance, which should not only be felt by the older people being cared for, but also the staff working with them.

REFLECTION AND LEARNING – WHAT NEXT?

- **Test** your knowledge by visiting the website and answering the multiple choice questions and critical thinking questions.

- **Consolidate** your learning by looking at some of the further reading suggestions, references and specialist websites.

- **Revisit** some of the additional material on the website.

- **Consider** what you have learnt and how this will help your professional development.

- **Reflect** on how you can apply this knowledge to the care of your patients.

- **Discuss** your learning with your mentor/supervisor, lecturer and colleagues.

REFERENCES

Adams J, Herbert RA: Redfern SJ, Ross FM, editors: *Nursing older people*, ed 4, Edinburgh, 2006, Churchill Livingstone.

Alzheimer's Society: *Washing and bathing*, London, 2010. Available online http://www.alzheimers.org.uk/factsheet/504.

Araujo AB, Mohr BA, McKinlay JB: Changes in sexual function in middle-aged and older men: longitudinal data from the Massachusetts Male Aging Study, *J Am Geriatr Soc* 52:1502–1509, 2004.

Armour D, Cairns C: *Medicines in the elderly*, London, 2002, Pharmaceutical Press.

Ashburner C, Meyer J, Johnson B, et al: Using action research to address loss of personhood in a continuing care setting, *Illness, Crisis and Loss* 12(1):23–37, 2004.

Bridges J, Flatley M, Meyer J, et al: *Best practice for older people in acute care settings. Guidance for nurses*, London, 2009, RCN Publishing Company/City University.

Bridges J, Flatley M, Meyer J: Older people's and relatives' experiences in acute care settings: Systematic review and synthesis of qualitative studies, *Int J Nurs Stud* 47:87–107, 2010.

British Society for Research on Ageing (BSRA): *Scientific aspects of ageing: response to the House of Lords Science and Technology Committee enquiry*, London, 2004, BSRA.

Carrigan M, Szmigin I: Advertising in an ageing society, *Ageing and Society* 20:217–234, 2000.

Cass E, Robbins D, Richardson A: *Social Care Institute of Excellence Guide 15: Dignity in Care*, London, 2009, SCIE.

Chang JT, Morton SC, Rubenstein LZ, et al: Interventions for the prevention of falls in older adults: systematic review and meta-analysis of randomised clinical trials, *Br Med J* 328:680, 2004.

Clay M: Oral health in older people, *Nurs Older People* 12(7):21–26, 2000.

Cunningham C, Archibold C: Supporting people with dementia in acute hospital settings, *Nurs Stand* 20(43):51–55, 2006.

Davenhill R: *Looking into later life, A psychoanalytic approach to depression and dementia in old age*, London, 2007, Karnac Books.

Davenhill R: Psychodynamic observation and emotional mapping. A tool for continuing professional development and research in services for older people, *Quality in Ageing* 10(1):32–39, 2009.

De la Cuesta C: The craft of care: family care of relatives with advanced dementia, *Qual Health Res* 15(7):881–896, 2005.

Denny A: Tackling malnutrition among older people in the community, *Br J Community Nurs* 12(3):98–106, 2007.

Department of Health: *National Service Framework for Older People*, London, 2001a, DH.

Department of Health: *Seeking consent: working with older people*, London, 2001b, DH.

Department of Health: *Medicines and older people: implementing medicine-related aspects of the NSF for older people*, London, 2001c, DH.

Department of Health: *About dignity in care*, London, 2006, DH.

Department of Health: *Living well with dementia: A national dementia strategy*, London, 2009, DH.

Erikson EH, Erikson JM, Kivnick HQ: *Vital involvement in old age: the experience of old age in our time*, New York, 1986, Norton.

Farley A, McLafferty E: Delirium part one: clinical features, risk factors and assessment, *Nurs Stand* 21(29):35–40, 2007.

Ferrini AF, Ferrini RL: *Health in the later years*, ed 4, New York, 2008, McGraw Hill.

Field D, Froggatt K: Issues for palliative care in nursing and residential homes. In Katz JS, Peace S, editors: *End of life in care homes. A palliative care approach*, Oxford, 2003, Oxford University Press.

Gates S, Fisher JD, Cooke MW, et al: Multifactorial assessment and targeted intervention for preventing falls and injuries among older people in community and emergency care settings: systematic review and meta-analysis, *Br Med J* 336:130–133, 2008.

Gott M, Hinchliff S: Sex and ageing: a gendered issue. In Arber S, Davidson K, Ginn J, editors: *Gender and ageing. Changing roles and relationships*, Berkshire, 2003, Open University Press.

Hallpike B: Promoting good nutrition with patients with dementia, *Nurs Stand* 22(29):37–43, 2008.

Health Advisory Service: *Not because they are old*, London, 2000, HAS.

Heath H, Sturdy D: *Nutrition and older people. Nutrition. Essential Guide*, London, 2009, RCN.

Heath T, Watson R: Mostly male. In Getliffe K, Dolman M, editors: *Promoting continence: a clinical research resource*, ed 2, London, 2003, Baillière Tindall.

Herbert RA: The biology of human ageing. In Redfern SJ, Ross FM, editors: *Nursing older people*, ed 4, Edinburgh, 2006, Churchill Livingstone.

Hockley J: Organizational structures for enhancing standards of palliative care. In Hockley J, Clark D, editors: *Palliative care for people in care homes*, Buckingham, 2002, Open University Press.

Holman C, Roberts S, Nicol M: Promoting good care for people with hearing impairment, *Nurs Older People* 17(2):31–32, 2005a.

Holman C, Roberts S, Nicol M: Promoting adequate hydration in older people, *Nurs Older People* 17(4):37–38, 2005b.

Holman C, Roberts S, Nicol M: Promoting adequate nutrition, *Nurs Older People* 17(6):31–32, 2005c.

Holman C, Crowhurst K: The importance of staff support in the provision of emotionally sensitive care. In Froggatt K, Davies S, Meyer J, editors: *Understanding care homes. A research and development perspective*, London, 2009, Jessica Kingsley Publishers.

Kelly A, Dowling M: Reducing the likelihood of falls in older people, *Nurs Stand* 18(49):33–40, 2004.

Kubler-Ross E, Kessler D: *On grief and grieving. Finding the meaning of grief through the five stages of loss*, London, 2005, Simon and Schuster.

Loretto W, Duncan C, White PJ: Ageism and employment: controversies, ambiguities and younger people's perceptions, *Ageing and Society* 20:279–302, 2000.

Markle-Reid M, Browne G: Conceptualizations of frailty in relation to older adults, *J Adv Nurs* 44:58–68, 2003.

McCreadie C, Penhale B: Abuse of older people. In Redfern SJ, Ross FM, editors: *Nursing older people*, ed 4, Edinburgh, 2006, Churchill Livingstone.

McGavock H: *How drugs work*, Oxford, 2003, Radcliffe Medical Press.

McKeith I, Fairbairn A: Biomedical and clinical perspectives. In Cantley C, editor: *A handbook of dementia care*, Buckingham, 2001, Open University Press.

McKevith B: Diet and nutrition issues relevant to older adults. In Stanners CH, Thompson R, Buttriss JL, editors: *Healthy ageing. The role of nutrition and lifestyle*, Chichester, 2009, Wiley-Blackwell for British Nutrition Foundation.

Minardi H, Blanchard M: Older people with depression: pilot study, *J Adv Nurs* 46(1):23–32, 2004.

National Institute for Health and Clinical Excellence (NICE): *The assessment and prevention of falls in older people*, Clinical Guideline 21. London, 2004, NICE.

Nicholson C: End of life care. In *National Care Homes Research and Development Forum and Help the Aged. My home life. Quality of life in care homes. A review of the literature*, London, 2007, Help the Aged.

NIH Consensus Development Panel on Osteoporosis Prevention, Diagnosis and Therapy: Osteoporosis prevention, diagnosis and therapy, *J Am Med Assoc* 285:758–795, 2001.

Nolan M, Davies S, Grant G: Quality of life, quality of care. In Nolan M, Davies S, Grant G, editors: *Working with older people and their families. Key issues in policy and practice*, Buckingham, 2001, Open University Press.

Norton C: Eliminating. In Redfern SJ, Ross FM, editors: *Nursing older people*, ed 4, Edinburgh, 2006, Churchill Livingstone.

Nursing and Midwifery Council: *Guidance for the care of older people*, London, 2009, NMC.

Ponto MT: The psychology of human ageing. In Redfern SJ, Ross FM, editors: *Nursing older people*, ed 4, Edinburgh, 2006, Churchill Livingstone.

Porter L: The bifurcated gift: Love and intimacy in drama psychotherapy, *The Arts in Psychotherapy* 27(2):309–320, 2000.

Royal College of Nursing (RCN): *Let's respect. The mental health needs of older people*, London, 2006, RCN.

Royal College of Nursing (RCN): *'Let's talk about restraint'. Rights, risk and responsibility*, London, 2008, RCN.

Royal Commission on Long Term Care: *With respect to old age*, London, 1999, TSO.

Schofield I: Promoting travel health for older people, *Elder Care* 12(2):15–19, 2000.

Schofield I: Delirium: challenges for clinical governance, *J Nurs Manag* 16:127–133, 2008.

Seers K: Pain and older people. In Redfern SJ, Ross FM, editors: *Nursing older people*, ed 4, Edinburgh, 2006, Churchill Livingstone.

Standing Nursing and Midwifery Advisory Committee (SNMAC): *Caring for older people: a nursing priority – integrating knowledge, practice and values*, London, 2001, DH.

Vincent J: *Old age*, London, 2003, Routledge.

Wagg A: *Urinary continence management in older people. Continence essential guide*, London, 2009, RCN.

Wang S, Wollin J: Falls among older people: identifying those at risk, *Nurs Older People* 15(10):14–16, 2004.

Watson R: Nursing older adults. In Brooker C, Nicol M, editors: *Nursing adults: the practice of caring*, Edinburgh, 2003, Mosby.

Watson R, Fawcett TN: *Pathophysiology, homeostasis and nursing*, London, 2003, Routledge.

Waugh A: Depression and older people, *Nurs Older People* 18(8):27–30, 2006.

White H, Getliffe K: Mostly male. In Getliffe K, Dolman M, editors: *Promoting continence: a clinical research resource*, ed 2, London, 2003, Baillière Tindall.

Wolf N: How does one define aging in relation to pathology? Lifespan, *The Journal of the British Society for Research on Ageing* 12(2):1–9, 2004.

World Health Organization: *ICD-10 Classification of mental and behavioural disorders*, London, 2003, Churchill Livingstone.

FURTHER READING

Aged and National Care Homes Research and Development Forum (NCHRDF): Owen T, editor: *My Home Life: Quality of Life in Care Homes*, London, 2006, Help the Aged.

Brown J, Nolan M, Davies S, et al: Transforming students' views of gerontological nursing: Realising the potential of 'enriched' environments of learning and care: A multi-method longitudinal study, *Int J Nurs Stud* 45:1214–1232, 2008.

Froggatt K, Davies S, Meyer J: *Understanding Care Homes. A Research and Development Perspective*, London, 2009, Jessica Kingsley Publishers.

Redfern SJ, Ross FM: *Nursing Older People*, Edinburgh, 2006, Churchill Livingstone.

USEFUL WEBSITES

Action on Elder Abuse: www.elderabuse.org.uk

Age Concern: www.ageconcern.org.uk

Alzheimer's Society: www.alzheimers.org.uk

Better Government for Older People: www.bgop.org.uk

British Society for Research on Ageing: www.bsra.org.uk

Cancer Research UK: www.cancerresearchuk.org

Carers UK: www.carersuk.org

For Dementia: www.fordementia.org.uk

Help the Aged: www.helptheaged.org.uk

My Home Life: www.myhomelife.org.uk

National Service Frameworks: www.dh.gov.uk/PublicationsAndStatistics/fs/en

Royal Bank of Scotland Centre for the Older Person's Agenda – Scottish Hub for Access to Research and Evidence: www.qmuc.ac.uk/opa/share

CHAPTER

35

Nursing patients with sexually transmitted infections and HIV/AIDS

Marsh Gelbart, Mark Jones

Introduction

Sexually transmitted infections (STIs), also known as sexually acquired infections (SAIs), are a long-established problem. SAIs have continued to expand in terms of incidence and impact throughout the early years of the twenty-first century. Over the last 25 years sexually acquired viral infections, in particular the human immunodeficiency virus (HIV), have wreaked havoc on an international scale. SAIs can loosely be grouped as being parasitical (e.g. pubic lice), bacterial (e.g. chlamydial) or viral (e.g. HIV). If the affected patient has access to appropriate treatment, remembering that many people living in the developing world do not, then parasitical infections are eradicable, bacterial infections are curable and viral infections are treatable.

Sexual infections have carried a significant social stigma throughout the ages; various acts of legislation, such as the Contagious Diseases Act 1864, confirmed abhorrence of these infections and sought to 'blame' individuals (usually women) for their spread (Cooper & Reid 2007). In the wake of an upsurge in sexual infections during the First World War, a different approach was adopted. In 1916 the Public Health (Venereal Diseases) Regulations heralded free and confidential SAI clinics for all (Clutterbuck 2008). As a result, gonorrhoea and syphilis became less common in the UK, compared with industrialised countries that still stigmatised these infections. The advent of penicillin was a major breakthrough in the treatment of SAIs. Treatment availability, along with the advent of the oral contraceptive pill, may have contributed to sexual freedom. Unfortunately the oral contraceptive pill led to a reduction in condom use

883

and consequential rise in the incidence of SAIs experienced in the 1960s. Since this time, HIV has appeared on the scene. Faced once more with a potentially fatal and incurable SAI, society has looked for scapegoats, often incorrectly blaming those on the periphery of society.

The current trends in SAIs show that cases are still rising despite public health programmes and the ready, and often free, availability of barrier contraceptives such as condoms. Those most at risk of acquiring SAI include: young, single people; those who have multiple sexual partners; those who do not use barrier contraceptives; and those who live in metropolitan areas. Structural gender inequality, where women are forced into having unsafe sex as a byproduct of social, economic and gender disparity, is an additional factor (Gupta et al 2008). The number of all episodes of SAIs continues to increase in the UK.

Of all the SAIs, HIV has the most significant impact and it is on HIV that much of this chapter is focused. HIV is a global pandemic and has had a devastating effect on the developing world, in particular sub-Saharan Africa, which bears the greatest burden. The World Health Organization (WHO) estimated that in December 2007 over 33 million people worldwide were living with HIV, of whom two thirds live in sub-Saharan Africa, which also bears the brunt of new infections and death from acquired immune deficiency syndrome – AIDS (WHO 2008). In the UK, although there is a relatively low incidence when compared to many countries in the developing world, HIV continues to be a growing problem. In 2007 the Health Protection Agency (HPA) estimated that 77 400 people were living with HIV, of whom 7734 were newly diagnosed, and an increasing percentage (23%) were heterosexually acquired cases originating within the UK (HPA 2008b).

The role of the nurse

The role of the nurse in a sexual health setting involves several key concepts, irrespective of the infection with which patients present. A diagnosis of any SAI can raise significant anxieties, not only from the diagnosis but also from the need for health care professionals to know the type of sexual act involved. It is also essential to provide open, non-judgemental care, responding to the needs of the patients. Counselling services and sexual health education are still seen as important for patient support, particularly when patients are deciding whether to have a test for HIV. However, with the advent of better treatment options for HIV, there is increased pressure that testing should be 'normalised' with less emphasis placed upon pre- and post test counselling. Whatever changes are made in approaching the screening for SAIs, sexual health centres maintain a policy of confidentiality that often allows previously undisclosed sexual expression from the patient or client.

Partner notification

One of the most important aspects of nursing patients in a sexual health setting is the provision of partner notification (Trelle et al 2007). Health advisors attached to sexual health clinics organise partner notification. Only by encouraging patients to contact their partners to inform them of the chance of infection and then screening and treating those

partners before further sexual activity, can the cycle of infection and re-infection be broken. In order to do this successfully, an accurate sexual history is of fundamental importance. Without a comprehensive and accurate history it can prove impossible to contact, screen and treat all affected parties. Although it is more effective if partner notification is performed by the patients themselves, health advisors may act in lieu of their patients and contact the patient's sexual partners on their behalf.

The common sexually acquired/transmitted infections are discussed below, with some generalised treatment strategies; however, since this field of health care is evolving (particularly so with HIV), the drugs indicated are a rough guide rather than fixed treatment regimens, since in this dynamic area therapies often change. The British Association for Sexual Health and HIV (www.bashh.org/guidelines) provides information on the latest treatment trends.

Taking a sexual history

Before examining the various SAIs in more detail, it is necessary to consider the patient's sexual history. This is an essential first step prior to screening a patient for SAIs. Obtaining a sexual history in the context of a sexual health centre is easier than with a general practitioner or family doctor. In the sexual health centre the patient is expecting to discuss sexual problems and infections. In a general practitioner or family doctor surgery, the patient might wish to discuss an embarrassing sexual problem but not know how to introduce it into the conversation. 'I have a little problem down below' can mean anything from genital warts to a prolapsed rectum. Conversely the patient attending a general practitioner or family doctor with a body rash might not understand why the doctor may wish to discuss their sexual history. This can be particularly uncomfortable if the doctor is seen as a family friend and may mean that the practice nurse needs to work in a more facilitative way and give the patient 'permission' to talk about intimate and possibly embarrassing issues. Also, the doctor's or nurse's own embarrassment may present an obstacle in identifying, treating and educating their patient about STIs (Box 35.1).

The term 'confidentiality' implies that only the client and the providers involved in direct care have access to the client's personal information. If there are any limitations to

Box 35.1 Reflection

Embarrassment as a barrier to information exchange

Embarrassment and discomfiture by either the patient or nurse in a sexual health setting can lead to inadequate information exchange and history taking.

Activity

- Reflect on how reading a patient's body language and paraverbal communication may help you understand what they are telling you.
- How might your own body language be interpreted by the patient?
- Think about how to explain treatment and health education issues, simply, accurately and without jargon.

the boundaries of confidentiality, these should be disclosed clearly at the outset, for example, issues relating to child protection.

The environment is important when taking a sexual history. Ideally the discussion should take place in a sound-proof room, preferably away from clinical areas, so that people can talk freely. The room should be comfortable and not harshly lit. Arrange comfortable seating, so that interviewer and patient are at an angle facing each other, not face on. Use the same type of chair as the patient to try and ensure a sense of equality and not of a power relationship of professional and patient. Remember, attending a sexual health clinic can be awkward and embarrassing.

Be aware of a patient's body language, it hints at their state of mind. The patient might be attending for a wide-ranging set of conditions ranging from Candida to erectile dysfunction. They can be under enormous stress. When taking a sexual history, it is important to be non-coercive, non-judgemental and non-punitive. Use language appropriately and make sure the patient is not confused by the use of technical terms or jargon. Take into account the patient's potential embarrassment, but make sure your meaning is clear.

History taking

Human sexuality is complex and presumptions are often wrong. Do not assume that the patient is gay or straight; it is important to ask. Use open, inclusive questions when discussing the patient's sexual activities. History taking needs to be systematic, incorporating questions appropriate for ascertaining risks and then provision of appropriate care. Consequently, whilst taking into account the individual patient, a sexual history should include the following questions (French 2007):

- When did you last have sex?
- Was it with a man or a woman?
- Was it with a regular partner?
- What kind of intercourse was it?
- Were barrier contraceptives (condoms or femidoms) used?
- Do you or your partner/s have any symptoms?
- Have you had any other partner in the past 12 weeks? (If so, double-check partner's gender.)
- Do you have pain during or after intercourse?
- Have you ever had a sexually transmitted infection before?
- Have you ever had a sexual health screen before? (If not, explain and reassure.)
- Have you ever been screened for hepatitis, syphilis or HIV before? (If not, explain that a blood test is involved.) It is important to reassure patients that their blood will not be tested for HIV without their informed consent. Anonymous and random testing for HIV is carried out in some clinical areas including sexual health centres; this is generally done to collect data for government health departments to measure the spread of the virus within the population and enable planning for future health care provision. There is usually an ability to 'opt out' if the patient is concerned but it is important to reassure the patient that they cannot be identified.
- Have you been vaccinated against hepatitis B? (If not, assess risk and offer vaccination if required.)

If the patient is symptomatic

- Identify the presenting complaint and ascertain its history.
- How does the patient perceive the problem?
- If there is a discharge, how much is there and what is the colour?
- Any associated bowel or bladder symptoms?
- How long have the symptoms been present?

Other useful information

- Determine if any of their sexual partners were from abroad and if so, which countries.
- Check if there are any allergies to medications.
- Past medical history – note serious medical conditions and operations.

If there has been a history of a previous sexually transmitted infection

- What was diagnosed and when?
- How was it treated?
- Did you and your partner(s) comply with treatment?
- Have you ever used recreational drugs? If so, what type of drugs?
- Have you ever worked in the sex industry or paid for sex?

Parasitical infections

Common parasitical infections that may affect the genital area include scabies and lice. In addition *Trichomonis vaginalis* and Candida will be discussed. Strictly speaking, Candida is an opportunistic fungal infection, which does not sit clearly within the classic 'trinity' (parasitical, bacterial and viral infections) found in SAIs. It is normally grouped with the parasitical sexual infections.

Scabies

The parasite *Sarcoptes scabiei* is a tiny skin mite that is almost impossible to see without a microscope. It causes a fiercely itchy skin condition known as scabies. Dermatologists estimate that more than 300 million cases of scabies occur worldwide every year. The disease can strike anyone of any race or age, poverty and over-crowding being more associated with the transmission of scabies than personal hygiene (McCarthy et al 2004).

The mite is a tiny eight-legged creature with a round body that burrows under the surface of the skin, forming shallow burrows of up to 4 mm in length. The normal colony is made up of 10–50 mites. The scabies mite is an arachnid 0.4 mm in length which tunnels approximately 2 mm a day. The burrows are 1–4 mm in length and contain 10–25 eggs plus the mites' waste products. The larvae take 3–4 days to hatch. The human body develops a reaction to the mite that results in severe itching that is often intense enough to keep sufferers awake at night, and frequently leads to skin infections.

Transmission

Human scabies is almost always contracted from close personal contact with someone who is already infested. Amongst adults the most common source of infection is a sexual partner (Walton & Currie 2007). Some people react more severely than others, and rarely an infected person may hardly itch at all. The mite is attracted to the warmth and odour of the body. The female mite is drawn to a new host, making a burrow, laying eggs and producing secretions that cause an allergic reaction. Larvae hatch from the eggs and travel to the skin surface, lying in shallow pockets where they will develop into adult mites. It may be 4–6 weeks before a newly infected person will notice the itching or swelling that can indicate the presence of scabies. In cases of reinfestation, established hypersensitivity may lead to symptoms within 1–3 days (Chosidow 2006).

Clinical presentation

The earliest and most common symptom of scabies is itching, particularly at night. An early scabies rash will present as little red bumps, like hives, tiny bites or pimples. In more advanced cases, the skin may be crusty or scaly. Scabies will usually begin in the folds and crevices of the body, particularly between the fingers, under the arms, on the wrists, buttocks or belt line and on the penis. Mites also tend to hide in, or on, the skin under rings, bracelets or watchbands or under the nails. The head and face are not affected, except in children or those with a compromised immune system.

Diagnosis of scabies is usually by means of direct examination of skin scrapings, epiluminescence microscopy, identification of the burrows or epidemiological diagnosis. An epidemiological diagnosis is one where all signs and symptoms point to a specific cause, but as yet there has been no laboratory confirmation.

 ## Nursing management and health promotion: scabies

The patient's household contacts and sexual contacts during the month prior to diagnosis will require treatment. All household contacts will be required to take treatment at the same time.

Two treatments are available:

- permethrin 5% dermal cream applied to the whole of the body below the neck and washed off after 8–24 h, according to the manufacturer's instructions
- malathion 0.5% in an aqueous lotion applied to the whole body below the neck and washed off after 24 h.

The cure rate is 95% with one application; however, it is important to warn patients that the intense itching might continue for several weeks. This is because proteins from the dead mites and the faecal waste left behind in their burrows can continue to trigger an immune response, even though the infestation has been successfully treated. Practitioners need to monitor treatment compliance, but should resist the automatic assumption of re-infestation and thus unnecessary re-treatment. Potentially contaminated clothing and bedding should be washed at a temperature of over 50°C as it is thought that mites may survive for up to 72 h when separated from their human host.

Crusted (Norwegian) scabies

Crusted or Norwegian scabies is caused by exactly the same mite as found in standard infestations, the main difference being simply the number of mites present on an infected person. In regular scabies, the number of mites on a host at any one time is, on average, 10–15 (with a range of 3–50). Persons with crusted scabies, on the other hand, will have thousands to millions of mites. Consequently their skin manifestations are much more severe, with thick, hyperkeratotic crusts that can occur on almost any area of the body. This form of scabies affects frail elderly people, often those in residential care, and patients who are immunosuppressed, such as those who are HIV positive (Johnston & Sladden 2005).

 ## Nursing management and health promotion: crusted (Norwegian) scabies

As with all types of scabies, the patient's household contacts and sexual contacts during the month prior to diagnosis will require treating. All household contacts will be required to take treatment at the same time. Crusted scabies can be treated with two doses of oral ivermectin, 2 weeks apart. The actual dosage required is dependent on body weight (Johnston & Sladden 2005).

Pediculosis

The most common parasitic infection pediculosis is an infestation by *Pthirus pubis*, otherwise known as the pubic louse or crab louse. The pubic or crab louse is quite distinct in appearance; it has pincer-like claws resembling those of sea crabs. These claws on their legs are adapted for feeding and clinging to hair or clothing. Lice are blood-sucking insects that move freely and quickly, which explains their ease of transmission. The eggs (nits) are attached to the hair shaft, close to the skin surface, where the temperature is optimal for incubation. The eggs hatch in about 8–10 days. Nits are cemented to the hair shaft and are very difficult to remove. The eggs themselves are encased in an armoured material known as chitin and are well protected.

Clinical presentation

Pubic lice may be found on the short hairs of the body, areolar hair (around the nipple), axillary hair, beard, scalp margins, eyebrows and eyelashes, in addition to pubic hair. Pubic lice are spread through sexual activity but can also be passed on through contact with infested clothing or objects, such as bedding, combs or hats. Pubic lice can only live for a short period of time away from their natural habitat, coarse body hair. Those found on bedding or clothing are often physically damaged and have lost their ability to grip. However, they can remain viable and active for several hours whilst off the host's body. Pubic lice cause the infected person to itch as the lice suck blood. The lice do not produce a rash, but constantly scratching the skin could cause irritation. In addition, some people have an inflammatory skin reaction to the louse's bite. The insect is about 2 mm in diameter and has a 30 day lifespan, feeding approximately 12 times a day. It lays up to 10 eggs per day. The chitinous envelope that makes up the egg casing is known as the nit. Larvae take 8–10 days to hatch and the larvae take another week to mature fully into adult lice.

The lice can be seen by the naked eye upon close inspection, and with a magnifying lens the eggs or nits can be seen; these are usually attached near to the base of the pubic hairs.

Nursing management and health promotion: pediculosis

Infestation with *Pthirus pubis* is on the whole a sexually transmitted infection, and 30% of these patients have a second STI. Therefore the nurse needs to bear in mind the need for a full sexual health screen (Varela et al 2003). If a patient has been infested with pubic lice they often feel 'unclean', particularly as the parasites are visible. The nurse needs to reassure the patient that the infestation, although easily acquired, is readily treatable and eradicable. It is important to remember that sexual partner(s) require treatment.

Pubic lice can be treated and destroyed with one application of a prescription medication or over-the-counter shampoo.

- Malathion 1% in a shampoo base (Derbac-M) is applied to pubic hair and body hair other than the scalp. It should be left on for 5 min and then rinsed. Application is repeated after 7 days.
- Permethrin 1% cream rinse in an alcohol base (Lyclear) is applied to pubic hair and body hair other than the scalp. It should be left on for 10 min and then rinsed and dried.

In the case of pediculosis of the eyelashes, treatment is with occlusive ophthalmic ointment, which is applied to the eyelid margins twice a day for 10 days. Occlusive ointment works by occluding or blocking the breathing holes found in the mites' skin, thus suffocating them.

Candidiasis (vaginal thrush)

The causative organism is usually *Candida albicans*. Most women will have an episode in their lifetime. The yeast normally lives in the gut, mouth and genital tract, thriving in warm, moist and dark environments. The vagina can be considered an ideal environment for growth of this infection, since semen, menstrual blood, pregnancy and feminine hygiene products can all change the pH of the vagina. Some cultures resort to vaginal douches with home-made or proprietary preparations immediately after penetrative intercourse, in an attempt to prevent conception or infection. They are also used as a means of 'improving' feminine hygiene. This practice should be discouraged as it adversely affects the pH values of the vagina. Changes in pH create an imbalance that predisposes to the development of thrush. Additional risk factors include diabetes mellitus, hormone replacement therapy (HRT), the oral contraceptive, antibiotic therapy and immunodeficiency (Barousse et al 2004).

Transmission can be by sexual intercourse, during foreplay and by oral–genital contact. Men are more likely to acquire the infection during sexual activity, whereas women are more likely to acquire it as a result of the factors identified above. The incubation period is between 2 and 5 days.

Clinical presentation

Signs and symptoms include intense pruritus (itching) that is often worse at night, vaginal soreness, white patches on the vulva/vagina, sometimes dysuria (pain when passing urine), creamy white vaginal discharge and balanitis (inflammation of the glans penis) in men, although these signs are non-specific. Diagnosis is by examination and microbiological investigation.

Nursing management and health promotion: candidiasis

Antifungal drugs such as clotrimazole, miconazole and nystatin are commonly used as creams and pessaries in the management of this condition. Systemic treatment by fluconazole capsules may be necessary if symptoms persist. Sexual partners with symptoms should also be treated as they may cause re-infection. Some patients prefer to use one of the many traditional and alternative therapies, e.g. oral garlic supplements and dietary changes.

Trichomoniasis

Trichomonas vaginalis (a protozoon) causes trichomoniasis and is exclusively a sexually acquired disease in adults. This is a very common infection. Trichomonas causes disease in the genital tract, affecting the vagina and urethra. Transmission is by contact with vaginal or seminal fluid; the protozoa can last for several hours outside the body.

Clinical presentation

The signs and symptoms include profuse vaginal discharge (offensive, yellow, thin, frothy and irritating), dysuria, vulval soreness and lower abdominal pain, although men can remain asymptomatic. The incubation period can be up to 4 weeks, although this can be dependent on the menstrual cycle. It can be difficult to diagnose in men due to the lack of distinct symptoms, and although there are difficulties, it is vital to trace sexual partners.

Nursing management and health promotion: trichomoniasis

Diagnosis is by examination (the vaginal walls and cervix may be inflamed). A high vaginal swab is taken for culture, microscopy or, where available, a screening test known as latex agglutination (Adu-Sarkodie et al 2004). Treatment options include the antibiotic metronidazole, given to both partners over 5 days. This should be taken with food, and alcohol and sexual activity should be avoided during the treatment programme.

Bacterial sexually acquired infection

Sexually acquired bacterial infections can range from the relatively innocuous to the life threatening. They encompass a wide range of symptoms and may even be symptom free.

If they have been screened for and detected, most bacterial infections can be successfully treated.

Bacterial vaginosis

This is a condition caused by overgrowth of the vaginal commensal microorganisms, associated with changes in the normal pH values of the vagina. If the mildly acidic environment of the vagina is subject to disturbance, the normal acid-producing lactobacilli of the vagina are supplanted by anaerobic bacteria. This initiates an increase in vaginal discharge and an increase in the pH of the vagina to above 4.5. Bacterial vaginosis (BV) may or may not be sexually transmitted; its aetiology remains unclear (Wilson 2004). The bacterium most associated with BV is *Gardnerella vaginalis* although it is suspected that several other organisms may be implicated. The presence of *Gardnerella vaginalis* does not necessarily mean the woman will be symptomatic (Smart et al 2004).

Clinical presentation

Women complain of a thin, grey-white vaginal discharge that has a 'fishy' odour. The nature of the discharge can be very distressing and women are embarrassed and acutely aware of the associated odour. The odour is caused by the release of amines, a product caused by changes in the pH value of the vagina and which releases the distinct smell of ammonia.

 ## Nursing management and health promotion: bacterial vaginosis

On microscopic examination of vaginal secretions, characteristic clue cells can be seen. These are epithelial cells covered in a profusion of mixed bacteria which obscures the outline of the normally clearly delineated cell wall. In conjunction with the distinctive smell of BV, a raised vaginal pH value and the presence of the offensive discharge, clue cells help diagnose the presence of BV (Keane et al 2005).

The causes of BV are not known for certain. The pH value of the vagina can be disturbed by the presence of seminal fluid. Similar untoward disturbances can be caused by the use of strongly scented soaps and feminine hygiene products. The practice of douching (washing out the vagina after penetrative sex), common in some cultures, should be discouraged by the nurse as this appears to alter vaginal pH balance.

There are potentially serious complications of BV. Its presence has been implicated in an increase in risk of acquiring and transmitting HIV as well as other SAIs such as *Trichomonas vaginalis* and chlamydia (Livengood 2009).

Treatment of BV is straightforward and consists of metronidazole for 5 days. Alcohol must be avoided during treatment, as should sexual intercourse.

Chlamydia

Chlamydia is caused by the bacterium *Chlamydia trachomatis*. It is the most common sexually acquired infection in the UK (HPA 2009). It is particularly common in young, sexually active women (16–19 years). It is thought that younger women tend to have more sexual partners than older women and perhaps lack the skills and experience to negotiate

safer sex, making them more vulnerable to infection. In men, the highest incidence of chlamydia is between the ages of 19 and 24.

Chlamydia is a potentially serious infection and has a number of complications; therefore early detection and treatment are important. However, many patients are asymptomatic (see below) making early investigation and detection less likely.

Testing for chlamydia now involves the use of molecular biological tests to detect chlamydial DNA in urine and vaginal, cervical and vulval swabs. A national screening service for chlamydial infection was introduced in the UK during 2002 to 2003. This offers screening in non-traditional venues, in an effort to increase the number of participants. The screening programme has adopted non-invasive or self-administered tests involving urine samples and vaginal swabs (LaMontagne et al 2004).

Clinical presentation

Many patients with chlamydia (80% of women and 50% of men) are asymptomatic. However, women may present with:

- postcoital or intermenstrual bleeding
- purulent vaginal discharge
- lower abdominal pain
- proctitis (inflammation of the rectum).

The presentation in men includes:

- urethral discharge
- dysuria
- testicular/epididymal pain
- proctitis.

Chlamydial infection leads to a number of major complications in women. These include pelvic inflammatory disease (PID), which can be defined as infection and resultant inflammation of the upper genital tract that may ascend to the fallopian tubes, ovaries and surrounding structures (Ross 2001). Commencing sexual activity under the age of 20, non-white ethnicity, and not having had children all increase the chances of developing PID (Simms et al 2006). PID can cause chronic pelvic pain and significantly increases the risk of ectopic pregnancy and infertility. Specific aspects of PID can include endometritis (infection of the lining of the womb) and even salpingitis (inflammation/infection affecting the uterine tubes). This is a consequence of ascending infection as described above and can cause acute abdominal pain. Long-term damage to pelvic organs can result, causing infertility.

In men, chlamydial infection can spread to the upper genital tract causing inflammation of the epididymis and testes (epididymo-orchitis) (Fenton et al 2001).

 ## Nursing management and health promotion: chlamydia

Sexual intercourse should be abstained from during the treatment programme. Antibiotics such as doxycycline can be used provided the patient is not breast feeding or at risk of pregnancy. A single dose of azithromycin is becoming a popular mode of treatment; giving a single dose of an antibiotic avoids the problems with patient compliance frequently experienced with treatment involving a week of doxycycline. An alternative treatment is erythromycin.

Partner notification must be discussed with patients. It is essential that all recent (previous 3 months or previous partner if longer) and current sexual partners should be informed and advised to attend for assessment. Without treatment the reproductive system of both sexes can be severely damaged, in addition to the continued transmission of the infection.

Non-specific urethritis (NSU)

This condition only affects men. It is an inflammation of the urethra and is called 'non-specific' because there are a range of different causes, of which chlamydia is the most common. Other sexually transmitted infections may be implicated; there is increasing evidence that *Mycoplasma genitalium* is associated with this condition (Moi et al 2009). Urine and/or bladder infection may cause NSU, but this is quite unusual, particularly in younger men. Another cause is injury during sexual activity; the urethra is delicate and may be damaged during vigorous sexual activity, leading to NSU.

Clinical presentation

Many men notice a clear (sometimes cloudy) discharge coming from the end of their penis which is associated with pain, irritation or discomfort on passing urine.

 ## Nursing management and health promotion: NSU

NSU can usually be successfully treated with doxycycline. It is important to ensure that sexual partners are also seen and examined and treated as necessary to prevent re-infection. Damage to the urethra takes a few weeks to heal and therefore it is best for patients to avoid sexual intercourse until there is no sign of the infection and sexual partners have also been treated.

Anxious patients should be discouraged from over-examination of their genitals following a diagnosis of NSU. Squeezing the penis or, for example, using disinfectants when worried about an unresolved infection might cause further inflammation of the urethra.

Gonorrhoea

Gonorrhoea is caused by the bacterium *Neisseria gonorrhoeae*, which infects the mucosal surfaces of the genital tract, rectum and oropharynx. The infection is always transmitted by sexual contact; however, eye infections can occur in infants during birth, and gonococcal vulvovaginitis in young girls can result from sexual abuse. The incubation period is around 24 h. Gonorrhoea is usually symptomatic within 3 days but can take up to 5 days. It is highly infectious. Currently gonorrhoea is most commonly seen in minority ethnic groups, homosexuals, women aged 16–19 and men aged 20–24. Uncomplicated gonorrhoea is the second most common bacterial SAI (HPA 2009).

Clinical presentation

The signs and symptoms of gonorrhoea depend on the site of infection but include urethritis (causing dysuria and purulent discharge), cervicitis (inflammation of the cervix causing vaginal discharge), proctitis with discharge and pharyngitis. However, many patients, especially women with uncomplicated infection, are asymptomatic. It is important to note that:

- 85% of men with urethral infection develop symptoms within 2 weeks
- rectal infection may be asymptomatic
- pharyngeal infection may be asymptomatic
- cervical infection in women is often asymptomatic.

Complications of gonorrhoea in men include formation of abscess, epididymitis, prostatitis and urethral strictures (see Ch. 8). Women may develop endometritis, ovarian abscesses, salpingitis and infertility, and bartholinitis (see Ch. 7). Gonorrhoea is diagnosed by microbiological examination of a swab of the discharge to identify the microorganism. In addition, patients should be screened for concurrent SAIs, especially chlamydia and trichomoniasis.

 ## Nursing management and health promotion: gonorrhoea

In the past *Neisseria gonorrhoeae* proved sensitive to penicillin. However, as resistant strains of gonorrhoea have become more common, treatment options have evolved. A single dose of intramuscular ceftriaxone or oral cefixime is the treatment of choice (British Association for Sexual Health and HIV Clinical Effectiveness Group [BASHH] 2005). Single-dose treatments are used wherever possible as they overcome problems of non-compliance with medication regimens. Patients are asked to abstain from sexual activity until a second test confirms that treatment has been effective. The opportunity should be taken to advise patients about the use of condoms in preventing the spread of SAIs.

Contact tracing with partner notification must be discussed with patients but it is essential that all recent (previous 2 weeks or previous partner if longer) and current sexual partners should be informed and advised to attend for assessment. After treatment, patients should be encouraged to return to clinic for a test of cure some 3–5 days after completing treatment.

Lymphogranuloma venereum (LGV)

LGV is caused by specific sub-types of *Chlamydia trachomatis* that attack regional lymph nodes rather than mucocutaneous tissue, which is more usual. Until recent years, LGV was an almost forgotten infection in the industrially developed world. However, it remained endemic in Africa, the Caribbean and parts of Asia. Since 2004 there has been an increase of LGV in the industrialised West, in particular, although not exclusively, amongst men who have sex with men (MSM) (Ward & Miller 2009).

Clinical presentation

LGV is normally associated with inflammation of the inguinal lymph nodes with possible abscess formation. In the current resurgence of LGV amongst MSM, proctitis (an inflammation of the rectal mucosa) is often the presenting condition. Currently, in the Western world, LGV diagnosis appears to be closely associated with co-infection by HIV and other SAIs (Sethi et al 2009). If left untreated LGV may cause inguinal bubo (a highly inflamed, infected lymph node) with fistula formation and significant scarring.

▷ Nursing management and health promotion: LGV

Nurses will need to ensure that patients understand the need to complete treatment, as a rather lengthy course (3 weeks) of oral doxycycline twice daily is required. Alternatively erythromycin may be used if a patient is allergic to doxycycline or pregnant (Klausner & Hook 2007). If a patient is diagnosed with LGV, it would be appropriate for the nurse to discuss HIV screening, given the association between the two infections.

Syphilis

Syphilis is a potentially lethal infection if left untreated and has a complex pattern of development (Box 35.2). Once thought to be in decline in industrialised countries, syphilis diagnoses have increased in recent years, generating concern (Simms et al 2005, Kerani et al 2007).

Box 35.2 Information

The stages of syphilis – clinical presentation (from Brooker & Nicol 2003)

Primary

Two to four weeks after exposure, a papule develops (at the site of infection) and ulcerates, becoming a hard, painless ulcer known as a chancre. There is swelling of local lymph nodes. The ulcer is highly infectious. It usually heals within a few weeks.

Secondary

A few months after the ulcer has healed, there may be a generalised 'flu-like illness with fever, sore throat and non-specific pain. Clinical signs of secondary syphilis may be present and include generalised lymph node enlargement, skin rashes, warty areas (condylomata lata) in the perianal and other moist body sites, and mucosal ulcers in the mouth/external genitalia (also called 'snail-track' ulcers).

Latent

The person is well but serological tests for syphilis are positive. This stage may last for years.

Tertiary

Tertiary syphilis is characterised by deep ulcers (gumma) affecting the skin, bones and organs, and further cardiovascular and neurological effects:

- Cardiovascular problems include aneurysm formation in the ascending aorta.
- Cerebral vascular changes increase the risk of strokes and dementia.
- Neurosyphilis may lead to tabes dorsalis (ataxia with loss of coordination and abnormal sensation in the legs) and general paralysis of the insane (GPI).

The causative organism is *Treponema pallidum*, a corkscrew-shaped motile bacterium that is transmitted sexually and vertically (in utero). *Treponema pallidum* enters the body via skin and mucous membranes through macroscopic and microscopic abrasions during sexual contact. The spirochaete, a bacterium, disseminates itself by travelling via the lymphatic system to regional lymph nodes and then throughout the body via the bloodstream.

Clinical presentation

Syphilis progresses in stages and without treatment remains chronic. The stages are known as primary, secondary and tertiary. Risk of infection after sexual exposure is about 30%; the disease is most contagious to sexual partners during the primary and secondary stages. Invasion of the central nervous system may occur in the case of untreated syphilis. Syphilis can also be vertically transmitted from mother to fetus.

Primary syphilis

A primary lesion or 'chancre' develops at the site of inoculation, usually the penis, vulva, anus or mouth, from 9 to 90 days after the patient has caught syphilis. The chancre itself is a painless ulcer with a raised, rubbery rim and heals spontaneously, usually without scarring, within 1–6 weeks. It is important to note that although the chancre itself is heavily colonised with *Treponema pallidum*, a serological (blood) test for syphilis may not be positive at this stage of syphilis.

Secondary syphilis

Secondary lesions of syphilis occur 3–6 weeks after the primary chancre appears, usually after it has healed. The patient experiences generalised lymphadenopathy (swelling of the lymph nodes). A skin rash may occur and, on occasion, this is followed by generalised or localised skin eruptions with mucosal lesions. These lesions may persist for weeks to months. Some patients are affected by a wart-like growth known as condylomata lata, often found around the perineum.

Serological testing for syphilis antibodies is positive during this stage of the disease. Relapses of secondary symptoms can occur in 25% of cases, usually within the first year of infection. Eventually, the host (the patient) suppresses the infection sufficiently that no lesions are clinically apparent. In about 70% of patients, the infection remains asymptomatic for the lifetime of the individual. Patients who have been symptom free for less than a year are referred to being in the early latent stage. If there are no symptoms beyond that period, the clinical stage is referred to as late latent syphilis.

Tertiary (late) syphilis disease progression

Approximately 30% of untreated patients progress to the tertiary stage within 1–20 years. Clinically, this final stage may manifest as encapsulated, necrotic lesions known as gummata. Gummata are found in soft tissue or viscera and can also erode bony surfaces. As well as involving the skin and bones, tertiary syphilis may also attack the cardiac and central nervous systems causing cardiovascular and cerebral vascular damage (Box 35.3). Cardiovascular syphilis often involves the aortic arch, causing aortic incompetence or a saccular aortic aneurysm. The usual period in untreated

Box 35.3 Information

Systemic complications of tertiary syphilis

Cardiovascular system

- Aortic aneurysm
- Coronary ostial stenosis, a narrowing of the coronary arteries
- Cerebral vascular accidents (CVA)

Central nervous system

- Dementia
- Syphilitic meningitis
- Degeneration of the nerve fibres, with muscle wastage and reduced mobility
- Ocular problems as nerves are attacked by the infection

syphilis from primary infection to development of the aneurysm is 10–15 years (Bossert et al 2004). Neurological manifestations of syphilis include meningovascular damage leading to strokes. In addition there may be the development of tabes dorsalis, a form of ataxia caused by syphilis attacking the neurological system, and possibly the development of general paresis (Goh 2005).

Congenital syphilis

Transmission to the fetus can occur during any stage of syphilis, but the risk is much higher during pregnancy with primary and secondary syphilis. Fetal infection can occur during any trimester of the pregnancy. Treatment of the mother during the last month of pregnancy cannot be considered adequate treatment for the fetus.

The manifestation of early lesions in infants less than 2 years old is usually inflammatory and may involve the development of blisters on the skin, mucous membranes and bones. In addition the spleen and lymph glands may be inflamed. Haematological abnormalities may include thrombocytopenia and anaemia (see Ch. 11). The manifestation of late lesions in infants older than 2 years tends to be immunological and destructive. A chronic inflammation of the middle layers of the cornea known as interstitial keratitis may occur. Less commonly nerve deafness or developmental abnormalities of the teeth and long bones may be found.

Diagnosing syphilis

Given the complexity of syphilis, a close examination and a careful medical history is required. Confirmation of diagnosis is dependent on serological tests that are used to detect the presence of antibodies. The tests include the fluorescent treponemal antibody absorbed test (specific test) and the rapid plasma reagin test (non-specific test). Primary syphilis may be diagnosed by confirmation of the presence of the microorganism in exudates obtained from the ulcer (chancre). This requires a nurse or technician who is familiar with dark ground microscopy.

Interaction between syphilis and HIV

The lesions associated with syphilis allow easier transmission of HIV. Syphilis and HIV infections commonly coexist and, in general, the clinical course is similar to non-HIV-infected patients. However, it has been suggested that in cases of co-infection with both syphilis and HIV, there is likely to be a higher viral load of HIV and a lower CD4 count (Buchacz et al 2004). The reasons why this should be are not fully understood; however, it has been demonstrated that successful treatment of syphilis is followed by a decrease in HIV viral load and a rise in the patient's CD4 count (Kofoed et al 2006). In addition, in cases of co-infection the chancre of primary syphilis may be multiple and deeper than the classic presentation (painless and solitary) (Zetola et al 2007). Some research notes that the symptoms of secondary syphilis are on occasion more severe and neurosyphilis more likely (Lynn & Lightman 2004). In the vast majority of patients serological tests for syphilis are equally sensitive in both HIV-infected and non-infected persons. However, if clinical suspicion is high for syphilis and the serological tests are negative, biopsy of the lesion or rash is recommended.

 ## Nursing management and health promotion: syphilis

In cases of co-infection, conventional therapy as given in syphilis alone is usually effective. However, some investigators believe in cases of co-infection, patients are more likely to present with or develop neurosyphilis and require a more intensive course of antibiotics (Goh 2005). The antibiotic chosen and duration of treatment depend on the disease stage: intramuscular procaine penicillin (or oral erythromycin if allergic to penicillin) or oral doxycycline and oxytetracycline are used. Patients having penicillin should be warned about the possibility of experiencing a Jarisch–Herxheimer reaction. This is characterised by fever, chills, nausea, muscle pain, dizziness and headache and is thought to be caused by toxins released when the microorganisms are destroyed (Pound & May 2005). The reaction occurs within a few hours of having the penicillin and is usually short-lived.

Patients should also abstain from sexual activity during antibiotic treatment and continue to use a barrier method (i.e. condoms) at least until blood tests show that the infection has passed. However, the benefits of condom use in preventing further infection should be stressed. As with all sexually acquired infections, patients found to be positive for syphilis require screening for other SAIs and should be encouraged to undergo screening for HIV.

Viral sexually acquired infections

As in the case of bacterial sexually acquired infections, viral infections can range from the relatively innocuous to the life threatening. However, in the case of viral infections our ability to cure is restricted. For most viral sexually acquired infections, at best we can ameliorate symptoms for what often becomes a chronic condition.

Genital herpes

This highly contagious viral disease is transmitted through close physical or sexual contact and is caused by the herpes simplex virus (HSV). Once acquired, HSV remains in the body, lying dormant within nerve roots. In most patients the virus intermittently works its way along the nerve root to the surface of the skin, where it may cause symptoms. There are two types of HSV, both of which infect the skin and mucous membranes: HSV-1 commonly causes cold sores, and HSV-2 infects the genital areas. In addition, HSV-1 is frequently the cause of genital herpetic lesions. If a person contracts HSV, they may be subject to repeated symptomatic episodes (Sen & Barton 2007).

Genital herpes is often asymptomatic; in fact, most cases are transmitted when the partner with HSV is symptom free (Box 35.4). The virus remains latent indefinitely and reactivation can be precipitated by multiple known and unknown factors which then induce viral replication. The efficiency of sexual transmission is greater from men to women than from women to men, although it is thought that the likelihood of transmission to others declines with increased duration of infection. The incubation period after acquisition is 2–12 days although the average is 4 days. Genital HSV infection will increase the risk of both acquisition and transmission of HIV infection.

Clinical presentation

The virus attacks the outer layer of the skin, forming characteristic blisters with clear fluid inside. Prior to the formation of these blisters, however, the skin often becomes 'tingly' or more sensitive. The period between infection and appearance of signs of the disease is approximately 7 days. In addition to the signs described above, patients may complain of fever, joint/muscle pain and cystitis. Viral culture of serous fluid obtained from lesions is used as a diagnostic tool.

- Primary episodes of herpes occur at the time of the initial infection with either HSV-1 or HSV-2. Symptoms are more severe than in any future recurrent episodes. There are no antibodies present when symptoms appear. Local symptoms include pain, itching, dysuria, urethral discharge and tender inguinal adenopathy. There are numerous bilateral painful genital lesions lasting an average of 11–12 days.

Box 35.4 Reflection

Viral shedding

When the virus moves along the nerves to the surface of the skin this is called 'viral shedding' or 'shedding'. During shedding, the virus can be passed on to others by direct skin-to-skin contact, especially from anal, oral or vaginal sex. Sometimes shedding is accompanied by symptoms, such as the characteristic herpes blisters, but sometimes shedding occurs without any noticeable symptoms; this is referred to as 'asymptomatic shedding'.

Asymptomatic shedding causes considerable problems in relationships. One partner with HSV, which may or may not have been previously diagnosed, may shed HSV whilst they themselves are symptom free. Consequently their sexual partner is exposed to and may catch HSV and perhaps become symptomatic. Both partners often wrongly assume that a third party is involved.

Activity

- Reflect upon how you could explain asymptomatic HSV shedding to people in a relationship where one person has unexpectedly become symptomatic.

- Recurrent symptomatic episodes, sometimes referred to as secondary episodes of HSV, are usually mild and short in duration, as antibodies are present when the symptoms appear. In approximately 50% of cases prodromal symptoms (localised tingling, irritation) begin 12–24 hours before lesions appear and the illness lasts from 5 to 10 days. The symptoms tend to be milder and less severe than in primary infection. HSV-2 primary infection is more prone to recur than HSV-1 primary infection.

Nursing management and health promotion: genital herpes

Systemic antiviral chemotherapy partially controls symptoms and signs of herpes episodes but does not eradicate latent virus. It does not affect the risk, frequency or severity of recurrences after the drug is discontinued. Systemic antiviral chemotherapy includes three oral medications: aciclovir, valaciclovir and famciclovir. Topical antiviral treatment has minimal clinical benefit and is not recommended (Sen & Barton 2007). Suppressive therapy, where the patient is given relatively low dosages of aciclovir, valaciclovir or famciclovir on a daily basis for a period of a year, is offered for recurrent genital herpes if a patient has more than six recurrences of episodic HSV in a year. It reduces frequency of recurrences and reduces but does not eliminate subclinical viral shedding. Periodically, at least once a year, the need for continued suppressive therapy should be reassessed.

There is no cure for HSV – once infected the individual is always a carrier of the virus. It lies dormant around nerve roots, but reactivates in the presence of a weakened immune system. Patients should be advised to use mild painkillers, e.g. paracetamol, rest and take extra fluids during the systemic disturbance associated with the primary infection. Blisters should be kept dry and clean, and treatment with aciclovir (topical or via the oral route) may help to prevent the formation of blisters. Since transmission of HSV is through close contact, a barrier (condom) method of contraception should be used. Even when there are no blisters or ulcers visible, the virus can be passed on during sexual intercourse, oral sex (from a cold sore to the genitals) and via the vulva during vaginal births.

It is important to remember that asymptomatic herpes can cause much distress. If, within a long-term partnership, one of the members suddenly develops herpes, it does not necessarily mean that a third party is involved sexually. It is quite possible that the long-term partner has asymptomatic herpes and that they have passed the virus on. Alternatively, the person who has suddenly developed symptoms may themselves have been previously an asymptomatic 'shedder' and, because stress or other factors have depressed their immune system, they are now symptomatic. It can be useful to offer asymptomatic partners serological screening to confirm the presence of HSV, but this is not done routinely as it can cause harm to some personal relationships. Nurses need to be sensitive and supportive to patients with HSV as it can have a dramatic impact on that person's life. Counselling should be offered and include natural history, sexual and perinatal transmission, and methods to reduce transmission.

As in the case of all sexual infections, patients should be assessed for their potential for behaviour change and prevention strategies should be discussed to develop an individualised risk-reduction plan. Prevention strategies include abstinence, mutual monogamy with an uninfected partner, use of condoms and limiting the number of sex partners. Nurses should also be aware that there is an intrinsic link between people contracting SAIs that produce genital ulceration, such as herpes and syphilis, and an increased risk of HIV (Freeman et al 2006).

Genital warts

External genital warts are caused by various types of human papillomavirus (HPV) and are very common. There are over 100 types of HPV, four of which are of most concern: types 6 and 11, which are responsible for the majority of genital warts, and types 16 and 18, which are associated with cervical cancer. HPV transmission is by close physical contact (skin to skin) and is almost always through genital contact, although warts in the oral cavity are not uncommon. The HPV attacks squamous epithelia and mucous membranes of the cervix, vagina, vulva, penis, anal cavity and oral cavity. The warts appear as pink or whitish lumps, either singly or in groups. These groups have been divided into three categories: pointed (acuminata), rounded (papula) and flat (macula) (Von Krogh 2001).

Clinical presentation

The signs and symptoms of genital warts include small growths around the genitals, bleeding, itchiness and sometimes hyperpigmentation; therefore diagnosis can be made visually. In some cases, however, the incubation period can be up to 18 months. Consequently for women, DNA testing on cells obtained by Pap screens (smear) of the cervix may be necessary. The DNA tests are able to identify the strain of HPV and identify whether types 16 and 18, which are associated with cervical cancer, are present. Patients with a diagnosis of genital warts should always be tested for other SAIs.

 ## Nursing management and health promotion: genital warts

A recent and exciting development involving the prevention of genital warts is the development of a number of effective vaccines against HPV and thus cervical cancer (Franco & Harper 2005). Two basic vaccine types have been developed. The one adopted in the UK as part of a national immunisation programme, launched in autumn 2008, protects against HPV types 16 and 18, those responsible for 70% of cervical carcinomas (Jit et al 2008). Immunisation is targeted at all girls aged 12–13 years and is most effective if the girl has not yet been sexually active and exposed to the virus. The second vaccine, which not only protects against types 16 and 18, but also types 6 and 11, has not been adopted in the UK.

It is impossible to eradicate the virus and so treatment is aimed at removing visible warts. The treatment options include cryotherapy (see below) or solutions and creams containing podophyllin or its major active constituent, podophyllotoxin. Podophyllin is a cytotoxic topical solution that is applied two to three times per week to the wart. The solution is left in situ for 4–6 h and then washed off. Care should

be taken to protect the surrounding skin by using a covering of soft paraffin, to reduce the risk of damaging the skin. Podophyllin should not be used in pregnancy or during breast feeding. Cervical warts may require colposcopy and/or cryotherapy, and oral warts are treated by cryotherapy. This technique freezes the wart with liquid nitrogen, resulting in cell necrosis.

There is a continuing trend to adopt self-administered wart treatments that can be applied at home rather than requiring patients to attend clinic at regular intervals. Self-administered treatments are more cost effective, less embarrassing for the patient and tend to result in better compliance. The different types of podophyllin-based creams and gels intended for self-administration have less active ingredient than clinic-applied creams. Despite this, better patient compliance means little difference in treatment success rates (O'Mahoney 2005).

Normally, contact tracing would form a routine part of the patient assessment, but since incubation may be delayed, this is often futile in these individuals.

Hepatitis

Hepatitis is a general term meaning inflammation of the liver. This inflammation can be caused by a variety of different viruses such as hepatitis viruses A, B, C, D and E. All can cause an acute disease with symptoms lasting several weeks including jaundice, dark urine, extreme fatigue, nausea, vomiting and abdominal pain. Since the development of jaundice is a characteristic feature of liver disease, a correct diagnosis can only be made by testing the patient's blood for the presence of specific antiviral antibodies. It can take several months to a year to make a full recovery. In the case of hepatitis B and C, the patient may have to endure a chronic illness which can cause severe liver damage or even liver cancer (see Ch. 4).

Hepatitis A

Hepatitis A (HAV) is one of the oldest diseases known to humankind. It is normally a self-limiting disease; however, it is a significant cause of morbidity and socio-economic loss in many parts of the world. On rare occasions HAV may lead to fulminant hepatitis with catastrophic liver failure which can prove fatal. This is usually associated with co-infection with hepatitis C.

The hepatitis A virus (HAV) is a non-enveloped, positive-stranded RNA virus, i.e. the virus is without the normal protective external envelope of lipids and proteins. The virus interferes with the liver's functions while replicating itself inside the hepatocytes (liver cells). The individual's immune system is then activated to produce a specific reaction to attack and possibly eradicate the infectious agent. As a consequence of pathological damage, the liver becomes inflamed.

Transmission

HAV is transmitted from person to person via the faecal–oral route as HAV is abundantly excreted in faeces and can survive in the environment for prolonged periods of time; it is typically acquired by ingestion of faeces-contaminated food or water. Direct person-to-person spread is common under poor hygienic conditions. Occasionally, HAV is also acquired through anal–oral sexual contact, particularly, although not exclusively, in men who have sex with men. HAV can also be transferred by blood transfusions, although this is rare as it will only occur if the donor is in the viraemic prodromal phase of infection at the time of blood donation.

In patients who develop clinically apparent hepatitis A, secretion of high titres of the virus in the faeces begins 1–3 weeks prior to onset of illness and may continue for several weeks at lower titres after jaundice appears. Although the level of virus shedding does not correlate with the severity of liver disease, faeces are highly infectious and therefore extremely contagious during all of this period. Oral–anal sex during this time would be extremely risky. As no specific treatment exists for hepatitis A, prevention in the form of vaccination is the most effective approach.

Prevention

Vaccination against HAV can be given either before or after exposure to the virus.

Pre-exposure prophylaxis Pre-exposure hepatitis A vaccination is recommended for those who are at increased risk of infection and for any person wishing to obtain immunity, particularly men who have sex with men. Those who seek immunological protection but are allergic to vaccine components should receive immune globulin (IG). The administration must be repeated if protection is required for periods exceeding 5 months. For those who require repeated IG, screening of their immune status will avoid unnecessary doses of IG.

Post-exposure prophylaxis Patients who have been exposed to HAV and have not previously been vaccinated should receive IG within 2 weeks of exposure. Patients who have received hepatitis A vaccine at least 2 weeks prior to exposure to HAV do not need IG.

Hepatitis B

Hepatitis B is a serious and common infectious disease of the liver, affecting millions of people throughout the world. Sexual transmission is through contact with infected sexual fluids and/or blood, mainly through unprotected anal sex. 'Rimming' (oral–anal sex) and 'fisting' (fist to anus) are also implicated. In some cases of high infectivity, transmission occurs through contact with saliva. Gay men, people with multiple partners, intravenous drug users and sex workers are most at risk. Hepatitis B is also transmitted through vertical transmission to the fetus.

Hepatitis B virus (HBV) infection is a global public health problem, with approximately 400 million people chronically infected. Each year it causes more than 500 000 deaths worldwide (Lavanchy 2004). The clinical presentation of acute HBV infection is most commonly asymptomatic subclinical infection (70%), with 30% developing symptomatic acute hepatitis; a small number (0.1–0.5%) develop fulminant (severe) hepatic failure. A proportion of people infected with HBV (5–10% among adults) progress to chronicity, defined as persistence of infection for more than 6 months. The rate of chronicity is much higher among neonates and children. The spectrum of chronic HBV infection ranges from the asymptomatic carrier state to chronic hepatitis B, liver cirrhosis and hepatocellular carcinoma (see Ch. 4).

Overall, chronic hepatitis progresses to end-stage liver disease in 15–40% of patients.

During the incubation phase of the disease (6–24 weeks), patients may feel unwell with possible nausea, vomiting, diarrhoea, loss of appetite and headaches. Patients may then become jaundiced although the low-grade fever and loss of appetite may improve. However, sometimes HBV infection produces neither jaundice nor obvious symptoms.

Pathogenesis

HBV infection has three possible outcomes:

- 90–95% of people experience an acute illness with complete recovery and subsequent immunity from re-infection.
- Fulminant hepatitis with liver failure and death occurs in less than 1% of those people infected.
- Chronic infection with carrier status and virus persistence is found in 5–10% of those affected.

Chronic carriers are identified by the presence of hepatitis B surface antigen (HBsAG) in the bloodstream. Those with highest infectivity have high levels of HBV DNA and hepatitis B e antigen (HBeAG). Given that there are around 350 million people who are HBV carriers worldwide, out of a world population of over 6 billion, approximately 5% of the global population are HBV carriers (Lavanchy 2004).

 ## Nursing management and health promotion: hepatitis B

Diagnosis is confirmed by serological tests for surface antigens (HBsAg) and/or antibodies (anti-HBc). HBsAg can be detected in the serum from several weeks before onset of symptoms to months after onset. HBsAg is present in serum during acute infections and persists in chronic infections (Shepard et al 2006). The presence of HBsAg indicates that the person is potentially infectious. The presence of HBeAg is associated with relatively high infectivity and severity of disease (Yim & Lok 2006). Anti-HBc is the first antibody to appear. Demonstration of anti-HBc in serum indicates HBV infection, current or past. IgM anti-HBc is present in high titre during acute infection and usually disappears within 6 months, although it can persist in some cases of chronic hepatitis. This test may therefore reliably diagnose acute HBV infection. IgG anti-HBc generally remains detectable for a lifetime.

Acute hepatitis B will often lead to nausea, anorexia and vomiting. Nurses will need to support patients through this period, administering prescribed antiemetics where possible. Hepatitis B can be prevented by vaccination and nurses need to ensure that the partners of those found to be hepatitis B positive are screened for the infection. If they are found to have no natural protection, they should be encouraged to accept vaccination.

Treatments are available including interferon, tenofovir, adefovir, and lamivudine for chronic disease. The aim of treatment is the suppression of viral replication and the reduction of liver injury and progression to cirrhosis. Treatment is expensive, imperfect and requires careful monitoring for side-effects such renal problems, further emphasising the importance of safe, cheap vaccination.

Hepatitis C

Hepatitis C virus (HCV) is usually spread by sharing contaminated needles, receiving an unscreened blood transfusion, and from accidental exposure to infected blood. Some people acquire the infection through non-parenteral means that have not been fully defined. These include sexual transmission, although transmission of HCV is much less common than that of HBV and HIV.

▷ **Nursing management and health promotion: hepatitis C**

Nurses should encourage those patients who have not been screened for hepatitis to do so. If they are found to have no natural immunity to hepatitis A and B, then vaccination should be actively promoted as co-infection with other hepatitides puts an intolerable burden on the liver and complicates the prognosis.

There are no vaccines currently effective against hepatitis C. Nurses need to promote harm-reduction strategies. Sharing of needles should be discouraged but, if it occurs, patients should be advised that not only clean, sterile needles, but clean 'works' (syringe, spoon, filter, etc.) should be always used to reduce the chance of HCV cross-infection. Those patients with a history of percutaneous drug usage should be offered a hepatitis C test and, if positive, further screens of liver function. Treatment, imperfect as it is, may prove advisable. Current treatment options incorporate antiviral drugs such as interferon and ribavirin and are not without considerable potential side-effects including clinical depression and anaemia. Treatment effectiveness is around 50%.

Human immunodeficiency virus (HIV)

HIV represents one of the most important health challenges facing the world today. There are two strains of this virus, HIV-1 and HIV-2, although the relatively uncommon HIV-2 is concentrated in West Africa and is rarely found elsewhere. Both destroy the immune system's CD4 defence cells, in particular targeting helper cells that help coordinate the body's response to infection. The immune system provides specific resistance or defence against harmful substances that have invaded the body. This involves a complex series of actions that includes recruitment of white blood cells or lymphocytes that respond to substances that actively harm the body, either by surrounding them so that no further damage can occur, or killing them. The activation of lymphocytes is prompted by the presence of viral antigens. By depleting the number of available T helper cells, HIV undermines the body's immune defences, leaving the infected person open to secondary infections, many of which can be life threatening (Figure 35.1).

HIV is a broad-spectrum disorder ranging from primary infection with the HIV retrovirus, through the asymptomatic state to advanced disease. In advanced disease, when the body's immune defences are collapsing, a person is considered to have acquired immune deficiency syndrome (AIDS, see p. 896). Transmission is via sexual activity after contact with infected body fluids, primarily ejaculate, vaginal lubrication, blood or blood products, or mother to infant peripartum or via breast milk. Patients may initially experience 'acute HIV syndrome' after the primary infection. However, this may go unnoticed because it mimics a 'flu-like illness.

The hallmark of the disease is immunodeficiency, from progressive reduction of CD4 cells. HIV infiltrates and destroys human helper T lymphocytes, which are necessary for the

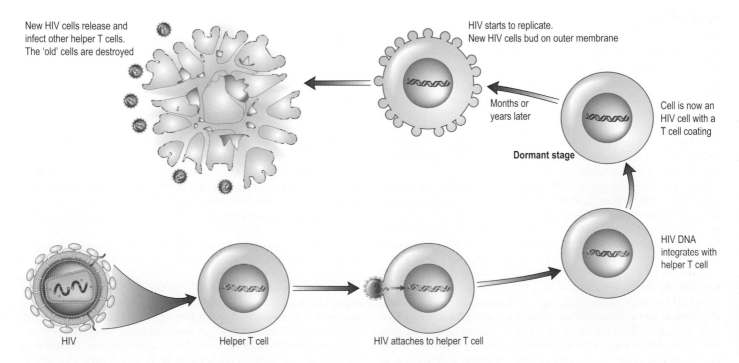

New HIV cells release and infect other helper T cells. The 'old' cells are destroyed

HIV starts to replicate. New HIV cells bud on outer membrane

Months or years later

Cell is now an HIV cell with a T cell coating

Dormant stage

HIV DNA integrates with helper T cell

HIV

Helper T cell

HIV attaches to helper T cell

Figure 35.1 The human immunodeficiency virus in action.

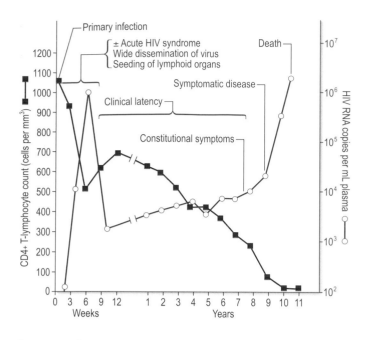

Figure 35.2 The course of HIV infection.

production of antibodies and the activation of killer T lymphocytes (CD8+ cytotoxic cells), which attack and kill those cells infected with viruses. Although HIV will become apparently latent for a variable period, it is associated with a gradual and progressive diminution in the CD4 count. Advanced HIV disease occurs when the CD4 T-cell count falls below 200/μL and renders the patient susceptible to opportunistic infections (Figure 35.2).

Treatment of HIV

Since HIV was first recognised, great advances have taken place in the treatment of people with the virus and its related illnesses. Undoubtedly, the main advance is in the expansion and sophistication of combination (multiple) therapies. Current treatment aims to block the cycle of viral replication throughout its various stages. The British HIV Association website (http://www.bhiva.org/) provides excellent information about HIV treatment guidelines. In the early days of the emergence of the disease, people diagnosed with AIDS were expected to live only weeks or months, whereas improved therapies have led to the survival of some patients for over 20 years, and to many more patients being cared for outside hospital (Fang et al 2007).

Currently, treatment for HIV is focused not only on reducing viral replication but also providing prophylaxis and treatment for the major opportunistic infections. HIV cannot be cured but it can be managed, and the disease process can be dramatically slowed by the use of a combination of anti-retroviral drugs. Prophylaxis against potentially lethal infections such as *Pneumocystis jiroveci* pneumonia (see p. 902) is now increasingly effective

Whilst treatment options of increased complexity and sophistication are becoming available, a fundamental problem remains. The majority of people living with HIV are from the developing world, where problems with available financial resources and medical infrastructure restrict access to treatment regimens. There is a renewed emphasis on the

practical implementation of treatment for the vast numbers of people with HIV and its related illnesses in financially poor and developing countries, particularly in Africa. Progress is slow, but gathering momentum. Although the World Health Organization's '3 by 5' campaign (WHO 2003a), which aimed to treat 3 million people by 2005, failed to meet its objectives, it did set a precedent.

HIV-2

Since the discovery of HIV, a major strain variation within the human immunodeficiency viruses, HIV-2, has been identified. It is most commonly found in certain countries on the west coast of Africa and in west India. HIV-2 is less able to be transmitted from an infected mother to her child (vertical transmission) and infection with HIV-2 is generally associated with a longer incubation period before the patient contracts an AIDS-defining illness (Adler 2001).

Acquired immune deficiency syndrome (AIDS)

The Centers for Disease Control's (CDC) 1993 recommendations (1992) state that the definition of AIDS is when a person with HIV develops a major opportunistic infection, or if asymptomatic, when the CD4 (T helper cell) count is less than 200/μL (Schneider et al 2008). It is important to understand the relationship between HIV antibodies and AIDS; everyone who has AIDS is HIV antibody positive, but not everybody who is HIV antibody positive has AIDS. A person is infected by HIV but develops AIDS as the virus slowly destroys their immune system. It should also be pointed out that an individual who has a positive HIV antibody status may sometimes become ill without being diagnosed as having AIDS. This may be because they have not yet contracted one of the infections or diseases on the classified list but are ill for some other reason, or because they are experiencing side-effects of, for instance, antiretroviral treatment.

When a person has been infected with HIV, over the course of time their immune system starts to become severely damaged. Microorganisms that generally inhabit the body harmlessly take the opportunity to replicate wildly, disseminate and cause clinical illness, e.g. *Pneumocystis jiroveci* pneumonia (PCP). Until the emergence of HIV, this infection was seen only occasionally in patients who were immunosuppressed with diseases such as leukaemia or whose immunity was suppressed as a side-effect of medication. These types of illness and neoplastic events, which only manifest themselves in those with a severely compromised immune system, are referred to as 'opportunistic diseases' and they are the hallmark of the syndrome now referred to as AIDS. As this immunosuppressed state was not a primary, e.g. congenital, but a secondary immunodeficiency, it was called acquired immune deficiency (the main linking clinical factor) syndrome, i.e. a group of recognised clinical signs. In time it would be recognised that this particular immunodeficiency was secondary to specific viral infection.

A patient is diagnosed as having AIDS only if they are HIV antibody positive and have one of the designated infections or diseases associated with AIDS. The classification of these diseases devised by the US CDC (1987), and

Box 35.5 Information

World Health Organization staging system for HIV infection and disease in adults and adolescents (WHO 2007)

Clinical stage I

1. Asymptomatic
2. Persistent generalised lymphadenopathy

Performance scale 1: asymptomatic, normal activity

Clinical stage II

3. Unexplained weight loss, <10% of body weight
4. Minor mucocutaneous manifestations, e.g. seborrhoeic dermatitis, prurigo, fungal nail infections, recurrent oral ulcerations, angular cheilitis
5. Herpes zoster
6. Recurrent upper respiratory tract infections, e.g. bacterial sinusitis

And/or performance scale 2: symptomatic, normal activity

Clinical stage III – advanced HIV disease

7. Unexplained severe weight loss, >10% of body weight
8. Unexplained chronic diarrhoea, >1 month
9. Unexplained prolonged fever >37.6°C (intermittent or constant), >1 month
10. Persistent oral candidiasis (thrush)
11. Oral hairy leucoplakia
12. Current pulmonary tuberculosis
13. Severe bacterial infections, i.e. pneumonia, pyomyositis, bone or joint infections

And/or performance scale 3: bedridden <50% of the day during the last month

Clinical stage IV – AIDS

14. HIV wasting syndrome, as defined by the Centers for Disease Control and Prevention – (involuntary weight loss >10% of

baseline body weight) associated with either chronic diarrhoea (≥2 loose stools per day ≥1 month) or chronic weakness and documented fever ≥1 month

15. *Pneumocystis jiroveci* pneumonia
16. CNS toxoplasmosis
17. Cryptosporidiosis with diarrhoea >1 month
18. Cryptococcosis, extrapulmonary
19. Cytomegalovirus disease of an organ other than liver, spleen or lymph nodes
20. Herpes simplex virus infection, mucocutaneous >1 month, or visceral any duration
21. Progressive multifocal leucoencephalopathy
22. Any disseminated endemic mycosis, i.e. histoplasmosis, coccidioidomycosis
23. Candidiasis of the oesophagus, trachea, bronchi or lungs
24. Atypical mycobacteriosis, disseminated
25. Non-typhoid *Salmonella* septicaemia
26. Extrapulmonary tuberculosis
27. Lymphoma
28. Kaposi's sarcoma
29. HIV encephalopathy, as defined by the Centers for Disease Control and Prevention

And/or performance scale 4: bedridden >50% of the day during the last month

Note: both definitive and presumptive diagnoses are acceptable.

HIV wasting syndrome: weight loss of >10% of body weight, plus either unexplained chronic diarrhoea (>1 month) or chronic weakness and unexplained prolonged fever (>1 month).

HIV encephalopathy: clinical findings of disabling cognitive and/or motor dysfunction interfering with activities of daily living, progressing over weeks to months, in the absence of a concurrent illness or condition other than HIV infection which could explain the findings.

---

later revised (Schneider et al 2008), is used globally. Also current is the WHO Clinical Staging System for HIV Infection and Disease (WHO 2003b), which has been recently revised (WHO 2007), see Box 35.5. This system attempts to address some of the anomalies presented by the CDC system. A helpful explanation of the staging system is given in Pratt (2003).

Nurses will meet many people who have at some time been diagnosed as having AIDS but who are presently well. A patient may have an AIDS-defining illness, be treated for it, recover and feel relatively healthy. This is increasingly common as people with the syndrome survive longer; 10–20 years is not uncommon. Thus the term 'AIDS' as an 'illness label' can be unhelpful and even misleading, because it does not necessarily reflect how the person is at a given moment. The terminology used when describing patients with HIV and AIDS has become deeply politicised. It is helpful if nurses avoid terms such as 'AIDS patients' or 'HIV patients' and instead use the term 'persons living with HIV infection'. The term conveys a continuum from the moment of infection to end-stage disease and death, with early, middle and late events and issues affecting individuals, and neither stigmatises nor gives offence.

Viruses and immunology

Viruses are not complete organisms. They can survive only as part of 'host' cells. Unlike bacteria, fungi, protozoa and other infective agents, all of which are complete and independently viable, viruses cannot replicate (multiply/reproduce) by themselves. They are also very small and cannot be seen by a light microscope. Viruses are made up of a core of nucleic acid, i.e. DNA or RNA, never both, and are enveloped in a protein shell (see Figure 35.1).

Retroviruses

HIV is a retrovirus, which is a type of virus that contains RNA. Retroviruses have the ability to infiltrate the DNA of the host cell and implant their genetic material there, after which the host cell will have the capability to reproduce the virus. In essence, the host cell has been 'hijacked' and its function changed to a 'factory' for the mass replication of virus.

DNA is present in all organisms. It plays a central part in heredity and, because of its structure, the two interwoven strands of nucleotides, connected by hydrogen bonds, can replicate, carrying the genetic blueprint to the next generation of cells. RNA is made up of a single strand of nucleotides and is involved in protein synthesis. It provides the genetic blueprint of some viruses, including HIV. HIV infects a variety of cells that contain the CD4 receptors, including T lymphocytes. The presence of additional host cell receptors is known to be necessary in order for HIV to attach itself to, and infect a cell.

The importance of this disruption of the T lymphocytes must be understood within the context of the normal immune response. The various types of white blood cell have interlinking but quite distinct cell-mediated responses to seek and destroy invading microorganisms and malignant cells (Box 35.6). Given the essential role played by helper T cells in the immune system, it is clear that their invasion and destruction by HIV will have devastating results. In a healthy HIV-negative individual the number of T cells per cubic mm of blood varies. For males the normal range is between 400 and 1200 T cells per cubic mm of blood and for females 500–1600. In the case of HIV, the lower the T-cell level drops, the more severe the damage to the immune system. If, in an HIV-infected individual, the T-cell count drops to 200 or below, then the damage is very serious. Indeed, for a person living with HIV, if their T-cell count drops below 200, they are classified as having developed AIDS. However, such an individual may still feel well, despite the severe damage to their immune system. For further information on retroviruses, see Pratt (2003, Chs 2 and 3).

Modes of transmission

The first stage of HIV infection occurs when the individual is infected through an exchange of body fluids and/or blood with an infected individual. Sexual contact and blood-to-blood contact are known as 'horizontal' methods of transmission, i.e. they move 'across' from one individual to another.

Box 35.6 Information

The normal immune response

Warning

In response to the invading microorganism, helper T cells orchestrate defences by releasing chemicals that stimulate other cells of the immune system.

Preparation

Activated by these chemical signals, other kinds of T cells (cytotoxic cells and lymphokine producers) begin to proliferate, while B lymphocytes multiply and become plasma cells that start to manufacture antibodies.

Attack

Activated T cells and antibodies are released into the circulation, where they specifically target and destroy the invading organism.

Stand down

Once the foreign organism is routed and the infection is under control, the activity of the immune system is reduced, perhaps partly through the action of suppressor T lymphocytes.

Transmission through sexual contact

Unprotected vaginal or anal intercourse is the most common means by which HIV can be transmitted from an infected to a non-infected person. It is difficult to determine absolutely whether other intimate sexual activities, e.g. oral sex, can transmit the virus as they do not often occur in isolation. However, some individual cases have been reported and it is possible that the number of cases transmitted through oral sex might have been understated (Hawkins 2001).There is much debate in the scientific and secular worlds about which sexual activities are the most 'dangerous'. Until recently, anal sex was considered to be most risky. Also, women were thought to be more at risk than men during penetrative vaginal sex. More recent findings are leading to a re-examination of these assumptions, and the scientific debate is not conclusive (Varghese et al 2002). It is important, therefore, to inform patients that they may be at risk from any intimate sexual contact.

Transmission through blood and blood products

Transmission of HIV through blood and blood products can occur in one of six ways.

- *Blood transfusion.* The spread of HIV in Western countries that have sophisticated blood transfusion services has been greatly reduced since the rigorous screening of donors was instituted in most countries in 1985. The best-known recipients of blood products are those suffering from haemophilia and those with other blood-clotting disorders. Before 1985, many thousands of such individuals became infected through blood products. Since 1985, these products have been heat treated.
- *Blood transmission through sharing of equipment.* HIV transmission can occur through the sharing of syringes, needles and other blood-giving equipment. In Western countries this commonly occurs through the illicit, intravenous (i.v.) use of drugs. Here the probability of infection is often increased by the user 'flushing' the syringe with their blood before injection. In poorer countries, it also occurs where there is reuse of medical equipment and insufficient sterilising facilities. The mode of transmission is the same in both cases.
- *Percutaneous 'needle stick' injuries.* There have been very few proven cases of infection by this mode. A study of 3000 incidents where individuals were exposed to HIV puts the risk of seroconversion from a contaminated needle stick at 0.3%. Only 109 cases of occupational infection with HIV have been reported worldwide (Jagger 2007). Five confirmed and 16 probable cases of HIV have been reported in UK health care workers following occupational exposure (HPA et al 2008a).
- *Transmission through skin piercing procedures.* Transmission is certainly a theoretical risk from procedures such as tattooing (Antoszewski et al 2006), and cases have been reported of transmission by body piercing (Armstrong 1998) and skin grafting.
- *Transmission through other bodily fluids.* Infection with HIV takes place only when there is sufficient concentration of the virus. Infection through saliva, for instance, is therefore considered unlikely. Worldwide retrospective studies have shown that the number of workers contracting the virus through urine, faeces or saliva, for example, has been extremely small (Jeffries 1997).

- *Mother to child transmission.* This form of transmission is known as 'vertical' transmission, i.e. 'from' an infected mother to her child in the womb or during delivery, when the mother's blood and the child's blood become mixed. In Europe and the USA the rate of transmission from a positive mother to her baby, unless there are therapeutic interventions such as antiretrovirals and precautionary measures such as elective caesarean section, is around 15–20%. This compares to about 30% in Africa. The difference in transmission rates is explained by breast feeding (Sharland et al 2003).

From birth until 11–18 months, the baby will carry the mother's antibodies including HIV. Therefore all babies born to HIV-infected mothers are found to be HIV antibody positive. At about 11–18 months, the baby will lose the mother's antibodies and go on either to be HIV antibody negative, i.e. not carrying the virus, or to develop their own antibodies, i.e. infected in their own right. A few of these babies go on to become HIV antibody negative but positive to another test which isolates antigen (particles of the actual virus), so that they are carrying the virus but not the antibodies. For further information, see Newberry & Kelsey (2003).

At the beginning of the HIV epidemic it appeared that approximately 50% of children born to HIV antibody-positive mothers became infected in their own right. In countries where there are good antenatal facilities and the mother remains well throughout pregnancy, the rate of transmission from mother to child is dramatically lower. If the mother's immune system is robust, if she is treated in the last trimester and has an early elective caesarean section, transmission is reduced to less than 1% (De Cock et al 2000, WHO 2000).

Infection prevention and control

The essence of infection prevention and control of HIV is the use of standard infection control precautions (see Ch. 16) to protect patients, who will be at increased risk of health care associated infection (HAI) (Wilson 2006). Care should be taken with all body fluids, and gloves and aprons should be used for all intimate procedures. Because of their damaged immune system, patients may be more at risk from the nurse than the other way round. For further information on HIV-related infection control, see Pratt (2003, Ch. 14). Disposal of clinical waste should be carried out in accordance with local nursing policies and procedures.

Stages of HIV infection

People with HIV disease rarely get all of the diseases associated with AIDS and often those that do occur manifest one at a time. The precise course of the illness in an individual is virtually impossible to predict, but the WHO (2007) has introduced a staging system for HIV (Table 35.1) so that the progress of the disease can be assessed and the appropriate medical and nursing intervention carried out in response.

Table 35.1 WHO criteria for HIV staging in adults using CD4+ T-lymphocyte count (WHO 2007 and CDC 2008)

WHO STAGE	CD4+ T-LYMPHOCYTE COUNT
Clinical stage I (HIV infection)	CD4 $\geq$500 cells/mm^3
Clinical stage II (HIV infection)	CD4 $\geq$350–499 cells/mm^3
Clinical stage III (advanced HIV infection)	CD4 $\geq$200–349 cells/mm^3
Clinical stage IV (AIDS)	CD4 <200 cells/mm^3

The natural history of HIV replication

In HIV-related illness, two main processes take place in the infected person's body:

- HIV destroys the helper T cells and replicates itself.
- The body's immunity is inexorably weakened and is attacked by other infections. The body becomes increasingly unable to combat these attacks.

Since viruses cannot multiply by themselves, they need to use the cell-building material of their host cells in order to reproduce. When HIV enters the bloodstream, it attaches itself to the outer cell membrane of the helper T lymphocyte. Following this, it breaks into the cell and releases its genetic blueprint, which has the ability to replicate itself.

The person infected with HIV may take 3 months or more to produce antibodies as part of the immune response (see Figure 35.2). If they have seroconverted and started to produce antibodies, they may or may not have become ill. If they did become ill with acute seroconversion illness (CDC phase A), the usually mild and very common 'flu-like symptoms were probably not recognised by the individual or their doctor as a sign of HIV infection. The helper T-lymphocyte blood count will still be within normal range and therefore the immune system will remain apparently unaffected. However, HIV is selectively taking over and eventually destroying key elements of the immune system, putting it under immense strain (Grossman et al 2006). This stage, often called the dormant stage, is referred to as 'Clinical stage I: 1-Asymptomatic' in the WHO staging system (see Box 35.5, WHO 2007).

In time, the infected T cells will start to replicate new HIV retroviruses. Although it is unclear what triggers this process, it seems that, if an individual keeps generally well and leads a healthy lifestyle, the stage at which HIV starts to replicate and destroy the T cells may be delayed. A clearer finding is that, in conditions of deprivation and poor health, the illness seems to progress more quickly.

At some point after HIV has been incorporated into the helper T lymphocyte, it begins to replicate itself within the cell walls using the cell's own material. The new viruses aggregate, start to destroy the outer cell membrane and break out of the helper T cell, encased in membrane stolen from the host cell and clinging onto the remnants of the cell. This is known as 'budding'. At this stage, the host cell dies. The new viruses then disperse throughout the bloodstream, infecting other helper T lymphocytes, and the process begins again.

The second process begins when helper T cells have been infected to the degree that the number of normal, healthy helper T cells begins to fall markedly. Patients diagnosed with HIV will have their T-cell count taken at regular intervals, as in conjunction with a check on the viral load of HIV within their bloodstream it provides an indication as to well their immune system is coping with the virus. Once the T-cell count begins to fall, the body's immune response to other infections will begin to be compromised. From the clinician's viewpoint, this is a significant stage, as the depletion of normal helper T cells can be measured in a blood sample. Also significant is the ratio between the helper T lymphocytes and the cytotoxic T lymphocytes, which is thought to assist in the 'stand down' phase of the normal immune response (see Box 35.6). Normally, the ratio is 1.5 helpers to 1.0 suppressor cytotoxic cells; however, as the number of healthy helper cells decreases, this ratio changes. This will have a detrimental effect on the immune system. It is also one of the diagnostic signs used to confirm the presence of HIV-related illness. In other forms of immune deficiency illnesses, both helper and suppressor cell levels fall, and so the ratio between them remains roughly the same.

As the helper T-cell level falls, the body will become more susceptible to other infections. The individual may at first experience rather vague symptoms, progressing to debilitating but not life-threatening conditions and finally to serious illness and death. Information on the specific diseases that may appear is given later in the chapter. A typical profile of HIV infection is shown in Figure 35.2. The way in which HIV/AIDS actually manifests itself will vary dramatically from one person to another. Many people with extremely low helper T-cell counts may seem healthy; others with what should be a 'good' T-cell count may be extremely ill. Nurses must rely on observations of and discussions with the patient in assessing their condition, rather than on abstract clinical indicators alone.

Clinical staging of HIV infection

The WHO (2007) states that HIV can be staged and AIDS diagnosed by two sets of criteria: acquiring one of the clinical conditions listed within Box 35.5, and/or the positive person's immune count, see Table 35.1.

In addition to the number of CD4+ T lymphocytes, viral load, i.e. the amount of HIV circulating in the bloodstream needs to be taken into account. In general, the higher the viral load the more infectious the patient and the greater the chance of HIV transmission. In addition, the higher the viral load, the greater the prospective damage to the immune system. HIV viral load is normally highest in primary infection, which the WHO (2007) refers to as clinical stage I, and in late-stage HIV (clinical stages III and IV). The times of highest infectivity are thought to be the 3 months after seroconversion and the period between 19 and 10 months before death (Hollingsworth et al 2008).

Measuring viral load demands complex laboratory facilities and is limited in resource-stretched areas of the developing world. For that reason, the WHO does not insist on its necessity for its staging protocols. If such facilities are available, then clinicians have a vital tool for measuring treatment efficacy and adherence and it is hoped that viral load screening will become increasingly available in resource-limited settings (Calmy et al 2007).

Clinical stage I HIV infection

After initial exposure to HIV, some people undergo an acute seroconversion illness. In most individuals this illness is not recognised. It may be seen 2–6 weeks after exposure to HIV. Not everyone infected with HIV gets this 'flu- or glandular fever-like condition. It may be associated with joint pain and other non-specific signs. A skin rash is sometimes seen, as are swollen lymph glands; these usually reduce after some time. At this stage the body will be producing HIV antibodies (seroconversion). A few individuals may also show early signs of HIV affecting the central nervous system, particularly the layers of the brain, causing for example encephalopathy or meningitis. Seroconversion, if symptomatic, may alert the doctor and nurse to the presence of HIV. However, the signs are very similar to those of many minor infections.

Patients who are classified as being in stage I of HIV infection either have one of the conditions listed above and/or have a CD4+ T-lymphocyte count of 500 or more.

Persistent generalised lymphadenopathy (PGL) or lymphadenopathy syndrome (LAS) is sometimes the condition that alerts medical services to investigate for HIV. The individual presents with swollen glands of more than 1 cm which persist for longer than 12 weeks. Although the individual may have swollen inguinal glands, they must also have other affected glands. Other reasons for swollen glands must be discounted before a diagnosis is given. It is at this stage that the individual may be tested for HIV for the first time. If positive, monitoring of helper T cells and suppressor T cells and other investigations may begin.

Clinical stage II HIV infection

Stage II HIV infection refers to a period in an individual's illness when they may contract a variety of well-known conditions, but not major, life-threatening, opportunistic infections or cancers. Common bacterial, viral and fungal infections, such as oral and genital herpes and athlete's foot, frequently occur and are often marked by their persistence and virulence. Another typical clinical symptom of clinical stage II is angular cheilitis, where the splits and fissures in the corner of the patient's mouth are related not to iron deficiency but to underlying fungal conditions. In a normally healthy person, these conditions would resolve within a few days. In stage II HIV infection, the duration of the infection is lengthened and the whole foot, for instance, may become affected.

Loss of weight of less than 10% of measured or presumed body weight may be seen at this stage (WHO 2007). This may be due to a specific mechanical problem, such as mouth ulcers, or to persistent low-grade attacks from infections. At this stage a significant drop may be seen in the helper T cells. In day-to-day practice, nurses should bear in mind that young healthy people should overcome common infections quickly without them becoming widespread. Any persistent condition, e.g. coughing, loss of weight, should be noted. While thrush (Candida albicans) is common in the vagina, it is very uncommon in the mouth of a young healthy person. Such an occurrence should immediately alert the practitioner to the fact that the individual may have an underlying condition such as HIV.

Nurse working with diagnosed patients should also be aware that, since the positive diagnosis, the individual will have been dreading the onset of illness. When weight loss, mouth ulcers or fungal infections occur, the patient may become acutely anxious, considering themselves to be in imminent danger of pain or death. Other professionals, such as clinical psychologists, can assist the patient during these periods. Involvement of the patient in all stages of decision making and treatment right from the start will assist them to take control of their condition and reduce any feeling of helplessness.

HIV patients classified as having stage II HIV infection either have one of the conditions listed above and/or a CD4+ T-lymphocyte count of 350–499.

Clinical stage III – advanced HIV disease

Clinical stage III is confirmed by the presence of any of a number of chronic constitutional and medical conditions associated with advanced HIV disease. Unexplained weight loss of more than 10% of body mass is associated with advanced HIV disease. This is often accompanied by chronic diarrhoea for which no specific cause has been determined and which lingers on for over a month. Such weight loss remains a problem even in the era of otherwise effective antiviral therapy and is often associated with other co-morbidities and generally sicker patients (Siddiqui et al 2009).

Persistent or intermittent pyrexia, which involves a fever of over 36.7°C and which lasts longer than a month, is one of the diagnostic conditions of stage III HIV. All too often in Africa such a pyrexia is indicative of undiagnosed tuberculosis, and if highly active antiretroviral therapy (HAART; see p. 904) is initiated without diagnosing and treating tuberculosis, the patient outcome is adversely affected (Bizuwork et al 2007).

Tuberculosis (TB), caused by *Mycobacterium tuberculosis*, is now increasingly seen in patients with HIV. It represents the most common cause of death amongst those patients who die of HIV-related opportunistic infections (Cahn et al 2003). People who are HIV positive and have current TB are classified as having clinical stage III. TB is often associated with poor social conditions and increasingly with vulnerable groups such as asylum seekers. Prisons around the world have seen an increase in TB prevalence, including potentially lethal strains of drug-resistant TB, particularly where there is a high prevalence of HIV (Wells et al 2007). Prisoners with HIV are affected, as are other vulnerable inmates.

Treatment is with rifampicin, isoniazid, ethambutol and pyrazinamide for a 2-month induction phase and with rifampicin and isoniazid for a 4-month continuation phase (Kaplan et al 2009). TB in the general population, when responsive to treatment, is not generally life threatening. However, patients with HIV and compromised immune systems face a greater risk (United Nations 2004). As treatment-resistant strains of TB evolve, countries such as those that made up the old Soviet Union have a particularly severe problem (Wright et al 2009). However, it is in sub-Saharan Africa, with its high incidence of HIV, that resistant strains of TB have the greatest capacity to wreak harm on vulnerable populations (Raviglione & Smith 2007).

Conditions that affect the mouth such as Candida or oral hairy leucoplakia are also characteristic of clinical stage III. Persistent oral Candida can be treated with topical preparations or by a systemic antifungal agent such as fluconazole.

Oral hairy leucoplakia appears in the form of linear, corrugated lesions on the sides of the tongue and is caused by Epstein–Barr virus. Although it can be unsightly, oral hairy leucoplakia is usually asymptomatic. Mucocutaneous conditions such as acute necrotising ulcerative stomatitis, gingivitis or periodontitis associated with HIV infection indicate that the patient has reached clinical stage III (Weinberg & Kovarik 2010).

Severe or persistent cases of infections such as pneumonia, empyema or meningitis are indicative of clinical stage III amongst HIV-positive populations. Whilst pneumonia can occur at any stage of HIV, it tends to be more common in stages III and IV as the patient's CD4 count tends to be lower. Bacteraemia can also be a feature of the pneumonia (Kaplan et al 2009). HIV-associated meningitis tends to be cryptococcal in nature. In the initial 3 months after contracting HIV-related meningitis, the mortality rate is as listed in the industrialised countries, 55% among low-income developing countries, and 70% in sub-Saharan Africa (Park et al 2009). Unexplained anaemia, neutropenia or thrombocytopenia in the presence of HIV indicates that clinical stage III has been reached.

HIV patients classified as having stage III of HIV infection either have one of the conditions listed above and/or a CD4+ T-lymphocyte count of 200–349.

Clinical stage IV – AIDS

The diagnosis of AIDS depends on an individual being diagnosed as HIV antibody positive, plus being diagnosed as having one of HIV wasting syndrome, life-threatening opportunistic infections or secondary cancers associated with clinical stage IV. HIV patients thus need to have one of the conditions listed below and/or a CD4+ T-lymphocyte count of less than 200 to be classified as having stage IV HIV infection.

Wasting syndrome

The appreciation of the importance of HIV wasting syndrome has arisen from the experience in Africa, where AIDS is called 'slim disease'. In the West, it is also increasingly recognised that some individuals become extremely ill, losing excessive amounts of weight, more than 10% body mass, and suffering from morbid weakness and loss of function. In the USA, 19% of adults with AIDS are diagnosed as having HIV wasting syndrome (Kirton 2003). The causes of HIV wasting syndrome may be mechanical or systemic. People lose weight if factors such as mouth ulcers and sickness deter them from eating. Malabsorption may also be seen and may be due to the presence of a lesion such as Kaposi's sarcoma in the gut or to a more generalised dysfunction. In all these cases the patient is starved of nutrients.

Wasting may also occur as a result of metabolic changes. As in cancerous conditions, the body may go from its normal balance of catabolism and anabolism into a catabolic crisis in which body mass is 'burnt up' at an increased and dangerous rate, often causing irreparable damage. These patients may recover some weight but they often do not recover muscle mass (Stine 2000, Shaw & Mahoney 2003). Supervised nutritional rehabilitation is therefore necessary. This may include nutritional supplements and more invasive therapy such as continuous or intermittent parenteral feeding. However, it is important to remember that nurses can play a life-saving role in the attention given to the ordinary nutritional service to the patient.

Opportunistic infections

Opportunistic infections may be protozoal, fungal, bacterial or viral.

Protozoal infections **Cryptosporidiosis** is a protozoal infection that has achieved some notoriety because of the sometimes devastating diarrhoea it causes. It is also because high levels of the organism in the general water supply are often reported in the news. The protozoon is normally present in small quantities in the water supply. In immunocompromised patients it multiplies within the gastrointestinal tract and causes diarrhoea. The loss of fluid can be as much as 10–20 L/day although less virulent attacks are also seen.

Cryptosporidiosis is generally seen only in patients who are already very ill and have suffered other infections. It is very difficult to manage this condition at home, as intravenous fluid replacement and constant bowel movements will need attention. For the patient, this condition may mean an extremely poor state of health and hospitalisation. In its worst form, it is an extremely distressing condition for both the patient and carers. There is no specific curative therapy for this infection but highly active antiretroviral therapy is associated with clinical improvement. Treatment with antidiarrhoeals, oral or intravenous rehydration and nutritional support will be required.

The causative protozoon of **toxoplasmosis** is sometimes present in cat faeces and in raw meat. Pregnant women who are HIV negative are vulnerable to this protozoon, although it does not generally manifest itself as a disease in healthy people. Its most common manifestation is cerebral toxoplasmosis. The organism causes space-occupying lesions in the brain. These create cerebral oedema and raised intracranial pressure. In the HIV-positive patient the observant nurse might notice subtle changes in the patient's cognitive function and personality, coupled with pyrexia, before the onset of more severe symptoms which include paralysis and unconsciousness. Toxoplasmosis is often fatal and treatment must be prolonged as relapses are almost inevitable. The main medication is co-trimoxazole, or dapsone with pyrimethamine. In the most serious cases constant nursing attention is needed as the patient's condition may deteriorate rapidly (Stine 2000, Adler 2001, Pratt 2003).

Fungal infections **Pneumocystosis or PCP** is the major fungal infection associated with HIV and AIDS. Once thought to be protozoal in nature and caused by *Pneumocystis carinii*, PCP is now known to be a fungal infection and the causative organism is referred to as *Pneumocystis jiroveci*. Although PCP was once one of the most common causes of death in AIDS, the organism responsible can be found, quite normally, in most humans. However, in health, the immune system keeps the population of the organism at an acceptable level. When the immune system is compromised, the level rises and causes severe, life-threatening pneumonia. PCP remains the most common opportunistic infection in patients with AIDS (Fujii et al 2007). Because the vast majority of people diagnosed as having AIDS have been unaware of their HIV status, many people who have contracted PCP

for the first time present not to specialist units but to emergency departments, GPs and other non-specialist areas.

The individual usually presents with a 2–5 week history of increasing shortness of breath, weakness and dry cough; cyanosis is often seen (Stine 2000, Adler 2001, Pratt 2003). A variety of drugs are used in the treatment of PCP: co-trimoxazole for mild to moderate episodes and aerosolised pentamidine isethionate for moderate to severe episodes. Pentamidine can be used either as a treatment for existing infection or as prophylaxis against further episodes.

Candidiasis is sometimes seen in virulent manifestations in people with advanced HIV illness (Box 35.7). To be indicative of clinical stage IV, candidiasis should be present in the oesophagus, trachea, bronchus or lungs. Infection may extend from the mouth to the alimentary tract.

Cryptococcosis is a systemic fungal condition. Treatment is with amphotericin and fluconazole. Two others are **histoplasmosis**, which affects the lungs, liver and gastrointestinal tract, and **coccidioidomycosis**, which affects any organ, including the brain (Pratt 2003).

Viral infections **Herpes simplex virus** has been mentioned in association with early phases of HIV, where it occurs in its less virulent forms. Serious and life-threatening forms, e.g. encephalitis, are sometimes seen, affecting the central nervous system (Pratt 2003). Aciclovir is used in treatment.

Cytomegalovirus (CMV) is encountered in general practice and in midwifery, where it is known to cause spontaneous abortion. In HIV-related illness it is most commonly seen causing damage to the retina, which appears as if molten cheese has fallen on its surface, hence the term 'pizza-pie retinopathy'. Deterioration of sight is rapid and blindness can occur in the space of a few days. Treatment with intravenous ganciclovir, foscarnet sodium or cidofovir is given (Kedhar & Jabs 2007). Treatment may be given in the hospital setting, but increasingly is given at home. Improvement is seen with treatment but relapse occurs in almost all cases. In recent years, intra-ocular medication in the form of tiny slow-release capsules of ganciclovir is implanted directly onto the inner surface of the eyeball.

Progressive multifocal leucoencephalopathy (PML) is an unusual disease caused by JC virus, a type of papovavirus, and results in demyelination of the nerve pathways. Conditions most likely to be seen are blindness, hemiparesis, ataxia and aphasia (Adler 2001). Antiretroviral therapy with

Box 35.7 Reflection

The psychological impact of 'minor' opportunistic infections

A patient contracted two serious bouts of PCP over a period of 2 years. He had borne these very well. However, he became severely depressed some time later when he was back at work. Having contracted oral thrush, he could not swallow properly and was losing weight. This made him feel powerless and he said it was worse than the 'serious' illnesses. Such examples serve to remind the practitioner that the seriousness of a condition cannot be judged strictly by clinical criteria. Moreover, by taking notice of even the smallest signs and taking action, nurses can help many patients remain alive. Many HIV-related conditions, if diagnosed early, respond well to treatment.

zidovudine-containing regimens may provide temporary improvement in this late-stage, crippling condition (Pratt 2003).

Bacterial infections As indicated when discussing clinical stage III HIV, **tuberculosis** is one of the main indicators of advanced HIV disease. If the TB is extrapulmonary in nature, it is indicative of clinical stage IV or the presence of AIDS.

Salmonellosis poses a particular danger to people with HIV. Scrupulous care should be taken in food preparation and delivery. Patients should avoid undercooking foods such as eggs and poultry. Hand hygiene is also important (see Ch. 16). Treatment is with chloramphenicol, ampicillin or amoxicillin.

People in advanced stages of HIV illness are sometimes found to have atypical mycobacteria – *Mycobacterium avium* **complex** (MAC) – in their lungs. Infection with MAC has become less common since the widespread use of combination antiretroviral therapy (HAART; see p. 904).

Secondary cancers

The immune system has the function not only of fighting infection, but also of fighting and inhibiting malignant cells. The following two forms of cancer are associated with HIV and an AIDS diagnosis.

Kaposi's sarcoma (KS) This purplish skin cancer was previously seen only in older men of certain ethnic origins, e.g. some Jewish men of Eastern European origin. Classically KS, in the era before HIV, was a slow-growing tumour usually restricted to the feet and shins (Vano-Galvan & Alonso-Jimenez 2007). With the advent of AIDS in the Western world, it was one of the first manifestations of the condition. Unlike KS prior to HIV, the tumours in the presence of HIV tend to be relatively aggressive, widely disseminated and life threatening (Schwartz et al 2008). As with opportunistic infections, it is not seen in all patients. As a skin condition it is very disfiguring, particularly when on the face. If it remains in small patches, treatment is often confined to cosmetic camouflage. However, it sometimes forms constricting bands on the skin, e.g. around the ankle. Internally, it may also lead to gastrointestinal obstruction and it is sometimes found in the lungs and other internal organs. Patients with visceral or advanced KS are treated with radiotherapy or systemic chemotherapy. With widespread adoption of safer sex practices and the introduction of HAART, the incidence of KS has declined dramatically (Adler 2001).

Non-Hodgkin's lymphomas (B-cell lymphomas, undifferentiated lymphomas) These are seen in much higher numbers among people with AIDS than in the general population. They are found in the central nervous system, the bone marrow and the gastrointestinal tract. They are often rapidly fatal and treatment is often not successful.

Neurological disease

HIV encephalopathy HIV neurological disease is not an opportunistic infection. It is the human immunodeficiency virus directly affecting the central nervous system, including the covering of the brain. It may manifest early on as peripheral neuropathy, in its many forms, and later progress to affect the individual's personality and lucidity. Eventually the person may suffer dementia. One of the problems in diagnosing this condition is that changes in computed tomograms (CT scans) do not necessarily accompany changes in behaviour; it is possible for a patient with a normal CT to experience dementia.

Acute viral encephalitis can occur in late symptomatic HIV disease caused by reactivation of latent cytomegalovirus (CMV) or herpes simplex virus (HSV) infection.

Nursing care of the various conditions associated with neurological disease and encephalopathy is often challenging in terms of both short- and long-term care. Remissions can occur but there can be periods of despair for the individual. On a more optimistic note, however, HIV neurological disease does appear to respond well to antiviral therapy. Many patients show a marked improvement as well as a slowing down of the advancement of the disease.

 ## Nursing management and health promotion: HIV/AIDS

At present there is no effective vaccine against AIDS. Vaccines have proved exceptionally difficult to develop as the virus has several different subtypes and tends towards mutation and change when replicating, even within an individual. Although there are various treatments that ameliorate the effects of viruses, there has never been anything in the nature of a cure. Efforts have concentrated on reducing the level of viral replication, preventing opportunistic infections and symptom control.

Antiretroviral therapy

For a medication regimen to be considered successful, the viral load of HIV within the patient's bloodstream must be undetectable after 6 months of treatment. In addition, a boost in the patient's CD4 count is advantageous. If a patient is taking antiviral medication, regular monitoring will be required of both the patient's viral load and immune system. The overall aim of care is to improve the patient's quality of life. There is thus a similarity between AIDS nursing and oncology and palliative care. At the beginning of the epidemic, the life expectancy of someone diagnosed as having AIDS ranged from a few weeks to 2 years. Patients receiving care, particularly those in affluent countries, can now live for 10 years or more. However, when compared with other life-threatening conditions such as cancer or diabetes mellitus, which similarly depend on symptomatic control but for which there is a much longer life expectancy, it becomes apparent that the care of HIV-related illness continues to be in a developing stage.

Treatment compliance

Treatment compliance is an important area of concern in HIV nursing. HIV treatment requires a strict schedule of medication at the correct time in order to ensure therapeutic levels. If the patient is unable to adhere to a medication regimen, the chance of their achieving a low viral load of HIV is reduced. The patient has to take a large variety of medications, often strictly to time and with consequent restrictions to their lifestyle. The nurse has to ensure patient compliance with often complex medication regimens. Much effort is expended in gaining patient concordance, rather than merely promoting adherence, actively involving the patient in helping to tailor their particular regimen to one that best matches their lifestyle, to maximise chances of compliance. Nurse-led clinics are now an important source of support, particularly around the time of starting HAART.

If patients do not adhere to their medication regimen, it allows the HIV within their bodies to build resistance to their current drugs, which is a major obstacle to successful treatment. HIV evolving resistance to medication is an ongoing problem, even when patients do comply with treatment. This is because HIV is a mutating virus. When exposed to medication, eventually only the sturdiest strains of HIV survive within the body, becoming the dominant strains within an individual. When this occurs, the patient's immune system will begin to deteriorate and require a change in HAART regimen.

Highly active antiretroviral therapy (HAART)

Since the mid 1990s, antiretroviral treatment has developed significantly, reducing HIV-related morbidity and mortality. The prognosis for people living with HIV improved markedly after the introduction of combination therapy involving the use of more than one antiviral medication to combat HIV. HAART takes the use of combination therapy further, normally involving a combination of three, four or five medications. Occasionally six medications may be given in 'salvage' therapy where a patient's treatment appears to be failing.

Treatment aims to reduce the plasma HIV RNA level, i.e. the viral load of HIV circulating in the patient's bloodstream. These medications target two specific viral enzymes necessary for HIV replication: reverse transcriptase and protease. In addition, the first experimental integrase inhibitors, which prevent the viral DNA copy from joining with a target cell's genome, are being trialled. Currently, fusion inhibitors that prevent HIV attaching to receptor sites on the surface of targeted host cells are being preserved for salvage therapy (Rockstroh & Mauss 2004) (Box 35.8).

The treatment of HIV is a rapidly changing field and readers are recommended to regularly consult the British HIV Association (BHIVA) treatment guidelines (http://www.bashh.org). Gazzard (2008) has collated the latest UK guidelines.

Side-effects associated with HAART A range of serious side-effects is associated with these medications, and adherence to HAART is a major issue. Adverse effects include kidney and liver toxicity, hyperglycaemia, raised plasma levels of triglycerides and cholesterol, lipodystrophy, hypersensitivity reactions and peripheral neuropathy. As the commitment to HAART is for life, GPs and practice nurses in particular have an important role in supporting patients in adhering to these challenging medication regimens. There have been advances to improve the pill burden, and once-daily regimens are now popular. Antiretroviral medications are also extremely expensive and ways of reducing costs are being explored. For further information on side-effects and adherence to antiretroviral therapy see Loveday (2003).

HIV care used to be delivered almost exclusively in the hospital inpatient setting. This was an expensive, labour-intensive and often arguably a 'patient unfriendly' option

Box 35.8 Information

Overview of highly active antiretroviral therapy (HAART)

A typical HAART regimen would include two nucleoside reverse transcriptase inhibitors (NRTIs) in combination with either a protease inhibitor (PI) or a non-nucleoside reverse transcriptase inhibitor (NNRTI).

Nucleoside reverse transcriptase inhibitors (NRTIs)

This group of drugs forms the backbone of HAART regimens. Two NRTIs are usually given in combination. These work by blocking viral replication within a CD4 (T helper) cell. The virus has to convert its own material into DNA by using the enzyme reverse transcriptase to make blueprints for further replication. NRTIs block the action of reverse transcriptase.

Non-nucleoside reverse transcriptase inhibitors (NNRTIs)

This group of drugs also blocks the action of the reverse transcriptase enzyme, thus stalling viral replication.

Nucleotide reverse transcriptase inhibitors (NtRTIs)

These work in the same way as NRTIs but have an extra phosphate attached to the drug molecule, which tends to make them more long acting.

Protease inhibitors (PIs)

Protease is an enzyme used by HIV to break up the long chains of proteins manufactured within infected cells. Protease inhibitors work by blocking this enzyme from cutting protein chains and thus preventing new copies of HIV being formed ready to infect other cells.

Fusion inhibitors

This group of drugs works by blocking HIV access to the cell, attacking the mechanism whereby the HIV can 'dock' to the cell wall, thus preventing replication.

as individuals would spend many days or weeks in hospital per year. The advent of HAART has transformed this pattern of care. HAART, although expensive, is cost effective as it delays the onset of the advanced stages of HIV disease (AIDS) for which care is very expensive (Adler 2003). The hospital setting is still used for seriously ill patients. However, day care units are now used extensively and often have flexible hours to facilitate patients' work commitments. Day care units and outpatient departments are used as places of treatment, monitoring, counselling and group work as well as traditional consultation.

Testing and screening

Given the fact that HIV can represent a 'silent infection', the timing of HIV screening is vital. HIV testing normally involves searching for the presence of HIV antibodies in a patient's blood. Testing for the actual virus, i.e. testing for HIV core antigen, particles of the virus, is used for clinical prognosis and management, not generally for diagnostic purposes. Blood samples are used at present for all forms of testing, although urine and saliva tests are being developed, especially for use in screening.

The term 'screening' is generally used, in the context of HIV, to refer to the process by which blood samples undergo laboratory analysis by enzyme-linked immunosorbent assay (ELISA). This procedure is carried out on several samples from different patients at once and is used to determine the prevalence of HIV antibodies in a batch of samples. While ELISA is an efficient method of mass screening it is far from satisfactory for testing an individual, for whom a false-positive result would be devastating. Therefore, in individual testing, the sample first undergoes ELISA and then immuno-blotting or the Western blotting method, accurate to within thousandths of 1%, to confirm the diagnosis. This method is more complex and is available only in sophisticated laboratories. In poorer countries, samples may undergo repeated ELISA procedures instead of Western blotting to achieve maximal accuracy in difficult circumstances.

Timing

Generally, HIV antibodies are produced between 3 weeks and 3 months after the individual becomes infected with HIV. The timing of a diagnostic test is important. Individuals who have a test that proves negative are often advised to come back for a repeat test. Because of this uncertainty and the personal impact of a positive result, there has been much recent controversy as to whether or not HIV antibody testing should take place only with pre- and post-test counselling. The accepted approach has been voluntary testing with pre- and post-test counselling. This occurs when an individual seeks a test following a specific high-risk activity or contact, or when the individual, for reasons of their own, wants to know their HIV status. It is available at genitourinary clinics and HIV units, and from some GPs and other community practitioners. People found to be positive are, with their consent, referred to medical/nursing services. It has been accepted that this form of testing is the most acceptable, both practically and ethically. However, as the treatment for HIV has improved, there has been a groundswell of support for the notion that testing should be 'normalised', performed on a wider basis without formal pre-test counselling, except for those cases where the individual to be tested has engaged in high-risk sexual activity (Manavi & Welsby 2005).

Counselling

Nurses are often expected to give pre- and post-test counselling and it is essential that nurses have these skills. Counselling in other clinical areas, especially oncology, genetics and palliative care, can provide very good experience. The counsellor must have sound clinical knowledge, as unusual questions that are worrying the patient will often be encountered. Nurses are bound to uphold the rights of the individual, but they also have a duty towards the community. These obligations are not mutually exclusive but require that the issues are considered from every viewpoint. The professional bodies provide guidelines on many of the more contentious issues. It may be fair to say, however, that nurses should generally 'err' on the side of the individual patient, for the nurse is sometimes their only advocate (Nursing and Midwifery Council 2003b).

Nurses have an extremely important role in HIV. Partner notification work, for example, requires a sensitive and expert approach. Given the limitations of mass communications in influencing behaviour, nurses must take every opportunity to make general messages relevant to the patients in their care. Nurses have always been involved in assisting patients to understand their treatment, and in answering their questions in terms that can be understood. In doing so, they require sound clinical knowledge together with an understanding of the patient's needs, lifestyle and expectations, as obtained from the nursing assessment. It is important to consider HIV in relation to the full range of services available to the (typically young) person living with HIV, particularly in the light of innovations in medication in the mid 1990s and the longer life expectancy.

Diarrhoea

Diarrhoea is one of the most common conditions associated with untreated HIV. It can be caused by a wide range of bacterial and viral infections as well as gut parasites. If a patient is on HAART there is less chance that they will have diarrhoea-causing gut pathogens. However, the treatment itself can cause diarrhoea, in particular if patients are taking protease inhibitors. In addition, some patients on HAART continue to have diarrhoea with no known aetiology which is difficult to prevent (Salminen et al 2004). Nursing interventions for the patient with HIV and diarrhoea are the same for any patient, to assist with hygiene needs whilst maintaining dignity and promoting independence. Immediate monitoring of hydration and nutrition should start with the help of a dietitian whilst stool specimens should be taken to exclude a treatable infection or infestation.

Weight loss

Weight loss is a feature of the HIV-related continuum from clinical stage II onwards (WHO 2007) into advanced HIV disease, clinical stages III and IV (Siddiqui et al 2009). Measurements of muscle and fat loss should be included in the care programme. Eating patterns should be discussed along with ways of increasing intake, e.g. taking frequent, smaller meals and perhaps supplementary feeds such as Ensure. Fluid and electrolyte replacement is essential. Codeine phosphate, loperamide hydrochloride and diphenoxylate hydrochloride may be useful, but it is emphasised that medication should always be given in combination with dietary monitoring and therapy.

Herpes

Herpes simplex is prevalent amongst people living with HIV, 70–90% of whom have contracted the infection (Malkin 2004). It is important to offer appropriate prophylactic antiviral therapy such as aciclovir, not only to alleviate but to prevent symptoms. It is important to understand that both clinical and subclinical episodes of herpes simplex appear to increase the rate of HIV replication through mechanisms not fully understood, whilst the ulceration associated with herpes makes HIV transmission more likely during sexual intercourse (Nagot et al 2008).

In the case of herpes zoster there are no prophylactic medications available. More common in HIV-positive people, herpes zoster mostly affects the back, chest and face, usually on one side of the body. Ensuring that the patient receives adequate analgesia is probably the most important nursing intervention. Mouth and lip care are important to prevent cracking and secondary infection. Soothing lotions and loose clothing may be appropriate for attacks of shingles. Sleep, fluid intake and diet should be monitored.

Dermatitis

Seborrhoeic dermatitis is associated with advanced HIV and is thought to be caused by the overgrowth of *Malassezia* species of fungus in those parts of the body rich in sebaceous glands (Schwartz et al 2007). These include the trunk, upper back and head. Nursing interventions focus on assisting with the application of topical skin preparations. Salicylic acid and tar-based lotions are used. Low-dose steroids and steroid/antibiotic/antifungal combinations, e.g. clobetasone butyrate (Trimovate), are sometimes used for short periods. The antifungal azoles may also be used locally where they are particularly useful, combining both antifungal and anti-inflammatory properties. Responding to the individual patient's discomfort is important; in the case of HIV-positive individuals the seborrhoeic lesions are often inflamed and weepy. Giving attention to small details in order to alleviate the irritation of skin conditions is one of the most appreciated of nursing services.

In the case of tinea pedis, miconazole and clotrimazole creams are used topically. Systemic griseofulvin or, more recently, either oral terbinafine or itraconazole is used if the infection is persistent (Elewski & Tavakkol 2005). Keeping the feet dry and comfortable can be helped by such measures as drying with a cool hair dryer and leaving the end of the bed covers loose.

Oral care

Oral candidiasis is associated with HIV infection. Nystatin antifungal topical drops may be used. However, oral thrush is often persistent in HIV illness, in which case systemic fluconazole is used. Mouth care is vital, as is a high fluid intake. Hypo-salivation is associated with Candida in HIV-infected individuals, and regular saline mouthwashes are thought to help with mechanical cleaning and help to prevent Candida adhering to the surface of the mucosa (Oji & Chukwuneke 2008). Some patients find mouth rinsing with benzydamine hydrochloride, which has anaesthetic properties, helpful. Others rinse with fizzy water or diet cola to relieve discomfort, a valued practice that is not yet supported by research evidence.

After Candida, oral hairy leucoplakia is the most common opportunistic infection associated with HIV. It is caused by Epstein–Barr virus and can be treated with regular mouth care and the application of podophyllin or aciclovir cream (Moura et al 2007).

Male circumcision

In recent years there has been a significant development in the field of HIV prevention and health promotion that does not involve antiviral drugs. In December 2006, new evidence from clinical trials demonstrated that male circumcision reduced the chances of HIV transmission by 50% (Gray et al 2007). Those nurses working in developing areas where antiretrovirals are difficult or impossible to obtain might find themselves advocating the practice of male clinical circumcision.

Social impact of HIV and AIDS

HIV has an enormous social impact on both the individual and carers. In order to provide the best possible care, it is essential to have an integrated, multidisciplinary service that addresses social as well as clinical concerns, particularly in discharge planning and follow-up (Pratt 2003). Creating an environment that enables an effective but confidential service is difficult, especially as more agencies become involved in care. More people are able to stay well for longer although, despite some remarkable survival stories, the long-term efficacy of combination therapy is unknown (Stine 2000). The move to establish combination therapy in poor and developing countries magnifies these challenges considerably (Lo & Bayer 2003, Mandela 2003, WHO 2003a).

🖱 **See website Critical thinking question 35.1**

The problems the patient experiences, as a stigmatised member of society, demand that nurses who seek to help are very clear about their own attitudes and professional philosophy. Central to any philosophy of nursing practice is the patient's right to 'quality health care in an atmosphere of human dignity without regard to age, ethnic or national origin, sex or sexual orientation, religion or presenting illness' (Pratt 2003). Coupled with this is the duty of nurses to look after all patients.

If one compares HIV therapy with another long-term disease and treatment, e.g. diabetes mellitus and insulin, where many individuals being treated from a young age may expect to live a fully functional life with normal longevity, the situation with HIV is still uncertain, especially as other factors, such as virus mutation with new disease patterns, manifest themselves (Shaw & Mahoney 2003). These patterns include drug resistance. Statistics from the HPA (2008b) show the cumulative total of cases reported for HIV and AIDS in the UK. Although the greatest proportion of people affected has been homosexual men, the most rapid increase is among heterosexuals. In the UK, heterosexual transmission outstripped homosexual transmission in 2004.

Political and social implications of HIV

Like other infectious diseases that have reached epidemic or pandemic proportions, HIV/AIDS has given rise to a great deal of fear and stigmatisation. In formulating health and social policies in response to AIDS, governments have a duty not only to safeguard the health and well-being of their populations as a whole, but also to protect the rights of those individuals affected by the disease.

The most intractable problem presented by HIV to policy makers is the length of time it takes for the disease to manifest itself after an individual becomes infected. This has the following profound epidemiological implications:

- Most people who are infected are not aware of it until they become ill.
- The government figures published regularly related to people with AIDS do not reflect the prevalence of HIV at that moment.

It is more difficult to gauge specifically who is at risk, although some 'high-risk' activities can be identified, e.g. intravenous drug use and unprotected sexual intercourse (Box 35.9).

Box 35.9 Reflection

HIV screening: opt-in or opt-out system?

In the industrially developed countries with easy access to HAART there has been much discussion about a switch from an opt-in system for HIV testing to an opt-out system. In the latter system, HIV screening would be done routinely in primary care and no longer primarily the remit of specialised services such as sexual health clinics. The aim is to achieve a greater uptake of screening and consequently earlier identification of HIV-positive individuals and, as a result, optimal treatment (Bartlett et al 2008). Newly emerging technology will allow rapid saliva-based HIV tests to be offered within primary care settings (Prost et al 2009). Less invasive than traditional blood-based testing and with results available in minutes, this will help normalise HIV screening.

Opt-out testing will both increase take-up of HIV screening and will help reduce associated stigma (Young et al 2009). Currently HIV screening tends to be opt-in and normally involves pre-test counselling. The opt-out system, with its larger number of patients being screened, makes it more difficult to identify and prioritise those patients who have been involved in high-risk activities and who require appropriate pre-test counselling. What happens if people who are at high risk of HIV are given a positive result without adequate, prior preparation? The question remains – even given the fact that our treatment regimens are becoming more effective, we still do not have a cure for HIV and the diagnosis is still associated with stigma.

Activity

• Given the advantages and disadvantages of normalising HIV screening, what do you think is the best option? Which form of testing would *you* opt for?

Health promotion

Health education and promotion are absolutely vital in combatting the spread of HIV. These general aims must be responsive to the physical, mental, emotional, spiritual and societal needs of the individual (Ewles & Simnett 2003). Health promotion in HIV/AIDS entails more than raising general public awareness through mass media campaigns. It can also involve such activities as providing assertiveness training for individuals affected and helping them to learn self-care and nurturing skills. HIV awareness also has implications for the workplace, raising concerns about working practice and hiring policies. Legal and ethical issues must also be grappled with by nurses working with people who are involved in illicit drug use and prostitution and who consequently face particular difficulties.

Nurses need to take great care when targetting people for health promotion interventions. There are no high-risk groups, only high-risk activities. A gay man, for example, is not at risk if he refrains from unprotected sexual intercourse. An intravenous drug user who does not share injecting equipment or practise unprotected penetrative sex is also not at risk from HIV. Health educators, however, are aware that certain groups have particular behaviour patterns in common. It makes sense, therefore, to target these groups with certain services and messages, always remembering that general patterns will not fully reflect the complexity of individuals.

One of the nurse's greatest advantages as a health educator lies in the opportunities to be with the patient for long periods of time in a position of trust. Nurses are particularly good at building and maintaining a therapeutic relationship with their patients (Sheldon 2008). Nevertheless, the nurse may still experience difficulty in discussing sexual matters and sexuality with patients. Public campaigns are restricted by legislation and 'public taste', and it may be left to the nurse to provide more explicit information.

Personal value judgements, embarrassment and questions of status may present obstacles. Answering questions on, for example, oral sex from a person of a different sexual persuasion to oneself may be difficult. Speaking to an underage person who is sexually active may be embarrassing and raise ethical questions. Many practitioners become expert at putting up verbal and non-verbal barriers so that such discussions are avoided. However, caring must be unconditional, answering to the patient's needs regardless of the nurse's personal values. By appreciating that HIV/AIDS is a clinical and a socio-political issue, nurses will be better able to develop a knowledgeable and empathetic mode of practice with people living with HIV.

Nurses are increasingly becoming involved in working with small groups, particularly in the community. By doing so, the nurse can make health education messages personally relevant. For further information on the formal and informal intricacies of setting up groups, agendas and action plans see Ewles & Simnett (2003).

SUMMARY: KEY NURSING ISSUES

• HIV and other sexually transmitted infections continue to be a major and growing worldwide problem. For HIV the situation has been further compounded by the emergence of widespread drug-resistant tuberculosis which, in cases of co-infection with HIV, increases patient morbidity.

• The nursing care of people with SAIs and HIV has seen a real growth in innovative practice. Working with drug users, prisoners, commercial sex workers and other marginalised people has meant that nurses are increasingly working in non-traditional areas, using new procedures.

• People with HIV may present with seemingly minor problems that cannot always be diagnosed or predicted. For example, an individual may suffer weight loss, difficulty in swallowing, anorexia, night sweats, lethargy, mouth ulcers, diarrhoea and/or constipation. In addition to this, they may become depressed and desperate, as such conditions, even if not life threatening, can be very distressing.

• Non-judgmental attitudes are essential. If people with sexually acquired infections are subject to prejudicial and punitive interaction with health care professionals, they will be reluctant to attend sexual health clinics. Consequently fewer people will obtain treatment and the cycle of infection and re-infection will become well established and difficult to break.

• Nurses specialising in HIV and SAIs have an extended role in health education and promotion. Nurses play an important role in ensuring their patients understand the need for treatment, for partner notification and for safer sex in order to break the cycle of infection and re-infection. Considerable effort has to be spent in engaging patients and ensuring treatment concordance.

- In the industrialised West, although a vaccine has proved elusive, treatment regimens mean that HIV has become a chronic illness rather than an inevitable death sentence. However, this situation needs to be emulated in the developing world, which with its inadequate resources and medical infrastructure bears the burden of the majority of cases of HIV.

→ REFLECTION AND LEARNING – WHAT NEXT?

- **Test** your knowledge by visiting the website 🖱 and answering the multiple choice questions and critical thinking questions.

- **Consolidate** your learning by looking at some of the further reading suggestions, references and specialist websites.

- **Revisit** some of the additional material on the website.

- **Consider** what you have learnt and how this will help your professional development.

- **Reflect** on how you can apply this knowledge to the care of your patients.

- **Discuss** your learning with your mentor/supervisor, lecturer and colleagues.

REFERENCES

Adler M: *ABC of AIDS*, ed 5, London, 2001, BMJ Publications.

Adler M: Sexual health – Report finds sexual health service to be a shambles [editorial], *Br Med J* 327:62–63, 2003.

Adu-Sarkodie Y, Opoku B, Danso K, et al: Comparison of latex agglutination, wet preparation, and culture for the detection of Trichomonas vaginalis, *Sex Transm Infect* 80:201–203, 2004.

Antoszewski B, Sitek A, Jedrzejczak M, et al: Are body piercing and tattooing safe fashions? *Eur J Dermatol* 16:572–575, 2006.

Armstrong ML: Body piercing: a clinical look, *Office Nurse* 11(3):26–29, 1998.

Barousse M, Van Der Pol B, Fortenberry D, et al: Vaginal yeast colonisation, prevalence of vaginitis, and associated local immunity in adolescents, *Sex Transm Infect* 80:48–53, 2004.

Bartlett J, Branson B, Fenton K, et al: Opt-out testing for human immunodeficiency virus in the United States, *J Am Med Assoc* 300(8): 945–951, 2008.

Bizuwork T, Makombe S, Kamoto K, et al: WHO Stage 3 disease conditions and outcomes in patients started on anti-retroviral therapy in Malawi, *The Journal of Infection in Developing Countries* 1(2):118–122, 2007.

Bossert T, Battellini R, Kotowicz V, et al: Ruptured giant syphilitic aneurysm of the descending aorta in an octogenarian, *J Card Surg* 19(4):356–357, 2004.

British Association for Sexual Health and HIV Clinical Effectiveness Group (BASHH): *National Guideline on the Diagnosis and Treatment of Gonorrhoea in Adults 2005*, London, 2005, BASHH.

Brooker C, Nicol M: *Nursing Adults. The Practice of Caring*, London, 2003, Mosby.

Buchacz K, Patel P, Taylor M, et al: Syphilis increases HIV viral load and decreases CD4 cell counts in HIV-infected patients with new syphilis infections, *AIDS* 18(15):2075–2079, 2004.

Cahn P, Perez H, Ben G, et al: Tuberculosis and HIV: A partnership against the most vulnerable, *J Int Assoc Physicians AIDS Care* 2(3):106–123, 2003.

Calmy A, Ford N, Hirschel B, et al: HIV viral load monitoring in resource-limited regions: optional or necessary? *Clin Infect Dis* 44:128–134, 2007.

Centers for Disease Control and Prevention (CDC): A report by Council of State and Territorial Epidemiologists; AIDS Program, Centre for Infectious Diseases, *MMWR* (Suppl 36):1–15, 1987.

Centers for Disease Control and Prevention (CDC): 1993 Revised classification system for HIV infection and expanded surveillance definition for AIDS among adolescents and adults, *MMWR* 41:1–19, 1992.

Centers for Disease Control and Prevention (CDC): Comparison of the revised World Health Organization and CDC surveillance case definitions and staging systems for HIV infection, *MMWR appendix B* 57(Recommendations and Reports 10):10–11, 2008.

Chosidow O: Scabies, *N Engl J Med* 354:1718–18127, 2006.

Clutterbuck F: Genitourinary medicine clinic and general practitioner contact: what do patients want? *Sex Transm Infect* 84:67–69, 2008.

Cooper R, Reid P: Sexually transmitted disease/HIV health-care policy and service provision in Britain, *Int J STD AIDS* 18(10):655–661, 2007.

De Cock KM, Fowler MG, Mercier E: Prevention of mother-to-child HIV transmission in resource poor countries: translating research into policy and practice, *J Am Med Assoc* 283(9):1175–1182, 2000.

Elewski B, Tavakkol: Safety and tolerability of oral antifungal agents in the treatment of fungal nail disease: a proven reality, *Therapeutics and Clinical Risk Management* 1(4):299–306, 2005.

Ewles L, Simnett I: *Promoting health: a practical guide*, ed 5, Edinburgh, 2003, Baillière Tindall.

Fang C, Chang Y, Hsu H, et al: Life expectancy of patients with newly-diagnosed HIV infection in the era of highly active antiretroviral therapy, *QJM* 100:97–105, 2007.

Fenton K, Korovessis C, Johnson A, et al: Sexual behaviour in Britain: sexually transmitted infections and prevalent Chlamydia trachomatis infection, *Lancet* 358:1851–1854, 2001.

Franco E, Harper D: Vaccination against human papillomavirus infection: a new paradigm in cervical cancer control, *Vaccine* 23(17–18): 2388–2394, 2005.

Freeman E, Weiss H, Glynn J, et al: Herpes simplex virus 2 infection increases HIV acquisition in men and women: systematic review and meta-analysis of longitudinal studies, *AIDS* 20(1):73–83, 2006.

French P: BASHH 2006 National Guidelines – consultations requiring sexual history-taking, *Int J STD AIDS* 18:17–22, 2007.

Fujii T, Nakamura T, Iwamoto A: Pneumocystis pneumonia in patients with HIV infection: clinical manifestations, laboratory findings and radiological features, *J Infect Chemother* 13(1):1–7, 2007.

Gazzard B: British HIV Association guidelines for the treatment of HIV-1-infected adults with antiretroviral therapy 2008, *HIV Med* 9:563–608, 2008.

Goh B: Syphilis in adults, *Sex Transm Infect* 81:448–452, 2005.

Gray R, Kigozi G, Serwadda D, et al: Male circumcision for HIV prevention in men in Rakai, Uganda: a randomised trial, *The Lancet* 369:657–666, 2007.

Grossman Z, Meir-Schellersheim M, Paul W, et al: Pathogenesis of HIV infection: what the virus spares is as important as what it destroys, *Nat Med* 12(3):289–295, 2006.

Gupta G, Parkhurst J, Ogden J, et al: Structural approaches to HIV prevention, *Lancet* 372:764–775, 2008.

Hawkins D: Oral sex and HIV transmission, *Sex Transm Infect* 77:307–308, 2001.

Health Protection Agency, Centre for Infections, National Public Health Service for Wales, CDSC Northern Ireland and Health Protection Scotland Eye of the needle: *United Kingdom surveillance of significant occupational exposures to bloodborne viruses in healthcare workers*, London, 2008a, HPA.

Health Protection Agency: *HIV in the United Kingdom 2008 Report*, London, 2008b, HPA. Available online http://www.hpa.org.uk/web/HPAwebFile/HPAweb_C/1227515298354.

Health Protection Agency: *Genital Chlamydia*, London, 2009, HPA. Available online http://www.hpa.org.uk/webw/HPAweb&Page&HPAwebAutoListName/Page/1191942172070?p=1191942172070.

Hollingsworth T, Anderson R, Fraser C: HIV-1 Transmission by stage of infection, *J Infect Dis* 198:687–693, 2008.

Jagger J: Caring for healthcare workers: a global perspective, *Infect Control Hosp Epidemiol* 28(1):1–4, 2007.

Jeffries DJ: Occupational exposure and treatment options, *Journal of HIV Combination Therapy* 2(3):44, 1997.

Jit M, Choi YH, Edmunds J: Economic evaluation of human papillomavirus vaccination in the United Kingdom, *Br Med J* 337:769, 2008.

Johnston G, Sladden M: Scabies: diagnosis and treatment, *Br Med J* 331:619–622, 2005.

Kaplan J, Benson C, Holmes K, et al: Guidelines for prevention and treatment of opportunistic infections in HIV-infected adults and adolescents, *MMWR* 58:1–206, 2009.

Keane F, Maw R, Pritchard C, et al: Methods employed by genitourinary medicine clinics in the United Kingdom to diagnose bacterial vaginosis, *Sex Transm Infect* 81:155–157, 2005.

Kedhar S, Jabs D: Cytomegalovirus retinitis in the era of highly active antiretroviral therapy. CMV and immune reconstitution on HAART, *HERPES* 14(3):66–71, 2007.

Kerani R, Handsfield H, Stenger M, et al: Rising rates of syphilis in the era of syphilis elimination, *Sex Transm Dis* 34(3):154–161, 2007.

Kirton C: *ANAC's core curriculum for HIV/AIDS nursing*, ed 2, Akron, OH, 2003, Association of Nurses in AIDS Care.

Klausner J, Hook E: *Current diagnosis and treatment of sexually transmitted diseases*, New York, 2007, McGraw-Hill Professional.

Kofoed K, Gerstoft J, Mathiesen L, et al: Syphilis and human immunodeficiency virus (HIV)-1 coinfection: Influence on CD4 T-cell count, HIV-1 viral load, and treatment response, *Sex Transm Dis* 33(3):143–148, 2006.

LaMontagne D, Fenton K, Randall S, et al: on behalf of the National Chlamydia Screening Steering Group: Establishing the National Chlamydia Screening Programme in England: results from the first full year of screening, *Sex Transm Infect* 80:335–341, 2004.

Lavanchy D: Hepatitis B virus epidemiology, disease burden, treatment, and current and emerging prevention and control measures, *J Viral Hepat* 11(2):97–107, 2004.

Livengood C: Bacterial vaginosis: an overview for 2009, *Obstet Gynecol* 2(1):28–37, 2009.

Lo B, Bayer R: Establishing ethical trials for treatment and prevention of AIDS in developing countries, *Br Med J* 327:337–339, 2003.

Loveday H: Adherence to antiretroviral therapy. In Pratt RJ, editor: *HIV and AIDS: a strategy for nursing care*, ed 6, London, 2003, Hodder-Arnold, Ch. 21.

Lynn W, Lightman L: Syphilis and HIV: a dangerous combination, *Lancet Infect Dis* 4(7):456–466, 2004.

Malkin J: Epidemiology of genital herpes simplex virus infection in developed countries, *Herpes* 11(Suppl 1):2A–23A, 2004.

Manavi K, Welsby PD: HIV testing should no longer be offered special status, *Br Med J* 330(7490):492–493, 2005.

Mandela N: *Conference speech*. London, 2003, The 2003 British Red Cross Humanity Lecture.

Moi H, Reinton N, Moghaddam A: Mycoplasma genitalium is associated with symptomatic and asymptomatic non-gonococcal urethritis in men, *Sex Transm Infect* 85:15–18, 2009.

McCarthy J, Kemp D, Walton S, et al: Scabies: more than an irritation, *Postgrad Med J* 80:328–387, 2004.

Moura M, Guimaraes T, Fonseca L, et al: A random clinical trial study to assess the efficiency of topical applications of podophyllin resin (25%) versus podophyllin resin (25%) together with acyclovir cream (5%) in the treatment of oral hairy leukoplakia, *Oral Surg Oral Med Oral Pathol Oral Radiol Endod* 103(1):64–71, 2007.

Nagot N, Ouedraoga A, Konate I, et al: Roles of clinical and subclinical reactivated herpes simplex virus type 2 infection and Human Immunodeficiency Virus type 1 (HIV-1) – induced immunosuppression on genital and plasma HIV-1 levels, *J Infect Dis* 298:241–249, 2008.

Newberry Y, Kelsey JJ: Mother to child transmission of HIV, *Journal of Pharmacy Practice* 16:182–190, 2003.

Nursing and Midwifery Council (NMC): *Anonymous testing for HIV*, London, 2003b, Register: Journal of the Nursing and Midwifery Council.

Oji C, Chukwuneke F: Evaluation and treatment of oral candidiasis in HIV/AIDS patients in Enugu, Nigeria, *J Oral Maxillofac Surg* 12:67–71, 2008.

O'Mahoney C: Genital warts: current and future treatment options, *Am J Clin Dermatol* 6(4):239–243, 2005.

Park B, Wannemuehler K, Marston B, et al: Estimation of the current global burden of cryptococcal meningitis among persons living with HIV/AIDS, *AIDS* 23(4):525–530, 2009.

Pound M, May D: Proposed mechanisms and preventative options of Jarisch–Herxheimer reactions, *J Clin Pharm Ther* 30(3):291–295, 2005.

Pratt R: *HIV and AIDS: a strategy for nursing care*, ed 6, London, 2003, Hodder Arnold.

Prost A, Griffiths C, Anderson J, et al: Feasibility and acceptability of offering rapid HIV tests to patients registering with primary care in London UK: a pilot study, *Sex Transm Infect* 85:326–329, 2009.

Raviglione M, Smith I: XDR Tuberculosis – implications for global public health, *N Engl J Med* 356:656–659, 2007.

Rockstroh J, Mauss S: Clinical perspective of fusion inhibitors for treatment of HIV, *J. Antimicrob Chemother* 53:700–702, 2004.

Ross J: Pelvic inflammatory disease, *Br Med J* 322(7287):658–659, 2001.

Salminen M, Tynkkynen S, Rautelin H, et al: The efficacy and safety of probiotic Lactobacillus rhamnosus GG on prolonged, non-infectious diarrhoea in HIV patients on antiretroviral therapy. A randomized, placebo-controlled crossover study, *HIV Clin Trials* 5(4):183–191, 2004.

Schneider E, Whitmore S, Glynn K, et al: Revised surveillance case definitions for HIV infection among adults, adolescents, and children aged <18 months and for HIV infection and AIDS among children aged 18 months to <13 years – United States, 2008, *MMWR Morb Mortal Wkly Rep* 57(RR10):1–8, 2008.

Schwartz R, Janusz C, Jenniger C: Seborrhoeic dermatitis: An overview, *South African Family Practice* 49(1):40–44, 2007.

Schwartz R, Micali G, Nasca M, et al: Kaposi sarcoma: a continuing conundrum, *J Am Acad Dermatol* 59(2):179–206, 2008.

Sen P, Barton S: Genital herpes and its management, *Br Med J* 334:1048–1052, 2007.

Sethi G, Allason-Jones E, Richens J, et al: Lymphogranuloma venereum presenting as genital ulceration and inguinal syndrome in men who have sex with men in London, *Sex Transm Infect* 85:165–170, 2009.

Sharland M, Gibb D, Tudor-Williams G: Advances in the prevention and treatment of paediatric HIV infection in the United Kingdom, *Sex Transm Infect* 79:53–55, 2003.

Shaw JK, Mahoney AM: *HIV/AIDS nursing secrets*, Philadelphia, 2003, Hanley and Belfus.

Sheldon L: *Communication for Nurses: Talking with Patients*, Philadelphia, 2008, Jones and Bartlett.

Shepard C, Simard E, Finelli L, et al: Hepatitis B virus infection: epidemiology and vaccination, *Epidemiol Rev* 28:12–25, 2006.

Siddiqui J, Phillips A, Freedland E, et al: Prevalence and cost of HIV-associated weight loss in a managed care population, *Curr Med Res Opin* 25:1307–1317, 2009.

Simms I, Fenton K, Ashton M, et al: The re-emergence of syphilis in the United Kingdom: the new epidemic phases, *Sex Transm Dis* 32(4):220–226, 2005.

Simms I, Stephenson J, Mallinson H, et al: Pelvic inflammatory disease: risk factors associated with pelvic inflammatory disease, *Sex Transm Infect* 82:452–457, 2006.

Smart S, Singal A, Mindel A: Social and sexual risk factors for bacterial vaginosis, *Sex Transm Infect* 80:58–62, 2004.

Stine GJ: *AIDS update 2000*, Upper Saddle River, NJ, 2000, Prentice Hall.

Trelle S, Shang A, Nartey L, et al: Improved effectiveness of partner notification for patients with sexually transmitted infections: systems review, *Br Med J* 334:332–334, 2007.

United Nations: *Report on the global AIDS epidemic*, 2004. Available online http://www.unaids.org/bangkok2004/report.html.

Vano-Galvan S, Alonso-Jimenez T: Classic Kaposi's sarcoma, *Isr Med Assoc J* 9:896, 2007.

Varela J, Otero L, Espinosa E, et al: Phthirus pubis in a Sexually Transmitted Disease Unit. A study of 14 years, *Sex Transm Dis* 30(4):292–296, 2003.

Varghese B, Maher J, Peterman T, et al: Reducing the risk of sexual HIV transmission: Quantifying the per-act risk for HIV on the basis of choice of partner, sex act, and condom use, *Sex Transm Dis* 29(1):38–43, 2002.

Von Krogh G: Management of anogenital warts (condylomata acuminata), *Eur J Dermatol* 11(6):598–604, 2001.

Walton S, Currie B: Problems in diagnosing scabies, a global disease in human and animal populations, *Clin Microbiol Rev* 20(2):268–279, 2007.

Ward H, Miller RF: Lymphogranuloma venereum: here to stay? *Sex Transm Infect* 85:157, 2009.

Weinberg J, Kovarik C: The WHO Clinical Staging System for HIV/AIDS, *American Medical Association Journal of Ethics* 12(3):202–206, 2010.

Wells C, Cegielski J, Nelson L, et al: HIV infection and multidrug-resistant tuberculosis – the perfect storm, *J Infect Dis* 196(Suppl 1):S86–S107, 2007.

Wilson J: Managing recurrent bacterial vaginosis, *Sex Transm Infect* 80:8–11, 2004.

Wilson J: *Infection control in clinical practice*, ed 3, London, 2006, Baillière Tindall.

World Health Organization: *Technical consultation on behalf of the UNFPA/UNICEF/WHO/UNAIDS interagency task team on mother-to-child transmission of HIV. New data on the prevention of mother-to-child transmission of HIV and their policy implications: conclusions and recommendations*, Geneva, 2000, WHO.

World Health Organization: *The 3 by 5 initiative*, Geneva, 2003a, WHO. Available online http://www.who.int/3by5/en/index.html.

World Health Organization: *Annex 1 World Health Organization staging system for HIV infection and disease in adults and adolescents*, Geneva, 2003b, WHO. Available online http://www.who.int/docstore/hiv/scaling/anex1.html.

World Health Organization: *WHO Case Definitions of HIV for Surveillance and Revised Clinical Staging and Immunological Classification of HIV-Related Disease In Adults and Children*, Geneva, 2007, WHO. Accessed March 18th, 2010. Available online http://www.who.int/hiv/pub/guidelines/HIVstaging150307.pdf.

World Health Organization: *HIV/AIDS epidemiological surveillance report for the WHO African Region: 2007 update*, Geneva, 2008, WHO.

Wright A, Zignoi M, Van Deun A, et al: Epidemiology of antituberculosis drug resistance 2002–2007; an updated analysis of the Global Project on Anti-tuberculosis Drug Resistance Surveillance, *Lancet* 373(9678):1861–1873, 2009.

Yim H, Lok S: Natural history of chronic hepatitis B virus infection: what we knew in 1981 and what we know in 2005, *Hepatology* 43(S1):173–181, 2006.

Young S, Monin B, Owens D: Opt-out testing for stigmatized diseases: a social psychological approach to understanding the potential effect of recommendations for routine HIV testing, *Health Psychol* 28(6):675–681, 2009.

Zetola N, Engelman J, Jensen T, et al: Syphilis in the United States: An update for clinicians with an emphasis on HIV coinfection, *Mayo Clin Proc* 82(9):1091–1102, 2007.

FURTHER READING

Adler M: *ABC of Sexually Transmitted Infections*, ed 5, London, 2004, BMJ Publishing Group.

Andrews G: *Women's Sexual Health*, ed 3, London, 2005, Baillière Tindall.

De Cock K, Gilks C, Ying-Ru L, et al: Can antiretroviral therapy eliminate HIV transmission? *Lancet* 373(9657):7–9, 2009.

Granich R, Gilks C, Dye C, et al: Universal voluntary HIV testing with immediate antiretroviral therapy as a strategy for elimination of HIV transmission: a mathematical model, *Lancet* 373(9657):48–57, 2009.

Grundy-Bowers M, Davies J, editors: *Advanced Clinical Skills for GU Nurses*, Chichester, 2007, John Wiley & Sons.

Hayes RJ: Herpes simplex virus 2 infection increases HIV acquisition in men and women: systematic review and meta-analysis of longitudinal studies, *AIDS* 20(1):73–83, 2006.

Holmes K, Sparling P, Stamm W, et al, editors: *Sexually Transmitted Diseases*, ed 4, New York, 2008, McGraw Hill.

McMillan A: *Sexually Transmissible Infections in Clinical Practice. A Problem Based Approach*, London, 2009, Springer.

Patterman R, Snow M, Handy P, et al: *Oxford Handbook of Genitourinary Medicine, HIV and AIDS*, vol 93, New York, 2005, Oxford University Press.

Thompson M, Aberg J, Cahn P, et al: Antiretroviral treatment of adult HIV infection. 2010. Recommendations of the International AIDS Society – USA Panel, *JAMA* 304(3):321–333, 2010.

Tomlinson J, editor: *ABC of Sexual Health*, London, 2005, Blackwell Publishing.

USEFUL WEBSITES AND HELPLINE

AVERT: www.avert.org
British Association for Sexual Health and HIV: www.bashh.org.uk
British HIV Association: www.bhiva.org
British National Formulary (BNF): www.bnf.org
Department of Health: www.dh.gov.uk
Haemophilia Society: www.haemophilia.org.uk
Health Protection Agency (England and Wales): www.hpa.org.uk
Health Protection Scotland: www.hps.scot.nhs.uk
Institute of Psychosexual Medicine: www.ipm.org.uk
Medical Foundation for Aids and Sexual Health: www.medfash.org.uk
National AIDS Map: www.aidsmap.com
National AIDS Helpline (24 hour): 0800 567 123
NICE: www.nice.org.uk
Royal College of Nursing Sexual Health Forum: www.rcn.org.uk
Terrence Higgins Trust: www.tht.org.uk

Appendix – normal values

Notes on International system of units/ Système International (SI) units

Base units

Length	metre (m)
Mass	kilogram (kg)
Amount of substance	mole (mol)
Time	second (s)
Electric current	ampere (A)
Thermodynamic temperature	kelvin (K)
Luminous intensity	candela (cd)

Derived units obtained by dividing or multiplying any two or more of the seven base units

Radioactivity	becquerel (Bq)
Absorbed dose of radiation	gray (Gy)
Frequency	hertz (Hz)
Work, energy, quantity of heat	joule (J)
Force	newton (N)
Pressure	pascal (Pa)
Dose equivalent	sievert (Sv)
Electrical potential, potential difference, electromotive force	volt (V)
Power	watt (W)

Examples of decimal multiples and submultiples of SI units

Factor	Prefix	Symbol
10^{12}	tera-	T
10^{9}	giga-	G
10^{6}	mega-	M
10^{3}	kilo-	k
10^{2}	hecto-	h
10^{1}	deca-	da
10^{-1}	deci-	d
10^{-2}	centi-	c
10^{-3}	milli-	m
10^{-6}	micro-	μ
10^{-9}	nano-	n
10^{-12}	pico-	p
10^{-15}	femto-	F
10^{-18}	atto-	a

Volume is calculated by multiplying length, width and depth. The SI unit for length, the metre (m), is not appropriate, as a cubic metre (1000 L) is not practical. Because of its convenience, the litre (L) (the volume of a 10 cm cube) is used as the unit of volume in laboratory work.

Amount of substance The mole (mol) is the SI base unit for amount of substance. The concentration of many substances is expressed in moles per litre (mol/L) or millimoles per litre (mmol/L), which replaces milliequivalents per litre (meq/L). Some exceptions exist and include: haemoglobin expressed in grams per litre (g/L) or grams per decilitre (g/dL), proteins and some enzymes and hormones (see below).

Mass concentration (e.g. g/L, μg/L) is used for all protein measurements, for substances which do not have a sufficiently well-defined composition and for serum vitamin B_{12} and folate measurements.

Enzymes and hormones Some hormones and enzymes are measured using bioassay, whereby hormone/enzyme activity is compared with a standard sample and expressed in standardised International Units or Units (IU, iu or U).

Pressure The pascal (Pa) is the SI unit for pressure, and the kilopascal (kPa) replaces millimetres of mercury pressure (mmHg) for blood gases. However, blood pressure continues to be measured in mmHg pressure.

Reference ranges

In common with previous editions the reference ranges provided draw heavily on those in *Davidson's Principles and Practice of Medicine* (Walker S W 2010 Laboratory reference ranges. In: Colledge N R, Walker B R, Ralston S H, eds. Davidson's Principles and Practice of Medicine, 21st edition. Churchill Livingstone, Edinburgh, pp 1293–1298) which are largely those used in the Departments of Clinical Biochemistry and Haematology, Lothian Health University Hospitals Division, Edinburgh, UK.

Reference ranges can vary from laboratory to laboratory, depending on the method used and other factors; this is especially the case for enzyme assays. Although the SI system of units is used in the UK, values for both SI and non-SI units are provided here.

Specific collection requirements, which may be critical to obtaining a meaningful result, are not included.

The reference ranges provided apply to adults. Reference ranges for infants and children may be different.

Biochemical values

Table A1.1 Arterial blood analysis

ANALYSIS	REFERENCE RANGE	
	SI UNITS	NON-SI UNITS
Bicarbonate	21–27.5 mmol/L	21–27.5 meq/L
Hydrogen ion	36–44 nmol/L	pH 7.36–7.44
$PaCO_2$	4.4–6.1 kPa	33–46 mmHg
PaO_2	12–15 kPa	90–113 mmHg
Oxygen saturation	Normally >97%	

Table A1.2 Cerebrospinal fluid

ANALYSIS	REFERENCE RANGE	
	SI UNITS	NON-SI UNITS
Cells	$<5 \times 10^6$ cells/L (all mononuclear)	<5 cells/mm³
Glucose*	2.5–4.0 mmol/L	45–72 mg/dL
IgG index**	<0.65	–
Total protein	140–450 mg/L	0.014–0.045 g/dL

*Interpret in relation to the level of glucose in the plasma.

**A crude index of increase in IgG attributable to intrathecal synthesis.

Table A1.3 Reference values in venous serum for the more common analytes in adults

ANALYSIS	REFERENCE RANGE	
	SI UNITS	NON-SI UNITS
α_1-antitrypsin	1.1–2.1 g/L	110–210 mg/dL
Alanine aminotransferase (ALT)	10–40 U/L	–
Albumin	36–47 g/L	3.6–4.7 g/dL
Alkaline phosphatase	40–125 U/L	–
Amylase	<100 U/L	–
Aspartate aminotransferase (AST)	10–45 U/L	–
Bilirubin (total)	2–17 µmol/L	0.12–1.0 mg/dL
Caeruloplasmin	0.2–0.6 g/L	15–60 mg/dL
Calcium	2.12–2.62 mmol/L	4.24–5.24 meq/L or 8.50–10.50 mg/dL
Carboxyhaemoglobin	0.1–3.0%	–
Chloride	95–107 mmol/L	95–107 meq/L

Cholesterol (total)
    Ideally (level varies and depends upon other cardiovascular risk factors)
    Mild increase
    Moderate increase
    Severe increase (as defined by European Atherosclerosis Society)
	
	  <5.2 mmol/L
	
	5.2–6.5 mmol/L
	6.5–7.8 mmol/L
	>7.8 mmol/L
		
		  <200 mg/dL
		
		200–250 mg/dL
		250–300 mg/dL
		>300 mg/dL

Continued

Table A1.3 Reference values in venous serum for the more common analytes in adults – cont'd

ANALYSIS	REFERENCE RANGE	
	SI UNITS	NON-SI UNITS
HDL-cholesterol (ideal level varies and depends upon other cardiovascular risk factors)	>1.0 mmol/L	>40 mg/dL
Copper	13–24 µmol/L	83–153 µg/dL
C-reactive protein	<5 mg/L	–

Creatine kinase CK (total)
  Male
  Female
	
	55–170 U/L
	30–135 U/L
		
		–
		–

Creatine kinase (MB isoenzyme)	Normally <6% of total CK	–
Creatinine	55–120 µmol/L	0.62–1.36 mg/dL
Ethanol	Not normally detectable 65–87 mmol/L (marked intoxication) 87–109 mmol/L (stupor) >109 mmol/L (coma)	 300–400 mg/dL 400–500 mg/dL >500 mg/dL

Gamma-glutamyl transferase (GGT)
  Male
  Female
	
	10–55 U/L
	5–35 U/L
		
		–
		–

Glucose (venous blood, fasting)	3.6–5.8 mmol/L	65–104 mg/dL
Glycated haemoglobin (HbA$_{1c}$)	4.0–6.0% 20–42 mmol/mol Hb	–
Immunoglobulin A	0.8–4.0 g/L	–
Immunoglobulin G	6.0–16.0 g/L	–
Immunoglobulin M	0.35–2.9 g/L	–
Iron	10–32 µmol/L	56–178 µg/dL
Iron-binding capacity	45–72 µmol/L	251–402 g/dL
Lactate (venous whole blood)	0.6–2.2 mmol/L	5.0–20.0 mg/dL
Lactate dehydrogenase (LDH) (total)	230–460 U/L	–
Lead	<1.0 µmol/L	<21 µg/dL
Magnesium	0.75–1.0 mmol/L	1.5–2.0 meq/L or 1.82–2.43 mg/dL
Phosphate (fasting)	0.8–1.4 mmol/L	2.48–4.34 mg/dL
Potassium (plasma)	3.3–4.7 mmol/L	3.3–4.7 meq/L
Potassium (serum)	3.6–5.1 mmol/L	3.6–5.1 meq/L
Protein (total)	60–80 g/L	6–8 g/dL
Sodium	135–145 mmol/L	135–145 meq/L
Triglycerides (fasting)	0.6–1.7 mmol/L	53–150 mg/dL
Troponins	Depends on whether troponin I or T is measured and the method used	

Urate
  Male
  Female
	
	0.12–0.42 mmol/L
	0.12–0.36 mmol/L
		
		2.0–7.0 mg/dL
		2.0–6.0 mg/dL

Urea	2.5–6.6 mmol/L	15–40 mg/dL
Zinc	11–22 µmol/L	72–144 µg/dL

Table A1.4 Reference values for the more common analytes in urine

ANALYSIS	REFERENCE RANGE SI UNITS	NON-SI UNITS
Albumin/creatinine ratio (ACR)	Less than 3.5 mg albumin/mmol creatinine	
Albumin excretion rate (AER)	Less than 20 µg albumin/min	
Calcium (normal diet)	Up to 7.5 mmol/24 h	Up to 300 mg/24 h
Copper	Up to 0.6 µmol/24 h	Up to 38 µg/24 h
Cortisol (24 h collection)	25–250 nmol/24 h	9.1–91 µg/24 h
Creatinine	10–20 mmol/24 h	1130–2260 mg/24 h
5-hydroxyindole-3-acetic acid (5-HIAA)	10–42 µmol/24 h	1.9–8.1 mg/24 h

Metadrenalines
  Normetadrenaline
  Metadrenaline
	
	0.4–3.4 µmol/24 h
	0.3–1.7 µmol/24 h
		
		73–620 µg/24 h
		59–335 µg/24 h

Oxalate	0.04–0.49 mmol/24 h	3.6–44 mg/24 h
Phosphate	15–50 mmol/24 h	465–1548 mg/24 h
Potassium*	25–100 mmol/24 h	25–100 meq/24 h
Protein	Up to 0.3 g/L	Up to 0.03 g/dL
Sodium*	100–200 mmol/24 h	100–200 meq/24 h
Urate	1.2–3.0 mmol/24 h	202–504 mg/24 h
Urea	170–600 mmol/24 h	10.2–36.0 g/24 h

*The urinary output of electrolytes such as potassium and sodium is normally a reflection of intake. This can vary widely, especially on a cultural, worldwide basis. The values quoted are more suitable to a 'Western' diet.

Table A1.5 Hormones in serum

HORMONE	REFERENCE RANGE SI UNITS	NON-SI UNITS
Adrenocorticotrophic hormone (ACTH) (plasma)	1.5–11.2 pmol/L (0700–1000 h)	7–51 pg/mL

Aldosterone
  Supine
  Erect
	
	30–440 pmol/L
	110–860 pmol/L
		
		1.09–15.9 ng/dL
		3.97–31.0 ng/dL

Follicle-stimulating hormone (FSH)
  Male
  Female
	
	1.0–10.0 U/L
	3.0–9.0 U/L (early follicular, luteal)
	<30 U/L (mid-cycle)
	>30 U/L (postmenopausal)
		
		0.2–2.2 ng/mL
		0.7–2.0 ng/mL
		<6.7 ng/mL
		>6.7 ng/mL

Gastrin (plasma, fasting)	<57 pmol/L	<120 pg/mL
Growth hormone (GH)	<0.5 µg/L excludes acromegaly (if insulin growth factor 1 [IGF1] in reference range) >6 µg/L excludes growth hormone (GH) deficiency	–
Insulin	Highly variable and interpretable only in relation to plasma glucose and body habitus	–

Continued

Table A1.5 Hormones in serum – cont'd

HORMONE	REFERENCE RANGE	
	SI UNITS	NON-SI UNITS
Luteinising hormone (LH) Female	2.5–9.0 U/L (early follicular, luteal) Up to 90 U/L (mid-cycle) >20 U/L (postmenopausal)	0.3–1.0 µg/L Up to 10 µg/L >2.2 µg/L
Male	1.0–9.0 U/L	0.11–1.0 µg/L
17β-Oestradiol Female	110–180 pmol/L (early follicular) 550–2095 pmol/L (mid-cycle) 370–770 pmol/L (luteal) <150 pmol/L (postmenopausal)	30–49 pg/mL 150–570 pg/mL 101–209 pg/mL <41 pg/mL
Male	<160 pmol/L	<43 pg/mL
Parathyroid hormone (PTH)	1.0–6.5 pmol/L	10–65 pg/mL

Progesterone
  Male
  Female
	<2.0 nmol/L
	<2.0 nmol/L (follicular)
	>15 nmol/L (mid-luteal)
	<2.0 nmol/L (postmenopausal)
		<0.63 ng/mL
		<0.63 ng/mL
		>4.7 ng/mL
		<0.63 ng/mL

Prolactin (PRL)	60–500 mU/L	–

Testosterone
  Male
  Female
	10–30 nmol/L
	0.4–3.0 nmol/L
		2.88–8.64 ng/mL
		0.12–0.87 ng/mL

Thyroid-stimulating hormone (TSH)	0.2–4.5 mU/L	–
Thyroxine (free) (free T_4)	9–21 pmol/L	700–1632 pg/dL
Triiodothyronine (T_3)	0.9–2.4 nmol/L	59–156 ng/dL

Notes

1. A number of hormones are unstable, and collection details are critical to obtaining a meaningful result. Refer to local hospital handbook.

2. Values in the table are only a guideline; hormone levels can often only be meaningfully understood in relation to factors such as gender (e.g. testosterone), age (e.g. FSH in women), time of day (e.g. cortisol) or regulatory factors (e.g. insulin and glucose, PTH and [Ca^{2+}]).

3. Also, reference ranges may be critically method-dependent.

Haematological values

Table A1.6 Haematological values

ANALYSIS	REFERENCE RANGE	
	SI UNITS	NON-SI UNITS
Bleeding time (Ivy)	Less than 8 min	–

Blood volume
  Male
  Female
	75 ± 10 mL/kg
	70 ± 10 mL/kg
		–
		–

Coagulation screen
  Prothrombin time
  Activated partial thromboplastin time
	10.5–13.5 s
	26–36 s
		–
		–

Continued

Table A1.6 Haematological values – cont'd

ANALYSIS	REFERENCE RANGE	
	SI UNITS	NON-SI UNITS
D-dimers		
To detect venous thromboembolism (VTE)	<500 µg/L	<500 ng/mL
To detect disseminated intravascular coagulation (DIC)	<200 µg/L	<200 ng/mL
Erythrocyte sedimentation rate*		
Adult male	0–10 mm/h	–
Adult female	3–15 mm/h	–
Ferritin		
Male	20–300 µg/L	20–300 ng/mL
Female	14–150 µg/L	14–150 ng/mL
Fibrinogen	1.5–4.0 g/L	0.15–0.4 g/dL
Folate		
Serum	5.0–20 µg/L	5.0–20 ng/mL
Red cell	257–800 µg/L	257–800 ng/mL
Haemoglobin		
Male	130–180 g/L	13–18 g/dL
Female	115–165 g/L	11.5–16.5 g/dL
Haptoglobin	0.4–2.4 g/L	0.04–0.24 g/dL
Leucocytes (adults)	$4.0–11.0 \times 10^9$/L	$4.0–11.0 \times 10^3$/mm^3
Differential white cell count		
Neutrophil granulocytes	$2.0–7.5 \times 10^9$/L	$2.0–7.5 \times 10^3$/mm^3
Lymphocytes	$1.5–4.0 \times 10^9$/L	$1.5–4.0 \times 10^3$/mm^3
Monocytes	$0.2–0.8 \times 10^9$/L	$0.2–0.8 \times 10^3$/mm^3
Eosinophil granulocytes	$0.04–0.4 \times 10^9$/L	$0.04–0.4 \times 10^3$/mm^3
Basophil granulocytes	$0.01–0.1 \times 10^9$/L	$0.01–0.1 \times 10^3$/mm^3
Mean cell haemoglobin (MCH)	27–32 pg	–
Mean cell volume (MCV)	78–98 fL	–
Packed cell volume (PCV) or haematocrit		
Male	0.40–0.54	–
Female	0.37–0.47	–
Platelets	$150–350 \times 10^9$/L	$150–350 \times 10^3$/mm^3
Red cell count		
Male	$4.5–6.5 \times 10^{12}$/L	$4.5–6.5 \times 10^6$/mm^3
Female	$3.8–5.8 \times 10^{12}$/L	$3.8–5.8 \times 10^6$/mm^3
Red cell lifespan (mean)	120 days	–
Red cell lifespan half-life (^{51}Cr)	25–35 days	–
Reticulocytes (adults)	$25–85 \times 10^9$/L	$25–85 \times 10^3$/mm^3
Transferrin	2.0–4.0 g/L	0.2–0.4 g/dL
Vitamin B$_{12}$	251–900 ng/L	–

*Higher values in older patients are not necessarily abnormal.

Source (with permission): Walker S W 2010 Laboratory reference ranges. In:
Colledge N R, Walker B R, Ralston S H, eds. Davidson's Principles and Practice of
Medicine, 21st edn. Churchill Livingstone, Edinburgh, pp 1293–1298.

Glossary

Abortion/miscarriage The legal definition of 'abortion' refers to the premature delivery of a non-viable fetus, spontaneously or by induction. Currently, in the UK, a fetus is considered viable from the 24th week of pregnancy. The term 'miscarriage' is recommended when the pregnancy loss is spontaneous and is generally more acceptable to women who lose a wanted pregnancy (RCOG 2006).

Acidaemia A high level of acid (hydrogen ions) in the blood which results in a below normal blood pH, less than 7.35 (greater than 44 nmol/L H^+).

Acidosis The processes that lead to excess acid in the body.

Acquired immune deficiency syndrome (AIDS) A specific stage of infection with the human immunodeficiency virus (HIV); the development of an AIDS-defining illness in a person with HIV infection.

Acute coronary syndrome A continuum of manifestations of coronary heart disease (CHD). It includes unstable angina and acute myocardial infarction which have as common underlying pathology the abrupt, total or subtotal occlusion of a coronary artery.

Acute pain Often described as being short lived, that is less than 6 weeks, and commonly nociceptive pain associated with surgery, trauma or acute disease.

Adaptive specific immunity The specific immune responses comprising the humoral (antibody-mediated) immune response, initiated by B lymphocytes, and the cell-mediated response, initiated by T lymphocytes.

Ageing The normal structural and physiological changes that occur with time. The process of growing old.

Age-related macular degeneration (AMD) Degenerative changes in the macular region of the retina that may lead to central vision loss. AMD may be described as 'dry' or 'wet'.

Albuminuria The presence of albumin in the urine.

Alkalaemia Low level of acid (hydrogen ions) in the blood and an above normal pH.

Alkalosis The processes that result in low levels of acid (excess of alkali) in the body.

Alzheimer's disease A neurodegenerative brain disorder characterised by progressive dementia. The onset is subtle and includes progressive memory loss (particularly short-term or recent), failing intellectual ability, confusion, restlessness, speech problems, motor retardation, depression and personality changes (Brooker 2010).

Ambulatory surgery (day surgery) Surgery undertaken on the day of admission. If recovery is problem free, the patient is discharged that day to the care of the primary care team. Procedures include cataract surgery, minor gynaecological and orthopaedic procedures and endoscopic examinations.

Amnesia Loss of memory.

Anaemia Decreased oxygen-carrying capacity of the blood, due to a reduced number of erythrocytes and/or the amount of haemoglobin within the erythrocytes.

Anaesthesia Loss of sensation.

Analgesics Drugs such as paracetamol or morphine that relieve pain.

Anaphylaxis Sudden life-threatening allergic reaction. An exaggerated type I hypersensitivity response to an antigen, such as peanuts or a penicillin.

Aneurysm A localised dilatation of a blood vessel. It usually occurs in an artery such as the aorta, carotid artery, cerebral arteries and popliteal artery.

Angina pectoris Part of the spectrum of acute coronary syndrome. Discomfort or pain felt in a variety of sites including the chest, throat and arms, resulting from a transient, reversible episode of inadequate coronary circulation.

Antibodies (immunoglobulins) Globular proteins able to recognise and bind to a specific antigen, usually a microorganism.

Antigen Foreign cell/substance that induces a specific immune response in the host.

Anuria Complete cessation of urine production by the kidneys.

Aphthous ulcers, aphthae Shallow, painful ulcers usually affecting the oral mucosa.

Apyrexia Without fever.

Arrhythmia A term used to imply an abnormality in either electrical impulse formation or electrical impulse conduction within the heart, e.g. atrial fibrillation.

Ascites (hydroperitoneum) An accumulation of fluid in the peritoneal cavity.

Aseptic technique Techniques and procedures that exclude pathogenic microorganisms, e.g. non-touch technique, sterile equipment.

Asthma An obstructive pulmonary disease characterised by chronic inflammation of the airways with bronchial wall hyperactivity leading to bronchospasm and airway narrowing.

Ataxia Uncoordinated voluntary movement.

Atelectasis Alveolar collapse.

Atheroma Plaques of fatty material in the lining of arteries. Eventually the build-up reduces the lumen of the artery which results in ischaemia. A thrombus may develop if a plaque ruptures, which leads to further blockage of the artery.

Atherosclerosis Coexisting atheroma and arteriosclerosis.

Autoantibodies Abnormal antibodies that bind to self-antigens of normal body cells.

Autoimmune disorders Those that occur when the normal tolerance to 'self' breaks down and autoantibodies against self-antigens are formed.

Autologous Describes a situation in which the person's own cells are used for a graft, such as blood transfusion, skin or bone marrow.

Biological response modifiers (BRMs) (immunotherapies) Substances that occur naturally in the body and can be used therapeutically. Most are involved in some way in the immune response. It may be possible to manipulate the immune system such that it recognises tumour cells as antigens and causes the body to reject them. Examples include cytokines and monoclonal antibodies.

Biopsy The procedure of obtaining a sample of tissue for examination from a specified area.

Body image The image held in the person's mind of their body.

Bradykinesia Slowness of movement.

Breast Screening Programme A national programme in the UK that invites women between the ages of 47 and 73 years to attend a screening unit for bilateral mammograms.

Breast ultrasound A scan using high-frequency sound waves to image the breast tissue.

Breathlessness *See Dyspnoea.*

Burn assessment Involves factors including extent (size), depth, location, complexity and the possibility of respiratory involvement. Patient-related factors such as age are also considered.

Burn injury Tissue damage caused by moist and dry heat, flame, electricity, friction, chemicals (acids and alkalis) and radiation (sunlight and ionising radiation).

Burn sequelae (long term) Include psychosocial problems, wound contracture and scarring, and loss of function.

Burns prevention Involves assessment of the incidence of burn injuries, the causative agents and any predisposing factors, followed by planning, implementation and evaluation of appropriate interventions.

Cancer Cancer initiation is a very complex process involving the disruption of the regulation of growth of normal cells in the body. 'Cancer' is a general term describing any malignant tumour, the growth of which is purposeless, parasitic and at the expense of the host. It has a tendency to destroy tissue locally, attack adjacent tissue and spread to distant sites (metastasise).

Candidiasis (thrush) Fungal infection caused by *Candida*, usually *Candida albicans*. Affected areas include the mouth and gastrointestinal tract, respiratory tract, nails, skin or genitourinary tract (balanitis, vulvovaginitis). Risk factors include debilitation, e.g. by cancer, or immunosuppression, and long-term or extensive treatment with antibiotics and other drugs, such as corticosteroids. Candidiasis is also associated with immunodeficiency conditions including HIV disease.

Cardiac arrest Failure of the heart to pump sufficient blood to maintain cerebral function. The main mechanisms of cardiac arrest are:

- pulseless ventricular tachycardia and ventricular fibrillation (VF)
- ventricular asystole
- pulseless electrical activity (PEA).

Cardiac output The volume of blood ejected from the ventricles in 1 minute.

Cardiogenic shock That caused by myocardial dysfunction such as following an extensive myocardial infarction.

Cardiovascular disease (CVD) Diseases of the heart and blood vessels. The main diseases are CHD and stroke, but CVD also includes congenital heart disease and peripheral vascular disease.

Carer A person who accepts the responsibility for caring for another (child, person with an illness or disability, or an older person). Usually describes unpaid family, friends and neighbours in the UK, and not paid helpers such as care workers or nurses.

Cast (1) Exudate or other matter that has been moulded to the shape of a structure in which it has collected. (2) Splinting device comprising layers of bandages impregnated with plaster of Paris, fibreglass or resin; used to immobilise and hold bone fragments in reduction and to support and stabilise weak joints.

Cataract Opacity of the crystalline lens. Usually age-related, but may be congenital, iatrogenic or due to inflammation, trauma or metabolic causes.

Cell-mediated immunity The adaptive specific immune response initiated by T lymphocytes important for dealing with intracellular organisms, such as viruses. Also causes graft rejection.

Central venous pressure (CVP) The blood pressure within the right atrium and vena cava. It provides information about blood volume or venous system capacity. It can also give an indication of vascular tone and pulmonary vascular resistance, as well as of the effectiveness of the right heart pump.

Chemotherapy Chemicals of various types, administered to delay or arrest growth of cancer cells.

Chlamydiae Microorganisms belonging to the genus *Chlamydia*. Subgroups of *Chlamydia trachomatis* lead to reproductive tract infections in adults which are sexually acquired. Men may be asymptomatic, but can have urethritis or epididymitis. Most chlamydial infections are symptomless in women; however, untreated women may develop pelvic inflammatory disease with damage to the uterine tubes with risk of ectopic pregnancy or infertility.

Chronic obstructive pulmonary disease (COPD) Chronic airflow limitation. There is increased airway resistance with impaired airflow, e.g. pulmonary emphysema, chronic bronchitis. Some authorities include asthma.

Chronic pain (persistent pain) Pain unresolved after 3 months. Subdivided into chronic non-malignant pain (nociceptive and or neuropathic pain) and malignant (life-threatening) pain.

Cirrhosis 'Hardening' of an organ with degenerative changes and fibrosis. For example, liver cirrhosis is caused by viruses, other microorganisms, toxins including alcohol and nutritional deficiencies.

Climacteric The normal changes that occur leading up to the menopause (cessation of menstruation). The changes of the climacteric are usually gradual and may occur over several years.

Colloid A non-crystalline substance. It is diffusible but insoluble in water, thus it does not pass through a semi-permeable membrane.

Coma See Deep coma.

Compartment syndrome Occurs when tissue pressure within a compartment increases to the point that circulation and function of tissues are compromised (Lucas & Davis 2004). This results in tissue death (necrosis) and permanent loss of function, which can occur within 6–8 h.

Computed tomography (CT) A computer-constructed imaging technique of a thin slice through the body, derived from X-ray absorption data collected during a circular scanning motion.

Concordance The making of decisions about treatment and management in negotiation and partnership with the patient. It is very different from compliance where the patient is expected to agree to treatment decisions made by a health care professional.

Consciousness Hickey (2003) defines consciousness as 'a state of general awareness of oneself and the environment' and includes the ability to orientate towards new stimuli. The individual is awake, alert and aware of their personal identity and of the events occurring in their surroundings.

Consent Informed consent to treatment, surgery and any intervention that requires physical contact is a legal requirement. Depending on the intervention, consent may be verbal, written or implied, i.e. by non-verbal communication.

Constipation The infrequent and difficult passing of hard stools.

Continence Having voluntary control over voiding urine and passing faeces.

Coping In a neutral sense, the term 'coping' refers to the way in which the individual responds to a stressful situation or to the perception of threat, by attempting consciously and unconsciously to maintain equilibrium.

Core body temperature See Deep body (core) temperature.

Coronary heart disease (CHD) Includes angina pectoris and myocardial infarction; caused by a deficient supply of oxygenated blood to the myocardium.

Corticosteroids Three types of hormones produced by the adrenal cortex: glucocorticoids, mineralocorticoids, sex hormones. Also applied to synthetic steroids such as prednisolone.

Creatinine A substance produced during the metabolism of creatine phosphate in muscle tissue. It is normally removed from the blood by the kidneys and excreted in the urine. Measurements of creatinine in blood and urine are used to assess renal function.

Critical care support See Levels of critical care support.

Crystalloid A clear solution containing molecules small enough to pass through semi-permeable membranes, i.e. between the blood and the interstitial fluid.

Cyanosis Bluish colour seen in hypoxic tissue, visible in the lips, skin and under the nails. Caused by lack of oxygen, it may be peripheral, affecting the digits, ear lobes or nose, or central such as the tongue or oral mucosa.

Debridement Removal of dead or devitalised tissue. This can be achieved in various ways including autolysis with dressings, or sharp or surgical debridement.

Deep body (core) temperature The temperature (close to 37°C) of the organs of the central cavities of the body, i.e. cranium, thorax and abdomen.

Deep coma Deep coma is the opposite of consciousness, it is defined as being unrousable and unresponsive to external stimuli; there are varied states of altered consciousness in between the two extremes.

Defecation The passage of faeces which may be involuntary or voluntary.

Dehiscence Breakdown of a surgical wound, most commonly due to infection or undue strain on wound edges.

Delirium An acute confusional state. A fluctuating mental state with disturbance of awareness and thought processes characterised by confusion, disorientation, fear, irritability and disturbed or agitated behaviour.

Dementia A progressive irreversible brain disorder leading to memory disturbance, impaired cognition, disorientation and personality changes. The many causes include Alzheimer's disease and vascular degeneration.

Dentition The natural teeth present in the dental arches of a person. The 20 primary teeth and later the 32 permanent teeth of the secondary dentition.

Detrusor The smooth muscle of the walls of the bladder, which contracts to empty the bladder.

Diabetes mellitus A metabolic disorder characterised by chronic hyperglycaemia with disturbances of carbohydrate, protein and fat metabolism which results from defects in insulin secretion, insulin action or both (World Health Organization [WHO] 1999).

Diabetic ketoacidosis (DKA) Uncontrolled lipolysis in the absence of insulin, gluconeogenesis, ketogenesis and glycogenolysis combine to raise the blood glucose level still further, increase osmotic diuresis, and exacerbate fluid imbalance and metabolic acidosis.

Dialysis Renal replacement therapy. A process involving diffusion, osmosis and filtration in which solutes (waste, electrolytes) and excess fluid are removed across a selectively permeable membrane in patients with renal failure.

Diarrhoea Loose, frequent watery stools.

Diffusion The passive (requiring no energy) movement of solutes from an area of higher concentration to an area of lower concentration, which results in an equal concentration in both areas.

Dignity A complex concept with many definitions. Dignified care is that which promotes the person's self-respect and usually involves respect. *See Person-centred care.*

Disability The *medical model* regards disability as a problem which is intrinsic to the person and caused directly by disease, a health condition or trauma. In this model, 'impairment' is not only used to describe disturbance in the body's structure and function. It is also seen as responsible for preventing the individual's participation in normal society and, therefore, disabling them. Conversely, the *social model* is based on the assumption that disability exists where attitudinal or environmental barriers exclude people with impairments from full engagement in mainstream activities. This defines it as a socially created problem which is distinct from and superimposed on impairment.

Donor area/site The area used to take a skin graft to treat a burn injury.

Dyspareunia Difficult or painful sexual intercourse for a woman.

Dyspepsia Indigestion. A feeling of fullness after eating and discomfort in the epigastrium. Causes include peptic ulcer, chronic cholecystitis and gallstones.

Dysphagia Difficulty swallowing. Causes include oesophageal stricture or tumour, stroke, motor neurone disease.

Dysphasia Loss of ability to understand/produce language.

Dyspnoea Difficulty in or laboured breathing. May be due to respiratory conditions, anaemia or cardiovascular conditions.

Dysuria Pain or discomfort on micturition. Often due to bacterial infection (urethritis, cystitis, prostatitis) but may be associated with bladder tumours or calculi, or changes to urethral mucosa during the climacteric.

Elective surgery Planned surgery rather than an emergency procedure.

Embolism Obstruction of a blood vessel by a mass of undissolved material. Usually caused by a thrombus (clot), but other causes include malignant cells, fat, amniotic fluid, gases, bacteria and parasites.

Emollient An agent that moisturises and lubricates the skin. Used as soap substitute/bath additive or 'leave on' preparations.

Encopresis The involuntary or voluntary passage of a normal consistency stool in a socially unacceptable place.

End-of-life care (terminal care/phase) Care delivered in the last days of life. The focus moves from achieving a quality of life and supporting the patient in 'living whilst dying' whilst their illness is progressing, to ensuring a peaceful death and supporting the family in coping with their impending loss. Readers should be aware that the terminology is sometimes used differently.

Enteral feeding The delivery of nutrients directly into the stomach or small intestine via a tube.

Enuresis Any involuntary loss of urine; it may be primary or secondary. Nocturnal enuresis is urinary incontinence occurring during sleep, in the absence of organic disease or infection.

Epilepsies A group of conditions resulting from intermittent, uncontrolled discharge of neurones within the CNS. Manifests seizures which can range from a major motor convulsion to a brief period of lack of awareness and can occur in any individual at any time.

Epistaxis Bleeding from the nose. Causes include nasal trauma, infection or tumour, hypertension, coagulation problems and sudden changes in atmospheric pressure.

Erectile dysfunction (ED) The inability to achieve and maintain an erection sufficient for sexual intercourse.

Erythema Skin redness due to vascular congestion or perfusion.

Escharotomy Incision(s) into eschar for decompression. Used in full-thickness burn injury occurring circumferentially around a limb, to prevent compression of the deeper structures, especially the blood vessels, or when full-thickness burn injury of the chest/upper abdomen inhibits respiratory movement.

Expert Patient Programme (EPP) The UK Government's EPP initiative stems from recognition that traditional cure-oriented services have not dealt comprehensively with problems faced by people with long-term conditions and that partnership enhances self-efficacy (Department of Health 2001a). EPPs are led by lay people rather than health care professionals, EPPs aim to increase people's confidence, resourcefulness and control, thereby improving quality of life and reducing service use.

External fixation Used to keep bone fragments in position by skeletal pins inserted into the bone on either side of the fracture and held in alignment by a scaffold or a ring fixator.

Exudate Wound fluid which ranges from a watery consistency to being thick and tenacious. It is serous fluid which is beneficial for moist wound healing and bringing growth factors to the wound. However, enzymes in exudate can cause wound and skin breakdown if not controlled.

Falls prevention A person-centred, multidisciplinary approach to care. Education, training and audit are integral to falls prevention strategies. People in contact with health professionals should be assessed for risk routinely. Assessment of risk of falling and interventions should be multifactorial.

Fever High deep/core body temperature due to an upward reset in the hypothalamic set-point temperature.

First aid The immediate management of a person following sudden illness or injury before the arrival of a qualified health professional. The aims are to preserve life, prevent deterioration and promote recovery.

Fluid replacement Various ways of replacing fluid lost from the body – oral, enteral, subcutaneous, rectal, parenteral.

Fracture A break in the continuity of a bone resulting from direct or indirect trauma, repetitive stress applied to a bone or disease affecting bone.

Frailty Weakness and/or infirmity occurring not only as the result of medical condition(s) but also as a result of the difficult losses sometimes experienced in later life.

Frequency Voiding of urine more often than is acceptable to the person. Usually it is more often than before and in smaller volumes.

Full-thickness burn injury Destroys the epidermis and all of the dermis; may also involve deeper structures such as fat, muscle and bone.

Gastritis Acute or chronic inflammation of the stomach lining.

Gingivitis Inflammation of the gingivae (gums).

Glasgow Coma Scale (GCS) A reliable rating scale of conscious level for trauma and neurological patients that assesses their best motor, verbal and eye opening response. The best response for each of the three aspects is recorded as a numerical score: best eye opening is 4, best verbal is 5 and the best motor is 6. The lowest response for each of the three parameters is a score of 1. Thus the highest total score is 15 and the lowest is 3.

Glomerular filtration rate (GFR) The volume of plasma filtered by the kidneys in one minute. In health it is typically around 120 mL per min.

Glucagon A catabolic pancreatic hormone secreted in response to falling blood glucose. It causes glycogenolysis and the release of glucose from the liver and increased fat and protein breakdown in order to provide an alternative source of glucose via lipolysis and gluconeogenesis.

Gonorrhoea Caused by the bacterium *Neisseria gonorrhoeae*, it is a sexually acquired infection in adults. Newborns may be infected during a vaginal delivery leading to gonococcal conjunctivitis. Gonococcal vulvovaginitis in prepubertal girls may point to sexual abuse. Most women with uncomplicated gonorrhoea are asymptomatic, whereas men have dysuria and purulent urethral discharge.

Grading A classification of cancers based on histopathological characteristics.

Granulation New red, moist tissue in a wound. Comprises new capillaries held in a matrix of collagen and other cells found in a healing wound.

Haematemesis Vomiting of blood. It is bright red in recent bleeding, darker in colour or resembling 'coffee grounds' due to the action of gastric acid in earlier bleeding. Bleeding usually originates from the upper gastrointestinal tract due to gastritis, peptic ulceration, oesophageal varices, tumour, drug-induced erosions or blood coagulation disorders. Blood swallowed following oral trauma, dental procedures or epistaxis may be vomited.

Haematopoiesis Formation of blood cells from pluripotent stem cells present in the red marrow.

Haematopoietic growth factors Substances controlling haematopoiesis. They include hormones, cytokines and growth factors including erythropoietin, colony-stimulating factors (CSFs), thrombopoietin and interleukins (Hoffbrand et al 2006).

Haematopoietic stem cell transplantation (HSCT) The transplantation of healthy haematopoietic progenitor cells to re-establish healthy bone marrow function in someone whose bone marrow has been destroyed or depleted by disease or its treatment.

Haematuria Blood present in the urine. It may be macroscopic, when it may be bright red, dark red or smoky in appearance; or microscopic when it is detected by dipstick urine tests or microscopy. Causes include urinary tract infection, glomerulonephritis, cancer, kidney trauma, urinary calculi, anticoagulant drugs or blood coagulation disorders.

Haemofiltration A form of renal replacement therapy in which the patient's blood is passed through a filter allowing separation of an ultrafiltrate containing fluid and solutes. This is discarded and replaced with an isotonic solution. It is usually continuous as in continuous venovenous haemofiltration (CVVH).

Haemophilias A group of inherited disorders in which an essential coagulation factor is either partly or completely missing. A person with haemophilia bleeds for longer than normal. Haemophilia is a recessive X-linked condition (sex-linked inheritance) which nearly always affects males while females carry the defective gene. However, it is possible for a female to have haemophilia or a bleeding tendency.

Haemoptysis Coughing up of blood or blood-stained sputum/mucus from the respiratory tract. The amount ranges from blood-streaked sputum up to a life-threatening haemorrhage. The blood may be bright red, pink and frothy or described as rusty looking. Causes include pneumonia, lung abscess, tuberculosis, chronic bronchitis, lung cancer, pulmonary infarction, left ventricular failure, anticoagulant drugs and blood coagulation disorders.

Hand hygiene Considered to be the most important step in preventing health care associated infection (HCAI). Recognising the times when hand hygiene is required is crucially important. These are: before touching a patient, before invasive procedures including aseptic tasks, after body fluid exposure risk, after touching a patient and touching patient surroundings. An effective hand hygiene technique is important in ensuring adequate hand hygiene standards. This includes ensuring thorough cleansing and drying of all areas of the hands and avoiding recontamination when closing taps and disposing of paper towels.

Health care associated infection (HCAI) Previously known as hospital acquired infection (HAI) or nosocomial infection. Refers to infection acquired during receipt of some form of health care.

Healthy diet One that provides the appropriate amounts of all nutrients in the correct proportions to meet body requirements.

Hearing loss (deafness) May be total or partial and can affect all age groups. It may be conductive (e.g. cerumen) or sensorineural (e.g. damage to the organ of Corti or the cochlear part of the VIIIth cranial nerve).

Heart failure A clinical syndrome that results from an inability of the heart to provide an adequate cardiac output for the body's metabolic requirements. It may be acute or chronic. Heart failure may involve either ventricle or both together.

Highly active antiretroviral therapy (HAART) Combination of three or more different types of antiretroviral drugs active against HIV at different stages of replication.

Histamine H$_2$-receptor antagonists Drugs such as ranitidine that reduce gastric acid production by blocking the histamine H_2 receptors. Used in gastro-oesophageal reflux disease and peptic ulceration.

Homeostasis The autoregulatory mechanisms whereby functions such as blood pH, glucose, body temperature, etc., are maintained within set parameters.

Hormone Chemical messenger secreted by endocrine glands, neurones and other structures. Usually travelling in the bloodstream, hormones maintain homeostasis by acting on and coordinating activity within target organs or tissues.

Hormone therapy The use of drugs to replace, manipulate or block the production and function of circulating hormones.

Hospice care Care provided for people with life-limiting illnesses and their families, including end-of-life care. Care may be offered at home, as daycare and in hospice premises.

Human immunodeficiency virus (HIV) The virus causing AIDS. There are two types: HIV-1 mainly responsible for HIV disease in Western Europe, North America and Central Africa, and HIV-2, causing similar disease mainly in West Africa.

Humoral (antibody-mediated) immunity Adaptive specific immune response initiated by B lymphocytes. The humoral response deals mainly with extracellular organisms through the production of antibodies (immunoglobulins).

Hypercalcaemia Excessive level of calcium in the blood.

Hypercapnia Increased carbon dioxide tension in arterial blood.

Hyperchloraemia Excessive level of chlorides in the blood.

Hyperglycaemia Increased level of glucose in the blood.

Hyperkalaemia Excessive level of potassium in the blood.

Hypermagnesaemia Excessive level of magnesium in the blood.

Hypernatraemia Excessive level of sodium in the blood.

Hyperphosphataemia Excessive level of phosphates in the blood.

Hyperpyrexia Core body temperature above 40–42°C due to an altered set-point.

Hypersensitivity and allergic reactions Abnormal and excessive immune responses following contact with an antigen (allergen). Effects range from local tissue damage to life-threatening anaphylaxis.

Hypertension An abnormally high arterial blood pressure involving systolic and/or diastolic readings.

Hyperthermia An abnormally high body deep/core temperature caused by loss of thermoregulatory control.

Hypertonic solutions Those with a higher osmotic pressure relative to another solution such as serum.

Hypertrophic scar Scar that appears red and is raised above the level of the surrounding skin. A complication of burn injury.

Hypervolaemia Increased volume of circulating blood.

Hypocalcaemia Decreased level of calcium in the blood.

Hypochloraemia Decreased level of chlorides in the blood.

Hypoglycaemia Decreased level of glucose in the blood.

Hypokalaemia Decreased level of potassium in the blood.

Hypomagnesaemia Decreased level of magnesium in the blood.

Hyponatraemia Decreased level of sodium in the blood.

Hypophosphataemia Decreased level of phosphates in the blood.

Hypothermia A state in which the deep/core body temperature is lower than the thermoregulatory set-point. Usually considered to be below 35°C.

Hypotonic solutions Those with a lower osmotic pressure relative to another solution such as serum.

Hypovolaemia Reduced volume of circulating blood.

Hypoxaemia Reduced oxygen content in arterial blood, evidenced by decreased PaO_2.

Hypoxia Reduced oxygen in the tissues.

Immunity An innate or acquired state of immune responsiveness to an antigen.

Immunodeficiency Defective immune responses, leading to increased susceptibility to infection, autoimmune diseases and cancer.

Immunoglobulins *See Antibodies.*

Immunosuppressants Drugs that suppress the immune responses, e.g. ciclosporin, tacrolimus.

Immunotherapy *See Biological response modifiers.*

Impaired glucose tolerance (IGT) and Impaired fasting glycaemia (IFG) Stages in the natural history of diabetes rather than a class of diabetes (WHO 1999).

Infection prevention Measures required routinely in order to minimise the risk of infection to patients, their relatives/carers and staff. These include standard precautions (e.g. hand hygiene, personal protective equipment, environmental cleaning), decontamination of reusable medical devices, transmission-based precautions, aseptic and clean techniques, use of evidence-based practice guidelines, antimicrobial stewardship and outbreak management.

Infertility A couple is said to be subfertile if they have been having unprotected sexual intercourse for 12 months without conception occurring. It may be primary or secondary where there has been a previous pregnancy, irrespective of the outcome.

Inflammation A non-specific defence mechanism initiated by tissue injury. The injury may be caused by trauma, microorganisms, extremes of temperature and pH, ultraviolet (UV) radiation, or ionising radiation. A phase in wound healing.

Insomnia Sleeplessness. An inability to initiate sleep or to stay asleep or waking in the early hours. Sleep is of poor quality and the person does not feel refreshed.

Insomnia treatments Include pharmacological solutions, alternative approaches, e.g. developing good sleep habits ('sleep hygiene'), complementary and alternative medicine therapies (CAM) and cognitive-behavioural therapies.

Insulin An anabolic pancreatic hormone secreted in response to a rising blood glucose level. Insulin has numerous effects on the metabolism of carbohydrate, fat and protein.

Internal fixation An operative fracture reduction whereby metal pins, plates, screws or nails are used to hold the bony fragments in position.

Intracranial pressure (ICP) Pressure exerted inside the skull by the brain, cerebrospinal fluid and blood volume contained within the cranium.

Intracranial pressure monitoring Invasive technique involving direct measurement of ICP. A typical system comprises a fibreoptic transducer-tipped catheter, which can be placed in the lateral ventricle, subdural or extradural space.

Ischaemia Lack of oxygenated (arterial) blood to an area of tissue, causing tissue destruction. Can be a result of a compromised vascular system due either to atherosclerosis or to localised pressure, both of which cause arterial occlusion.

Isotonic Having equal tension. Any solution which has the same osmotic pressure as the fluid with which it is being compared.

Jaundice Yellow discolouration of the skin, sclerae and mucosae. It is due to an increase in the level of bilirubin in the blood. It may be accompanied by pruritus.

Joint arthroplasty (joint replacement) The surgical insertion of inert prostheses of similar shape into joints, such as hip, knee and shoulder. May be total, as in replacing the head of femur and acetabulum, or partial.

Laxatives (aperients) Drugs used to prevent or relieve constipation. Administered orally or rectally (suppositories or enema).

Leg ulcer The major cause in the UK is chronic venous insufficiency associated with venous hypertension (70–75%). Between 20 and 30% of patients with a leg ulcer have some degree of ischaemia, with diabetes, vasculitis and trauma accounting for other causes of leg ulceration (Moffatt et al 2007).

Lesion An area of skin with changes to texture, elevation or colour which is bordered by normal skin.

Leukaemia A group of blood disorders in which there is abnormal and excessive proliferation of malignant leucocytes. Typically divided into acute and chronic types, and further subdivided into myeloid or lymphoid types depending on the type of leucocytes affected.

Levels of critical care support *Level 0* Patients whose needs can be met through normal ward care in an acute hospital. *Level 1* Patients at risk of their condition deteriorating, or those recently relocated from a higher level of care, whose needs can be met on an acute ward with additional advice and support from the critical care team. *Level 2* Patients requiring more detailed observation or intervention including support for a single failing organ system or postoperative care and those 'stepping down' from a higher level of care. *Level 3* Patients requiring advanced respiratory support alone or basic respiratory support together with support of at least two organ systems. This level includes all complex patients requiring support for multi-organ failure (Department of Health 2000).

Life-limiting illness A progressive and ultimately fatal condition. Includes inherited diseases such as muscular dystrophy as well as cancer, chronic respiratory and cardiovascular disease, stroke and dementia.

Locked in syndrome Damage to the pons in the brain stem, resulting from cerebral vascular disease or trauma, paralyses voluntary muscles without interfering with consciousness and cognitive functions. The patient is unable to speak and is sometimes unable to breathe spontaneously. However, they are able to control vertical eye movements and blinking and may be able to use these movements to develop a simple communication system.

Lund and Browder's charts Used to calculate more accurately a burn area. They allow for the changing proportions of different age groups and show which percentages are applicable to smaller, more specific areas of the body surface.

Lymphoma A group of malignant disorders characterised by a proliferation of lymphoid cells originating in the lymph nodes or lymphoid tissue. Traditionally divided into two groups: Hodgkin's lymphoma (HL) and non-Hodgkin lymphoma (NHL).

Magnetic resonance imaging (MRI) A non-invasive imaging technique that uses a powerful magnetic field combined with radiofrequency pulses to excite hydrogen nuclei in the body. When the hydrogen nuclei settle, the signal from the body is measured and reconstructed, using computer software, into two-dimensional or three-dimensional images.

Major incident preparedness (emergency planning) The emergency preparedness for major incidents within the NHS to ensure that all the emergency services are able to work collaboratively and provide an effective response to any type of incident.

Mammogram Breast X-ray that involves compression of the breast tissue both laterally and medial-obliquely before the X-ray is taken.

Mastectomy Surgical removal of the breast.

Mechanical ventilation Artificial support of, or assistance with, breathing when adequate gaseous exchange and tissue perfusion can no longer be maintained. Respiratory support may be invasive through an endotracheal tube or tracheostomy or non-invasive through a mask or hood.

Mechanism of injury Classified into four main groups (Greaves et al 2001): blast, blunt, penetrating or thermal.

Melaena Black stools with tar-like consistency with a distinctive odour. They contain digested blood and are evidence of upper gastrointestinal bleeding, such as from oesophageal varices, peptic ulceration, stomach cancer, or small bowel disease.

Menopause The cessation of menstruation, a single event occurring during the climacteric.

Menstrual (uterine) cycle The endometrial changes caused by the ovarian hormones. They correspond to the hormonal events of the ovarian cycle and can be divided into three phases: proliferative phase (follicular or pre-ovulatory), secretory phase (luteal or post-ovulatory) and menstrual phase.

Mouth care *See Oral hygiene.*

Multidisciplinary team (MDT) A team of health care professionals assigned to plan, treat, care and meet the needs of the individual with a particular condition or need, such as a woman with breast cancer when the team would usually include surgeons, pathologists, radiologists, specialist nurses, radiographers, etc.

Multiple organ dysfunction syndrome (MODS) A syndrome in critically ill patients in which more than one organ system (e.g. renal, coagulation, respiratory and gastrointestinal) fails to function normally and may progress to multiple organ failure. It requires appropriate organ support such as mechanical ventilation and haemofiltration (Brooker 2010).

Myeloma (multiple myeloma) An uncommon malignant disorder characterised by abnormal and unregulated proliferation of plasma cells which develop from mature B lymphocytes.

Myocardial infarction (MI) Part of the spectrum of acute coronary syndrome. There is death (necrosis) of part of the myocardium (heart muscle) from deprivation of oxygenated blood following occlusion of a coronary artery.

Nasal obstruction Results from a number of causes, e.g. infection, polyps. The most common symptoms are obstructed breathing and increased nasal discharge

Negative feedback A homeostatic mechanism whereby increased levels, for example, of a specific hormone in the blood 'turn off' or cancel the stimulus causing hormone secretion. Once hormone levels are below the normal range, the stimulus is 'turned on' and again causes the hormone to be secreted

Neurogenic shock A type of distributive shock, which is due to altered vascular resistance.

Neurological assessment Includes the Glasgow Coma Scale, vital signs – blood pressure, pulse rate, respirations, temperature, and also pupil size and reaction and limb movements.

Neuropathic pain Describes pain that persists beyond the original cause, such as a nerve injury or infective cause.

Neutropenia A decrease in the number of circulating neutrophils to below $1.0 \times 10^9/L$.

Nociceptive pain Somatic or visceral pain that results from stimulation of nociceptors following tissue damage or inflammation, e.g. surgery, infection or trauma.

Nocturia Waking up to void urine at night.

Non-rapid eye movement (NREM) sleep Four sleep stages associated with differing electrical activity of the brain.

Non-specific immunity Natural non-specific immunity includes intact skin/mucosae, specialised epithelial surfaces, body secretions containing antibacterial substances such as lysozyme and immunoglobulins (Storey & Jordan 2008) and the microorganisms of the normal flora. The inflammatory process and phagocytosis are also included. Additionally, natural killer (NK) cells detect and destroy damaged or malignant cells and virus-infected cells, and undertake non-specific immunosurveillance.

Nutritional science The science of the macronutrients and micronutrients needed to maintain health.

Obesity The condition of excessive accumulation of fat in the body, leading to an increase in weight beyond that considered desirable.

Oedema Abnormal collection of fluid in the tissues, such as around the ankles. Fluid may also collect in the pericardial or pleural cavities or in the abdominal cavity.

Oliguria Reduced urine output.

Oral assessment Thorough examination to assess the condition of the oral cavity, preferably using a valid and reliable tool for the care setting.

Oral cancers Cancers affecting the lips, floor of the mouth and tongue, the palate and the salivary glands. In 2006 over 5000 people were diagnosed with oral cancer and there were 1805 deaths in 2007 (Cancer Research UK 2009a).

Oral candidiasis *See Candidiasis.*

Oral hygiene Measures required to ensure the mouth is clean and healthy, including a thorough oral assessment, sufficient fluid intake (especially oral fluids), teeth and oral surface cleaning and regular dental examination.

Orodental disease Includes both conditions of the teeth (plaque, calculus, caries) and periodontal conditions affecting the supporting structures of the teeth (gingivitis, periodontitis).

Orofacial trauma Soft tissue injuries range from simple lacerations, knife wounds and bites to multiple injuries resulting in tissue loss. Bone injuries include fracture of the mandible and fracture of the maxillae, malar (zygomatic) and nasal bones (middle third fracture). Causes include violence, road traffic accidents, work accidents, sport, falls and burns.

Osmolality The concentration of a solution expressed as osmoles of solute per kilogram of solvent.

Osmolarity The concentration of a solution expressed as osmoles of solute per litre of solvent.

Osmosis Passive movement of fluid from an area of lower concentration (of solutes) to an area of higher concentration, in an attempt to dilute the 'stronger' solution and achieve an equal balance on both sides of the membrane.

Osteoarthritis (OA) Slow deterioration of the articular cartilage in a synovial joint. OA may be primary or secondary; the former is more common in older people, especially females.

Oxygen therapy A potent drug used to relieve breathlessness and manage hypoxaemia.

Pain management (palliative care) Analgesic medications, given regularly to prevent the recurrence of pain, are central to effective pain management in palliative care. An adequate, regular dose is calculated and administered, enabling the patient to be as comfortable as possible without being drowsy.

Pain threshold 'The least experience of pain which a subject can recognize' (International Association for the Study of Pain [IASP] 1994).

Pain tolerance 'The greatest level of pain which a subject is prepared to tolerate' (IASP 1994).

Paraesthesia Abnormal sensation, e.g. tingling or 'pins and needles'.

Parenteral nutrition Nutrients in solution infused directly into the venous system.

Partial thickness burn injury Injury involving the epidermis and part of the dermis. Classified as 'superficial' or 'deep', depending on the amount of dermis involved.

Perioperative care Care throughout the surgical experience from pre-admission, pre-operative period, anaesthesia and surgery, recovery to postoperative period.

Peripheral vascular disease (PVD) Pathological processes affecting both the peripheral arterial and venous circulations.

Personal protective equipment (PPE) The disposable, single use clothing and equipment, e.g. disposable gloves, aprons/gowns, goggles/visors and masks/respirators, available to health care workers, and at times visitors, to protect them from exposure to microorganisms no matter in which setting they are working.

Person-centred care Care in which nurses and carers get to know the person in a more intimate way. It is still important to plan care to meet the clinical needs of the older person, but this is in the context of the whole person, including their life history (Ashburner et al 2004). Communication and care interactions are more likely to prioritise the older person's needs rather than those of the care organisation.

Pneumonia Lower respiratory tract infection. Characterised by inflammation of the lung parenchyma, usually resulting from bacterial or viral infection, but may be fungal or parasitic.

Positron emission tomography (PET) scan Imaging technique that produces three-dimensional images illustrating metabolic activity in particular areas of the body. It employs cyclotron-produced isotopes of extremely short half-life that emit positrons which are introduced into the patient. As positrons react with electrons in the body gamma rays are emitted, which are detected by a specialist gamma camera.

Pressure ulcer 'An area of localized skin damage caused by disruption of the blood supply to the area, usually caused by pressure, shear or friction, or a combination of any of these' (Dealey 1999).

Primary and secondary surveys Assessment and management of the trauma patient includes the initial assessment (primary survey) which has five components ('A, B, C, D, E'):

- **A**irway with cervical spine control
- **B**reathing and ventilation
- **C**irculation and haemorrhage control
- **D**isability and dysfunction
- **E**xposure and environmental control.

The secondary survey only commences when the primary survey is complete and the patient's condition is stabilised. The secondary survey may not take place in the ED, as the critically injured patient is likely to require surgical intervention to stabilise their condition. If the patient's condition does permit, then the secondary survey involves a full head-to-toe examination and gives the nurse the opportunity to complete a thorough assessment including documenting wounds (location, surface area and depth), skin integrity, tetanus status, allergies.

Protein pump inhibitors (PPIs) Drugs such as lansoprazole that inhibit gastric acid production by blocking the 'proton pump' in the parietal cells of the stomach. Used with antibacterials to eliminate *Helicobacter pylori*, for gastro-oesophageal reflux disease, peptic ulceration.

Proteinuria Protein in the urine.

Pruritus Intense itching. Generalised pruritus may be associated with jaundice, cancer, renal failure or Hodgkin's lymphoma. Localised pruritus affecting the vulva or peri-anal area may be due to a number of causes, e.g. vaginal candidiasis.

Pubic ('crab') louse *Pthirus pubis*, a parasitic insect that infests the pubic area, can be sexually acquired.

Public health nutrition The promotion of good nutritional health and the prevention of diet-related illness in groups of people, rather than the nutritional care of individuals.

Pyrexia Deep/core body temperature above normal.

Quality adjusted life year (QALY) A measurement that attempts to provide an objective estimate of the costs and benefits of a health intervention. A QALY is a measure of years of life gained through a health intervention adjusted for the quality of life (on a scale 0 to 1).

Radiotherapy The use of ionising radiation to kill dividing cells in a therapeutic approach.

Rapid eye movement (REM) sleep Sleep characterised by dreaming, muscular relaxation and high levels of physiological arousal.

Rapid/premature ejaculation (PE) Persistent or recurrent ejaculation with minimal stimulation that causes marked interpersonal distress.

Rash A skin eruption. A collection of numerous lesions with some coalescing.

Reconstructive breast surgery A surgical method using implants or autologous tissue flaps to re-create the breast once a mastectomy has been performed.

Re-feeding syndrome The term 're-feeding syndrome' is applied to the problems arising from sudden feeding in a very malnourished patient. This is caused by a rapid shift of electrolytes, glucose and water from extracellular to intracellular compartments, causing deficits in the extracellular fluid.

Rehabilitation Definitions vary, in line with the perceived purpose, but it is best described as an ongoing process which begins as soon as individuals are clinically stable, is independent of the location of care, reflects a transferable underpinning philosophy and involves shifting degrees and forms of support.

Relationship-centred care Nolan et al (2001) identified a relationship-centred care framework that acknowledges the needs of those delivering care. This shifts the focus to the organisation of care rather than just the individuals providing it. Nolan et al (2001) suggest that where care delivery is of an optimal standard, the culture of an organisation provides a certain atmosphere or feeling. They suggest the organisation should promote a sense of security, continuity, belonging, purpose, fulfilment and significance. Importantly, these senses should not only be felt by the older people being cared for, but also the staff working with them.

Respiratory failure Results from a situation where the lungs fail to oxygenate the blood sufficiently or excrete waste carbon dioxide.

Reticular activating system (RAS) A diffuse functional area of the reticular formation. It has connections with other brain areas including the thalamus, hypothalamus, cerebral cortex and ocular motor nuclei. Involved in levels of consciousness, cortical arousal and sleep/wake cycles.

Reticular formation (RF) A network of neurones within the brain stem that connect with the spinal cord, cerebellum, thalamus and hypothalamus. Involved in the coordination of skeletal muscle activity, including voluntary movement, posture and balance, as well as automatic and reflex activities that link with the limbic system.

Retinopathy Disease of the retina. Associated with hypertension, diabetes mellitus, abnormal retinal vessels and sun damage.

Rheumatoid arthritis (RA) A systemic autoimmune disease of connective tissue. There is joint inflammation due to inflammatory changes in the synovial membrane. The synovium becomes thicker, very vascular and there may be joint effusion. As proliferative tissue spreads as a 'pannus' over the articular cartilage, the cartilage is slowly eroded. Systemic inflammatory effects include pericarditis, alveolitis, pleuritis, eye involvement and bowel vasculitis, as well as general malaise, fever and anaemia.

Rigidity Increased resistance to passive movement; it is not velocity-dependent.

Scabies A parasitic skin disease caused by the itch mite (*Sarcoptes scabiei*). Highly contagious, scabies spreads in situations where there is frequent intimate personal contact.

Screening Secondary preventive measure to identify potential or incipient disease at an early stage when it may be more easily treated.

Sepsis State of being infected with pus-forming (pyogenic) microorganisms.

Seroconversion Conversion from a negative blood test where specific antibodies are not present to a positive test in which specific antibodies present in the serum confirm that a response to an antigen has taken place.

Sexually acquired infections (SAI) Infections which are usually acquired through sexual contact, but not exclusively so. They include gonorrhoea, syphilis, HIV/AIDS, candidiasis, chlamydial infection, genital herpes, genital warts, trichomoniasis, scabies and pubic lice.

Shock A state in which there is inadequate flow of oxygenated blood to the tissues, which results in cell hypoxia and inadequate tissue perfusion.

Sickle cell disease An inherited haemoglobinopathy.

Sinusitis Inflammation of one or more paranasal sinuses.

Skin graft A sheet of skin containing dermis and epidermis applied to a raw surface such as burn injury.

Sleep A naturally periodic altered state of consciousness occurring in humans in a 24 h biological rhythm. Provides rest for both body and mind. Sleep state is characterised by cyclical brain wave patterns with periods of dreaming.

Sleep assessment Requires the nurse's observations of sleep and their communication skills, both questioning patients carefully and listening to what they tell them. Assessment should take into account the patient's age, gender, diet, medical diagnosis and medical/surgical treatments, as well as paying specific attention to issues related to sleep (Fordham 1996) and the patient's immediate environment and how that might impact on their dignity and privacy (Department of Health 2001b).

Sleep disorders Include insomnia (most common), sleep apnoea, sleep-induced nocturnal myoclonus, narcolepsy, sleep walking, night terrors and nightmares.

Sleep hygiene The pre-sleep routines that relax and promote sleep. These may include going to bed at the same time, a milky drink and putting on nightclothes.

Spasticity Increased muscle tone; there is velocity-dependent increase in tonic stretch reflexes.

Staging (of cancer) The process whereby the extent of disease is established. One of two methods are used: (1) the TMN system – tumour (T) size, nodal (N) status and metastases (M) present/absent; (2) the number system – I, II, III, IV, which denotes the degree of spread with IV being the most advanced with distant metastases.

Standard precautions The measures applied at all times when performing health care activities in order to minimise the risk of spreading microorganisms to patients, health care staff and others, including hand hygiene, dealing with blood and body fluid spillages, PPE, prevention of exposure to infection. Applied routinely in all situations, whether or not an infection has been identified.

Stoma An opening, such as a colostomy.

Stomatitis Inflammation of the mouth.

Stress Can be viewed as a disturbed homeostasis that manifests itself via certain physiological and psychological imbalances (Watson & Fawcett 2003). The impact of stress occurs only when the cumulative effects of stressors surpass the individual's ability easily to return to equilibrium.

Stress management The methods used to manage stress include deep breathing, improving diet and regular exercise.

Stroke (cerebrovascular accident) Sudden loss of blood supply to an area of the brain causing a neurological defect lasting more than 24 h.

Stroke volume The volume of blood ejected from the heart by each ventricular contraction.

Superficial burn injury A type of partial thickness burn injury in which there is limited dermal involvement.

Swallowing (deglutition) A process initiated voluntarily but completed through involuntary reflex action. It has three stages: the voluntary oral stage, pharyngeal stage (reflex) and oesophageal.

Symptom management in palliative care Effective symptom management requires a thorough assessment of each symptom, e.g. pain, nausea and vomiting, breathlessness, cough, hiccup and constipation, before discussing causes and options with the patient. Management is planned in consideration of the patient's expectations and priorities and evaluated regularly.

Terminal care Care in the last stage of a patient's illness, where there is increasing disability, dependence and death is anticipated in the near future. *See End-of-life care.*

Testicular cancer Cancers of the testes are divided in to two groups: germ cell tumours (the majority) or stromal tumours. The two basic groups are further subdivided. Testicular cancer is a relatively rare cancer (less than 1% of all cancers in the UK), but is the most common cancer in males aged 15–44 years (Cancer Research UK 2009b). It is one of the most curable solid tumours.

Thalassaemia An inherited haemoglobinopathy.

Thermogenesis Production of body heat, either chemically by the release of noradrenaline (non-shivering thermogenesis [NST]) or physically by skeletal muscle contraction (shivering thermogenesis).

Thrombocytopenia Decrease in the number of platelets (thrombocytes) in the blood.

Thrombosis The formation of a thrombus (clot) in the heart, artery or vein.

Tinnitus Usually a subjective sensation of sound in the ear. It is often accompanied by vertigo and/or deafness.

Tonsillectomy Surgical removal of the palatine tonsils.

Tracheostomy An opening through the skin and structures of the neck into the trachea.

Traction A pulling force applied to a part or parts of the body; counter-traction, a pulling force in the opposite direction, is also applied (Lucas & Davis 2004). Counter-traction is usually supplied by the patient's body weight. Traction may be skeletal or skin traction, balanced/sliding or fixed.

Transmission-based precautions (TBP) Incorporating isolation procedures, previously often known as 'barrier nursing'. Should be applied in addition to standard precautions when highly transmissible or antimicrobial-resistant microorganisms are present in a patient. The procedures are commonly categorised by the organism's main route of transmission, the most common being contact, droplet and airborne.

Trauma nursing Includes several roles: initial care in the Emergency Department, care of relatives, involvement in organ and tissue donation, health promotion/injury prevention and rehabilitation.

Tremor Rhythmic, involuntary movement – may occur at rest or on movement.

Trichomoniasis Inflammation of the vagina (vaginitis) or urethritis in males caused by the motile protozoan *Trichomonas vaginalis* (TV). Usually sexually acquired.

Tuberculosis (TB) A chronic granulomatous infection caused by the bacterium *Mycobacterium tuberculosis*. Mainly affects the lungs (pulmonary TB) but may affect the kidneys, uterine tubes, bones and joints, gastrointestinal tract and lymph nodes, or cause meningitis.

Uraemia (azotaemia) Increased levels of waste products including urea and other nitrogenous substances in the blood. It leads to electrolyte and acid–base imbalance. Caused by severely impaired renal function or renal failure.

Urgency The sensation of an immediate need to pass urine, it may have a motor or sensory cause.

Urinary catheterisation The passage of a tube through the urethra or suprapubically through the abdominal wall into the bladder to drain urine. Also required for certain investigations, e.g. cystometry, and to administer intravesical medication.

Vegetative state (VS) Describes a condition that may occur following a severe brain injury, where there is extensive damage to the cerebral cortex. Although the patient has sleep/waking cycles, the higher centres of the brain are destroyed. The brain stem is functioning but the cerebral cortex is not and patients can survive for several years requiring full-time nursing care.

Venous disease Includes venous insufficiency, venous ulcers, venous thromboembolism (VTE) (deep vein thrombosis, pulmonary embolism), and varicose veins.

Ventilator acquired pneumonia (VAP) Pneumonia diagnosed more than 48 h following the insertion of an endotracheal tube and the commencement of mechanical ventilation.

Vertigo A disturbance of equilibrium in the absence of an external cause which creates a sensation of rotating motion of oneself or one's surroundings. Often described as a whirling sensation, but rocking and swaying sensations are also reported. May be accompanied by pallor, nausea and vomiting.

Visual impairment (VI) Some degree of low vision, sight impairment or total blindness. Important causes worldwide include cataract, trachoma caused by *Chlamydia trachomatis*, onchocerciasis (river blindness – caused by *Onchocerca volvulus*, a parasitic microfilarial worm), xerophthalmia (vitamin A deficiency), glaucoma, macular degeneration, diabetic and other retinopathies and trauma.

Wallace's rule of nines A simple method of assessing the percentage of body surface area affected by a burn injury, using standard body maps. In adults, the head and upper limbs each equal 9%, while the anterior trunk, the posterior trunk and the lower limbs each equal 18%. The remaining 1% is usually applied to the perineum.

Weaning The gradual transition from mechanical ventilatory support to spontaneous ventilation (self-ventilation).

Wound assessment The state of the wound and surrounding skin is assessed using a range of wound criteria. Wound assessment charts will usually collect information around key parameters which suggest if the wound is healing, deteriorating or static. Key parameters include: cause and location of the wound, size of wound, pain, condition of surrounding skin, volume of exudate, odour and type and amount of tissue, e.g. necrotic tissue, slough, granulation, epithelialisation.

Wound dressing Product applied to surgical or medical wounds, e.g. pressure ulcers. Dressings should be permeable to water vapour and gases but not to bacteria or liquids, thus retaining serous exudate. Vitally they do not adhere to the wound surface, thereby reducing damage to new tissue during dressing change.

Wound healing A complex series of events comprising haemostasis, inflammation, proliferation and maturation. The events depend on many patient and environmental factors and can easily be disrupted by inappropriate care.

REFERENCES

Ashburner C, Meyer J, Johnson B, et al: Using action research to address loss of personhood in a continuing care setting. *Illn Crises Loss* 12(1):23–37, 2004.

Brooker C, editor: *Mosby's Dictionary of Medicine, Nursing and Health Professions*, Edinburgh, 2010, Mosby.

Cancer Research UK: *Oral Cancer Statistics*, 2009a. Available online http://info.cancerresearchuk.org/cancerstats/types/oral/index.htm?script=true.

Cancer Research UK: *UK Testicular Cancer Statistics*, 2009b. Available online http://info.cancerresearchuk.org/cancerstats/types/testis/index.htm?script=true.

Dealey C: The management of patients with chronic wounds. In *The care of wounds*, Oxford, 1999, Blackwell Science.

Department of Health: *Comprehensive Critical Care. A review of adult critical care services*, 2000. Available online http://www.dh.gov.uk/prod_consum_dh/groups/dh_digitalassets/@dh/@en/documents/digitalasset/dh_4082872.pdf.

Department of Health: *The expert patient: a new approach to chronic disease management for the 21st century*, London, 2001a, DH.

Department of Health: *Essence of Care: Patient-focused benchmarking for health care practitioners*, London, 2001b, DH.

Fordham M: *Patient problems: a research base for nursing*, Edinburgh, 1996, Churchill Livingstone.

Greaves I, Porter KM, Ryan JM, editors: Mechanism of injury. In *Trauma Care Manual*, London, 2001, Arnold, pp 99–114.

Hickey JV: *The clinical practice of neurological and neurosurgical nursing*, ed 5, New York, 2003, Lippincott Williams and Wilkins.

Hoffbrand AV, Moss PAH, Pettit JE: *Essential Haematology*, ed 5, Oxford, 2006, Blackwell Publishing.

International Association for the Study of Pain (IASP) Task Force on Taxonomy: IASP pain terminology. In Merskey N, Bogduk N, editors: *Classification of chronic pain*, ed 2, Seattle, 1994, IASP Press.

Lucas B, Davis PS: Why restricting movement is important. In Kneale J, Davis P, editors: *Orthopaedic and trauma nursing*, ed 2, Edinburgh, 2004, Churchill Livingstone, pp 105–139.

Moffatt CJ, Franks PJ, Morison MJ: Models of service provision. In Morison MJ, Moffatt CJ, Franks PJ, editors: *Leg ulcers: A problem based learning approach*, Edinburgh, 2007, Mosby.

Nolan M, Davies S, Grant G: Quality of life, quality of care. In Nolan M, Davies S, Grant G, editors: *Working with older people and their families. Key issues in policy and practice*, Buckingham, 2001, Open University Press.

Royal College of Obstetricians and Gynaecologists (RCOG): Green-top Guideline No 25. *The management of early pregnancy loss*, 2006. Available online http://www.rcog.org.uk/files/rcog-corp/uploaded-files/GT25ManagementofEarlyPregnancyLoss2006.pdf.

Storey M, Jordan S: An overview of the immune system, *Nurs Stand* 23(15–17):47–56, 2008.

Watson R, Fawcett TN: *Pathophysiology, homeostasis and nursing*, London, 2003, Routledge.

World Health Organization (WHO): *Values for diagnosis of diabetes mellitus and other categories of hyperglycaemia*, 1999. Available online http://www.who.int/diabetesactiononline/diabetes/basics/en/index4.html.

Index

stroke patients, 319, 321
terminal illness, 862
tinnitus, 458
tracheostomy, 467–468
wound healing, 637–638
see also anxiety; boredom; dignity;
psychogenic factors; self-esteem;
stigma; stress
psychosomatic problems, 525–528
psychotherapy, stress, 529
puberty
breast development, 249
menstruation onset delay, 212
pubic louse (pediculosis pubis), 886–887
public awareness campaigns of long-term
conditions, 826
public health nurses, orodental health
promotion, 479
public health nutrition, 599–600
definition, 925
public health programmes, pain
management and palliative care,
552
pubocervical ligament, 144
pulmonary artery catheter in critical care,
762–763
pulmonary artery wedge pressure
(PAWP), 763
pulmonary embolism (PE)
characteristics of pain, 23*t*
myocardial infarction complicated by,
27
traumatic/surgical causes, 341
pulmonary non-vascular tissue *see* lung
pulmonary valve, 11
pulse
as fluid/electrolyte status indicator,
587*t*
peripheral arterial disease, 43
pressure narrowing in hypovolaemic
shock, 538
trauma patient, 726*t*
burns, 781
unconscious patient, 745
pulse contour cardiac output index,
critical care, 763
pulse oximetry, 57–58
shock, 547
pupil
constriction *see* miosis
reactions to light, unconscious patient,
745
brain stem death assessment, 753
significance of clinical features on
examination, 425*t*
size, unconscious patient, 745
purpura, idiopathic thrombocytopenia,
393
pustular psoriasis, 403
pyelogram, intravenous, 280*b*
pyelolithotomy, 283
pyelonephritis, 279*t*, 280

pyramidal tracts, 308
pyrexia *see* fever
pyridoxine *see* vitamin B₆

Q

Q wave (ECG), 12
QRS complex, 12
quality-adjusted life year (QALY),
definition, 925
quality improvement in infection control,
506–507
quality of life (QoL)
assessment
growth hormone deficiency,
134–135
hypothyroidism, 140
skin disorders, 397
improvement in heart failure, 34
Queyrat's erythroplasia, 238
quinsy, 470–471

R

R wave (ECG), 12
race/ethnicity
breast cancer in ethnic minorities, 266,
266*b*
diabetes type 2 and, 152–153
testicular cancer and, 233
see also cultural issues
radial fractures, distal (= Colles'
fracture), 348–349
radiation
ionising *see* ionising radiation
non-ionising *see* non-ionising radiation
exposure
thermal, heat loss by, 620, 621*t*
radiography *see* X-ray radiography
radioiodine *see* iodine-131
radiology
diagnostic *see* imaging
interventional, stroke, 320
radionuclide imaging (scintigraphy),
myocardial perfusion in stable
angina, 17
radiotherapy, 801–808
bladder cancer, 290
breast cancer
adjuvant, 261–262, 263
metastatic disease, 269
side effects, 261–262
cervical cancer, 213–214
colorectal cancer, 96
intent, 803
large field, 803
liver cancer, 109
myeloma, 390
oral cancer, 491
for pain management, 569
penile cancer, 239
physics and biology, 801

pituitary tumours, 131, 133, 134
prostate cancer, 296, 297
protection from radiation, 803
side-effects (in general), 800*f*, 803–807
sources, 802–803
testicular cancer, 235
see also chemoradiotherapy
rapid eye movement sleep, 676
Raynaud's disease, 44–45, 629
Raynaud's phenomenon, 629
reabsorption, renal, 274–275
reassurance, critically ill patient, 770
recoil, lung, 54
reconstructive phase of wound healing, 635
reconstructive surgery (repair)
bladder cancer, 290
breast cancer, 261, 261*b*, 266
definition, 925
heart valve, 37
oral cancer, 491, 491*t*
recovery room, 703–704
nurse, roles, 704
rectum
administration via
analgesics, 568
enemas and suppositories, 861
fluids/electrolytes, 589
anatomy and physiology, 75
digital examination, in incontinence,
663–664
disorders, 97–99
constipation related to, 98
malignant *see* colorectal cancer
painful, incontinence due to, 663
peristalsis (stimulation to empty
contents), 659
prolapse, 214, 219
see also proctitis
red blood cells *see* erythrocytes
red eye, 435–438
redness, allergic contact dermatitis, 407
reduction of fractures, 341
re-epithelialisation of wounds, 635, 640
refeeding syndrome, 602, 925
reference ranges, laboratory, 912–916
referrals
incontinence, 671
for surgery, 691
minor surgery, increasing numbers,
690
reflective practice, 4
reflex(es), assessment for brain stem
death, 753–754
reflex centres (brainstem), 305
reflex incontinence, 660
reflexology, depression, 528
reflux nephropathy, 280
refraction, 424
errors
laser treatment, 432
terminology associated with, 423
refractory shock, 537–538